COMPREHENSIVE GYNECOLOGY

COMPREHENSIVE GYNECOLOGY

ARTHUR L. HERBST, M.D.

Joseph Bolivar DeLee
Distinguished Service Professor and Chairman,
Department of Obstetrics and Gynecology,
University of Chicago,
Chicago, Illinois

DANIEL R. MISHELL, JR., M.D.

Lyle G. McNeile Professor and Chairman,
Department of Obstetrics and Gynecology,
University of Southern California School of Medicine,
Los Angeles, California

MORTON A. STENCHEVER, M.D.

Professor and Chairman,
Department of Obstetrics and Gynecology,
University of Washington School of Medicine,
Seattle, Washington

WILLIAM DROEGEMUELLER, M.D.

Robert A. Ross Distinguished Professor and Chairman,
Department of Obstetrics and Gynecology,
University of North Carolina School of Medicine,
Chapel Hill, North Carolina

SECOND EDITION

with 818 illustrations

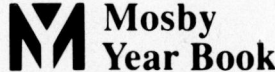

Mosby
Year Book

St. Louis   Baltimore   Boston   Chicago   London   Philadelphia   Sydney   Toronto

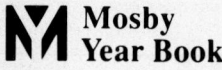
Mosby
Year Book
Dedicated to Publishing Excellence

Editor: Stephanie Manning
Developmental Editor: Elaine Steinborn
Assistant Editor: Jo Salway

SECOND EDITION

Mosby-Year Book, Inc.
11830 Westline Industrial Drive
St. Louis, Missouri 63146

Library of Congress Cataloging–in–Publication Data

Comprehensive gynecology / Arthur L. Herbst ... [et al.]. 2nd ed.
    p. cm.
    Includes bibliographical references and index.
    ISBN 0-8016-6244-3
    1. Gynecology. I. Herbst, Arthur L.
    [DNLM: 1. Genital Diseases, Female. 2. Genital Neoplasms, Female.
WP 140 C737]
RG101 . C726 1991
618.1--dc20
DNLM/DLC
for Library of Congress   91-35012
                                             CIP

92 93 94 95 96 CI/MY 9 8 7 6 5 4 3 2 1

Preface

This second edition of *Comprehensive Gynecology* maintains the high standards of the first edition. Great efforts have been made to update the material completely and retain our goal of providing comprehensive contemporary information. As stated in the preface to the first edition, the book is primarily intended for the resident training in gynecology, but provides sufficient detail to be used by the practitioner, and will also serve as a reference for medical students. We have kept the needs of these diverse readers in mind as we prepared this new edition.

The basic chapters have been updated and contemporary clinically relevant material added as appropriate. We believe that in relating basic science to clinical relevance the reader will have a better understanding of the disease processes involved. In chapters dealing with diagnostic methods, we have eliminated minimally used techniques and substituted the latest procedures. In addition, all terminology reflects most current usage. Throughout we have tried to maintain the reader's awareness that the patient is a complex individual with distinct and personal needs and rights that merit our respect. All of this has been substantiated with over 850 illustrations and a total of 3300 references, 1700 of which are new to this edition.

As in the first edition, each chapter begins with a list of key terms and concludes with a listing of the key points covered. This allows the reader quick reference in studying the chapter and affords an easy review.

As outlined in the first edition, authorship among equals means there is no senior author. As we initially planned, our names have been rotated through the alphabetical cycle to reflect our equivalent contributions.

Again, we thank our families for the patience and loving support that they have provided as we undertook this task. The publication of this new edition reflects their tolerance as much as our hard work, and we are grateful for their continuing endurance. We also thank our staff, who worked long hours in preparing the final manuscript drafts. Finally, we have remained close friends throughout this process. We are proud of this accomplishment, as well as our new text.

Arthur L. Herbst
Daniel R. Mishell, Jr.
Morton A. Stenchever
William Droegemueller

Contents

COMPREHENSIVE
GYNECOLOGY

BASIC SCIENCES

Embryology

KEY TERMS AND DEFINITIONS

Acrosome Reaction. The process by which the cap over the head of the sperm, the acrosome, is removed to expose the portion of the sperm head containing the hydrolytic enzymes, which makes it possible for the sperm to penetrate the cells and structures investing the egg. This process is involved in capacitation but is not necessarily the same response as capacitation.

Anlage. The cell mass that gives rise to a specific organ or structure.

Bivalent. Homologous chromosomes that become paired during meiosis.

Blastula. The stage of embryonic development that follows the morula stage. At this stage a cyst (blastocyst) forms within the cell mass and early differentiation begins.

Capacitation. The morphologic, physiologic, and biochemical changes that a sperm goes through to be capable of penetrating the cumulus oophorus, corona radiata, and zona pellucida of the egg. It involves the sequentially timed release of a series of hydrolytic enzymes, which allows the sperm to digest a passage through the aforementioned structures.

Chiasmata. Points of attachment of homologous chromosomes during meiosis, where the exchange of genetic material occurs.

Cleavage. The first cell division of the fertilized ovum (zygote).

Cumulus Oophorus. The cell mass that invests the egg. It is a remnant of the primitive sex cords of the embryonic ovary.

Gartner's Duct. Remnants of the mesonephric (wolffian) duct system often found in the broad ligament and beside the uterus, cervix, and vagina of the adult woman.

H-Y Antigen. A cell surface antigen that leads to male differentiation of the gonad.

Implantation. The process by which the early embryo burrows within the endometrial lining of the uterus.

Mesonephros. The mesodermal anlage of the male sexual duct system.

Metanephros. The anlage of the adult kidney.

Morula. A ball of cells composing the early embryo that produces both the embryo and the placenta and membranes. Each cell is totipotential.

Oogenesis. The development of the ovum from an oogonium by meiosis.

Paramesonephric (Müllerian) Duct. The anlage of the female sex duct system that gives rise to the fallopian tube, uterus, and cervix in the adult woman.

Polar Body. The daughter cell produced during oogenesis at first and second meiotic division (first and second polar body); it contains a nucleus and minimal cytoplasm. For each polar body the nuclear material is similar to the nucleus of the ovum at the same stage.

Primordium. An early embryonic structure that further differentiates into an adult structure.

Sister Chromatid Exchange. The exchange of chromosomal material between the homologous arms of a chromosome that has already divided all of its structure except its centromere.

Spermatogenesis. The development of mature sperm from spermatogonia by meiosis.

Synapsis. The pairing process that brings together homologous chromosomes of maternal and paternal origin during meiosis.

Teratogen. An endogenous or exogenous substance that causes the formation of an anomaly.

Teratogenesis. The process of developing an anomaly of an organ or organs.

Zona Pellucida. The translucent belt consisting of a noncellular layer of mucopolysaccharide that is deposited at the periphery of the ovum while it is in the ovary and continues to surround the egg, the conceptus, and the morula until the stage of implantation.

Two areas of investigation within the field of gynecology have refocused attention on the process of fertilization and embryonic development: teratology and in vitro fertilization. The process under which eggs and sperm are produced and fertilization occurs is gaining close scrutiny. Likewise, the preimplantation, implantation, and embryonic stages of development in the human can be studied because of the development of newer techniques and pursuits. This chapter considers the processes of oocyte meiosis, fertilization and early cleavage, implantation, development of the genitourinary system, and sex differentiation.

OOCYTE MEIOSIS

The oocyte is a unique and extremely specialized cell. During the process of oocyte meiosis, genetic variability of the species is ensured. Later the oocyte develops the ability to facilitate fertilization and to provide the energy system to support the early embryonic development of the new individual.

Primordial germ cells in both males and females are large eosinophilic cells derived from endoderm in the wall of the yolk sac. These cells migrate to the germinal ridge by way of the dorsal mesentery of the hind gut by ameboid action. Here they undergo a period of intense mitotic activity in which their numbers increase to 6 to 7 million. By 20 weeks' gestation, this rapid multiplication has ended, and indeed the numbers rapidly fall off, being about 2 to 4 million at birth and about 400,000 at menarche. By 5 months' gestation, surviving oocytes enter the process of meiosis and progress to the prophase of the first meiotic division before entering an arrest period that lasts many years. After puberty a few oocytes mature during each ovarian cycle. The numbers vary from species to species, being one or two in the human. Maturation then continues to the second meiotic metaphase, when once again arrest of meiosis occurs unless the oocyte is activated by fertilization.

Figure 1-1 illustrates the steps of meiosis through both the first and second meiotic divisions. Prophase of the first meiotic division is divided into several phases. The earliest, the leptotene stage, is associated with condensation of the chromatin, which becomes visible as single elongated, threadlike structures. The next stage, zygotene, features the migration of these single threadlike chromosomes toward the equatorial plate of the nucleus. Homologous chromosomes arrange themselves close to one another to form bivalents. At the end of this stage, tight pairing of the chromosomes along their entire length, synapsis, takes place. The pachytene stage follows, during which the chromosome pairs contact one another and become shorter and thicker. During this stage each chromosome splits longitudinally, and two chromatids are produced that are united at the centromere. Thus the bivalent is now a structure composed of four closely opposed chromatids, or tetrads. The human ovum at pachytene demonstrates 23 tetrads. In the next stage, diplotene, the member chromosomes of the bivalents are held together only at certain points. At these terminal bridges, called chiasmata, the crossing over of genetic material takes place. The sister chromatids are still joined at the centromere, and crossing takes place only between the chromatids of homologous chromosomes and not between identical sister chromatids. The ovum then enters the dictyate stage and meiosis is arrested. Ova at this stage usually form germinal vesicles. Initiation of the meiotic process occurs because of stimulation by meiotic-inducing substance, which originates in the rete cords derived from the developing mesonephric tubules. Meiosis-

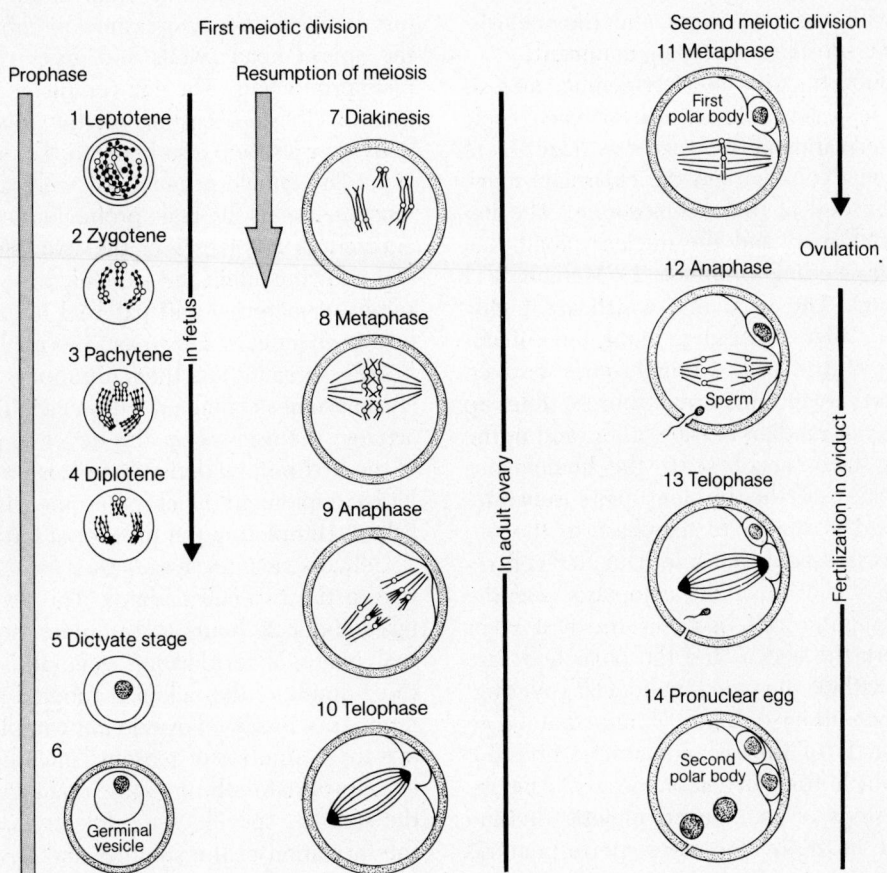

FIGURE 1-1

Diagram of oocyte meiosis. For simplicity, only three pairs of chromosomes are depicted. *1-4*, Prophase stages of the first meiotic division, which occur in most mammals during fetal life. The meiotic process is arrested at the diplotene stage ("first meiotic arrest"), and the oocyte enters the dictyate stages *(5-6)*. When meiosis is resumed, the first maturation division is completed *(7-11)*. Ovulation occurs usually at the metaphase II stage *(11)*, and the second meiotic division *(12-14)* takes place in the oviduct only after sperm penetration. (From Tsafriri A: Oocyte maturation in mammals. In Jones RE, editor: The vertebrate ovary, New York, 1978, Plenum Publishing Corp.)

preventing substance, probably produced by the granulosa cells of the differentiated ovarian follicle, acts as a countersubstance to inhibit meiosis. Apparently the interaction of these two substances regulates meiosis in the developing gonad. Once the ovum at the dictyate stage is encapsulated in granulosa cells, oogenesis is arrested because of the interruption of contact with the rete ovarii and the meiosis-preventing substance becomes dominant.

After puberty, with follicle ripening, meiosis resumes in a few follicles during each cycle with the formation of the diakinesis stage. Here the bivalents contract and the chiasmata move toward the end of the chromosomes. The homologs pull apart and the nuclear membrane disappears, ending prophase I. Metaphase I then occurs. The bivalents, which are highly contracted, align themselves along the equatorial plate of the cell. Chromosomes derived from paternal and maternal sources line up completely at random to each other, and in the following stage, anaphase I, the homologous chromosomes of the bivalent pairs separate. Telophase I is similar to telophase in the mitotic process except that one daughter cell receives the majority of the cytoplasm and the second daughter cell becomes the first polar body. Both the oocyte and the polar body are present within the zona pellucida covering. The oocyte then advances immediately to metaphase II of the second meiotic division, during which time ovulation occurs. The remaining steps of the second meiotic division take place in the oviduct after sperm penetration takes place.

FERTILIZATION AND EARLY CLEAVAGE

In humans and most other mammals, the egg is released from the ovary in the metaphase II stage. At the time it enters the fallopian tube, it is surrounded by a cumulus of granulosa cells (cumulus oophorus) and intimately surrounded by a clear zona pellucida. Within the zona pellucida are both the egg and the first polar body. Meanwhile, spermatozoa are transported through the cervical mucus and the uterus and into the fallopian tubes. During this transport period they undergo two changes, capacitation and acrosome reaction, which essentially activate enzyme systems within the sperm head and make it possible for the sperm to trans-

gress the cumulus oophorus and the zona pellucida. Once the sperm has passed the barrier of the zona pellucida, it attaches to the cell membrane of the egg and enters the cytoplasm. When the sperm enters the cytoplasm, intracytoplasmic structures, the coronal granules, arrange themselves in an orderly fashion around the outermost portion of the cytoplasm just beneath the cytoplasmic membrane, and the sperm head swells and gives rise to the male pronucleus. The egg completes its second meiotic division, casting off the second polar body to a position also beneath the zona pellucida. The female pronucleus swells as well. In most mammals the male pronucleus can be recognized as the larger of the two. The pronuclei, which contain the haploid sets of chromosomes of maternal and paternal origin, do not fuse in mammals. However, the nuclear membranes surrounding them disappear, and the chromosomes contained within each membrane arrange themselves on the developing spindle of the first mitotic division. In this way the diploid complement of chromosomes is reestablished, completing the process of fertilization.

Cell division (cleavage) then occurs, giving rise to the two-cell embryo. The first division takes about 20 hours to complete, and the actual phase of fertilization generally occurs in the ampulla of the fallopian tube. A significant number of fertilized ova do not complete cleavage for a number of reasons, including failure of appropriate chromosome arrangement on the spindle, specific gene defects that prevent the formation of the spindle, and environmental factors. Teratogens acting at this point are usually either completely destructive or cause little or no effect. Twinning may occur by the separation of the two cells produced by cleavage, each of which has the potential to develop into a separate embryo. Twinning may occur at any stage until the formation of the blastula, since each cell is totipotential. Both genetic and environmental factors are probably involved in the causation of twinning.

Morula and Blastula Stage: Early Differentiation

After the first mitotic division the cells continue to divide as the embryo passes along the fallopian tube and enters the uterus. This process takes 3 to 4 days after fertilization in the human, and the embryo may arrive at the uterus in any form, from 32 cells to the early blastula stage. In the human, implantation generally takes place 3 days after the embryo enters the uterus.

Implantation depends on the development of early trophoblastic cells during the blastula stage. These cells digest away the zona pellucida and allow the embryo to fix to the wall of the uterus and subsequently to burrow within the endometrium. The development of the blastula and the separation of the embryonic disk cells from the developing trophoblastic cells together make up the first stage of differentiation in the embryo. Again, at this stage of development, teratogens are generally either completely destructive or have little or no effect, since each of the cells of the early embryonic disk is multipotential. Differentiation within the embryonic disk, however, proceeds fairly rapidly, and if separation of cells and twinning occur at this point, the twins are frequently conjoined in some fashion. Figure 1-2 presents photomicrographs of several fresh human embryos obtained during in vitro fertilization. Various early cleavage stages are depicted as well. Figure 1-3 schematically demonstrates the process of follicle growth, ovulation, sperm capacitation, fertilization, and preimplantation.

IMPLANTATION

Implantation has been noted to occur in the human embryo as early as day 6 after ovulation. For implantation to take place, the zona pellucida must be removed from the developing blastocyst, which occurs because of enzyme action produced either by cells of the blastocyst or by some endometrial enzymes. Endometrial capillaries in contact with the invading syncytiotrophoblast are engulfed to form venous sinuses at or about 7½ days after conception and are seen abundantly by day 9. Endometrial spiral arteries are not invaded at this point. The endoplasmic reticulum of the syncytiotrophoblast is probably responsible for the synthesis of chorionic gonadotrophin, which is well developed by 11 days after ovulation. Transfer is probably through the venous sinuses before intact circulation to the developing embryo has been established. It is important that chorionic

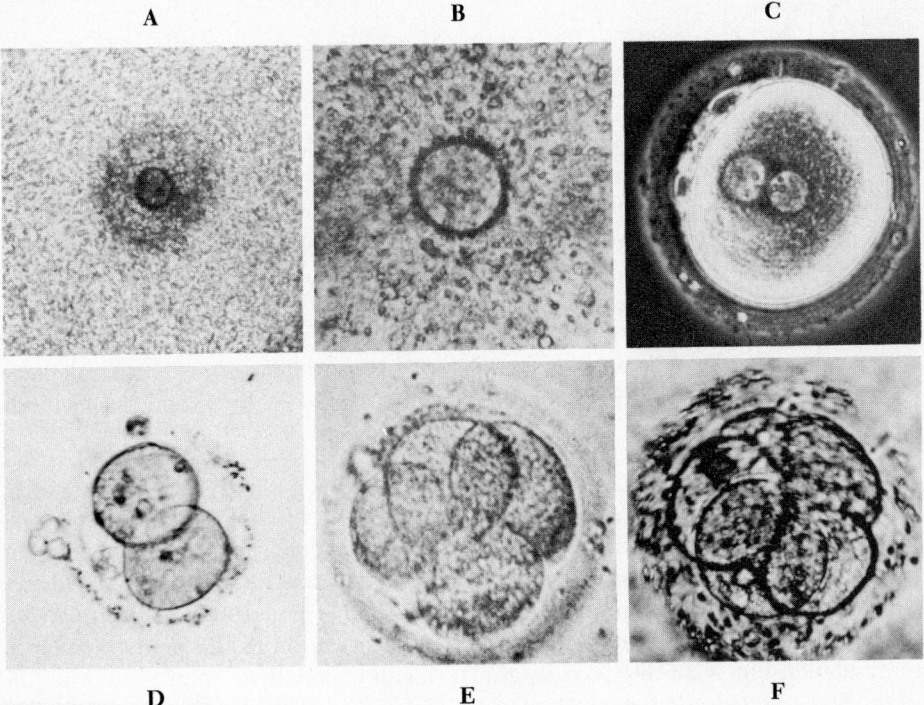

FIGURE 1-2
Six photo micrographs of fresh, unmounted human eggs and embryos. **A,** Early maturing oocyte. **B,** Mature oocyte surrounded by granulousal cells, zona pellucida visible. **C,** Fertilized oocyte demonstrating male and female pronuclei and both polar bodies. **D,** Two-cell zygote. **E,** Four-cell embryo. **F,** Eight-cell embryo.

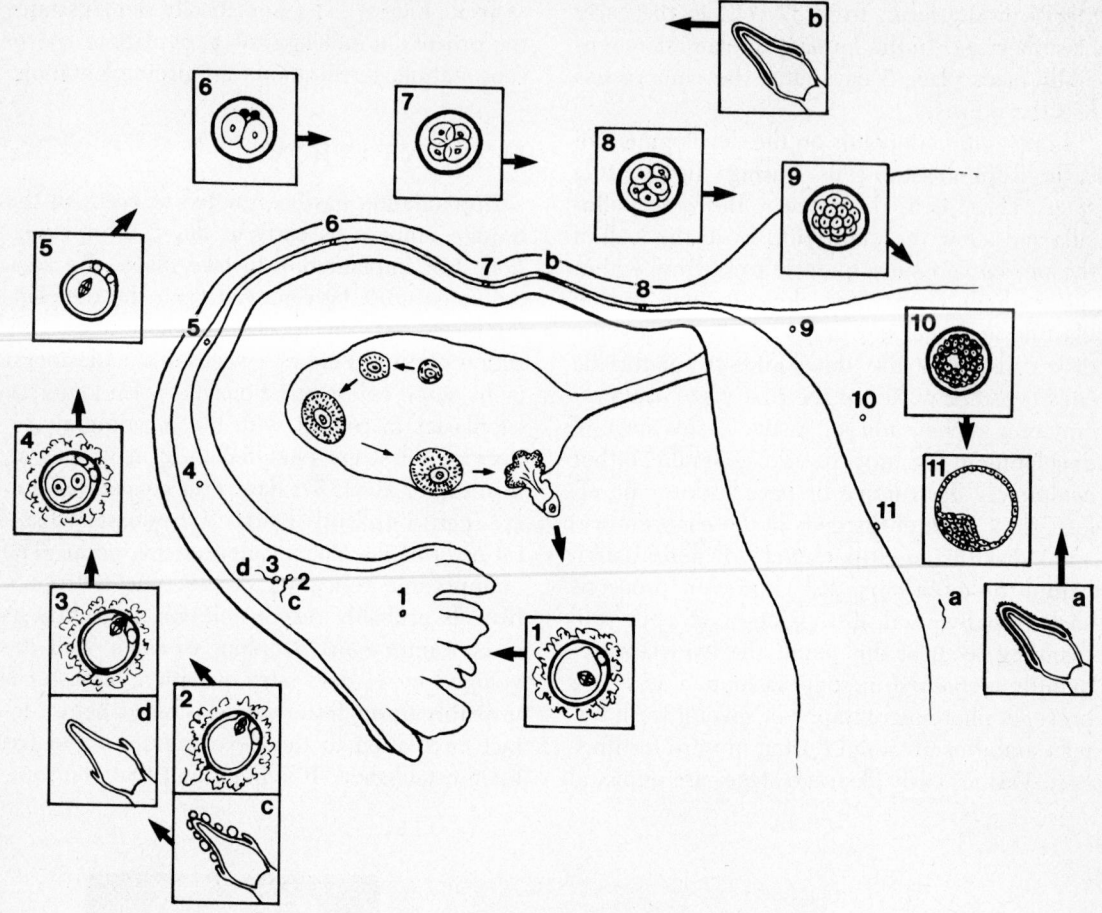

FIGURE 1-3

Diagrammatic representation of follicle growth, ovulation, sperm migration and maturation, fertilization, and preimplantation. *a-d,* Demonstrate sperm during migration through female tract accomplishing capacitation and acrosome reaction. *1,* Egg in meiosis enters fallopian tube after ovulating. *2,* Capacitated sperm penetrates cumulus cells and zona pellucida. *3,* Fertilization occurs; second meiotic division is complete. *4,* Male and female pronucleui are seen within the cytoplasm of egg; both polar bodies are present beneath the zona pellucida. *5,* First mitotic division takes place. *6,* Cleavage is complete. *7,* Four-cell stage. *8,* Eight-cell stage. *9,* Morula. *10,* Early blastocyst formation. *11,* Blastocyst formation; implantation occurs.

gonadotrophin be transmitted to maternal circulation by one means or another, since it is responsible for maintaining the corpus luteum. Chorionic gonadotrophin has been detected in the peripheral blood of the mother as early as 6 days after ovulation but is always seen by the twelfth day. The concentration doubles every 1.2 to 2 days, reaching its highest point at 7 to 9 weeks of pregnancy.

Discussion of implantation is not complete without at least considering why the fetus is not immunologically rejected by the mother.

Although it is not completely understood why rejection does not occur, some theories have been advanced. One theory suggests that some substance or substances suppress lymphocyte transformation in the mother. Such substances could be any that are produced by the embryo, including chorionic gonadotrophin, or by the decidua. Other theories include the production of suppressor T lymphocytes by the fetus, which could inhibit maternal lymphocyte transformation by secreting an inhibitory substance that crosses the placenta. Alternately, the phe-

TABLE 1-1
Events of Implantation

Event	Days After Ovulation
Zona pellucida disappears	4-5
Blastocyst attaches to epithelial surface of endometrium	6
Trophoblast erodes into endometrial stroma	7
Trophoblast differentiates into cytotrophoblastic and syncytial trophoblastic layers	7-8
Lacunae appear around trophoblast	8-9
Blastocyst burrows beneath endometrial surface	9-10
Lacunar network forms	10-11
Trophoblast invades endometrial sinusoids, establishing a uteroplacental circulation	11-12
Endometrial epithelium completely covers blastocyst	12-13
Strong decidual reaction occurs in stroma	13-14

nomenon of enhancement, which states that weakly antigenic sites on the trophoblast are blocked by maternal antibodies, thereby rendering them unavailable to circulating T cells, is also a possibility. Finally, the trophoblast may prevent entry of maternal lymphocytes to the fetus by virtue of features of its cell membrane molecular structure or by substances secreted by it to block the action of maternal antibodies.

Table 1-1 describes the events of implantation.

Early Organogenesis in the Embryonic Period

During the third week after fertilization the primitive streak forms in the caudal portion of the embryonic disk and the embryonic disk begins to grow and change from a circular to a pear-shaped configuration. At that point the epithelium facing superiorly is considered ectoderm and will eventually give rise to the developing central nervous system, and the epithelium facing downward toward the yolk sac is endoderm. During this week the neuroplate develops with its associated notochordal process. By the sixteenth day after conception the

third primitive germ layer, the intraembryonic mesoderm, begins to form between the ectoderm and endoderm. Early mesoderm migrates cranially, passing on either side of the notochordal process to meet in front in the formation of the cardiogenic area. The heart soon develops from this area. Later in the third week extraembryonic mesoderm joins with the yolk sac and the developing amnion to contribute to the developing membranes. An intraembryonic mesoderm develops on each side of the notochord and neural tube to form longitudinal columns, the paraxial mesoderm. Each paraxial column thins laterally into the lateral plate mesoderm, which is continuous with the extraembryonic mesoderm of the yolk sac and the amnion. The lateral plate mesoderm is separated from the paraxial mesoderm by a continuous tract of mesoderm called the intermediate mesoderm. By the twentieth day, paraxial mesoderm begins to divide into paired linear bodies known as somites. About 38 pairs of somites form during the next 10 days. Eventually a total of 42 to 44 pairs will develop, and these will give rise to body musculature.

Angiogenesis, or blood vessel formation, can be seen in the extraembryonic mesoderm of the yolk sac by day 15 or 16. Embryonic vessels can be seen about 2 days later and develop when mesenchymal cells known as angioblasts aggregate to form masses and cords called blood islands. Spaces then appear within these islands, and the angioblasts arrange themselves around these spaces to form primitive endothelium. Isolated vessels form channels and then grow into adjacent areas by endothelial budding. Primitive blood cells develop from endothelial cells as the vessels develop on the yolk sac and allantois. However, blood formation does not begin within the embryo until the second month of gestation, occurring first in the developing liver and later in the spleen, bone marrow, and lymph nodes. Separate mesenchymal cells surrounding the primitive endothelial vessels differentiate into muscular and connective tissue elements. The primitive heart forms in a similar manner from mesenchymal cells in the cardiogenic area. Paired endothelial channels called heart tubes develop by the end of the third week and fuse to form the primitive heart. By the twenty-first day, this primitive heart has linked up with blood vessels of the embryo, forming a primitive cardiovascular system. Blood circulation starts

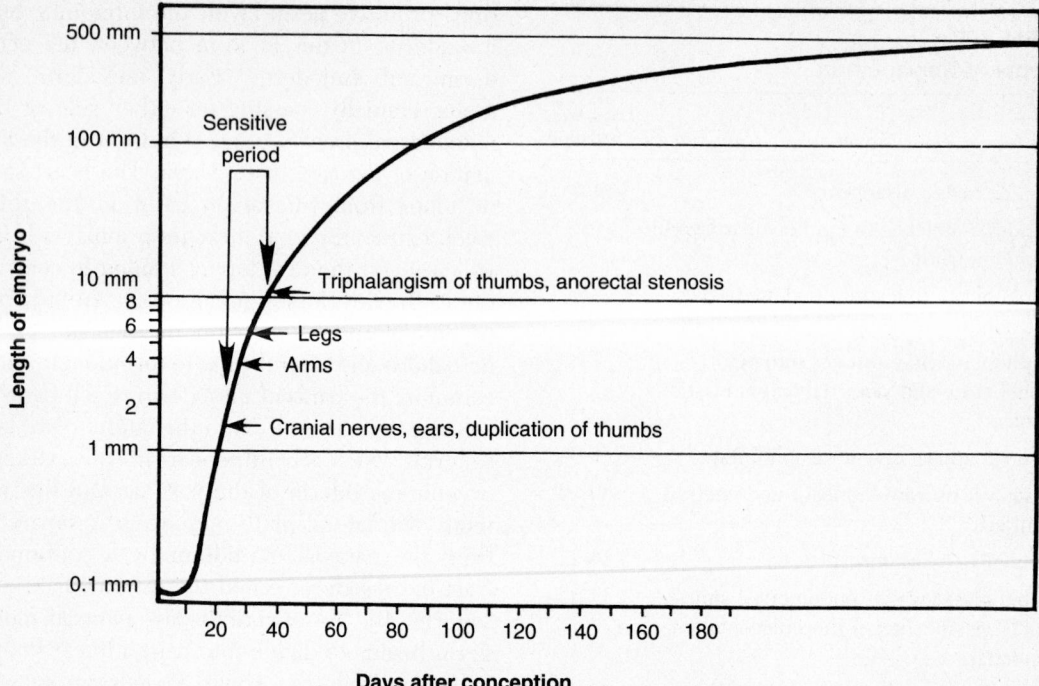

FIGURE 1-4

Schematic drawing of sensitive period for teratogenic effect of thalidomide with corresponding length of embryo. (From Lenz W: Chemicals and malformations in man. In Fishbein M, ed: Second International Conference on Congenital Malformations, New York, 1964, International Medical Congress.)

about this time, and the cardiovascular system becomes the first functioning organ system within the embryo.

From the fourth to the seventh week of gestation all the organ systems are formed. Only the genitourinary system is considered in detail later in this chapter.

A teratogenic event that takes place during the embryonic period gives rise to a constellation of malformations related to the organ systems that are actively developing at that particular time. Thus cardiovascular malformations tend to occur because of teratogenic events early in the embryonic period, whereas genitourinary abnormalities tend to occur because of events that occur later. Figure 1-4 demonstrates the malformations that were seen when thalidomide was applied to a human population during gestational days 35 to 50. Teratogenic effects before implantation often cause death but not malformations.

In general, the effects of a given teratogen depend on the genetic makeup of the individual, other environmental factors in play at the time, the stage during embryonic development that the teratogen is applied, and in some cases the dose of the teratogen and the duration that

it is allowed to act. Some teratogens in and of themselves are harmless, but their metabolites cause the damage. Teratogens may be chemical substances and their by-products, or they may be physical entities, such as temperature elevation and irradiation. Teratogenic agents applied after the forty-ninth day of gestation may injure or kill the embryo or cause developmental and growth retardation but usually will not be responsible for specific malformations. The period of embryonic development is said to be complete when the embryo attains a crown-rump length of 30 mm. It corresponds in most cases to day 49 after conception.

DEVELOPMENT OF THE GENITOURINARY SYSTEM

Excretory System

Nephrogenic cords develop from the intermediate mesoderm as early as the 2 mm embryo stage, beginning in the more cephalad portions of the embryo. Three sets of excretory ducts and tubules develop, each bilaterally. The first, the pronephros, with its pronephric ducts, forms in the most cranial portion of the embryo at about the beginning of the fourth week after conception. The tubules associated with the duct probably have no excretory function in the human. Late in the fourth week a second set of tubules, the mesonephric tubules, and their accompanying mesonephric ducts begin to develop. These are associated with tufts of capillaries, or glomeruli, and tubules for excretory purposes. Thus the mesonephros functions as a fetal kidney, producing urine for about 2 or 3 weeks. As new tubules develop, those derived from the more cephalad tubules degenerate. Usually about 40 mesonephric tubules function on either side of the embryo at any given time.

The metanephros, or permanent kidney, begins its development early in the fifth week of gestation and starts to function late in the seventh or early in the eighth week. The metanephros develops both from the metanephrogenic mass of mesoderm, which is the most caudal portion of the nephrogenic cord, and from its duct system, which is derived from the metanephric diverticulum (ureteric bud). It is a cranially growing outpouching of the mesonephric duct close to where it enters the cloaca. The latter gives rise to the ureter, the renal pelvis, the calyces, and the collecting tubules of the adult kidney. A critical process in the development of the kidney requires that the cranially growing metanephric diverticulum meet and fuse with the metanephrogenic mass of mesoderm so that formation of the kidney can take place. Originally the metanephric kidney is a pelvic organ, but by differential growth it becomes located in the lumbar region.

The fetus produces urine throughout all the periods of gestation, but the placenta handles the excretory functions of the fetus. The urine produced by the fetus contributes to the amniotic fluid. The fetus may swallow the amniotic fluid and recirculate it through the digestive system. This seems to be an important factor in regulating the amount of amniotic fluid present in the fetus. Agenesis of the kidneys generally results in little or no amniotic fluid, and gastrointestinal malformations or the inability of the fetus to swallow the amniotic fluid may lead to hydramnios.

Bladder and Urethra

The embryonic cloaca is divided by the urorectal septum into a dorsal rectum and a ventral urogenital sinus. The urogenital sinus, in turn, is divided into three parts: the cranial portion—the vesicourethral canal, which is continuous with the allantois; a middle pelvic portion; and a caudal urogenital sinus portion, which is closed over externally by the urogenital membrane. The epithelium of the developing bladder is derived from the endoderm of the vesicourethral canal. The muscular layers and serosa of the bladder develop from adjacent splanchnic mesenchyme. As the bladder develops, the caudal portion of the mesonephric ducts is incorporated into its dorsal wall. The portion of the mesonephric duct distal to the points where the metanephric duct is taken up into the bladder becomes the trigone of the bladder. Although this portion is mesoderm in origin, it is probably epithelialized eventually by endodermal epithelium from the urogenital sinus. In this way the ureters, derived from the metanephric duct, come to open directly into the bladder.

In the male the mesonephric ducts open into the urethra as the ejaculatory ducts. Also in the male, mesenchymal tissue surrounding the developing urethra where it exits the bladder develops into the prostate gland, through which the ejaculatory ducts traverse. Figure 1-5 demonstrates graphically the development of the male and female urinary systems.

The epithelium of the female urethra is derived from endoderm of the vesicourethral canal.

Genital Duct System

Early in embryonic life, two sets of paired genital ducts develop in each sex: the mesonephric (wolffian) ducts and the paramesonephric (müllerian) ducts. The mesonephric duct development precedes the paramesonephric duct development. The paramesonephric ducts develop on each side of the mesonephric ducts from the evaginations of the coelomic epithelium. The more cephalad ends of the ducts open directly into the peritoneal cavity, and the distal ends grow caudally, fusing in the lower midline to form the uterovaginal primordium. This tubular structure joins the dorsal wall of the urogenital sinus and produces an elevation, the müllerian tubercle. The mesonephric ducts enter the urogenital sinus on either side of the tubercle.

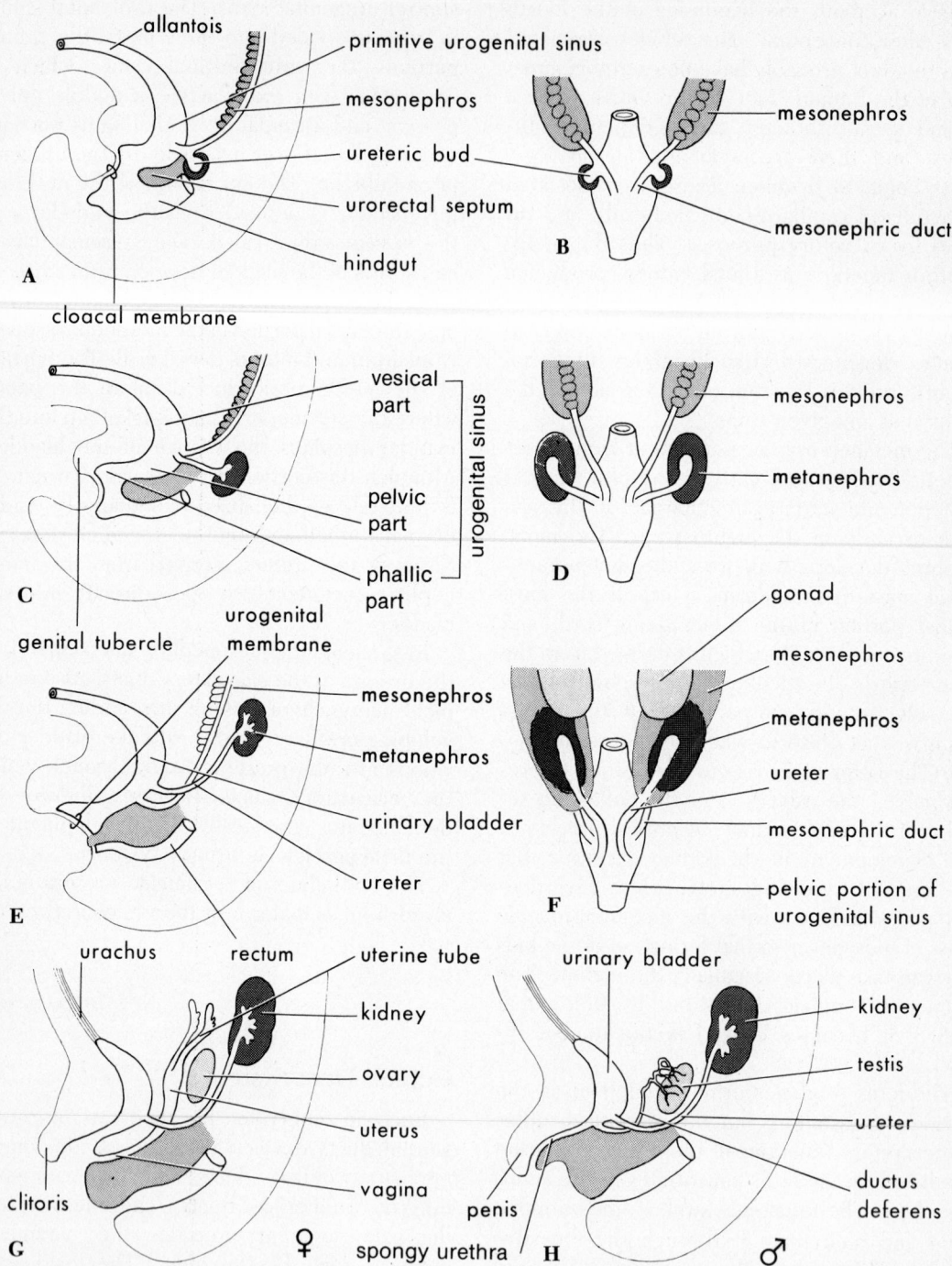

FIGURE 1-5

Graphic development of the urinary system in the male and female. Diagrams showing (1) division of the cloaca into urogenital sinus and rectum, (2) absorption of the mesonephric ducts, (3) development of the urinary bladder, urethra, and urachus, and (4) changes in the location of the ureters. **A**, Lateral view of the caudal half of 5-week-old embryo; **B, D,** and **F**, dorsal views; **C, E, G,** and **H,** lateral views. The stages shown in **G** and **H** are reached at about 12 weeks. (From Moore KL: The developing human: clinically oriented embryology, ed 3, 1982. Courtesy WB Saunders Co.)

Male Genital Ducts

Some seminiferous tubules are produced in the fetal testes during the seventh and eighth weeks after conception, and in the eighth week interstitial (Leydig) cells differentiate and begin to produce testosterone. At this point the mesonephric duct differentiates into the vas deferens, epididymis, and seminal vesicles, and the müllerian anlage is suppressed by the action of a substance known as müllerian inhibiting factor (MIF), produced by the Sertoli cells of the testes. The development of the prostate gland was referred to earlier. The bulbourethral glands, which are small structures that develop from outgrowths of endodermal tissue from the membranous portion of the urethra, incorporate stroma from the adjacent mesenchyme.

The most distal portion of the paramesonephric duct remains, in the male, as the appendix of the testes. The most proximal end of the paramesonephric duct remains as a small outpouching within the body of the prostate gland, known as the prostatic utricle. Occasionally the prostatic utricle is developed to the point where it will excrete a small amount of blood and cause hematuria in adult life.

Female Genital Ducts

In the presence of ovaries or of no gonads at all, the mesonephric ducts regress and the paramesonephric ducts develop into the female genital tract. This process begins at about 6 weeks and proceeds in a cephalad and caudal fashion. The more cephalad portions of the paramesonephric ducts, which open directly into the peritoneal cavity, form the fallopian tubes. The fused portion, or uterovaginal primordium, gives rise to the epithelium and glands of the uterus and cervix. Endometrial stroma and myometrium are derived from adjacent mesenchyme.

Failure of development of the paramesonephric ducts leads to agenesis of the cervix and the uterus. Failure of fusion of the caudal portion of these ducts may lead to a variety of anomalies of the uterus, including complete duplication of the uterus and cervix or partial duplication of a variety of types, which are outlined in Chapter 9.

Peritoneal reflections in the area adjacent to the fusion of the two paramesonephric ducts give rise to the formation of the broad ligaments. Mesenchymal tissue here develops into the parametrium.

The vagina develops from paired solid outgrowths of endoderm of the urogenital sinus, the sinovaginal bulbs. These grow caudally as a solid core toward the end of the uterovaginal primordium. This core constitutes the fibromuscular portion of the vagina. The sinovaginal bulbs then canalize to form the vagina. However, abnormalities in this process may lead to either transverse or horizontal vaginal septa. The junction of the sinovaginal bulbs with the urogenital sinus remains as the vaginal plate, which forms the hymen. This remains imperforate until late in embryonic life, although occasionally, perforation does not take place normally (imperforate hymen).

Failure of the sinovaginal bulbs to form leads to agenesis of the vagina. The precise boundary between the paramesonephric and urogenital sinus portions of the vagina has not been established.

Auxiliary genital glands in the female form from buds that grow out of the urethra. The buds derive contributions from the surrounding mesenchyme and form the urethral glands and the paraurethral glands (Skene's glands). These glands correspond to the prostate gland in males. Similar outgrowths of the urogenital sinus form the vestibular glands (Bartholin's glands), which are homologous to the bulbourethral glands in the male.

The remnants of the mesonephric duct in the female include a small structure called the appendix vesiculosa, a few blind tubules in the broad ligaments, the epoophoron, and a few blind tubules adjacent to the uterus collectively called the paroophoron. Remnants of the mesonephric duct system are often present in the broad ligaments or are adjacent to the uterus or the vagina as Gartner's duct cysts. The epoophoron or paroophoron may develop into cysts. Cysts of the epoophoron are known as paraovarian cysts.

Remnants of the paramesonephric duct in the female may be seen as a small, blind cystic structure attached by a pedicle to the distal end of the fallopian tube, the hydatid of Morgagni. Table 1-2 categorizes the adult derivatives and residual remnants of the urogenital structures in both the male and the female. Figure 1-6 outlines schematically the development of the internal sexual organs in both sexes.

TABLE 1-2
Male and Female Derivatives of Embryonic Urogenital Structures

Embryonic Structure	Derivatives	
	Male	Female
Labioscrotal swellings	Scrotum	Labia majora
Urogenital folds	Ventral portion of penis	Labia minora

Phallus	Penis
	   Glans, corpora cavernosa penis, and
	      corpus spongiosum
		Clitoris
		   Glans, corpora cavernosa, bulb of
		      the vestibule

Urogenital sinus	Urinary bladder Prostate gland Prostatic utricle Bulbourethral glands Seminal colliculus	Urinary bladder Urethral and paraurethral glands Vagina Greater vestibular glands Hymen
Paramesonephric duct	Appendix of testes	Hydatid of Morgagni Uterus and cervix Fallopian tubes
Mesonephric duct	Appendix of epididymis Ductus epididymis Ductus deferens Ejaculatory duct and seminal vesicle	Appendix vesiculosis Duct of epoophoron Gartner's duct —
Metanephric duct	Ureter, renal pelvis, calyces, and col- lecting system	Ureter, renal pelvis, calyces, and col- lecting system
Mesonephric tubules	Ductuli efferentes Paradidymis	Epoophoron Paroophoron
Undifferentiated gonad	Testis	Ovary
Cortex	Seminiferous tubules	Ovarian follicles
Medulla	— Rete testis	Medulla Rete ovarii
Gubernaculum	Gubernaculum testis	Round ligament of uterus

External Genitalia

In the fourth week after fertilization, the genital tubercle develops at the ventral tip of the cloacal membrane. Two sets of lateral bodies, the labioscrotal swellings and urogenital folds, develop soon after on either side of the cloacal membrane. The genital tubercle then elongates to form a phallus in both males and females. By the end of the sixth week, the cloacal membrane is joined by the urorectal septum. The septum separates the cloaca into the urogenital sinus ventrally and the anal canal and rectum dorsally. The point on the cloacal membrane where the urorectal septum fuses becomes the location of the perineal body in later development. The cloacal membrane is then divided into the ventral urogenital membrane and the dorsal anal membrane. These

membranes then rupture, opening the vulva and the anal canal. Failure of the anal membrane to rupture gives rise to an imperforate anus. With the opening of the urogenital membrane, a urethral groove forms on the undersurface of the phallus, completing the undifferentiated portion of external genital development. Differences between male and female embryos can be noted as early as the ninth week, but the distinct final forms are not noted until 12 weeks.

Androgens produced by the testes are responsible for the masculinization of the undifferentiated external genitalia. The phallus grows in length to form a penis, and the urogenital folds are pulled forward to form the lateral walls of the urethral groove on the undersurface of the penis. These folds then fuse to

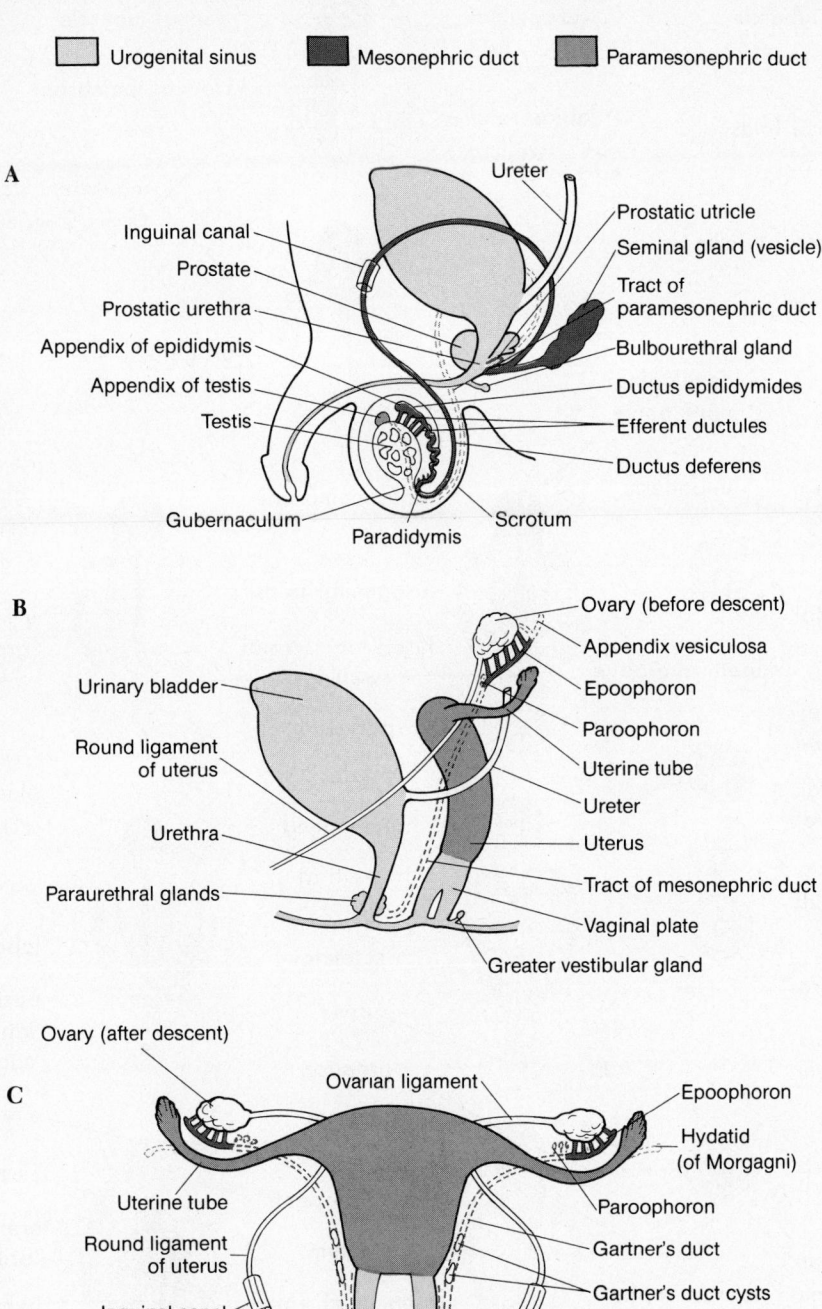

Urogenital sinus   Mesonephric duct   Paramesonephric duct

A

Ureter
Prostatic utricle
Seminal gland (vesicle)
Inguinal canal
Prostate
Prostatic urethra
Tract of paramesonephric duct
Appendix of epididymis
Appendix of testis
Bulbourethral gland
Ductus epididymides
Testis
Efferent ductules
Ductus deferens
Gubernaculum
Scrotum
Paradidymis

B

Ovary (before descent)
Appendix vesiculosa
Urinary bladder
Epoophoron
Round ligament of uterus
Paroophoron
Uterine tube
Ureter
Urethra
Uterus
Paraurethral glands
Tract of mesonephric duct
Vaginal plate
Greater vestibular gland

C

Ovary (after descent)
Ovarian ligament
Epoophoron
Hydatid (of Morgagni)
Uterine tube
Paroophoron
Round ligament of uterus
Gartner's duct
Gartner's duct cysts
Inguinal canal
Vagina
Labium majus   Hymen

FIGURE 1-6
Schematic drawings illustrating development of male and female reproductive systems from the primitive genital ducts. Vestigial structures are also shown. **A,** Reproductive system in a newborn male. **B,** Reproductive system in a female fetus at 12 weeks. **C,** Reproductive system in a newborn female. (From Moore KL: The developing human: clinically oriented embryology. Philadelphia, 1973, WB Saunders Co.)

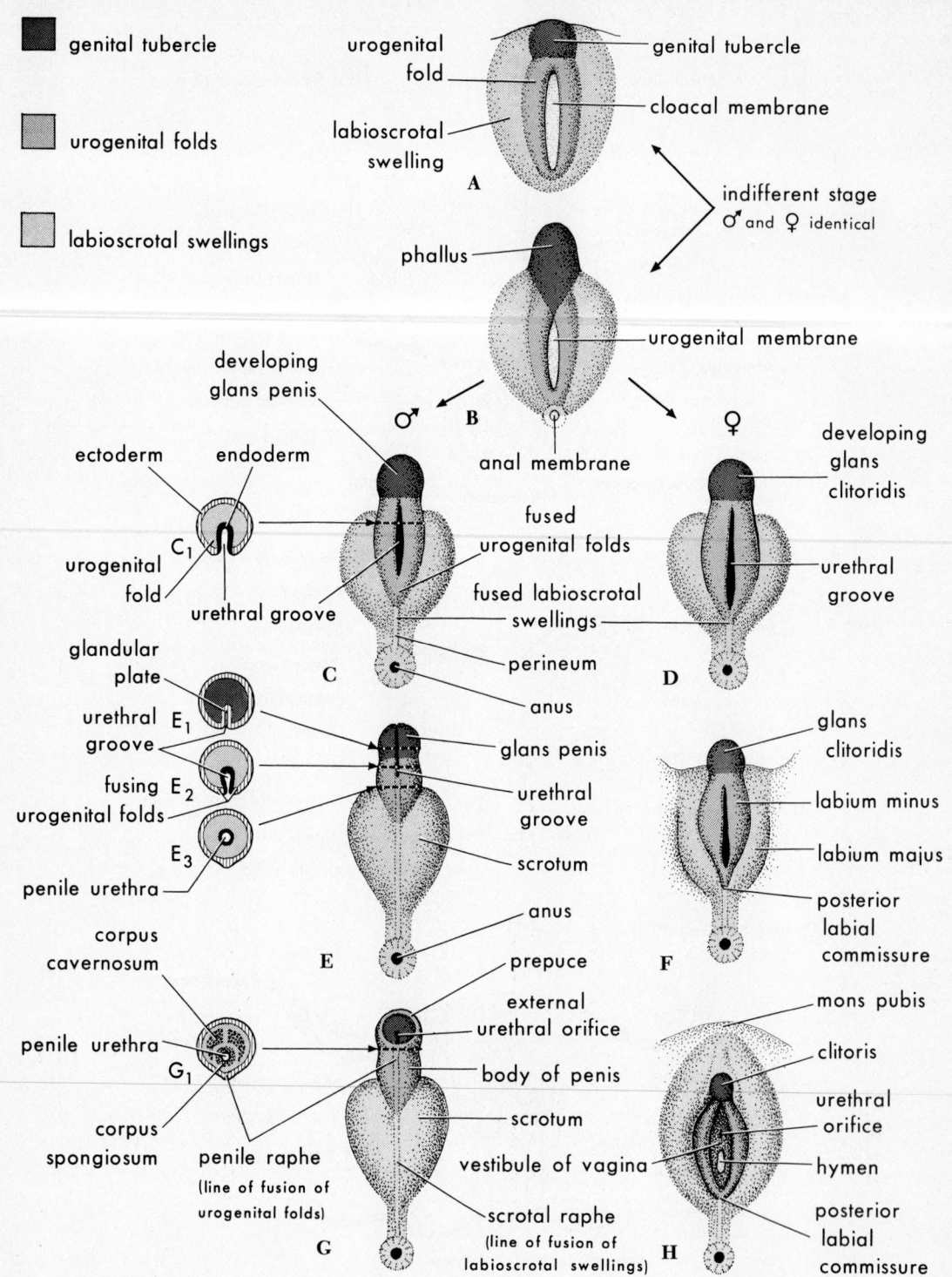

FIGURE 1-7

A and **B,** Development of the external genitalia in different stages (4 to 7 weeks). **C, E,** and **G,** Stages in the development of the external male genitalia at about 9, 11, and 12 weeks, respectively. To the left are schematic transverse sections (C_1, E_1 to E_3, and G_1) through the developing penis, illustrating formation of the penile urethra. **D, F,** and **H,** Stages in the development of the female external genitalia at 9, 11, and 12 weeks, respectively. (From Moore KL: The developing human: clinically oriented embryology, ed 3, 1982. Courtesy WB Saunders Co.)

form the penile urethra. Defects in fusion of various amounts give rise to various degrees of hypospadias. The skin at the distal margin of the penis grows over the glans to form the prepuce (foreskin). The vascular portion of the penis (corpora cavernosa penis and corpus cavernosum urethrae) arises from the mesenchymal tissue of the phallus. Finally, the labioscrotal swellings grow toward each other and fuse in the midline to form the scrotum. Later in embryonic life, usually at about the twenty-eighth week, the testes descend through the inguinal canal guided by the gubernaculum.

In the absence of androgen stimulation, feminization of the undifferentiated external genitalia occurs. The embryonic phallus does not demonstrate rapid growth and becomes the clitoris. Urogenital folds do not fuse except in front of the anus. The unfused urogenital folds form the labia minora. The labioscrotal folds fuse posteriorly in the area of the perineal body but laterally remain as the labia majora. The labioscrotal folds fuse anteriorly to form the mons pubis. A portion of the urogenital sinus between the level of the hymen and the labia develops into the vestibule of the vagina, into which the urethra, the vagina, and the ducts of Bartholin's glands enter.

The ovaries do not descend into the labioscrotal folds. A structure similar to the gubernaculum develops in the inguinal canal, giving rise to the round ligaments, which suspend the uterus in the adult. Figure 1-7 summarizes the development of the external genitalia in each sex.

SEX DIFFERENTIATION

Genetic sex is determined at the time of conception. In general, a Y chromosome is necessary for the development of the testes, and the testes are responsible for the organization of the sexual duct system to a male configuration and for the suppression of the paramesonephric system. In the absence of a Y chromosome, indeed, in the absence of a gonad, development will be female in nature. General phenotypic development of the female seems to be a neutral event.

One theory on sex differentiation is that genes coded on the Y chromosome are responsible for either the development of a cell-specific protein, the H-Y antigen, or the activator genes that stimulate the gene for the H-Y antigen on another chromosome. In rare cases a Y chromosome may be absent, but the H-Y antigen may express itself. In theory, one could speculate that in such cases the H-Y antigen was indeed present on another chromosome, most likely the X chromosome, and that either an activator gene or some other gene that acts as an activator is capable of stimulating its response.

Recently Amice et al. noted H-Y–positive lymphocytes in women with both idiopathic hirsutism and hirsute women with polycystic ovaries. These authors concluded that women can produce H-Y antigen in the same way as men and that hirsutism is associated with an increase in H-Y antigen.

New evidence suggests an alternative theory, which uses evidence that at least two genes are involved. The first is a testis-determining gene probably coded on the Y chromosome and designated Tdy. The second is an ovary-determining gene present on either the X chromosome or an autosome and designated Od. These genes are believed to interact and initiate either testis or ovary development, depending on their presence and time of expression in development. Thus in a normal XY male the Tdy gene is probably expressed earlier than the Od gene and may be responsible for Od inactivation. With a lack of Tdy in the normal XX female, the Od gene is expressed and the ovary develops. Sinclair et al. have recently described a 35-kilobase region on the human Y chromosome necessary for the male sex determination. This gene shows homology with other mammals, including the mouse, and is a candidate to be the Tdy gene.

During the fifth week after conception, coelomic epithelium, later known as germinal epithelium, thickens in the area of the medial aspect of the mesonephros. As germinal epithelial cells proliferate, they invade the underlying mesenchyme, producing a prominence known as the gonadal ridge. In the sixth week the primordial germ cells, which have formed at about week 4 in the wall of the yolk sac, migrate up the dorsal mesentery of the hind gut and enter the undifferentiated gonad. For the formation of a testis, H-Y antigen must be activated. A gene or genes in the area of the centromere of the Y chromosome cause the somatic cells of the primitive gonadal ridge to differentiate into interstitial cells (Leydig cells) and Sertoli cells. As they do so, the primordial

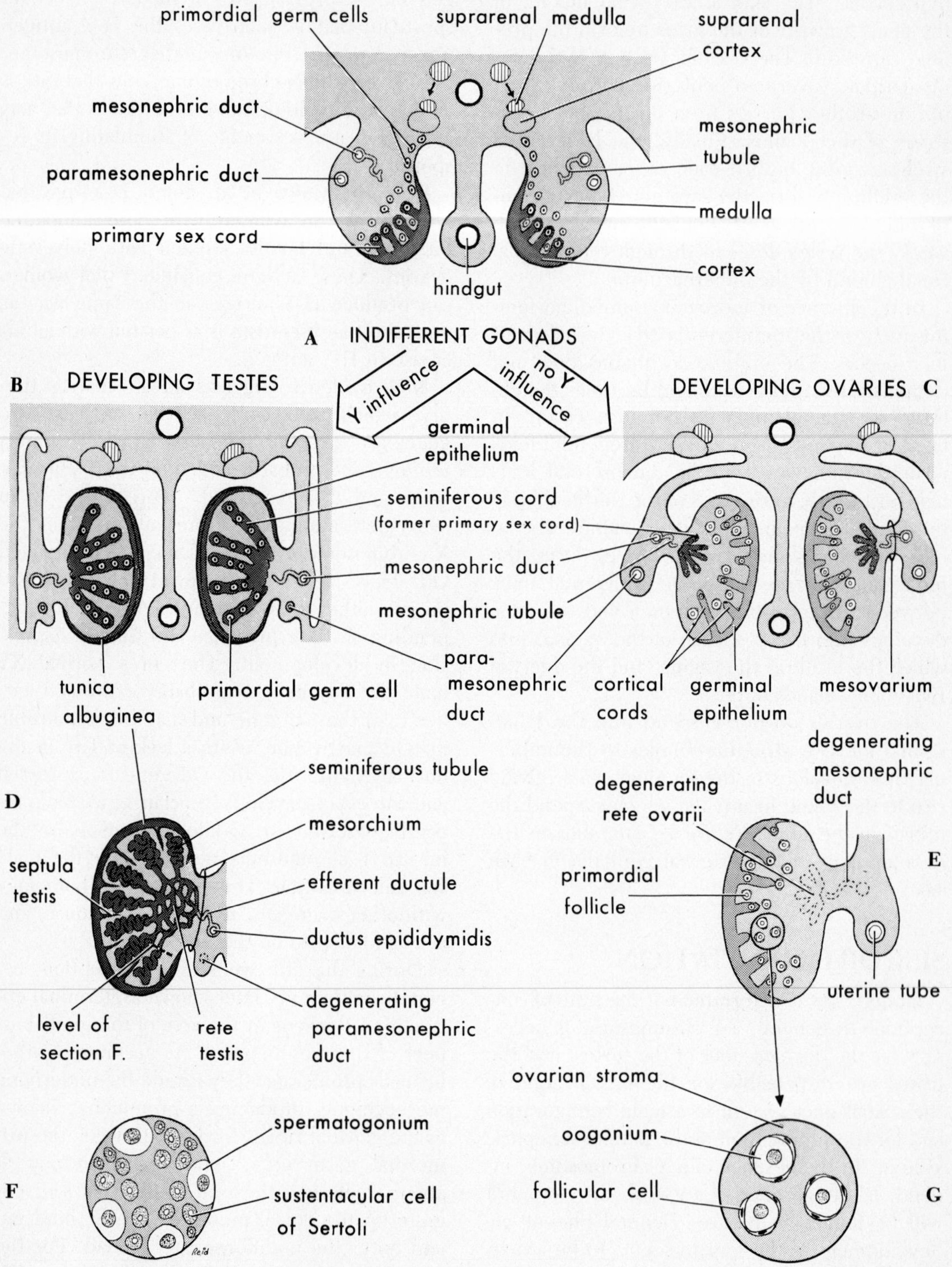

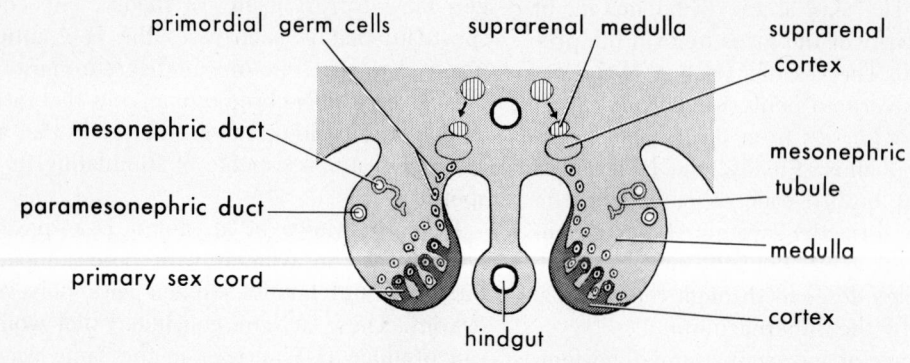

primordial germ cells   suprarenal medulla   suprarenal cortex

mesonephric duct

paramesonephric duct

primary sex cord

mesonephric tubule

medulla

cortex

hindgut

A   INDIFFERENT GONADS

B   DEVELOPING TESTES

Y influence   no Y influence

DEVELOPING OVARIES   C

germinal epithelium

seminiferous cord (former primary sex cord)

mesonephric duct

mesonephric tubule

para-mesonephric duct

tunica albuginea

primordial germ cell

cortical cords

germinal epithelium

mesovarium

D

seminiferous tubule

mesorchium

efferent ductule

ductus epididymidis

degenerating paramesonephric duct

septula testis

level of section F.

rete testis

degenerating rete ovarii

degenerating mesonephric duct

primordial follicle

uterine tube

E

ovarian stroma

F

spermatogonium

sustentacular cell of Sertoli

oogonium

follicular cell

G

FIGURE 1-8
Differences in development in gonads of each sex. (From Moore KL: The developing human: clinically oriented embryology, ed 3, 1982. Courtesy WB Saunders Co.)

germ cells and Sertoli cells become enclosed within seminiferous tubules, and the interstitial cells remain outside these tubules. H-Y antigen can be demonstrated in Sertoli cells at this stage but not in the developing germ cells. However, the H-Y antigen activity is passed to the germ cells by Sertoli cells when they are encased in the seminiferous tubules in the seventh and eighth weeks. In the eighth week Leydig cells differentiate and begin to produce testosterone. At this point the mesonephric (wolffian) duct differentiates into the vas deferens, epididymis, and seminal vesicles while the paramesonephric duct is suppressed because of the action of MIF.

Primary sex cords, meanwhile, have condensed and extended to the medullary portion of the developing testes. They branch and join to form the rete testis. The testis therefore is primarily a medullary organ, and eventually the rete testis connects with the tubules of the mesonephric system and joins the developing epididymal duct.

In specific androgen target areas, testosterone is converted to 5-α-dihydrotestosterone by the microsomal enzyme Δ-4-5-α-reductase. Data suggest that two androgens, testosterone and its metabolite, dihydrotestosterone, are involved in sexual differentiation in the male fetus, with selective roles for each hormone during embryogenesis; that is, dihydrotestosterone stimulates the testes and scrotum, and testosterone stimulates the prostate gland.

Androgen action must be initiated at the target areas. Testosterone enters the cell and either is bound to a cytoplasmic receptor or, in certain target tissue, is converted to dihydrotestosterone. Dihydrotestosterone in such cells would then bind to a cytoplasmic receptor. Afterward, the androgen-receptor complex gains access to the nucleus, where it binds to chromatin and initiates the transcription of messenger ribonucleic acid. This leads to the metabolic process of androgen action.

For normal male development in utero, the testes must differentiate and function normally.

At a critical point, MIF, produced by Sertoli cells, and testosterone, secreted by Leydig cells, must be produced in sufficient amounts. MIF acts locally in suppressing the müllerian duct system, and testosterone acts systemically, causing differentiation of the mesonephric duct system and affecting male development of the urogenital tubercle, urogenital sinus, and urogenital folds. Thus the masculinization of the fetus is a multifactorial process under a variety of genetic controls. Genes on the Y chromosome are responsible for testicular differentiation. Enzymes involved in testosterone biosynthesis and conversion to dihydrotestosterone are regulated by genes located on autosomes. The ability to secrete MIF is a recessive trait coded on either an autosome or the X chromosome, and genes for development of cytoplasmic receptors of androgens seem to be coded on the X chromosome.

Development of the ovary occurs at about the eleventh or twelfth week. Two functional X chromosomes seem necessary for optimal development of the ovary. The effect of an X chromosome deficiency is most severe in species in which there is a long period between the formation and use of oocytes (i.e., the human). Thus in 45,X and 46,XY females, the ovaries are almost invariably devoid of oocytes. On the other hand, germ cells in the testes do best when only one X chromosome is present; rarely do they survive in the XX or XXY condition.

When non-Y-bearing oocytes enter the differentiating gonad, the primary sex cords do not become prominent but, instead, break up and encircle the oocytes in the cortex of the gonad. This occurs at about 16 weeks, and the isolated cell clusters derived from the cortical cords that surround the oocytes are called primordial follicles. No new oogonia form after birth, and many of the oogonia degenerate before birth. Those that remain grow and become primary follicles to be stimulated after puberty. Figure 1-8 illustrates the differences in development in the gonads of each sex.

KEY POINTS

- Oocyte meiosis is arrested at prophase I from the fetal period until the time of ovulation.

- Fertilization occurs in the ampulla of the fallopian tube before the second polar body is cast off.

- After fertilization, first cell division leading to the two-cell embryo takes 20 hours.

- The human embryo enters the uterus somewhere between 3 and 4 days after conception. At this point it will be between the 32-cell and blastocyst stages of development.

- Implantation occurs when trophoblastic cells contact endometrium and burrow beneath the surface by enzymatic action. This generally takes place 3 days after the embryo enters the uterus.

- Twinning may occur at any time until the formation of the blastula, after which time each cell is no longer multipotential.

- The earliest fetal epithelium to develop is the ectoderm; the second is the endoderm; and the third is the mesoderm.

- Chorionic gonadotrophin is secreted by the syncytiotrophoblast at about the time of implantation. It doubles in quantity every 1.2 to 2 days until 7 to 9 weeks of gestation.

- Angiogenesis is seen by day 15 or 16. Embryonic heart function begins in the third week of gestation.

- Organogenesis is complete by day 49.

- The mesonephric duct system gives rise in the male to the epididymis, vas deferens, and seminal vesicles. Remnants of the mesonephric duct system in the female remain as parovarian cysts and Gartner's duct.

- The paramesonephric duct system develops in the female to give rise to the fallopian tube, uterus, and cervix. Remnants give rise to the hydatid of Morgagni at the end of the fallopian tubes. Remnants in the male remain as the appendix of the testes and prostatic utricle.

- The vagina develops from the sinovaginal bulbs, which are outgrowths of the urogenital sinus. Failure of these bulbs to form leads to agenesis of the vagina.

- The adult kidney develops from the metanephros, and its collecting system (ureter and calyceal system) develops from the metanephric (ureteric) bud from the mesonephric duct.

- The urinary bladder develops from the urogenital sinus.

- A Y chromosome is responsible for the development of testes. Without the presence of a Y chromosome, the gonadal development is usually that of an ovary or is undifferentiated. If no testicular tissue is present, the paramesonephric duct system develops into a phenotypic female configuration and the mesonephric duct system is suppressed.

- The genital tubercle elongates to form the penis in the male and the clitoris in the female.

- Two functional X chromosomes are necessary for optimal development of the ovary.

BIBLIOGRAPHY

Amice B, Bercovic JP, Nahoul K, et al: Increase in H-Y antigen-positive lymphocytes in hirsute women: Effects of cyproterone acetate and estradiol treatment, J Clin Endocrinol Metab 68:58, 1989.

Billington WD: Maternal immune response in pregnancy, Reprod Fertil Dev 1:183, 1989.

Hartman CG: Science and the safe period: A compendium of human reproduction, Huntington, NY, 1972, RE Krieger Publishing Co.

Heap RV, Flint AP, and Gadsby JE: Role of embryonic signals in the establishment of pregnancy, Br Med J 35:129, 1979.

Lenz W: Chemicals and malformations in man. In Fishbein M, ed: Second International Conference on Congenital Malformations, New York, 1964, International Medical Congress.

Mohr LR, Trounson AO, Leeton JF, and Wood C: Evaluation of normal and abnormal human embryo development during procedures in vitro. In Beier HM and Lindner HR, eds: Fertilization of human egg in-vitro, Berlin, 1983, Springer-Verlag.

Moor RM and Warnes RM: Meiosis in mammalian oocytes, Br Med Bull 35:97, 1979.

Moore KL: The developing human: Clinically oriented embryology, Philadelphia, 1973, WB Saunders Co.

Parhar RS, Yagel S, and Lala PK: PGE-2-mediated immunosuppressive by first trimester: human decidual cells block activation of maternal leukocytes in the decidua with potential antitrophoblast activity, Cell Immunol 120:61, 1989.

Patton HD, Fuchs AF, Hill EB, et al: Textbook of physiology, vol 2, Philadelphia, 1989, WB Saunders.

Short RV: Sex determination in differentiation, Br Med Bull 35:121, 1979.

Sinclair AH, Berta P, Palmer MS, et al: A gene from the human sex-determining region encodes a protein with homology to a conserved DNA-binding motif, Nature 346:240, 1990.

Tsafriri A: Oocyte maturation in mammals. In Jones RE, ed: The vertebrate ovary, New York, 1978, Plenum Publishing Corp.

Tsafriri A, Bar-Ami S, and Lindner HR: Control of the development of meiotic competence in an oocyte maturation in mammals. In Beier HM and Lindner HR, eds: Fertilization of human egg in-vitro, Berlin, 1983, Springer-Verlag.

Whittingham DG: In-vitro fertilization, embryo transfer and storage, Br Med Bull 35:105, 1979.

Mosaicism. The presence of two or more genetically different cell types within the same individual.

Mutation. An alteration in DNA leading to a phenotypic change. A dominant characteristic is one expressed phenotypically when the gene on only one chromosome of the pair is affected. A recessive characteristic requires the same mutant gene on both paired chromosomes for expression.

Nondisjunction. The failure of a pair of chromosomes to separate during meiosis or mitosis. In meiosis, if one daughter cell receives both members of the chromosome pair, after fertilization a triple number of the chromosome, or a trisomic state, exists in each cell.

Oncogenes. A gene normally important in cell skeleton structure or vital cell functions, which when mutated may convert the cell to a cancer cell.

Penetrance. The percentage of individuals in a population with a mutation that actually demonstrates a phenotypic change.

Restriction Endonucleases. Bacterial enzymes that recognize and cut specific nucleotide sequences in the double-stranded DNA molecule at specific sites. More than 200 different ones are known.

Restriction Fragment Length Polymorphism (RFLP). The study of DNA fragments produced by restriction endonucleases has demonstrated that normal individuals may have variations in the DNA sequences without the presence of an abnormality. In addition, differences are often seen in individuals with specific diseases, such as sickle cell anemia. Thus polymorphism exists with respect to the presence or absence of restriction sites, and this has been defined as restriction fragment length polymorphism.

Ribonucleic Acid (RNA). A single-helix nuclear protein that serves several purposes in the cell. It is composed of a sugar (ribose), a phosphate, and a purine or pyrimidine base.

Translocation. The rearrangement of two chromosomes involving the exchange of chromosome material. Balanced translocation is one in which no active genetic material is lost.

A number of illnesses and conditions have a genetic basis. In some cases the problem arises from a single-point mutation within a gene, whereas others may involve changes in multiple genes or in an interreaction of genes and environmental factors. Finally, some conditions are the result of chromosome abnormalities of a variety of types. Although this chapter cannot provide a complete course in genetics, it attempts to offer an understanding of the genetic basis of conditions of particular interest to the gynecologist.

GENES AND GENE ACTION

Genes consist of deoxyribonucleic acid (DNA) molecules, which are made up of a linear sequence of nucleotides, each of which is composed of a pentose sugar, a phosphate, and a nitrogenous base. Four such bases are found in a DNA molecule. They are two purines, adenine (A) and guanine (G), and two pyrimidines, thymine (T) and cytosine (C). It has been shown that the total amount of purine in DNA molecules equals the total amount of pyrimidine, and the pairings of A to T and G to C always occur in the two strands of the double helix. These associations allow for accuracy both in the replication of the DNA molecule and in the translation of a genetic message from the DNA molecule to the development of a single-strand ribonucleic acid (RNA) molecule known as messenger RNA. The message is transmitted in such a fashion that a configuration with three bases in sequence represents a code, known as the *genetic code*, for an amino acid. With the message of the gene encoded on the messenger RNA, the latter leaves the nucleus of the cell, attaches to a cytoplasmic structure (the ribosome), and then attracts amino acids by means of smaller RNA molecules known as *transfer RNA*. Transfer RNA molecules each carry a specific amino acid and have three bases, which match the code of the

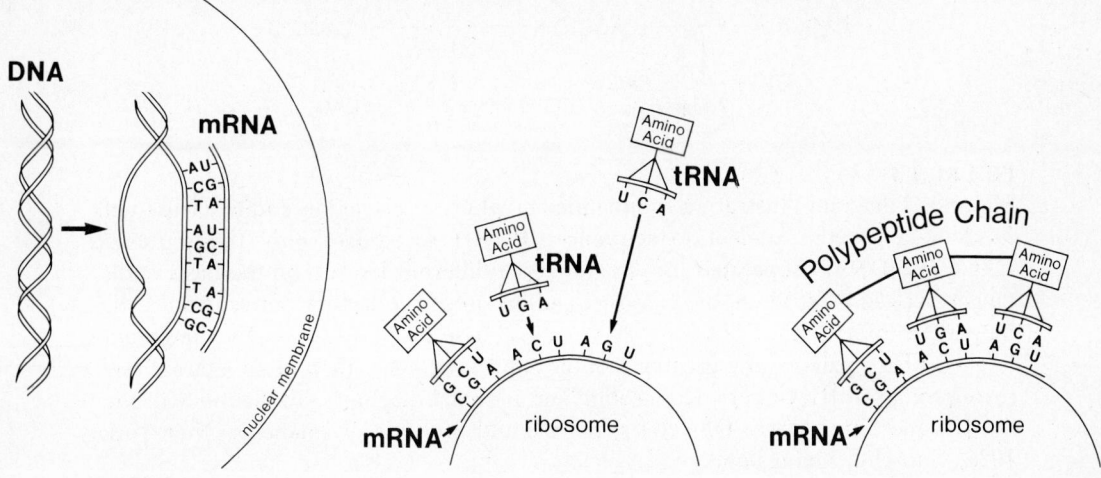

FIGURE 2-1
Schematic representation of protein production from genetic message on the DNA molecule to the final product.

messenger RNA, following the A to T and G to C pairings. In the RNA molecule, uracil (U) is substituted for thymine. When all segments of the message are covered, the amino acids are spliced together and the protein determined by the message is complete and free for use in the cell and for transport from the cell. Figure 2-1 schematically demonstrates this process.

GENE MUTATION

Conditions that change the sequence of bases in the genetic code may cause a mutation. The mutation may involve a single point, that is, the changing of a single base, or a larger segment, in which the bases are removed or replaced. Mutation may occur spontaneously by the accidental replacement of one base with another during replication of DNA, by the incorporation of an inappropriate base during repair of a DNA molecule, or by an intermediate replacement with a substance similar to a usual base but capable of entering the DNA molecule and later attracting an inappropriate base in the next replication. Agents such as x-rays or other forms of irradiation may break a DNA strand, leading to the loss of one or more bases and a complete change in the sequence or to a replacement with an inappropriate base during healing. Even a single-point mutation will lead to the production of a modified protein that may be responsible for an abnormal expression of a trait. Figure 2-2 demon-

	Possible Mutation 1	Possible Mutation 2
Hgb A (glutamic acid)	CTT	CTC
Hgb S (valine)	CAT	CAC
Hgb C (lysine)	TTT	TTC

FIGURE 2-2
Point mutation in a DNA molecule causing a single amino acid substitution and conversion of hemoglobin A to hemoglobin S or hemoglobin C.

strates such an occurrence for a group of hemoglobinopathies caused by the substitution of a single base at a single point.

Recent studies using molecular genetic techniques have made it possible not only to isolate and amplify genes responsible for specific characteristics, but also to evaluate the biochemical nature of a mutation. The key to the localization of genetic information on the DNA molecule has been the discovery of a group of more than 200 bacterial enzymes, restriction endonucleases, that recognize and cut specific nucleotide sequences in the double-stranded DNA molecule. The sites of their action are known as restriction sites. Each enzyme recognizes a unique sequence of nucleotides. Figure 2-3 demonstrates the action of one such enzyme, Pvu II, to separate the nucleotide junc-

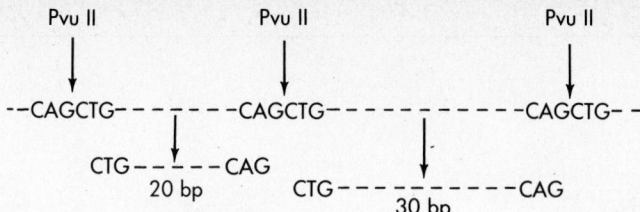

FIGURE 2-3

Simplified diagram illustrating the manner in which a restriction endonuclease cuts DNA at a specific nucleotide sequence. Pvu II recognizes only the sequence CAGCTG. DNA is separated into fragments of different lengths on the basis of distances between restriction enzyme recognition sites. The farther between sites, the longer the intervening DNA (i.e., 20 versus 30 base pairs). Shorter DNA fragments (e.g., 20 base pairs) show greater mobility and migrate farther in an agarose cell. (From Simpson JL: Genetic Counseling and prenatal diagnosis. In Gabbe SG, Niebyl JR, and Simpson JL: Obstetrics: normal and problem pregnancies, New York, 1986, Churchill Livingstone.)

TABLE 2-1

Genetic Diseases Associate with Restriction Fragment Length Polymorphism (RFLP)

Disease	Chromosome	Disease	Chromosome
Huntington's disease	4	Ornithine transcarbamoylase deficiency	X
Cystic fibrosis	7		
Polycystic kidney disease	16	Lesch-Nyhan syndrome	X
Familial Alzheimer's disease	21	Choroideremia	X
Myotonic muscular dystrophy	19	Lowe's oculocerebrorenal syndrome	X
Wilms' tumor	11	Wiskott-Aldrich syndrome	X
Sickle cell anemia	11	Coffin-Lowry syndrome	X
Thalassemia	11	Andersen-Fabry disease (alpha-galactosidase A deficiency)	X
Acute intermittent porphyria	11		
Retinoblastoma	13	Adrenoleukodystrophy	X
von Recklinghausen's neurofibromatosis	17	Fragile X syndrome (X-linked metal retardation)	X
Bilateral acoustic neurofibromatosis	22	Steroid sulphatase deficiency (X-linked ichthyosis)	X
Systemic amyloidosis in juvenile arthritis	1	Charcot-Marie-Tooth disease (X-linked neuropathy)	X
Osteogenesis imperfecta	7		
Multiple endocrine neoplasia type 2A	10	X-linked spinal muscular atrophy	X
Familial adenomatous polyposis (colon cancer)	5	X-linked anhidrotic ectodermal dysplasia	X
Manic-depressive illness	11	X-linked retinitis pigmentosa	X
Tuberous sclerosis	9	X-linked retinoschisis	X
Phenylketonuria	12	X-linked chronic granulomatous disease	X
von Willebrand's disease	12		
Alpha-antitrypsin deficiency	14	X-linked hypophosphatemia	X
Spinocerebellar ataxia	6	X-linked nephrogenic diabetes insipidus	X
Congenital and adrenal hyperplasia (steroid 21-hydroxylation deficiency)	6		
Duchenne's muscular dystrophy	X	X-linked spastic paraplegia	X
Becker-type muscular dystrophy	X	X-linked cleft palate	X
Emery-Dreifuss muscular dystrophy	X	X-linked myotubular myopathy	X
Hemophilia A	X	X-linked dysplasia gigantism syndrome	X
Hemophilia B (factor IX deficiency)	X		

From Watkins PC: Restriction fragment length polymorphism (RFLP): applications in human chromosome mapping and genetic disease research, BioTechniques 6:310, 1988.

tion GC in the sequence CAGCTG. Using these techniques it has been possible to define the specific genetic material related to almost 100 disease states, such as sickle cell anemia, the thalassemias, and cystic fibrosis. Identification of an affected individual or carrier may be accomplished by specifically identifying the mutant gene or by identifying a closely linked gene known to be associated with the mutant gene in one of the parents. This linkage study is an indirect means of identifying whether the mutant gene is present and is based on the fact that closely linked genes rarely separate during the process of meiotic crossover. These techniques have been helpful in the prenatal diagnosis of several conditions and in the identification of carrier states.

The study of DNA fragments produced by restriction endonucleases has identified a number of normal individuals with variations in DNA sequences but without any specific abnormality. Likewise, DNA fragment differences have been discovered in different individuals with the same condition. Therefore it is known that polymorphism exists with respect to the presence or absence of restriction sites, referred to as *restriction fragment length polymorphism (RFLP)*. A number of genetic diseases have been identified as associated with RFLPs (Table 2-1). These molecular techniques continue to be useful tools in the prenatal diagnosis of an increasing number of conditions but will also aid in the development of our understanding of many disease states and conditions. Eventually they will play a role in our ability to find therapies for conditions whose roots are in genetic mutation.

TYPES OF INHERITANCE

Autosomal Dominant Trait

If only one gene of a pair is mutated and if the altered protein produced by the mutated gene brings about a phenotypic change, the condition is said to be *autosomal dominant*. If both genes of a pair must carry the mutation for the phenotypic characteristic to occur, the condition is said to be *autosomal recessive*. Usually, if 50% of the protein produced by the gene pair is enough to give the usual phenotype, the condition is dominant. However, phenotypic expression of a mutation may occasionally occur under unusual circumstances.

For example, a patient with sickle cell trait usually does not experience red blood cell sickling at sea level with normal oxygen saturation but may do so at high altitudes or in cases of decreased oxygen saturation, which may occur with pneumonia. Thus the presence of hemoglobin S in the red blood cell in equal proportions to hemoglobin A does not usually lead to the expression of sickling unless oxygen saturation is decreased.

With respect to autosomal dominant conditions, the concept of *penetrance* and *expressivity* must be introduced to explain some variations noted. Penetrance is the percentage of individuals in a population with the mutation that actually demonstrates the phenotypic change. Expressivity is the degree to which the phenotypic change occurs in the affected individual, that is, the degree to which the gene expresses itself. Penetrance and expressivity are dependent on the action of other genes and on environmental factors that may modify the action of the mutated gene.

The following general statements can be made about autosomal dominant mutations:

1. Phenotypic expression appears with equal frequency in both sexes.
2. For inheritance to take place, at least one parent must be affected unless a new mutation has occurred.
3. When an individual who is homozygous for the mutation (mutation occurs on both genes of the pair) is mated with a normal individual, all offspring will carry the trait. When a heterozygous individual is mated with a normal individual, 50% of the offspring will demonstrate the trait.
4. If the trait is rare in the population, most individuals demonstrating it will be heterozygous.

The following is a list of a number of autosomal dominant conditions:

Achondroplasia
Angioedema, hereditary
Craniofacial dysostosis
Dupuytren's contracture
Ehlers-Danlos syndrome
Facial palsy, congenital
Huntington's chorea
Intestinal polyposis
Keloid formation
Marfan's syndrome
Mitral valve prolapse
Muscular dystrophy

Neurofibromatosis (von Recklinghausen's disease)
Night blindness
Otosclerosis
Pectus excavatum
Renal disease, polycystic, adult type
Tuberous sclerosis
von Willebrand's disease
Wolff-Parkinson-White syndrome (some cases)

When one parent demonstrates one of these conditions, appropriate counseling would be that 50% of future offspring could be expected to demonstrate the condition as well. When neither parent demonstrates the condition but when a child is born with such a condition, it can be assumed that the problem is caused by a new mutation. In such cases, future progeny of the couple would be expected to be no more likely to have the condition than would occur by chance mutation.

Autosomal Recessive Trait

The following general statements can be made about an autosomal recessive trait:
1. The characteristic will occur equally in both sexes.
2. For the characteristic to be present, both parents must demonstrate or be carriers of the recessive trait.
3. If both parents are homozygous for the trait, all offspring will demonstrate it.
4. If both parents are heterozygous (carrier) for the trait, 25% of the offspring will have the trait and 50% will be carriers. The remaining 25% will be free of the trait.
5. Consanguinity is often present in families demonstrating frequent occurrences of rare recessive traits.

The following is a list of a number of common autosomal recessive conditions:

Acid maltase deficiency
Alkaptonuria
Ataxia-telangiectasia
Bloom's syndrome
Color blindness (total)
Cystic fibrosis
Cystinosis
Cystinuria
Deafness (many variants)
Dysautonomia
Galactosemia
Gaucher's disease
Glaucoma (congenital)
Homocystinuria
11β-hydroxylase deficiency

21-hydroxylase deficiency
Maple syrup urine disease
Mucolipidosis I, II, III
Mucopolysaccharidosis I-H, I-S, III, IV, VI, VII
Muscular dystrophy (autosomal recessive)
Niemann-Pick disease
Phenylketonuria
Sickle cell anemia
Tay-Sachs disease
Wilson's disease

In counseling a couple who have produced a child with such a characteristic, it is appropriate to tell them that 25% of future offspring will have the condition and 50% will be carriers. If a prenatal diagnostic test is available, it should be offered. One autosomal recessive condition, Tay-Sachs disease, is the subject of a large national screening program to determine carriers. Because the condition usually occurs in Jews of Eastern European origin, such individuals should certainly be offered screening. Another major screening program is aimed at discovering sickle cell anemia in blacks.

X-Linked Trait

Most X-linked conditions are recessive in type, since female carriers do not demonstrate the trait. A few conditions belie this rule, however, and are really X-linked dominant conditions. For the X-linked recessive trait the following statements are true:
1. The condition is more common in males.
2. If both parents are free of the trait and a male is produced with the trait, it must be assumed that the mother is a carrier.
3. If the father is affected and an affected male is produced, it must be assumed that the mother is at least a carrier of the trait.
4. If a female is produced who exhibits the X-linked trait, she may do so for one of two reasons. First, she may have received the mutant gene from both the mother and father and thereby is homozygous for the trait. Generally this would imply the father is affected and the mother is a carrier. Second, she may exhibit the trait as a function of the Lyon hypothesis, which states that in a female heterozygous for the trait, each cell of the developing embryo from about the time of implantation selects and uses one X chromosome only. Thereafter all developing cells from these particular cells use the same X chromo-

some. Thus a female is mosaic for her two X chromosomes, with some cells using the paternal X chromosome and some using the maternal X chromosome. Because this selection occurs on a random basis, some females will be produced who use an X chromosome predominantly from one parent. If the X chromosome has the mutation, the female will exhibit the trait because of the quantitative influence of that chromosome. Thus the female may be genotypically heterozygous but still exhibit the trait.

In the case of X-linked dominant traits the following may be said:

1. They occur in both males and females with equal frequency.
2. An affected male mated to a normal female will produce offspring with the trait 50% of the time, but all female offspring will be affected.
3. An affected homozygous female mated to a normal male will produce offspring with the trait 100% of the time.
4. Occasional heterozygous females will not exhibit the trait on the basis of the Lyon hypothesis.

The following is a list of several X-linked recessive conditions:

Agammaglobulinemia, X-linked, infantile
Androgen insensitivity syndrome, complete
Androgen insensitivity syndrome, incomplete
Color blindness, several varieties
Diabetes insipidus, some varieties
Fabry's disease
Glucose-6-phosphate dehydrogenase deficiency
Gonadal dysgenesis, XY type (probable)
Gout, some types
Factor VIII disease
Factor IX disease
Lesch-Nyhan syndrome
Mucopolysaccharidosis II
Muscular dystrophy, Duchenne type

Some X-linked dominant conditions are as follows:

Aeroosteolysis, dominant type
Cervicooculoacoustic syndrome
Hyperammonemia
Orofaciodigital syndrome I
Tubular stenosis (possible)

Multifactorial Inheritance

Multifactorial inheritance is defined as traits or characteristics produced by the action of several genes, with or without the interplay of environmental factors. A number of structural abnormalities such as cleft palate and harelip, open neural tube disease (including anencephaly and spina bifida), and several orthopedic and cardiac defects are examples of such conditions. When both parents are normal and an affected child is produced, the chance of recurrence is generally between 2% and 5% for any given pregnancy. These risk rates, however, are modified when one or both parents are affected with the condition or when close relatives are also affected. Many multifactorial diseases and conditions are more common in offspring when transmitted via the mother, and in general, when more than one offspring is affected in a family, the chances that subsequent offspring will be affected are greater.

Open neural tube disease (NTD) is a good example of a multifactorial defect. When a couple produces a child with such a defect, appropriate counseling is important. In this condition the observation that alpha-fetoprotein is increased both in the amniotic fluid and in the maternal serum in affected offspring is helpful in making a prenatal diagnosis of the condition. Ultrasound examination is also helpful in making a specific diagnosis. Although the diagnosis can be made prenatally if sought, 9 of 10 cases occur spontaneously in the offspring of couples who have no family or personal history. This observation has led to the suggestion that all pregnancies be screened with maternal serum alpha-fetoprotein determinations to uncover such cases antenatally. At present, screening programs are common. In fact, California has developed a state-wide screening program for all pregnancies. Patients should probably be offered the option of being studied even if there is no family history of open neural tube disease.

The screening of 1000 pregnant women will uncover about 50 who have maternal serum alpha-fetoprotein determinations in excess of 2.5 times the mean for values considered normal for their specific week of gestation. Although a number of instances of multiple gestation, Turner syndrome, other anomalies, and fetal demise may be uncovered, only about 1 of these 50 women will actually prove to be carrying a fetus with NTD.

Chromosome Abnormalities

A variety of chromosome abnormalities may occur during meiosis or mitosis (see Chapter

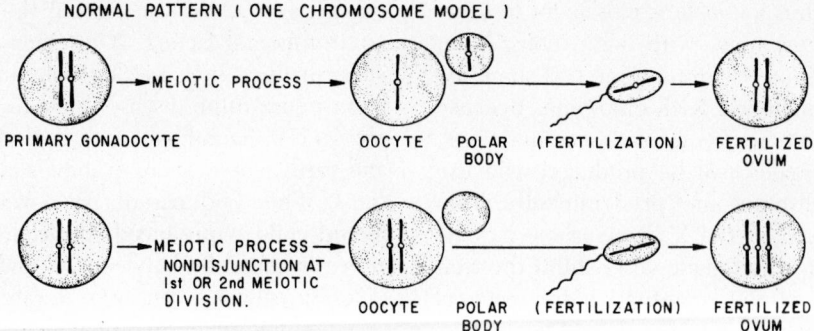

NORMAL PATTERN (ONE CHROMOSOME MODEL)

FIGURE 2-4
Meiotic nondisjunction, graphic representation. (Reproduced with permission from Stenchever MA: Human cytogenetics: a workbook in reproductive biology, Chicago, 1973, Mosby–Year Book, Inc.)

1). They fall into several general categories, and many clinical conditions are associated with each type. Although it is impossible within the scope of this chapter to discuss every clinical condition associated with a known chromosome abnormality, an attempt is made to categorize the specific types of anomalies and the more common problems seen by obstetricians and gynecologists that relate to these anomalies. Several conditions are dealt with in more detail in other chapters of this book.

Nondisjunctional Events and Deletion

A nondisjunctional event is the faulty separation of chromosome pairs at anaphase in either meiosis or mitosis. The result in meiosis is that the daughter cell receives either both chromosomes of the pair or neither. At the time of fertilization, with the addition of another haploid set of chromosomes, the resulting individual will have either three chromosomes at that particular position or only one (Figure 2-4). In normal mitosis, after division of the chromosomes at anaphase, a complete pair goes to each daughter cell. If nondisjunction occurs, three chromosomes go to one daughter cell and one to the other.

Deletion is the simple loss of a chromosome at anaphase because of either anaphase lag or nondisjunction. In this instance the new cell receives only one chromosome of the pair and is essentially monosomic for that chromosome. Monosomic states involving autosomes are extremely rare and generally lethal. With respect to the sex chromosomes, monosomy of the Y chromosome without the presence of an X

chromosome is likewise lethal and has never been seen in a clinical situation or even in an abortus. Monosomy of the X chromosome, however, is the typical finding in the condition known as *Turner syndrome.* This condition is likewise lethal, with as many as 24 of each 25 of such conceptuses being aborted. When an infant is born alive with a 45,X karyotype (Figure 2-5), the common denominators of shortness of stature and sexual infantilism are seen, and many abnormalities involving most of the organ systems may likewise occur. One frequent occurrence (about 50% of cases) is webbing of the neck, which is the end product of hygromas seen during embryologic development (Figure 2-6).

Nondisjunctional events involving the autosomes have been seen in abortus material in all but chromosomes 1 and 17. However, in infants born alive, only trisomic states of chromosomes 13, 18, 21, and 22 and an occasional C group chromosome have been seen. Trisomy of chromosome 13 (Patau's syndrome) results in gross multiple structural defects that are usually incompatible with extended life. Trisomy of chromosome 18 likewise leads to a syndrome (Edwards' syndrome) that has a characteristic group of structural abnormalities, again generally not compatible with long life. Trisomy 21 is classic Down syndrome, and trisomy 22 has been seen in a few live-born individuals but is associated with severe retardation.

Trisomy involving the sex chromosomes has been seen in circumstances relating to both the X and the Y chromosome. Nondisjunctional events involving both oogenesis and spermatogenesis can be responsible, as in autosomal trisomy.

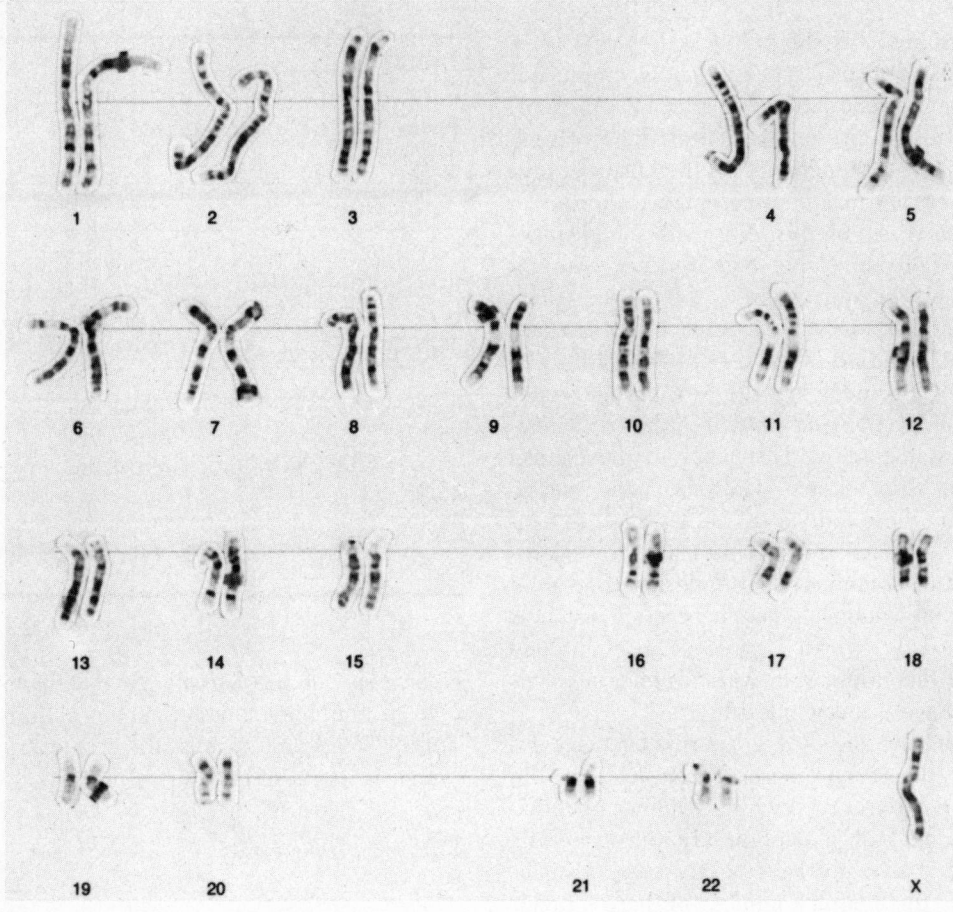

FIGURE 2-5
Example of a karyotype from a newborn patient with Turner syndrome showing the presence of a single X chromosome (45,X).

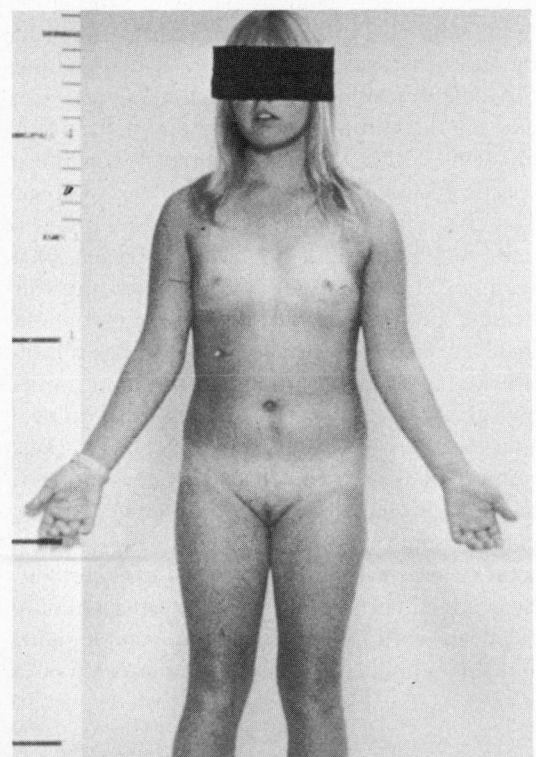

FIGURE 2-6
A 17-year-old patient with Turner syndrome demonstrating short stature, poor sexual development, and increased carrying angles at elbows. Patient also has webbing of the neck.

If trisomy X is the result, a female with a reasonably normal phenotype is produced. Mild mental retardation is occasionally present, but fertility is present in at least 50% of such individuals. Although most of the offspring produced are normal chromosomally, there is a slight increase of offspring with nondisjunctional events involving both the sex chromosomes and the autosomes.

Individuals with a 47,XXY karyotype are likewise produced as the result of a nondisjunctional event involving the sex chromosomes that may occur by an error in either oogenesis or spermatogenesis. This leads to the clinical state of Klinefelter's syndrome. The classic finding in these individuals is that they are usually tall and have azoospermia caused by sclerosis of the seminiferous tubules. Other mild phenotypic anomalies may be present, such as gynecomastia, which is present in about one third of the cases. Men with Klinefelter's syndrome have primary infertility.

Nondisjunction during spermatogenesis involving the Y chromosome can lead to the karyotype 47,XYY. Such individuals may be entirely normal phenotypically but generally are tall, and many have aggressive personalities. For this reason a number of these individuals have been found in prisons and mental hospitals, but just as many have been found among the normal population. Although such men are fertile, their female partners often have repetitive abortion and other reproductive wastage problems, and this may be the means of identifying such cases. In addition, they often produce offspring with normal karyotypes but may produce conceptuses with trisomic problems involving both autosomes and the sex chromosomes.

Nondisjunctional events during mitosis in the early embryo frequently produce individuals with cell populations containing different chromosome numbers. This condition, known as *mosaicism*, may involve any of the members of the autosome complement or the sex chromosomes. The actual phenotype produced depends on the number of cells present with an abnormal complement and on the tissue in which these cells have the opportunity to express themselves.

Turner syndrome has afforded an excellent opportunity to evaluate the various chromosomal mechanisms that can lead to the same (or similar) phenotypic finding. Table 2-2 summarizes many of the karyotypes that have been detected in patients with the clinical findings of Turner syndrome. Thus the clinical picture can occur because of an error in meiosis or mitosis or because of chromosome rearrangements.

Chromosome Breaks and Rearrangements

Chromosome breaks and rearrangements may be brought about by damage to the chromosome caused by irradiation of many different types, by viruses, or by other changes within the cell or within its environment that can damage the chromosome structure or the DNA molecule within the chromosome. When these breaks occur, a number of things can happen. The break may simply heal, with or without a point mutation at the point of breakage. If a segment of the chromosome is lost during this healing process, partial deletion of chromatin material may take place. If two chromosomes break, they may exchange chromosome arms and give rise to a translocation. In karyotypes, translocations have been seen involving various combinations of all the chromosomes. Although they are probably a chance occurrence, there may be some active areas on various chromosomes that make such events more common. Rearranged chromosomes at first are generally balanced with respect to gene complement, and the individual so affected is referred to as a *carrier* of the translocation and can expect in

TABLE 2-2
Karyotypes Discovered in Patients with Phenotypic Characteristics of Turner Syndrome

Karyotype	Error
45,X	Deletion X
45,Xi (Xq)	Deletion Xp, Isochromosome Xq
45,X,Xq	Deletion Xp
45,X/46,XX	Mosaicism
45,X/46,XX/47,XXX	Mosaicism
45,X/46,XY	Mosaicism
45,X/46,XY/47,XYY	Mosaicism
45,XringX	Ring chromosome
46,XX	Phenotype with normal karyotype

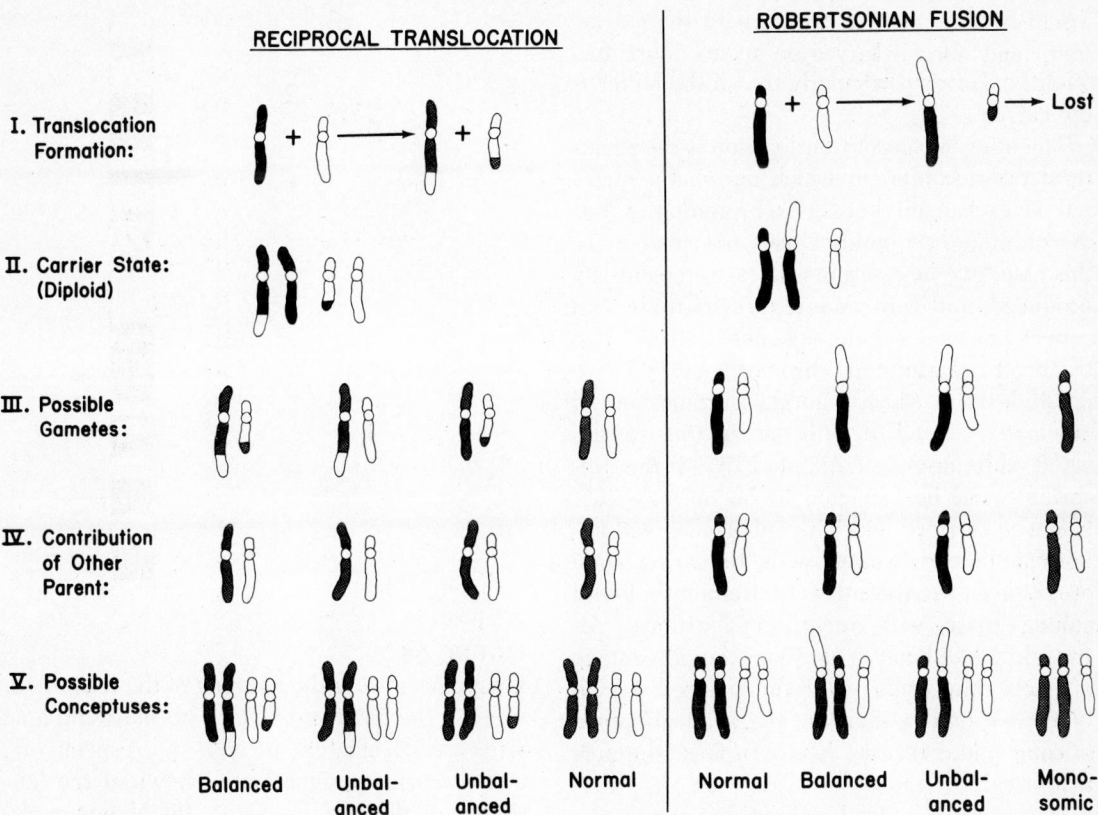

RECIPROCAL TRANSLOCATION

ROBERTSONIAN FUSION

I. Translocation Formation:

II. Carrier State: (Diploid)

III. Possible Gametes:

IV. Contribution of Other Parent:

V. Possible Conceptuses:

Balanced | Unbalanced | Unbalanced | Normal | Normal | Balanced | Unbalanced | Monosomic

Lost

FIGURE 2-7

Schematic representation of translocation formation, including reciprocal translocation and Robertsonian fusion. (From Stenchever MA: Contemp OB/GYN 16:24, 1980.)

most cases to be phenotypically normal. About 10% of new translocations, even though balanced, are associated with mental retardation and other mild anomalies. These carrier individuals, however, have difficulty when meiosis occurs in gametogenesis. With the production of the gametes, the stage might be set for reassortment of chromosomes in such a way that normal chromosomes pair with abnormal chromosomes, leading to partial trisomy or partial monosomy of various chromatin materials. Such individuals are said to be unbalanced and generally have severe phenotypic abnormalities. Roughly 3% to 4% of all abortuses have unbalanced chromosome rearrangements, and some live-born infants have unbalanced translocations.

Figure 2-7 demonstrates two possible ways that such translocations can come about. The first involves the fusion of two acrocentric chromosomes in which the short arms of both and the centromere of one are lost, with the pro-

duction of a chromosome that essentially has the long arm of each of these two chromosomes and an overall reduction of the chromosome number by one. Thus the balanced carrier has 45 chromosomes with the loss of one normal chromosome from each pair involved and the formation of one translocated chromosome, which is known as *Robertsonian fusion.* Gametes produced by such an individual are normal in chromosome configuration, balanced as in the parent, unbalanced because the translocated chromosome and one or the other of the normal chromosomes of the pairs involved are included, or monosomic because only one of the chromosomes is present and not the translocated chromosome. After fertilization, the following are possible: 25% of the offspring should be normal; 25%, carriers; 25%, unbalanced and affected; and 25%, monosomic and probably aborted. In actual experience with reproduction in such carriers, the unbalanced karyotype in offspring seems to occur less frequently than would be expected by chance with the carrier state, and normal karyotype occurs more frequently. This is particularly true if the father is the carrier.

The other means of translocation is the reciprocal translocation, in which chromatin material is exchanged between chromosomes but the chromosome number does not change. In this case, two new chromosomes are essentially produced, and with gamete formation one can expect a normal gamete, a gamete with the two balanced translocated chromosomes, or two possibilities in which a normal chromosome of one pair is matched with one of the translocated chromosomes. About 25% of the offspring could be expected to be normal, 25% balanced carriers, and 50% unbalanced and abnormal. Indeed, women with the carrier state of reciprocal translocation are frequently found among those with recurrent abortions. Although it is difficult to ascertain the percentage of such conceptuses with unbalanced karyotypes that end in abortion, the preponderance of conceptions that are live born favor the normal or carrier state.

If one chromosome breaks at two points, the broken segment may turn on its axis, leading to an *inversion*. If the centromere is present in the broken segment, a *pericentric inversion* is seen. Although this, too, will allow the individual to be phenotypically normal, problems involved in meiosis are such that infants with unbalanced chromosome components may be produced.

Finally, a break may lead to the actual loss of a small segment of the chromosome, a *partial deletion*. With the loss of the genes on that segment, the infant produced usually is extremely abnormal. A few such partial deletions have been seen in individuals born alive. The resulting abnormalities include Wolf's syndrome, with the deletion of a portion of the short arm of chromosome 4, which leads to severe retardation problems; cri-du-chat syndrome, which involves the loss of a portion of the short arm of chromosome 5, again leading to gross retardation in an individual in whom laryngeal changes result in a cry that sounds like the plaintive cry of a cat; and gross abnormalities resulting from the deletion of the short arm of chromosome 18.

Partial deletions of both the X and Y chromosomes have been seen. With the loss of part or all of the short arm (Xp−) of the X chromo-

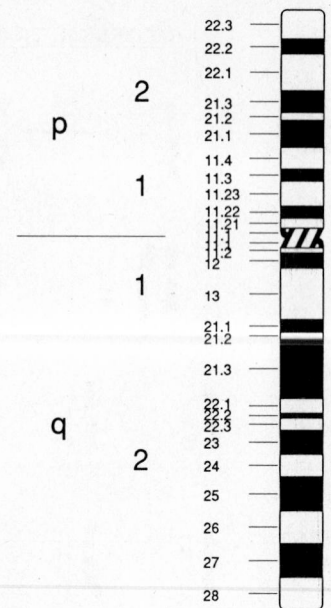

FIGURE 2-8
Diagram showing the banding of the X chromosome at the 550-band level. The short and long arms are designated "p" and "q," respectively, and the band designation is shown at the left. (Diagram derived from the ISCN nomenclature, as prepared by D. Adler, Arrowpoint, Bainbridge Island, Wash.)

some, many of the findings of Turner syndrome, including shortness of stature, have been noted. With the loss of all or part of the long arm of the X chromosome (Xq−), some of the findings of Turner syndrome have been seen but not shortness of stature. Figure 2-8 depicts the X chromosome divided by arms and bands.

Chromosome Abnormalities and Abortion

Hertig and Rock observed, as early as 1949, that many early gestations were obviously defective and that a genetic defect might be responsible. When it became possible to karyotype these abortuses, a number of investigators verified this theory by finding specific chromosome anomalies of a variety of types. Now with banding techniques, specific chromosomes can be identified, and the abnormalities can be more accurately categorized.

With the use of the data from a number of different studies, it has been estimated that about 15% of ova penetrated by sperm fail to divide. Another 15% fail to implant, and 25% to 30% are aborted spontaneously at previllous stages. Of the roughly 40% of fertilized ova that survive the first missed menstrual period, as many as one fourth are aborted spontaneously, so that only about 30% to 35% of all ova penetrated by sperm actually result in live-born infants.

From the work of many, it has been estimated that between 30% and 60% of early pregnancy losses that are recognizable as having been gestations are associated with chromosome abnormalities and many of the rest probably have other genetic defects.

Of those abortuses with chromosome abnormalities, roughly 50% have autosomal trisomy. Trisomies have been defined in abortus material for all autosomes except chromosomes 1 and 17. A trisomy of chromosome 16 has been noted in about one third of the cases, and since this has never been seen in living individuals, it must be considered universally lethal. Autosomal trisomies such as those of chromosomes 13, 18, and 21 do occur in live-born babies but may be seen in abortus material as well. It is of interest that as many as 80% of trisomy 21 fetuses are aborted. The error itself is that of nondisjunction of the chromosome pair at anaphase in either the first or the second meiotic division. Because the risk of repeating a nondisjunctional event is greater than in the general population, a woman who is known to have produced a trisomic abortus should be offered prenatal diagnosis by amniocentesis or chorionic villus sampling in much the same fashion as she would be if she had previously produced a live-born infant with a trisomy. In women who have produced a conceptus that is trisomic, the risk of subsequent trisomy is 1% to 2%, being somewhat less for women under the age of 35 and higher for women over the age of 35.

Roughly 20% of the chromosomally aborted abnormal fetuses have the karyotype 45,X. Only about 5% of such conceptuses are born alive, and these have the characteristic findings of Turner syndrome. The mechanism responsible for this condition seems to be the loss of a sex chromosome at zygote formation, but the loss of a chromosome via the mechanism of nondisjunction is also possible. The error leading to the problem may occur in either male or female meiosis, and a variety of mosaic patterns have been seen, indicating that errors in mitosis after fertilization may also occur. Data obtained from studies using as a marker the Xg blood group, which is coded on the X chromosome, suggest that about three fourths of living 45,X individuals use the X chromosome derived from the mother.

Sex chromosome trisomies such as 47,XXX, 47,XXY, and 47,XYY are rarely found in abortus material. The relative lethality of such karyotypes is probably minor, and most individuals are born alive. Each birth occurs about once per thousand live births of infants of the appropriate sex.

Triploidy occurs in between 14% and 19% of abortuses with chromosome abnormalities and apparently results from errors in meiosis or from double fertilization of a single ovum. It has been seen in live-born infants only as a mosaic when a normal cell line is also present. Using special chromosome banding techniques, Kajii and Nikawa demonstrated that triploidy occurs by a variety of mechanisms. This phenomenon has been seen in artificially bred cattle and in other animals as well and is thought to be the result of late insemination in some cases. In such situations, double fertilization in an egg that has lost its selectivity for penetration by normal sperm may be the mechanism. Triploid abortuses frequently are associated with multiple anomalies as well as hydropic degeneration of the placenta (Figure 2-9). Some hydatidiform moles therefore have a triploid karyotype.

Tetraploidy, or a mean chromosome count of 92, occurs in 3% to 6% of all chromosomally abnormal abortuses. This condition is undoubtedly lethal, since it has never been seen in living individuals. It probably occurs when chromosome division is not followed by cytoplasmic division in the initial cell division of the zygote.

Rearrangements, primarily translocations and inversions, are noted in about 3% of all chromosomally abnormal abortuses. According to Creasy and associates, most but definitely not all of these are unbalanced translocations. Although most unbalanced translocations in conceptuses result in abortion, some individuals are born alive.

A discussion of chromosome abnormalities among early abortuses is not complete without mentioning the findings in a series of stillbirths. Shepard and Fantel noted that of 283 stillborn infants, 17 had chromosome abnor-

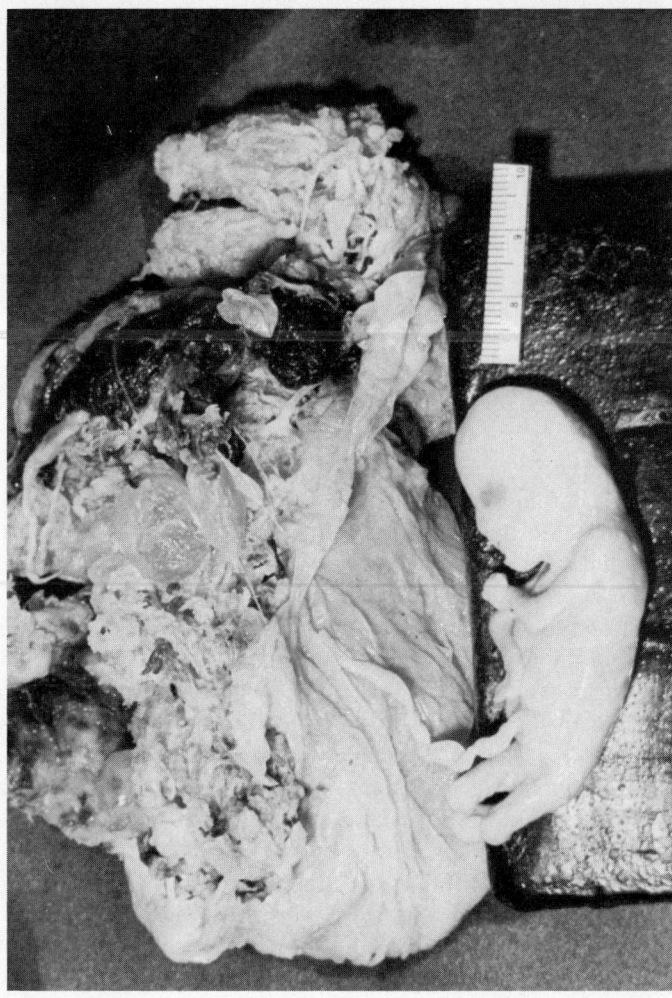

FIGURE 2-9
Abortus with triploid karyotype. Note hydropic degeneration of the placenta.
(From Stenchever MA: Contemp OB/GYN 17:38, 1981.)

malities, a rate of 6%. Trisomies occurred in 58.8% of these chromosomally abnormal fetuses. Sex chromosome abnormalities occurred in 29.4%, but none had a karyotype of 45,X. There was one instance of translocation and one of triploidy among the stillborn infants.

It is interesting to compare the findings of chromosome abnormalities among spontaneous abortuses with those among live-born infants. In a series of 43,558 live-born infants reported by Ratcliff, 247 (0.56%) had chromosome abnormalities. Of these, two (0.8%) had a karyotype of 45,X, 36.8% had other sex chromosome abnormalities, and 21.1% had autosomal trisomies of chromosomes 13, 18, and 21. The latter abnormality was by far the most common. Balanced chromosomal translocations were found

in 32.4% of chromosomally abnormal individuals, and unbalanced translocations were present in 3.2%. The remaining abnormalities were classified as miscellaneous. In a comparison of chromosome abnormalities in live-born infants with those in abortuses and stillborn infants, a concept of lethality can be noted.

Recurrent Abortion

Roughly 1 in every 200 couples has multiple abortions or multiple pregnancy wastage. Depending on how the problem is defined, one individual of the couple is found to have a chromosome abnormality in somewhere between 6% and 25% of couples. A review of the world literature by Simpson revealed that the

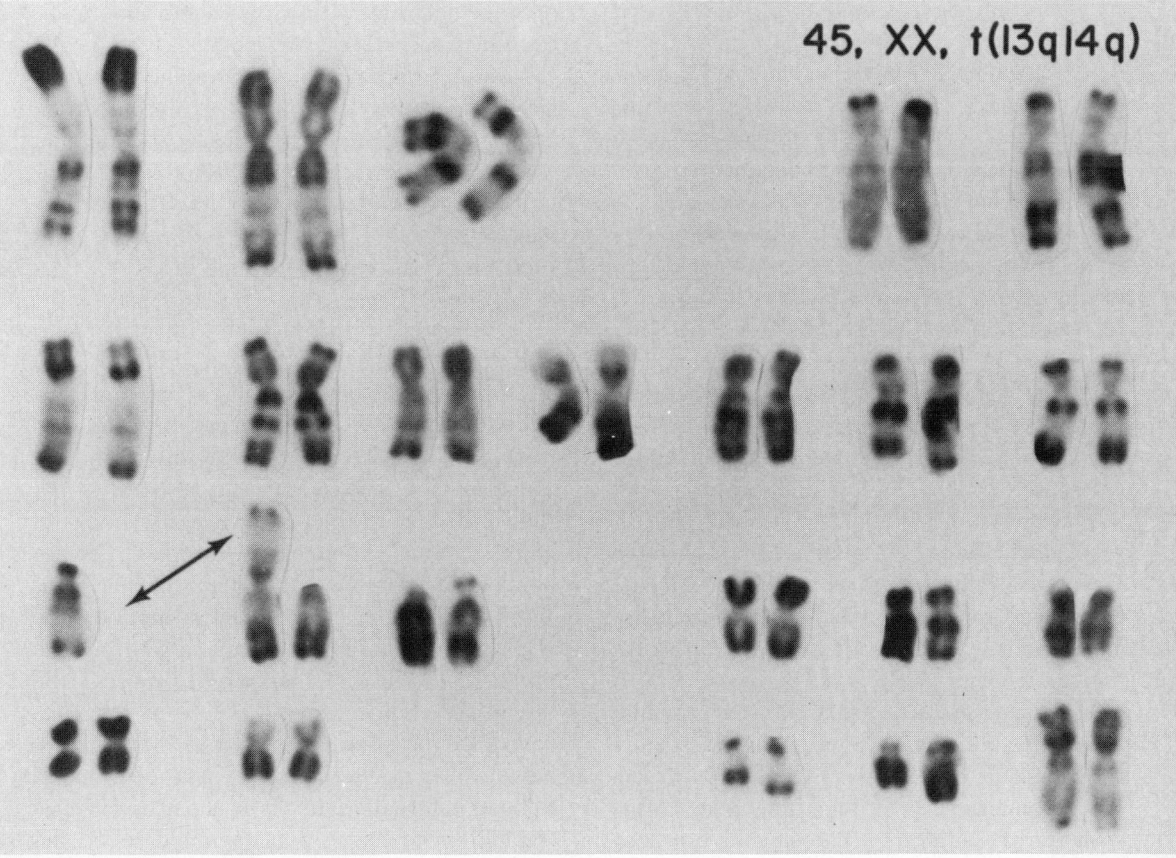

FIGURE 2-10
Karyotype of patient with 13 to 14 translocation (45,XX,+[13q 14q]) who had a history of three spontaneous first-trimester abortions. (From Stenchever MA: Contemp OB/GYN 17:38, 1981.)

prevalence of chromosome abnormalities in women with chronic spontaneous abortion problems was about twice that in men (4.8% versus 2.4%). Although occasional sex chromosome abnormalities such as 47,XXX and 47,XYY, as well as a variety of mosaic representations, are seen among such couples, the majority demonstrate either balanced reciprocal translocations or Robertsonian fusion problems (Figure 2-10).

Fortuny et al. studied the karyotypes of 445 couples who demonstrated repetitive (two or more) abortions and detected a balanced translocation in 19 (4.7%) of the couples, pericentric inversions in 8 (1.8%) of the couples, and polymorphisms in 52 (11.4%) of the couples. Significantly higher frequencies of translocations and polymorphism were found in these couples than in a control group of 600 consecutively delivered live-born infants (0.33% and 2.3%, re-

spectively). No differences were noted in the incidence of inversions. Of the translocations in the study group, 16 were reciprocal and 3 were Robertsonian. Of the couples with chromosome rearrangements, 17 underwent subsequent prenatal testing. Of 11 fetuses with parent carriers of a Robertsonian-type translocation, 9 were carriers of the balanced translocation, 2 were normal, and none were unbalanced. Of the 4 who had a carrier parent with a reciprocal translocation, 3 fetuses had a balanced translocation and 1 had a normal karyotype. Again, no unbalanced karyotypes were noted in offspring. Two carriers of inversions underwent prenatal diagnosis; one fetus carried the inversion and the other was normal. Although balanced carriers and normals seem to have the advantage over the unbalanced state, it is still not known whether there are fewer conceptions of fetuses with unbalanced karyotypes or that such conceptuses frequently end in early abortion.

In a large collaborative study of 71 European prenatal diagnosis centers reported by Boue and Gallano, when parents carried Robertsonian translocations, all unbalanced fetuses were detected when the mother was the carrier of the translocation. When the translocation involved chromosome 21, the risk that the fetus would have Down syndrome was 10% to 15%. In contrast, when the mother is a carrier of a Robertsonian translocation that does not include a chromosome 21 or when the father is the carrier of any type of Robertsonian translocation, the risk of producing a fetus with an unbalanced karyotype is low. This work is supported by the observations of several other investigators. Table 2-3 summarizes the risk of Down syndrome based on specific risk factors and is an example of the risks for producing chromosomally abnormal fetuses when risk factors are known.

The diagnosis of a chromosome abnormality in couples with chronic pregnancy wastage is important for two reasons. The first is to rule out an abnormality incompatible with normal gestation. Examples are homologous translocations between identical members of the same group of chromosomes, such as 13-13, 14-14, 15-15, 21-21, and 22-22. Individuals with other types of reciprocal translocations or Robertsonian fusion may have a normal pregnancy in which the chromosome makeup reflects either a normal karyotype or a balanced carrier state. However, such individuals may produce a conceptus with an unbalanced translocation, which would not be normal. In addition, chromosomally abnormal individuals are more likely to produce offspring with chromosome abnormalities. In some cases in which the father is the carrier of a chromosome abnormality, particularly when the abnormality is incompatible with normal gestation, artificial insemination with donor sperm may be offered. The techniques of ovum donation or embryo transplant may offer potential help to the woman with such a chromosomal problem.

Hydatidiform Mole

The two most common karyotypes noted in hydatidiform moles, and indeed in other trophoblastic disease, are 46,XX and triploidy. The use of Q and R banding techniques has shown that most moles have a karyotype of 46,XX, and all homologous chromosomes are homozygous for banding polymorphism. Thus although the moles are diploid in number, the chromosomes arise from a haploid set from one parent. In each case that parent proved to be the father. Some moles have been found to have a karyotype of 46,XY, but in all cases both haploid sets of chromosomes have been found to be of paternal origin. Even the occasional tetraploid mole has also been noted to be derived from a diploid set of chromosomes, all of which are of paternal origin. Thus it appears that in the formation of a hydatidiform mole, the female nucleus is lost and all chromosomes are of paternal origin either by the duplication of a haploid set or by the presence of two separate haploid sets of paternal origin. Therefore all of the genetic material of the mole is foreign to the mother (Figure 2-11).

The other type of chromosome abnormality seen in hydatidiform moles is triploidy. Frequently a fetus is present, and the problem is represented by a hydropic degeneration of the placenta. Although most choriocarcinomas are derived from 46,XX moles, triploidy has occasionally been seen. Triploidy may occur because of extra haploid chromosome sets from either parent, but molar degeneration seems to occur when at least two haploid sets are of paternal origin.

Genetic Abnormalities in Cancer

A number of tumors have demonstrated aneuploidy, and many have been seen with marker chromosomes specific for that particular tumor. The best example is the Philadelphia chromo-

---

TABLE 2-3

Risk of Producing a Down Syndrome Offspring by Specific Risk Factors

Risk Factor	Risk (%)
Previous trisomy-21, normal parental karyotypes	1-2
D-G (21) Robertsonian translocation	
Mother is carrier	10-15
Father is carrier	1-2
G-G heterologous translocation (21-22)	15
G-G homologous translocation (21-21)	100

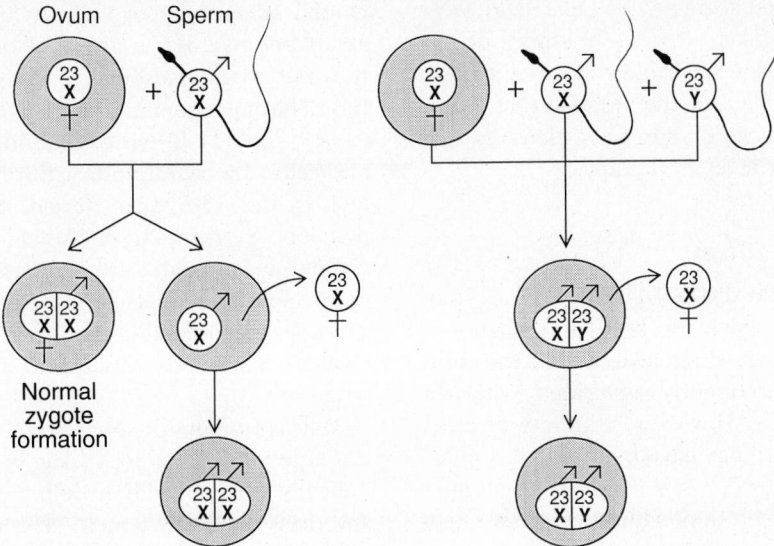

FIGURE 2-11

Diagram demonstrating potential mechanisms for developing a hydatidiform mole. All genetic material is derived from the father.

some, seen in chronic myelogenous leukemia. This minute chromosome disappears from peripheral circulation and from the bone marrow when therapy is effective and the patient's cancer is in remission. Space does not allow a categorization of each tumor that can occur in the human and its chromosome experience. It should be noted, however, that premalignant (dysplastic) cells of the cervix are generally aneuploid, as are the cells that compose invasive squamous cell carcinomas. This aneuploid distribution has been observed in cancers that arise in other organs as well but frequently is not observed in tumors arising in endocrine organs (including endometrium, breast, and thyroid).

A variety of cancers occur in individuals who have fragile chromosomes and may be associated with chromosome breaks and rearrangements or with mutations that occur when breaks take place and healing is faulty. Such conditions are seen in families with Bloom's syndrome, Fanconi's anemia, and ataxia-telangiectasia. In each case there is an increased percentage of individuals with a variety of cancers, and chromosome breaks are commonly seen in the cells of these individuals.

Current theories suggest that the majority of human cancers arise from a genetic change in a single cell. Such genetic alterations may be of a variety of types but essentially involve either (1) the somatic activation of cell oncogenes through point mutations, rearrangements, or amplifications or (2) the inactivation of tumor-suppressor genes by point mutation or deletion in either germ or somatic cells. For example, Fearon et al., using cloning techniques, have identified an allelic deletion in a gene on chromosome 18q (long arm) in 70% of studied colorectal tumors. This gene, thought to be a tumor-suppressor gene, may play a role in the pathogenesis of the cancer, perhaps through the alteration of normal cell-cell interactions controlling growth.

Oncogenes seem to fall into two general categories: those related to the structure of the cell's skeleton and those related to the transmission and transduction of growth regulatory signals. Watson et al. demonstrated that a nuclear-associated protein product of the C-myc gene, $P62^{C-myc}$, is of a significantly higher level in serous papillary carcinomas of the ovary than in normal ovarian tissue. Borderline tumors demonstrated levels between normal and cancer cell levels, and the differences between normal cells and borderline cancer cells were significantly different, but no significant differences were noted between the cells of the borderline and frank tumors. The majority of these carcinomas were also noted to be aneuploid.

The C-myc gene seems to be related to DNA synthesis. It is likely that the methods of molecular biology now available will make it possible to identify the genetic systems that, when altered, lead to cancer transformation and may eventually offer clues to therapy.

Hermaphroditism

TRUE HERMAPHRODITISM. True hermaphroditism, which involves the presence of both male and female gonads within the same individual, is frequently associated with the karyotype 46,XX. However, a variety of other chromosome findings have been noted. One of these, 46,XX/46,XY, is a condition that most likely occurs when the fertilization of two eggs is followed by their fusion, resulting in chimerism within the individual. Chimerism is defined as the presence of two different cell populations from two separate conceptuses within the same individual. Other chromosome anomalies associated with true hermaphroditism include various mosaicisms involving 45,X/46,XY and 45,X/47,XYY karyotypes, as well as karyotypes with various translocations and deletions of the X and Y chromosomes. The influence of these chromosomes in the development of hermaphroditism is discussed in detail elsewhere.

PSEUDOHERMAPHRODITISM. Female pseudohermaphroditism occurs when a female is androgenized during embryonic life. The most common such case is associated with congenital adrenal hyperplasia, which may come about because of a number of enzyme defects transmitted as autosomal recessive characteristics. The most common is 21-hydroxylase deficiency, but 11-β-hydroxylase deficiency may also cause the syndrome. A third and rarer defect is the 18-hydroxysteroid dehydrogenase deficiency, which leads to aldosterone deficiency but no genital tract anomalies. In every case, such individuals have a 46,XX karyotype unless other conditions are associated by chance. These are discussed in detail elsewhere.

Male pseudohermaphroditism occurs when the individual has a 46,XY karyotype and is genetically and gonadally male but phenotypically and psychologically female. The most common condition in which this is found is the androgen insensitivity syndrome (testicular feminization syndrome).

In this condition the genetic error is transmitted as an X-linked recessive characteristic leading to a faulty androgen receptor on the cell membranes, preventing the cell from transporting testosterone or dihydrotestosterone into the cell. Both complete and incomplete forms exist. A related condition, 5α-reductase deficiency, prevents the conversion of testosterone to dihydrotestosterone. Because the latter is the form of testosterone that enters most cells, a defect of the enzyme mimics the findings of androgen insensitivity.

_____ **KEY POINTS** _____

- Base pairing in DNA molecules is always A-T and G-C, and in RNA molecules is always A-U and G-C.

- Endonuclease enzymes cleave specific nucleotide pairs, making DNA fragment evaluation and gene cloning possible. More than 200 different endonucleases exist.

- When a heterozygous individual who has an autosomal dominant trait mates with a normal individual, 50% of their offspring will have the trait.

- When two individuals who carry an autosomal recessive trait mate, 25% of their offspring will demonstrate the trait and 50% will be carriers.

- X-linked recessive characteristics are transmitted from maternal carriers to male offspring and will affect 50% of such male offspring.

- In general, if a couple produces an offspring with a multifactorial defect, and the problem has never occurred in the family, it can be expected to be repeated in 2% to 5% of subsequent pregnancies.

- The findings always present in 45,X Turner syndrome are shortness and sexual infantilism.

- A variety of different karyotypes have been discovered in individuals with the phenotype of Turner syndrome.

- Nondisjunctional events have been described in every autosome except chromosomes 1 and 17. The risk of producing a second conceptus with a nondisjunctional event is 1% to 2%.

- Conditions always seen in individuals with Klinefelter's syndrome (47,XXY) are tallness and azoospermia. One third of these individuals have gynecomastia.

- Of ova penetrated by sperm, 15% fail to implant and 25% to 30% are aborted spontaneously at a previllous stage. Of the 40% that survive the first missed menstrual period, as many as one fourth abort spontaneously. From 30% to 35% of ova penetrated by sperm end in live-born individuals.

- Between 30% and 60% of known aborted conceptuses have chromosome abnormalities. Half of these have autosomal trisomies; 20%, 45,X; 14% to 19%, triploidy; 3% to 6%, tetraploidy; and 3% to 4%, chromosome rearrangements.

- Of live-born infants with chromosome abnormalities, about 0.8% to 1% have 45,X; 36.8% have other sex chromosome abnormalities; 21% have autosomal trisomies; and balanced chromosome translocations occur in 32.4%. About 3.2% have unbalanced translocation abnormalities.

- One in 200 women has recurrent (three or more) abortions, with chromosome abnormalities occurring in about 4.8% of the mothers and 2.4% of the fathers.

- When chromosome 21 is present as part of a Robertsonian translocation with a D group chromosome, the chance of transmission of an unbalanced karyotype (leading to a Down syndrome offspring) is 10% to 15% if the mother is the carrier and 1% to 2% if the father is the carrier.

• Hydatidiform moles are either diploid (46,XX or 46,XY) or triploid. The chromosomes of the diploid type, usually seen in true moles, are completely derived from paternal chromosomes. Triploidy moles have at least two haploid sets derived from paternal origin.

• Oncogenes fall into two general categories: those related to the cell skeleton and those related to the transmission or transduction of growth-regulating signals. Mutations in these genes by a variety of genetic mechanisms may lead to loss of normal cell controls, resulting in transformation of the cell to cancer.

BIBLIOGRAPHY

Boue J, Boue A, and Lazar P: Retrospective and prospective epidemiological studies of 1500 karyotyped spontaneous human abortions, Teratology 12:11, 1975.

Boue A and Gallano P: A collaborative study of the segregation of inherited chromosome structural rearrangements in 1356 prenatal diagnoses, Prenat Diagn 4:45, 1984.

Creasy MR, Crolla JA, and Alberman ED: A cytogenetic study of human spontaneous abortion using banding techniques, Hum Genet 31:177, 1976.

Dewhurst J: Fertility in 47,XXX and 45,X patients, J Med Genet 15:132, 1978.

Fearon ER, Cho KR, Nigro JM, et al: Identification of a chromosome 18q gene that is altered in colorectal cancers, Science 247:49, 1990.

Ford EHR: Human chromosomes, New York, 1973, Academic Press.

Fortuny A, Carrio A, Soler A, et al: Detection of balanced chromosome rearrangements in 445 couples with repeated abortion and cytogenetic prenatal testing in carriers, Fertil Steril 49:774, 1988.

Hamerton JL, Canning N, Ray M, and Smith S: A cytogenetic survey of 14,069 newborn infants. I. Incidence of chromosome abnormalities, Clin Genet 8:223, 1975.

Harnden DG and Klinger HP, editors: An international system for human cytogenetic nomenclature, published in collaboration with Cytogenet Cell Genet, Basel, Switzerland, 1985, S Karger Medical and Scientific Publishers.

Jones HW Jr and Scott WM: Hermaphroditism: genital anomalies and related endocrine disorders, Baltimore, 1971, Williams & Wilkins.

Kajii T and Nikawa N: Origin of triploidy and tetraploidy in man: cases with chromosome markers, Cytogenet Cell Genet 18:109, 1977.

Kajii T and Ohama K: Androgenetic origin of hydatidiform mole, Nature 268:633, 1977.

King CR: Prenatal diagnosis of genetic disease with molecular genetic technology, Obstet Gynecol Surv 43:493, 1988.

Lubinsky MS: Female pseudohermaphroditism and associated anomalies, Am J Med Genet 6:123, 1980.

McKusick VA: Mendelian inheritance in man, Baltimore, 1978, The Johns Hopkins Press.

Ratcliffe S: Postnatal chromosome abnormalities. In Boyce HJ, editor: Chromosome variations in human evolution, London, 1975, Taylor & Francis.

Schmike RN: Genetics and cancer in man, Edinburgh, 1980, Churchill Livingstone.

Shepard TH and Fantel AG: Embryonic and early fetal loss, Clin Perinatol 6:219, 1979.

Simpson JL: Disorders of sexual differentiation: etiology and clinical delineation, New York, 1976, Academic Press.

Simpson JL: True hermaphroditism: etiology and phenotypic considerations, Birth Defects 14:9, 1978.

Simpson JL: Repeated suboptimal pregnancy outcome, Birth Defects 17:113, 1981.

Simpson JL, Globus MS, Martin AO, and Sarto GE: Genetics in obstetrics and gynecology, New York, 1982, Grune & Stratton.

Stene J, Stene E, and Mikkelsen M: Risk for chromosome abnormality at amniocentesis following a child with a non-inherited chromosome aberration, Prenat Diagn 4:81, 1984.

Vejerslev LO, Fisher RA, Surti U, and Walke N: Hydatidiform mole: cytogenetically unusual cases and their implications for the present classification, Am J Obstet Gynecol 157:180, 1984.

Watkins PC: Restriction fragment length polymorphism (RFLP): applications in human chromosome mapping and genetic disease research, BioTechniques 6:310, 1988.

Watson EJ, Hernandez E, and Miyazawa K: Partial hydatidiform moles: a review, Obstet Gynecol Surv 42:540, 1987.

Watson JD, Hopkins NH, Roberts WJ, et al: Molecular biology of the gene, ed 4, Menlo Park, 1987, Benjamin–Cummings Publishing Co.

Watson JV, Curling OM, Munn CF, and Hudson CN: Oncogene expression in ovarian cancer: a pilot study of C-myc oncoprotein in serous papillary ovarian cancer, Gynecol Oncol 28:137, 1987.

Anatomy

_____ KEY TERMS AND DEFINITIONS _____

Auerbach's Plexus. A network of twin vessels within the tunica muscularis of the ureters.

Apocrine Gland. A gland that produces secretions formed partially from the secreting cells of the gland itself.

Bladder Neck. That part of the bladder that is continuous with the urethra.

Canal of Nuck. A tubular process of peritoneum that accompanies the round ligament into the inguinal canal. It is generally obliterated in the adult but sometimes remains patent.

Carunculae Myrtiformes. Small nodules of fibrous tissue at the vaginal orifice that are remnants of the hymen.

Cornua. The superolateral aspects of the uterine cavity; the anatomic areas where the oviducts enter the uterine cavity.

Cul-de-sac of Douglas. A deep pouch formed by the most caudal extent of the parietal peritoneum. It is anterior to the rectum, separating the uterus from the large intestine.

Eccrine Gland. A simple sweat-producing gland in which the secreting cells are maintained intact during production of secretions.

Fimbria Ovarica. One of the largest fingerlike projections of the distal end of the oviducts. The fimbria ovarica usually attaches the oviducts to the ovary.

Frankenhäuser's Plexus. An extensive concentration of both myelinated and nonmyelinated nerve fibers located in the uterosacral ligaments and supplying primarily the uterus and the cervix.

Fundus. The dome-shaped top of the uterus.

Genitocrural Fold. The skin line dividing the external female genitalia and the medial aspects of the thigh.

Isthmus. The short area of constriction in the lower uterine segment.

Parametria. The extraperitoneal fatty and fibrous connective tissue immediately adjacent to the uterus. The parametria lie between the leaves of the broad ligament and in the contiguous area anteriorly between the cervix and the bladder.

Pelvic Diaphragm. A thin, muscular layer of tissue that forms the inferior border of the abdominal pelvic cavity. The primary muscles of the pelvic diaphragm are the levator ani and coccygeus muscles.

Perineum. The region between the thighs bounded anteriorly by the vulva and posteriorly by the anus.

Plexus. A mixture of preganglionic and postganglionic fibers, small, inconsistently placed nerve ganglia, and afferent sensory fibers. In the female pelvis a plexus also may be termed a *nerve*.

Plicae Palmatae. Longitudinal folds in the mucous membrane of the endocervical canal. The secondary branching folds are called *arbor vitae*.

Posterior Fourchette. The fold of skin that joins the labia minora at their inferior margins.

Presacral Nerve. Found in the retroperitoneal connective tissue from the fourth lumbar vertebra to the hollow over the sacrum. (Also termed the *superior hypogastric plexus*.)

Rugae. Numerous transverse folds of the vagina in women of reproductive age.

Space of Retzius. The area lying between the bladder and symphysis pubis, bounded laterally by the obliterated hypogastric arteries.

Urachus. The adult remnant of the embryonic allantois.

Urogenital Diaphragm. A strong, muscular membrane that occupies the area between the symphysis pubis and the ischial tuberosities. Posteriorly, the urogenital diaphragm inserts into the central point of the perineum.

Vestibular Bulbs. Two elongated masses of erectile tissue situated on either side of the vaginal orifice. They are homologous to the bulb of the penis in the male.

The organs of the female reproductive tract are classically divided into the external and the internal genitalia. The external genital organs are present in the vulvar region and include the mons pubis, clitoris, urinary meatus, labia majora, labia minora, vestibule, Bartholin's glands, and periurethral glands. The internal genital organs are located in the true pelvis and include the vagina, uterus, cervix, oviducts, ovaries, and surrounding supporting structures. This chapter attempts to integrate the basic anatomy of the female pelvis with clinical situations.

Embryologically the urinary, reproductive, and gastrointestinal tracts develop in close proximity. This relationship continues throughout a woman's life span. In the adult the reproductive organs are in intimate contact with the lower urinary tract and large intestines. Because of the anatomic proximity of the genital and urinary systems, altered pathophysiology in one organ often produces symptoms in the other, adjacent organ. The gynecologic surgeon masters the intricacy of these anatomic relationships to avoid major surgical complications.

This chapter does not duplicate the completeness of anatomic texts or surgical atlases; it concentrates on the norms of human anatomy. The reader must appreciate that wide individual differences in anatomic detail exist among patients. Understanding these variations is one of the greatest challenges of clinical medicine.

EXTERNAL GENITALIA
Vulva

The vulva, or pudendum, is a collective term for the external genital organs that are visible in the perineal area. The vulva consists of the following: the mons pubis, labia majora, labia minora, hymen, clitoris, vestibule, urethra, Skene's glands, Bartholin's glands, and vestibular bulbs (Figure 3-1).

The boundaries of the vulva extend from the mons pubis anteriorly to the rectum posteriorly and from one lateral genitocrural fold to the other. The entire vulvar area is covered by keratinized, stratified squamous epithelium. The farther from the vagina, the thicker, more pigmented, and more keratinized is the skin. The skin closest to the vagina is the thinnest and has the least keratin.

Mons Pubis

The mons pubis is a rounded, cushionlike eminence that becomes hairy after puberty. It is directly anterior and superior to the symphysis pubis. The hair pattern, or escutcheon, of most women is triangular. Genetic and racial differences produce a variety of normal hair patterns, with approximately one in four women having a modified escutcheon that has a diamond (malelike) pattern.

Labia Majora

The labia majora are two large, longitudinal, cutaneous folds of adipose and fibrous tissue. Each labium majus is approximately 7 to 8 cm in length and 2 to 3 cm in width. The labia extend from the mons pubis anteriorly to become lost in the skin between the vagina and the anus in the area of the posterior fourchette. The skin of the outer convex surface of the labia majora is pigmented and covered with hair follicles. The thin skin of the inner surface does not have hair follicles but has many sebaceous glands. Histologically, the labia majora have both sweat and sebaceous glands (Figure 3-2). The apocrine glands are similar to those of the breast and axillary areas. The size of the labia is related to fat content. Usually the labia atrophy

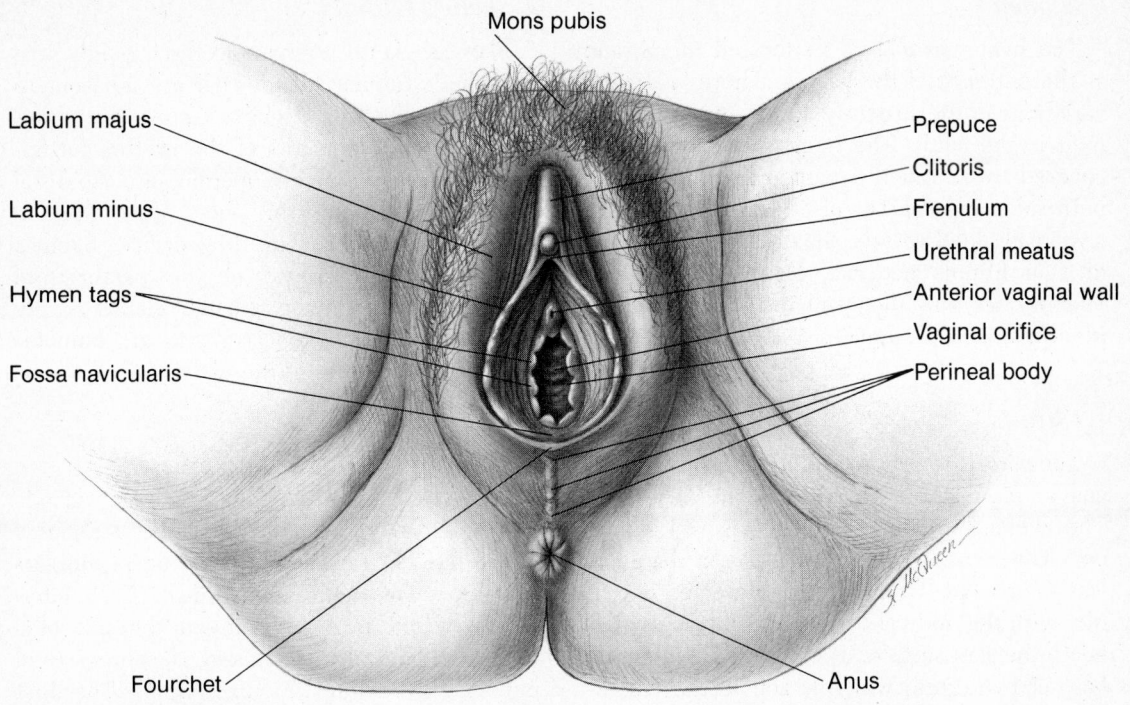

Mons pubis

Labium majus

Labium minus

Hymen tags

Fossa navicularis

Fourchet

Prepuce

Clitoris

Frenulum

Urethral meatus

Anterior vaginal wall

Vaginal orifice

Perineal body

Anus

FIGURE 3-1
The structures of the external genitalia that are collectively called the *vulva*. (Redrawn from Pritchard JA, MacDonald PC, and Gant NF: Williams' obstetrics, ed 17, New York, 1985, Appleton-Century-Crofts, p 8.)

after menopause. The labia majora are homologous to the scrotum in the male.

Labia Minora

The labia minora, or nymphae, are two small, red cutaneous folds that are situated between the labia majora and the vaginal orifice. They are more delicate, shorter, and thinner than the labia majora. Anteriorly, they divide at the clitoris to form superiorly the prepuce and inferiorly the frenulum of the clitoris. Histologically, they are composed of dense connective tissue with erectile tissue and elastic fibers, rather than adipose tissue. The skin of the labia minora is less cornified and has many sebaceous glands but no hair follicles or sweat glands. The labia minora and the breasts are the only areas of the body rich in sebaceous glands without hair folicles. Among women of reproductive age, there is considerable variation in the size of the labia minora. They are relatively more prominent in children and postmenopausal women. The labia minora are homologous to the penile urethra and part of the skin of the penis in males.

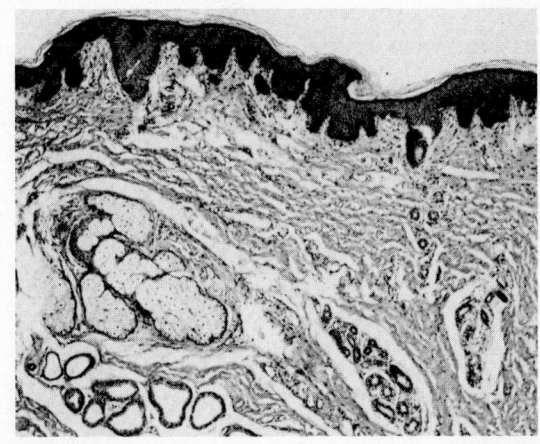

FIGURE 3-2
A histologic section from the labium majus. A cornified squamous epithelium covers the dermis, which contains eccrine, apocrine, and sebaceous glands. (H&E stain; ×77.) (Reproduced with permission from Kaufman RH: Anatomy of the vulva and vagina. In Gardner HL and Kaufman RH, editors: Benign disease of the vulva and vagina, ed 2, Chicago, 1981, Mosby–Year Book, Inc.)

Hymen

The hymen is a thin, perforated membrane at the entrance of the vagina. There are many variations in the structure and shape of the hymen in the adult. The hymen histologically is covered by stratified squamous epithelium on both sides and consists of fibrous tissue with a few small blood vessels. Small tags, or nodules, of firm fibrous material, termed *carunculae myrtiformes,* are the remnants of the hymen identified in adult females.

Clitoris

The clitoris is a short, cylindrical, erectile organ at the superior portion of the vestibule. The average length of the clitoris is 1.5 to 2 cm. The normal adult clitoris has a diameter less than 1 cm. Usually, only the glans is visible, with the body of the clitoris positioned beneath the skin surface. The clitoris consists of a base of two crura, which attach to the periosteum of the symphysis pubis. The body has two cylindrical corpora cavernosa composed of thin-walled, vascular channels that function as erectile tissue. The distal one third of the clitoris is the glans, which has many nerve endings. The clitoris is the female homologue of the penis in the male.

Vestibule

The vestibule is the lowest portion of the embryonic urogenital sinus. It is the cleft between the labia minora that is visualized when the labia are held apart. The vestibule extends from the clitoris to the posterior fourchette. The orifices of the urethra and vagina and the ducts from Bartholin's glands open into the vestibule. Within the area of the vestibule are the remnants of the hymen and numerous mucinous glands.

Urethra

The urethra is a membranous conduit for urine from the urinary bladder to the vestibule. The female urethra measures 3.5 to 5 cm in length. The mucosa of the proximal two thirds of the urethra is composed of stratified transitional epithelium, whereas the distal one third is stratified squamous epithelium. The distal orifice is 4 to 6 mm in diameter, and the mucosal edges grossly appear everted.

Skene's Glands

Skene's glands, or paraurethral glands, are branched, tubular glands that are adjacent to the distal urethra. Usually Skene's ducts run parallel to the long axis of the urethra for approximately 1 cm before opening into the distal urethra. Sometimes the ducts open into the area just outside the urethral orifice. Skene's glands are the largest of the paraurethral glands; however, many smaller glands empty into the urethra. Skene's glands are homologous to the prostate in the male.

Bartholin's Glands

Bartholin's glands are vulvovaginal glands that are located beneath the fascia at about 4 and 8 o'clock, respectively, on the posterolateral aspect of the vaginal orifice. Each lobulated, racemose gland is about the size of a pea. Histologically the gland is composed of cuboidal epithelium (Figure 3-3, *A*). The duct from each gland is lined by transitional epithelium and is approximately 2 cm in length (Figure 3-3, *B*). Bartholin's ducts open into a groove between the hymen and the labia minora. Bartholin's glands are homologous to Cowper's glands in the male.

Vestibular Bulbs

The vestibular bulbs are two elongated masses of erectile tissue situated on either side of the vaginal orifice. Each bulb is immediately below the bulbocavernosus muscle. The distal ends of the vestibular bulbs are adjacent to Bartholin's glands. They are homologous to the bulb of the penis in the male.

Clinical Correlations

The skin of the vulvar region is subject to both local and general dermatitis. The intertriginous areas of the vulva remain moist, and obese women are particularly susceptible to chronic infection. The vulvar skin of a postmenopausal woman is sensitive to topical cortisone and testosterone but insensitive to topical estrogen. In general, cortisone cream is prescribed for hyperplastic vulvar skin disease, whereas testosterone cream is given for atrophic skin changes.

The vulvar vestibule is an area where small mucous glands sometimes become cystic. The most common large cystic structure of the

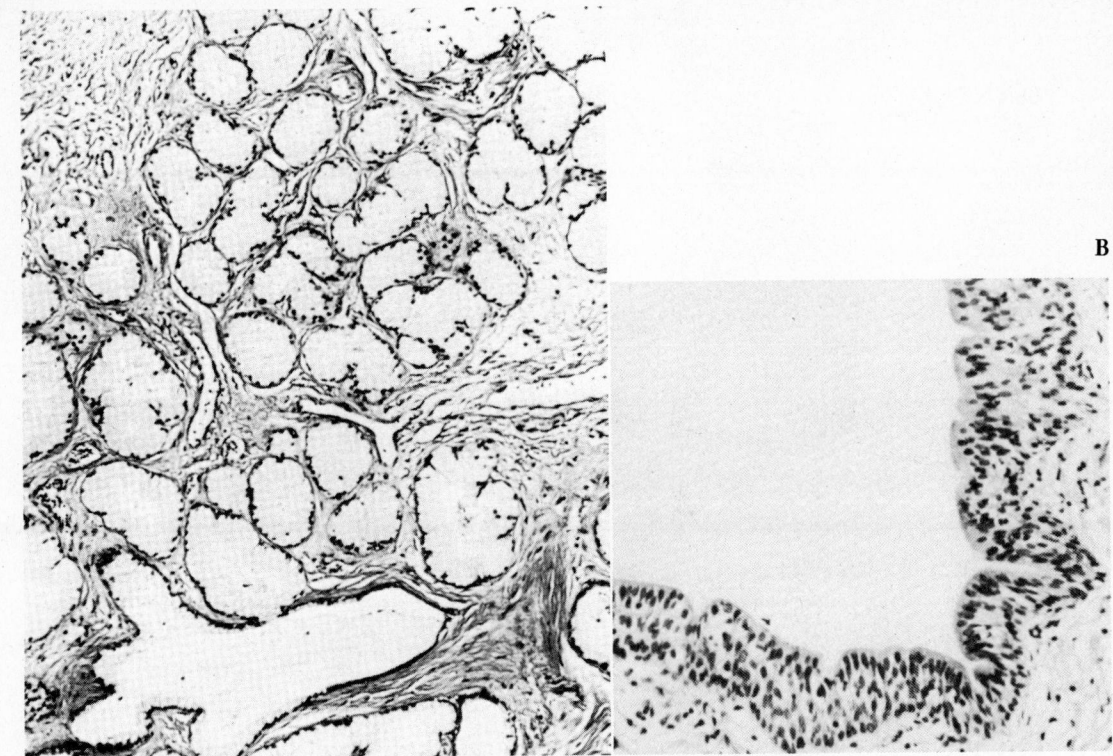

FIGURE 3-3
A, A histologic section of a Bartholin's gland, showing cuboidal epithelium lining acinar structures. (H&E stain; ×117.) **B,** A histologic section of the duct of the Bartholin's gland. The lining of the duct is transitional epithelium. (H&E stain; ×286.) (Reproduced with permission from Kaufman RH: Anatomy of the vulva and vagina. In Gardner HL and Kaufman RH, editors: Benign diseases of the vulva and vagina, ed 2, Chicago, 1981, Mosby–Year Book, Inc.)

vulva is a Bartholin's duct cyst. This condition may become painful if the cyst develops into an acute abscess. Chronic infections of the periurethral glands may result in one or more urethral diverticula. The most common symptoms of a urethral diverticulum are similar to the symptoms of a lower urinary tract infection: urinary frequency, urgency, and dysuria.

Vulvar trauma frequently results in a large hematoma or profuse external hemorrhage. The richness of the vascular supply and the absence of valves in vulvar veins contribute to this complication. However, the abundant vascularity of the region promotes rapid healing, with an associated low incidence of wound infection in episiotomies or obstetric tears of the vulva.

VAGINA

The vagina is a thin-walled, distensible, fibromuscular tube that extends from the vesti-bule of the vulva to the uterus. The potential space of the vagina is larger in the middle and upper thirds. The walls of the vagina are normally in apposition and flattened in the anteroposterior diameter. Thus the vagina has the appearance of the letter H in cross section (Figure 3-4).

The axis of the upper portion of the vagina lies close to the horizontal plane when a woman is standing, with the upper portion of the vagina curving toward the hollow of the sacrum. In most women an angle of at least 90 degrees is formed between the axis of the vagina and the axis of the uterus. The vagina is secured in its position by the surrounding endopelvic fascia and ligaments.

The lower third of the vagina is in close relationship with the urogenital and pelvic diaphragms. The middle third of the vagina is supported by the levator ani muscles and the lower portion of the cardinal ligaments. The upper third is supported by the upper portions

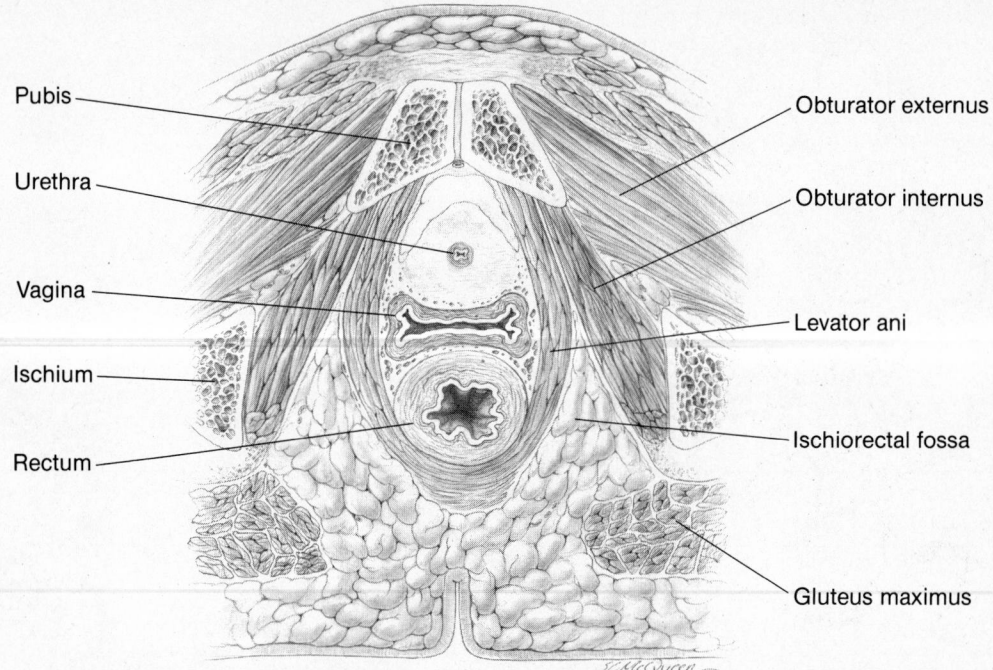

Pubis

Urethra

Vagina

Ischium

Rectum

Obturator externus

Obturator internus

Levator ani

Ischiorectal fossa

Gluteus maximus

FIGURE 3-4
A schematic drawing of a cross section of the female pelvis, demonstrating the H shape of the vagina. Note the surrounding levator ani muscle. (Redrawn from Pritchard JA, MacDonald PC, and Gant NF: Williams' obstetrics, ed 17, New York, 1985, Appleton-Century-Crofts, p 12.)

of the cardinal ligaments and the parametria.

The vagina of reproductive-age women has numerous transverse folds, termed *rugae*. They help provide accordion-like distensibility and are more prominent in the lower third of the vagina. The cervix extends into the upper part of the vagina. The spaces between the cervix and attachment of the vagina are called *fornices*. The posterior fornix is considerably larger than the anterior fornix; thus the anterior vaginal length is approximately 6 to 9 cm in comparison with a posterior vaginal length of 8 to 12 cm.

Histologically, the vagina is composed of four distinct layers. The mucosa consists of a stratified, nonkeratinized squamous epithelium. If the environment of the vaginal mucosa is modified, as in uterine prolapse, then the epithelium may become keratinized. The squamous epithelium is similar microscopically to the exocervix, although the vagina has larger and more frequent papillae that extend into the connective tissue. The normal vagina does not have glands. The next layer is the lamina propria, or tunica. It is composed of fibrous connective tissue. Throughout this layer of collagen and elastic tissue is a rich supply of vascu-

lar and lymphatic channels. The density of the connective tissue in the endopelvic fascia varies throughout the longitudinal axis of the vagina. The muscular layer has many interlacing fibers. However, an inner circular layer and an outer longitudinal layer can be identified. The fourth layer consists of cellular areolar connective tissue and a large plexus of blood vessels.

The vascular system of the vagina is generously supplied with an extensive anastomotic network throughout its length. The vaginal artery originates either directly from the uterine artery or as a branch of the internal iliac artery arising posterior to the origin of the uterine and inferior vesical arteries. The vaginal artery may be multiple arteries on each side of the pelvis. There is an anastomosis with the cervical branch of the uterine artery to form the azygos arteries. Branches of the internal pudendal, inferior vesical, and middle hemorrhoidal arteries also contribute to the interconnecting network and the longitudinal azygos arteries.

The venous drainage is complex and accompanies the arterial system. Below the pelvic floor the principal venous drainage occurs via the pudendal veins. The vaginal, uterine, and vesical veins, as well as those around the rectosigmoid, all provide venous drainage of the venous plexuses surrounding the middle and upper vagina.

The nerve supply of the vagina comes from the autonomic nervous system's vaginal plexus, and sensory fibers come from the pudendal nerve. Pain fibers enter the spinal cord in sacral segments 2 to 4.

The lymphatic drainage is characterized by its wide distribution and frequent crossovers between the right and left sides of the pelvis. In general the primary lymphatic drainage of the upper third of the vagina is to the external iliac nodes, the middle third of the vagina drains to the common and internal iliac nodes, and the lower third has a wide lymphatic distribution, including the common iliac, superficial inguinal, and perirectal nodes.

Clinical Correlations

In clinical practice anatomic descriptions of pelvic organs are derived from Latin roots, such as "vagina," from the Latin word for sheath. In contrast, the names for surgical procedures of pelvic organs are derived from Greek roots. *Colpectomy, colporrhaphy*, and *colposcopy* are derived from *kolpos* (fold), the Greek word for the vagina.

Clinicians must consider the H shape of the vagina when they insert a speculum and inspect the walls of the vagina. The posterior fornix is an important surgical landmark, since it provides direct access to the cul-de-sac of Douglas. The distal course of the ureter and the changes in anatomic relationships produced by uterine prolapse are important considerations in vaginal surgery. Ureteral injury has occurred as a result of vaginally placed sutures to obtain hemostasis with vaginal lacerations. The anatomic proximity and interrelationships of the vascular and lymphatic networks of the bladder and vagina are such that inflammation of one organ will often produce symptoms in the other. For example, vaginitis often produces urinary tract symptoms, such as frequency and dysuria.

Gartner's duct cyst, a cystic dilation of the embryonic mesonephros, is usually present on the lateral wall of the vagina. However, in the lower third of the vagina these cysts are present anteriorly and may be difficult to distinguish from a large urethral diverticulum.

An interesting phenomenon discovered by recent interest in sexual medicine is the source of vaginal lubrication during intercourse. For years there was speculation on how an organ without glands is able to "secrete" fluid. Vaginal lubrication occurs from a transudate produced by engorgement of the vascular plexuses that encircle the vagina. The anatomic relationship between the long axis of the vagina and other pelvic organs may be altered by pelvic relaxation resulting from the trauma of childbirth. Atrophy or weakness of the endopelvic fascia and muscles surrounding the vagina may result in the development of a cystocele, rectocele, and/or enterocele.

CERVIX

The lower, narrow portion of the uterus is the cervix. The word *cervix* originates from the Latin word for neck. The Greek word for neck is *trachēlos*, and when the cervix is removed, the surgical procedure is termed *trachelectomy*. The cervix may vary in shape from cylindrical to conical. It is predominantly fibrous and is separated from the muscular corpus of the uterus by the internal os.

The vagina is attached obliquely around the middle of the cervix; this attachment divides the cervix into an upper, supravaginal portion and a lower segment in the vagina called the *portio vaginalis* (Figure 3-5). The supravaginal segment is covered by peritoneum posteriorly and is surrounded by loose, fatty connective tissue, the parametrium, anteriorly.

The canal of the cervix is fusiform, with the widest diameter in the middle. The length and width of the endocervical canal varies; it is usually 2.5 to 3 cm in length and 7 to 8 mm at its widest point. The width of the canal varies with changing hormonal levels. The cervical canal opens into the vagina at the external os of the cervix, which is small and round in nulliparous women. The os is wider and gaping following vaginal delivery. Often lateral or stellate scars are residual marks of previous cervical lacerations. In the majority of women the external os is in contact with the posterior vaginal wall.

The mucous membrane of the endocervical canal of nulliparous women is arranged in longitudinal folds, plicae palmatae, with secondary branching folds, the arbor vitae (Figure 3-6). These folds, which form a herringbone pattern, disappear following vaginal delivery.

A single layer of columnar epithelium lines

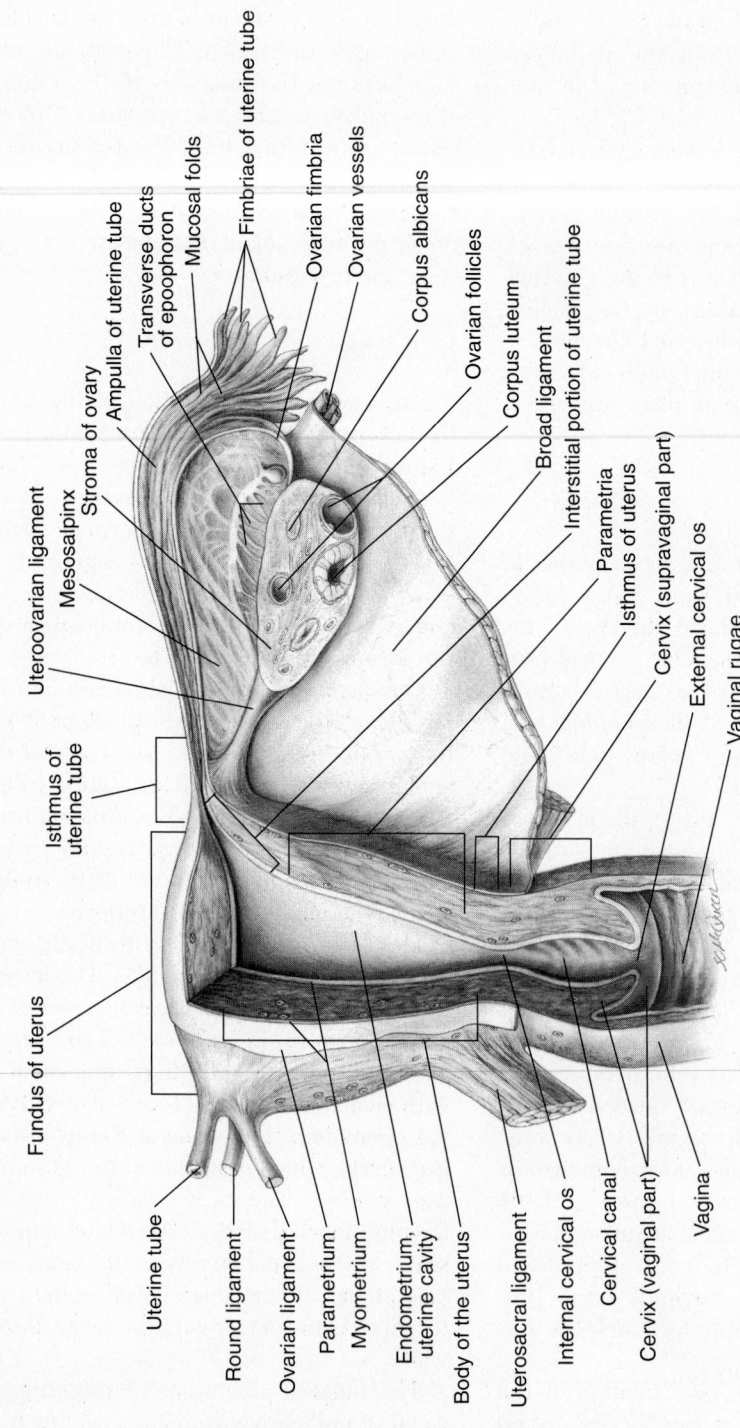

FIGURE 3-5

A schematic drawing of a posterior view of the cervix, uterus, fallopian tube, and ovary. Note that the cervix is divided by the vaginal attachment into an external portio segment and a supravaginal segment. Note that the uterus is composed of the dome-shaped fundus, the muscular body, and the narrow isthmus. Note the fimbria ovarica, or ovarian fimbria, attaching the oviduct to the ovary. (Redrawn from Clemente CD: Anatomy: a regional atlas of the human body, Baltimore-Munich, 1987, Urban & Schwarzenberg.)

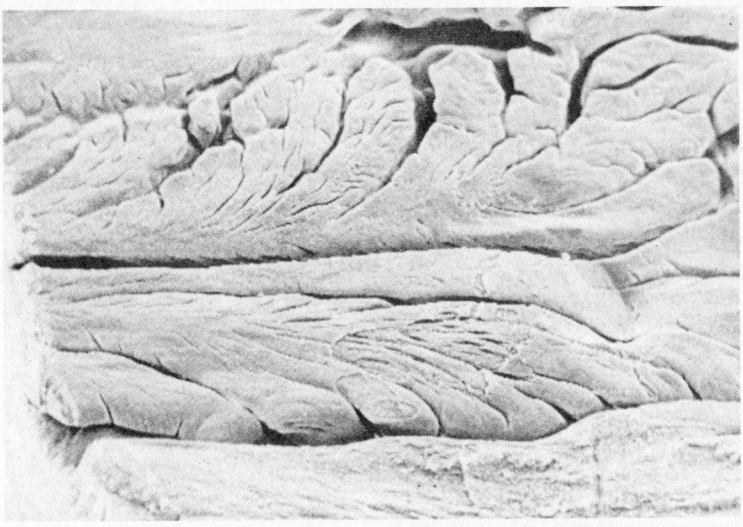

FIGURE 3-6
An electron micrograph of the endocervical canal, demonstrating the "arbor vitae." These folds and crypts provide a reservoir for sperm. (From Singer A and Jordan JA: The anatomy of the cervix. In Jordan JA and Singer A, editors: The cervix, Philadelphia, 1976, WB Saunders Co, p 18.)

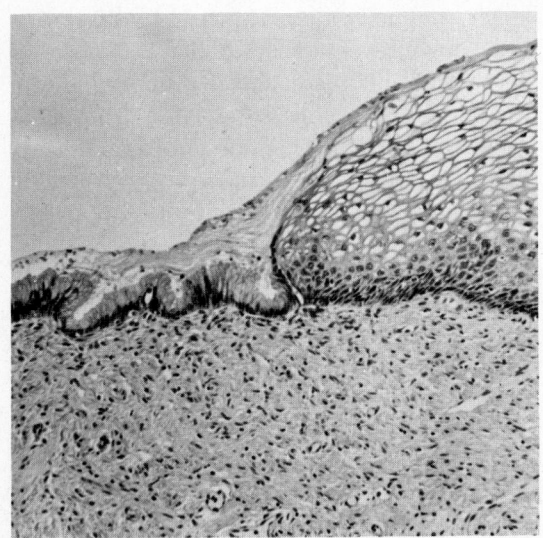

FIGURE 3-7
A histologic section through the squamocolumnar junction of the cervix. Note the abrupt transformation from squamous to columnar epithelium. (From Ferenczy A: Anatomy and histology of the cervix. In Blaustein A, editor: Pathology of the female genital tract, ed 2, New York, 1982, Springer-Verlag, p 127.)

the endocervical canal and the underlying glandular structures. This specialized epithelium secretes mucus, which facilitates sperm transport. Anatomically arranged crypts and villi provide a reservoir for spermatozoa immediately after coitus. This epithelium contains two types of columnar cells: nonciliated secretory cells and ciliated cells. An abrupt transformation usually is seen at the junction of the columnar epithelium of the endocervix and the nonkeratinized stratified squamous epithelium of the portio vaginalis (Figure 3-7). The stratified squamous epithelium of the exocervix is identical to the lining of the vagina.

The dense, fibromuscular cervical stroma is composed primarily of collagenous connective tissue and mucopolysaccharide ground substance. The connective tissue contains approximately 15% smooth muscle cells and a small amount of elastic tissue. However, there are few muscle fibers in the distal portions of the cervix.

Because the cervix is the lower portion of the uterus, it is not surprising that the cervical and uterine vascular supplies are interrelated. The arterial supply of the cervix arises from the descending branch of the uterine artery. The cervical arteries run on the lateral side of the cervix and form the coronary artery, which encircles the cervix. The azygos arteries run longitudinally in the middle of the anterior and posterior aspects of the cervix and the vagina. There are numerous anastomoses between these vessels and the vaginal and middle hemorrhoidal arteries. The venous drainage accompanies these arteries. The lymphatic drainage of the cervix is complex, involving multiple chains of nodes. The principal regional lymph nodes are the obturator, common iliac, internal iliac, external iliac, and visceral nodes of the parametria. Other possible lymphatic drainage includes the following chains of nodes: superior and inferior gluteal, sacral, rectal, lumbar, aortic, and visceral nodes over the posterior surface of the urinary bladder. The stroma of the endocervix is rich in free nerve endings. Pain fibers accompany the parasympathetic fibers to the second, third, and fourth sacral segments.

Clinical Correlations

The major arterial supply to the cervix is located on the lateral cervical walls at the 3 and 9 o'clock positions, respectively. Therefore a deep figure-of-eight suture through the vaginal mucosa and cervical stroma at 3 and 9 o'clock helps to reduce blood loss during procedures such as cone biopsy. If the gynecologist is overzealous in placing such a hemostatic suture high in the vaginal fornix, it is possible to compromise the course of the distal ureter. In rare cases, after large cone biopsies, a woman may become infertile because of the loss of sufficient cervical mucus to facilitate sperm transport from the exocervix to the uterine cavity.

The transformation zone of the cervix is an important anatomic landmark for clinicians. This area encompasses the transition from stratified squamous epithelium to columnar epithelium. Dysplasia of the cervix develops within this transformation zone. The position of a woman's transformation zone, in relation to the long axis of the cervix, depends on her age and hormonal status.

The endocervix is rich in free nerve endings. Occasionally, women experience a vagovagal response during transcervical instrumentation of the uterine cavity. Serial cardiac monitoring during insertion of intrauterine devices demonstrates a reflex bradycardia in some women. The sensory innervation of the exocervix is not as concentrated or sophisticated as that of the endocervix or external skin. Therefore the exocervix may be cauterized by either cold or heat with only minor discomfort to the patient.

UTERUS

The uterus is a thick-walled, hollow, muscular organ located centrally in the female pelvis. Adjacent to the uterus are the urinary bladder anteriorly, the rectum posteriorly, and the broad ligaments laterally (Figure 3-8). The uterus is globular and slightly flattened anteriorly; it has the general configuration of an inverted pear. The short area of constriction in the lower uterine segment is termed the *isthmus* (see Figure 3-5). The dome-shaped top of the uterus is termed the *fundus*. The lower edge of the fundus is described by an imaginary line drawn between the site of entrance of each oviduct. The size and weight of the uterus depend on previous pregnancies and the hormonal status of the individual. The uterus of a nulliparous woman is approximately 8 cm long, 5 cm wide, and 2.5 cm thick and weighs 40 to 50 g. In contrast, in a multiparous woman, each measurement is approximately 1.2 cm larger, and normal uterine weight is 20 to 30 g heavier. A recent study at the University of Southern California defines the upper limit for weight of a normal uterus as 110 g. The capacity of the uterus to enlarge during pregnancy results in a 10- to 20-fold increase in weight at term. After menopause the uterus atrophies in both size and weight.

The cavity of the uterus is flattened and triangular. The oviducts enter the uterine cavity at the superolateral aspects of the cavity in the areas designated the cornua. In the majority of women, the long axis of the uterus is both anteverted in respect to the long axis of the vagina and anteflexed in relation to the long axis of the cervix. However, a retroflexed uterus is a normal variant found in approximately 25% of women.

The uterus has three layers, similar to other hollow abdominal and pelvic organs. The thin, external serosal layer comprises the visceral peritoneum. The peritoneum is firmly attached to the uterus in all areas except anteriorly at the level of the internal os of the cervix. The wide middle muscular layer is composed of three indistinct layers of smooth muscle. The outer longitudinal layer is contiguous with the muscle layers of the oviduct and vagina. The middle layer has interlacing oblique, spiral bundles of smooth muscle and large venous

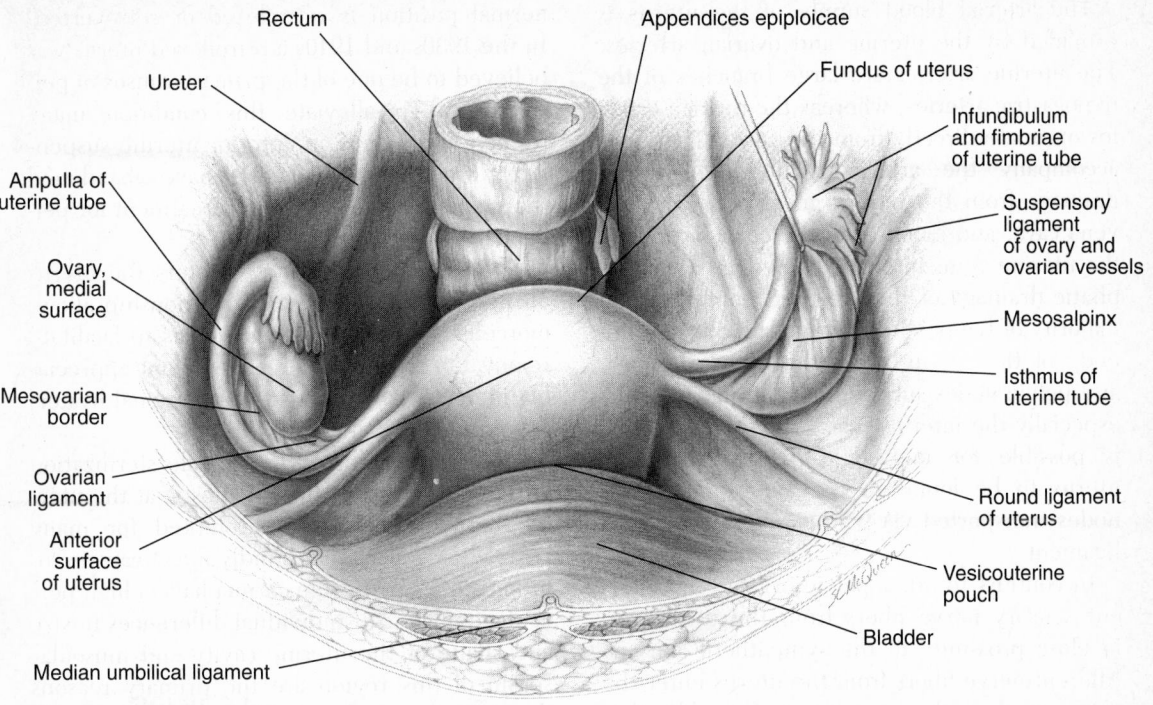

Rectum

Appendices epiploicae

Fundus of uterus

Ureter

Infundibulum
and fimbriae
of uterine tube

Ampulla of
uterine tube

Suspensory
ligament
of ovary and
ovarian vessels

Ovary,
medial
surface

Mesosalpinx

Isthmus of
uterine tube

Mesovarian
border

Ovarian
ligament

Round ligament
of uterus

Anterior
surface
of uterus

Vesicouterine
pouch

Median umbilical ligament

Bladder

FIGURE 3-8
The organs of the female pelvis. The uterus is surrounded by the bladder anteriorly, the rectum posteriorly, and the folds of the broad ligaments laterally. (Redrawn from Clemente CD: Anatomy: a regional atlas of the human body, Baltimore-Munich, 1987, Urban & Schwarzenberg.

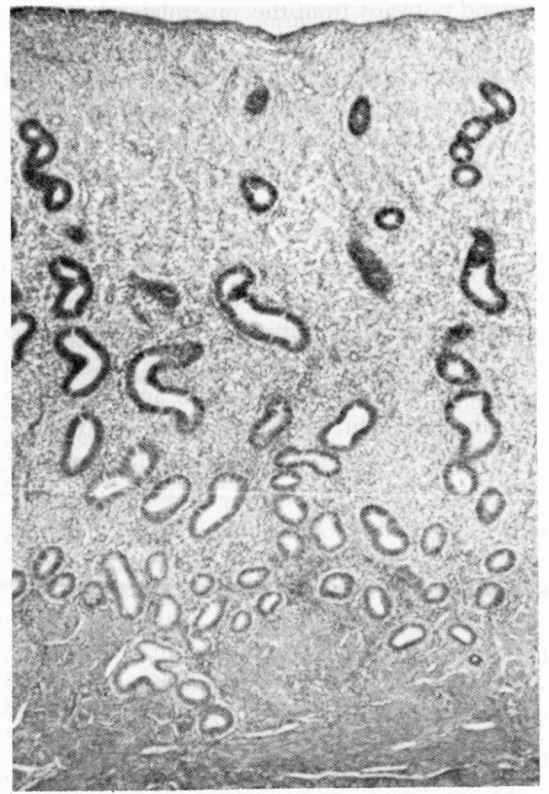

FIGURE 3-9
A histologic view of the endometrium during the proliferative phase, demonstrating the strata in the endometrium. (From Demopoulos RI: Normal endometrium. In Blaustein A, editor: Pathology of the female genital tract, ed 2, New York, 1982, Springer-Verlag, p 216.)

plexuses. The inner muscular layer is also longitudinal. The endometrium is a reddish mucous membrane that varies from 1 to 6 mm in thickness, depending on hormonal stimulation. The uterine glands are tubular and composed of tall columnar epithelium. The cells of the endometrial stroma resemble embryonic connective tissue with scant cytoplasm and large nuclei. The endometrium may be divided into an inner stratum basale and an outer stratum functionale. The stratum functionale may be further subdivided into an inner compact stratum and a more superficial spongy stratum. Only the stratum functionale responds to fluctuating hormonal levels (Figure 3-9).

the epithelium and muscular layers. The smooth muscle of the tube is arranged into inner circular and outer longitudinal layers. Between the peritoneal surface of the tube and the muscular layer is an adventitial layer that contains blood vessels and nerves.

The arterial blood supply to the oviducts is derived from terminal branches of the uterine and ovarian arteries. The arteries anastomose in the mesosalpinx. Blood from the uterine artery supplies the medial two thirds of each tube. The venous drainage runs parallel to the arterial supply. The lymphatic system is separate and distinct from the lymphatic drainage of the uterus. Lymphatic drainage includes the internal iliac nodes and the aortic nodes surrounding the aorta and the inferior vena cava at the level of the renal vessels.

The tubes are innervated by both sympathetic and parasympathetic nerves from the uterine and ovarian plexuses. Sensory nerves are related to spinal cord segments T11, T12, and L1.

Clinical Correlations

The vast majority of ectopic pregnancies occur in the oviduct. The acute abdominal and pelvic pain that women with an ectopic pregnancy experience is believed to be caused by hemorrhage resulting in acute distention of the oviduct. The most catastrophic bleeding associated with ectopic pregnancy occurs when the implantation site is in the intramural segment of the tube.

The isthmic segment of the oviduct is the preferred site to apply an occlusive device, such as a clip or band, for female sterilization. The right oviduct and appendix are often adjacent. Clinically it may be difficult to differentiate inflammation of the tube and acute appendicitis. Accessory tubal ostia are discovered frequently and always connect with the lumen of the tube. These accessory ostia are usually found in the ampullary portion of the tube.

The wide mesosalpinx of the ampullary segment of the tube allows torsion of the tube, which occasionally results in ischemic atrophy of the ampullary segment. Paratubal or paraovarian cysts can reach 5 to 10 cm in diameter and occasionally are confused with ovarian cysts before surgery.

Although a definitive anatomic sphincter has not been identified at the uterotubal junction,

a temporary physiologic obstruction has been identified at hysterosalpingography. Sometimes clinicians may alleviate this temporary obstruction by giving the patient intravenous sedation, a paracervical block, or intravenous glucagon.

OVARIES

The paired ovaries are light gray and approximately the size and configuration of a large almond. The surface of the ovary of adult women is pitted and indented from previous ovulations. The ovaries contain approximately 1 to 2 million oocytes at birth. During a woman's reproductive lifetime, about 8000 follicles begin development. The growth of many follicles is blunted in various stages of development, but approximately 300 ova eventually are released. The size and position of the ovary depend on the woman's age and parity. During the reproductive years, ovaries weigh 3 to 6 g and measure approximately 1.5 cm × 2.5 cm × 4 cm. As the woman ages, the ovaries become smaller and firmer in consistency.

In a nulliparous woman who is standing, the long axis of the ovary is vertical. The ovary in nulliparous women rests in a depression of peritoneum named the ovarian fossa. Immediately adjacent to the ovarian fossa are the external iliac vessels, the ureter, and the obturator vessels and nerves.

There are three prominent ligaments that determine the anatomic mobility of the ovary (see Figure 3-5). The posterior portion of the broad ligament forms the mesovarium, which attaches to the anterior border of the ovary. The mesovarium contains the arterial anastomotic branches of the ovarian and uterine arteries, a plexus of veins, and the lateral end of the ovarian ligament. The ovarian ligament is a narrow, short, fibrous band that extends from the lower pole of the ovary to the uterus. The infundibular pelvic ligament, or suspensory ligament of the ovary, forms the superior and lateral aspect of the broad ligament. This ligament contains the ovarian artery, ovarian veins, and accompanying nerves. It attaches the upper pole of the ovary to the lateral pelvic wall.

The ovary is subdivided histologically into an outer cortex and an inner medulla (Figure 3-12). The ovarian surface is covered by a single layer of cuboidal epithelium, termed the *germinal epithelium*. The latter term is a misnomer because the cells are similar to those of

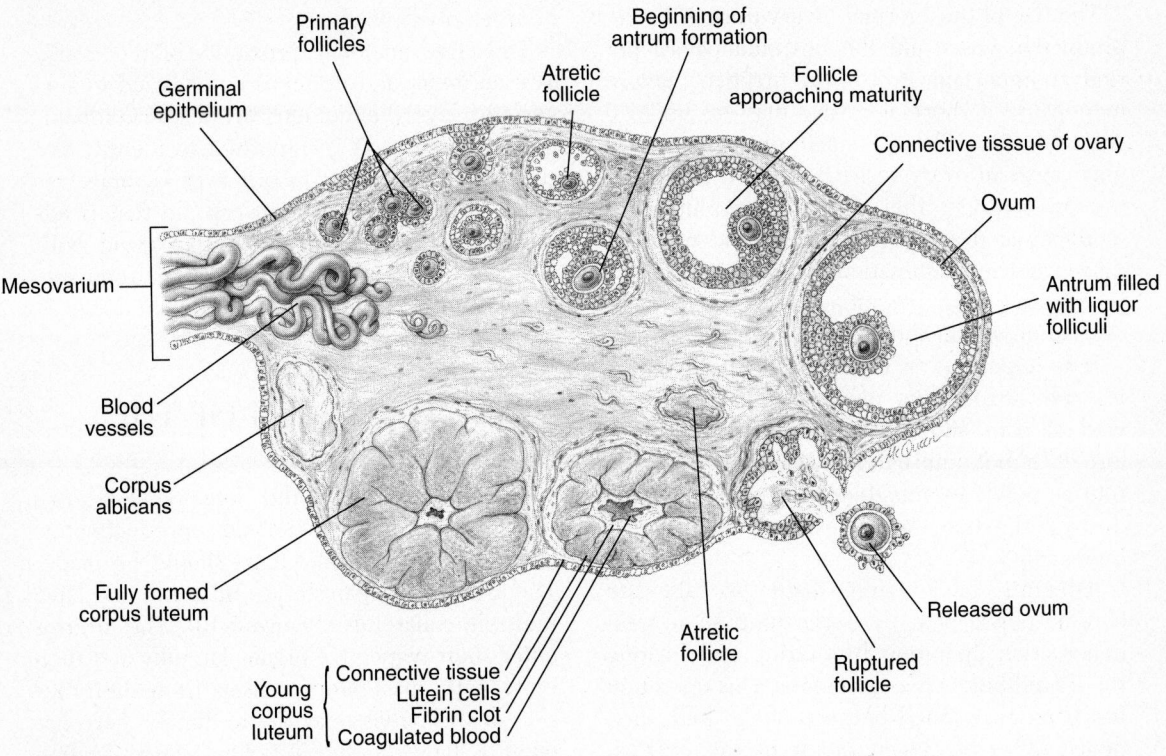

Primary follicles

Germinal epithelium

Beginning of antrum formation

Atretic follicle

Follicle approaching maturity

Connective tisssue of ovary

Ovum

Antrum filled with liquor folliculi

Mesovarium

Blood vessels

Corpus albicans

Fully formed corpus luteum

Young corpus luteum { Connective tissue / Lutein cells / Fibrin clot / Coagulated blood

Atretic follicle

Ruptured follicle

Released ovum

FIGURE 3-12
A schematic drawing of the ovary. Note the single layer of cuboidal epithelium called the *germinal epithelium.* Note the graafian follicles in different stages of development. Note the inner medullary region of stroma and blood vessels. (Adapted from Gray's Anatomy of the human body, ed 35, Philadelphia, 1973, Lea & Febiger. Redrawn from Blaustein A: Anatomy and histology of the human ovary. In Blaustein A, editor: Pathology of the female genital tract, ed 2, New York, 1982, Springer-Verlag, p 417.)

the coelomic mesothelium, which forms the peritoneum, and because the germinal epithelium is not related to the histogenesis of graafian follicles. If the ovary is transected, numerous transparent, fluid-filled cysts are noted throughout the cortex. Microscopically these are graafian follicles in various stages of development, active or regressing corpus luteum, and atretic follicles. The stroma of the cortex is composed primarily of closely packed cells around the follicles. These specialized connective tissue cells form the theca. The medulla contains the ovarian vascular supply and a loose stroma. The specialized polyhedral hilar cells are similar to the interstitial cells of the testis.

Each of the ovarian arteries arises directly from the aorta just below the renal arteries. They descend in the retroperitoneal space, cross anterior to the psoas muscles and internal iliac vessels, and enter the infundibulopelvic

ligaments, reaching the mesovarium in the broad ligament. The ovarian blood supply enters through the hilum of the ovary. The venous drainage of the ovary collects in the pampiniform plexus and consolidates into several large veins as it leaves the hilum of the ovary. The ovarian veins accompany the ovarian arteries, with the left ovarian vein draining into the left renal vein, whereas the right ovarian vein connects directly with the inferior vena cava.

The lymphatic drainage of the ovaries is primarily to the aortic nodes adjacent to the great vessels at the level of the renal veins. Metastatic disease from the ovary occasionally takes a shorter course to the iliac nodes. The autonomic and sensory nerve fibers accompany the ovarian vasculature in the infundibulopelvic ligament. They connect with the ovarian, hypogastric, and aortic plexuses.

Clinical Correlations

The size of the "normal" ovary during the reproductive years and the postmenopausal period is important in clinical practice. Before menopause a "normal" ovary may be up to 5 cm in length. Thus a small physiologic cyst may cause an ovary to be 6 to 7 cm in diameter. In contrast, the "normal" atrophic postmenopausal ovary usually cannot be palpated during pelvic examination. If an adnexal mass is palpated in a postmenopausal woman, an ovarian neoplasm should be suspected.

It is important to emphasize that the ovaries and surrounding peritoneum are not devoid of pain and pressure receptors. Therefore it is not unusual for a woman during a routine pelvic examination to experience some discomfort when normal ovaries are palpated bimanually.

Attempts have been made to alleviate chronic pelvic pain by performing an ovarian denervation operation by cutting and ligating the infundibulopelvic ligaments. This operation has been abandoned because of the high incidence of cystic degeneration of the ovaries, which resulted from the interruption of their primary blood supply that accompanied the neurectomy procedure.

The close anatomic proximity of the ovary, ovarian fossa, and ureter is emphasized in surgery for severe endometriosis or pelvic inflammatory disease. It is important to identify the course of the ureter in order to facilitate removal of all of the ovarian capsule that is adherent to the peritoneum and to avoid both ureteral injury and residual ovarian remnants in the future.

VASCULAR SYSTEM OF THE PELVIS

In a description of the network of arteries that bring blood to the female reproductive organs, several generalizations should be made. The arteries are paired, are bilateral, and have multiple collaterals (Figure 3-13). The arteries enter their respective organs laterally and then unite with anastomotic vessels from the other side of the pelvis near the midline. There has been a long-standing teaching generalization that the pelvic reproductive viscera lie within a

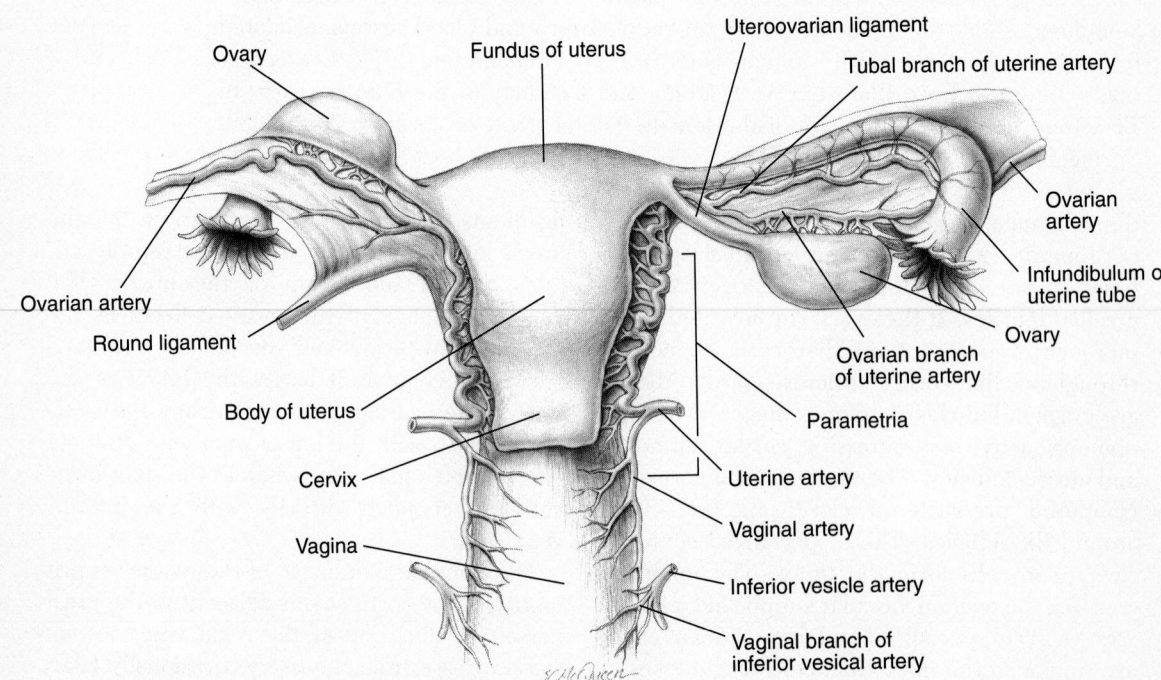

FIGURE 3-13

The arteries of the reproductive organs. Note the paired arteries entering laterally and freely anastomosing with each other. (Redrawn from Clemente CD: Anatomy: a regional atlas of the human body, Baltimore-Munich, 1987, Urban & Schwarzenberg.)

loosely woven basket of large veins with numerous interconnecting venous plexuses. The arteries thread their way through this interwoven mesh of veins to reach the pelvic reproductive organs, giving off numerous branching arcades to provide a rich blood supply.

Arteries

Inferior Mesenteric Artery

The inferior mesenteric artery, a single artery, arises from the aorta approximately 3 cm above the aortic bifurcation. It supplies part of the transverse colon, the descending colon, the sigmoid colon, and the rectum and terminates as the superior hemorrhoidal artery. The inferior mesenteric artery is occasionally torn during node dissections performed in staging operations for gynecologic cancer. Because of the rich collateral circulation from the middle and inferior hemorrhoidal arteries, the inferior mesenteric artery can be ligated without compromise of the distal portion of the colon.

Ovarian Artery

The ovarian arteries originate from the aorta just below the renal vessels. Each one courses in the retroperitoneal space, crosses anterior to the ureter, and enters the infundibulopelvic ligament. As the artery travels medially in the mesovarium, numerous small branches supply the ovary and oviduct. The ovarian artery unites with the ascending branch of the uterine artery in the mesovarium just under the suspensory ligament of the ovary.

Common Iliac Artery

The bifurcation of the aorta occurs at the level of the fourth lumbar vertebra, forming the two common iliac arteries. Each common iliac artery is approximately 5 cm in length before the vessel divides into the external iliac and hypogastric arteries.

Hypogastric Artery (Internal Iliac Artery)

The hypogastric arteries are short vessels, each approximately 3 to 4 cm in length. Throughout their course they are in close proximity to the ureters, which are anterior, and to the hypogastric veins, which are posterior. Each hypogastric artery branches into an anterior and a posterior division (or trunk). The posterior trunk gives off three parietal branches: the iliolumbar, lateral sacral, and superior gluteal arteries. The anterior trunk has nine branches. The three parietal branches are the obturator, internal pudendal, and inferior gluteal arteries. The six visceral branches include the umbilical, middle vesical, inferior vesical, middle hemorrhoidal, uterine, and vaginal arteries. The superior vesical artery usually arises from the umbilical artery. The individual branches of the hypogastric artery may vary from one woman to another.

Uterine Artery

The uterine artery arises from the anterior division of the hypogastric artery and courses medially toward the isthmus of the uterus. Approximately 2 cm lateral to the endocervix, it crosses over the ureter and reaches the sidewall of the uterus. The ascending branch of the uterine artery courses in the broad ligament, running a tortuous route to finally anastomose with the ovarian artery in the mesovarium (Figure 3-14). Through its circuitous route in the parametrium, the uterine artery gives off numerous branches that unite with arcuate arteries from the other side. This series of arcuate arteries develops radial branches that supply the myometrium and the basalis layer of the endometrium. The arcuate arteries also form the spiral arteries of the functional layer of the endometrium. The descending branch of the uterine artery produces branches that supply both the cervix and the vagina. In each case the vessels enter the organ laterally and anastomose freely with vessels from the other side.

Vaginal Artery

The vaginal artery may arise either from the anterior trunk of the hypogastric artery or from the uterine artery. It supplies blood to the vagina, bladder, and rectum. There are extensive anastomoses with the vaginal branches of the uterine artery to form the azygos arteries of the cervix and vagina.

Internal Pudendal Artery

This artery is the terminal branch of the hypogastric artery and supplies branches to the rectum, labia, clitoris, and perineum.

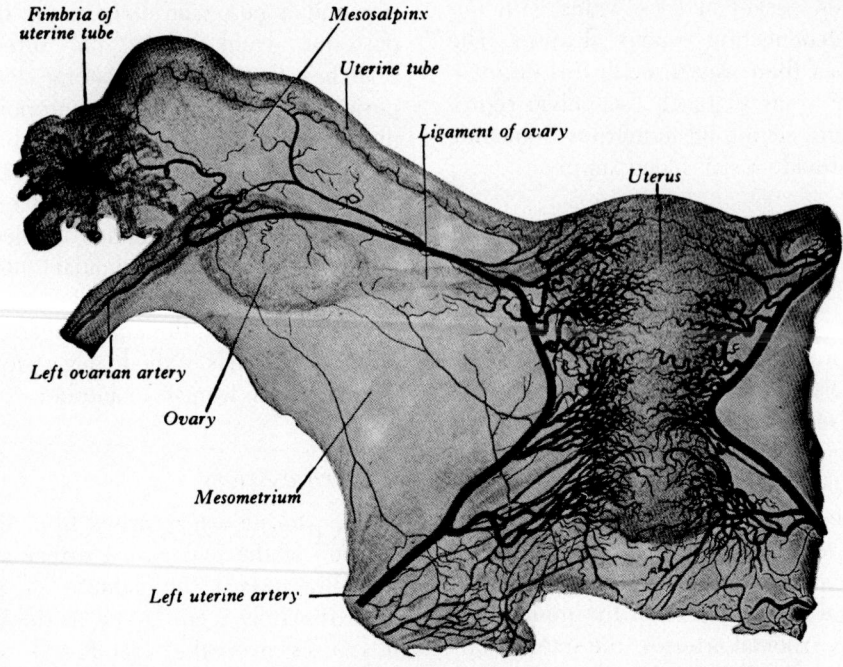

FIGURE 3-14

A photograph of an injected specimen demonstrating the rich anastomoses of the uterine and ovarian arteries. (From Warwick R and Williams PL: Gray's anatomy, ed 35, Edinburgh, 1973, Churchill Livingstone, p 1361.)

Veins

The venous drainage of the pelvis begins in small sinusoids that drain to profuse venous plexuses contained within or immediately adjacent to the pelvic organs. Invariably there are numerous anastomoses between the parietal and visceral branches of the venous system. In general, the veins of the female pelvis and perineum are thin walled and have few valves.

The veins that drain the pelvic plexuses follow the course of the arterial supply. Their names are similar to those of the accompanying arteries. Often multiple veins run alongside a single artery. The leading exception to these generalizations is the venous drainage of the ovaries. The left ovarian vein empties into the left renal vein, whereas the right ovarian vein connects directly with the inferior vena cava.

Clinical Correlations

Although the external iliac artery and its branches do not supply blood directly to the pelvic viscera, they are important landmarks in surgical anatomy. The fact that the external iliac artery gives rise to the obturator artery in 15% to 20% of women must be considered in radical cancer operations with associated node dissections of the obturator fossa. The external iliac artery also gives rise to the inferior epigastric artery. The inferior epigastric artery must be avoided when performing paracentesis or amniocentesis.

In certain clinical situations associated with profuse hemorrhage from the female pelvis, hypogastric ligation is performed. Because of the extensive collateral circulation, this operation does not produce hypoxia of the pelvic viscera but reduces hemorrhage by decreasing the pulse pressure. The extent of collateral circulation after hypogastric artery ligation depends on the site of ligation and may be divided into three groups (Table 3-1).

In cases of intractable pelvic hemorrhage, it may be necessary to supplement the effects of bilateral hypogastric artery ligation with ligation of the anastomotic sites between the ovarian and uterine vessels. Ligation of the terminal end of the ovarian artery preserves the direct blood supply to the ovaries, and there is no fear of the subsequent cystic degeneration of the ovaries that may occur after ligation of

TABLE 3-1
Collateral Arterial Circulation

Branches from aorta

Ovarian artery—anastomoses freely with uterine artery

Inferior mesenteric artery—continues as superior hemorrhoidal artery to anastomose with middle and inferior hemorrhoidal arteries from hypogastric and internal pudendal

Lumbar and vertebral arteries—anastomose with iliolumbar artery of hypogastric

Middle sacral artery—anastomoses with lateral sacral artery of hypogastric

Branches from external iliac artery

Deep iliac circumflex artery—anastomoses with iliolumbar and superior gluteal of hypogastric

Inferior epigastric artery—gives origin to obturator artery in 25% of cases, providing additional anastomoses of external iliac with medial femoral circumflex and communicating pelvic branches

Branches from femoral artery

Medial femoral circumflex artery—anastomoses with obturator and inferior gluteal arteries from hypogastric

Lateral femoral circumflex artery—anastomoses with superior gluteal and iliolumbar arteries from hypogastric

Reprinted with permission from Mattingly RF and Thompson JD: Te Linde's operative gynecology, ed 6, Philadelphia, 1985, JB Lippincott Co.

the vessels in the infundibulopelvic ligaments. An alternative approach to ligation is to embolize the bleeding vessel with Gelfoam, small coils of plastic, absolute alcohol, a detachable balloon, or Ivalon particles. This is accomplished by direct canalization with fluoroscopy.

Treatments for repetitive embolization from the female pelvis are either the placement of a vascular umbrella or ligation of the inferior vena cava. Collateral circulation exists between the portal venous system of the gastrointestinal tract and the systemic venous circulation through anastomosis in the pelvis, especially in the hemorrhoidal plexus. The pelvic veins also anastomose with the presacral and lumbar veins. Therefore patients may develop trophoblastic emboli to the brain without the trophoblast being filtered by the capillary system in the lungs.

LYMPHATIC SYSTEM

External Iliac Nodes

The external iliac nodes are immediately adjacent to the external iliac artery and vein (Figures 3-15 and 3-16). There are two distinct groups, one situated lateral to the vessels and the other posterior to the psoas muscle. The distal portion of the posterior group is enclosed in the femoral sheath. The majority of lymphatic channels to this group of nodes originate from the vulva, but there are also channels from the cervix and lower portion of the uterus. The external iliac nodes receive secondary drainage from the femoral and internal iliac nodes.

Internal Iliac Nodes

The internal iliac nodes are found in an anatomic triangle whose sides are composed of the external iliac artery, the hypogastric artery, and the pelvic sidewall. Included in this important area for biopsy are nodes with special designation, including the nodes of the femoral ring, the obturator nodes, and the nodes adjacent to the external iliac vessels. This rich collection of nodes receives channels from every internal pelvic organ and the vulva, including the clitoris and urethra.

Common Iliac Nodes

The common iliac nodes are a group of nodes located adjacent to the vessels that bear their name and are between the external iliac and aortic chains. Most of these nodes are found lateral to the vessels. To remove this chain, it is necessary to dissect the common iliac vessels away from their attachments to the psoas muscle. This group receives lymphatics from the cervix and the upper portion of the vagina. Secondary lymphatic drainage from the internal iliac, external iliac, superior gluteal, and inferior gluteal nodes is to the common iliac nodes.

Inferior Gluteal Nodes

A small group of lymph nodes, the inferior gluteal nodes, are located in the anatomic proximity of the ischial spines and are adjacent to the sacral plexus of nodes. It is difficult to remove these nodes surgically, and often they are considered inaccessible. The nodes receive

FIGURE 3-15
Schematic view of the pelvic lymph nodes. (From Plentl AA and Friedman EA: Lymphatic system of the female genitalia, Philadelphia, 1971, WB Saunders Co, p 13.)

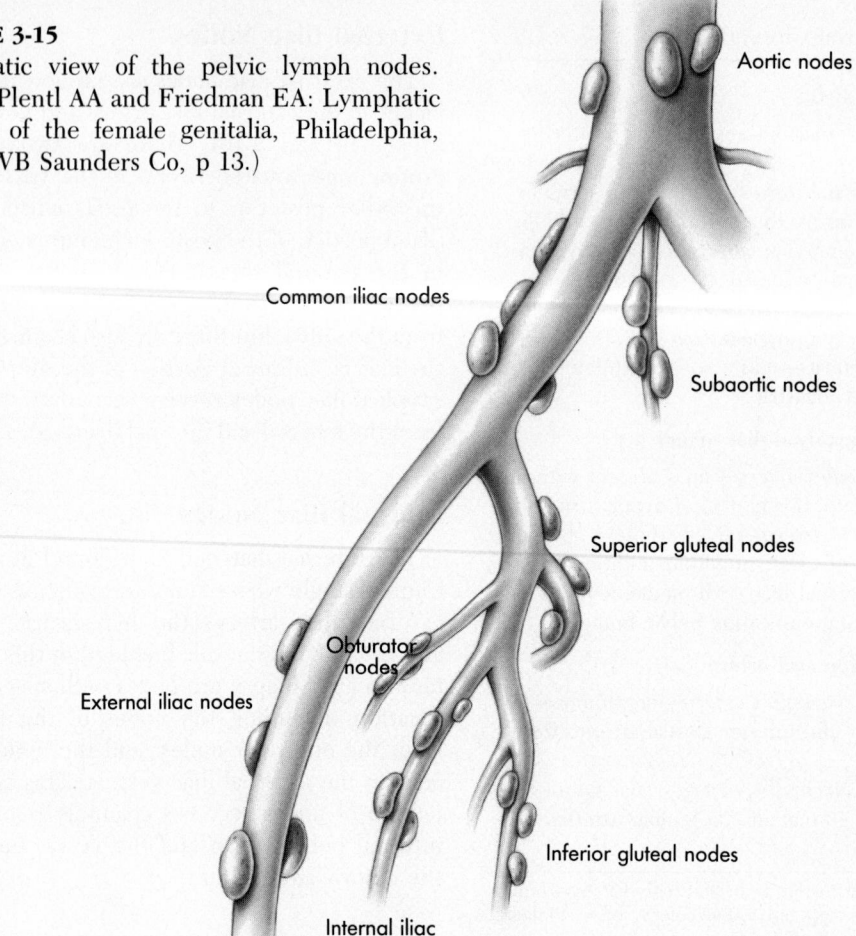

Aortic nodes

Common iliac nodes

Subaortic nodes

Superior gluteal nodes

Obturator nodes

External iliac nodes

Inferior gluteal nodes

Internal iliac nodes

lymphatics from the cervix, the lower portion of the vagina, and Bartholin's glands. This group of nodes secondarily drains to the internal iliac, common iliac, superior gluteal, and subaortic nodes.

Superior Gluteal Nodes

The superior gluteal nodes are a group of nodes found near the origin of the superior gluteal artery and adjacent to the medial and posterior aspects of the hypogastric vessels. The superior gluteal nodes receive primary lymphatic drainage from the cervix and the vagina. Efferent lymphatics from this chain drain to the common iliac, sacral, or subaortic nodes.

Sacral Nodes

The sacral nodes are found over the middle of the sacrum in a space bounded laterally by the sacral foramina. These nodes receive lym-

phatic drainage from both the cervix and the vagina. Secondary drainage from these nodes runs in a cephalad direction to the subaortic nodes.

Subaortic Nodes

The subaortic nodes are arranged in a chain and are located below the bifurcation of the aorta, immediately anterior to the most caudal portion of the inferior vena cava and over the fifth lumbar vertebra. The primary drainage to this chain of nodes is from the cervix, with a few lymphatics from the vagina. This group is the first secondary chain to receive the efferent lymphatics as lymph flow progresses in a cephalad direction from the majority of other pelvic nodes.

Aortic Nodes

The many aortic nodes are immediately adjacent to the aorta on both its anterior and lateral

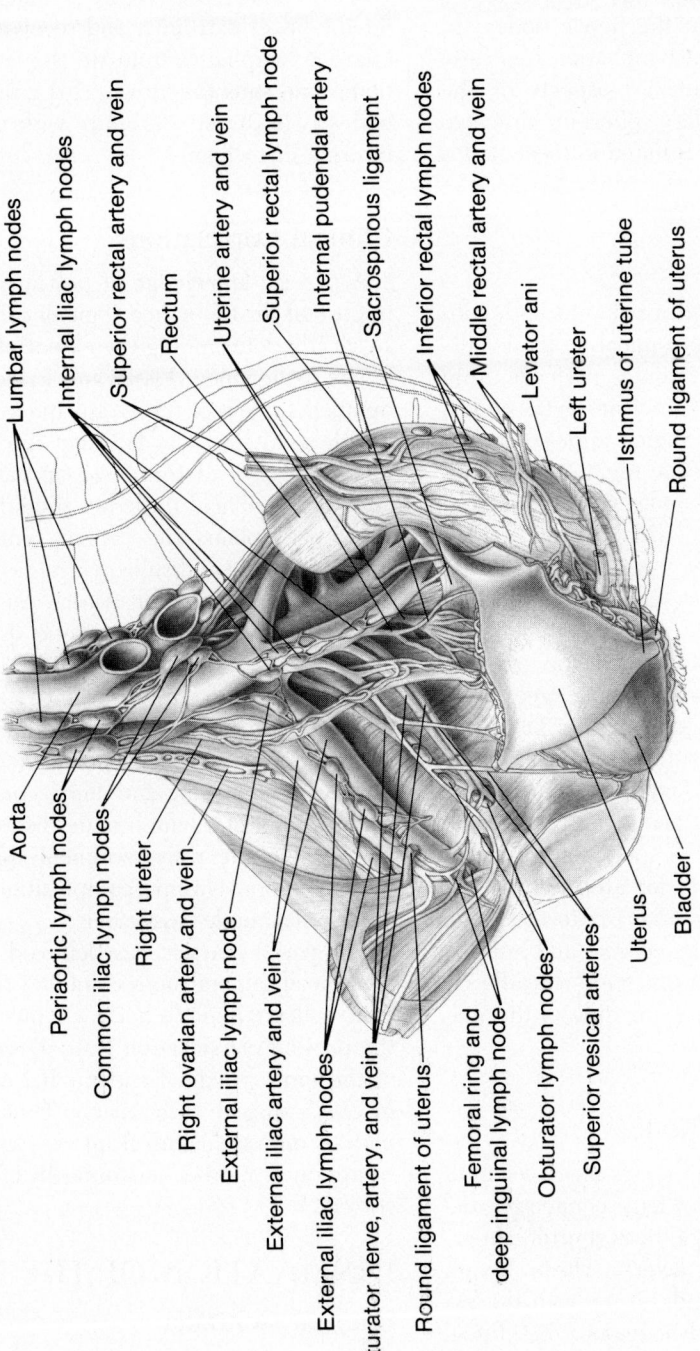

Lumbar lymph nodes

Internal iliac lymph nodes

Superior rectal artery and vein

Rectum

Uterine artery and vein

Superior rectal lymph node

Internal pudendal artery

Sacrospinous ligament

Inferior rectal lymph nodes

Middle rectal artery and vein

Levator ani

Left ureter

Isthmus of uterine tube

Round ligament of uterus

Aorta

Periaortic lymph nodes

Common iliac lymph nodes

Right ureter

Right ovarian artery and vein

External iliac lymph node

External iliac artery and vein

Obturator nerve, artery, and vein

Round ligament of uterus

Femoral ring and
deep inguinal lymph node

Obturator lymph nodes

Superior vesical arteries

Uterus

Bladder

FIGURE 3-16

A lateral view of the female pelvis demonstrating the extensive lymphatic network. Note that most of the lymphatic channels follow the courses of the major vessels. (Redrawn from Clemente CD: Anatomy: a regional atlas of the human body, Baltimore-Munich, 1987, Urban & Schwarzenberg.)

aspects, predominantly in the furrow between the aorta and inferior vena cava. Primary lymphatics drain from all the major pelvic organs, including the cervix, uterus, oviducts, and especially the ovaries. The aortic chain receives secondary drainage from the pelvic nodes. In general, primary afferent lymphatics drain into the nodes over the anterior aspects of the aorta, whereas secondary efferent drainage from other pelvic nodes is found in those nodes situated lateral and posterior to the aorta.

Rectal Nodes

The chain of rectal nodes is found both subfascially and in the loose connective tissue surrounding the rectum. Primary drainage from the cervix flows to the superior rectal nodes, and drainage from the vagina appears in the rectal nodes in the anorectal region. Secondary drainage from the rectal nodes goes to the subaortic and aortic groups.

Parauterine Nodes

The number of lymph nodes in the group of parauterine nodes is small; most frequently there is a single node immediately lateral to each side of the cervix and close to the pelvic course of the ureter. Though anatomists frequently do not comment about the parauterine nodes, the group receives special attention in radical surgical operations for uterine or cervical malignancy. Primary drainage to this node originates in the vagina, cervix, and uterus. Secondary drainage from this node is to the internal iliac nodes on the same side of the pelvis.

Superficial Femoral Nodes

The superficial femoral nodes are a group of nodes found in the loose, fatty connective tissue of the femoral triangle between the superficial and deep fascial layers. These lymph nodes receive lymphatic drainage from the external genitalia of the vulvar region, the gluteal region, and the entire leg, including the foot. Efferent lymphatics from this group of nodes penetrate the fascia lata to enter the deep femoral nodes. Plentl and Friedman have stated that this area undoubtedly represents the greatest concentration of lymph nodes in the female (Figure 3-17).

Deep Femoral Nodes

The deep femoral nodes are located within the femoral sheath, adjacent to both the femoral artery and the vein within the femoral triangle. This chain receives the primary lymphatics for the lower extremity and receives secondary efferent lymphatics from the superficial lymph nodes and thus the vulva. This group of lymph nodes is in direct continuity with the iliac and internal iliac chains.

Clinical Correlations

A precise knowledge of pelvic lymphatics is important for the gynecologic oncologist who is surgically determining the extent of spread of a pelvic malignancy. Plentl and Friedman give a detailed review of the lymphatic system of the female genitalia. The fact that most lymphatic metastatic spread from ovarian carcinoma occurs in a cephalad direction should be emphasized; it explains the primary importance of sampling aortic and subaortic nodes during second-look operations for ovarian cancer. In carcinoma of the vulva, lymphatic drainage may occur in either side of the pelvis. Thus bilateral node dissections are important. Because most pelvic lymph nodes are in anatomic proximity to major pelvic vessels, pelvic hemorrhage is the most important and most common acute complication of a lymph node dissection. Lymphocysts in the retroperitoneal space are the most common chronic complication associated with radical node dissections.

For many years it was believed that all the superficial femoral nodes drained to a sentinel node called *Cloquet's node*. Cloquet's node, by the present classification system, would be one of the most proximal and medial of the nodes in the external iliac chain. Thus, Cloquet's node is only of historical interest, since the assumption is neither anatomically nor clinically correct.

INNERVATION OF THE PELVIS
Internal Genitalia

The innervation of the internal genital organs is supplied primarily by the autonomic nervous system. The sympathetic portion of the autonomic nervous system originates in the thoracic and lumbar portions of the spinal cord, and sympathetic ganglia are located adjacent to the central nervous system. In contrast, the para-

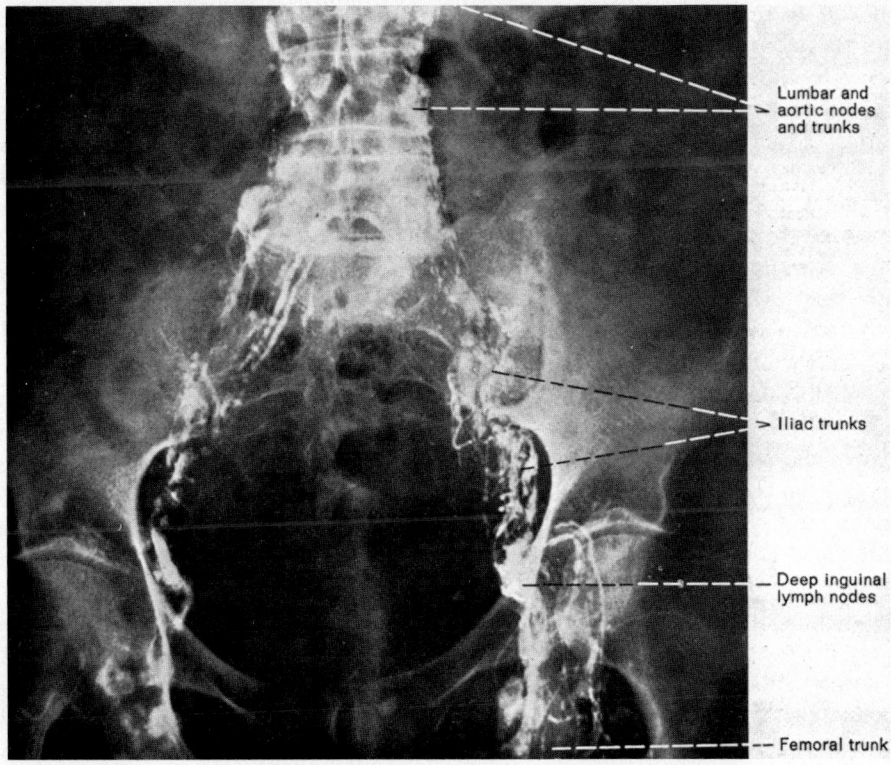

Lumbar and aortic nodes and trunks

Iliac trunks

Deep inguinal lymph nodes

Femoral trunk

FIGURE 3-17
A lymphangiogram of the pelvis and lumbar areas. This x-ray film shows the course of the lymphatics from the deep femoral nodes into the iliac nodes. Note the extensive network of nodes in the inguinal region. (From Clemente CD: A regional atlas of the human body, ed 3, Baltimore-Munich, 1987, Urban & Schwarzenberg.)

sympathetic portion originates in cranial nerves and the middle three sacral segments of the cord, and the ganglia are located near the visceral organs. Although the fibers of both subdivisions of the autonomic nervous system frequently are intermingled in the same peripheral nerves, their physiologic actions are usually directly antagonistic. As a broad generalization, sympathetic fibers in the female pelvis produce muscular contractions and vasoconstriction, whereas parasympathetic fibers cause the opposite effect on muscles and vasodilation.

The semantics of pelvic innervation are confusing and imprecise. A plexus is a mixture of preganglionic and postganglionic fibers; small, inconsistently placed ganglia; and afferent (sensory) fibers. Throughout both the anatomic and surgical literature, a plexus may also be termed a *nerve*. For example, the superior hypogastric plexus is also called the *presacral nerve*.

Although autonomic nerve fibers enter the pelvis by several routes, the majority are con-

tained in the superior hypogastric plexus, which is a caudal extension of the aortic and inferior mesenteric plexuses. The superior hypogastric plexus is found in the retroperitoneal connective tissue. It extends from the fourth lumbar vertebra to the hollow over the sacrum. In its lower portion the plexus divides into two parts to form the two hypogastric nerves, which run laterally and inferiorly. These nerves fan out to form the inferior hypogastric plexus in the area just below the bifurcation of the common iliac arteries. The nerve trunks then descend farther into the base of the broad ligament, where they join with parasympathetic fibers to form the pelvic plexus. Both motor fibers and accompanying sensory fibers reach the pelvic plexus from S2, S3, and S4 via the pelvic nerves, or nervi erigentes. From the pelvic plexus secondary plexuses are adjacent to all pelvic viscera, namely, the rectum, anus, urinary bladder, vagina, and Frankenhäuser's plexus in the uterosacral ligaments. Frankenhäuser's plexus is extensive and contains both myelinated and nonmyelinated fibers passing primarily to the uterus and cervix, with a few fibers passing to the urinary bladder and vagina. The ovarian plexus, like the blood supply to the ovaries, is not part of the hypogastric system. The ovarian plexus is a downward extension of the aortic and renal plexuses.

It is impossible to separate afferent, sensory fibers from pelvic organs into morphologically independent tracts. The majority of fibers accompany the vascular system from the organ and then enter plexuses of the autonomic nervous system before eventually entering white rami communicates to the cell bodies in dorsal root ganglia of the spinal column. The major sensory fibers from the uterus accompany the sympathetic nerves, which enter the nerve roots of the spinal cord in segments T11 and T12. Thus referred uterine pain is often felt in the lower abdomen. In contrast, afferents from the cervix enter the spinal cord in nerve roots of S2, S3, and S4. Referred pain from cervical inflammation is characterized as low back pain in the lumbosacral region.

External Genitalia

The pudendal nerve and its branches supply the majority of both motor and sensory fibers to the muscles and skin of the vulvar region. The pudendal nerve arises from the second, third, and fourth sacral roots. It has a complicated course in which it initially leaves the pelvis via the greater sciatic foramen. Next, it crosses beneath the ischial spine, running on the medial side of the internal pudendal artery. The pudendal nerve then reenters the pelvic cavity and travels in Alcock's canal, which runs along the lateral aspects of the ischial rectal fossa. As the nerve reaches the urogenital diaphragm, it divides into three branches: the inferior hemorrhoidal, the deep perineal, and the superficial perineal (Figure 3-18). The dorsal nerve of the clitoris is a terminal branch of the deep perineal nerve.

The skin of the anus, clitoris, and medial and inferior aspects of the vulva is supplied primarily by distal branches of the pudendal nerve. The vulvar region receives additional sensory fibers from three nerves. The anterior branch

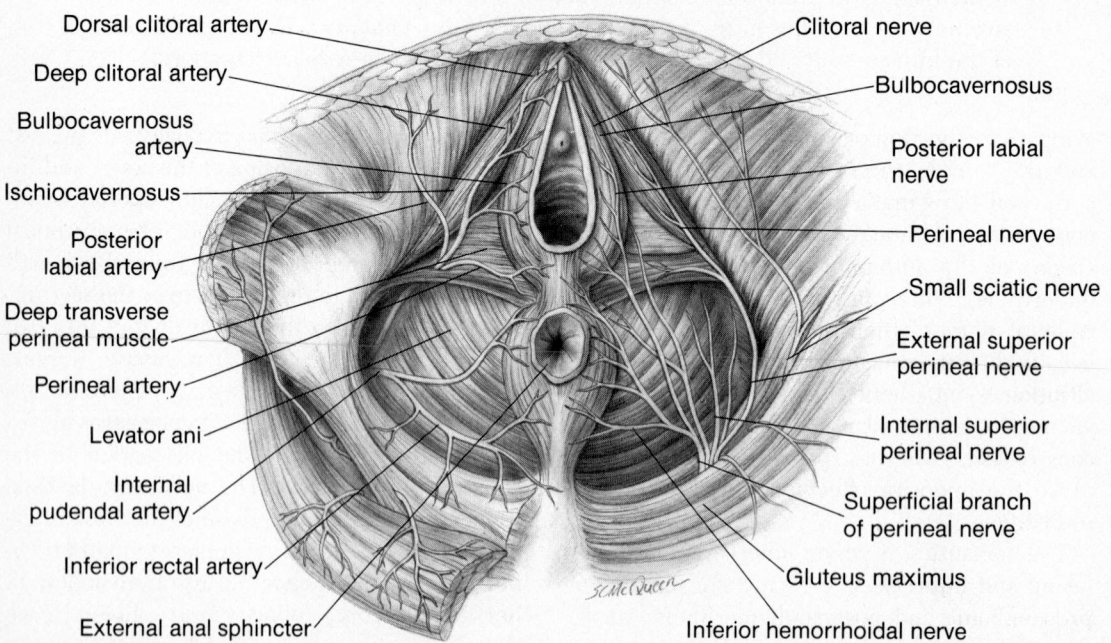

FIGURE 3-18

A posterior view of the female perineum, demonstrating the pudendal nerve emerging externally. The nerve divides into three segments as it passes out of the pelvis: the inferior hemorrhoidal nerve and the deep and superficial perineal nerves. The clitoral nerve is the terminal branch of the deep perineal nerve. (Redrawn from Mattingly RF and Thompson JD: Te Linde's operative gynecology, ed 6, Philadelphia, 1985, JB Lippincott Co, p 49.)

of the ilioinguinal nerve sends fibers to the mons pubis and the upper part of the labia majora. The genital femoral nerve supplies fibers to the labia majora, and the posterior femoral cutaneous nerve supplies fibers to the inferoposterior aspects of the vulva.

Clinical Correlations

An unusual but troublesome postoperative complication of gynecologic surgery is injury to the femoral nerve. During abdominal hysterectomy the femoral nerve may be compromised by pressure from the lateral blade of a self-retaining retractor in the area adjacent to where the femoral nerve penetrates the psoas muscle. During vaginal hysterectomy the femoral nerve may be injured from exaggerated hyperflexion of the legs in the lithotomy position, since hyperflexion produces stretching and compression of the femoral nerve as it courses under the inguinal ligament.

Because of the low density of nerve endings in the upper two thirds of the vagina, women are unable to determine the presence of a foreign body in this area. This explains how a "forgotten tampon" may remain unnoticed for several days in the upper part of the vagina until its presence results in a symptomatic discharge, abnormal bleeding, or odor. Infrequent but serious complications of pudendal nerve block are hematomas from trauma to the pudendal vessels and intravascular injection of anesthetic agents. The vessels and nerves are in close anatomic proximity to the ischial spine.

The fallopian tube is one of the most sensitive of the pelvic organs when crushed, cut, or distended, a fact that is appreciated in performing tubal ligations with the patient under local anesthesia. Damage to the obturator nerve during radical pelvic operations does not affect the pelvis directly. Although the nerve has an extensive pelvic course, its motor fibers supply the adductors of the thigh and its sensory fibers innervate skin over the medial aspects of the thigh.

DIAPHRAGMS AND LIGAMENTS

Pelvic Diaphragm

The pelvic diaphragm is a wide but thin muscular layer of tissue that forms the inferior border of the abdominopelvic cavity. Composed of a broad, funnel-shaped sling of fascia and muscle, it extends from the symphysis pu-

bis to the coccyx and from one lateral sidewall to the other. The primary muscles of the pelvic diaphragm are the levator ani and the coccygeus (Figure 3-19). This structure is the evolutionary remnant of the tail-wagging muscles in lower animals.

The muscles of the pelvic diaphragm are interwoven for strength, and a continuous muscle layer encircles the terminal portions of the urethra, vagina, and rectum. The levator ani muscles constitute the greatest bulk of the pelvic diaphragm and are divided into three components, which are named after their origin and insertion: pubococcygeus, puborectalis, and iliococcygeus. The coccygeus is a triangular muscle that occupies the area between the ischial spine and the coccyx. The fascia of the pelvic diaphragm divides the extraperitoneal space around the rectum from the lower ischiorectal spine.

The paired levator ani muscles act as a single muscle and functionally are important in the control of urination, in parturition, and in maintaining fecal continence. The pelvic diaphragm is important in supporting both abdominal and pelvic viscera and facilitates equal distribution of intraabdominal pressure during activities such as coughing.

Urogenital Diaphragm

The urogenital diaphragm, also called the *triangular ligament,* is a strong, muscular membrane that occupies the area between the symphysis pubis and ischial tuberosities (Figure 3-20) and stretches across the triangular anterior portion of the pelvic outlet. The urogenital diaphragm is external and inferior to the pelvic diaphragm. Anteriorly, the urethra is suspended from the pubic bone by continuations of the fascial layers of the urogenital diaphragm. The free edge of the diaphragm is strengthened by the superficial transverse perineal muscle. Posteriorly, the urogenital diaphragm inserts into the central point of the perineum. Situated farther posteriorly is the ischiorectal fossa. Located more superficially are the bulbocavernosus and ischiocavernosus muscles.

The urogenital diaphragm has two layers that enfold and cover the striated, deep transverse perineal muscle. The latter muscle surrounds both the vagina and the urethra, which pierce the diaphragm. The pudendal vessels and nerves, the external sphincter of the membra-

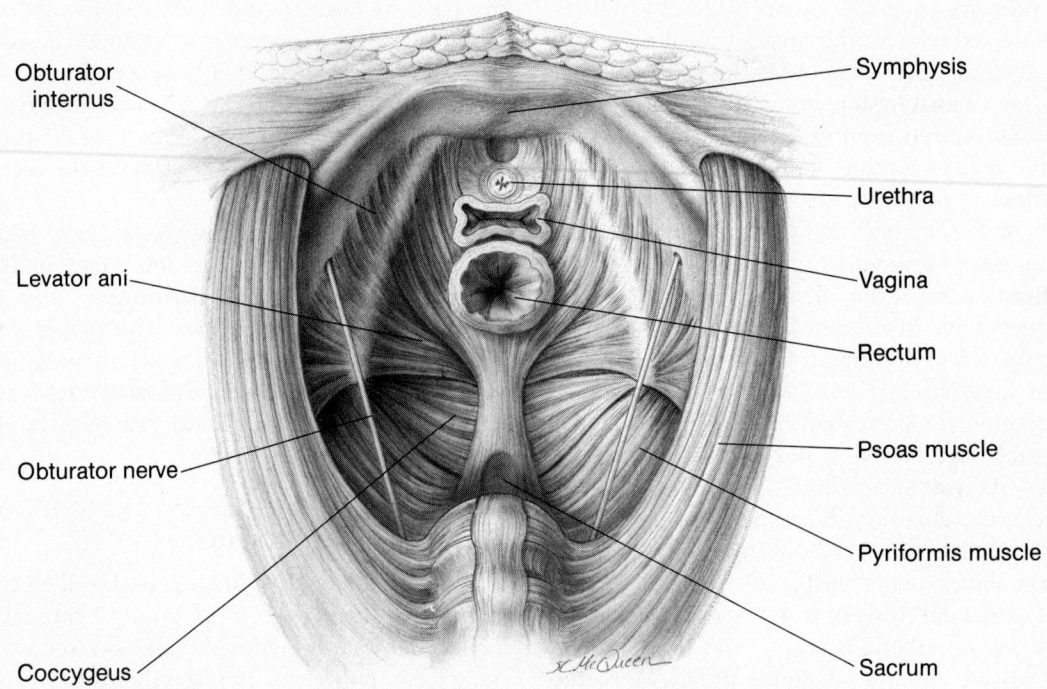

Obturator internus

Symphysis

Urethra

Levator ani

Vagina

Rectum

Obturator nerve

Psoas muscle

Pyriformis muscle

Coccygeus

Sacrum

FIGURE 3-19
A superior view of the pelvic diaphragm of the pelvic floor. The primary muscles that compose this funnel-shaped sling are the coccygeus and the levator ani. (Redrawn from Mattingly RF and Thompson JD: Te Linde's operative gynecology, ed 6, Philadelphia, 1985, JB Lippincott Co, p 41.)

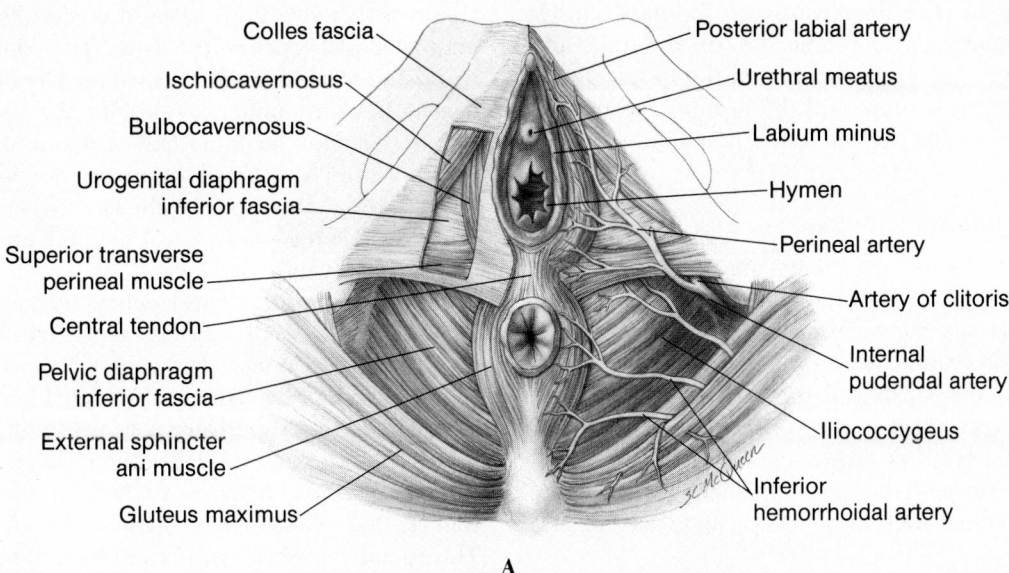

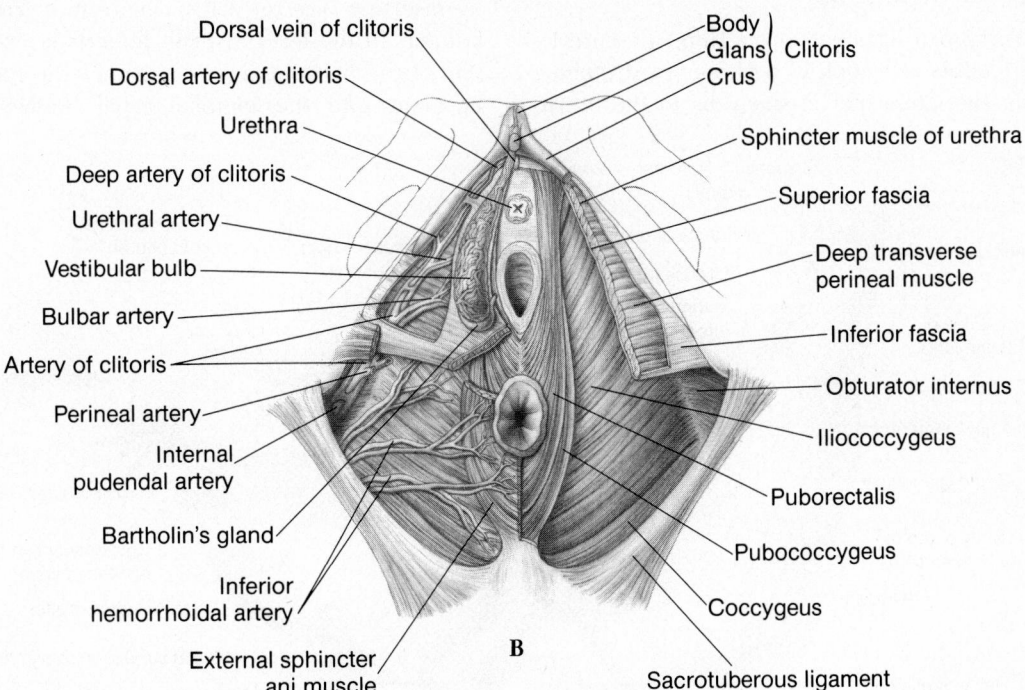

FIGURE 3-20

A, Schematic views of the perineum demonstrating superficial structures. Note the two layers of the urogenital diaphragm enfolding the deep transverse perineal muscle. **B,** Schematic views of the perineum demonstrating superficial structures and deeper structures. Note the pelvic diaphragm deep to the perineum, composed primarily of the levator ani and the coccygeus muscles. (Redrawn from Pritchard JA, MacDonald PC, and Gant NF: Williams' obstetrics, ed 17, New York, 1985, Appleton-Century-Crofts, p 14.)

nous urethra, and the dorsal nerve to the clitoris are also found within the urogenital diaphragm. The deep transverse perineal muscle is innervated by branches of the pudendal nerve. The major function of the urogenital diaphragm is support of the urethra and maintenance of the urethrovesical junction.

Ligaments

The pelvic ligaments are not classic ligaments but are thickenings of retroperitoneal fascia and consist primarily of blood and lymphatic vessels, nerves, and fatty connective tissue. Anatomists call the retroperitoneal fascia *subserous fascia,* whereas surgeons refer to this fascial layer as *endopelvic fascia.* The connective tissue is denser immediately adjacent to the lateral walls of the cervix and the vagina.

Broad Ligaments

The broad ligaments are a thin, mesenteric-like double reflection of peritoneum stretching from the lateral pelvic sidewalls to the uterus (Figure 3-21). They become contiguous with the uterine serosa, and thus the uterus is contained within two folds of peritoneum. These peritoneal folds enclose the loose, fatty connective tissue termed the *parametrium.* The broad ligaments afford minor support to the uterus but are conduits for important anatomic structures. Within the broad ligaments are found the following structures: oviducts; ovarian and round ligaments; ureters; ovarian and uterine arteries and veins; parametrial tissue; embryonic remnants of the mesonephric duct, wolffian body, and secondary ligaments; mesovarium; and mesosalpinx. The round ligament is composed of fibrous tissue and muscle fibers. It attaches to the superoanterior aspect of the uterus, anterior and caudal to the oviduct, and runs via the broad ligament to the lateral pelvic wall. It, too, offers little support to the uterus. The round ligament crosses the external iliac vessels and enters the inguinal canal, ending by inserting into the labia majora in a fanlike fashion. In the fetus a small, fingerlike projection of the peritoneum accompanies the round ligament into the inguinal canal, known as

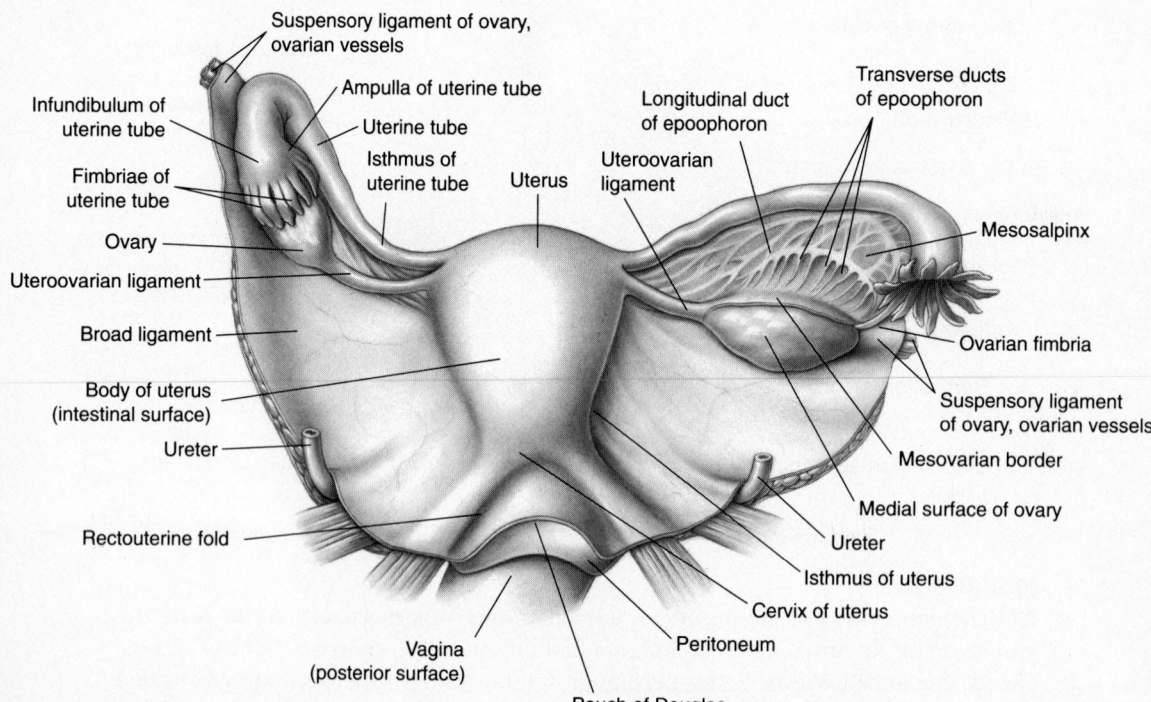

FIGURE 3-21

A schematic drawing of the broad ligament, posterior view. Note the many structures contained within the broad ligament. Note the posterior aspect of the rectouterine fold, called the cul-de-sac, or pouch, of Douglas. (Redrawn from Clemente CD: Anatomy: a regional atlas of the human body, Baltimore-Munich, 1987, Urban & Schwarzenberg.)

Nuck's canal. Generally it is obliterated in the adult woman.

Cardinal Ligaments

The cardinal, or Mackenrodt's, ligaments extend from the lateral aspects of the upper part of the cervix and the vagina to the pelvic wall. They are a thickened condensation of the subserosal fascia and parametria between the interior portion of the two folds of peritoneum. The cardinal ligaments form the base of the broad ligaments, laterally being attached to the fascia over the pelvic diaphragm and medially merging with fibers of the endopelvic fascia. Within these ligaments are found blood vessels and smooth muscle. The cardinal ligaments help to maintain the anatomic position of the cervix and the upper part of the vagina and provide the major support of the uterus and cervix.

Uterosacral Ligaments

The uterosacral ligaments extend from the upper portion of the cervix posteriorly to the third sacral vertebra. They are thickened near the cervix and then run a curved course around each side of the rectum and subsequently thin out posteriorly. The external surface of the uterosacral ligaments is formed by an inferoposterior fold of peritoneum at the base of the broad ligaments. The middle of the uterosacral ligaments is composed primarily of nerve bundles. The uterosacral ligaments serve a minor role in the anatomic support of the cervix.

Clinical Correlations

The posterior fibers of the levator ani muscles encircle the rectum at its junction with the anal canal, thereby producing an abrupt angle that reinforces fecal continence. Surgical repair of a displacement or tear of the levator ani muscles resulting from childbirth is important during posterior colporrhaphy. Coccygodynia, a form of chronic low back pain, may be related to tearing of muscle fibers during childbirth.

An apron of omentum has been used to create a replacement for portions of the pelvic diaphragm removed during radical pelvic surgery.

The round ligament is an important surgical landmark in making the initial incision into the parietal peritoneum to gain access to the retroperitoneal space. Direct visualization of the retroperitoneal course of the ureter is an important step in many pelvic operations, including dissections in women with endometriosis, pelvic inflammatory disease, large adnexal masses, broad ligament masses, and pelvic malignancies. A cyst of Nuck's canal may be confused with an indirect inguinal hernia. When a large amount of fluid is placed in the abdominal cavity, postoperative bilateral labial edema develops in 10% to 20% of women because of patency of the canal of Nuck.

During pelvic surgery, traction on the uterus makes the uterosacral and cardinal ligaments more prominent. There is a free space approximately 2 to 4 cm below the anterior edge of the broad ligament. In this free space there are no blood vessels, and the two sides of the broad ligament are in close proximity. Gynecologic surgeons utilize blunt dissection of this area to facilitate clamping of the anastomosis between the uterine and ovarian arteries.

NONGENITAL PELVIC ORGANS

Ureters

The ureters are whitish, muscular tubes, 28 to 34 cm in length, extending from the renal pelves to the urinary bladder. The ureter is divided into abdominal and pelvic segments. The diameters vary. The abdominal segment is approximately 8 to 10 mm in diameter. The pelvic segment is approximately 4 to 6 mm. A congenital anomaly of a double, or bifid, ureter occurs in 1% to 4% of the population. Ectopic ureteral orifices may occur in either the urethra or the vagina.

The abdominal portion of the right ureter is lateral to the inferior vena cava. Four arteries and accompanying veins cross anterior to the right ureter: the right colic artery, the ovarian vessels, the ileocolic artery, and the superior mesenteric artery. The course of the left ureter is similar to its counterpart on the right side in that it runs downward and medially along the anterior surface of the psoas major muscle.

The iliopectineal line serves as the marker for the pelvic portion of the ureter. The ureters run along the common iliac artery and then cross over the iliac vessels as they enter the pelvis. There is a slight variation between the two sides of the female pelvis. The right ureter tends to cross at the bifurcation of the common

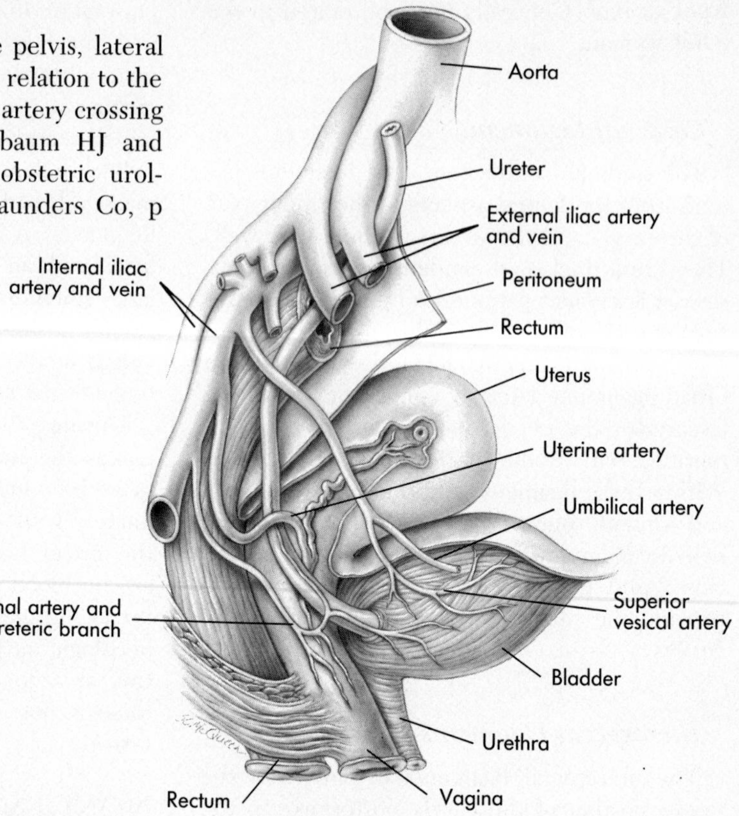

FIGURE 3-22
A schematic drawing the female pelvis, lateral view, demonstrating the ureter's relation to the major arteries. Note the uterine artery crossing over the ureter. (From Buchsbaum HJ and Schmidt JD: Gynecologic and obstetric urology, Philadelphia, 1978, WB Saunders Co, p 24.)

iliac artery, whereas usually the left ureter crosses 1 to 2 cm above the bifurcation.

The ureters then follow the descending, convex curvature of the posterolateral pelvic wall toward the perineum. Throughout its course the ureter is retroperitoneal in location. The ureter can be found on the medial leaf of the parietal peritoneum and in close proximity to the ovarian, uterine, obturator, and superior vesical arteries (Figure 3-22). The uterine artery lies on the anterolateral surface of the ureter for 2.5 to 3 cm. At approximately the level of the ischial spine, the ureter changes its course and runs forward and medially from the uterosacral ligaments to the base of the broad ligament. There the ureter enters into the cardinal ligaments. In this location the ureter is approximately 1 to 2 cm lateral to the uterine cervix and is surrounded by a plexus of veins. The ureter then runs upward and medially in the vesical uterine ligaments to obliquely pierce the bladder wall. Just before entering the base of the bladder, the ureter is in close contact with the anterior vaginal wall.

The ureter has a rich arterial supply with numerous anastomoses from many small vessels that form a longitudinal plexus in the adventitia of the ureter. Parent vessels that send branches to this arterial plexus surrounding the ureter include the renal, ovarian, common iliac, hypogastric, uterine, vaginal, vesical, middle hemorrhoidal, and superior gluteal arteries. The ureter is resistant to injury resulting from devascularization unless the surgeon strips the adventitia from the muscular conduit.

Urinary Bladder

The urinary bladder is a hollow muscular organ that lies between the symphysis pubis and the uterus. The size and shape of the bladder vary with the volume of urine it contains. Similarly, the anatomic proximity to other pelvic organs depends on whether the bladder is full or empty. The superior surface of the bladder is the only surface covered by peritoneum. The inferior portion is immediately adjacent to the uterus. The urachus is a fibrous cord extending from the apex of the bladder to the umbilicus. The urachus, which is the adult remnant of the embryonic allantois, is occasionally patent for part of its length. The base of the bladder lies directly adjacent to the endopelvic fascia over the anterior vaginal wall. The bladder neck and connecting urethra are attached to the symphysis pubis by fibrous ligaments. The prevesical or retropubic space of Retzius is the area lying between the bladder and symphysis pubis and is bounded laterally by the obliterated hypogastric arteries. This space extends from the fascia covering the pelvic diaphragm to the umbilicus between the peritoneum and transversalis fascia.

The mucosa of the anterior surface of the bladder is light red and has numerous folds. The inferoposterior surface delineated by the two ureteral orifices and the urethral orifice is the trigone. The trigone is a darker red than the rest of the bladder mucosa and is free of folds. When the bladder is empty, the ureteral orifices are approximately 2.5 cm apart. This distance increases to 5 cm when the bladder is distended. The muscular wall of the bladder, the detrusor muscles, is arranged in three layers. The arterial supply of the bladder originates from branches of the hypogastric artery: the superior vesical, inferior vesical, and middle hemorrhoidal arteries. The nerve supply to the bladder includes sympathetic and parasympathetic fibers, with the external sphincter supplied by the pudendal nerve.

Rectum

The rectum is the terminal 12 to 14 cm of the large intestine. The rectum begins over the second or third sacral vertebra , where the sigmoid colon no longer has a mesentery. After the large intestine loses its mesentery, its anatomic posterior wall is in close proximity to the curvature of the sacrum. Anteriorly, peritoneum covers the upper and middle thirds of the rectum. The lowest one third is below the peritoneal reflection and is in close proximity to the posterior wall of the vagina.

The rectum empties into the anal canal, which is 2 to 4 cm in length. The anal canal is fixed by the surrounding levator ani musculature of the pelvic diaphragm (Figure 3-4). The external sphincter of the anal canal is a circular band of striated muscle. The rectum, unlike other areas of the large intestine, does not have teniae coli or appendices epiploicae. The arterial supply of the rectum is rich, originating from five arteries: the superior hemorrhoidal artery, which is a continuation of the inferior mesenteric; the two middle hemorrhoidal arteries; and the two inferior hemorrhoidal arteries. At least 10% of carcinomas of the large bowel occur within the rectum. Therefore an annual rectal examination with special emphasis to palpate the entire circumference of the rectum, not just the area of the rectovaginal septum, is an important part of screening for colon cancer.

Clinical Correlations

The anatomic proximity of the ureters, urinary bladder, and rectum to the female reproductive organs is a major consideration in most gynecologic operations. Surgical compromise of the ureter may occur during clamping or ligating of the infundibulopelvic vessels, clamping or ligating of the cardinal ligaments, reperitonealization of the lateral wall after hysterectomy, or wide suturing in the endopelvic fascia during an anterior repair. Two of the classical ways to differentiate a ureter from a pelvic vessel are (1) visualization of peristalsis after stimulation by a surgical instrument and (2) visualization of Auerbach's plexuses, which are numerous, wavy, small vessels that, anastomose over the surface of the ureter.

For years teachers have referred to the area in the base of the broad ligament near the cervix where the uterine artery crosses the ureter as the area where "water flows under the bridge." A ureter may be differentiated from a large vessel in the retroperitoneal space by touching the wall of the ureter with a surgical instrument and observing for characteristic peristalsis.

The urinary bladder, if properly drained, will heal rapidly after a surgical insult if the blood supply to the bladder wall is not compromised. This capacity allows the gynecologist to insert a suprapubic cystostomy tube blindly without fear of fistula formation.

One of the surgical approaches for urinary stress incontinence is to suspend the periurethral tissue to either the symphysis pubis or Cooper's ligaments. Occasionally, this surgical approach is complicated by a significant amount of postoperative venous bleeding. If the space of Retzius is not properly drained, a subfascial hematoma may extend as high as the umbilicus.

Rectal injury occurs most frequently during vaginal hysterectomy with associated posterior colporrhaphy. In the middle third of the vagina the distance between vaginal and rectal mucosa is only a few millimeters, and the connective tissue is densely adherent and must be separated by sharp dissection.

CUL-DE-SAC OF DOUGLAS

The cul-de-sac of Douglas is a deep pouch formed by the most caudal extent of the parietal peritoneum. The cul-de-sac is a potential space and is also called the *rectouterine pouch* or *fold* (see Figure 3-21). It is anterior to the rectum, separating the uterus from the large intestine. The parietal peritoneum of the cul-de-sac covers the cervix and upper part of the posterior vaginal wall, then reflects to cover the anterior wall of the rectum. The pouch is bounded on the lateral sides by the peritoneal folds covering the uterosacral ligaments.

Parametria

The parametria are the extraperitoneal fatty and fibrous connective tissues adjacent to the uterus. The parametria lie between the leaves of the broad ligament and in the contiguous area anteriorly between the cervix and bladder. This connective tissue is thicker and denser adjacent to the cervix and vagina, where it becomes part of the connective tissue of the pelvic floor. The parametria may also thicken in response to radiation, pelvic cancer, infection, or endometriosis.

Clinical Correlations

The parametria and cul-de-sac of Douglas are important anatomic landmarks in advanced pelvic infection and neoplasia. Intrauterine infec-

tion, cervical carcinoma, and endometrial carcinoma may penetrate the endocervical stroma or the myometrium and secondarily may invade the loose connective tissue of the parametria. Bleeding resulting from an anterior perforation of the lower uterine segment during dilation and curettage may produce a pelvic hematoma involving both broad ligaments because of the anatomic continuity of the two areas.

The pouch of Douglas is easily accessible in performing transvaginal surgical procedures. Vaginal tubal ligation may be the procedure of choice in massively obese women. The most common diagnostic procedure involving this space for the purpose of aspirating peritoneal fluid is culdocentesis. Identification of peritoneal fluid helps determine the presence or absence of a tubal pregnancy or ruptured tubalovarian abscess. Posterior colpotomy is frequently chosen for drainage of a pelvic abscess occurring in the posterior cul-de-sac.

Many women with uterine prolapse have an associated enterocele, which is a hernial sac of parietal peritoneum that protrudes between the uterosacral ligaments. Surgical repair of an enterocele includes removal of the sac of peritoneum and plication of the uterosacral ligaments. Occasionally the cul-de-sac of Douglas is obliterated by the inflammatory process associated with either endometriosis or advanced malignancy.

KEY POINTS

- The labia majora are homologous to the scrotum in the male. Skene's glands are homologous to the prostate gland in the male.

- The vulvar skin of a postmenopausal woman is sensitive to topical testosterone and cortisone but is insensitive to topical estrogens.

- The average length of the clitoris is 1.5 to 2 cm. Clinically, width is more important and should be less than 1 cm, for it is difficult to actually measure the length of the clitoris.

- The female urethra measures 3.5 to 5 cm in length. The mucosa of the proximal two thirds of the urethra is composed of stratified transitional epithelium, and the distal one third is stratified squamous epithelium.

- The middle third of the vagina is supported by the levator ani muscles and the lower portion of the cardinal ligaments.

- The primary lymphatic drainage of the upper third of the vagina is to the external iliac nodes, the middle third of the vagina drains to the common and internal iliac nodes, and the lower third has a wide lymphatic distribution, including the common iliac, superficial inguinal, and perirectal nodes.

- In a description of the clinical practice of gynecology, descriptive terms for pelvic organs are derived from the Latin root, whereas terms relating to surgical procedures are derived from the Greek root.

- The transformation zone of the cervix, encompassing the border of the squamous epithelium and columnar epithelium, changes position on the cervix depending on a woman's hormonal status.

- The fibromuscular cervical stroma is composed primarily of collagenous connective tissue and ground substance. The connective tissue contains approximately 15% smooth muscle cells and a small amount of elastic tissue.

- The major arterial supply to the cervix is located on the lateral cervical walls at the 3 and 9 o'clock positions.

- The pain fibers from the cervix accompany the parasympathetic fibers to S2, S3, and S4.

- The uterus of a nulliparous woman is approximately 8 cm long, 5 cm wide, and 2.5 cm thick and weighs 40 to 50 g. In contrast, in a multiparous woman each measurement is approximately 1.2 cm larger and normal uterine weight is 20 to 30 g heavier. The maximal weight of a normal uterus is 110 g.

- In the majority of women, the long axis of the uterus is both anteverted in respect to the long axis of the vagina and anteflexed in relation to the long axis of the cervix. However, a retroflexed uterus is a normal variant found in approximately 25% of women.

- The cardinal ligaments provide the major support to the uterus.

- Afferent nerve fibers from the uterus enter the spinal cord at the eleventh and twelfth thoracic segments.

- The femoral nerve may be compromised by pressure on the psoas muscle during abdominal surgery and by hyperflexion of the leg during vaginal surgery.

- The oviducts are 10 to 14 cm in length and are composed of four anatomic sections. Closest to the uterine cavity is the interstitial segment, followed by the narrow isthmic segment, then the wider ampullary segment, and distally the trumpet-shaped infundibular segment.

- During the reproductive years the ovaries measure approximately 1.5 cm × 2.5 cm × 4 cm.

- The ovary in nulliparous women rests in a depression of peritoneum named the *fossa ovarica*. Immediately adjacent to the ovarian fossa are the external iliac vessels, the ureter, and the obturator vessels and nerves.

- The arterial supply of the pelvis is paired, bilateral, and has multiple collaterals and numerous anastomoses.

- The pudendal nerve and its branches supply the majority of both motor and sensory fibers to the muscles and skin of the vulvar region.

- The pelvic diaphragm is important in supporting both abdominal and pelvic viscera and facilitates equal distribution of intraabdominal pressure during activities such as coughing.

- The major function of the urogenital diaphragm is support of the urethra and maintenance of the urethrovesical junction.

- A congenital anomaly of a double, or bifid, ureter occurs in 1% to 4% of the population.

- Two ways of distinguishing the ureter from pelvic vessels are (1) identification of peristalsis after stimulation with a surgical instrument and (2) identification of Auerbach's plexuses.

- The distal ureter enters into the cardinal ligament. In this location the ureter is approximately 1 to 2 cm lateral to the uterine cervix and is surrounded by a plexus of veins.

- Surgical compromise of the ureters may occur during clamping or ligating of the infundibulopelvic vessels, clamping or ligating of the cardinal ligaments, reperitonealization of the lateral wall after hysterectomy, or wide suturing in the endopelvic fascia during an anterior repair.

BIBLIOGRAPHY

Aspden RM: The importance of a slit-like lumen cross-section for the mechanical function of the cervix, Br J Obstet Gynaecol 94:915, 1987.

Boss JH, Scully RE, Wegner JH, et al: Structural variations in the adult ovary: clinical significance, Obstet Gynecol 25:747, 1965.

Burchell RC: Physiology of internal iliac artery ligation, J Obstet Gynaecol Br Commnw 75:642, 1968.

Carpenter MB and Sutin J: Human neuroanatomy, ed 8, Baltimore, 1983, Williams & Wilkins.

Clemente CD: Gray's anatomy, ed 30, Philadelphia, 1985, Lea & Febiger.

Cruikshank SH: Retroperitoneal dissection in gynecologic surgery for benign disease, South Med J 80:296, 1987.

Cruikshank SH and Stoelk EM: Surgical control of pelvic hemorrhage: method of bilateral ovarian artery ligation, Am J Obstet Gynecol 147:724, 1983.

Demopoulous RI: Normal endometrium. In Blaustein A, ed: Pathology of the female genital tract, ed 2, New York, 1982, Springer-Verlag.

Farrer-Brown G, Beilby JOW, and Tarbit MH: The blood supply of the uterus, J Obstet Gynaecol Br Commnw 77:673, 1970.

Ferenczy A and Richart RM: Female reproductive system: dynamics of scan and transmission microscopy, New York, 1974, John Wiley & Sons.

Finn CA and Porter DG: The uterus, Acton, Mass, 1975, Publishing Sciences Group.

Gosling JA: The structure of the female lower urinary tract and pelvic floor, Urol Clin North Am 12:207, 1985.

Grant JCB: An atlas of anatomy, ed 8, Baltimore, 1983, Williams & Wilkins.

Hahn L: Clinical findings and results of operative treatment in ilioinguinal nerve entrapment syndrome, Br J Obstet Gynaecol 96:1080, 1989.

Jordan JA and Singer A: The cervix, Philadelphia, 1976, WB Saunders Co.

Koelbl H, Strassegger H, Riss PA, and Gruber H: Morphologic and functional aspects of pelvic floor muscles in patients with pelvic relaxation and genuine stress incontinence, Obstet Gynecol 74:789, 1989.

Krantz KE: The anatomy of the urethra and anterior vaginal wall, Am J Obstet Gynecol 62:374, 1951.

Krantz KE: Innervation of the human vulva and vagina, Obstet Gynecol 12:382, 1958.

Kuhn RJP and Hollyock VE: Observations on the anatomy of the rectovaginal pouch and septum, Obstet Gynecol 59:445, 1982.

Mahran M: The microscopic anatomy of the round ligament, J Obstet Gynaecol Br Commnw 72:614, 1965.

Milley PS and Nichols DH: The relationship between the pubo-urethral ligaments and the urogenital diaphragm in the human female, Anat Rec 170:281, 1971.

Neilson D, Jones GS, Woodruff JD, et al: The innervation of the ovary, Obstet Gynecol Surv 25:889, 1970.

Netter FH: Reproductive system, vol 2, The CIBA collection of medical illustrations, Summit, NJ, 1983, CIBA Pharmaceutical Products.

Nichols DH and Milley PS: Surgical significance of the rectovaginal septum, Am J Obstet Gynecol 108:215, 1970.

Nichols DH and Randall CL: Vaginal surgery, ed 3, Baltimore, 1989, Williams & Wilkins.

Novak ER and Woodruff JD: Gynecologic and obstetric pathology, ed 8, Philadelphia, 1979, WB Saunders Co.

Pauerstein CJ: The fallopian tube: a reappraisal, Philadelphia, 1974, Lea & Febiger.

Plentl AA and Friedman EA: Lymphatic system of the female genitalia: the morphologic basis of oncologic diagnosis and therapy. Philadelphia, 1971, WB Saunders Co.

Roberts WH, Habenicht J, and Krishinger G: The pelvic and perineal fasciae and their neural and vascular relationships, Anat Rec 149:707, 1964.

Stulz P and Phfeiffer KM: Peripheral nerve injuries resulting from common surgical procedures in the lower portion of the abdomen, Arch Surg 117:324, 1982.

Tanagho EA: Anatomy of the lower urinary tract. In Walsh PC, Gittes RF, Perlmutter AD, and Stamey TA, eds: Campbell's urology, ed 5, Philadelphia, 1986, WB Saunders Co.

Wynn RM and Jollie WP: Biology of the uterus, ed 2, New York, 1989, Plenum Publishing Co.

Zacharin RF: The suspensory mechanism of the female urethra, J Anat 97:423, 1963.

Zacharin RF: Abdominoperineal urethral suspension in the management of recurrent stress incontinence of urine—a 15-year experience, Obstet Gynecol 62:644, 1983.

CHAPTER

4

Reproductive Endocrinology

KEY TERMS AND DEFINITIONS

Activin. Peptide witha similar structure to inhibin but an opposite action. Activins stimulate pituitary follicle-stimulating hormone (FSH) release and ovarian estradiol production.

Affinity (K). Degree to which a hormone binds to its receptor. Affinity is determined by the degree to which the hormone structurally fits, or interlocks, with the receptor.

Arcuate Nucleus. A group of nerve cells lying in the medial portion of the hypothalamus just above the median eminence. Nerve cells in the arcuate nucleus are the major source of gonadotrophin-releasing hormone (GnRH) secretion.

Aromatization. Synthesis of a phenolic, or aromatic, benzene ring, as occurs during conversion of testosterone to estradiol.

Atresia. Process of regression of preantral follicles.

Autocrine. Producing hormonal effects by intracellular communication.

Bioassay. Measurement of the amount of hormone present in a substance by determining its effect on a target organ in an animal and comparing it with the effect produced by a known (standard) amount of hormone.

Catecholestrogens. Steroids that structurally resemble both estrogens and catecholamines and have only a weak estrogenic action.

Coefficient of Variation (CV). Mathematical technique to measure precision of assay after results of measurement of same substance are calculated several times in one assay (interassay CV) or in several assays (intraassay CV).

Cortical Granules. Particles in ooplasm that are released into the surface membrane after one sperm penetrates the ovum. They may act to block further sperm penetration.

Cross-reaction. Interference in immunoassay by a substance that is not being measured but reacts with the antibody to a lesser degree than the hormone being measured. It thus alters the results of the assay.

Desensitization (Down Regulation). The condition wherein a hormone is secreted or administered for a prolonged period and produces an inhibitory instead of a stimulatory response because of saturation of its receptor.

Dominant Follicle. Follicle that enlarges to about 2 cm in diameter and eventually ovulates.

Eicosanoids. Class of fatty acid derivatives containing prostaglandins, thromboxanes, and leukotrienes. Eicosanoids are derived from the unsaturated fatty acid form of eicosanoic acid and have a high degree of biologic activity. The most important precursor of the eicosanoids is arachidonic acid.

β-Endorphin. A potent opioid peptide—more potent than morphine—that is concentrated in the hypothalamus and pituitary. It inhibits luteinizing hormone (LH) secretion.

Extraglandular Conversion. Process whereby one steroid is converted to another steroid in tissue other than an endocrine organ.

Follicle-Stimulating Hormone (FSH). A glycoprotein with a molecular weight of 33,000 that is composed of a nonspecific α subunit and a specific β subunit. The primary action of FSH in the female is to stimulate granulosa cell synthesis.

Germinal Vesicle. Nuclear material that is surrounded by a membrane, visible histologically, and that is present in the primary oocyte.

Gonadotrophin-Releasing Hormone (GnRH). A decapeptide synthesized in and secreted by the hypothalamus at periodic intervals to stimulate gonadotrophin release from the pituitary gland.

Gonadotrophin-Releasing Hormone Analogue (GnRH Analogue). GnRH analogues are proteins composed of the 10 amino acids found in the parent molecule of GnRH, but with substitutions at amino acids 6 and 10 to increase potency and half-life.

Growth Factors. Growth-promoting polypeptide hormones secreted by gonadal cells. They are classified into groups (families) based on their protein sequence.

Hormone Receptors. Proteins on the cell membrane or within the cell of the target tissue that bind to a specific molecule of the hormone (ligand) for the purpose of eliciting a biologic response. Hormone receptors bind only with ligands of a specific hormone and thus are hormone specific.

Hypothalamus. Portion of the base of the brain that is located just below the optic chiasm and that has a major role in regulating the hormones involved in reproductive endocrinology.

Inhibin. A polypeptide dimer composed of an α and a β subunit joined by disulfide bonds. This hormone is produced by ovarian granulosa cells and inhibits FSH secretion.

Leukotrienes. Derivatives of unsaturated eicosanoic acid, particularly arachidonic acid, which do not have a closed ring structure but have a similar system of assignment of letters and numeric subscripts. Their biologic effects are not completely understood but appear to stimulate smooth muscle.

Luteinizing Hormone (LH). A glycoprotein with a molecular weight of 28,000 that is composed of a nonspecific α subunit and a specific β subunit. The primary action of LH in the female is to stimulate ovarian steroid synthesis.

Median Eminence (Infundibulum). The portion of the neurohypophysis lying in the midline at the base of the hypothalamus. It is connected to the infundibular stalk and the posterior (neural) lobe of the pituitary gland.

Metabolic Clearance Rate (MCR). Volume of plasma, serum, or blood that is cleared of the steroid per unit of time (liters per day).

Monoclonal Antibody. Single type of antibody produced by the spleen cell of a mouse that was injected with antigen. The spleen cell is subsequently fused with a myueloma cell to form a hybridoma cell in order to produce large quantities of the antibody.

Neurohypophysis. The portion of the hypothalamus consisting of the median eminence, infundibular stalk, and posterior lobe of the pituitary.

Neuromodulator. A substance that affects the action of a neurotransmitter.

Neurotransmitter. Biogenic amines secreted by a nerve cell that produce an action on another cell.

Nonradioactive immunoassays. Assays that do not use a radioactive marker but act by the same principle. These include the chemiluminescent immunoassay, fluoroimmunoassay, and enzyme immunoassay (which use excess antigen) and the enzyme-linked immunosorbent assay (ELISA), which uses excess antibody.

Oogonia. Primordial female germ cells with a full chromosomal complement that are present in the fetal ovary.

Paracrine. Producing hormonal effects by diffusion to contiguous cells.

Primary Follicle (Preantral Follicle). Immature oocyte covered by multiple layers of granulosa cells but without an antrum.

Primary Oocyte. Female germ cell in the diplotene stage of first meiotic division.

Primordial Follicle. Immature oocyte covered by a single layer of granulosa cells.

Production Rate. Amount of steroid that enters the circulation per unit of time (usually measured in milligrams or micrograms per day).

Prostaglandins. Prostanoids with a cyclopentane ring and two side chains. The different letters assigned to the various prostaglandins refer to different substitutions in the cyclopentane ring, and the numbers in the subscript of the letter indicate the number of double bonds in the side chain.

Prostanoids. Family of closely related lipids that include prostaglandins and thromboxanes. They have the basic structure of prostanoic acid, which consists of 20 carbon atoms arranged in a ring structure with two side chains.

Radioimmunoassay (RIA). Technique of measurement of hormone using a specific antibody raised against it and a radioactive-labeled hormone (antigen) in an antigen-antibody reaction.

Second Messenger. A substance, usually a cyclic nucleotide, that is activated when a protein hormone attaches to its receptor to induce changes within the cell.

Sex Hormone–Binding Globulin (SHBG). A serum globulin that has a high affinity for estrogens and androgens (also called testosterone-estrogen–binding globulin [TeBG]).

Standard Curve. Curved line that results from connecting the endpoints derived from assay of different amounts of known (standard) hormone plotted graphically against the amount of hormone present.

Stratum Basale. Thin, lowermost portion of endometrium that overlies muscularis and consists of primordial glands and densely cellular stroma.

Stratum Functionale. Thick, uppermost portion of endometrium that grows under the influence of estrogen. It is composed of a thin superficial stratum compactum and an underlying broader stratum spongiosum.

Thromboxanes. Prostanoids with an oxane ring instead of an cyclopentane ring. Letters and numeric subscripts are assigned similar to those used with prostaglandins.

Transcription. Generation of messenger RNA from a segment of DNA produced by the hormone-receptor complex in the nucleus.

Transformation. The change in receptor configuration produced by a steroid that allows the receptor-hormone complex to undergo translocation.

Zona Pellucida. Mucopolysaccharide coat surrounding oocyte that allows only sperm of the same species to penetrate the ovum.

The endocrinologic regulation of the reproductive system is extremely complex. Much information has been accumulated in the past two decades, and new information is constantly becoming available. Entire books have been written about each aspect of reproductive endocrinology. In this chapter, only the basic information required for an understanding of this complex process will be presented.

No single organ that secretes hormones involved in the reproductive process acts independently. Nevertheless, for ease of understanding, each organ and its principal hormones will be discussed as a unit. Information in this chapter will include the central nervous system control of gonadotrophin-releasing hormone (GnRH) secretion, GnRH action on gonadotrophin secretion, gonadotrophin effects on the ovary, and ovarian steroid effects on the uterus. The positive and negative feedback control of the various organs involved in human reproduction will be presented. The regulation of prolactin secretion is discussed in Chapter 37. Because of space limitations, even though the adrenal and thyroid hormones have a profound influence on the reproductive system, a discussion of adrenal and thyroid endocrinology will not be included in this text.

NEUROENDOCRINOLOGY OF GnRH SECRETION

The hypothalamic hormone that controls gonadotrophin release is GnRH. GnRH is a decapeptide whose structural formula was first determined by Schally et al. (Figure 4-1). The most biologically active amino acids in the GnRH molecule are pyroglutamic acid, hista-

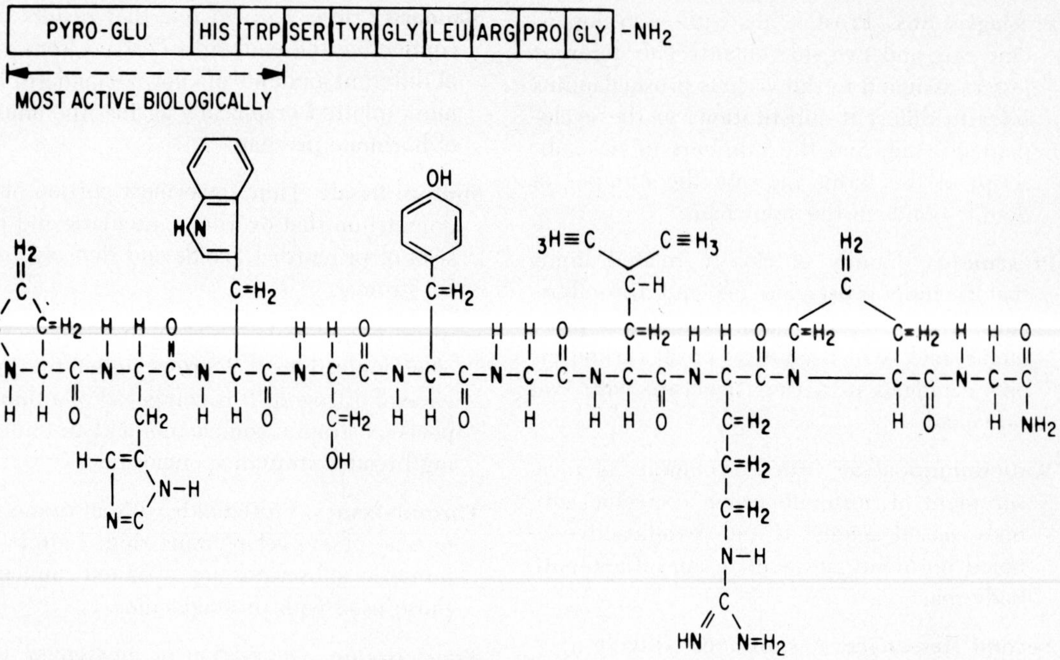

FIGURE 4-1

Amino acid sequence of gonadotrophin-releasing hormone (GnRH). (From Kletzky OA and Lobo RA: Reproductive neuroendocrinology. In Mishell DR Jr, Davajan V, and Lobo RA, editors: Infertility, contraception and reproductive endocrinology, ed 3, Cambridge, Mass, 1991, Blackwell Scientific Publications.)

dine, and tryptophan, as well as the amino terminal group.

The cell bodies of the hypothalamic neurons that produce GnRH are concentrated mainly in two areas: the anterior hypothalamus and the medial basal (tuberal) hypothalamus. In the latter area, the greatest number of GnRH-producing neurons are in the arcuate nucleus (Figure 4-2). From these areas, GnRH is transported along the axons of these neurons, which terminate in the median eminence around the capillaries of the primary portal plexus. The nerve cells that transport GnRH from the arcuate nucleus to the median eminence are called the tuberoinfundibular tract.

The median eminence, or infundibulum, together with the infundibular stalk and posterior (neural) lobe of the pituitary, make up the neurohypophysis. The three components of the neurohypophysis share a common capillary network and have a direct arterial blood supply from the hypophyseal arteries. The capillaries of the median eminence have a fenestrated epithelium similar to that of peripheral tissue, which allows passage of large molecules. These capillaries differ from those present in the brain, and thus the median eminence is outside the blood-brain barrier.

The nerve cell terminals of the tuberoinfundibular tract secrete GnRH directly into the portal circulation, which carries the hormone to the gonadotrophin-containing cells in the anterior lobe of the pituitary. The pars tuberalis of the anterior lobe of the pituitary (adenohypophysis) receives its vascular supply from pituitary portal vessels and is located adjacent to the base of the hypothalamus and the pituitary stalk (Figure 4-2). Unlike the neurohypophysis, the adenohypophysis has no direct arterial blood supply and receives all of its blood from the portal vessels. After leaving the pituitary gland, the circulation returns to the neurohypophyseal capillary plexus, allowing pituitary hormones to help regulate the secretion of GnRH from the median eminence.

In addition to this major route of GnRH transport, an alternative route may exist. Axons of the tuberoinfundibular tract may transport GnRH directly into the third ventricle. A specialized ependymal cell, the tanycyte, extends from the lumen of the third ventricle into the outermost zone of the median eminence (Fig-

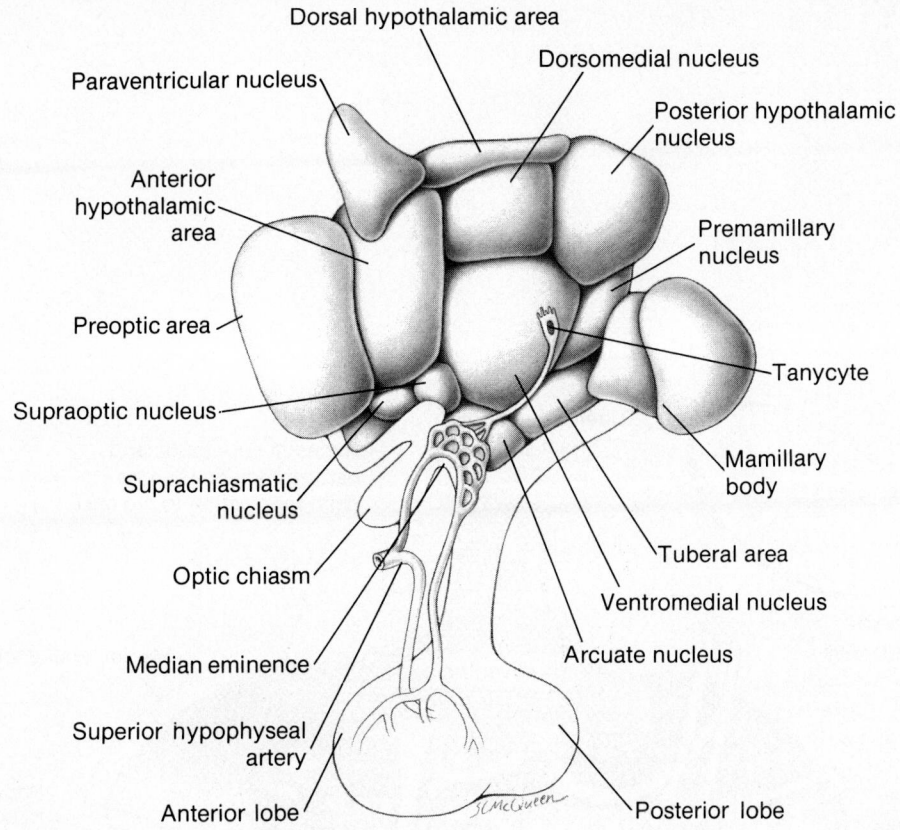

Dorsal hypothalamic area

Dorsomedial nucleus

Paraventricular nucleus

Posterior hypothalamic nucleus

Anterior hypothalamic area

Premamillary nucleus

Preoptic area

Tanycyte

Supraoptic nucleus

Mamillary body

Suprachiasmatic nucleus

Tuberal area

Optic chiasm

Ventromedial nucleus

Median eminence

Arcuate nucleus

Superior hypophyseal artery

Anterior lobe

Posterior lobe

FIGURE 4-2

Nuclear organization of hypothalamus, shown diagrammatically in sagittal plane as it would appear from third ventricle. Rostral area is to left and caudal to right. Pituitary gland is shown ventrally. *AL,* Anterior lobe; *MB,* mamillary body; *ME,* median eminence; *NL,* neural lobe; *OC,* optic chiasm. (Redrawn from Moore RY: Neuroendocrine mechanisms: cells and systems. In Yen SSC and Jaffe R, editors: Reproductive endocrinology: physiology, pathophysiology and clinical management, Philadelphia, 1986, WB Saunders Co.)

ure 4-3). Since, when GnRH is administered into the third ventricle, it is transported into the portal system, it has been postulated that transport occurs via the tanycytes and their microvilli. Thus GnRH can be released both in large amounts periodically via the tuberoinfundibular tract (cyclic release) and in a low-grade continuous transependymal manner (tonic release) via the tanycytes.

In humans, GnRH is secreted in a pulsatile manner. The amplitude and frequency of the pulse vary throughout the menstrual cycle, with the frequency being more rapid in the follicular phase, about one pulse per hour, and slower in the luteal phase, about one pulse in 2 to 3 hours.

Knobil et al. performed a series of elegant experiments using an oophorectomized mon-

key model in which endogenous GnRH secretion had been abolished by a lesion in the hypothalamus. These investigators showed that altering the interval of GnRH pulses interferes with gonadotrophin secretion. If exogenous GnRH pulses were administered every hour, a midcycle gonadotrophin surge occurred (Figure 4-4). However, when the pulse frequency was increased to five pulses per hour, gonadotrophin secretion was inhibited (Figure 4-5). Decreasing GnRH pulse frequency to once every 3 hours decreased the levels of luteinizing hormone (LH) and increased those of folliclestimulating hormone (FSH); in addition, no gonadotrophin surge occurred. Decreasing the amount of exogenous GnRH also inhibited gonadotrophin release.

Crowley et al. have demonstrated that some

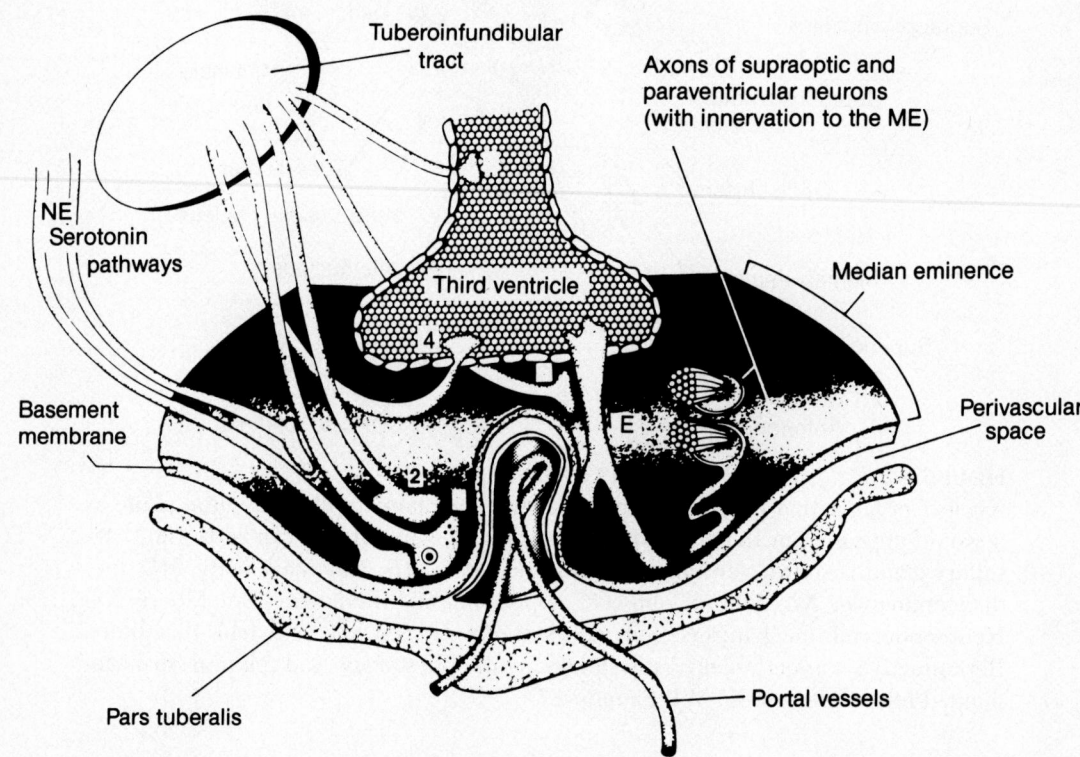

FIGURE 4-3

Schematic diagram showing tanycytes *(E)*, stretching between third ventricle and outer portion of median eminence. (From Reichlin S: Neural control of the pituitary gland: normal physiology and pathophysiologic implications. In Current concepts, Kalamazoo, Mich, 1978, Upjohn Publications.)

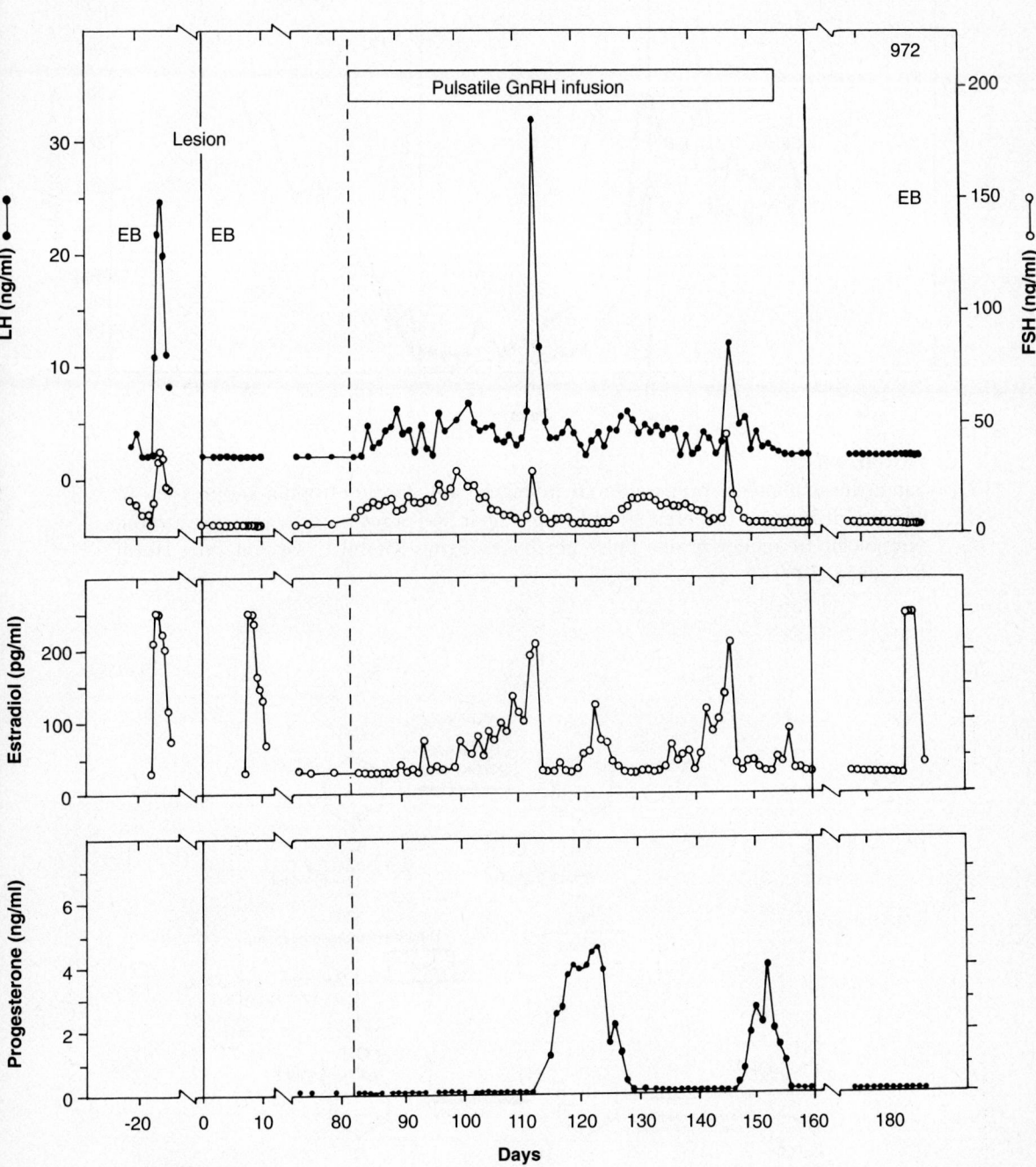

FIGURE 4-4

Induction of two ovulatory menstrual cycles by administration of pulsatile GnRH replacement (1 μg/min for 6 minutes, once every hour) in rhesus monkey with hypothalamic lesion that had abolished endogenous GnRH secretion. Estradiol benzoate *(EB)* elicited gonadotrophin response before placement of lesion but not afterward. (Redrawn from Knobil E, Plant TM, Wildt L, et al: Science 207:1371, 1980.)

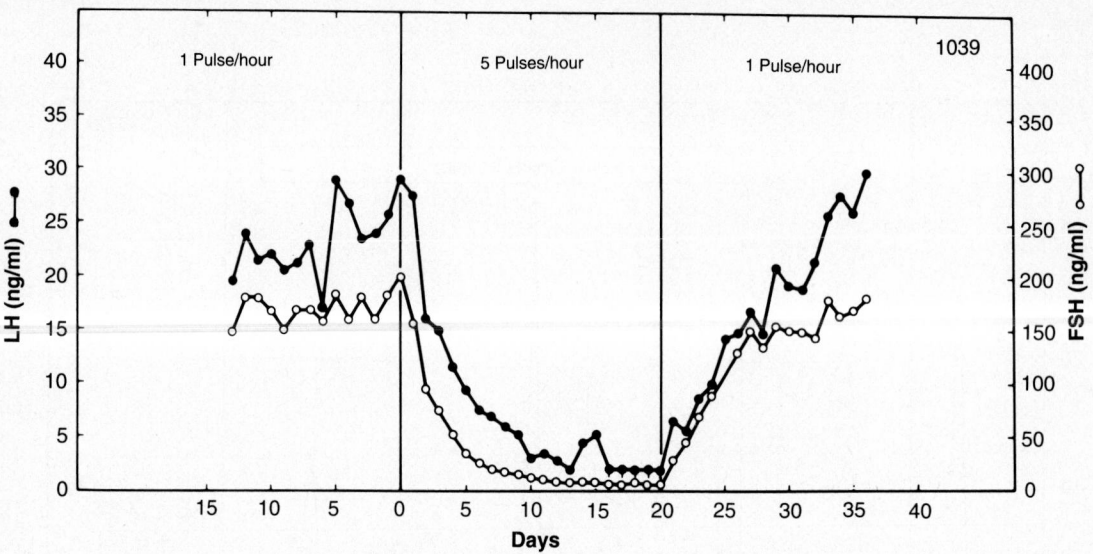

FIGURE 4-5

Same rhesus monkey preparation as in Figure 4-4. Gonadotrophin suppression in which GnRH pulse is increased to five per hour and is restored by returning to the physiologic frequency of one pulse per hour. (From Knobil E: Recent Prog Horm Res 36:53, 1980.)

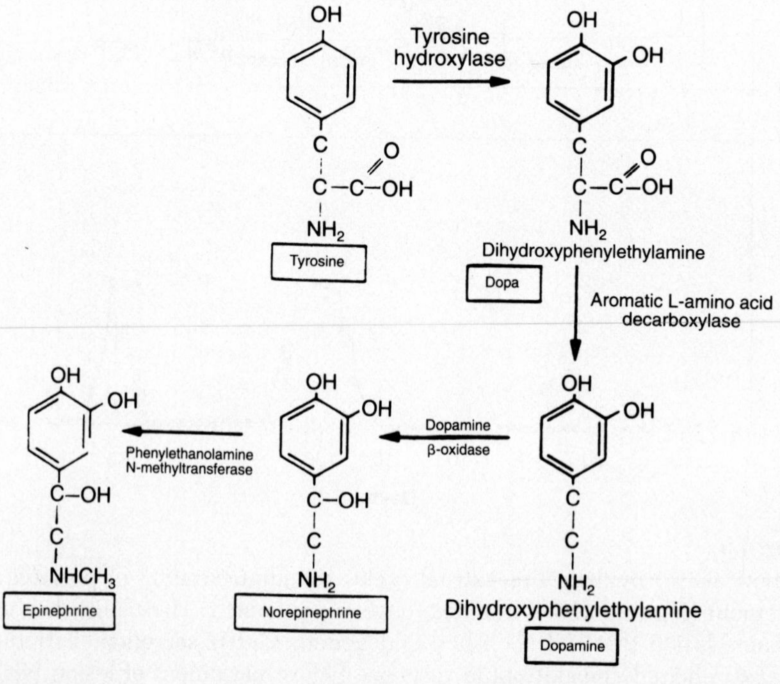

FIGURE 4-6

Metabolic pathways of dopamine, norepinephrine, and epinephrine synthesis. (From Kletzky OA and Lobo RA: Reproductive neuroendocrinology. In Mishell DR Jr, Davajan V, and Lobo RA, editors: Infertility, contraception and reproductive endocrinology, ed 3, Cambridge, Mass, 1991, Blackwell Scientific Publications.)

women with anovulation (hypothalamic amen-orrhea) and amenorrhea without a known cause have altered pulse frequency or amplitude of GnRH secretion or both. Thus the control of episodic GnRH secretion is extremely important for the maintenance of normal ovulatory cyclicity. The amplitude and frequency of GnRH secretion by the hypothalamus not only are regulated by the feedback of two ovarian steroids, estradiol and progesterone, but by gonadotrophins as well through the humoral input pathway. Amplitude and frequency also are modulated by several neurotransmitters and neuromodulators within the brain through a neural input pathway.

Neurotransmitters

The most important neurotransmitters involved in reproductive neuroendocrinology are two catecholamines, dopamine and norepinephrine, as well as an indolamine, serotonin. All three of these neurotransmitters are monoamines. Dopamine and norepinephrine are produced by conversion of tyrosine in the midbrain (Figure 4-6). The enzyme tyrosine hydroxylase converts tyrosine to dopa, which is then decarboxylated to dopamine. Pyridoxine is an important coenzyme in this process. Dopamine oxidase converts dopamine to norepinephrine. Norepinephrine is then converted to epinephrine by the addition of a methyl group by a methyl transferase enzyme.

Dopamine is a neurotransmitter itself, as well as the precursor of another neurotransmitter, norepinephrine. Dopamine, in addition to stimulating prolactin-inhibiting factor and thus decreasing prolactin release, acts in the median eminence and appears to inhibit the release of GnRH. Several studies have demonstrated that dopamine inhibits LH secretion in humans. The role of norepinephrine is less clear. It may stimulate the release of GnRH. Epinephrine has little effect on the hypothalamic release of reproductive hormones.

The precursor of serotonin is tryptophan, which is first converted to 5-hydroxytryptophan by the enzyme tryptophan-hydroxylase (Figure 4-7). This substance is then decarboxylated to form serotonin. The principal metabolite of serotonin is 5-hydroxyindoleacetic acid (5-HIAA), which can be measured in urine. Serotonin has not been shown to affect GnRH release, but it does stimulate the release of prolactin, proba-bly by stimulating the release of the hypothalamic prolactin-releasing factor.

Mechanism of Action and Pharmacologic Effects

The effects of neurotransmitters on the secretion of hypothalamic hormones probably are exerted by different mechanisms. One possible mechanism is through a direct cell-to-cell connection or a multisynaptic communication whereby the neurotransmitter is released by the terminal nerve and depolarizes the receptor site on a hypothalamic cell (Figure 4-8). Depolarization results in the release of a specific hormone from the hypothalamic cell.

These specific effects of neurotransmitters on hypothalamic cells can be altered by the systemic administration of certain drugs. For example, methyldopa and α-methyl-*p*-tyrosine can block dopamine and norepinephrine synthesis by inhibiting tyrosine hydoxylase. Reserpine and chlorpromazine interfere with norepinephrine, dopamine, and serotonin binding and storage. Finally, and clinically important, the frequently prescribed tricyclic antidepressants inhibit the reuptake of neurotransmitters, whereas other medications such as propranolol, phentolamine, haloperidol, and cyproheptadine act by blocking the receptors at the level of the hypothalamus.

As a consequence of receiving such medications, many patients develop such disorders as galactorrhea and oligoamenorrhea. These clinical entities are a result of either hyperprolactinemia or alterations in GnRH-gonadotrophin secretion.

Neuromodulators

Opioids

Receptors for the opioid peptides are present in the brain. There are three subgroups of opiates: enkephalins, endorphins (α, β, γ), and dynorphins. β-Endorphin (β-EP) contains 31 amino acids, is 5 to 10 times as potent as morphine, and is concentrated mainly in the arcuate nucleus and median eminence of the hypothalamus, as well as the pituitary gland. β-EP has also been localized in the placenta, pancreas, gastrointestinal (GI) tract, and in seminal fluid. The concentrations of endorphins are about 1000 times higher in the pituitary than in the hypothalamus. Infusion of β-EP results in

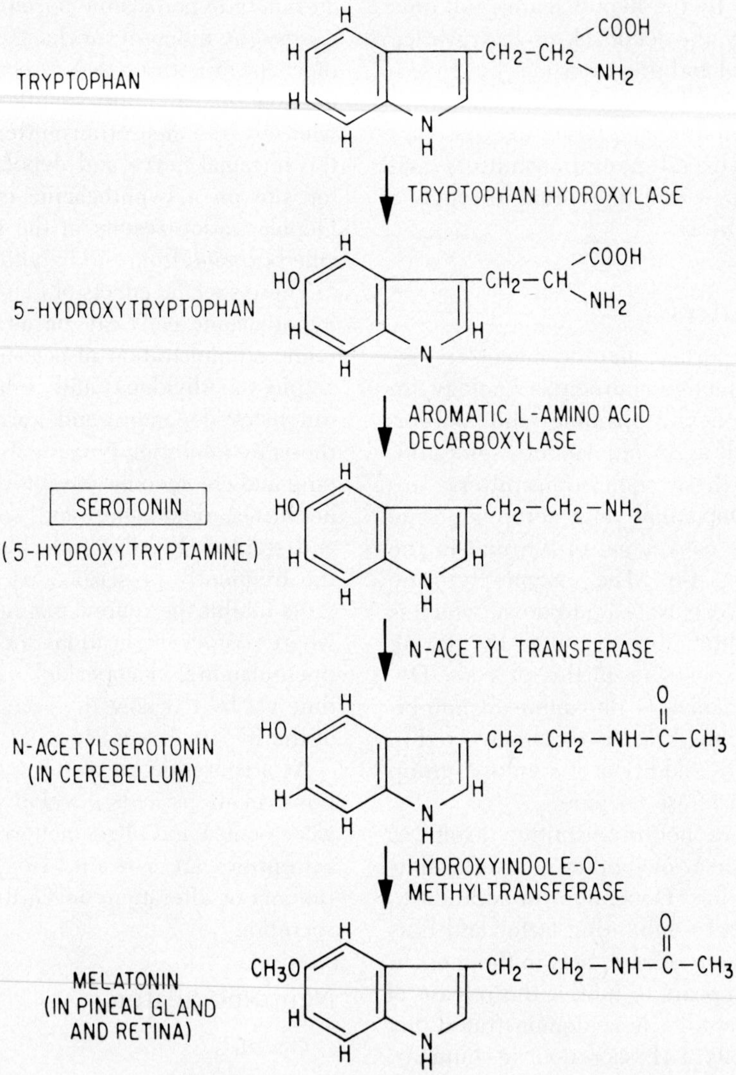

FIGURE 4-7

Metabolic pathway of serotonin synthesis. (From Kletzky OA and Lobo RA: Reproductive neuroendocrinology. In Mishell DR Jr, Davajan V, and Lobo RA, editors: Infertility, contraception and reproductive endocrinology, ed 3, Cambridge, Mass, 1991, Blackwell Scientific Publications.)

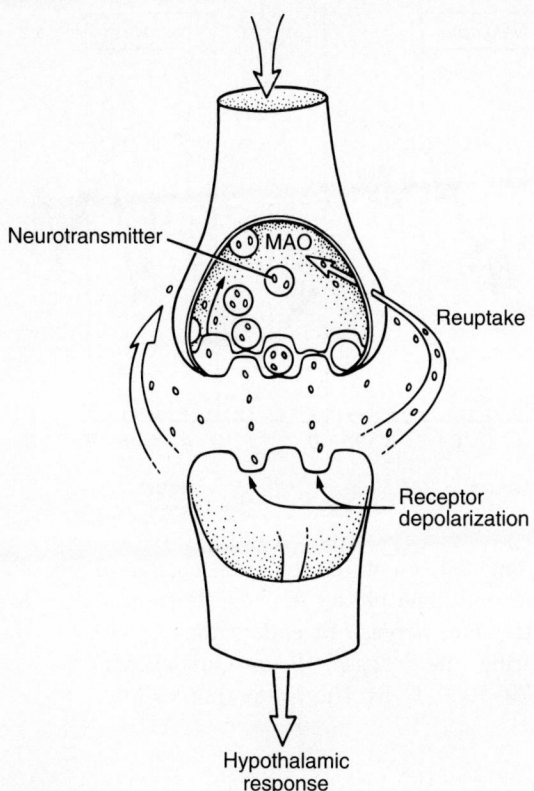

Neurotransmitter

MAO

Reuptake

Receptor
depolarization

Hypothalamic
response

FIGURE 4-8

A stimulus induces release of stored neurotransmitter by exocytosis. Most of it is taken up again; the rest binds to a specific receptor, resulting in hypothalamic response. *MAO*, Monoamine oxidase. (From Kletzky OA and Lobo RA: Reproductive endocrinology. In Mishell DR Jr, Davajan V, and Lobo RA, editors: Infertility, contraception and reproductive endocrinology, ed 3, Cambridge, Mass, 1991, Blackwell Scientific Publications.)

an increase in prolactin and a decrease in LH, the latter occurring by an inhibitory effect on GnRH neurons in the hypothalamus.

Peripheral measurement of plasma β-EP is difficult to interpret because it does not reflect levels in the central nervous system (CNS) circulation. Specifically, the pituitary and/or peripheral pool of β-EP appears to be separate from the pool within the hypothalamus. Therefore peripheral measurements of β-EP reflect pituitary and non-CNS secretions rather than those from the hypothalamus. Another difficulty results from the low peripheral concentration of β-EP. In addition, cross-reactivity with β-lipotropins occurs in the immunoassays currently used for β-EP.

Therefore, to study β-EP action, experiments are performed using infusions of naloxone, an opioid antagonist. Infusion of greater than 1 mg per hour blocks brain opioid activity and results in an increase of LH in the late follicular and luteal phases but not in the early follicular phase or postmenopausally. This suggests that both estrogen and progesterone increase levels of β-EP in the brain (Figure 4-9). The increase in β-EP may account for the decreased frequency of GnRH pulses in the luteal phase.

Prostaglandins

Hypothalamic levels of prostaglandins may modulate the release of GnRH. Administration of prostaglandin E_2 significantly increases GnRH levels in the portal blood. Furthermore, a physiologic role of prostaglandins in regulating or modulating the secretion of GnRH is supported by experiments demonstrating that the midcycle surge of LH can be abolished in the rat and ewe by the administration of aspirin or indomethacin, which blocks the synthesis of prostaglandins. No information is available at present concerning the effects of prostaglandin, or of inhibitors of prostaglandin synthesis, on gonadotrophin secretion in the human.

Catechol Estrogens

The compounds 2-hydroxyestradiol and 2-hydroxyestrone, as well as their 3-methyl derivatives, are present in higher concentrations in the hypothalamus than are prostaglandins E_1 and E_2. It has been hypothesized that these compounds may act as neuromodulators by modulating the function of catecholamines through inhibition of tyrosine hydroxylase and competition for the enzyme catechol-O-methyltransferase. However, the evidence that catechol estrogens have a major effect on neuromodulating reproductive function is insufficient.

GnRH ACTION

GnRH, when it reaches the anterior lobe of the pituitary, stimulates the synthesis and release of both LH and FSH from the same cell in the pituitary gland. Thus, whereas the hypothalamic control of prolactin is both inhibitory (dominant) and stimulatory, the hypothalamic

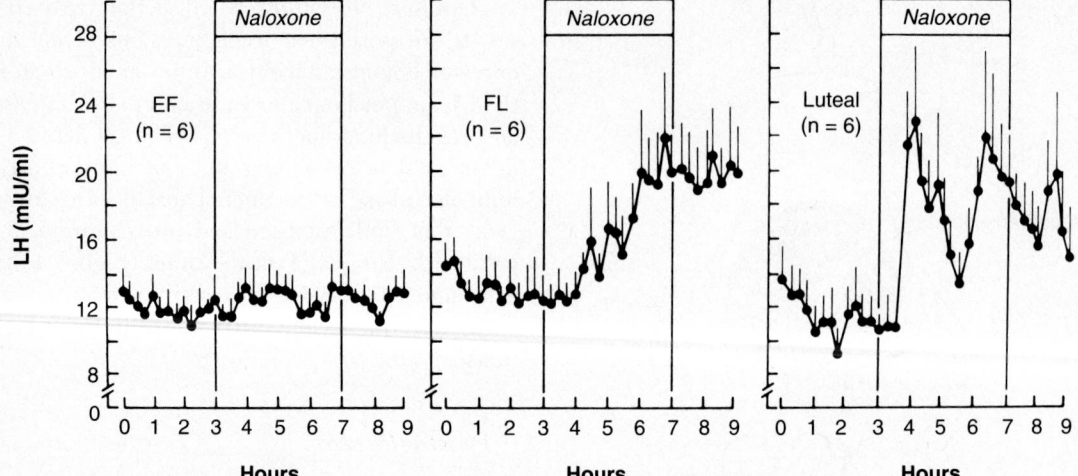

FIGURE 4-9
Infusion of naloxone, an opiate receptor antagonist, elicits incremental change of LH in subjects during late follicular *(LF)* and midluteal phases of cycle (but not in early follicular *[EF]* phase), indicating progressive increase in endogenous opioid inhibition of GnRH secretion, especially during luteal phase. (From Quigley ME and Yen SSC: J Clin Endocrinol Metab 51:179, 1980. © by The Endocrine Society, 1980.)

control of gonadotrophins is only stimulatory. The peptide hormones, such as GnRH, bind to specific receptors on the surface membrane of the target cell, in contrast to steroid hormones, which pass through the cell membrane to bind to intracellular receptors.

Protein hormone receptors are of high molecular weight (200,000 to 300,000 daltons), and each receptor binds a single molecule of the protein. Peptide hormones, including LH, FSH, and prolactin, although highly soluble in aqueous media, have low solubility in lipids and thus do not readily pass the lipid barrier of the target cell's plasma membrane. After the protein hormone binds to its receptor, the hormone receptor complex may be brought through the cell membrane to protect it from other interactions. This process is called *internalization*. In addition to hormone-receptor complex internalization, the hormone message may be transmitted into the cell by transmembrane signaling via at least three known pathways: (1) production of an intracellular second messenger, which increases phosphorylation of regulatory proteins to produce a cellular response; (2) production of a membrane-bound second messenger; or (3) membrane-bound cystosolic phosphorylation activity triggered by hormone binding at the extracellular interface (Figure 4-10).

When a protein hormone binds to its specific receptor, it activates or inhibits the enzyme adenylate cyclase, the second messenger, which in turn changes the concentration of adenosine 3'5'-cyclic monophosphate (cyclic AMP, cAMP). The cAMP then activates protein kinase in the cytoplasm by binding its regulatory subunit and thus dissociating this subunit from its catalytic subunit. When the regulatory subunit of the protein kinase is freed from the catalytic subunit, the latter subunit is able to transfer a phosphate from adenosine triphosphate (ATP) to the protein substrate. This action modifies the biologic function of the protein to produce a cellular response.

At the pituitary gonatrophin cell membrane, GnRH binding is facilitated by the action of calcium and prostaglandin. The hormone-receptor complex activates membrane-bound adenylate cyclase, which stimulates cAMP production and activates a protein kinase by dissociating its regulatory component from the catalytic subunit. The catalytic subunit then phosphorylates the membrane protein to increase calcium permeability. This change allows calcium to enter the cell. Calcium activates the release of stored LH and FSH, producing a stimulus-secretion coupling analogous to muscle excitation-contraction coupling. Enhanced LH and FSH synthesis is also seen and may in-

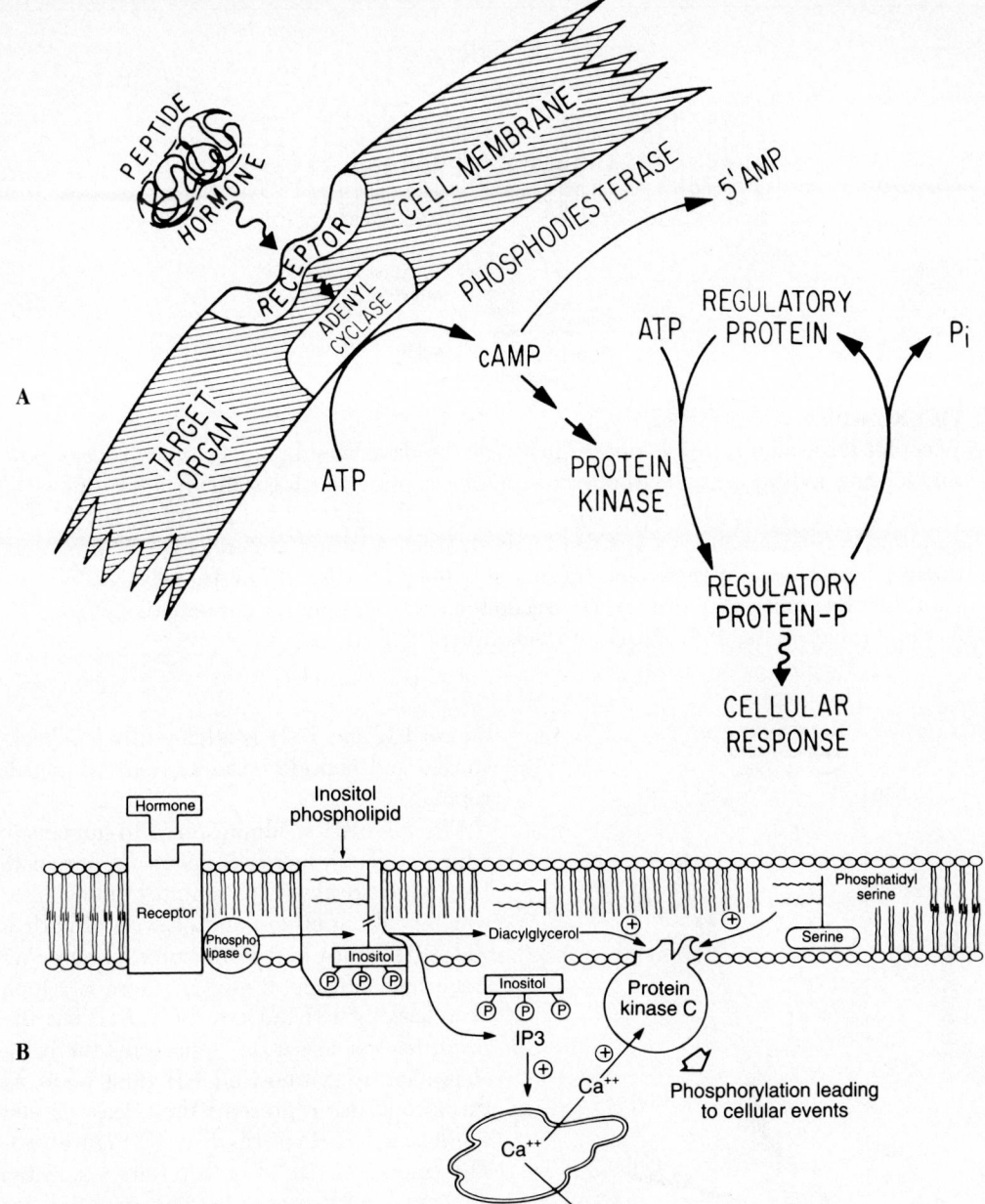

FIGURE 4-10

A, Second messenger model of peptide hormone action. Interaction of hormone
with receptor leads to activation of membrane-bound adenylate cyclase, resulting in
conversion of adenosine triphosphate *(ATP)* to cyclic AMP (cAMP). cAMP then interacts with cAMP-dependent protein kinase, causing activation of the enzyme and
phosphorylation of intracellular regulatory protein substrates, with ATP as phosphate donor. *P,* Phosphate group; P_i, inorganic phosphate. cAMP is inactivated by
conversion to 5′-AMP by phosphodiesterase. **B,** Phospholipase C−protein kinase C
pathway. Peptide hormone binds to its receptor on external surface, which activates
the enzyme phospholipase C within membrane. This enzyme hydrolyzes phosphati-
dylinositol-4,5-bisphosphate to produce two second messengers: inositol triphosphate *(IP3)* and 1,2-diacyglycerol (DG). IP3 is soluble in cystol, where it binds to
receptors on endoplasmic reticulum, causing an opening of Ca^{++} channels and an
increase of cytosolic Ca^{++}. DG remains in membrane, where it activates protein
kinase C (PKC). Ca^{++} is also necessary for full activation of PKC. Activation of
PKC causes phosphorylation and cellular responses. *Continued.*

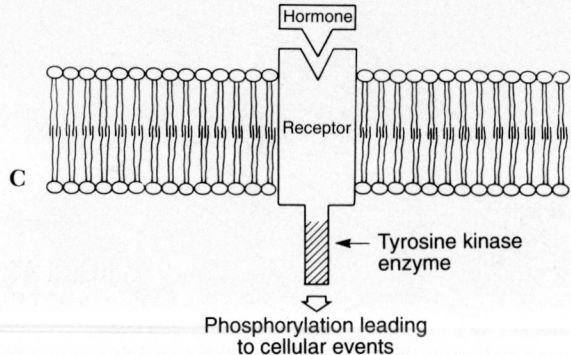

FIGURE 4-10, C

Receptor-associated tyrosine kinase. Hormone binds to membrane-spanning receptor, causing activation of a cytosolic domain of receptor, which is actually a tyrosine kinase enzyme. Once activated, tyrosine residues on proteins are phosphorylated, resulting in cellular actions. (**A**, **B**, and **C** from Hylka VW and di Zerega GS: Reproductive hormones and their mechanisms of action. In Mishell DA Jr, Davajan V, and Lobo RA, editors: Infertility, contraception and reproductive endocrinology, ed 3, Cambridge, Mass, 1991, Blackwell Scientific Publications.)

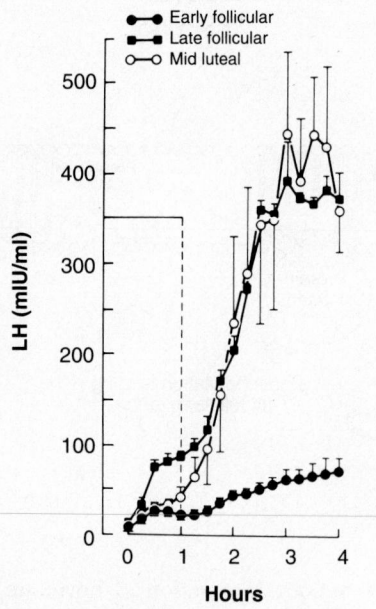

FIGURE 4-11

Quantitative LH release within first and second pool during GnRH infusion. Dotted line separates two pools. (From Hoff JD, Lasley BL, Wang CF, et al: J Clin Endocrinol Metab 44:302, 1977. © by The Endocrine Society, 1977.)

volve altering ribosomal phosphorylation to increase messenger ribonucleic acid (mRNA) translation. GnRH receptor synthesis is also stimulated by GnRH action. Differential secretion of LH and FSH is attained by feedback of steroid and peptide hormones on the gonadotrophs.

When GnRH is administered to humans in a bolus, a rapid increase occurs in circulating LH, which peaks at 30 minutes, and in FSH, which peaks at 60 minutes. Levels of both LH and FSH return to baseline after 3 hours. With a constant infusion of GnRH, there is a biphasic release of LH but not FSH. Yen has theorized that the initial rise represents the release of previously synthesized LH (first pool), and the second rise represents the release of newly synthesized LH (second pool)(Figure 4-11). The combined size of both pituitary sensitivity (first pool) and reserve (second pool) has been called the functional capacity of the gonadotrophs. However, if GnRH continues to be infused, gonadotrophin secretion is inhibited, probably because the receptors are saturated and are unable to continue to stimulate release of the second messenger (Figure 4-12). Even though maximal hormonal stimulation occurs when only a small percentage of the target cell receptors are bound by hormone, when stimulation is maximal the unoccupied receptors become refractory to hormone binding for 12 to 72 hours. This phenomenon has allowed frequent administration of GnRH analogues to be used clinically.

GnRH analogues are synthesized by substitution of amino acid 6 in the parent molecule with a *d*-amino acid and/or replacement of amino

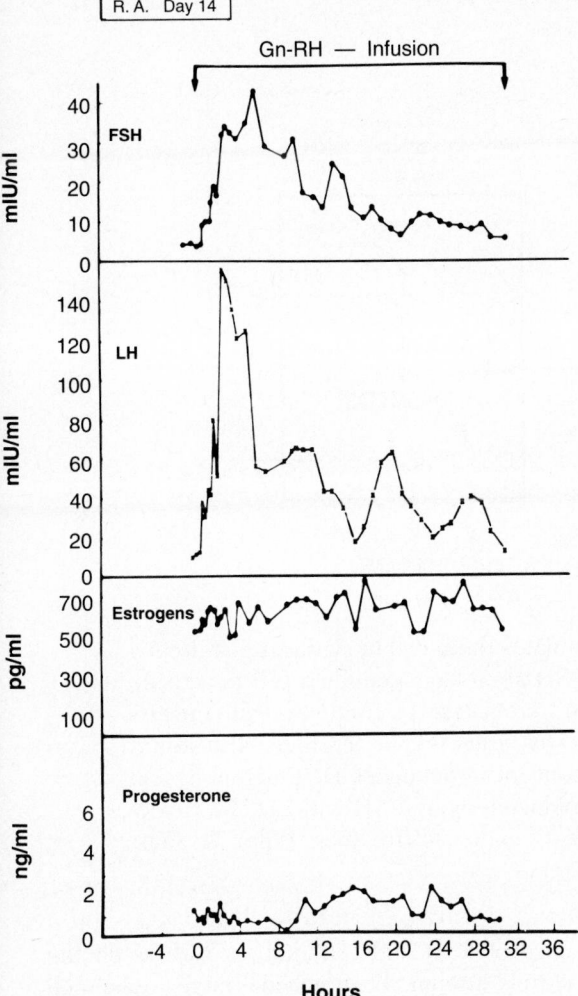

FIGURE 4-12
Mean serum FSH, LH, estrogen, and progesterone levels during 30-hour continuous infusions of GnRH at midcycle phase in three normal women. (From Jewelewicz R, Ferin M, Dyrenfurth I, et al: Long-term LH, RH infusions at various stages of the menstural cycle in normal women. In Beling CG and Wenitz AC, editors: The LH-releasing hormone, New York, 1980, Masson Publishing.)

acid 10 with an *N*-ethylamide ($Na-CH_2-CH_3$) or Aza-Gly ($NHNHCO$) moiety. The various agonists have greater potencies (15 to 200 times) and longer half-lives (1, 3, 6 hours) than GnRH. The agonists initially simulate gonadotrophic release (flare). This effect lasts from 1 to 3 weeks. After this time, as the GnRH receptors become saturated with the constantly administered analogue the stimulatory effect of the periodic release of endogenous GnRH on the pituitary gland is

USE OF GnRH AND GnRH ANALOGUES IN GYNECOLOGY

> Stimulation of pituitary-gonadal function
> (GnRH)
> Delayed puberty
> Induction of ovulation
> Suppression of pituitary-gonadal function
> (GnRH analogues)
> Precocious puberty
> Endometriosis
> Breast cancer
> Uterine leiomyomas
> Ovarian androgen excess

blocked. The process is called *desensitization* or *down regulation*. Therefore these analogues are used clinically to treat various steroid hormone–dependent entities (see box above).

In 1985 the GnRH agonist leuprolide acetate was approved for the palliative treatment of prostate cancer. Leuprolide is also available in the depot form (7.5 mg), which allows for the monthly intramuscular administration of 3.75 to 7.5 mg for women with endometriosis and leiomyomata uteri. Although therapy has been shown to be effective, bone mineral content has decreased and hot flashes occur as a result of low estradiol levels. Presently, investigators are using combinations of leuprolide with conjugated estrogens or progestins ("add back" therapy) to minimize these side effects.

Recently, although not yet approved for clinical use, a potent GnRH-antagonist, Nal-Glu, has demonstrated many promising features. Nal-Glu has been shown to decrease serum LH levels effectively in a single dose (in a dose- and time-dependent manner) in both men and women without a flare effect. Nal-Glu acutely inhibits ovulation and affects LH more than FSH while decreasing estradiol levels at midcycle.

GONADOTROPHIN STRUCTURE AND FUNCTION

LH and FSH are glycoproteins of high molecular weight, 28,000 and 37,000 daltons, respectively. They each have the same α subunit (14,000 daltons) of about 90 amino acids, which is similar in structure to the α subunit of thy-

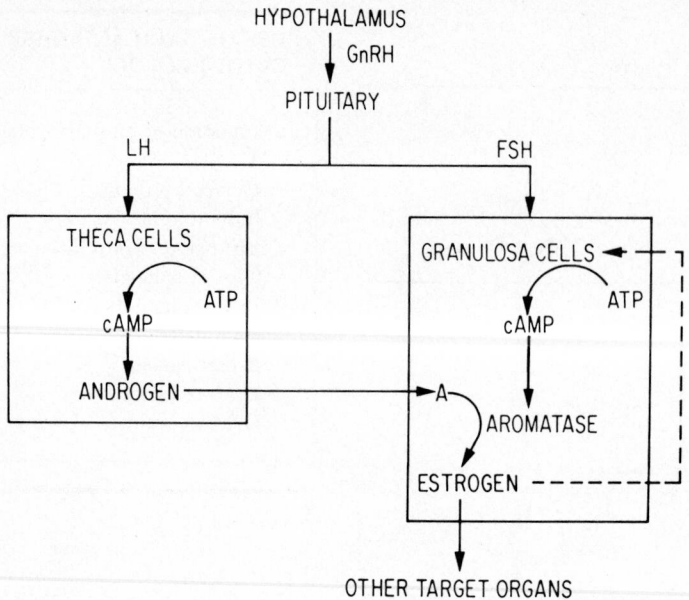

FIGURE 4-13

Action of gonadotrophins on ovary: LH stimulates theca cell to synthesize androgen by cyclic AMP (cAMP)–mediated action. FSH stimulates granulosa cell to activate aromatase via cyclic AMP–mediated action. Aromatase in granulosa cell converts androgen to estrogen, which is then utilized by target organs. Estrogen also stimulates granulosa cell proliferation. (From a concept in Schulster D, Burstein S, and Cooke BA, editors: Control of gonadal steroidogenesis by FSH and LH. In Molecular endocrinology of the steroid hormones, London, 1976, John Wiley & Sons, Ltd.)

roid-stimulating hormone and human chorionic gonadotrophin. The β subunits of all these hormones have different amino acids and carbohydrates and provide specific biologic activity. The α and β subunits are joined by disulfide bonds. The sialic acid content of each hormone increases with the duration of biologic action from one or two molecules in LH, which has a half-life of 30 minutes, to five molecules in FSH, which has a half-life of 3.9 hours. In the female, although the two gonadotrophins act synergistically, LH acts primarily on the theca cells to induce steroidogenesis, whereas FSH acts primarily on the granulosa cells to stimulate follicular growth. FSH release is greater than LH release until puberty, when the normal menstrual cycle is established and LH secretion overtakes that of FSH. After menopause the LH/FSH ratio is again reversed. This preferential inhibition of FSH release during the reproductive years results from increasing levels of both estradiol and inhibin.

Receptors for LH exist on the theca cells at all stages of the cycle; they are on granulosa cells after the follicle matures under the influ-

ence of FSH and estradiol, as well as on the corpus luteum. Each gonadal target tissue cell contains between 2000 and 30,000 membrane receptors. Maximal stimulation of hormonal activity occurs when less than 5% of these receptors are bound with hormone. The main action of LH is to stimulate androgen synthesis by the theca cells and progesterone synthesis by the corpus luteum through stimulation of intracellular cAMP production (Figure 4-13). The precise action of LH on granulosa cells has not been determined, but it probably acts synergistically with FSH to help follicular maturation. LH stimulates several other metabolic events in the ovary, such as amino acid transport and RNA synthesis. LH may also induce ovulation by stimulating a plasminogen activator that decreases tensile strength of the follicle wall before follicular rupture occurs.

FSH receptors exist primarily on the granulosa cell membrane. In addition to stimulating LH receptors on this cell memberane, FSH activates the aromatase and the 3-hydroxysteroid dehydrogenase enzymes within the cell by increasing cAMP. FSH stimulation of isolated granulosa cells in vitro produces only small amounts of estrogen; however, when androgens or theca cells are added, large amounts of estrogen are produced. These data support the two-cell hypothesis of estrogen production. This hypothesis proposes that LH acts on the theca to produce androgens (androstenedione and testosterone), which are then transported to the granulosa cells, where they are aromatized to estrogens (estrone and estradiol) by the action of FSH (see Figure 4-13). The aromatase enzyme catalyzes this conversion.

Concomitant with increased estrogen production, mitosis is stimulated in granulosa cells, augmenting cell number. Estradiol and FSH receptor production is increased as well, maintaining intracellular cAMP levels as circulating FSH decreases. In granulosa cells primed by exposure to large amounts of estradiol and FSH, LH acts synergistically with FSH to increase LH receptors and induces luteinization of the follicle, increasing progesterone production. Premature delivery of LH will disrupt the process, resulting in premature luteinization, whereas the capacity of the follicle to respond to estrogen appears to determine whether it will mature or become atretic.

LH also stimulates prostaglandin synthesis by intracellular production of cAMP. Prostaglandin may play a role in follicle rupture, since the prostaglandin content of preovulatory follicles increases at the time of the gonadotrophin surge and may stimulate smooth muscle contraction. Plasminogen activator (PA) concentration also increases in the midcycle follicle, and its action is enhanced by LH. Follicle rupture is blocked by administration of PA inhibitors in vivo.

GONADAL REGULATION BY GROWTH FACTORS

Growth factors provide traditional hormonal, autocrine, and paracrine effects within the ovary, as summarized in Table 4-1.

Insulin-like Growth Factors (IGFs)

The two polypeptide hormones in this family, IGF-I and IGF-II, have structural homology to proinsulin. At physiologic concentrations they bind to their specific receptors, but in higher concentrations they cross-react with the other receptor.

IGF-I stimulates basal and gonadotrophin-in-duced steroidogenesis in both theca and granulosa cells. It enhances FSH-induced increases in cAMP, LH receptors, proteoglycan, and basal inhibin synthesis in granulosa cells. Granulosa cells appear to secrete IGF-I, whereas the receptor is made in both granulosa and theca cells, suggesting a plausible regulatory mechanism for the two compartments of ovarian steroidogenesis.

IGF-II is secreted by granulosa cells and enhances steroidogenesis in both theca and granulosa cells. Receptors have been found in the granulosa cell. Insulin, although not produced by the ovary, modulates steroidogenesis by interaction with granulosa cell receptors and may bind to IGF-I receptors in high concentration.

Inhibin and Activins

Inhibin consists of one type of alpha (α) and two types of beta (β) subunits (Figure 4-14). Inhibin A contains the A β subunit, whereas inhibin B contains the B β subunit. Both subunits stimulate progesterone and inhibit estradiol in the ovarian follicle, and both are potent inhibitors of pituitary FSH release (Figure 4-15). Activins are composed of two inhibin β subunits. These are called activin A if two A β subunits are present, activin B if two B β subunits are present, and activin if both an A and B β subunit are present. These peptides stimulate pituitary release of FSH without affecting LH output, but their effects can be overridden by inhibin. Activins also oppose the action of inhibin in the ovary.

Other Growth Factors

Follistatin is a distinct class of hormone found in follicular fluid that has only one-third the potency of inhibin in blocking FSH secretion. Follistatin antagonizes FSH action in the granulosa cell, reducing estradiol synthesis.

Epidermal growth factor (EGF) appears to be made in theca cells but acts in the granulosa cells, where it stimulates growth and thymidine incorporation and increases FSH binding. EGF also inhibits steroid production and delays induction of LH receptors.

Transforming growth factor alpha (TGFα) binds to EGF receptors. As yet, no separate function or receptor for this factor has been identified. Transforming growth factor beta (TGFβ), made in theca cells, promotes growth and cAMP accumulation in granulosa cells and

TABLE 4-1
Role of Growth Factors in Ovarian Function

Factor	Granulosa Cells	Theca Cells	Corpus Luteum	Other
Insulin	Has receptors Augments basal and HCG-induced P Enhances prostaglandin E_2–stimulated P	Enhances LH/HCG-induced Adione, E_2, P, T Increases basal secretion of E_2, P, T, Adione	Enhances secretion of oxytocin and P	Receptors present in stroma
IGF-I (somatomedin C)	Has type I receptors that are increased by FSH Made here Enhances cAMP-induced P Enhances FSH-induced P, E_2, cAMP, adenylate cyclase, luteinization, LH receptors, proteoglycans Enhances PMSG-induced aromatase and P Stimulated by LH, FSH, cAMP, GH, EGF Enhances HDL-induced P Enhances P and inhibin production	Has type I receptors Increases HCG-induced E_2, P, T, Adione Increases basal secretion of P	Increases secretion of oxytocin and P	Stimulated by GH in whole ovary Enhances aromatase in luteinized granulosa cells Enhances androsterone from theca-interstitial cells Stimulated in ovary by HCG
IGF-II (MSA)	Made here Enhances steroidogenesis Has type II receptors Stimulated by LH and FSH Increases ornithine decarboxylase	Enhances HCG-induced P, T, E_2		Stimulated by GH, HCG, HPL, PRL, and FSH in luteinized granulosa cells

TGFβ	Inhibits EGF-induced growth Enhances FSH-induced LH receptors, aromatase, EGF receptors, and inhibin Inhibits EGF-induced IGF-I Inhibits basal and FSH-stimulated P Increases production of E_2, cAMP, inhibin Increases growth	Produced here Increases basal and HCG-induced E_2 production Inhibits HCG-induced P, T, Adione Inhibits basal P, Adione	Augments basal and HCG-induced P in luteinized granulosa cells Present in theca-interstitial cells
EGF/TGFα	Inhibits FSH-induced aromatase, E_2 Stimulates growth/mitosis Has receptors Receptors are stimulated by FSH and inhibited by LH Stimulates P and E_2 Enhances FSH-receptor binding Inhibits LH-receptor binding, inhibin secretion	TGFα made here (not EGF) Decreases basal and HCG-stimulated E_2 Stimulates growth	
FGFa	Produced here Inhibits FSH-induced LH receptors Inhibits FSH-induced cAMP, E_2	Produced here	

From Hylka VW and di Zerega GS: Reproductive hormones and their mechanisms of action. In Mishell DR Jr, Davajan V, and Lobo RA, editors: Infertility, contraception and reproductive endocrinology, ed 3, Cambridge, Mass, 1991, Blackwell Scientific Publications.

P, Progesterone; T, testosterone; PMSG, pregnant mare serum gonadotrophins; HDL, high density lipoprotein; HPL, human placental lactogen; Adione, androstenedione, TGF, transforming growth factor; MSA, multiplication stimulating activity; HCG, human chorionic gonadotrophin; GH, growth hormone; EGF, epidermal growth factor; FGFa, acidic fibroblast growth factor.

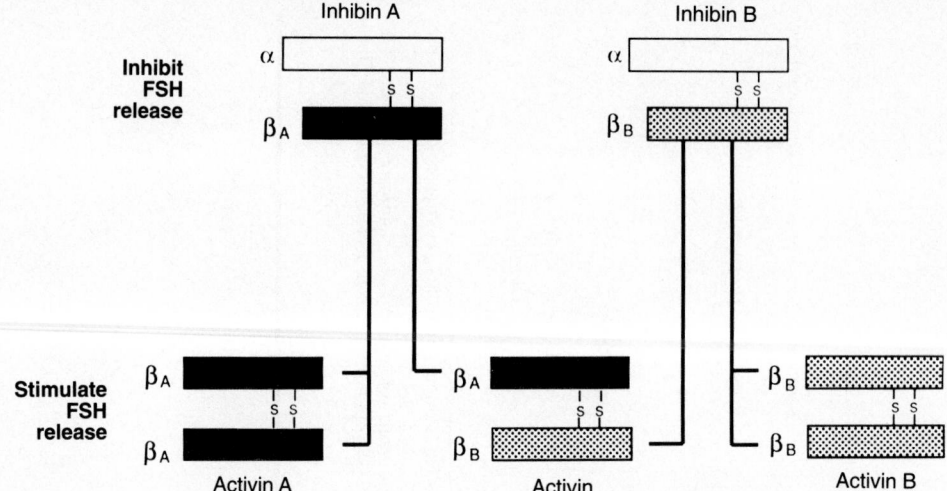

FIGURE 4-14
Chemical relationships of inhibins and activins. *S,* Disulfide bond. (From Hylka VW and di Zerega GS: Reproductive hormones and their mechanisms of action. In Mishell DR Jr, Davajan V, and Lobo RA, editors: Infertility, contraception and reproductive endocrinology, ed 3, Cambridge, Mass, 1991, Blackwell Scientific Publications.)

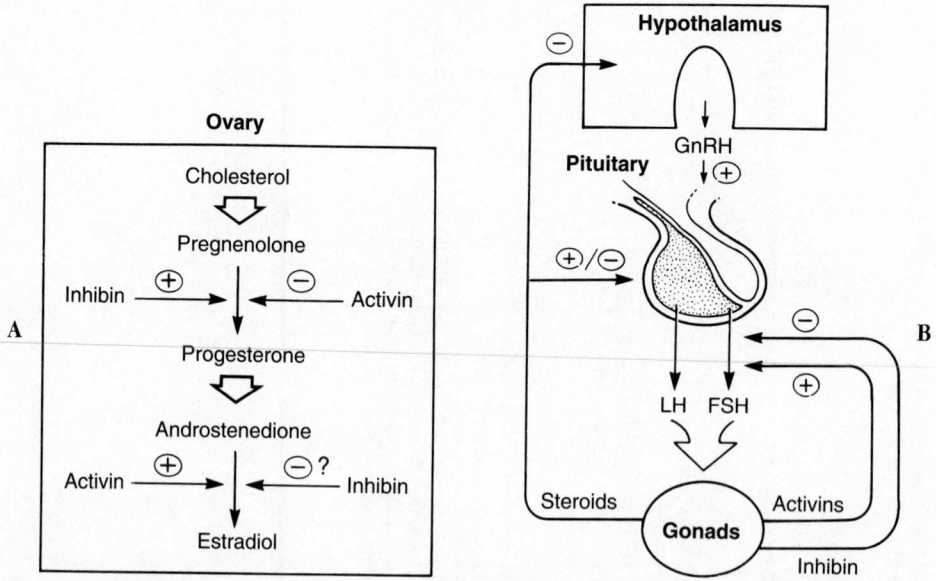

FIGURE 4-15
Generalized schemata showing involvement of activins and inhibins **A,** in hypothalamic-hypophyseal-gonadal axis and **B,** when activins and inhibins regulate steroidogenesis intragonadally. (From Hylka VW and di Zerega GS: Reproductive hormones and their mechanisms of action. In Mishell DR Jr, Davajan V, and Lobo RA, editors: Infertility, contraception and reproductive endocrinology, ed 3, Cambridge, Mass, 1991, Blackwell Scientific Publications.)

enhances FSH-induced increases in aromatase and LH receptors.

Acidic fibroblast growth factor (FGFa) is made in granulosa cells and promotes their growth in culture. FGFa inhibits steroidogenesis and induction of LH receptors in these cells.

Other ovarian regulators include follicle regulatory protein (FRP), oocyte maturation inhibitor (OMI), substance P, plasminogen activators (PAs), FSH-binding inhibitor, and GnRH-like protein. These and other factors are listed in Table 4-2 with a short description of their functions.

PROSTAGLANDINS AND RELATED COMPOUNDS

Arachidonic acid, the most abundant and important precursor for the biosynthesis of eicosanoids in humans, is formed from linoleic acid and is supplied in the diet. Arachidonic acid is released from membrane phospholipids by lipases, which are activated by various stimuli.

The biosynthesis of prostanoids takes place through the cyclic endoperoxides prostaglandin G (PGG) and prostaglandin H (PGH) (Figure 4-16). PGG, through which all prosanoids are formed, is itself formed from one of the three

TABLE 4-2
Local Nonsteroidal Intrafollicular Regulators

Factor	Description
Oxytocin	Pituitary hormone produced in granulosa cells and corpus luteum that regulates progesterone production, particularly in the corpus luteum. May be regulated by prostaglandin $F_{2\alpha}$.
Plasminogen activators (PAs)	Serine proteases that cleave plasminogen to form plasmin, which activates collagenase. Granulosa cells produce tissue-type plasminogen activator (tPA), whereas theca cells or macrophages produce urokinase type PA (uPA). Activated collagenase is thought to have a role in dissolution of the basal lamina for effective ovulation (rupture). Both gonadotrophins and prostaglandins stimulate PA activity.
Renin/angiotensin	Proteins that help promote angiogenesis and that may be found in theca cells. Necessary for the formation of new blood vessels during follicular growth.
Follicle regulatory protein (FRP)	Protein made by granulosa cells that inhibits aromatase activity and may counteract FSH to promote atresia.
Oocyte maturation inhibitor (OMI)	A protein of ovarian origin that maintains meiotic arrest of the oocyte and inhibits cumulus growth and progesterone production.
Substance P	A small neurotransmitter molecule found in nerve terminals invading the thecal layer. It may alter ovarian blood flow.
FSH-binding inhibitor	Low-molecular-weight protein (5000) isolated from follicular fluid. It inhibits FSH binding in the ovary and testis.
Glycosaminoglycans (GAGs)	GAGs are composed of repeating disaccharide units, usually hexuronic acid or hexosamine. They are the outer shell of proteoglycans. GAGs are regulated by FSH. They inhibit LH receptor number and inhibit FSH-stimulated progesterone. They are found in follicular fluid. The most prevalent are chonoroitin sulfate (CS), heparin sulfate, and dermatan sulfate. High levels of CS are found in atretic follicles.
GnRH-like protein	Protein of ovarian origin that competes with GnRH for GnRH receptors. Recently identified as histone 2A.

From Hylka VW and diZerega GS: Reproductive hormones and their mechanisms of action. In Mishell DR Jr, Davajan V, and Lobo RA, editors: Infertility, contraception and reproductive endocrinology, ed 3, Cambridge, Mass, 1991, Blackwell Scientific Publications.

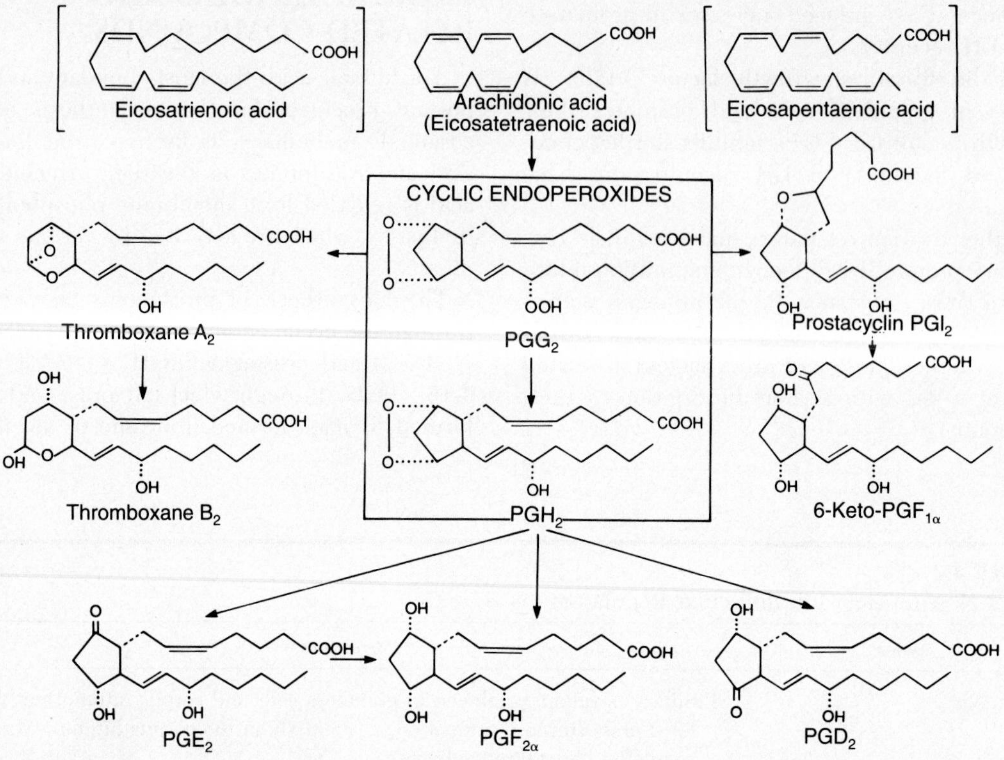

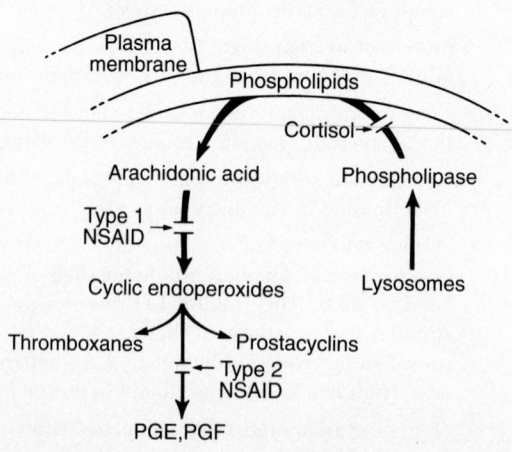

FIGURE 4-16

Biosynthesis of prostanoids. (From Hylka VW and di Zerega GS: Reproductive hormones and their mechanisms of action. In Mishell DR Jr, Davajan V, and Lobo RA, editors: Infertility, contraception and reproductive endocrinology, ed 3, Cambridge, Mass, 1991, Blackwell Scientific Publications.)

FIGURE 4-17

Inhibition of enzymes involved in biosynthesis of prostanoids. *NSAID*, Nonsteroidal antiflammatory drug. (From Stanczyk FZ: Prostaglandins and related compounds. In Mishell DR Jr, Davajan V, and Lobo RA, editors: Infertility, contraception and reproductive endocrinology, ed 3, Cambridge, Mass, 1991, Blackwell Scientific Publications.)

precursor fatty acids by the microsomal enzyme prostaglandin synthetase. The formation of endoperoxides and their subsequent conversion to prostanoids is very rapid. Since prostanoids are then released immediately from the cell, measurement of tissue or serum levels of prostanoids does not accurately reflect in vivo levels before biopsy or blood collection.

The biosynthesis of prostanoids can be inhibited by several groups of compounds, including the nonsteroidal antiinflammatory drugs (NSAIDs) type 1 (aspirin and indomethacin, which inhibit endoperoxide formation) and type 2 (phenylbutazone), which inhibit action of endoperoxide isomerase and reductase. Corticosteroids can also inhibit prostanoid formation by decreasing precursor phospholipid hydrolysis and release (Figure 4-17).

In contrast to steroid hormones, which are stored and act at target organs distant from their source, prostanoids are produced intracellularly shortly before they are released and generally act locally. Specific prostanoids can have variable effects on different tissues as well as variable effects on the same organ, even when relaesed in the same concentration (Table 4-3). One important effect is their ability to modulate the responses of endogenous stimulators and inhibitors, such as ovarian stimulation by LH, which is modulated by $PGF_{2\alpha}$, which in turn regulates ovarian receptor availability.

Eicosanoids have a wide variety of biologic effects throughout the body and an important role in reproductive system function. Prostaglandins have an important role in ovarian physiology. They help control early follicular growth by increasing blood supply to certain follicles and inducing FSH receptors on granulosa cells of preovulatory follicles. Both PGE_2 and $PGF_{2\alpha}$ are concentrated in the follicular fluid of preovulatory follicles. $PGF_{2\alpha}$ may reduce synthesis of collagen in the preovulatory follicular wall and thus assist in the process of follicular rupture. Prostaglandins may help regulate the life span of the corpus luteum. PGE_2 is probably luteotrophic, and $PGF_{2\alpha}$ results in luteolysis.

Prostaglandins also have potent effects on oviductal motility, mediating the stimulatory estrogen effect and the inhibitory progesterone effect on oviductal muscular contractility. Prostaglandins also act to delay passage of the fertilized ovum into the uterus by influencing uterotubal junction activity. In the cervix, PGE_2 relaxes the smooth muscle, whereas $PGF_{2\alpha}$

TABLE 4-3
Effects of Eiconsanoids

Prostaglandins	Effects
PGI_2, PGE_2, PGD_2	Vasodilation
	Cytoprotection
	Platelet aggregation
	Leukocyte aggregation
	Cyclic AMP formation
	IL-1 and IL-2 formation
$PGF_{2\alpha}$	Vasoconstriction
	Bronchoconstriction
	Smooth muscle contraction
TXA_2	Vasoconstriction
	Platelet aggregation
	Lymphocyte proliferation
	Bronchoconstriction
LTB_4	Vascular permeability
	Leukocyte aggregation
	IL-1 formation
	IL-2 formation
	Natural killer cell cytotoxicity
	Chemoattractant
LTC_4, LTD_4	Bronchoconstriction
	Vascular permeability

PGI_2, Prostacyclin; PG, prostaglandin; TX, thromboxane; LT, leukotriene; IL, interleukin.

causes the muscle to contract.

Many prostanoids are produced by the endometrium. These include PGE_2, $PGF_{2\alpha}$, PGI_2 and thromboxane A_2 (TXA_2). Concentrations of PGE_2 and $PGF_{2\alpha}$ increase progressively from the proliferative to the secretory phase. The highest levels are found during menstruation. These prostaglandins help regulate myometrial contractility and appear to be important in regulating the process of menstruation.

OVARIAN STEROIDS

Chemistry

Steroids are lipids that have a basic chemical structure or nucleus. The nucleus consists of three 6-carbon rings (A, B, and C) joined to a 5-carbon atom D ring that is called cyclopentanoperhydrophenantherene, or gonane (Figure 4-18). The molecular weight of most steroid hormones is in the range of 250 to 550 daltons. Steroids such as progesterone and estradiol are insoluble in water but dissolve readily in organic solvents such as diethyl ether and chloroform. In contrast, steroids have a sulfate or glu-

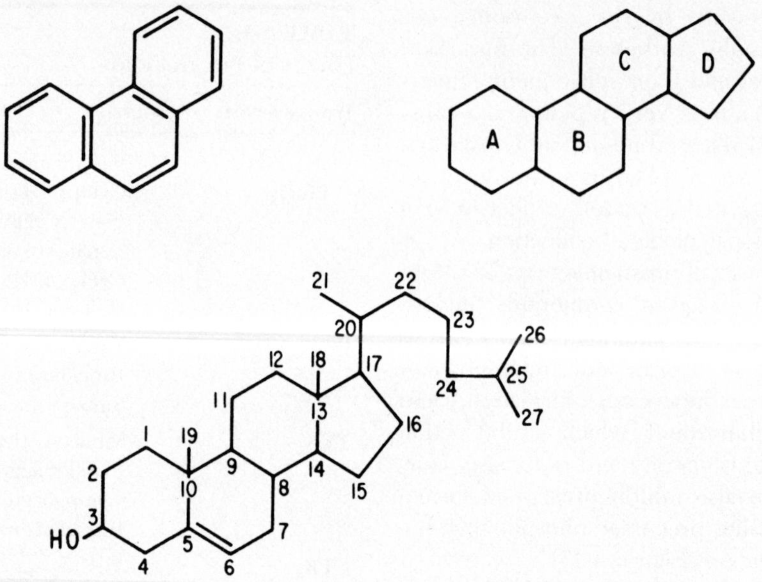

FIGURE 4-18

Phenanthrene *(top left).* Cyclopentanoperhydrophenanthrene nucleus *(top right),* in which the three 6-carbon rings *(A, B,* and *C)* resemble the phenanthrene ring system and the 5-carbon ring *(D)* resembles cyclopentane. Cholesterol *(bottom)* is the common biosynthetic precursor of steroid hormones. Numbers *1* to *27* indicate conventional numbering system of carbon atoms in steroids. (From Stanczyk FZ: Steroid hormones. In Mishell DR Jr, Davajan V, and Lobo RA, editors: Infertility, contraception and reproductive endocrinology, ed 3, Cambridge, Mass, 1991, Blackwell Scientific Publications.)

curonide group attached (conjugated steroids), such as pregnanediol glucuronide and estrone sulfate, and are water soluble.

Steroids are named according to a generally accepted convention that is used to determine their systemic (scientific) names. Most steroid hormones have common (trivial) names, such as progesterone and estradiol, which are generally used instead of the scientific names. The carbon atoms of steroids are numbered as shown in Figure 4-18. Functional groups above the plane of the molecule are preceded by the β symbol and shown in the structural formula by a solid line, whereas those below the plane are indicated by an α symbol and a dotted line. The symbol Δ indicates a double bond, and those steroids with a double bond between carbon atoms 5 and 6 (cholesterol, pregnenolone, 17-hydroxypregnenolone, and dehydroepiandrosterone) are called Δ^5 steroids, whereas those with a double bond between carbon atoms 4 and 5 (progesterone, all mineralocorticoids and glucocorticoids, androstenedione, and testosterone) are Δ^4 steroids.

Biosynthesis

All steroids in the body are formed from acetate, a 2-carbon compound. The first step in its conversion to a variety of steroids is the formation of cholesterol, a 27-carbon steroid, via a complex series of reactions (11 steps). All sex steroids and corticosteroids are derived by stepwise degradation of cholesterol. Corticosteroids, progesterone, pregnenolone, 17-hydroxypregnenolone, and 17-hydroxyprogesterone have 21 carbon atoms; androgens (testosterone and androstenedione) have 19 carbon atoms; and natural estrogens have 18 carbon atoms and a phenolic or aromatic ring A.

The first step in ovarian steroid biosynthesis is the reduction of cholesterol to pregnenolone by hydroxylation of C-20 and C-22 and cleavage between these atoms. This process reduces the C-27 compound cholesterol to the C-21 compound pregnenolone. From pregnenolone, ovarian steroid biosynthesis proceeds along two major pathways under the influence of specific enzymes: (1) the Δ^5 pathway through 17-hydroxypregnenolone and dehydroepiandrostenedione (DHEA) to Δ^5 androstenediol and (2) the Δ^4 pathway through progesterone and 17-hydroxyprogesterone to androstenedione and testosterone (Figure 4-19). LH stimulates this synthesis. Androstenedione and testosterone are interconverted, and the former can be converted to estrone and the latter to estradiol, respectively, by 19-hydroxylation. This enzymatic process results in loss of the C-19 group and development of the phenolic, or aromatase A, ring (aromatization) in the C-18 steroid.

The ovary secretes three primary steroids: estradiol, progesterone, and androstenedione. It also secretes pregnenolone, 17-hydroxyprogesterone, testosterone, DHEA, and estrone. Because the ovaries lack 21-hydroxylase, 11β-hydroxylase, and 18-hydroxylase activity, they are unable to synthesize mineralocorticoids or glucocorticoids. Each day the ovary secretes between 100 and 500 μg of estradiol, with the amount being lowest during menses and highest just before ovulation. Daily progesterone production varies from 0.5 mg in the follicular phase to 20 mg in the luteal phase. During the follicular phase, almost all progesterone is secreted from the adrenal gland and very little from the ovary. The ovary secretes between 1 and 2 mg of androstenedione, less than 1 mg of DHEA, and about 0.1 mg of testosterone daily. Androgen metabolism and corticosteroid synthesis are discussed in Chapter 38.

In addition to gonadal steroid biosynthesis, extraglandular steroid metabolism occurs. Interconversion of androstenedione and testosterone, as well as estrone and estradiol, takes place outside the ovaries, mainly by oxidation of the latter steroids to the former, thus reducing their biologic potency. Estrone is then converted to estrone sulfate, which has a long half-life and is the largest component of the pool of circulating estrogens (Figure 4-20). Estrone sulfate in turn may be converted to estrone and, to a lesser extent, to estradiol.

MacDonald et al. showed that androstenedione is peripherally converted to estrone in adipose tissue. The greater the amount of fat tissue present, the greater the percentage of androstenedione that is converted to estrone. In a normal individual about 1.3% of the daily 3000 μg of androstenedione produced is converted to estrone (40 μg), whereas in an obese individual as much as 7% (200 μg) of the 3000 μg is converted.

Transport

After they are secreted into the circulation, steroids bind to either specific proteins, such as sex hormone–binding globulin (SHBG) and corticosteroid-binding globulin (CBG) or to nonspecific proteins, such as albumin. The bound form of a steroid hormone represents approximately 95% of the total circulating concentration of the hormone; the remainder is unbound ("free"). For example, in premenopausal women approximately 65% and 30% of circulating testosterone is bound to SHBG and albumin, respectively; less than 2% is unbound. SHBG and CBG have a low capacity for steroids but bind them with high affinity ($K_a = 1 \times 10^8$ to 1×10^9), whereas albumin has a high capacity but binds with low affinity ($K_a = 1 \times 10^4$ to 1×10^6). Albumin binds all steroids. SHBG primarily binds dihydrotestosterone, testosterone, and estradiol (in order of decreasing affinity). CBG binds with highest affinity to cortisol, corticosterone, and 11-deoxycortisol, and, to a lesser extent, to progesterone. Circulating levels of each of the globulins are increased by estrogen; SHBG levels are also increased by obesity and hyperthyroidism and lowered by androgens and hypothyroidism.

Metabolism

The liver and, to a small extent, the kidney are the major sites of inactivation of steroids in the body. Inactivation mechanisms include hydroxylation of carbons on different sites of the steroid nucleus, reduction of ketone groups and double bonds, and conjugation (formation of sulfates and glucuronides). The process by which steroids are conjugated involves the transformation of lipophilic compounds, which are only sparingly soluble in water, into metabolites that are readily water soluble and can therefore be eliminated in urine. Examples of conjugation include the following. About 10% to 15% of progesterone is transformed to pregnanediol-3-glucuronide, which is the major urinary metabolite of progesterone. Estradiol and estrone are converted in the liver to estriol. These three estrogens are often referred to as the *classic* estrogens because they were the first ones to be isolated. These estrogens are conjugated by the liver and intestinal mucosa into different forms of estrogen sulfates and glucuronides, such as estrone

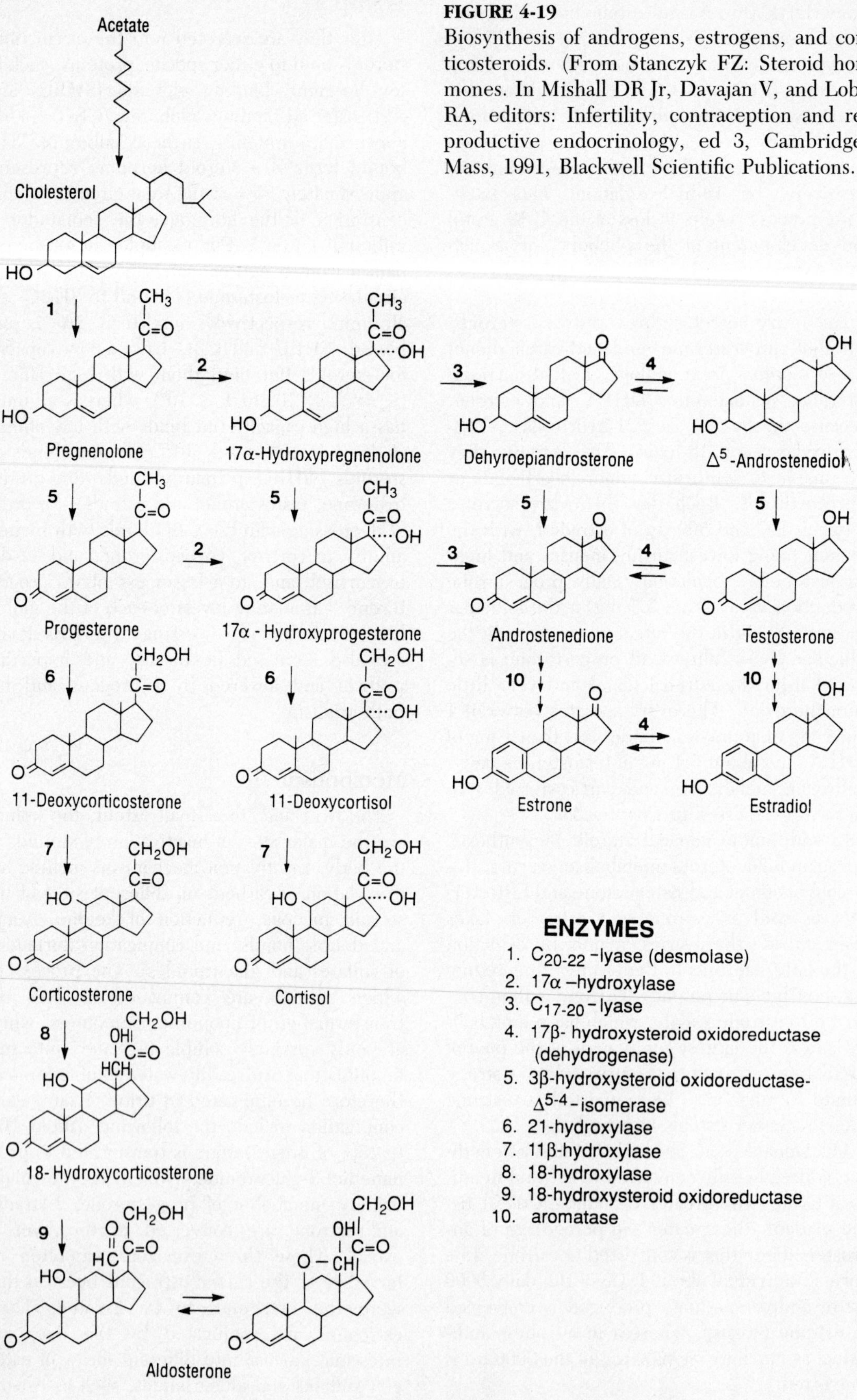

Acetate

Cholesterol

FIGURE 4-19
Biosynthesis of androgens, estrogens, and corticosteroids. (From Stanczyk FZ: Steroid hormones. In Mishall DR Jr, Davajan V, and Lobo RA, editors: Infertility, contraception and reproductive endocrinology, ed 3, Cambridge, Mass, 1991, Blackwell Scientific Publications.)

Pregnenolone

17α-Hydroxypregnenolone

Dehyroepiandrosterone

Δ⁵-Androstenediol

Progesterone

17α - Hydroxyprogesterone

Androstenedione

Testosterone

11-Deoxycorticosterone

11-Deoxycortisol

Estrone

Estradiol

Corticosterone

Cortisol

18- Hydroxycorticosterone

Aldosterone

ENZYMES

1. C_{20-22} –lyase (desmolase)
2. 17α –hydroxylase
3. C_{17-20} – lyase
4. 17β- hydroxysteroid oxidoreductase (dehydrogenase)
5. 3β-hydroxysteroid oxidoreductase-$Δ^{5-4}$ – isomerase
6. 21-hydroxylase
7. 11β-hydroxylase
8. 18-hydroxylase
9. 18-hydroxysteroid oxidoreductase
10. aromatase

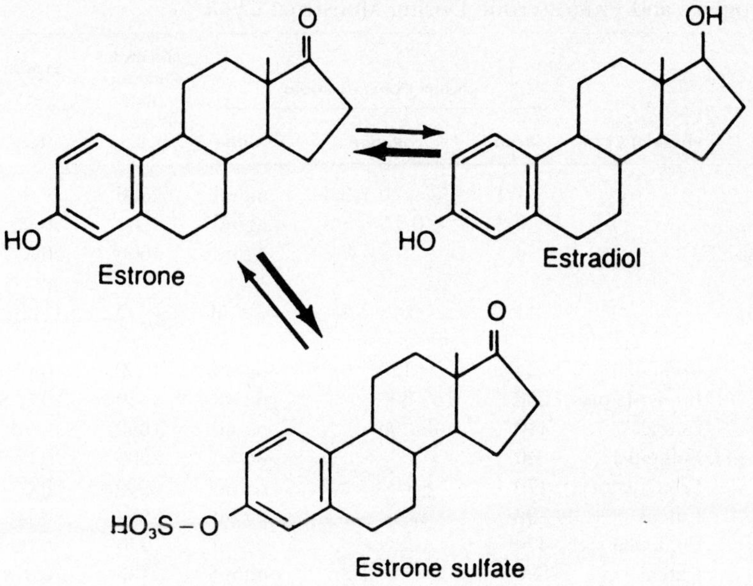

FIGURE 4-20

Interconversion of three principal circulating estrogens. (From Stanczyk FZ: Steroid hormones. In Mishall DR Jr, Davajan V, and Lobo RA, editors: Infertility, contraception and reproductive endocrinology, ed 3, Cambridge, Mass, 1991, Blackwell Scientific Publications.)

sulfate, estradiol-17-glucuronide, and estriol-16-glucuronide.

Dynamics of Hormone Production and Metabolism

The concentration of a steroid hormone in serum or plasma is dependent on its production rate (PR) and metabolic clearance rate (MCR). The MCR is determined by infusing a radioactively labeled steroid in tracer amounts at a constant rate over several hours. The MCR is calculated according to the following formula:

$$MCR = \frac{\text{Tracer administered/time}}{\text{Tracer concentration}}$$
$$= \frac{\text{Counts/min/day}}{\text{Counts/min/liter}} = \text{Liters/day}$$

The concentration (C) of steroid can be measured by radioimmunoassay, and when both MCR and C are known, the PR is determined by multiplying the MCR by C: PR = MCR × C = liters/day × amount/liter = amount/day. Normal C, MCR, and PR of androgens, estrogens, and progesterone at different phases of the menstrual cycle have been calculated (Table 4-4).

Hormone Action

In contrast to the membrane receptors of protein hormones, steroid hormone receptors are intracellular. Steroid hormone receptors will bind a specific class of steroids. Thus estrogen receptors will bind natural and synthetic estrogens but not gestagens or androgens. The affinity of a receptor for a steroid correlates with steroid potency. Thus the estrogen receptor has a greater affinity for estradiol than estrone or estriol. After the steroid hormone (S) is bound to its receptor (R), a hormone-receptor (SR) complex forms. The steroid induces a change in receptor conformation that allows it to pass through the nuclear membrane (transformation). It was previously thought that the hormone receptor complex passes from the cytoplasm through the nuclear membrane into the nucleus (translocation), but current information indicates that all steroid receptors are located in the nucleus. After transformation, mRNA is then generated from a segment of DNA (transcription). The mRNA migrates into the cytoplasm, where it attaches to ribosomes and translates information so that they synthesize new protein (Figure 4-21).

The magnitude of the signal to the cell depends on the concentration of both hormones

TABLE 4-4
Plasma Concentrations (C), Metabolic Clearance Rates (MCR), and Production Rates (PR) of Androgens, Estrogens, and Progesterone During Menstrual Cycle

Steroid Hormone	Phase of Cycle	Plasma Concentration*			Metabolic Clearance Rate Plasma* (L/day)	Production Rate (mg/day) (PR = C × MCR)	
		Mean	Range	Units		Mean	Range
Androstenedione	†	1.4	0.7-3.1	ng/ml	2000	2.8	1.4-6.2
Testosterone	†	0.35	0.15-0.55	ng/ml	700	0.25	0.1-0.4
Dehydroepiandros-terone	†	4.2	2.7-7.8	ng/ml	1600	6.7	4.8-12.5
Dehydroepiandros-terone sulfate	†	1.6	0.8-3.4	µg/ml	7	11.2	5.6-23.8
Estradiol	Follicular	44	20-120	pg/ml	1350	0.059	0.027-0.162
	Preovulatory	250	150-600	pg/ml	1350	0.338	0.203-0.810
	Luteal	110	40-300	pg/ml	1350	0.149	0.054-0.405
Estrone	Follicular	40		pg/ml	2200	0.088	
	Preovulatory	170		pg/ml	2200	0.374	
	Luteal	92		pg/ml	2200	0.202	
Estrone-sulfate	Follicular	470		pg/ml	146	0.069	
	Luteal	890		pg/ml	146	0.130	
Progesterone	Follicular	0.2	0.06-0.37	ng/ml	2300	0.46	0.14-0.85
	Luteal	8.9	4.3-19.4	ng/ml	2300	20.5	9.9-45.0

From Stanczyk FZ: Steroid hormones. In Mishell DR, Davajan V, and Lobo RA, editors: Infertility, contraception and reproductive endocrinology, ed 3, Cambridge, Mass, 1991, Blackwell Scientific Publications.
*These values may vary somewhat depending on investigator and method.
†Unspecified. No major changes during menstrual cycle.

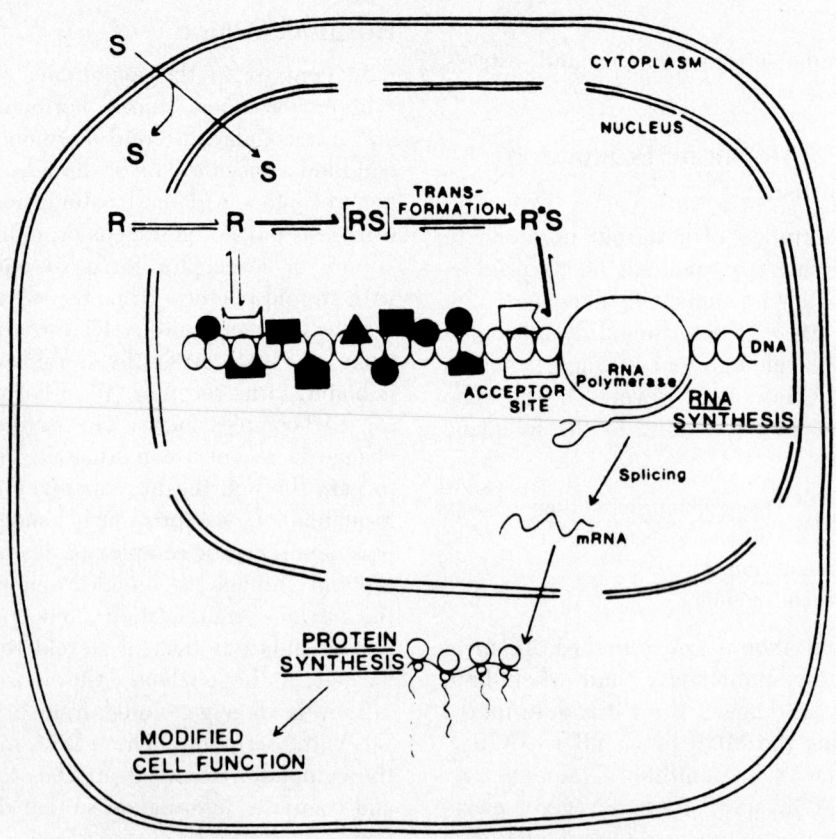

FIGURE 4-21
Revised model of steroid-receptor interaction and induction of cellular response. For simplicity, molecular aspects of receptor structure have been omitted. (From Walters MR: Endocrinol Rev 6:512, 1985.)

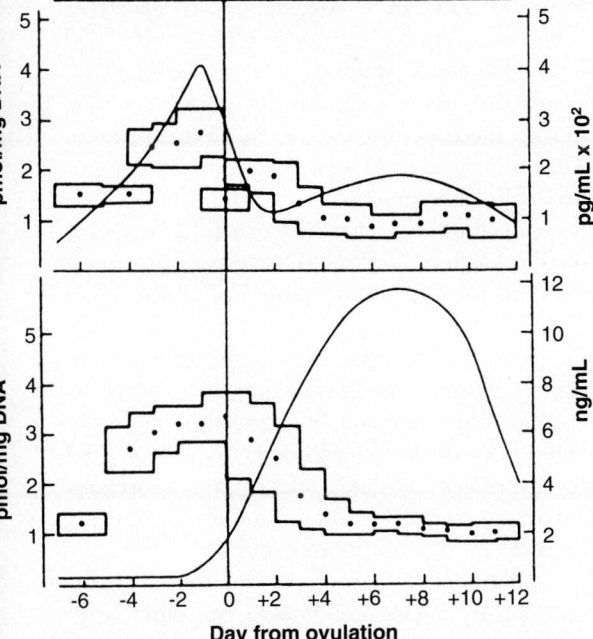

FIGURE 4-22
Estradiol and progesterone receptors in endometrial cells during normal menstrual cycle. Concentrations of estradiol receptor *(upper panel)* and of total progesterone receptor *(lower panel)* for each day of cycle were pooled with those of adjacent days. Each point represents the mean of pooled values. It is surrounded by a rectangle, with its abscissa extending from preceding to following day to account for imprecision of dating and with its ordinate equal to twice the standard error of the mean. Curves represent mean values of plasma estradiol *(upper panel)* and progesterone *(lower panel)*. (From Levy C, Robel P, Gautray JP, et al: Am J Obstet Gynecol 136:646, 1980.)

(S) and receptors (R), as well as on the affinity (K) of the receptor for hormone. Thus the hormone effect may be altered by receptor concentration and affinity, as well as by concentration of the hormone in the circulation. Affinity is quantitatively characterized by a constant derived from the law of mass action.

$$S + R \underset{k_d}{\overset{k_a}{\rightleftharpoons}} SR$$

The association constant, K_a, is determined by dividing the rate constant for association, k_a, by the rate constant for dissociation, k_d. The dissociation constant, K_d, is the inverse of K_a;

therefore, $K_d = 1/K_a$. The K_d is equal to the concentration of the hormone when half the receptor sites are occupied. Receptor affinity is correlated with the physiologic concentration of the hormone. Steroid hormones are present in concentrations of 10^{-10} to 10^{-8} M, and most steroid receptors have a K_d of 10^{-9}.

Estrogen stimulates the synthesis of both estrogen and progesterone receptors in target tissues such as the endometrium. Progestins inhibit the synthesis of both estrogen and progesterone receptors. Thus receptor content in the endometrium peaks about midcycle and then decreases (Figure 4-22). Mitotic activity and endometrial growth rates therefore peak at midcycle. Progestins also increase the intracellular synthesis of estradiol dehydrogenase, which converts the more potent estradiol to the less potent estrone, further decreasing estrogenic activity in the target cell.

Antiestrogens, such as clomiphene or tamoxifen, bind to the estrogen receptor but initiate little transcription. Thus estrogen receptors are depleted without new receptor synthesis or estrogenic action.

EFFECTS OF HORMONES ON SPECIFIC REPRODUCTIVE FACTORS

Ovarian Gametogenesis (Oogenesis)

Oogenesis begins in fetal life when the primordial germ cells migrate to the genital ridge. These germ cells, oogonia, increase in number by mitotic division from about 600,000 in the second month to 7 million in the seventh month of fetal life. The oogonia then begin meiotic division and are called primary oocytes. Just prior to birth the primary oocytes, which now number 2 to 4 million, reach the diplotene stage of development, also called the germinal vesicle stage. At this stage they stay quiescent or undergo atresia until puberty, at which time some of the oocytes mature and complete their meiotic division.

The primary oocyte that is still in the diplotene stage of its first meiotic division is covered by a single layer of granulosa cells and constitutes the primordial follicle. Even without gonadotrophin stimulation, some primordial follicles develop into (primary) preantral follicles, which are oocytes covered by multiple layers of granulosa cells (Figure 4-23). This process occurs in all premenopausal women during

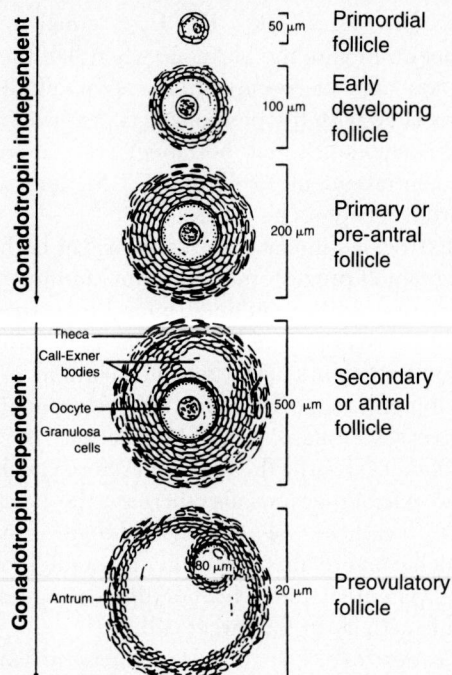

Gonadotropin independent

Gonadotropin dependent

50 μm   Primordial follicle

100 μm   Early developing follicle

200 μm   Primary or pre-antral follicle

Theca
Call-Exner bodies
Oocyte
Granulosa cells
500 μm   Secondary or antral follicle

Antrum
80 μm
20 μm   Preovulatory follicle

FIGURE 4-23
Follicle development. Progress beyond primary follicle stage depends on FSH stimulation. (From Paulson RJ: Oocytes: from development to fertilization. In Mishell DR Jr, Davajan V, and Lobo RA, editors: Infertility, contraception and reproductive endocrinology, ed 3, Cambridge, Mass, 1991, Blackwell Scientific Publications.)

the nonovulatory states of childhood, pregnancy, and oral contraceptive use, as well as during ovulatory cycles. Nearly all these follicles become atretic, but under the influence of FSH in ovulatory cycles, some of them develop to the antrum stage.

Under the influence of FSH the number of granulosa cells in the primordial follicle increases dramatically, and the follicle matures into a primary (preantral) follicle. As the number of granulosa cells increases under the influence of LH and FSH, there is a concomitant parallel increase in estradiol production and secretion. Estradiol stimulates preantral follicle growth, reduces follicle atresia, and increases FSH action on the granulosa cells. Testosterone, on the other hand, increases follicle atresia and prevents preantral follicle growth. Ross et al. suggested that local concentration of estrogens and androgens within the follicle de-

termines whether a specific follicle grows or becomes atretic.

The follicle destined to become dominant secretes the greatest amount of estradiol, which in turn increases the density of FSH receptors. Thus mitotic activity and the number of granulosa cells also increase. In addition, the rising concentration of estradiol exerts a negative feedback effect of FSH release from the pituitary, which halts development of all the other follicles so that they become atretic. In addition, granulosa cells secrete a nonsteroidal substance, inhibin, which also suppresses FSH secretion. The dominant follicle continues to develop because it has a greater density of FSH receptors, and its theca cells become more vascularized than the other follicles, allowing more FSH to reach its receptors.

As the oocyte develops, it becomes surrounded by the zona pellucida, and fluid accumulates in the follicle. The zona pellucida is a mucopolysaccaride coat containing specific protein sites that allow only spermatozoa of the same species to penetrate and fertilize the ovum. Underneath the zona pellucida is the vitelline membrane, which surrounds the ooplasm. Cortical granules form just below this membrane as the oocyte matures. Once the zona pellucida has been penetrated by a single sperm cell, these granules are released and block further sperm penetration (Figure 4-24). The follicular fluid contains estrogens, androgens, and various proteins. Granulosa cells are not just recipients of regulatory protein hormones. As mentioned earlier, granulosa cells have also been shown to secrete various peptides such as inhibin and activin, which regulate hormone synthesis in the ovary and hormone release from the pituitary gland. Several of the proteins in follicular fluid are now being characterized, and they, in addition to the steroids, appear to help regulate follicle maturation by acting within the follicle to alter gonadotrophin action. As the granulosa cells proliferate, LH receptors appear on their surface membrane; when LH binds to these receptors, granulosa cell proliferation ceases and the cells begin to secrete progesterone.

The pattern of follicular growth, as determined by ultrasonography, has been correlated with the endocrine pattern in several studies. Eissa et al., as well as Zegers-Hochschild et al., correlated these parameters in 43 cycles in which conception occurred. Both these groups

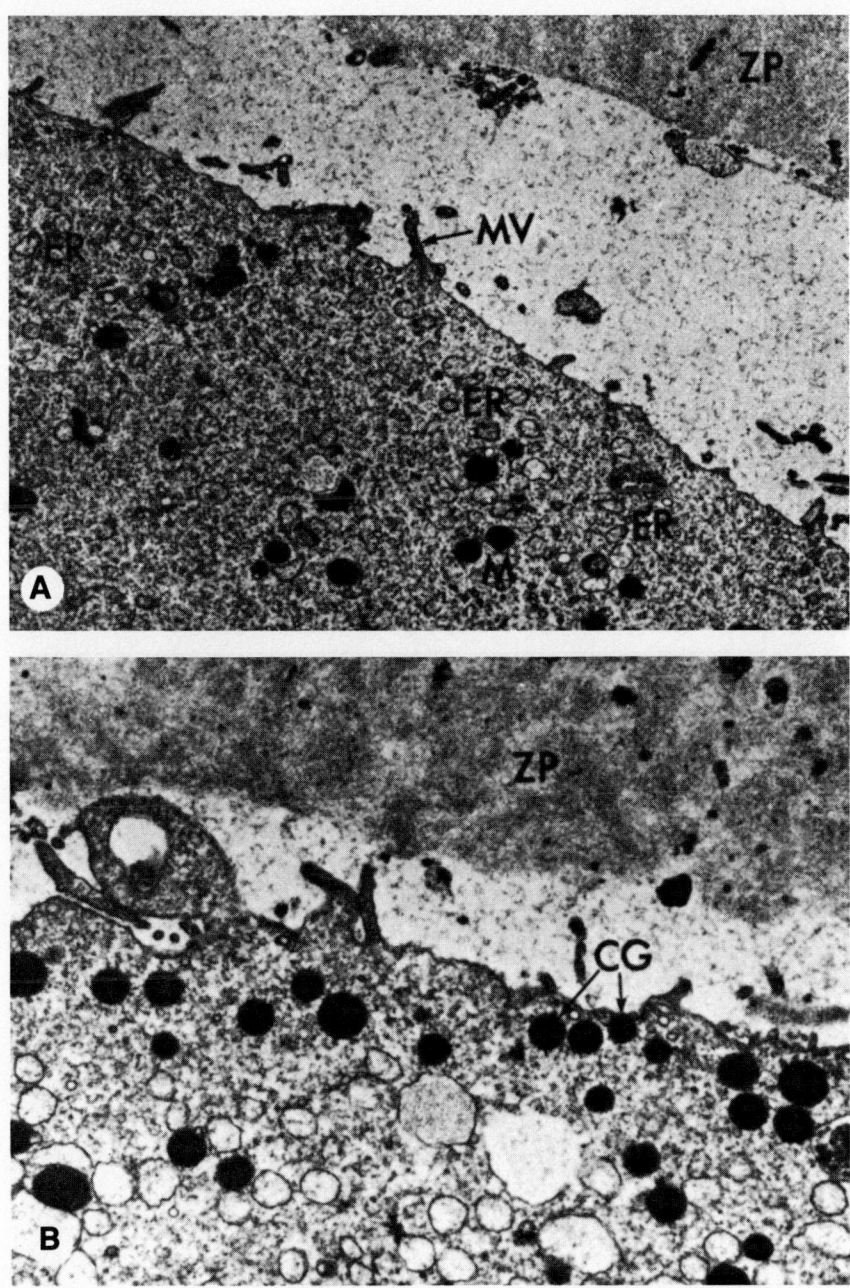

FIGURE 4-24

A, Surface of fertilized ovum, showing absence of cortical granules. A few microvilli *(MV)* are projecting into perivitelline space, which has been widened by retraction of ooplasm from zona pellucida *(ZP)*. Dense mitochondria *(M)* and large vesicular components of endoplasmic reticulum *(ER)* are visible in ooplasm. The egg was fixed 3 hours after insemination in vitro. (×15,400.) **B,** Surface of unfertilized ovum that had been inseminated for 3 hours. Numerous extremely electron-dense cortical granules *(CG)* are present beneath vitelline membrane. Zona pellucida *(ZP)* has a fine fibrillar appearance. (×19,600.) (From Lopata A, Sathananthan AM, McBain JC, et al: Fertil Steril 33:12, 1980. Reproduced with permission of the publisher, The American Fertility Society.)

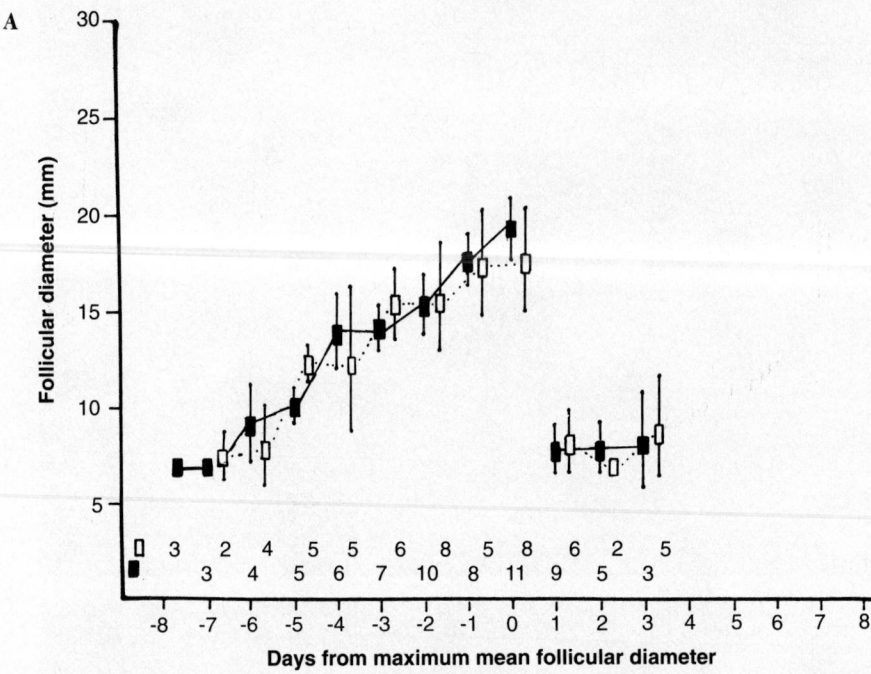

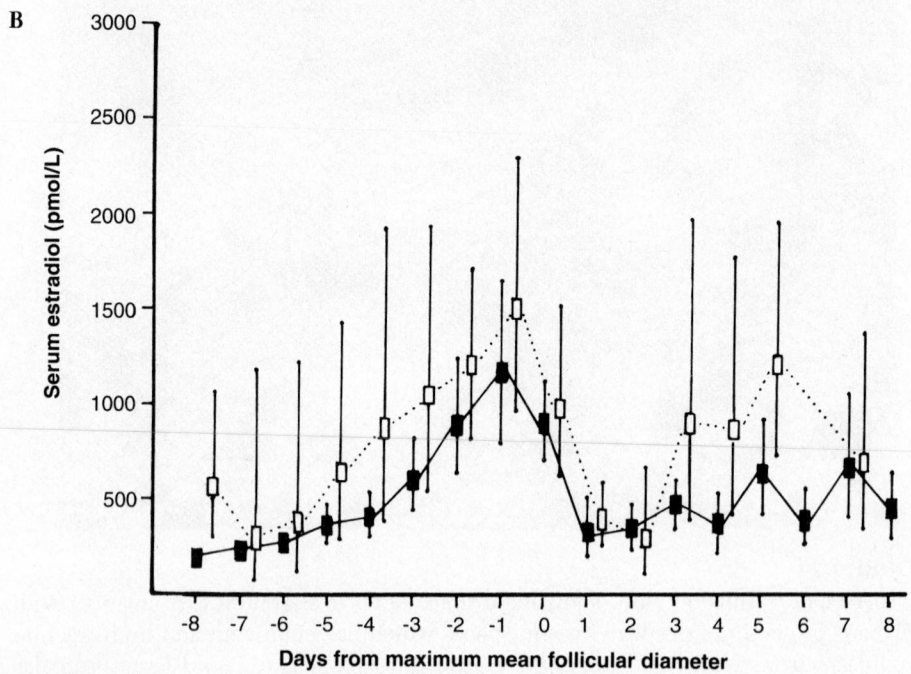

FIGURE 4-25
Correlation of follicular diameter with follicular growth and volume with estradiol in 11 spontaneous and 8 induced conception cycles. (Redrawn from Eissa MK, Obhrai MS, Docker MF, et al: Fertil Steril 45:191, 1986. Reproduced with permission of the publisher, The American Fertility Society.)

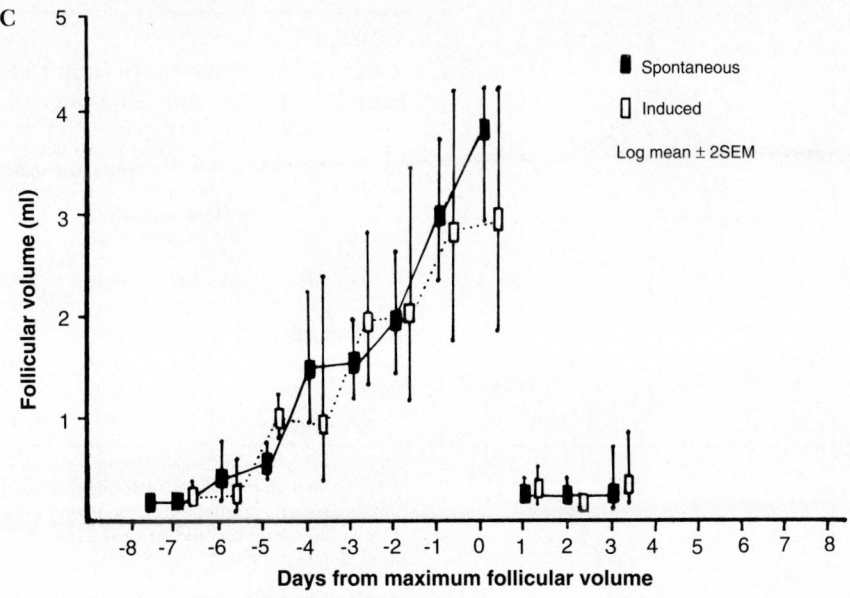

FIGURE 4-25, cont'd
For legend see opposite page.

found a steady increase in follicular diameter and volume that parallels the rise in estradiol (Figure 4-25).

As determined by ultrasonography, the dominant follicle has a maximal mean diameter of about 19.5 mm, with a range of 18 to 25 mm just before ovulation. The mean maximal follicular volume is 3.8 ml, with a range of 3.1 to 8.2 ml. The investigators just mentioned, as well as others, have shown that the maximal size of the dominant follicle can vary among different women. LeMay et al. have shown that the mean maximal diameter of the preovulatory follicle can vary in the same woman in different cycles.

About 80% of the approximately 500 mg of estradiol produced daily just before ovulation comes from the dominant follicle. The rapidly rising estradiol levels, in combination with a small but significant increase in progesterone produced by the dominant follicle, serve as the signal to the hypothalamic-pituitary axis that the follicle is ready to ovulate. When estradiol levels rise substantially at midcycle, to about 200 pg/ml or higher for 2 or more days, LH secretion is stimulated (positive feedback) (Figure 4-26). Apparently the small preovulatory increase in progesterone also stimulates the release of LH and may be responsible for the midcycle FSH surge. Thus by a positive feedback, these steroids elicit a surge in LH and FSH release from the pituitary. The midcycle LH surge initiates the ovulatory process.

A task force of the World Health Organization correlated the temporal relation of changes in hormone levels with the time of ovulation as determined by histologic examination of the maturity of the corpus luteum, which had been removed at the time of subsequent laparotomy in 78 women. With the use of those parameters, it was determined that ovulation occurs about 24 hours after the estradiol peak. Ovulation occurs about 32 hours after the initial rise in LH levels and about 12 to 16 hours after the peak of LH levels in serum (Table 4-5). Using ultrasonography to detect the time of ovulation, LeMay et al. reported that ovulation occurs between 18 and 48 hours after the initial rise in LH levels. With serial ultrasound definition and LH measurements, Eissa et al. and Zegers-Hochschild et al. reported that in conception cycles, ovulation usually occurs within 24 hours and always within 48 hours after the LH peak.

The midcycle LH surge initiates germinal vesicle disruption, and metaphase I is completed. As the oocyte enters metaphase II, the first polar body appears. Completion of meiosis

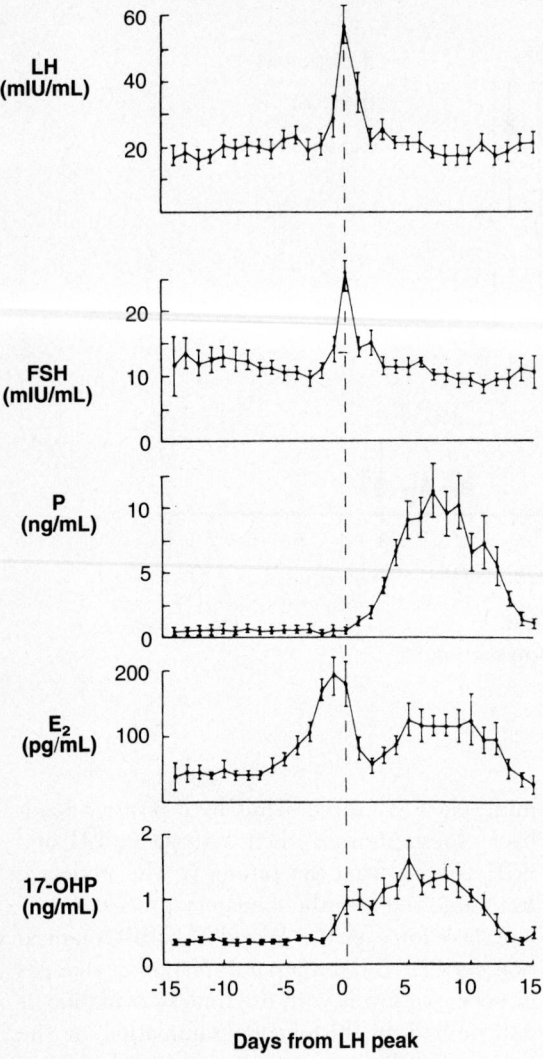

FIGURE 4-26
Means and standard errors of serum *LH*, *FSH*, progesterone *(P)*, estradiol *(E₂)*, and 17-hydroxyprogesterone *(17-OHP)* levels measured in nine women daily during entire ovulatory menstrual cycle. Individual daily results were grouped according to day of midcycle LH peak and averaged. (From Thorneycroft IH, Mishell DR Jr, Stone SC, et al: Am J Obstet Gynecol 111:947, 1971.)

and extrusion of the second polar body occur only when a spermatozoon penetrates the ovum. In preparation for follicular rupture, LH stimulates synthesis of both $PGF_{2\alpha}$ and PGE and proteolytic enzymes (collagenase). The rise in FSH levels stimulates production of a plasminogen activator, which converts plasminogen to the proteolytic enzyme plasmin. Plasmin helps to detach the cumulus from the parietal granulosa cells and thus aids in the process of

TABLE 4-5
Range of Observed Times from Defined Hormonal Events and Time of Ovulation

| Hormone | Time of Ovulation (hours) from Rise to Peak | | | |
| | First Significant Rise | | Peak | |
	Median	Range	Median	Range
17β-Estradiol	82.5	48-168	24.0	0-48
LH	32.0	24-56	16.5	8-40
FSH	21.1	8-24	15.3	8-40
Progesterone	7.8	0-32	—	—

From World Health Organization: Temporal relationships between ovulation and defined changes in the concentration of plasma estradiol-17β, luteinizing hormone, follicle-stimulating hormone, and progesterone, Am J Obstet Gynecol 138:383, 1980.

extrusion of the egg and cumulus at the time of follicle rupture.

After the oocyte is extruded, the amount of follicular fluid is markedly reduced, the follicular wall becomes convoluted, and the follicular diameter and volume greatly decrease. These changes are detectable by ultrasonography (Figure 4-27). As the granulosa and theca cells become luteinized, they take up lipids and lutein pigment, giving them a yellow coloration. The granulosa cell layer becomes vascularized only after ovulation. Under the influence of LH, the corpus luteum produces progesterone in amounts of about 20 mg/24 hours and also secretes estradiol.

Levels of progesterone steadily increase in the serum after ovulation and plateau about 1 week later, after which they decline unless pregnancy occurs. The increasing levels of progesterone and estradiol exert a negative feedback on FSH and LH secretion. Estradiol inhibits mainly FSH (negative feedback), whereas progesterone inhibits mainly LH. There is also evidence that the luteal estradiol production exerts a local luteolytic action. It is postulated that increased intraovarian progesterone concentration prevents follicle maturation in that ovary in the subsequent cycle.

As luteolysis occurs and estradiol and progesterone levels decline, there is less negative feedback. Therefore FSH and LH levels begin to rise before the onset of menstruation to stimulate follicular growth for the next cycle.

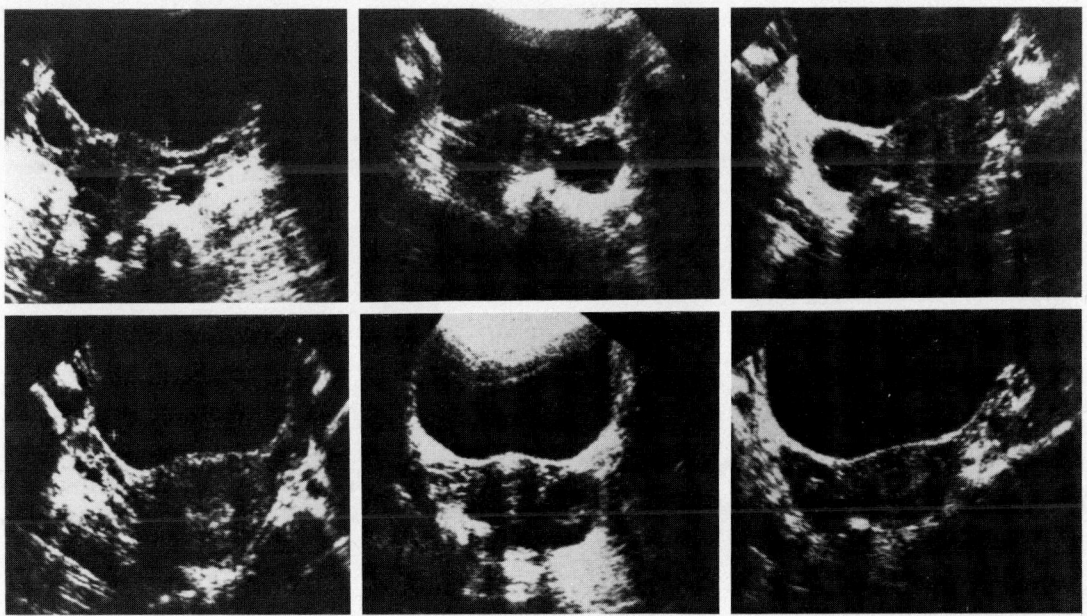

FIGURE 4-27
Ultrasonographic signs of ovulation: complete disappearance *(left)*, loss of volume and thickening of wall *(middle)*, and replacement by irregular spongy area *(right)*. (From Wetzels LCG and Hoogland HJ: Fertil Steril 37:336, 1982. Reproduced with permission of the publisher, The American Fertility Society.)

Estradiol and progesterone exert both a direct inhibitory effect on pituitary gonadotrophin synthesis and secretion and an effect on GnRH release, altering the frequency as well as the amplitude of GnRH pulses. The steroid feedback on GnRH release occurs by a direct effect on the neurotransmitters (dopamine and norepinephrine) and the neuromodulators (β-endorphin) in the arcuate nucleus.

Three studies by Reame et al., Crowley et al., and Filicori et al. have shown that the frequency of LH peaks, and presumably of GnRH pulses, when blood sampling was performed every 10 minutes, changes throughout the menstrual cycle. In sleep there is a close relationship between the frequency of GnRH pulses in portal blood and the frequency of LH pulses in the peripheral circulation. In the early follicular phase, LH pulses occur about once every 90 minutes, with an absence of pulsation during sleep (Figure 4-28). The frequency of LH pulses significantly increases in the middle and late follicular phases to about one pulse per hour throughout the day and night. The amplitude of LH pulses is low and decreases somewhat between the early and middle follicular phases; however, during the late follicular (preovulatory) phase, LH ampli-

tude significantly increases (Figure 4-29). LH pulse frequency progressively slows in the luteal phase from about one pulse every 90 minutes in the early luteal phase to about one every 3 hours in the late luteal phase (Figure 4-30). The amplitude of LH pulses varies after ovulation, with a bimodal distribution of small and large pulses. Overall mean LH levels are higher in the luteal phase than the follicular phase (Figure 4-31). Similar changes in FSH pulsation in peripheral blood do not occur, probably because of its longer half-life.

The increase in frequency of LH pulses during the late follicular phase is probably important in stimulating follicular secretion of estradiol, since 80% of LH pulses are followed by a rise in circulating estradiol levels. An increased amplitude of LH pulses is observed during the midcycle LH surge, probably because of either an increased frequency of GnRH pulsations or the positive feedback effect of increasing levels of estradiol and progesterone on increasing gonadotrophin responsiveness to GnRH. Middle to late luteal LH pulses stimulate progesterone production. Bächström et al. and Filicori et al. have shown that beginning in the midluteal phase, progesterone is secreted in a pulsatile manner, with increases occurring immediately

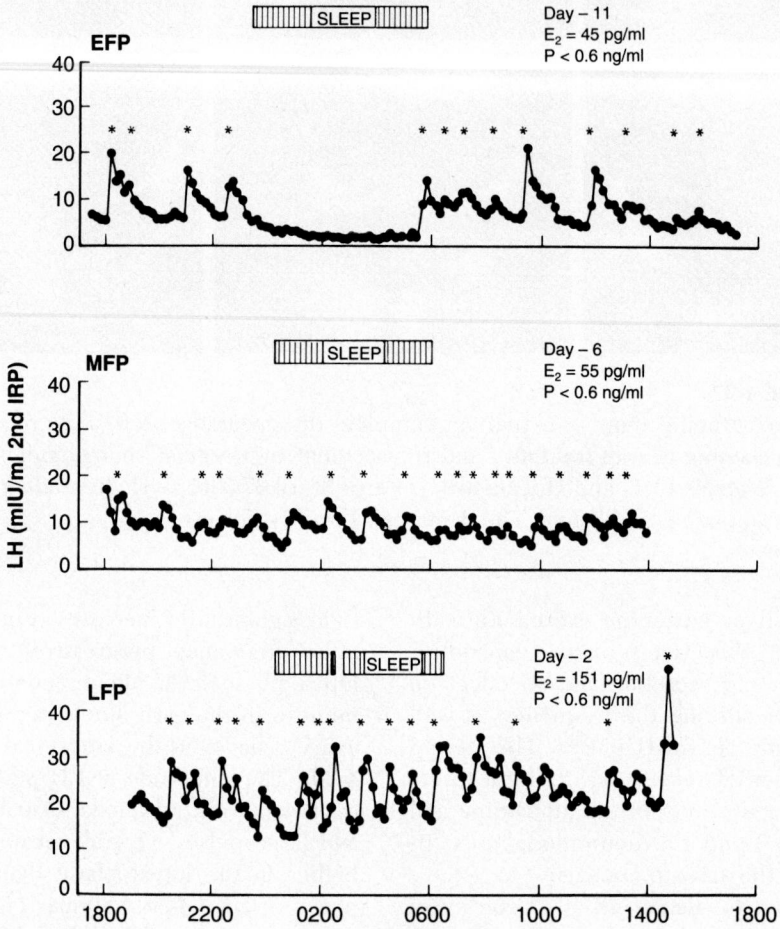

FIGURE 4-28

Patterns of episodic LH secretion throughout follicular phase of menstrual cycle. Representative examples of early follicular phase *(EFP)*, midfollicular phase *(MFP)*, and late follicular phase *(LFP)* series are shown. Stage of follicular phase is indicated from Day 0. LH pulsations are indicated by asterisks. Levels of prostaglandin E_2 and progesterone represent mean of samples obtained at 6-hour intervals. Sleep is indicated by hatched bars. *P*, Progesterone. (From Filicori M, Santoro N, Merriam GR, et al: J Clin Endocrinol Metab 62:1136, 1986.)

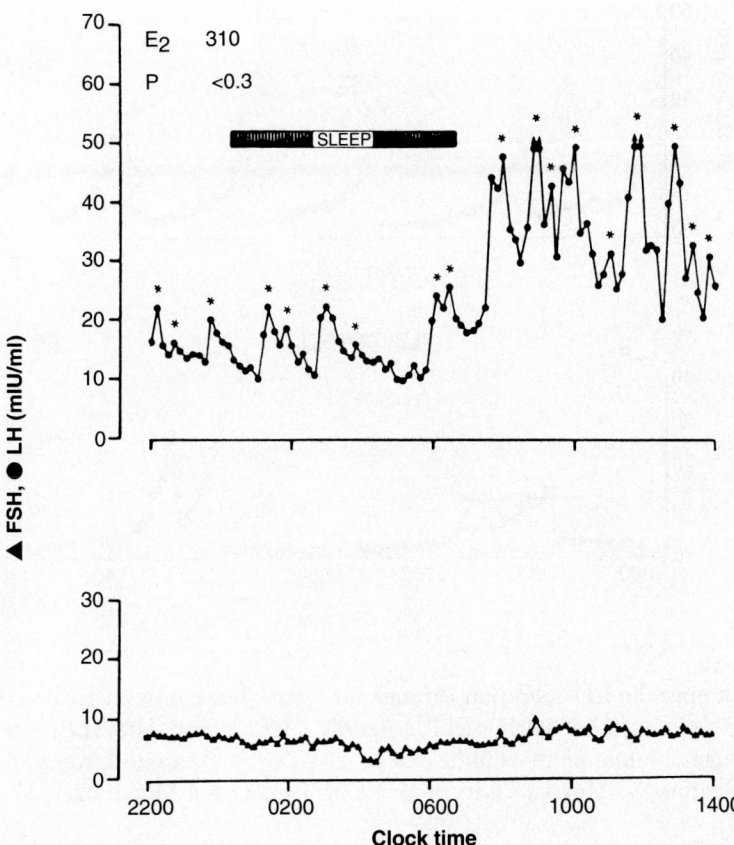

FIGURE 4-29
LH secretory response in normal woman studied on day of LH surge. Note increase in amplitude and frequency of GnRH secretion, absence of any day-night
variation, and discernible FSH pulsations. (From Crowley WF, Filicori M, Spratt
DI, et al: Recent Prog Horm Res 41:473, 1985.)

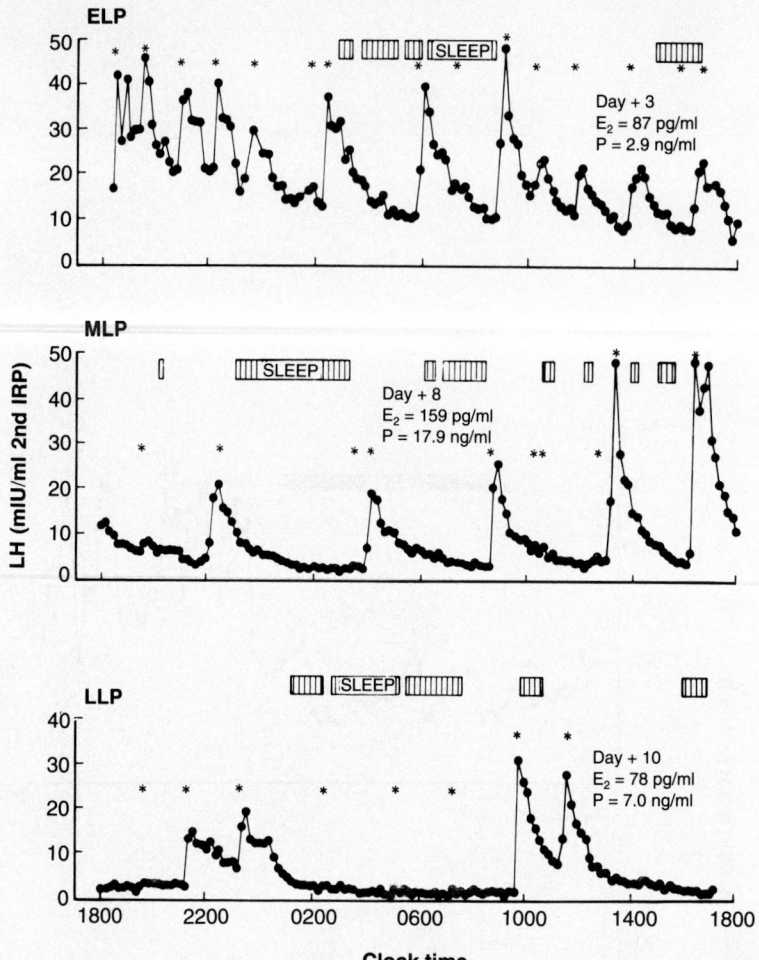

FIGURE 4-30
Patterns of episodic LH secretion throughout luteal phase of menstrual cycle. Representative examples of early *(ELP)*, middle *(MLP)*, and late *(LLP)* series are shown. Stage of luteal phase is indicated as post-Day 0. *P*, progesterone. (From Filicori M, Santoro N, Merriam GR, et al: J Clin Endocrinol Metab 62:1136, 1986.)

following an LH pulse (see Figure 4-30). The variations in LH pulse amplitude and the slower frequency in the midluteal phase are probably caused by the negative feedback effects of progesterone and estradiol. Filicori et al. have postulated that the decrease in LH frequency is due to an action of progesterone on hypothalamic release of GnRH, possibly being mediated through increased levels of β-endorphin, whereas the decrease in amplitude of LH pulses is due to a negative feedback effect of progesterone on the pituitary.

The patterns of FSH and LH levels obtained by radioimmunoassay (RIA) measurement in serum are similar to the patterns observed by bioassay of urinary extracts except that the midcycle FSH peak occurs 2 days later and is

more pronounced, probably because of the longer half-life of FSH in serum (Figure 4-32). The amounts of urinary FSH and LH excretion are about 1 to 10 IU/24 hr, whereas serum levels fluctuate between 1 and 100 mIU/ml.

Excretion of the three classic estrogens, estrone, estradiol, and estriol, is lowest during the early follicular phase, peaks just before LH peaks, decreases shortly thereafter, and rises in the luteal phase, after which it falls again. The luteal-phase rise of these estrogens is of smaller amplitude but longer duration than the preovulatory peak (Figure 4-33). Midcycle peak urinary excretion of all three estrogens is about 50 to 75 μg/24 hours. Serum levels of estradiol follow a similar pattern throughout the cycle, rising from less than 50 pg/ml in the early follicu-

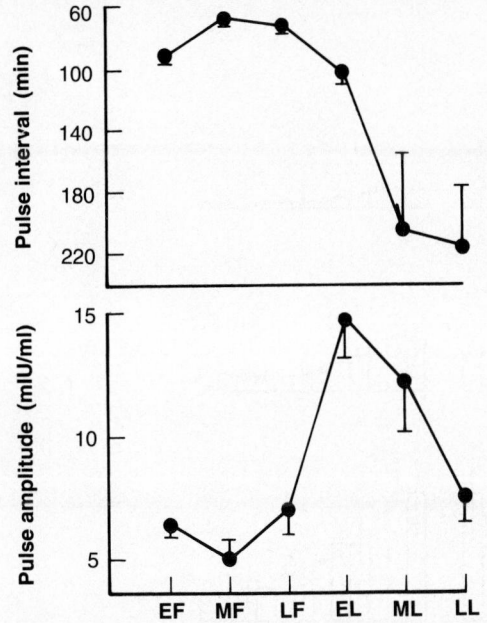

FIGURE 4-31

LH interpulse interval and amplitude during different stages of menstrual cycle. Data shown were obtained by pulse analysis and are expressed as means and standard errors. *EF*, Early follicular phase; *MF*, midfollicular phase; *LF*, late follicular phase; *EL*, early luteal phase; *ML*, midluteal phase; *LL*, late luteal phase. (From Filicori M, Santoro N, Merriam GR, et al: J Clin Endocrinol Metab 62:1136, 1986.)

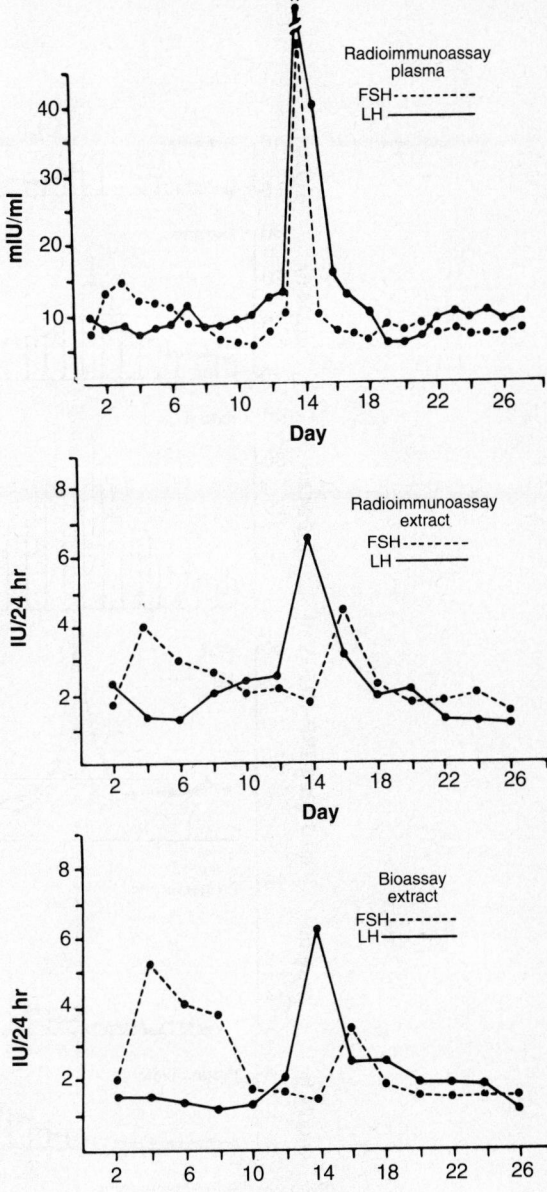

FIGURE 4-32

Serum FSH and LH measured by radioimmunoassay (RIA) and urinary FSH and LH measured by both RIA and bioassay through an entire ovulatory menstrual cycle. (From Stevens VC: J Clin Endocrinol Metab 29:904, 1969. © by The Endocrine Society, 1969.)

lar phase to 200 to 500 pg/ml at midcycle and having a broad luteal-phase peak level of about 100 to 150 pg/ml (see Figure 4-26).

The major metabolite of progesterone excreted in the urine is pregnanediol (PD). Levels of pregnanediol are less than 0.9 µg/24 hours before ovulation (mean, 0.4 µg/24 hours) and consistently greater than 1 µg/24 hours (mean, 3 to 4 µg/24 hours) after ovulation (Figure 4-34). Progesterone levels in serum are less than 1 ng/ml before ovulation and reach midluteal levels of 10 to 20 ng/ml. In cycles followed by conception, several investigators have reported that progesterone levels are always greater than 9 mg/ml. However, as progesterone is secreted in a pulsatile manner with wide fluctuations in its serum levels, a single low serum value may not be indicative of a lack of corpus luteum formation or an inadequate corpus luteum.

Levels of the steroid metabolite 17-hydroxyprogesterone increase concomitantly with the increase of the LH surge, indicating a shift of steroidogenesis from the Δ^5 to the Δ^4 pathway (see Figure 4-26). Levels of 17-hydroxyprogesterone then fall and rise again in the midluteal phase as progesterone and estradiol levels increase. About 4 to 6 days before the onset of menses, levels of estradiol, progesterone, and

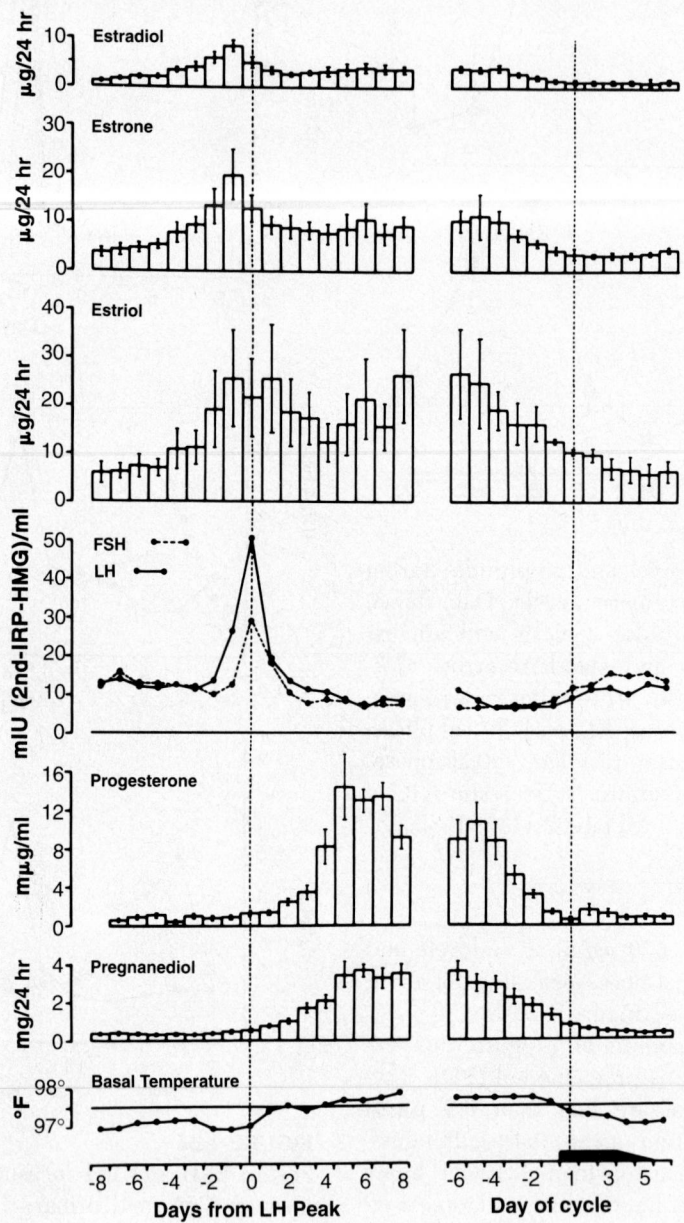

FIGURE 4-33
Mean serum FSH and LH levels, urinary estrogen levels, pregnanediol excretion, and basal body temperatures measured daily in five women during ovulatory menstrual cycle. Bars depict standard errors. Individual results were grouped according to day of midcycle LH surge *(left)* or first day of menstruation *(right)* and averaged. (From Goebelsmann UT, Midgey AR Jr, and Jaffe RB: J Clin Endocrinol Metab 29:1222, 1969. © by The Endocrine Society, 1969.)

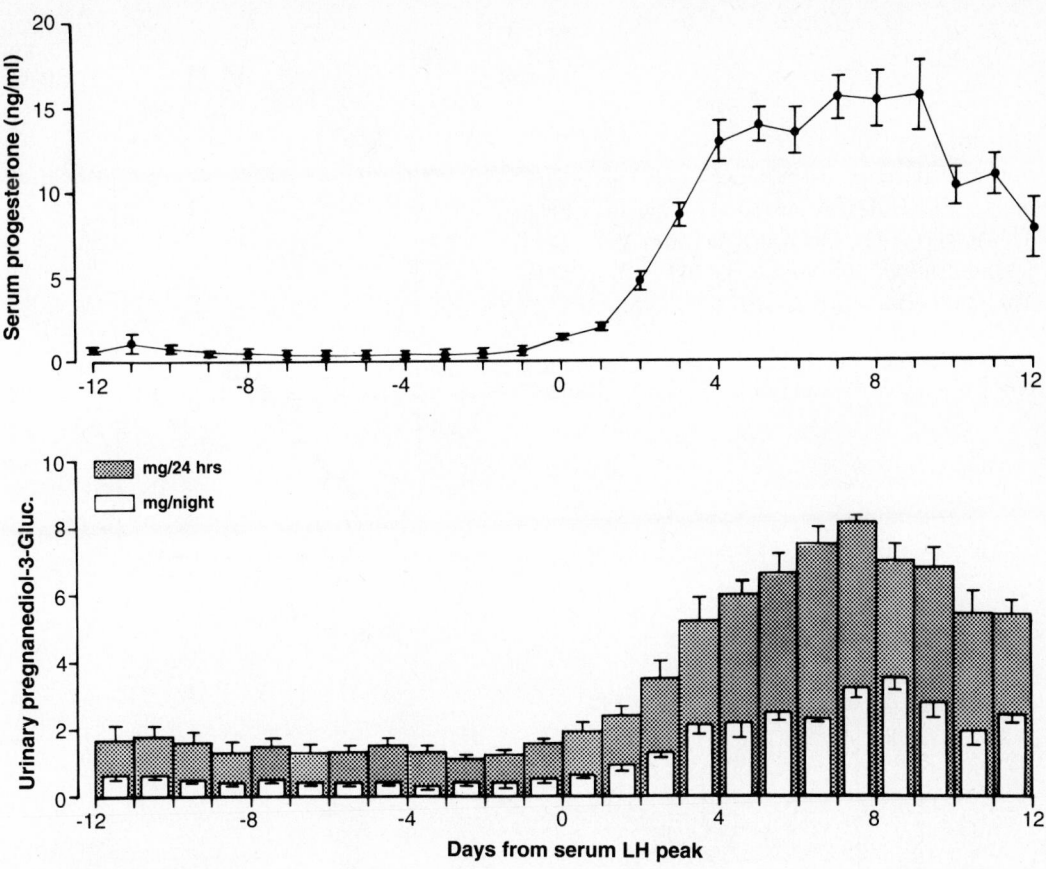

FIGURE 4-34

Means and standard errors of daily 8 AM serum progesterone concentrations and 24-hour (8 AM to 8 AM) and overnight urinary excretion of radioimmunoassayable pregnanediol-3-glucuronide in seven women during entire menstrual cycle. Data obtained in individual subjects were grouped according to day of midcycle LH peak and averaged. (From Stanczyk FZ, Miyakama I, and Goebelsmann UT: Am J Obstet Gynecol 137:443, 1980.)

17-hydroxyprogesterone all begin to decline.

During midcycle the first event is a rise in estradiol. When estradiol reaches peak levels, there is an abrupt increase (surge) in LH and FSH (Figure 4-35). The increase in LH reaches a peak in about 18 hours, and peak levels plateau for about 14 hours, after which there is a decline. The mean duration of the LH surge is about 24 hours. Beginning about 12 hours before the onset of the LH surge, there is an increase of both progesterone and 17-hydroxyprogesterone. With the occurrence of the LH peak there is a decline in estradiol and a further increase in progesterone. This shift in steroidogenesis in favor of progesterone instead of estradiol production is brought about by the luteinization of the granulosa cells produced by LH.

Levels of numerous other hormones have been measured in serum throughout the cycle and summarized in the excellent review by Diczfalusy and Landgren. Serum levels of androstenedione and testosterone change little during the cycle, but mean levels are slightly higher during the follicular than the luteal phase (Figure 4-36). Serum thyroid-stimulating hormone (TSH) levels also remain relatively constant, while adrenocorticotropic hormone (ACTH) and growth hormone (GH) have a preovulatory peak. Prolactin levels appear to be slightly higher in the luteal phase. Steroid hormone metabolites of estradiol, progesterone, and 17-hydroxyprogesterone follow cyclic changes similar to those of the parent hormone. Pregnenolone, 17α-hydroxypregnenolone, and dehydroepiandrostenedione all have a circadian variation, but only pregnenolone rises during the luteal phase. Cortisol, cortico-

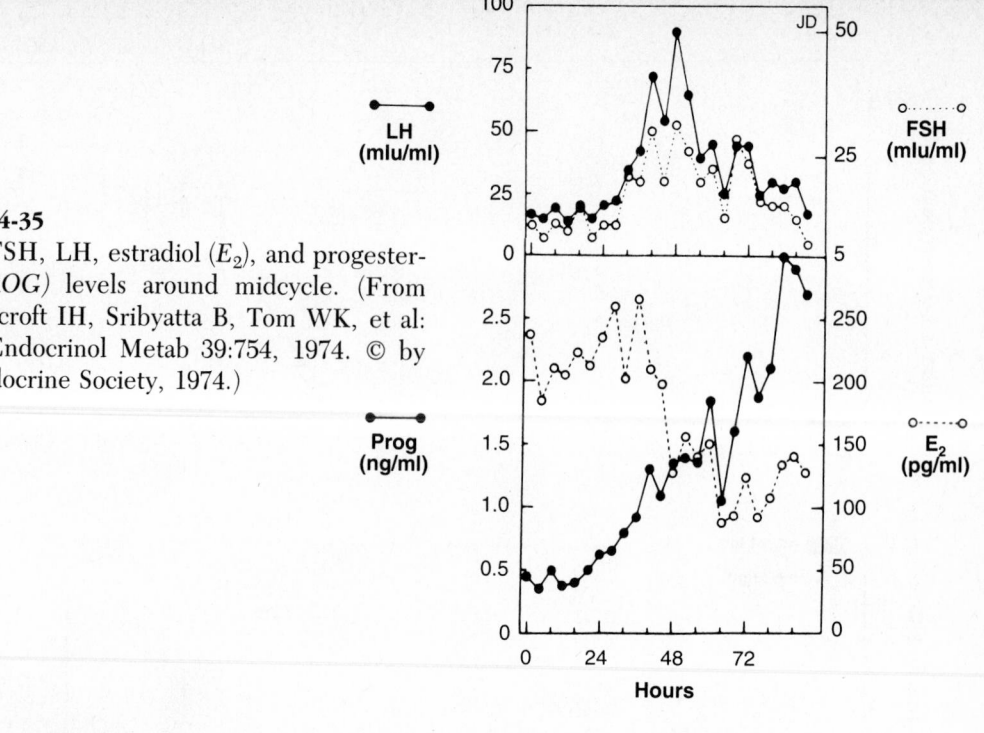

FIGURE 4-35
Serum FSH, LH, estradiol (E_2), and progesterone *(PROG)* levels around midcycle. (From Thorneycroft IH, Sribyatta B, Tom WK, et al: J Clin Endocrinol Metab 39:754, 1974. © by The Endocrine Society, 1974.)

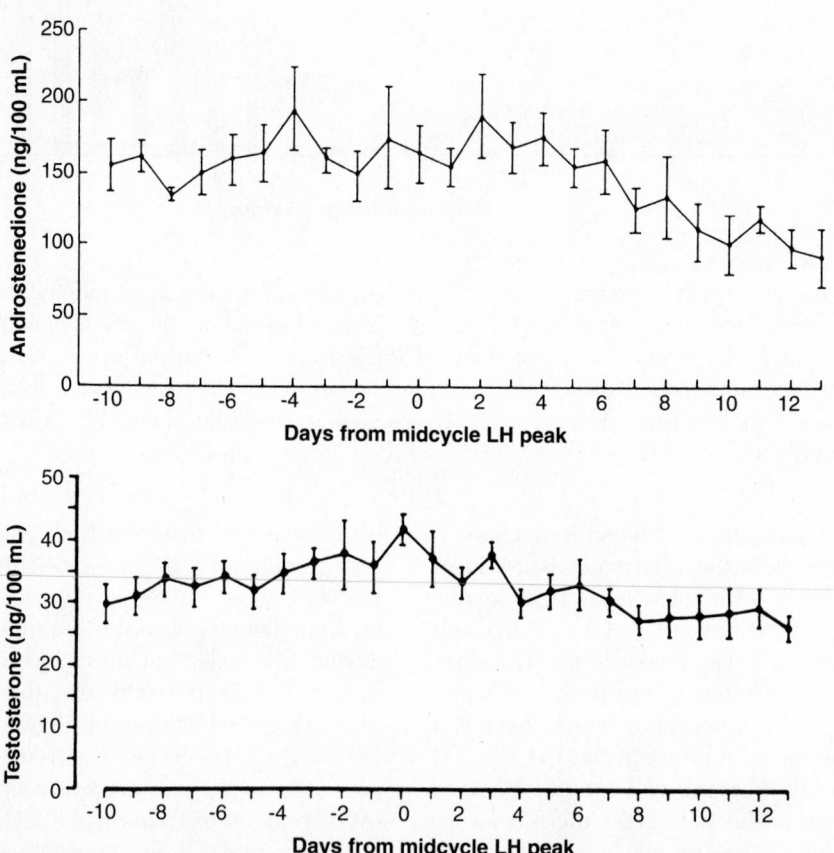

FIGURE 4-36
Upper panel: Means and standard errors of serum androstenedione concentrations measured in six women daily during entire ovulatory menstrual cycle. Individual daily results were grouped according to day of preovulatory serum estradiol peak and averaged. *Lower panel:* Means and standard errors of serum testosterone concentrations measured daily in eight women during entire ovulatory menstrual cycle. Individual daily results were grouped according to day of midcycle LH peak and averaged. (From Ribeiro WO, Mishell DR Jr, and Thorneycroft IH: Am J Obstet Gynecol 119:1026, 1974; and Goebelsmann UT, Arce JJ, Thorneycroft IH, et al: Am J Obstet Gynecol 119:445, 1974.)

steroid, and aldosterone, in addition to having a circadian variation, also increase during the luteal phase.

Menstrual Cycle Length

The mean age of menarche is about 13 years, and the mean age of menopause is about 51 years. Therefore women have menses for a duration of about 38 years. Menstrual cycle length varies among different women and for an individual woman at different times of her life. The most information regarding menstrual cycles comes from the classic study of Treloar et al., who analyzed 275,947 menstrual intervals recorded by more than 2700 women over prolonged periods. Analysis of these data revealed that menstrual cycle length is most irregular in the 2 years after menarche and the 3 years before menopause, times of life during which anovulatory cycles are most frequent (Table 4-6). During these times of life, both shortened and prolonged cycle lengths are common, with the latter being more frequent (Figure 4-37).

Menstrual cycle length is least variable between the ages of 20 and 40 years. During this time there is a gradual decrease of mean cycle length. However, between these ages, menstrual cycle length still varies in an individual woman, as shown by the variation in cycle length recorded by the women, with the most regular duration of menstrual cycles among the several thousand studied by Vollman for many years (Figure 4-38). It is generally accepted that the mean duration of menstrual cycle length is 28 ± 7 days, with the occurrence of shorter cycles (<21 days) being called polymenorrhea and that of longer cycles (>35 days) being called oligomenorrhea. The mean duration of menstrual flow is 4 ± 2 days.

Endometrial Histology

The human endometrium is made up of two basic layers: the stratum basale, which lies above the myometrium, and the stratum functionale, lying between the stratum basale and the uterine lumen. The stratum basale consists of primordial glands and densely cellular stroma, which changes little throughout the menstrual cycle and does not desquamate at the time of menstruation. The stratum functionale is divided into two layers. The superficial,

TABLE 4-6
Means and Standard Deviations in Days for Menstrual Intervals at Selected Ages

Age	Mean (Days)	Standard Deviation (Days)
2 yr after menarche	32.20	8.38
20 yr	30.09	3.94
25 yr	29.84	3.45
30 yr	29.30	3.16
35 yr	28.22	2.67
40 yr	27.26	2.83
3 yr before menopause	33.20	14.24

Data from Treloar AE, Boynton RE, Borghild BG, et al: Variation of the human menstrual cycle through reproductive life, Int J Fertil 12:77, 1967.

narrow stratum compactum consists of the necks of the glands and densely populated stromal cells. The underlying, broader stratum spongiosum consists primarily of glands with less densely populated stroma and large amounts of interstitial tissue. The stratum functionale grows during the cycle, and a portion of it desquamates at the time of menses.

After menstruation the endometrium is only 1 to 2 mm thick and consists mainly of the stratum basale and a portion of the spongiosum. Under the influence of estrogen the stratum functionale proliferates greatly by multiplication of both glandular and stromal cells. Mitotic figures are abundant. In the late follicular phase, glycogen begins to be stored in the glands, which become more tortuous in appearance. Just before ovulation, as estrogen levels peak, the cells lining the gland lumina undergo pseudostratification (Figure 4-39).

Just after ovulation, glycogen-rich subnuclear vacuoles appear in the base of the cells lining the glands (Figure 4-40). This subnuclear vacuolization is the first histologic indication of the effect of progesterone but is not evidence that ovulation has occurred. As progesterone levels increase in the early luteal phase, the glycogen-containing vacuoles ascend toward the gland lumina. Soon thereafter the contents of the glands are released into the endometrial cavity to provide energy to the free-floating blastocyst, which reaches the endometrial cavity about 3½ days after fertilization but does not implant until 1 week after fertilization.

In the midluteal phase the glands become in-

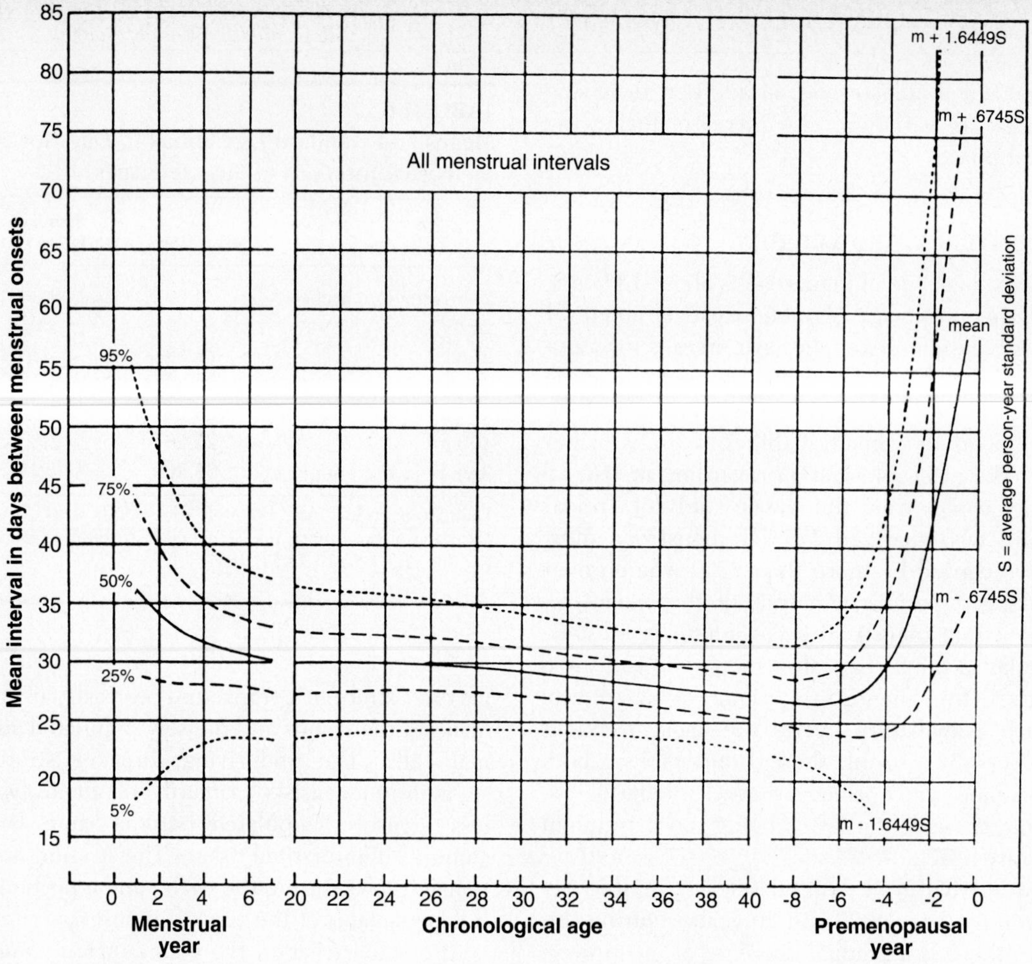

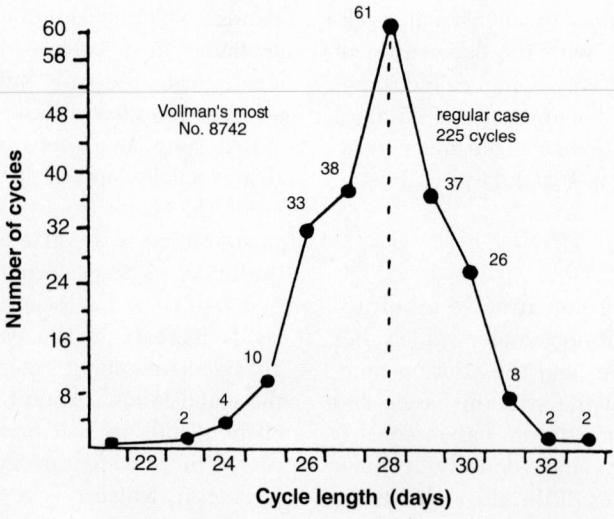

FIGURE 4-37
Normal curve contours for distribution of menstrual intervals in three zones of menstrual life. (From Treloar AE, Boynton RE, Borghild BG, et al: Int J Fertil 12:77, 1967.)

FIGURE 4-38
Frequency distribution of cycle lengths of Vollman's "most regular" subject. (From Hartman CG: The irregularity of the menstrual cycle. In Science and the safe period, Huntington, NY, 1972, RE Krieger Publishing Co.)

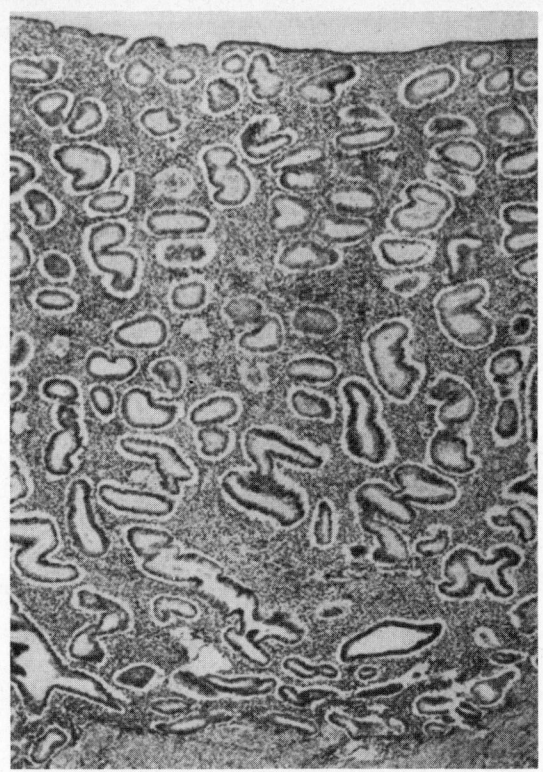

FIGURE 4-39
Early-interval endometrium. (From Novak E and Novak ER, editors: Textbook of gynecology, ed 4, Baltimore, 1952, Williams & Wilkins.)

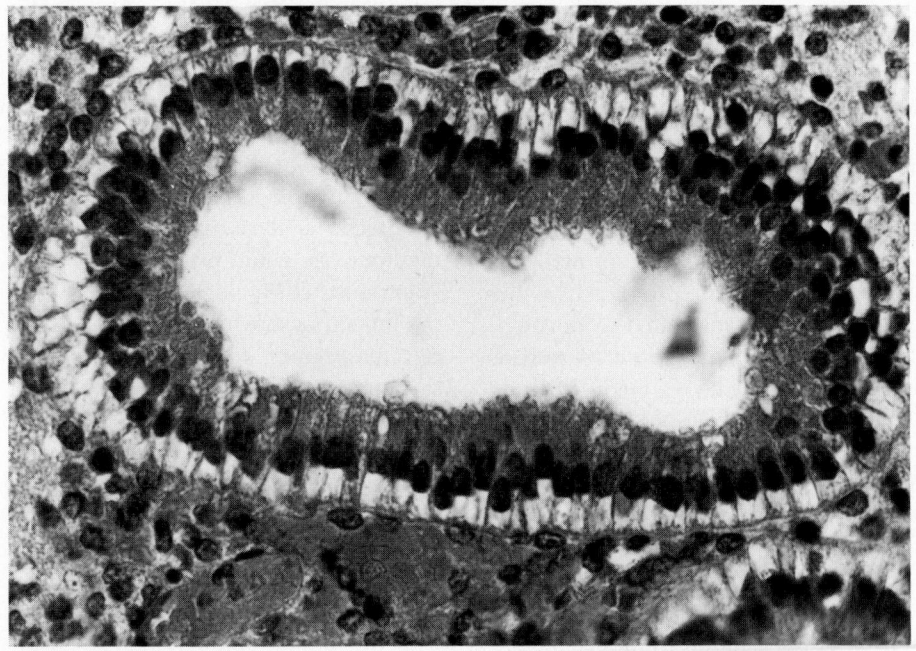

FIGURE 4-40
Subnuclear vacuoles lining base of endometrial gland 2 to 3 days after ovulation. (×500; reduced by 22%.) (From March CM: The endometrium in the menstrual cycle. In Mishell DR Jr, Davajan V, and Lobo RA, editors: Infertility, contraception and reproductive endocrinology, ed 3, Cambridge, Mass, 1991, Blackwell Scientific Publications.)

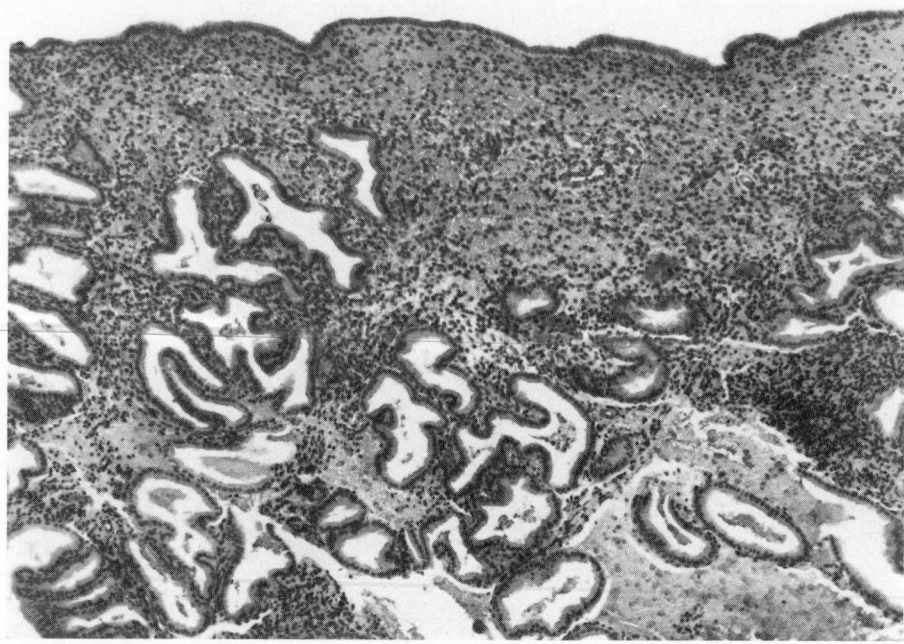

FIGURE 4-41
Maximal secretory activity characteristic of 7 to 8 days after ovulation. (×90; reduced by 22%.) (From March CM: The endometrium in the menstrual cycle. In Mishell DR Jr, Davajan V, and Lobo RA, editors: Infertility, contraception and reproductive endocrinology, ed 3, Cambridge, Mass, 1991, Blackwell Scientific Publications.)

creasingly tortuous and the stroma becomes more edematous and vascular (Figure 4-41). During the secretory phase a specific protein, progestogen-dependent endometrial protein (PEP), is produced by the glandular cells. Circulating levels of this protein correlate with serum progesterone levels, but the exact purpose of PEP has not been determined. In addition to PEP, other peptide hormones, growth factors, and prostaglandins are produced by the endometrium and have roles in the development of decidualized endometrium as well as menstruation. As steroid levels begin to wane in the late luteal phase, if implantation of the blastocyst does not occur and human chorionic gonadotrophin (HCG) is not produced to maintain the corpus luteum, the glands begin to collapse and fragment, and infiltration of the glands and stroma by polymorphonuclear leukocytes and monocytes occurs. Autolysis of the functional zone of the endometrium occurs and desquamation begins. The histologic pattern of the endometrium has been correlated with the phase of the menstrual cycle in the classic study of Noyes et al. (Figure 4-42).

This subjective method of correlating the de-gree of maturation of the endometrium is relatively imprecise. Several blind studies have demonstrated wide variability of both interobserver interpretation and interpretation by the same observer at different intervals. Recently, hormonal levels have been correlated with endometrial indices based on quantitative morphometric analysis. Li et al. noted that this methodology could produce a significant correlation with chronologic dating of the length of the luteal phase when only 5 of 17 morphometric measurements were used. These five measurements were (1) the frequency of mitosis per 1000 gland cells, (2) the amount of secretion in gland lumen, (3) the amount of gland cell pseudostratification, (4) the proportion of glands infused by gland cells, and (5) the amount of predecidual reaction. These authors concluded that use of these objective morphometric criteria resulted in better correlation with the actual length of the luteal phase than did histologic dating by the method of Noyes et al. Numerous authors have now confirmed the day of LH surge is a more appropriate dating correlate than the onset of the next menstrual cycle (Figure 4-43).

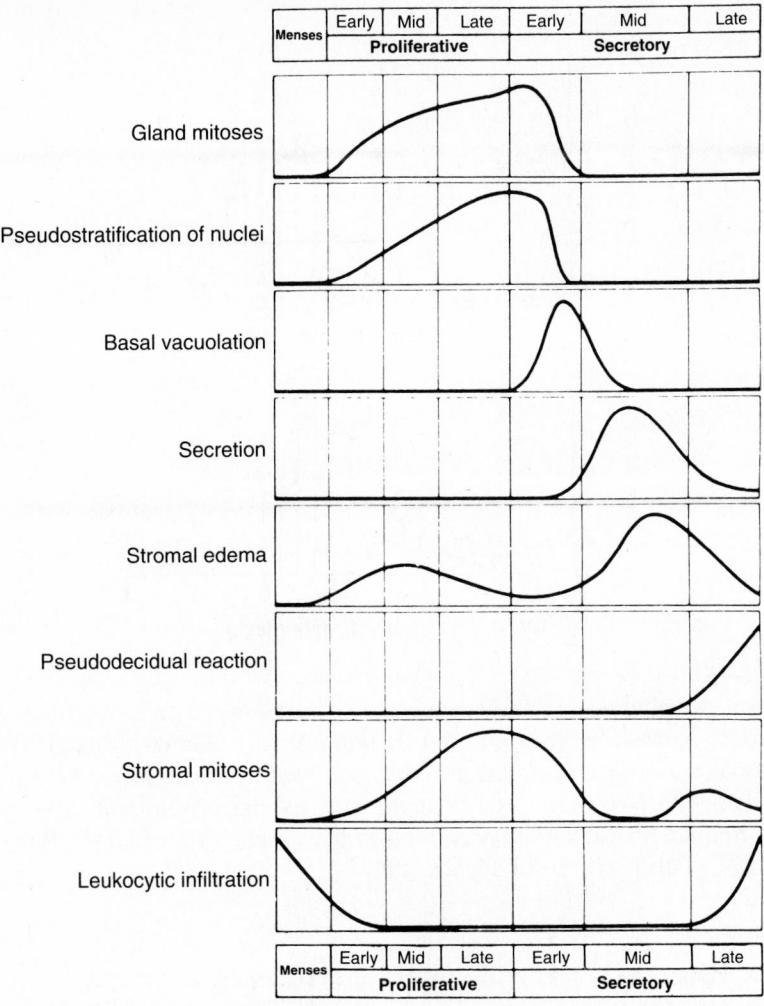

FIGURE 4-42
Patterns of histologic changes throughout menstrual cycle. (Modified from Noyes RW, Hertig AT, and Rock J: Fertil Steril 1:3, 1950. Reproduced with permission of the publisher, The American Fertility Society.)

Menstruation

There has been relatively little research regarding the mechanism of menstruation since the classic studies of Markee and those of Bartelmez in the 1930s and 1940s. In Markee's classic study, endometria from rhesus monkeys were transplanted into the anterior chamber of the eye of the same animal from which the tissue was obtained. He observed that during the cycle the transplants underwent four periods of change: (1) the period of rest (occurring just after menses), (2) the first period of growth (in the follicular phase, during which the size of the transplant doubled), (3) the second period of growth (after ovulation, during which the transplants doubled in size again), and (4) the period of regression (during which menstruation occurred) (Figure 4-44). Markee noted that as steroid levels fell several days before menstruation, there was regression in size of the transplants, resulting in coiling of the spiral arteries and slowing of the blood flow within them. This vascular stasis was followed 4 to 24 hours before menstruation by vasoconstriction of the coiled arteries. About 4 to 24 hours after vasoconstriction began, the coiled arteries relaxed, blood escaped from them, and menstruation began. Only the spiral arteries that supply the upper two thirds of the endometrium became coiled and constricted. The straight ar-

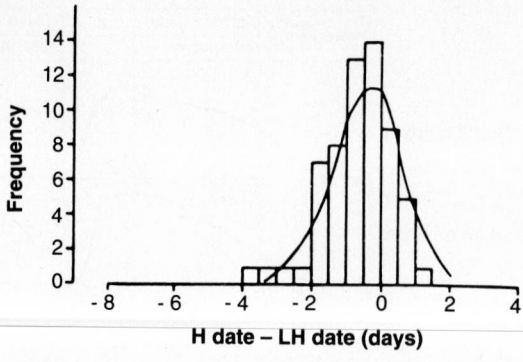

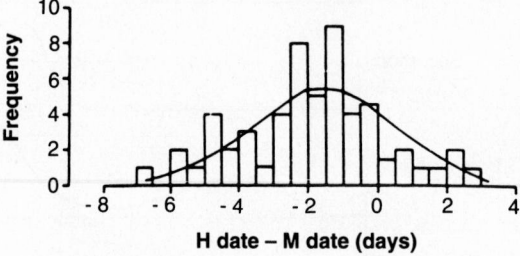

FIGURE 4-43

Frequency distribution of difference between histologic dating *(top)* and chronologic dating *(bottom)* by each method. *H date*, Mean value of histologic dating by two observers. *LH date*, Chronologic dating derived from LH surge. *M date*, Chronologic dating derived from onset of next menstrual period. Normal curve has been fitted to frequency distribution according to bar chart. (From Li T-C, Rogers AW, Lenton EA, et al: Fertil Steril 48:928, 1987.)

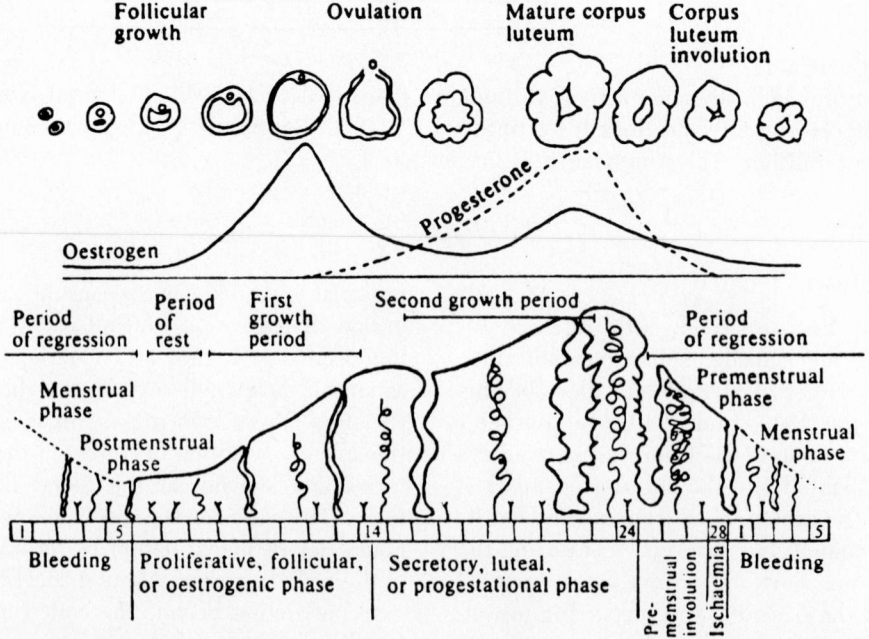

FIGURE 4-44

Diagram of changes in normal human ovarian and endometrial cycles. (From Shaw ST Jr and Roche PC: Menstruation. In Finn CA, editor: Oxford reviews of reproduction and endocrinology, vol 2, London, 1980, Oxford University Press.)

teries supplying the stratum basale did not constrict.

Thus the regression in size of the endometrium brought about by decreasing steroid levels leads to increased coiling and constriction of the spiral arteries, possibly because of decreased cellular monoamine oxidase levels. The resultant decreased blood flow to the functional portion of the endometrium causes ischemia of this tissue. The epithelial and stromal cells show ultrastructural changes of degeneration and autodegradation. With this autolysis, hydrolases and other lysosomal enzymes are released into the interstitium. These enzymes degrade the substances that make up the supporting growth substance of the endometrium, the mucopolysaccharides, collagen, and reticulum. The resulting degraded endometrial tissue is desquamated into the uterine cavity.

Both Markee and Bartelmez, who performed histologic studies on uteri removed by hysterectomy in the 1930s, concluded that menstruation begins in different areas of the uterus at different times and that all the extravasation of blood begins in the first 2 days of menses.

Although the classic belief that all tissue of the stratum functionale is exfoliated, leaving only the stratum basale remaining at the end of menstruation, is written in many textbooks of gynecology, Bartelmez reported that only the entire stratum compactum is uniformly shed, with variable amounts of the stratum spongiosum being desquamated. McLennan and Rydell confirmed this finding in their 1965 study and showed that regeneration of the endometrium comes from cells in the spongiosum that were previously a portion of the secretory endometrium, and not from the stratum basale, as was previously believed. These investigators also found extreme variations in the amount of endometrial shedding in different areas of the same uterus, as well as variations among different uteri removed by hysterectomy.

Nogales-Ortiz et al. also found extreme variability in the extent of endometrial exfoliation. In their study they found that usually only the entire compactum and some parts of the spongiosum were shed, but in some areas nearly the entire endometrium was desquamated. Desquamation of the endometrium occurs mainly in the fundus, not in the isthmus or cornual areas. As early as 36 hours after the onset of menses, regeneration of surface epithelium from the glandular stumps begins and continues to occur at the same time as endometrial shedding occurs.

Ferenczy, using scanning as well as transmission electron microscopy, also reported that the endometrium remained intact in the cervical and isthmic areas. His studies revealed that reepithelialization of the desquamated endometrium began 2 to 3 days after menses began and was completed in 48 hours. He concluded that repair of the desquamated endometrium occurred by both epithelial outgrowth from the mouths of the basal glands and by ingrowth from the endometrium in the cervical and isthmic areas that had not been desquamated. Ferenczy and co-workers also performed historadioautography studies that resulted in these findings: they believe that regeneration of the endometrial surface occurs as a local reaction to injury and is not mediated by ovarian steroid hormones. Circulatory estrogen levels are very low at this time of the cycle.

In 1978 Flowers and Wilborn performed a histologic, histochemical, and ultrastructural study of endometrial biopsy specimens obtained from a group of menstruating women. In these detailed studies they also found that the only cells that become desquamated are from the compactum and upper spongiosum layers and that very few endometrial cells undergo necrosis. Instead, the majority of cells in the endometrium survive, but they undergo regression in size by autophagocytosis, heterophagocytosis, and release of enzymes. Endometrial autophagocytosis is carried out by lysosomes, which digest the cytoplasm; heterophagocytosis is performed by macrophages, which phagocytose debris from stromal tissue; and the enzymes digest reticular fibers. After the regression of cell size, the cells are reorganized in structure and participate in the new proliferative process. Thus the same cells that previously formed the secretory endometrium also form the new proliferative endometrium. It has been postulated that a process called apoptosis is the mechanism whereby controlled cell deletion and tissue regression are followed by reorganization of cells so that large secretory glands revert to small glands found in the proliferative endometrium.

Thus menstruation in humans is probably a combination of (1) some superficial tissue shedding, brought about by ischemia and the presence of hydrolytic enzymes and possibly relaxin, (2) tissue regression (mainly), and (3) reorganization of the endometrial cells.

TECHNIQUE OF HORMONE ASSAY

Bioassay

Measurement (assay) of reproductive hormones was initially done by bioassay techniques. These hormones, usually gonadtrophins, were measured in urine. Bioassays measure the biologic response (growth) of target organs of certain animals (usually rats, rabbits, or mice), which is produced by administering different concentrations of the substances to be assayed, such as in urinary extracts. First, various dilutions of a known (standard) preparation of hormone are administered. The varying increases in weight of the target organ in the animal are then used to develop a dose-response curve against which the response of the substance being assayed is determined.

Chemical Methods

Chemical methods were developed to measure sex steroid levels in women. Before chemical assay, three basic preparatory steps are performed. First, the steroids need to undergo hydrolysis to remove the conjugate. Second, they need to be extracted by organic solvents from the urinary hydrolysate. The final basic step is purification of the steroid by column chromatography. The amount of steroid is then quantitated by measurement of the color reaction, using either colorimetry or the more sensitive fluorimetry. The most sensitive chemical method of measurement of steroids is gas chromatography, an extremely tedious procedure.

Radioimmunoassay

In 1959 Yalow and Berson developed the technique of radioimmunoassay, which provided the method of measuring extremely small amounts of hormone in serum or plasma. Use of this technique has greatly increased the knowledge of reproductive endocrinology. Radioimmunoassay allows a much greater number of assays to be performed than does bioassay or chemical assay, in addition to having much greater sensitivity and needing less than 1 ml of serum or plasma for testing. However, this technique measures only the immunologic property of a hormone, not its biologic effects. The two effects frequently differ in magnitude.

The basic principle of radioimmunoassay involves the competition between a radioactively labeled and an unlabeled antigen, both of which are present in excess, for binding sites on a limited amount of antibody. To produce a standard curve that permits measurement of a hormone in the serum or plasma, the investigator uses a standard preparation of the hormone to be measured (antigen). Varying known amounts of the unlabeled (cold) antigen and the labeled (hot) antigen are incubated for a time with an antibody raised specifically against the antigen to be measured, and an antigen-antibody complex is formed (Figure 4-45). Since there is always an excess of labeled and unlabeled antigen in the reaction, some of each type of antigen is always bound to the antibody and some always remains free in solution after the incubation. After the bound complex is separated from the excess free antigen in solution, usually by the addition of an antibody (second antibody) raised against the first antibody, the amount of tracer present in either the bound or free component, usually the bound complex, is measured by a radioactive analyzer (counter). A standard curve is then constructed by plotting the counts per minute measured in the various dilutions of the standard preparation against the mass of antigen used. The type of curve varies with the scale of the abscissa (Figure 4-46).

For measurement of the amount of hormone in the unknown specimen, excess labeled antigen and a limited amount of antibody are added to an aliquot of the unknown specimen. After incubation and separation, the amount of tracer that is bound in the antigen-antibody complex is counted. The number of counts per minute measured in the complex is located on the ordinate, and from this point a line is intersected on the standard curve. A perpendicular is dropped to the abscissa to determine the amount of hormone in the unknown specimen.

Antibodies

In contrast to steroid hormones, protein hormones themselves are antigenic and can produce antibody formation. Since steroids are haptens and are not antigenic by themselves, they need to be attached to a carrier protein (usually bovine serum albumin) to induce antibody formation. Even with the injection of purified antigens, there is a degree of cross-reaction of most hormone antibodies (polyclonal)

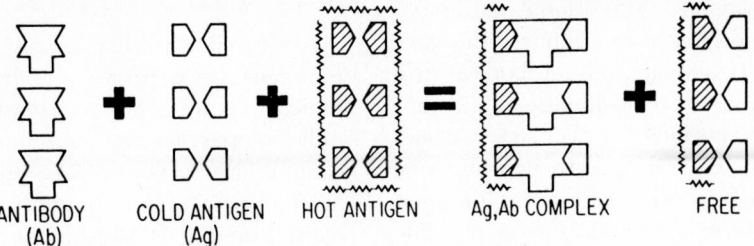

ANTIBODY (Ab)   COLD ANTIGEN (Ag)   HOT ANTIGEN   Ag,Ab COMPLEX   FREE

FIGURE 4-45

Schematic representation of antigen-antibody reaction in radioimmunoassay. For final analysis, free component must be separated from the antigen-antibody complex. (From Kletzky OA and Nakamura RM: Measurement of hormones. In Mishell DR Jr, Davajan V, and Lobo RA, editors: Infertility, contraception and reproductive endocrinology, ed 3, Cambridge, Mass, 1991, Blackwell Scientific Publications.)

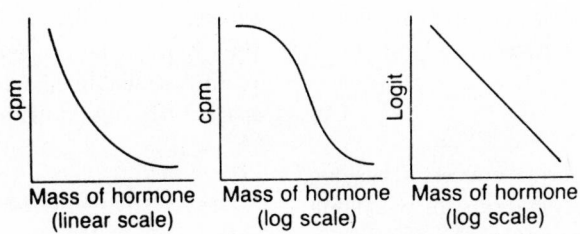

FIGURE 4-46

Standard curve using linear scale *(left)* or log scale *(center and right)* for the abscissa and linear *(left and center)* or logit *(right)* for the ordinate. *cpm*, Counts per minute. (From Kletzky OA and Nakamura RM: Measurement of hormones. In Mishell DR Jr, Davajan V, and Lobo RA, editors: Infertility, contraception and reproductive endocrinology, ed 3, Cambridge, Mass, 1991, Blackwell Scientific Publications.)

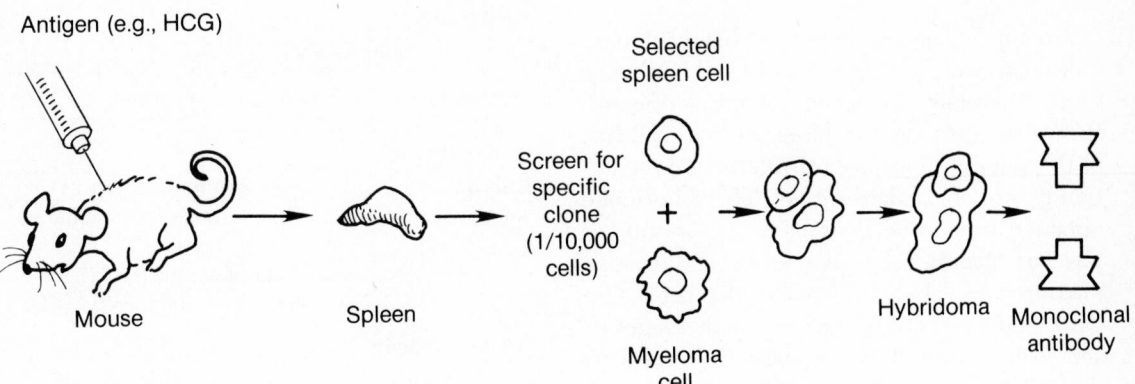

FIGURE 4-47

Schematic representation of monoclonal antibody production. (From Kletzky OA and Nakamura RM: Measurement of hormones. In Mishell DR Jr, Davajan V, and Lobo RA, editors: Infertility, contraception and reproductive endocrinology, ed 3, Cambridge, Mass, 1991, Blackwell Scientific Publications.)

with other hormones. Monoclonal antibodies are now being produced to eliminate the variability and heterogeneity of antibodies produced by several injections of antigen and thus to increase the specificity of the assay. Monoclonal antibodies are produced by first injecting the antigen into a mouse to induce an immunologic reaction in its spleen (Figure 4-47). The spleen cells are screened to find those particular ones (clones) capable of secreting a single antibody type. These cells are then fused with a myeloma cell from the same species to form a hybrid or hybridoma cell. Because of the immortality of the myeloma cell in culture, the hybridoma continually secretes antibodies characteristic of the selected spleen cell. This clone line is maintained in culture to provide homogenous monoclonal antibody molecules, which are used for sensitive and specific immunoassays of protein hormones.

Antigens

To produce standard curves, varying amounts of known preparations of hormone need to be utilized. Since steroid hormones are available as chemically pure preparations, the amount added to form the standard curve and determine the amount in the unknown can be expressed in terms of absolute mass or weight, such as nanograms (10^{-9}) or picograms (10^{-12}). Thus the results obtained from different laboratories should be constant. However, most European laboratories express the results in terms of nanomoles instead of nanograms. For most steroids, about 3 nmol/L is equivalent to 1 ng/ml.

Protein hormones, however, being of high molecular weight, are not circulated in pure form. Therefore the results of measuring unknown samples need to be expressed in terms of the amount of a standard reference preparation by use of standard extracts of the hormone obtained from collections of urine, serum, or pituitary glands. Thus the levels of hormone measured by laboratories using different standards do not always agree, and clinicians should be aware of the normal levels used by these laboratories. The protein standard is frequently an international reference preparation, and the results are usually expressed in international units.

Assay Markers

As described earlier, quantitation in a radioimmunoassay is carried out by measuring the radioactive antigen (assay marker). The use of radioisotopes for radioimmunoassay has become a negative factor in recent years because of the problems associated with radioactive waste disposal. During the past few years, major advances have occurred in both the development of new instruments and the identification of new nonradioactive markers. When coupled to the assay antigens, these instruments and markers are almost as sensitive as radioimmunoassay and sometimes are as sensitive as the most sensitive radioimmunoassay. The use of these markers has rejuvenated the field of immunoassays by allowing individuals without training in the use of radioisotopes to perform these assays. One can easily extend this use to the home, and "homekits" are becoming readily available. Examples of nonradioactive markers are given in the next section.

Types of Immunoassays

Because of the advances made in the development of nonradioactive markers to replace the radioactive markers used in radioimmunoassays, many new types of assays, some related and others not related, to radioimmunoassays, have been established. All these assays, however, use the antigen-antibody interaction and thus are now usually referred to as immunoassays. Immunoassays can be catego-

TABLE 4-7
Types of Immunoassays

Assay Type	Examples
Excess antigen	
Radioactive	Radioimmunoassay (RIA)
Nonradioactive	Chemiluminescent immunoassay (CIA)
	Fluoroimmunoassay (FIA)
	Enzyme immunoassay (EIA)
Excess antibody	
Radioactive	Immunoradiometric assay (IRMA)
Nonradioactive	Enzyme-linked immunosorbent assay (ELISA)

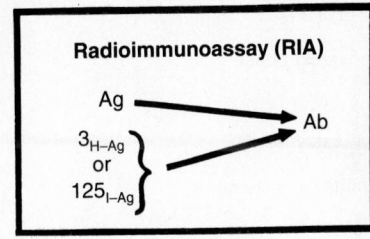

1. Fluoroimmunoassay (FIA)

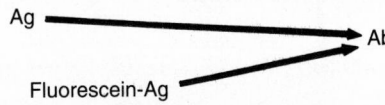

2. Chemiluminescent assay (CIA)

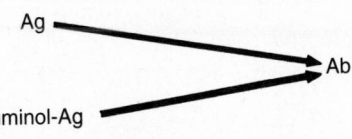

3. Enzyme immunoassay (EIA)

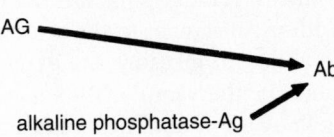

FIGURE 4-48
Competition between excess antigen *(Ag)* (analyte or standard) and excess radioactive or non-radioactive antigen (marker) for a limited amount of antibody *(Ab)*. (From Stanczyk FZ: Immunoassays. In Mishell DR Jr, Davajan V, and Lobo RA, editors: Infertility, contraception and reproductive endocrinology, ed 3, Cambridge, Mass, 1991, Blackwell Scientific Publications.)

rized not only on the basis of whether they use excess antigen or excess antibody, but also according to whether they use a radioactive tracer. A categorization of some of the most frequently used types of immunoassays in reproductive endocrinology laboratories is shown in Table 4-7.

The basic principle of the nonradioactive immunoassays that use antigen excess is the same as that of radioimmunoassay (Figure 4-48). The nonradioactive immunoassay uses a nonradioactive tag, such as fluorescein in the fluorometric immunoassay (FIA), luminol in the chemiluminescent immunoassay (CIA), and an alkaline phosphatase conjugate in the enzyme immunoassay (EIA). Quantification of these tags is achieved by use of a fluorometer luminometer in the FIA and a luminometer in the CIA. In the EIA, quantification is carried out by addition of a specific substrate. For example, *p*-nitrophenylphosphate is used with alkaline phosphatase, and the product formed, *p*-nitrophenol, can be measured spectrophotometrically.

Two of the most widely used excess-antibody assays in clinical reproductive endocrinology laboratories are the immunoradiometric assay (IRMA) and the enzyme-linked immunosorbent assay (ELISA). In the IRMA the principle involves the use of excess radiolabeled antibody that binds to the antigen, followed by removal of excess antibody. At present the two-site IRMA (Figure 4-49) is often employed. It requires the addition of a second antibody attached to a solid phase, such as a bead. The

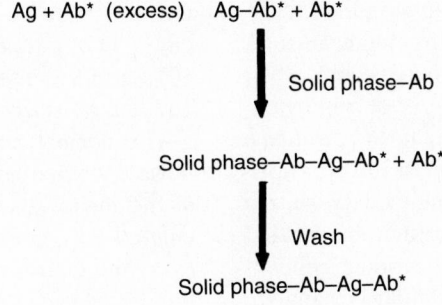

FIGURE 4-49
Principle of the immunoradiometric assay. *Ag*, Antigen; *Ab*, antibody. (From Stanczyk FZ: Immunoassays. In Mishell DR Jr, Davajan V, and Lobo RA, editors: Infertility, contraception and reproductive endocrinology, ed 3, Cambridge, Mass, 1991, Blackwell Scientific Publications.)

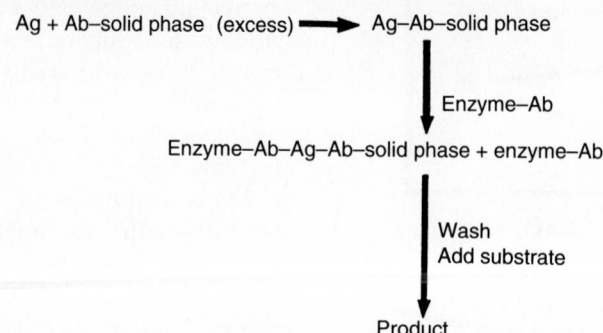

FIGURE 4-50

Principle of the enzyme-linked immunosorbent assay. *Ag*, Antigen; *Ab*, antibody. (From Stanczyk FZ: Immunoassays. In Mishell DR Jr, Davajan V, and Lobo RA, editors: Infertility, contraception and reproductive endocrinology, ed 3, Cambridge, Mass, 1991, Blackwell Scientific Publications.)

second antibody differs from the first one in that the second is not radioactive and recognizes a different site on the antigen. Since the complex formed is attached to a solid phase, it can be readily separated from the excess radioactive antibody by centrifugation. The amount of radioactivity measured in the final complex is directly proportional to the concentration of standard used to prepare the standard curve and the concentration of analyte in the specimen. This is in contrast to the inverse relationship between the "bound" radioactivity and standard concentrations observed in a radioimmunoassay.

In the ELISA, antigen is bound to an excess of antibody, which is attached to a solid phase, such as a plastic tube or plate (Figure 4-50). Once the antigen-antibody complex is formed, an antibody-enzyme conjugate is added. The antibody in this conjugate is directed against an antigenic site different from that recognized by the first antibody. The result is a "sandwich" type of complex; thus the term *sandwich ELISA*. Following the addition of the appropriate substrate for the enzyme, the resulting product is measured spectrophotometrically. The relationship between the product concentration and concentration of standard or analyte is similar to that obtained by IRMA.

Four characteristics of assays apply to each of these techniques: sensitivity, specificity, accuracy, and precision. Sensitivity is the least amount of substance that can be measured in the assay. Specificity is the ability of the assay to measure only one substance and not allow the measurement to be altered by the presence of other substances (cross-reaction). Accuracy is the ability to measure the exact amount of substance in the sample; thus specimens containing known low and high values of the substance to be measured are always included in each assay. Precision is the ability of the assay to consistently reproduce the same results. Precision is determined by measuring the within-assay, or intraassay, coefficient of variation (CV) and the between-assay, or interassay, CV. The intraassay CV is calculated by determining the amounts of a known sample measured in about 10 replicates in the same assay.

$$CV = \frac{\text{Standard deviation}}{\text{Mean}} \times 100$$

The interassay CV is determined by measuring the same unknown sample on different days. The intrassay CV should be less than 10%, and the interassay CV should be less than 15% for satisfactory precision of the assay.

The normal range of values of hormones in normal women is frequently expressed in terms of the mean level plus the mathematically calculated 95% confidence limits (±2 SD). However, the distributions of hormone levels in the menstrual cycles of a group of women with normal ovulation follow a log-normal distribution instead of a gaussian (normal) distribution. Although results of normal values usually vary from laboratory to laboratory, the 95% confidence limits of measurement of reproductive hormones among women in our laboratory are listed in Table 4-8 as a guide of normality.

TABLE 4-8
95% Confidence Limits of Hormones Used in Reproduction

Hormone	Phase of Menstrual Cycle			
	Follicular	Midcycle	Luteal	Menopause
LH (mIU/ml)	4.0-20.0	43-145	3-18	>40
FSH (mIU/ml)	3.2-9.0	10-18	3-9	>30
Prolactin (ng/ml)	8.0-20.0	0-22	10-30	8-25
Estradiol (pg/ml)	30-140	150-480	50-250	10-30
Progesterone (ng/ml)	0.5-1.0	0.8-2.0	3.0-31	0.5-1.0
Testosterone (ng/dl)	20-85	20-85	20-85	8-30*
Free testosterone (ng/dl)	1.2-9.9	1.2-9.9	1.2-9.9	3-13†
DHEA-S (µg/ml)	0.5-2.8	0.5-2.8	0.5-2.8	0.2-1.5

From Kletzky OA and Nakamura RM: Measurement of hormones. In Mishell DR Jr, Davajan V, and Lobo RA, editors: Infertility, contraception and reproductive endocrinology, ed 3, Cambridge, Mass, 1999, Blackwell Scientific Publications.
*In oophorectomized women the range is 4 to 18 ng/dl.
†In oophorectomized women the range is 1 to 10 ng/dl.

KEY POINTS

- The hypothalamic hormone that controls gonadotrophin release is a decapeptide, gonadotrophin-releasing hormone (GnRH).

- The cell bodies of the hypothalamic neurons that produce GnRH are concentrated mainly in two areas: the anterior hypothalamus and the medial basal (tuberal) hypothalamus.

- GnRH can be released both in large amounts periodically via the tuberoinfundibular tract (cyclic release) and in a low-grade continuous transependymal fashion (tonic release) via the tanycytes.

- GnRH is secreted in a pulsatile manner. The amplitude and frequency of the pulse vary throughout the menstrual cycle. The frequency is rapid in the follicular phase, about one pulse per hour, and slower in the luteal phase, about one pulse every 2 or 3 hours.

- The most important neurotransmitters involved in reproductive neuroendocrinology are two catecholamines, dopamine and norepinephrine, as well as an indolamine, serotonin.

- Infusion of β-endorphin results in an increase in prolactin and a decrease in luteinizing hormone (LH), the latter occurring by an inhibitory effect on GnRH neurons in the hypothalamus.

- Peripheral measurement of plasma β-endorphin levels does not reflect levels in the central nervous system circulation.

- The peptide hormones, such as GnRH, bind to specific receptors on the surface membrane of the target cell, in contrast to steroid hormones, which pass through the cell membrane to bind to intracellular receptors.

- When a protein hormone binds to its specific receptor, it activates or inhibits the enzyme adenyl cyclase, the second messenger, which in turn changes the concentration of adenosine 3′, 5′-cyclic monophosphate (cyclic AMP, cAMP).

- The various growth factors provide hormonal effects within the ovary by both autocrine and paracrine mechanisms.

- Inhibin inhibits pituitary follicle-stimulating hormone (FSH) release, whereas in the ovarian follicle inhibin stimulates progesterone and inhibits estradiol production. Activins have an opposite action to inhibins by stimulating pituitary FSH release and opposing ovarian action by inhibiting progesterone and stimulating estradiol.

- Biosynthesis of prostanoids from arachidonic acid and other precursors takes places via the cyclic endoperoxides prostaglandins G and H (PGG and PGH). Prostanoids are produced intercellularly shortly before they are released and generally act locally, in contrast to steroids.

- Following a single intravenous bolus of GnRH, the LH levels peak in 30 minutes and FSH in 60 minutes.

- With a constant infusion of GnRH there is a biphasic release of LH but not FSH. The initial increase of LH occurs 30 minutes and the second 90 minutes after the start of the infusion.

- When stimulation by hormone is maximal, the unoccupied receptors become refractory to hormone binding for 12 to 72 hours. This phenomenon has allowed frequent administration of GnRH analogues to be used clinically to inhibit FSH and LH levels and thus decrease steroidogenesis.

- GnRH analogues are synthesized by substitution of amino acids in the parent molecule at the 6 and 10 positions. The various agonists have greater potencies and longer half-lives than the parent GnRH.

- LH and FSH have the same α subunit, which is similar in structure to the α subunit of thyroid-stimulating hormone and human chorionic gonadotrophin (HCG). The β subunits of all these hormones have different amino acids and carbohydrates, which provide specific biologic activity.

- The half-life of LH is more rapid (30 minutes) than that of FSH (60 minutes).

- LH acts primarily on the theca cells to induce steroidogenesis, whereas FSH acts primarily on the granulosa cells to stimulate follicular growth.

- LH acts on the theca cells to produce androgens, which are then transported to the granulosa cells, where they are aromatized to estrogens.

- After sufficient LH receptors have been produced by the action of FSH and estradiol, LH acts directly on the granulosa cells to cause luteinization and production of progesterone.

- The ovary secretes three principal steroid hormones: estradiol from the follicle, progesterone from the corpus luteum, and androstenedione from the stroma.

- Corticosteroids, progesterone, pregnenolone, 17-hydroxypregnenolone, and 17-hydroxyprogesterone have 21 carbon atoms; androgens (testosterone and androstenedione) have 19 carbon atoms; and natural estrogens have 18 carbon atoms and a phenolic or aromatic ring A.

- Because the ovaries lack 21-hydroxylase, 11β-hydroxylase, and 18-hydroxylase reductase activity, they are unable to synthesize mineralocorticoids or glucocorticoids.

- Estradiol and estrone are interconverted outside the ovary. Estrone is then converted to estrone sulfate, which has a long half-life and is the largest component of the pool of circulating estrogens.

- The greater the amount of fat tissue present, the greater is the percentage of androstenedione that is converted to estrone. In a normal individual, about 1.3% of the daily 3000 μg of androstenedione produced is converted to estrone (40 μg), whereas in an obese individual as much as 7% of the 3000 μg is converted (20 μg).

- Before excretion, estrogens are conjugated by the liver and intestinal mucosa into sulfates, glucuronides, or other conjugates so that they can be excreted, and progesterone is conjugated to pregnanediol glucuronide.

- The process by which steroids are conjugated involves the transformation of lipophilic compounds, which are only sparingly soluble in water, into metabolites that are readily water soluble and can therefore be eliminated in urine. Conjugation of progesterone provides pregnanediol-3-glucuronide. The natural estrogens are converted into sulfates and glucuronides.

- Sex hormone–binding globulin (SHBG) primarily binds dihydrotestosterone, testosterone, and estradiol. About 65% of circulating testosterone is bound to SHBG and 30% to albumin. Less than 2% remains unbound or free.

- Corticosteroid-binding globulin (CBG) binds with highest affinity to cortisol, corticosterone, and 11-deoxycortisol, and to a lesser extent to progesterone.

- Estrogen stimulates the synthesis of both estrogen and progesterone receptors in target tissues, and progestins inhibit the synthesis of both estrogen and progesterone receptors.

- Just before birth the primary oocytes, which now number 2 to 4 million, reach the diplotene stage, also called the germinal vesicle stage of development.

- Estradiol stimulates preantral follicle growth, reduces follicular atresia, and increases FSH action on the granulosa cells. Testosterone increases follicular atresia and prevents preantral follicle growth.

- The follicle destined to become dominant secretes the greatest amount of estradiol, which in turn increases the density of FSH receptors.

- With ultrasound it has been found that there is a steady increase in follicular diameter and volume that parallels the rise in estradiol. The dominant follicle has a maximal mean diameter of about 19.5 mm, with a range of 18 to 25 mm just before ovulation. The mean maximal follicular volume is 3.8 ml, with a range of 3.1 to 8.2 ml.

- Ovulation occurs about 24 hours after the estradiol peak, as well as 32 hours after the initial rise in LH and about 12 to 16 hours after the peak of LH levels in serum.

- The midcycle LH surge initiates germinal vesicle disruption, and metaphase I is completed. As the oocyte enters metaphase II, the first polar body appears. Completion of meiosis and extrusion of the second polar body occur only when a sperm penetrates the ovum.

- By serial ultrasound observation and LH measurements, ovulation usually occurs within 24 hours and always within 48 hours after the peak in LH.

- Beginning in the midluteal phase, progesterone is secreted in a pulsatile manner, occurring immediately following an LH pulse.

- Serum levels of estradiol rise from less than 50 pg/ml in the early follicular phase to 200 to 500 pg/ml at midcycle and have a broad luteal-phase peak level of about 100 to 300 pg/ml.

- Progesterone levels in serum are less than 1 ng/ml before ovulation and reach midluteal levels of 10 to 20 ng/ml.

- During a normal ovulatory cycle at midcycle, the first event is a rise in estradiol. When estradiol reaches peak levels, there is an abrupt increase (surge) in LH and FSH. The increase in LH reaches a peak in about 18 hours, and peak levels plateau for about 14 hours, after which there is a decline. The mean duration of the LH surge is about 24 hours. Beginning about 12 hours before the onset of the LH surge, there is an increase of both progesterone and 17-dihydroxyprogesterone.

- With the occurrence of the LH peak, there is a decline in estradiol and a further increase in progesterone. This shift in steroidogenesis in favor of progesterone instead of estradiol production is brought about by the luteinization of the granulosa cells produced by LH.

- Menstrual cycle length is most irregular in the 2 years after menarche and the 3 years before menopause, times of life during which anovulatory cycles are most frequent.

- The mean duration of menstrual cycle length is 28 ± 7 days, with menstruation in which cycles occur at more frequent intervals (<21 days) being called polymenorrhea and that in which cycles are less frequent (>35 days) being called oligomenorrhea. The mean duration of menstrual flow is 4 ± 2 days.

- Only the spiral arteries that supply the upper two thirds of the endometrium become coiled and constrict.

- After menstruation, regeneration of the endometrium comes from cells in the spongiosum that were previously a portion of the secretory endometrium and not from the stratum basale, as previously believed.

- The endometrium produces growth factors, prostaglandins, and peptide hormones, including a specific peptide called progestogen-dependent endometrial protein.

- The subjective method of correlating the degree of maturation in the endometrium by histologic visualization is relatively imprecise, and more precise indices based on quantitative morphometric analysis have been developed. To date the endometrium most accurately, the maturation should be correlated with the days after LH peak, not the number of days before the onset of the next menstrual period.

- There are extreme variations in the amounts of endometrial shedding in different areas of the same uterus, as well as variations among different uteri removed by hysterectomy.

- Menstruation in humans is probably a combination of some superficial tissue shedding, brought about by ischemia and the presence of hydrolytic enzymes and possibly relaxin, as well as mainly by tissue regression and reorganization of the endometrial cells.

- Just after ovulation, glycogen-rich subnuclear vacuoles appear in the base of the cells lining the glands. This subnuclear vacuolization is the first histologic indication of the effect of progesterone but is not evidence that ovulation has occurred.

- Enzyme-linked immunosorbent assay (ELISA), or "sandwich," techniques have been developed to measure protein hormones with the use of monoclonal antibodies against the α and β subunits. The endpoint is a color reaction and can be read in a spectrophotometer.

- There are four characteristics of assays of hormones: sensitivity, specificity, accuracy, and precision.

BIBLIOGRAPHY

Bächström CT, McNeilly AS, Leask RM, et al: Pulsatile secretion of LH, FSH, prolactin, oestradiol and progesterone during the human menstrual cycle, Clin Endocrinol 17:29, 1982.

Borth R: Generic names for steroid hormones and related substances (guest editorial), Contraception 12:373, 1975.

Brannstrom M and Janson PO: The biochemistry of ovulation. In Hillier SG, editor: Ovarian endocrinology, Cambridge, Mass, 1991, Blackwell Scientific Publications.

Chan L and O'Malley BW: Mechanism of action of the sex steroid hormones (first of three parts), N Engl J Med 294:1322, 1976.

Crowley WF Jr, Filicori M, Spratt DI, et al: The physiology of gonadotropin-releasing hormone (GnRH) secretion in men and women, Recent Prog Horm Res 41:501, 1985.

Diczfalusy E and Landgren BM: Hormonal changes in the menstrual cycle. In Diczfalusy E and Diczfalusy A, editors: Regulation of human fertility. Copenhagen, 1977, Scriptor.

di Zerega GS and Hodgen GD: The interovarian progesterone gradient: a trial and temporal regulator of folliculogenesis in the primate ovarian cycle, J Clin Endocrinol Metab 54:495; 1982.

Eissa MK, Obhrai MS, Docker MF, et al: Follicular growth and endocrine profiles in spontaneous and induced conception cycles, Fertil Steril 45:191, 1986.

Ferenczy A: Studies on the cytodynamics of human endometrial regeneration, Am J Obstet Gynecol 124:64, 1976.

Filicori M, Butler J, and Crowley WF: Neuroendocrine regulation of the corpus luteum in the human, J Clin Invest 73:1638, 1984.

Filicori M, Santoro N, Merriam GR, et al: Characterization of the physiological pattern of episodic gonadotropin secretion throughout the human menstrual cycle, J Clin Endocrinol Metab 1136, 1986.

Flowers CE and Wilborn WH: New observations on the physiology of menstruation, Obstet Gynecol 51:16, 1978.

Gibbons WE, Battin DA, and di Zerega GS: Mechanisms of action of reproductive hormones. In Mishell DR Jr, Davajan V, and Lobo RA, editors: Infertility, contraception, and reproductive endocrinology, ed 3, Cambridge, Mass, 1991, Blackwell Scientific Publications.

Goebelsmann UT, Arce JJ, Thorneycroft IH, et al: Serum testosterone concentrations in women throughout the menstrual cycle and following HCG administration, Am J Obstet Gynecol 119:445, 1974.

Goebelsmann UT, Midgey AR Jr, and Jaffe RB: Regulation of human gonadotropins. VII. Daily individual urinary estrogens, pregnanediol and serum luteinizing and follicle-stimulating hormones during the menstrual cycle, J Clin Endocrinol Metab 29:1222, 1969.

Goebelsmann UT and Mishell DR Jr: The menstrual cycle. In Mishell DR Jr, Davajan V, and Lobo RA, editors: Infertility, contraception and reproductive endocrinology, ed 3, Cambridge, Mass, 1991, Blackwell Scientific Publications.

Hartman CG: The irregularity of the menstrual cycle. In Science and the safe period, Huntington, NY, 1972, Robert E. Krieger Publishing Co.

Hasegawa Y: Changes in serum concentrations of inhibin in mammals. In Hodgen G, Rosenwales F Sr, and Spieler JM, editors: Physiological roles and possibilities in contraceptive development, Norfolk, Va, 1988, The Jones Institute Press.

Hoff JD, Lasley BL, Wang CF, et al: The two pools of pituitary gonadotropin, J Clin Endocrinol Metab 44:302, 1977.

Housep D, Mishell DR Jr, et al: Correlation of endometrial maturation with four methods of estimating day of ovulation, Obstet Gynecol 73:88, 1989.

Hylka VW and di Zerega GS: Reproductive hormones and their mechanisms of action. In Mishell DR Jr, Davajan V, and Lobo RA, editors: Infertility, contraception, and reproductive endocrinology, ed 3, Cambridge, Mass, 1991, Blackwell Scientific Publications.

Jewelewicz R, Ferin M, Dyrenfurth I, et al: Long-term LH, RH infusions at various stages of the menstrual cycle in normal women. In Beling CG and Wenitz AC, editors: The LH-releasing hormone, New York, 1980, Masson Publishing Co.

Jockenhovel F, Bhasin S, et al: Hormonal effects of single gonadotropin-releasing hormone antagonist doses in men, J Endocrinol Metab 66:1065, 1988.

Johannissoon E, Parket RA, Landgren BNM, and Duiczfalusy E: Morphometric analysis of the human endometrium in relation to peripheral hormone levels, Fertil Steril 38:564, 1982.

Joshi SG, Rao R, et al: Luteal phase concentrations of progestagen-associated endometrial protein (PEP) in the serum of cycling women with adequate or inadequate endometrium, J Clin Endocrinol Metab 63:1247, 1986.

Katt JA, Duncan JA, et al: The frequency of gonadotropin-releasing hormone stimulation determines the number of pituitary gonadotropin-releasing hormone receptors, Endocrinology 116:2112, 1985.

Kletzky OA and Lobo RA: Reproductive neuroendocrinology. In Mishell DR Jr, Davajan V, and Lobo RA, editors: Infertility, contraception and reproductive endocrinology, ed 3, Cambridge, Mass, 1991, Blackwell Scientific Publications.

Kletzky OA and Nakamura RM: Measurement of hormones. In Mishell DR Jr, Davajan V, and Lobo RA, editors: Infertility, contraception and reproductive endocrinology, ed 3, Cambridge, Mass 1991, Blackwell Scientific Publications.

Knobil E: The neuroendocrine control of the menstrual cycle, Recent Prog Horm Res 36:53, 1980.

Knobil E, Plant TM, Wildt L, et al: Control of the rhesus monkey menstrual cycle: permissive role of hypothalamic gonadotropin-releasing hormone, Science 207:1371, 1980.

Lemay A, Maheux R, et al: Reversible hypogonadism induced by a LH-RH agonist (Buserelin) as a new therapeutic approach for endometriosis, Fertil Steril 41:863, 1984.

Levy C, Robel P, Gautray JP, et al: Estradiol and progesterone receptors in human endometrium: normal and abnormal menstrual cycles and early pregnancy, Am J Obstet Gynecol 136:647, 1980.

Li T-C, Rogers AW, Lenton EA, et al: A comparison between two methods of chronological dating of human endometrial biopsies during the luteal phase, and their correlation with histologic dating, Fertil Steril 48:928, 1987.

Li T-C, Rogers AW, et al: A new method of histologic dating of human endometrium in the luteal phase, Fertil Steril 50:52, 1988.

Li T-C, Dockery P, et al: How precise is histologic dating of endometrium using the standard dating criteria? Fertil Steril 51:759, 1989.

Lobo RA: The menstrual cycle: In Mishell DR Jr, Davajan V, and Lobo RA, editors: Infertility, contraception, and reproductive endocrinology, ed 3, Cambridge, Mass, 1991, Blackwell Scientific Publishers.

Lopata A, Sathananthan AM, McBain JC, et al: The ultrastructure of the preovulatory human egg fertilized in vitro, Fertil Steril 33:12, 1980.

MacDonald PC, Rombaut RP, and Siiteri PK: Plasma precursors of estrogen. I. Extent of conversion of plasma Δ^4-adrenalectomized females, J Clin Endocrinol Metab 27:1103, 1967.

March CM: The endometrium in the menstrual cycle. In Mishell DR Jr, Davajan V, and Lobo RA, editors: Infertility, contraception and reproductive endocrinology, ed 3, Cambridge, Mass, 1991, Blackwell Scientific Publications.

McLennan CE and Rydell AH: Extent of endometrial shedding during normal menstruation, Obstet Gynecol 26:605, 1965.

Moore RY: Neuroendocrine mechanisms: cells and systems. In Yen SSC and Jaffe R, editors: Reproductive endocrinology: physiology, pathophysiology and clinical management, Philadelphia, 1986, WB Saunders Co.

Nippoldt TB, Reame NE, Kelch RP, et al: The roles of estradiol and progesterone in decreasing luteinizing hormone pulse frequency in the luteal phase of the menstrual cycle, J Clin Endocrinol Metab 69:67, 1989.

Nogales-Ortiz F, Puerta J, and Nogales FF Jr: The normal menstrual cycle, J Obstet Gynecol 51:259, 1978.

Novak E and Novak ER, editors: Textbook of gynecology, ed 4, Baltimore, 1952, Williams & Wilkins.

Noyes RW, Hertig AT, and Rock J: Dating the endometrial biopsy, Fertil Steril 1:3, 1950.

Orczyk GP and Behrman OR: Ovulation blockade by aspirin or indomethacin: in vivo evidence for a role of prostaglandins in gonadotropin secretion, Prostaglandins 1:3, 1972.

Paulson RJ: Oocytes: from development to fertilization. In Mishell DR Jr, Davajan V, and Lobo RA, editors: Infertility, contraception, and reproductive endocrinology, ed

3, Cambridge, Mass, 1991, Blackwell Scientific Publications.

Quigley ME and Yen SSC: The role of endogenous opiates on LH secretion during the menstrual cycle, J Clin Endocrinol Metab 51:179, 1980.

Reame N, Sauder SE, Kelch RP, et al: Pulsatile gonadotropin secretion during the human menstrual cycle: evidence for altered frequency of gonadotropin-releasing hormone secretion, J Clin Endocrinol Metab 59:328, 1984.

Reichlen S: Neural control of the pituitary gland: normal physiology and pathophysiologic implications. In Current concepts, Kalamazoo, Mich, 1976, Upjohn Publications.

Ribeiro, WO, Mishell DR Jr, and Thorneycroft IH: Comparison of the patterns of androstenedione, progesterone and estradiol during the human menstrual cycle, Am J Obstet Gynecol 119:1026, 1974.

Ross GT, Cagrille CM, Lipsett MB, et al: Pituitary and gonadal hormones in women during spontaneous and induced ovulatory cycles, Recent Prog Horm Res 26:1, 1970.

Schulster D, Burstein S, and Cooke BA, editors: Control of gonadal steroidogenesis by FSH and LH. In Molecular endocrinology of the steroid hormones, London, 1976, John Wiley & Sons, Ltd.

Shaw ST Jr and Roche PC: Menstruation. In Finn CA, editor: Oxford reviews of reproduction and endocrinology, vol 2 London, 1980, Oxford University Press.

Shea BF, Baker RD, and Latour JPA: Oogenesis, folliculogenesis and maturation of follicular oocytes. In Hafez ED, editor: Human ovulation: mechanism, prediction, detection, and induction, New York, 1979, Elsevier-North Holland.

Stanczyk FZ: Immuno assays. In Mishell DR Jr, Davajan V, and Lobo RA, editors: Infertility, contraception, and reproductive endocrinology, ed 3, Cambridge, Mass, 1991, Blackwell Scientific Publications.

Stanczyk FZ: Prostaglandins and related compounds. In Mishell DR Jr, Davajan V, and Lobo RA, editors: Infertility, contraception, and reproductive endocrinology, ed 3, Cambridge, Mass, 1991, Blackwell Scientific Publications.

Stanczyk FZ: Steroid hormones. In Mishell DR Jr, Davajan V, and Lobo RA, editors: Infertility, contraception, and reproductive endocrinology, ed 3, Cambridge, Mass, 1991, Blackwell Scientific Publications.

Stanczyk FZ, Miyakama I, and Goebelsmann UT: Direct radioimmunoassay of urinary estrogen and pregnanediol glucuronides during the menstrual cycle, Am J Obstet Gynecol 137:443, 1980.

Stevens VC: Comparison of FSH and LH patterns in plasma urine and urinary extracts during the menstrual cycle, J Clin Endocrinol Metab 29:904, 1969.

Thorneycroft IH, Mishell DR Jr, Stone SC, et al: The reaction of serum 17-hydroxyprogesterone and estradiol-17β levels during the human menstrual cycle, Am J Obstet Gynecol 111:947, 1971.

Thorneycroft IH, Sribyatta B, Tom WK, et al: Measurement of serum LH, FSH, progesterone 17-hydroxyprogesterone and estradiol-17β levels at 4-hour intervals during the periovulatory phase of the menstrual cycle, J Clin Endocrinol Metab 39:754, 1974.

Tonetta SA and Di Ze Rega GS: Intragonadal regulation of follicular maturation, Endocrinol Rev 10:205, 1989.

Treloar AE, Boynton RE, Borghild BG, et al: Variation of the human menstrual cycle through reproductive life, Int J Fertil 12:77, 1967.

Waites GT, Wood PL, et al: Immunohistological localization of human endometrial secretory protein, pregnancy-associated endometrial α_2-globulin (α2-PEG), during the menstrual cycle, J Reprod Fertil 82:665, 1988.

Walters MR: Steroid hormone receptors and the nucleus, Endocr Rev 6:512, 1985.

Wetzels LCG and Hoogland HJ: Relation between ultrasonographic evidence of ovulation and hormonal parameters: luteinizing hormone surge and initial progesterone rise, Fertil Steril 37:336, 1982.

World Health Organization: Temporal relationships between ovulation and defined changes in the concentration of plasma estradiol-17β, luteinizing hormone, follicle-stimulating hormone, and progesterone, Am J Obstet Gynecol 138:383, 1980.

Yalow RS and Berson SA: Assay of plasma insulin in human subjects by immunological methods, Nature 184:1648, 1959.

Ying S-Y, Becker A, et al: A inhibin and beta type transforming growth factor (TGFβ) have opposite modulating effects on the follicle stimulating hormone (FSH) induced aromatase activity of cultured rat granulosa cells, Biochem Biophys Res Commun 126:969, 1986.

Zegers-Hochschild F, Lira CG, Parada M, et al: A comparative study of the follicular growth profile in conception and nonconception cycles, Fertil Steril 41:244, 1984.

APPROACH TO
THE PATIENT

History and Examination of the Patient

CHAPTER 5

KEY TERMS AND DEFINITIONS

Anovulatory Cycle. Menstrual cycle when ovulation does not occur.

Dyspareunia. Painful intercourse.

Ectropion. The presence of endocervical (glandular) epithelium on the portio vaginalis of cervix. It may result from scarring of the external os or may be congenital.

LMP. Last menstrual period.

Menstrual Formula. Age of menarche × number of days of cycle × number of days of menstrual flow (e.g., 13 × 28 × 5).

Normal Transformation Zone. Area of columnar epithelium and squamous metaplasia in the vagina or on the cervix that has normal colposcopic patterns.

PMP. Previous menstrual period.

Sexual Dysfunction. A psychologic or physiologic problem or condition that prevents the usual full participation and enjoyment of coitus.

The first contact a physician has with a patient is critical. It allows an initial bond of trust to be developed on which the future relationship may be built. The patient will share sensitive information, feelings, and fears. The physician will gain her confidence and establish rapport by the understanding and nonjudgmental manner in which he or she collects these data.

The first contact generally involves taking a complete history, performing a complete physical examination, and ordering appropriate initial laboratory tests. In such a way the physician gains impressions of the patient's problems and needs and develops a plan for solutions. A gynecologic history includes a complete general history and adds information of gynecologic importance. In like manner the physical examination should be complete; no corners should be cut. The physician practicing obstetrics and gynecology should not assume that the patient's general medical needs are cared for by others, even if the patient has a personal family physician.

This chapter focuses on the appropriate manner that a gynecologic physician should use to conduct a history and physical examination.

DIRECT OBSERVATIONS BEFORE SPEAKING TO PATIENT (NONVERBAL CLUES)

When meeting a patient it is important to *look* at her even before speaking. Some experienced physicians observe patients sitting in their waiting rooms before actually beginning personal contact. The general demeanor of the patient should be evaluated. Basically five general impressions can be transmitted both by facial expression and by posture, including happiness, apathy, fear, anger, and sadness.

A patient who is happy, self-assured, and in good personal control generally has a relaxed face with a smile and a sparkle in her eyes. She is generally sitting relaxed and will offer the physician a warm and friendly greeting. Many new patients are apprehensive about meeting a new physician, and this apprehension may modify their usual expression of good spirits. Even under these circumstances, however, their warmth shows. Happy patients returning for visits after having established a relationship with a physician are usually warm, relaxed, and responsive.

Apathetic patients generally have a blank facial expression. The eyes lack sparkle, there is little muscular movement of the face, and the mouth is generally thin and in a neutral position, neither turned up nor down. The posture may be somewhat slouched, the handshake may be weak, and answers to verbal questions are short and unemotional. Although apathetic patients may have severe emotional illness, they may also be demonstrating resignation to an imagined or serious condition or they may be responding to multiple problems, which make them feel overwhelmed.

The frightened patient frequently has a tense expression on her face; her mouth is tight and the eyes are darting and narrow. She may be perspiring but have a dry mouth. Her posture demonstrates forward leaning, and there is often endless hand activity. When she reacts, it may be grossly out of proportion to offered stimuli.

The angry patient frequently has narrowed eyes, furrowed brows, and narrow, tight lips. She may be sitting on the edge of her chair, leaning forward as if to pounce. Unlike the frightened patient, whose pose may be defensive, the angry patient radiates aggression. Her voice is usually harsh, and her overreaction to questions usually involves short, threatening phrases.

The sad patient generally sits with slouched shoulders, large, sad eyes, and a turned-down mouth. The eyes may glisten, and there may be tears. This patient is most likely depressed, and her speech reflects remorse and hopelessness.

By observing these nonverbal clues, the physician determines the appropriate style for conducting the interview. Often an opening remark appropriate to the patient's demeanor may be useful, such as, "You seem sad today, Ms. Jones," or, "I detect a note of anger in your voice, Ms. Smith. Can you tell me why that is?" By so doing, the physician projects sensitivity to the patient's feelings and genuine care with respect to her circumstances.

ESSENCE OF THE GYNECOLOGIC HISTORY

Chief Complaint

The patient should be encouraged to tell the physician why she has sought help. Questions such as, "What is the nature of the problem that brought you to me?" or, "How may I help you?" are good ways to begin. The patient should be able to present the problem as she sees it, in her own words, and should be interrupted only for specific clarification of points or to offer direction if she digresses too far. During the interview the physician should face the patient with direct eye contact and acknowledge important points of the history either by nodding or by a word or two. Such an approach allows the physician to be involved in the problem and demonstrates a degree of caring to the patient. When the patient has completed the history of her current problem, pertinent open-ended questions should be asked with respect to specific points made by the patient. This process allows the physician to develop a more detailed data base. Directed questions may be asked where pertinent to clarify points. In general, however, the patient should be encouraged to tell her story as she sees it rather than to react with short answers to very specific questions. Under the latter circumstance the physician may get the answers he or she is looking for, but they may not be accurate answers.

A general outline for a gynecologic and general history is given in the box on p. 145. The outline is given in a specific order for general orientation. The information, however, may be collected through any comfortable discussion with the patient that seems appropriate in the circumstances. It is important that all aspects be covered.

Pertinent Gynecologic History

A pertinent gynecologic history can be divided into several parts. It begins with a menstrual history, in which the age of menarche, duration of each monthly cycle, number of days during which menses occur, and regularity of the menstrual cycles should be noted. The dates of the last menstrual period and previous menstrual period should be obtained. In addition, the characteristics of the menstrual flow, including the color, the amount of flow, and accompanying symptoms, such as cramping, sweating, headache, or diarrhea, should be noted. In general, menstruation that occurs monthly (range 21 to 40 days), lasts 4 to 7 days, is bright red, and is often accompanied by cramping on the day preceding and the first day of the period is characteristic of an ovulatory cycle. Menstruation that is irregular, often dark in color, painless, and frequently short or very long may indicate lack of ovulation. The first few cycles in teenagers or cycles in premenopausal women are frequently anovulatory and as a result may come at irregular intervals.

The second pertinent point in the gynecologic history is that of previous pregnancies. The patient should be asked specifically to list pregnancies that she has experienced, including the year of the pregnancy, the duration, the type of delivery, the size, sex, and current condition of the baby, any complications that may have occurred, and whether the infant was breast fed and, if so, for how long. Elective terminations of pregnancy and spontaneous abortions should also be noted, including the time of gestation that they occurred and the circumstances under which they took place. Ectopic or molar pregnancies should also be noted, including the type of therapy that was given. When such events have occurred, obtaining old records for review is appropriate. Any pregnancy should be discussed with respect to excessive bleeding, chills, fever, known infection, or other complicating events. It is also appropriate to ask the patient about the individual who fathered each of these pregnancies so that the physician may determine the number of sexual partners the patient has had.

A history of vaginal and pelvic infections should be obtained. The patient should be asked what types of infection she has had in the past, what treatment was received, and what complications were experienced. Risk factors for human immunodeficiency virus (HIV) infection, such as intravenous drug abuse or coitus with drug abusers or bisexual men, should be sought by direct questioning and HIV screening offered where appropriate. All hospitalizations should be reviewed as to cause and outcome.

All instances of gynecologic surgical procedures should be noted, including minor operations, such as endometrial biopsies; vulvar, vaginal, or cervical biopsies; dilation and curettage; laparoscopic examinations; and any major procedure that the patient may have undergone. When such data are elicited, dates, types of procedures, diagnosis, and significant complications should be noted. In cases where pertinent, past records should be sought.

A careful urologic history should be taken. A history of bladder dysfunction, loss of urine,

HISTORY OUTLINE

I. Observation—nonverbal clues
II. Chief complaint
III. History of gynecologic problem(s)
  A. Menstrual history—LMP, PMP
  B. Pregnancy history
  C. Vaginal and pelvic infections
  D. Gynecologic surgical procedures
  E. Urologic history
  F. Pelvic pain
  G. Vaginal bleeding
  H. Sexual status
  I. Contraceptive status
IV. Significant health problems
  A. Systemic illnesses
  B. Surgical procedures
  C. Other hospitalizations
V. Medications, habits, and allergies
  A. Medications taken
  B. Medication and other allergies
  C. Smoking history
  D. Alcohol usage
  E. Illicit drug usage
VI. Bleeding problems
VII. Family history
  A. Illnesses and causes of death of first-order relatives
  B. Congenital malformations, mental retardation, and reproductive wastage
VIII. Occupational and avocational history
IX. Social history
X. Review of systems
  A. Head
  B. Cardiovascular-respiratory
  C. Gastrointestinal
  D. Genitourinary
  E. Neuromuscular
  F. Psychiatric
    1. Physical abuse
    2. Sexual abuse
      a. Incest
      b. Rape

acute or chronic bladder or kidney infections, or other urologic problems, such as hematuria or the passage of urinary stones, should be noted.

Symptoms of pelvic pain or discomfort should be discussed fully. The pain should be described, noting the presence or absence of a relationship to the menstrual cycle and its association with other events, such as coitus or bleeding.

IMPORTANT POINTS OF SEXUAL HISTORY

1. Sexual activity (presence of)
2. Types of relationships
3. Individual(s) involved
4. Satisfaction? Orgasmic?
5. Dyspareunia
6. Sexual dysfunction
   a. Patient
   b. Partner

Any vaginal bleeding not related to menses should be noted, as well as its relationship to the menstrual cycle and to other events, such as coitus, the use of tampons, or the use of a contraceptive device.

A complete sexual history should be obtained (see box above), and specific problems should be evaluated. The history should include whether the patient is sexually active, the types of relationships she has, whether she is orgasmic, whether she experiences pain or discomfort with coitus (dyspareunia), and whether she or her partner is experiencing problems with sexual performance (sexual dysfunction). It is important that the physician review or rehearse the types of questions that will be asked and consider the response he or she will give to less typical answers (e.g., responses concerning homosexuality or less common sexual practices). This helps prevent the physician from demonstrating surprise and thus transmitting an attitude of disapproval.

Finally, the patient's contraceptive history should be investigated, including methods used, length of time they have been used, and any complications that may have arisen.

General Health History

The patient should be asked to list any significant health problems that she has had during her lifetime, including all hospitalizations and operative procedures. It is reasonable for the physician to ask about specific illnesses, such as diabetes, hepatitis, tuberculosis, or rheumatic fever, that seem likely based on what is known about the patient or about the patient's situation. Some physicians use a history checklist of the most common conditions, but a careful physician who questions appropriately can be equally effective.

Medications taken and reasons for doing so should be noted, as should allergic responses to medications.

The patient should be questioned for evidence of a bleeding or clotting problem, such as a history of hemorrhage with minor procedures, easy bruisability, or bleeding from mucous membranes.

A smoking history should be obtained in detail, including amount and time she has smoked. She should be questioned about the use of illicit drugs, including marijuana and cocaine. Any affirmative answers should be followed by specific questions concerning length of use, types of drugs used, and side effects that may have been noticed. Her use of alcohol should be detailed carefully, including the number of drinks per day and any history of binge drinking or previous therapy for alcoholism.

Family History

A detailed family history of first-order relatives (mother, father, sisters, brothers, children, and grandparents) should be taken and a family tree constructed (Figure 5-1). Serious illnesses or causes of death for each individual should be noted. Also, an inquiry should be made about any congenital malformations, mental retardation, or pregnancy wastage in either the patient's or her husband's family. Such information may offer clues to hereditarily determined causes of reproductive problems.

Occupational and Social History

The patient should be asked to detail her and her husband's occupational histories, including jobs held and work performed. It is also useful to elicit a history of hobbies and other avocations that might affect health or reproductive capacity.

A social history should be obtained. This involves where and with whom the patient lives, other individuals in the household, areas of the world where the patient and her husband have lived or traveled, and unusual experiences that either may have had.

Review of Systems

A complete review of systems is necessary to uncover symptoms from other areas that relate

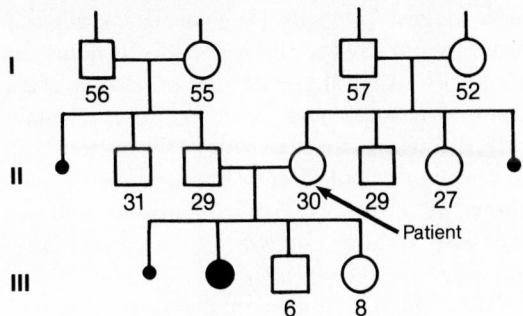

- ● Spontaneous miscarriage
- ○ Living females
- ☐ Living males
- ● Female who died neonatally because of prematurity (30 weeks)

FIGURE 5-1
Family tree of typical gynecologic patient.

to reproduction and gynecologic problems (e.g., serious headaches, epileptic seizures, dizziness, or fainting spells). Such a history also may indicate exposure to medications that may be injurious should a pregnancy occur in the future.

It is important to obtain a good cardiovascular/respiratory history, as well as a history of hypertension, heart disease, or chest problems, such as asthma. Each of these may have an immediate effect on the patient and may also influence a future pregnancy.

Of importance to the gynecologist is a history of gastrointestinal disorders, such as functional bowel problems or hepatitis. Affirmative answers should be fully investigated with respect to specific illnesses and potential residuals that may affect the patient's current health.

Questions about the genitourinary system are important both from the standpoint of bladder function and as an indication of whether renal function has been or is impaired.

Neurologic or neuromuscular impairment may be important from the standpoint of the ability of the patient to carry and deliver a child without difficulty.

A history of vascular disease, including thrombophlebitis with or without pulmonary embolism, varicose veins, or other vascular problems, should be sought. If a positive history of thrombophlebitis is obtained, possible relationship to a hormonal exposure, such as pregnancy or oral contraceptive use, should be sought.

The psychiatric history should be detailed carefully for any emotional or mental disease processes. In addition, the patient should be asked specifically whether she has been sexually abused in adult life, in childhood, by a stranger, or incestuously, or raped. This is further discussed in Chapter 12.

ESSENCE OF COMPLETE PHYSICAL EXAMINATION

The gynecologist should perform a complete physical examination on every patient at the first visit and at each annual checkup, particularly if the gynecologist is the primary physician caring for the patient. Physical examination is a time to both gather information about the patient and teach the patient information she should know about herself and her body.

The patient should disrobe completely and be covered by a hospital gown that ensures warmth and modesty. During each step of the examination she should be allowed to maintain personal control by being offered options whenever possible. These options begin with the presence or absence of a chaperone. The chaperone, a third party, usually a woman, serves a variety of purposes. She may offer warmth, compassion, and support to the patient during uncomfortable or potentially embarrassing portions of the examination. She may help the physician to carry out procedures, such as the Papanicolaou (Pap) smear, and in some cases she offers the physician protection from having his intentions misunderstood by a naive or suspicious individual. Although the presence of a chaperone is not absolutely imperative in every physician-patient relationship, the availability of one for the specific instance where it is deemed advisable should be ensured. Many clinics insist on the presence of a chaperone, and it is wise for the physician to follow local custom.

The examination should begin with a general evaluation of the patient's appearance and posture. Her weight and her blood pressure should be taken initially, and postmenopausal women should have their height measured routinely to document evidence of osteoporosis, which causes vertebral compression fractures.

The patient's eyes, ears, nose, and throat should be examined. Funduscopic examination should be performed at least annually to inspect the blood vessels of the retina and to observe the lens for evidence of early cataract formation. The gynecologist should either measure intraocular pressures in women over age 40 or suggest that they be seen by an ophthalmologist for this purpose. The patient should be inspected for evidence of upper lip or chin hair, which may indicate increased androgen activity.

The thyroid gland should be palpated for irregularities or increase in size (goiter). Discrete areas of enlargement, hardness, and tenderness should be described. The patient's neck should be palpated for evidence of adenopathy along the supraclavicular and posterior auricular chains.

The chest should be inspected for symmetry of movement of the diaphragm, percussed for areas of consolidation, and auscultated bilaterally for breath and adventitious sounds.

The heart should be examined by palpation for points of maximum impulse, percussed for size, and auscultated for irregularities of rate and evidence of murmurs and other adventitious sounds. An older woman's neck should be auscultated for evidence of vascular bruits. The patient's heart should be auscultated in both the lying and the sitting positions.

A careful breast examination should be carried out in a systematic fashion as described in Chapter 13. At this time the patient should be taught breast self-examination and encouraged to perform this each month.

The abdomen should be systematically examined in the following fashion.

Inspection. The abdomen should be inspected for symmetry; scars, protuberance, or discoloration of the skin; and striations, which may suggest previous pregnancies or adrenal gland hyperactivity. The hair pattern should be noted. The typical female pattern is that of an inverted triangle over the mons pubis. A male pattern involves hair growth between the area of the mons pubis and the umbilicus, also known as a diamond pattern and may indicate excessive androgen activity in the patient (Figure 5-2).

Palpation. The abdomen should be palpated for organomegaly (enlarged organs), particularly involving the liver, spleen, kidneys, and uterus, and for adnexal masses, which may be palpated abdominally. Palpation also affords the possibility of noting a fluid wave, which would suggest either ascites or hemoperitoneum. Palpation also yields evidence for rigidity of the abdomen, which would imply spasm in the rectus muscles secondary to intraabdominal irritation. Where the irritation is caused by intraabdominal hemorrhage or infection, this rigidity is often evidence of an acute abdomen. During the palpation of the abdomen the physician should elicit the phenomenon of *rebound*, which also signifies intraabdominal irritation, by gently pressing the abdomen and then releasing. The release may cause pain either under the spot (direct rebound) or in a different portion of the abdomen (referred rebound). It should be noted, however, that sudden, rough pressure may cause pain even in a normal patient.

Percussion. Percussion affords the ability to differentiate fluid waves and to outline solid organs and masses.

Auscultation. The physician should listen for

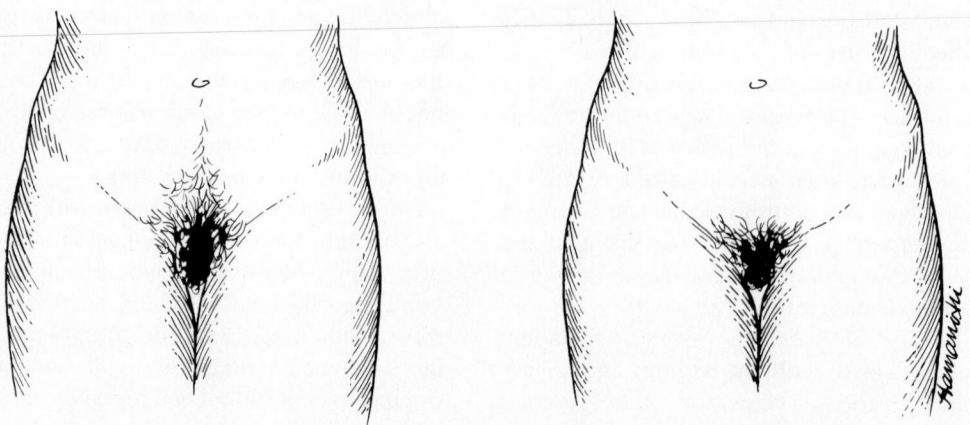

FIGURE 5-2
Normal female pubic hair pattern (*right*) and hair pattern of female showing male (androgenized) pattern (*left*).

bowel sounds. Hypoactive or absent bowel sounds may imply an ileus caused by peritoneal irritation of the bowel. Hyperactive bowel sounds may imply intrinsic irritation of the bowel or partial or complete bowel obstruction.

The groins should be palpated for adenopathy and inguinal hernias. The physician should also elicit the femoral pulses beneath the groin in the femoral triangles, and when these are present, the differences that may exist between the two femoral areas should be noted.

Legs should be examined for evidence of varicose veins, edema, and other lesions. In addition, it is reasonable to judge arterial circulation to the extremities by palpating pedal pulses on the dorsum of the foot.

PELVIC EXAMINATION

The pelvic examination is conducted with the patient lying supine on the examining table with the legs in stirrups. The patient may or may not desire to be draped with a sheet. Because the physician should be pointing out aspects of the patient's pelvic anatomy where possible, many patients prefer to have the head of the table elevated and to use a small hand mirror to follow the examination with the physician. In such instances, a sheet may be cumbersome. The physician should be sure the patient is as relaxed as possible and should take a few minutes to describe the procedure and allow the shy or nervous patient to prepare herself. Suggesting that the patient allow her legs to fall wide apart and concentrate on relaxing her abdominal muscles may be helpful.

Inspection

The perineum should be carefully inspected beginning with the mons pubis. The quality and pattern of the hair on the mons and the labia majora should be noted. Areas of alopecia should be noted, because they may imply a skin abnormality. In general, as a woman ages, the pubic hair becomes less dense and may turn gray. During the inspection of the pubic hair the physician should look for evidence of body lice (pediculosis). Next, the skin of the perineum is inspected for redness, excoriation, discoloration, or loss of pigment and for the presence of vesicles, ulcerations, pustules, warty growths, or neoplastic growths. In addition, pigmented nevi or other pigmented le-

sions should be noted, as should varicose veins. Skin scars denoting previous episiotomy or other obstetric lacerations should be noted.

Next the specific structures of the perineum should be systematically evaluated. The clitoris should be noted and its size and shape described. Normally it is 1 to 1.5 cm in length. Any irregularities or abnormalities of the labia majora or minora should be noted and carefully described. At times these areas are injured by trauma related to coitus, accidental injury, or childbearing. The patient should be questioned about evidence of trauma when appropriate.

The introitus should be observed closely. Whether the hymen is intact, imperforate, or marital and whether the perineum gapes or remains closed in the usual lithotomy position should be noted.

The perineal body, the area at the posterior aspect of the labia where the muscles of the superficial perineal compartment come together, should be inspected. It represents the focal point of support for the perineum and is between the vagina and the rectum. The perianal area is then inspected for evidence of hemorrhoids, sphincter continence, and other lesions (Figure 5-3).

Palpation

The next step in the examination of the perineum involves palpation. With the second and fourth fingers of the gloved hand separating the labia minora, the urethra is inspected and the length of the urethra is palpated and "milked" with the middle finger. In this way, irregularities and inflammation of Skene's glands (periurethral glands), pus or mucus expressed, or a suburethral diverticulum can be noted. Any pus expressed from the urethra should be submitted to Gram stain and cultured, since it is frequently found to contain gonococci. The gloved hand then palpates the area of the posterior third of the labia majora, placing the index finger inside the introitus and the thumb on the outside of the labium. In this way, enlargements or cysts of Bartholin glands are noted. This exercise should be performed on each side.

With the gloved hand holding the labia apart, the opening of the vagina should be inspected. The presence of a cystocele or a cystourethrocele should be noted. This would be seen as a bulging of vaginal mucosa downward

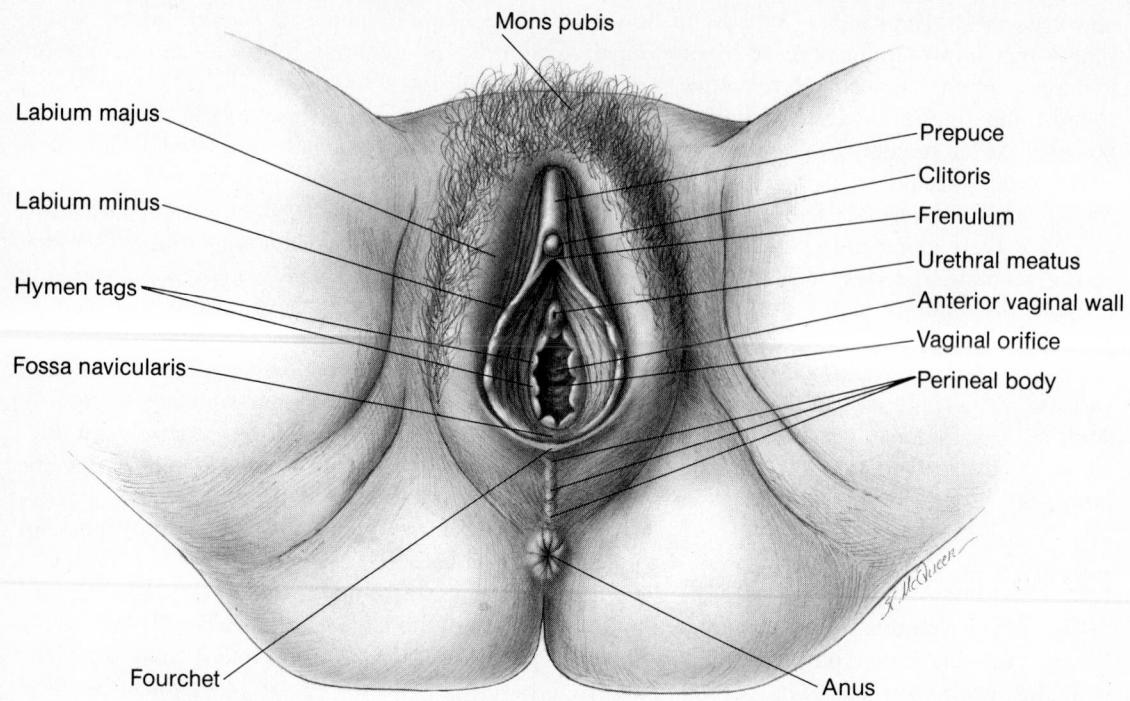

FIGURE 5-3
Normal female perineum. (Redrawn from Krantz KE: Anatomy of the female reproductive system. In Benson RC, editor: Current obstetric and gynecologic diagnosis and treatment, editor 5, Los Altos, Calif, 1984, Lange Medical Publications.)

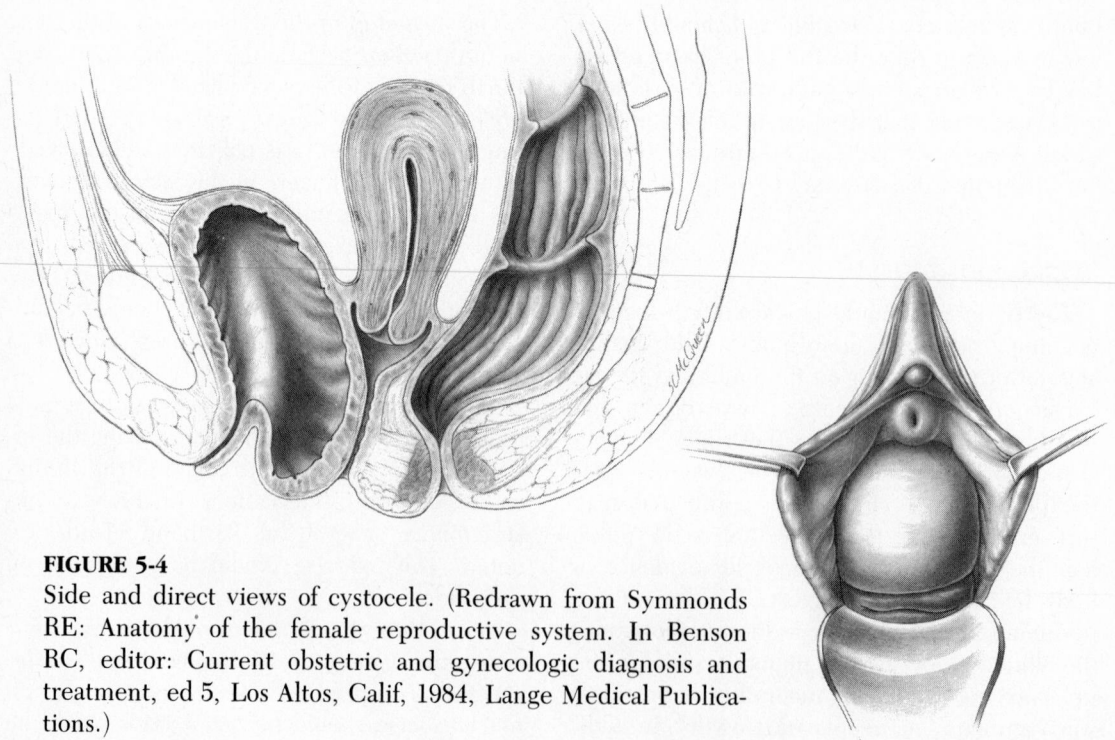

FIGURE 5-4
Side and direct views of cystocele. (Redrawn from Symmonds RE: Anatomy of the female reproductive system. In Benson RC, editor: Current obstetric and gynecologic diagnosis and treatment, ed 5, Los Altos, Calif, 1984, Lange Medical Publications.)

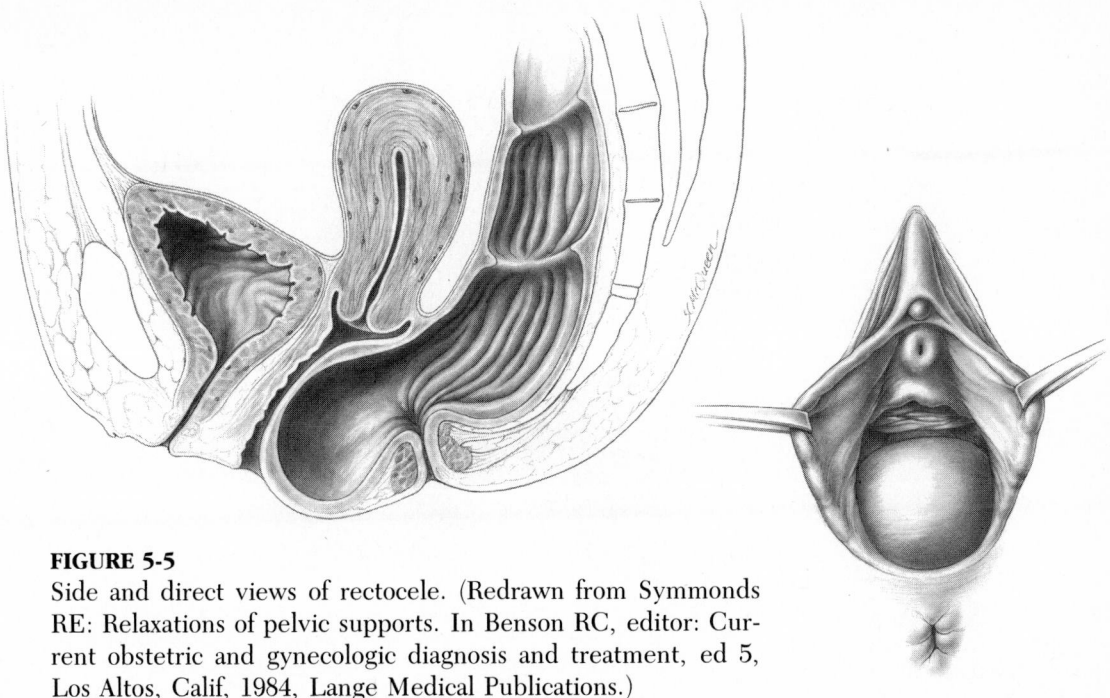

FIGURE 5-5
Side and direct views of rectocele. (Redrawn from Symmonds RE: Relaxations of pelvic supports. In Benson RC, editor: Current obstetric and gynecologic diagnosis and treatment, ed 5, Los Altos, Calif, 1984, Lange Medical Publications.)

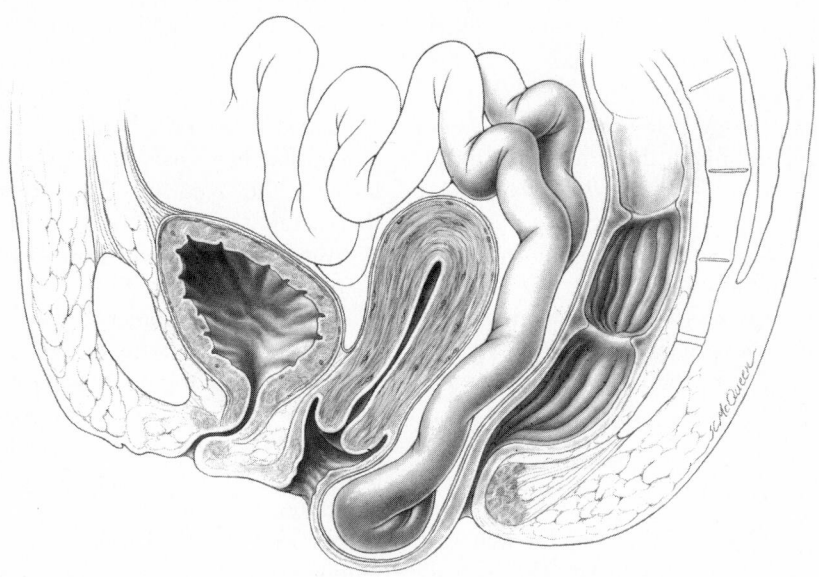

FIGURE 5-6
Lateral view of enterocele. (Redrawn from Symmonds RE: Relaxations of pelvic supports. In Benson RC, editor: Current obstetric and gynecologic diagnosis and treatment, ed 5, Los Altos, Calif, 1984, Lange Medical Publications.)

from the anterior wall of the vagina. The presence of this abnormality may be noted either by simply observing or by asking the patient to bear down (Figure 5-4). Likewise, the posterior wall should be noted for a bulging upward, which would represent a rectocele (Figure 5-5).

Also, with the patient bearing down, the cervix may become visible, indicating prolapse of the uterus. A cystic bulge in the cul-de-sac may represent an enterocele (Figure 5-6). Each of these observations is evidence for relaxation of the pelvic supports and should be graded 1+

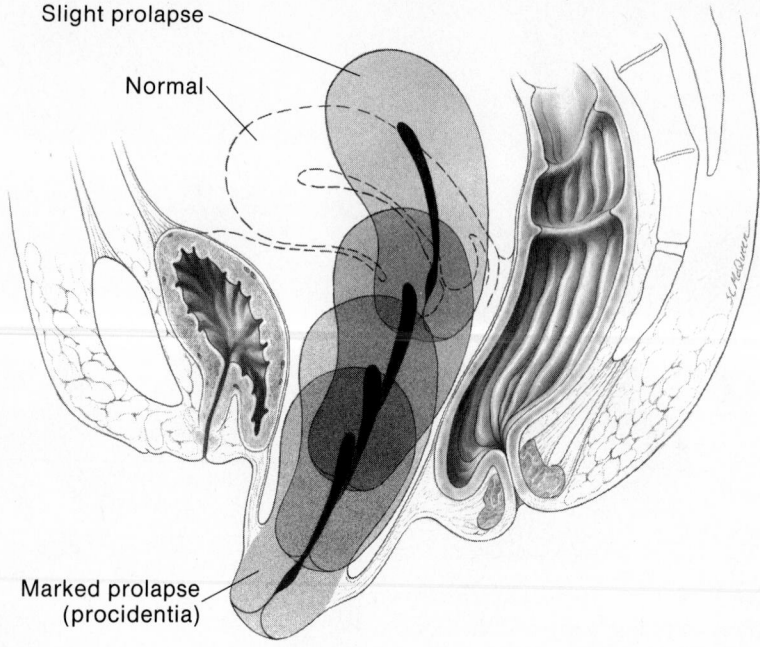

Slight prolapse

Normal

Marked prolapse
(procidentia)

FIGURE 5-7
Depiction of prolapse of uterus. (Redrawn from Symmonds RE: Relaxations of pelvic supports. In Benson RC, editor: Current obstetric and gynecologic diagnosis and treatment, ed 5, Los Altos, Calif, 1984, Lange Medical Publications.)

to 4+, with 1+ being a minimum bulge and 4+ being a bulge through the introitus. A prolapse of the cervix and uterus downward into the uterine canal can be graded in stages I, II, and III, with stage I being a minimum descent of the cervix into the vaginal canal, stage II being a descent of the cervix to the introitus, and stage III being the prolapse of the cervix or uterus through the introitus (total descensus) (Figure 5-7).

Speculum Examination

After palpation the physician chooses the appropriate speculum for the patient. The typical Graves speculum generally is of three sizes: small, which is used in young children, women who have undergone tight perineal repair, or occasionally in the aged patient who has undergone severe involution; medium, used for most women; and large, which is useful in large or obese women or those who are grand multiparas. Also available is the narrow Pederson speculum, which is the length of the Graves speculum but is narrow, for women who have not become active sexually, have never become pregnant, or have not used tampons. It is also of value for women who have undergone operations that have narrowed the vaginal diameter. For the majority of women the length of the vagina is similar, approximately 6 to 7 cm, and the Pederson or medium Graves speculum is appropriate (Figure 5-8).

The speculum should be warmed, either by a warming device or by being placed in warm water, and then touched to the patient's leg to see if the temperature is appropriate and comfortable. The speculum is then inserted by placing the transverse diameter of the blades in the anteroposterior position and guiding the blades through the introitus in a downward motion with the tips pointing toward the rectum. Because the anterior wall of the vagina is backed by the pubic symphysis, which is rigid, pressure upward causes the patient discomfort. This is avoided by following the described method of introducing the speculum. Also, in the resting state the vagina lies on the rectum and actually extends posteriorly from the introitus. The procedure may be facilitated by placing two fingers into the introitus and pressing down.

Once the blades are inserted, the speculum should be turned so that the transverse

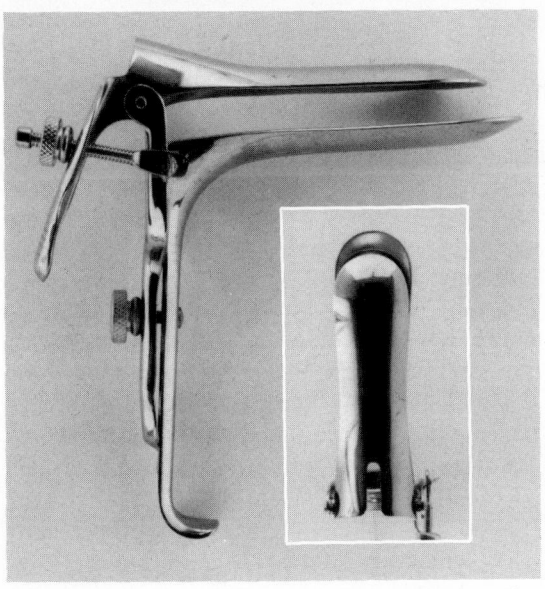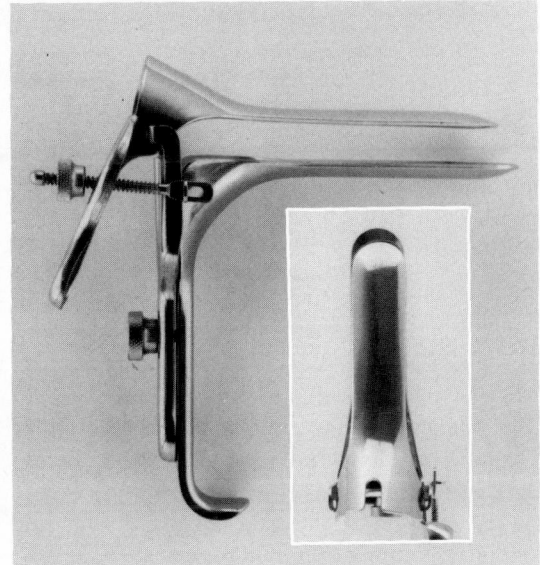

FIGURE 5-8
Graves *(left)* and Pederson *(right)* specula.

axis of the blades is in the transverse axis of the vagina. The blades should be inserted to their full length and then opened so that the physician may inspect for the position of the cervix. The cervix generally fits into the open blades with ease. If this does not occur, the physician should inspect for the position of the cervix with his or her finger and then reinsert the speculum accordingly. Once the blades are inserted and the cervix is visualized, the speculum should be opened and the introitus widened so that the cervix can be adequately inspected and a Pap smear taken. This can be done by using the screw adjustment on the base of the speculum. When inserted properly the speculum generally stays in place.

The physician then inspects the vagina and cervix. The vaginal canal is inspected during the insertion of the speculum or on its removal. The vaginal epithelium should be noted for evidence of erythema or lesions. Fluid discharge should be evaluated on slides prepared in the following fashion. One drop of vaginal secretion is placed in one drop of sodium chloride solution, cover-slipped, and inspected for unicellular flagellated protozoa, *Trichomonas vaginalis*. The vaginal epithelial cells should also be inspected. The cells should have sharp borders and normal-appearing nuclei. Any variation from the normal appearance of cells may

imply infection (see Chapter 21). A drop of potassium hydroxide is placed on another slide, and a drop of vaginal secretion is placed within this. The potassium hydroxide causes lysis of the epithelial cells and trichomonads but leaves intact the mycelium of *Monilia*. Thus the presence of mycelium is helpful in diagnosing vaginal moniliasis. Vaginal lesions, such as areas of adenosis (see DES, Chapter 14), clear cystic structures (Gartner's cysts), or inclusion cysts on the lines of scars or episiotomy incisions, should be noted.

The cervix is inspected next. It should be pink, shiny, and clear. In a nulliparous individual, the external os should be round. When a woman is parous, the external os takes on a fishmouth appearance, and if there have been cervical lacerations, healed stellate lacerations may be noted (Figure 5-9). Normally the transformation zone (i.e., the junction of squamous and columnar epithelium) is just barely visible inside the external os. Occasionally glandular epithelium may be present on the portio vaginalis, moving the transformation zone onto the portio. This is common in teenage girls, women who have been exposed to diethylstilbestrol in utero, some women with vaginitis, or women immediately postpartum or postabortion. Generally, this is cleared by a process of metaplasia, in which squamous epithelium covers the columnar epithelium. This process,

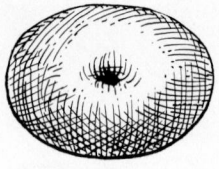
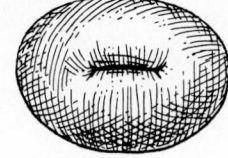
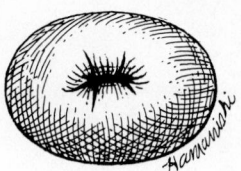

Nulliparous   Parous   Stellate

FIGURE 5-9
Nulliparous, parous, and stellate lacerations of cervix.

however, may leave small areas of irregularities and inclusion cysts, called *nabothian cysts*, which may be seen in various sizes and shapes. They are of no clinical significance. Often after a women has delivered a baby, there is lateral scarring at the 3 and 9 o'clock positions, causing an eversion of the external os so that the reddened columnar epithelium is visible on the anterior and posterior lips of the cervix. If the observer looks closely, the transitional zone can be seen along the edges of this area of eversion and may be perfectly healthy. This is called an *ectropion* and is not evidence of a pathologic condition.

Any lesions of the cervix should be noted and, where appropriate, a biopsy should be performed. In a patient with acute herpes progenitalis, vesicles or ulcers may be noted. In a patient infected with human papillomavirus, warts (condyloma acuminata) on the cervix may also be observed.

Papanicolaou Smear

At this point in the examination a Pap smear is usually taken. In 1943 Papanicolaou and Trout published their now classic monograph demonstrating the value of vaginal and cervical cytology as a screening tool for cervical neoplasm. With the use of the Pap smear in screening programs, the incidence of invasive cervical cancer has been reduced 50%. Recently, programs focusing on cost-effectiveness have suggested that the screening interval may be extended from the usual 1 year to 3 years in certain low-risk individuals. Because low risk is often difficult to define, the American College of Obstetricians and Gynecologists suggested in 1984 that annual screening was appropriate for most American women. Initial screening should begin at age 18 or when the individual becomes sexually active. High-risk women, those with a history of early sexual activity and multiple partners, should be screened annu-

ally. Those patients with later exposure to coitus who have only one sexual partner and who have had two successive negative annual smears may be considered low-risk and should be screened every 1 to 3 years at the discretion of the physician. A recent case-control study by Shy et al. questioned the wisdom of extending the screening interval beyond 2 years. Although no significant increase was noted in the incidence of cervical cancer in women screened every 2 years compared with annually, the risk increased 3.9 times if the interval was 3 years and 12.3 times in women not screened for 10 years. The presence of risk factors did not influence these results.

A Pap smear can be performed in a number of ways. The major objective is to sample secretions from the endocervical canal and to scrape the transitional zone. It is also useful to sample the vaginal pool, although this does not usually yield as high an incidence of cervical disease as does sampling of the canal and the transitional zone. One way of performing the Pap smear is as follows:

1. After excess mucus is gently removed, the endocervical canal is sampled with either a cotton-tipped applicator or a cytobrush, which is placed into the canal and rotated. Although both instruments generally dislodge adequate numbers of cells for study, the cytobrush appears to give more accurate results and higher yields of positive findings. The material obtained is then smeared thinly on a microscope slide by rotation of the swab or brush on the glass surface. This is labeled *endocervix* and fixed immediately either by use of a spray fixative or by immersion of the slide into a fixative solution (Figure 5-10).

2. With an Ayers spatula or some variation thereof, the entire transformation zone is scraped and smeared thinly on a second slide, which is immediately fixed. If the physician wishes a sample of the vaginal

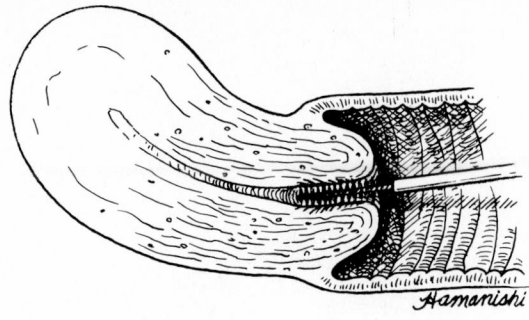

FIGURE 5-10
Obtaining cells from endocervix using a cytobrush.

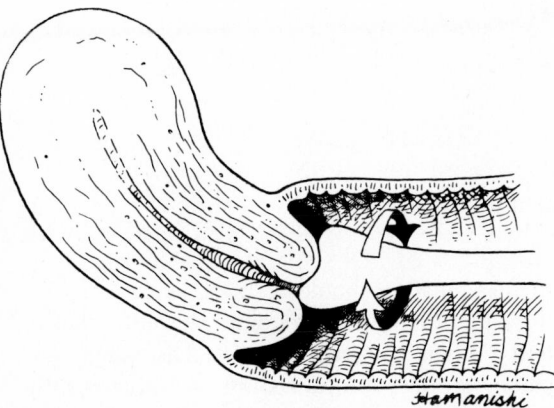

FIGURE 5-11
Obtaining cells from transformation zone using Ayers spatula.

pool, this may be taken with the reverse side of the Ayers spatula and smeared on a third slide or on a second portion of the slide containing the transformation zone material (Figure 5-11).

A number of fixatives are available, but it is important that they be applied immediately before drying and distortion of the cells takes place. Pap smears are currently reported using the following descriptive system:

Normal
Atypical
  Inflammation
  Possible dysplasia
Metaplasia
Mild dysplasia
Moderate dysplasia
Severe dysplasia—
  carcinoma in situ
Invasive cancer

In most instances, particularly with new patients, it is appropriate to culture for gonorrhea and *Chlamydia* using swabs that sample secretions from the endocervical canal. This step may be performed after the Pap smear.

Bimanual Examination

The bimanual examination allows the physician to palpate the uterus and the adnexa. The index and middle fingers of the dominant hand are placed within the vagina, and the thumb is folded under so as not to cause the patient distress in the area of the mons pubis, clitoris, and pubic symphysis. The fingers are inserted deeply into the vagina so that they rest beneath the cervix in the posterior fornix. The physician should be in a comfortable position at this point, generally with the leg on the side of the vaginal examining hand on a table lift and the elbow of that arm resting on the knee. The opposite hand is placed on the patient's abdomen above the pubic symphysis. The flat of the fingers are used for palpation. The physician then elevates the uterus by pressing up on the cervix and delivering the uterus to the abdominal hand so that the uterus may be placed between the two hands, thereby identifying its position, size, shape, consistency, and mobility. In the normal and nonpregnant state the uterus is approximately 6 by 4 cm and weighs about 70 g. It may be somewhat larger in a woman who has had children (Figure 5-12).

Enlargement of the uterus should be described in detail. Size may be estimated in centimeters or by comparing with weeks of normal gestational age.

The uterus in two thirds of instances is anteflexed so that the abdominal hand is palpating the posterior wall of the uterus and the vaginal fingers the anterior wall. The uterus may be retroverted. If it is positioned in a straight line with the vagina, it is said to be midposition or first-degree retroverted; if it lies backward in the cul-de-sac off the direct line of the vagina, it is said to be second-degree retroverted; if it is flexed deeply into the cul-de-sac pressing toward the rectum, it is third-degree retroverted. A third-degree retroverted uterus that cannot be brought forward by manipulation is best examined by rectovaginal examination, which is described later in the chapter. The general shape of the uterus is that of a pear, with the broadest portion at the upper pole of

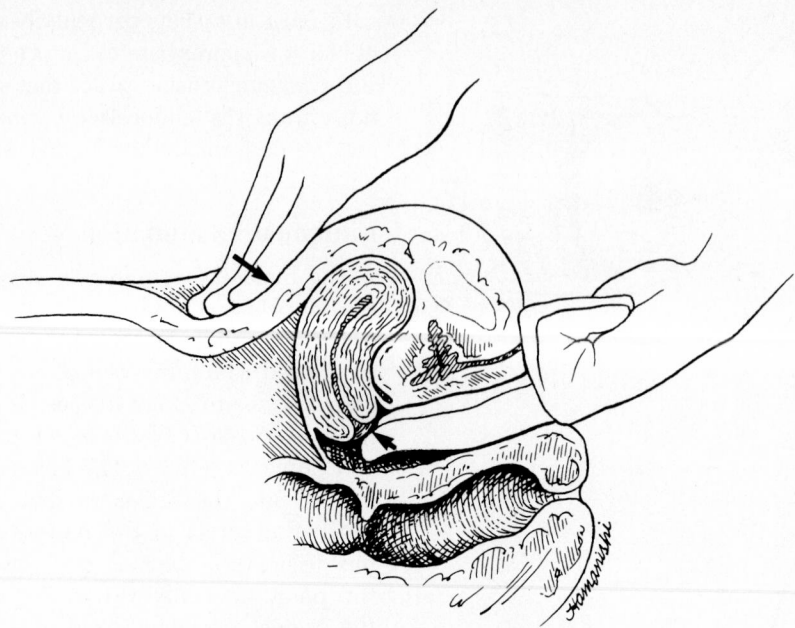

FIGURE 5-12
Bimanual examination of uterus.

the fundus. Generally the uterus is mobile, and if it fails to move, it may be fixed by adhesions. The surface should be smooth; irregularities may indicate the presence of uterine leiomyomas (fibroids).

The shape of the uterus should also be described in detail. The consistency of the uterus is generally firm but not rock-hard, and this should be noted in the examination. Any undue tenderness caused by palpation or movement of the uterus should be noted, since it may imply an inflammatory process.

Attention is then turned to examination of the adnexa. If the right hand is the pelvic hand, the first two fingers of the right hand are then moved into the right vaginal fornix as deeply as they can be inserted. The abdominal hand is placed just medial to the anterior superior iliac spine on the right, the two hands are brought as close together as possible, and with a sliding motion from the area of the anterior superior iliac spine to the introitus, the fingers are swept downward, allowing for the adnexa to be palpated between them. A normal ovary is approximately 3 by 2 cm (about the size of a walnut) and will sweep between the two fingers with ease unless it is fixed in an abnormal position by adhesions. When the adnexa is palpated, its size, mobility, and consistency should be described. However, this portion of

the examination should be brief, since it causes the patient a mild to moderate sickening sensation. When the right adnexa has been palpated, the left adnexa should be palpated in a similar fashion by turning the vaginal hand to the left vaginal fornix and repeating the exercise on the left side (Figure 5-13). Adnexa are usually not palpable in postmenopausal women because of involution and retraction of the ovary to a position higher in the pelvis. A palpable organ in such an individual should be further investigated for ovarian pathology.

Rectovaginal Examination

After completing the vaginal portion of the bimanual examination, the middle finger is re-lubricated with a water-soluble lubricant and placed into the rectum. Many physicians think the glove should be changed so as not to contaminate the rectum with vaginal organisms. The index finger is reinserted into the vagina. In this fashion the rectovaginal septum is palpated between the two fingers, and any thickness or mass is noted. The finger should also attempt to identify the uterosacral ligaments, which extend from the posterior wall of the cervix posteriorly and laterally toward the sacrum. Any thickening or beadiness of these

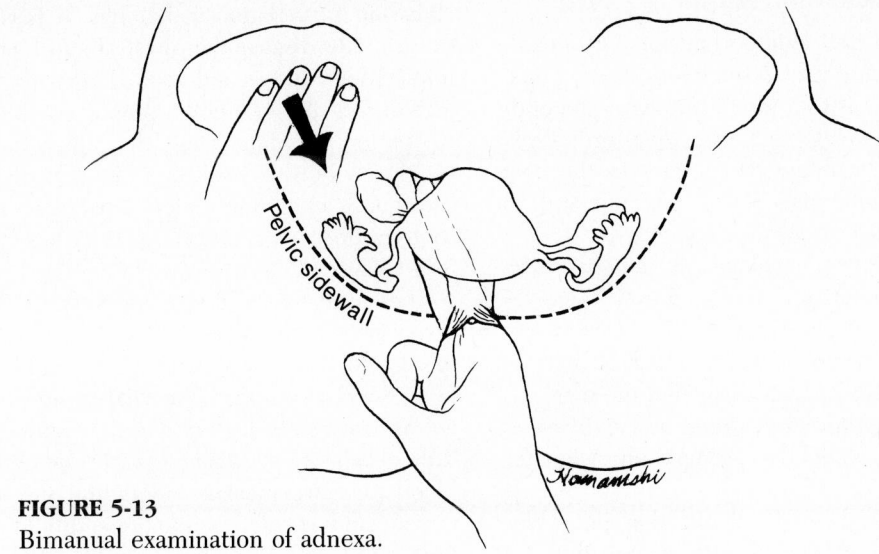

FIGURE 5-13
Bimanual examination of adnexa.

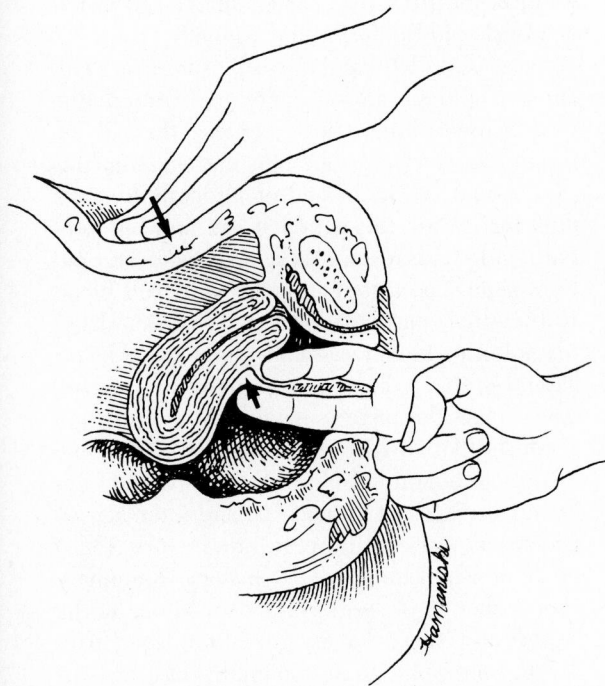

FIGURE 5-14
Rectovaginal examination.

Rectal Examination

The rectum is then palpated in all dimensions with the rectal examining finger. It should be possible to palpate as many as 70% of bowel lesions with the rectal finger. Because bowel cancer is common in women, particularly after the age of 35, this part of the examination should not be overlooked. The physician should also note the tone of the anal sphincter and any other anal abnormalities, such as hemorrhoids, fissures, or masses. Finally, a stool sample is taken on the examining finger and tested for occult blood. This is particularly important in women past the age of 35 who may be at risk for bowel cancer.

At the end of the examination the physician should give the patient some facial tissue so that she may remove the lubricating jelly from her perineum before she dresses.

It is important that each step of the examination be explained to the patient and that she be reassured about all normal findings. Wherever possible, abnormal findings should be pointed out to the patient either by allowing her to palpate the pathologic condition or by demonstrating it to her using a hand mirror. It is also appropriate to demonstrate normal structures to the patient, such as the cervix and portions of the vagina that she may be able to see with her hand mirror. The physician should use the examination as a vehicle for teaching the patient about her body.

structures may imply an inflammatory reaction or endometriosis. If the uterus is retroverted, that organ should be outlined for size, shape, and consistency at this point. It may be examined appropriately using the fingers inserted into the vagina and the rectum, as well as using the abdominal hand (Figure 5-14).

THE ANNUAL VISIT

The annual visit is important for both health maintenance and preventive medicine reasons. Although the visit varies in emphasis depending on the patient's age, the long-term goals should be to maintain the patient in the best health and functional status possible and to promote high-quality longevity.

Although the gynecologist is generally the primary physician for women during their reproductive years, until recently this was not necessarily the case for postmenopausal women. However, it has become clear that the gynecologist with appropriate training and motivation can continue being the primary physician for older women as well.

Byyny recently pointed out that poor lifestyle is often at least partly responsible for chronic disease, disability, and premature mortality. In 1973 Belloc reported that in a study of women past the age of 45 the life expectancy was 7 years greater for those who routinely practiced six of seven important health habits as compared with those who practiced three or fewer (see box below). During the annual visit physicians should therefore discuss nutrition regarding (1) proper caloric intake to maintain the patient's weight near her optimum and avoid obesity, (2) restricting saturated fat and cholesterol, and (3) understanding the need for adequate calcium in the diet.

At each checkup the physician should also encourage the patient to develop an exercise program appropriate for her abilities and to avoid smoking and excessive alcohol use (if she has these habits). The physician should discuss possible stressors in the patient's life, such as her relationship with her husband and other family members, her satisfaction or dissatisfaction with her job, and other social problems that she may be experiencing. It is appropriate to ask questions that assess her sexual activity and gratification and questions that detect

---

GOOD HEALTH HABITS

Eat moderately
Eat regularly
Eat breakfast
Avoid smoking
Exercise regularly
Use alcohol in moderation or not at all
Sleep 7 to 8 hours per night

---

abuse or intimidation in her life. It is also appropriate to discuss the physical and emotional implications of loss and grief. Everyone suffers loss during his or her lifetime, and the older the patient the more likely that this is the case. Grief may be the result of a loss of a spouse or loved one, a pet, a job, a body part, or the ability to perform activities the patient has enjoyed (see Chapter 7).

The annual visit is an opportunity for the physician to screen for a variety of illnesses affecting not only the reproductive organs but all of the organ systems. The visit should include an interim health history and a complete physical examination. The weight, height, and blood pressure measurements and the breast, pelvic, and rectal examinations should all be performed and recorded so that comparisons may be made from year to year. A gross assessment of the patient's hearing ability and visual acuity should be performed annually.

Screening laboratory tests such as Pap smear, lipid profile, sexually transmitted disease screen, tuberculosis screen, thyroid assessment, electrocardiogram, and mammography should be performed at intervals that are appropriate for the patient's age and are recommended based on risk assessment. The patient should be tested annually for occult blood in the stool, particularly after age 35, and hemoglobin or hematocrit and blood sugar levels should probably be tested annually after age 40 or earlier if the history or physical examination suggests that this would be useful. A baseline electrocardiogram is generally ordered between the ages of 40 and 50, and after age 50 proctoscopy should be performed every 3 to 4 years or when indicated by history. Mammography should be performed according to the American Cancer Society guidelines (see Chapter 13) and ophthalmic tonometry and funduscopy should be performed at least every few years after age 35.

The physician should keep a history of the patient's immunizations and recommend booster shots for tetanus and diphtheria every 10 years and annual influenza immunizations in women who have a history of chest disease or those over age 60. Women at high risk for hepatitis B should be advised to undergo vaccination.

Promoting good health is a continuing responsibility for both the physician and the patient. It represents a challenge that includes education and observation on the physician's part and motivation on the part of the patient.

_____ KEY POINTS _____

- Five general impressions of patients may be gleaned nonverbally (by observation): happiness, apathy, fear, anger, and sadness.

- Menstrual history includes age of menarche, number of days of cycle, number of days of flow, presence of bleeding between menstrual periods, the date of the last menstrual period, and the date of the previous menstrual period.

- Menstrual cycles occurring just after puberty and just before menopause are frequently anovulatory and may be irregular in frequency.

- Pregnancy history should include the details of term and premature labors, spontaneous abortion, ectopic pregnancies, molar pregnancies, and terminations.

- A complete gynecologic evaluation should always include a sexual history, contraceptive history, and history of physical or sexual abuse.

- A detailed family history includes inquiry about congenital malformations, mental retardations, or pregnancy wastage in the families of the patient and her husband.

- Occupational and avocational activity should be investigated for the presence of potential hazards to the patient's health.

- Pap smears should be performed every 1 to 3 years, depending on the patient's risk level.

- Sexually active women should be evaluated at appropriate intervals for sexually transmitted diseases.

- The physician should use the occasion of the history and physical examination to teach the patient important aspects of self-evaluation.

- Goals of preventive medicine are to maintain good health and function and promote high-quality longevity.

BIBLIOGRAPHY

American College of Obstetricians and Gynecologists: Cervical cytology: evaluation and management of abnormalities, Tech Bull 81, 1984.

Belloc NB: Relationship of health practices and mortality, Prev Med 2:67, 1973.

Byyny RL: Establishing guidelines for preventive medicine, Contemp Obstet Gynecol 31:43, 1988.

Papanicolaou GN and Trout HF: Diagnosis of uterine cancer by vaginal smears, New York, 1943, The Commonwealth Fund.

Shy K, Chu J, Mandelson M, et al: Papanicolaou smear screening interval and risk of cervical cancer, Obstet Gynecol 74:838, 1989.

Taylor PT, Andersen WA, Barber SR, et al: The screening Papanicolaou smear: contribution of the endocervical bush, Obstet Gynecol 70:734, 1987.

Significant Symptoms and Signs in Different Age Groups

KEY TERMS AND DEFINITIONS

Hematocolpos. Distention of an obstructed vagina (caused by imperforate hymen or transverse septum) with blood and blood products.

Hematometria. A uterus distended with blood, secondary to partial or complete obstruction of any portion of the lower genital tract.

Levator Spasm. Spasm of the levator ani muscles frequently associated with chronic pelvic pain or vaginismus.

Pain. An unpleasant sensory or emotional experience associated with actual or potential tissue damage or described in terms of such damage.

Pelvic Congestion Syndrome. Vascular engorgement of the uterus and the vessels of the broad ligament and lateral pelvic walls, which may lead to chronic pelvic pain.

Trigger Points. Painful spasm of local muscle bundles or areas of scar tissue within the abdominal wall, at times associated with chronic pelvic and lower abdominal pain.

The gynecologist will evaluate a variety of women at different periods of life for relatively few specific symptoms and signs. Perhaps the three most common of these are unusual vaginal bleeding, pelvic pain, and pelvic or abdominal mass. Although each of these complaints will be of concern to the individual patient, their diagnostic implications may vary greatly depending on the patient's age. This chapter considers unusual vaginal bleeding, pelvic pain, and pelvic or abdominal mass from the standpoint of differential diagnosis, emphasizing the differences seen at different periods of a woman's life, and includes a detailed consideration of the problem of chronic pelvic pain.

VAGINAL BLEEDING

Abnormal vaginal bleeding includes prepubertal bleeding, menorrhagia, metrorrhagia or postcoital bleeding, and postmenopausal bleeding. Although the cause of the bleeding will frequently determine the characteristics that it exhibits, the physician should develop a systematic approach to the differential diagnosis of

abnormal vaginal bleeding. The box on p. 162 offers an outline that can be followed in considering a patient with abnormal vaginal bleeding. In addition, Chapter 35 considers this topic in detail.

Pregnancy

The possibility of a pregnancy must be considered in any woman in the reproductive years. This possibility can be rapidly ruled out using a sensitive serum pregnancy test. If the patient is found to be pregnant and vaginal bleeding is noted, the diagnostic possibilities include implantation bleeding; threatened, inevitable, complete, or incomplete abortion; ectopic pregnancy; and molar pregnancy.

Implantation bleeding is quite common. It usually consists of minimal bleeding at about the time of the first missed menstrual period and generally lasts a very short time. Occasionally it may be present for 1 to 2 days with a flow similar to that of a menstrual period. Often implantation bleeding is not perceptible to the patient but can be seen by the physician as

ETIOLOGY OF ABNORMAL VAGINAL BLEEDING

Pregnancy
    Abortion
        Threatened
        Inevitable
        Complete
        Incomplete
    Ectopic
    Molar—trophoblastic disease
Dysfunctional uterine bleeding
    Postpuberty
    During reproductive years
    Perimenopausal
Neoplastic
    Vulva and vagina
    Cervix
    Uterine corpus
    Fallopian tube
    Ovary
    Other
Inflammatory
    Vulvitis and vaginitis
    Cervicitis
    Endometritis
    Pelvic inflammatory disease
Traumatic
    Foreign body
    Direct trauma
Systemic diseases
    Coagulopathies
    Blood dyscrasias
    Endocrinopathy
    Drug effects
    Others

a brownish-tinged cervical mucus if a pelvic examination is performed. Bleeding in excess of a normal menstrual flow is quite rare, and prolonged bleeding does not usually occur.

Bleeding in the first trimester of pregnancy is not uncommon. About 20% to 25% of all pregnant women will spot or bleed in the first trimester. If the bleeding can be observed to be coming from the cervix and the cervix is closed, a diagnosis of threatened abortion can be made (Chapter 15). The size of the uterus should be consistent with what is normal for the dates of the pregnancy and may or may not be contracting and tender to the touch. A threatened abortion becomes inevitable when the cervix dilates and products of conception pass through the internal os or when the bleeding is profuse.

A complete abortion is noted when the uterus has expelled its contents, the internal os is closed, the bleeding is minimal, and the uterus has returned to near normal size. It is unusual for a patient who has a complete abortion to experience significant pelvic cramping or to cramp when a uterotonic agent such as ergonovine maleate (Ergotrate) or methylergonovine maleate (Methergine) is administered.

Incomplete abortion occurs when a part of the products of conception has been expelled but some remains within the uterus. The cervix is generally dilated, and there is usually bleeding, which may be profuse. The uterus is generally enlarged, and the patient may experience cramping pain. Most gestations of 6 weeks or less from the time of the last menstrual period will abort completely. Incomplete abortions become more common after 6 weeks of gestation.

A missed abortion occurs when the embryo dies but the products of conception are not expelled from the uterus. Generally the uterus involutes so that it is smaller than expected by dates. There may be dark red or brown vaginal bleeding, often minimal in amount. Pregnancy tests may remain positive for quite some time in the face of a missed abortion. Such conditions are more common when progestational agents have been given in the hopes of supporting the pregnancy.

Ectopic pregnancies are quite common and seem to be becoming more prevalent (Chapter 16). Currently about 1% of all pregnancies end as ectopic pregnancies, but these figures vary from group to group. An ectopic pregnancy is defined as one that is implanted outside of the endometrial cavity. Thus an ectopic pregnancy may exist in the cervix, within various portions of a fallopian tube, in the ovary, in the peritoneal cavity, and, in some rare instances, within the myometrium or a distant organ such as the spleen. A primary ectopic pregnancy in a specific organ implies that the pregnancy was implanted directly within that organ. A secondary ectopic pregnancy implies that the pregnancy ruptured from the fallopian tube and reimplanted completely or partially on another organ.

Ectopic pregnancies cause vaginal bleeding because of the separation of the decidua from the endometrium as the ectopic pregnancy dies or because of direct bleeding from the site of the ectopic pregnancy, with the blood being transported to the uterus and through the cervix. In most but not all cases the patient misses at least one menstrual period, begins to bleed from scant to significant amounts, and generally experiences pelvic pain. The pain may be limited to one side, in the case of a fallopian tube pregnancy, or may present as a more generalized pelvic pain. The pain may be similar to that experienced with pelvic inflammatory disease, but the patient with an ectopic pregnancy has a low-grade fever or is afebrile.

If the ectopic pregnancy is ruptured, intraperitoneal hemorrhage may occur and the patient may exhibit signs and symptoms of hypovolemia. Such an acute situation requires rapid intervention.

Ectopic pregnancies become a diagnostic problem when they are unruptured. Vaginal bleeding occurs in about 90% of early ectopic pregnancies that are unruptured, and almost all such patients experience pain. The uterus may be slightly enlarged or seem to be normal in size. If the ectopic pregnancy is tubal or ovarian, an adnexal mass may be noted. However, adnexal masses are not uncommon in normal pregnancies, representing the corpus luteum of pregnancy, and this may make the differential diagnosis somewhat more difficult.

With the availability of serum pregnancy tests, rapidly ascertaining that the patient is pregnant is possible. When a pregnancy is diagnosed, it becomes necessary to establish whether it is intrauterine or ectopic. A vaginal ultrasound examination may be of help. If the pregnancy has progressed beyond 6 weeks' gestation, it is frequently possible to see a pregnancy sac within the uterine cavity. Occasionally such a sac may be seen outside the uterine cavity in an adnexa.

Several authors have attempted to compare the levels of human chorionic gonadotrophin (HCG) with the gestational age of the pregnancy and determine from this whether a normal pregnancy is developing. However, it is not yet possible to differentiate with certainty between an intrauterine and an ectopic pregnancy by relating levels of HCG to the presence or absence of a sac. DiMarchi et al. recently noted that in their series of 131 cases, ectopic pregnancies were identified with HCG levels of 15,000 to 100,000 mIU. A combination of HCG and vaginal ultrasound observations helped make the diagnosis, often because of poor correlation of findings referable to interuterine pregnancy. Tubal rupture rarely occurred if the HCG level was below 100 mIU/ml unless the pregnancy was in a region of the fallopian tube other than the ampulla. Although 83% of their pregnancies were ampullary, the remainder were more difficult to diagnose before rupture because the rupture often occurred with lower levels of HCG and before good ultrasound findings could be obtained. This is discussed more completely in Chapter 16.

In a patient experiencing vaginal bleeding and pelvic pain who has a positive pregnancy test and who does not exhibit a gestational sac within the uterus on ultrasound, the physician should consider laparoscopy for a definitive diagnosis. A gestational sac appearing outside the uterine cavity may be suggestive of an ectopic pregnancy, but frequent error has been noted in such diagnoses and often the gestational sac does turn out to be intrauterine. Nonetheless, when there is an element of doubt the physician may wish to consider laparoscopy for definitive diagnosis.

If the patient appears to have intraperitoneal bleeding, a culdocentesis may help. The presence of unclotted blood within the peritoneal cavity is evidence for intraperitoneal hemorrhage. Either a laparotomy or a laparoscopy should be undertaken. This procedure may be preceded by dilation and curettage (D&C) with evaluation of the curetting for evidence of products of conception. If this is not noted by visualizing fetal parts, by seeing villi when tissue is floated on water, or by frozen section and microscopic evaluation, further operative intervention is required.

Several types of patients are at high risk for ectopic pregnancy. These include women who have had previous ectopic pregnancies, those who have undergone tubal reparative procedures, those who have had previous pelvic infections, and those who have been exposed to in utero DES. Ectopic pregnancy should also be considered in users of intrauterine devices (IUDs), since IUDs only partially protect from tubular implantation.

Another cause of abnormal vaginal bleeding associated with pregnancy is trophoblastic disease (Chapter 33). Most trophoblastic tumors are hydatidiform moles, which occur about once in every 1000 gestations in nonoriental women. Although they may present in a variety of ways, the classic molar pregnancy may include vaginal bleeding and a uterus enlarged beyond the size expected for gestational age.

These findings may be associated with the passage of grapelike structures per vaginum, representing hydropic villi. At times hypertension, edema, and proteinuria occur. Some molar pregnancies are associated with uteri that are small or normal for gestational age. In these cases the diagnosis may be suspected by an elevation of quantitative chorionic gonadotrophin greater than 100,000 mIU/ml. Molar pregnancy must be differentiated from normal gestation, multiple gestation, and uterine enlargements caused by other factors, such as uterine myoma. Bleeding that occurs in the second trimester and is associated with hydatidiform mole may also be associated with a uterus that is large for gestational age; this will also need to be differentiated from hydramnios. An ultrasound examination in the late first trimester or early second trimester generally will detect hydatidiform mole and help in the differential diagnosis of other conditions, such as multiple gestation, hydramnios, and other uterine disorders.

Dysfunctional Uterine Bleeding

The endocrinology of dysfunctional uterine bleeding is discussed in Chapter 35. The frequency with which dysfunctional uterine bleeding occurs, however, is such that it is an important consideration in the differential diagnosis of abnormal vaginal bleeding. The common denominator in most patients with dysfunctional uterine bleeding is anovulation or short ovulatory cycle. It is most commonly seen in the postpubertal period when normal hypothalamic function is not well established. In most instances, menstrual periods occur irregularly, often with long gaps between menses. When menses occurs, it may vary from very heavy flow to scanty flow and may continue for a number of days. The bleeding in most instances is from a nonsecretory endometrium. Occasionally the bleeding is profuse with associated signs and symptoms of hypovolemia, requiring emergency care. Endometrial sampling will generally yield scanty nonsecretory endometrium. Rarely is any other pathologic condition noted.

Women in the perimenopausal period who are undergoing some early evidence of ovarian failure may also experience dysfunctional uterine bleeding. Again the pattern may be one of irregularity, and the flow may vary from one that is increased in amount with clots to a scant

flow with prolonged spotting. Endometrial biopsy or D&C may yield a diagnosis of nonsecretory endometrium, a histologic section, but hyperplasia of the endometrium may also be noted. In perimenopausal women it is important to differentiate dysfunctional uterine bleeding from other intrauterine disease, and endometrial sampling is indicated. An endometrial biopsy is generally sufficient to establish the appropriate diagnosis and rule out more serious conditions.

Dysfunctional uterine bleeding may also occur during the reproductive years. It may be associated with polycystic ovarian disease or as a secondary symptom to stress, excessive weight change, or increased exercise performance. In such instances amenorrhea, oligomenorrhea, menorrhagia, or metrorrhagia may all be seen. Endometrial sampling generally produces nonsecretory endometrium; rarely is specific disease seen. In patients with polycystic ovarian disease, hyperplastic endometrium may be present. This is discussed more fully in Chapter 35.

Neoplastic Conditions

Although vaginal bleeding can be caused by a wide variety of neoplastic lesions, both benign and malignant and affecting the various organs of the female reproductive tract, there are specific patterns that are typical of many of these (Table 6-1). In addition, knowledge of occurrence rates of specific neoplasms in various age groups may help the physician in developing a differential diagnosis.

Cancers of the vulva and vagina may present with vaginal bleeding and usually occur in women who are in the latter reproductive years or in the postmenopausal period. Should they occur in women during the reproductive years, the bleeding is generally intermittent and therefore presents as metrorrhagia or postcoital bleeding rather than with any specific relationship to the menstrual cycle. The bleeding is generally minimal, although in advanced cases it can become profuse. An unusual vaginal tumor that may occur in teenage or young women is clear-cell cancer of the vagina, which is most often seen in women who have been exposed in utero to diethylstilbestrol (DES). Since this condition was first described by Herbst et al. in 1971, the actual incidence has been found to be quite low in such women (Chapter 14). In addition, rare cases of clear-

TABLE 6-1

Bleeding Pattern Seen in Tumors of the Reproductive Tract

Condition	Menorrhagia	Metrorrhagia	Postmenopausal Bleeding
Vulvar cancer	−	+ +	+ +
Vaginal cancer	−	+ +	+ +
Cervical cancer	−	+ +	+ +
Cervical polyp	−	+ +	+
Uterine myoma	+ +	+	−
Carcinoma of endometrium	−	−	+ +
Fallopian tube cancer	−	−	+
Ovarian cancer	−	±	±

+ +, Usually occurs; +, occasionally occurs; ±, occurs rarely.

cell cancer of the vagina have been found in women who were not exposed to DES.

Tumors of the cervix are most often squamous cell carcinomas, although as many as 10% are adenocarcinomas and may be present within the endocervical canal (Chapter 27). Such lesions will generally bleed eventually, and the bleeding pattern will be one of metrorrhagia or postcoital staining. With larger lesions the bleeding may be quite profuse. Other cervical lesions, such as endocervical polyps, may also cause metrorrhagia.

The most common lesions of the uterine corpus that cause abnormal bleeding during the reproductive years are leiomyomas (fibroids). Although these are generally benign, they may become quite large and may cause menorrhagia or menometrorrhagia (Chapter 17). Submucous myomata are generally associated with severe menorrhagia. Leiomyomas rarely cause vaginal bleeding in postmenopausal women. Endometrial carcinoma, generally an adenocarcinoma but occasionally a sarcoma, carcinosarcoma, or some intermediate variety, will cause vaginal bleeding (Chapter 28). Most of these occur in postmenopausal women and therefore would present as postmenopausal bleeding. The bleeding may be scant or profuse. Approximately 5% of endometrial adenocarcinomas occur in premenopausal women. These women most often are exposed to continuous endogenous estrogen stimulation and are often found to have polycystic ovarian disease or a functioning ovarian tumor, such as a granulosal cell tumor or a thecoma. When adenocarcinoma occurs in premenopausal women, these diagnostic possibilities should be considered.

Vaginal bleeding in association with fallopian

tube cancer is quite rare and generally occurs in the postmenopausal woman. Nonetheless, scant vaginal bleeding associated frequently with a watery discharge, crampy pain, and occasionally with an adnexal mass should alert the physician to the possibility of this condition (Chapter 32).

Ovarian cancers may present with vaginal bleeding, which is most often the result of intraperitoneal blood finding its way through the fallopian tube and through the uterus into the vagina. In the case of functioning ovarian tumors such as granulosal cell tumor or thecoma, the bleeding may be caused by either a hyperplastic endometrium or an endometrial cancer secondary to the estrogen stimulation.

Rarely, other intraperitoneal tumors may cause intraperitoneal bleeding with eventual vaginal bleeding from secondary passage of the blood through the reproductive tract. This is an unusual occurrence but should be considered in the differential diagnosis of unexplained vaginal bleeding.

Inflammatory Conditions

Although bleeding is not common as a symptom in inflammatory conditions, severe inflammation in tissue will often lead to capillary oozing or a small blood vessel erosion. Thus vulvitis, vaginitis, cervicitis, and endometritis may all be associated with vaginal bleeding or spotting, generally without relationship to menses. At times patients with acute salpingitis or tuboovarian abscess may also experience vaginal bleeding. This most likely comes from endometrial inflammation or abnormal uterine bleeding secondary to ovarian dysfunction. The symptoms and signs of inflammation, including discharge, pain and tenderness, and generalized signs and symptoms of infection, will help in the differential diagnosis.

Traumatic Conditions

Direct trauma to the female external genitalia and internal reproductive tract may occur secondary to accidental injury, the placement of foreign bodies within the vagina, and traumatic coitus. Direct lacerations secondary to one of these causes may lead to scant or profuse bleeding, depending on the extent of the injury. Often the bleeding is arterial and requires suture ligations. In children the insertion of foreign bodies into the vagina may lead to vaginal discharge with or without bleeding. Pencils, crayons, pieces of chalk, wads of paper, hairpins, and other items may be found. This is discussed more fully in Chapter 10.

Coital lacerations may occur because of rape or as part of normal sexual function. Tears of the hymen or lacerations of the vagina when tissue is rigid may lead to severe vaginal bleeding. Occasionally, bleeding occurs from the vaginal vault after a hysterectomy. Although this often occurs shortly after the operation, there are reports of dehiscence of the upper vault years later.

Systemic Diseases

A number of systemic diseases are associated with clotting defects and therefore may present with vaginal bleeding or have vaginal bleeding associated with the natural history of the disease. These include various coagulopathies, blood dyscrasias, and endocrinopathies. In addition, patients who take medications that interfere with the normal clotting mechanism may suffer vaginal bleeding. Examples of such medications are heparin and sodium warfarin (Coumadin), which may affect the clotting mechanism directly, or agents that interfere with normal platelet function, such as salicylates and other prostaglandin synthetase inhibitors. Many such conditions can be suspected or diagnosed by history and physical examination. General laboratory studies such as complete blood count, cell smear, and assessment of the clotting mechanism will usually help discover such problems if they exist.

Postmenopausal Bleeding

Although postmenopausal bleeding may be associated with a number of different conditions, it must always be investigated because many causes are premalignant or malignant. The most common premalignant and malignant causes are atypical adenomatous hyperplasia and carcinoma of the endometrium. These disorders are present in as many as one third of the patients evaluated for postmenopausal bleeding in many series.

Dewhurst described the benign causes of postmenopausal bleeding in 249 women seen at the Chelsea Hospital for Women in London. These are listed in Table 6-2. A large variety of lesions were noted, and the commonest single cause proved to be atrophic vaginitis. Dewhurst wisely counsels that even though an apparent benign cause of bleeding is found, women with postmenopausal bleeding deserve a thorough evaluation to rule out a malignancy that may *also* be present.

Although many other lesions of the reproductive tract, both benign and malignant, may be discovered, one fourth to one third of the patients evaluated may demonstrate no obvious pathologic condition other than an atrophic endometrium.

TABLE 6-2

Benign Conditions Causing Postmenopausal Bleeding Found in Patients Seen at the Chelsea Hospital for Women, London

Cause	Number
Atrophic vaginitis	129
Cervical polyps	65
Leiomyomata uteri	24
Endometrial hyperplasia	13
Cervical erosion	5
Trichomoniasis	3
Hematuria	2
Trauma	1
Vaginal endometriosis	1
Hemorrhoids	1
Moniliasis	1
Bartholin gland abscess	1
Vulvar warts	1
Urethral caruncle	1
TOTAL	248

(Modified from Dewhurst J: Clin Obstet Gynecol 26:769, 1983.)

PELVIC AND ABDOMINAL PAIN

In 1979 the Taxonomy Committee of the International Association for the Study of Pain defined pain as "an unpleasant sensory and emotional experience associated with actual or potential tissue damage or described in terms of such damage." The committee further stated that pain is always subjective, with each individual learning the application of the word through experience related to injury in early life. It is always unpleasant and is, therefore, an emotional experience. They recognize that people may report pain in the absence of tissue damage or any likely pathophysiologic cause and that this may be secondary to psychological or psychosocial reasons. Blendis points out that most children and adults have experienced abdominal pain that is often short-lived and rarely associated with physical or organic cause. In many cases, both physical and psychogenic elements exist, making it impossible to tell which was the cause.

Acute Abdomen

A number of intraabdominal conditions can lead to the findings of an acute abdomen. These findings include acute pain, generally of sudden onset, tenderness to palpation, rebound tenderness, and diminished or absent bowel sounds. The pain may be caused by infection, hemorrhage, infarction of tissue, or obstruction of bowel. In the case of bowel obstruction, bowel sounds may be hyperactive. It is important to construct a differential diagnosis when signs and symptoms of acute abdomen are noted. Table 6-3 lists the more common causes of an acute abdomen and identifies the quadrant of the abdomen where findings are more likely to be positive. It should be remembered, however, that the abdominal cavity is a continuum and overlap of signs is extremely common. Disease within a tubular viscus, such as the bowel, fallopian tube, or ureter, may cause crampy pain. Frequently patients complain of paroxysms of sharp, crampy pain interspaced with no pain at all or with periods of dull ache. Inflammatory conditions involving the ovary are frequently associated with continuous pain often described as sharp and throbbing.

Acute appendicitis, mesenteric lymphadenitis, and occasionally torsion of an adnexa may be found in preadolescent and adolescent girls.

TABLE 6-3
Conditions That May Cause Signs and Symptoms of Acute Abdomen and Abdominal Quadrants in Which They Most Often Occur

Condition	Quadrant			
	Right Upper	Right Lower	Left Upper	Left Lower
Salpingitis	−	+	−	+
Tuboovarian abscess	±	+	±	+
Ectopic pregnancy	−	+	−	+
Torsive adnexa	−	+	−	+
Ruptured ovarian cyst	−	+	−	+
Acute appendicitis	−	+	−	−
Mesenteric lymphadenitis	−	+	−	−
Crohn's disease	−	+	−	−
Acute cholecystitis	+	±	−	−
Perforated peptic ulcer	+	±	+	±
Acute pancreatitis	+	−	+	−
Acute pyelitis	+	±	+	±
Renal calculus	+	+	+	+
Splenic infarct	−	−	+	−
Splenic rupture	−	−	+	−
Acute diverticulitis	−	−	−	+

+, More frequently; ±, may occur.

Appendicitis is, of course, a possible differential diagnosis in all age groups. It often presents initially as periumbilical pain that localizes to the right lower quadrant and is accompanied by anorexia or nausea and vomiting. Salpingitis, tuboovarian abscess, ectopic pregnancy, and ruptured ovarian cysts are common findings in those patients of reproductive age who have an acute abdomen. Patients with salpingitis tend to have a higher fever than those with appendicitis, but great variability may be observed. Although their pain may be severe, they tend to be less ill than those with appendicitis. However, these women may have Crohn's disease, acute cholecystitis, perforated peptic ulcer, acute pyelitis, renal calculi, splenic infarct, and splenic rupture. Occasionally, they may also suffer from acute pancreatitis, which usually presents as epigastric pain often radiating to the back.

Acute abdomen in older women suggests torsion or rupture of an adnexa, acute cholecystitis, perforated ulcer, or acute diverticulitis. Pelvic inflammatory disease is less common in older women, and acute exacerbations are rare in those who have had tubal ligation.

Acute Pelvic Pain

Acute pain of gynecologic origin presents as both pelvic and lower abdominal pain. Diseases and dysfunction of the genitourinary tract, gastrointestinal tract, and musculoskeletal system may also cause pain in these regions. The box at right lists a number of gynecologic and nongynecologic conditions that can cause acute onset of pelvic or lower abdominal pain.

Threatened, inevitable, or incomplete abortion generally is accompanied by midline or bilateral lower abdominal pain, usually of a crampy, intermittent nature. In such instances vaginal bleeding is generally present. When infection occurs concurrently (septic abortion), there is generally temperature elevation, systemic symptoms of chills and malaise, and often an elevated white cell count and erythrocyte sedimentation rate (ESR). Rapid serum pregnancy tests are generally positive.

Ectopic pregnancy generally is associated with unilateral, continuous, crampy pain, although there may be some bilaterality to the presentation. Most ectopic pregnancies are associated with vaginal bleeding. Temperature elevation, if present, is usually minimal, and

---

POSSIBLE CAUSES OF ACUTE PELVIC AND LOWER ABDOMINAL PAIN

Pregnancy-related
  Abortion
  Ectopic
Disorders of the uterus and cervix
  Cervicitis
  Endometritis
  Degenerating myoma
Disorders of the adnexa
  Salpingitis
  Tuboovarian abscess
  Endometriosis (endometrioma)
  Torsion of adnexa
  Torsion of hydatid of Morgagni
  Rupture of follicle or corpus luteum cyst
  Ovarian hyperstimulation syndrome
  Degenerating ovarian tumor
Nongynecologic disorders
  Appendicitis
  Mesenteric lymphadenitis
  Diverticulitis
  Functional bowel syndrome
  Cystitis
  Trigonitis
  Renal calculus
  Musculoskeletal disorders

---

white cell count and ESR are generally normal but may be slightly elevated, particularly if there is intraperitoneal hemorrhage. Serum β-HCG is positive, and ultrasound examination may help in the diagnosis either by revealing a gestational sac in an adnexa or by ruling out the diagnosis through demonstration of a gestational sac within the uterus. Physical examination frequently demonstrates the presence of a mass in the adnexal region. Intraperitoneal bleeding may be diagnosed by culdocentesis and definitive diagnosis made by laparoscopy.

Acute cervicitis, often caused by *Neisseria gonorrhoeae* or *Chlamydia trachomatis*, may frequently be associated with lower abdominal and pelvic pain. The pain is often of a dull, aching nature and may radiate to the low back or to the upper thighs. There is generally a cervical and vaginal discharge, and there may be a low-grade fever, slight leukocytosis, and slight increase in ESR. Definitive diagnosis is made by specific culture for the organism.

Endometritis is generally transient and occurs in *Neisseria* or *Chlamydia* infections as part of their natural history. Occasionally, vigorous chemical douching will lead to a chemical endometritis. The pain is generally midline, pelvic, or lower abdominal and often aching in type.

Degenerating myoma will frequently cause acute, sharp, or aching pain in the region of the myoma. Diagnosis is aided by the facts that the uterus is irregular and enlarged and that there is tenderness to palpation. There may be a mild leukocytosis, but generally laboratory parameters are normal.

Salpingitis and tuboovarian abscess have been discussed under Acute Abdomen. Endometriosis is discussed in detail in Chapter 18. The pain pattern depends on the location of the endometrial implants and varies from dysmenorrhea and dyspareunia to continuous, generalized pelvic discomfort.

Torsion of an adnexa with or without an ovarian cyst or tumor may lead to acute, crampy, or continuous pain and has been discussed under Acute Abdomen. It can be confused with appendicitis or pelvic inflammatory disease (PID). Occasionally a hydatid of Morgagni will undergo torsion and give similar symptoms.

Rupture of an ovarian cyst may cause a sudden onset of pain. Leaking from a corpus luteum cyst generally occurs midcycle and, if it is on the right side, may be misdiagnosed as appendicitis. Ovarian hyperstimulation syndrome is a rare entity that may occur in women being treated with follicle-stimulating hormone (Pergonal) to stimulate ovulation; it is most likely to occur if pregnancy ensues. In such instances the gestation is generally found to be multiple. Ovarian hyperstimulation-like conditions may occur in women suffering from trophoblastic disease and, rarely, in women with severe isoimmunization disease such as Rh isoimmunization. It is often seen in women undergoing in vitro fertilization procedures because of the ovulation-stimulating drugs.

Degenerating adnexal tumors that have outgrown their blood supply may also cause acute-onset lower abdominal or pelvic pain.

Appendicitis, mesenteric lymphadenitis, and diverticulitis have all been discussed under Acute Abdomen. Appendicitis and mesenteric lymphadenitis generally present as right lower quadrant or right pelvic pain, and diverticulitis most often presents as a left-sided pain. Young women suffering from functional bowel syndrome will often present with a crampy severe left lower quadrant pain generally made worse by emotional tension and stress.

Patients suffering from cystitis and trigonitis may complain of lower abdominal or pelvic pain, generally midline in nature, accompanied by dysuria. Women suffering from renal calculus will generally have severe, intermittent flank pain on the side of the stone; this pain often radiates toward the lower abdomen.

A variety of musculoskeletal disorders may also present as pelvic pain, lower abdominal pain, or backache. Slocumb has recently called attention to the presence of "trigger points" discernible by palpation in the abdominal wall, lower back, and in the vaginal vault. Touching or stimulating these may simulate the pain about which the patient is complaining. Slocumb noted relief in several patients after the injection of these points with a local anesthetic such as 0.25% bupivacaine on one or several occasions. He notes that the pain often disappears for longer periods than the drug would be expected to cause. Because of this he speculates that in some instances chronic pelvic pain may be caused by a neurologic reflex that can be interrupted by the injection. Certainly irritation of the musculoskeletal system by exercise or injury can produce pain that can cause the patient to believe she has internal organ disease. Perhaps the injection of "trigger points" contributes to a reassurance that this is not the case.

Pain emanating from the uterus, such as with dysmenorrhea or that associated with adenomyosis and occasionally adnexal disease, may radiate to the anterior thigh. Rarely are the inner or outer aspects of the thigh involved, and the posterior thigh is never involved with such conditions. Pain radiating to the posterior thigh generally denotes sciatic nerve involvement, and this is commonly seen with cervical cancer of an advanced nature. Occasionally, endometriosis may cause such pain by irritating the sciatic nerve.

Most pain that is limited to the lower back but not to the abdominal region is generally of musculoskeletal origin rather than from gynecologic disease.

Chronic Pelvic Pain

Chronic and recurrent pelvic pain is one of the major problems seen by the gynecologist.

Dysmenorrhea (see Chapter 34) is perhaps the commonest example of recurrent pelvic pain. In addition, incompletely treated pelvic infections, recurrent pelvic infections, endometriosis, and possibly postoperative pelvic adhesions and diseases of the urinary tract and bowel may all be responsible for recurrent or persistent pelvic pain. Many who complain of chronic pelvic pain have no demonstrable pelvic disorder. Cunanan et al. reviewed 1194 charts of consecutive pelvic pain patients who had undergone diagnostic laparoscopy and discovered that in 355 cases a normal pelvis was found. Interestingly, of the 1194 patients, 749 had a normal pelvic examination before the diagnostic laparoscopy and, of these, 479 (63%) had abnormal findings on diagnostic laparoscopy. Of the 445 patients who had been thought to have an abnormal pelvic examination before laparoscopy, 78 (17.5%) actually had normal findings on diagnostic laparoscopy.

Kresch et al. reported the laparoscopic findings of 100 women who complained of constant pelvic pain in the same location for a minimum of 6 months. These authors compared the findings in this group with those of 50 women who were asymptomatic but who were undergoing laparoscopic tubal ligation. Overall, 83% of the group with pelvic pain had abnormal pelvic findings, whereas only 29% of the asymptomatic group demonstrated such findings. Pelvic adhesions were the most common pathologic finding, accounting for 38% of the abnormalities seen. Pelvic endometriosis accounted for 32% of the abnormal findings in the symptomatic group. These authors pointed out that when chronic pelvic pain exists in the same area for a minimum of 6 months, it is usually associated with specific pathologic conditions. However, even in this group of patients, 17% had no pelvic disorder at the time of diagnostic laparoscopy.

The question of whether pelvic adhesions are a frequent cause of chronic pelvic pain is as yet unanswered. Rapkin reviewed 100 consecutive laparoscopies performed because of chronic pelvic pain and compared the pelvic findings with those noted in 88 laparoscopies performed in infertility patients. A total of 26 (26%) of the pain group and 34 (39%) of the infertility group demonstrated pelvic adhesions as the only pathology seen. However, only 4 of the 34 patients in the infertility group complained of pain.

Patients presenting with chronic pelvic pain deserve an adequate workup. In most cases this would include a laparoscopic examination. The box below offers an outline of a workup

---

WORKUP OF A PATIENT WITH CHRONIC PELVIC PAIN

History
  Description and timing of pain (menstrual, intermittent, continuous, related to stress, etc.)
  Presence of pain in other parts of the body (headache, backache, etc.)
  Menstrual history and history of abnormal bleeding
  Sexual history
    Dyspareunia
  Work and leisure habits
  Problems involving other organ systems (urinary tract, GI tract)
  Previous pelvic and abdominal infections
  Previous operative procedures or diagnostic procedures
  Other gynecologic disorders (e.g., endometriosis)
  Social history (marital status; children; stresses in life as a child, an adolescent, and an adult; history of physical or sexual abuse or intimidation)

Physical examination
Laboratory evaluation
  CBC
  ESR
  VDRL
  Urinalysis and culture
  Evaluation of GI and GU tracts (where appropriate)
  Pap smear
Other studies (where appropriate)
  Psychiatric evaluation
  Social work evaluation
  Psychological testing (e.g., MMPI)
  Laparoscopy
  Ultrasound
  CT scan, magnetic resonance imaging
  Biopsies if indicated
  Cultures of cervix

for a patient with chronic pelvic pain. It is important that the physician determine not only the specific nature of the pain itself but acquire a good understanding of the patient's basic physical, mental, and social status to determine what factors may be influencing the patient's symptom complex.

A complete physical examination with emphasis on the effects of previous operations, infections, injuries, and, of course, a complete pelvic examination should be carried out. Cervical cultures for gonococcus and *Chlamydia*, as well as a Pap smear, are appropriate.

Laboratory data for patients with chronic pelvic pain should include CBC, ESR, serologic tests for syphilis, urine analysis, and urine culture where appropriate. When indicated by history and physical findings, radiologic or ultrasound evaluation of the gastrointestinal (GI) and genitourinary (GU) tracts should be ordered.

Other studies that may be appropriate, depending on the history and physical examination, include psychiatric evaluation, social work evaluation, psychological testing, such as the Minnesota Multiphasic Personality Index (MMPI), and biopsies if indicated. Laparoscopic examination is indicated in such patients to discover or rule out pathologic conditions.

After completing the workup the physician may still be unable to find a cause for the chronic pelvic pain. In the past a variety of explanations were offered, including abnormal positioning of the uterus, laceration of the uterine supports, and vascular congestion of the pelvic organs. However, many of these patients have a psychosomatic disorder and benefit from counseling.

Perhaps as many as 20% of all women demonstrate retroversion or retroflexion of the uterus at any given time. Rarely is the condition pathologic, and in most cases the uterus can be displaced from its posterior position in the pelvis to its normal anterior position by bimanual examination or by positioning the patient in the knee-chest position. When such anterior displacement of the uterus has been effected, the physician may place a Smith-Hodge pessary into the vagina to hold the uterus in an anterior position. If this maneuver alleviates the pain, the patient may continue to wear the pessary or may be offered a uterine suspension procedure. In most cases, however, retrodisplacement of the uterus does not appear to be a cause of pelvic pain, and replacement will make no difference in the patient's symptoms. Occasionally the uterus is fixed in the posterior pelvis by postinflammatory or postoperative adhesions or by endometriosis. In these instances, the primary disease, not the retrodisplacement, may be responsible for the pain.

Allen and Masters defined the problem of traumatic lacerations of the uterine supports in 1955. They theorized that lacerations of the posterior leaf of the broad ligament or of the uterosacral ligament may have occurred at the time of a traumatic obstetrical delivery and that with healing a greater rotation was allowed for the uterus. This condition has been called the *universal joint syndrome*, since it was theorized that the uterus could rotate freely, as with a universal joint. Many physicians have attempted to repair these so-called lacerations, and they are visible in some patients on laparoscopic examination. However, it is difficult to demonstrate a cause-and-effect relationship with pelvic pain, and a placebo effect may be responsible for occasional apparently successful outcomes.

Pelvic vascular engorgement has been observed on many occasions. Taylor defined the pelvic congestion syndrome as pain and heaviness in the pelvis that occurs after arising and becomes worse as the day progresses. On laparoscopic examination the uterus usually appears to be dusky blue and mottled, and often varicosities of the veins of the broad ligament are noted. Not all women with such findings complain of pelvic pain, and it is difficult to prove an actual cause. Beard et al. recently offered some evidence that pelvic varicosities might be a source of chronic pelvic pain. They compared 45 patients with chronic pelvic pain and no obvious pathology with 10 patients with pelvic pathology and 8 who were scheduled for tubal ligations. Each patient underwent a pelvic venogram, and the pelvic vein varicosities were graded by a radiologist blinded to the patients' complaints. A definite difference was noted in the increased diameters of the ovarian veins associated with a slower emptying time in the pelvic pain group.

Some patients do appear to suffer from psychosomatic disease with pelvic pain as a manifestation. Patients with chronic pelvic pain who do not seem to have obvious pathologic conditions will often reveal chaotic social histories involving both early and present life. Many of these individuals will be depressed and suffer from stress and anxiety, and some will suffer from borderline personality disorders. It is difficult to draw specific conclusions in this respect, however. Renaer demonstrated multiple symptom complaints in 12 of 24 patients with chronic pelvic pain without obvious disease. But only 1 of 22 patients suffering from chronic pelvic pain and endometriosis had such multiple symptoms. However, personality profiles developed by psychometric testing in each group failed to show differences between the two groups. A number of previous authors have pointed out that personality examinations in patients with chronic pain do not differentiate between psychogenic and organic pain.

Some investigators have recently noted a relationship between a history of childhood and later-life physical and sexual abuse and chronic pelvic pain. Harrop-Griffiths et al. ascertained a greater prevalence of lifetime major depression, current major depression, lifetime substance abuse history, sexual dysfunction, somatization, and an increased incidence of childhood and adult sexual abuse in a group of chronic pelvic pain patients at the time of laparoscopy compared with a group of patients without pain undergoing laparoscopy for tubal ligation or infertility.

Physicians should evaluate chronic pelvic pain patients in a holistic fashion, investigating past social and emotional problems along with the physical evaluation. This makes it possible to offer specific multidiscipline therapy without suggesting to the patient that the problem is "all in her head." Placing the pain in the context of the patient's total life situation rather than as a specific isolated entity often makes a holistic approach possible.

Patients with chronic pain who do not demonstrate apparent organic causes will frequently have levator ani muscle spasm or spasm of other groups of muscle within the pelvis. Occasionally trigger points may be defined in the anterior abdominal wall by deep digital pressure. These probably also represent spasm in local muscle bundles. These patients may also suffer from tenderness of the uterus and adnexa, which conceivably could be caused by vascular engorgement or adenomyosis. They pose difficult and demanding diagnostic and treatment challenges.

If no pathologic condition is evident but pain is persistent, physicians and patients alike have often yielded to the temptation of treating with a total hysterectomy and bilateral salpingo-oophorectomy. There is no evidence that this therapy relieves the pain in such patients and, indeed, failure to relieve the pain may lead to anger and frustration. Slocumb has shown that hysterectomy was successful in relieving pelvic pain only if dysmenorrhea was part of the symptom complex. Therefore patients without obvious pelvic disease who have pelvic pain but not dysmenorrhea should not be offered hysterectomy. In such cases the physician should seek and treat psychosocial problems, depression, or other psychological disease with medications, counseling, or referral to a psychiatrist or other mental health worker where appropriate.

PELVIC AND LOWER ABDOMINAL MASSES

Pelvic and lower abdominal masses may be cystic or solid and occur in any age group. They may originate from the cervix, the uterus, or the adnexa; from other organs, such as the GU tract or the bowel; or from the musculoskeletal system, vascular-lymphatic system, or nervous system. In this section the relevant incidence of pelvic and lower abdominal tumors in the various age groups will be considered and, where appropriate, means of differential diagnosis will be discussed.

Before discussing relative frequencies and types of abdominal and pelvic tumors found in different age groups, some comparisons of the more common adnexal tumors by age group are appropriate. During the reproductive years the majority of adnexal masses are follicle cysts. These tumors are functional in nature and generally disappear in 1 to 3 months. They vary in size from just a few centimeters to as much as 8 to 10 cm in diameter. They are thin-walled and frequently rupture during pelvic examination. In and of themselves they are of no clinical significance. It is likely that most women develop follicle cysts from time to time, and discovery may be related to the chance of performing a pelvic examination at the time when they exist. They rarely cause symptoms; however, when they do become large, they may cause some heaviness in the lower pelvis or in the leg. Because they are filled with follicular fluid, their rupture rarely causes any pathologic problem. A cystic adnexal mass of 5 to 8 cm that develops in a woman during the reproductive years is usually followed for at least one menstrual cycle, since functional cysts are common and the risk of malignancy is small. Ultrasound

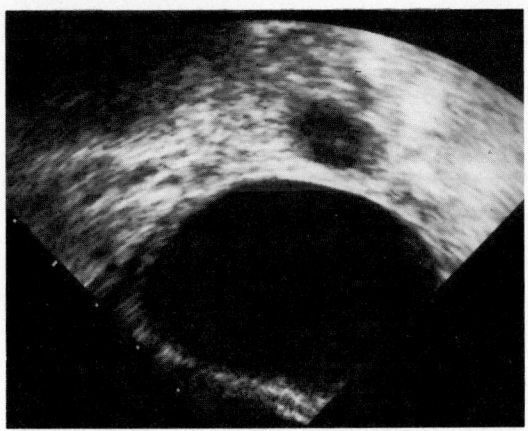

FIGURE 6-1
Large simple follicle cyst detected by vaginal ultrasound examination.

studies, particularly using a vaginal probe, can be very helpful in establishing a diagnosis and following the progress of a cyst, and can be reassuring to the patient and the doctor alike. It can help differentiate between a simple and a multiloculated cyst and can rule out a solid tumor. Figure 6-1 is an example of a simple follicle cyst seen with vaginal ultrasound.

Also common during the reproductive years are hemorrhagic corpora lutea. These masses rarely become larger than 5 cm in diameter and frequently are somewhat tender to palpation. If they leak blood, they may mimic an ectopic pregnancy. They generally regress within a few weeks.

There are a number of benign and malignant neoplasms of the ovary that occur quite frequently and do have special incident relationships to various age groups (Chapters 17 and 29). In 1968 Bennington et al. reviewed 443 benign and 106 malignant neoplasms of the ovary discovered in a period from 1951 to 1963 at the Oakland Kaiser Foundation Hospital. During those years, between 61,000 and 83,500 women were served annually. Because the Kaiser enrollees represented a cross section of the population in that area of California, this study made it possible to observe the relative frequency of different ovarian neoplasms within the general population. Most other studies were reported by referral institutions, and therefore the data from the standpoint of prevalence was clouded. Bennington et al. noted that serous cystadenoma and benign cystic teratoma (dermoid cyst) were the most commonly observed benign neoplasms of the adnexa. In addition, mucinous cystadenoma, Brenner tu-

mors, and thecoma fibromas were also seen. Table 6-4 demonstrates the age distribution and occurrence of bilaterality of 443 benign ovarian neoplasms observed by Bennington et al. Although benign ovarian neoplasms were uncommon in the group up to 19 years of age, the most commonly seen neoplasm in this age group was the benign cystic teratoma. In the 20-to-44-year age group, serous cystadenomas were the most common neoplasm, with benign cystic teratomas and mucinous cystadenomas next in frequency. The serous cystadenomas occurred in all age groups but less commonly in women over 75. Mucinous cystadenomas occurred sporadically in all age groups, but none were seen after age 75. The majority of mucinous cystadenomas, however, occurred in women in the reproductive years. Similarly, benign cystic teratomas occurred in all age groups until age 75, but the majority occurred in the reproductive years. Brenner tumors occurred sporadically; however, none were seen after age 55. Thecomas and fibromas occurred in all age groups from 20 to beyond 75, but again the majority were in women between the ages of 20 and 64.

Malignant tumors of the ovary were not seen in the 19-and-younger age group of the Kaiser population except for one tumor that was metastatic to the ovary from another site. Serous cystadenocarcinoma occurred in all age groups from 20 to beyond 75 and was the most common malignant tumor seen in all age groups, but ovarian carcinomas are rare before age 40 (Figure 6-2). Metastatic tumors to the ovary were the second most common ovarian malignant neoplasm seen in this study. Of the serous cystadenocarcinomas, 40% were bilateral, and roughly 50% of metastatic neoplasms were bilateral in all age groups. Mucinous cystadenocarcinoma was seen in all age groups from 20 to beyond 75. In general the chance of malignancy seemed to be greater in these tumors in the older age groups. Endometrioid carcinoma occurred in a few patients in the series, as did granulosal cell carcinoma. Few other tumors were seen in this study. Table 6-5 summarizes the 106 patients with malignant ovarian neoplasm in the Bennington study by age distribution, laterality, and cell type.

Figure 6-3 plots the incidence of a number of the tumors noted in the Bennington study per 100,000 woman-years. Although their numbers of cases were relatively small, the incidence figures do demonstrate the prevalence

TABLE 6-4

Age Distribution and Laterality of 443 Benign Ovarian Neoplasms

Type	Age						Total
	0-19	20-44	45-54	55-64	65-74	75+	
Serous cystadenoma							
U*	4	124	35	23	10	2	198
B	1	17	3	4	2	0	27
Mucinous cystadenoma							
U	1	42	5	5	1	0	54
B	0	1	0	0	0	0	1
Benign teratoma							
U	8	93	12	7	2	0	122
B	0	9	1	0	0	0	10
Brenner							
U	1	4	1	0	0	0	6
B	0	0	0	0	0	0	0
Thecoma-fibroma							
U	0	11	3	8	1	1	24
B	0	0	0	1	0	0	1
TOTAL							
U	14	274	56	43	14	3	404
B	1	27	4	5	2	0	39

From Bennington JL, Ferguson BR, and Haber SL: Obstet Gynecol 32:627, 1968. Reprinted with permission from The American College of Obstetricians and Gynecologists.
*Location of neoplasm: U, unilateral; B, bilateral.

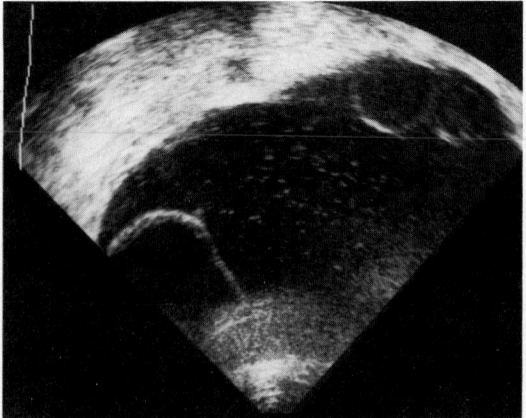

FIGURE 6-2

Multiloculated ovarian cyst detected by vaginal ultrasound. Pathology proved to be serous cystadenocarcinoma.

TABLE 6-5

Age Distribution and Laterality of 80 Primary and 26 Secondary Malignant Ovarian Neoplasms

Type	0-19	20-44	45-54	55-64	65-74	75+	Total
Serous cystadenocarcinoma							
U*	0	8	9	10	1	2	30
B	0	7	11	3	2	1	24
Mucinous cystadenocarcinoma							
U	0	1	0	4	1	1	7
B	0	0	0	2	1	0	3
Endometrioid carcinoma							
U	0	2	0	0	0	0	2
B	0	0	1	1	1	0	3
Granulose carcinoma							
U	0	2	0	2	1	1	6
B	0	0	0	0	0	0	0
Other							
U	0	1†	4‡	0	0	0	5
B	0	0	0	0	0	0	0
Metastases							
U	1	3	7	1	0	0	12
B	0	7	4	3	0	0	14
Total							
U	1	17	20	17	3	4	62
B	0	14	16	9	4	1	44

From Bennington JL, Ferguson BR, and Haber SL: Obstet Gynecol 32:627, 1968. Reprinted with permission from The American College of Obstetricians and Gynecologists.
*Location of neoplasm: U, unilateral; B, bilateral.
†Squamous carcinoma arising in a cystic teratoma.
‡One arrhenoblastoma, 1 germinoma, 1 malignant Brenner tumor, and 1 mesonephric carcinoma.

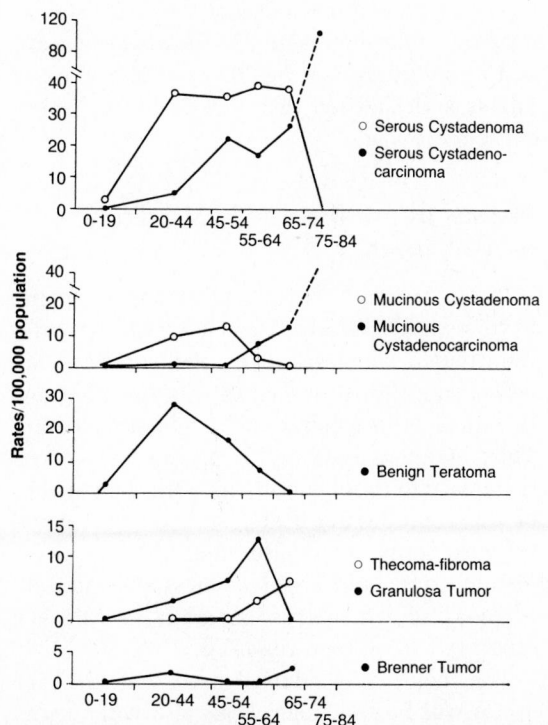

FIGURE 6-3

Incidence rates for ovarian tumors by age group per 100,000 women at each age interval. (From Bennington JL, Ferguson BR, and Haber SL: Obstet Gynecol 32:627, 1968. Reprinted with permission from The American College of Obstetricians and Gynecologists.)

TABLE 6-6
Surgical Findings in 540 Patients Evaluated for Leiomyomata/Pelvic Masses at St. Lukes-Roosevelt
Hospital 1984-1985

Surgical Diagnosis	Number of Patients in Each Age Group							
	10-20	21-30	31-40	41-50	51-60	61-70	>70	Total
Leiomyomata	0	13	99	142	19	3	0	276
Benign/functional cysts	1	24	32	23	8	9	7	104
Cancer	2	0	3	11	7	12	9	44
Benign cystic teratoma	4	17	9	3	0	3	1	37
Endometriosis	0	7	16	7	2	0	0	32
Miscellaneous	1	4	11	2	1	4	2	25
Tubo-ovarian abscess/ pelvic inflammatory disease	2	7	9	4	0	0	0	22
Total	10	72	179	192	37	31	19	540

(From Killackey MA and Neuwirth RS: Obstet Gynecol 71:319, 1988.)

by age of these various tumors.

Killackey and Neuwirth evaluated pelvic masses in 540 patients admitted to St. Lukes-Roosevelt Hospital in New York in 1984-85. Of 249 patients admitted with a diagnosis of uterine myomata, 235 (94.4%) diagnoses proved to be correct, whereas benign adnexal masses were found in 7 (2.8%), cancers in 4 (1.6%), and miscellaneous findings in 3 (1.2%). Of 291 patients evaluated for "pelvic mass," benign ovarian or tubal cysts were noted in 98 (33.7%), uterine myoma in 42 (14.4%), cancers in 40 (13.7%), benign cystic teratomas in 38 (13.1%), endometriosis in 28 (9.6%), miscellaneous in 23 (7.9%), and pelvic inflammatory disease in 22 (7.6%). Table 6-6 demonstrates these diagnostic findings by patient age.

Masses in Childhood

Occasionally babies are born with adnexal cysts that present as abdominal masses. These are generally follicular cysts secondary to maternal hormone stimulation of fetal ovaries. The cysts generally regress within the first few months of life. Thereafter cysts and all tumors of the female pelvic organs are quite rare during childhood. Abdominal masses found in the young child are more likely to be Wilms' tumors or neuroblastomas. Tumors of the GI tract, musculoskeletal system, or lymphatic system may also occur occasionally. Solid or mixed solid and cystic adnexal masses are rare, but when they do occur are almost always dys-

germinomas or teratomas. Mueller et al. reviewed 427 cases of dysgerminoma in 1950 and noted that 6.89% of the tumors occurred in the 1-to-10-year age group. Asadourian and Taylor, reviewing 105 cases of dysgerminoma in the Armed Forces Institute of Pathology experience, noted that only seven of these patients were 9 years of age or younger.

Although benign and malignant teratomas have been reported in childhood, they are quite rare before the age of 10. Caruso et al., reporting on 305 teratomas of the ovary, found none in children under 10. However, Costin and Kennedy, reviewing 200 ovarian tumors in infants and children, found 25% to be benign cystic teratomas.

Masses in Adolescence (Menarche to 19 Years)

Once menses begins, obstruction of the lower reproductive tract, such as with imperforate hymen, agenesis of the vagina with intact cervix and uterus, or vaginal septum, may give rise to a hematocolpos or a hematometrium. Thus abdominal or pelvic masses may occur secondary to these conditions. Other anomalies of the reproductive tract, such as obstructed uterine horns, may also give rise to a hematometrium and a pelvic mass (Chapter 9). Myomas of the uterus are rare in this age group but have been reported.

The majority of adnexal masses in this age group will be functional cysts and will vary in size from 3 to 10 cm. Of neoplastic ovarian tumors found, the most common is benign cystic teratoma of the ovary. In Caruso's study of 305 teratomas of the ovary, 8.5% occurred in this age group. These tumors are generally between 5 and 10 cm in diameter, are slow-growing, and are frequently asymptomatic. Some benign cystic teratomas are larger than 10 cm. In Caruso's series of 305 teratomas, 49 measured 10 to 14 cm; 21, 15 to 19 cm; and 11, between 20 and 39 cm. They are generally found because a mass is detected on abdominal or pelvic examination. However, benign cystic teratomas may cause adnexal torsion and present as an acute abdomen. Rarely, the tumor may rupture, spilling oily, irritating contents into the peritoneal cavity and creating evidence of an acute abdomen. These tumors frequently have a thickened capsule, and rupture is unusual. Because benign cystic teratomas may contain bone or teeth, abdominal roentgenograms or ultrasound may identify these.

Solid or solid and cystic adnexal tumors, although rare in adolescence, are almost always dysgerminomas or malignant teratomas.

In 137 women younger than 21 years who were found to have ovarian enlargement reported by Diamond et al., 82 had ovarian neoplasms, of which 8 were borderline or malignant. All six malignant lesions were germ cell in origin. Likewise, in a study by Norris and Jensen of 353 primary ovarian neoplasms in women younger than 20 years, germ cell tumors represented 58% of cases. Of these 205 patients, 71 had benign cystic teratomas, 54 malignant teratomas, 48 dysgerminomas, and 32 embryonal carcinomas. Of the remaining cases, 67 (19%) were of epithelial origin, 62 (18%) stromal, and 19 (5%) miscellaneous.

Dysgerminomas and teratomas can vary from just a few centimeters to an extremely large size. In 117 dysgerminomas reviewed by Asadourian and Taylor, 12 were found to have other germ cell elements, including embryonal carcinoma, teratocarcinoma, and choriocarcinoma.

Cystic adnexal masses derived from mesonephric elements, such as paraovarian and paratubal cysts, are also seen in this age group. They may vary in size from 1 to 2 cm to quite large. They are thin-walled, benign entities without solid components.

Masses emanating from other organ systems in the pelvis and abdomen also occur in this age group and must be considered.

Masses During the Reproductive Years (20 to 44 Years)

Masses seen in women of reproductive age may develop from the uterus and cervix, the adnexa, and other organ systems. Intrauterine pregnancy, ectopic pregnancy, and trophoblastic disease should always be considered in women of reproductive years who develop such masses. These conditions can often be ruled in or out by use of a serum pregnancy test and ultrasound. Ectopic pregnancy is generally associated with an adnexal mass, vaginal bleeding, and pelvic pain, as discussed earlier in this chapter. Trophoblastic disease may be associated with inappropriate uterine size for menstrual dates, vaginal bleeding, pelvic pain, and symptoms of toxemia of pregnancy. Adnexal enlargements caused by thecalutein cysts of the ovaries may be associated with trophoblastic disease.

Myomas of the uterus, the cervix, the round ligament, or other pelvic organs are quite common in this age group. As many as 30% of women in the reproductive years may develop myomas of the uterus and accessory organs, and by age 50, perhaps as many as 40% will have developed such tumors. These tumors occur 3 times more frequently in blacks than in whites. The majority are benign and vary in size from very small to large enough to fill the entire abdominal cavity. These tumors are composed of smooth muscle cells in concentric whorls and are generally benign. Leiomyosarcoma occurring in such tumors is rare (0.1% to 0.5%). The tumors are usually solid but with degeneration may give the impression of a cystic consistency. Ultrasound and CT scan may be helpful in making a specific diagnosis.

Rarely, myomas of the uterus occur in the cervix or lower uterine segment. They may become quite large and may put pressure on the bladder neck, causing acute urinary retention. Myomas tend to enlarge premenstrually and in pregnancy. Occasionally cervical or lower uterine segment myomas have caused intermittent urinary retention premenstrually or during early pregnancy.

Adnexal masses in the reproductive years may involve any known ovarian tumor, as well as cysts of mesonephric origin. In this age group functional cysts of the ovary are still the most common adnexal masses found, and benign cystic teratomas are the most common neoplastic adnexal masses. During the reproductive years, endometriosis occurs, and ovarian endometrial cysts develop reasonably frequently in this age group. They generally are accompanied by the usual symptoms for endometriosis in association with a tender adnexal mass.

Tumors emanating from other organ systems should also be considered in the differential diagnosis as in other age groups. One of the more common of these is not a tumor at all but a pelvic kidney. An intravenous pyelogram should be useful in differentiating this entity from other pathologic conditions.

Masses in the Perimenopausal and Postmenopausal Years

In this age group it is once again appropriate to consider masses originating from the uterus and cervix, from the adnexa, and from other organ systems. In general, myomas of the uterus regress postmenopausally even in the face of estrogen hormone replacement. Therefore a uterus that is growing in size should be investigated for the possibility of malignancy. Adenocarcinoma of the endometrium, sarcomas, and mixed tumors of the uterus are all more common in the postmenopausal period, and many will be responsible for enlargement of uterine size, as well as postmenopausal bleeding.

TABLE 6-7
Adnexal Masses in 150 Women ≥50 Years

Pathology	<5 cm	5-10 cm	>10 cm
Benign disease			
Epithelial tumors	12	26	15
Stromal and germ cell tumors	7	12	4
Nonneoplastic ovarian cysts	2	1	0
Uterine myomas	3	3	4
Nonovarian adnexal lesions	2	6	0
Absence of true mass	5	1	0
Malignant disease			
Epithelial carcinomas	1	3	29
Borderline tumors	0	2	2
Other ovarian carcinomas	0	0	4
Nonovarian carcinoma	0	1	5
TOTAL	32	55	63

(From Rulin MC and Preston AL: Obstet Gynecol 70:578, 1987.)

Adnexal masses occurring in postmenopausal women may still be benign, but the chance of malignancy increases with age. The presence of ascites and the detection of the tumor bilaterally suggest malignancy. Rulin and Preston analyzed 150 adnexal tumors in women over the age of 50 and noted 103 benign tumors and 47 malignant ones. Table 6-7 summarizes these tumors by size and pathologic findings. Only 1 tumor of 32 that were less than 5 cm proved to be malignant, whereas 6 of 55 tumors 5 to 10 cm and 40 of 63 tumors larger than 10 cm were malignant. The majority of the malignant tumors were epithelial in this age group, and most were greater than 10 cm. Thus size appears to be a reasonable indicator of malignancy in this age group.

Endometriosis occurs primarily in women in the reproductive years; however, as many as 5% of cases do occur postmenopausally, particularly in women on hormone replacement therapy. Therefore endometriosis of the ovaries should be part of the differential diagnosis in such women (Chapter 18).

Masses from other organ systems are quite common in this age group. Diverticulitis may be responsible for a painful left adnexal mass. Bowel tumors may present as abdominal masses, as may tumors of the kidney, the musculoskeletal system, and the lymphatic system. Blood dyscrasias and lymphomas are more common in this age group. Lymphomas may present as rapidly growing, firm masses, at times accompanied by ascites. They may develop from any abdominal or pelvic organ, including lymph nodes.

Special Considerations

A number of findings associated with abdominal mass may help direct the physician to the appropriate diagnosis. If ascites is present, as detected by physical examination or ultrasound, a malignant tumor, frequently of the ovary, is strongly suspected. A needle aspiration with cell block of the fluid obtained may be diagnostic.

Defeminization or masculinization of the patient may suggest a rare masculinizing tumor of the ovary, such as a Sertoli-Leydig tumor. In the preadolescent female, precocious puberty of a heterosexual type may be the presenting symptom. In the postpubertal girl, cessation of menses and early masculinization may occur.

These may also be the presenting symptoms in women in the reproductive years.

Feminizing tumors, such as granulosal cell tumors and thecomas, are more common. In the prepubertal girl they may present as precocious puberty. In the menstruating woman they may cause menometrorrhagia, and in the postmenopausal woman they may present with postmenopausal bleeding. In a granulosal cell tumor a solid or cystic mass is readily detected. Thecomas are solid tumors and are also readily detected. Occasionally other ovarian stromal tumors, such as a Brenner tumor, may produce sex steroids and present in a similar fashion.

Struma ovari, a teratoma with thyroid elements, may present by developing signs of hyperthyroidism in the patient.

General Diagnostic Considerations

Specific differential diagnosis of abdominal and pelvic masses is often aided by ultrasound and CT scan. In addition, special radiographic studies, such as intravenous pyelogram, barium enema, and upper GI series, may be helpful in identifying the site of the tumor. Because metastatic cancer to the ovaries is common, investigation of the patient for another primary source is often fruitful.

Tumor markers may be elevated, such as Ca-125 in epithelial tumors, serum HCG and alpha fetoprotein in germ cell tumors, and androgens or estrogens in specific hormone-producing tumors. These tests have frequent false-positive and false-negative findings and should be used only in conjunction with other diagnostic procedures.

KEY POINTS

- Bleeding in early pregnancy usually implies threatened or inevitable abortion, ectopic pregnancy, or trophoblastic disease.

- Bleeding at the time of the missed menstrual period may represent implantation bleeding.

- About 90% of all ectopic pregnancies are associated with vaginal bleeding.

- Vaginal bleeding in a patient with a positive pregnancy test, lower abdominal pain, adnexal mass, and failure to demonstrate a gestational sac by ultrasound beyond 6 weeks of gestational age should suggest the possibility of an ectopic pregnancy.

- Incidence of ectopic pregnancy is increased in women who have had previous ectopic pregnancies, have undergone tubal reparative procedures, have had previous pelvic infections, wear an IUD, or were exposed to DES in utero.

- Molar pregnancies are suggested by vaginal bleeding, uteri larger than gestational age, and serum HCG levels of 100,000 mIU/ml or greater.

- Molar pregnancy must be differentiated from normal gestation, multiple gestation, uterine enlargement because of uterine pathology, and hydramnios.

- Molar pregnancies are best diagnosed with the aid of ultrasound examination.

- Dysfunctional uterine bleeding is generally associated with anovulation or short ovulatory cycle.

- Dysfunctional uterine bleeding is most commonly seen in the postpubertal period, perimenopausally, or in women during their reproductive years who have undergone excessive weight change, who are under stress, or who have embarked on a strenuous exercise program.

- A patient presenting with symptoms or signs of PID who is afebrile or has a low-grade fever should be suspected of having an ectopic pregnancy.

- Appendicitis is characterized by periumbilical pain that radiates to the right lower quadrant accompanied by loss of appetite, nausea, and vomiting. Patients with PID can have similar pain but usually have a higher fever and mild gastrointestinal symptoms and appear less ill.

- Dysfunctional uterine bleeding is often associated with polycystic ovarian syndrome and functioning ovarian tumors.

- Endometrial biopsy with dysfunctional uterine bleeding in younger women will generally demonstrate nonsecretory endometrium.

- Clear-cell cancer of the vagina is often associated with intrauterine DES exposure.

- Myomas of the uterus often are associated with vaginal bleeding; submucous myomas are most commonly associated with this problem.

- Of all adenocarcinomas of the endometrium, 95% occur in postmenopausal women.

- Adenocarcinoma of the endometrium found in premenopausal women is most often associated with polycystic ovarian syndrome or a functioning ovarian tumor.

- Systemic diseases that cause abnormal vaginal bleeding include coagulopathies, blood dyscrasias, and certain endocrinopathies.

- In a study of 1194 patients with chronic pelvic pain, 749 had normal pelvic examinations.

- In 749 patients with chronic pelvic pain who had normal pelvic examinations, 63% had abnormal findings at diagnostic laparoscopy.

- Of 445 patients who had abnormal pelvic examinations and a history of chronic pelvic pain, 17.5% had normal findings at the time of diagnostic laparoscopy.

- Of 100 women who reported constant pelvic pain in one place for at least 6 months, 83% had abnormal findings at diagnostic laparoscopy. Pelvic adhesions and endometriosis accounted for the majority of abnormalities seen.

- Pelvic adhesions may not be the cause of chronic pelvic pain. Whereas 26% of 100 such patients were found to have adhesions on laparoscopy, 39% of 88 patients undergoing laparoscopy for tubal ligation or infertility also had adhesions, and only 4 of these 34 patients complained of pain.

- A total of 20% of all women demonstrate retroversion or retroflexion of the uterus. This anatomic variation usually does not cause symptoms.

- Of patients with chronic pelvic pain, 50% demonstrated multiple symptom complaints.

- Personality examinations in patients with chronic pelvic pain frequently define psychosocial problems, but such testing does not determine whether the pain is psychogenic or organic in nature.

- Chronic pelvic pain patients have been found to have a greater prevalence of lifetime major depression, current major depression, lifetime substance abuse, sexual dysfunction, somatization, and a greater incidence of childhood and adult sexual abuse.

- The majority of adnexal masses in women in the reproductive years are follicle cysts of the ovary.

- The most common benign neoplastic tumors of the ovary are serous cystadenoma and benign cystic teratoma.

- The most common benign cystic neoplasms of the ovary in the 20- to-44-year age group are benign cystic teratoma, serous cystadenoma, and mucinous cystadenoma.

- Serous cystadenocarcinoma is the most common malignant tumor in all age groups from 20 to 75 years.

- Wilms' tumor and neuroblastoma are the most common abdominal tumors in childhood.

- Dysgerminoma and teratoma are the most common solid adnexal tumors in young women.

- Most benign cystic teratomas are 10 cm or less in diameter, but about one sixth will be larger.

- Of women in the reproductive years, 30% develop myoma of the uterus. By age 50, 40% will have developed such tumors.

- A total of 95% of all endometriosis occurs in women in the reproductive years.

- Of 150 adnexal tumors in women over 50, 103 were benign. Of the malignant tumors in this age group, most were epithelial tumors. Tumors less than 5 cm were usually benign, but 40 of 63 tumors larger than 10 cm were malignant.

- Postmenopausal bleeding may be caused by a premalignant or malignant lesion of the uterus or cervix, but is often associated with an atrophic endometrium.

- The most common cause of vaginal bleeding in childhood is foreign bodies in the vagina.

BIBLIOGRAPHY

Allen WM and Masters WH: Traumatic lacerations of uterine support, Am J Obstet Gynecol 70:500, 1955.
Asadourian LA and Taylor HB: Dysgerminoma: an analysis of 105 cases, Obstet Gynecol 33:370, 1969.
Beard RW, Pearce S, Highman JH, and Reginald RW: Diagnosis of pelvic varicosities in women with chronic pelvic pain, Lancet 2:946, 1984.
Bennington JL, Ferguson BR, and Haber SL: Incidence and relative frequency of benign and malignant ovarian neoplasms, Obstet Gynecol 32:627, 1968.

Blendis LM: Abdominal pain. In Wall DP and Melzack R, eds: Textbook of pain, New York, 1984, Churchill Livingstone.
Bond M: The relation of pain to the Eysenck personality inventory, Cornell Medical Index and Whiteley Index of Hypochondriasis, Br J Psychol 119:671, 1971.
Buttram VC and Reiter RC: Uterine leiomyomata: etiology, symptomatology, and management, Fertil Steril 36:433, 1981.

Caruso PA, Marsh MR, Minkowitz S, and Karten G: An intense clinical pathologic study of 305 teratomas of the ovary, Cancer 27:343, 1971.

Costin ME and Kennedy RLJ: Ovarian tumors in infants and children, Am J Dis Child 76:127, 1948.

Cunanan RG, Courey NG, and Lippes J: Laparoscopic findings in patients with pelvic pain, Am J Obstet Gynecol 146:589, 1983.

Dewhurst J: Postmenopausal bleeding from benign causes, Clin Obstet Gynecol 26:769, 1983.

DiMarchi JM, Kosasa TS, and Hale RW: What is the significance of the human chorionic gonadotropin value in ectopic pregnancy? Obstet Gynecol 74:851, 1989.

Fraiz J and Jones RB: Chlamydial infections, Ann Rev Med 39:357, 1988.

Harrop-Griffiths J, Katon W, Walker E, et al: The association between chronic pelvic pain, psychiatric diagnoses, and childhood sexual abuse, Obstet Gynecol 71:589, 1988.

Herbst AL, Ulfelder H, and Poskanzer DC: Adenocarcinoma of the vagina: Association of maternal stilbestrol therapy with tumor appearance in young women, N Engl J Med 284:878, 1971.

Killackey MA and Neuwirth RS: Evaluation and management of the pelvic mass: a review of 540 cases, Obstet Gynecol 71:314, 1988.

Kistner RW: Gynecology principles and practice, ed 4, Chicago, 1986, Mosby–Year Book, Inc.

Kresch A, Seifer DB, Sachs LD, and Barrese I: Laparoscopy in 100 women with chronic pelvic pain, Obstet Gynecol 64:672, 1984.

Merskey H, Albe-Fessard DG, Bonica JJ, et al: Definitions and notes on usage recommended by the IASP Subcommittee on Taxonomy, Pain 6:249, 1979.

Mueller CW, Tompkins P, and Lapp WA: Dysgerminoma of the ovary: an analysis of 427 cases, Am J Obstet Gynecol 60:153, 1950.

Norris HJ and Jensen RD: Relative frequency of ovarian neoplasms in childhood and adolescence, Cancer 30:713, 1972.

Paavonen J, Kiviat N, Brunham RC, et al: Prevalence and manifestations of endometritis among women with cervicitis, Am J Obstet Gynecol 152:280, 1985.

Peterson WF, Prevost EC, Edmunds FT, et al: Benign cystic teratomas of the ovary: a clinico-statistical study of 1007 cases with review of the literature, Am J Obstet Gynecol 70:368, 1955.

Pritchard JA, MacDonald PC, and Gant NF: Williams Obstetrics, ed 7, Norwalk, Conn, 1985, Appleton-Century-Crofts.

Rapkin AJ: Adhesions and pelvic pain: a retrospective study, Obstet Gynecol 68:13, 1986.

Renaer M: Gynecological pain. In Wall DP and Melzack R, eds: Textbook of pain, New York, 1984, Churchill Livingstone.

Renaer MJ, Vertommen H, Nijs P, et al: Psychic aspects of pelvic pain in women, Am J Obstet Gynecol 134:75, 1979.

Rulin MC and Preston AL: Adnexal masses in postmenopausal women, Obstet Gynecol 70:578, 1987.

Slocumb JC: Neurological factors in chronic pelvic pain: trigger points and the abdominal pelvic pain syndrome, Am J Obstet Gynecol 149:536, 1984.

Stenchever MA: Symptomatic retrodisplacement, pelvic congestion, universal joint, and peritoneal defects: fact or fiction? Clin Obstet Gynecol 33:161, 1990.

Sternbach RA, Wolf SR, Murphy RW, and Akeson WH: Aspects of chronic low back pain, Psychosomatics 14:52, 1973.

Taylor HC: Vascular congestion and hyperemia. I. Physiologic basis in history of the concept, Am J Obstet Gynecol 57:211, 1949.

Taylor HC: Vascular congestion and hyperemia. II. The clinical aspects of congestion-fibrosis syndrome, Am J Obstet Gynecol 57:637, 1949.

Woodforde JM and Merskey H: Personality traits of patients with chronic pain, J Psychosom Res 16:167, 1972.

Counseling the Patient

_____ KEY TERMS AND DEFINITIONS _____

Agitated Depression. A severe and rare grief reaction in which the bereaved develops tension, agitation, insomnia, feelings of worthlessness, and fantasies of the need for punishment, at times including suicide.

Anhedonia. Loss of feelings of joy and pleasure.

Anorexia Nervosa. A psychiatric disease associated with a food aversion, fear of weight gain or obesity, and a distorted body image in which the individual limits caloric intake to starvation levels. In addition to severe weight loss, there is a decreased metabolic rate and amenorrhea.

Behavior Modification. A treatment program using reward and punishment techniques to change behavior.

Binge Drinking. The consumption of five or more drinks on a specific occasion or drinking until intoxicated.

Bulimia. A symptom of anorexia nervosa that features binge eating and self-induced purging using both vomiting and diarrhea as methods.

Cognitive Behavior Therapy. The technique of behavior change that attempts to modify beliefs, assumptions, and thinking styles.

Delayed Grief Reaction. The postponement of the grief reaction for various reasons and for a period from days to years.

Distorted Grief Reaction. The assumption of the characteristics of the deceased by the bereaved for a prolonged period and at times in a distorted fashion, during which the bereaved often evidences no sense of loss.

Dyspareunia. Painful intercourse.

Excessive Alcohol Consumption. The consumption of 45 or more alcoholic drinks per month or 5 or more alcoholic drinks on a specific occasion.

G-spot. An area on the anterior vaginal wall beneath the urethra defined by Grafenberg as analogous to the male prostate gland and which during sexual arousal may be stimulated to the point of orgasm with ejaculation into the urethra of fluid similar in nature to prostatic fluid.

Grief Reaction. A group of symptoms associated with loss, which generally resolves in 6 to 18 months.

Obesity. An eating disorder in which the individual's weight is 20% or more above the mean weights for individuals of the same sex and height. Mild obesity is defined as 20% to 40% overweight; moderate obesity as 41% to 100% overweight; and severe obesity as greater than 100% overweight.

Orgasmic Dysfunction. Difficulty or inability in reaching orgasm.

Sexual Dysfunction. A psychologic or physiologic problem or condition that prevents the usual full participation and enjoyment of coitus.

Sexual Response Curve. The graphic expression of sexual response as defined by Masters and Johnson involving four phases: excitement, plateau, orgasm, and resolution.

Vaginismus. Involuntary spasm of vaginal, introital, and levator ani muscles causing painful sexual intercourse or preventing penetration.

During a lifetime the individual faces several tasks and challenges. Perhaps the first is the development of an identity and the building of a self-esteem. This begins in early childhood and continues through adolescence. Such development is aided by positive and nurturing forces. On the other hand, attacks against the young individual's mental or physical well-being may have a distorting influence. The quality of her self-esteem and self-perception will influence the choices she makes in life situations and will affect her personal development.

All individuals experience loss throughout their lifetime. The scope of such loss may be quite varied, including lack of accomplishment or loss of opportunity in career, the loss of a body organ or a body part, the loss of a friend or a loved one through separation or death, the loss of a relationship, or the loss of a physical or mental ability because of illness or accident. In general, loss is managed by a grieving process. The way in which the individual grieves and resolves grief often determines the degree of success in the next stage of life. The inability to handle grief appropriately may lead to lost opportunities, poor choices, and poorly developed future relationships.

The gynecologist is in an important position to help the young woman develop her self-image and to help her manage the losses that she will inevitably face. The gynecologist has the opportunity to participate with the patient in critical life events from adolescence to late in life and to provide or obtain counseling for her as she works her way through these problems.

This chapter will outline the major social problems that can arise during a woman's lifetime and will offer suggestions as to how the physician can aid the patient.

CHILDHOOD COUNSELING PROBLEMS

Self-esteem begins to develop in early childhood and is the result of positive efforts of parents and others in the child's immediate environment. Continuous reinforcement of a child's worth as an individual, by verbal and nonverbal means, should be encouraged. Touching, talking to the child in gentle ways, positively praising the child's actions, and, as the child becomes older, setting limits that are socially acceptable within the framework of the family are all reasonable steps. Punishment should be limited to reinforcing the needs for the limits set. Intimidation by verbal or physical means should be avoided. The physician may have the opportunity to suggest help for parents by offering reading material, discussing the issue directly with them, or referring them to parenting classes. In general, positive reinforcement of the child's worth as an individual mixed with appropriate warmth and love tends to build self-esteem, whereas negative statements or actions tend to tear it down. The child has little with which to compare, and if she is given negative information about herself, the tendency is to believe it.

Physical or sexual abuse in childhood can have serious consequences for the child's development. These are extreme influences and must be handled energetically when they occur or as soon afterwards as they are noted. The health care professional must communicate to the child that she is a victim and in no way responsible for what has happened. Any contrary statements may have a lasting effect on the child's developing self-esteem. Issues of abuse are discussed more fully in Chapter 12.

Parental Loss in Childhood

A serious threat to normal emotional development in childhood is the loss of a parent by death or permanent separation. Laajus reviewed a large number of studies addressing this problem. Because the study methodology is complex, it is difficult to draw comparisons between different reports. However, a number of general observations were made. In Laajus's experience parental loss was a common finding in children referred for psychiatric treatment and was associated with a variety of pathologic and behavior disturbances. The period between the loss of a parent and the onset of the disorder is often quite long.

Tennant et al., applying multiple regression analysis, believe that the earlier the separation and the longer its duration, the more maladjustment is likely to occur. The risk of developing a psychiatric disorder seems greatest if the child is younger than 5 years or an adolescent and if the child loses a parent of the same sex. Males seem more susceptible to the loss of a father than the loss of a mother and seem to be more affected by this loss than are females. In general, their major reaction is to develop antisocial tendencies. On the other hand, loss of a father during adolescence seems to influence the emotional development of females, although the problems may not be manifested for a number of years. Loss of a mother in girls under age 11 seems to significantly affect development.

Some of the difficulty in clarifying the role of the loss of a mother or father in young children relates to the way parent substitutes are developed. Because maternal loss usually necessitates the finding of a care provider, often a female, the effect of maternal loss may be blunted. On the other hand, male substitution after paternal loss may not occur rapidly or at all. Tennant et al. showed a consistent relationship between parental loss and the development of psychiatric illness in all ages. Children between the ages of 5 and 10 years seem to be the most susceptible to behavior changes. But adolescence was also a time of important vulnerability in cases of schizophrenia, depression, and a variety of medical illnesses occurring in adolescence. The loss of a parent early in life was a frequent and significant finding in such patients, with the loss of a father being noted more frequently than the loss of a mother.

Gregory has demonstrated that parental loss is often associated with antisocial disorders, especially delinquency. The highest rates seem to occur among males who have lost their father. One study shows a 3.5-fold increase of severe crimes in a group of males who had lost one or more parents before the age of 5 years. On the other hand, the perpetration of severe crimes was less frequent among males who had experienced parental losses later in life. Anderson compared a group of delinquent and nondelinquent boys who had suffered parental loss between the ages of 4 and 7 years and demonstrated that a father substitution had occurred more frequently in the group that was not delinquent.

Counseling considerations for children and adolescents who have suffered parental loss should include attention to the child's bereavement with active help in working through the acute phase of grief followed by the incorporation of an individual into the child's life who is of the same sex as the lost parent. If the mother is deceased or absent, a loving, nurturing, and supportive female or group of females should be identified to participate in the child's care and development. This may be a grand-parent, an aunt, a hired nanny, or an effective childcare program. Eventually it may be a stepmother. If the father is lost, older brothers, grandfathers, uncles, or males volunteering as "big brothers" may all be considered. In addition, surviving parents should be encouraged to protect the child as much as possible from their own grieving process and to maintain the integrity of the family unit.

Similar observations have been made with respect to the loss of a parent through separation or divorce. Hostile marital relationships seem to be more detrimental to child development than does the permanent absence of a parent by divorce or separation. Continuous discord within the family has been shown by Rutter to be associated with an increase of antisocial disorders in boys but not in girls. Tennant et al. investigated individuals with psychiatric disorders and looked at four causes of separation from parents during childhood. These include illness of the individual, wartime evacuation, parental illness, and marital discord. They found that parental illness and marital discord had a statistically significantly greater association with the development of psychiatric diseases than did separation because of the individual's illness or wartime evacuation.

PROBLEMS IN ADOLESCENCE AND ADULTHOOD

Eating Disorders

Anorexia nervosa, bulimia, and obesity are the major eating disorders affecting adolescents and young adults. On the one hand, eating is one of the major gratifications of life and is also a readily available substitute for other forms of gratification that cannot be achieved. Today a young woman is bombarded by two very different signals stemming primarily from advertising campaigns presented on television and radio and in magazines and books. The first of these involves food. Citizens of the Western world are offered foods of vast variety and unusual quantity presented in an appealing and almost demanding fashion. Stimuli to eat are seductive and almost continuous. On the other hand, the image of the American woman as depicted by the media is one of thinness. Garner et al., in discussing the cultural expectations of American women, noted that a definite trend for decrease in body weight was noted between 1959 and 1978 in *Playboy* centerfold models and participants in the Miss America pageant. In both instances these women weighed significantly less than the average American woman. Further, the weights of the finalists in the Miss America pageant were noted to be significantly below those of other contestants during the years 1970 through 1978. The image that these "ideal women" create is in severe contrast to the reality that the average weight of American women increased by several pounds during that same period.

Johnson et al. recently reported that in a survey of 1200 high school girls, 48% believed that they were either overweight or very overweight, whereas only 8% considered themselves underweight. Interestingly, the mean weight of these young women was within the normal range. Because the majority believed they were overweight, 50% of those who were 14 years or older and 70% who were 18 years or older were actively dieting. Many reported the use of diuretics, diet pills, laxatives, and self-induced vomiting to lower their weight. In another survey in 1978, 56% of women between the ages of 24 and 54 were found to be dieting, and 75% of the dieters stated that they did so for cosmetic reasons.

The effects of dieting may bring women to the attention of the gynecologist and may be responsible for symptoms that may not seem readily related to dieting. For instance, Pirke et al. studied 13 healthy women of normal weight who volunteered to lose 1 kg/week on an 800-calorie vegetarian diet for an average weight loss of 4.9 ± 0.7 kg. At the completion of the study, their body mass index was 99% of ideal body weight (Metropolitan Life Insurance standards). During their control cycles, each demonstrated normal gonadal function, but during the dietary cycles only two remained normal. Seven did not develop dominant follicles, and four others who did demonstrated impaired progesterone secretion by the corpus luteum. Dieting altered episodic luteinizing hormone (LH) secretion during the follicular phase, and LH concentrations and the frequency of episodic secretions were significantly reduced during the follicular phase but not during the luteal phase. Follicle-stimulating hormone (FSH) was unaltered by dieting.

Likewise, Kreipe et al. studied two groups of women who had clinical or subclinical eating disorders classified as restrictive anorexia nervosa, bulimic anorexia nervosa, normal weight bulimia nervosa, and other subclinical eating disorders and compared these with control subjects. None had weights above 110% of ideal body weight. Of 48 women with a diagnosed eating disorder, 45 (93.7%) had a menstrual abnormality consisting of amenorrhea or oligomenorrhea. Of the 22 patients with subclinical eating disorders, 21 gave a history of amenorrhea although none had this problem at present. Nine complained of oligomenorrhea. Most of these women reported weight fluctuations of 10% to 20% of ideal body weight in the past. Of the 37 controls, only 1 had a history of amenorrhea and 4 of oligomenorrhea. Thus an eating disorder apparently can present with menstrual abnormalities even in the subclinical stages and can probably affect reproductive efficiency.

Johnson and Schlundt stated that stress on women in the 1980s is accentuated by the double role they must play. Not only are they expected to fill the traditional roles of wives and mothers, but also they are expected to compete in the marketplace for contemporary careers. On the traditional side they must compete with women, whereas on the contemporary side they must compete with men as well.

Anorexia Nervosa and Bulimia

Although anorexia nervosa is quite uncommon in the general population (0.24 to 1.6 per 100,000 people), it is quite common in middle-class adolescent girls, occurring in about 1 in every 100. The incidence in professional ballet dancers varies from 5% to 20% depending on the level of competition of the ballet company, the weight standards imposed, and the number of hours of exercise required. The condition is 9 times more common in women than in men. It does occur among men who must restrict their weights in training for competitive athletic events.

Although various clinical signs and symptoms occur in the patient with anorexia nervosa, it basically concerns food aversion, fear of weight gain or obesity, and a distorted body image. There is often an associated amenorrhea, which frequently disappears with weight gain. The central nervous system and endocrine considerations are discussed in Chapter 36.

Bulimia occurs in about 50% of anorectic patients and is defined as binge eating and self-induced purging. Not all bulimics have low body weight. Bulimic persons may have more severe psychological problems and be more difficult to treat. In a study by Casper et al. 57% of bulimic patients reported vomiting after meals, in contrast to only 18% of patients with anorexia without bulimia. Bulimic persons in this series tended to be more extroverted and demonstrated symptoms of depression and anxiety, particularly with sleep disturbances. They also were more obsessional about food than were anorectics without bulimia.

Gershen et al. described an incidence of anorexia nervosa and bulimia 6 times greater in first-degree relatives of anorectic probands than in first-degree relatives of controls (6% and 1.1% respectively). Strober et al. looked at the incidence of anorexia nervosa, bulimia, and subclinical anorexia nervosa in first- and second-degree relatives of anorectic patients and demonstrated that eating disorders are familial. They were, however, unable to demonstrate mechanisms responsible for these familial relationships. They suggested that genetically transmitted defects in the neurobiologic processes that control feeding behavior may be present but could not rule out specific psychological or familial vulnerabilities, common exposure to psychologically determined environmental experiences, cotransmission, or personality traits or psychopathologic disorders that may involve eating disturbances. They also could not rule out some important combinations of all of these factors.

An interesting association between eating disorders and an adverse sexual experience was noted by Oppenheimer et al. Two thirds of 78 patients with eating disorders reported such experiences and stated that thoughts of previous sexual abuse were often stressing and significant to the individuals. A total of 80% of the events occurred in childhood or adolescence, and most involved a significantly older male, usually a person known to the subject. In most cases both social taboo and personal trust were violated. The authors felt that given the nature of their study questionnaire, the incidence of such adverse sexual experience among anorectics may have been underreported.

Johnson and Schlundt in commenting on therapy for anorexia nervosa pointed out that the general modalities have included medication, hospitalization, nutritional support, and behavior therapy. To evaluate any therapy it is important to understand what the spontaneous remission rate might be among untreated patients. Hsu et al. compared three groups of patients with anorexia nervosa who were evaluated between 1968 and 1973 and were followed for 4 to 6 years. Within the group there were those treated as inpatients and as outpatients, and those not treated. Evaluation included weight gain and menstrual function. Good or fair outcomes were observed in 88% of those treated as inpatients, 77% of those treated as outpatients, and 59% of those not treated. In general, inpatient therapy consisted of hospitalization, nutritional support, various medications, and often individual or family counseling and psychotherapy. Most studies report excellent weight gain in such patients. Agres and Kraemer, in reviewing a number of studies, found that the therapy lasted 2½ to 3½ months, with an average weight gain of 4.1 kg per month noted.

A number of medications have been tried with varying success. These medications have included insulin, lithium, tricyclics, and phenothiazides, as well as high-potency vitamins. In many case control studies these have not been found to be more effective than placebo. It is often difficult to separate the effect of a medication from the effects of counseling and psychotherapy given simultaneously.

In severe cases, patients have been fed intravenously, given total parenteral nutrition, or given nasogastric tube feedings. Generally, these methods are used when normal feeding attempts in inpatient therapy have not been associated with weight gain. Such extreme measures are generally used in the most severe and life-threatening situations.

In the 1960s and 1970s therapy was often tailored to the technique of behavior modification. When controlled studies were carried out, it seemed apparent that hospitalization per se would allow for reasonable weight gain, but when behavior modification was added, the hospital course could be shortened because of accelerated weight gain. Behavior modification was based on the reward and punishment program used for a number of behavior and habituation problems.

More recently, however, cognitive behavior therapy has been used in the treatment of anorexia. This therapy is aimed at bringing to the attention of the individual the fact that her or his beliefs, assumptions, and style of thinking have brought about distorted body image, food aversion, phobias, and unreasonable fears of weight gain. In short, the therapy is aimed at reshaping patients' thinking processes with respect to themselves and to their body images. No specific studies have been done to compare one method with another, but cognitive behavior therapy appears to be directed toward the specific thinking disorder rather than merely to its effect.

Finally, it is important to consider ultimate outcome in groups of patients with anorexia nervosa and bulimia. Theander, in a recent discussion of outcome, reviewed three long-term follow-up studies and discussed the results of his own study in Sweden. In three British studies a 5- to 6-year follow-up demonstrated good to intermediate results in 74% of patients. However, 23% of patients experienced a poor outcome, with 3% dying of the disease. In the Swedish study described by Theander with a mean observation time of 33 years, good to fair outcomes were noted in 76% of patients, poor outcomes in 6%, and death in 18%. Deaths were the result of starvation or suicide. Isager et al. recently analyzed survival data in 151 cases of anorexia nervosa, considering specifically death and relapse rates. Follow-up was from 4 to 22 years. The authors calculated the

hazard of death as 0.5% per year and the hazards of relapse at 3% per year. Both hazards, however, declined steadily after therapeutic contact.

Obesity

Stunkard has suggested a classification for obesity in which mild designates individuals who are 20% to 40% overweight; moderate, 41% to 100% overweight; and severe, greater than 100% overweight. By these standards, 35% of women in the United States are considered obese. U.S. vital health statistics in 1983 suggest that of women who qualify as obese by these guidelines, 90.5% of the cases are classed as mild, 9% as moderate, and 0.5% as severe. Table 7-1 is the 1983 Metropolitan Life Insurance Company height and weight table.

Severe obesity is a health hazard that carries a twelvefold increase in mortality for persons between the ages of 25 and 34 years. Often these individuals suffer complicating factors, such as hypertension, diabetes, hyperlipedemias, arthritis, increased operative morbidity and mortality, and compromised pulmonary function. According to Stunkard, severe obesity may also be associated with hypertrophic

TABLE 7-1
Height and Weight Table for Women*

Height		Weight (lbs)		
Feet	Inches	Small Frame	Medium Frame	Large Frame
4	10	102-111	109-121	118-131
4	11	103-113	111-123	120-134
5	0	104-115	113-126	122-137
5	1	106-118	115-129	125-140
5	2	108-121	118-132	128-143
5	3	111-124	121-135	131-147
5	4	114-127	124-138	134-151
5	5	117-130	127-141	137-155
5	6	120-133	130-144	140-159
5	7	123-136	133-147	143-163
5	8	126-139	136-150	146-167
5	9	129-142	139-153	149-170
5	10	132-145	142-156	152-173
5	11	135-148	145-159	155-176
6	0	138-151	148-162	158-179

*Weights at ages 25 to 29 based on lowest mortality. Weight in pounds according to frame (in indoor clothing weighing 3 pounds; shoes with 1-inch heels). (From 1983 Metropolitan Height & Weight Tables, Metropolitan Life Insurance Company, Health and Safety Division.)

adipose tissue cells with an increased proliferation of adipose tissue and thus an increasing severity of obesity.

Stunkard suggests that diet and behavior modification provided by lay supervision is appropriate for those suffering from mild obesity; diet and behavior modification under medical supervision is appropriate for those suffering from moderate obesity; and operative intervention is appropriate for those suffering from severe obesity. Patients suffering from severe obesity almost always have medical complications, and these often improve with weight reduction. In previous years jejunoileal bypass procedures were the treatment of choice. These, however, had many complications. Currently procedures that reduce gastric size and narrow the outlet of the stomach seem to be the most appropriate approaches taken (Table 7-2).

When dietary and pharmacologic therapy has been used for treating severe obesity, 15% of patients suffer from severe depression and 26% from moderate depression. Depression is much less common in patients who undergo gastric reduction operations. Of these individuals, 75% report elation and a feeling of well-being. In addition, 91% of these patients state that before operation they had required a good deal of willpower to keep from overeating, and indeed, 33% stated that they could eat another full meal after eating most of their meals. Only 14% ever felt satisfied after eating. After the operation 10% state that they require willpower to keep from eating more, and only 1% state that they could eat another full meal after eating. On the other hand, 94% feel that they could eat no more after completing the usual meal.

Moderately obese patients will lose weight on diets of 1200 to 1500 calories and generally find this approach comfortable. However, weight loss under these circumstances takes a long time. On very low-calorie diets (400 to 700 calories), which consist mostly of protein (fish, fowl, or lean meat), dramatic change in weight can usually be accomplished in 3 months. The patient will lose 1.5 to 2.3 kg per week depending on the amount of body fat at the beginning of dieting. The major problem with such individuals is maintaining weight loss.

Craighead et al. point out that unless behavior is modified, weight loss is usually not maintained. These workers studied 145 patients who were approximately 60% overweight and divided them into three groups. Treatment continued for 6 months, and there was at least 1 year of follow-up in 99% of those who completed the therapy. Group 1 underwent behavior modification using Ferguson's *Learning to Eat* manual. They lost an average of 11.4 kg and regained only 1.8 kg during the follow-up year. Group 2 received medication therapy with an appetite suppressant, fenfluramine hydrochloride (Pondimin). They lost an average of 14.5 kg but regained 8.6 kg during the follow-up period. The third group was treated with a combination of behavior modification and medication and lost an average of 15.0 kg but regained 9.5 kg during the follow-up period. The authors concluded that behavior modification without medication was the most appropriate therapy for moderate obesity.

Mild obesity seems to respond best to dieting and behavior modification under lay supervision. Such individuals will generally embrace fad diets and look for magic cures. However, if placed on a nutritionally appropriate limited-caloric diet, they will generally do well if their attitudes toward eating and response to various stimuli are modified. Lay groups, such as Weight Watchers or Take Off Pounds Sensibly (TOPS), are usually quite successful for motivated individuals. Currently there are many commercial diet centers available for referral. Most prescribe or sell low-fat foods in an attempt to achieve a diet containing about 20% fat. Because fat represents 9 calories/gram and protein and carbohydrate represent 4 calories/gram, it is possible by changing eating habits to allow a patient a considerable quantity of food without high numbers of calories. Educating patients to change eating habits in this fashion is the key not only to losing weight, but to maintaining the weight loss.

TABLE 7-2
Recommended Therapy in Obesity

Degree of Obesity	Percent Above Normal Weight	Therapy
Mild	20-40	Diet and lay supervision
Moderate	41-100	Low-calorie diet and medical supervision
Severe	>100	Gastric reduction operation

Obesity in adolescence is a variant of the problem in the general population. Because the risk for progression with increasing morbidity and mortality is great, prompt support and behavior modification are most important. School and parental involvement are important aspects of controlling the problem. Where an obese parent is also present, best results seem to be achieved when both the parent and the child undergo therapy but in separate counseling sessions. In a study by Brownell et al. using 16 weeks of treatment of 42 obese adolescents ages 12 through 16, three groups were studied. When the child alone attended group therapy, there was an average 3.3 kg weight loss; when the child and mother were treated together there was an average 5.3 kg weight loss; and when the child and mother were both treated but separately, there was an 8.4 kg weight loss. After 1 year of follow-up the group in which the mother and child were treated separately maintained their weight loss at a mean of 7.7 kg, whereas the other two groups had regained their previous baseline levels.

Obviously, counseling and behavior modification are important in the management of both the adolescent and adult obese patient.

Sexual Function and Dysfunction

Sexual satisfaction is one of the more important human experiences, yet it has been estimated that as many as 50% of all married couples experience some sexual dissatisfaction or dysfunction. Although there is a strong physiologic basis for sexual function, it is impossible to separate sexual response from the many emotional and other contributing factors that may influence a relationship.

In 1966 Masters and Johnson published their now famous book, *Human Sexual Response*, which was a discussion of observations made on the sexual cycles of 700 subjects. It is on this important work that our current understanding of the female sexual response is based. Masters and Johnson described four phases of the sexual response: excitement, plateau, orgasm, and resolution (Figure 7-1).

The excitement or seduction phase may be initiated by a number of internal or external stimuli. Physiologically it is associated with deep breathing, increase in heart rate and blood pressure, a total body feeling of warmth associated often with erotic feelings, and an increase in sexual tension. There is generalized vasocongestion, which leads to breast engorgement and the development of a maculopapular erythematous rash on the breasts, the chest, and the epigastrium, which is called the *sex flush*. There is also engorgement of the labia majora (seen particularly in multiparous women) and of the labia minora. The clitoris generally swells and becomes erect, causing it to be tightly applied to the clitoral hood. The vagina "sweats" a transudative lubricant, and the Bartholin glands may secrete small amounts of liquid. With the increasing deep breathing the uterus may tent up into the pelvis, perhaps as a result of the Valsalva maneuver. There is also a myotonic effect, which is most notable in nipple erection. Much of the response in the excitement phase is caused by stimulation of the parasympathetic fibers of the autonomic nervous system. In some cases anticholinergic drugs may interfere with a full response in this stage.

Next is the plateau stage, which is the culmination of the excitement phase and is associated with a marked degree of vasocongestion throughout the body. Breasts and their areolae are markedly engorged, as are the labia and the lower third of the vagina. The vasocongestion in the lower third of the vagina is such that it forms what has been called the *orgasmic platform*, causing a decrease in the diameter of the vagina by as much as 50% and thus allowing for greater friction against the penis. At this stage the clitoris retracts tightly against the pubic symphysis, and the vagina lengthens, with dilation of the upper two thirds. Uteri in the normal anteflex position tend to tent up more. Retroverted uteri do not.

The next stage is orgasm, in which the sexual tension that has been built up in the entire body is released. A myotonic response involves muscle systems of the entire body. Individuals may experience carpal spasm. Rarely, a grand mal type seizure may be observed. There is contraction of the muscles surrounding the vagina, as well as the anal sphincter. The uterus also contracts. Muscle contraction occurs 2 to 4 seconds after the woman begins to experience the orgasm and repeats at 0.8-second intervals. The actual number and intensity of contractions vary from woman to woman. Some women observed to have orgasmic contractions are not aware that they are having an orgasm. Masters and Johnson feel that prolonged stimu-

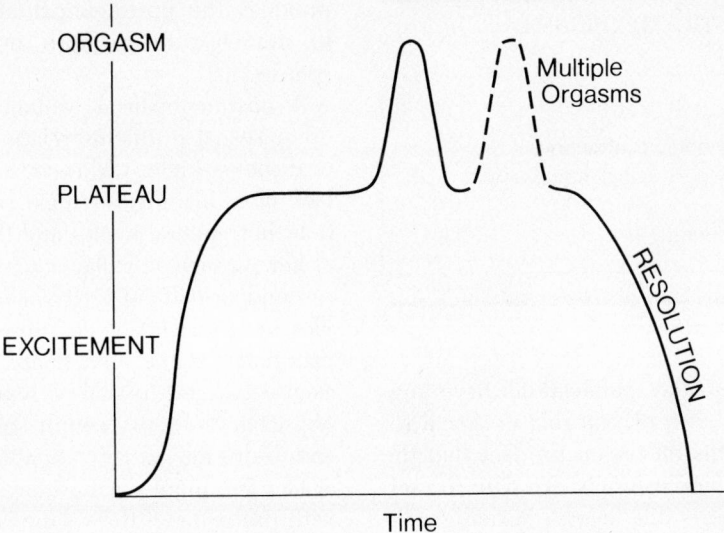

FIGURE 7-1
Sexual response cycle defined by Masters and Johnson. (From Masters WH and Johnson VE: Human sexual response, Boston, 1966, Little, Brown & Co.)

CHARACTERISTICS OF EXCITEMENT PHASE OF SEXUAL RESPONSE CYCLE IN THE FEMALE

Deep breathing
Increased pulse
Increased blood pressure
Warmth and erotic feelings
Increased tension
Generalized vasocongestion
Skin flush
Breast engorgement
Nipple erection
Engorgement of labia and clitoris
Vaginal transudation
Uterine tenting

lation during the excitement phase, during masturbation, or in conjunction with the use of a vibrator may lead to more pronounced orgasmic activity. Whereas the excitement phase is under the influence of the parasympathetic portion of the autonomic nervous system, orgasm seems to be related to the sympathetic portion. Medication such as antihypertensive drugs may affect orgasmic response.

The resolution stage is last and represents a return of the woman's physiologic state to the preexcitement level. Although a refractory period is typical of the sexual response cycle in the male, no such refractory periods have been identified in women. Therefore new sexual excitement cycles may be stimulated at any time after orgasm. During the resolution phase the woman generally experiences a feeling of personal satisfaction and well-being.

Masters and Johnson identified the clitoris as the center of sexual satisfaction in the female. However, recently Whipple and Perry have rediscovered some work first suggested by Ernest Grafenberg that suggests that there is an anatomic position on the anterior wall of the vagina suburethrally that when stimulated becomes engorged and during orgasm is associated with an ejaculation of prostatic-like fluid into the urethra. Whipple and Perry have designated this the *G-spot* after Grafenberg and believe that it is analogous to the male prostate gland. Their concept that the G-spot is intimately involved in the orgasmic process is based on their observation that when this area is stimulated in women, a feeling of sexual excitement is produced, and when the area is stimulated to the point of orgasm, ejaculation of fluid from the urethra occurs. Analysis of this fluid has shown it to have some of the qualities of prostatic fluid. Whipple and Perry believe that this evidence supports the G-spot thesis. It has been difficult for other authors to reproduce their work, and at present the significance of and necessity for the G-spot is still unclear.

CHARACTERISTICS OF ORGASM IN THE FEMALE

> Release of tension
> Generalized myotonic contractions
> Contractions of perivaginal muscles and anal sphincter
> Uterine contractions

Recently several lay publications have suggested that the cervix plays a role in sexual response, basing this theory on the fact that the cervix has a rich nerve supply. To date, no scientific data supports this theory. Sexual gratification and orgasmic behavior definitely seem to be associated with nerve endings in the clitoris, mons pubis, labia, and possible pressure receptors in the pelvis. In a recent study by Andersen et al., 42 women aged 31 to 81 (average 50.3) who had been treated for in situ vulvar carcinoma were compared with a group of comparable women aged 30 to 61 (average 44.3) with respect to sexual function. Six of the women had undergone local therapy with laser or chemotherapy, 26 had wide excision of lesions, 9 had undergone simple vulvectomy, and 1 had undergone a radical vulvectomy. Sexual behavior patterns and desires were maintained after therapy, but a specific disruption of the phases of excitement and resolution, and to a lesser extent orgasm, were noted. There was 2 to 3 times greater incidence of sexual dysfunction in the patient group, and 30% became sexually inactive. Loss or disruption of the clitoris seemed to be the single most important factor.

Sexual Response and Menopause

The postmenopausal woman who is not on hormone replacement experiences progressive atrophy of vaginal epithelium, a change in vaginal pH, a decrease in quantity of vaginal secretions, and a decrease in the general circulation to the vagina and uterus. She may also have pelvic relaxation, including cystocele, rectocele, or prolapse of the uterus, and a general loss of vaginal tone. Women on replacement hormone therapy have been shown by Semmens and Semmens not to suffer the problems of vaginal atrophy and poor circulation. It is likely that hormone replacement, therefore, prolongs the postmenopausal woman's ability to demonstrate a more normal sexual response.

A postmenopausal woman may experience other sexual problems relating to her partner, or if she is single, widowed, or divorced, to her lack of availability of male partners. In addition, her general health and the general health of her partner will play a role in her ability to respond sexually in a satisfactory manner. Couples with marital or communication problems may find that the menopause is an appropriate excuse to cease sexual activities. A concerned physician can help a couple sort out their needs and desire for sexual compatibility at this stage of life. Frequently counseling aimed at dealing with problems of the relationship will alleviate sexual response difficulties.

Male partners of older women may suffer from medical illnesses or be affected by medications they must take, with resultant decrease in arousal, difficulties in maintaining an erection, or complete impotence. The physician should ask women about sexual function and if male dysfunction is evident, should make suggestions for appropriate referral to physicians or other health care workers who may deal with the male sexual dysfunction problems. Table 7-3 lists several drugs that can affect sexual function.

Sexual Dysfunction

Sexual dysfunction is quite common. Masters and Johnson estimated that it exists in 50% of marriages. Higher percentages of dysfunction are seen in couples presenting for marital therapy. That sexual dysfunction is not necessarily incompatible with a happy marriage was noted in a study by Frank et al. who surveyed couples felt to be well adjusted who were selected from general community groups. Of these couples, 83% rated their marriages as happy or very happy, but 63% of the women and 40% of the men gave a history of sexual dysfunction. A total of 48% of the women stated that they had difficulties becoming sexually excited, and 33% found difficulty in maintaining excitement. Of the total group, 46% of the women experienced difficulty in reaching orgasm, and 15% had never had an orgasm. Finally, 35% of the women expressed disinterest in sex. These workers' experience implies that physicians caring for women should make a special effort to uncover sexual dysfunction or poor sexual

TABLE 7-3
Drugs That May Affect Sexual Function

Drug	Adverse Effect	Drug	Adverse Effect
Acetazolamide (Diamox and others)	Loss of libido; decreased potency	Danazol (Danocrine)	Increased or decreased libido
Alprazolam (Xanax)	Inhibition of orgasm; delayed or no ejaculation	Desipramine (Norpramin and others)	Decreased libido; impotence; difficult ejaculation and painful orgasm
Amiloride (Midamor)	Impotence; decreased libido	Diazepam (Valium and others)	Decreased libido; delayed ejaculation; retarded or no orgasm in women
Amiodarone (Cordarone)	Decreased libido		
Amitriptyline (Elavil and others)	Loss of libido; impotence; no ejaculation	Dichlorphenamide (Daranide and others)	Decreased libido; impotence
Amoxapine (Asendin)	Loss of libido; impotence; retrograde, painful, or no ejaculation	Digoxin	Decreased libido; impotence
Amphetamines and related anorexic drugs	Chronic abuse; impotence; delayed or no ejaculation in men; no orgasm in women	Disopyramide (Norpace and others)	Impotence
		Disulfiram (Antabuse and others)	Impotence
Anticholinergics	Impotence	Doxepin (Adapin Sinequan)	Decreased libido; ejaculatory dysfunction
Atenolol (Tenormin)	Impotence	Estrogens	Decreased libido in men
Baclofen (Lioresal)	Impotence; inability to ejaculate	Ethionamide (Trecator-SC)	Impotence
Barbiturates	Decreased libido; impotence	Ethosuximide (Zarontin)	Increased libido
Carbamazepine (Tegretol)	Impotence	Ethoxzolamide (Ethamide)	Decreased libido
Chlorpromazine (Thorazine and others)	Decreased libido; impotence; no ejaculation; priapism	Fenfluramine (Pondimin)	Loss of libido (frequent in women with large doses or long-term use); impotence
Chlorprothixene (Taractan)	Inhibition of ejaculation; decreased intensity of orgasm	Fluphenazine (Prolixin, Permitil)	Changes in libido; erection difficulties; inhibition of ejaculation
Chlorthalidone (Hygroton and others)	Decreased libido; impotence	Guanabenz (Wytensin)	Impotence
Cimetidine (Tagamet)	Decreased libido (men and women); impotence	Guanadrel (Hylorel)	Decreased libido; delayed or retrograde ejaculation; impotence
Clofibrate (Atromid-S)	Decreased libido; impotence	Guanethidine (Ismelin)	Decreased libido; impotence; delayed, retrograde, or no ejaculation
Clomipramine (Anafranil)	Decreased libido; impotence; retarded or no ejaculation (men) or orgasm (women); spontaneous orgasm associated with yawning		
		Guanfacine (Tenex)	Impotence
		Haloperidol (Haldol and others)	Impotence; painful ejaculation
Clonidine (Catapres and others)	Impotence; delayed or retrograde ejaculation; inhibition of orgasm (women)	Hydralazine (Apresoline and others)	Impotence; priapism

From Med Lett Drugs Ther 29:65, 1987.

Continued.

TABLE 7-3
Drugs That May Affect Sexual Function—cont'd

Drug	Adverse Effect	Drug	Adverse Effect
Hydroxyprogesterone caproate (Delalutin and others)	Impotence	Methyldopa (Aldomet and others)	Decreased libido; impotence; delayed or no ejaculation (men) or orgasm (women)
Imipramine (Tofranil and others)	Decreased libido; impotence; painful, delayed ejaculation; delayed orgasm in women	Metoclopramide (Reglan and others)	Impotence; decreased libido
		Metoprolol (Lopressor)	Decreased libido; impotence
Indapamide (Lozol)	Decreased libido; impotence	Metyrosine (Demser)	Impotence; failure of ejaculation
Interferon (Roferon-a)	Decreased libido; impotence	Mexiletine (Mexitil)	Impotence; decreased libido
Isocarboxazid (Marplan)	Impotence; delayed ejaculation; no orgasm (women)	Molindone (Moban)	Priapism
		Naltrexone (Trexan)	Delayed ejaculation; decreased potency
Isocarboxazid (Marplan)	Impotence; delayed ejaculation; no orgasm (women)	Naproxen (Anaprox, Naprosyn)	Impotence; no ejaculation
Ketoconazole (Nizoral)	Impotence	Norethindrone (Norlutin and others)	Decreased libido; impotence
Labetalol (Trandate, Normodyne)	Priapism; impotence; delayed or no ejaculation; decreased libido	Nortriptyline (Aventyl, Pamelor)	Impotence; decreased libido
Levodopa (Dopar and others)	Increased libido	Pargyline (Eutonyl)	No ejaculation; impotence
Lithium (Eskalith and others)	Decreased libido; impotence	Perphenazine (Trilafon)	Decreased or no ejaculation
Maprotiline (Ludiomil)	Impotence; decreased libido	Phenelzine (Nardil)	Impotence; retarded or no ejaculation; delayed or no orgasm (men and women)
Mazindol (Sanorex, Mazanor)	Impotence; spontaneous ejaculation; painful testes	Phenytoin (Dilantin and others)	Decreased libido; impotence
Mecamylamine (Inversine)	Impotence; decreased libido	Pimozide (Orap)	Impotence; no ejaculation; decreased libido
Mepenzolate bromide (Cantil)	Impotence	Pindolol (Visken)	Impotence
Mesoridazine (Serentil)	No ejaculation; impotence; priapism	Prazosin (Minipress)	Impotence; priapism
		Primidone (Mysoline and others)	Decreased libido; impotence
Methadone (Dolophine and others)	Decreased libido; impotence; no orgasm (men and women); retarded ejaculation	Progesterone	Decreased libido; impotence
Methandrostenolone (Dianabol)	Decreased libido	Propantheline bromide (Pro-Banthine and others)	Impotence
Mathantheline bromide (Banthine)	Impotence	Propranolol (Inderal and others)	Loss of libido; impotence
Methazolamide (Neptazane)	Decreased libido (men and women); impotence; delayed or no ejaculation (men) or orgasm (women)	Protriptyline (Vivactil)	Loss of libido; impotence; painful ejaculation

TABLE 7-3
Drugs That May Affect Sexual Function—cont'd

Drug	Adverse Effect	Drug	Adverse Effect
Ranitidine (Zantac)	Loss of libido; impotence	Timolol (Blocadren, Timolide, Timoptic)	Decreased libido; impotence
Reserpine	Decreased libido; impotence; decreased or no ejaculation	Tranylcypromine (Parnate)	Impotence
Spironolactone (Aldactone and others)	Decreased libido; impotence	Trazodone (Desyrel)	Priapism; increased libido (women); retrograde ejaculation
Thiazide diuretics	Impotence	Trifluoperazine (Stelazine and others)	Decreased, painful, or no ejaculation; spontaneous ejaculations
Thioridazine (Mellaril and others)	Impotence; priapism; delayed, decreased, painful, retrograde, or no ejaculation	Verapamil (Calan and others)	Impotence
Thiothixene (Navane and others)	Spontaneous ejaculations; impotence; priapism		

response in their patients even when the patients demonstrate general marital satisfaction. Obviously, assembling a careful history by asking general and directed questions is appropriate when dealing with a patient in a gynecologic visit. The patient should be asked if she is sexually active, if intercourse is comfortable and enjoyable (if heterosexual), and if orgasm is experienced. If she answers no to any of these questions, more specific questioning should follow with the objective of outlining the extent of the problem and the basis for it.

Sexual response problems may be the result of a previous negative sexual experience or may be secondary to emotional or physical illness. The problem may also be related to difficulties in the current relationship or to alcohol or drug abuse. Although an occasional alcohol drink may decrease inhibitions and improve sexual response, in general, alcohol is a depressant and decreases the woman's ability to become sexually aroused and to become vaginally lubricated. Drugs with antihypertensive and anticholinergic activity, as well as those active at the alpha and beta receptor sites, may decrease arousal or inhibit sexual interest. Narcotics and sedatives may also depress sexual responsiveness.

Inhibited sexual desire is the most common sexual dysfunction. Because each individual has his or her own libidinal drive, it is not surprising that couples may have some incompatibility of needs. It is important, however, that these

needs and desires be discussed openly and that reasons for lack of sexual arousal that may involve experiences or problems inherent in the relationship be resolved. At times the problem may be merely a failure to set aside appropriate time for intimacy. The couple should be encouraged to give sexual activity a high priority within their relationship rather than leaving it last on the list after the 11 o'clock news. Couples should be encouraged to use arousal and seduction techniques that are appropriate for their relationship. Satisfactory foreplay of a mutually enjoyable nature should be encouraged.

Vaginismus is a condition that is secondary to involuntary spasm of vaginal introital and levator ani muscles. Because of this spasm penetration is either painful or impossible. Lamont has attempted to classify the degrees of vaginismus and, in a group of 80 patients, noted that 27 (34%) had first-degree vaginismus, defined as perineal and levator spasm relieved by reassurance during pelvic examination. Another 21 (26%) had second-degree vaginismus, defined as perineal spasm maintained throughout the pelvic examination. Another 18 (22.5%) demonstrated third-degree vaginismus, defined as levator spasm and elevation of the buttocks. A total of 10 (12.5%) had fourth-degree vaginismus, defined as levator and perineal spasm with withdrawal and retreat. Four of the 80 patients refused pelvic examination.

These patients frequently complain not only

of pain or fear of pain with coitus or pelvic examination, but also difficulty in inserting a tampon or vaginal medication. The condition may be primary, in which case the individual has never experienced successful coitus. This problem is generally based on either early sexual abuse or aversion to sexuality in general. This leads to a form of conversion hysteria or to a lack of appropriate learning about sex secondary to cultural or familial teaching that sex is evil, painful, or undesirable. When the underlying cause for the vaginismus is understood, the matter may be discussed frankly with the patient and her partner to effect a relearning process that is conducive to relieving the symptoms. The actual vaginal spasm then may be relieved by teaching the patient self-dilation techniques, using fingers or dilators, in which she and her partner can participate. The period of therapy is usually short and the results good.

Orgasmic dysfunction is quite common. As many as 10% to 15% of women have never experienced an orgasm through any form of sexual stimulation, and another 25% to 35% will have difficulty reaching an orgasm on any particular occasion. Many women may be orgasmic secondary to masturbation or oral sex but may not be orgasmic with penile intercourse. It is important to discern by history the extent of the patient's problem and to place it into proper perspective. If the patient is anorgasmic during intercourse but has experienced orgasms, communication with her partner may aid in bringing about an orgasm during intercourse by allowing her or her partner to stimulate her clitoral area with the intensity and timing necessary to bring about an orgasm. If the woman is anorgasmic, she may be taught masturbatory techniques to demonstrate an orgasm to her, and then these techniques may be applied to the coital situation, thereby developing the desired response during coitus. Couples should be encouraged to communicate their sexual needs so that appropriate stimulation is offered during the arousal period and during intercourse. Developing this type of dialogue is often difficult but can be aided by counseling with a sensitive physician.

Dyspareunia is a sexual dysfunction that frequently has an organic basis. The physician should obtain a careful history of when the dyspareunia occurs (i.e., on insertion of the penis, at the mid-vagina during thrusting, or with deep penetration of the vault), since facts obtained by this history may point to organic causes, such as poor lubrication, urethritis, cystitis, trigonitis, poorly healed vaginal lacerations or episiotomy, and disease such as pelvic inflammatory disease or endometriosis. When no organic cause can be found for the dyspareunia, techniques similar to those used in evaluating and managing vaginismus are appropriate. Specific pathologic conditions should, of course, be treated. At times dyspareunia can be relieved by changing coital position. Couples should be encouraged to experiment with female-dominant and side-by-side positions to see if the pain can be prevented.

Tobacco, Alcohol, and Drug Use

The use of tobacco, alcohol, marijuana, cocaine, and other drugs is quite common in the United States, and the abuse of these substances is not unusual. The prevalence of their use among women is variable and often age-dependent. In 1970 one third of American women of childbearing age were cigarette smokers. However, only 20% to 25% of pregnant women were actually believed to smoke during their pregnancies.

Sokol found in a study of pregnant women in Cleveland that only 1.2% would state that they had an alcohol problem; however, on careful questioning about alcohol consumption, 11% were noted to be heavy drinkers.

In a detailed history of marijuana use, Nahas reviewed the work of several other authors and noted that in 1970 between 7% and 20% of college students were using marijuana. In addition, he pointed out that 15% of adolescents between the ages of 12 and 17 in one series were found to be using marijuana, with an incidence of 17% among boys and 14% among girls. Recent data imply that the percentages of users are higher. The prevalence of cocaine, heroin, and other drug use is variable from group to group, but overall these uses are quite common.

It is beyond the scope of this book to discuss the health hazards of these various agents, the problems of habituation, or the social and legal considerations. It is appropriate, however, to recognize that each of these agents adversely affects the reproductive process, causes a variety of illness, and influences the health and social relationships of the users.

The obstetrician and gynecologist is in an excellent position to discourage young women from beginning to use these substances by offering educational information at the time of visits for routine check-ups, for treatment of simple problems such as dysmenorrhea or vaginitis, or during consultations for contraception. The obstetrician and gynecologist may also influence women contemplating reproduction by pointing out the potential dangers of these substances to the fetus. As the primary physician for women, the obstetrician and gynecologist has the opportunity to periodically define activities that may be affecting the individual's health and offer education and counseling to modify these activities. Where appropriate, referrals to other health care specialists may be made.

To modify behavior in patients who abuse tobacco, alcohol, and other drugs, the physician must first identify their use. A history at the time of a routine check-up should include the following:

1. Smoking history. Does the patient smoke? For how long has she smoked? What substances are smoked and in what quantity? Moderate cigarette smokers (1 to 10 cigarettes per day) may be influenced to stop by simply discussing health hazards and suggesting that the practice be terminated. If the individual smokes fewer than 10 cigarettes a day, stopping without tapering off is appropriate and if motivated, the individual is usually successful. If the individual smokes more than 10 cigarettes a day, habituation may be a problem. Reducing the number of cigarettes to 10 per day and then stopping may be successful. If not, consultation with health care professionals who may use behavioral modification therapy is appropriate. Organized behavior modification programs to aid individuals to quit smoking are available in most communities. Fiore et al. have demonstrated, however, that 90% of successful quitters and 80% of unsuccessful quitters used individual methods similar to those described above. In their series, 47.5% of individuals who had tried to quit on their own in the previous 10 years were successful, whereas only 23.6% of those who used organized cessation methods were successful. These programs, however, were shown by the authors to aid a small group of smokers who were primarily heavy smokers.

2. Alcohol use. Cahalan et al. defined high-volume alcohol use as the consumption of 45 drinks a month or at least 5 drinks on some occasions (binge drinking). To describe a particular patient's drinking habits it is necessary to take a detailed history of how many drinks per day the patient takes and the type of substance consumed (whiskey, beer, or wine). One ounce of whiskey, a wineglass of wine, and 12 ounces of beer are interchangable. Binge drinking, which is defined as five drinks or more per day or periodic drinking to intoxication, should be noted as should its frequency. If a patient consumes more than 45 drinks per month or is a binge drinker, the physician should attempt to obtain behavior modification help for the patient. Generally, attendance at an Alcoholics Anonymous program with or without other specialized health care is indicated. If the patient does not consume large amounts of alcohol but does drink regularly, educational literature and counseling should be provided.

3. Marijuana use. Marijuana is an illegal substance and has many biological side effects. Its use should be discouraged among all patients. If marijuana is used daily, the patient's habituation must be recognized and behavior modification therapy offered.

4. Other drug use. Patients are frequently habituated to illegal drugs, such as cocaine and heroin, and often to prescription drugs as well (i.e., tranquilizers, barbiturates, and amphetamines). The physician should identify the quantity and type of drug used by history and should make the appropriate referral to a health care agency. Cocaine is a major problem in the United States at present. It is addicting and gives users a sense of power and strength that they find rewarding. Because of this and the fact that users can often function reasonably well under its influence, stopping its use can be very difficult. Cocaine use and possible addiction should be sought by the physician in all patients and treatment vigorously suggested when it is discovered. For instance, individuals habituated to cocaine are often treated in a fashion similar to alcoholics, using such help groups as Cocaine Anonymous.

Depression

Depression is a common symptom in a variety of conditions. Patients suffering loss or grief are often depressed. However, depression as a symptom is quite common in the general population. In a recent review, Ripley offered evidence from the world literature to indicate that as many as 10% of all individuals are depressed. Depression associated with psychoses such as is seen in manic-depressive (bipolar) psychosis may occur as often as 3 to 4 per 1000 people. Dorpat and Ripley noted that 9.3% of patients suffering from personality disorders, 26.9% of patients suffering from alcoholism, and 12.0% of schizophrenics had depression as a major symptom. Unfortunately, patients who suffer from depression are more prone to suicide, and psychiatric patients who commit suicide are more likely to have a depressive component to their illness.

Depression in infants and young children is frequently the result of deprivation, particularly maternal deprivation. It is frequently characterized by crying and behavior disorders and later by despair and withdrawal. The child may fail to eat and may eventually starve to death. If the child does not die, strong depressive symptomatology may continue into adulthood. Ripley cites the work of several authors who have shown a significantly higher rate of bereavement or broken homes in childhood among adult depressive patients.

It is useful for a gynecologist to understand the way in which depression may present in patients. Early symptoms include chronic fatigue, anxiety and irritability, anhedonia (loss of feelings of joy and pleasure), decreased interest in usual pursuits including sexual activity and personal appearance, and mental changes, including poor concentration and lack of decisiveness. The individual may complain of loss of recent memory; insomnia, especially occurring shortly after falling asleep; a pessimistic outlook about the future, often associated with feelings of guilt; and a number of physical complaints including loss of appetite or a great increase in appetite; change in bowel habits, including constipation or diarrhea; headache; various aches and pains; and general lability.

Late in the disease the patient may experience deep feelings of hopelessness with difficulty in presenting ideas. The patient may also complain of generalized weakness, fear of impending doom from a serious illness or fear that serious problems will befall a close family member, suicidal thoughts, and occasionally, delusions.

The physician should be alert to patients who have suffered personal loss or grief but who are still deeply depressed after 6 to 18 months of grieving. Although depression is normal in a grief situation, it should not last for a prolonged period.

The diagnosis is often suspected by simply assessing the patient's appearance and asking the usual questions concerning the patient's mood and health. Several psychological tests have been developed to assess depression and can be used in subtle cases. The physician should assess the degree to which the patient is depressed and whether the reason for the depression is appropriate. If the patient is grieving because of a real life situation, the physician should demonstrate concern and offer appropriate assurance that the problem will be relieved with time.

If the degree of depression is inappropriate for the life situation, the physician should determine whether the individual has suicidal thoughts and assess whether these thoughts are likely to be put into practice. Such questions as, "Have you considered harming yourself or taking your own life?" are appropriate in this situation. If the patient states that she has had such thoughts, the degree to which she is contemplating them may be assessed by asking if she has considered how she would carry out the suicide or what circumstances deterred her from attempting this act. If the patient seems to be seriously considering suicide, prompt referral to a mental health worker or facility should be made.

Patients who are depressed but give no evidence for psychoses may be helped by medication. Currently the tricyclic drugs are the most useful in usual clinical practice. Table 7-4 lists a group of these drugs by generic and trade names. Most of the tricyclic drugs have a parasympathomimetic effect. Therefore dryness of the mouth, blurred vision, hesitancy of urination or dribbling, some menstrual disorders (i.e., amenorrhea or irregularities), and a decrease in sexual arousal are complaints often associated with their use. Each of the tricyclics acts slightly differently, and undesirable side effects in a specific patient may be alleviated by switching to a different medication. Although patients may note reduction of symptoms of depression after 1 to 2 weeks of drug use, real improvement may take as long as 1

TABLE 7-4
Tricyclic Antidepressants

Generic Name	Trade Names
Amitriptyline	Amitril, Elavil, Amitid, Amitriptyline, Endep, SK-Amitriptyline
Amoxapine	Asendin
Desipramine	Norpramin, Pertofrane
Doxepin	Sinequan, Adapin
Imipramine	Tofranil, Antipress, Imavate, Imipramine, Janimine, SK-pramine, Presamine
Nortriptyline	Pamelor
Protriptyline	Vivactil
Trimipramine	Surmontil

month. Dosage of these medications will need to be varied depending on the patient's response.

Lithium salts have been used to treat depression and are most useful in the treatment of manic-depressive psychosis. Monamine oxidase inhibitors are also in common clinical use but frequently have serious side effects and should be administered only by individuals well experienced in their use.

Many patients will have complete relief of symptoms in 1 to 3 months of tricyclic therapy. However, some patients will require counseling as an adjunct to the therapy to work out serious emotional and social problems. Frequently drug therapy is necessary to bring the patient's depression under control to an extent that allows psychotherapy to be useful. Many patients can use tricyclic drugs intermittently when symptomatology warrants.

Loss and Grief

Loss is a common human experience and may affect women of all ages. The loss of a child, a spouse, or a close relative should and probably will precipitate an acute grief reaction. However, the physician must remember that a similar reaction will be precipitated by a spontaneous abortion, by the loss of a body part or organ, or by the realization that infertility and childlessness face the couple. It may also be part of a syndrome in women undergoing separation or divorce.

Lindemann points out that acute grief is a definite syndrome with both psychological and somatic components. In his vast experience with grieving patients he has observed that the syndrome may appear immediately after the loss or be delayed. If it is delayed, grief may appear to be absent only to occur at a future time, often in a more exaggerated fashion. At times the syndrome may occur in a distorted fashion. For successful resolution of grief, the individual must be helped to transform these distorted reactions into normal grief.

Lindemann points out that the symptomatology of normal grief is quite uniform. The individual often complains of tightness in the throat and chest, a choking sensation, a feeling of shortness of breath, and frequent sighing. There is often reported an empty feeling in the abdomen, muscle weakness, and a feeling of tension and mental pain. These symptoms frequently come in waves lasting from minutes to an hour and are often dreaded by the sufferer.

Lindemann further points out that the bereaved experience disorders of the sensorium often involving a sense of unreality, a tendency to place emotional distance between themselves and other people, and a preoccupation with imagery of the deceased. At times the bereaved will assume the mannerisms of the deceased or even attempt to perform the work of the lost loved one. If the mother has died, the bereaved daughter may see the mother's face when she looks at herself in the mirror and may assume the mother's mannerisms in her speech and gestures. There is often the perception that the deceased is nearby and can communicate.

In the immediate grief period the bereaved often feels guilt. This may directly involve the events of the death or of tasks left unfinished before the individual died. The bereaved often feels a lack of warmth and may demonstrate feelings of hostility toward others.

The burden of the grief is often so great that the individual can barely handle the maintenance activities of living, and has little energy left over for social contact or growth and development.

Most authorities feel that a normal grief reaction takes 6 to 18 months and ends when the individual has appropriately experienced the pain and suffering, placed the memory of the deceased in a proper place within the bereaved's life, and established new relationships and new life directions.

Lindemann notes, however, that abnormal grief reactions are possible and divides these into several categories. The first is the delay of reaction, which essentially is a postponement of grieving. This may be seen in an individual who is injured in an accident that kills the person to be grieved. The individual may be preoccupied with personal survival and recuperation and may not have the opportunity to grieve until this has passed. In other instances the individual may delay grieving for a long period, often years. There are often psychological reasons why this occurs, but when the grieving is finally precipitated, it may appear quite pathological and out of context for current life situations.

A second variant is a distorted reaction. In this situation the bereaved may take on the characteristics of the deceased without evidencing a sense of loss. The bereaved may actually take on the symptoms of the lost person if that individual had experienced a prolonged illness before death.

A third abnormal reaction to grieving may be the development of a psychosomatic condition. Ulcerative colitis, rheumatoid arthritis, and asthma have all been noted to occur in approximation to bereavement. Lindemann points out that some patients suffering from these problems may improve when the grief reaction is resolved.

Other types of abnormal grief reactions include pathological alterations in relationships with friends and relatives, inappropriate hostility toward others, behavior patterns resembling psychoses, continuing inability to make decisions or to take initiative, and performance of activities that have destructive social and economic outcomes. Finally, Lindemann notes that in the reaction of agitated depression the bereaved develops tension, agitation, insomnia, feelings of worthlessness, and fantasies of a need for punishment. In such situations suicide may be a danger. Fortunately, agitated depression is quite unusual. Lindemann feels that it may be more common in individuals who have experienced a previous depression or in those who have been intensely involved with the deceased, such as mothers who have lost young children.

Loss of a Child by Abortion, Stillbirth, or Neonatal or Infant Death

Obstetricians and gynecologists may need to counsel patients experiencing grief related to several areas of reproduction. Leppert and Pahlka counseled 22 women who had experienced spontaneous abortion. The study format was to hold a counseling session immediately after abortion and again in 4 to 6 weeks. These authors report that all women demonstrated the classic stages of grief, but that guilt was the stage that appeared the most difficult for them and their spouses to resolve. The authors thought that the unexpressed emotions relating to pregnancy loss might affect the relationship of the couple unless they are explored and defused. They suggested that the obstetrician and gynecologist make it a point to add such counseling to his or her practice routines. Bruhn and Bruhn point out that a predictable pattern of grief follows every stillbirth and perinatal death and urge physicians to work with their patients in resolving these feelings.

In addition to the physician's offering understanding and counseling, there are many self-help groups that offer aid to parents who have lost children either in the perinatal period or in infancy. The physician should become aware of the agencies or groups within the community that offer group and self-help therapy in neonatal and infant loss. It is reasonable for the physician to learn the techniques used by these groups and to assess whether their approach fits the needs of the patient before making referrals.

The physician should also be aware of the fact that each member of the couple may grieve differently and, indeed, the style of grieving that one may exhibit may be in conflict with that of the other. Pointing out these differences and helping the couple to express their true feelings to each other may be very beneficial during this process.

An important issue in understanding the management of grief in couples who have lost infants was demonstrated in an evaluation of a group of patients by Estok and Lehman. They found that such individuals wished health care providers to acknowledge the couple's feelings of shock, guilt, and grief and to recognize the importance of their memories of the birth and of the baby. In essence, they wished the health care providers to help them sharpen the reality of the death of the child and provide support through the postloss period rather than focus on other life events, such as the next pregnancy.

Certain aspects of bereavement should be

understood by the physician in dealing with patients who are suffering grief. The loss of a child is always a serious problem. Even the loss of an adult child can have long-term sequelae. Shanfield and Swain noted that parents who have lost adult children in traffic accidents continued to grieve intensely for a prolonged period and had a higher than expected level of psychiatric symptoms and health complaints. Families that were unstable and in which problems had existed with these children suffered more guilt and more psychiatric symptoms. In addition, factors that intensified the bereavement experience were a mother losing a daughter, parents losing children who lived at home, the loss of children born early in the birth order, and the loss of multiple children in a single-car, single-driver accident. A protecting factor seemed to be a prior bereavement experience.

These observations were supported by Lundin, who used the Texas Inventory of Grief to study first-degree relatives 8 years after bereavement. He noted that relatives of persons who had died suddenly or unexpectedly suffered a more pronounced grief reaction than those who had lost someone in a death that was expected. He also noted that bereavement was greater in parents after the loss of a child than in widows or widowers who lost a spouse.

Unplanned Pregnancy

A special counseling challenge involves the care of a woman with an unplanned pregnancy. Such individuals often suffer conflicting feelings, which may include shame and guilt for their predicament, a genuine desire to have a child, fear of social consequences, and fear for their own future and physical well-being. In addition, they may suffer from guilt about the destruction of the pregnancy if abortion is considered. Although many such women have good support groups (e.g., family, significant other, friends, and religious counselors), others will rely on the physician entirely for advice and direction. The physician should discuss all possible options with the patient, including having and raising the child, offering it for adoption, or terminating the pregnancy. Issues involving the role of the baby's father, the effect of any decision on the future life of the patient, and the risks of the procedure should be considered. The patient should be aided in reaching the most appropriate decision for her needs and then should be supported in carrying out her plan. Where necessary, appropriate referrals to social agencies (e.g., adoption, abortion counseling, or welfare services) should be made.

Infertility

The inability to reproduce leads to a major life frustration and often generates a series of symptoms similar to the grief reaction. Many sequelae may occur that stress the couple's relationship. Guilt, anger, and shame may be components, depending on the social forces at play in the relationship. Sexual dysfunction may result because of the stresses imposed by the requirements of a treatment regimen or because of general dysfunction within the relationship brought about by the infertility. At times the problems associated with the infertility (e.g., endometrial implants in the cul-de-sac) may cause dyspareunia and lead to sexual dysfunction. External stresses from family and friends who continuously refer to the couple's childlessness may contribute to the tension as well.

The physician must be complete in the medical evaluation of the couple, as well as supportive of their emotional needs. The physician should discuss fully all treatment options and the chances for success. He or she should also continuously help the couple to accentuate the positives of their relationship and to consider referring them to self-help groups for infertile couples or to health care counselors who can help with the maintenance of their relationship and self-images.

Death of a Spouse

Holmes and Rahe rate the death of a spouse as one of the major life stresses among survivors independent of age and cultural background, and state that it may contribute to a decline in physical and mental well-being of the survivor. Gallagher et al. recently reported the effects of acute bereavement on the indicators of mental health in widows and widowers beyond the age of 55. These workers evaluated a group from the standpoint of past grief, present grief, depression, somatic symptomatology, and self-rating of mental health status. They noted that these individuals in the early stages of their bereavement were suffering from considerable psychological distress compared with individuals of similar age who were not bereaved. They demonstrated that the degree of effect of bereavement on the patient's mental health did not vary by sex. Those conditions that were more likely to occur in one sex rather than the other occurred with incidence equal to those individuals of the same sex in the study group. Thus findings in women, who tend to have a higher incidence of depression in the general population than do men, demonstrated this to be the case in the same proportions among the study group.

CROSS-CULTURAL DIFFERENCES. Eisenbruch has pointed out that there are significant cross-cultural differences in bereavement, whereas there are great similarities in the grief reaction between different ethnic and cultural groups. Individuals from different backgrounds tend to experience difficulty with their grief when they attempt to respond in a fashion specific for the majority within the culture in which they now reside. Specific rituals, attitudes toward widowhood, mores with respect to length and type of grieving, the way in which the deceased is remembered, and the appropriate length of time for grieving and mourning may be quite different in various minority groups when compared with the general white majority of the United States. Physicians dealing with minority groups are urged to consider the points raised by Eisenbruch in his review to be better able to help the minority patients through their grieving period.

Separation and Divorce

Currently the number of divorces occurring annually in the United States is about 40% of the number of marriages. There are many reasons for this increase, including the emerging of women to a level of self-support, changing attitudes toward a desire to remain married, and an increased public awareness of family dysfunction, such as spouse and child abuse. Often one or both members of a divorcing couple will demonstrate evidence of grief, as well as anger, shame, and guilt. Counseling can be very useful in restoration of self-esteem and in helping the individual to emerge from the experience with the ability to survive in new relationships. Although physicians should recognize these needs in their patients who are go-

ing through separation and divorce, their primary role should be to make appropriate referrals to counselors who have the time and the skills to deal with the patient in this area.

Loss of an Organ or Body Part

Loss of a body part can be expected to bring about a grief reaction with accompanying symptoms of an emotional and somatic nature. Depression is frequently a strong component. Workers who have investigated the loss of limbs have noted this, and it is reasonable to expect that the loss of such organs as the breast or the uterus would evoke a similar reaction.

Several workers have reported depression among posthysterectomy patients with an incidence ranging from 4% to as high as 70%. In a recent review, Drummond and Field point out that the stages of the process of incorporating the loss of a uterus into the individual's self-image is similar to that of the loss of other body parts. They refer to the four stages of incorporation listed by Roberts: impact, retreat, acknowledgment, and reconstruction.

The impact stage occurs when the individual becomes aware that she has a problem with her uterus. If she is symptomatic this may be obvious. If she has been told she must lose her uterus because it is diseased, such as with cancer, she will need to make a mental adjustment to this fact. Steiner and Aleksandrowicz have pointed out that when the disease that requires operation is life-threatening or serious, the likelihood of depression is minimized. Richards has pointed out that when disease of the uterus is absent, depression is more likely to occur.

The second stage of organ loss is retreat. This is the period in which the patient accepts the need for the loss of an organ and depersonalizes it in her thinking. If denial occurs at this period, the depression that she notes later may be quite severe. The desire for a second opinion often occurs in this phase. It is a healthy response and should be encouraged.

The third stage is acknowledgment. The physician will recognize this stage because it involves the woman's repeated discussion of the procedure, the need for the procedure, and the meaning of the loss of the uterus postoperatively. It is the woman's attempt to place the procedure and the need for the procedure within the appropriate context of her life and her self-image.

The final phase is reconstruction. This involves the redefinition of her self-image without the organ. It will require acceptance by her spouse or significant other and by other members of her community of importance in this event. The physician should attempt to discuss the need for and the likely sequelae of the hysterectomy before it is performed. This discussion should include the significant other in the woman's life so that any fantasies or fears that may arise can be discussed at this point. Some men have difficulty continuing an active sexual experience with a woman who has lost her uterus. These points should be discussed ahead of time so that each realizes the implication of the operation. On the other hand, some women feel that sex is for procreation only and after the removal of the uterus may respond quite differently from what the significant other has known in the past. These points, too, should be discussed before the fact.

If the individual cannot work through the four stages of loss of an organ, disruption of relationships and depression may be sequelae. Newton and Baron have noted that between 20% and 40% of couples stop having sexual intercourse after hysterectomy. They do not state whether this is a direct effect of the hysterectomy and the inability to work out feelings related to this procedure or whether other problems may have been in existence, allowing for the hysterectomy to be an excuse to stop experiencing intercourse. Physicians should consider these points, however, and discuss them with the patient and her significant other before embarking on an operative procedure, particularly if it is elective and the time is available for discussion.

Loss of a Pet

A final bereavement situation often overlooked by physicians but frequently important to patients is the grief associated with the death of a pet. Quackenbush reviewed the subject and concluded that animals play an important role in the human social system and may contribute greatly to the quality of life of many pet owners. In some cases where the individual lives alone and may be elderly, the animal may be the only living thing in close daily contact with the individual. It is, therefore, not unusual that when the pet dies, the owner suffers grief. Quackenbush states that understanding and sensitivity to the feelings and sense of loss that the pet owner experiences will help to facilitate the resolution of the grief.

Counseling the Dying

Elizabeth Kubler-Ross revolutionized our understanding of the death process with her classic book on the subject in 1969. An important paragraph taken from the first chapter describing the fear of death is quite revealing:

When we look back in time and study old cultures and people, we are impressed that death has always been distasteful to man and will probably always be. From the psychiatrist's point of view this is very understandable and can perhaps best be explained by our basic knowledge that, in our unconscious, death is never possible in regard to ourselves. It is inconceivable for our unconscious to imagine an actual ending of our own life here on earth and if the life of ours has to end the ending is always attributed to a malicious intervention from the outside by someone else. In simple terms, in our unconscious mind we can only be killed; it is inconceivable to die of a natural cause or of old age. Therefore, death in itself is associated with a bad act, a frightening happening, something that in itself calls for retribution and punishment.*

Kubler-Ross describes five stages through which an individual progresses in the acceptance of the inevitability of death. They are denial, anger, bargaining, depression, and acceptance. *Denial* and isolation is a temporary state brought about by the shock of learning that the individual suffers from a problem from which he or she cannot recover. The transition from denial to partial acceptance will depend on the nature of the patient's illness, how long he or she has left before death will occur, and the way in which he or she has prepared throughout life to cope with such serious situations. Kubler-Ross notes that when confronted with multiple health care providers who are likely to express the inevitable in a variety of ways, the dying person often chooses to accept the individual style of presentation that most fits her need. During this period of adjustment, therefore, a number of different opinions may be sought and specific interpretations questioned. Inevitably the individual may be depressed and may isolate herself from those with whom she would normally associate. Frequently the indi-

---

*From Kubler-Ross, E: On death and dying, New York, 1969, Macmillan Co.

vidual may appear confused and in some cases may deny that any information about the impending death has ever been given. Most patients, according to Kubler-Ross, will go through this period long before death occurs. However, in 3 of 200 patients that she studied, acceptance of the inevitable did not occur until the very time of death.

Hospital personnel must guard against avoiding patients after having given the initial information. They must not interpret the period of the patient's denial as a distasteful circumstance with which they cannot cope. Instead they should help the patient work through this period by patiently repeating information, answering questions, and offering comfort. Terms that remove all hope, such as *terminal* or *hopeless*, should be avoided.

The second stage described by Kubler-Ross is *anger*. Staff and family members find this the most difficult one with which to cope, since the anger felt by the patient may be inappropriately displaced to everyone and everything in the environment. The physician or nurse caring for the patient falls into the unenviable position of the messenger who is hated because of the bad news he or she has brought. The health care worker who tries to make the patient comfortable may be accused of being overly solicitous, whereas the health care worker who attempts to give the patient the privacy that it is believed she seeks may be accused of being uncaring. Likewise, family members who attempt to be cheerful in visiting the patient may be accused of being glib and uncaring, whereas if they are more somber, they may be accused of being depressing. In such cases the health care worker or family member will probably experience guilt and possibly shame, and may adjust to the problem by avoiding the dying person altogether.

During the anger period the dying individual will be irritated by all stimuli. Happiness depicted on television may upset her because she feels that she is not included in it. Discussion of future plans of friends or family members will be equally depressing because the dying individual realizes that she will not be around to participate. The anger period ends when the individual can reconcile the fact that she is different from every healthy person but is still capable of being loved and accepted.

The third stage is *bargaining*. This is an attempt to postpone the inevitable by offering concessions, presumably to God. It is essentially the hope of getting more time for good behavior. In this period the individual may do charitable acts, correct past misdeeds, or reconcile damaged relationships. It is a time for relieving guilt and defusing the feeling of required punishment. It may, in many ways, be an opportunity to "put one's house in order."

The fourth stage described by Kubler-Ross is *depression*. Although symptoms of depression may occur in the earlier stages, depression at this stage may occur because the patient has had to cope with a number of factors associated with the illness. For instance, she may be concerned about the expenses of her care, loss of wages, and the simple fact that she feels poorly, added to the fact that she now realizes she is going to die. In addition, fears that her death will adversely affect other members of her family who depend on her may also add to her depression. Health care workers should be comfortable in allowing the patient to know that they understand the reasons for the depression. They should do everything possible to eliminate the feelings of guilt that the patient may have because of the conditions in which she finds herself. She should be made to realize that the financial burdens that may be developing or the effect that her death may have on family members and their lives are not a result of specific actions that she may have taken. In other words, she is not responsible for the condition she is in and the resulting circumstances are not legitimate reasons for her to feel guilt. Family members can be helpful by accentuating the positive aspects of the patient's life, the love they feel for her, and the happiness they have experienced with her. They should downplay the burdens that the patient's illness and death will create for them. Essentially the patient is working through a period of grief, in this case, grief for herself.

The fifth and final stage is *acceptance*. At this point the individual has worked through the anger that she has felt for her misfortune and for those healthy individuals who do not have to die at this time and has also passed the period of depression and into a period of accepting her fate. This step will most often be achieved if there is a long enough period for the individual to work through the previous stages. Unfortunately, many die before all of these stages have been reconciled. In a very ill patient acceptance is frequently a giving in to the symptoms she has had to bear and a looking forward to peace from these symptoms that the death will bring. However, Kubler-Ross points out that the acceptance stage is not necessarily this alone, because patients who are not physically suffering also will go through this stage. This is often a time when the individual takes comfort in having quality visits with family members in which positive experiences are remembered. She may also obtain comfort from interacting with representatives of her religious faith.

A new innovation in the care of the terminally ill and their families was introduced with the hospice concept during the 1970s. There are currently more than 800 hospice organizations in the United States, offering psychosocial support to both patients and families. The service includes postdeath follow-up with the families to help them through the grieving period. Hospice organizations include free-standing institutions that offer inpatient services; community-based home programs that include both professional and volunteer services; hospital-based hospice teams, which may include physicians, nurses, social workers, chaplains, and volunteers who are in a position to minister to any patient in any bed; and hospital-based hospice units that are geographically separate from other patients and often are coordinated with a home care program.

Godkin et al. studied 58 bereaved spouses and their families whose loved ones had recently died of late-stage cancer after care in a hospital-based hospice service. These families in general rated hospice care significantly better than that received in prior experiences, stating that the hospice services contributed to an improved family function, greater individual well-being, and the ability of family members to cope with the situation. Over three quarters of the families reported that they were emotionally prepared and prepared in a practical sense for the death of the victim. Health problems were reported by these family members in about the same proportion as was experienced in other bereaved groups, but when these problems occurred they were dealt with within the framework of the program.

Physicians who care for chronically ill and terminal patients, particularly those suffering from cancer, should consider availing themselves of the services of such organizations within their geographic area.

KEY POINTS

- The risk of developing a psychiatric disorder seems greatest if the child loses a parent before age 5 or in adolescence.

- The risk of developing a psychiatric disorder is greatest if the child loses a parent of the same sex.

- The highest rate of delinquency seems to occur in males who have lost their fathers unless father substitution occurs.

- Separation from parents in childhood is more likely to cause psychiatric illness when the separation is necessitated by parental illness or marital discord than when it is necessitated by the child's illness or because of wartime evacuation.

- The ideal of thinness for the American woman has increased at the same time that her actual weight has increased.

- More than half of the women between ages 24 and 54 are dieting even though they are not overweight; 75% state they do it for cosmetic reasons.

- Anorexia nervosa occurs in 1% of middle-class adolescent girls.

- Anorexia nervosa occurs in 5% to 20% of ballet dancers.

- When anorexia nervosa occurs in men, it is usually in those individuals training for competitive athletic events.

- Bulimia occurs in about 50% of anorectic patients.

- Vomiting after meals is 3 times as common in bulimics as it is in patients with anorexia nervosa without bulimia.

- Anorexia nervosa and bulimia occur 6 times more frequently in first-degree relatives than in the general population.

- Two thirds of patients with the eating disorders of anorexia nervosa and bulimia have been sexually molested in childhood.

- Good to fair outcomes were observed in 88% of anorexia nervosa patients treated as inpatients, 77% of those treated as outpatients, and 59% of those not treated at all.

- Medications have not been useful in treating anorexia nervosa; counseling and behavior modification programs seem to be more effective.

- Long-term follow-ups of patients with anorexia nervosa calculate the hazard of death as 0.5% per year and of relapse as 3% per year. Treatment reduces these.

- Patients between the ages of 25 and 34 who suffer from severe obesity have a mortality 12 times greater than the general population in that age group.

- Of patients with severe obesity who are treated with nonsurgical management, 15% suffer severe depression and 26% suffer moderate depression.

- Behavior modification without medication is the most successful therapy for moderate obesity.

- Diet modification in the treatment of obesity involves lowering fat content to 20%.

- Obesity in adolescence responds best when parents and children are given behavior modification therapy in separate counseling groups.

- Half of all married couples experience some sexual dysfunction or dissatisfaction.

- The sexual response cycle includes excitement, plateau, orgasm, and resolution.

- Sexual arousal is under the control of the parasympathetic portion of the autonomic nervous system.

- Orgasm is under the control of the sympathetic portion of the autonomic nervous system.

- A total of 15% of healthy women have never experienced orgasm.

- A total of 35% of healthy women in a large survey expressed disinterest in sex.

- Inhibited sexual desire is the most common sexual dysfunction.

- Heavy drinking of alcohol among pregnant women may be 10 times higher than that stated in patient histories. In one study, 11% were noted to be heavy drinkers of alcohol.

- Roughly 7% to 20% of college students use marijuana.

- Smoking more than 10 cigarettes per day is evidence for habituation.

- Most smokers who successfully quit do so without behavior modification programs, but such programs seem to benefit heavy smokers.

- High-volume alcohol use is defined as 45 alcoholic drinks per month or 5 drinks or more on specific occasions.

- A total of 10% of all individuals suffer depression.

- Manic depressive (bipolar) psychoses occur in a ratio of approximately 3 to 4 per 1000 people.

- Acute grief reaction lasts 6 to 18 months.

- Currently the number of divorces occurring annually in the United States is about 40% of the number of marriages.

- Posthysterectomy depression occurs in 4% to 70% of women, depending on the indication for the operation and the preparation offered.

- Roberts's four stages of incorporation as an individual response to organ or body part loss are *impact, retreat, acknowledgment,* and *reconstruction.*

- Kubler-Ross defines the stages of individual progress to acceptance of the inevitability of death as *denial, anger, bargaining, depression,* and *acceptance.*

- Hospice programs are support groups for both dying patients and their families.

BIBLIOGRAPHY

Agres WS and Kraemer HC: The treatment of anorexia nervosa: do different treatments have different outcomes? In Stunkard AJ and Stellar E, eds: Eating and its disorders, New York, 1984, Raven Press.

Anderson RE: Where's Dad? parental deprivation in delinquency, Arch Gen Psychiatry 18:641, 1968.

Andersen BL, Turnquist D, LaPolla J, and Turner D: Sexual functioning after treatment of in situ vulvar cancer: preliminary report, Obstet Gynecol 71:15, 1988.

Barker MG: Psychiatric illness after hysterectomy, Br Med J 2:91, 1968.

Barnes GE and Prosen H: Parental death and depression, J Abnorm Psychol 94:64, 1985.

Birtchnell J: Early parent death in relation to size and constitution of sibship, Acta Psychiatr Scand 47:250, 1971.

Birtchnell J: Early parent death in psychiatric diagnosis, Soc Psychiatry 7:202, 1972.

Brown GW, Harris T, and Copeland JR: Depression and loss, Br J Psychiatry 130:1, 1977.

Brownell KD: New developments in the treatment of obese children in adolescence. In Stunkard AJ and Stellar E, eds: Eating and its disorders, New York, 1984, Raven Press.

Brownell KD, Kelman JH, and Stunkard AJ: Treatment of obese children with and without their mothers: changes in weight and blood pressure, Pediatrics 71:515, 1983.

Bruhn DF and Bruhn P: Stillbirth: a humanistic response, J Reprod Med 29:107, 1984.

Casper RC, Eckert ED, Halmi KA, et al: Bulimia: its incidence and clinical importance in patients with anorexia nervosa, Br J Psychiatry 27:1030, 1980.

Craighead LW, Stunkard AJ, and O'Brien R: Behavior therapy and pharmacotherapy of obesity, Arch Gen Psychiatry 38:763, 1981.

DeGraaf R: New treatise concerning the generative organs of women. In Ladas AK, Whipple B, and Perry JD, eds: The G-spot and other recent discoveries about human sexuality, New York, 1983, Holt, Rinehart & Winston.

Dietrich DR: Psychological health of young adults who experienced early parent death: MMPI trends, J Clin Psychol 40:901, 1984.

Dorpat TL and Ripley HS: A study of suicide in the Seattle area, Compr Psychiatry 1:349, 1960.

Drummond J and Field PA: Emotional and sexual sequelae following hysterectomy, Health Care Women Int 5:261, 1984.

Earls F: The fathers (not the mothers): their importance and influence with infants and young children. In Chess S and Thomas A, eds: Annual progress in child psychiatry and child development 1977, vol 10, New York, 1977, Brunner/Mazel, Publishers.

Eisenbruch M: Cross cultural aspects of bereavement. II. Ethnic and cultural variations in the development of bereavement practices, Cult Med Psychiatry 8:315, 1984.

Estok P and Lehman A: Perinatal death: grief support for families, Birth 10:17, 1983.

Ferguson JM: Learning to eat: leader's manual and patient manual, Palo Alto, Calif, 1975, Bull Publishing Co.

Fiore MC, Novotny TE, Pierce JP, et al: Methods used to quit smoking in the United States, JAMA 263:2760, 1990.

Frank E, Anderson C, and Rubinstein D: Frequency of sexual dysfunction in "normal" couples, N Engl J Med 299:111, 1978.

Gallagher DE, Breckenridge JN, Thompson LW, and Peterson JA: Effects of bereavement on indicators of mental health in elderly widows and widowers, J Gerontol 38:565, 1983.

Garrow JS: Treat obesity seriously: a clinical manual, New York, 1982, Churchill Livingstone, Inc.

Godkin MA, Krant MJ, and Doster NJ: The impact of hospice care on families, Int J Psychiatry Med 13:153, 1983-84.

Grafenberg E: The role of the urethra in female orgasm, Int J Sexol 3:145, 1950.

Green BL: A clinical approach to marital problems, Springfield, Ill, 1970, Charles C Thomas, Publishers.

Gregory I: Anterospective data following childhood loss of a parent. I. Pathology, performance, and potential among college students, Arch Gen Psychiatry 13:110, 1965.

Halmi KA, Stunkard AJ, and Mason EE: Emotional responses to weight reduction by three methods: diet, jejunoileal bypass and gastric bypass, Am J Clin Nutr 33:446, 1980.

Hamilton LH, Brooks-Gunn J, and Warren MP: Sociocultural influences on eating disorders in professional female ballet dancers, Int J Eating Disorders 4:465, 1985.

Hammond DC: Screening for sexual dysfunction, Clin Obstet Gynecol 27:732, 1984.

Holmes TH and Rahe RH: The social adjustment rating scale, J Psychosom Res 11:213, 1967.

Hsu LKG, Crisp AH, and Harding B: Outcome of anorexia nervosa, Lancet 1:61, 1979.

Isager T, Brinch M, Kreiner S, and Tolstrup K: Death and relapse in anorexia nervosa: survival analysis of 151 cases, J Psychiatr Res 19:515, 1985.

Johnson CL, Lewis C, Love S, et al: Incidence and correlates of bulimic behavior in a female high school population, J Youth Adolescence 13:6, 1984.

Johnson WG and Schlundt DG: Eating disorders: assessment and treatment, Clin Obstet Gynecol 28:598, 1985.

Kalucy RC, Crisp AH, Lacy JH, and Harding B: Prevalence and prognosis of anorexia nervosa, Aust NZ J Psychiatry 11:251, 1977.

Kaplan HS: The new sex therapy, New York, 1974, Brunner/Mazel, Inc.

Kendell RE, Hall DJ, Harley A, and Babigan HM: The epidemiology of anorexia nervosa, Psychol Med 2:200, 1973.

Kline NS: From sad to glad, New York, 1974, GP Putnam's Sons.

Kreipe RE, Strauss J, Hodgman CH, and Ryan RM: Menstrual cycle abnormalities and subclinical eating disorders: preliminary report, Psychosom Med 51:81, 1989.

Kubler-Ross E: On death and dying, New York, 1969, Macmillan Publishing Co.

Laajus S: Parental losses, Acta Psychiatr Scand 69:1, 1984.

LaFerla JJ: Inhibited sexual desire and orgasmic dysfunction in women, Clin Obstet Gynecol 27:738, 1984.

Lamont J: Vaginismus, Am J Obstet Gynecol 131:632, 1978.

Leppert PC and Pahlka BS: Grieving characteristics after spontaneous abortion: a management approach, Obstet Gynecol 64:119, 1984.

Lindemann E: Symptomatology and management of acute grief, Am J Psychiatry 101:141, 1944.

Lundin T: Long-term outcome of bereavement, Br J Psychiatry 145:424, 1984.

Masters WH and Johnson VE: Human sexual response, Boston, 1966, Little, Brown & Co.

Masters WH and Johnson VE: Human sexual inadequacy. Boston, 1970, Little, Brown & Co.

Melody GF: Depressive reactions following hysterectomy, Am J Obstet Gynecol 83:410, 1962.

Munro A and Griffiths AB: Some psychiatric nonsequelae of childhood bereavement, Br J Psychiatry 115:305, 1969.

Nahas GG: Marijuana: deceptive weed, New York, 1973, Raven Press.

Newton N and Baron E: Reactions to hysterectomy—fact or fiction, Prim Care 3:781, 1976.

Oppenheimer R, Howells K, Palmer RL, and Chaloner DA: Adverse sexual experience in childhood and clinical eating disorders: a preliminary description, J Psychiatr Res 19:357, 1985.

Parker C and Hadzi-Pavlovic D: Modification of level of depression in mother-bereaved women by parental and marital relationships, Psychol Med 14:125, 1984.

Pirke KM, Schweiger U, Strowitzki T, et al: Dieting causes menstrual irregularities in normal weight young women through impairment of episodic luteinizing hormone secretion, Fertil Steril 51:263, 1989.

Quackenbush J: The death of a pet: how it can affect owners, Vet Clin North Am [Small Anim Pract] 15:395, 1985.

Richards DH: Depression after hysterectomy, Lancet 2:430, 1973.

Richards DH: A posthysterectomy syndrome, Lancet 2:983, 1974.

Ripley HS: Depression and the life span—epidemiology. In Usdin G, ed: Depression: clinical, biological and psychological perspectives, 1977, New York, Brunner/Mazel, Inc.

Roberts SL: Behavioral concepts in the critically ill patient, Englewood Cliffs, NJ, 1976, Prentice-Hall.

Rutter M: Parent child separation: psychological effects on the child, J Child Psychol Psychiatry 12:233, 1971.

Sager CJ: Sexual dysfunction in marital discord. In Kaplan HS, ed: The new sex therapy. New York, 1974, Brunner/Mazel, Inc.

Semmens JP, and Semmens EC: Sexual function in the menopause, Clin Obstet Gynecol 27:717, 1984.

Semmens JP and Wagner G: Estrogen deprivation and vaginal function in menopausal women (a study of menopausal vaginal physiology and the effect of exogenous estrogen therapy, JAMA 248:445, 1982.

Shanfield SB and Swain BJ: Death of adult children in traffic accidents, J Nerv Ment Dis 172:533, 1984.

Smith NJ: Excessive weight loss and food aversion in athletes simulating anorexia nervosa, Pediatrics 66:139, 1980.

Sokol RJ: Alcohol in pregnancy: clinical research problems, Neurobehav Toxicol Teratol 2:157, 1980.

Steege JF: Dyspareunia in vaginismus, Clin Obstet Gynecol 27:750, 1984.

Steiner M and Aleksandrowicz DR: Psychiatric sequelae to gynecological operations, Israel Ann Psychiatr Related Disciplines 8:186, 1970.

Streissguth AP, Darby BL, and Barr HM, et al: Comparison of drinking and smoking patterns during pregnancy over a 6-year interval, Am J Obstet Gynecol 145:716, 1983.

Strober M, Morrell W, Burroughs J, et al: A controlled family study of anorexia nervosa, J Psychiatr Res 19:239, 1985.

Stunkard AJ: Current status of treatment for obesity in adults. In Stunkard AJ and Stellar E, eds: Eating and its disorders. New York, 1984, Raven Press.

Tennant C, Smith A, Bebbington P, and Hurry J: Parental loss in childhood: relationship to adult psychiatric impairment and contact with psychiatric services, Arch Gen Psychiatry 38:309, 1981.

Tennant C, Bebbington P, and Hurry J: Social experience in childhood and adult psychiatric morbidity: a multiple regression analysis, Psychol Med 12:321, 1982.

Theander S: Outcome and prognosis in anorexia nervosa and bulimia: some results of previous investigations compared with those of a Swedish longterm study, J Psychiatr Res 19:493, 1985.

Theander S: Anorexia nervosa, Acta Psychiatr Scand (Suppl) 214:1, 1970.

The health consequences of smoking, US Department of Health, Education and Welfare, Jan, 1973.

Thompson M: Cultural expectation of thinness of women. Psychol Rep 47:483, 1980.

Wadden TA, Stunkard AJ, and Brownell KD: Very low calorie diets: their efficacy, safety and future, Ann Intern Med 99:675, 1983.

Warren MP: Anorexia nervosa and the related eating disorders, Clin Obstet Gynecol 28:588, 1985.

Weiner L, Rosett HL, Edelin KC, et al: Alcohol consumption by pregnant women, Obstet Gynecol 61:6, 1983.

Weisberg M: Physiology of female sexual function, Clin Obstet Gynecol 27:697, 1984.

Diagnostic Procedures

_____ KEY TERMS AND DEFINITIONS _____

Adhesiolysis. The cutting or lysis of adhesions.

Computed Tomography (CT). An imaging technique to detect soft tissue abnormalities that uses a computer to integrate differences in x-ray beam attenuation resulting from varying densities in adjacent tissue.

Contact Hysteroscopy. Visualization of the endometrial cavity by directly touching the surface to be viewed.

Culdocentesis. The transvaginal aspiration of fluid from the cul-de-sac of Douglas.

Discriminatory HCG Zone. A blood level of human chorionic gonadotrophin (HCG) at which an intrauterine pregnancy may be visualized by ultrasound.

Endometrial Sampling. Obtaining either a tissue biopsy of the endometrial lining by abrasion or a sample of cells for cytologic screening by placing an instrument transcervically into the endometrial cavity.

Hysterosalpingography. An x-ray imaging technique whereby the uterine cavity and lumina of the fallopian tubes are visualized by injecting contrast material through the cervical canal.

Hysteroscopy. The direct visualization of the endometrial cavity using an endoscope, a light source, and a medium to distend the uterus.

Laparoscopy. Examination and inspection of the peritoneal cavity and pelvic organs by means of an endoscope and a light source.

Magnetic Resonance Imaging (MRI). Previously _nuclear magnetic resonance (NMR)_. Technique of soft tissue imagery using resonance of hydrogen nuclei in a static magnetic field exposed to low-frequency radiowaves.

Nondiagnostic Culdocentesis. A procedure wherein neither peritoneal fluid nor injected saline can be withdrawn from the cul-de-sac.

Tubal Ring. A circular, clear-appearing ultrasound finding within the area of the adnexa, representing an early ectopic pregnancy.

Ultrasound. A noninvasive imaging technique using acoustic waves; modern equipment includes linear array and sector scan.

This chapter will present an overview of eight frequently used diagnostic procedures in gynecology. Indications, contraindications, and complications are included for each procedure. For those unfamiliar with the procedures, the diagnostic and therapeutic uses are also detailed. The chapter spans a wide spectrum as it discusses one of the oldest and simplest diagnostic techniques in gynecology, _culdocentesis_, and also one of the newest, _magnetic resonance imaging_. During the past 3 decades there have been significant changes in the use of endos-

copy in gynecologic practice. The fiberoptic bundle and more versatile light sources, as well as the incorporation of laser technology, have dramatically increased the diagnostic and therapeutic capabilities of the hysteroscope and laparoscope. Colposcopy is discussed in Chapter 27.

There are two directly conflicting trends in present medical care. One is the increasing use of noninvasive diagnostic imaging. For example, the applications of magnetic resonance imaging appear limitless. The conflicting trend stems from society's emphasis on cost containment, which curtails the impetus for ordering imaging procedures. As we face the future, cost will be one of the foremost issues in the physician's mind. Thus the average cost of each procedure has been included.

ULTRASOUND

Ultrasound, or sonography, is a noninvasive imaging technique utilizing acoustic waves similar to sonar. Since the early 1950s, major improvements in equipment, from crude waterbath immersion tanks to modern highly developed gray-scale instruments, have resulted in revolutionary and fundamental changes in the practice of high-risk obstetrics. The clinical applications of ultrasound in gynecology, other than the diagnosis of early pregnancy, are less frequent and less specific and often only confirm the clinical findings of a bimanual pelvic examination.

For transabdominal gynecologic examinations, a sector scanner is preferable. It provides greater resolution of the pelvis and an easier examination than the linear array. During pelvic ultrasound it is important for the patient to have a full bladder. This helps to elevate the uterus and ovaries and serves as an acoustic window for the high-frequency sound waves (Figures 8-1 and 8-2). Ultrasound is approximately 90% accurate in recognizing the presence of a pelvic mass, but rarely does it establish a tissue diagnosis. In several comparison studies, ultrasound was not as reliable as a bimanual examination in the diagnosis of pelvic disease.

Ultrasound transducers fitted on endovaginal probes are useful in the examination of very early pregnancy before visualization by abdominal pelvic scans. The vaginal probes are inserted into a sterile sheath, usually a glove or condom, before patient use. The transducer is inserted a few centimeters into the vagina while the woman is in a dorsal lithotomy position. Because the transducer is closer to the pelvic organs than when a transabdominal approach is employed, the resolution is often superior. However, if the pelvic structures in question extend into the patient's abdomen, the organs are difficult to visualize with an endovaginal probe. Most ultrasound machines are fitted with both types of transducers.

Ultrasonography employs an acoustic pulse echo technique. The transducer of the ultrasound machine is made up of piezoelectric crystals. When the crystals receive an electric charge, they vibrate and emit acoustic pulses, vibrations in the form of pulsed sound waves. Acoustic echoes return from the tissues being scanned and cause the piezoelectric crystals to vibrate again and release an electric charge. These electric charges are then integrated by a computer within the ultrasound machine to form a two-dimensional display image. Present equipment provides resolution between 0.5 and 1 mm.

With this pulse echo technique, anatomic structures are identified by measuring the time for the sound wave to reach the structure and return. With Doppler ultrasound techniques the frequency of returning sound echoes is analyzed to determine the velocity of moving structures. Many images per second may be developed, allowing direct measurement of blood flow. For the gynecologist, this technique provides a noninvasive method of diagnosing deep vein thrombophlebitis of the legs. A disadvantage of ultrasound is its poor penetration of bone and air; thus the pubic symphysis and air-filled small and/or large intestine often inhibit visualization.

One of the most reassuring facts concerning sonography is the absence of adverse clinical effects in humans from the energy levels used in diagnostic studies. A select committee of the National Institutes of Health reviewed the potential harmful effects studied in laboratory experiments. These in vitro biologic experiments discovered a reduction in immune response, changes in sister chromatid exchange frequency, cell death, changes in the function of cell membranes, and degradation of macromolecules. However, these experiments used ultrasound with higher energy levels than those used in diagnostic studies, and the concerns of these basic scientists must be balanced by 30 years of clinical practice without documented harmful effects.

The usefulness of ultrasound in gynecology depends largely on the pathologic conditions involved. It is most useful for infertility studies and less so for oncologic evaluation or benign gynecology. For example, ultrasound has greatly improved the efficiency of ovulation induction by its ability to document when ovulation is about to occur or has already occurred. Serial examinations have aided in determining

FIGURE 8-1
Normal pelvis on transverse ultrasonic scan demonstrating uterus *(u)* lying behind bladder *(b)*. Both ovaries *(o)* are seen in angle between bladder and pelvic side wall. Round ligaments *(arrows)* are defined. (From Morley P and Barnett E: The ovarian mass. In Sanders RC and James AE Jr, editors: The principles and practice of ultrasonography in obstetrics and gynecology, ed 2, New York, 1980, Appleton-Century-Crofts.)

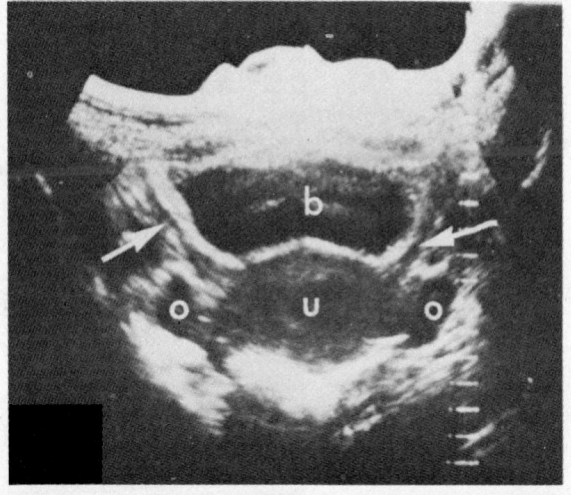

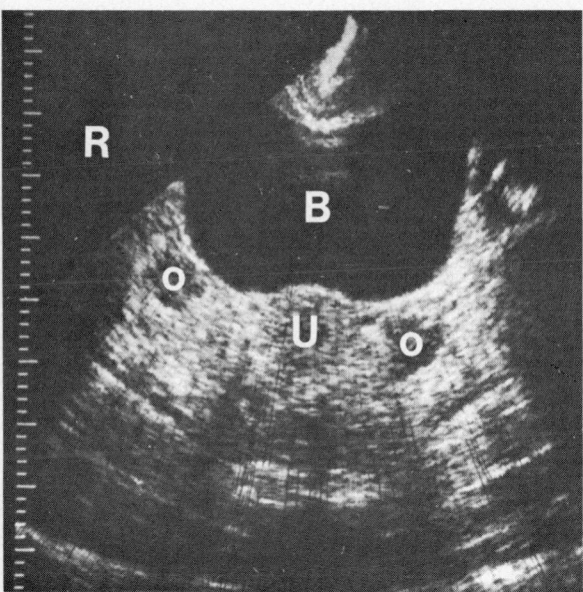

A

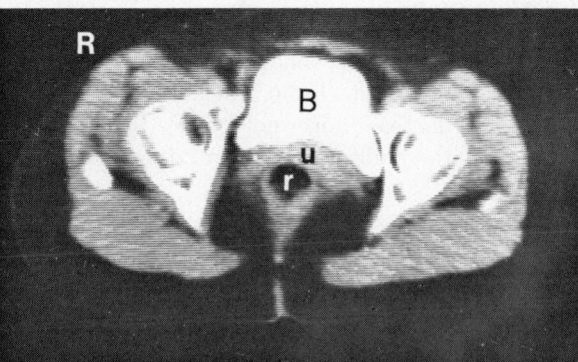

B

FIGURE 8-2
A, Transverse sonogram, and **B,** CT scan of normal female pelvis. In sonogram, normal ovaries *(o)* and uterus *(U)* are seen posterior to bladder. On CT scan gas is seen in the rectum *(r)* posterior to uterus; ovaries are not imaged *(R,* right; *B,* bladder). (From Sommer FG, Walsh JW, Schwartz PE, et al: J Reprod Med 27:47, 1982.)

the appropriate timing of artificial insemination and in identifying the best time for human chorionic gonadotrophin (HCG) administration. Sonography has also been invaluable in assessing the time for oocyte retrieval for in vitro fertilization, as well as for human menopausal gonadotrophin use (Figure 8-3). During induced cycles, several follicles develop, in contrast to the "dominant" follicle of a normal cycle. Serial ultrasound scans and plasma estrogen levels complement each other in the clinical management of ovulatory induction and prevention of

the hyperstimulation syndrome. Oocyte retrieval with ultrasonic guidance can be performed in several repetitive cycles with the patient given local anesthesia. The pregnancy rate using this technique with in vitro fertilization approaches pregnancy rates when the oocytes are retreived by laparoscopy.

In contrast to its usefulness in reproductive endocrinology, ultrasound has limited value in gynecologic oncology. The major limitation of this technique is its inability to differentiate a benign from a malignant process. One advan-

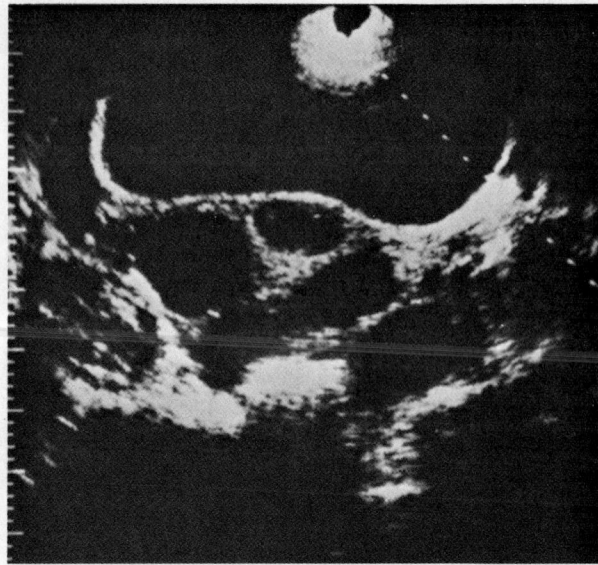

FIGURE 8-3
Transverse sonogram demonstrating multiple ovarian cysts in Pergonal-induced ovulation. (From DeCherney AH, Romero R, and Polan ML: Ultrasound in reproductive endocrinology, Fertil Steril 37:323, 1982. Reproduced with permission of the publisher, The American Fertility Society.)

tage of ultrasound over computed tomography is its ability to identify normal ovaries. The sagittal view obtained with a sector scanner facilitates differentiation of the ovaries from the uterus. Ultrasound easily recognizes such advanced manifestations of pelvic neoplasm as ascites and hydronephrosis.

Ultrasound is clinically useful in the differential diagnosis of abnormalities of early pregnancy. The characteristic "snowstorm" pattern of ill-defined echogenic areas inside the uterus is pathognomonic of hydatidiform mole. Ultrasound may be of value in differentiating an intrauterine from an ectopic pregnancy. In early pregnancy the single ring inside the uterus may be either a gestational or a pseudogestational sac. The pseudogestational sac is formed by the decidual reaction that accompanies an ectopic pregnancy. However, when the serum HCG titer reaches 6000 to 6500 mIU/ml (the discriminating HCG zone), this dilemma can be resolved with an abdominal-pelvic ultrasound, since above this titer signs of an intrauterine pregnancy should be visualized. With an endovaginal ultrasound, intrauterine pregnancies may be visualized as early as 4 weeks after the last menstrual period with an HCG titer of approximately 1000 mIU/ml. A pregnancy should be routinely visualized by 5 postmenstrual weeks, when the gestational sac is 4 mm in diameter. A yolk sac should be clearly visible by the time the gestational sac is 8 mm. If not, the viability of the pregnancy is in question. The finding during ultrasonography of fluid in the cul-de-sac or hepatorenal space is a helpful sign. As little as 5 to 10 ml of fluid can be seen with modern ultrasound transducers. In addition, a cystic mass in the adnexa may be a corpus luteum that can be sonographically confused with ectopic pregnancy. Endovaginal scanning can help differentiate the tubal ring, a clear, circular adnexal structure that represents an ectopic gestation, from the corpus luteum.

Sonography is the method of choice to locate a "missing" intrauterine device (IUD) (Figure 8-4). It will help in diagnosing perforation of the uterus or unrecognized expulsion of the device. Ultrasonography facilitates surgical procedures such as chorionic villus biopsy. Endovaginal ultrasound transducers equipped with needle guides are frequently used for oocyte aspiration as part of in vitro fertilization. Success rates are equal to those with laparoscopic oocyte retrieval, with less cost, time, and risk.

The use of ultrasonography in women with pelvic infection has been disappointing. Swayne et al. discovered that not only was sonography unable to delineate the severity of

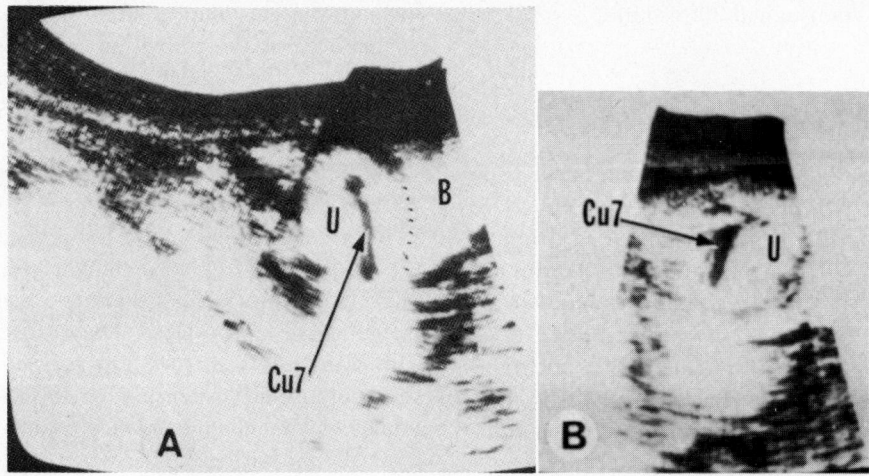

FIGURE 8-4
A, Sonographic longitudinal scan of uterus displaying Copper-7 intrauterine device (IUD) in its longitudinal axis. **B,** Transverse scan through fundus of uterus displaying characteristic "7" configuration of IUD (*B*, bladder; *Cu-7*, Copper-7; *U*, uterus). (From Cochrane WJ: The value of ultrasound in the management of intrauterine devices. In Sanders RC and James AE Jr. editors: The principles and practice of ultrasonography in obstetrics and gynecology, ed 2, New York, 1980, Appleton-Century-Crofts.)

this disease, but it produced images similar to those seen in many other pelvic abnormalities. The lack of specificity in gynecology is a major limitation of ultrasonography. Gas- or fluid-filled intestines are commonly misinterpreted as gynecologic problems. It is possible to differentiate fluid-filled bowel by giving a water enema simultaneously with the scan. However, because this technique is cumbersome, it is not frequently used.

Ultrasound is often used to follow growth and resolution of myomas. The use of ultrasound as a screening tool to evaluate the ovaries of postmenopausal women is being investigated.

Recommendations and Cost Information

In summary, ultrasound should be used selectively in gynecology. It is excellent for monitoring ovulation induction. It is helpful in evaluating the different abnormalities of early pregnancy. It is useful in identifying pelvic masses in women in whom pelvic examination is difficult. The latter group includes massively obese women, those who are distended, and those with extreme pelvic tenderness.

Ultrasound adds little to the clinical manage-

ment of a patient in whom a distinct mass has been palpated on bimanual examination. Although it may describe the size and internal consistency and can distinguish between solid and cystic masses, the technique lacks sensitivity and specificity in establishing the diagnosis. If the clinician is unsure, obtaining an ultrasound scan will confirm the presence of a mass.

Ultrasound should not alter clinical decisions in the management of a pelvic mass. Most important, there is no reason to routinely perform ultrasonography if the mass can be palpated on pelvic examination. In a comparison study, O'Brien et al. found ultrasonography inferior to clinical examination. The large number of false positive diagnoses by ultrasound was especially disturbing. In this series the pelvic diagnosis advanced by ultrasound was correct in only 42% of cases when compared to operative findings at laparoscopy or celiotomy. One can only condemn the practice of substituting a pelvic ultrasound for a pelvic examination.

Ultrasound in gynecology is caught between the two conflicting trends of increasing reliance on noninvasive imaging techniques and greater cost containment, with an emphasis on decreasing the overuse of diagnostic procedures. The average cost of a pelvic ultrasound examination is between $150 and $250. The cost of an endovaginal ultrasound is $175 to $300.

COMPUTED TOMOGRAPHY

High-resolution computed tomography (CT) is a leading example of advanced technology in gynecology. CT is a major advance in diagnostic imaging that provides detailed, two-dimensional images. The ability to image anatomic areas in a cross section a few millimeters thick has varied clinical applications. CT is most popular in studies of the central nervous system and is claimed to have revolutionized the clinical practice of neurology and neurosurgery. The critics of CT cite the expense of the equipment and its impact on cost containment. Proponents counter that CT scans reduce the need for other imaging techniques.

A CT scan identifies gross distortions in local anatomy by using the difference in x-ray beam attenuation that results from different densities in adjacent tissues. For example, this technique is excellent in discovering extension of pelvic cancer into the fat of the retroperitoneal space. Even so, CT definitely has its limitations. Abnormal masses are visualized, yet a definitive pathologic diagnosis cannot be established until a surgical biopsy is performed, because most masses do not have distinctive enough anatomic shapes or unique density characteristics. The CT scan may recognize a group of enlarged lymph nodes adjacent to pelvic vessels but cannot differentiate between benign hyperplasia or metastatic carcinoma. However, CT facilitates needle placement in percutaneous biopsy of suspicious nodes.

There have been several improvements in machinery for CT since its introduction into clinical medicine. The machine rotates the x-ray beam in an arc of 180 degrees perpendicular to the long axis of the body. A group of crystal detectors are directly opposite the narrow beam, only 2 to 10 mm wide. These crystals are capable of photon detection efficiencies of approximately 80%. The detectors measure the amount of tissue absorption, and a computer then develops two-dimensional images of the cross-sectional planes under investigation. The newer equipment provides more sophisticated density determinations, which increases diagnostic accuracy.

Before the scan, contrast medium is given intravenously, orally, or rectally to outline the urinary and gastrointestinal tracts. In gyneco-logic studies, a tampon often is placed in the vagina because the gas within the tampon helps to delineate the vaginal cavity. Some investigators place a small Foley catheter in the uterine cavity to increase diagnostic landmarks.

One of the leading indications in gynecology for a CT scan is the assessment of a prolactin-secreting microadenoma of the pituitary gland. CT has virtually replaced standard tomography of the sella turcica in evaluating a woman with elevated serum prolactin levels (Figure 8-5). The scans are used to follow patients with either suprasellar expansion or intrasellar adenomas. Women who develop visual field defects should have a CT scan performed to determine the degree of suprasellar extension.

CT has been used extensively in gynecologic oncology. In general, it is more useful to the clinician in staging than in diagnosis (Figure 8-6). It is more accurate in diagnosing retroperitoneal metastases than intraperitoneal ones. Often a CT scan helps in the initial evaluation of a pelvic neoplasm. Walsh et al. found CT scans accurate in staging advanced cervical carcinoma in 92% of cases. In a companion study, he found CT to be true positive in 17 of 20 cases (85%) with metastatic disease, false negative in 3 of 20 (15%), and false positive for lymph node metastasis in 5 of 15 (33%). Although imperfect, CT scans are a valuable noninvasive technique to screen patients for retroperitoneal metastatic disease. A CT scan is able to identify a node when it reaches a diameter of 1.5 to 2 cm (Figure 8-7). Moldofsky et al. developed a technique of discovering metastatic carcinoma in normal-size retroperitoneal lymph nodes by using monoclonal antibody imaging.

Women with endometrial carcinoma have been studied by CT. Following injection of intravenous contrast material, a hypodense or low-attenuation area in the uterus is specific for endometrial carcinoma. It is possible to predict the depth of penetration into the myometrium. Walsh and Goplerud documented an accuracy of 86% in diagnosing extrauterine spread of the endometrial carcinoma.

In patients with ovarian carcinoma, the primary use of CT scans is in evaluating the extent of the disease. It is an excellent technique to discern small collections of ascites (Figure 8-8). CT scans give further information of retroperitoneal involvement and ureteral obstruction. However, CT scans definitely do not re-

A   B   C

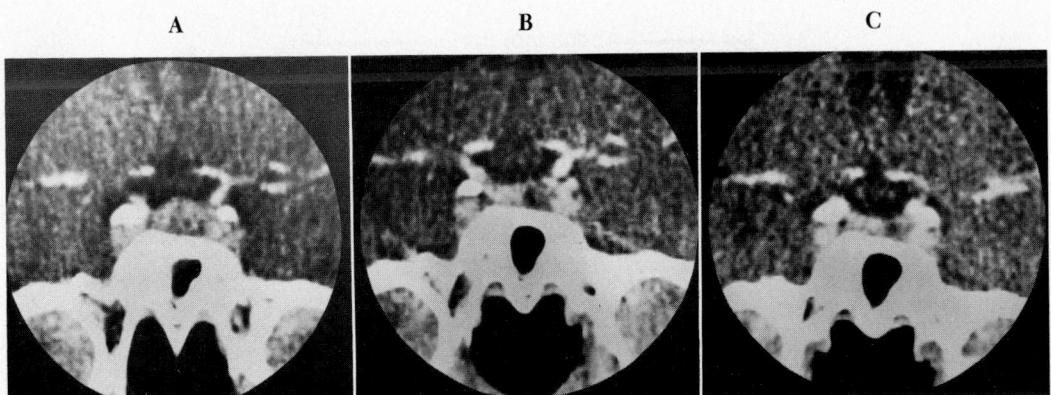

FIGURE 8-5

A 17-year-old woman with amenorrhea, galactorrhea, and hyperprolactinemia. **A,** Coronal CT scan after intravenous injection of contrast medium shows heterogeneous enhancement of pituitary, bulging of sellar diaphragm, and depression of left sellar floor. **B,** Six months after bromocriptine therapy, patient had restoration of ovulatory cycles, disappearance of galactorrhea, and normal prolactin level, CT scan shows decrease in size of content of pituitary fossa; adenoma appears as rounded defect in enhancement, 6 mm in diameter. **C,** One year after initiation of bromocriptine treatment, sellar diaphragm is now in a normal position; adenoma measures less than 4 mm in diameter. (From Bonneville JF, Poulignot D, Cattin F, et al: Radiology 143:454, 1982.)

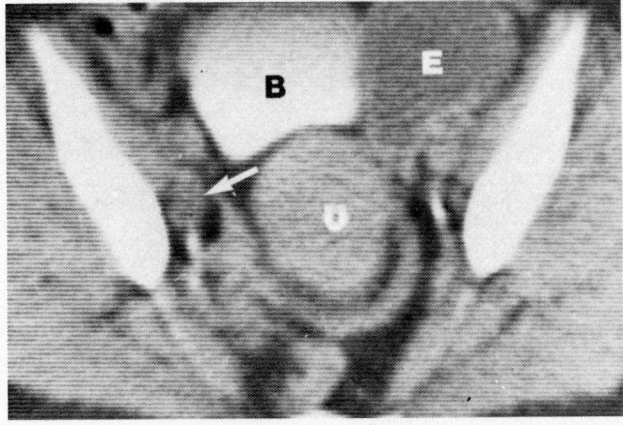

FIGURE 8-6

Stage IIB cervical carcinoma, CT scan through bladder *(B)* and uterine corpus *(U)*. Right obturator lymph node metastasis *(arrow)*, 2 cm in diameter, and left ovarian endometrioma *(E)* confirmed at laparotomy. (From Walsh JW and Goplerud DR: Prospective comparison between clinical and CT staging in primary cervical carcinoma, AJR 137:1000, 1981. Copyright © by American Roentgen Ray Soc, 1981.)

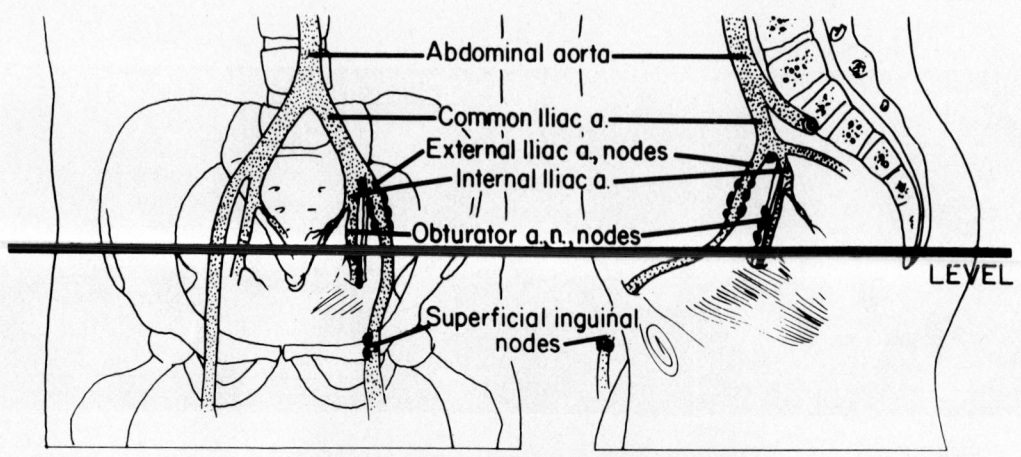

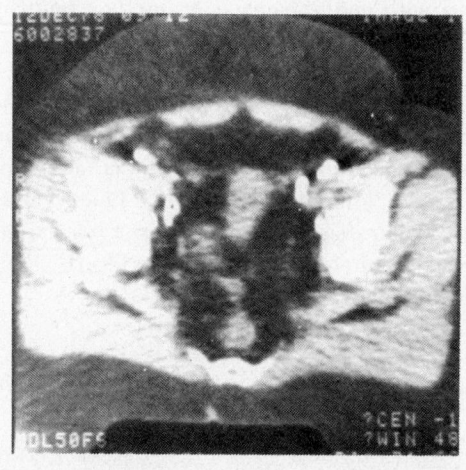

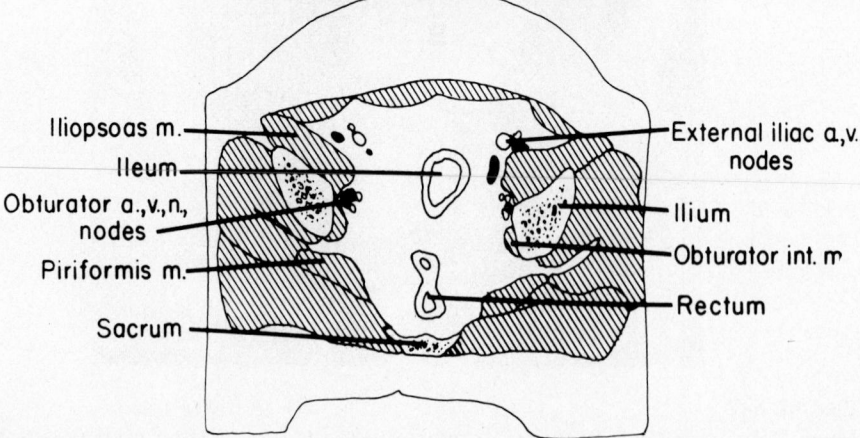

FIGURE 8-7

Illustrations and corresponding CT section after lymphangiography, demonstrating normal anatomic features of pelvic vessels, nerves, and lymph nodes. (From Walsh JW, Amendola MA, Konerding KF, et al: Radiology 137:158, 1980.)

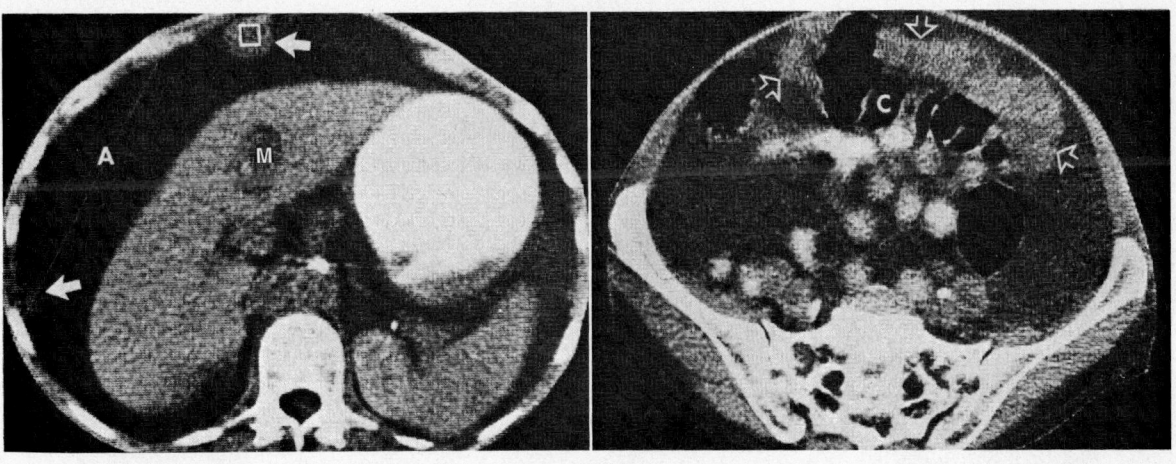

A   B

FIGURE 8-8
Metastatic ovarian carcinoma demonstrated by CT scan. **A,** Recurrent carcinoma is evident in this patient by ascites *(A)*, liver metastases *(M)*, and peritoneal metastatic implants *(arrows)*. **B,** Omental metastases are also seen as a flattened mass *(arrows)* lying on top of transverse colon *(C)* in this patient. (From Federle MP: Female Patient 9:45, 1984.)

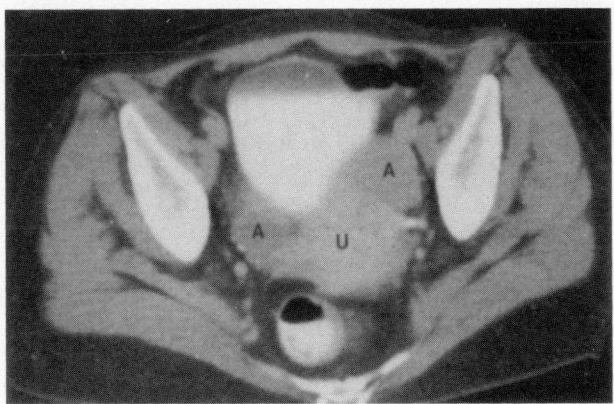

FIGURE 8-9
CT scan of patient with pelvic inflammatory disease with bilateral adnexal masses *(A,* tuboovarian abscesses; *U,* uterus). (From Gross BH, Moss AA, Mihara K, et al: Computed tomography of gynecologic diseases, AJR 141:771, 1983. Copyright © by American Roentgen Ray Soc, 1983.)

place the second-look operation. A scan misses small areas of metastatic spread, especially along serosal surfaces. If the area of carcinoma is less than 1 cm in diameter and is on a visceral surface, it is unlikely to be visualized by the imaging technique. Buy et al. have shown that subphrenic metastatic disease surrounded by ascites is more frequently visualized than metastatic lesions in the mesentery.

CT scans have been used for other intraabdominal and pelvic problems in gynecology (Figure 8-9). Wittenberg cites several studies with an accuracy of CT in locating intraabdominal abscesses of over 90%. Because of differences between fat, hair, and bone, CT is very accurate in the diagnosis of cystic teratoma. It is an excellent technique to confirm the diagnosis of ovarian vein thrombophlebitis (Figure

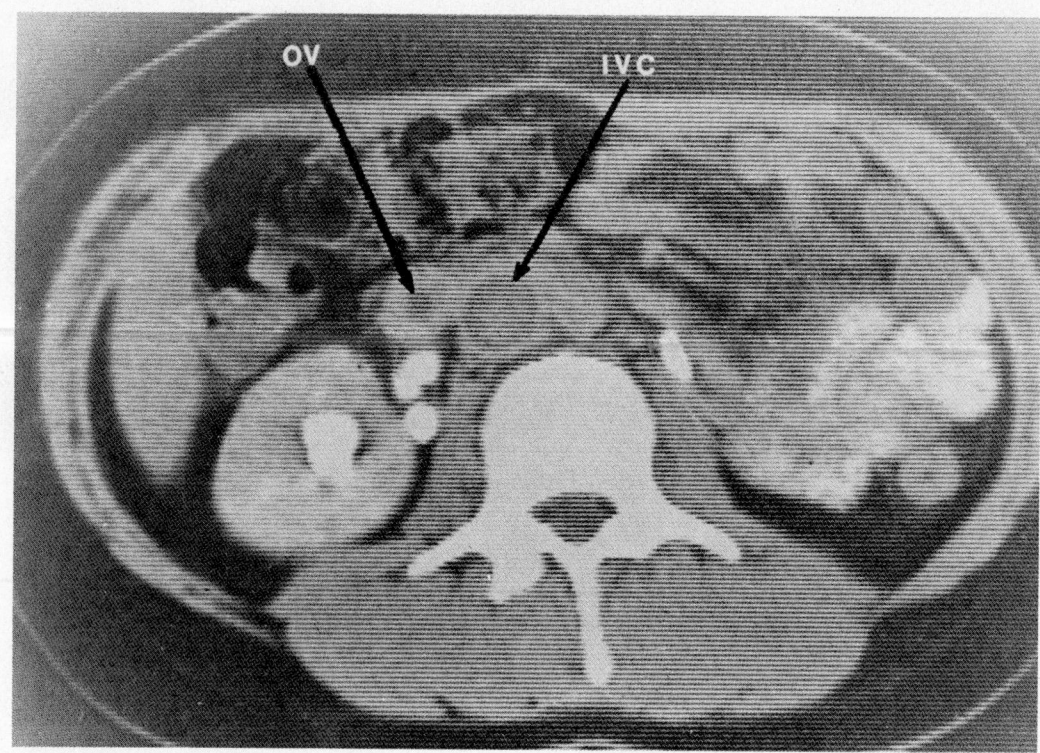

FIGURE 8-10
CT image of abdomen. Note thrombus within lumen of right ovarian *(OV)* and inferior vena cava *(IVC)*. Right ovarian vein is markedly enlarged. (From Angel JL and Knuppel RA: Obstet Gynecol 63:62, 1984. Reprinted with permission from The American College of Obstetricians and Gynecologists.)

8-10). When a linear mass is identified from the adnexal area to the vena cava or renal vein, the diagnosis is established and appropriate medical therapy can be started. Ultrasonography is the first choice to locate a lost IUD. However, CT scans have been able to diagnose partial perforations of the uterus missed by ultrasound.

Recommendations and Cost Information

In summary, the major use of CT scans in gynecology has been in evaluating pituitary tumors and in identifying retroperitoneal disease during the initial evaluation of pelvic carcinoma. CT scans also facilitate the percutaneous needle biopsy of suspicious lymph nodes.

State-of-the-art CT equipment costs approximately $1 million. The average cost of an individual scan is $350 to $450, which is comparable to the combined cost of an intravenous py-

elogram and a barium enema. The average CT scan of the abdomen and pelvis takes between 30 and 45 minutes to perform, and the surface radiation dose is between 2 and 10 rads. The dose to the midpelvis is approximately 50% of the surface dose. This radiation exposure is similar to that of a barium enema.

CT has been an important and helpful addition to gynecologists' diagnostic armamentarium. However, in competition is magnetic resonance imaging, for which comparative studies with CT are just beginning.

MAGNETIC RESONANCE IMAGING

Magnetic resonance imaging is predicted to be the greatest advance in radiology in the past 3 decades. The phenomenon of nuclear magnetic resonance was first discovered in 1945 and was renamed magnetic resonance imaging (MRI) to avoid misinterpretation of the word

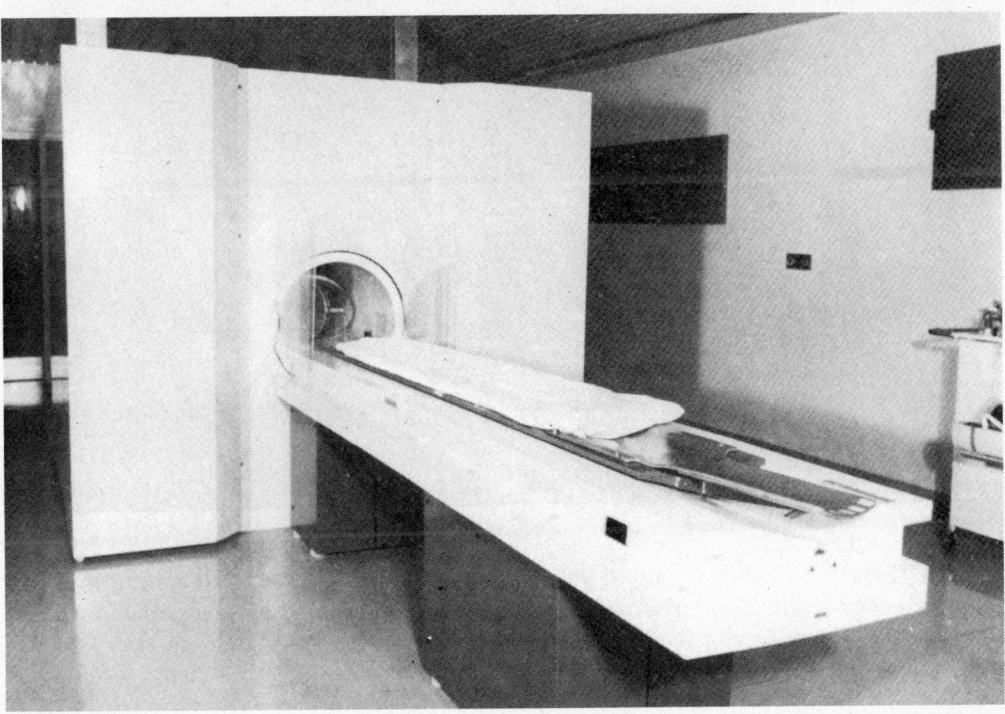

FIGURE 8-11
Magnetic resonance imager. Movable bed and patient access tube are shown and, within latter, RF coil. (From Johnson IR, Symonds EM, Worthington BS, et al: Br J Obstet Gynaecol 91:261, 1984.)

nuclear by the public. Clinical studies using MRI are relatively new in the gynecologic literature because most major university centers have had MRI facilities for less than 10 years.

MRI is a technique that uses radio frequency radiation and a varying magnetic field. The patient is placed within the machine, and a magnetic field is produced (Figure 8-11). The image depends on the resonant absorption and emission of radio waves by the atomic nuclei in the various tissues being observed. Because of their intrinsic magnetism, the nuclei act like small bar magnets and are influenced by the machine's magnetic field. The summation of the resonance of the vast number of atomic nuclei in a single thin slice of tissue provides the overall result. Intensity of image can be modified by varying the magnetic field.

Images are tomographic (in thin slices) and may be visualized in coronal, sagittal, or transverse planes. The radio waves penetrate bone and air without attentuation. Thus MRI allows identification of soft tissue lesions inaccessible to other imaging techniques.

MRI uses nonionizing radiation. Extensive basic investigations have demonstrated no evidence of mutagenic effects in studies of bacteria, and no chromosomal changes were produced in human lymphocytes. No adverse or harmful effects have been reported from repetitive examinations.

MRI can differentiate normal from malignant tissue and also can identify areas of abnormal tissue metabolism. MRI is most specific in the diagnosis of conditions associated with edema. Edema prolongs the spin-spin proton relaxation time (T_2), thereby producing a stronger image. Investigators have discovered significant prolonged proton relaxation times or spin lattice relaxation times (T_1) for the atoms in most carcinomas. The T_1 and T_2 properties of tissues affect the intensity of the image produced.

In an early study of three-dimensional MRI, Mann et al. demonstrated that imaging could identify the exact area of a vulvar neoplasm (Figure 8-12). MRI correctly identified microscopic tumor at the surgical margin of the vulvectomy incision. This technique also holds promise for measurement of the amount of blood flow to a specific organ.

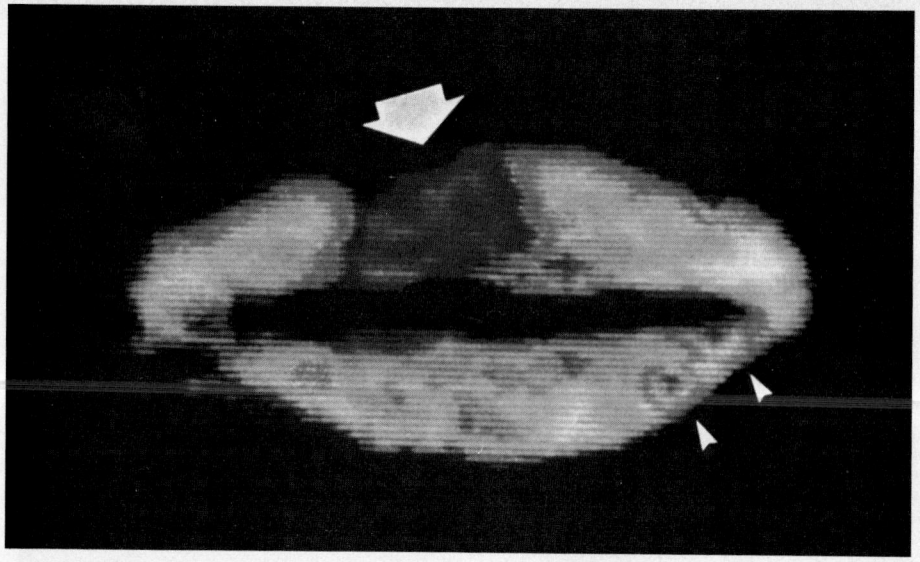

FIGURE 8-12
MRI of transverse slice of radical vulvectomy specimen. Large arrow indicates primary vulvar lesion; smaller arrows indicate two nodes containing metastatic disease that measured 0.7 and 1.0 cm in diameter. (From Mann WJ, Mendonca-Dias MH, Lauterbur PC, et al: Am J Obstet Gynecol 148:93, 1984.)

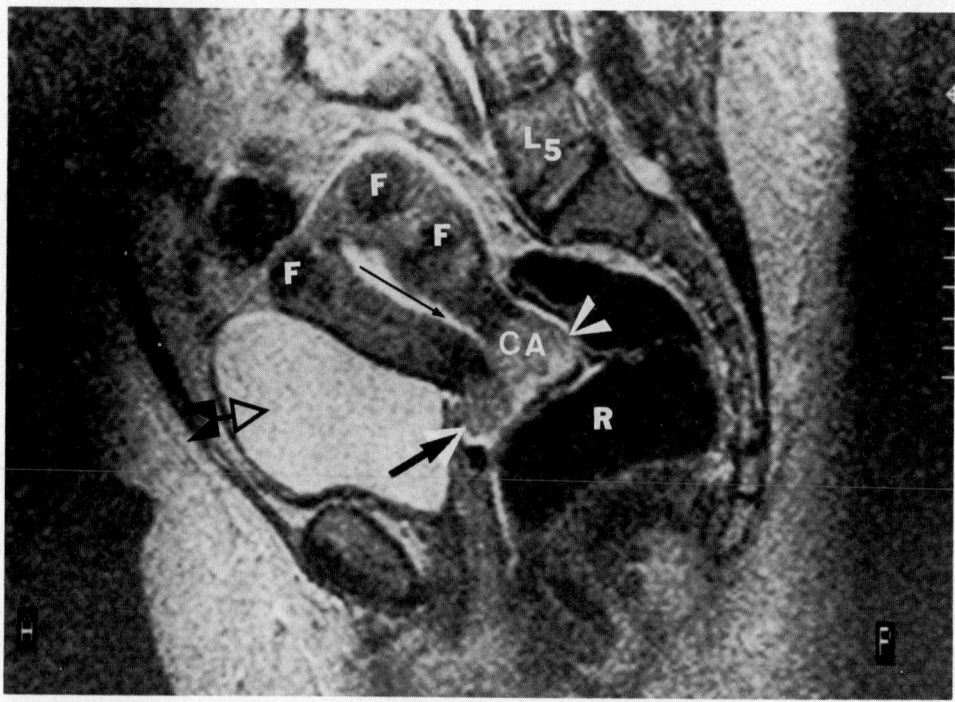

FIGURE 8-13
Sagittal MRI of woman with cervical cancer. Cancer *(CA)* is area of higher signal intensity within cervix (between *black arrows* on *white arrowheads*). Rectum *(R)* can be seen immediately posterior and inferior to enlarged cervical mass. Endometrial canal is slightly enlarged and contains fluid *(thin black arrow)*. Three leiomyomata *(F)* can be seen scattered throughout myometrium. Bladder is seen internally as fluid-filled structure *(open black arrow)*. Parameters for this examination were spin echo sequence of TR 2500/TE 80, 256 × 198 matrix, and 1 signal average. (Courtesy Mark L. Schiebler, M.D.)

MRI has been found to be accurate in evaluating vaginal anatomy and congenital defects of the müllerian system. Chang et al. found MRI to have a 95% sensitivity and 90% specificity in evaluating vaginal malignancy. Several reports in the past 5 years have documented the advantages of MRI in diagnosing and evaluating disease processes of adenomyosis, myomas, endometrial cancer (including myometrial invasion), and cervical carcinoma, both local and distant spread. MRI is more accurate than CT scans in evaluating the spread of uterine and cervical malignancy (Figure 8-13). MRI has been employed, although to a lesser degree, also in the evaluation of endometriosis and the evaluation of adnexal disease.

Recommendations and Cost Information

The future and potential clinical impact of MRI is limited only by availability, patient acceptance, and physician familiarity. It is anticipated that equipment will be able to produce images of tissue slices 1 mm thick. Three-dimensional studies from surgical specimens have demonstrated that MRI can definitely distinguish a normal node from a node of the same size involved with metastatic disease.

MRI has several distinct advantages over other forms of imaging. It does not use ionizing radiation; therefore there are no known hazards. Radio frequency electromagnetic radiation penetrates calcified material without significant attenuation. Unlike ultrasound, MRI can penetrate through gas, thus allowing visualization of the bowel and vagina. MRI has the ability to add coronal and sagittal sections to the transverse sections visualized on CT scans. In addition, MRI does not require the use of contrast agents required with CT scans. Most important, it has the abilitiy to differentiate areas of neoplastic growth from normal tissue on the basis of proton relaxation times.

The two limitations to MRI are expense and patient acceptance. Many patients feel trapped and claustrophobic in the machine. State-of-the-art equipment with superconductive magnets costs between $1.5 and $2 million. The additional expense of a special structure to enclose the equipment must also be considered in the overall cost. Clinical studies involving pelvic organs take from 30 minutes to more than an hour to complete. The fee is between $300 and $700 and depends on the time involved in the study. The cost is usually comparable with CT scans.

CULDOCENTESIS

Culdocentesis is the transvaginal aspiration of peritoneal fluid from the cul-de-sac of Douglas. This minor procedure is a rapid and simple technique to establish the presence of intraperitoneal bleeding. It is a standard procedure in the diagnostic evaluation of a woman with a suspected ectopic pregnancy. Culdocentesis can be performed in the office or in the emergency room to aid in diagnosing patients with abnormal bleeding and pelvic pain.

Although suspected ectopic pregnancy is the leading indication for culdocentesis, intraperitoneal bleeding from other causes, such as hemorrhage from a corpus luteum, can be confirmed. Peritoneal fluid can be obtained in suspected cases of pelvic infection. The aspiration of turbid fluid with inflammatory cells and bacteria helps to establish the diagnosis. Cultures of peritoneal fluid obtained via culdocentesis cannot be used for selecting antibiotic therapy. Just as sputum cultures may be contaminated by bacteria in the oropharynx, cul-de-sac cultures obtained transvaginally may not be "pure" cultures, because it is virtually impossible not to contaminate the needle while inserting it through the vaginal canal. Twenty-five years ago there was brief interest in attempting to diagnose ovarian carcinoma by peritoneal cytology obtained from culdocentesis. These programs of yearly cytologic screening have been abandoned.

There are few contraindications to culdocentesis, the major ones being a bleeding diathesis or a large adnexal mass in the cul-de-sac. In the latter instance, culdocentesis could result in contamination of the peritoneal cavity by an ovarian carcinoma or purulent fluid from an abscess.

Culdocentesis is performed with the patient in the dorsal lithotomy position. The table is tilted to position the pelvis in the most dependent portion of the body and allow intraperitoneal fluid to pool in the posterior cul-de-sac. Then a bimanual examination is done to rule out the presence of a large adnexal mass in the cul-de-sac. A speculum is placed in the vagina, and the posterior cervical lip is secured with a single-toothed tenaculum (Figure 8-14). Traction on the tenaculum is used to lift the cervix anteriorly, exposing the uterosacral ligaments.

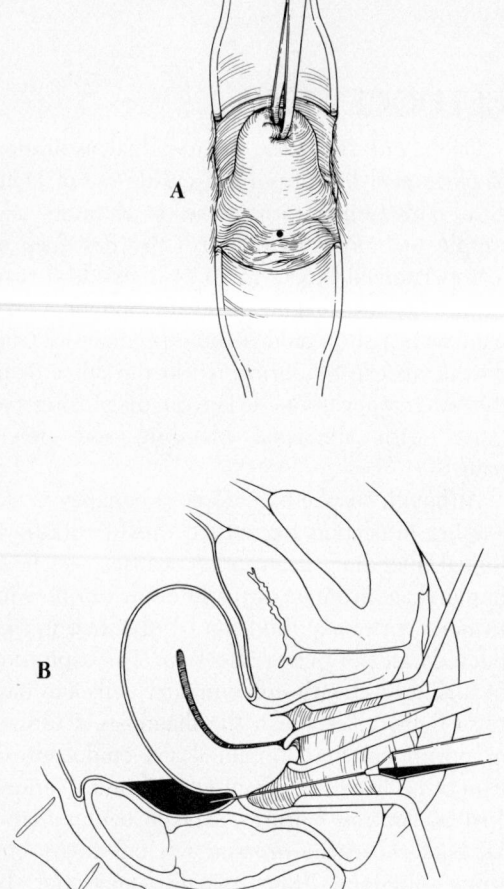

FIGURE 8-14

Culdocentesis. **A,** Traction on posterior lip of cervix exposes posterior cul-de-sac. Black dot indicates site of needle insertion. **B,** Syringe containing 3 to 5 ml of saline is attached to 18-gauge, 3½-inch needle. Needle is introduced into posterior cul-de-sac. Fluid is injected to clear tissue from needle, followed by aspiration of cul-de-sac contents. Needle is introduced parallel to sacrum to avoid entry into uterus or rectum. (From Bowes WA and Droegemueller W: Female genitourinary tract and obstetrics outpatient gynecological surgery. In Hill GJ, editor: Outpatient surgery, Philadelphia, 1973, WB Saunders Co.)

The area of insertion is in the midline, approximately 2 cm below the attachment of the ligaments.

Culdocentesis is performed with an 18-gauge spinal needle attached to a 20 ml syringe. Prior to the procedure, 3 to 5 ml of saline solution is aspirated into the syringe. The needle is inserted into the posterior cul-de-sac with a rapid, deliberate thrust. Injecting local anesthesia and slowly puncturing the cul-de-sac increases, rather than decreases, patient discomfort. Once the needle is positioned in the cul-de-sac, the saline solution in the syringe is injected to help confirm correct needle placement. A sample of the pooled intraperitoneal fluid is then aspirated. Normal peritoneal fluid is clear and resembles plasma. The diagnosis of intraperitoneal bleeding is confirmed if nonclotting blood is obtained. Blood that escapes into the peritoneal cavity initially undergoes clotting and subsequently undergoes fibrinolysis. If the aspirated blood forms a solid clot, the needle has inadvertently sampled blood directly from the vascular system, most frequently from a uterine vein.

An important step is performing a hematocrit on the unclotted blood. The hematocrit exceeds 15% with significant bleeding, such as with an ectopic pregnancy or hemorrhage from a corpus luteum. The hematocrit is low, 2% to 8%, with blood-tinged fluid from a ruptured ovarian cyst or pelvic inflammation.

A positive culdocentesis should be obtained in over 90% of ruptured ectopic pregnancies. A nondiagnostic, or "dry," tap occurs when neither peritoneal fluid nor injected saline solution can be withdrawn. This indicates either poor positioning of the needle or a cul-de-sac obliterated by adhesions. It is important to take into consideration that virtually all women experience retrograde menstruation. Therefore culdocentesis just before menstruation or after a dilation and curettage (D&C) may give a false positive test. Inadvertent entry into the lumen of the bowel is not associated with morbidity.

Recommendations and Cost Information

In summary, culdocentesis is a rapid and simple means of confirming the presence of intraperitoneal bleeding. A positive culdocentesis with dark, nonclotting blood and a hematocrit greater than 15% is an absolute indication for surgical therapy. The incidence of a false positive test is less than 2%. The cost of culdocentesis is the cost of a disposable syringe and needle, which is minimal. Culdocentesis remains an important gynecologic procedure.

ENDOMETRIAL SAMPLING

Endometrial biopsy is one of the diagnostic tests most frequently performed by gynecologists. This rapid, safe, and inexpensive sampling of the endometrial lining is a standard procedure in the clinical workup of women with infertility or abnormal perimenopausal bleeding. The renowned gynecologist Howard Kelly was an enthusiast for outpatient endometrial biopsy in the 1920s, and in the past decade there has been an increase in its popularity. This increase reflects the recent emphasis on cost containment in medical practice. Instruments have now been developed that abrade, scrape, lavage, brush, and aspirate the endometrium.

There are four common indications for endometrial sampling. It is useful in the investigation of an infertile couple. The biopsy gives indirect evidence of ovulation. Endometrial sampling is frequently performed to evaluate the cause of abnormal uterine bleeding. The third indication has evolved because of the increasing use of hormonal replacement therapy to prevent osteoporosis in postmenopausal women. This practice may include the periodic sampling of the uterine lining to rule out endometrial carcinoma. Endometrial biopsy is the standard diagnostic test to confirm a chronic uterine infection. If pelvic tuberculosis is suspected, sampling of the endometrial lining is performed late in the menstrual cycle. This gives the pathologist the best opportunity to discover the classic giant cells and tubercles.

There are only a few contraindications to endometrial biopsy. Acute pelvic infection and profuse bleeding are relative contraindications. Endometrial biopsy should not be performed more than 14 to 16 days after ovulation because of the possibility of interfering with an early pregnancy. In contrast, endometrial biopsy 10 to 14 days following the temperature rise is optimal for evaluation of corpus luteum function and does not interfere with implantation during that cycle.

Although there are many different models and modifications of devices used for endometrial sampling, they can be subdivided into two groups. The first group aspirates a tissue biopsy of the endometrial lining following abrasion or scraping with a small, sharp curette (Figures 8-15, 8-16, and 8-17). The second group obtains a small sample of cells for cytologic screening by rotating a plastic or metal brush or sponge inside the endometrial cavity.

Endometrial biopsy is performed on an outpatient basis, usually without anesthesia. It is helpful to explain to the patient that she will experience uterine cramping for the 1 or 2 minutes that the biopsy instrument is inside the uterus. A bimanual examination is performed to note the size of the uterus and direction of the uterine cavity. A single-toothed tenaculum may be used to secure the anterior cervical lip. The exocervix is then cleaned of mucus and bacteria. If the biopsy is performed as part of an infertility investigation, a single strip of endometrium from the

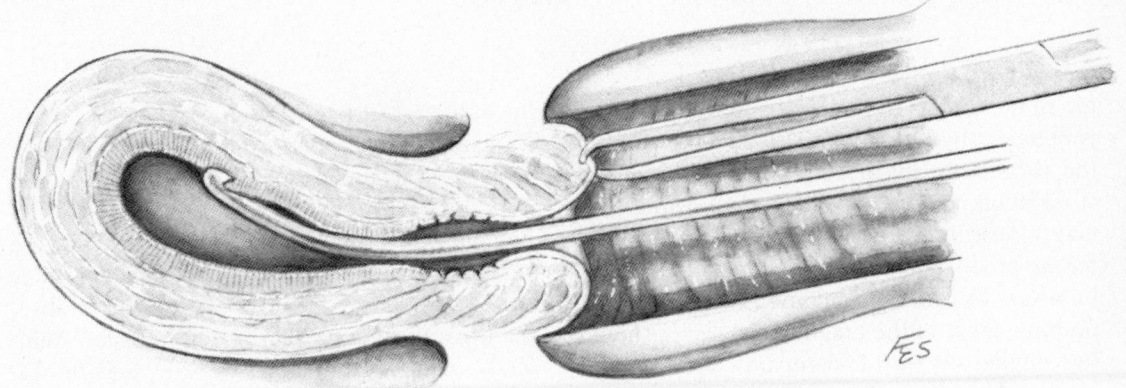

FIGURE 8-15
Office endometrial aspiration with 3 mm Randall suction curette. (From Copenhaver EH: *Surgery of the vulva and vagina: a practical guide*, Philadelphia, 1981, WB Saunders Co.)

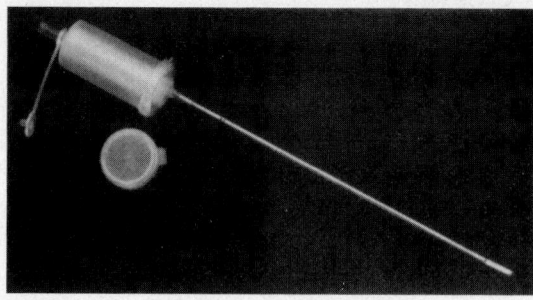

FIGURE 8-16
Vabra aspirator. (From Einerth Y: Acta Obstet Gynecol Scand 61:374, 1982.)

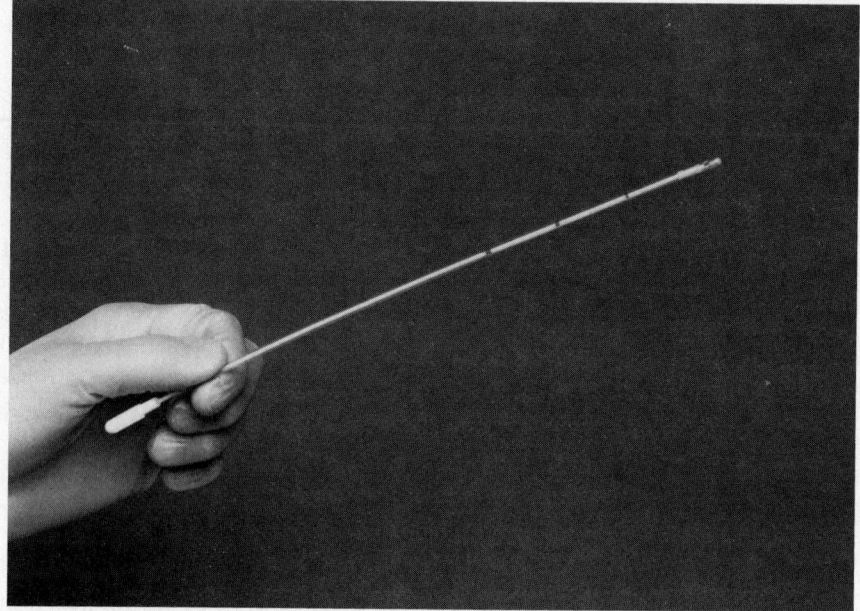

FIGURE 8-17
Pipelle endometrial suction curette. Note small diameter and flexible nature. Suction is produced by partly withdrawing inner stem.

top of the fundus to the lower uterine segment is obtained by aspiration. The endometrium of the isthmus is not as responsive to hormonal stimulation, and a sample from this area may give a false impression of inadequate progesterone production. When the indication for the biopsy is to rule out endometrial hyperplasia, multiple areas of the endometrial cavity should be sampled. At least four separate areas should be abraded. If copious or necrotic tissue is discovered, a fractional diagnostic D&C should be considered.

The most frequent problem in obtaining tissue is cervical stenosis or spasm. When this is encountered, a paracervical block with 1% xylocaine should be performed. Occasionally the endocervical application of viscous 2% to 4% lidocaine may decrease discomfort. Twenty percent benzocaine gel applied topically to the cervical os with a cotton-tipped applicator may also serve as an effective anesthetic. Subsequently, the cervix then can be dilated painlessly, with narrow metal dilators, and the biopsy completed.

There are many modifications of the original Novak and Randall endometrial biopsy instruments. Most cannulas are 2 to 4 mm in diameter and are either metal or plastic. Aspiration of

Suction pressure
(mm Hg)

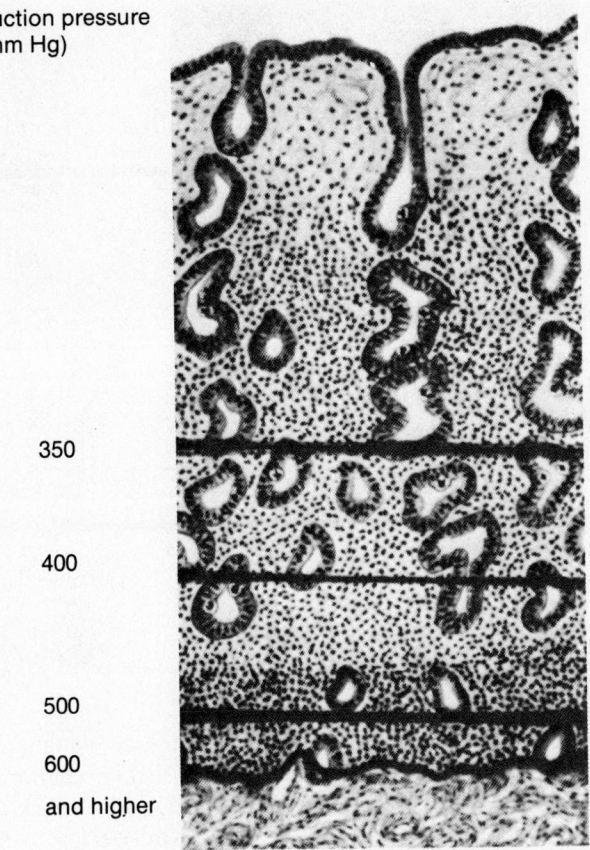

350

400

500

600
and higher

FIGURE 8-18

Schematic interpretation of effects of negative pressures used for vacuum aspiration and depth of cleavage planes in endometrium. (From Marik JJ and Tataryn IV: Dilatation, fractural curettage, and nonpregnant vacuum aspiration. In Symonds EM and Zuspan FP, editors: Clinical and diagnostic procedures in obstetrics and gynecology. Part B. Gynecology, New York, 1984, Marcel Dekker, Inc. Reprinted from Gynecology, p 206, by courtesy of Marcel Dekker, Inc.)

the endometrium is accomplished by a syringe or a portable pump. The Vabra aspirator has a reservoir similar to a sputum collection trap. The suction pump with the Vabra aspirator facilitates collection of an adequate sampling of the endometrium in approximately 1 minute. Optimal pressure is 500 to 600 mm Hg. The pressure used determines the depth of the cleavage plane in the endometrium (Figure 8-18). The thin, flexible polypropylene Pipelle cannula (see Figure 8-17) is as effective as the Vabra aspirator and Novak curettes in obtaining endometrial specimens, often with less discomfort. Most clinicians use the Pipelle as the intrument of first choice for endometrial sampling. Other flexible plastic cannulas (Milex)

have been recently introduced, and preliminary reports find them equally effective as earlier models.

Complications following endometrial biopsy are exceedingly rare. The major complication is uterine perforation, with an incidence of 1 or 2 cases per 1000. Infection and postoperative bleeding are very rare. Some women develop a severe vasovagal reflex from instrumentation of the uterine cavity. This reflex can be diminished by either giving the patient intravenous atropine or performing a paracervical block. Some clinicians pretreat women with prostaglandin synthetase inhibitors to decrease the pain associated with this procedure.

Cancer of the endometrium is the most com-

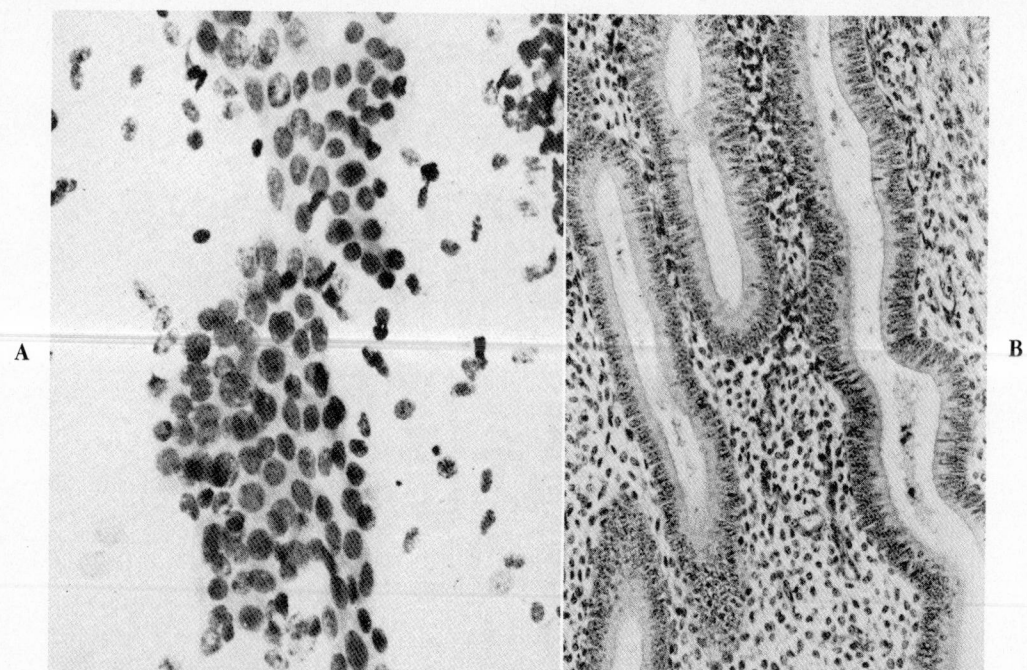

FIGURE 8-19
Cyclic proliferative endometrium. **A,** Endocyte cytology containing sheets of epithelial cells in which nuclei have uniform size and regular contour. Cellular cohesion and orientation are regular (Papanicolaou; × 500). **B,** Kevorkian biopsy of normal proliferative endometrium (hematoxylin and eosin [H&E]); × 250). (From Ferenczy A and Gelfand MM: Obstet Gynecol 63:298, 1984. Reprinted with permission from the American College of Obstetricians and Gynecologists.)

mon pelvic malignancy. Statistically, 2 to 3 women out of 100 will develop endometrial carcinoma. The increasing incidence of endometrial carcinoma and the increasing popularity of hormonal treatment of menopause have focused research on innovative means of mass screening for endometrial hyperplasia and carcinoma. Several different instruments, including the Endocyte brush, Mimark Helix, Zelsmyr cytobrush, and the Isaac's sampler, have been developed. These instruments are designed to obtain cells for cytologic screening. The cellular material obtained should be put into Bouin's solution rather than formalin. Bouin's solution preserves cytonuclear characteristics, while nuclear detail may be distorted by formalin. Examples of tissues obtained by endometrial sampling are shown in Figures 8-19 and 8-20.

Direct cytologic material from the endometrial cavity has a false negative rate between 5% and 15% when compared to material from D&C or hysterectomy. Although this rate is

substantial, it is virtually identical to the false negative rate of cytologic screening associated with invasive carcinoma of the cervix. Cytologic sampling obtained only from the vaginal pool and endocervical canal is able to diagnose approximately 25% of endometrial carcinomas.

Recommendations and Cost Information

For mass screening, endometrial cytologic sampling has several advantages over endometrial biopsy. The various instruments designed for obtaining endometrial cells for cytology are of a smaller diameter and generally a softer material than biopsy instruments. The majority of procedures performed with the narrow plastic cytologic devices do not require the use of a tenaculum. The foundation of the success or failure of any screening program is patient acceptance, and cytologic screening causes less discomfort than endometrial biopsy. In one comparison study, Ferenczy and Gelfand reported

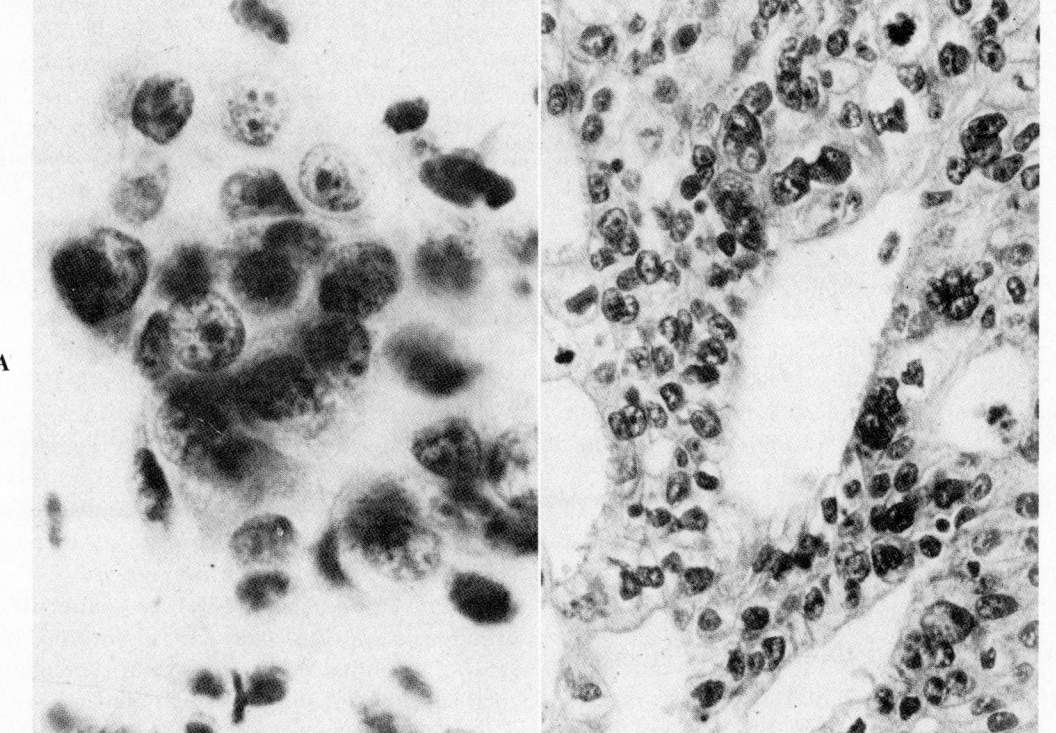

FIGURE 8-20
Adenocarcinoma of endometrium. **A,** Endocyte cytology of highly atypical epithelial cells with large, round pleomorphic nuclei and prominent nucleoli. There is
severe cellular crowding and overlapping (Papanicolaou; × 1000). **B,** Kevorkian
biopsy of well-differentiated adenocarcinoma with cribriform glandular pattern.
Cells have distributed cohesion and organization and pleomorphic nuclei (H&E; ×
500). (From Ferenczy A and Gelfand MM: Obstet Gynecol 63:300, 1984. Reprinted with permission from The American College of Obstetricians and Gynecologists.)

that 100% of the women returned who had undergone sampling of the endometrium with a
brush, while only 40% of the women who had
endometrial biopsies would consent to a subsequent biopsy procedure. The disadvantages of
endometrial cytology as compared to endometrial biopsy are common to most screening procedures. They include decreased accuracy and
decreased sensitivity in identifying endometrial
hyperplasia.

The major advantages to the patient of the
endometrial biopsy over D&C are convenience
and cost saving. An endometrial biopsy is an
estimated $500 to $750 less than an outpatient
D&C.

Endometrial biopsy costs between $100 and
$200. Cytologic aspiration of cells from the en-
dometrial cavity costs $30 to $60. The interpre-

tation of a cytologic smear from the endometrium is more complex and takes 3 to 4 times
longer than interpretation of a cervical cytology
smear.

Although multiple instruments are designed
for both endometrial biopsy and cytologic sampling, none is superior. The clinical results obtained depend on two factors, the patient's acceptance and the physician's skill and persever-
ance. The patient's acceptance is higher with
narrow cannulas made of plastic. Liberal use of
paracervical block in difficult procedures allows
the physician to be successful in obtaining tissue in over 95% of cases.

The accuracy of endometrial biopsy in diagnosing malignancy is 90% to 98% when compared to subsequent findings at D&C or hysterectomy. Therefore, if abnormal perimeno-

pausal or menopausal bleeding recurs following an endometrial biopsy, a D&C should be performed to rule out carcinoma. Routine preoperative endometrial biopsy in asymptomatic women undergoing hysterectomy has not proved necessary. Most physicians perform a D&C if the endometrial biopsy demonstrates an advanced endometrial hyperplasia. However, in a retrospective review of 223 patients, Daniel and Peters found that 16% of tumors had a more advanced grade of endometrial carcinoma at hysterectomy than after office curettage. Also, 10% of tumors had a higher grade after operating room D&C, not a significant difference compared with office sampling. Regardless of how meticulously and aggressively endometrial biopsy is performed, dilation of the cervix improves the ability to sample a larger area of the endometrial lining.

HYSTEROSALPINGOGRAPHY

Hysterosalpingography (HSG) is an x-ray imaging technique in which the uterine cavity and lumina of the fallopian tubes are visualized by injecting contrast material through the cervical canal. This test was first described by two investigators, Rubin and Cary, working independently in 1914. There have been numerous recent refinements in techniques and contrast material. The most dramatic advance has been the addition of image intensification with screen fluoroscopy, which provides more precise visualization and reduces radiation exposure. HSG is a safe and rapid means of investigating abnormalities in the uterus and fallopian tubes (Figure 8-21). Often an inference of abnormal function can be postulated from an abnormal HSG. These judgments should not be absolute; for example, approximately 15% of women who have "obstructed" fallopian tubes diagnosed by HSG subsequently become pregnant without further treatment.

The leading indications for HSG are primary and secondary infertility. This imaging technique gives evidence of tubal patency, tubal mobility, and sometimes peritubal disease (Figure 8-22). Laparoscopy is a more sophisticated and expensive method of diagnosing the tubal factor during an infertility investigation. Chromopertubation with an innocuous dye, such as indigo carmine, demonstrates tubal patency during laparoscopy. Comparative studies have documented that HSG discovers only 50% of the peritubal disease diagnosed by direct visualization via the laparoscope. Tubal obstruction via HSG has a false positive rate of approximately 15%. The etiology of this false reading is thought to be tubal spasm. The study by Hutchins of 409 infertile patients who had sequential HSG and laparoscopy under general anesthesia enriched our understanding of tubal spasm. In this series, HSG showed 93 women to have blocked tubes, and 30 of these were patent by chromopertubation. Pain relief does not invariably alleviate tubal spasm. Tubal anomalies, including diverticula and accessory ostia, can be diagnosed by HSG. In summary, HSG is useful in diagnosing intrinsic disease of the fallopian tubes, while laparoscopy is more effective in identifying extrinsic disease.

Uterine cavity abnormalities, present in 10% of infertile women, may be discovered by HSG. Congenital müllerian system anomalies, such as bicornuate, septate, arcuate, and T-shaped uteri (associated with in utero diethylstilbestrol exposure), may be diagnosed (Figure 8-23). Malformations such as synechiae of the endometrial cavity may also be discovered (Figure 8-24). HSG is a basic and essential tool in the evaluation of patients with poor reproductive histories. It is specifically applicable for women with repetitive second-trimester losses. The technique is frequently performed preoperatively and postoperatively in patients undergoing tubal or plastic surgery to correct tubal obstruction or uterine anomalies or to remove myomas.

HSG has been used to diagnose an incompetent internal cervical os by measuring its diameter (Figure 8-25). The maximum normal diameter of the isthmus and internal cervical os is reported to be between 0.7 and 1.0 cm. The anatomic changes in the diameter of the internal os in the nonpregnant state may have little predictive value for future competency in pregnancy because of the dynamic changes during pregnancy that affect cross-linking of collagen and water content of the ground substance in the cervical stroma.

Women with amenorrhea and a history of curettage who do not respond to a hormonal challenge should have an HSG, hysteroscopy, or both. Uterine synechiae are identified by

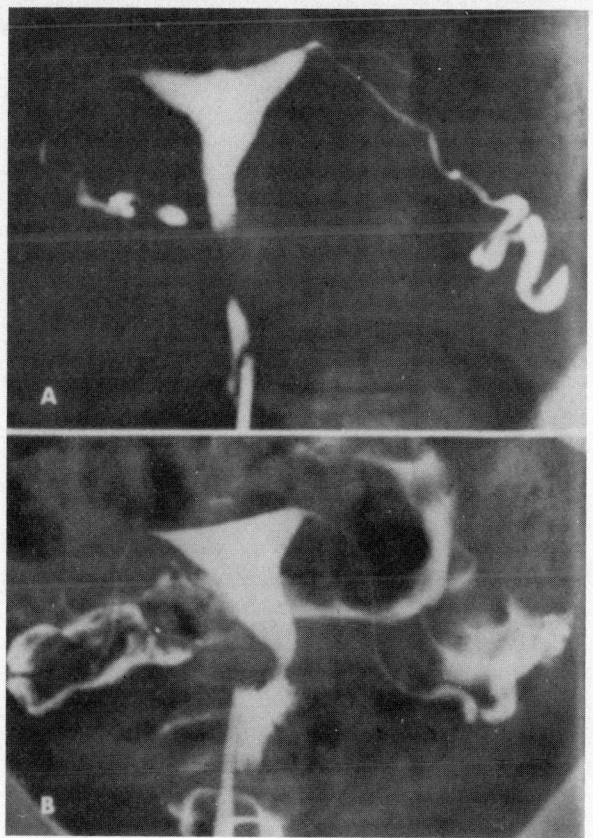

FIGURE 8-21
Two normal hysterosalpingograms. (From Soules MR and Spadoni LR: Oil versus aqueous media for hysterosalpingography: a continuing debate based on many opinions and few facts, Fertil Steril 38:1, 1982. Reproduced with permission of the publisher, The American Fertility Society.)

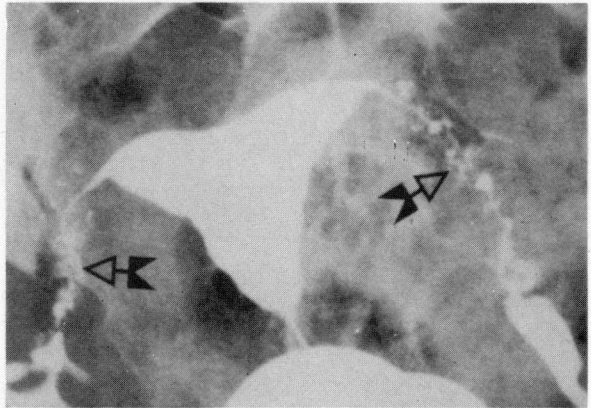

FIGURE 8-22
Hysterosalpingogram from patient with tubal endometriosis. Flecks of contrast material *(arrows)* are seen about isthmus without central linear pattern. Distal ends appear normally patent. (From Siegler AM: Hysterosalpingography, Fertil Steril 40:139, 1983. Reproduced with permission of the publisher, The American Fertility Society.)

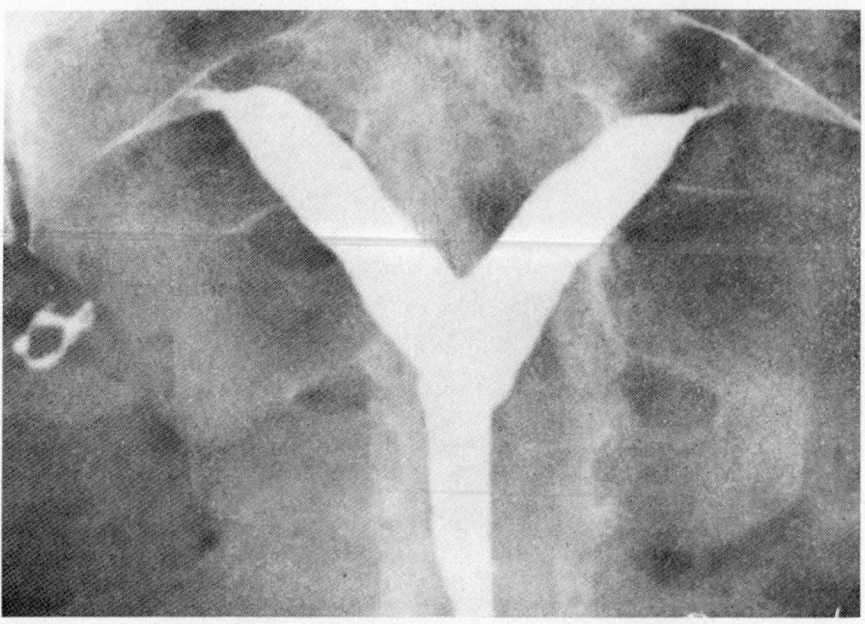

FIGURE 8-23
Hysterosalpingogram from 34-year-old, nulliparous woman who had regular menses and no dysmenorrhea. V-shaped fundal defect with single cervix proved to be bicornuate uterus. (From Siegler AM: Hysterosalpingography, New York, 1967, Harper & Row, Publishers, Inc.)

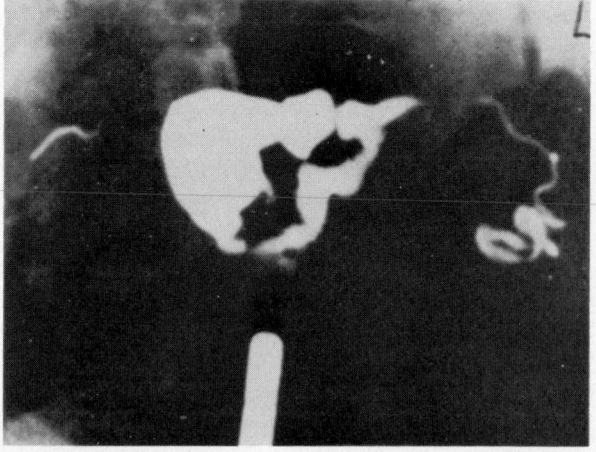

FIGURE 8-24
Hysterosalpingogram demonstrating intrauterine adhesions, grade 3, after repeated curettage for missed abortion. (From Schenker JG and Margalioth EJ: Intrauterine adhesions: an updated appraisal, Fertil Steril 37:593, 1982. Reproduced with permission of the publisher, The American Fertility Society.)

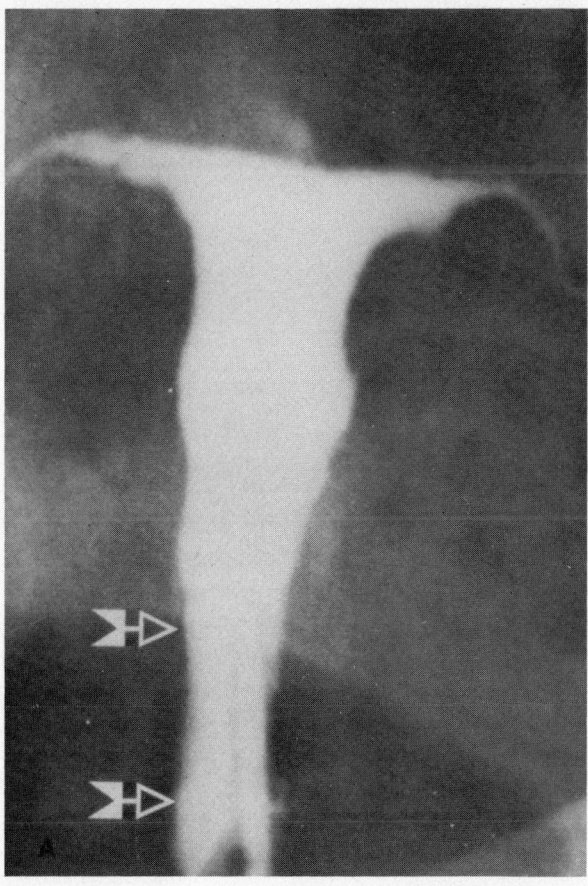

FIGURE 8-25

Hysterosalpingogram demonstrating dilated lower uterine segment *(arrows)* associated with previous second-trimester abortion suggesting incompetent cervix. (From Siegler AM: Hysterosalpingography, Fertil Steril 40:139, 1983. Reproduced with permission of the publisher, The American Fertility Society.)

slowly injecting a water-soluble medium. If the patient has synechiae, tubal obstruction, and pelvic calcifications, a diagnosis of pelvic tuberculosis should be strongly suspected. HSG will also discover polyps or small submucous myomas in refractory cases of abnormal uterine bleeding.

Contraindications to HSG include the obvious: acute pelvic infection, active uterine bleeding, pregnancy, and allergy to iodine.

The choice of using a small Foley catheter or an adjustable rubber or plastic acorn and cannula for injection depends on physician preference. This decision does not seem to bias results as long as all air in the system is replaced by the liquid contrast medium. The choice of water-soluble versus oil-based contrast medium depends on the primary indication for the test and physician preference. The advantages and disadvantages of various contrast media have

been reviewed by Soules and Spadoni. Water-soluble iodine is preferred for documenting intrauterine filling defects and identifying the severity of mucosal damage in chronic tubal infection. Lipid-based material provides a more distinct and clearer radiographic image. Periodically the opinion has been expressed that the pregnancy rate after HSG is 2 to 3 times greater with oil-soluble media. It is difficult to control the multiple variables associated with this finding. However, DeCherney et al. have suggested instillation of 5 ml of oil-based material for its therapeutic effect immediately following a normal diagnostic study with water-based material.

The endpoint of an x-ray examination for tubal patency is either tubal filling with intraperitoneal spilling or increasing pelvic pain secondary to uterine distention associated with tubal obstruction. Tubal spasm may sometimes be

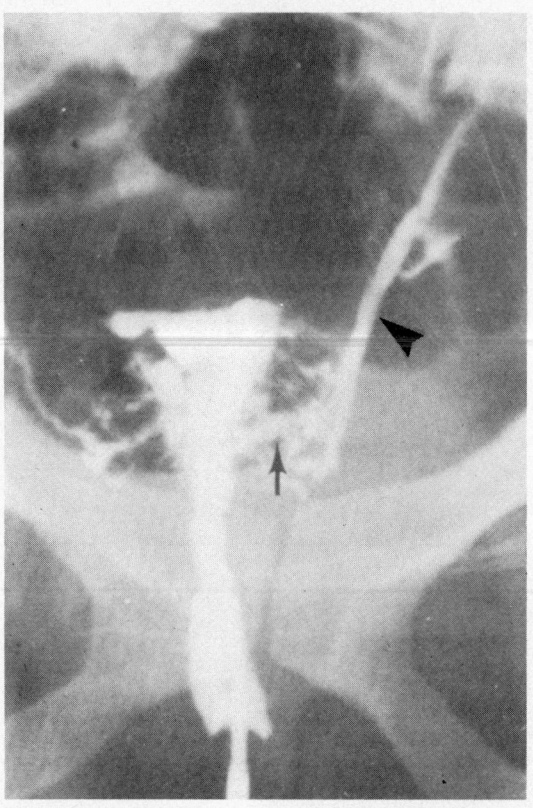

FIGURE 8-26
Hysterosalpingogram showing both lymphatic (*small arrow*) and venous (*large arrow*) intravasation. (From Soules MR and Spandoni LR: Oil versus aqueous media for hysterosalpingography: a continuing debate based on many opinions and few facts, Fertil Steril 38:1, 1982. Reproduced with permission of the publisher, The American Fertility Society.)

overcome by glucagon (2 mg intravenously), which produces atony of smooth muscle. Glucagon is effective in about one of three women with tubal spasm.

Complications of HSG are rare, but serious when they happen. Acute pelvic infection serious enough to require hospitalization develops in 0.3% to 3.1% of patients. This incidence of pelvic infection is directly related to the population studied, that is, more common in women with dilated tubes. The use of prophylactic antibiotics (tetracycline) may reduce the incidence of acute infection following instrumentation of the uterus. As with surgical procedures that invade the uterus, pelvic pain, uterine perforation, and vasovagal vasomotor reactions do occur. Allergic reactions, particularly to the

iodine dye, are a possibility. Intravasation of the dye into the vascular system occurs with high injection pressures, partial perforation of the cannula, and endometrial defects associated with synechiae (Figure 8-26). Embolic phenomena have been observed with oil-based contrast material. Pelvic peritonitis and granuloma formation with oil-based dye is a very rare complication.

Recommendations and Cost Information

In summary, HSG is a rapid and relatively safe imaging technique. Its major uses are in the evaluation of patients with infertility or poor pregnancy outcomes. The procedure can diagnose uterine and tubal abnormalities with success. Both oil- and water-based dyes are used. Recent advances in office hysteroscopy may lead to a substantial decrease in the use of HSG.

With a TV screen image intensifier, the average HSG takes 10 minutes to perform. This procedure involves approximately 90 seconds of fluoroscopic time and an average radiation exposure to the ovaries of 1 to 2 rads. The average cost of this outpatient test is between $125 and $175.

HYSTEROSCOPY

Hysteroscopy, the oldest gynecologic endoscopic procedure, is the direct visualization of the endometrial cavity using an endoscope and a light source. The earliest hysteroscope was nothing more than a hollow tube with an alcohol lamp and mirror for a light source. In 1869 Pantalloni reported the successful removal of an endometrial polyp through the scope. Modern hysteroscopes are modifications of cystoscopes with a channel for a fiberoptic light, a channel to introduce surgical instruments, and a channel to introduce various media to distend the uterus.

Twenty years ago interest in hysteroscopy increased as a result of both improved instrumentation and the use of dextran (Hyskon) as a distending medium. The popularity of hysteroscopy has also been enhanced by the fact that it is a simple technique, much easier to master than laparoscopy. The diagnostic and therapeutic indications for hysteroscopy are also rapidly expanding. Women with recurrent abnormal bleeding, repetitive abortion, uterine synechiae, abnormal HSGs, and infertility are candidates for hysteroscopy. Surgical procedures, which usually require anesthesia, performed under hysteroscopic guidance include location and removal of intact or fragmented IUDs, resection of submucous myomas, lysis of synechiae, incision of uterine septa, removal of endometrial polyps, laser ablation of the endometrium, and placement of silicone plugs into the tubes for sterilization.

Hysteroscopes vary from 4 to 8 mm in diameter (Figure 8-27). The smaller-caliber scopes, 4 to 5 mm, are used for diagnostic purposes. The angle of view is 30 degrees. Similar to that of a cystoscope, the outer sleeve contains several channels that extend the full length of the instrument, as described earlier.

The cavity of the uterus is a potential space. The success of hysteroscopy depends on the medium used to expand this space. The three most popular choices for diagnostic hysteroscopy are 32% dextran, 5% dextrose and water, and carbon dioxide gas. High-molecular-weight dextran (average molecular weight, 70,000 in 10% glucose) is preferred by the majority of investigators, especially if a surgical procedure is contemplated. This extremely viscous fluid is biodegradable, nontoxic, and nonconductive and has good optical qualities. Most important, dextran is immiscible with blood; this helps to keep the field clear during intrauterine surgery. Dextran has two drawbacks: it is antigenic, and anaphylaxis has been reported. It also rapidly crystallizes; thus endoscopic instruments must be cleaned shortly after the procedure. Carbon dioxide must be infused with special equipment that carefully limits flow to less than 100 ml per minute and maintains the pressure at approximately 60 to 70 mm Hg. The major precaution with 5% dextrose and water is the monitoring of total fluid intake so as not to produce fluid overload.

Hysteroscopy is usually an office procedure. A local anesthetic may be applied to the endocervix, or a paracervical block may be used. Anxious patients may be pretreated with diazepam and/or a nonsteroidal antiinflammatory agent.

Hysteroscopy is ideal to directly visualize and remove partially perforated or broken IUDs. Women with repetitive abortions should have a diagnostic hysteroscopic procedure. Congenital abnormalities that interfere with the success of early pregnancies, such as septa of the uterus, may be seen (Figure 8-28). Women with recurrent abnormal uterine bleeding may also benefit from this procedure. Often endometrial polyps or small submucous myomas are discovered and may be removed. The extent and location of the uterine synechiae are best described by hysteroscopic examination.

In Europe, endometrial carcinoma is staged by hysteroscopy. In one series, 26% of stage I carcinomas of the endometrium were upgraded to stage II by direct visualization of spread from the fundus to the cervix. Hysteroscopy is helpful in differentiating between adenocarcinoma of the endometrium and endocervix. The theoretic concerns of washing viable malignant cells from the endometrial cavity into the peritoneal cavity and increasing pelvic metastatic disease has not been demonstrated. In the future, hysteroscopy may replace many diagnostic D&C procedures. No matter how meticulous the surgeon is, he or she may miss a focal lesion, particularly pedunculated structures. D&C is a blind, hit-or-miss procedure. With the hysteroscope the gynecologist may visually

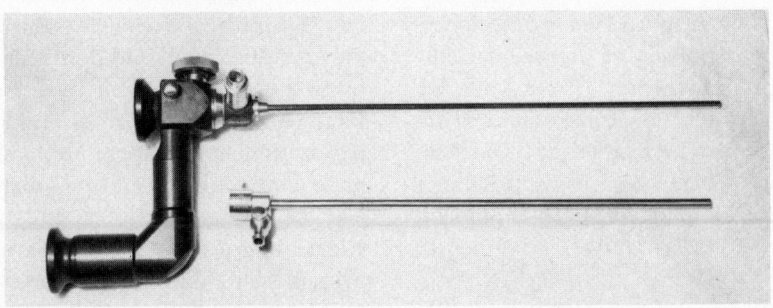

FIGURE 8-27
A 5 mm hysteroscope (Storz Instruments).

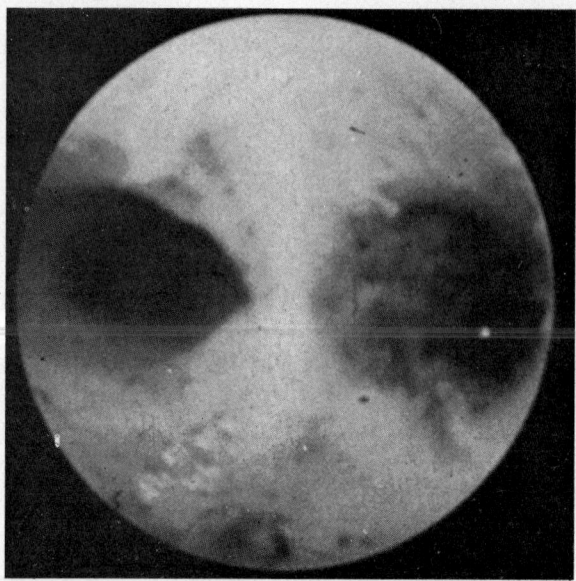

FIGURE 8-28
Intraoperative hysteroscopic view of septate uterus showing inferior point of septum and each uterine horn. (From Israel R and March CM: Am J Obstet Gynecol 149:67, 1984.)

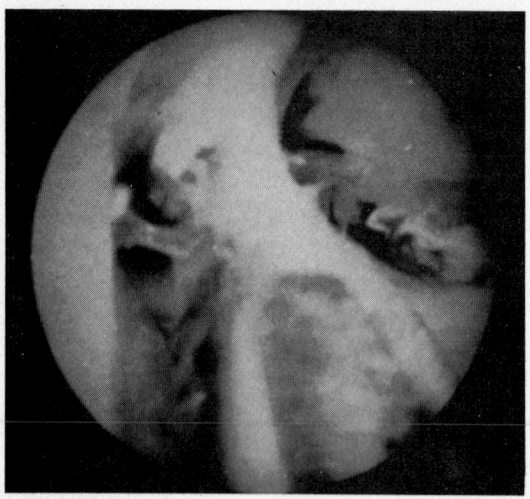

FIGURE 8-29
Hysteroscopic view of intrauterine adhesion in right lateral upper portion of uterus, partially occluding uterotubal junction. (From Valle RF and Sciarra JJ: Hysteroscopic treatment of intrauterine adhesions. In Siegler AM and Lindemann HJ, editors: Hysteroscopy: principles and practice, Philadelphia, 1984, JB Lippincott Co.)

direct the biopsy forceps to the suspicious area.

Hysteroscopy is superior to HSG in discovering intrauterine disease. In comparative studies the use of hysteroscopy revealed synechiae, polyps, or myomas in 40% of patients with normal HSGs (Figure 8-29). These abnormalities were undetected and unsuspected using x-ray techniques. The false positive rate of HSG is 33% when compared to hysteroscopy. One in three women diagnosed as having an intrauterine filling defect by x-ray imaging will have a normal cavity directly visualized with the hysteroscope.

Recently contact hysteroscopy has become more popular because of its simplicity, since a distending medium is not needed. The contact hysteroscope touches the surface to be viewed, and blood and debris are pushed away from the field of vision by gentle tissue contact. The interpretation of endometrial pathology is similar to colposcopy in that it depends on color, contour, and vascular pattern. The contact hysteroscope is the instrument of choice to examine the vagina of an infant or prepubertal child. Hamou developed a microhysteroscope that does not require cervical dilation. This instrument has interchangeable lenses that produce magnifications of ×1, ×20, ×60, and ×150. He uses the higher magnifications to perform contact microcolposcopy of the endocervical canal. This necessitates staining with a vital stain, such as Waterman's blue ink.

The variety and extent of surgery performed transcervically with the hysteroscope have expanded significantly with technologic advances. Endoscopic procedures have progressed from snaring a small polyp to ablating the entire endometrial lining with a laser.

Operative hysteroscopy may be performed with mechanical devices such as small operating scissors, electrocautery, and modified resectoscopes and lasers. Laser hysteroscopy with carbon dioxide or neodymium:yttrium-argon-garnet (Nd:YAG) lasers requires more expensive equipment and expertise and to date has not proved more advantageous than simpler techniques. Operative hysteroscopy usually requires general anesthesia and is best performed in the operating room. The uterine synechiae of a woman with Asherman's syndrome can be cut with microscissors, gradually reestablishing the endometrial cavity. Following the operation, a large plastic IUD is placed in the cavity as a stent. For the next 2 months the patient should receive 7.5 mg of conjugated estrogen per day to facilitate regeneration and reepithelialization of the endometrium. An oral progestogen should be given during the last 10 days of estrogen therapy. By performing this operation on an outpatient basis and transcervically, major morbidity and expense can be avoided. Valle and Sciarra reported a series of 187 patients who underwent hysteroscopy for intrauterine pathologic conditions and infertility. Postoperatively, 88% resumed normal menstruation. Seventy-six percent of women became pregnant, 80% of whom carried pregnancies to term.

Hysteroscopic metroplasty of intrauterine septa has been successful and is safer with less complications than laparotomy. However, concurrent laparoscopy is advocated by most investigators to evaluate the rest of the pelvis. Transabdominal metroplasty involves a uterine incision, necessitating that future pregnancies be delivered by cesarean section. Daly et al. reported 70 consecutive hysteroscopic metroplasties. Subsequently, 51 patients become pregnant; 80% went to viability, and 73% went to term. The primary cesarean delivery rate was 20%.

Neuwirth has pioneered a method of removing submucous myomas with a modified uro-

logic resectoscope. He uses a cutting electric current and shaves the myoma until it is flat with the surrounding endometrial lining. An inflatable balloon is inserted into the uterine cavity and left for 24 hours, facilitating hemostasis. After the procedure, endometrial regeneration is stimulated with oral estrogen.

Many groups have attempted to develop a method of outpatient transcervical sterilization. The most sophisticated technique uses a hyst-

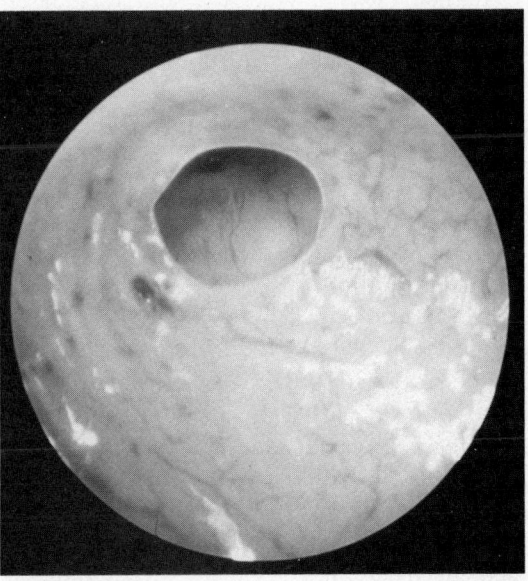

FIGURE 8-30
Hysteroscopic view of tubal ostium. (From Hamou JE: Clin Obstet Gynecol 26:290, 1983.)

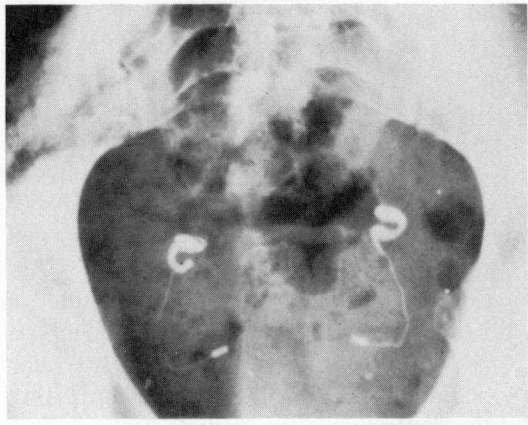

FIGURE 8-31
Normal silicon plugs on pelvic flat-plate radiograph. (From Houck RM, Cooper JM, and Rigberg HS: Obstet Gynecol 62:588, 1983. Reproduced with permission from The American College of Obstetricians and Gynecologists.)

eroscope to inject liquid silicone into the tubal ostia (Figures 8-30 and 8-31). A special catalyzer causes the liquid to form a plug within a few minutes. The silicone contains radiopaque silver powder so it may be visualized by a pelvic radiograph. The procedure is still in the experimental stages. Approximately 85% of women have plugs successfully placed. In preliminary studies, failure rates have been similar to those for other methods of female sterilization.

Carbon dioxide, Nd:YAG, and KTP lasers may be used for removal of adhesions, septa, or myomas and for the ablation of the endometrium.

Goldrath et al. pioneered the ablation of the endometrial lining using the hysteroscopic-directed laser. The laser photovaporizes the epithelium. This procedure is performed in women with severe dysfunctional uterine bleeding who are not candidates for hysterectomy. The procedure usually takes 1 hour and is most effective in producing amenorrhea in women over age 40. Hysterograms following laser treatment have demonstrated contraction, scarring, and dense adhesion formation. Electrocoagulation with a resectoscope or a rollerball may also be used for endometrial ablation. Although these procedures are generally safe and effective, long-term follow-up and information concerning the potential for endometrial carcinoma to develop in unablated foci have not been determined. Endometrial ablation, by either electrocautery or laser, produces amenorrhea in approximately half of patients, with substantially decreased bleeding in another 40%.

There are few contraindications to hysteroscopy. Acute pelvic infection is the leading one because of the potential of spreading the disease by the media used for uterine distention. Active bleeding is a relative contraindication. If the bleeding is brisk, the hysteroscopic procedure will be unsatisfactory. Pregnancy is a contraindication.

Complications of hysteroscopy are noted in less than 2% of the procedures. The complications include uterine perforation, pelvic infection, and bleeding. The potential complications of the distending media include anaphylaxis to dextran, circulatory overload with 5% dextrose and water, and the potential of gas embolism with carbon dioxide. Cardiac arrests have been reported with uterine insufflation with carbon dioxide when unmonitored amounts of gas were used.

Recommendations and Cost Information

In summary, hysteroscopy is a simple technique for the evaluation of intrauterine pathology. The use of the hysteroscope for intrauterine surgery is rapidly expanding. The cost of a diagnostic hysteroscopic procedure is between $250 and $500, depending on whether therapeutic instruments are used. Operative hysteroscopic costs vary and depend on the time involved and the specific procedure performed.

LAPAROSCOPY

Laparoscopy has radically changed the clinical practice of gynecology over the past 25 years. This outpatient surgical technique provides a window to directly visualize pelvic anatomy as well as a technique to perform many operations with less morbidity than laparotomy (Figure 8-32). Today laparoscopy has replaced D&C as the most frequently performed operation by the gynecologic service of university hospitals.

Laparoscopy was first performed in the early 1900s. Two events of the early 1960s renewed interest in this surgical technique, the first being the development of fiberoptic cables and the second the change in society's attitude toward overpopulation and sterilization. Patrick Steptoe is considered the "father" of modern laparoscopy for his work in the mid-1960s with laparoscopic sterilization. By the mid-1970s laparoscopy had been adopted as the method of choice for female sterilization.

The advantages of low cost, convenience, and shorter stay are obvious when laparoscopy is compared to celiotomy (laparotomy). Minilaparotomy in a thin woman may be competitive in time and cost to laparoscopy. However, if a woman is moderately obese, there is no comparison.

There are several indications for laparoscopy, both diagnostic and therapeutic. The most common indication is female sterilization. Laparoscopy is an essential step in the diagnostic workup of a couple with infertility or a woman with chronic pelvic pain. In the past decade, gynecologists have progressed from using the laparoscope to perform such simple surgical tasks as removal of a perforated IUD to more complicated surgery, such as evacuating unruptured ectopic pregnancies, adhesiolysis (cutting of adhesions), and treatment of endometriosis.

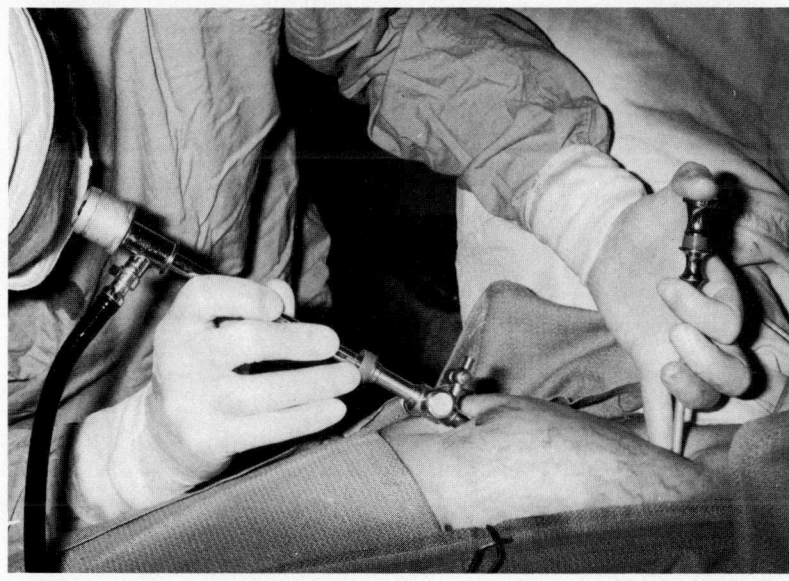

FIGURE 8-32
Insertion of accessory trocar for laparoscopy is made under direct visual control of operator. (From Cibils LA: Gynecologic laparoscopy, Philadelphia, 1975, Lea & Febiger.)

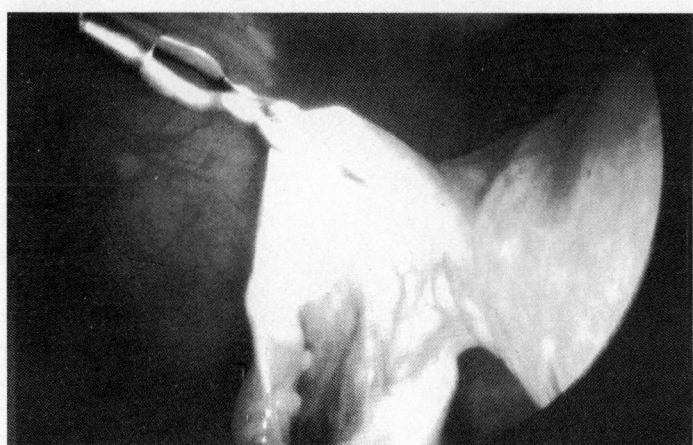

FIGURE 8-33
Laparoscopic view of bipolar coagulation. Kleppinger bipolar forceps has been used to coagulate isthmic-ampullary junction of this tube in three contiguous places. (From Hulka JF: Textbook of laparoscopy, Orlando, Fla, 1985, Grune & Stratton, Inc.)

Laparoscopy has made outpatient sterilization available to women throughout the world. The failure rate is approximately 1 in 250 to 1 in 500 cases. Sterilization is accomplished with electric cauterization, Silastic bands, or spring-loaded clips. Because of the serious complications with unipolar cautery, most cautery sterilization procedures are performed with bipolar coagulation of approximately 2 cm of the tube without division (Figure 8-33). Of the nonelectric alternatives, the Silastic bands have a lower failure rate than the clips (Figure 8-34). However, with the bands, 2 to 3 procedures per 100 result in acute transection of the tube with bleeding from the tube or mesosalpinx. Hemostasis can be obtained by applying another

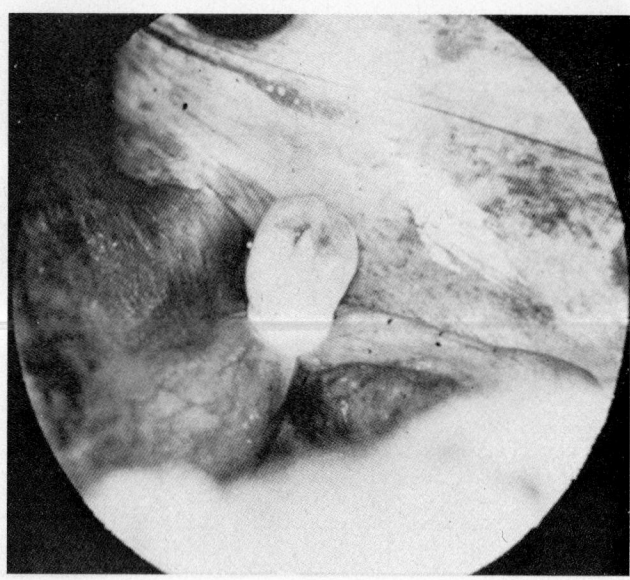

FIGURE 8-34
Laparoscopic view of a Falope-Ring applied to fallopian tube. (From Yoon I: Silicone ring. In Phillips JM, ed: Laparoscopy. Copyright © 1977 by The Williams & Wilkins Co, Baltimore.)

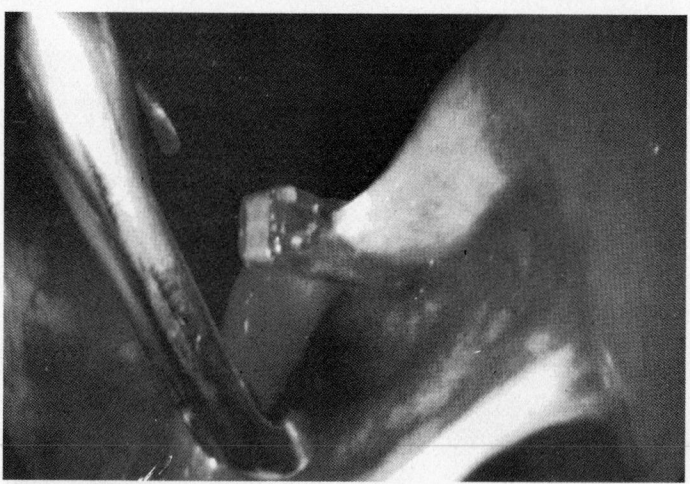

FIGURE 8-35
Laparoscopic view of clip application. Clip has been correctly applied within 1 to 2 cm of uterine fundus. (From Hulka JF: Textbook of laparoscopy, Orlando, Fla, 1985, Grune & Stratton, Inc.)

band or with cautery. The spring-loaded clip causes necrosis of less than 1 cm of tube and is the easiest sterilization procedure to successfully reverse (Figure 8-35). The clip or the band should be placed on the narrow isthmus so the size of the appliance conforms to the diameter of the fallopian tube.

There are several indications for laparoscopy in infertile women, both diagnostic and thera-

peutic. Tubal patency and mobility can be directly observed via the laparoscope (Figure 8-36). Laparoscopy is able to confirm or rule out intrinsic pelvic disorders, such as endometriosis or chronic pelvic inflammatory disease. It is possible not only to describe and stage the extent of endometriosis or pelvic adhesions but to treat them. Adhesions can be lysed and areas of endometriosis can be ablated by electro-

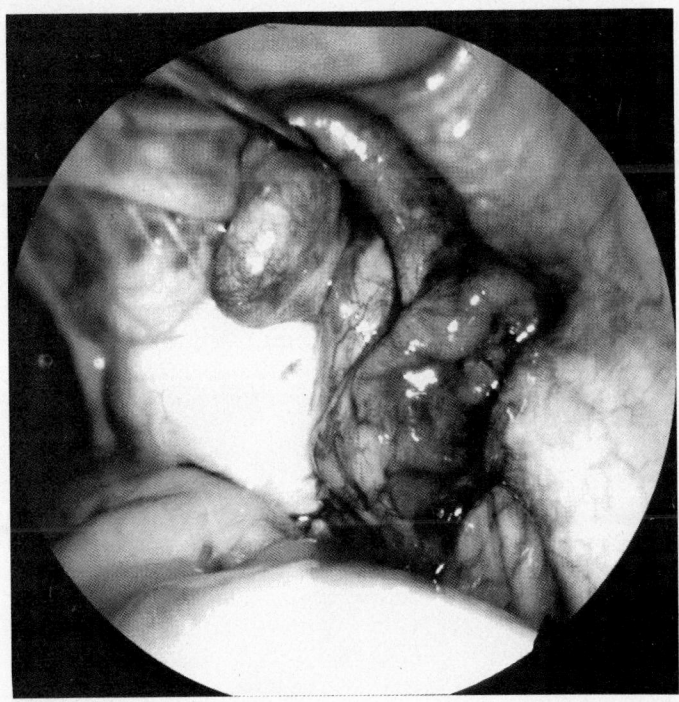

FIGURE 8-36
Laparoscopic view of normal patient tube. (From Hulka JF: Textbook of laparoscopy, Orlando, Fla, 1985, Grune & Stratton, Inc.)

cautery or laser. Oocyte recovery for in vitro fertilization has been performed by direct aspiration of the developing follicle under laparoscopic direction.

The management of a patient with pelvic pain has been dramatically changed by the laparoscope. The differential diagnosis of acute pain may be defined by direct visualization of the fallopian tubes, ovaries, and appendix. Several centers include laparoscopy in the management of acute pelvic infection, taking direct bacterial cultures of purulent material from the tubes. These direct transabdominal cultures have changed our opinions concerning the clinical management of polymicrobial pelvic infections. The enigma of chronic pelvic pain may be solved by the findings at laparoscopy (Figure 8-37). Following the procedure, a plan for long-term management of the pain can be discussed with the patient.

Besides diagnostic uses, the laparoscope can be utilized for therapeutic indications (Figure 8-38). Intraperitoneal intrauterine devices are best retrieved with the laparoscope. Laparoscopic ovarian biopsy (for karyotyping in certain endocrine disorders) is possible. Lysis of adhesions, evacuation of small ec-

topic pregnancies, and treatment of endometriosis are therapeutic uses of the laparoscope. The limits and indications of surgical procedures via the laparoscope depend on the experience and judgment of the surgeon. At some point, celiotomy is the more reasonable decision.

Absolute contraindications to laparoscopy include intestinal obstruction, significant hemoperitoneum, anticoagulation therapy, advanced malignancy, large abdominal masses, severe cardiovascular disease, and tuberculous peritonitis. Relative contraindications, in which each case must be individualized, include extensive obesity, hiatal hernia, advanced pregnancy, generalized peritonitis, and extensive intraabdominal scarring.

Laparoscopy may be performed under local or general anesthesia. Many prefer local anesthesia for its safety. The risks associated with general anesthesia are one of the major hazards of laparoscopy. However, when operative laparoscopy is contemplated, general anesthesia is recommended. As Gomel has summarized, the requirements of operative laparoscopy include general anesthesia to ensure adequate muscle relaxation, patient comfort, and the ability to

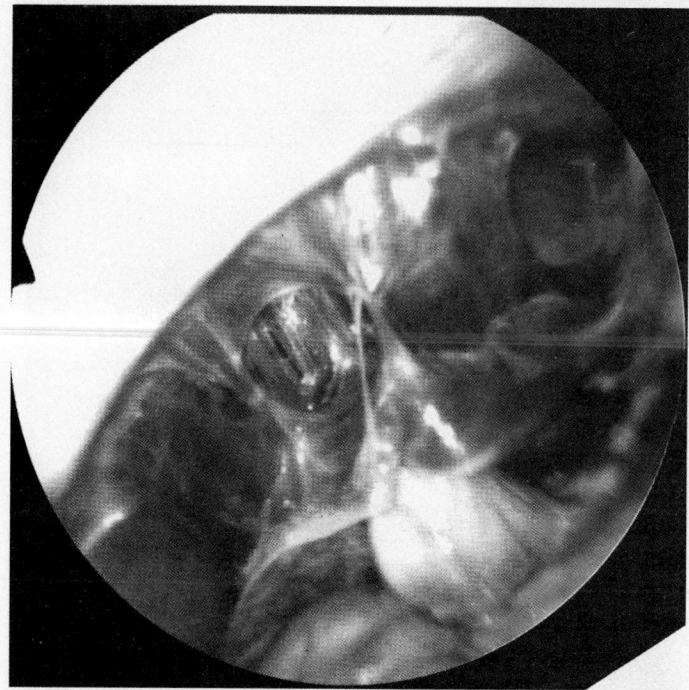

FIGURE 8-37
Laparoscopic view of Fitz-Hugh Curtis syndrome. (From Hulka JF: Textbook of laparoscopy, Orlando, Fla, 1985, Grune & Stratton, Inc.)

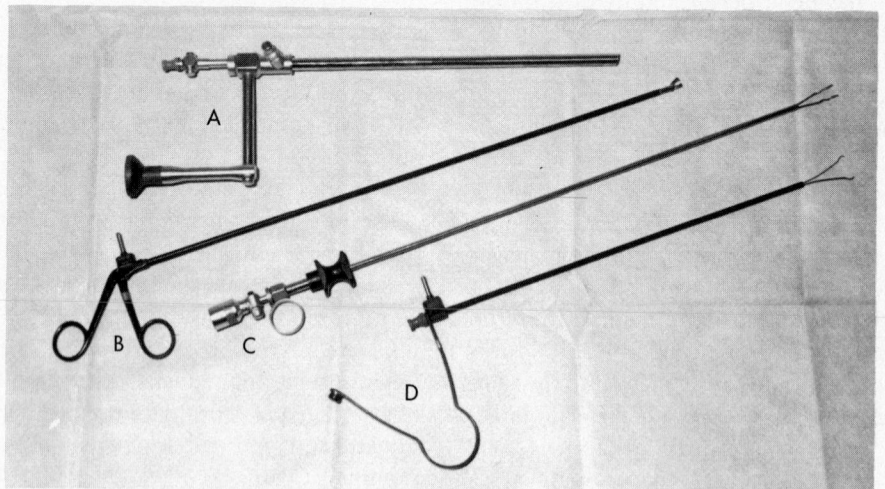

FIGURE 8-38
A, Operating laparoscope with instruments: **B,** scissors; **C,** cautery; and **D,** forceps.

manipulate intraabdominal organs. The most frequent complication of laparoscopy is hypercarbia associated with hypoventilation. The standard diagnostic laparoscope is 10 mm in diameter. Secondary puncture trochars vary from 5 mm (bipolar forceps) to 7 or 8 mm in width (spring-loaded clip and Silastic band). A laparoscope is 30 cm long and provides

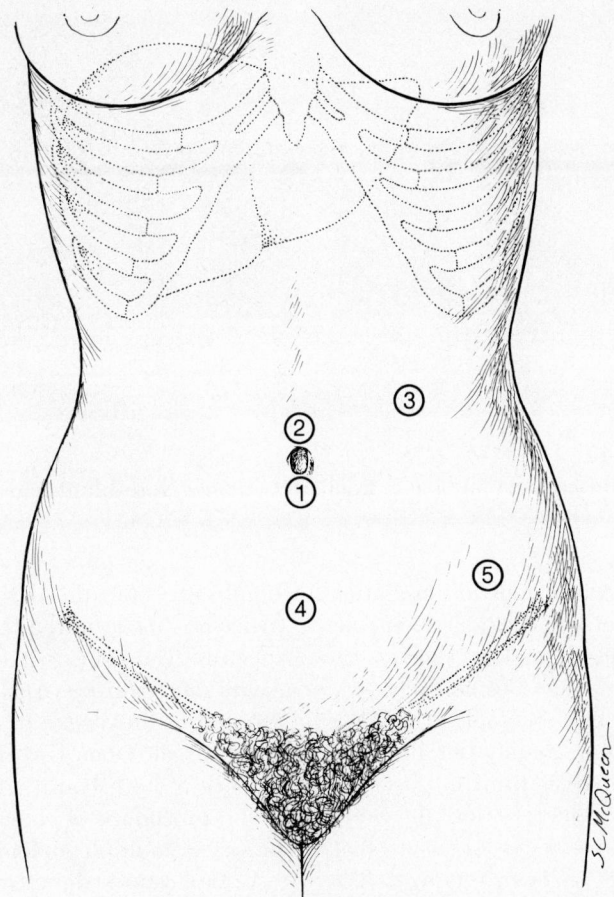

FIGURE 8-39
Usual sites for insertion of insufflating needle in laparoscopy: (1) infraumbilical fold,
(2) supraumbilical fold, (3) left costal margin, (4) midway between umbilicus and
pubis, and (5) left McBurney's point. (From Corson SL: Operating room preparation and basic techniques. In Phillips JM, editor: Laparoscopy. Copyright © 1977
by the Williams & Wilkins Co, Baltimore.)

a field of vision of 60 to 75 degrees. The
inferior margin of the umbilicus is the preferred site of entry, as this is the thinnest area
of the abdominal wall. Alternative sites are
detailed in Figure 8-39. The choice of gas to
develop the pneumoperitoneum depends on
the choice of anesthesia. Nitrous oxide is preferable with local anesthesia, while carbon dioxide is the choice with general anesthesia. Nitrous oxide is nonflammable but does support
combustion. Carbon dioxide quickly forms car-
bonic acid on the moist parietal peritoneal
surface, which results in considerable discomfort to a patient without regional or general
anesthesia.

Operative laparoscopy may be performed
with mechanical instruments, including an extensive variety of scissors, scalpels, endoscopic
syringes, manipulators, suture devices (en-
doloops), electrocautery instruments (both unipolar and bipolar), and laser instruments. During operative laparoscopy, stabilization of the
pelvic organ is essential, such as traction on the
edges of an adhesion. Thus third and fourth
puncture sites are often required. Because
each puncture site is a potential gas leak, high-
flow insufflation equipment is necessary. In addition, video cameras are usually employed so
that both surgeon and assistant can work effectively. Unlike the short time needed for diagnostic laparoscopy, operative laparoscopy may
require 1 to 1½ hours. The constant use of the
eyepiece for intraabdominal visualization produces operator eyestrain and interruption of

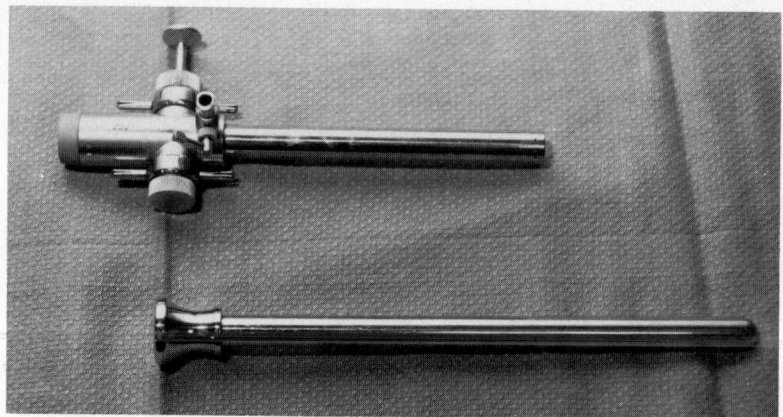

FIGURE 8-40
Open laparoscopy cannula and trochar *(bottom)*. Note blunt end of trochar.

surgical technique. Advantages of operative laparoscopy over celiotomy include decreased postoperative adhesion formation, shorter recovery time, and less, if any, hospital stay.

Laparoscopic treatment of ectopic pregnancy most often involves salpingotomy but also may include salpingectomy. HCG titers must be followed after conservative surgery until the titers fall to zero (usually 3 to 4 weeks) to ensure that all trophoblastic tissue has been removed. Tubal patency and subsequent pregnancy rates are comparable between laparoscopic techniques and celiotomy. Laparoscopic treatment of endometriosis includes lysis of adhesions, ablation of endometriomas, and removal of endometrial cysts. Operative laparoscopy has been used for myomectomy, ovarian biopsy and wedge resection, salpingo-oophorectomy, salpingostomy and fimbrioplasty, appendectomy, uterosacral ligament ligation, and presacral neurectomy. The relative advantages of laparoscopy over celiotomy for these indications, as well as the long-term success, remain under investigation.

The major categories of complications with laparoscopy are laceration of vessels, intestinal injuries, and cardiorespiratory problems arising from the pneumoperitoneum. Since abdominal wall hematomas are usually subfascial in location, care must be taken to avoid the epigastric vessels. Laceration of the aorta, inferior vena cava, or iliac vessels is a surgical emergency. Intestinal injuries may be produced by the Veress needle or the trochar.

Hasson has advocated open laparoscopy to avoid intestinal injury (Figure 8-40). Instead of blind entry into the peritoneal cavity, a small incision is made in the fascia and parietal peritoneum. The cone is placed in the abdominal cavity under direct visual control. The fascia is secured to the sleeve of the cone to obtain an airtight seal. Open laparoscopy reduces the incidence of both bowel and vascular trauma. It is the procedure of choice if the patient has a history of multiple abdominal operations.

Complications directly related to the pneumoperitoneum include pneumothorax, diminished venous return, gas embolism, and cardiac arrhythmias. It is important not to develop pressures greater than 20 mm Hg in establishing the pneumoperitoneum. High pressures impede venous return and limit excursion of the diaphragm. A rare but life-threatening complication of laparoscopy is gas embolism, which produces hypotension and the classical "mill wheel" murmur, which can be heard over the entire precordium. The patient with this complication should be turned on her left side and the frothy blood aspirated by a central venous catheter directed into the right side of the heart.

Recommendations and Cost Information

In summary, laparoscopy, more than any other advance, has changed the clinical practice of gynecology over the past 3 decades. Today's residents have a difficult time contemplating the practice of the specialty prior to the introduction of the "silver tube." Laparoscopy provides a window for the diagnosis of infertil-

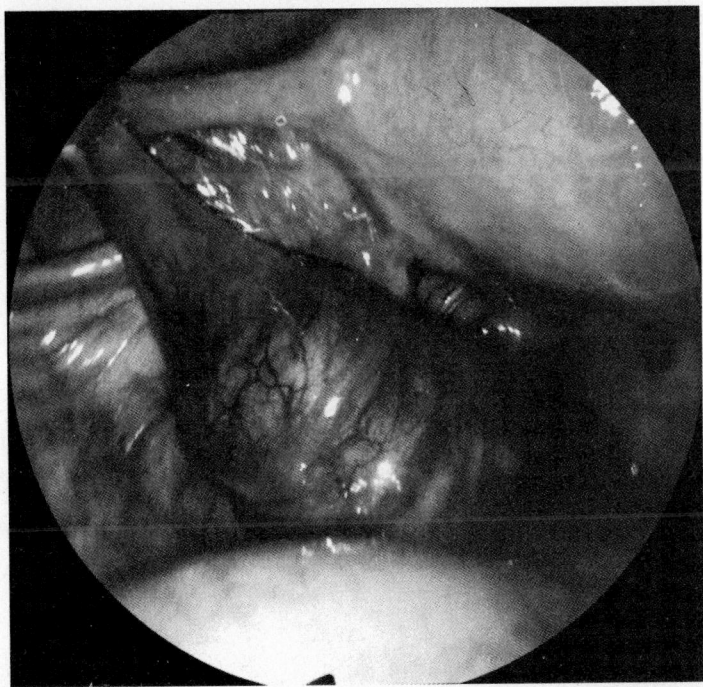

FIGURE 8-41
Laparoscopic view of unruptured ectopic pregnancy. (From Hulka JF: Textbook of laparoscopy, Orlando, Fla, 1985, Grune & Stratton, Inc.)

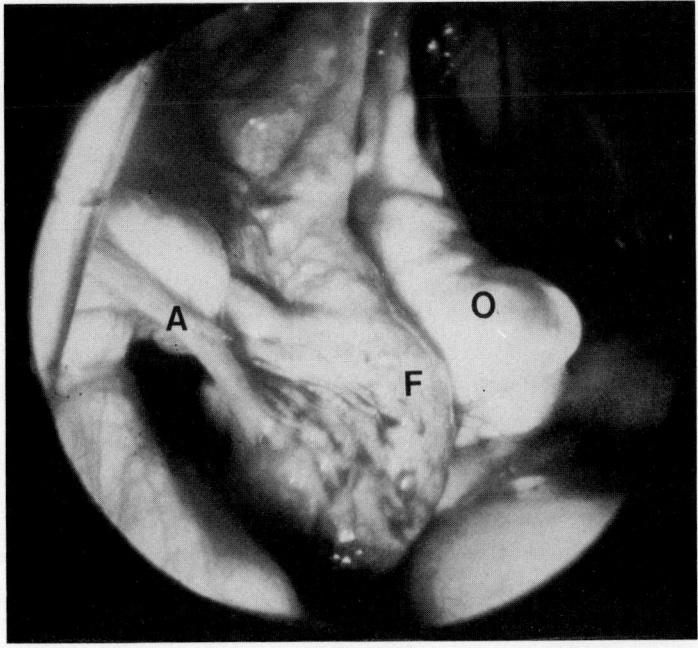

FIGURE 8-42
Laparoscopic view of acute salpingitis. The ovary (*O*) is normal in appearance 12 days postmenstrual with a developing follicle. The fallopian tube (*F*) is indurated inflamed, and erythematous. There is an adhesion (*A*) from the fallopian tube to the pelvic sidewall. (Courtesy Jaroslav Hulka, M.D.)

ity, pelvic pain, ectopic pregnancy, abdominal and pelvic trauma, staging the extent of pelvic disease, and the visual diagnosis of abnormal anatomy. Therapeutically the uses of the laparoscopy include female sterilization, biopsy of abnormal tissue, lysis of adhesions, aspiration of oocytes, retrieval of lost IUDs, and treatment of endometriosis and early ectopic pregnancies (Figure 8-41). The total cost of a diagnostic laparoscopic procedure is between $700 and $1000, which is approximately 25% of the cost of a celiotomy.

KEY POINTS

- A sector scanner is preferable for transabdominal gynecologic ultrasound examinations, as it provides greater visualization of the pelvis than a linear array.

- Endovaginal transducers may provide greater visualization of the pelvic organs than transabdominal ultrasound.

- Sonography has not been found to cause adverse clinical effects in humans with the energy levels used in diagnostic studies.

- Endovaginal ultrasound may be used to visualize an intrauterine pregnancy by 5 weeks after the last normal menstrual period.

- Computed tomography (CT) is useful in discovering extension of pelvic cancer into the fat of the retroperitoneal space and the detection of enlarged lymph nodes.

- For CT the surface radiation dose is between 2 and 10 rads. This radiation exposure is similar to that of a barium enema.

- The major use of CT scans in gynecology has been in evaluating women with pituitary tumors and in identifying retroperitoneal disease during the initial evaluation of pelvic carcinoma.

- Magnetic resonance imaging (MRI) penetrates bone and air without attenuation. Therefore this technique allows identification of soft tissue disease inaccessible to other imaging techniques.

- MRI uses radio frequency radiation, which is nonionizing radiation.

- MRI has the capacity to differentiate normal from malignant tissue and also may identify areas of abnormal tissue metabolism.

- The hematocrit of unclotted blood obtained during culdocentesis will be over 15% when bleeding emanates from an ectopic pregnancy.

- The incidence of false positive culdocentesis in the diagnosis of ectopic pregnancy is less than 2%.

- The diagnostic accuracy of endometrial biopsy is 90% to 98% when compared to subsequent findings at dilation and curettage or hysterectomy.

- The evaluation of direct cytologic material from the endometrial cavity has a false negative rate for malignancy between 5% and 15%.

- Fifteen percent of women who have obstructed fallopian tubes, as determined by hysterosalpingography (HSG), subsequently become pregnant without further treatment.

- Pain relief does not invariably alleviate tubal spasm during HSG.

- Acute pelvic infection develops in 0.3% to 3.1% of patients following HSG.

- Major indications for diagnostic hysteroscopy include abnormal uterine bleeding, infertility, and recurrent abortion.

- Indications for operative hysteroscopy include resection of submucous myomas, polyps, adhesions, and septa, as well as ablation of the endometrium.

- Hysteroscopy is superior to HSG in discovering and diagnosing intrauterine pathology.

- Dextran is an extremely viscous fluid used to distend the uterus during hysteroscopy. Dextran is nontoxic, nonconductive, and immiscible with blood.

- Hysteroscopic resection of uterine septa is superior to transabdominal resection in allowing vaginal delivery and avoidance of celiotomy.

- The failure rate with laparoscopic sterilization is between 1 in 250 and 1 in 500 cases.

- Absolute contraindications to laparoscopy include significant hemoperitoneum, anticoagulation therapy, advanced malignancy, large abdominal masses, severe cardiovascular disease, and tuberculous peritonitis.

- Major complications of laparoscopy are laceration of vessels, intestinal injuries, and cardiorespiratory problems arising from the pneumoperitoneum. The incidence of major complications in diagnostic laparoscopy is less than 1 in 1000 patients.

- Patients with ectopic pregnancies treated by laparoscopic salpingotomy should have subsequent human chorionic gonadotrophin titers until the titers fall to zero.

BIBLIOGRAPHY

Angel JL and Knuppel RA: Computed tomography in diagnosis of puerperal ovarian vein thrombosis, Obstet Gynecol 63:61, 1984.

Arrive L, Hricak H, and Martin MC: Pelvic endometriosis: MR imaging, Radiology 171:687, 1989.

Baggish MS and Barbot J: Contact hysteroscopy, Clin Obstet Gynecol 26:219, 1983.

Baggish MS, Barbot J, and Valle RF: Diagnostic and operative hysteroscopy: a text and atlas, Chicago, 1989, Mosby–Year Book, Inc.

Bamford DS, Hall EW, and Newman MR: The Isaacs endometrial cell sampler: an evaluation in 100 patients with postmenopausal bleeding, Acta Cytol 28:101, 1984.

Bhiwandiwala PP, Mumford SD, and Feldblum PJ: A comparison of different laparoscopic sterilization occlusion techniques in 24,439 procedures, Am J Obstet Gynecol 144:319, 1982.

Blumenfeld Z, Yoffe N, and Bronshtein M: Transvaginal sonography in infertility and assisted reproduction, Obstet Gynecol Surv 46:36, 1991

Bourne TH, Campbell S, Whitehead MI, et al: Detection of endometrial cancer in postmenopausal women by transvaginal ultrasonography and colour flow imaging, Br Med J 301:369, 1990

Brooks PG, Loffer FD, and Serden SP: Resectoscopic removal of symtomatic intrauterine lesions, J Reprod Med 34:435, 1989.

Buy JN, Ghossain MA, Moss AA, et al: Cystic teratoma of the ovary: CT detection, Radiology 171:697, 1989.

Buy JN, Moss AA, Ghossain MA, et al: Peritoneal implants from ovarian tumors: CT findings, Radiology 169:691, 1988.

Cacciatore B, Stenman UH, and Ylostalo P: Comparison of abdominal and vaginal sonography in suspected ectopic pregnancy, Obstet Gynecol 73:770, 1989.

Carlson JA Jr, Arger P, Thompson S, et al: Clinical and pathologic correlation of endometrial cavity fluid detected by ultrasound in the postmenopausal patient, Obstet Gynecol 77:119, 1991.

Chang YCF, Hricak H, Thurnher S, et al: Vagina: evaluation with MR imaging. Part II. Neoplasms, Radiology 169:175, 1988.

Check JH, Chase JS, Nowroozi K, et al: Clinical evaluation of the Pipelle endometrial suction curette for timed endometrial biopsies, J Reprod Med 34:218, 1989.

Chen SS, Rumancik WM, and Spiegel G: Magnetic resonance imaging in stage I endometrial carcinoma, Obstet Gynecol 75:274, 1990.

Cohen HL, Tice HM, and Mandel FS: Ovarian volumes measured by US: bigger than we think, Radiology 177:189, 1990.

Council on Scientific Affairs: Medical diagnostic ultrasound instrumentation and clinical interpretation: report of the Ultrasonography Task Force, JAMA 265:1155, 1991.

Council on Scientific Affairs: Magnetic resonance imaging of the abdomen and pelvis, JAMA 261:420, 1989.

Council on Scientific Affairs, American Medical Association: Gynecologic sonography: report of the Ultrasonography Task Force, JAMA 265:2851, 1991.

Crooks LE, Hoenninger J, Arakawa M, et al: High-resolution magnetic resonance imaging, Radiology 150:163, 1984.

Daly DC, Maier D, and Soto-Albors C: Hysteroscopic metroplasty: six years' experience, Obstet Gynecol 73:201, 1989.

Daniel AG and Peters WA III: Accuracy of office and operating room curettage in the grading of endometrial carcinoma, Obstet Gynecol 71:612, 1988.

DeCherney AH, Romero R, and Polan ML: Ultrasound in reproductive endocrinology, Fertil Steril 37:323, 1982.

Diamond MP, Lavy G, and DeCherney AH: Hysteroscopic use of dextran 70, Contemp OB/GYN, 30:29, 1989.

Einerth Y: Vacuum curettage by the Vabra® method, Acta Obstet Gynecol Scand 61:373, 1982.

Federle MP: Computed tomography in obstetrics and gynecology, Female Patient 9:39, 1984.

Ferenczy A and Gelfand MM: Outpatient endometrial sampling with endocyte: comparative study of its effectiveness with endometrial biopsy, Obstet Gynecol 63:295, 1984.

Goldrath MH, Fuller TA, and Segal S: Laser photovaporization of endometrium for the treatment of menorrhagia, Am J Obstet Gynecol 140:14, 1981.

Goldstein SR, Snyder JR, Watson C, et al: Very early pregnancy detection with endovaginal ultrasound, Obstet Gynecol 72:200, 1988.

Gomel V: Operative laparoscopy: time for acceptance, Fertil Steril 52:1, 1989.

Grimes DA: Diagnostic dilation and curettage: a reappraisal, Am J Obstet Gynecol 142:1, 1982.

Gross BH, Moss AA, Mihara K, et al: Computed tomography of gynecologic diseases, AJR 141:765, 1983.

Hamou JE: Microhysteroscopy, Clin Obstet Gynecol 26:285, 1983.

Houck RM, Cooper JM, and Rigberg HS: Hysteroscopic tubal occlusion with formed-in-place silicone plugs: a clinical review, Obstet Gynecol 62:587, 1983.

Hricak H, Chang YCF, and Thurnher S: Vagina: evaluation with MR imaging. Part I. Normal anatomy and congenital anomalies, Radiology 169:169, 1988.

Hulka JF: Textbook of laparoscopy, Orlando, Fla, 1985, Grune & Stratton, Inc.

Hutchins CJ: Laparoscopy and hysterosalpingography in the assessment of tubal patency, Obstet Gynecol 49:325, 1977.

Israel R and March CM: Hysteroscopic incision of the septate uterus, Am J Obstet Gynecol 149:66, 1984.

Iversen OE and Segadal E: The value of endometrial cytology: a comparative study of the Gravlee Jet-Washer, Isaacs cell sampler, and endoscan versus curettage in 600 patients, Obstet Gynecol Surv 40:14, 1985.

Johnson IR, Symonds EM, Kean DM, et al: Imaging the pregnant human uterus with nuclear magnetic resonance, Am J Obstet Gynecol 148:1136, 1985.

Johnson IR, Symonds EM, Worthington BS, et al: Imaging ovarian tumors by nuclear magnetic resonance, Br J Obstet Gynaecol 91:260, 1984.

Kaunitz AM, Masciello A, Ostrowski M, et al: Comparison of endometrial biopsy with the endometrial Pipelle and Vabra aspirator, J Reprod Med 33:427, 1988.

Lewis BV: Hysteroscopy in gynaecological practice: a review, J R Soc Med 77:235, 1984.

Mann WJ, Mendonca-Dias MH, Lauterbur PC, et al: Preliminary in vitro studies of nuclear magnetic resonance spin-lattice relaxation times and three-dimensional nuclear magnetic resonance imaging in gynecologic oncology, Am J Obstet Gynecol 148:91, 1984.

Mawhinney RR, Powell MC, Worthington BS, et al: Magnetic resonance imaging of benign ovarian masses, Br J Radiol 61:179, 1988.

McLucas B: Hyskon complications of hysteroscopic surgery, Obstet Gynecol Surv 46:196, 1991.

Mendonca-Dias MH, Mann WJ, Chumas J, et al: Three-dimensional nuclear-magnetic-resonance zeugmatographic imaging of surgical specimens, Biosci Rep 2:713, 1982.

Moldofsky PJ, Sears HF, Mulhern CB, et al: Detection of metastatic tumor in normal-sized retroperitoneal lymph nodes by monoclonal-antibody imaging, N Engl J Med 311:106, 1984.

Neuwirth RS: Hysteroscopic management of symptomatic submucous fibroids, Obstet Gynecol 62:509, 1983.

Nunley WC Jr, Bateman BG, Kitchin JD III, et al: Intravasation during hysterosalpingography using oil-base contrast medium—a second look, Obstet Gynecol 70:309, 1987.

O'Brien WF, Buck DR, and Nash JD: Evaluation of sonography in the initial assessment of the gynecologic patient, Am J Obstet Gynecol 149:598, 1984.

Oldendorf WH: NMR imaging: its potential clinical impact, Hosp Pract 17:114, 1982.

Partain CL, James AE Jr, Rollo FD, et al: Nuclear magnetic resonance imaging, Philadelphia, 1983, WB Saunders Co.

Perino A, Mencaglia L, Hamou J, et al: Hysteroscopy for metroplasty of uterine septa: report of 24 cases, Fertil Steril 48:321, 1987.

Peterson HB, DeStefano F, Rubin GL, et al: Deaths attributable to tubal sterilization in the United States, 1977-1981, Am J Obstet Gynecol 146:131, 1983.

Pittaway DE, Winfield AC, Maxson W, et al: Prevention of acute pelvic inflammatory disease after hysterosalpingography: efficacy of doxycycline prophylaxis, Am J Obstet Gynecol 147:623, 1983.

Rabin JM, Spitzer M, Dwyer AT, et al: Topical anesthesia for gynecologic procedures, Obstet Gynecol 73:1040, 1989.

Reich H, Wilkie WL, DeCaprio J, et al: Peritoneal trophoblastic tissue implants after laparoscopic treatment of tubal ectopic pregnancy, Fertil Steril 52:337, 1989.

Rodriguez MH, Platt LD, Medearis AL, et al: The use of transvaginal sonography for evaluation of postmenopausal ovarian size and morphology, Am J Obstet Gynecol 159:810, 1988.

Romero R, Kadar N, Castro D, et al: The value of adnexal sonographic findings in the diagnosis of ectopic pregnancy, Am J Obstet Gynecol 158:52, 1988.

Sanfilippo JS and Levine RL, editors: Operative gynecologic endoscopy. In Buchsbaum HJ, editor: Clinical perspectives in obstetrics and gynecology, New York, 1989, Springer-Verlag, New York, Inc.

Sauer MV, Agnew C, Worthen N, et al: Reliability of ultrasound in predicting uterine leiomyoma volume, J Reprod Med 33:612, 1988.

Schenker JG and Margalioth EJ: Intrauterine adhesions: an updated appraisal, Fertil Steril 37:593, 1982.

Shapiro BS and DeCherney AH: Ultrasound and infertility, J Reprod Med 34:151, 1989.

Siegler AM: Hysterosalpingography, Fertil Steril 40:139, 1983.

Siegler AM and Lindemann HJ: Hysteroscopy: principles and practice, Philadelphia, 1984, JB Lippincott Co.

Siegler AM and Valle RF: Therapeutic hysteroscopic procedures, Fertil Steril 50:685, 1988.

Sommer FG, Walsh JW, Schwartz PE, et al: Evaluation of gynecologic pelvic masses by ultrasound and computed tomography, J Reprod Med 27:45, 1982.

Soules MR and Spadoni LR: Oil versus aqueous media for hysterosalpingography: a continuing debate based on many opinions and few facts, Fertil Steril 38:1, 1982.

Stovall TG, Solomon SK, and Ling FW: Endometrial sampling prior to hysterectomy, Obstet Gynecol 73:405, 1989.

Swayne LC, Love MB, and Karasick SR: Pelvic inflammatory disease: sonographic-pathologic correlation, Radiology 151:751, 1984.

Symonds EM and Zuspan FP: Clinical and diagnostic procedures in obstetrics and gynecology, New York, 1984, Marcel Dekker, Inc.

Thickman D, Kressel H, Gussman D, et al: Nuclear magnetic resonance imaging in gynecology, Am J Obstet Gynecol 149:835, 1984.

Timbos-Kemper TCM and Veering BT: Anaphylactic shock from intracavitary 32% dextran-70 during hysteroscopy, Fertil Steril 51:1053, 1989.

Timor-Tritsch IE and Rottem S: Transvaginal ultrasonographic study of the fallopian tube, Obstet Gynecol 70:424, 1987.

Togashi K, Nishimura K, Itoh K, et al: Adenomyosis: diagnosis with MR imaging, Radiology 166:111, 1988.

Togashi K, Nishimura K, Sagoh T, et al: Carcinoma of the cervix: staging with MR imaging, Radiology 171:245, 1989.

Togashi K, Ozasa H, Konishi I, et al: Enlarged uterus: differentiation between adenomyosis and leiomyoma with MR imaging, Radiology 171:531, 1989.

Valle RF and Sciarra JJ: Intrauterine adhesions: hysteroscopic diagnosis, classification, treatment, and reproductive outcome, Am J Obstet Gynecol 158:1459, 1988.

Voss SC, Lacey CG, Pupkin M, et al: Ultrasound and the pelvic mass, J Reprod Med 28:833, 1983.

Waggenspack GA, Amparo EG, and Hannigan EV: MR imaging of uterine cervical carcinoma, J Comput Assist Tomogr 12:409, 1988.

Walsh JW, Amendola MA, Konerding KF, et al: Computed tomographic detection of pelvic and inguinal lymph-node metastases from primary and recurrent pelvic malignant disease, Radiology 137:157, 1980.

Walsh JW and Goplerud DR: Prospective comparison between clinical and CT staging in primary cervical carcinoma, AJR 137:997, 1981.

Wentz AC: Endometrial biopsy in the evaluation of infertility, Fertil Steril 33:121, 1980.

Wittenberg J: Computed tomography of the body, I, N Engl J Med 309:1160, 1983.

Wittenberg J: Computed tomography of the body, II, N Engl J Med 309:1224, 1983.

Worthington BS: Clinical prospects for nuclear magnetic resonance, Clin Radiol 34:3, 1983.

Worthington JL, Balfe DM, Lee JKT, et al: Uterine neoplasms: MR imaging, Radiology 159:725, 1986.

Yoder IC: Hysterosalpingography and pelvic ultrasound: imaging in infertility and gynecology, Boston, 1989, Little, Brown & Co.

Zawin M, McCarthy S, Scoutt L, et al: Endometriosis: appearance and detection at MR imaging, Radiology 171:693, 1989.

CHAPTER 9

Congenital Abnormalities

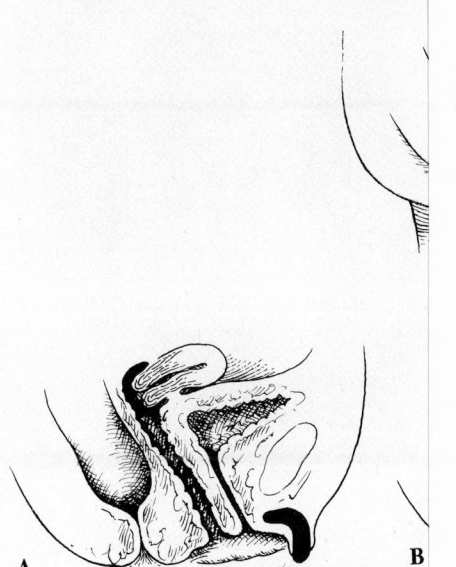

FIGURE 9-1
Sagittal views of genital defor[...]
Minimal masculinization wit[...]
and more marked enlargeme[...]
ment of the clitoris, and fo[...]
Verkauf BS and Jones HW Jr[...]

malities are unusual, although the c[...]
be enlarged because of androgen s[...]
In such circumstances the shaft of [...]
may be quite enlarged, and partia[...]
ment of a penile urethra may have[...]
Extreme cases of androgen stimulati[...]
erally associated with fusion of the l[...]
findings occur in infants with conge[...]
nal hyperplasia and in those expose[...]
to exogenous or endogenous androg[...]
9-1).

Labial Fusion

Although labial fusion may result[...]
sure to exogenous androgens or be[...]
with defects of the anterior abdomir[...]
most common cause is congenital [...]
perplasia. The most common form i[...]
an inborn error of metabolism invol[...]
zyme 21-hydroxylase. This conditi[...]
mitted as an autosomal recessive [...]
on chromosome 6, and because of [...]
21-hydroxylase metabolism, the m[...]
thesis pathway to cortisol is dimir[...]
mozygous individuals occur at a r[...]
490 to 1 per 67,000 of the populati[...]

KEY TERMS AND DEFINITIONS

Accessory Ovary. Excess ovarian tissue near a normally placed ovary and connected to it.

Ambiguous Genitalia. Anatomic modification of the external genitalia, which makes specific determination of gender difficult.

Androgen Insensitivity Syndrome. An X-linked condition of a testosterone receptor defect in a 46,XY individual with testes and normal male testosterone levels. These individuals have absent uterus, normal female phenotype, and scanty body hair.

Arcuate Uterus. A minimum septate uterus; probably of no clinical importance.

Bicornuate Uterus. A partial lack of fusion of two uterine corpora to varying degree. A single cervix is present.

Didelphic Uterus. Complete duplication of the uterus and cervix without fusion of the two cavities. One fallopian tube joins each fundal cavity. This condition may be associated with a septate vagina.

Hematocolpos. Distention of an obstructed vagina (caused by imperforate hymen or transverse septum) with blood and blood products.

Hydrocolpos. Distention of an obstructed vagina (caused by imperforate hymen or transverse septum) with fluid.

Labial Fusion. Fusion of the labia minora in the midline, closing the introitus.

Mucocolpos. A vagina blocked by an imperforate hymen or transverse septum and filled with mucus.

Ovotestes. Gonads that contains both ovarian and testicular remnants.

Repetitive Spontaneous Abortion. The loss of three or more pregnancies before 20 weeks' gestation. Functionally, however, many physicians will do a workup for repetitive spontaneous abortion after two or more pregnancy losses.

Rokitansky-Küster-Hauser Syndrome. A 46,XX female with müllerian failure, usually showing absence of all or most of vagina, cervix, uterus, and fallopian tubes.

Rudimentary Uterine Horn. A structure that develops from one müllerian duct and does not communicate with the uterine cavity. The contralateral fallopian tube communicates with the uterine cavity. The ipsilateral fallopian tube communicates with that horn.

Septate Uterus. The presence of a septum that separates the uterine cavity either partially or completely into two separate cavities.

Supernumerary Ovary. The presence of a third ovary separated from the normally situated ovaries.

Unicolic (Unicornuate) Uterus. A uterus and cervix that develop from a single müllerian duct joined at the top of the fundus by only one fallopian tube. It represents complete arrest of one müllerian duct.

Vaginal Agenesis. Absence of the vagina.

Congenital abnormalities of th[e repro]ductive tract can be caused by [genes] or by a teratologic event during [de]velopment. Minor abnormalitie[s are of lit]tle consequence, but major ab[normalities] lead to severe impairment of m[any re]productive functions. This cha[pter considers] a number of such abnormalitie[s and their] diagnosis and treatment. For d[iscussion of the] etiology of these problems, th[e reader is re]ferred to Chapter 1, Embryolog[y.]

EXAMINATION OF TH[E] NEWBORN FOR SEXU[AL] AMBIGUITIES

The first major diagnostic dec[ision the ob]stetrician or neonatal physician [makes when] the newborn is gender assign[ment. In most] cases the designation is clear [but for the] newborns with ambiguous gen[italia it is a] potentially serious problem for [the physician] and parents. The female who ha[s been viril]enized may appear similar to th[e male pseudo]hermaphrodite suffering from [an]drogen insensitivity syndrome. [Still] var abnormalities may resemble [viril]enization. It is therefore approp[riate to system]atically evaluate the newborn's g[enitalia for] the appropriate gender assignme[nt.]

The first and probably most i[mportant part] of the examination is inspection[. The physician] should systematically observe [the] perineum, beginning with the [mons. The] clitoris should be noted for a[ny en]largement, the opening of the [urethra should] be identified, and the labia shou[ld be separated] to see if the introitus can be vi[sualized. If the] labia are fused, this maneuver [is not possi]ble. At times the labia are joi[ned by ad]hesions; these generally separat[e in child]hood or respond to the applicat[ion of estrogen] cream. If it is possible to separa[te them, the] hymen may be observed. Gen[erally it is par]tially perforate, revealing the e[ntrance to the] vagina. Posteriorly the labia fus[e to join] at the posterior fourchette of [the perineum.] Posterior to the perineal body [the anus should] be visualized, and it should b[e checked to en]sure that it is perforate. Mec[onium staining] about the rectum is evidence fo[r patency. If] there is doubt, the rectum ma[y be probed] with a cotton-tipped swab or, if [necessary, with] the little finger encased in a [rubber] finger cot.

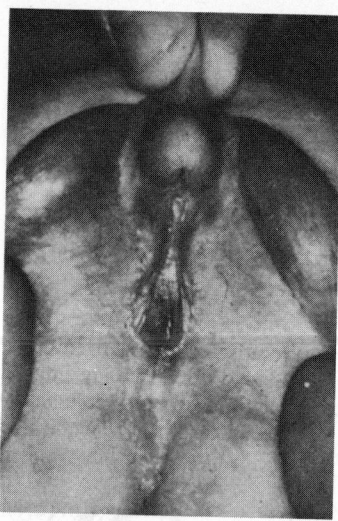

FIGURE 9-2
External genitalia of female with congenital adrenal hyperplasia showing clitoral enlargement and labial fusion. (From Jones HW Jr and Scott WW: Hermaphroditism, genital anomalies and related endocrine disorders, ed 2, Baltimore, 1971, Williams & Wilkins.)

hydroxyprogesterone in the serum. This test has been used in screening newborns for 21-hydroxylase deficiency, particularly in known high-risk populations, such as Alaskan Eskimos. Using a 3 mm filter paper disk elution technique to study the presence of 17-hydroxyprogesterone in capillary blood of these day-old newborns, these authors determined levels in normal infants to be less than 40 pg/3 mm disk. Affected infants had 17-OHP levels of 57 to 980 pg/disk.

Treatment of congenital adrenal hyperplasia involves replacement cortisol. This suppresses adrenocorticotropic hormone (ACTH) output and therefore decreases the stimulation of the cortisol-producing pathways of the adrenal cortex.

Imperforate Hymen

The hymen represents the junction of the sinovaginal bulbs with the urogenital sinus and therefore is composed of endoderm from the urogenital sinus epithelium. Ordinarily the hymen is perforated during embryonic life to establish a connection between the lumen of the vaginal canal and the vestibule. If this perforation does not take place, the hymen is imperforate (Figure 9-3).

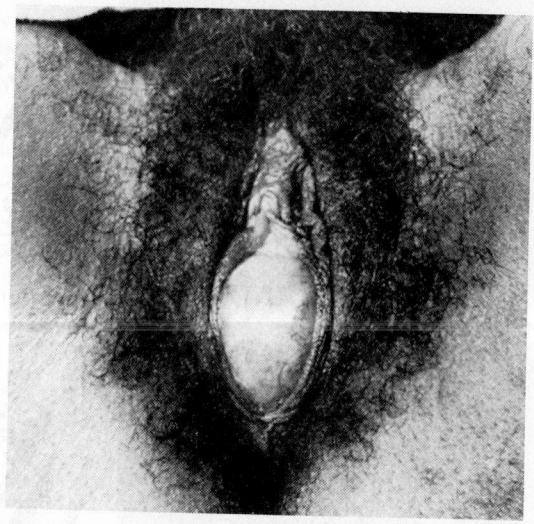

FIGURE 9-3
Imperforate hymen distended by hematocolpos. (From Baramki TA: J Reprod Med 29:376, 1984.)

It is rare to make the diagnosis of imperforate hymen before puberty, at which point primary amenorrhea is the major symptom. Occasionally in childhood a hydrocolpos or mucocolpos may occur. This is caused by a collection of secretions behind the hymen, which in rare cases may build up to form a mass that obstructs the urinary tract. If such is discovered, the hymen should be incised to release the build-up.

At puberty the patient may experience cyclic cramping but no menstrual flow. Over time the patient may develop a hematocolpos and a hematometrium. In more advanced cases the fallopian tubes may be distended with menstrual flow, and the flow may back up through the tubes and form endometrial implants in the peritoneal cavity. Quite surprisingly, many patients are free of symptoms.

The diagnosis can be determined by history and by the presence of a bulging membrane at the introitus. Therapy consists of a cruciate incision into the hymen extending to the 10, 2, and 6 o'clock positions. In dense hymens a triangular section may be excised, although this is rarely necessary. Hemostasis is secured by fine suture, and evolution to normal usually occurs rapidly.

Vaginal Agenesis

Vaginal agenesis is usually associated with the Rokitansky-Küster-Hauser syndrome (Fig-

throug
consid
bicycle
the di
minute
day. T
ties w
month
this te

Surg
evolve
the m
betwee
placed
such a
membr
ness sl
dure,
form b
will us
and sh
the ne
becom

An a
Willian
and re:
rectly
cally si
of the
functio
by pati
reporte

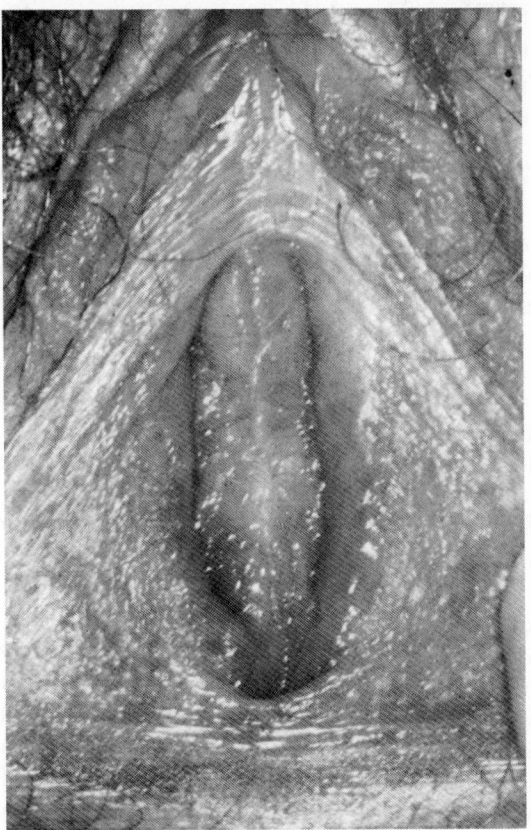

FIGURE 9-4
External genitalia of patient with congenital absence of vagina. (From Baramki TA: J Reprod Med 29:376, 1984.)

ure 9-4). This syndrome is characterized by congenital absence of the vagina and uterus, although small masses of smooth muscular material resembling a rudimentary bicornuate uterus may be noted. These masses rarely have an epithelial lining and rarely menstruate, although occasionally this does occur, giving rise to monthly cyclic cramping. The ovaries are normal, and the fallopian tubes are usually present. Complete vaginal agenesis is discovered in 75% of patients with Rokitansky-Küster-Hauser syndrome. Approximately 25% of patients have a short vaginal pouch. These individuals have a 46,XX karyotype. The disorder seems to be an accident of development and not an inherited condition.

The androgen insensitivity syndrome (testicular feminization syndrome) demonstrates a 46,XY karyotype. While vaginal agenesis or the presence of a short pouch vagina is usually found, these patients have undescended testicles and male sex ducts. They usually exhibit

minimal pubic hair after puberty. The testes should be removed after puberty to prevent the development of seminomas. The ovaries of the patient with Rokitansky-Küster-Hauser syndrome are normal and should not be removed.

Phelan reported that of 72 patients with vaginal agenesis, 25% had urologic abnormalities noted on intravenous pyelography. A later study by Baramki demonstrated that 40% of 92 patients had urologic abnormalities. Further, Turunen and Unnerus found that 25 of 200 such patients had skeletal anomalies, usually involving congenital fusion or absence of vertebrae.

Diagnosis of Rokitansky-Küster-Hauser syndrome is demonstrated by the presence of primary amenorrhea at the time of puberty, physical examination that demonstrates the absence of a vaginal opening or the presence of a short vaginal pouch, and failure to palpate a uterus on rectal examination, coupled with the finding of a normal karyotype. Laparoscopic examination may be performed in cases where the diagnosis is not clear or where there is some concern over the presence of a functioning uterus. In most cases, however, laparoscopic diagnosis is not necessary. Ultrasound examination may verify the presence of normal ovaries and the absence of the uterus. Basal body temperature curves and serial progesterone determinations may also be used to verify ovarian function.

Therapy involves the creation of a vagina when the patient wishes to become sexually active. There are several therapeutic choices. The first, which is time consuming but nonsurgical, requires the use of progressive vaginal dilators. This can be accomplished in a well-motivated patient over a period of several months, and functioning vaginas have been achieved in many patients in this manner.

Using the concept of vaginal dilators, Ingram has devised a useful technique. He used three sets of Lucite dilators. The first set contains 10 that are 1.5 cm in diameter and that increase in length from 1.5 to 10 cm; the second set contains 5 that are 2.5 cm in diameter and that increase in length from 3 to 10 cm; and the third set has 8 dilators, 3.5 cm in diameter and from 3 to 10 cm long. A racing bicycle seat is mounted on a stool and is used to maintain dilator pressure on the introital dimple just posterior to the urethra. The patient holds the dilators in place with a pad or girdle and works

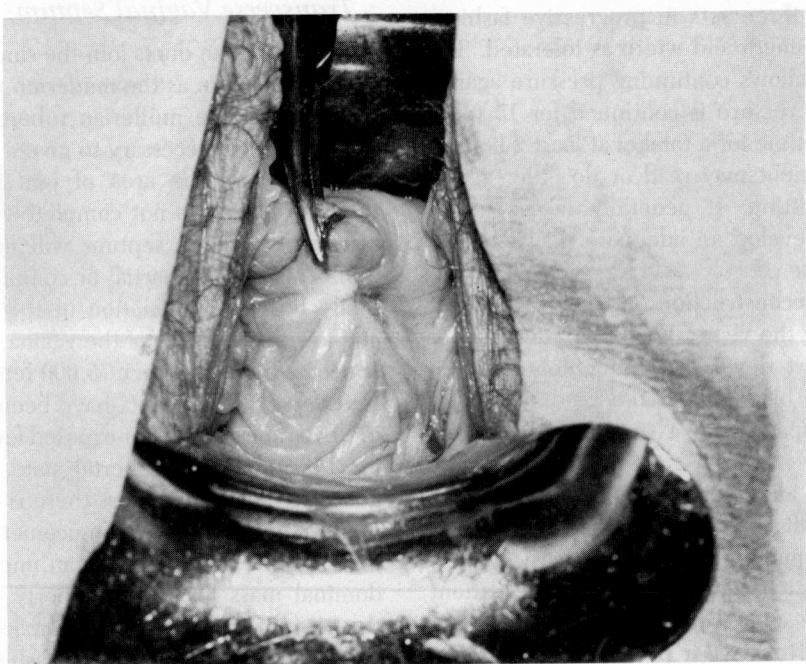

FIGURE 9-7
Patient with complete transverse vaginal septum.

sion, with suturing of the edges of the vagina on either side. Occasionally the septum is thick, and the two areas of the vagina are quite distantly separated. In such a case excision may require the implantation of a split-thickness skin graft in a fashion similar to the McIndoe procedure.

Longitudinal septa of the vagina will be discussed with duplication of the uterus and cervix.

Vaginal Adenosis

In the female exposed to DES in utero the junction between the müllerian ducts and the sinovaginal bulb may not be sharply demonstrated. If müllerian elements invade the sinovaginal bulb, remnants may remain as areas of adenosis in the adult vagina. They are generally palpated submucosally, although they may be observable at the surface. These anomalies are discussed more fully in Chapter 14.

Abnormalities of the Cervix and Uterus

Embryologic Considerations

Between the third and fifth weeks of gestation the metanephric ducts develop and join the cloaca. By the fifth week two ureteric buds develop from the mesonephric ducts close to the distal ends. These grow cephalad toward the mesonephric mass. The müllerian or paramesonephric duct forms from a cleft between the mesonephros and the forming gonad. These ducts are bilateral and grow caudally just lateral to and intimately associated with the mesonephric ducts. The fate of these various elements is therefore closely entwined. Damage to one usually affects the others. The paramesonephric ducts grow caudally, meet in the midline, and descend into the pelvis, reaching the urogenital sinus at an elevation known as the *müllerian tubercle*.

Musset analyzed 133 cases of genitourinary malformation and described a three-stage process for fusion of the two müllerian ducts into the uterus and cervix. The first stage is described as short, taking place at the beginning of the tenth week. The medial aspect of the more caudal portions of the two ducts fuse, starting in the middle and proceeding simultaneously in both directions. In this way a median septum is formed. The second stage continues from the tenth to the thirteenth week and occurs because of a rapid cell proliferation and the filling in of the triangular space between the two uterine cornua. In this way a thick upper median septum is formed. This is wedgelike and gives rise to the usual external contour of the fundus. At the same time the lower portion of the median septum is resorbed, unifying the cervical canal first and then the upper vagina. The third stage lasts from the thirteenth to about the twentieth week. In this stage the degeneration of the upper uterine septum occurs, starting at the isthmic region and proceeding cranially up to the top of the fundus. In this way a unified uterine cavity is formed.

The vagina develops from a combination of the müllerian tubercles and the urogenital sinus. Cells proliferate from the upper portion of the urogenital sinus to form solid aggregates known as the *sinovaginal bulbs*. These cell masses develop into a cord, the vaginal plate, which extends from the müllerian ducts to the urogenital sinus. This plate canalizes, starting at the hymen, which is where the sinovaginal bulb attaches to the urogenital sinus, and proceeding cranially to the developing cervix, which has by this time already canalized. The process is completed at about the twenty-first week of intrauterine life.

Toaff et al. have pointed out from their review of the literature that the type of communicating abnormality of the uterus depends on a teratogenic process active at different stages in the embryonic development. Most symmetric communicating uteri have a normal urinary system, indicating that normal growth of the two mesonephric ducts had taken place before the fusion problem occurred. They point out, however, that all patients with communicating uteri with atretic hemivagina who were studied had ipsilateral renal agenesis. Likewise, in patients with anomalies wherein a hemicervix was absent, ipsilateral renal agenesis occurred. They inferred from these findings that an early teratogenic process active during the fourth week of gestation resulted in arrested growth of one mesonephric duct, agenesis of the ureteric bud, and therefore renal agenesis.

Genetic Studies of Müllerian Fusion Difficulties

Elias et al. reviewed the cases of sisters, mothers, and aunts of 24 women with known müllerian fusion abnormalities. Only 1 sister out of 37 (2.7%) was found to have a similar abnormality. No such abnormalities were found among 24 mothers, 45 maternal aunts, or 50 paternal aunts. However, the data in this study were accumulated by history and medical records and not by direct uterine examination. Nonetheless, Elias et al. concluded that the major genetic transmission mechanism could be only polygenic or multifactorial.

Incidence

It is difficult to estimate the incidence of uterine fusion anomalies because the data in most reports are derived from study groups rather than from the general population. The incidence is reported as 0.1% in retrospective studies and from 2% to 3% in observations of uteri at the time of delivery. Most uteri in the latter study, however, fit into the category of arcuate uterus or subseptate uterus.

Symptoms and Signs

Complete duplication of the vagina, uterus, and cervix may be asymptomatic until the woman begins to menstruate. Frequently the earliest symptom brought to the attention of the gynecologist is the fact that tampons do not obstruct menstrual flow. What occurs is that the patient inserts a tampon into one vagina but the other vagina is still open. The second most common way the diagnosis is made is by observation at the time of the first pelvic examination.

Obstructive vaginal lesions often lead to cyclic pain at the time of menstruation or to the presence of a mucus-filled or blood-filled mass in the vagina. This may be mistaken for a paravaginal tumor.

A noncommunicating uterine horn may be indicated in one of two fashions. The first may be pain or a mass exacerbated cyclically at the time of menses, which occasionally is associated with symptoms and signs of endometriosis in a teenage woman. The early onset of signs and symptoms of endometriosis should alert the physician to this possibility. A mass is often noted on physical examination. Olive and Henderson noted that 10 of 13 women (77%) with anomalies associated with outflow obstruction had endometriosis, whereas only 16 of 43 (37%) who did not have outflow obstruction had evidence from endometriosis.

The second way such a problem may present is as an ectopic pregnancy. Because sperm may migrate through the patent horn and because the rudimentary horn may have a normal tube attached to it, pregnancy can occur in the rudimentary horn. But because such horns are frequently small, rupture or pain caused by the obstruction may point to the diagnosis.

One of the major presenting symptoms is reproductive wastage. Didelphic uteri are usually not associated with this complaint. Musset estimated that abnormalities of the uterus may occur in as many as 15% to 25% of women with a history of repetitive abortion. Most patients with pregnancy wastage, however, had a variation of septate uterus. Whereas pretherapy pregnancy wastage rates were as high as 85% to 90%, improvement of pregnancy efficiency to as much as 80% occurred after metroplasty. Table 9-1 summarizes the results of a number of such reports. It is important to thoroughly evaluate such patients before exposing them to an operative procedure, since other problems may cause pregnancy wastage.

Uterine dysfunction and incoordinate uterine action are complicating problems seen in labor in women with septate and bicornuate uteri. Likewise, breech presentations and transverse lies occur more commonly in women with such abnormal uteri.

Diagnosis

Diagnosis of a uterine anomaly may be indicated by history of spontaneous abortion, especially in the second trimester, but is best proved by hysterosalpingography, hysteroscopy, and at times, laparoscopy. Valdes et al. in 1984 reviewed the use of ultrasound for diagnosing female genital tract anomalies. A group of 64 patients with an ultrasound diagnosis of an anomaly were studied retrospectively to determine the accuracy and usefulness of the sonographic examination in such cases. Of these patients, 64% were pregnant; 36% were not. Of 46 patients who had ultrasound diagnoses, 21 cases were diagnosed as bicornuate/septate uterus, 18 cases as didelphia, 3 cases as vaginal and cervical atresia, 2 cases as obstructed lower but normal upper genital tract, and 2 cases as abnormal-appearing uterus. Ultrasound diagnosis was compared with hysterosalpingographic and operative findings in 43 patients and with physical examination in three patients. Scan results were classified as diagnostic in 26%, confirmatory in 63%, and incorrect in 11%.

Fedele et al. studied 43 infertile patients with hysterosalpingographic evidence for bifid uterus, using ultrasound and laparoscopy/hysteroscopy. They were able to adequately visualize the uteri of 39, and they correctly identified with ultrasound: 1 of 2 uteri didelphys, all 11 bicornuate uteri, and all 4 totally and 22 partially septate uteri. In a separate report Fedele et al. studied 14 women with a hysterosalpingographic diagnosis of uterus unicornis. Ultrasound achieved an 85.7% sensitivity and 100% specificity for diagnosing the presence of a rudimentary horn that existed in 7 cases.

Ultrasound is a reasonable diagnostic procedure in such cases but should not be considered diagnostic until supplementary studies are

TABLE 9-1

Results of Studies Evaluating Reproductive Success in Women Who Have Had Repair of Septate Uterus

Author(s) (Year)	Number	Live Births	Abortions	Ectopic Pregnancy
Musich and Behrman (1978)	21	9	2	0
Buttram (1979)	46	23	1	1
Palmer (1981)	100	67	4	0
Rochet and Dargert (1981) (per Audebert, Cittadini, and Cognat [1983])	38	29	2	0
Cardiani and Fedele (1981)	68	31	2	0
Audebert, Cittadini, and Cognat (1983)	54	19	3	0
Perino, Mencaglia, Hamou, and Cittadini (1987)	24	10	1	0
TOTAL	351	188	15	1

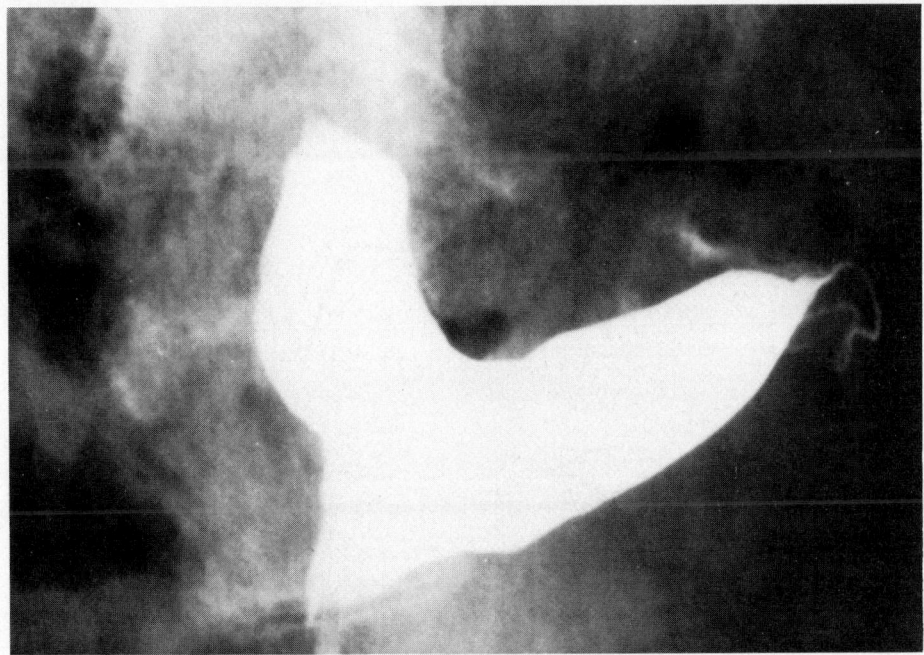

FIGURE 9-8
Hysterosalpingogram of bicornuate uterus seen in patient with repetitive abortions.

performed. Hysterosalpingography and direct observation via hysteroscopy are the perferred methods of diagnosis. Laparoscopy and laparotomy may be useful in unusual cases (Figure 9-8).

Specific Anomalies

ABSENCE OF CERVIX AND UTERUS. As discussed under Rokitansky-Küster-Hauser syndrome, the cervix and uterus are often not completely absent; the fallopian tubes and possibly some fibrous tissue are usually present. Absence is frequently associated with urinary tract anomalies.

UNICORNUATE UTERUS. Destruction of one müllerian duct may occur for various embryonic reasons. It is often related to lack of development of the mesonephric system on one side associated with lack of the appropriate development of the müllerian system. When this is the case, there is almost always a missing kidney and ureter on the same side. A single cervix and a single horn of the uterus with the fallopian tube of the side entering it are seen. The ovary may be present on the opposite side. Such a uterus usually supports a pregnancy. Unicornuate uterus may not be di-

agnosed unless the patient is evaluated with a hysterosalpingogram or is subjected to an operative procedure.

In a review of the literature consisting of 31 patients, Buttram found a 48% spontaneous abortion rate, a 17% prematurity rate, and a 40% live birth rate in patients with this anomaly.

ANOMALIES OF LATERAL FUSION OF MÜLLERIAN DUCTS. Partial or complete duplication of the vagina, cervix, and uterus may be seen clinically. These may be classified as didelphic, which may involve a complete duplication of vagina, uterus, and cervix; bicornuate, which consists of a single-chamber vagina and cervix with a complete or partial septate uterus and two uterine bodies (see Figure 9-8); septate, in which the uterus appears as a single organ but contains a midline septum that is either partial or complete; or arcuate, which demonstrates a small septate indentation at the upper end of the fundus. Figure 9-9 graphically depicts these.

Toaff et al. reviewed the subgroup of malformed uteri that includes duplication of the vagina, cervix, and uterus with communication between the horns. Nine subcategories have been described and are depicted in Figure

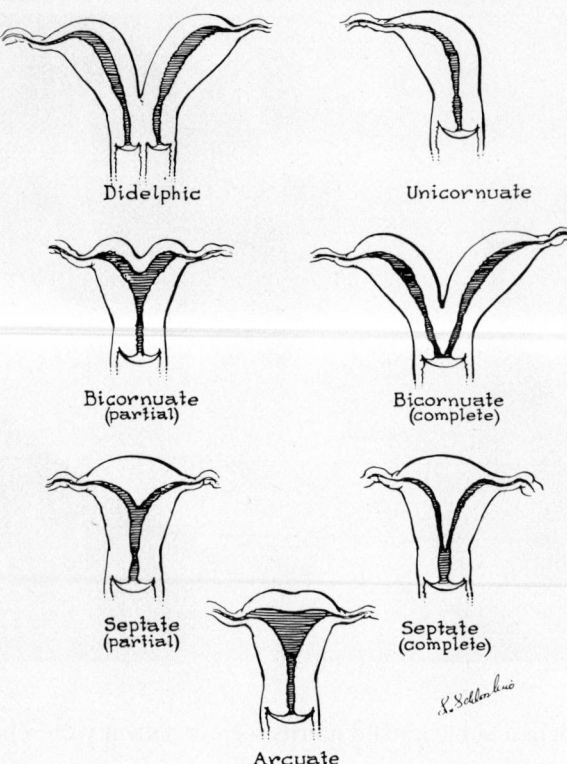

Didelphic

Unicornuate

Bicornuate
(partial)

Bicornuate
(complete)

Septate
(partial)

Septate
(complete)

Arcuate

FIGURE 9-9
Nonobstructive maldevelopment of the Müllerian system. (From Baramki TA: J Reprod Med 29:376, 1984.)

9-10. Some involve septate uteri and others didelphic uteri. Some involve obstructive areas of the vagina. Because of the structural differences the clinical findings may be quite different from case to case.

Finally, obstructive varieties of duplication may be noted, again involving the uterus or the vagina.

Management

For patients with nonobstructed abnormalities, no therapy may be indicated. This is particularly true for women with unicornuate and didelphic uteri. On the other hand, septate uteri are frequently associated with reproductive wastage problems, and correction may be necessary to relieve these situations. A number of metroplasty procedures are available. The first was described by Strassman and involved the removal of the septum by a wedge incision and the reunification of the two cavities. However, a number of other means have been de-

vised to eliminate the septum. Table 9-2 summarizes some of these and outlines their differences.

Recently septate uteri have been treated by division of the septum through the hysteroscope. To perform this procedure, a laparoscope should first be introduced into the peritoneal cavity so that the uterus can be directly visualized during the procedure. This will also allow differentiation of a septate uterus from a bicornuate or didelphic uterus. An operating hysteroscope is then used to progressively cut the septum with scissors, until a cavity with normal appearing contour is achieved. Little or no bleeding generally occurs, since the septum is fibrous and poorly vascularized. After operation some surgeons may insert a Lippes-type IUD for 30 days, and the patient may be treated with a conjugated estrogen (1.25 mg per day) for 1 month. This step has not been proved to be necessary and often can be withheld. This vaginal approach eliminates the need for an abdominal procedure and thus lim-

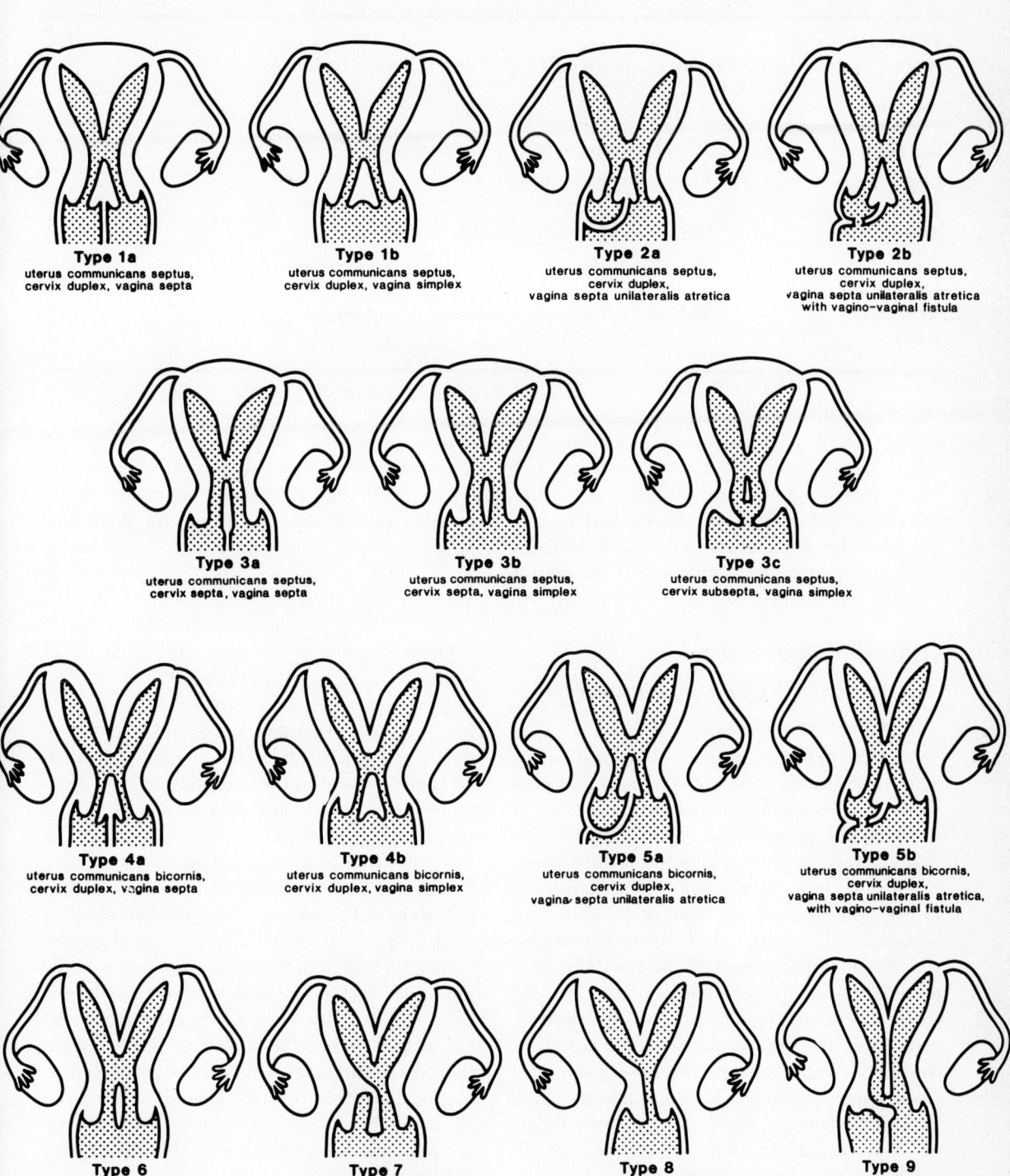

Type 1a
uterus communicans septus,
cervix duplex, vagina septa

Type 1b
uterus communicans septus,
cervix duplex, vagina simplex

Type 2a
uterus communicans septus,
cervix duplex,
vagina septa unilateralis atretica

Type 2b
uterus communicans septus,
cervix duplex,
vagina septa unilateralis atretica
with vagino-vaginal fistula

Type 3a
uterus communicans septus,
cervix septa, vagina septa

Type 3b
uterus communicans septus,
cervix septa, vagina simplex

Type 3c
uterus communicans septus,
cervix subsepta, vagina simplex

Type 4a
uterus communicans bicornis,
cervix duplex, vagina septa

Type 4b
uterus communicans bicornis,
cervix duplex, vagina simplex

Type 5a
uterus communicans bicornis,
cervix duplex,
vagina septa unilateralis atretica

Type 5b
uterus communicans bicornis,
cervix duplex,
vagina septa unilateralis atretica,
with vagino-vaginal fistula

Type 6
uterus communicans bicornis,
cervix septa, vagina simplex

Type 7
uterus communicans bicornis,
cervix septa unilateralis atretica,
vagina simplex

Type 8
uterus communicans bicornis,
hemicervix una, vagina simplex

Type 9
uterus bicornis, cervix communicans
septa unilateralis atretica,
vagina septa

FIGURE 9-10
Morphologic classification of communicating uteri. All have an isthmic communication except type 9, which has a low cervical communication. (From Toaff ME, Lev-Toaff AS, and Toaff R: Communicating uteri: review and classification with introduction of two previously unreported types, Fertil Steril 41:661, 1984. Reproduced with permission of the publisher, The American Fertility Society.)

TABLE 9-2
Procedures for Performing Metroplasty on Uteri with Müllerian Fusion Anomalies

Procedure	Technique
Strassman	Wedge excision of septum—reunification of cavity
Jones	Cone resection of septum
Tompkins Bret Palmer	Sagittal incision with severance of septum
Chervenak Neuwirth Perino	Hysteroscopically controlled severance of septum

its the risk of pelvic adhesions, which may in themselves interfere with fertility. Israel and March recently noted that no serious complications occurred in 72 such treated patients reported in the world literature. In the future, laser beams may replace scissors for incision of the septum.

Ovarian Abnormalities

Accessory Ovary and Supernumerary Ovary

In 1959 Wharton defined *accessory ovary* and *supernumerary ovary*. The former term is used when excess ovarian tissue is noted near a normally placed ovary and connected to it. Supernumerary ovary occurs when a third ovary is separated from the normally situated ovaries. Printz et al. pointed out that such ovaries may be found in the omentum or retroperitoneally, and Hogan et al. reported the presence of a dermoid cyst in a supernumerary ovary that occurred in the greater omentum. Wharton estimated that the occurrence of either accessory ovary or supernumerary ovary was quite rare, finding approximately 1 case of accessory ovary per 93,000 patients and 1 case of supernumerary ovary in 29,000 autopsies. In fact, only 13 reported cases of supernumerary ovary have been found to date in the world literature. In

Wharton's review, 3 of 4 patients with supernumerary ovary and 5 of 19 patients with accessory ovary had additional congenital defects, most frequently abnormalities of the genitourinary tract.

Ovotestes

Ovotestes are present in individuals with ovaries that have an HY antigen present. The majority are true hermaphrodites. The degree to which müllerian and mesonephric development occurs depends on the amount of testicular tissue present in the ovotestes and the proximity to the developing duct system. Where a considerable amount of testicular tissue is present within the organ, there is a tendency for descent toward the labial scrotal area. Thus palpation of the gonad in the inguinal canal or within the labial scrotal area is fairly common. Ovulation and menstruation may occur if the müllerian system is appropriately developed. In a similar fashion, spermatogenesis may occur as well. Where testicular tissue is present, there is an increased risk for malignant degeneration, and these gonads should be removed after puberty. Germ cell tumors, such as dysgerminomas, have been reported in the ovarian portion of ovotestes.

_____ **KEY POINTS** _____

- Gender identification in a newborn infant has such emotional impact that it should be considered an emergency procedure.

- Congenital adrenal hyperplasia is an autosomal recessive condition most commonly the result of an inborn error of metabolism involving the enzyme 21-hydroxylase. Homozygous individuals occur in 1 of every 490 to 67,000 births. Heterozygote carriers are present in 1 in 20 to 1 in 250 individuals. Differences depend on ethnic background of people tested.

- The hymen is the junction of the sinovaginal bulb with the urogenital sinuses and is derived from endoderm.

- Vaginal agenesis is most often associated with Rokitansky-Küster-Hauser syndrome. From 25% to 40% of these will have urologic abnormalities. Approximately one eighth will have skeletal abnormalities as well.

- Abnormalities of the uterus and cervix may be transmitted as a polygenic or multifactorial pattern of inheritance. They occur in about 2% to 3% of the female population.

- From 15% to 20% of women with repetitive abortion histories may be found to have anomalies of the uterus.

- Pretherapy pregnancy wastage rates in women with anomalies of the uterus may be as high as 85% to 90%. After surgical repair the pregnancy efficiency rate may be as high as 80%.

- Accessory ovaries occur in approximately 1 per 93,000 patients. Supernumerary ovaries occur in approximately 1 of every 29,000 women.

BIBLIOGRAPHY

Abrego D and Ibrahim AA: Mesenteric supernumerary ovary, Obstet Gynecol 45:352, 1975.

Audebert AJM, Cittadini E, and Cognat M: Habitual abortion in uterine malformations, Acta Eur Fertil 14:273, 1983.

Baramki TA: The treatment of congenital anomalies in girls and women, J Reprod Med 29:376, 1984.

Beheshti M, Hardy BE, Churchill BM, et al: Gender assignment in male pseudo hermaphrodite children, Urology 22:604, 1983.

Blair RG: Pregnancy associated with congenital malformations of the reproductive tract, J Obstet Gynaecol Br Emp 67:36, 1960.

Buttram VC: Müllerian anomalies and their management, Fertil Steril 40:159, 1983.

Buttram VC, Zanotti L, Acosta AA, et al: Surgical correction of septate uterus, Fertil Steril 25:373, 1974.

Cardiani GB and Fedele L: Clinical management of uterine anomalies, Acta Eur Fertil 12:83, 1981.

Cruikshank SH and VanDrie DM: Supernumerary ovaries: update and review, Obstet Gynecol 60:126, 1982.

Daly DC, Walters CA, Soto-Albers CE, et al: Hysteroscopic metroplasty: surgical technique and obstetric outcome, Fertil Steril 39:623, 1983.

Dillon WP and Dewey M: A case of accessory ovary, Obstet Gynecol 58:660, 1981.

Elias S, Simpson JL, Carson SA, et al: Genetic studies in incomplete müllerian fusion, Obstet Gynecol 63:276, 1984.

Emans SJ, Grace E, Fleischnick E, et al: Detection of late onset 21-hydroxylase deficiency congenital adrenal hyperplasia in adolescents, Pediatrics 72:690, 1983.

Fedele L, Dorta M, Vercellini P, et al: Ultrasound in the diagnosis of subclasses of unicornuate uterus, Obstet Gynecol 71:274, 1988.

Fedele L, Ferranzzi E, Dorta M, et al: Ultrasonography in the differential diagnosis of "double" uteri, Fertil Steril 50:361, 1988.

Fleischnick E, Rum D, Alosco SM, et al: Extended MHC haplotypes in 21-hydroxylase deficiency congenital adrenal hyperplasia: shared genotypes in unrelated patients, Lancet 1:152, 1983.

Greiss FC and Mauzy CH: Congenital anomalies in women: an evaluation of diagnosis, incidence, and obstetric performance, Am J Obstet Gynecol 82:330, 1961.

Hahn-Pedersen J and Larsen PM: Supernumerary ovary, Acta Obstet Gynecol Scand 63:365, 1984.

Hauser GA and Schreiner WE: Das Mayer-Rokitansky-Küster-Syndrom, Schweiz Med Wochenschr 91:381, 1961.

Hay D: Uterus unicornis and its relationship to pregnancy, J Obstet Gynaecol Br Emp 68:371, 1961.

Hogan ML, Barber DD, and Kaufmann RH: Dermoid cyst in supernumerary ovary: the greater omentum: report of a case, Obstet Gynecol 29:405, 1967.

Israel R and March CM: Hysteroscopic incision of the septate uterus, Am J Obstet Gynecol 149:66, 1984.

Kaufman RH, Noller K, Adam E, et al: Upper genital tract abnormalities and pregnancy outcome in diethylstilbestrol-exposed progeny, Am J Obstet Gynecol 148:973, 1984.

McIndoe A: Treatment of congenital absence and obliterative conditions of vagina, Br J Plast Surg 2:254, 1950.

Muller U, Mayerova A, Debus B, et al: Correlation between testicular tissue and HY phenotype in intersex patients, Clin Genet 23:49, 1983.

Musich JR, and Behrman SJ: Obstetric outcome before and after metroplasty in women with uterine anomalies, Obstet Gynecol 52:63, 1978.

Musset R: Classification globale des malformations uterines, Gynécol Obstét 66:145, 1967.

Olive D and Henderson DY: Endometriosis and müllerian anomalies, Obstet Gynecol 69:412, 1987.

Palmer R: Anomalies uterines congenitales. In Boury-Heyler C, Maulbeon P, Rochet Y, et al: Uterus et fécondité, vol 1, Paris, 1981, Masson.

Pang S, Hotchkiss J, Drash AL, et al: Microfilter paper method for 17-hydroxyprogesterone radioimmunoassay: its application for rapid screening for congenital adrenal hyperplasia, J Clin Endocrinol Metab 45:1003, 1977.

Pang S, Murphey W, Levine LS, et al: A pilot newborn screening for congenital adrenal hyperplasia in Alaska, J Clin Endocrinol Metab 55:413, 1982.

Perino A, Mencaglia L, Hamou J, and Cittadini E: Hysteroscopy for metroplasty of uterine septa: report of 24 cases, Fertil Steril 48:321, 1987.

Phelan JT, Counseller VS, and Greene LF: Deformities of the urinary tract with congenital absence of the vagina, Surg Gynecol Obstet 97:1, 1953.

Printz JL, Choate JW, Townes PL, et al: The embryology of supernumerary ovaries, Obstet Gynecol 41:246, 1973.

Semens JP: Congenital anomalies of the female genital tract: functional classification based on a review of 56 personal cases and 5 unreported cases, Obstet Gynecol 19:328, 1962.

Toaff ME, Lev-Toaff AS, and Toaff R: Communicating uteri: review and classification with introduction of two previously unrecorded types, Fertil Steril 41:661, 1984.

Turunen A and Unnerus CE: Spinal changes in patients with congenital aplasia of the vagina, Acta Obstet Gynecol Scand 46:99, 1967.

Valdes C, Malini S, and Malinak LR: Ultrasound evaluation of female genital tract anomalies: a review of 64 cases, Am J Obstet Gynecol 149:285, 1984.

Wharton LR: Two cases of supernumerary ovary and one of accessory ovary within an analysis of previously reported cases, Am J Obstet Gynecol 78:1101, 1959.

Pediatric Gynecology

KEY TERMS AND DEFINITIONS

Adhesive Vulvitis. A self-limiting consequence of chronic vulvitis in which denuded epithelium of adjacent labia minora agglutinates and fuses the two labia together.

Adolescence. The period of life during which an individual matures physiologically and psychologically from a child into an adult.

Factitious Precocious Puberty. The result when a young girl has used or has been given hormonal creams or has ingested adult medications such as oral estrogens or birth control pills.

Gelastic Seizures. An unusual neurologic symptom sometimes associated with precocious puberty. It involves seizures with inappropriate laughter.

Heterosexual Precocious Puberty. Premature virilization in a female child, including development of secondary sexual characteristics.

Incomplete or Pseudoprecocious Puberty. Premature female sexual maturation and uterine bleeding without associated ovulation.

McCune-Albright Syndrome (Polyostotic Fibrous Dysplasia). A rare triad of café-au-lait spots, fibrous dysplasia, and cysts of the skull and long bones.

Precocious Puberty. The appearance of signs of secondary sexual maturation at an age more than 3.0 standard deviation below the mean for the population to which the child belongs. In girls in North America, precocious puberty is defined as initiation of signs of sexual maturation occurring before 8 years of age.

Premature Adrenarche. Isolated early development of axillary hair without other signs of secondary sexual maturation.

Premature Pubarche. Isolated early development of pubic hair without other signs of secondary sexual maturation.

Premature Thelarche. Isolated early unilateral or bilateral breast development without other signs of secondary sexual maturation.

Puberty. The process of biologic and physical development after which sexual reproduction first becomes possible.

$\mathbf{G}$ynecologic diseases are uncommon in children, especially in comparison with the incidence of diseases in women of reproductive age. This chapter considers gynecologic diseases of children from infancy until the completion of puberty. Congenital anomalies and neoplasia of infants are covered in other chapters. The evaluation of children's gynecologic problems involves considerations of physiology, psychology, and treatments that are different from those of adult gynecology.

An outpatient visit by a prepubertal or pu-

bertal child to a gynecologist should be structured differently from a gynecologic visit by a woman of reproductive age. Considerable time must be devoted to gaining the child's confidence and establishing rapport. If the interaction is poor during the first visit, the negative experience will detract from future physician-patient interactions. In addition, a child's visit to a gynecologist usually focuses on a perceived problem rather than on preventive medicine, such as occurs with the usual appointment with the pediatrician. Also, the vast majority of children's gynecologic problems are treated by medical rather than surgical means.

The most frequent gynecologic disease of children is *vulvovaginitis*. Vulvitis is the primary problem, with vaginitis of secondary importance unless there is associated vaginal bleeding, a foreign body, sexual abuse, or a sexually transmitted disease.

Adolescence is the period of life during which an individual matures physiologically and psychologically from a child into an adult. This period of transition involves important physical and emotional changes. Before puberty, the child's female organs are in a resting, dormant state. Puberty produces dramatic alterations in both the external and the internal female genitalia. The range of normality of pubertal changes is emphasized in Chapter 36. Because the changes are frequently a cause of concern for adolescent females and their parents, the gynecologist must offer the adolescent female a kind, patient, and gentle approach. These interactions between the physician and the adolescent female will allow the physician an opportunity to instruct the pubertal teenager about pelvic anatomy and establish a trusting relationship. Thus at the appropriate time, contraceptive counseling may occur.

GYNECOLOGIC EXAMINATION OF A CHILD

A successful gynecologic examination of a child demands that the physician adopt a slow pace, take ample time, and show gentleness and patience. The examination should not be hurried or rushed. The components of a complete pediatric examination include a history, inspection with visualization of the vagina and cervix, appropriate cultures of the vagina, and a rectal examination if the patient has vaginal bleeding or abdominal or pelvic pain. To accomplish each step of the examination, the clinician and nurse must establish rapport with the child. A child's reaction will depend on her age, emotional maturity, and previous experience with health care providers. The child's anxiety should be assessed during the general physical examination. Sometimes it is best to defer the pelvic examination until a second visit. This is a difficult decision and is based on the extent of the child's anxiety in relation to the severity of the clinical symptoms. A physician may elect to treat the primary symptoms

of vulvovaginitis for 2 to 3 weeks before searching for a foreign body. However, Capraro warned that physicians should not share parents' reluctance to have the female child examined. He emphasized that in the field of pediatric gynecology most errors are errors of omission rather than commission.

Obtaining a history from a child is not an easy process. Children are not skilled historians and will often ramble, introducing many unrelated facts. Much of the history must be obtained from the parents. However, both the child and the parents are often reluctant to report genital symptoms. Consequently, most gynecologic symptoms in children are chronic when first seen by the physician.

After the history has been obtained, the parents and the child should be reassured that the examination will not hurt. To successfully examine a child, one needs the cooperation of the patient, her mother, and a skilled nurse with empathy for children. The nurse must be a reassuring influence on the child during the examination.

During the history and most of the general physical examination, the child should sit on the edge of the examination table. A helpful technique is to place the child's hand on top of the physician's hand as the abdominal examination is being performed. This will give the child a sense of control as well as diverting the child's attention if she is ticklish or is moving or squirming. For the pelvic examination a young child is best examined on her mother's lap. An older child may be examined in the supine position with her knees apart and her feet together or in the knee-chest position. Draping for the gynecologic examination produces more anxiety than it relieves and should be avoided for the preadolescent child. The most important step to ensure cooperation is to involve the child as a partner.

A child should never be restrained for a gynecologic examination. If a child is extremely anxious, mild sedation may be helpful. The combination of 50 mg (1 ml) meperidine (Demerol), 12.5 mg (0.5 ml) chlorpromazine hydrochloride (Thorazine), and 12.5 mg (0.5 ml) promethazine hydrochloride (Phenergan) may be given in a dose of 1 ml intramuscularly for every 20 pounds, to a maximum of 2 ml. In rare circumstances it may be necessary to use general anesthesia to examine an extremely apprehensive child.

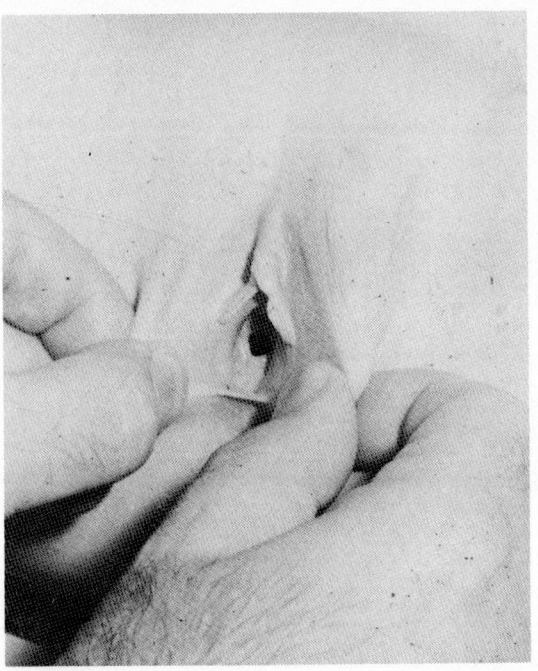

FIGURE 10-1
Pulling labia gently laterally and toward examiner reveals hymenal opening and permits visualization of vaginal canal. (From Capraro VJ: Pediatric gynecology. In Danforth DN, editor: Obstetrics and gynecology, ed 4, Philadelphia, 1982, Harper & Row, Publishers, Inc.)

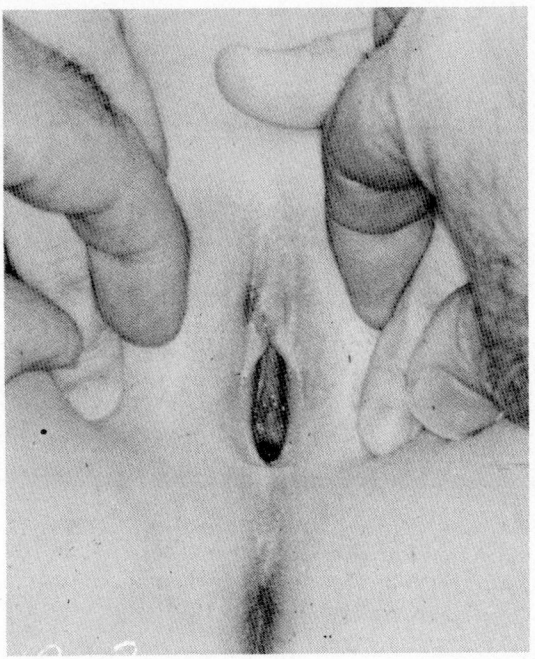

FIGURE 10-2
Child helps examiner by separating labia. This not only assures her that she will not be hurt but also distracts her, permitting examiner to use fingers without her realizing it. (From Capraro VJ: Pediatric gynecology. In Danforth DN, editor: Obstetrics and gynecology, ed 4, Philadelphia, 1982, Harper & Row, Publishers, Inc.)

The initial phase of the pelvic examination involves inspection of the vulvar area. The child and the nurse may facilitate inspection of the distal vagina by exerting pressure laterally and posteriorly on the inferior portion of the labia and surrounding skin (Figures 10-1 and 10-2). The vaginal epithelium of the prepubertal child appears redder and thinner as compared with the vagina of a woman in her reproductive years. The vagina is 4 to 6 cm long, and the secretions have a neutral pH. Emans and Goldstein (1990) have found that the knee-chest position usually allows the physician to visualize the vagina and cervix of a child after age 2 years without instrumentation. Inspection is facilitated by the vagina being filled with air in the knee-chest position (Figure 10-3). The child is encouraged to lie on her "tummy" with her buttocks in the air. The nurse holds the buttocks apart, and with relaxation of the abdominal muscles and a few deep inspirations,

the vaginal orifice opens and the canal fills with air. A bright light helps to illuminate the upper vagina and cervix. The cervix appears as a transverse ridge or pleat that is redder than the vagina. Following inspection of the vagina and cervix, vaginal secretions may be obtained for microscopic examination and culture, with either a plastic medicine dropper or a saline-saturated, cotton-tipped applicator. Dry cotton-tipped applicators are abrasive and may cause discomfort to the child. Pokorny has described a new method for collecting fluid from a child's vagina using a catheter within a catheter. This easily assembled adaptation uses a no. 12 red rubber bladder catheter for the outer catheter and the hub end of an intravenous butterfly catheter for the inner catheter (Figure 10-4). The outer catheter serves as an insulator, and the inner catheter is used to instill a small amount of saline and aspirate the vaginal fluid.

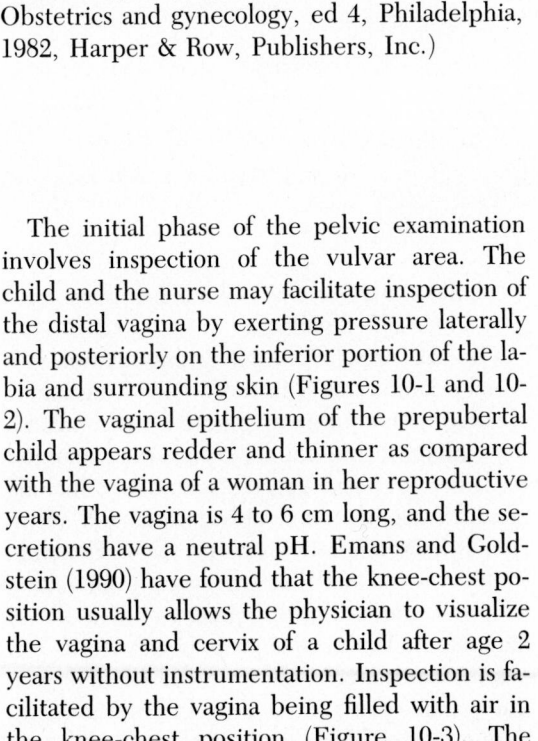

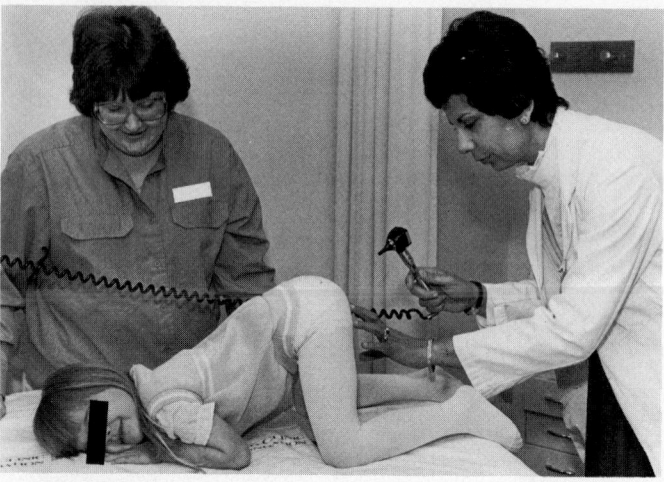

FIGURE 10-3
Knee-chest position used to examine child to visualize cervix and vagina. Otoscope head is usually longer than one shown in photograph. (From Gidwani GP: Clin Obstet Gynecol 30:643, 1987.)

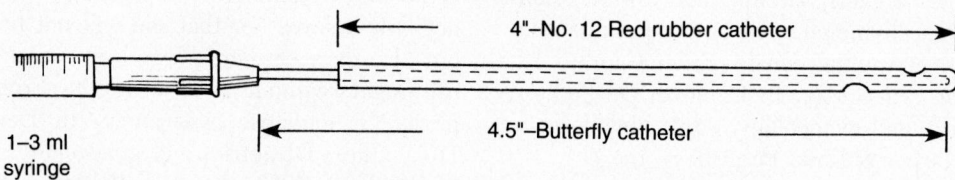

FIGURE 10-4
Assembled catheter-within-a-catheter, as used to obtain samples of vaginal secretions from prepubertal patients. (Redrawn from Pokorny SF and Stormer J: Am J Obstet Gynecol 156:581, 1987.)

Recurrent vulvovaginitis, persistent bleeding, suspicion of a foreign body or neoplasm, and congenital anomalies are indications for vaginoscopy. Introduction of any instrument into the vagina of a young child takes patience and time. The prepubertal vagina is narrower, thinner, and lacking in the distensibility of the vagina of a woman in her reproductive years. There are many narrow-diameter endoscopes that will suffice, including the Kelly air cystoscope, contact hysteroscopes, pediatric cystoscopes, small-diameter laparoscopes, plastic vaginoscopes, and special virginal speculums designed by Huffman and Pederson (Figure 10-5). A nasal speculum or otoscope is usually too short. The physician can divert the child's attention from the endoscope in the vagina by simultaneously gently compressing one of the patient's buttocks. Sometimes, one can divert the child's attention by having her blow up a latex glove like a balloon.

The last step in the pelvic examination is a rectal examination. This most distressing aspect of the examination may sometimes be omitted, depending on the child's symptoms. Common reasons to perform a rectal examination include genital tract bleeding, pelvic pain, and suspicion of a foreign body or pelvic mass. The child should be warned that the rectal examination will feel similar to the pressure of a bowel movement. The normal prepubertal uterus and ovaries are nonpalpable on rectal examination. The relative size ratio of cervix to uterus is two to one in a child, in contrast to the larger fundus in the adult. Any mass discovered on rectal examination except the cervix of an older child should be considered abnormal. At the conclusion of the rectal examination the child should

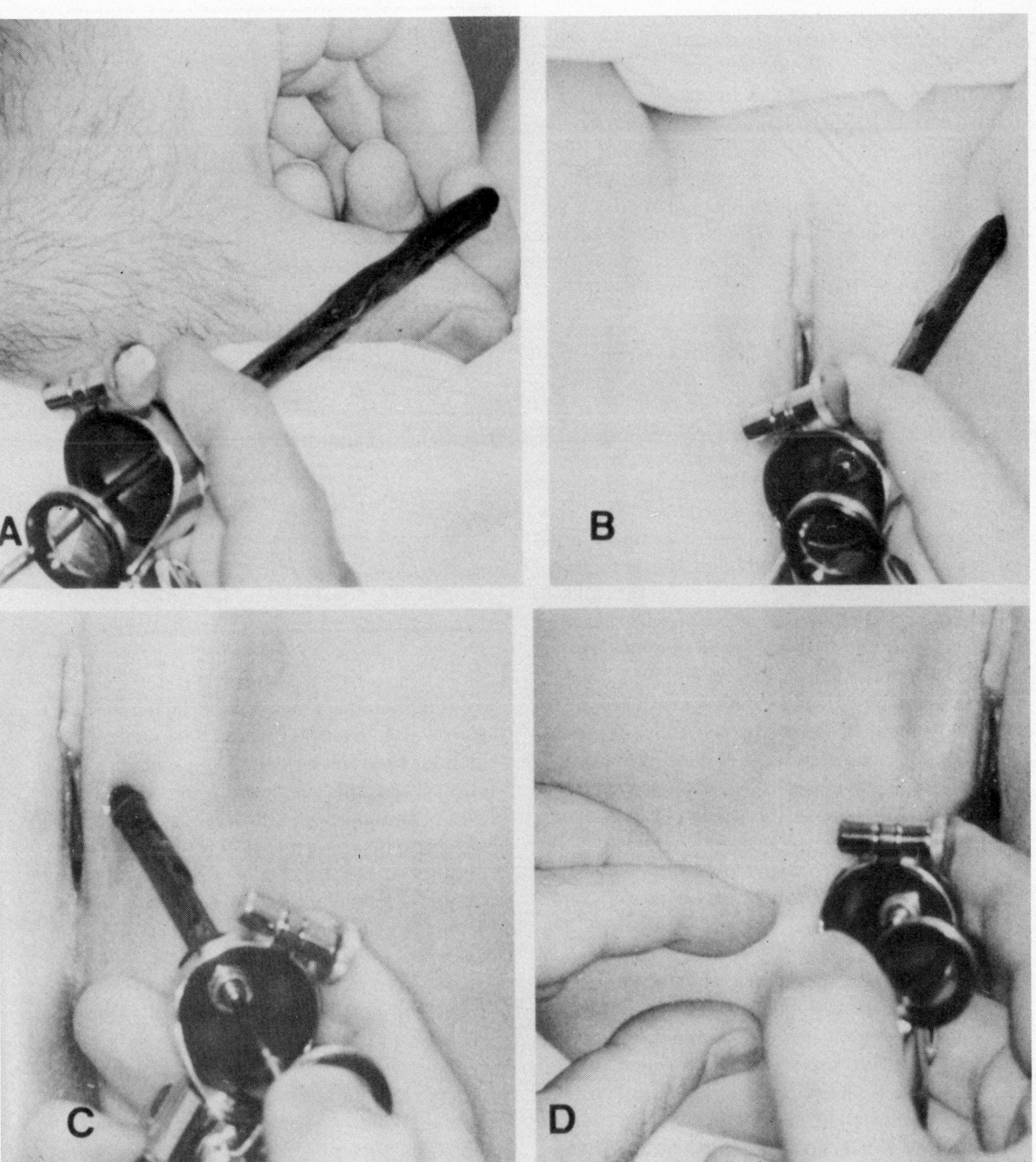

FIGURE 10-5

Vaginoscopic examination. **A,** Child touches well-lubricated vaginoscope with her index finger; examiner points out that it feels "funny," slippery, and cool. **B,** Speculum is then placed against inner left thigh, and examiner repeats that it feels slippery and cool. **C,** Speculum next touches left labium majus, and examiner makes same remarks. **D,** When speculum is passed through hymenal opening, patient does not jump because previous three steps have conditioned her to feel speculum. Note that examiner's left hand simultaneously presses patient's right buttock firmly to distract her from speculum as it is passing painlessly through hymenal orifice. (From Capraro VJ: Pediatric gynecology. In Danforth DN, editor: Obstetrics and gynecology, ed 4, Philadelphia, 1982, Harper & Row, Publishers, Inc.)

be praised for her cooperation.

The critical factors surrounding the pelvic examination of a female adolescent are different than examinations of younger children 2 to 8 years old. Many female adolescents do not want other observers in the examining room. In one study at a university hospital clinic, 24% of inner-city youths did not want a chaperone present. Also 60% to 80% of private adolescent patients request no chaperone, even when the examining gynecologist is a man.

VULVOVAGINITIS

Vulvovaginitis is the most common gynecologic problem of the premenarcheal female. It is estimated that 80% to 90% of outpatient visits of children to gynecologists involve the classic symptoms of vulvovaginitis: introital irritation and discharge. Although the severity of these symptoms varies widely from child to child, usually the parents express great concern. The pathophysiology of the majority of instances of vulvovaginitis in children involves a primary irritation of the vulva with secondary involvement of the lower one third of the vagina. Approximately 75% of children with vulvovaginitis have a nonspecific etiology; that is, cultures are similar to the flora of the gastrointestinal tract. One in four cultures of the discharge from vulvovaginitis will identify a specific organism, such as *Neisseria gonorrhoeae, Trichomonas vaginalis, Chlamydia trachomatis,* herpes simplex virus, *Shigella boydii,* or mycotic or bacterial vaginosis (Table 10-1). The vulvar irritation may be secondary to a topical allergy, skin or respiratory infection, foreign body, urinary tract infection, vulvar skin disease, ectopic ureter, pinworms, or sexual abuse (see box on p. 277). Positive identification of *Trichomonas,* gonorrhea, or *Chlamydia* in a child with premenarcheal vulvovaginitis often indicates sexual molestation.

There are both physiologic and behavioral reasons why a child is susceptible to vulvar infection. Physiologically, the child's vulva and vagina are exposed to bacterial contamination more frequently than are the adult's. Because the child lacks the labial fat pads and pubic hair of the adult, when a child squats, the lower one third of the vagina is unprotected and open. The vulvar and vaginal epithelium lack the protective effects of estrogen and thus are sensitive to irritation or infection. The thin vag-

TABLE 10-1

Etiology and Age Distribution for 500 Cases of Vulvovaginitis

Cause	Number	Average Age (Years)
Nonspecific (mixed)	213	8.8
Monilia (Candida)	63	12.5
Foreign body	55	7.2
Streptococcus	45	10.4
Physiologic	33	11.5
Staphylococcus	30	6.9
Gonococcus	24	9.9
Trichomonas	15	11.9
Pinworms	8	6.3
Congenital anomalies	6	6.2
Escherichia coli	5	4.6
Other	2	5.0
4-degree tear	1	14.0

From Capraro VJ: Pediatric gynecology. In Danforth DN, editor: Obstetrics and gynecology, ed 4, Philadelphia, 1982, Harper & Row, Publishers, Inc, p 892.

inal epithelium of a prepubertal child has a neutral pH, which provides an excellent medium for bacterial growth. The vagina of a child lacks glycogen, lactobacilli, and a sufficient level of antibodies to help resist infection. The normal vagina of a prepubertal child is colonized by an average of nine different species of bacteria—four aerobic and facultative anaerobic species and five obligatory anaerobic species.

The major factor in childhood vulvovaginitis is poor perineal hygiene. This results from the anatomic proximity of the rectum and vagina coupled with the fact that following toilet training, most youngsters are unsupervised when they defecate. Many youngsters wipe their anus from posterior to anterior and thus inoculate the vulvar skin with intestinal flora. A minor vulvar irritation may result in a scratch-itch cycle, with the possibility of secondary seeding because children rarely wash their hands. Similarly, a child with an upper respiratory tract infection may autoinoculate her vulva, especially with group A beta-hemolytic streptococci. Children's clothing is often tight fitting, which keeps the vulvar skin warm and moist and prone to vulvovaginitis.

There is nothing specific about the symptoms or signs of childhood vulvovaginitis. Often the first awareness comes when the mother no-

ETIOLOGIC FACTORS IN PREMENARCHEAL VULVOVAGINAL INFECTIONS AND INFLAMMATIONS

Bacterial causes
  Nonspecific mixed infections secondary to:
    Poor perineal hygiene
    Respiratory infections
    Skin infections
    Intestinal parasitic invasion of vagina
    Foreign bodies in vagina
    Urinary tract infection
    Unknown avenues of infection
  Specific nongonorrheal infection caused by:
    The exanthemas
    Haemophilus vaginalis (Corynebacterium vaginalis)
    Hemolytic streptococci
    Corynebacterium diphtheriae
    Neisseria meningitidis
    Neisseria sicca
    Diplococcus pneumoniae
    Shigella boydii
    Chlamydia
  Gonorrhea
Protozoal infections
  Trichomoniasis
  Amebiasis
  Other

Mycotic causes
  Candida albicans
  Other candidal organisms
  Other mycotic organisms
Mycoplasmas
Helminthiasis
Hirudiniasis
Viral infections
  Chickenpox
  Smallpox
  Vaccinia
  Condyloma acuminatum
  Herpes
Physical agents
  Sandbox
  Other agents
Chemical agents
  Bubble bath preparations
  Medications
  Deodorant vulvar sprays
Allergenic agents
  Nylon or rayon underclothing
  Medications
  Soaps, laundry detergents
  Other allergens
  Neurogenic factors
Neoplasia
Granulomatous diseases
Syphilis

From Huffman JW: The gynecology of childhood and adolescence, ed 2, Philadelphia, 1981, WB Saunders Co, p 123.

tices staining of the child's underpants. There is a wide range in the quantity of discharge, from minimal to copious. The color ranges from white or gray to yellow or green. Symptoms associated with vulvovaginitis include pain, pruritus, irritation, and occasionally dysuria. A discharge that is both bloody and foul smelling strongly suggests the presence of a foreign body. Signs are variable and not diagnostic but include vulvar erythema, edema, and excoriation.

The differential diagnosis of persistent or recurrent vulvovaginitis should include considerations of a foreign body, pinworms, primary vulvar skin disease, ectopic ureter, and child abuse. A history of a foul, bloody vaginal discharge is highly indicative of a foreign body; however, the discharge associated with a foreign body is not invariably bloody or foul smelling. Approximately 20% of female chil-

dren infected with pinworms *(Enterobius vermicularis)* develop vulvovaginitis. The classic symptom of pinworms is nocturnal vulvar and perianal itching. At night the milk-white, pin-sized adult worms migrate from the rectum to the skin of the vulva to deposit eggs. They may be discovered by means of a flashlight or by dabbing of the vulvar skin with clear cellophane adhesive tape. The tape is subsequently examined under the microscope. The vulvar skin of children may also be affected by systemic skin diseases, including lichen sclerosus, seborrheic dermatitis, psoriasis, and atopic dermatitis. An ectopic ureter emptying into the vagina may only intermittently release a small amount of urine; thus this rare congenital anomaly should be considered in the differential diagnosis.

In the period from 6 to 12 months before menarche, children often develop a physiologic vaginal discharge secondary to the increase in circulating estrogen levels. This gray-white discharge is nonirritating. When the physiologic discharge is examined with the microscope, sheets of vaginal epithelial cells are identified. The only treatment necessary is reassurance of both mother and child that this is a normal physiologic process that will subside with time.

The foundation of treating childhood vulvovaginitis is the improvement of local perineal hygiene. Both mother and child should be instructed that the vulvar skin should be kept clean, dry, and cool. For acute weeping lesions, wet compresses of Burow's solution should be prescribed. An alternative is a sitz bath containing 2 tablespoons of baking soda in the water. The child should be taught to wipe from front to back after defecation. Loose-fitting cotton undergarments should be worn. Chemicals that may produce topical allergies, such as bubble bath, must be discontinued. Harsh soaps and chemicals should be avoided, and dryness of the vulva should be maintained with calamine lotion or a nonirritating talcum powder. Approximately one in four episodes of childhood vulvovaginitis is cured by improved local hygiene. The vast majority of cases of nonspecific vulvovaginitis respond to a combination of topical estrogen cream and oral antibiotics given for 10 to 14 days. Estrogen cream is applied to the vulvar area each night. It is not necessary to place hormonal cream into the vagina. The parent should be cautioned that the vulvar skin will become darker and not to use the cream for longer than 3 to 4 weeks because of systemic absorption. Vaginal cultures help to determine the choice of oral broad-spectrum antibiotics; usually a tetracycline, depending on the child's age, or ampicillin is appropriate (dosage depends on the child's weight). If the child has intense pruritus, 0.5% hydrocortisone cream may be applied.

Appropriate treatment of pinworms is the anthelmintic agent mebendazole (Vermox). The dosage is one chewable tablet for each family member over the age of 2 years (one dose only). Vermox is contraindicated in pregnancy.

Foreign Bodies

Symptoms secondary to a vaginal foreign body are responsible for approximately 4% of pediatric gynecologic outpatient visits. The history is usually not helpful because the mother has not witnessed, nor does the child remember, putting a foreign object into the vagina. Many types of foreign bodies have been discovered; however, the most common are small wads of toilet paper. Other common foreign objects include small, hard objects, such as hairpins, parts of a toy, crayons, and small pebbles of sand or gravel. As emphasized previously, the classic symptom is a foul, bloody vaginal discharge. Large objects may be removed by means of bayonet forceps; small objects such as sand may be washed out of the vagina by irrigation. It is frustrating to parents and physicians alike that often the child places another foreign body into the vagina several months later.

Vaginal Bleeding

Persistent vaginal bleeding is an extremely rare symptom in a preadolescent female. The differential diagnosis of vaginal bleeding includes neoplasia, precocious puberty, urethral prolapse, trauma, sexual assault, vulvar vaginitis, and possible exposure to exogenous estrogens either from oral preparations or skin creams. The differential diagnosis of a bloody vaginal discharge includes the consideration of two bacterial infections of the vagina: Shigella and group A beta-hemolytic streptococcus. The latter usually occurs 7 to 10 days after a sore throat or upper respiratory tract infection. Because of the serious sequelae of some of these diseases, it is mandatory to adequately visualize the entire lower reproductive tract. Usually, endoscopy for vaginal bleeding is performed with the patient under general anesthesia.

In a recent 20-year review of vaginal bleeding, 52 cases were identified in girls 10 years and younger from the Chelsea Hospital for Women. Genital tumors, precocious puberty, vulvar lesions, and urethral prolapse were the four leading causes in this series (Tables 10-2 and 10-3). This report by Hill et al. was from a referral center and therefore may not truly represent the cases seen in the practitioner's office. The authors of this series could not explain the absence of the diagnosis of sexual abuse in their study.

ADHESIVE VULVITIS

Adhesive vulvitis is a self-limiting consequence of chronic vulvitis in which denuded

TABLE 10-2
Age at Presentation of Vaginal Bleeding

Age (Years)	Number of Girls
0-1	6
1-2	7
2-3	4
3-4	2
4-5	8
5-6	5
6-7	3
7-8	4
8-9	2
9-10	5
10	6

From Hill NCW, Oppenheimer LW, and Morton KE: Br J Obstet Gynecol 96:467, 1989.

TABLE 10-3
Etiology of Vaginal Bleeding

	Number	Percentage
Genital tumours	11	21
Precocious puberty	11	21
Vulval lesions	5	10
Urethral prolapse	5	10
Trauma	4	8
Vulvovaginitis	3	6
Unknown aetiology	13	25

From Hill NCW, Oppenheimer LW, and Morton KE: Br J Obstet Gynecol 96:467, 1989.

epithelium of adjacent labia minora agglutinates and fuses the two labia together. This condition is usually not a serious one; however, it may be mistaken for congenital absence of the vagina. This condition is most common in young girls between 2 and 6 years of age. In one large study the average age of a child with agglutination of the labia was 2½ years; 90% of cases appeared before age 6. The labia minora stick together in the midline, forming a translucent vertical line. This thin, narrow line in an anteroposterior direction is pathognomonic for a diagnosis of adhesive vulvitis. In mild or early stages of the process, agglutination occurs only in the posterior aspects of the labia (Figure 10-6). There is considerable variation in the length of agglutination of the two labia minora. In the most advanced cases, there is fusion over both the urethral and the vaginal orifices. Most children are free of symptoms. If the urethra is covered, there may be difficulty in voiding and associated urinary tract infections.

No treatment is necessary for adhesive vulvitis unless the child has problems in voiding. Jenkinson and Mackinnon published results of a series of 10 girls who had no therapy and noted spontaneous separation of the adhesive vulvitis within 6 to 18 months. Most mothers prefer active treatment of the condition. Topical estrogen cream dabbed onto the labia once a day will result in spontaneous separation within 2 to 4 weeks. Forceful separation is un-

necessarily traumatic and should not be done. Recurrent adhesive vulvitis occurs in one of five children. A familial form of true posterior labial fusion has been reported by several authors. Analysis of the pedigrees of these children suggests that this congenital defect may be an autosomal dominant trait with incomplete penetrance.

McCann et al. (1988) emphasized the association between injuries of the posterior fourchette and labial adhesions in sexually abused children. Labial agglutination alone is so common that suspicion of child abuse is unwarranted. However, the combination of labial adhesions and scarring of the posterior fourchette obligates the gynecologist to consider sexual abuse in the differential diagnosis.

GENITAL TRAUMA

The usual cause of genital trauma during childhood is an accidental fall. Most of these traumas involve straddle injuries. If the vulva strikes a blunt object, a hematoma usually results. If the object is sharp, such as a fence post, the injury may be a laceration with the potential for penetration of the perineum and injury to internal pelvic organs. Other common causes of vulvar and vaginal trauma include sexual molestation, automobile and bicycle accidents, being kicked in a fight, and self-inflicted wounds (Figure 10-7). Sexual molestation is discussed in Chapter 12.

The size of vulvar and vaginal hematomas varies widely. Initially there is bleeding into the loose connective tissue. When the pressure

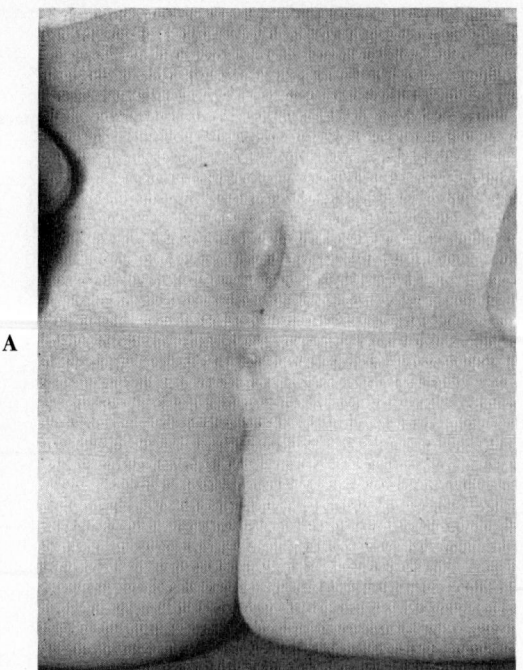

A

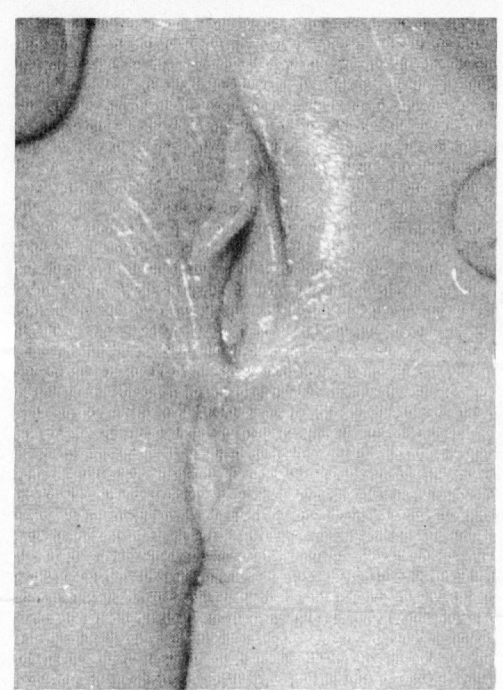

B

FIGURE 10-6
A, Labial adhesions in 2½-year-old girl. Two tiny openings exist, one beneath clitoris and another near middle of line of fusion. **B,** Appearance in same child after 10 days of local application of estrogen ointment. (From Dewhurst CJ: Gynaecological disorders of infants and children, Philadelphia, 1963, FA Davis Co.)

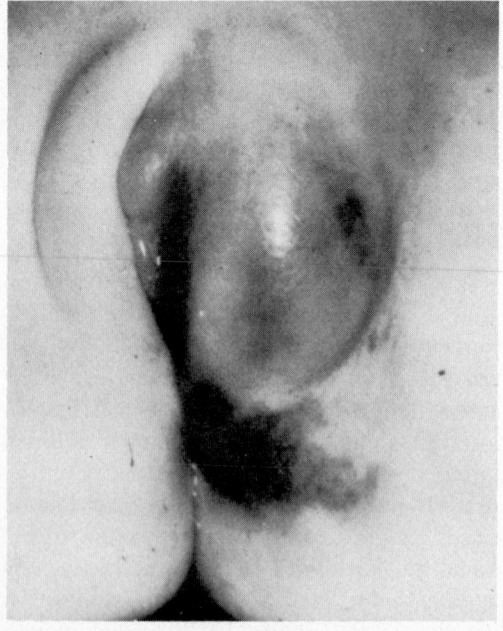

FIGURE 10-7
Vulvar hematoma resulting from a kick in 2-year-old child. (From Huffman JW: The gynecology of childhood and adolescence, ed 2, Philadelphia, 1981, WB Saunders Co.)

from the expanding hematoma exceeds the venous pressure, in most cases the hematoma will stop growing. In lacerations when an artery has been traumatized, bleeding may continue until the artery is ligated.

The diagnosis of a vulvar or vaginal hematoma is straightforward with a history of trauma and the appearance of a bluish red mass. The extent of the hematoma should be determined by both visualization and palpation. The extent of injury with a laceration is more difficult to assess. The depth of most lacerations is usually more extensive than suspected on initial inspection. Vaginal lacerations are almost always associated with corresponding vulvar injuries. The extent of the penetrating injury to the lateral vaginal wall may be more serious than the patient's symptoms indicate, as these injuries are associated with minor symptoms. With penetrating lacerations, trauma to the bladder, intestines, and peritoneal cavity must be ruled out. If gross hematuria is discovered, the child should undergo cystoscopy. General anesthesia is usually required to investigate the extent and depth of all vaginal lacerations and the majority of extensive vulvar lacerations.

The treatment of nonexpanding vulvar hematomas is the use of an ice pack or ice sitz bath. Rarely a hematoma will continue to increase in size necessitating evacuation and ligation of bleeding vessels. The identification of a bleeding vessel is difficult at best, and conservative therapy is preferable. As stated previously, general anesthesia is usually required for diagnosis of extensive lacerations. During this anesthesia the laceration should be irrigated and debrided, the vessels ligated, and the injuries repaired. Occasionally it is necessary to perform an exploratory celiotomy for a suspected retroperitoneal hematoma. Children with vulvar trauma should have a booster injection of tetanus toxoid if the last immunization was more than 5 years before the trauma.

PELVIC MASS

Recurrent abdominal pain is a frequent complaint of grammar school children. From 10% to 15% experience this symptom. The young child does not differentiate lower abdominal pain from pelvic pain. Often, because of the smallness of the preadolescent female pelvis, the ovaries are abdominal organs. Ovarian tumors constitute approximately 1% of all neoplasias in premenarcheal children. Thus ovarian neoplasia must be considered in the differential diagnosis of children with persistent or recurrent abdominal pain. Pediatricians used to order an intravenous pyelogram as one of the first diagnostic tests in investigating abdominal pain of unknown origin. Recently, ultrasound and abdominal computed tomography (CT) have been more useful in establishing the diagnosis. Calcifications in an ovarian mass indicate a diagnosis of an ovarian teratoma. The increased use of ultrasound in young females complaining of abdominal pain has led to the discovery of echolucent areas within the ovary. Follicular cysts greater than 20 mm in diameter are frequently discovered; however, almost all will disappear spontaneously within 4 to 6 weeks.

The most common clinical manifestation of an ovarian tumor is lower abdominal pain or the presence of a mass. Some ovarian tumors in children produce only vague discomfort, such as abdominal fullness or bloating. The latter tumors are sometimes discovered by diagnostic radiologic techniques or ultrasound. However, adnexal masses in children are more frequently associated with acute complications, such as torsion, hemorrhage, and rupture, than are similar tumors in adults. Torsion of a normal ovary or fallopian tube is a rare but serious problem in children. Often the symptoms caused by a reduction of the ovarian blood supply produced by torsion is subclinical, with the process progressing to aseptic necrosis of the involved adnexa. The etiology of torsion of normal adnexa in children is not understood. McCrea and other researchers have suggested suspension of the uninvolved ovary to prevent subsequent torsion of the remaining adnexa.

Shawis et al. reviewed 71 premenarcheal females with ovarian tumors hospitalized during a 33-year period in Liverpool (Table 10-4). In this series an abdominal mass was palpated in 20 children, and eight masses were discovered by means of rectal examination. Fifteen of the 71 patients had adnexal torsion. Ten of the tumors (14%) were malignant, with dysgerminoma being the most common malignant neoplasm. Benign teratoma was the most common tumor in children. Conservative surgery, cystectomy, was accomplished in 16 of the 61 benign lesions.

Ehren et al. published the results of a similar series of 63 children with benign and malignant ovarian neoplasms in a review of 21 years' experience from The Children's Hospital in Los Angeles. The histologic diagnosis in 47 children was benign neoplasms—41 teratomas and 6 ovarian cystadenomas. More than 75% of the children had a history of chronic abdominal pain. The percentages of torsion (41%), palpable abdominal masses (83%), and calcifications on x-ray examination (54%) were all higher than those in the Shawis et al. series. However, only 6 of the 47 children with benign tumors had cystectomy with preservation of ovarian tissue. Again, cystic teratoma was the most common benign tumor in these children.

The most common differential diagnosis of an abdominopelvic mass in children that is not an ovarian mass is a benign cyst of the mesentery or omentum. Benign uterine tumors are rare in children. However, functional luteal cysts of the ovary are not uncommon in neonates secondary to maternal gonadotrophins. These cysts do not need operative intervention as they will regress spontaneously.

In summary, approximately 75% of ovarian neoplasms that necessitate surgery, in premenarcheal females, are benign teratomas, and ap-

TABLE 10-4
Pathology of Tumors and Cysts of the Ovary

Type	Classification	Number
Benign neoplasms	Teratoma	30
	Cystadenoma	6 (one bilateral)
	Granulosa cell tumor	2
	Brenner's disease	1
Malignant neoplasms	Dysgerminoma	8
	Anaplastic carcinoma	2 (one bilateral)
"Functional" neoplasms	Luteal cysts	8 (one bilateral)
	Follicular cyst	7
Neoplasms of indeterminate histology (hemorrhage or infarction)		8

From Shawis RN, El Gohary AE, and Cook RCM: Ann R Coll Surg Engl 67:18, 1985.

proximately 25% are malignant tumors. Abdominal pain is the most common symptom, and an abdominopelvic mass is the most frequent sign of an ovarian tumor in childhood. Even though ovarian neoplasia is rare in children, this diagnosis must be considered in a young girl with abdominal pain and a palpable mass.

PRECOCIOUS PUBERTY

Puberty in the female is the process of biologic change and physical development after which sexual reproduction becomes possible. This is a time of accelerated linear skeletal growth and development of secondary sexual characteristics, such as breast development and the appearance of axillary and pubic hair. The usual sequence of the physiologic events of puberty begins with breast development, the subsequent appearance of pubic and axillary hair, followed by the period of maximal growth velocity, and lastly, menarche. Menarche may occur before the appearance of axillary or pubic hair in 10% of normal females. Normal puberty occurs over a wide range of ages (Chapter 36). Precocious puberty is arbitrarily defined as the appearance of any signs of secondary sexual maturation at an age more than 3.0 standard deviations below the mean. Thus, in females in North America, precocious puberty is initiation of secondary sexual characteristics before the age of 8 years or menarche beginning before 9 years. Precocious puberty is associated with a wide range of disorders (see box on p. 283). When it is diagnosed, the physician should undertake a detailed investigation of the etiology of the condition in order not to overlook a potentially correctable pathologic lesion. The two primary concerns of parents of children with precocious puberty are the social stigma associated with the child being physically different from her peers and the diminished ultimate height caused by the premature closure of epiphyseal growth centers.

Puberty is a time of accelerated growth, skeletal maturation, and resulting epiphyseal closure. Although precocious puberty occurs early in a child's life, it usually develops in the normal sequence. This produces the paradox of precocious puberty. Early in the course of the disease the girls are taller and heavier than their chronologic peers who have not experienced the growth spurt (Figure 10-8). However, although the patient is tall as a child, her eventual adult height will be shorter than normal. Without therapy, approximately 50% of females with precocious puberty will not reach a height of 5 feet. The pathophysiology of this short stature is related to the limited duration of the rapid growth spurt. There is accelerated bone maturation and premature closure of the distal epiphyseal growth centers.

The syndrome of precocious puberty is subdivided into complete (true) or incomplete (pseudo) and isosexual and heterosexual disorders. These definitions are of clinical value only after the eventual diagnosis has been estab-

DIFFERENTIAL DIAGNOSIS OF PRECOCIOUS PUBERTY

I. Complete or true precocious puberty
   A. Idiopathic or constitutional causes
   B. Neurogenic, cerebral lesions
      1. Tumors of hypothalamus, pineal gland, or cortex, including hamartoma, craniopharyngioma, glioma
      2. Infections, including toxoplasmosis, encephalitis, meningitis
      3. Neurocutaneous syndromes, neurofibromatosis
      4. Developmental defects, including microcephaly, tuberous sclerosis, aqueductal stenosis, craniostenosis
      5. Trauma
      6. Miscellaneous causes: Sturge-Weber syndrome, diffuse encephalopathy, idiopathic epilepsy
   C. McCune-Albright syndrome
   D. Juvenile primary hypothyroidism
   E. Silver's syndrome (craniofacial disproportion, small stature, retarded bone age, increased gonadotrophin levels)
II. Incomplete or pseudoprecocious puberty
   A. Premature pubarche
   B. Premature thelarche
   C. Adrenal lesions: congenital adrenal hyperplasia, Cushing syndrome, tumors
   D. Ovarian tumors: estrogen producing, granulosa-theca cell, luteoma
   E. Iatrogenic causes: androgen or estrogen administration, vitamins, oral contraceptives
III. Extrapituitary gonadotrophin production
   A. Gonadotrophin-secreting tumors: choriocarcinoma, teratoma, hepatoblastoma, dysgerminoma
   B. Exogenous gonadotrophin administration

Adapted from Goldfarb AF: Endocrine disturbance of puberty. In Lavery JP and Sanfilippo JS, editors: Pediatric and adolescent obstetrics and gynecology, New York, 1985, Springer-Verlag, p 176.

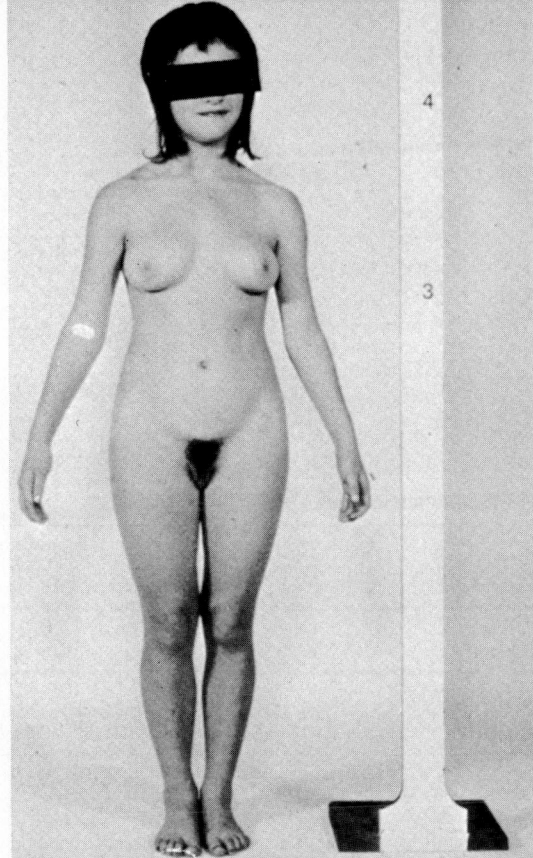

FIGURE 10-8
Child aged 7 years with constitutional precocious puberty. Note increased height for age. (From Dewhurst CJ: Practical pediatric and adolescent gynecology, New York, 1980, Marcel Dekker, Inc. Reprinted courtesy of Marcel Dekker, Inc.)

lished. The pathophysiology of precocious puberty is divided into two distinct categories: a normal physiologic process occurring at an abnormal time or an abnormal physiologic process independent of an integrated hypothalamic-pituitary-ovarian axis. Complete or true precocious puberty involves premature matura-

tion of the hypothalamic-pituitary-ovarian axis and includes normal menses, ovulation, and the possibility of pregnancy. Incomplete or pseudoprecocious puberty involves premature female sexual maturation and uterine bleeding but without associated ovulation. In the latter syndrome, secretion of estrogens is independent of hypothalamic-pituitary control. Obviously, depending on when the patient is first seen in relationship to the natural history of her disease, it may be necessary to observe her at regular intervals for 2 to 3 years to distinguish one syndrome from another (Tables 10-5 and 10-6). Prolonged follow-up is sometimes necessary to rule out subtle, slow-growing lesions of the brain, ovary, or adrenal gland. The

TABLE 10-5

Physical Findings Among Patients with Various Syndromes of True Precocious Puberty

| | | | True Precocious Puberty | | | |
Findings	Premature Thelarche	Premature Adrenarche	Idiopathic	Central Nervous System Tumor	McCune-Albright Syndrome	Hypothyroid
Breast enlargement	Yes	No	Yes	Yes	Yes	Yes
Pubic hair	No	Yes	Yes	Yes	Yes	Unusual
Vaginal bleeding	No	No	Yes	Yes	Yes	Yes
Virilizing signs	No	No	No	No	No	No
Bone age	Normal	Normal to minimally advanced	Advanced	Advanced	Advanced	Normal or retarded
Neurologic deficit	No	No	No	Yes	Yes	No
Abdominopelvic mass	No	No	Occ'l	No	No	Occasionally

From Ross GT: Disorders of the ovary and female reproductive tract. In Wilson JD and Foster DW, editors: Williams textbook of endocrinology, ed 7, Philadelphia, 1985, WB Saunders Co, p 230.

TABLE 10-6

Physical Findings Among Patients with Various Syndromes of Pseudoprecocious Puberty

| | Isosexual | | | Heterosexual | | |
Findings	Ovarian Tumors	Adrenal Tumors	Factitious	Ovarian Tumors	Adrenal Tumors	Adrenal Hyperplasia
Breast enlargement	Yes	Yes	Yes	Yes	Yes	Yes
Pubic hair	Yes	Yes	Yes	Yes	Yes	Yes
Vaginal bleeding	Yes	Yes	Yes	Yes	Yes	Yes
Virilizing signs	No	Yes	No	Yes	Yes	Yes
Bone age	Advanced	Advanced	Advanced	Advanced	Advanced	Advanced
Neurologic deficit	No	No	No	No	No	No
Abdominopelvic mass	Usually	No	No	Occ'l	No	No

From Ross GT: Disorders of the ovary and female reproductive tract. In Wilson JD and Foster DW, editors: Williams textbook of endocrinology, ed 7, Philadelphia, 1985, WB Saunders Co, p 230.

exact etiology of the majority of cases of true precocious puberty is unknown (constitutional); however, approximately 10% are secondary to life-threatening central nervous system disease. A definitive diagnosis is established more often for pseudoprecocious puberty, and it is usually related to an ovarian or adrenal disorder. Both true precocious puberty and pseudoprecocious puberty are rare; however, true precocious puberty is 5 to 6 times more frequent than pseudoprecocious puberty. If the secondary sex characteristics are discordant with the genetic and phenotypic sex, the condition is termed *heterosexual precocious puberty*. This is premature virilization in a female child and includes development of masculine secondary sexual characteristics. The androgens that cause heterosexual precocious puberty usually come from the adrenal gland.

Premature Thelarche

Premature thelarche is defined as isolated unilateral or bilateral breast development as the only sign of secondary sexual maturation. It is not accompanied by other associated evidence of pubertal development, such as axillary or pubic hair or changes in vaginal epithelium. Breast hyperplasia is a normal physiologic phenomenon in the neonatal period, and it may persist for up to 6 months of age. Premature thelarche usually occurs between 2 and 4 years of age. Nipple development is absent. This is a benign, self-limiting condition that does not require treatment. Often the breast enlargement spontaneously regresses. It is important to observe these children closely for other signs of precocious puberty. The etiology of premature thelarche is not understood. However, it is postulated to be related either to a slight increase in circulating estrogen levels or an increased end-organ sensitivity of breast tissue to endogenous estrogens. This condition frequently occurs in female infants who had extremely low birth weights.

Premature Pubarche or Adrenarche

Premature pubarche is early isolated development of pubic hair without other signs of secondary sexual maturation. Premature adrenarche is isolated early development of axillary hair. Neither of these conditions is progressive, and the girls do not have clitoral hypertrophy. However, it is important to differentiate premature pubarche from the adrenogenital syndrome. Some children with premature pubarche have abnormal electroencephalograms (EEGs) without significant neurologic disease. The bone age should not be advanced. The etiology is poorly understood but believed to be related to increased androgen production by the adrenal glands.

True Precocious Puberty

Etiology

Idiopathic (constitutional) development is responsible for approximately 70% of the cases of true precocious puberty. Some of these children are simply at the earliest limits of the normal distribution of the biologic curve. Most idiopathic cases are sporadic in distribution; however, a few are familial. The mode of inheritance is believed to be autosomal recessive.

A high incidence of abnormal EEGs in children with idiopathic precocious puberty has raised the question of potential central nervous system disease. With increasing use of high-resolution imaging techniques, such as cranial CT scan and magnetic resonance imaging (MRI), the number of idiopathic cases is declining.

These girls have no genital abnormality except early development. Occasionally they de-

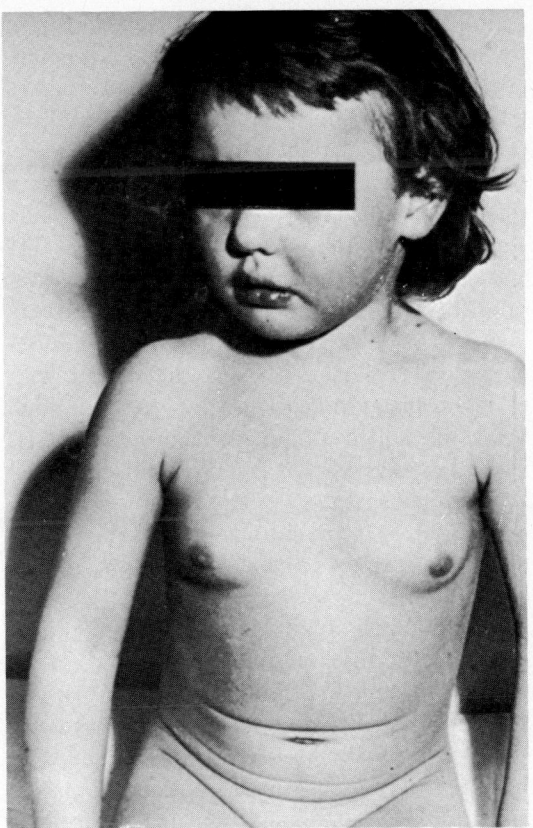

FIGURE 10-9
Precocious puberty in young girl. Child had large lower abdominal swelling, which at operation was shown to be bilateral follicular cysts (result of premature ovarian stimulation and not cause of condition). (From Dewhurst CJ: Practical pediatric and adolescent gynecology, New York, 1980, Marcel Dekker, Inc. Reprinted courtesy of Marcel Dekker, Inc.)

velop follicular cysts of the ovaries secondary to increased levels of pituitary gonadotrophins (Figure 10-9). In these cases the cysts are a result, not the cause, of precocious puberty. Gonadotrophin levels, sex steroid levels, and response of luteinizing hormone (LH) after administration of gonadotrophin-releasing hormone (GnRH) are similar to those in normal puberty. The cause of premature maturation of the hypothalamic-pituitary-ovarian axis is unknown. The syndrome may appear as early as age 3 to 4 years. When observed for several decades, these women have normal menopausal ages. Emotional problems are a concern because the young girls suffer from extreme social pressures. The intellectual and psychologic development of girls with precocious puberty is appropriate for their chronologic age. Most are shy and withdrawn from their peers. The diagnosis of idiopathic or constitutional precocious puberty is made by exclusion. A report by Cacciari et al. stimulated the hypothesis that many cases of idiopathic puberty may be related to small hamartomas of the hypothalamus. They studied 15 children who underwent cranial CT, and 6 had subsequent pneumoencephalography. In their series, 33% of the children were found to have small hamartomas of the tuber cinereum. This series selected children with early onset of precocious puberty and high levels of follicle-stimulating hormone (FSH) and LH. The current hypothesis is that the harmartoma secretes GnRH, but this secretion is not subject to the normal physiologic inhibition of GnRH secretion that occurs during childhood.

A wide range of inflammatory, degenerative, or neoplastic diseases that involve the central nervous system may produce true precocious puberty. Usually, symptoms of a neurologic disease, especially headaches and visual disturbances, precede the manifestations of precocious puberty. A most unusual neurologic symptom that may be associated with precocious puberty is seizures with inappropriate laughter (gelastic seizures). Anatomically, most central nervous system lesions are located near the hypothalamus in the region of the third ventricle, tuber cinereum, or mamillary bodies. Major central nervous system diseases associated with true precocious puberty include tuberculosis, encephalitis, trauma, secondary hydrocephalus, neurofibromatosis, granulomas, harmartomas, teratomas, craniopharyngiomas, and congenital brain defects, such as hydrocephalus and cysts in the area of the third ventricle. These children have markedly fluctuating estrogen levels and low gonadotrophin concentrations that are independent of GnRH stimulation. They may have either complete (true) or incomplete (pseudoprecocious) puberty. These central nervous system space-occupying masses are most difficult to successfully treat surgically.

McCune-Albright syndrome (polyostotic fibrous dysplasia) is a rare triad of café-au-lait spots, fibrous dysplasia, and cysts of the skull and long bones (Figure 10-10). These patients also have definite facial asymmetry. Approximately 40% of girls with McCune-Albright syndrome have associated isosexual true precocious puberty.

Hypothyroidism most commonly is associ-

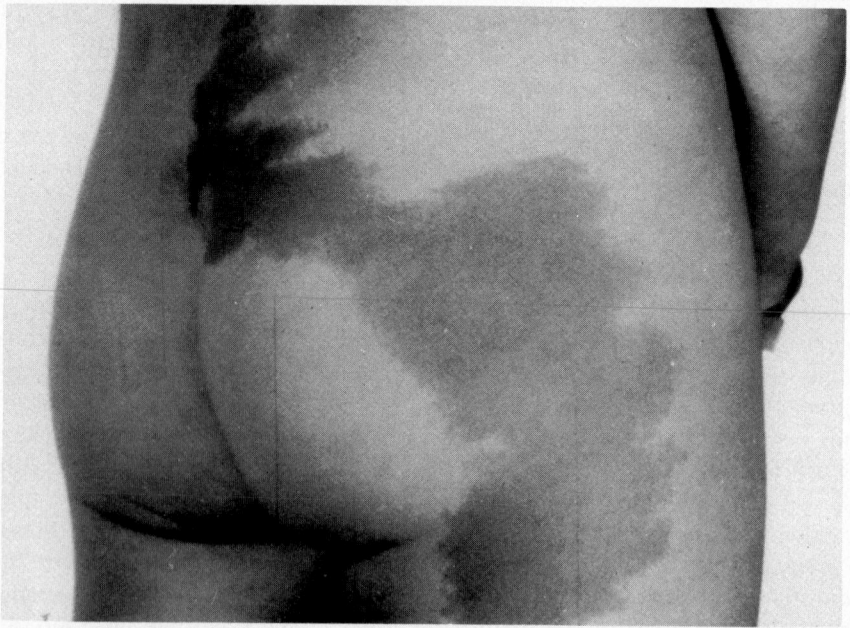

FIGURE 10-10
Large café-au-lait spot in child with precocious puberty as result of McCune-Albright syndrome. (From Dewhurst CJ: Practical pediatric and adolescent gynecology, New York, 1980, Marcel Dekker, Inc. Reprinted courtesy of Marcel Dekker, Inc.)

ated with delayed pubertal development. However, in rare instances untreated hypothyroidism results in either isosexual, true, or pseudoprecocious puberty. The hypothyroidism associated with precocious puberty is due to primary thyroid insufficiency, not a deficiency in pituitary thyroid-stimulating hormone (TSH). The pathophysiology of this syndrome is caused by the diminished negative feedback of thyroxine, resulting in an increased production of TSH. There appears to be a hormone overlap with an associated increase in production of gonadotropins. Interestingly, hypothyroidism is the only etiology of precocious puberty in which the bone age is retarded. This syndrome is seen usually in girls between the ages of 6 and 8 years.

Silver's syndrome is a rare congenital disease with multiple anomalies, including low birth weight, asymmetry of the body, abnormal jaw, café-au-lait spots, abnormal and short little fingers, and a tendency for the corner of the mouth to turn down. Recent reports have documented that most young females with Silver's syndrome have normal sexual maturation. Therefore Silver's syndrome is another rare cause of precocious puberty.

The relationship between congenital adrenal hyperplasia and puberty depends on the time of initial diagnosis and therapy. If the disease is diagnosed in the neonatal period and treated, normal puberty ensues. If the disease is untreated, the girl usually develops heterosexual precocious puberty from the adrenal androgens. However, if congenital adrenal hyperplasia is diagnosed late in childhood, isosexual precocious puberty may follow initial treatment of the adrenal disease.

The most common cause of pseudoprecocious puberty is a functioning ovarian tumor. Granulosa cell tumors are the most common type, accounting for approximately 60%. These tumors are usually greater than 8 cm when associated with precocious puberty; 80% can be palpated abdominally. Other ovarian tumors that may be associated with precocious puberty include thecomas, luteomas, teratomas, Sertoli-Leydig tumors, choriocarcinomas, and benign follicular cysts. Thecomas and luteomas are much smaller than granulosa tumors and usually cannot be palpated abdominally. Overall, these tumors are rare during childhood; only 5% of granulosa cell tumors and 1% of thecomas occur before puberty. On rare occa-

sions follicular cysts of the ovary enlarge and secrete enough estrogen to be the cause rather than the result of precocious puberty. It is speculated that the benign cysts function in an autonomous fashion. The ability of many tumors, to secrete human chorionic gonadotrophin (HCG) or estrogen, including teratomas, choriocarcinomas, and dysgerminomas, has been established by radioimmunoassay. Rarely do these tumors produce precocious puberty. Adrenocortical neoplasms usually produce heterosexual precocious puberty, although isosexual precocity is seen occasionally. Congenital adrenal hyperplasia usually produces virilization and heterosexual precocious puberty.

Iatrogenic or factitious precocious puberty results when a young female has used hormonal cream or ingested adult medication such as oral estrogen or birth control pills. The secondary sexual characteristics regress after discontinuation of the medication.

Wierman et al. identified a new subset of children with precocious puberty. They found a small number of children with gonadotrophin-independent precocity. Gametogenesis and steroidogenesis may occur in these individuals despite the absence of pubertal patterns of gonadotrophin release. When the children were tested with an analogue of GnRH, there was no effect on the pattern or mean levels of gonadotrophins or circulating sex steroids.

Diagnosis

The diagnostic workup of a young child with precocious puberty begins with a meticulous history and physical examination. The height of the girl and exact stage of pubertal development should be recorded. Similar to other syndromes with a long list of etiologies, a battery of tests, including imaging studies of the brain, serum estradiol levels, FSH levels, and thyroid function tests, may be needed to establish the diagnosis. Acceleration of growth is one of the earliest clinical features of precocious puberty. Thus bone age should be determined by hand-wrist films and compared with standards for a patient's age (Figure 10-11). Usually these films are repeated at 6-month intervals to evaluate the rate of skeletal maturation and correspondingly the necessity of active treatment of the disease. Advancement of bone age more than 95% of the norm for the child's chrono-

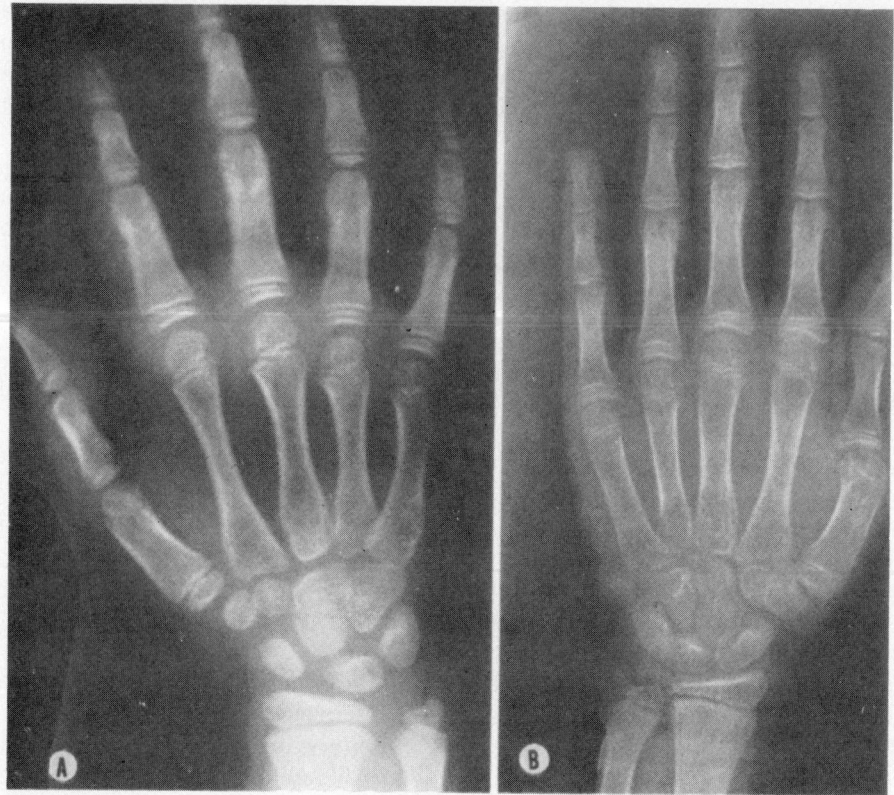

FIGURE 10-11
X-ray films demonstrating bone age. **A,** Normal for 7 years of age. **B,** Advanced bone age in girl 7 years of age who also shows other signs of isosexual precocity. (From Huffman JW: The gynecology of childhood and adolescence, ed 2, Philadelphia, 1981, WB Saunders Co.)

logic age documents a peripheral estrogen effect.

Diseases of the central nervous system are confirmed or excluded by a series of tests, including neurologic and ophthalmologic examinations, EEGs, skull x-ray films, and subsequent cranial CT and/or MRI.

Recent improved radiologic diagnosis of subtle central nervous system abnormalities with use of cranial CT, pneumoencephalography, and MRI has increased the sensitivity and frequency of discovery of the underlying cause of true precocious puberty. Ultrasound and/or CT of the abdomen should be performed to discover enlargement of the ovaries, uterus, or adrenal glands.

Serum levels of FSH, LH, prolactin, TSH, estradiol, testosterone, dehydroepiandrosterone (DHEA) or DHEA-S, HCG, triiodothyronine, and thyroxine all may be of value in establishing the differential diagnosis. Sometimes a GnRH stimulation test is diagnostic in differentiating incomplete from true precocious puberty, but this test does not specifically identify children with central nervous system lesions. The LH responses to gonadotrophin stimulation after reaching a basal level are similar in cases of true precocious puberty to the responses of a mature adult. In contrast, a child with precocious puberty secondary to a feminizing ovarian neoplasm does not have a significant elevation in LH response to gonadotrophins.

Management

The treatment of precocious puberty depends on the cause, the extent and progression of precocious symptoms, and whether the cause may be removed operatively. For example, extirpation of a granulosa cell tumor and subtotal removal of a hypothalamic hamartoma are successful treatments because they remove hormone-secreting tumors. Because most cases involve premature maturation of the hypothalamic-pituitary-ovarian axis without a lesion, this discussion focuses on medical management

TABLE 10-7

Gonadotrophin and Estradiol Levels in Girls with Precocious Puberty Before and After Administration of 100 μg GnRH

	Number	LH (IU/L, mean ± SD)		FSH (IU/L, mean ± SD)		Estradiol (pmol/L)	
		Basal	Peak	Basal	Peak	Mean	Range
Idiopathic precocious puberty	18	2.4 ± 2.0	36.9 ± 20.0	3.0 ± 1.8	16.3 ± 7.9	91.2	22-318
Intracranial lesion	9	2.6 ± 2.0	30.7 ± 17.3	4.4 ± 3.0	24.6 ± 5.1	107	22-240

From Lyon AJ, De Bruyn R, and Grant DB: Acta Pediatr Scand 74:953, 1985.

of these patients. Girls with menarche before age 8 years, progressive thelarche and pubarche, and bone age more than 2 years greater than their chronologic ages definitely should be treated. The goals of therapy are to reduce gonadotrophin secretions and reduce or counteract the peripheral actions of the sex steroids, decrease growth rate to normal, and slow skeletal maturation.

The present drug of choice for true precocious puberty is one of the potent agonists or analogues of GnRH (Table 10-7). The development of GnRH agonists and analogues was a major advance in the treatment of true precocious puberty, and even conservative endocrinologists have called this type of medication the "ideal drug" for this condition. The long-acting analogues were developed by inserting a D-amino acid in place of the naturally occurring L-amino acid at critical enzyme cleavage sites of the hormone. These drugs may be given by the intranasal route or by daily subcutaneous injection. Most recently, agonists have been combined with microcapsules that allow monthly injections. They are rapid, safe, and effective treatments for children with the disease secondary to disturbances in the hypothalamic-pituitary-ovarian axis. Wierman et al., using daily injections of the agonist, observed involution of secondary sexual characteristics, with menstruation ceasing and breast development and pubic hair regressing. In their series of nine children, spontaneous LH and FSH pulsations were abolished. Most importantly the drug not only reversed the ovarian cycle but changed the growth pattern. Growth velocity was decreased approximately 50% (Figure 10-12). In this series the predicted adult height increased a mean of 3.3 cm. The potent agonist inhibits gonadotrophin secretion by increasing the down regulation of GnRH receptors. This inhi-

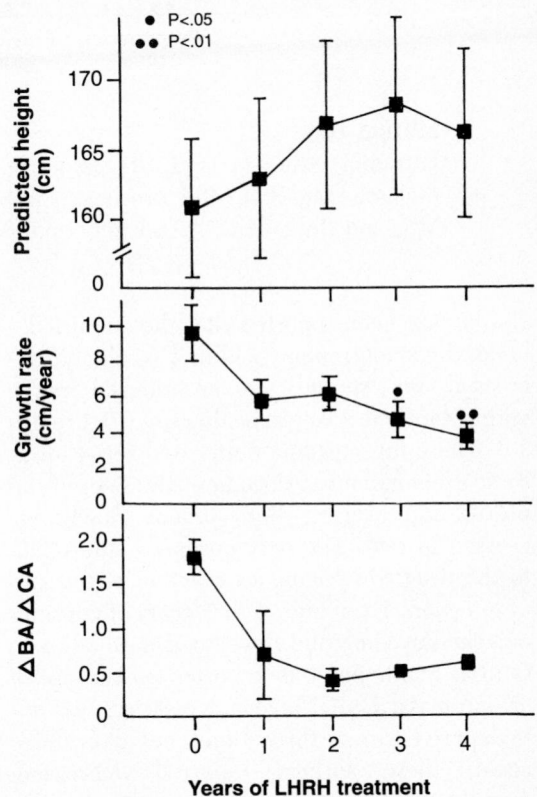

FIGURE 10-12

Predicted height, growth rate, and rate of bone age advancement in six children with central precocious puberty who have received 4 years of therapy with the long-acting analogue of luteinizing hormone releasing hormone (LHRH). Asterisks indicate significant differences compared with pretreatment value. (Redrawn from Comite F, Cassorla F, Barnes KM, et al: JAMA 255:2615, 1986.)

bition of the pituitary secretion and release of gonadotrophins through continuous therapy is readily reversible by discontinuing the medication.

Styne et al. reported results of a similar se-

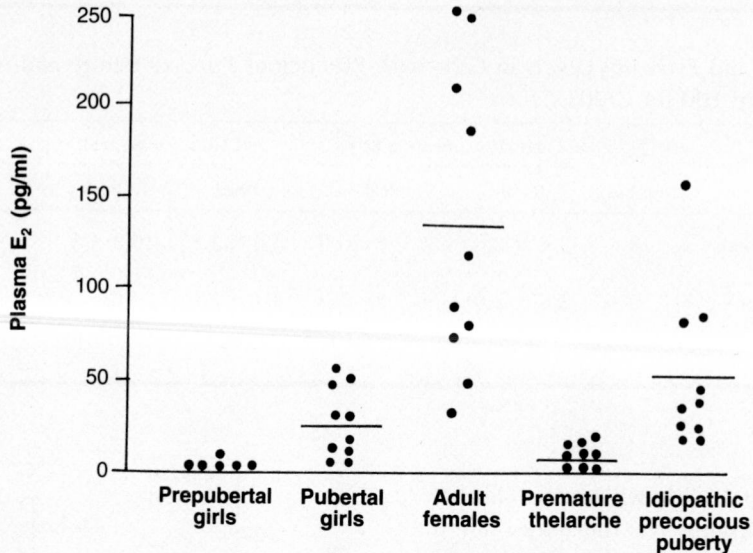

FIGURE 10-13
Estradiol values (x = 1 SD) in normal females and in patients with premature
thelarche and idiopathic precocious puberty. (Redrawn from Escobar ME, Rivarola
MA, and Bergada C: Acta Endocrinol 81:351, 1976.)

ries. It has been reported that the agonist decreased gonadotrophins within 1 week and decreased sex steroids to prepubertal range within the first 2 weeks of therapy (Figure 10-13). These investigators performed serial ultrasonic examinations to document the sizes of the uterus and ovaries. Both organs slowly regressed in size. The only observed side effect to the drug was cutaneous reaction at the site of injection. Even after 4 to 5 years of continuous therapy, no child developed antibodies to GnRH. Stanhope et al. reported on the use of an intranasal GnRH analogue; 100 μg was administered two or three times per day. Once again, these authors reported decreasing growth rate to normal and the ability to slow the process of skeletal maturation. Pescovitz et al. from the National Institutes of Health recently reported the largest series. Ninety-five girls were treated for at least 6 months with a long-acting GnRH analogue. Their positive findings were similar; however, they found the analogue ineffective in patients with McCune-Albright syndrome. The effects of these new drugs are quickly reversible when the drugs are discontinued after normal adult height is achieved. Patients with McCune-Albright syndrome may be treated with testolactone, an aromatase inhibitor, which prevents the conversion of estrogen precursors to biologically active estrogens. This treatment leads to diminished circulating estrogen levels, diminished frequency of menses, and a decreased rate of growth and skeletal maturation.

Before the introduction of agonists or analogues to GnRH, most children with true precocious puberty were treated with medroxyprogesterone acetate (Depo-Provera) at a dosage of 100 to 200 mg weekly. High levels of this progestin did suppress menstruation and produce regression of breast development. However, medroxyprogesterone did not change skeletal growth rates. Danazol has also been used in selected cases. It produced amenorrhea and inhibited further breast development; however, once again, there was no effect on growth rate or skeletal maturation. Cyproterone acetate is an antiandrogen that has been prescribed for precocious puberty in doses of 70 and 150 mg/m² per day in Europe. The results are similar to those obtained with medroxyprogesterone and danazol.

Both the child with precocious puberty and her family need intensive counseling. The child may be exposed to ridicule by her peers and to sexual exploitation. Thus the child needs extensive sex education and help in anticipating and confronting various social experiences. Often it is possible to dress the child in clothes that diminish the appearance of her advanced sexual maturation until the effects of her disease are inhibited by drug therapy.

_____ **KEY POINTS** _____

- The most frequent gynecologic problem of children is vulvovaginitis.

- In the field of pediatric gynecology, most diagnostic errors result from errors of omission during the examination rather than errors of commission.

- If a child is anxious about the physical examination, mild sedation may be helpful: the combination of 50 mg meperidine, 12.5 mg chlorpromazine hydrochloride, and 12.5 mg promethazine hydrochloride given in a dose of 1 ml intramuscularly for every 20 pounds, up to a maximum of 2 ml.

- The vaginal epithelium of the prepubertal child appears redder and thinner than the vaginal epithelium of a woman in her reproductive years. The prepubertal vagina is also narrower, thinner, and lacking in the distensibility of the vagina of a woman in her reproductive years. The vagina of a child is 4 to 5 cm long and has a neutral pH.

- During the physical examination and rectal examination, no pelvic masses should be felt. The normal prepubertal uterus and ovaries are nonpalpable. The relative size ratio of cervix to uterus is 2 to 1 in a child.

- It is estimated that 80% to 90% of outpatient visits of children to gynecologists involve the classic symptoms of vulvovaginitis: introital irritation and discharge.

- One in four cultures of the discharge from vulvovaginitis identifies mycotic or bacterial vaginosis or a specific organism, such as *Neisseria gonorrhoeae, Trichomonas vaginalis, Chlamydia trachomatis*, herpes simplex virus, or *Shigella boydii*.

- Identification of vaginal infection by *Trichomonas,* gonorrhea, or *Chlamydia* organisms in a child often indicates sexual molestation.

- The normal vagina of the prepubertal child is colonized by an average of nine different species of bacteria—four aerobic and facultative anaerobic species and five obligatory anaerobic species.

- In the period from 6 to 12 months before menarche, children often develop a physiologic discharge secondary to the increase in circulating estrogen levels.

- A vaginal discharge that is both bloody and foul smelling strongly suggests the presence of a foreign body.

- The vast majority of patients with nonspecific vulvovaginitis respond to a combination of topical estrogen cream and oral antibiotics given for 10 to 14 days.

- Adhesive vulvitis does not require treatment unless voiding is compromised. If necessary, small amounts of daily topical estrogen to the labia may be used.

- The classic symptom of pinworms *(Enterobius vermicularis)* is nocturnal vulvar and perianal itching, the treatment for which is the antihelmintic agent mebendazole (Vermox).

- The usual cause of genital trauma during childhood is an accidental fall. The majority of such trauma involves straddle injuries.

- The treatment of nonexpanding vulvar hematomas consists of an ice pack or ice sitz bath.

- Small follicular cysts are common in preadolescent females and are usually self-limiting.

- Ovarian tumors constitute approximately 1% of all neoplasms in premenarcheal children. Approximately 75% of ovarian neoplasms necessitating surgery are benign, with cystic teratomas being the most common.

- Precocious puberty is the appearance of signs of sexual maturation before 8 years of age. Physiologic development in females with precocious puberty usually follows the normal sequence of changes of secondary sexual characteristics.

- Without therapy, approximately 50% of females with true precocious puberty will not reach a height of 5 feet.

- The exact etiology of the majority of cases of true precocious puberty is unknown; however, approximately 10% of cases are secondary to life-threatening central nervous system disease.

- Idiopathic (constitutional) development is responsible for approximately 70% of the cases of true precocious puberty.

- Breast hyperplasia is a normal phenomenon in neonates and may persist up to 6 months of age.

- The most common cause of pseudoprecocious puberty is a functioning ovarian tumor. Granulosa cell tumors are the most common type, accounting for approximately 60%.

- The goals of therapy of precocious puberty are to reduce gonadotrophin secretions and reduce or counteract the peripheral actions of sex steroids, decreasing growth rate to normal, and slowing skeletal maturation. This is best accomplished by agonists or analogues to GnRH.

BIBLIOGRAPHY

Altchek A: Pediatric vulvovaginitis, J Reprod Med 29:359, 1984.

Altchek A: Vulvovaginitis in adolescents and younger girls, Contemp OB/GYN, 27:85, 1986.

Brämswig JH, Fasse M, Holthoff ML, et al: Adult height in boys and girls with untreated short stature and constitutional delay of growth and puberty: accuracy of five different methods of height prediction, J Pediatr 117:886, 1990.

Brenner PF: Precocious puberty in the female. In Mishell DR, Davajan V, and Lobo R, editors: Infertility, contraception and reproductive endocrinology, ed 3, Oradell, NJ, 1990, Medical Economics Books.

Buchta RM: Use of chaperones during pelvic examinations of female adolescents, Am J Dis Child 141:666, 1987.

Bump RC: *Chlamydia trachomatis* as a cause of prepubertal vaginitis, Obstet Gynecol 65:384, 1985.

Cacciari E, Frejaville E, Cicongnani A, et al: How many cases of true precocious puberty in girls are idiopathic? J Pediatr 102:357, 1983.

Capraro VJ: Pediatric gynecology. In Danforth DN, editor: Obstetrics and gynecology, ed 4, Philadelphia, 1982, Harper & Row, Publishers, Inc.

Clark SJ, Van Dop C, Conte FA, et al: Reversible true precocious puberty secondary to a congenital arachnoid cyst, Am J Dis Child 142:255, 1988.

Comite F, Cassorla F, Barnes KM, et al: Luteinizing hormone releasing hormone analogue therapy for central precocious puberty: long-term effect on somatic growth, bone maturation, and predicted height, JAMA 255:2613, 1986.

Dattel BJ, Landers DV, Coulter K, et al: Isolation of *Chlamydia trachomatis* from sexually abused female adolescents, Obstet Gynecol 72:240, 1988.

De Jong AR: Sexually transmitted diseases in children, Am Fam Physician 30:185, 1984.

Dewhurst CJ: Gynaecological disorders of infants and children, Philadelphia, 1963, FA Davis Co.

Dewhurst CJ: Practical pediatric and adolescent gynecology, New York, 1980, Marcel Dekker, Inc.

Duffy TJ: Torsion of the fallopian tube in a premenarchal girl, Postgrad Med J 56:267, 1981.

Ehren IM, Mahour GH, and Isaacs H: Benign and malignant ovarian tumors in children and adolescents, Am J Surg 147:339, 1984.

Ehrhardt AA and Meyer-Bahlburg HFL: Idiopathic precocious puberty in girls: long-term effects on adolescent behavior, Acta Endocrinol 279:247, 1986.

Emans SJ and Goldstein DP: The gynecologic examination of the prepubertal child with vulvovaginitis: use of the knee-chest position, Pediatrics 65:758, 1980.

Emans SJH and Goldstein DP: Pediatric and adolescent gynecology, ed 3, Boston, 1990, Little, Brown & Co.

Emans SJ, Woods ER, Flagg NT, and Freeman A: Genital findings in sexually abused symptomatic and asymptomatic girls, Pediatrics 79:778, 1987.

Feuillan PP, Foster CM, Pescovitz OH, et al: Treatment of precocious puberty in the McCune-Albright syndrome with the aromatase inhibitor testolactone, N Engl J Med 315:1115, 1986.

Fleischer AC and Shawker TH: The role of sonography in pediatric gynecology, Clin Obstet Gynecol 30:735, 1987.

Galatzer A and Laron Z: Behavior in girls with true precocious puberty, J Pediatr 108:790, 1986.

Gidwani GP: Approach to evaluation of premenarchal child with a gynecologic problem, Clin Obstet Gynecol 30:643, 1987.

Goff CW, Burke KR, Rickenback C, and Buebendorf DP: Vaginal opening measurement in prepubertal girls, Am J Dis Child 143:1366, 1989.

Goldberg CC and Yates A: The use of anatomically correct dolls in the evaluation of sexually abused children, Am J Dis Child 144:1334, 1990.

Golladay ES and Mollitt DL: Ovarian masses in the child and adolescent, South Med J 76:954, 1983.

Haney PJ and Whitley NO: CT of benign cystic abdominal masses in children, AJR 142:1279, 1984.

Herman-Giddens ME, Sandler AD, and Friedman NE: Sexual precocity in girls: an association with sexual abuse? Am J Dis Child 142:431, 1988.

Hibi I and Fujiwara K: Precocious puberty of cerebral origin: a cooperative study in Japan, Prog Exp Tumor Res 30:224, 1987.

Hill NCW, Oppenheimer LW and Morton KE: The aetiology of vaginal bleeding in children: a 20-year review, Br J Obstet Gynecol 96:467, 1989.

Huffman JW: The gynecology of childhood and adolescence, ed 2, Philadelphia, 1981, WB Saunders Co.

Huffman JW: Premenarchal vulvovaginitis, Clin Obstet Gynecol 20:581, 1977.

Jenkinson SD and Mackinnon AE: Spontaneous separation of fused labia minora in prepubertal girls, Br Med J 289:160, 1984.

Jones JG, Yamauchi T, and Lambert B: *Trichomonas vaginalis* infestation in sexually abused girls, Am J Dis Child 139:846, 1985.

Kaplan SL and Grumbach MM: Clinical review 14: pathophysiology and treatment of sexual precocity, J Clin Endocrinol 71:785, 1990.

Kennedy LA, Pinckney LE, Currarino G, et al: Amputated calcified ovaries in children, Radiology 141:83, 1981.

Kingsbury A: The clinical importance of vaginal discharge in childhood, Aust NZ J Obstet Gynaecol 24:135, 1984.

Klein VR, Willman SP, and Carr BR: Familial posterior labial fusion, Obstet Gynecol 73:500, 1989.

Knorr D, Bidlingmaier F, Holler W, et al: Is heterozygosity for the steroid 21-hydroxylase deficiency responsible for hirsutism, premature pubarche, early puberty, and precocious puberty in children? Acta Endocrinol 279:284, 1986.

Kosloske AM, Goldthorn JF, Kaufman E, et al: Treatment of precocious pseudopuberty associated with follicular cysts of the ovary, Am J Dis Child 138:147, 1984.

Kreiter M, Burstein S, Rosenfield RL, et al: Preserving adult height potential in girls with idiopathic true precocious puberty, J Pediatr 117:364, 1990.

Lacson AG, Gillis DA, and Shawwa A: Malignant mixed germ cell–sex cord–stromal tumors of the ovary associated with isosexual precocious puberty, Cancer 61:2122, 1988.

Lavery JP and Sanfilippo JS: Pediatric and adolescent obstetrics and gynecology, New York, 1985, Springer-Verlag New York, Inc.

Lee PA, Page JG, and the Leuprolide Study Group: Effects of leuprolide in the treatment of central precocious puberty, J Pediatr 114:321, 1989.

Levine MD and Rappaport LA: Recurrent abdominal pain in school children: the loneliness of the long-distance physician, Pediatr Clin North Am 31:969, 1984.

Liapi C and Evain-Brion D: Diagnosis of ovarian follicular cysts from birth to puberty: a report of twenty cases, Acta Paediatr Scand 76:91, 1987.

Lin T-H, LePage ME, Henzl M, and Kirkland JL: Intranasal nafarelin: an LH-RH analogue treatment of gonadotropin-dependent precocious puberty, J Pediatr 109:954, 1986.

Lyon AJ, De Bruyn R, and Grant DB: Isosexual precocious puberty in girls, Acta Paediatr Scand 74:950, 1985.

Mansfield MJ, Beardsworth DE, Loughlin JS, et al: Long-term treatment of central precocious puberty with a long-acting analogue of luteinizing hormone–releasing hormone, N Engl J Med 309:1286, 1983.

McCann J, Voris J, and Simon M: Labial adhesions and posterior fourchette injuries in childhood sexual abuse, Am J Dis Child 142:659, 1988.

McCann J, Voris J, Simon M, and Wells R: Comparison of genital examination techniques in prepubertal girls, Pediatr 85:182, 1990.

McCrea RS: Uterine adnexal torsion with subsequent contralateral recurrence, J Reprod Med 25:123, 1980.

Mishell DR and Davajan V: Infertility, reproductive endocrinology and contraception, ed 3, Oradell, NJ, 1990, Medical Economics Books.

Muram D: Child sexual abuse—genital tract findings in prepubertal girls. I. The unaided medical examination, Am J Obstet Gynecol 160:328, 1989.

Muram D and Elias S: Child sexual abuse—genital tract findings in prepubertal girls. II. Comparison of colposcopic and unaided examinations, Am J Obstet Gynecol 160:333, 1989.

Orsini LF, Salardi S, Pilu G, et al: Pelvic organs in premenarcheal girls: real-time ultrasonography, Radiology 153:113, 1984.

Paradise JE, Campos JM, Friedman HM, et al: Vulvovaginitis in premenarcheal girls: clinical features and diagnostic evaluation, Pediatrics 70:193, 1982.

Paradise JE and Willis ED: Probability of vaginal foreign body in girls with genital complaints, Am J Dis Child 139:472, 1985.

Pasquino AM, Tebaldi L, Cives C, et al: Precocious puberty in the McCune-Albright Syndrome, Acta Paediatr Scand 76:841, 1987.

Pescovitz OH, Comite F, Hench K, et al: The NIH experience with precocious puberty: Diagnostic subgroups and response to short-term luteinizing hormone releasing hormone analogue therapy, J Pediatr 108:47, 1986.

Pescovitz OH, Hench KD, Barnes KM, et al: Premature thelarche and central precocious puberty: the relationship between clinical presentation and the gonadotropin response to luteinizing hormone–releasing hormone, J Clin Endocrinol Metab 67:474, 1988.

Pokorny SF: Configuration of the prepubertal hymen, Am J Obstet Gynecol 157:950, 1987.

Pokorny SF and Stormer J: Atraumatic removal of secretions from the prepubertal vagina, Am J Obstet Gynecol 156:581, 1987.

Root AW and Shulman I: Isosexual precocity: current concepts and recent advances, Fertil Steril 45:749, 1986.

Salardi S, Orsini LF, Cacciari E, et al: Pelvic ultrasonography in girls with precocious puberty, congenital adrenal hyperplasia, obesity, or hirsutism, J Pediatr 112:880, 1988.

Scott JR, editor: Danforth's obstetrics and gynecology, ed 5, Philadelphia, 1990, JB Lippincott Co.

Shawis RN, El Gohary AE, and Cook RCM: Ovarian cysts and tumours in infancy and childhood, Ann R Coll Surg Engl 67:17, 1985.

Singleton AF: Vaginal discharge in children and adolescents, Clin Pediatr 19:799, 1980.

Sonis WA, Comite F, Pescovitz OH, et al: Biobehavioral aspects of precocious puberty, J Am Acad Child Psychiatry 25:674, 1989.

Stanhope R, Adams J, and Brook CGD: The treatment of central precocious puberty using an intranasal LHRH analogue (Buserelin), Clin Endocrinol 22:795, 1985.

Styne DM, Harris DA, Egli CA, et al: Treatment of true precocious puberty with a potent luteinizing hormone–releasing factor agonist: effect on growth, sexual maturation, pelvic sonography, and the hypothalamic-pituitary-gonadal axis, J Clin Endocrinol Metab 61:142, 1985.

Swischuk LE and Hayden CK: Abdominal masses in children, Pediatr Clin North Am 32:1281, 1985.

Takeuchi J and Hajime H: Pubertas praecox and hypothalamic hamartoma, Neurosurg Rev 8:225, 1985.

Widholm O: Genital bleeding during childhood, Pediatr Ann 10:170, 1981.

Wierman ME, Beardsworth DE, Mansfield MJ, et al: Puberty without gonadotropins, N Engl J Med 312:65, 1985.

Wilson JD and Foster DW: Williams textbook of endocrinology, ed 7, Philadelphia, 1985, WB Saunders Co.

Contraception, Sterilization, and Pregnancy Termination

KEY TERMS AND DEFINITIONS

Contraception. The temporary avoidance of pregnancy.

Contraceptive Failure Rate. Pregnancy rates with various types of contraceptives at different intervals, usually yearly. This is frequently expressed as a failure per 100 women at 1 year or per 100 woman-years.

Induced Abortion. Intentional medical or surgical termination of pregnancy before 20 weeks' gestation. Also called *elective pregnancy termination* if performed for the woman's desires or *therapeutic abortion* if performed for reasons of maintaining the mother's health.

Intrauterine Device (IUD). A small foreign body, usually made of plastic with or without copper, placed into the endometrial cavity to provide an effective method of contraception.

IUD Event Rates. Incidence of adverse effects, such as expulsion, removal for medical reasons, and pregnancy, at various times after insertion of an IUD.

Life Table Method. An actuarial technique for determining rates of occurrence of events, such as pregnancy and discontinuation, at various intervals after starting any type of contraceptive.

Method Effectiveness. The rate of effectiveness when the contraceptive method is always used correctly.

Natural Family Planning. Periodic abstinence from intercourse during the periovulatory time of the cycle. Also known as *rhythm*.

Norplant. Polysiloxane capsules containing levonorgestrel that are implanted subdermally and release relatively constant amounts of levonorgestrel continuously. They provide excellent contraceptive effectiveness for at least 5 years.

Oral Contraceptive Steroids (OCs). Formulations of synthetic progestins and usually estrogens that are ingested orally to prevent conception.

Pearl Index. A nonactuarial method used for determining the pregnancy (failure) rate of any contraceptive technique:

$$\text{Pregnancy rate} = \frac{\text{No. of pregnancies} \times 1200}{\text{Woman-months of use}}$$

Postcoital Contraception. Administration of steroids or insertion of an IUD within 3 days after a single episode of unprotected, midcycle sexual intercourse.

Progestin. A class of sex steroids having progestational activity. The terms *progestagen* and *gestagen* are synonymous.

Spermicide. A local contraceptive containing the agent nonoxynol 9, which is toxic to sperm.

Sterilization. The permanent prevention of pregnancy.

Use Effectiveness. Overall effectiveness rate in actual use for a specific contraceptive method.

CONTRACEPTIVE USE AND EFFECTIVENESS

An ideal method of contraception for all individuals is not now available and most probably will never be developed. A variety of very effective methods of contraception is currently available, each with certain advantages and disadvantages. Therefore, when giving advice about contraception, the clinician should explain to the couple the advantages and disadvantages of each method so that they will be fully informed and can rationally choose the method most suitable for them. Because no contraceptive method other than the condom has been developed as yet for use by the male, the contraceptive provider generally counsels the female partner and should inform her if medical reasons contraindicate the use of certain methods and should offer her alternatives.

Contraceptive Use in the United States

Data from the 1988 National Survey of Family Growth revealed that about one third of the 57.9 million U.S. women in the reproductive age group (15 to 44), or 19.2 million women, were not exposed to unwanted pregnancy. These women were not having sexual inter-course, had a hysterectomy for reasons other than sterility (noncontraceptively sterile), or were infertile, pregnant, or attempting to conceive. Of the remaining 38.7 million women exposed to the risk of pregnancy, all but 3.8 million (9.7%) used a method of contraception. Approximately twice as many unmarried exposed women as married women failed to use a contraceptive method.

The remaining 35 million women, approximately 60% of those in the reproductive age group, were using a method of contraception in 1988. Sterilization was the most common method used by these women. A total of 13.7 million women, 35% of those exposed to unwanted pregnancy, used sterilization of one member of the couple, 9.6 million women (17%) and 4.1 million men (7%), to prevent pregnancy. Use of sterilization among married U.S. women has increased dramatically in the past 25 years (Figure 11-1). In 1973 approximately one fourth of married women of reproductive age practicing contraception used sterilization as their method of preventing pregnancy. By 1988 more than half of married women of reproductive age exposed to the risk of unwanted pregnancy were using sterilization.

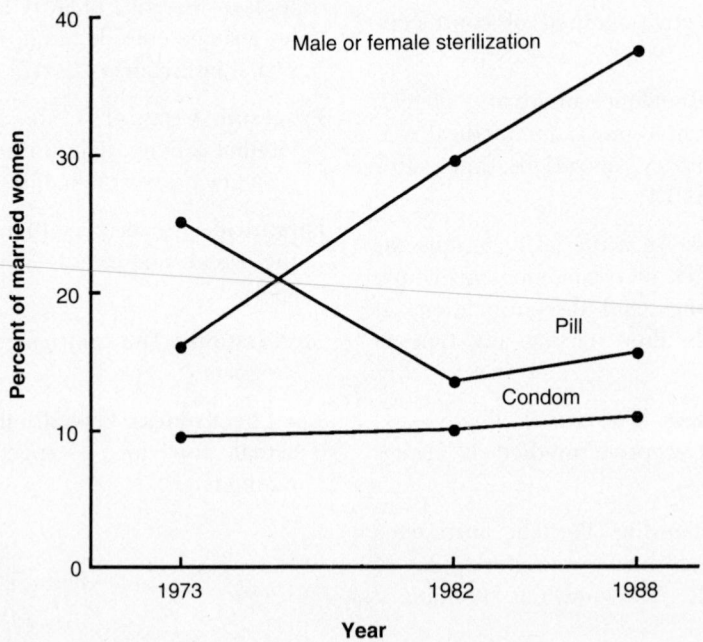

FIGURE 11-1

Percent of married women (15 to 44 years of age) using sterilization, the pill, and the condom: United States, 1973, 1982, and 1988. (From Mosher WD and Pratt WF: Contraceptive use in the United States, 1973-88, Patient Educ Couns 16:163, 1990.)

Of the nonsurgical, reversible methods of contraception, oral contraceptives (OCs) were most popular in 1988, used by 10.7 million women, 18.5% of all women in this age group. OCs were followed in frequency of use by the condom, periodic abstinence, withdrawal, diaphragm, intrauterine device (IUD), and spermicides alone (Table 11-1). Overall, approximately one fourth of women of reproductive age exposed to unwanted pregnancy (27%) used OCs, about half of the exposed unmarried women and one fifth of exposed married women. More women using reversible contraceptive methods used OCs, 50.4%, than all the other methods combined.

Oral contraceptives were first marketed in the United States in 1960, and their use steadily increased until 1973. Pharmacy purchases of OCs began declining in 1975. Among married U.S. women practicing contraception, OC use peaked at 36% in 1977 but declined to 23% by 1982. Since 1982, however, this trend has reversed; by 1988, 27% of all women exposed to unwanted pregnancy used OCs. Condom use increased between 1982 and 1988, mainly because of greater use by unmarried women. During this time, IUD use decreased by about two thirds, diaphragm use declined among unmarried but not married women, and use of the other techniques remained relatively stable.

Contraceptive Effectiveness

It is difficult to determine the actual effectiveness of various methods of contraception because of the many factors that affect contraceptive failure. The terms *method effectiveness* and *use effectiveness* (or *method failure* and *patient failure*) have been used to differentiate whether conception occurred while the contraceptive method was being used correctly or incorrectly. In general, methods used at the time of coitus, such as the diaphragm, condom, spermicides, and withdrawal, have a much greater method effectiveness than use effectiveness. With use of the methods in which coitus-related activities are not needed, such as the OCs and IUD, less difference exists between method and use effectiveness, and thus their overall effectiveness is greater than that of the coitus-related methods.

The overall value of a contraceptive method as used by a couple (correctly or incorrectly) is determined by calculation of actual effectiveness, as well as the continuation rate. To determine these rates, actuarial methods such as the log-rank life table method should be used in-

TABLE 11-1

Contraceptive Use of 57.9 Million U.S. Women 15 to 44 Years Old (1988 National Survey of Family Growth)

Exposure and Contraceptive Method	Number (Millions)	Percentage of Exposed Women	Percentage of All Women Aged 15-44
Exposed users	34.7	90.0	60.3
Sterilization	13.7	35.5	23.6
Female	9.6	24.9	16.6
Male	4.1	10.6	7.0
Oral contraceptives	10.7	27.7	18.5
Condom	5.1	13.2	8.8
Spermicides	0.3	0.7	0.6
Withdrawal	0.8	2.1	1.3
Diaphragm	2.0	5.2	3.5
Periodic abstinence	0.8	2.1	1.4
IUD	0.7	1.8	1.2
Douche	0.05	0.1	0.1
Exposed nonusers	3.8	9.8	6.5
Not exposed	19.2	49.6	33.2
TOTAL	57.9		

From Mosher WD and Pratt WF: Contraceptive Use in the United States, Patient Educ Couns 16:163, 1990.

TABLE 11-2

Lowest Expected, Typical, and Lowest Reported Failure Rates During First Year of Use of Contraceptive Method and First-Year Continuation Rates in United States

Method	Percentage of Women Experiencing Accidental Pregnancy in First Year of Use			Percentage of Women Continuing Use at 1 Year[4]	
	Lowest Expected[1]	Typical[2]	Lowest Reported[3]	Excluding Pregnancy	Including Pregnancy
Chance[5]	85	85	43.1		
Spermicides[6]	3	21	0.0	55	43
Periodic abstinence		20		84	67
Calendar method	9		14.4[7]		
Ovulation method	3		10.5[7]		
Sympto-thermal[8] method	2		12.6		
Postovulation	1		2.0[7]		
Withdrawal	4	18	6.7[7]		
Cap[9]	6	18	8.0	77	63
Sponge					
Parous women	9	28	27.7	73	53
Nulliparous women	6	18	13.9	73	60
Diaphragm[9]	6	18	2.1	69	57
Condom[10]	2	12	4.2	73	64
IUD		3		75	73
Progestasert	2.0		1.9		
Copper T 380A	0.8		0.5		
Oral contraceptives	3		75	73	
Combined	0.1		0.0		
Progestin only	0.5		1.1		
Injectable progestin[11]				70	70
DMPA	0.3	0.3	0.0		
NET	0.4	0.4	0.0		
Implants				90	90
Norplant (6 capsules)	0.04	0.04	0.0		
Norplant-2 (2 rods)	0.03	0.03	0.0		
Female sterilization	0.2	0.4	0.0		
Male sterilization	0.1	0.15	0.0		

From Trussell J, et al: Stud Fam Plann 21(1):51, 1990. Reprinted with permission of the Population Council.

[1] Among couples who initiate use of a method (not necessarily for the first time) and who use it *perfectly* (both consistently and correctly), the authors' best guess of the percentage expected to experience an accidental pregnancy during the first year if they do not stop use for any other reason.

[2] Among *typical* couples who initiate use of a method (not necessarily for the first time), the percentage who experience an accidental pregnancy during the first year if they do not stop use for any other reason.

[3] In the literature on contraceptive failure, the *lowest reported* percentage who experienced an accidental pregnancy during the first year following initiation of use (not necessarily for the first time) if they did not stop use for any other reason. However, see Note 8.

[4] Among couples attempting to avoid pregnancy, the percentage who continue to use a method for 1 year, under the alternative assumptions that no one becomes pregnant (Excluding Pregnancy column) and that the proportion becoming pregnant is given by Lowest Expected column (Including Pregnancy column).

[5] The lowest expected and typical percentages are based on data from populations where contraception is not used and from women who cease using contraception to become pregnant. These represent our best guess of the percentage who would conceive among women now relying on reversible methods of contraception if they abandoned contraception altogether. The lowest reported percentage is based on U.S. women who use no contraception even though they do not wish to become pregnant. This group is selected for low fecundity or low coital frequency, and some fraction may use an unreported variant of periodic abstinence.

[6] Foams and vaginal suppositories.

[7] Too low, because rate is based on more than 1 year of exposure.

[8] Cervical-mucus (ovulation) method supplemented by calendar method in the preovulatory and basal body temperature in the postovulatory phases.

[9] With spermicidal cream or jelly.

[10] Without spermicides.

[11] DMPA, Depo-medroxyprogesterone acetate; NET, norethindrone.

stead of the less accurate Pearl index.

Even with the use of these excellent statistical techniques, it is difficult to determine the effectiveness of the various methods in actual practice. Most studies undertaken to determine effectiveness of a contraceptive method are performed under carefully controlled clinical trials during which frequent patient contact with supportive clinical personnel results in lower failure rates and higher continuation rates than occur in normal use. Furthermore, these clinical trials are infrequently performed in a comparative randomized manner, so clinicians cannot compare trial results of one type of contraceptive method with those of another type.

Several other factors influence contraceptive failure rates. One of the most important is the couple's motivation. Contraceptive failure is more likely to occur in couples seeking to delay a wanted birth than in couples seeking to prevent any more births, especially for coitus-related methods. The woman's age has a strong negative correlation with the failure of a contraceptive method, as does the socioeconomic class and level of education. In addition, failure rates of prospective studies are consistently lower than those of retrospective interview studies. Finally, for all methods, failure rates are greater during the first year of use than in subsequent years, but most studies report only first-year failure rates. Thus one must consider many variables when evaluating the effectiveness of any contraceptive method for an individual woman.

In 1987 Trussell and Kost performed a comprehensive critical review of the existing scientific literature concerning effectiveness of the various contraceptive methods. After analyzing the entire data base, they calculated the lowest expected (method) and typical (use) failure rates of the various contraceptive methods during their first year of use. In 1990 Trussell et al. published a revised estimate of first-year failure rates based on recently reported data. OCs, the IUD, and Norplant had the lowest method and use failure rates (Table 11-2).

Vessey et al. (1982) analyzed failure rates of various contraceptive methods among more than 17,000 women enrolled in the Oxford/Family Planning Association Contraceptive Study. This study included only married women, 25 to 39 years of age, who had been using the diaphragm, IUD, or OCs for at least 5 months before enrollment. Most of the

TABLE 11-3

Contraceptive Failures with Various Methods (Oxford Family Planning Association Contraceptive Study)

Method	Failure Rate (per 100 Woman-Years)
Sterilization	
Male	0.02
Female	0.13
Oral contraceptives	
<50 μg estrogen	0.27
50 μg estrogen	0.16
>50 μg estrogen	0.32
Progesterone only	1.2
IUD	
Copper T	1.2
Copper 7	1.5
Dalkon Shield	2.4
Loop A	6.8
Loop B	1.8
Loop C	1.4
Loop D	1.3
Saf-T-Coil	1.3
Not known	1.8
Diaphragm	1.9
Condom	3.6
Withdrawal	6.7
Spermicides	11.9
Rhythm	15.5

From Vessey M, Lawless M, and Yeates D: Lancet 1:841, 1982.

women were well educated and of higher socioeconomic status. This select population comprised women who were motivated to attend family planning clinics and who had been under observation for an average of 9.5 years. Failure rates per 100 woman-years were very low for several contraceptive methods: approximately 0.3 for OCs, 1.3 for the IUD, 1.9 for the diaphragm, 3.6 for the condom, 11.9 for spermicides, and 15.5 for the rhythm method (Table 11-3). Failure rates declined with increasing age and increasing duration of use, especially for barrier methods and the IUD. However, except for the diaphragm, no substantial difference occurred in failure rates among women wishing to delay or prevent a pregnancy.

Further data from national surveys indicate that 1-year continuation rates for the various contraceptive methods are highest for the IUD, which necessitates a visit to a health care facility to discontinue use, and lowest for the diaphragm, condom, and spermicide.

SPERMICIDES: INTRAVAGINAL SPONGE, FOAMS, CREAMS, AND SUPPOSITORIES

All spermicidal agents contain a surfactant, usually nonoxynol 9, which immobilizes or kills sperm on contact. They also provide a mechanical barrier and must be placed into the vagina before each coital act. The effectiveness of these agents, except for the sponge, increases with increasing age of the woman and is similar to effectiveness of the diaphragm for all age and income groups.

The most popular spermicide is a contraceptive sponge, which is a cylindric piece of soft polyurethane impregnated with 1 mg of nonoxynol 9. In contrast to other spermicidal methods, the sponge does not have to be inserted into the vagina before each act of intercourse and is effective for 24 hours. In large clinical trials, the 1-year failure rate for the sponge was slightly but significantly higher than that for the diaphragm, approximately 15%. A study by McIntyre and Higgins indicated that the increased risk of pregnancy occurred only in women who had already had a child. In nulliparous women, the first-year failure rate was similar to that for the diaphragm, about 13%; in parous women, the first-year failure rate with the sponge was 28%, more than twice as high as that for diaphragm users. However, the latest study by the original investigators, Edelman and North, using the same data base, did not confirm the differences in failure rates according to parity and has created some controversy.

The incidence of toxic shock syndrome appears to be slightly increased in users of the sponge, especially if used during the menses or the puerperium or if left in place for more than 24 hours. Both these risk factors are contraindications for use of the sponge. The overall incidence of toxic shock syndrome in women using the sponge is low, estimated at one infection per 2 million sponges.

Although a few early studies linked the use of a spermicide at the time of conception with an increased risk of some congenital malformations, these studies were probably flawed by recall bias. Studies by Bracken and Vita, Linn et al., and Louik et al. have shown no increased risk of congenital malformations in newborns or of karyotypic abnormalities in the spontaneous abortuses of women who conceived while using spermicides.

BARRIER TECHNIQUES

Diaphragm

A diaphragm must be carefully fitted by the physician or nurse. The largest size that does not cause discomfort or undue pressure on the vaginal mucosa should be used. After the fitting, the patient should remove the diaphragm and reinsert it herself. She should then be examined to make sure the diaphragm is covering the cervix. The diaphragm should be used with contraceptive cream or jelly and be left in place for at least 8 hours after coitus. If repeated intercourse takes place or coitus occurs more than 8 hours after insertion of the diaphragm, additional contraceptive cream or jelly should be used. Although advisable, it may not be necessary to use a spermicide with the diaphragm, since it has not been conclusively demonstrated that pregnancy rates are lower when a spermicide is used. The number of urinary tract infections in women who use diaphragms is significantly higher than in nonusers, probably because of the mechanical obstruction of urine outflow by the diaphragm.

Diaphragm users should also be cautioned not to leave the device in place for more than 24 hours, since ulceration of the vaginal epithelium may occur with prolonged usage.

Data from the Oxford Family Planning Association Contraceptive Study indicated that the diaphragm is an effective method of contraception in married motivated women and that failure rates decline with increasing age and increasing use. In this cohort study of married women who had been using a diaphragm for more than 5 months before enrollment, the pregnancy rates were 4.1 per 100 woman-years for those 25 to 29 years of age and 1.1 for those 35 to 39. However, in a cohort study by Kovacs et al. of both married and unmarried diaphragm users, most of whom were young, the pregnancy rate at 1 year was 21%. This rose to 37% at 2 years, mainly because the women did not use the method consistently.

Cervical Cap

The cervical cap, a cup-shaped plastic or rubber device that fits around the cervix, has

been used as a barrier contraceptive for decades, mainly in Great Britain and other parts
of Europe.

Interest in this older method has recently
grown, since the cervical cap can be left in
place longer than the diaphragm and is more
comfortable. Each type of device is manufactured in different sizes and should be fitted to
the cervix by a clinician. The cervical cap
should not be left in place for more than 48
hours because of possible ulceration, unpleasant odor, and infection.

The Prentif cavity-rim cervical cap was approved in 1988 for general use in the United
States. Product labeling stipulates that the cap
should be left on the cervix for no more than
48 hours and that a spermicide should always
be placed inside the cap before use. The cap is
manufactured in four sizes and requires more
training, both for the provider in fitting it and
for the user in placing it correctly, than does
the diaphragm. Failure rates are similar to
those observed with the diaphragm. In a large
randomized clinical trial, 1-year pregnancy
rates were 17.4% for the cap and 16.7% for the
diaphragm. Of the pregnancies with the cap,
one third were method failures and two thirds
were user-related failures. In other studies,
pregnancy rates at 1 and 2 years with the cervical cap ranged from 8% to 17% and 14% to
38%, respectively, with good continuation
rates. Because of concern about its possible adverse effect on cervical tissue, the cervical cap
should be used only by women with a normal
cervical cytologic examination. Also, it is recommended that users have another cervical cytology examination 3 months after starting this
method.

Condom

Individuals with multiple sex partners should
be encouraged to use the condom. It is the
contraceptive method most effective in preventing sexually transmitted diseases. The condom should not be applied tightly. The tip
should extend beyond the end of the penis by
about ½ inch to collect the ejaculate.

In the Oxford Study, one of the largest that
has published findings on condom use, all couples using condoms had previously used another method, mainly OCs. During 12,497
woman-years of exposure, 449 unplanned pregnancies occurred, for a use-pregnancy rate of
3.6 per 100 woman-years. The pregnancy rate

increased linearly over time: from 0.7 per 100
woman-years at 3 months to 8.4 at 24 months.
Accidental pregnancy rates were slightly lower
among women over age 35 and among women
who had completed their families, even when
these factors were standardized for other characteristics. These results are consistent with
those of several previous studies, which show a
similarly high level of effectiveness for the condom when used by strongly motivated couples.

Barrier techniques are effective methods of
contraception in women age 30 and older. In
the analysis by Trussell and Kost, the first-year
failure rates for condom use among women
wishing no more pregnancy ranged from 3% to
6% for those over age 30, but from 8% to 10%
for those under 25.

Barrier Techniques and Sexually Transmitted Diseases

Barrier methods have the advantage of reducing the rate of sexually transmitted diseases. Several epidemiologic studies have
shown that spermicides reduce the frequency
of clinical infection with these diseases, both
bacterial and viral. In vitro studies by Conant
et al. have demonstrated that condoms prevent
the transmission of viruses, specifically the
herpesvirus and the human immunodeficiency
virus, as well as *Chlamydia trachomatis* bacteria, which is a frequent cause of salpingitis.
Several epidemiologic studies, both case control and cohort, indicate that the use of the
condom or diaphragm protects both men and
women from clinically apparent gonorrheal infection.

An epidemiologic study by Cramer et al.
(1985) of women with infertility caused by tubal
obstruction found that the past use of barrier
techniques protected women against tubal
damage. The greatest protection occurred with
the use of diaphragms or condoms with spermicides. The incidence of cervical neoplasia was
also greatly diminished among women in couples using condoms or diaphragms, probably
because of the decreased transmission of human papillomavirus (HPV). This antiviral action
may explain why women who use spermicides
are only one-third as likely to have cervical
cancer as members of a control group. Certain
strains of HPV have been causally linked to the
later development of cervical neoplasia.

Unfortunately, the failure rates of diaphragm
or condom users are highest for persons

younger than age 25, who are most likely to become infected with sexually transmitted disease. Therefore, to prevent the transmission of these diseases, as well as unwanted pregnancy, in this age group, the use of a barrier technique together with the most effective reversible method, the oral contraceptive, is advisable.

PERIODIC ABSTINENCE

The avoidance of sexual intercourse during the days of the menstrual cycle when the ovum can be fertilized is used by many highly motivated couples as a means of preventing pregnancy. Four techniques of periodic abstinence are now used. With the oldest of these, the *calendar rhythm method,* the period of abstinence is determined solely by calculating the length of the individual woman's previous menstrual cycle. The rationale for the rhythm method is based on three assumptions: (1) the human ovum is capable of being fertilized for only about 24 hours after ovulation; (2) spermatozoa retain their fertilizing ability for only about 48 hours after coitus; and (3) ovulation usually occurs 12 to 16 days (14 ± 2 days) before the onset of the subsequent menses. According to these assumptions, after the woman records the length of her cycles for several months, she establishes her fertile period by subtracting 18 days from the length of her previous shortest cycle and 11 days from her previous longest cycle. Then, in each subsequent cycle, the couple abstain from coitus during this calculated fertile period.

This method requires abstinence by most women with regular menstrual cycles for almost half the days of each cycle and cannot be used by women with irregular menstrual cycles. Although calendar rhythm is the most widely used technique of periodic abstinence, pregnancy rates are high, ranging from 14.4 to 47 per 100 woman-years, mainly because most couples fail to abstain for the relatively long periods required. The use of the calendar rhythm method alone is currently not advocated or taught to couples interested in practicing periodic abstinence.

In the past 2 decades, new techniques have been developed whereby women rely on physiologic changes during each cycle to determine the fertile period. The term *natural family planning* has been used instead of *rhythm* to describe these new techniques. They include the temperature method, the cervical-mucus method, and the sympto-thermal method. Each of these techniques requires much motivation and training. In most reports on use of these methods, pregnancy rates are relatively high and continuation rates are low.

The *temperature method* relies on measuring basal body temperature daily. The woman is required to abstain from intercourse from the onset of the menses until the third consecutive day of elevated basal temperature. Because abstinence is required for the entire preovulatory period in ovulatory cycles and for the entire cycle in anovulatory cycles, the temperature method alone is seldom used.

The *cervical-mucus method* requires that the woman be taught to recognize and interpret cyclic changes in the presence and consistency of cervical mucus; these changes occur in response to changing estrogen and progesterone levels. Abstinence is required during the menses and every other day after the menses ends (because of the possibility of confusing semen with ovulatory mucus) until the first day that copious, slippery mucus is observed. Abstinence is required every day thereafter until 4 days after the last day when the characteristic mucus is present, called the *peak mucus day.* In two well-designed, randomized clinical trials by Medina et al. and Wade et al., the pregnancy rates for new users of this method in the first year after 3 to 5 months of training were 20% and 24%, with discontinuation rates of 72% to 74%. In a five-country study of 725 highly motivated couples sponsored by the World Health Organization (WHO) (1981, 1983), the use failure rate during the first year after three cycles of training was 19.6%, with a method failure rate of 3.5%. Most of the pregnancies (15.4% of the 19.6%) resulted from conscious deviation from the rules of the method. The mean length of the fertile period in this study was 9.6 days, and abstinence was therefore required for about 17 days in each cycle. In this study the continuation rate after 1 year was high, 64.4%.

The *sympto-thermal method,* rather than relying on a single physiologic index, uses several indices to determine the fertile period. These usually include calendar calculations and changes in the cervical mucus to estimate the onset of the fertile period and changes in mucus or basal temperature to estimate its end.

Because several indices need to be monitored, this method is more difficult to learn than the single-index methods, but it is more effective than the cervical-mucus method alone. In the studies by Medina et al. and Wade et al. comparing these methods, the pregnancy rates at the end of 1 year of use after training were 10.9% and 19.8% with the sympto-thermal method, compared with 20% and 24% for the cervical-mucus method. In addition, the continuation rate among the women who used the sympto-thermal method was higher after 1 year (approximately 50% in each study) than that among those who used the cervical-mucus method (26% and 40%).

The major reason for the lack of acceptance of natural family planning, as well as the relatively high pregnancy rates among users of these methods, is the need to avoid having sexual intercourse for many days during each menstrual cycle. To overcome this problem, many women use barrier methods or spermicides during the fertile period. In a study by Rogow et al. of women who used the sympto-thermal method with barrier contraceptives or withdrawal during the fertile period, the failure rate during the first year was 9.9%, with a discontinuation rate of 33%.

Because the use of any method of contraception other than abstinence is unacceptable to many couples, simple, self-administered tests to detect hormonal changes have been developed to reduce the number of days of abstinence required in each cycle to a maximum of 7. Enzyme immunoassays for urinary estrogen and pregnanediol glucuronide have recently been developed that can easily be used at home and require minimal cost and time. Such tests must be performed by the woman about 12 days each month, but they should reduce the days of abstinence required. It remains to be determined to what extent this aid to natural family planning will be used when it becomes generally available.

ORAL STEROID CONTRACEPTIVES

Oral steroid contraceptives (OCs) were initially marketed in the United States in 1960. Because of their extremely high rate of effectiveness and ease of administration, they soon became one of the most widely used methods of reversible contraception in developing countries among both married and unmarried women. The initially marketed formulations of OCs contained 150 μg of the estrogen component, mestranol, and 9.85 mg of the progestin component, norethynodrel. The minor side effects produced by each of these steroids, such as nausea, breast tenderness, and weight gain, were common and occasionally severe enough to cause discontinuation of use. During the past 30 years many other formulations were developed and marketed with steadily decreasing dosages of both the estrogen and the progestin components. All the formulations initially marketed after 1975 contain less than 50 μg of ethinyl estradiol and 1 mg or less of several progestins. The use of these agents is associated with very low pregnancy rates, similar to those for formulations with higher doses of steroid, and a significantly lower incidence of adverse metabolic effects.

Data compiled by the U.S. Food and Drug Administration (FDA) indicate that the use of formulations containing less than 50 μg of estrogen has steadily increased in the United States since they were first marketed in 1973, from about 10% of prescriptions in 1976 to 82% in 1988 (Figure 11-2). Prescriptions for formulations with more than 50 μg of estrogen have been steadily decreasing since 1964, and in 1988 only 1.6% of OC prescriptions were for these high-dose compounds. Because these higher-dose estrogen formulations are associated with a greater incidence of adverse effects without greater efficacy, they are no longer marketed for contraceptive use in the United States, Canada, and Great Britain.

Pharmacology

The three major types of OC formulations are fixed-dose combination, combination phasic, and daily progestin. The combination formulations are the most widely used and most effective. They consist of tablets containing both an estrogen and a progestin given continuously for 3 weeks. The original sequential type, which is no longer marketed, provided a regimen of estrogen alone given for about 2 weeks, followed by 1 week of combination estrogen/progestin tablets. The combination phasic formulations contain two or three different amounts of the same estrogen and progestin. Each of the tablets containing one of these various dosages is given for intervals varying from

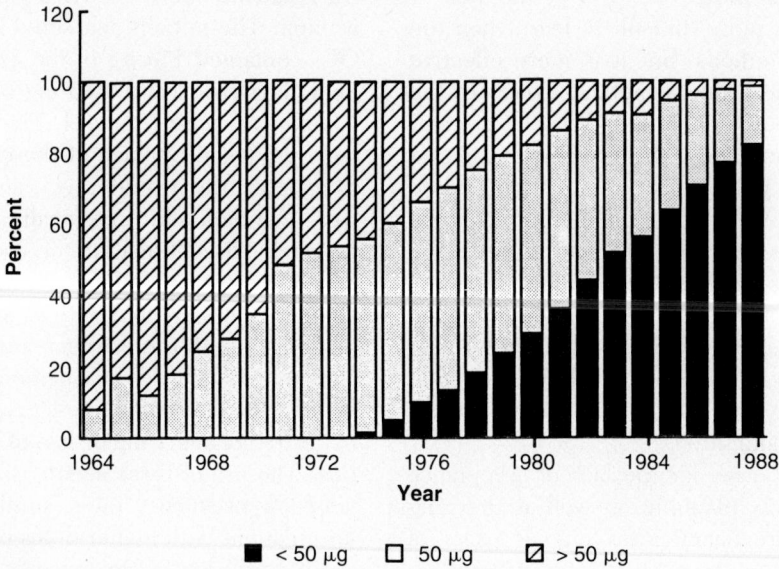

FIGURE 11-2
Percentage of oral contraceptive prescriptions in the United States by estrogen strength. (From Diane Kennedy, US Food and Drug Administration [FDA], personal communication.)

5 to 11 days during the 21-day medication period. These formulations have been described as biphasic or triphasic and are generally referred to as *multiphasic*. The rationale for this type of formulation is that a lower total dose of steroid is administered without increasing the incidence of breakthrough bleeding. In the usual regimen for combination OCs, no medication is given for 1 week out of 4 to allow withdrawal bleeding to occur. The third type of contraceptive formulation, consisting of tablets containing a progestin without any estrogen, is designed to be taken daily without a steroid-free interval.

OCs currently being used are formulated from synthetic steroids and contain no natural estrogens or progestins. The two major types of synthetic progestins are (1) derivatives of 19-nortestosterone and (2) derivatives of 17α-acetoxyprogesterone. The second group are C_{21} progestins, consisting of such steroids as medroxyprogesterone acetate and megestrol acetate. In contrast to the 19-nortestosterone derivatives, when high dosages of the C_{21} progestins were given to female beagle dogs, the animals developed an increased incidence of mammary cancer. Because of this carcinogenic effect, contraceptives containing these progestins are no longer being made.

All OC formulations now available in the United States consist of varying dosages of one of the following four 19-nortestosterone progestins: norethindrone, norethindrone acetate, ethynodiol diacetate, or norgestrel (Figure 11-3). The parent compound of the latter steroid, *dl*-norgestrel, consists of two isomeres, only one of which is biologically active. Currently, formulations containing only the active isomere of *dl*-norgestrel, levonorgestrel, are primarily being produced. In Europe, formulations containing three additional progestins—desogestrel, gestodene, and norgestimate—have been marketed for several years (Figure 11-4). These have greater progestational activity but are less androgenic than the currently used progestins. Clinical testing with these formulations in the United States is now being done or has been completed, and approval for their use is expected shortly.

With the exception of two daily progestin-only formulations, the progestins are combined with varying dosages of two estrogens, ethinyl estradiol and ethinyl estradiol 3-methyl ether, also known as mestranol (Figure 11-5). All the previous higher-dosage formulations contained mestranol, and this steroid is still present in some 50 μg formulations. All formulations with less than 50 μg of estrogen contain the parent

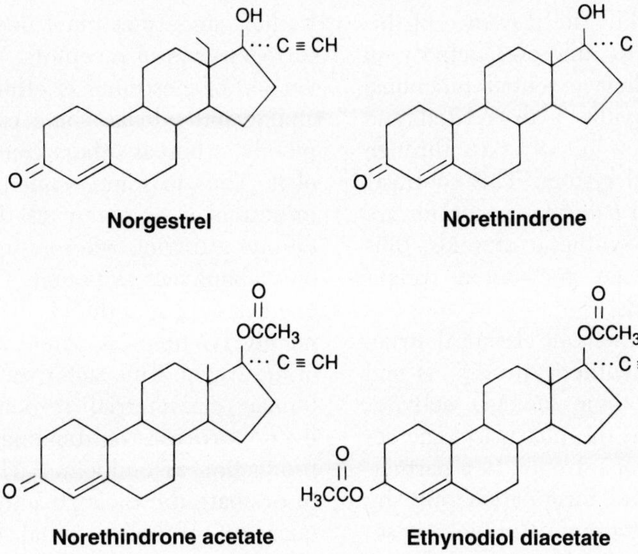

FIGURE 11-3
Structural formulas of the four progestins in oral contraceptives manufactured in the United States in 1990.

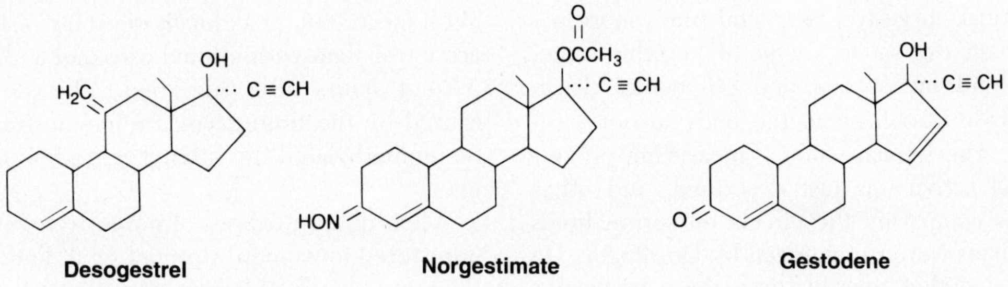

FIGURE 11-4
Structural formulas of three new progestins used in oral contraceptive formulations.

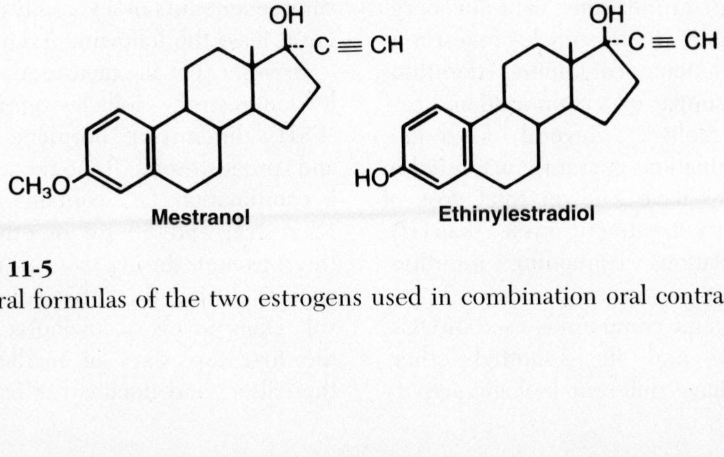

FIGURE 11-5
Structural formulas of the two estrogens used in combination oral contraceptives.

compound, ethinyl estradiol. All the synthetic estrogens and progestins in OCs have an ethinyl group at position 17. The presence of this ethinyl group enhances the oral activity of these agents, since their essential functional groups are not as rapidly hydroxylated and then conjugated as they initially pass through the liver via the portal system. This contrasts with what occurs when natural sex steroids are ingested orally. The synthetic steroids thus have greater oral potency per unit of weight than the natural steroids.

The various modifications in chemical structure of the different synthetic progestins and estrogens also affect their biologic activity. Thus one cannot judge the pharmacologic activity of the progestin or estrogen in a particular contraceptive steroid formulation only by the amount of steroid present. The biologic activity of each steroid must also be considered. Using established tests for progestational activity in animals, it has been found that a given weight of norgestrel is several times more potent than the same weight of norethindrone. Studies in humans, using delay of menses or endometrial histologic alterations such as subnuclear vacuolization as endpoints, also conclude that norgestrel is several times more potent than the same weight of norethindrone. Norethindrone acetate and ethynodiol diacetate are metabolized in the body to norethindrone. The human studies, measuring progestational activity as just described, and other studies comparing the effects on serum lipids in humans were summarized by Dorflinger. He concluded that each of these three progestins has approximately equal potency per unit of weight, whereas levonorgestrel is 10 to 20 times as potent. Thus, when considering which contraceptive to prescribe, the physician should consider both the dose and the potency of each steroid. The currently marketed triphasic contraceptive formulations with levonorgestrel contain about 10% as much progestin as triphasic formulations containing norethindrone and have similar effects on lipid and carbohydrate metabolism. Several fixed-dose monophasic formulations currently marketed in the United States have a lower total dose of norethindrone per treatment cycle than the triphasic formulations containing norethindrone.

The two estrogenic compounds used in OCs, ethinyl estradiol and its 3-methyl ether, mestranol, also have different biologic activity

in women. To become biologically effective, mestranol must be demethylated to ethinyl estradiol, since mestranol does not bind to the estrogen cytosol receptors. The degree of conversion of mestranol to ethinyl estradiol varies among individuals; some can convert it completely, whereas others convert only a portion of it. Thus in some women a given weight of mestranol is as potent as the same weight of ethinyl estradiol, whereas in other women it is only about half as potent. Overall it has been estimated that ethinyl estradiol is approximately 1.7 times as potent as the same weight of mestranol. This factor was determined using human endometrial response and effect on liver corticosteroid-binding globulin (CBG) production as endpoints. Thus it is important to evaluate the biologic activity, as well as the quantity, of both steroid components when comparing potency of the various formulations.

Radioimmunoassay methods have been developed to measure blood levels of these synthetic estrogens and progestins. Peak plasma levels of ethinyl estradiol occur about 1 hour after ingestion, then rapidly decline. However, measurable amounts of ethinyl estradiol are still found in plasma 24 hours after ingestion. With mestranol, peak levels of ethinyl estradiol are lower than with ethinyl estradiol and occur 2 to 4 hours after ingestion. This delay is caused by the time necessary for mestranol to be demethylated to ethinyl estradiol in the liver.

When different doses of norgestrel were administered to women, Brenner et al. found that the serum levels of levonorgestrel were related to the dosage. Peak serum levels were found ½ to 3 hours after oral administration, followed by a rapid, sharp decline. However, 24 hours after ingestion, 20% to 25% of the peak level of levonorgestrel was still present in the serum. After 5 days of norgestrel administration, measurable amounts of levonorgestrel were present for at least the following 5 days.

Brenner et al. measured serum levels of levonorgestrel, follicle-stimulating hormone (FSH), luteinizing hormone (LH), estradiol, and progesterone 3 hours after ingestion of a combination OC containing 0.5 mg of *dl*-norgestrel and 50 μg of ethinyl estradiol in three women during two consecutive cycles, as well as during the intervening pill-free interval. Daily levels of levonorgestrel rose during the first few days of medication, plateaued thereafter, and declined after ingestion of the

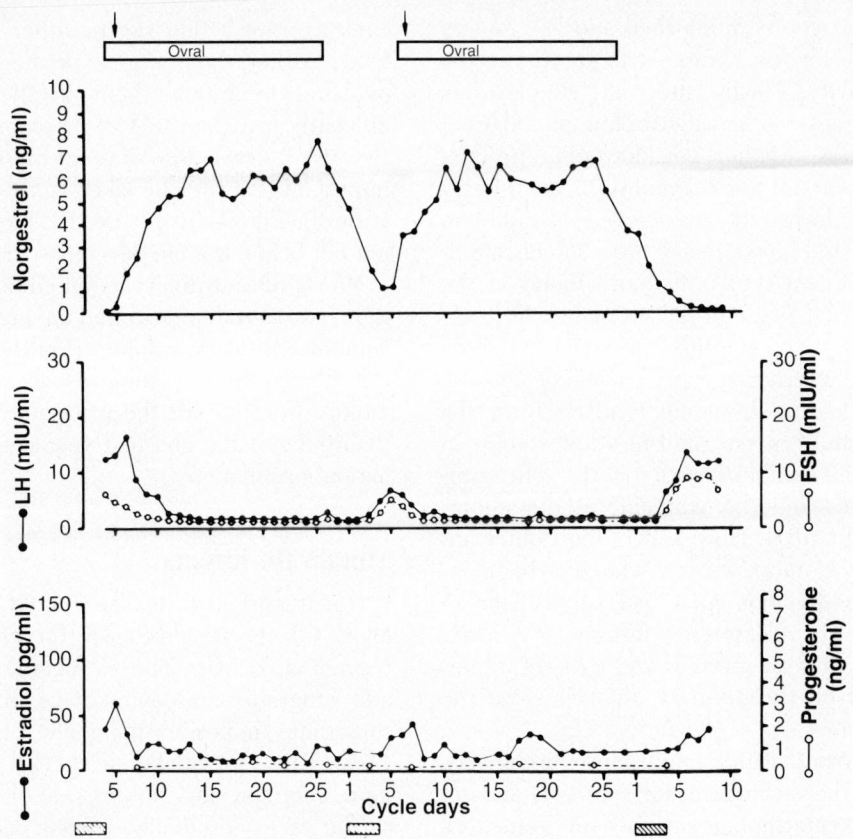

FIGURE 11-6

Serum *d*-norgestrel, FSH, LH, estradiol, and progesterone levels in patient during and after oral administration of 500 μg of *dl*-norgestrel and 50 μg of ethinyl estradiol (Ovral) for two subsequent 21-day periods interrupted by a pill-free interval of 6 days. (From Brenner PF, Mishell DR Jr, Stanczyk FZ, et al: Am J Obstet Gynecol 129:133, 1977.)

last pill (Figure 11-6). Nevertheless, substantial amounts of levonorgestrel remained in the serum for at least the first 3 to 4 days after the last pill was ingested. These steroid levels were sufficient to suppress gonadotrophin release; thus follicle maturation, as evidenced by rising estradiol levels, does not occur during the pill-free interval.

From these data it seems reasonable to conclude that accidental pregnancies during OC use probably do not occur because of a failure to ingest one or two pills more than a few days after a treatment cycle is initiated, but rather because initiation of the next cycle of medication is delayed for a few days. Therefore it is important that the pill-free interval be limited to no more than 7 days. This is best accomplished by administering either a placebo or iron pill daily during the steroid-free interval (the so-called 28-day package). Alternatively, treatment may be started on the first Sunday

after menses begins instead of the first or fifth day of the cycle; it is easier to remember to start the new package on a Sunday. Patients should be warned that the most important pill to remember to take is the first one of each cycle.

Mechanism of Action

The estrogen/progestin combination is the most effective type of OC formulation, since these preparations consistently inhibit the mid-cycle gonadotrophin surge and thus prevent ovulation. Such formulations also act on other aspects of the reproductive process. They alter the cervical mucus, making it thick, viscid, and scanty, which thus retards sperm penetration. They also alter motility of the uterus and oviduct, thus impairing transport of both ova and sperm. Furthermore, combination OCs alter the endometrium so that its glandular production of glycogen is diminished and less energy is available for the blastocyst to survive in the uterine cavity. Finally, they may alter ovarian responsiveness to gonadotrophin stimulation. Nevertheless, neither gonadotrophin production nor ovarian steroidogenesis is completely abolished. Levels of endogenous estradiol in the peripheral blood during ingestion of combination OCs are similar to those found in the early follicular phase of the normal cycle.

Contraceptive steroids prevent ovulation mainly by interfering with release of gonadotrophin-releasing hormone (GnRH) from the hypothalamus. In rats, and in a few studies in humans, this inhibitory action of the contraceptive steroids could be overcome by the administration of GnRH. However, in most other human studies, most women who had been ingesting combination OCs had suppression of LH and FSH release after infusion of GnRH, indicating that the steroids had a direct inhibitory effect on the pituitary, as well as on the hypothalamus.

When hypothalamic inhibition is prolonged, however, the mechanism for synthesis and release of gonadotrophins may become refractory to the normal amount of GnRH stimulation. Nevertheless, in a few OC users studied, a refractory response to a GnRH infusion still occurred after serial daily administration of GnRH. Thus the combination OCs probably do have a direct inhibitory effect on the gonadotrophin-producing cells of the pituitary, in addition to affecting the hypothalamus. This effect occurs in approximately 80% of women ingesting combination OCs. Although unrelated to the age of the patient or the duration of steroid use, this effect is related to the potency of the preparations. The effect is more pronounced with formulations containing a more potent progestin and with those containing 50 μg or more of estrogen than with 30 to 35 μg formulations. It has not been demonstrated that the amount of pituitary suppression is related to post-OC amenorrhea, but if a relationship exists, the lower-dose formulations should be associated with a lower frequency of this condition. Bracken et al. reported that the delay in the resumption of ovulation after discontinuation of OC use is shorter in women ingesting preparations with less than 50 μg of estrogen than in those ingesting formulations with 50 μg or more.

The daily progestin-only preparations do not consistently inhibit ovulation. They exert their contraceptive action via the other mechanisms listed earlier, but because of the inconsistent ovulation inhibition, their effectiveness is significantly less than that of the combined type. Because a lower dose of progestin is used, it is important that they be taken consistently at the same time of day to ensure that blood levels do not fall below the effective contraceptive level.

No significant difference in clinical effectiveness has been demonstrated among the various combination formulations currently available in the United States (Table 11-4). Provided no tablets are omitted, the pregnancy rate is less than 0.2% at the end of 1 year with all combination formulations.

Metabolic Effects

It is important to realize that OCs have metabolic effects, in addition to the effects on the reproductive axis. The estrogenic component and progestin component have different, and sometimes opposite, metabolic effects (Table 11-5). These metabolic effects can produce the more common, less serious side effects, as well as the rare, potentially serious complications. The magnitude of these effects is directly related to the dosage and potency of the steroids in the formulations. Fortunately, in most instances the more common adverse effects are relatively mild.

The symptoms most frequently produced by the estrogenic component include nausea (a central nervous system effect), breast tenderness, and fluid retention from decreased sodium excretion, which usually does not exceed 3 to 4 pounds of body weight. Minor, clinically insignificant changes in circulating vitamin levels also have occurred after ingestion of the higher-dosage OCs. These changes include a decrease in levels of the B-complex vitamins and ascorbic acid and increases in vitamin A levels. Even with use of the high-dose OCs, dietary vitamin supplementation is not necessary, since the changes in circulating vitamin levels are small and clinically insignificant. Estrogen can also cause chloasma (pigmentation of the malar eminences), which is accentuated by sunlight and usually takes a long time to disappear after OCs are discontinued. The incidence of all these estrogenic side effects is much lower now than in the past because formulations today contain only one-fifth as much estrogen as those used in the 1960s.

The estrogen component of OC agents also

TABLE 11-4
Estrogen and Progestin Components of Oral Contraceptives

Manufacturer/Product		Type*	Progestin	Estrogen
Berlex Laboratories, Inc.				
Levlen		Comb.	0.15 mg levonorgestrel	30 μg ethinyl estradiol
Tri-Levlen 6/		Comb.-triphasic	0.05 mg levonorgestrel	30 μg ethinyl estradiol
5/			0.075 mg levonorgestrel	40 μg ethinyl estradiol
10/			0.125 mg levonorgestrel	30 μg ethinyl estradiol
GynoPharma, Inc.				
Norcept-E 1/35		Comb.	1 mg norethindrone	35 μg ethinyl estradiol
Mead Johnson Laboratories				
Ovcon-35		Comb.	0.4 mg norethindrone	35 μg ethinyl estradiol
Ovcon-50		Comb.	1.0 mg norethindrone	50 μg ethinyl estradiol
Ortho Pharmaceutical Corp.				
Micronor		Prog.	0.35 mg norethindrone	
Modicon		Comb.	0.5 mg norethindrone	35 μg ethinyl estradiol
Ortho-Novum 1/35		Comb.	1.0 mg norethindrone	35 μg ethinyl estradiol
Ortho-Novum 1/50		Comb.	1.0 mg norethindrone	50 μg mestranol
Ortho-Novum 7/7/7	7/	Comb.-triphasic	0.5 mg norethindrone	35 μg ethinyl estradiol
	7/		0.75 mg norethindrone	35 μg ethinyl estradiol
	7/		1.0 mg norethindrone	35 μg ethinyl estradiol
Ortho-Novum 10/11	10/	Comb.-biphasic	0.5 mg norethindrone	35 μg ethinyl estradiol
	11/		1.0 mg norethindrone	35 μg ethinyl estradiol
Parke-Davis				
Loestrin 1/20		Comb.	1.0 mg norethindrone acetate	20 μg ethinyl estradiol
Loestrin 1.5/30		Comb.	1.5 mg norethindrone acetate	30 μg ethinyl estradiol
Norlestrin 1/50		Comb.	1.0 mg norethindrone acetate	50 μg ethinyl estradiol
Norlestrin 2.5/50		Comb.	2.5 mg norethindrone acetate	50 μg ethinyl estradiol
Rugby Laboratories, Inc.				
Genora 1/35		Comb.	1 mg norethindrone	35 μg ethinyl estradiol
Genora 1/50		Comb.	1 mg norethindrone	50 μg ethinyl estradiol
Genora 0.5/35		Comb.	5 mg norethindrone	35 μg ethinyl estradiol
Schiapparelli Searle				
Norethin 1/35E		Comb.	1 mg norethindrone	35 μg ethinyl estradiol
Norethin 1/50M		Comb.	1 mg norethindrone	50 μg ethinyl estradiol
Searle Laboratories				
Demulen 1/35		Comb.	1.0 mg ethynodiol diacetate	35 μg ethinyl estradiol
Demulen 1/50		Comb.	1.0 mg ethynodiol diacetate	50 μg ethinyl estradiol
Syntex Laboratories, Inc.				
Brevicon		Comb.	0.5 mg norethindrone	35 μg ethinyl estradiol
Norinyl 1 + 35		Comb.	1.0 mg norethindrone	35 μg ethinyl estradiol
Norinyl 1 + 50		Comb.	1.0 mg norethindrone	50 μg mestranol
Nor-Q D		Prog.	0.35 mg norethindrone	

*Comb., Combination; Prog., progestin only.

Continued.

TABLE 11-4
Estrogen and Progestin Components of Oral Contraceptives—cont'd

Manufacturer/Product	Type*	Progestin	Estrogen
Syntex Laboratories, Inc.—cont'd			
Tri-Norinyl 7/	Comb.-triphasic	0.5 mg norethindrone	35 μg ethinyl estradiol
9/		1 mg norethindrone	35 μg ethinyl estradiol
5/		0.5 mg norethindrone	35 μg ethinyl estradiol
Wyeth-Ayerst Laboratories			
Lo/Ovral	Comb.	0.3 mg norgestrel	30 μg ethinyl estradiol
Nordette	Comb.	0.15 mg levonorgestrel	30 μg ethinyl estradiol
Ovral	Comb.	0.5 mg norgestrel	50 μg ethinyl estradiol
Ovrette	Prog.	75 μg norgestrel	
Triphasil 6/	Comb.-triphasic	50 μg levonorgestrel	40 μg ethinyl estradiol
5/		75 μg levonorgestrel	40 μg ethinyl estradiol
10/		125 μg levonorgestrel	30 μg ethinyl estradiol

*Comb., Combination; Prog., progestin only.

accelerates the development of the symptoms of gallbladder disease in young women but does not increase the overall incidence of cholelithiasis. In a very large, retrospective cohort study by Strom et al., the risk ratio for gallbladder disease in OC users was only 1.14, which barely achieved statistical significance. Among women using formulations with less than 50 μg of estrogen, the risk ratio for gallbladder disease was 0.97.

It was previously postulated that high dosages of the synthetic estrogens could also produce changes in mood and depression, a result of tryptophan metabolism being diverted from its minor pathway in the brain to its major pathway in the liver. The end product of tryptophan metabolism, serotonin, is thus decreased in the central nervous system. The theory was that the resultant lowering of serotonin could produce depression in some women and sleepiness and mood changes in others. Analysis of the data from the Royal College of General Practitioners' (RCGP) Oral Contraception Study indicated that OC use was positively correlated with the incidence of depression, which in turn was directly related to the dose of estrogen in the formulation. Users of OCs containing less than 50 μg of estrogen reported no excessive depression in this cohort study. Data from studies of postmenopausal women receiving estrogen therapy alone, as well as estrogen-progestin sequential therapy, indicate that estrogen alone improves the mood of women,

whereas the addition of a progestin increases the amount of depression, irritability, tension, and fatigue. These studies also indicate that the progestin component may be the major cause of the adverse mood changes and tiredness observed in some women after ingestion of OCs. It has not been definitely established, however, whether estrogen or progestin is the major factor in producing adverse mood changes. Possibly both are involved.

The progestins, because they are structurally related to testosterone, also produce certain adverse androgenic effects, including weight gain, acne, and a symptom perceived by some women as nervousness. Some women taking OCs gain considerable weight, caused by the anabolic effect of the progestin component. Although estrogens decrease sebum production, progestins increase sebum production and can cause acne to develop or worsen. Thus patients who have acne should be given a formulation with a low progestin/estrogen ratio. A final symptom produced by the progestin component is failure of withdrawal bleeding, or amenorrhea. Because the progestins decrease the synthesis of estrogen receptors in the endometrium, endometrial growth is decreased, and some women have failure of withdrawal bleeding. This symptom is not important medically; however, since bleeding serves as a signal that the woman is not pregnant, it is desirable to have some periodic withdrawal bleeding during the days she is not taking these steroids.

TABLE 11-5

Metabolic Effects of Contraceptive Steroids

	Effects	
	Chemical	Clinical
Estrogen—ethinyl estradiol		
Proteins*		
Albumin	↓	None
Amino acids	↓	None
Globulins	↑	
Angiotensinogen		↑ Blood pressure
Factors VII and X		Hypercoagulability
Carrier proteins (CBG, TBG, transferrin, ceruloplasmin)		
Carbohydrate		
Plasma insulin	None	None
Glucose tolerance	None	None
Lipids†		
Cholesterol	None	None
Triglyceride	↑	None
HDL cholesterol	↑	None
LDL cholesterol	↓	None
Electrolytes		
Sodium excretion	↓	Fluid retention
		Edema
Vitamins		
B complex	↓	None
Ascorbic acid	↓	None
Vitamin A	↑	None
Target tissues		
Breast	↑	Breast tenderness
Endometrial receptors	↑	Hyperplasia
Skin	↓	Sebum production
	↑	Facial pigmentation
Progestins—19-nortestosterone derivatives		
Proteins	None	None
Carbohydrate		
Plasma insulin	↑	None
Glucose tolerance	↓	None
Lipids†		
Cholesterol	↓	None
Triglyceride	↓	None
HDL cholesterol	↓ ⎫	? ↑ Cardiovascular disease
LDL cholesterol	↑ ⎭	
Nitrogen retention	↑	↑ Body weight
Skin—sebum production	↑	↑ Acne
Central nervous system effects	↑	Nervousness, fatigue, depression
Endometrial receptors	↓	Amenorrhea

*CBG, Corticosteroid-binding globulin; TBG, thyroxine-binding globulin.
†HDL, High-density lipoprotein; LDL, low-density lipoprotein.

TABLE 11-6

Mean Factor VII and Fibrinogen Levels* in Relation to Oral Contraceptive Use
and Estrogen Dose

	Not Taking OCs	OC Estrogen Dose	
		30 μg	50 μg
No. of patients	243	15	65
Factor VII (%)	83.0	96.6	121.1
Fibrinogen (g/L)	2.52	2.84	2.89

From Meade TW: Am J Obstet Gynecol 142:758, 1982.
*Age-adjusted values.

Both steroid components can act together to produce irregular bleeding. Breakthrough bleeding (usually produced by insufficient estrogen, too much progestin, or a combination of both), as well as failure of withdrawal bleeding, can be alleviated by increasing the amount of estrogen in the formulation or by switching to a more estrogenic formulation. Many women taking OCs complain of increased headaches. The exact relation, if any, between OC use and headaches has not been determined.

Protein

The synthetic estrogens used in OCs increase the hepatic production of several globulins, some of which are involved in the coagulation process. Another globulin, angiotensinogen, may be converted to angiotensin and may increase blood pressure in some users. The circulating levels of each of these globulins correlate directly with the amount of estrogen in the OC formulation (Table 11-6). Epidemiologic studies have shown that the incidence of both venous and arterial thrombosis is also directly related to the dose of estrogen (Table 11-7 and 8).

Angiotensinogen levels are lower in women who ingest formulations with 30 to 35 μg of ethinyl estradiol than in those who ingest formulations with 50 μg. However, Wilson et al. still observed a significant increase in blood pressure in women who receive the lower dosage. Thus blood pressure should be monitored in all users of OCs. Indirect evidence suggests that the progestin component may also affect blood pressure. However, women who receive progestins without estrogen do not have an increase in blood pressure over time, indicating

that the estrogen component is the major factor in causing elevated blood pressure in certain users of OCs.

Carbohydrate

When formulations with a high dose of progestin are administered, 4% to 16% of women (depending on their age) have an abnormal response on the glucose tolerance test. The incidence of abnormal test results is related to the dose and potency of the progestin, since estrogen does not affect carbohydrate metabolism. Some studies have shown that formulations with a low dose of progestin (even one containing levonorgestrel) do not significantly alter levels of glucose, insulin, or glucagon after a glucose load in healthy women or in those with a history of gestational diabetes. However, other studies indicate that the multiphasic formulations with norgestrel, but not those with norethindrone, produce some deterioration of glucose tolerance in normal women, as well as in those with a history of gestational diabetes.

When prescribing OCs for women with a history of glucose intolerance, one should choose formulations with a low dose of a norethindrone-type progestin and monitor glucose tolerance periodically to reduce the possible risk of accelerating the onset of permanent diabetes. Data from 20 years' experience with use of mainly high-dose formulations in the large RCGP study revealed no increased risk of developing diabetes mellitus among current OC users (relative risk, 0.80) or former OC users (relative risk, 0.82), even among those women who had used OCs for 10 years or longer.

TABLE 11-7

Ratio of Observed to Expected Embolism and Thrombosis in Relation to Type and Dose of Estrogen in Combined Oral Contraceptives

	Estrogen					
	Mestranol Dose (μg)				Ethinyl Estradiol Dose (μg)	
	150	100	75-80	50	100	50
Fatal pulmonary embolism*	2.8	1.5	0.9	0.6	1.0	0.5
Nonfatal pulmonary embolism†	2.3	1.2	0.9	1.0	1.8	0.7
Cerebral thrombosis‡	3.2	1.2	0.7	0.5	—	0.8
Coronary thrombosis*	2.6	1.2	0.3	1.1	1.8	0.9

Modified from Mann JI: Am J Obstet Gynecol 142:752, 1982.
*Linear trend test: $P < 0.05$.
†Linear trend test: $P < 0.01$.
‡Linear trend test: $P < 0.001$.

TABLE 11-8

Ratio of Observed to Expected Cardiovascular Events in Relation to Estrogen Dose in Oral Contraceptives (United Kingdom, 1974-1977)

Event	Ethinyl Estradiol	
	50 μg	30 μg
Venous deaths	1.40	0.65
Nonvenous deaths	1.52	0.53*
Ischemic heart disease	1.48	0.54*
Cerebrovascular accident (stroke)	1.20	0.80

Adapted from Meade TW, Greenberg G, and Thompson SG: Br Med J 280:1157, 1980.
*Linear trend test: $P < 0.05$.

Lipids

Adverse alterations in high-density lipoprotein (HDL) cholesterol and low-density lipoprotein (LDL) cholesterol are produced by all the progestins currently used in OCs available in the United States. The degree of change in the levels of these cholesterols is related to the amount and potency of the progestin. Because estrogen has the opposite effect of progestin, a decrease in HDL cholesterol levels after ingestion of various formulations containing 50 μg of estrogen has been noted only for a formulation containing norgestrel. Studies have measured lipid levels before and after the ingestion of several low-dose estrogen-progestin formulations, including the triphasic formulation containing levonorgestrel. These found no adverse alterations in the levels of HDL or LDL cholesterol or in the ratio of total cholesterol to HDL cholesterol. In two studies the triphasic formulation with norgestrel, but not the triphasic formulation with norethindrone, still significantly lowered the level of the HDL_2, which is believed to be the cardioprotective fraction of HDL cholesterol. In a prospective randomized study of the three triphasic formulations, two with norethindrone and one with levonorgestrel, currently being marketed in the United States, Patsch et al. reported that each had similar effects on carbohydrate and lipid metabolism, including changes in HDL, HDL_2 and LDL cholesterol. Another prospective randomized study by Notelovitz et al. compared the effects of a norethindrone and a levonorgestrel triphasic formulation on serum lipid levels. They also found no statistically significant difference between the two formulations.

Cardiovascular Effects

One must be concerned about the adverse changes in lipid levels produced by the progestin component of certain high-progestin OC formulations. However, the cause of the increased incidence of both venous and arterial cardiovascular disease, including myocardial infarction (MI), in users of OCs appears to be thrombosis and not atherosclerosis.

Estrogens can increase blood viscosity by raising plasma fibrinogen levels, as well as the hematocrit. The synthetic progestins also increase blood viscosity by raising the hematocrit and decreasing erythrocyte deformability. Increased blood viscosity, produced by either of these dose-related steroid mechanisms, could cause an increased incidence of thrombosis. This could explain the findings in several epidemiologic studies, including the RCGP study, that the incidence of both venous and arterial thrombotic events are directly related independently to both the estrogen dose and the progestin dose.

Neither epidemiologic studies of humans nor experimental studies with subhuman primates have observed an acceleration of atherosclerosis with the ingestion of OCs. Three large epidemiologic studies by Layde et al., Stampfer et al., and Rosenberg et al. (1990) found no increased risk of MI among former users of OCs (Table 11-9). The incidence of cardiovascular disease is also not correlated with the duration of OC use. A study with cynomolgus macaque monkeys by Adams et al. found that the ingestion of an OC containing high doses of norgestrel and ethinyl estradiol lowered HDL cholesterol levels significantly. After 2 years of ingesting this formulation and being fed an atherogenic diet, however, the animals had a significantly smaller area of coronary artery atherosclerosis than a control group of female monkeys fed the same diet. Another group of monkeys who received levonorgestrel without estrogen also had lowered HDL cholesterol levels. In this group the extent of coronary atherosclerosis was significantly increased as compared with that of the controls. The results of this study have since been confirmed in a larger study by Clarkson et al. with two high-dose estrogen-progestin formulations. In this study the mean coronary artery placque extent of the high-risk control group of female animals was more than 3 times greater than that found in animals ingesting a high-dose norgestrel compound and more than 10 times greater than those ingesting a high-dose norethindrone

TABLE 11-9
Age-Adjusted Relative Risks of Cardiovascular Diseases Among Past Users of Oral Contraceptives, According to Duration of Use and as Compared with Those Who Never Used Oral Contraceptives, in the Nurses' Health Study, 1976 Through 1984

Duration of Use (Months)	Major Coronary Disease		Total Stroke		Fatal Cardiovascular Disease		Major Cardiovascular Disease	
	RR	95% CI	RR	95% CI	RR	95% CI	RR	95% CI
None	1.0	—	1.0	—	1.0	—	1.0	—
1-11	1.0	0.7-1.4	0.8	0.5-1.3	1.1	0.7-1.7	1.0	0.8-1.2
12-35	1.0	0.7-1.4	0.8	0.5-1.3	0.5	0.3-1.1	0.9	0.7-1.2
36-59	1.0	0.6-1.7	1.1	0.6-2.0	0.7	0.3-1.5	1.1	0.8-1.5
60-119	0.8	0.5-1.2	1.4	0.9-2.1	1.0	0.6-2.5	1.0	0.7-1.3
≥120	0.7	0.4-1.2	1.3	0.7-2.3	1.3	0.6-2.5	0.9	0.6-1.3
Chi trend	−1.51		1.36		−0.18		−0.61	
P value		0.13		0.17		0.86		0.54
Overall age-adjusted RR	0.91	0.74-1.12	1.01	0.78-1.12	0.98	0.73-1.32	0.95	0.81-1.1
Multivariate RR	0.80	0.64-0.99	0.96	0.74-1.25	0.90	0.67-1.21	0.85	0.72-1.0

From Stampfer MJ, Willett WC, Colditz GA, et al: N Engl J Med 319:1313, 1988.
RR, Relative risk; CI, confidence interval.

compound. Both these compounds lowered the HDL cholesterol levels by half and tripled the cholesterol/HDL cholesterol ratio. These studies suggest that the estrogen component of OCs may have a protective effect on coronary atherosclerosis that would otherwise be accelerated by decreased levels of HDL cholesterol.

The epidemiologic studies that reported an increased incidence of MI in older users of OCs were published in the late 1970s and thus used as a data base women who ingested only formulations with 50 μg or more of estrogen. In these case-control and cohort studies, a significantly increased incidence of MI was found mainly among older users who had risk factors that caused arterial narrowing, such as smoking, preexisting hypercholesterolemia, hypertension, or diabetes mellitus.

Data accumulated during the first 10 years of the RCGP study, 1968 to 1978, in which most users ingested formulations with more than 50 μg of estrogen and high doses of progestin, showed that a significantly increased relative risk of death from circulatory disease occurred only among women over age 35 who also smoked. A more recent analysis of data obtained during the first 20 years of this study, 1968 to 1988, revealed no significant increased relative risk of acute MI among current or former OC users of who did not smoke cigarettes (Table 11-10). Even though most of the women in this study used high-dose formulations, a significantly increased risk of MI occurred only among both mild (less than 15 cigarettes a day) and heavy cigarette smokers, with the latter group having a greater relative risk. In this and other studies, cigarette smoking was an independent risk factor for MI, but the use of OCs by cigarette smokers greatly en-

hanced their risk of developing an MI, with the two factors acting synergistically.

The mechanism whereby cigarette smoking increases the risk of arterial thrombosis in OC users appears to be caused by nicotine's effect on the coagulation process. Although OCs increase the concentration of factors involved in producing blood coagulation, they also affect the activity of factors inhibiting coagulation. Notelovitz et al. (1985) found that smokers who ingested low-dose OCs had a significantly greater decrease in levels of endogenous coagulation inhibitors, mainly antithrombin III, than did nonsmoking OC users. Dynamic tests of coagulation and fibrinolysis by these investigators showed an altered procoagulant activity only among the OC users who also smoked. Mileikowsky et al. reported that platelet aggregation was increased only among OC users who also smoked, and not among women who smoked and did not use OCs. This thrombotic effect was probably related to prostacyclin inhibition, since prostacyclin formation was reduced only among the women in the study who smoked and used OCs. The usual balance of prostacyclin and thromboxane is thus altered when OC users smoked, producing a relative excess of thromboxane. The results of this study therefore suggest that the synergistic effect of OCs and smoking on the results of arterial thrombosis, such as MI and cerebral thrombosis, are produced by activation of the thromboxane A_2–mediated mechanism of platelet aggregation brought about by prostacyclin reduction.

Although epidemiologic data from studies performed in the 1970s indicated that a possible causal relation existed between ingestion of high-dose OC formulations and cerebrovascular

TABLE 11-10

Relative Risk of Myocardial Infarction in Relation to Smoking and Oral Contraceptive Use (RCGP Study, 1968-1987) (n = 158)

	Oral Contraceptive Use		
Smoking	Never (CL)	Previously (CL)	Current (CL)
Never	1.0	1.1(0.6-2.2)	0.9(0.3-2.7)
<15/day	2.0(1.0-3.9)	1.3(0.6-2.8)	3.5(1.3-9.5)
≥15/day	3.3(1.6-6.7)	4.3(2.3-8.0)	20.8(5.2-83.1)

Modified from Croft P and Hannaford PC: Br Med J 298:165, 1989.
CL, Confidence limits.

TABLE 11-11

Relative Risk of Breast Cancer in Women Who Ever Used Oral Contraceptives

Author	Year	RR Estimate (95% CI)
Case-control studies		
Henderson et al.	1974	0.7 (0.5–1.2)
Paffenbarger et al.	1977	1.1 (0.9–1.4)
Sartwell et al.	1977	0.9 (0.5–1.5)
Kelsey et al.	1978	1.6 (0.8–2.4)
Ravnihar et al.	1979	0.9 (0.6–1.5)
Pike et al.	1981	1.2 (0.7–1.9)
Kelsey et al.	1981	0.9 (0.6–1.3)
Brinton et al.	1982	1.1 (0.8–1.4)
Harris et al.	1982	1.0 (0.6–1.4)
Vessey et al.	1983	1.0 (0.8–1.2)
Hennekens et al.	1984	1.0 (0.9–1.2)
Rosenberg et al.	1984	0.9 (0.8–1.1)
Talamini et al.	1985	0.7 (0.4–1.4)
CASH study	1986	1.0 (0.9–1.1)
Paul et al.	1986	0.9 (0.9–1.25)
LaVecchia et al.	1986	1.1 (0.8–1.5)
SUMMARY RR	—	1.0 (0.9–1.1)
Cohort studies		
Vessey et al.	1981	1.0 (0.6–1.6)
Trapido	1981	0.8 (0.7–1.2)
RCGP	1981	1.2 (0.8–1.7)
Lipnick et al.	1986	1.0 (0.8–1.3)
SUMMARY RR	—	1.0 (0.8–1.1)

From Prentice RL and Thomas DB: Adv Cancer Res 49:285, 1987.
RR, Relative risk; CI, confidence interval.

studies is the Cancer and Steroid Hormone (CASH) study performed by the U.S. Centers for Disease Control. Because hormones are considered to be promoters, not initiators, of cancers, any adverse oncologic effects of these steroids should show a dose-response relationship, as demonstrated by an increased risk occurring with increased duration of use. In 1989 Schlesselman addressed this issue by reviewing all the epidemiologic studies reported since 1980 that analyzed the effect of OCs according to their duration of use on cancer of the breasts and female reproductive organs.

Breast Cancer

No study has reported a significant increase or decrease in the risk of developing breast cancer among the entire population of OC users. The combined risk estimate of the 16 case-control studies and 4 cohort studies summarized by Prentice and Thomas in 1987 was 1.0 (Table 11-11). In Schlesselman's review of 17 different studies in which the risk of developing breast cancer in women under age 60 was compared with the duration of OC use, no overall dose-response relationship was found to exist, and long-term use did not increase the risk of developing breast cancer (Figure 11-8).

The issue of latency, time since first use of OCs, and risk of breast cancer has also been studied. In groups of women using OCs more than 10 years, no changes in risk of breast cancer were found with increasing duration of time since first use. Thus no evidence supports a long-term latent effect. Several studies have presented data regarding the risk of developing breast cancer under age 45 by duration of OC use before age 25. The combined data fail to show a dose-response relationship, indicating that early age of first OC use is not by itself a risk factor for development of breast cancer. The preponderance of data in studies estimating risk of breast cancer in women under age 60 by duration of OC use before the first term pregnancy also failed to show an increased risk

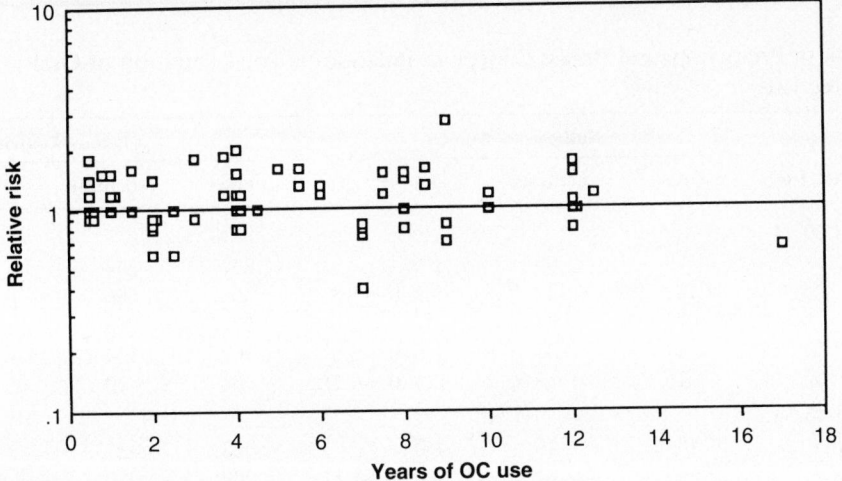

FIGURE 11-8
Breast cancer in women younger than age 60. Relative risk by total years of oral contraceptive use in 17 studies. (From Schlesselman JJ: Contraception 40:1, 1989.)

or a dose-response relationship. However, analysis of the studies that estimated the relative risk of developing breast cancer in women under age 45 suggested that there was a trend of increasing risk with increasing duration of overall use, as well as with increasing duration of use before the first term pregnancy. The increased risk in both groups became most evident after 8 years of use.

Three large studies suggested that prolonged use of OCs might increase the risk of developing breast cancer, but only when initially diagnosed at an early age. Analysis of data from the cohort RCGP study, begun in 1968 by Kay and Hannaford, revealed that increased risk of breast cancer among OC users occurred only among those women who developed breast cancer between the ages of 30 to 34, not in other age categories. A large British case-control study found that prolonged use of OCs more than 5 years increased the risk of developing breast cancer under age 36, with the risk increasing with more than 8 years of use. This study reported a lower risk associated with low-estrogen (less than 50 µg) formulations and stated that data from national breast cancer registries did not show increased rates of the disease after OCs were widely used. A detailed analysis by Stadel et al. of the CASH study data indicated that the only subset of women with an increased risk of developing breast cancer were nulliparous women whose menarche was before age 13 and who used OCs for more than 8 years. To provide a rational basis to explain observations of these studies, Stadel et al.

performed additional analysis of the data in the CASH studies. They found no overall change in the risk of developing premenopausal breast cancer in women under age 55 with increasing duration of OC use. They also found no change in risk among parous women who used OCs and developed breast cancer under age 45 or between ages 45 and 54 (Table 11-12).

However, when data from nulliparous women were analyzed, there was an OC duration–dependent increased risk of developing breast cancer if the disease occurred under age 45, but a duration-dependent decreased risk of developing breast cancer if the disease was initially found between ages 45 and 54 (Table 11-12). These data are consistent with the belief that long-term use of high-dose OCs could have promoted the age at which breast cancer was diagnosed clinically among susceptible nulliparous women. This promotional effect was transient, not persistent, and thus had no appreciable effect on the aggregate lifetime risk of developing breast cancer in the population despite the widespread use of OCs. These findings could also provide an explanation for the findings that prolonged OC use before the first pregnancy increased the risk of developing breast cancer under age 45, but not under age 60, since total duration of use in nulliparous women is equivalent to their use before the first term pregnancy.

Because formulations with low-dose estrogen have been used by most women ingesting OCs only since 1983, the effect of these agents, if any, on early development of breast cancer can

TABLE 11-12

Relative Risk of Premenopausal Breast Cancer in Relation to Total Duration of Oral Contraceptive Use

Total Years of OC Use	Nulliparous Women			Parous Women		
	Cases	Controls	RR (95% CI)	Cases	Controls	RR (95% CI)
Women aged 20-44						
Never	88	93	1.0 (—)	232	234	1.0 (—)
>0-3	109	133	1.2 (0.8-1.8)	598	596	1.1 (0.9-1.4)
4-7	73	64	1.7 (1.0-2.8)	292	273	1.2 (0.9-1.5)
8-11	43	35	1.6 (0.9-2.8)	162	134	1.3 (1.0-1.7)
≥12	16	6	2.5 (0.9-6.7)	64	70	0.9 (0.6-1.3)
Women aged 45-54						
Never	134	48	1.0 (—)	523	421	1.0 (—)
<0-3	35	21	0.6 (0.3-1.1)	269	270	0.8 (0.6-1.0)
4-7	8	2	1.2 (0.2-6.0)	105	79	1.1 (0.8-1.5)
8-11	2	3	0.3 (0.0-1.6)	76	62	1.0 (0.7-1.4)
≥12	4	4	0.3 (0.1-1.4)	48	51	0.8 (0.5-1.2)

From Stadel BV, Schlesselman JJ, and Murray PA: Lancet 1:1257, 1989.
RR, Relative risk; CI, confidence interval.

be determined only several years from now. However, the latest review of this data by the U.S. FDA resulted in a statement that no change in OC use or prescribing practice was warranted. Finally, there have been several studies of OC use and breast cancer risk in women at increased risk of developing the disease, those with a family history of breast cancer, as well as those with existing benign breast disease. The results of these studies indicate that OC use by each of these high-risk groups is not associated with any increased risk of developing breast cancer.

Cervical Cancer

The epidemiologic data obtained thus far indicate that long-term use of OCs is associated with an increased risk of preinvasive cervical neoplasia, as well as both epidermoid and adenocarcinoma of the cervix, when compared with matched control groups. Confounding factors, such as the woman's age at first sexual intercourse, the number of sexual partners, exposure to human papillomavirus (possibly greater among users of OCs), cytologic screening (more frequent among OC users), and the use of barrier contraceptives or spermicides (primarily by women in the control group), as well as cigarette smoking (an independent risk factor for this disease), could have influenced these results. Most of these studies made statistical cor-

rections for these confounding factors, and in many the control group did not use barrier methods of contraception.

As shown in Schlesselman's review, the overall pattern of epidemiologic results suggests an approximate doubling of risk of development of carcinoma in situ with use of OCs for more than 1 year, with three studies showing increasing risk with increasing duration of use. The data for invasive cervical cancer suggest no increased risk with less than 5 years of OC use, but a gradually increasing risk after 5 years of use, resulting in a twofold increase with 10 years of use (Figure 11-9). Data from the RCGP cohort study by Beral et al. support the results of these case-control studies, since there was a steadily increasing risk of both preinvasive and invasive cervical cancer with increasing duration of OC use. Thus, although it is uncertain whether OCs themselves increase the risk of cervical cancer, act as a cocarcinogen, or have no effect, OC users as a group are at high risk for cervical neoplasia and require at least annual screening of cervical cytology, especially if they have used OCs for more than 5 years.

Endometrial Cancer

As summarized in the 1987 CASH study and the review by Schlesselman, at least 11 studies have been published on the relation between

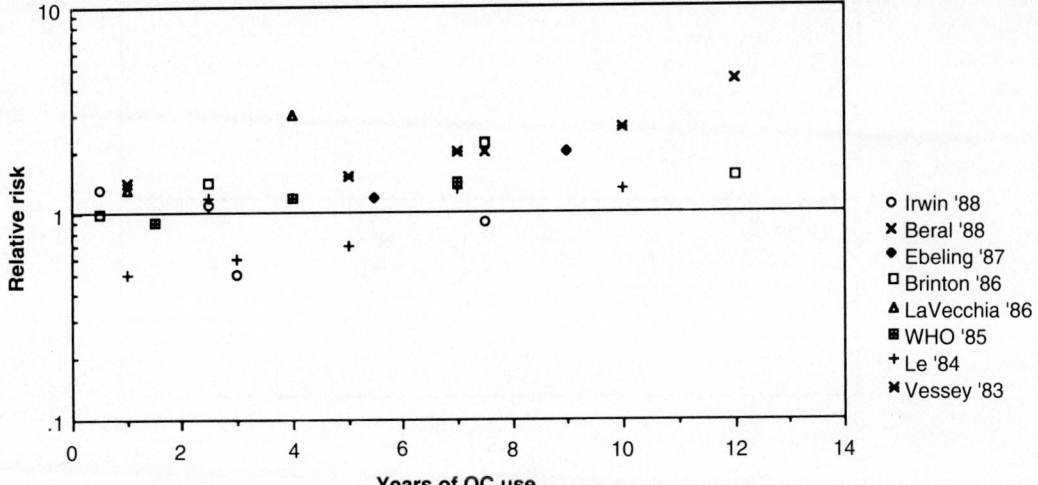

FIGURE 11-9

Invasive cervical cancer in women younger than age 60. Relative risk by years of oral contraceptive use. (From Schlesselman JJ: Contraception 40:1, 1989.)

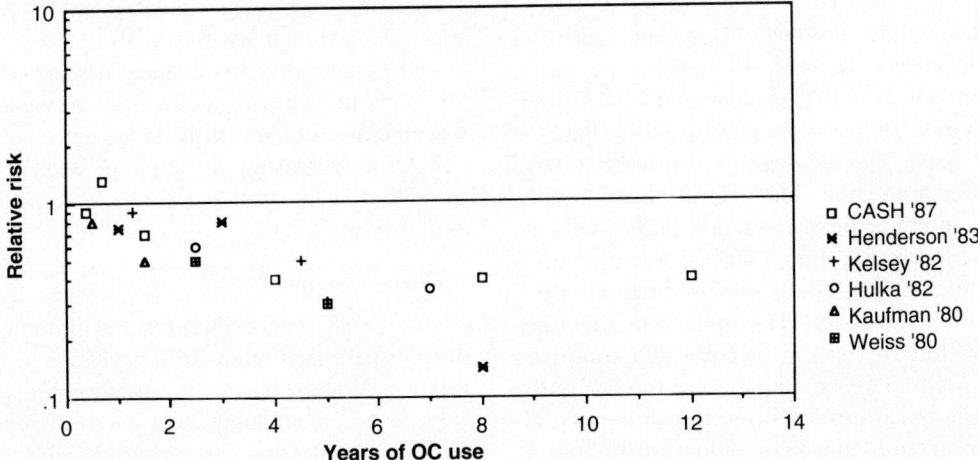

FIGURE 11-10

Endometrial cancer in women younger than age 60. Relative risk by years of combined oral contraceptive (COC) use. (From Schlesselman JJ: Contraception 40:1, 1989.)

OCs and endometrial cancer, and 9 have indicated that the use of these agents has a protective effect against endometrial cancer, the third most common cancer among U.S. women. Women who use OCs for at least a year have an age-adjusted relative risk of 0.5 of developing endometrial cancer between ages 40 and 55 as compared with nonusers. This protective effect is related to duration of use, increasing from a 20% reduction in risk with 1 year of use, to a 40% reduction with 2 years of use, to 60% reduction with 4 years of use (Figure 11-10). This protective effect appears within 10 years

of initial use and persists for at least 15 years after stopping use of OCs. The greatest protective effect is in nulliparous women (relative risk, 0.2) or women of low parity, who have the greatest risk of acquiring this disease.

Ovarian Cancer

As summarized by Schlesselman, 14 published reports have related the use of OCs with subsequent development of ovarian cancer, and each shows a reduction in risk, specifically of the most common type, epithelial ovarian

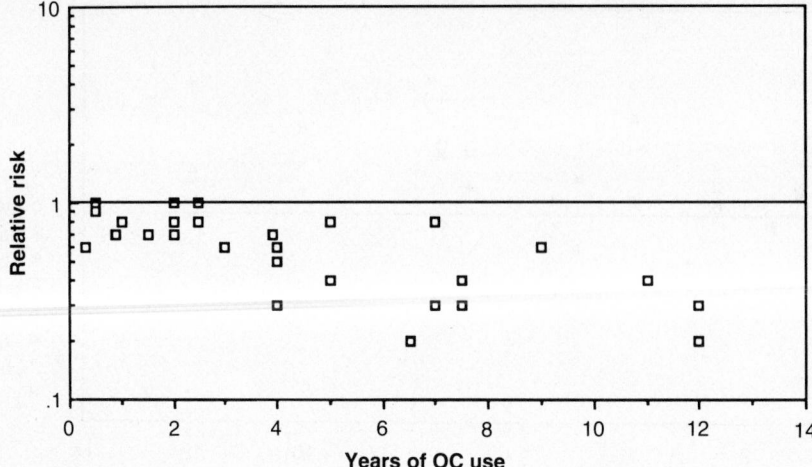

FIGURE 11-11
Epithelial ovarian cancer in women younger than age 60. Relative risk by years of oral contraceptive use in nine studies. (From Schlesselman JJ: Contraception 40:1, 1989.)

cancers (Figure 11-11). OCs reduce the risk of the four main histologic types of epithelial ovarian cancer: serous, mucinous, endometrioid, and clear cell. The relative risk of ovarian cancer is 0.6 for women who use OCs for 3 or more years, and as little as 6 months of use provides protection. The magnitude of the decrease in risk is directly related to the duration of use, increasing from a 50% reduction with 4 years of use to a 60% to 80% reduction with 7 or more years of use. The protective effect begins within 10 years of first use and continues for at least 15 years after the use of OCs ends. As with endometrial cancer, the protective effect occurs only in women of low parity (four or less), who are at greatest risk for this type of cancer.

Liver Adenoma and Cancer

The development of a benign hepatocellular adenoma is a rare occurrence in long-term users of OCs. The increased risk of this tumor was associated with prolonged use of high-dose formulations, particularly those containing mestranol. Although two British studies reported an increased risk of liver cancer among OC users, the number of patients was small and the results could have been influenced by confounding factors. The rate of death from this disease has remained unchanged in the United States over the past 25 years, a period when millions of women have used these agents.

Data from a large multicenter epidemiologic study coordinated by the WHO (1989) found no increased risk of liver cancer associated with OC users in countries with a high prevalence of this neoplasm. This study found no change in risk with increasing duration of use or time since first or last use.

Pituitary Adenoma

OCs mask the predominant symptoms produced by prolactinoma, amenorrhea, and galactorrhea. When OC use is discontinued, these symptoms occur, suggesting a causal relation. However, data from three studies indicate that the incidence of pituitary adenoma among users of OCs is not higher than that among matched controls.

Malignant Melanoma

Several epidemiologic studies have been undertaken to assess the relation of OC use and the development of malignant melanoma. The results are conflicting, since an increased risk, a decreased risk, and no effect have all been reported. In the review by Prentice and Thomas the summary relative risk for eight case-control studies was 1.0 and for three cohort studies 1.4, an insignificant increase. Thus no convincing evidence suggests that OC use increases the risk of developing malignant melanoma.

Oral Contraceptive Use and Overall Mortality

In 1989 Vessey et al. reported the cause of mortality through 1987 among OC users and nonusers enrolled in the Oxford Family Planning Association Contraceptive Study between 1968 and 1974. During this 20-year follow-up of 17,032 women, 238 deaths occurred. The overall risk of death among the OC users was 0.9 (confidence limits, 0.7 to 1.2) compared with the women of similar age and socioeconomic status using a diaphragm or condom for contraception. The risk of death from breast cancer in OC users was 0.9 (0.5 to 1.4); from cervical cancer, 3.3 (0.9 to 17.9); and from ovarian cancer, 0.4 (0.1 to 1.2). These cancer mortality rates are consistent with the other epidemiologic data reported earlier. The death rate from circulatory disease was 1.5 (0.7 to 3.0), and nearly all these deaths in OC users occurred in women who were also smokers. Thus the risk of death from circulatory disease was less than that reported for the first 10 years of the RCGP study, when higher-dose formulations were used and women with cardiovascular risk factors were using OCs. It thus appears that OC use has no appreciable risk on overall mortality. With exclusive use of low-dose formulations given to women without cardiovascular risk factors who have frequent cervical cytologic screening, an overall beneficial effect on mortality with OC use may be expected.

Contraindications to Oral Contraceptive Use

OCs can be prescribed for most women of reproductive age because these women are young and generally healthy; however, certain absolute contraindications exist. These include a present or past history of vascular disease, including thromboembolism, thrombophlebitis, atherosclerosis, and CVA; or systemic disease that may affect the vascular system, such as lupus erythematosus or hemoglobin SS disease. Cigarette smoking by users over age 35, hypertension, diabetes mellitus with vascular disease, and hyperlipidemia are also contraindications, since high-dose OC use in women with these disorders was reported to increase the risk of CVA or MI. One of the contraindications listed by the FDA is cancer of the breast or endometrium, although no data indicate OCs are harmful to women with these diseases.

Pregnant women should not ingest OCs because of the theoretic masculinizing effect of the 19 norprogestins on the external genitalia of female fetuses. As mentioned, concerns that OCs might produce other deleterious fetal effects, such as limb reduction and heart defects, have not proved valid.

Patients with functional heart disease should not use OCs because the fluid retention they produce could result in congestive heart failure. No evidence, however, suggests that those with an asymptomatic prolapsed mitral valve should not use OCs. Patients with active liver disease should not take OCs because the steroids are metabolized in the liver. However, women who have recovered from liver disease, such as viral hepatitis, and whose liver function tests have returned to normal can safely take OCs.

Relative contraindications to OC use include heavy cigarette smoking under age 35, migraine headaches, amenorrhea, and depression. Migraine headaches can be worsened by OC use, and patients who develop CVAs have been reported to have an increased incidence of headaches of the migraine type, fainting, temporary loss of vision or speech, or paresthesias before the CVA. If any of these symptoms develop in an OC user, the use of OCs should be stopped.

Patients who are amenorrheic for a cause other than polycystic ovary syndrome should probably not take OCs because a pituitary microadenoma may be present. Because OC use may mask the symptoms produced by a prolactin-secreting adenoma, amenorrhea, and galactorrhea, amenorrheic patients should not receive OCs until the diagnosis for this symptom is established. If galactorrhea develops during OC use, the OCs should be discontinued, and after 2 weeks the serum prolactin level should be measured. If elevated, further diagnostic evaluation is indicated. Patients with gestational diabetes can take low-dose OC formulations because, as reported by Kjos et al., these agents do not affect glucose tolerance or accelerate the development of diabetes mellitus. Insulin-dependent diabetes without vascular disease is a relative contraindication to OC use.

Beginning Oral Contraceptives

Adolescents

In deciding whether a sexually active pubertal girl should use OCs for contraception, the clinician should be more concerned about compliance with the regimen than about possible physiologic harm. Provided she has demonstrated maturity of the hypothalamic-pituitary-ovarian axis with at least three regular, presumably ovulatory, menstrual cycles, it is safe to prescribe OCs without concern that permanent damage to the reproductive process will result. It is probably best not to prescribe OCs for women of any age with oligomenorrhea, except those with polycystic ovary syndrome, because of their increased likelihood of developing post-OC amenorrhea. Oligomenorrhea is more common in adolescence than in later life. Post-OC amenorrhea that lasts more than 6 months is not produced by OCs but becomes manifest after discontinuing OCs, since OCs will mask the development of the symptoms of amenorrhea. It is not necessary to be concerned about accelerating epiphyseal closure in the postmenarcheal female. Endogenous estrogens have already initiated the process a few years before menarche, and the OCs will not hasten it.

After Pregnancy

A difference exists in the relationship of the return of ovulation and bleeding in the post-abortal woman and one who has had a term delivery. The first episode of menstrual bleeding in the postabortal woman is usually preceded by ovulation. After a term delivery, the first episode of bleeding is usually, but not always, anovulatory. Ovulation occurs sooner after an abortion, usually between 2 and 4 weeks, than after a term delivery, when ovulation is usually delayed beyond 6 weeks but may occur as early as 4 weeks in a woman who is not breastfeeding.

Thus, after spontaneous or induced abortion of a fetus of less than 12 weeks' gestation, OCs should be started immediately to prevent conception after the first ovulation. For patients who deliver after 28 weeks and are not nursing, the combination OCs (those containing both estrogen and progestin) should be initiated 2 to 3 weeks after delivery. If the termination of pregnancy occurs between 21 and 28 weeks, OCs should be started 1 week later. The reason for delay in the latter instances is that the normally increased risk of thromboembolism occurring postpartum may be further enhanced by the hypercoagulable state associated with OC ingestion. Because the first ovulation is delayed for at least 4 weeks after a term delivery, there is no need to expose the patient to this increased risk.

Because estrogen inhibits the action of prolactin in breast tissue receptors, the use of combination OCs diminishes the amount of milk produced by OC users who breast-feed their babies. Although the diminution of milk production is directly related to the amount of estrogen in the contraceptive formulation, only one study by Lönnerdal et al. has been published in which the amount of breast milk was measured by breast pump in women using formulations with less than 50 μg of estrogen. In this study the use of this low dose of estrogen reduced the amount of breast milk. Thus it is probably best for women who are nursing not to use combination OCs.

Women who are breast-feeding every 4 hours, including at night, will not ovulate until at least 10 weeks after delivery and thus do not need contraception before that time. Because only a small percentage of totally breast-feeding women will ovulate as long as they continue full nursing and remain amenorrheic, either a barrier method or a progestin-only OC can be used. The latter does not diminish the amount of breast milk and is effective in this group of women. Once supplemental feeding is introduced, ovulation can resume promptly and effective contraception is then needed.

All Patients

At the initial visit, after a history and physical examination have determined that no medical contraindications for OCs are present, the patient should be informed about the benefits and risks. For medicolegal reasons it is best to note on the patient's medical record that the benefits and risks have been explained to her.

Type of Formulation

In determining which formulation to use, it is best to prescribe initially a formulation with less than 50 μg of ethinyl estradiol, since these agents are associated with less cardiovascular risk, as well as less estrogenic side effects. It would also appear reasonable to use formulations with the lowest dosage of a particular progestin because less progestogenic metabolic and clinical adverse effects would be associated with their use. The development of multiphasic formulations has allowed the total dose of progestin to be reduced compared with some monophasic formulations without increasing the incidence of breakthrough bleeding. However, several monophasic formulations have a lower total dose of progestin per cycle than the multiphasic formulations.

The FDA has stated that the product prescribed should be one that contains the least amount of estrogen and progestin that is compatible with a low failure rate and the needs of the individual patient. Because few randomized studies have been performed comparing the different marketed formulations, until large-scale comparative studies are performed, the clinician must decide which formulation to use based on which formulations have the least adverse effects among patients in his or her practice. If estrogenic or progestogenic side effects occur with one formulation, a different agent with less estrogenic or progestogenic activity can be given.

The contraceptive formulations containing progestins without estrogen have a lower incidence of adverse metabolic effects than the combination formulations. Because the factors that predispose to thromboembolism are caused by the estrogen component, the incidence of thromboembolism in women ingesting these compounds is probably not increased. Furthermore, blood pressure is not affected, nausea and breast tenderness are eliminated, and milk production and quality are unchanged. Despite these advantages, these agents have the disadvantages of a high frequency of intermenstrual and other abnormal bleeding patterns, including amenorrhea, and a lower rate of effectiveness. The use failure rate of these preparations is higher than with the combined formulations, and a relatively high percentage of the pregnancies that do occur are ectopic. Because nursing mothers have reduced fertility and are amenorrheic, the major disadvantages of these preparations are minimized for these patients. Furthermore, because milk production and quality are unaffected, in contrast to the changes produced by combination OCs, the formulations with only a progestin may be offered to these women while they are nursing. However, a small portion of these synthetic steroids have been detected in breast milk. The long-term effects (if any) of these progestins on the infant are not known, but none has been detected to date. A long-term follow-up study by Nilsson et al. of breast-fed children, in which mothers ingested 50 μg of estrogen in combined OCs while they were lactating, revealed no difference in weight gain or height increase up to 8 years of age when compared with breast-fed children whose mothers did not ingest OCs. Also, the occurrence of disease or intellectual or psychologic behavior was no different between the two groups.

Follow-up

If the patient has no contraindications to OC use, the only routine laboratory tests indicated are a complete blood count, urinalysis, and cervical cytology. At the end of 3 months, the patient should be seen again; at this time a nondirected history should be obtained and the blood pressure measured. After this visit the patient should be seen annually, at which time a nondirected history should again be taken, blood pressure and body weight measured, and a physical examination (including breast, abdominal, and pelvic examination with cervical cytology) performed. It is important to perform annual cervical cytologic examinations on OC users, since they are a relatively high-risk group for development of cervical neoplasia. The routine use of other laboratory tests is not indicated unless the patient has a family history of diabetes or vascular disease. Routine use of these tests in women is not indicated because the incidence of positive results is extremely low. However, if the patient has a family history of vascular disease, such as MI occurring in family members under age 50, it would be advisable to obtain a lipid panel before OC use is started, since hypertriglyceridemia may be present and OC use will further raise triglycerides. Since the low-dose formulations do not alter the lipid profile except for triglycerides, it is not necessary to measure lipids, other than the routine cholesterol screening every 5 years, in women without cardiovascular risk factors even if they are over age 35. If the patient has a family history of diabetes or evidence of diabetes during pregnancy, a 2-hour postprandial blood glucose test should be performed before OCs are started and, if elevated, a glucose tolerance test performed. If the patient has a history of liver disease, a liver panel should be obtained to ensure that liver function is normal before OCs are started.

Drug Interactions

Although synthetic sex steroids can retard the biotransformation of certain drugs (e.g., phenazone, meperidine) as a result of substrate competition, such interference is not important clinically. OC use has not been shown to inhibit the action of other drugs. However, some drugs can clinically interfere with the action of OCs by inducing liver enzymes that convert the steroids to more polar and less biologically active metabolites. Certain drugs have been shown to accelerate the biotransformation of steroids in humans. These include barbiturates, sulfonamides, cyclophosphamide, and rifampicin. Back et al. have reported a relatively high incidence of OC failure in women ingesting rifampicin, and these two agents should not be given concurrently. The clinical data concerning OC failure in users of other antibiotics (e.g., penicillin, ampicillin, sulfonamides), analgesics (e.g., phenytoin), and barbiturates are less clear. A few anecdotal studies have appeared in the literature, but reliable evidence for a clinical inhibitory effect of these drugs, such as occurs with rifampicin, is not available. Until controlled studies are performed, it would appear prudent when both agents are given simultaneously to suggest use of a barrier method in addition to the OCs because of possible interference with OC action by the action of the antibiotic or the gut flora. In addition, women with epilepsy requiring medication possibly should be treated with formulations containing 50 µg of estrogen, since a higher incidence of abnormal bleeding has been reported in these women with the use of formulations with lower doses of estrogen.

Noncontraceptive Health Benefits

In addition to being the most effective method of contraception, OCs provide many other health benefits. Some occur because the combination OCs contain a potent, orally active progestin, as well as an orally active estrogen, and there is no time when the estrogenic target tissues are stimulated by estrogens without a progestin (unopposed estrogen).

Both natural progesterone and the synthetic progestins inhibit the proliferative effect of estrogen, the so-called antiestrogenic effect. Estrogens increase the synthesis of both estrogen and progesterone receptors, whereas progesterone decreases their synthesis. Thus one mechanism whereby progesterone exerts its antiestrogenic effects is by decreasing the synthesis of estrogen receptors. Relatively little progestin is needed to do this, and the amount present in OCs is sufficient. Another way progesterone produces its antiestrogenic action is by stimulating the activity of the enzyme estradiol-17β-dehydrogenase within the endometrial cell. This enzyme converts the more potent estradiol to the less potent estrone, reducing estrogenic action within the cell.

Benefits from Antiestrogenic Action of Progestins

As a result of the antiestrogenic action of the progestins in OCs, the height of the endometrium is less than in an ovulatory cycle, and less proliferation of the glandular epithelium occurs. These changes produce several substantial benefits for the OC user. One is a reduction in the amount of blood loss at the time of endometrial shedding. In an ovulatory cycle the mean blood loss during menstruation is about 35 ml, compared with 20 ml for women ingesting OCs. This decreased blood loss makes the development of iron deficiency anemia less likely. Data from the RCGP study showed that OC users were about half as likely to develop iron deficiency anemia as the controls. Moreover, the beneficial effect persisted to a similar degree in women who had previously used OCs and then stopped them, probably because of an increase in the iron stores that remained for several years after the drug was discontinued.

Because the OCs produce regular withdrawal bleeding, it would be expected that OC users would have fewer menstrual disorders than controls. The results of the RCGP study confirmed that OC users were significantly less likely to develop menorrhagia, irregular menstruation, or intermenstrual bleeding. Because these disorders are frequently treated by curettage and/or hysterectomy, OC users require these procedures less frequently.

Because progestins inhibit the proliferative effect of estrogens on the endometrium, as mentioned, women who use OCs have been found to be significantly less likely to develop adenocarcinoma of the endometrium.

Estrogen exerts a proliferative effect on

breast tissue, which also contains estrogen receptors. Progestins probably inhibit the synthesis of estrogen receptors in this organ as well, exerting an antiestrogenic action on the breast. Several studies have shown that OCs reduce the incidence of benign breast disease, and two prospective studies by Ory and Brinton et al. have indicated that this reduction is directly related to the amount of progestin in the compounds.

Data from the Oxford study indicated that current users of OCs had an 85% reduction in the incidence of fibroadenomas and 50% reductions in chronic cystic disease and nonbiopsied breast lumps, as compared with controls using IUDs or diaphragms. The risk of developing these three diseases decreased with increased duration of OC use and persisted for about 1 year after discontinuation of OCs, after which no reduction in risk was observed.

Benefits from Inhibition of Ovulation

Other noncontraceptive medical benefits of OCs result from their main action, inhibition of ovulation. Some disorders, such as dysmenorrhea and premenstrual tension, occur much more frequently in ovulatory than anovulatory cycles. In fact, inhibition of ovulation by exogenous steroids has been used as therapy for severe dysmenorrhea for decades. The RCGP study showed that OC users had 63% less dysmenorrhea and 29% less premenstrual tension than controls. Another study by Warner and Bancroft indicated that OC users were less likely to have varying degrees of a feeling of well-being throughout the cycle than non-OC users.

Another serious adverse effect of ovulatory menstrual cycles is the development of functional ovarian cysts—specifically, follicular and luteal cysts—that frequently require laparotomy because of enlargement, rupture, or hemorrhage. When ovulation is inhibited, functional cysts do not usually develop. In a survey performed by the Boston Collaborative Drug Surveillance Program, less than 2% of women with a discharge diagnosis of functional ovarian cysts were taking OCs, in contrast to 20% of control subjects. However, 20% of women with nonfunctional cysts were taking OCs, an incidence similar to that observed in the control subjects. Although authors of one small case series postulated that the formation of functional ovarian cysts may be increased in users of mul-

tiphasic OCs, the rate of hospitalization for ovarian cysts in the United States has remained unchanged after the widespread use of multiphasic formulations.

Another disorder linked to incessant ovulation is ovarian cancer. As mentioned, the development of ovarian cancer is significantly reduced in OC users, with a duration-dependent decrease in risk.

Other Benefits

Several European studies, including the RCGP study, showed that the risk of developing rheumatoid arthritis in OC users was only about half that in control subjects. Another benefit is protection against salpingitis, often referred to as pelvic inflammatory disease (PID). At least 11 published epidemiologic studies have estimated the relative risk of developing PID among OC users. Seven of these studies compared OC use with nonuse of any other contraception. As summarized by Sennayake et al., the relative risk of developing PID among OC users in most of these studies was approximately 0.5%. It has been estimated that 15% to 20% of women with cervical gonorrheal infection will develop PID. In a Swedish study by Rydén et al., all cases of suspected PID were confirmed by laparoscopic visualization 1 day after hospital admission. Of women who used contraception other than the IUD and OCs, 15% developed PID; only about half as many, 8.8%, of those who used OCs developed PID. The results of this study indicate that OCs reduce the clinical development of PID in women infected with gonorrhea. Although the incidence of cervical infection with *Chlamydia trachomatis* is increased in OC users compared with control subjects, Wølner-Hanssen et al. reported that the incidence of chlamydial PID in OC users was only half that in control subjects. This protection may be related to the decreased duration of menstrual flow, which permits a smaller number of organisms to ascend to the upper genital tract and allows the body's defenses to eliminate them more easily. One sequela of PID is ectopic pregnancy, an entity that has tripled in incidence in the past 15 years. OCs reduce the risk of ectopic pregnancy by more than 90% in current users and may reduce the incidence in former users by decreasing their chance of developing PID.

Ory (1982) estimated that of 100,000 women

TABLE 11-13
Hospitalizations Prevented Annually by Oral Contraceptive Use

Disease	Rate (per 100,000 OC Users)	No. of Hospitalizations*
Benign breast disease	235	20,000
Ovarian retention cysts	35	3000
Iron deficiency anemia†	320	27,200
Pelvic inflammatory disease (first episodes)		
Total episodes†	600	51,000
Hospitalizations	156	13,300
Ectopic pregnancy	117	9900
Rheumatoid arthritis†	32	2700
Endometrial cancer‡	5	2000
Ovarian cancer‡	4	1700

From Ory HW: Fam Plann Perspect 14:182, 1982.
*Except where noted, figures refer to hospitalizations prevented among the estimated 8.5 million OC users in the United States in 1982.
†Episodes prevented regardless of whether hospitalizations occurred.
‡Based on the estimated 39 million U.S. women who have ever used OCs.

in the United States using OCs each year, their use will prevent 320 from developing iron deficiency anemia, 32 from developing rheumatoid arthritis, and 450 from developing PID that does not require hospitalization. In addition, 150 fewer women will be hospitalized for PID, 235 fewer hospitalized for breast disease, 35 fewer hospitalized for ovarian tumors, and 117 fewer hospitalized for tubal pregnancies (Table 11-13). Ory estimated that each year about 1 of every 750 women taking OCs will not require hospitalization for a serious disease she would have developed if she had not taken this drug and that use of OCs prevents 50,000 women from being hospitalized in the United States each year. Although this study was based on data obtained with higher-dose formulations, since the lower-dose agents contain a progestin that inhibits estrogenic mitotic activity and also inhibits ovulation, the scope and magnitude of beneficial effects should be similar with all combination formulations currently marketed. Unfortunately, the infrequent adverse effects of OCs have received widespread publicity, whereas the more common noncontraceptive health benefits have attracted little attention.

LONG-ACTING CONTRACEPTIVE STEROIDS

Injectable Suspensions

Three types of injectable steroid formulations are currently in use for contraception throughout the world: (1) depo-medroxyprogesterone acetate (DMPA), given in a dose of 150 mg every 3 months; (2) norethindrone enanthate (NET-EN), given in a dose of 200 mg every 2 months; and (3) several once-a-month injections of combinations of different progestins and estrogens. It is estimated that about 5 million women are currently using injectable steroid formulations, twice the number who used them in 1985.

Depo-Medroxyprogesterone Acetate (DMPA)

DMPA is the most widely used injectable contraceptive and also the most widely studied. It is estimated that more than 15 million women have used DMPA since it was first made available for contraceptive use in the mid-1960s, and currently there are approximately 3.5 million users in the world. More than 1000 scientific articles have been written about DMPA. DMPA is approved for use as a contraceptive in more than 90 countries, including Sweden, France, West Germany, and the United Kingdom, but not the United States. In the United States the drug is approved only for the treatment of endometrial cancer; however, with physician and patient consent it can be used for contraception.

DMPA is extremely effective. The failure rates in various studies range from 0.0 to 1.2 per 100 woman-years. In a large WHO (1983)

TABLE 11-14

Net Termination Rates per 100 Women in WHO Study of DMPA and NET-EN

Reason for Termination	1-Year Net Cumulative Event Rates			2-Year Net Cumulative Event Rates		
	DMPA	NET-EN 60	NET-EN 60-84	DMPA	NET-EN 60	NET-EN 60-84
Pregnancy	0.1	0.4	0.6	0.4	0.4	1.4
Amenorrhea	11.9	6.8	8.4	24.2	14.7	14.6
Bleeding	15.0	13.6	13.7	18.8	18.4	21.8
Medical	11.8	13.7	12.7	15.0	16.0	16.7
Personal	20.7	24.5	22.8	38.8	42.6	40.2
TOTAL	51.4	49.7	50.3	73.5	70.7	72.4

From World Health Organization Expanded Programme of Research, Development and Research Training in Human Reproduction Task Force on Long-Acting System Agents for the Regulation of Fertility: Contraception 28:1, 1983.
DMPA, Depo-medroxyprogesterone acetate; NET-EN, norethindrone enanthate.

multiclinic study of 1587 users of DMPA, the failure rate at the end of 1 year was only 0.1% and at the end of 2 years, 0.4% (Table 11-14).

DMPA is formulated as a crystalline suspension. It should be given by injection in the upper outer quadrant of the gluteal region. The area should not be massaged so that the drug is released slowly into the circulation. Administering the drug by this method should result in a very low failure rate.

Ortiz et al. found that for a few days after the injection, MPA levels in the serum range from 1.5 to 3 ng/ml and gradually declined thereafter, reaching 0.2 ng/ml during the sixth month, and become undetectable about 7½ to 9 months after administration.

Serum estradiol levels remained at early follicular phase levels for 4 to 6 months after the DMPA injection. When serum levels of MPA fell below 0.5 ng/mL, estradiol rose to preovulatory levels. Ovulation, however, as evidenced by elevated serum progesterone levels, did not occur, apparently because the LH peak was suppressed by inhibition of the positive feedback of estrogen on its release. When serum MPA levels fell below 0.1 ng/mL, approximately 7 to 9 months after the injection, cyclic ovulatory ovarian function resumed. Thus the delay in ovulation after receiving injections of DMPA is caused by prolonged MPA release and persists until serum levels of MPA become very low. The time required for the drug to disappear from the circulation after the last of several injections should be approximately the same as that after a single injection, since MPA is rapidly cleared from the bloodstream. The prolonged presence in serum is related to the slow release from the injection site.

MPA acts by inhibiting the midcycle gonadotrophin surge. Levels of LH and FSH remain in the follicular-phase range and are not completely suppressed. Mean estradiol levels remain relatively constant, approximately 40 pg/ml, for as long as 5 years of treatment. These estradiol levels are higher than menopausal levels, and patients receiving DMPA do not develop signs or symptoms of estrogen deficiency, such as vaginal atrophy, hot flushes, or decreased bone density. As a result of the high progestin and low estrogen levels, the endometrium becomes low lying and atrophic. The glands are narrow and widely spaced with deciduoid stroma. With this atrophic type of endometrium, most women treated with DMPA develop amenorrhea.

The major side effect of DMPA is complete disruption of the menstrual cycle. In the first 3 months after the first injection, approximately 30% of the women are amenorrheic and another 30% have irregular bleeding and spotting more than 11 days per month. As duration of therapy increases, the incidence of frequent bleeding steadily declines and the incidence of amenorrhea steadily increases, so that at the end of 2 years about 70% of the women treated with DMPA are amenorrheic (Figure 11-12).

After treatment with DMPA is discontinued, about half the women resume a regular cyclic menstrual pattern within 6 months, and about three-fourths have regular menses within 1 year. When bleeding does resume after the effect of the last injection is dissipated, it is initially regular in approximately half the women and irregular in the remainder.

Additional side effects include slight weight gain, and because of the long duration of action

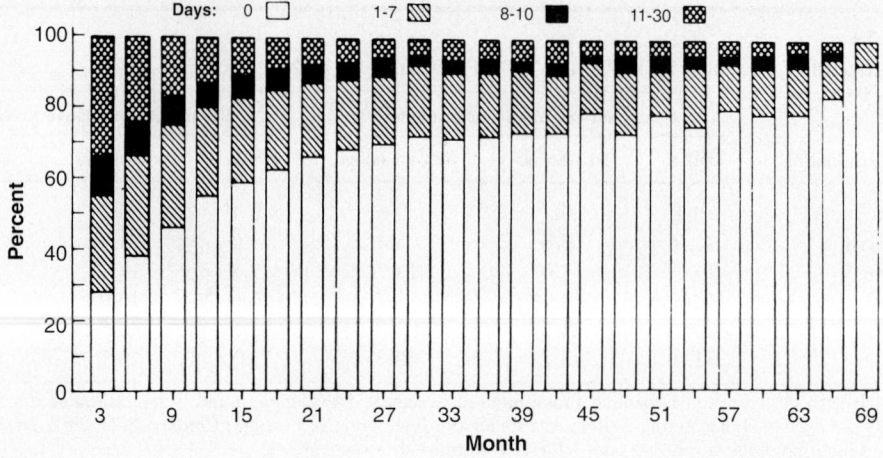

FIGURE 11-12
Percentage of patients with bleeding or spotting on days 0, 1 to 7, 8 to 10, or 11 to 30 per 30-day cycle while receiving injectable DMPA, 150 mg, every 3 months. (From Schwallie PC and Assenzo JR: Fertil Steril 24:331, 1973.)

of the drug, return of fertility is delayed.

Fertility rates have been calculated for fertile couples discontinuing various methods of contraception other than DMPA in order to conceive. At the end of 3 months, about 50% of these women are pregnant; at the end of a year, about 90% are pregnant. For DMPA users, the curve is shifted to the right, so the 50% pregnancy rate does not occur until about a year, a delay of approximately 9 months compared with women discontinuing barrier methods.

Therefore use of DMPA does not cause sterility but causes a temporary period of infertility. A major benefit of the drug's prolonged effect is that when patients do not return for their scheduled injection on time, but delay for 1 or 2 months, pregnancy rates remain very low. The incidence of failure to conceive, as well as the interval to conception after stopping DMPA, was similar among women who had used DMPA for various periods and received many or few injections of the drug.

Because DMPA does not increase liver globulin production, as does the estrogen component of OCs (ethinyl estradiol), no alteration in blood clotting factors or angiotensinogen levels is associated with its use. Thus, unlike OCs, DMPA has not been associated with increases in hypertension or thromboembolism. A WHO study (1983) reported that blood pressure measurements were unchanged in DMPA users after 2 years of injections.

When glucose tolerance tests were per-

formed on long-term DMPA users, a slight statistically significant but clinically insignificant impairment in glucose tolerance was observed when compared with a control group of women.

Another long-term cross-sectional study by Deslypere et al. reported that long-term DMPA users have altered levels of serum lipids. Levels of triglycerides and HDL cholesterol, but not total cholesterol, were significantly lower in long-term users compared with control subjects of similar age. However, no significant difference occurred in LDL cholesterol levels.

Concern has also been raised that DMPA may be associated with an increased incidence of abnormal cervical cytology. In a multinational case-control study conducted by WHO (1986), the adjusted relative risk for cervical cancer among women who had ever used DMPA compared with users of no contraception was 1.2, with confidence intervals of 0.4 to 1.5. This insignificantly increased risk showed no trend of increasing with increasing duration of use of DMPA, as has been observed in several studies of the relation between OC use and cervical neoplasia. Thus the increased incidence of abnormal cervical cytology reported among DMPA users appears to be related to confounding factors, such as failure to use a diaphragm or many sexual partners, since no evidence shows that the drug itself causes an increase in cervical dysplasia or carcinoma.

DMPA has been associated with an increased incidence of two types of carcinoma in animals but not in humans. When given in high doses to beagle dogs, it is associated with an increase in mammary cancer; however, the beagle is a poor model for study of steroid action in the human because progestins are metabolized differently in the two species. Beagles develop a high incidence of breast carcinoma after receiving various types of progestins. After 25 years of study with this agent in humans, no evidence shows an increased incidence of breast carcinoma. In the large WHO study just mentioned, the relative risk of developing breast cancer among women ever using DMPA was 1.0.

In long-term monkey studies, two monkeys developed adenocarcinoma of the endometrium when treated with high doses of DMPA for 10 years; however, no evidence suggests that DMPA produces endometrial cancer in humans. DMPA produces an atrophic endometrium and actually is used to treat metastatic endometrial carcinoma. In the WHO study the relative risk of developing endometrial cancer was 0.3. Nevertheless, concern about carcinogenicity in the animal studies has prevented approval of this drug for use as a contraceptive in the United States, despite DMPA's apparent noncontraceptive health benefits, similar to those of OCs. These benefits include a reduction in menstrual blood loss and thus anemia; a probable decreased incidence of developing PID, since most users are amenorrheic; and a decreased risk of developing endometrial and ovarian cancer, since DMPA is progestational and inhibits ovulation.

Norethindrone Enanthate (NET-EN)

NET-EN is another injectable progestogen approved for contraceptive use in more than 40 countries but not in the United States. It is administered in an oily suspension and thus has different pharmacodynamics from DMPA.

Goebelsmann et al. measured levels of norethindrone, FSH, LH, estradiol, and progesterone in a group of women for 6 months after a single injection of 200 mg of NET-EN. Approximately 1 week after the injection, peak serum levels of norethindrone of 12 to 17 ng/ml were reached. These high serum levels lasted for about 3 weeks and decreased thereafter, first precipitously and then gradually. Serum levels of norethindrone of 4 ng/ml or more suppressed gonadotrophin levels and follicular de-

velopment. Norethindrone levels in this range persisted for approximately 1 to 2 months after the injection. With a further fall in norethindrone levels, follicular maturation, as determined by estradiol peaks, occurred. Nevertheless, these peaks were not followed by ovulation because of inhibition of the positive feedback of estrogen as long as the serum norethindrone levels stayed above 1.8 ng/ml. Ovulation occurred at variable intervals in the subjects when their norethindrone concentrations ranged from 0.1 to 1.8 ng/ml. Thus variability in norethindrone levels, as well as inhibition of positive feedback, was observed among different women. These findings indicate why some women conceive in the last few weeks of NET-EN therapy with an injection interval of 12 weeks.

Furthermore, if the woman does not return exactly when scheduled for a subsequent injection, the possibility of pregnancy increases greatly. In a comparative study done by the WHO in 10 centers around the world in 1977, at the end of 1 year the pregnancy rate with DMPA treatment was 0.7%, whereas that with NET-EN given every 12 weeks was 3.6%—significantly higher. Because the rate of discontinuation of therapy was higher with DMPA than with NET-EN, mainly because of amenorrhea, it was decided to administer NET-EN at more frequent intervals in an attempt to lower the pregnancy rate.

In a subsequent comparative study using DMPA and NET-EN, NET-EN was given every 60 days to one group of subjects; a second group received NET-EN every 60 days for the first 6 months, followed by every 84 days thereafter. With both these regimens, at the end of 1 year the pregnancy rates with NET-EN were more comparable to the 0.1% rate found with DMPA: 0.4% for the 60-day regimen and 0.6% for the 60/84-day regimen (see Table 11-14). At the end of 2 years, the pregnancy rate for the 60-day regimen was still 0.4%, the same as with DMPA, whereas with the 60/84-day regimen it was 1.4%. For this reason, it is now recommended that NET-EN be given every 60 days for at least the first 6 months and no less often than every 12 weeks thereafter. WHO recommends that the drug be given at intervals no shorter than 46 days and no longer than 74 days.

NET-EN is also associated with irregular menstrual bleeding and few systemic effects other than weight gain. In the WHO study, mean weight gain with both DMPA and NET-EN was approximately 1.8 kg at the end of 1 year and 3.3 kg at the end of 2 years. Fewer NET-EN users than DMPA users became amenorrheic and, at the end of 1 year, more women discontinued the use of DMPA for this reason than NET-EN. Approximately 55% of DMPA users were amenorrheic at 1 year and 62% at 2 years, in contrast with about 30% and 40% of NET-EN users after the same periods. Nevertheless, total discontinuation rates for the two methods were similar at the end of 1 and 2 years, approximately 50% and 75%, respectively.

Progestin-Estrogen Injectable Formulations

Various injectable combinations of estrogen and progestogens have been investigated. The two formulations most widely studied have been dihydroxyprogesterone acetophenide, 150 mg, with estradiol enanthate, 10 mg (Deladroxate, Perlutal), and medroxyprogesterone acetate, 50 or 25 mg, with estradiol cypionate, 10 or 5 mg (Cyclo-Provera). All these formulations have an extremely high rate of effectiveness, with no pregnancies being reported in almost 23,000 cycles of use of the former formulation. These formulations cause less abnormal bleeding than do the injectable contraceptives without estrogen; however, not all subjects have regular cycles, and irregular bleeding and amenorrhea do occur in some. Because of concerns about the toxicity of high doses of estrogen, as well as the need for monthly injections, these formulations are not available for use in most countries; however, they are widely used in Mexico and some other countries in Latin America. It is reported that other monthly injectable formulations, including one with 250 mg of 17α-hydroxyprogesterone caproate and 5 mg of estradiol valerate, are used in the People's Republic of China.

Subdermal Implants: Norplant

Subdermal implants of capsules made of polydimethylsiloxane (Silastic) containing levonorgestrel have been developed and patented by the Population Council as Norplant. Clinical trials of this long-acting, effective, reversible method of contraception were initiated in 1975. To date Norplant has been used by more than 500,000 women in 45 countries. It is currently approved for use by regulatory agencies of 15 countries, and the U.S. FDA approved Norplant in 1991. As with all steroid-containing Silastic devices, the rate of steroid delivery is directly proportional to the surface area of the capsules, whereas duration of action depends on the amount of steroid within the capsules. To produce effective blood levels of norgestrel, it was found necessary to use six capsules filled with crystalline levonorgestrel. The cylindric capsules are 3.4 cm long and 2.4 mm in outer diameter, with the ends sealed with Silastic medical adhesive. Each capsule contains 36 mg of crystalline levonorgestrel, for a total amount of 216 mg in each six-capsule set.

Insertion is performed on an outpatient basis, and the entire procedure takes about 5 minutes. After infiltration of the skin with local anesthesia, a small (3 mm) incision is made with a scalpel, usually in the upper arm, although the lower arm and the inguinal and gluteal regions have also been used. The capsules are implanted into the subcutaneous tissue in a radial pattern through a large (10- to 12-gauge) trocar, and the incision is closed with adhesive. Stitches are not necessary. Because polydimethylsiloxane is not biodegradable, the capsules have to be removed through another incision when desired by the user or at the end of 5 years, which is the duration of maximal contraceptive effectiveness.

After insertion, blood levels of levonorgestrel rise rapidly to reach levels between 400 and 500 pg/ml in 24 hours. The serum levels remain relatively constant during the first year of use, with a mean of about 400 pg/ml, which is usually sufficient to inhibit ovulation (Figure 11-13). When the amount of steroid was measured in capsules removed from patients after various times, it was found that the rate of release was fairly constant during the first year of use, averaging about 50 μg of levonorgestrel per day from the six-capsule set. From about the end of the first year of use until 8 years of use, release rates declined to approximately 30 μg per day but remained constant during this interval. Mean serum levels of levonorgestrel also declined slightly beyond the third year of use and averaged about 300 pg/ml.

With this low level of levonorgestrel, gonadotrophin levels are not completely suppressed, and follicular activity results in peri-

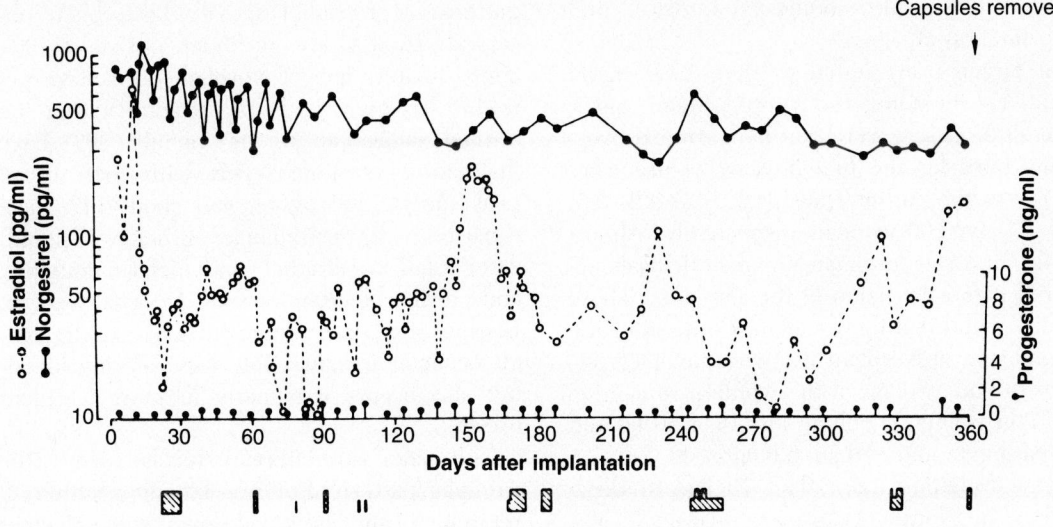

FIGURE 11-13
Serum levels of estradiol, progesterone, and *d*-norgestrel in a subject with six poly-siloxane capsules, each containing 33.9 mg of *d*-norgestrel, implanted on day 0. Hatched bars represent uterine bleeding. (From Moore DE, Roy S, Stanczyk FZ, et al: Contraception 17:315, 1978.)

odic peaks of estradiol. Because the level of circulating levonorgestrel is usually sufficient to inhibit the positive feedback effect of these estradiol peaks with LH release, LH levels are lower, even in Norplant users with regular cycles, and ovulation occurs infrequently.

It is difficult to determine the exact incidence of ovulatory cycles in Norplant users, since different investigators have used different minimal levels of serum progesterone as a definition of presumptive ovulation and serum samples have been obtained at various intervals. Using the finding of serum progesterone level above 3 ng/ml with twice-weekly blood sampling as a definition of presumptive ovulation, Brache et al. (1985) reported that about one third of the cycles of Norplant users are ovulatory, with the incidence of luteal activity increasing beyond the second year of use. However, this incidence of ovulation is an overestimate, since the mean peak progesterone level, duration of elevated progesterone levels, and thus total luteal amount of progesterone is significantly less in Norplant users than in control cycles, indicating a high incidence of luteal deficiency and/or anovulatory luteinized follicles. Daily ultrasonographic scanning of ovaries of Norplant users with regular cycles and elevated luteal phase progesterone levels revealed that only about one third of

these cycles had ovarian morphologic changes consistent with a normal ovulatory pattern. Because only about half the cycles of Norplant users have a fairly regular pattern, probably less than 20% of the cycles are ovulatory, and a high percentage of these have deficient progesterone production.

Thus inhibition of ovulation is one of the major mechanisms of action of this method of contraception. The consistently elevated levels of norgestrel also prevent the normal midcycle thinning of the cervical mucus to occur. The cervical mucus remains scanty and viscid, and normal sperm penetration does not take place, as demonstrated by both in vivo and in vitro studies. These two mechanisms of action result in a very high level of contraceptive effectiveness. In the clinical studies initiated before 1980 involving 992 women, Sivin (1988) reported that gross annual pregnancy rates for the first 5 years of use were 0.3, 0.2, 0.5, 1.6, and 0.0 per 100 women, respectively, for an average gross annual pregnancy rate of approximately 0.6. In the sixth and seventh year of study the annual gross pregnancy rates were 3.0 and 4.2 per 100 women, respectively. Because these annual rates exceeded the cumulative pregnancy rate for the preceding 5 years, it was concluded that the Norplant contraceptive method was effective for 5 years and that a new set of capsules should be inserted after that duration of use.

In larger trials initiated after 1980 in 11 countries, including the United States, more than 10,000 users were enrolled. Annual pregnancy rates for the first 5 years of use were similar to the earlier trials: 0.2, 0.2, 0.9, 0.5, and 1.1 per 100 women, respectively. Almost all the first-year pregnancies in both trials occurred before insertion of the implants. These studies found that the pregnancy rates after the second year of Norplant use were inversely related to body weight of the women, remaining at 0.2 in women weighing less than 50 kg and increasing to more than 6.0 after 3 years in women weighing more than 70 kg. In these studies the Norplant capsules were made of a denser type of tubing than is now being used, and serum levels of norgestrel were slightly lower than occur with the currently used less dense tubing. In ovulatory cycles of Norplant users, mean serum norgestrel levels are lower than in anovulatory cycles. Thus the higher serum levels of norgestrel associated with the less dense tubing should result in a lower incidence of ovulation and greater efficacy.

This relation has been found to be valid in clinical trials involving the less dense tubing. In studies performed to date, the gross cumulative pregnancy rate at the end of 5 years in a group of women using Norplant made of the less dense tubing was only 1.1. Furthermore, no relation was found between the incidence of pregnancy and the body weight of the user, since the pregnancy rate was not increased in women weighing more than 70 kg. Thus, with the less dense tubing, annual pregnancy rates for the first 5 years of use are approximately 0.2 per 100 women, making Norplant one of the most effective methods of reversible contraception available. As with all progestin-only methods of contraception, when pregnancies occur with Norplant, a high percentage (about 20%) are ectopic. Because of its high rate of effectiveness, however, the overall rate of ectopic pregnancies in Norplant users, 0.28 per 1000 woman-years of use, is less compared with ectopic pregnancy rates in the entire U.S. population of women of reproductive age, 1.5 per 1000 women annually.

Mean estradiol levels in Norplant users, whether they are ovulatory or anovulatory, are about the same as in women with regular ovulatory cycles who used IUDs, and three patterns of estradiol activity have been observed. In a study by Brache et al. (1990), approximately half of Norplant users have periodic, irregular peaks of estradiol within the normal range (up to 400 pg/ml), 30% have fluctuating estradiol levels with high broad peaks above 400 pg/ml, and about 10% have consistently low estradiol levels below 75 pg/ml. After a fall in estradiol, endometrial sloughing and uterine bleeding or spotting usually occur. Because the peaks and declines in estradiol levels occur at irregular intervals, uterine bleeding also occurs irregularly in most Norplant users.

The major side effect of Norplant use is the irregular pattern of uterine bleeding. Other alterations in uterine blood flow involve changes in duration and volume, with most bleeding episodes involving scanty amounts. Approximately half the bleeding episodes can be characterized as fairly regular, and the interval between episodes ranges from 21 to 35 days. About 40% of users have irregular episodes with intervals outside this range, and about 10% are amenorrheic with no bleeding for more than 3 months. Because of the high incidence of bleeding irregularities, potential Norplant users must be thoroughly counseled about this potential problem before insertion. Bleeding episodes tend to be more prolonged and irregular during the first year of use, after which greater frequency of a more regular pattern occurs. The mean number of days of bleeding also declines steadily with time, from 54.3 days in the first year to 44.1 days in the fifth year. Mean total blood loss in Norplant users is approximately 25 ml per month, slightly less than the average monthly blood loss of normally cycling women. Several clinical studies have shown that the mean hemoglobin concentration in the first 3 years of Norplant use tends to rise slightly. Sivin (1988) reported that even women who stop using the method because of bleeding problems have been found to have increased mean hemoglobin levels. When pregnancies occur in Norplant users, they usually occur in women with a recent history of regular cyclic uterine bleeding. Thus women who are amenorrheic or have infrequent episodes of uterine bleeding do not need to be monitored by periodic pregnancy tests.

Other problems associated with this method of contraception include infection, local irritation, or painful reaction at the insertion site.

Occasionally, expulsion of a capsule occurs, usually in association with infection. The incidence of insertion site infection is less than 1%. Headache is the single most frequent medical problem causing removal of the implants, accounting for approximately 30% of the medical reasons for removal. Weight gain was a typical reason for medical removal in U.S. studies, whereas weight loss occurred more often in the Dominican Republic. Other medical problems among Norplant users include acne, mastalgia, and mood changes, including anxiety, depression, and nervousness. Because ovarian follicular development without subsequent ovulation typically occurs among Norplant users, adnexal enlargement caused by persistent unruptured follicles has been noted during routine bimanual pelvic examination of many users. These enlarged follicles, which may reach 5 to 7 cm in diameter, usually spontaneously regress in 1 to 2 months without therapy.

Many metabolic studies have been performed among Norplant users in various population groups. Studies of carbohydrate metabolism, serum chemistries, liver function, serum cortisol levels, thyroid function, and blood coagulation have revealed only minimal changes that remain within the normal range. Several studies have been performed in different countries in which lipoproteins were measured before and after Norplant insertion. In most of these studies, levels of triglycerides, total cholesterol, and LDL cholesterol declined, whereas HDL cholesterol declined slightly or increased. Little change occurred in the cholesterol/HDL cholesterol ratio, indicating that Norplant should not enhance the development of atherosclerosis.

As with the insertion procedure, the removal process is performed using local anesthesia and a small skin incision. Removal of Norplant is a more difficult process than insertion because fibrous tissue develops around the capsule and must be cut before removing the capsule. It is important that the capsules are inserted superficially to enhance the ease of removal. Deeply implanted capsules are more difficult to remove.

After removal, the incision is closed without stitches and a pressure dressing applied for about 24 hours. If the woman wishes to continue use, another set can be inserted through the same incision or in the opposite arm. If another set of Norplant is not inserted after re-

moval, the steroid is rapidly cleared from the circulation, and serum levels of norgestrel fall rapidly, reaching nearly undetectable levels in 96 hours. If pregnancy is desired, return of ovulation is prompt and is similar to that in women discontinuing other nonhormonal methods of reversible contraception, reaching 50% at 3 months and 86% at 1 year.

Continuation rates with the Norplant method of contraception are very high, ranging from 76% to 99% at 1 year in different countries and from 33% to 78% at 5 years. These high continuation rates are similar to those observed with IUDs and result largely because these methods require the user to return to the clinic to discontinue use. This is the main reason why Norplant implants and the IUD have the highest continuation rates of any methods of contraception in use today.

Manufacture of the capsules is complicated, and placing or removing six capsules creates some difficulties; therefore norgestrel has been fabricated into solid rods that are a homologous mixture of Silastic and crystalline levonorgestrel covered with Silastic tubing. The rods are easier to manufacture, insert, and remove than the capsules. Because of different properties of diffusion, higher blood levels of norgestrel are achieved with a smaller total surface area using the rods. Thus, with two 4 cm covered rods with the same diameter as the capsules, the same release rate for norgestrel, approximately 50 μg per day, can be achieved as with placement of six 3 cm capsules. During a 2-year clinical study comparing rods and capsules, the serum norgestrel levels, bleeding patterns, and incidence of elevated progesterone levels were similar. Thus, if large-scale clinical studies confirm these findings, the two covered rods may be used instead of six capsules.

POSTCOITAL CONTRACEPTION (PCC)

Morris and Van Wagenen suggested in 1966 that high doses of estrogen administered in the early postovulatory period will prevent implantation in women. Various estrogenic compounds have been used for postcoital contraception (PCC), or what is usually referred to as the "morning-after pill." The estrogen compounds that have been used most often by various investigators for this purpose include di-

TABLE 11-15

Observed and Expected Pregnancies According to Various Methods of Postcoital Contraception

Treatment	Number of Studies	Total Number of Patients Considered	Number of Observed Pregnancies	Pregnancy Rate (%)
Ethinyl estradiol—high dosage	4	3168	19	0.6
Other estrogens—high dosage	2	975	11	1.1
Ethinyl estradiol plus *dl*-norgestrel	11	3802	69	1.8
Danazol	3	998	20	2.0
IUD	9	879	1	0.1

From Fasoli M, Parazzini F, Cecchetti G, et al: Contraception 39:459, 1989.
Xy^2 for heterogeneity = 35.31; $P < 0.001$.

ethylstilbestrol (DES), 25 to 50 mg/day; ethinyl estradiol, 5 mg/day; and conjugated estrogens, 30 mg/day. Treatment is continued for 5 days. If it is begun within 72 hours after an isolated midcycle act of coitus, its effectiveness is very good. If more than one episode of coitus has occurred or if treatment is initiated later than 72 hours after coitus, the method is much less effective.

Fasoli et al. performed a comprehensive literature review in 1989 and summarized the results of the 21 articles published in English, Italian, and French between 1975 and 1977 on the subject of PCC. In the six studies of high-dose estrogen, 4143 women were included, and the most (3168) received ethinyl estradiol. Pregnancy rates among the women treated with ethinyl estradiol were 0.6%; with DES, 0.7%; and with conjugated estrogen, 1.6% (Table 11-15). None of these rates was significantly different from the overall mean failure rate of 0.7%. None of the trials included a control group, but it has been estimated that the clinical pregnancy rate after midcycle coitus is approximately 7%. Thus high-dose estrogen is an effective method of PCC.

Side effects associated with this high-dose estrogen therapy are common and severe. They include nausea, vomiting, breast soreness, and menstrual irregularities, which tend to reduce compliance. The U.S. Centers for Disease Control performed a five-center study comparing use of ethinyl estradiol, 5 mg/day, with conjugated estrogens, 30 mg/day, for 5 days. The pregnancy rate was slightly lower with

ethinyl estradiol (0.7%) than with conjugated estrogens (1.6%). However, patients treated with ethinyl estradiol had a greater incidence of nausea and vomiting, indicating that its potency may have been greater. If treatment was begun 2 days after coitus, the pregnancy rate was 1.7 times greater than if it was begun the day after coitus. Thus it appears best to start treatment within 24 hours of coitus.

Because the side effects of high-dose estrogens cause many women to fail to complete the 5-day treatment course, a regimen of four tablets of an ethinyl estradiol, 0.05 mg, and *dl*-norgestrel, 0.5 mg, combination OC, (Ovral), given in doses of two tablets 12 hours apart, was initially tested in Canada. This regimen was found to be effective, with a shorter duration of adverse symptoms.

Fasoli et al. summarized the results of 11 studies with this treatment regimen involving 3802 women. Failure rates varied widely, from a low of 0.2% in a Canadian study to a high of 7.4% in an Italian study. The total pregnancy rate in the 11 studies was 1.8%, which was similar to the individual failure rate in the largest studies in this review. In one large Canadian study, 30% of the subjects treated with this regimen reported having nausea without vomiting, and another 20% had nausea with vomiting. These investigations included an antiemetic, 50 mg tablet of dimenhydrate, in the package and instructed the women to take it together with the second dose of contraceptive steroid if they experienced nausea after the first dose. They also reported the time to onset of the subsequent menses was slightly shortened in the users of this regimen.

Thus the effectiveness of this method appears to be slightly less than that of higher dosages of estrogen alone, but a lower incidence of abnormal bleeding, delayed menses, and gastrointestinal side effects occur with this regimen than with high-dose estrogen. Also, because of the 1-day treatment regimen, patient compliance is greater with this technique. Thus this method is more widely used than the high-dose estrogens.

Another method of PCC, the administration of danazol, 400 to 600 mg in two doses separated by 12 hours, has been tried by two groups of investigators. A total of 998 women were treated in these trials, and the pregnancy rate of 2.0% was similar to that with the two doses of combined OCs. However, the incidence of side effects, particularly nausea, was less with danazol, and thus patient acceptability was high. If the patient has a continuing need for contraception after the cycle in which either of these techniques is used, one of the conventional methods should be prescribed.

Several authors have advocated that intrauterine insertion of a copper IUD within 5 to 10 days of midcycle coitus is an effective method to prevent continuation of the pregnancy. Fasoli et al. summarized the results of nine published studies in four countries involving 879 women. Only one pregnancy occurred after a copper IUD was inserted in these women. As summarized in Table 11-15, one can see that insertion of a copper IUD and administration of high-dose estrogens are the most effective methods of PCC. However, side effects limit acceptance of high-dose estrogens, and cost and concern about introducing pathogens into the upper genital tract with IUD insertion limit its widespread use.

Antiprogestins

A few years ago Baulieu synthesized a progestogenic steroid compound that had weak progestational activity but great affinity for progesterone receptors in the endometrium. This compound was called RU 486, or mifepristone (Figure 11-14). Because of its high receptor affinity, RU 486 prevented progesterone from binding to its receptors and thus had an antiprogesterone action. In clinical trials it was found that if a single 600 mg dose of RU 486

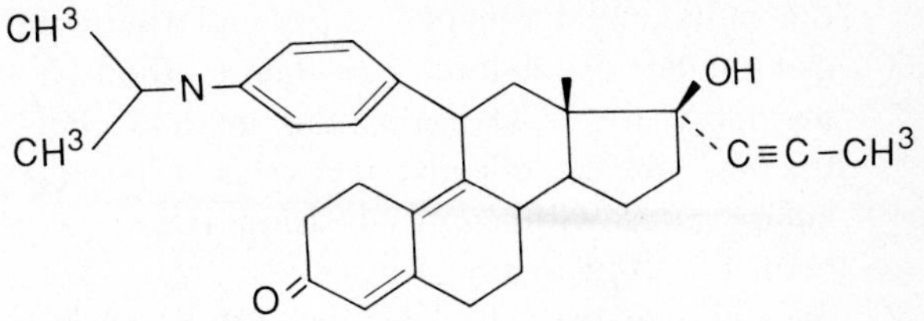

FIGURE 11-14
Molecular structure of RU 486. Molecular weight is 430, and empirical formula is $C_{29}H_{35}NO_2$. (From Healy DL, Baulieu EE, and Hodgen GD: Fertil Steril 40:253, 1983.)

was administered orally in early pregnancy, before 6 weeks after the onset of the last menses, approximately 85% of the pregnancies spontaneously terminated. When this treatment was combined with administration of a prostaglandin 36 to 48 hours later, the efficacy of pregnancy termination increased to 96%.

Side effects of RU 486 include nausea, vomiting, and abdominal pain. The main disadvantage of this method is prolonged and sometimes heavy vaginal bleeding that occasionally can cause anemia, necessitating a blood transfusion and possibly curettage. The mean duration of bleeding after administration of this drug is about 12 days when administered alone and 9 days when used with a prostaglandin. Currently, distribution of this drug is limited to France, but compounds with similar activity and steroid enzymatic inhibitors that prevent progesterone synthesis are also being studied.

INTRAUTERINE DEVICES

The main benefits of IUDs are (1) a high level of effectiveness, (2) a lack of associated systemic metabolic effects, and (3) the need for only a single act of motivation for long-term use. In contrast to other types of contraception, no need exists for frequent motivation to ingest a pill daily or to use a coitus-related method consistently. These characteristics, as well as the necessity for a visit to a health care facility to discontinue the method, account for IUDs having the highest continuation rate of all currently available reversible methods of contraception. All women should make at least annual visits to a health care facility, but in some areas of the world this is not possible.

Unlike other contraceptives, such as the barrier methods, which rely on frequent use by the individual for effectiveness and therefore have higher use failure rates than method failure rates, the IUD has similar method effectiveness and use effectiveness rates. First-year failure rates with copper-bearing IUDs have been reported to range from less than 1% to 3.7%. Pregnancy rates are related to the skill of the clinician inserting the device. With experience, correct high-fundal insertion occurs more frequently, and there is a lower incidence of partial or complete expulsion, with resultant lower pregnancy rates. Furthermore, the annual incidence of accidental pregnancy decreases steadily after the first year of IUD use. The incidence of all major adverse events with IUDs, including pregnancy, expulsion, or removal for bleeding and/or pain, also steadily decreases with increasing age. Thus the IUD is especially suited for older parous women who wish to prevent further pregnancies.

Mechanism of Action

The IUD's main mechanism of contraceptive action in the human is spermicidal, produced by a local sterile inflammatory reaction caused by the presence of the foreign body in the uterus. Moyer and Mishell found a nearly 1000% increase in the number of leukocytes in washings of the human endometrial cavity 18 weeks after the insertion of an IUD, compared with washings obtained before insertion. Tissue breakdown products of these leukocytes are toxic to all cells, including sperm and the blastocyst. Small IUDs do not produce as great an inflammatory reaction as larger ones do. There-

fore women using smaller IUDs have higher pregnancy rates than those using larger devices of the same design. The addition of copper increases the inflammatory reaction. Tredway et al. found that sperm transport from the cervix to the oviduct in the first 24 hours after coitus was greatly impaired in women wearing IUDs. Because of the spermicidal action of IUDs, very few, if any, sperm reach the oviducts, and the ovum usually does not become fertilized.

Further evidence for this spermicidal action of IUDs was recently reported by Alvarez et al. These investigators performed oviductal flushing in 56 women with IUDs and in 45 using no method of contraception. All women were sterilized by salpingectomy soon after ovulation and also had unprotected sexual intercourse shortly before ovulation. Normally cleaving, fertilized ova were found in the tubal flushings of about half the women not wearing IUDs, whereas no eggs with the microscopic appearance of a normally fertilized and developing preimplantation embryo were found in the oviducts of the women wearing IUDs.

In rabbits the sterile inflammatory reaction changes the receptiveness of the endometrium to the nidation of the blastocyst, preventing implantation. The same effect is believed to occur in humans if fertilization does take place. The presence of copper ions increases in locally released prostaglandins, and enzymatic changes within the endometrial cavity also probably act to prevent the normal process of implantation.

On removal of both copper-bearing and non-copper-bearing IUDs, the inflammatory reac-

---

TABLE 11-16
Fertility Rates (Mean % ± SE) of Parous Women Remaining Undelivered of Live Birth or Stillbirth at Given Intervals After Stopping Contraception to Plan Pregnancy

Method of Contraception Stopped	Mean Age (Years)	% Women Remaining Undelivered by Months Since Discontinuation					
		12	18	24	30	36	42
IUD	31.4	48.8 ± 2.4	18.1 ± 1.9	10.6 ± 1.6	9.3 ± 1.5	6.7 ± 1.4	6.3 ± 1.4
Oral contraceptives	30.6	60.7 ± 1.2	20.4 ± 1.0	10.8 ± 0.8	7.6 ± 0.7	5.4 ± 0.6	4.5 ± 0.6
Diaphragm	30.9	36.8 ± 1.5	13.8 ± 1.1	8.2 ± 0.9	6.2 ± 0.9	4.6 ± 0.8	4.2 ± 0.8
Other method	31.8	39.4 ± 1.5	16.2 ± 1.3	10.6 ± 1.1	7.8 ± 1.0	6.2 ± 0.9	5.0 ± 0.9
IUD users in past, stopped for medical reasons	32.7	49.3 ± 4.7	19.1 ± 4.1	13.6 ± 3.8			

From Vessey MP, Lawless M, McPherson K, and Yeates D: Br Med J 286:106, 1983.

tion rapidly disappears. Resumption of fertility after IUD removal is not delayed and occurs at the same rate as resumption of fertility after discontinuation of mechanical methods of contraception, such as the condom and diaphragm. Tietze and Lewit reported that of 378 women who had IUDs removed in order to conceive, 59.4% had conceived at the end of 3 months and 88.2% at the end of 1 year. These rates are similar to those found with women discontinuing barrier methods.

Another study by Vessey et al. (1983) reported that pregnancy rates of women who discontinued using IUDs were similar to those of women who discontinued barrier methods at 1 and 2 years. The only exception was for women discontinuing IUDs for medical problems, including infection, who had a slightly lower pregnancy rate at these intervals (Table 11-16).

Types of IUDs

In the past 25 years many types of IUDs have been designed and used clinically. The devices developed and initially used in the 1960s were made of a plastic polyethylene impregnated with barium sulfate to make them radiographic. In the 1970s smaller plastic devices covered with copper wire, such as the copper T, were developed and widely used. In the 1980s devices bearing a larger amount of copper, including sleeves on the horizontal arm, such as the copper T 380A and the copper T 220C, were developed. These devices had a longer duration of high effectiveness and thus had to be reinserted at less frequent intervals than the devices bearing a smaller amount of copper. Although many types of IUDs developed are still available for use in Europe, Canada, and elsewhere, at present only the copper T 380A and a progesterone-releasing IUD are being marketed in the United States (Figure 11-15). Although the barium-impregnated plastic loop and the copper-bearing copper 7 and copper T 200B are still approved by the FDA for use in the United States, they are no longer being sold. Production and distribution of the shield device with a multifilament tail were discontinued in 1974. Because of the increased risk of infection reported with shield IUDs, if any are still in place, they should be removed. All IUDs now approved for distribution by the FDA have monofilament tails.

The T- and 7-shaped plastic devices are smaller than most noncopper-bearing types of IUDs. When T-shaped devices without copper underwent clinical trials, women were found to have a much higher pregnancy rate than those using the larger loops and coils. With the addition of copper wire, the effectiveness of these IUDs was increased by the mechanism previously described and was comparable or higher than that of the nonmedicated IUDs.

Because of the constant dissolution of copper, which amounts daily to less than that ingested in the normal diet, all copper IUDs have to be replaced periodically. The copper T 380A is approved for use in the United States

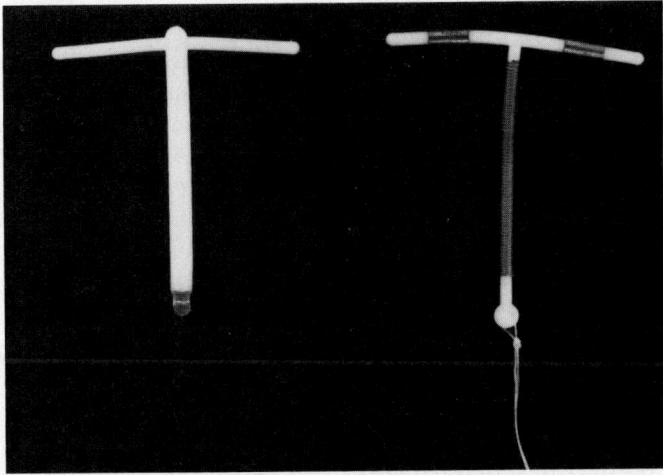

FIGURE 11-15
Intrauterine devices currently being marketed in the United States. (Left, progesterone-releasing IUD; right, copper T 380A.

for 4 years. However, a large, ongoing clinical trial by the WHO indicates that this device retains its contraceptive effectiveness for at least 7 years. At the scheduled time of removal, the device can be removed and another inserted during the same office visit.

Adding a reservoir of progesterone to the vertical arm also increases the effectiveness of the T-shaped devices. The currently marketed progesterone IUD releases 65 mg of progesterone daily. This amount is sufficient to prevent pregnancy by local action within the endometrial cavity, but it is not enough to cause a measurable increase in peripheral serum progesterone levels. The currently approved progesterone-releasing IUD needs to be replaced annually, since the reservoir of progesterone becomes depleted after about 18 months of use.

A T-shaped device containing a reservoir of levonorgestrel on the vertical arm has been developed, undergone extensive clinical testing, and has recently been approved for use in Finland. A large comparative trial by Sivin et al. of the Cu T 380A and the levonorgestrel-releasing IUD has found that the effectiveness and complication rates of both devices were similar. Because of the slower rate of release of levonorgestrel than progesterone, the levonorgestrel-releasing IUD has an estimated duration of use of at least 5 years.

Unlike the medicated IUDs, there is no need to change a nonmedicated plastic IUD unless the patient develops increased bleeding after it has been in place for more than a year. Calcium salts are deposited on the plastic over time, and their roughness can cause ulceration and bleeding of the endometrium. If increased bleeding develops after a noncopper-bearing IUD has been in the uterus for a year or more, the IUD should be removed and a new device inserted.

Time of Insertion

Although it is widely believed that the optimal time for insertion of an IUD is during the menses, data indicate that if a woman is not pregnant, the IUD can be safely inserted on any day of the cycle. White et al. analyzed 2-month event rates of about 10,000 women who had copper T 200 IUDs inserted on various days of the cycle. Rates of expulsion were lower when insertion occurred during the week

after menses stopped, whereas rates of removal for bleeding and pain, as well as pregnancy, were higher with insertions after cycle day 18. However, the differences were small and of little clinical relevance.

It has also been recommended that IUDs not be inserted until more than 2 to 3 months have elapsed after completing a term pregnancy. However, Mishell and Roy analyzed event rates in their clinic among women who had copper T IUDs inserted between 4 and 8 weeks postpartum and more than 8 weeks postpartum. The 1- and 2-year event rates for all causes were similar for the two groups, indicating that copper T IUDs can be safely inserted at the routine postpartum visit. No perforations occurred in this series, in which the withdrawal technique of insertion was used.

Although one report suggested that the perforation rate may be higher if the IUD is inserted when a woman is lactating, this finding has not been confirmed in other studies. The effect of breastfeeding on performance of the copper T 380A IUD was evaluated from data obtained from a large multicenter clinical trial by Chi et al. in which the device was inserted into 559 breastfeeding women and 590 nonbreastfeeding women, all of whom were at least 6 weeks postpartum. Significantly less pain and bleeding problems occurred at insertion in the breastfeeding group. The expulsion rate, which was low, and continuation rate, which was high, were lower in the breastfeeding and nonbreastfeeding groups 6 months after insertion.

Adverse Effects

Incidence

In general, in the first year of use most IUDs have about a 2% pregnancy rate, a 10% expulsion rate, and a 15% rate of removal for medical reasons, mainly bleeding and pain. The incidence of each of these events, especially expulsion, diminishes steadily in subsequent years.

The copper T 380A IUD, which has copper on the horizontal as well as the vertical arm, has a higher rate of effectiveness. In a U.S. multicenter study, Sivin and Tatum reported a net cumulative pregnancy rate of only 1.9% with this copper T device at the end of 4 years. In the ongoing WHO study of this device, termination rates for adverse effects continued to decline annually following the first year after

TABLE 11-17
Cumulative Discontinuation Rate for
Copper T 380A IUD

Event	Years Since Insertion		
	3	**5**	**7**
Pregnancies	1.0	1.4	1.6
Expulsions	7.0	8.2	8.6
Medical removals	14.6	20.8	25.8
Nonmedical removals	13.8	25.6	34.4
Loss to follow-up	10.2	15.5	22.1
All discontinuations	32.2	46.7	56.3
Woman-months	38,571	56,010	67,885

Modified from World Health Organization (WHO): Contraception 42:141, 1990.

insertion for each of the 7 years in which sufficient data has accumulated to date. In this study the cumulative discontinuation rate for pregnancy, bleeding and pain, and expulsion at the end of 7 years was 1.6, 22.7, and 8.6, respectively (Table 11-17). Thus the addition of copper on the horizontal arm of the T-shaped device appears to lower the pregnancy rate and increase the estimated duration of action to at least 7 years.

Uterine Bleeding

Most women discontinue the use of IUDs for medical reasons. Almost all the medical reasons accounting for IUD removal involve one or more types of abnormal bleeding: heavy and/or prolonged menses or intermenstrual bleeding. The IUD does not affect the pattern or level of circulating gonadotrophins and steroid hormones during the menstrual cycle. However, it does exert a local effect on the endometrium, causing menses to begin about 2 days earlier than normal, when steroid levels are higher than in control cycles. This early onset of menses may be produced by a premature increased rate of local release of prostaglandins because of the presence of the intrauterine foreign body. The stimulation of uterine contractions by excessive levels of prostaglandins may prolong the duration of the menstrual flow, which is significantly longer in women wearing IUDs.

The amount of blood loss in each menstrual cycle is significantly greater in women wearing inert as well as copper-bearing IUDs than in nonwearers. In a normal menstrual cycle the mean amount of menstrual blood loss (MBL) is about 35 ml. After insertion of a loop IUD, mean MBL increases to 70 to 80 ml. The increase is less with copper-bearing devices. With the copper 7 IUD, mean MBL has been found to vary from 50 to 55 ml, whereas with the copper T 200, mean MBL varies from 50 to 60 ml. In contrast, with the progesterone-releasing IUD, the amount of blood loss is significantly reduced, to approximately 25 ml per cycle.

After insertion of both copper and inert IUDs, a greater percentage of women have MBL in excess of 80 ml, an amount that has been shown to produce severe iron deficiency, than before insertion. In a study by Guillebaud et al. of English women using either the loop or copper 7 IUD, mean hemoglobin levels decreased after 1 year, and the percentage of women with hemoglobin levels below 12 g/dl significantly increased. As expected, because the mean MBL increase and the percentage of women losing more than 80 ml were greater with the loop than with the copper 7, the decrease in mean hemoglobin levels and the incidence of anemia were less with the copper 7 than with the loop. In a study by Rybo of Swedish women using the copper 7 or copper T 200, no significant change occurred in mean values for hemoglobin concentration, serum iron, and total iron-binding capacity 6 and 12 months after IUD insertion when compared with mean values before insertion. Blood loss studies with the copper T 380A have not been published to date.

A sensitive indicator of tissue iron stores is the serum ferritin level. Both copper-bearing IUDs and nonmedicated plastic IUDs are associated with significant decreases in serum ferritin levels overall, as well as with an increase in the percentage of women with extremely low ferritin levels (less than 16 mg/L), indicating an absence of iron in bone marrow. Low serum ferritin levels are a good predictor of the development of anemia. Therefore, ideally, both ferritin and hemoglobin levels should be measured annually in all women wearing nonsteroid-releasing IUDs. If either level decreases significantly, supplemental iron should be administered.

The exact mechanism whereby IUDs cause increased MBL is not completely understood, despite extensive investigative efforts. Histologic studies of endometrium obtained by biopsy and hysterectomy have demonstrated two types of lesions in association with IUDs. Vascular erosions have been seen in areas of direct contact with the IUD, and evidence of increased vascular permeability has been found in areas not in direct contact with the IUD. Both types of lesions could cause increased MBL, as well as intermenstrual bleeding. An increased concentration of proteolytic enzymes and plasminogenic activators that may lead to increased fibrinolytic activity has been found in the endometrial tissue adjacent to the device. This increase in fibrinolytic activity adversely affects hemostasis and increases MBL.

Excessive bleeding in the first few months after IUD insertion should be treated with reassurance and supplemental oral iron. The bleeding may diminish with time as the uterus adjusts to the presence of the foreign body. Excessive bleeding that continues or develops several months or more after IUD insertion may be treated by systemic administration of one of the prostaglandin synthetase inhibitors.

Mefenamic acid, 500 mg three times a day during the days of menstruation, has been shown by Anderson et al. to reduce MBL significantly in IUD users. If excessive bleeding continues despite this treatment, the device should be removed. After 1 month, another type of device may be inserted if the patient still wishes to use an IUD for contraception. Consideration should be given to using a progesterone-releasing IUD, since this device is associated with less blood loss than the copper-bearing IUDs.

Perforation

Although uncommon, one of the potentially serious complications associated with use of the IUD is perforation of the uterine fundus. Perforation initially occurs at insertion. It can best be prevented by straightening the uterine axis with a tenaculum and then probing the cavity with a uterine sound before IUD insertion. Sometimes only the distal portion of the IUD penetrates the uterine muscle at insertion. Then uterine contractions over the next few months force the IUD into the peritoneal cavity. IUDs correctly inserted entirely within the endometrial cavity do not wander through the uterine muscle into the peritoneal cavity. The incidence of perforation is generally related to the shape of the device and/or amount of force used during its insertion, as well as the experience of the clinician performing the insertion.

Perforation rates for the copper 7 and the copper T 200 were found to be about 1 in 1000 insertions. The clinician should always suspect perforation if a patient says she cannot feel the appendage but did not notice that the device was expelled. One should not assume that an unnoticed expulsion has occurred when the appendage is not visualized. Sometimes the IUD is still in its correct position in the uterine cavity, but the appendage has been withdrawn into the cavity as the position of the IUD within the cavity has changed. In this situation, after pelvic examination has been performed and the possibility of pregnancy excluded, the uterine cavity should be probed.

If the device cannot be felt with a uterine sound or biopsy instrument, a pelvic sonogram or x-ray film should be obtained. If the device is not visualized with pelvic ultrasonography, an x-ray film of the entire abdominal cavity should be performed, since IUDs that have been pushed through the uterus may be located anywhere in the peritoneal cavity, even in the subdiaphragmatic area.

Any type of IUD found to be outside the uterus, even if asymptomatic, should be removed from the peritoneal cavity because complications such as adhesions and bowel obstruction have been reported. Both the copper IUDs and the shields have been found to produce severe peritoneal reactions. Therefore it is best to remove these devices as soon as possible after the diagnosis of perforation is made. Unless severe adhesions have developed, most intraperitoneal IUDs can be removed by means of laparoscopy, avoiding the need for laparotomy.

Perforation of the cervix has also been reported with devices having a straight vertical arm, such as the copper T or 7. The incidence of downward perforation into the cervix has been reported to range from about 1 in 600 to 1 in 1000 insertions. When follow-up examinations are performed on patients with these devices, the cervix should be carefully inspected and palpated, since perforations often do not extend completely through the ectocervical epithelium. Cervical perforation is not a major problem, but devices that have perforated downward should be removed through the endocervical canal with uterine packing forceps.

Their downward displacement is associated with reduced contraceptive effectiveness.

Complications Related to Pregnancy

Congenital Anomalies

When pregnancy occurs with an IUD in place, implantation takes place away from the device itself, so the device is always extraamniotic. Although few published data exist, so far no evidence shows an increased incidence of congenital anomalies in infants born with an IUD in utero. In a study by Poland of spontaneously aborted tissue, 21% of the embryos conceived with an IUD in situ had evidence of abnormalities. This was considerably less than the 44% incidence of abnormalities in abortuses of women using no contraception and was similar to the incidence of embryonic abnormalities in abortuses of women having induced abortions. This suggests that the presence of an IUD has no influence on embryonic development and that the increased incidence of spontaneous abortion in IUD users is not caused by a greater incidence of embryonic abnormalities.

Tatum et al. reported that of 166 embryos conceived with an intrauterine copper T in place and large enough to permit adequate examination, only one had a congenital anomaly, a fibroma of the vocal cords. Guillebaud reported that in a series of 167 pregnancies that reached viability with the copper 7 in place, 159 normal babies were born. No details were given regarding three infants in this series, and the other five had a variety of anomalies. Therefore the incidence of congenital defects, 3%, was similar to the expected rate. Thus no evidence from these studies indicates that the presence of a copper IUD in the uterus exerts a deleterious effect on fetal development. Although relatively few infants have been born with a progesterone-releasing IUD in the uterus, careful examination of these infants has revealed no increased incidence of cardiac or other anomalies.

Spontaneous Abortion

In all reported series of pregnancies with any type of IUD in situ, the incidence of fetal death was not significantly increased; however, a significant increase in spontaneous abortion has been consistently observed. Three studies indicate that if a patient conceives while wearing an IUD that is not subsequently removed, the incidence of spontaneous abortion is about 55%, approximately 3 times greater than would occur without an IUD.

After conception, if the IUD is spontaneously expelled or if the appendage is visible and the IUD is removed by traction, the incidence of spontaneous abortion is significantly reduced. Of women who conceived with copper T devices in place, the incidence of spontaneous abortion was only 20.3% if the device was removed or spontaneously expelled. This figure is similar to the normal incidence of spontaneous abortion and significantly less than the 54.1% incidence of abortion reported in the same study among women retaining the devices in utero. Thus if a woman conceives with an IUD in place and wishes to continue the pregnancy, the IUD should be removed if the appendage is visible. This will significantly reduce the chance of spontaneous abortion. If the appendage is not visible, probing of the uterine cavity may increase the chance of abortion, as well as sepsis. However, two recent reports indicate that with careful ultrasonography and meticulous technique, it is possible to remove intrauterine IUDs without a visible appendage during pregnancy and have a normal outcome of gestation.

Septic Abortion

If the IUD cannot be easily removed, some evidence suggests that the risk of septic abortion may be increased if the IUD remains in place. Most of the evidence is based on data from women who conceived while wearing the shield type of IUD. This device, with its multifilament tail, was widely used from 1971 to 1974. It has been shown that the structure of the shield's appendage allowed bacteria to enter the spaces between the filaments of the tail underneath the sheath. This contrasts with the inability of bacteria to enter the monofilament tails of other devices. During pregnancy, when the shield was drawn upward into the uterus as gestation advanced, the bacteria in the tail had the potential for causing a severe and sometimes fatal uterine infection, usually in the second trimester of pregnancy.

Although theoretic and actual evidence suggests an increased risk of septic abortion if a patient conceives with a shield IUD in place, no conclusive evidence shows an increased risk if a patient conceives with a device other than the shield in place. In the Oxford study, there was no significant difference in the incidence of septic abortion among women who conceived with an IUD in place and those who conceived while using other methods. None of the women with septic abortions was seriously ill, and all responded promptly to treatment. In a study of 918 women who conceived with the copper T in situ, only two cases of septic abortion occurred, both in the first trimester. This evidence does not suggest an increase in sepsis in pregnancy caused by the presence of an IUD, except that about 2% of all spontaneous abortions are septic, and IUDs increase the rate of spontaneous abortion.

Although no conclusive evidence shows an increased incidence of sepsis with IUDs other than the shield, the patient should be informed of the possibility of a greater chance of sepsis and, if she wishes to continue the pregnancy, of the need to report symptoms of infection promptly. If an intrauterine infection does occur during pregnancy with an IUD in place, treatment should proceed in the same manner as if the IUD were absent. In such a situation, the endometrial cavity should be evacuated after a short interval of appropriate antibiotic treatment.

Ectopic Pregnancy

As stated earlier, the IUD's main mechanism of contraceptive action is the production of a continuous sterile inflammatory reaction in the uterine cavity because of foreign body presence. As the large numbers of leukocytes stimulated to enter the uterine cavity by the inflammatory reaction are catabolized, their breakdown products exert a toxic effect on sperm and the ovaries. If the egg is fertilized, effects of this foreign body reaction act to prevent implantation of the embryo into the endometrium. Because more inflammatory reaction is present in the endometrial cavity than the oviducts, the IUD prevents intrauterine pregnancy more effectively than it prevents ectopic pregnancy.

Several epidemiologic studies have confirmed that if pregnancy occurs with an IUD in place, it is more likely to be ectopic than if pregnancy occurs in the absence of an IUD. Despite the increased incidence of ectopic pregnancy in women conceiving with an IUD in place, overall the IUD reduces the incidence of ectopic pregnancy. A Centers for Disease Control (CDC) study reported that women using IUDs have only about 40% as great a chance of developing ectopic pregnancy as women using no method of contraception. This is similar to the protection against ectopic pregnancy provided by barrier methods, but not as effective as that provided by OCs.

If a patient conceives with an IUD in place, her chances of having an ectopic pregnancy range from 3% to 9%. This incidence is approximately 10 times greater than the reported ectopic pregnancy frequency of 0.3% to 0.7% of total births in similar populations. In two large Population Council studies, the ectopic pregnancy rate in IUD wearers was about 1.0 to 1.2 per 1000 woman-years.

Thus if a patient conceives with an IUD in place, ectopic pregnancy should be suspected. There appears to be a higher frequency of ectopic pregnancy with the progesterone-releasing IUD. Patients conceiving while wearing any IUD device should have sonography performed early in gestation. In addition, the possibility of ovarian pregnancy should always be considered, since the incidence of ovarian pregnancy is greater in women conceiving with an IUD in place than those conceiving while not wearing an IUD. IUD users with a clinical diagnosis of ruptured corpus luteum may have an unrecognized ovarian pregnancy. If any patient with an IUD has an elective termination of pregnancy, the evacuated tissue should be examined histologically to be certain that the gestation was intrauterine.

The effect of the IUD on increased development of ectopic pregnancy while it is in place appears to be temporary and does not persist after removal of the IUD. In two large European studies, women wishing to conceive after they had an ectopic pregnancy had a much greater chance of having a successful intrauterine pregnancy if they were using an IUD at the time of their ectopic pregnancy than those who had an ectopic pregnancy without an IUD.

Prematurity

Several studies indicate that the rate of preterm delivery is higher if an IUD remains in the uterus throughout gestation. If a pregnant patient has an IUD in place and the device cannot be removed but the patient wishes to continue her gestation, she should be warned of the increased risk of prematurity, as well as that of spontaneous abortion and ectopic pregnancy. She should also be informed of the possible increased risk of septic abortion and advised to report promptly the first signs of pelvic pain or fever. No evidence suggests that pregnancies with IUDs in utero are associated with an increased incidence of other obstetric complications. Also, no evidence shows that prior use of an IUD results in a greater incidence of complications in pregnancies occurring after its removal.

Infection in the Nonpregnant IUD User

In the 1960s, despite great concern among clinicians that use of the IUD would greatly increase the incidence of salpingitis (PID), little evidence supported such an increase. During that decade the IUD was inserted mainly into parous women, and the incidence of sexually transmitted disease was not as high as occurred subsequently. In 1966 Mishell et al. prepared aerobic and anaerobic cultures of homogenates of endometrial tissue obtained transfundally from uteri removed by vaginal hysterectomy at various intervals after insertion of the loop IUD. During the first 24 hours the normally sterile endometrial cavity was consistently infected with bacteria. Nevertheless, in 80% of cases the women's natural defenses destroyed these bacteria within the following 24 hours. In this study the endometrial cavity, the IUD, and the portion of the thread within the cavity were consistently found to be sterile when

transfundal cultures were obtained more than 30 days after insertion (Figure 11-16). These findings support the belief that development of PID more than a month after insertion of the loop IUD results from infection with a sexually transmitted pathogen and is unrelated to the presence of the device.

These findings agree with the incidence of clinically diagnosed PID found in a group of 23,977 mainly parous women wearing noncopper-bearing IUDs. When PID rates were computed according to the duration of IUD use, the rates were highest in the first 2 weeks after insertion and then steadily diminished. Rates after the first month were in the range of 1 to 2.5 per 100 woman-years.

The results of both of these studies indicate that an IUD should not be inserted into a patient who may have been recently infected with gonococci or *Chlamydia*. Insertion of the device will transport these pathogens into the upper genital tract. If there is clinical suspicion of infectious endocervicitis, cultures should be obtained and the IUD insertion delayed until the results reveal no pathogenic organisms are present. It does not appear to be cost-effective to administer systemic antibiotics routinely with every IUD insertion, but the insertion procedure should be as aseptic as possible.

After the introduction and widespread use of the shield device, particularly among nulliparous women (in whom IUDs were previously inserted only occasionally), several studies published in the late 1970s suggested that IUD use

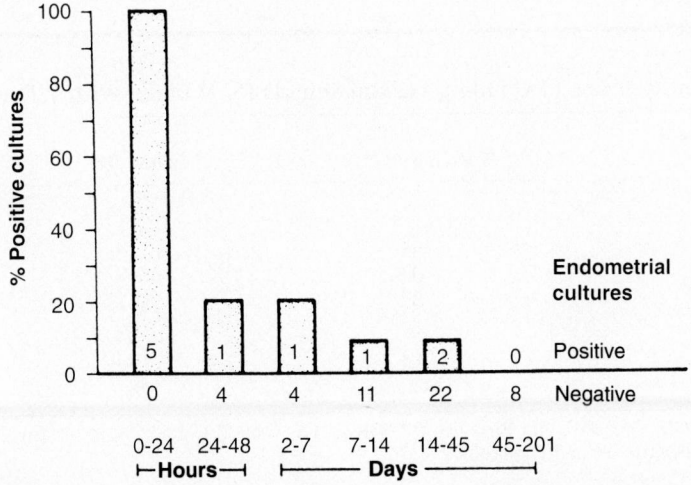

FIGURE 11-16
Relationship between incidence of positive endometrial cultures and duration of IUD use before hysterectomy. (From Mishell DR Jr, Bell JH, Good RG, et al: Am J Obstet Gynecol 1966:96:116.)

increased the relative risk of PID from three-fold to sevenfold.

Several problems accompany these studies. One is that uniform guidelines were not used for the diagnosis of PID (or salpingitis). Differences in diagnostic criteria may have increased the frequency of the diagnosis among IUD users. Patients with lower abdominal pain and only minimal or no elevation in temperature may have been given the diagnosis of PID more often when an IUD was in the uterus.

A second problem is the evidence that use of OCs, condoms, and diaphragms provides protection against development of PID. The data from numerous studies indicate that the incidence of both febrile and nonfebrile PID occurs about half as often in women using OCs and barrier methods as in women using no method of contraception. Most sexually active women use contraception, mainly OCs, barriers, or the IUD. The increased risk of infection reported with the IUD is largely caused by the protective effect of the other contraceptives.

A third problem is that in most of the studies performed in the 1970s, a high percentage of IUD wearers were using the shield. This device was more likely than other types to have a causal relationship to PID. Examination of the sheaths of the appendages of both new shields in their sterile packages and shields removed from patients showed that 9% of the new shields and 34% of the used shields had breaks in the sheath around the knot attaching it to the device. These breaks could allow bacteria to have continuous access from the vagina to the endometrial cavity and thus increase the risk of upper genital tract infection.

Finally, none of these studies differentiated between episodes of PID developing in the first few months after IUD insertion (previously shown to be related to the insertion itself) and episodes developing later. In 1987 CDC investigators reported results from a multicenter case-control study of the relationship between the IUD and PID. They found the overall risk of PID in IUD users versus non-contraceptive users to be 1.9. The risk in shield users was 8.3; in other IUD users, it was only 1.6. When the risk of PID in IUD users (other than shield users) was correlated with duration of use, it was found that a significantly increased risk of PID with the loop and copper 7 was present only during the first 4 months after insertion (Table 11-18). Beyond 4 months of use, there was no significantly increased risk in IUD users other than those with shields. Thus this report is in agreement with our bacteriologic study and the 1970 summary of 23,977 IUD users mentioned earlier. These data provide additional evidence that aside from the insertion process, the IUD with monofilament tail strings does not itself alter the incidence of PID. Additional support for this statement is provided from results of an epidemiologic study investigating the incidence of tubal infertility among former IUD users. It was reported that nulliparous women with a single sexual partner who had previously used an IUD had

---

TABLE 11-18

Duration of Current IUD Use (Excluding Dalkon Shield) for Women with PID and Controls

Duration of Use of Current IUD (Months)*	Women with PID†	Controls†	RR‡ (95% CL)
≤1	27	17	3.8 (2.1-6.8)
2-4	22	32	1.7 (1.1-3.1)
5-12	33	90	1.1 (0.7-1.7)
13-24	32	81	1.2 (0.7-1.8)
25-60	23	62	1.2 (0.7-2.0)
>60	13	40	1.4 (0.7-2.7)
No method	250	763	1 (Referrent)

From Lee NC, Rubin GL, Ory HW, and Burkman RT: Obstet Gynecol 62:1, 1983. Reprinted with permission from The American College of Obstetricians and Gynecologists.

PID, Pelvic inflammatory disease.

*IUD used in the 3 months before interview.

†Limited to women who reported no past history of PID.

‡Relative risk (RR) adjusted for age, marital status, and number of sexual partners within previous 6 months. CL, Confidence limits.

no increased risk of tubal infertility, whereas women with multiple sexual partners who used an IUD did have an increased risk of tubal infertility (Table 11-18).

A more detailed analysis of data from the CDC study was published in 1988. This analysis produced information about risk factors for developing PID, such as number of sexual partners and frequency of intercourse among IUD users and users of no method of contraception. They found that married women were less likely to have more than one sexual partner in the previous 6 months before data were gathered than previously married or never married women. Among women in each of these groups as well as those cohabiting but not married, who reported having only one sexual partner, the risk of developing PID in women wearing an IUD was significantly increased only in the previously married or never married group (Table 11-19). The authors postulated that this was probably because the partners of such women had an increased risk of transmitting a pathogen responsible for PID. In the group of married or cohabiting women who had an IUD inserted more than 4 months earlier, the relative risk of developing PID compared with users of no method was 1.0, with confidence limits of 0.6 to 1.6, whereas those who had it inserted within 4 months had a nonsignificant increased risk of developing PID of 1.8. Thus analysis of these data indicates that PID occurring more than a few months after insertion of loop or copper devices is caused by a sexually transmitted disease and not related to the IUD.

The populations at high risk for PID include those with a history of PID, nulliparous women under age 25, and women with multiple sexual partners. The FDA has recommended that women with these characteristics be especially advised about the risk of developing PID during IUD use and the possibility of subsequent loss of fertility. They should be told to watch for the early symptoms of PID so that treatment can be started before complications occur. These data, as well as those of two epidemiologic studies showing an increased risk of tubal causes of infertility in nulliparous women who had used an IUD, indicate that the clinician should avoid using IUDs in nulliparous women who may want to conceive in the future. The increased risk of impairment of future fertility from PID in the first few months after IUD insertion, as well as the possibility of ectopic pregnancy, must be considered when deciding whether to use an IUD in a nulliparous woman.

Symptomatic PID can usually be successfully treated with antibiotics without removing the IUD until the patient becomes symptom free. In patients with clinical evidence of a tuboovarian abscess or with a shield in place, the IUD should be removed only after a therapeutic serum level of appropriate parenteral antibiotics has been reached, and preferably after a clinical response has been observed. An alternative method of contraception should be substituted in those patients who develop PID with an IUD in place (or in those with a history of PID).

Evidence suggests that IUD users may have an increased risk for colonizing actinomycosis organisms in the upper genital tract. The relationship of actinomycosis to PID is unclear, since many women without IUDs have actinomycosis in their vagina. If these organisms are identified on the routine annual cytologic smear of IUD users, their existence should be confirmed by culture, since cytologic diagnosis of actinomycosis is not very precise. If the culture confirms their presence in the cervix, appropriate antimicrobial therapy should be used to eradicate the organisms, but the IUD does not have to be removed.

Overall Safety

Several long-term studies have indicated that the IUD is not associated with an increased incidence of endometrial or cervical carcinoma. Nevertheless, the IUD does produce morbidity that may result in hospitalization. The main causes of hospitalization among IUD users are

TABLE 11-19
Risk of PID Associated with IUD Use Versus No Method, by Marital Status Among Women with Only One Recent Sexual Partner

Marital Status	RR (95% CL)
Currently married	1.2 (0.7-1.9)
Cohabiting	1.0 (0.4-2.4)
Previously married	1.8 (1.0-3.2)
Never married	2.6 (1.6-4.3)

From Lee NC and Rubin GL: Obstet Gynecol 72:1, 1988. PID, Pelvic inflammatory disease; RR, relative risk; CL, confidence limits.

complications of pregnancy, uterine perforation, and hemorrhage, as well as pelvic infection. Despite the increased morbidity with IUDs, the actual incidence of these problems is very low. IUDs are not being inserted in women at risk for developing PID, and physicians are aware of the potential complications associated with IUDs in pregnancy. The IUD is a particularly useful method of contraception for women who have completed their families and do not wish permanent sterilization and have contraindications to or do not wish to use OCs.

STERILIZATION

In 1988 in the United States, sterilization of one member of a couple was the most widely used method of preventing pregnancy. The popularity of sterilization was greatest if (1) the wife was over age 30, (2) the couple had been married more than 10 years, and (3) the couple desired no further children. In contrast to the other methods of contraception, which are re-

versible or temporary, sterilization should be considered permanent. Although reanastomosis after vasectomy or tubal ligation is possible, the reconstructive operation is much more difficult than the original sterilizing procedure and the results are variable. Pregnancy rates after reanastomosis of the vas range from 45% to 60%, whereas those after oviduct reanastomosis range from 50% to 80%, depending on the amount of tissue damage associated with the original procedure, as well as technical competency.

Voluntary sterilization is legal in all 50 states, and the decision to be sterilized should be made solely by the patient in consultation with the physician. Because all currently available sterilization procedures require surgical techniques, patients who request sterilization should be counseled regarding both the risks and the irreversibility of the procedures. It is advisable to inform the patient fully, and the spouse if possible, of the benefits and risks of these surgical procedures. In addition, it has been useful to have more than one counselor

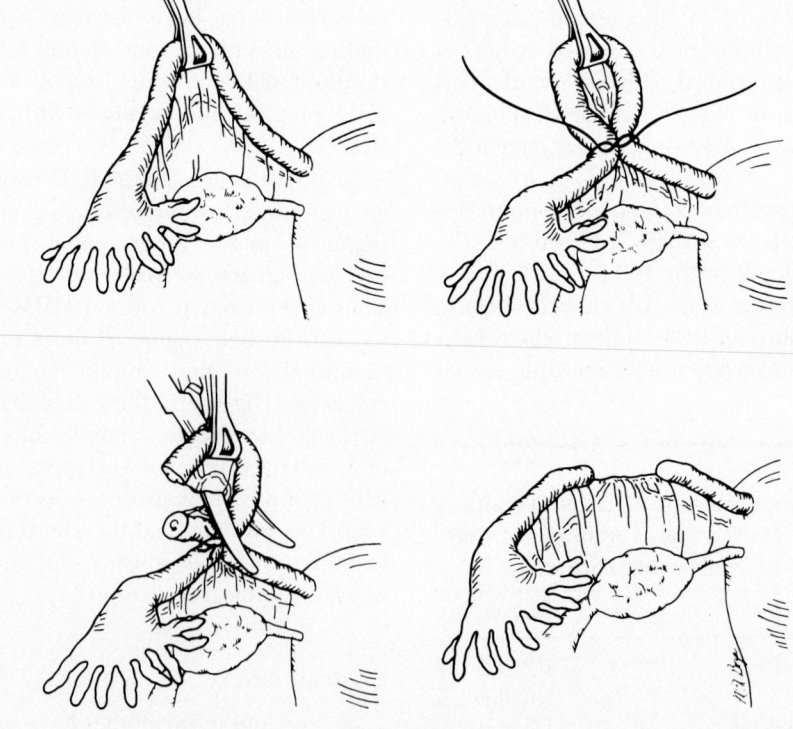

FIGURE 11-17
Modified Pomeroy technique of female sterilization. (From Sciarra JJ: Surgical procedures for tubal sterilization. In Sciarra JJ, Zatuchni GI, and Daly MJ: Gynecology and obstetrics, vol 6, Philadelphia, 1984, Harper & Row, Publishers, Inc.)

when sterilization is requested by a woman younger than age 25, as well as a woman older than age 40 without any children.

The rationale for such careful scrutiny of younger candidates for sterilization is that they tend to change their minds more often, their attitudes may be less fixed, and they face a longer period of reproductive life during which divorce, remarriage, or death among their children can occur. About 1% of sterilized women subsequently request reversal. In the United States approximately 7000 women request reversal each year.

The most effective, least destructive method of tubal occlusion is the most desirable in younger patients, since ovarian dysfunction and adhesion formation are diminished, while the incidence of successful reversal procedures is increased. The effective laparoscopic band techniques or the modified technique (Figure 11-17) should be used in patients younger than age 25. Reversal after this method of sterilization is followed by pregnancy in approximately 75% of women, a rate that is higher than that reported after most laparoscopic fulgurations, where more tube is destroyed.

Male Sterilization

Sterilization in the male is performed by vasectomy, an outpatient procedure that takes about 20 minutes and requires only local anesthesia. The vas deferens is isolated and cut. The ends of the vas are closed, either by ligation or by fulguration; they are then replaced in the scrotal sac, and the incision is closed. Complications of vasectomy include hematoma (in up to 5% of subjects), sperm granulomas (inflammatory responses to sperm leakage), and spontaneous reanastomosis (if this is to occur, it usually does so within a short time after the procedure). Hematoma is best prevented by ligating all small vessels in the scrotal wall. The occurrence of sperm granuloma is minimized by cauterizing or fulgurating the ends of the vas instead of ligating them. After the procedure the man is not considered sterile until two sperm-free ejaculates have been produced. Semen analysis should be performed 1 and 2 months after the procedure. Usually about 15 to 20 ejaculations are required after the operation before the man is sterile. Although in the United States requests range from 6% to 7%, vas reanastomosis is a difficult and meticu-

lous procedure that has a success rate of about 50%.

Female Sterilization

Sterilization of the female is more complicated, requiring a transperitoneal incision and usually general anesthesia. Postpartum sterilization is performed by making a small infraumbilical incision and performing either a Pomeroy or modified Irving type of tubal ligation. These simple and rapid procedures can be performed either in the delivery room immediately after delivery or in the operating room the following day without prolonging the patient's hospital stay. The same operative techniques can be used for female sterilization at times other than the puerperium, but additional techniques are also used for what has been termed *interval sterilization*. Ligation of the oviducts by the Pomeroy technique can be easily and rapidly performed through a small abdominal incision; this has been termed *minilaparotomy*. On occasion a colpotomy incision may also be used, but this incision is associated with a higher incidence of postoperative infection.

The development of fiberoptic light sources has made laparoscopy a popular gynecologic operative technique. By using various accessories in addition to the laparoscope, the operator can fulgurate and cut the oviducts without making an intraperitoneal incision other than one or two small punctures. Most gynecologists find the two-puncture technique for laparoscopy sterilization easier to learn and perform than the single-puncture technique. General anesthesia is usually employed for laparoscopic sterilization, but overnight hospitalization is unnecessary. The failure rate after this technique is about 1 per 1000 procedures. Because the pregnancy rate after fulguration and transection is similar to that after fulguration alone, it is now recommended that the oviducts not be cut after fulguration. The incidence of complications after laparoscopic fulguration ranges from 1% to 6%; major complications (hemorrhage, puncture, or cautery of bowel) occur in about 0.6% of patients.

In an attempt to eliminate the problem of bowel injury, bipolar forceps were developed to replace the unipolar apparatus, which has a grounding plate attached to the patient through which the current passes. In the bipolar system the current passes from one prong of the forceps, through the tissue, to the other prong, thus producing a limited coagulation with destruction of a small segment of the oviduct. After coagulation, if division is to be performed, scissors are introduced to cut the oviduct. If division is not to be performed, some operators perform a coagulation of two or three contiguous burns on each oviduct to ensure adequate obliteration of the lumen. When the unipolar apparatus is used, a single 1 cm burn on each oviduct is sufficient. However, even with this small amount of coagulation, local tissue damage after unipolar coagulation is extensive, and attempts at reanastomosis have a very low rate of success. Because bipolar coagulation not only is safer but also is associated with a higher success rate after a reanastomosis procedure, this technique is now preferred.

Because of the problems of electrocoagulation, efforts have been made to develop safer methods that destroy less tissue. Nonelectrical tubal occlusion techniques that may be performed through the laparoscope are those using the tantalum, plastic, spring-loaded clips, and the Silastic band (Falope ring). All these techniques require a modification of the conventional laparoscope, as well as specialized training in their use. The failure rate for the clip and band techniques averages about 2 per 1000 procedures, with a range of 1 to 6 per 1000.

INDUCED ABORTION

Induced abortion is one of the most common gynecologic operations performed in the United States and in many other countries. As determined by the landmark *Roe v. Wade* Supreme Court decision, the state may not interfere with the practice of abortion in the first trimester. In the second trimester, states may regulate abortion services in the interest of preserving the health of the woman. However, restrictions limiting the performance of second-trimester abortions to hospitals have been declared unconstitutional.

From 1973 through 1980, legal abortions performed annually in the United States steadily increased but have remained relatively stable since then. The annual variation has been less than 3% each year from 1980 to 1988.

In 1988 an estimated 1.6 million elective abortions were performed in the United States. The abortion ratio (number of abortions per 100 pregnancies) was 28.8, whereas the abortion rate (number of abortions per 1000 women of reproductive age) was 27.3. Approximately one third of abortions are performed in women under age 20, another third in women ages 20 to 24, and the remaining third among women 25 and older. Only one fourth of abortions are obtained by married women. Ninety percent of abortions are performed within the first 12 weeks of pregnancy, and about 50% of abortions are performed during the first 8 weeks of pregnancy.

Methods

Three principal methods are used for elective abortion: transcervical evacuation, induction of labor, and major operations. Suction curettage is the predominant method of performing abortion in the United States, accounting for approximately 85% of all abortion procedures; the remainder are performed by dilation and evacuation (curettage techniques in the second trimester), labor induction, and major operations.

Curettage Methods

Curettage by vacuum aspiration is the predominant method of performing abortion in the first trimester. Very early in pregnancy, *endometrial aspiration*, also termed *menstrual extraction*, can be done with a small, flexible plastic cannula without dilation or anesthesia. Abortions performed 8 weeks or more after the last menstrual period generally require dilation of the cervix and some type of anesthesia, either local or general.

Dilation of the cervix can be facilitated by use of osmotic dilators. These are usually placed in the cervical canal for several hours to overnight to produce gradual dilation. The traditional method has been use of *Laminaria japonica*, made of seaweed sticks. Synthetic osmotic dilators include a polyvinyl alcohol sponge impregnated with magnesium sulfate and a hygroscopic plastic polymer. Use of such osmotic dilators in nulliparous women substantially reduces the risk of uterine trauma, such as perforation and cervical injury.

Dilation and evacuation (D&E) is the predominant method of abortion used beyond the first trimester. Because larger cervical dilation is usually needed, osmotic dilators are usually inserted for several hours or several days before the procedure. Although recent data are lacking, early studies suggested that D&E was substantially safer than induction of labor or major operations for abortions at 13 to 16 weeks' gestation. For later abortions, D&E and induction of labor appear to have comparable risks of morbidity and mortality, although the range of complications varies by technique. Disadvantages of D&E include the greater technical expertise required, the emotional burden for participating physicians and medical personnel, and possible long-term effects on the cervix. Advantages include less emotional stress for the patient, avoidance of the need for hospitalization, greater convenience, and lower cost.

Induction of Labor

Second-trimester abortion is also performed by induction of labor. One technique involved instillation of hypertonic solutions into the amniotic cavity. The solution most frequently used was hypertonic saline (200 ml of 20% saline), although hypertonic glucose and urea were also employed. Labor usually started within 12 to 24 hours, and abortion occurred within a few hours thereafter. Use of ancillary agents such as *Laminaria* or oxytocin facilitated the procedure. However, instillation of hypertonic solutions is infrequently done today.

Two prostaglandin compounds have been increasingly used for inducing labor in the second trimester. One, prostaglandin E_2, is administered as a vaginal suppository, and the other, 15-methyl prostaglandin $F_{2\alpha}$, is administered as an intramuscular injection. Both techniques have the advantage of easy administration. Each compound is given at 2- to 3-hour intervals until evacuation of the gestational material is achieved. Disadvantages include gastrointestinal side effects and, with the prostaglandin E_2 suppositories, fever and chills.

Major Operations

Hysterotomy and hysterectomy are infrequently used for performing abortion in the United States. Both procedures have a much higher risk of morbidity and mortality than alternative methods. Hysterectomy should be reserved for those cases in which preexisting gynecologic pathology, such as carcinoma in situ of the cervix or large leiomyomata, also exist.

Ancillary Techniques

Pregnancy tests should be performed on all patients before abortion is carried out unless there is sonographic evidence of pregnancy. Performing a qualitative pregnancy test 2 weeks after the procedure will ensure that the pregnancy has been successfully aborted. In the first trimester, ultrasonography is usually reserved for determining gestational age when a substantial discrepancy occurs between menstrual history and clinical examination or when other uterine pathology, such as leiomyomata, is present. Routine preoperative ultrasound before second-trimester abortions has avoided the problem of misestimation of gestational age, which is an important cause of complications. Performing ultrasonography during D&E may facilitate the procedure.

Complications

Elective abortion in the United States is a very safe operation. Complications are infrequent, and the overall mortality is less than 1 per 100,000 procedures. Two important determinants of complications are the gestational age and method of abortion chosen. Abortions at 6 weeks and less have slightly higher complication rates than do abortions at 7 to 10 weeks. Thereafter, abortion complication rates increase progressively with gestational age. Suction curettage is the safest method of abortion, followed by D&E, induction of labor, and major operations.

The most common complication is infection, and the routine use of preoperative antibiotic prophylaxis has proved to be effective in reducing this risk. Other complications include hemorrhage, the consequences of uterine perforation, and anesthetic hazards.

_____ KEY POINTS _____

- In 1988, of the 58 million women in the United States aged 15 to 44 years, approximately one third were not exposed to pregnancy. Of the remaining 38.7 million women, all but 3.8 million (9.8%) were using a method of contraception.

- The most frequently used method to prevent conception in the United States is male and female sterilization. Of the nonsurgical methods of contraception, oral contraceptives (OCs) are most popular, being used by 18.5% of all women in this age group, followed by the condom (8.8%), diaphragm (3.5%), periodic abstinence (1.4%), withdrawal (1.3%), intrauterine device (IUD) (1.2%), and spermicide (0.6%).

- First-year use failure rates are the same for OCs and for the IUD (3%); higher for the condom (12%), diaphragm (18%), and periodic abstinence; and highest for spermicides (21%).

- Contraceptive failure rates are increased in inverse relation to the user's age, level of education, and socioeconomic class.

- Long-term failure rates among married motivated women are, per 100 women-years, 0.3% for OCs, 3.6% for the condom, 1.3% for the IUD, 11.9% for spermicides, 1.9% for the diaphragm, and 15.5% for periodic abstinence.

- Pregnancy results from failure of spermicide use are not associated with an increased risk of fetal malformations.

- The active ingredient in spermicides is a surfactant, usually nonoxynol 9, which immobilizes or kills sperm on contact.

- Barrier techniques reduce the rate of transmission of sexually transmitted diseases, both bacterial and viral.

- Pregnancy (failure rates) with the cervical cap are similar to those with the diaphragm.

- The most effective type of periodic abstinence is the sympto-thermal method.

- OC formulations in the United States consist of varying dosages of one of the following four 19-nortestosterone progestins—norethindrone, norethindrone acetate, ethynodiol diacetate, and norgestrel (or its active isomere, levonorgestrel)—and either of two estrogens: ethinyl estradiol or ethinyl estradiol-3-methyl ether. Newer, more potent progestins are now being used clinically in Europe and will be marketed in the United States. These are desogestrel, gestodene, and norgestimate.

- A given weight of norgestrel is 5 to 10 times more potent than the equivalent weight of norethindrone, whereas norethindrone acetate and ethinyl estradiol are similar in potency to norethindrone.

- Metabolic effects of the estrogen component of OCs include an increase in serum globulins and altering of the lipid profile to increase triglycerides and HDL cholesterol and lower LDL cholesterol.

- Metabolic effects of the progestin component of OCs include peripheral insulin resistance and lowering HDL cholesterol and raising LDL cholesterol.

- Ethinyl estradiol is approximately 1.7 times as potent as an equivalent weight of mestranol.

- No significantly increased risk of breast cancer exists in the overall population of OC users or in various high-risk subgroups of OC users.

- OC users have an increased risk of developing cervical dysplasia and invasive cervical cancer compared with users of no contraception, but a causal relation has not been established.

- The rate of return of fertility after stopping OCs is delayed, but eventually the percentage of women who conceive after stopping all methods of contraception, including OCs, is the same.

- Babies born to women who discontinue OCs or who conceive while ingesting OCs have no greater incidence of any type of birth defect.

- A significantly increased risk of developing cardiovascular disease occurs only in current OC users over age 35 who smoke or in women of any age who use OCs and also have some type of preexisting vascular disease, such as hypertension.

- The cause of myocardial infarction in older OC users who smoke is arterial thrombosis.

- Adverse effects produced by the estrogenic component of OCs include nausea, breast tenderness, fluid retention, temporary increase in blood pressure, thrombosis, changes in mood, and chloasma. Progestins produce certain androgenic adverse effects, including weight gain, nervousness, depression, tiredness, and acne, as well as failure of withdrawal bleeding or amenorrhea.

- Absolute contraindications for OC use include history of vascular disease (e.g., thromboembolism or thrombophlebitis), hypertension, diabetes mellitus with vascular disease, smoking after age 35, cancer of the breast or endometrium, pregnancy, and active liver disease. Relative contraindications to OC use include heavy cigarette smoking under age 35, migraine headaches, amenorrhea, and depression.

- In an ovulatory cycle the mean blood loss during menstruation is approximately 35 ml, compared with 20 ml for women ingesting OCs.

- OC users are about half as likely to develop iron deficiency anemia as are control subjects.

- OC users are significantly less likely to develop menorrhagia, irregular menstruation, or intermenstrual bleeding than nonusers.

- The risk of developing endometrial cancer, as well as ovarian cancer, in OC users is only half that in control subjects. OC users also have a 50% reduction in the incidence of benign breast disease.

- OC users have approximately 60% less dysmenorrhea and 39% less premenstrual tension than control subjects.

- Functional ovarian cysts occur infrequently in OC users.

- OCs reduce the clinical development of salpingitis (pelvic inflammatory disease [PID]) in women infected with gonorrhea or *Chlamydia* by 50%, and the overall incidence of PID in OC users is reduced 50%.

- OCs reduce the risk of ectopic pregnancy by more than 60% in women currently using them.

- OCs prevent approximately 50,000 women from being hospitalized in the United States each year as a result of their noncontraceptive health benefits.

- The three types of injectable contraception, depo-medroxyprogesterone acetate (DMPA), norethindrone enanthate, and progestin-estrogen combinations, are very effective but not approved for contraceptive use in the United States.

- Women using injectable DMPA (150 mg every 3 months) have a first-year pregnancy rate of 0.1%.

- Patients treated with injectable progestins for contraception have complete disruption of the normal menstrual cycle and a totally irregular bleeding pattern.

- Norplant releases sufficient amounts of levonorgestrel daily to maintain blood levels of 300 to 400 pg/ml for 5 years. The annual pregnancy rate with this method is approximately 0.2%, and its major side effect is abnormal bleeding.

- The most effective method of postcoital contraception is ingestion of high-dose estrogen for 5 days, whereas the most widely used is four tablets of ethinyl estradiol and norgestrel taken in doses of two tablets 12 hours apart.

- The cumulative incidence of accidental pregnancy with the copper T 380A IUD is 1.5% after 7 years of use.

- The incidence of adverse events with IUDs steadily decreases with increasing age of the patient.

- The main mechanism of contraceptive action of IUDs (other than the progesterone-releasing IUD) is production of a local sterile inflammatory reaction of leukocytes, which destroys sperm and prevents fertilization.

- Resumption of fertility after IUD removal is not delayed and occurs at the same rate as resumption after discontinuation of use of mechanical contraceptive methods.

- Several types of IUDs are approved for use in the United States—the plastic loop, the copper-bearing copper 7, the copper T 200, the copper T 380A, and the progesterone-releasing T-shaped device—but only the last two are currently marketed.

- During removal of a copper or progesterone-releasing IUD, the device can be removed and reinserted at the same clinic visit. The IUD can be safely inserted on any day of the cycle.

- In the first year of use, IUDs have approximately a 1% pregnancy rate, a 10% expulsion rate, and a 15% rate of removal for medical reasons, and the incidence of each of these events diminishes steadily in subsequent years.

- In women wearing a copper T IUD, 50 to 60 ml of blood is lost per cycle; with the progesterone-releasing IUD, the amount of blood loss is 25 ml per cycle.

- Mefenamic acid, 500 mg twice daily, significantly reduces menstrual blood loss in IUD users.

- IUD fundal perforation rates are about 1 in 1000 insertions. The incidence of cervical perforation by copper IUDs ranges from about 1 in 600 to 1 in 1000 insertions.

- No evidence shows an increased incidence of congenital anomalies in infants born with any type of IUD in utero.

- If a patient conceives with an IUD in place and the IUD is not removed, the incidence of spontaneous abortion is about 55%, approximately 3 times greater than would occur without an IUD. If, after conception, the IUD appendage is visible and the IUD is removed by traction, the incidence of spontaneous abortion is reduced to about 20%.

- If a patient conceives with an IUD in place, her chances of having an ectopic pregnancy range from 3% to 9%, approximately 10 times greater than occurs in conception without an IUD.

- Patients using an IUD have approximately a 60% lower overall risk of having an ectopic pregnancy than women using no method of contraception.

- The rate of prematurity among live births occurring with an IUD in situ is increased 2 to 4 times.

- The overall risk of PID in users of IUDs, excluding the shield type, is about 1.5 times that in control subjects, and a significantly increased risk of PID for the loop and copper IUDs is present only during the first 4 months after insertion.

- Pregnancy rates after reanastomosis of the vas range from 45% to 60%, whereas those after oviduct reanastomosis range from 50% to 80%.

- About 1% of sterilized women request reversal. In the United States approximately 7000 women request reversal each year.

- Usually about 15 to 20 ejaculations are required after vasectomy before a man is sterile.

- After vasectomy, two aspermic ejaculates are required before the male is considered sterile.

- The failure rate after laparoscopic fulguration of the oviducts is approximately 1 in 1000 procedures; with the clip and band techniques it is about 2 in 1000 procedures.

- In 1988 an estimated 1.6 million legal abortions were performed in the United States, and 29% of all pregnancies were terminated by induced abortion.

- Approximately 90% of elective abortions in the United States were performed at 12 weeks' gestation or less, and 50% during the first 8 weeks of pregnancy.

- Complication rates are 3 to 4 times higher for second-trimester abortions than for first-trimester abortions.

BIBLIOGRAPHY

Adams MR, Clarkson TB, Koritnik DR, and Nash HA: Contraceptive steriods and coronary artery atheroselerosis in cynomolgus macaques, Fertil Steril 47:1010, 1987.

Alvarez F, Guiloff E, Brache V, et al: New insights on the mode of action of intrauterine contraceptive devices in women, Fertil Steril 49:768, 1988.

Anderson ABM, Haynes PJ, Guillebaud J, et al: Reduction of menstrual blood loss by prostaglandin synthetase inhibitors, Lancet i:774, 1976.

Austin H, Louv WC, and Alexander WJ: A case-control study of spermicides and gonorrhea, JAMA 251:2822, 1984.

Back DJ, Breckenridge AM, Crawford FE, et al: The effects of rifampicin on the pharmacokinetics of ethinylestradiol in women, Contraception 21:135, 1980.

Beral V, Hannaford PC, and Kay C: Oral contraceptive use and malignancies of the genital tract, Lancet 2:1331, 1988.

Bowes WA, Katta LR, Droegemueller W, et al: Triphasic randomized clinical trial: comparison of effects on carbohydrate metabolism, Am J Obstet Gynecol 161:1402, 1989.

Brache V, Alvarez-Sanchez, Faundes A, et al: Ovarian endocrine function through 5 years of continuous treatment with Norplant® subdermal contraceptive implants, Contraception 41:169, 1990.

Brache V, Faundes A, Johansson E, et al: Anovulation, inadequate luteal phase and poor sperm penetration in cervical mucus during prolonged use of Norplant® implants, Contraception 31:261, 1985.

Bracken MB, Hellenbrand KG, and Holford TR: Conception delay after oral contraceptive use: the effect of estrogen dose, Fertil Steril 53:21, 1990.

Bracken MB and Vita K: Frequency of non-hormonal contraception around conception and association with congenital malformations in offspring, Am J Epidemiol 117:281, 1983.

Brenner PF and Mishell DR Jr: Progesterone and estradiol patterns in women using an intrauterine contraceptive device, Obstet Gynecol 46:456, 1975.

Brenner PF, Mishell DR Jr, Stanczyk FZ, et al: Serum levels of *d*-norgestrel, luteinizing hormone, follicle-stimulating hormone, estradiol, and progesterone in women during and following ingestion of combination oral contraceptives containing *dl*-norgestrel, Am J Obstet Gynecol 129:133, 1977.

Brinton LA, Vessey MP, Flavel R, et al: Risk factors for benign breast disease, Am J Epidemiol 113:203, 1981.

Brown JB, Blackwell LF, Billings JJ, et al: Natural family planning, Am J Obstet Gynecol 157:1082, 1987.

Cagen R: The cervical cap as a barrier contraceptive, Contraception 33:487, 1986.

The Cancer and Steroid Hormone Study of the Centers for Disease Control and the National Institute of Child Health and Human Development: Oral-contraceptive use and the risk of breast cancer, N Engl J Med 315:405, 1986.

The Cancer and Steroid Hormone Study of the Centers for Disease Control and the National Institute of Child Health and Human Development: The reduction in risk of ovarian cancer associated with oral-contraceptive use, N Engl J Med 316:650, 1987.

Celentano DD, Klassen AC, Weisman CS, and Rosenshein NB: The role of contraceptive use in cervical cancer: The Maryland Cervical Cancer Case-Control Study, Am J Epidemiol 126:592, 1987.

Centers for Disease Control: Combination oral contraceptive use and risk of endometrial cancer, JAMA 257:796, 1987.

Chi I-c, Potts M, Wilkens LR, et al: Performance of the Copper T-380A intrauterine device in breastfeeding women, Contraception 39:603, 1989.

Clarkson TB, Shively CA, Morgan TM, et al: Oral contraceptives and coronary artery atherosclerosis of cynomolgus monkeys, Obstet Gynecol 47:1010, 1990.

Conant MA, Spicer DW, and Smith CD: Herpes simplex virus transmission: condom studies, Sex Transm Dis 11:94, 1984.

Couzinet B, Le Strat N, Ulmann A, et al: Termination of early pregnancy by the progesterone antagonist RU 486 (mifepristone), N Engl J Med 315:1565, 1986.

Craig S and Hepburn S: The effectiveness of barrier methods of contraception with and without spermicide, Contraception 26:347, 1982.

Cramer DW, Goldman MB, Schiff I, et al: The relationship of tubal infertility to barrier method and oral contraceptive use, JAMA 257:2446, 1987.

Cramer DW, Schiff I, Schoenbaum SC, et al: Tubal infertility and the intrauterine device, N Engl J Med 312:941, 1985.

Croft P and Hannaford PC: Risk factors for acute myocardial infarction in women: evidence from the Royal College of General Practitioners' oral contraception study, Br Med J 298:165, 1989.

Crooij MJ, de Nooyer CCA, Rao BR, et al: Termination of early pregnancy by the 3b-hydroxysteroid dehydrogenase inhibitor epostane, N Engl J Med 319:813, 1988.

Croxatto HB, Diaz S, Pavez M, et al: Clearance of levonorgestrel from the circulation following removal of Norplant® subdermal implants, Contraception 38:509, 1988.

Croxatto HB, Diaz S, Pavez M, et al: Estradiol plasma levels during long-term treatment with Norplant® subdermal implants, Contraception 38:465, 1988.

Croxatto HB, Diaz S, Salvatierra AM, et al: Treatment with Norplant® subdermal implants inhibits sperm penetration through cervical mucus in vitro, Contraception 36:193, 1987.

Daling JR, Weiss NS, Metch BJ, et al: Primary tubal infertility in relation to the use of an intrauterine device, N Engl J Med 312:937, 1985.

Deslypere JP, Thiery M, and Vermeulen A: Effect of long-term hormonal contraception on plasma lipids, Contraception 31:633, 1985.

Diamond MP, Greene JW, Thompson JM, et al: Interaction of anticonvulsants and oral contraceptives in epileptic adolescents, Contraception 31:623, 1985.

Dixon GW, Schlesselman JJ, Ory HW, et al: Post-coital contraception: medical and social factors of the morning after pill, Contraception 15:445, 1977.

Dorflinger L: Relative potency of progestins used in oral contraceptives, Contraception 557:31, 1985.

Edelman DA and North BB: Updated pregnancy rates for the Today contraceptive sponge, Am J Obstet Gynecol 157:1164, 1987.

Fasoli M, Parazzini F, Cecchetti G, et al: Post-coital contraception: an overview of published studies, Contraception 39:459, 1989.

Fihn SD, Latham RH, Roberts P, et al: Association between diaphragm use and urinary tract infection, JAMA 254:240, 1986.

Forrest JD and Fordyce RR: U.S. women's contraceptive attitudes and practice: how have they changed in the 1980's? Fam Plann Perspect 20:112, 1988.

Glass R, Vessey M, and Wiggins P: Use-effectiveness of the condom in a selected family planning clinic population in the United Kingdom, Contraception 10:591, 1974.

Goebelsmann U, Stanczyk FZ, Brenner PF, et al: Serum norethindrone (NET) concentrations following intramuscular NET enanthate injection: effect upon serum LH, FSH, estradiol and progesterone, Contraception 19:283, 1979.

Grimes DA and Hughes JM: Use of multiphasic oral contraceptives and hospitalizations of women with functional ovarian cysts in the United States, Obstet Gynecol 73:1037, 1989.

Guillebaud J: Copper IUCDs and pregnancy (letter), Br J Fam Plann 7:88, 1981.

Guillebaud J, Barnett MD, and Gordon YB: Plasma ferritin levels as an index of iron deficiency in women using intrauterine devices, Br J Obstet Gynaecol 86:51, 1979.

Hall PE: Long-acting injectable formulations. In Diczfalusy E and Bygdeman M, eds: Fertility regulation today and tomorrow, vol 36, New York, 1987, Raven Press, p 119.

Hannaford PC and Kay CR: Oral contraceptives and diabetes mellitus, Br Med J 299:315, 1989.

Harlap S, Shiono PH, and Ramcharan S: Congenital abnormalities in the offspring of women who used oral and other contraceptives around the time of conception, Int J Fertil 30:39, 1985.

Hazes JMW, Dijkmans BAC, Vandenbroucke JP, et al: Reduction of the risk of rheumatoid arthritis among women who take oral contraceptives, Arthritis Rheum 33:173, 1990.

Healy DL, Baulieu EE, and Hodgen GD: Induction of menstruation by an antiprogesterone steroid (RU 486) in primates: site of action, dose-response relationships, and hormonal effects, Fertil Steril 40:253, 1983.

Hicks DR, Martin LS, Getchell JP, et al: Inactivation of HTLV-III/LAV-infected cultures of normal human lymphocytes by nonoxynol-9 in vitro, Lancet 2:1422, 1985.

Janerich DT, Piper JM, and Glebatis DM: Oral contraceptives and birth defects, Am J Epidemiol 112:73, 1980.

Jick H, Hanna MT, Stergachis A, et al: Vaginal spermicides and gonorrhea, JAMA 248:1619, 1982.

Kalkhoff RK: Relative sensitivity of postpartum gestational diabetic women to oral contraceptive agents and other metabolic stress, Diabetes Care 3:421, 1980.

Kay CR: Progestins and arterial disease—evidence from the Royal College of General Practitioners' study, Am J Obstet Gynecol 142:762, 1982.

Kay CR: The Royal College of General Practitioners' Oral Contraception Study: some recent observations, Clin Obstet Gynaecol 11:759, 1984.

Kay CR and Hannaford PC: Breast cancer and the pill—a further report from the Royal College of General Practitioners' Oral Contraception Study, Br J Cancer 58:676, 1988.

Kelaghan J, Rubin GL, Ory HW, and Layde PM: Barrier-method contraceptives and pelvic inflammatory disease, JAMA 248:184, 1982.

Khaw K-T and Peart WS: Blood pressure and contraceptive use, Br Med J 285:403, 1982.

Kjos SL, Shoupe D, Douhan S, et al: Effect of low-dose oral contraceptives on carbohydrate and lipid metabolism in women with recurrent gestational diabetes: results of a controlled randomized prospective study, Am J Obstet Gynecol 163(6):1822, 1990.

Klaus H: Natural family planning: a review, Obstet Gynecol Surv 37:128, 1982.

Klitsch M: FDA approval ends cervical cap's marathon, Fam Plann Perspect 20:137, 1988.

Kloosterboer HJ, van Wayjen RG, and van den Ende A: Comparative effects of monophasic desogestrel plus ethinyloestradiol and triphasic levonorgestrel plus ethinyloestradiol on lipid metabolism, Contraception 34:135, 1986.

Knopp RH, Walden CE, Wahl PW, and Hoover JJ: Effects of oral contraceptives on lipoprotein triglyceride and cholesterol: relationships to estrogen and progestin potency, Am J Obstet Gynecol 142:725, 1982.

Koetsawang S: The effects of contraceptive methods on the quality and quantity of breast milk, Int J Gynaecol Obstet 25(suppl):115, 1987.

Kovacs GT, Jarman H, Dunn K, et al: The contraceptive diaphragm: is it an acceptable method in the 1980's? Aust NZ J Obstet Gynaecol 26:76, 1986.

Kung AW, Ma JT, Wong VC, et al: Glucose and lipid metabolism with triphasic oral contraceptives in women with history of gestational diabetes, Contraception 35:257, 1987.

Larsson B, Hamberger L, and Rybo G: Influence of copper intrauterine devices (Cu-7-IUD) on the menstrual blood-loss, Acta Obstet Gynecol Scand 54:315, 1975.

Layde PM, Ory HW, and Schlesselman JJ: The risk of myocardial infarction in former users of oral contraceptives, Fam Plann Perspect 14:78, 1982.

Lee NC and Rubin GL: The intrauterine device and pelvic inflammatory disease revisited: new results from the women's health study, Obstet Gynecol 72:1, 1988.

Lee NC, Rubin GL, Ory HW, et al: Type of intrauterine device and the risk of pelvic inflammatory disease, Obstet Gynecol 62:1, 1983.

Liedholm P, Rybo G, Sjöjberg N-O, et al: Copper IUD—influence on menstrual blood loss and iron deficiency, Contraception 12:317, 1975.

Liew DFM, Ng CSA, Yong YM, et al: Long-term effects of depo-provera on carbohydrate and lipid metabolism, Contraception 31:51, 1985.

Linn S, Schoenbaum SC, Monson RR, et al: Lack of association between contraceptive usage and congenital malformations in offspring, Am J Obstet Gynecol 147:923, 1983.

Lipson A, Stoy DB, LaRosa JC, et al: Progestins and oral contraceptive–induced lipoprotein changes: a prospective study, Contraception 34:121, 1986.

Liskin L and Fox G: Periodic abstinence: how well do new approaches work? Popul Rep (I) 9:33, 1981.

Lönnerdel B, Forsum E, and Hambraeus L: Effect of oral contraceptives on composition and volume of breast milk, Am J Clin Nutr 33:816, 1980.

Louik C, Mitchell AA, Werler MM, et al: Maternal exposure to spermicides in relation to certain birth defects, N Engl J Med 317:474, 1987.

Luukkainen T, Allonen H, Haukkamaa M, et al: Five years' experience with levonorgestrel-releasing IUDs, Contraception 33:139, 1986.

Luyckx AS, Gaspard UJ, Romus MA, et al: Carbohydrate metabolism in women who used oral contraceptives containing levonorgestrel or desogestrel: a 6-month prospective study, Fertil Steril 45:635, 1986.

Makinen JI, Salmi TA, Nikkanen VPJ, et al: Encouraging rates of fertility after ectopic pregnancy, Int J Fertil 34:46, 1989.

Mant D, Villard-Mackintosh L, Vessey MP, et al: Myocardial infarction and angina pectoris in young women, J Epidemiol Community Health 41:215, 1987.

McIntyre SL and Higgins JE: Parity and use-effectiveness with the contraceptive sponge, Am J Obstet Gynecol 155:796, 1986.

Meade TW: Oral contraceptives, clotting factors, and thrombosis, Am J Obstet Gynecol 142:758, 1982.

Meade TW, Greenberg G, and Thompson SG: Progestogens and cardiovascular reactions associated with oral contraceptives and a comparison of the safety of 50- and 30-μg oestrogen preparations, Br Med J 280:1157, 1980.

Medina JE, Cifuentes A, Abernathy JR, et al: Comparative evaluation of two methods of natural family planning in Columbia, Am J Obstet Gynecol 138:1142, 1980.

Mileikowsky GN, Nadler JL, Huey F, et al: Evidence that smoking alters prostacyclin formation and platelet aggregation in women who use oral contraceptives, Am J Obstet Gynecol 159:1547, 1988.

Mishell DR Jr: Noncontraceptive health benefits of oral steroidal contraceptives, Am J Obstet Gynecol 142:809, 1982.

Mishell DR Jr, Bell JH, Good RG, et al: The intrauterine device: a bacteriologic study of the endometrial cavity, Am J Obstet Gynecol 96:119, 1966.

Mishell DR Jr, Kletzky OA, Brenner PF, et al: The effect of contraceptive steroids on hypothalamic-pituitary function, Am J Obstet Gynecol 128:60, 1977.

Mishell DR Jr and Roy S: Copper intrauterine contraceptive device event rates following insertion 4 to 8 weeks postpartum, Am J Obstet Gynecol 143:29, 1982.

Mishell DR Jr, Thorneycroft IH, Nakamura RM, et al: Serum estradiol in women ingesting combination oral contraceptive steroids, Am J Obstet Gynecol 114:923, 1972.

Moore DE, Roy S, Stanczyk FZ, et al: Bleeding and serum d-norgestrel, estradiol, and progesterone patterns in women using d-norgestrel subdermal polysiloxane capsules for contraception, Contraception 17:315, 1978.

Mosher WD and Pratt WF: Contraceptive use in the United States, 1973-88, Patient Educ Couns 16:163; 1990.

Moyer DL and Mishell DR Jr: Reactions of human endometrium to the intrauterine foreign body. II. Long-term effects on the endometrial histology and cytology, Am J Obstet Gynecol 111:66, 1971.

Murray PP, Stadel BV, and Schlesselman JJ: Oral contraceptive use in women with a family history of breast cancer, Obstet Gynecol 73:977, 1989.

Nilsson CG and Holma P: Menstrual blood loss with contraceptive subdermal levonorgestrel implants, Fertil Steril 35:304, 1981.

Nilsson S, Mellbin T, Hofvander Y, et al: Long-term follow-up of children breast-fed by mothers using oral contraceptives, Contraception 34:443, 1986.

Notelovitz M, Feldman EB, Gillespy M, et al: Lipid and lipoprotein changes in women taking low-dose, triphasic oral contraceptives: a controlled, comparative, 12-month clinical trial, Am J Obstet Gynecol 160:1269, 1989.

Notelovitz M, Levenson I, McKenzie L, et al: The effects of low-dose oral contraceptives on coagulation and fibrinolysis in two high-risk populations: young female smokers and older premenopausal women, Am J Obstet Gynecol 152:995, 1985.

Ortiz A, Hiroi M, Stanczyk FZ, et al: Serum medroxyprogesterone acetate (MPA) concentrations and ovarian function following intramuscular injection of depo-MPA, J Clin Endocrinol Metab 44:32, 1977.

Ory HW: Functional ovarian cysts and oral contraceptives, JAMA 228:68, 1974.

Ory HW: Ectopic pregnancy and intrauterine contraceptive devices: new perspectives, The Women's Health Study, Obstet Gynecol 57:137, 1981.

Ory HW: The noncontraceptive health benefits from oral contraceptive use, Fam Plann Perspect 14:182, 1982.

Pardthaisong T: Return of fertility after use of the injectable contraceptive Depo Provera: updated data analysis, J Biosoc Sci 16:23, 1984.

Patsch W, Brown SA, Gotto AM, et al: The effect of triphasic oral contraceptives on plasma lipids and lipoproteins, Am J Obstet Gynecol 161:1396, 1989.

Percival-Smith RKL and Abercrombie B: Postcoital contraception with dl-norgestrel/ethinyl estradiol combination: six years experience in a student medical clinic, Contraception 36:287, 1987.

Percival-Smith RK, Morrison BJ, Sizto R, et al: The effect of triphasic and biphasic oral contraceptive preparations on HDL-cholesterol and LDL-cholesterol in young women, Contraception 35:179, 1987.

Perlman JA, Russell-Briefel R, Ezzati T, et al: Oral glucose tolerance and the potency of contraceptive progestins, J Chron Dis 38:857, 1985.

Persson E, Holmberg K, Dahlgren S, et al: Actinomyces Israelii in genital tract of women with and without intrauterine contraceptive devices, Acta Obstet Gynecol Scand 62:563, 1983.

Piedras J, Cordova MS, Perez-Toral MC, et al: Predictive value of serum ferritin in anemia development after insertion of T Cu 220 intrauterine device, Contraception 27:289, 1983.

Pituitary Adenoma Study Group: Pituitary adenomas and oral contraceptives: a multicenter case-control study, Fertil Steril 39:753, 1983.

Poland B: Conception control and embryonic development, Am J Obstet Gynecol 106:365, 1970.

Porter JB, Hunter JR, Danielson DA, et al: Oral contraceptives and nonfatal vascular disease—recent experience, Obstet Gynecol 59:299, 1982.

Porter JB, Hunter JR, Jick H, et al: Oral contraceptives and nonfatal vascular disease, Obstet Gynecol 66:1, 1985.

Porter JB, Jick H, and Walker AM: Mortality among oral contraceptive users, Obstet Gynecol 70:29, 1987.

Powell MG, Mears BJ, Deber RB, et al: Contraception with the cervical cap: effectiveness, safety, continuity of use, and user satisfaction, Contraception 33:215, 1986.

Prentice RL and Thomas DB: On the epidemiology of oral contraceptives and disease, Adv Cancer Res 49:285, 1987.

Rogow D, Rintoul EJ and Greenwood S: A year's experience with a fertility awareness program: a report, Adv Planned Parenthood 15:27, 1980.

Rosenberg L, Palmer JR, Lesko SM, et al: Oral contraceptive use and the risk of myocardial infarction, Am J Epidemiol 131:1009, 1990.

Rosenberg MJ, Rojanapithayakorn W, Feldblum PJ, et al: Effect of the contraceptive sponge on chlamydial infection, gonorrhea, and candidiasis, JAMA 257:2308, 1987.

Rothman KJ and Louik C: Oral contraceptives and birth defects, N Engl J Med 299:522, 1978.

Roy S, Robertson D, Krauss RM, et al: Long-term reversible contraception with levonorgestrel-releasing Silastic rods, Am J Obstet Gynecol 148:1006, 1984.

Rybo G: The IUD and endometrial bleeding, J Reprod Med 20:175, 1978.

Rydén G, Fåhraeus L, Molin L, et al: Do contraceptives influence the incidence of acute pelvic inflammatory disease in women with gonorrhoea? Contraception 20:149, 1979.

Sandvei R, Ulstein M, and Wollen A-L: Fertility following ectopic pregnancy with special reference to previous use of an intra-uterine contraceptive device (IUCD), Acta Obstet Gynecol Scand 66:131, 1987.

Schlesselman JJ: Cancer of the breast and reproductive tract in relation to use of oral contraceptives, Contraception 40:1, 1989.

Scott JA, Kletzky OA, Brenner PF, et al: Comparison of the effects of contraceptive steroid formulations containing two doses of estrogen on pituitary function, Fertil Steril 30:141, 1978.

Sennayake P and Kramer DG: Contraception and the etiology of pelvic inflammatory disease: new perspectives, Am J Obstet Gynecol 138:852, 1980.

Shalev E, Edelstein S, Engelhard J, et al: Ultrasonically controlled retrieval of an intrauterine contraceptive device (IUCD) in early pregnancy, J Clin Ultrasound 15:525, 1987.

Shively CA, Kaplan JR, and Clarkson TB: Carotid artery atherosclerosis in cholesterol-fed female cynomolgus monkeys, Arteriosclerosis 10:358, 1990.

Silvestre L, Dubois C, Renault M, et al: Voluntary interruption of pregnancy with mifepristone (RU 486) and a prostaglandin analogue, N Engl J Med 322:645, 1990.

Sinei SKA, Schultz KF, Lamptey PR, et al: Preventing IUCD-related pelvic infection: the efficacy of prophylactic doxycycline at insertion, Br J Obstet Gynecol 97:412, 1990.

Sivin I: Copper T IUD use and ectopic pregnancy rates in the United States, Contraception 19:151, 1979.

Sivin I: International experience with Norplant® and Norplant®-2, Stud Fam Plann 19:81, 1988.

Sivin I, Mahgoub SE, McCarthy T, et al: Long-term contraception with the Levorgestrel 20 mcg/day and the Copper T 380Ag intrauterine devices: a five-year randomized study, Contraception 42(4):361, 1990.

Sivin I and Tatum HJ: Four years of experience with the T Cu 380A intrauterine contraceptive device, Fertil Steril 36:159, 1981.

Skouby SO, Kühl C, Mølsted-Pedersen L, et al: Triphasic oral contraception: metabolic effects in normal women and those with previous gestational diabetes, Am J Obstet Gynecol 153:495, 1985.

Spector TD, Roman E, and Silman AJ: The pill, parity, and rheumatoid arthritis, Arthritis Rheum 33:782, 1990.

Stadel BV, Lai S, Schlesselman JJ, et al: Oral contraceptives and premenopausal breast cancer in nulliparous women, Contraception 38:287, 1988.

Stadel BV, Schlesselman JJ, and Murray PA: Oral contraceptives and breast cancer, Lancet 1:1257, 1989.

Stampfer MJ, Willett WC, Colditz GA, et al: A prospective study of past use of oral contraceptive agents and risk of cardiovascular diseases, N Engl J Med 319:1313, 1988.

Stone KM, Grimes DA, and Magdar LS: Personal protection against sexually transmitted diseases, Am J Obstet Gynecol 155:180, 1986.

Strobino B, Kline J, Lai A, et al: Vaginal spermicides and spontaneous abortion of known karyotype, Am J Epidemiol 123:431, 1986.

Strom BL, Tamragouri RN, Morse ML, et al: Oral contraceptives and other risk factors for gallbladder disease, Clin Pharmacol Ther 39:335, 1986.

Stubblefield PG, Fuller AF, and Foster SC: Ultrasound-guided intrauterine removal of intrauterine contraceptive devices in pregnancy, Obstet Gynecol 72:961, 1988.

Swyer GIM: Potency of progestogens in oral contraceptives—further delay of menses data, Contraception 26:23, 1982.

Tatum HJ, Schmidt FH, and Jain AK: Management and outcome of pregnancies associated with the Copper T intrauterine contraceptive device, Am J Obstet Gynecol 126:869, 1976.

Tietze C and Lewis S: Evaluation of intrauterine devices: ninth progress report of the Cooperative Statistical Program, Stud Fam Plann 1:55, 1970.

Tredway DR, Umezaki CU, and Mishell DR Jr: Effect of intrauterine devices on sperm transport in the human being: preliminary report, Am J Obstet Gynecol 123:734, 1975.

Treiman K and Liskin L: IUDs—a new look, Popul Rep (B) 5:2, 1988.

Trussell J, Hatcher RA, Cates W Jr, et al: Contraceptive failure in the United States: an update, Stud Fam Plann 21:51, 1990.

Trussell J and Kost K: Contraceptive failure in the United States: a critical review of the literature, Stud Fam Plann 18:237, 1987.

UK National Case Control Study Group: Oral contraceptive use and breast cancer risk in young women, Lancet 1:973, 1989.

van der Vange N, Kloosterboer HG, and Haspels AA: Effect of seven low-dose combined oral contraceptive preparations on carbohydrate metabolism, Am J Obstet Gynecol 156:918, 1987.

Vessey MP, Johnson B, Doll R, et al: Outcome of pregnancy in women using an intrauterine device, Lancet i:495, 1974.

Vessey MP, Lawless M, McPherson K, et al: Fertility after stopping use of intrauterine contraceptive device, Br Med J 286:106, 1983.

Vessey M, Lawless M, and Yagi J: Contraceptive failure in the United States: estimates from the 1982 National Survey of Family Growth, Fam Plann Perspect 18:200, 1986.

Vessey M, Lawless M, and Yeates D: Efficacy of different contraceptive methods, Lancet 1:841, 1982.

Vessey M, Meisler L, Flavel R, et al: Outcome of pregnancy in women using different methods of contraception, Br J Obstet Gynaecol 86:548, 1979.

Vessey M, Metcalfe A, Wells C, et al: Ovarian neoplasma, functional ovarian cysts, and oral contraceptives, Br Med J 294:1518, 1987.

Vessey MP, Villard-Mackintosh L, McPherson K, et al: Mortality among oral contraceptive users: 20 year follow up of women in a cohort study, Br Med J 299:1487, 1989.

Vessey MP, Wright NH, McPherson K, et al: Fertility after stopping different methods of contraception, Br Med J 1:265, 1978.

Wade ME, McCarthy P, Abernathy JR, et al: A randomized prospective study of the use-effectiveness of two methods of natural family planning. Presented at the International Federation for Family Life Promotion Second International Congress, Navan, Ireland, Sept 24-Oct 1, 1980.

Wahl P, Walden C, Knopp R, et al: Effect of estrogen/progestin potency on lipid/lipoprotein cholesterol, N Engl J Med 308:862, 1981.

Warner P and Bancroft J: Mood, sexuality, oral contraceptives and the menstrual cycle, J Psychosom Res 32:417, 1988.

White MK, Ory HW, Rooks JB, et al: Intrauterine device termination rates and the menstrual cycle day of insertion, Obstet Gynecol 55:220, 1980.

Williams P, Johnson B, and Vessey M: Septic abortion in women using intrauterine devices, Br Med J 4:253, 1975.

Wilson ESB, Cruickshank J, McMaster M, et al: A prospective controlled study of the effect on blood pressure of contraceptive preparations containing different types and dosages of progestogen, Br J Obstet Gynaecol 91:1254, 1984.

Wilson JG and Brent RL: Are female sex hormones teratogenic? Am J Obstet Gynecol 141:567, 1981.

Wølner-Hanssen P, Svensson L, Mårdh P-A, et al: Laparoscopic findings and contraceptive use in women with signs and symptoms suggestive of acute salpingitis, Obstet Gynecol 66:233, 1985.

World Health Organization: A prospective multicentre trial of the ovulation method of natural family planning. II. The effectiveness phase, Fertil Steril 36:591, 1981.

World Health Organization: A prospective multicentre trial of the ovulation method of natural family planning. III. Characteristics of the menstrual cycle and of the fertile phase, Fertil Steril 40:773, 1983.

World Health Organization: Depo-medroxyprogesterone acetate (DMPA) and cancer: memorandum from a WHO meeting, Bull WHO 64:375, 1986.

World Health Organization: Combined oral contraceptives and liver cancer, Int J Cancer 43:254, 1989.

World Health Organization (WHO): The TCu220C, multiload 250 and Nova T IUDs at 3, 5, and 7 years of use: results from three randomized multicentre trials, Contraception 42:141, 1990.

World Health Organization Expanded Programme of Research, Development and Research Training in Human Reproduction Task Force on Long-Acting Systemic Agents for the Regulation of Fertility: Multinational comparative clinical evaluation of two long-acting injectable contraceptive steroids: norethisterone enanthate and medroxyprogesterone acetate. I. Use-effectiveness, Contraception 15:5, 1977.

World Health Organization Expanded Programme of Research, Development and Research Training in Human Reproduction Task Force on Long-Acting Systemic Agents for the Regulation of Fertility: Multinational comparative clinical evaluation of two long-acting injectable contraceptive steroids: norethisterone enanthate and medroxyprogesterone acetate—final report, Contraception 28:1, 1983.

World Health Organization Task Force on Oral Contraceptives: A randomized, double-blind study of two combined and two progestogen-only oral contraceptives, Contraception 25:243, 1982.

12 | Rape, Incest, and Abuse

――――――― KEY TERMS AND DEFINITIONS ―――――――

Abuse. This may be defined as aggressive behavior including acts of a sexual or physical nature, verbal belittling, or intimidation. The act may be premeditated, as when one individual wishes to gain control over another, or spontaneous, as a spontaneous response to anger or frustration.

Battered Wife Syndrome. A symptom complex occurring as a result of violence in which a woman has at any time received deliberate, severe, or repeated (more than three times) physical abuse from her husband, with minimal injury of severe bruising.

Battered Woman. Any woman over the age of 16 with evidence of physical abuse on at least one occasion at the hands of an intimate male partner.

Cycle of Battering. Three phases in the cycle of battering are noted: The first is tension building; the second is the act of violence; and the third is the apology and forgiveness phase. As cycles are repeated, the second phase tends to become more violent and the third less intensive.

Domestic Violence. Violence occurring between partners in an ongoing relationship regardless of whether or not they are married.

Incest. Sexual intimacy with or without coitus involving a close family member. The act may include fondling, exposure, or the penetration of an orifice by the phallus.

Rape. Any act of sexual intimacy performed by one person on another without mutual consent by force, by threat of force, or by the inability of the victim to give appropriate consent.

Rape-Trauma Syndrome. A set of behaviors that occur after a rape. The immediate response (acute phase) lasts hours to days and reflects a distortion or paralysis of the individual's coping mechanisms, but the outward responses vary from complete loss of emotional control to an apparently well-controlled behavior pattern. The delayed (or organization) phase involves flashbacks, nightmares, and a need for reorganization of thought process. It may occur months to years after the event and may involve major life-style adjustments.

Rape, incest, and other forms of physical and sexual abuse are very common. Physicians in general and obstetricians and gynecologists in particular are in a position to detect these problems and offer treatment and counsel when their patients have been found to be victims. In the acute state, a careful history using a compassionate and nonjudgmental approach will often allow an accurate story to be obtained. When the patient seeks medical advice at a time remote from the experience or when the experience is ongoing, the presenting chief complaint may have little to do with the actual problem. For the physician to elicit a clear picture, it is necessary to resort to open-ended questions and interviewing techniques that allow the patient to comfortably discuss truthfully the actual problem.

These patients are at risk for severe physical and emotional distress, and as victims they may suffer psychological damage to their self-image, which in turn may lead to many long-term poor choices in important life situations. Although rape, incest, and abuse will be discussed separately, there is frequently a relationship in the social pathology involved, as well as in the long-term effects that the patient must endure. In each instance appropriate physician response and physician responsibility will be discussed.

RAPE

Rape, or the sexual assault of children, women, and men, is a common act. Only recently has society identified the real scope of this problem. In 1978 an FBI report indicated that nearly 200,000 rapes were reported nationwide each year and that this could likely represent no more than 50% of the actual rapes committed. Victims, even today, are reluctant to report rapes to authorities because of embarrassment, fear of retribution, feelings of guilt, or simply lack of knowledge of their rights.

In the past, society has held many misconceptions about the rape victim, particularly a female. These included the notion that the individual encouraged the rape by specific behavior or dress and that no person who did not wish to be raped could be raped. Further, the feeling that rape was an indication of basic promiscuity was widely held. In many instances sexual assault victims were accused of lying to cause problems for otherwise innocent men. To some extent many of these societal misconceptions are held today.

Sexual assault happens to people of all ages and races in all socioeconomic groups. The very young, the mentally and physically handicapped, and the very old are particularly susceptible. Although the perpetrator may be a stranger, he or she is often an individual well known to the victim.

In submitting, the victim loses control over his or her life for that period and frequently experiences anxiety and fear. When the attack is life threatening, shock with associated physical and psychological symptoms may occur. Burgess and Holmstrom identify two phases of the rape-trauma syndrome.

The immediate or acute phase lasts from hours to days and may be associated with a paralysis of the individual's usual coping mechanisms. Outwardly, the victim may demonstrate manifestations ranging from complete loss of emotional control to a well-controlled behavior pattern. The actual reaction may depend on a number of factors, including the relationship of the victim to the attacker, whether force was used, and the length of time the victim was held against his or her will. Generally, the victim appears disorganized and may complain of both physical and emotional symptoms. Physical complaints include specific injuries or general complaints of soreness, eating problems, headaches, and sleep disturbances. Behavior patterns may include fear, mood swings, irritability, guilt, anger, depression, and difficulties in concentrating. Frequently the victim will complain of flashbacks to the attack. Medical care is often sought during the acute period, and at this point it is the physician's responsibility to assess the specific medical problems and also to offer a program of emotional support and reassurance.

The second phase of the rape-trauma syndrome involves long-term adjustment and is designated the reorganization phase. During this time flashbacks and nightmares may continue, but phobias may also develop. These may be directed against members of the opposite sex, the sex act itself, or nonrelated circumstances, such as a newly developed fear of crowds or heights. During this period the victim may institute a number of important lifestyle changes, including changes of job, residence, friends, and significant others. If major complications such as the contraction of a sexually transmitted disease or a pregnancy occurs, resolution may be more difficult. The reorganization period may last from months to years and generally involves an attempt on the part of the victim to regain control over his or her life. During this time medical care and counseling must be nonjudgmental, sensitive, and anticipatory. When the physician realizes that the patient is contemplating a major life-style change during this period, it is probably appropriate to point out to the patient the reasons why the change is being contemplated and the complicating effects it may have on the patient's overall well-being.

Physician's Responsibility in the Care of a Rape Victim

Although any individual may become a rape victim, this discussion will be limited to the care of a female, as is appropriate for a gynecology textbook. The physician's responsibility may be divided into three categories: medical, medical-legal, and supportive, as shown in the box on the facing page.

Medical

The physician's medical responsibilities are to treat injuries and to perform appropriate tests for, to prevent, and to treat infections and pregnancies. Experience derived at the Sexual Assault Center in Seattle, Washington, demonstrated that between 12% and 40% of victims who are sexually assaulted have injuries. Most of these, however, are minor and require simple reparative therapy. Only about 1% require hospitalization and major operative repair. Nonetheless, the victim will perceive the experience as life threatening, as in many cases it may have been. Many injuries occur when the victim is restrained or physically coerced into the sexual act. Thus the physician should seek bruises, abrasions, or lacerations about the neck, back, buttocks, or extremities. Where a knife was used as a coercive tactic, small cuts may also be found. Erythema, lacerations, and edema of the vulva and/or rectum may occur because of manipulation of these areas with the hand or the penis. These are particularly common in children or virginal victims but may occur in any woman and should be sought. Superficial or extensive lacerations of the hymen and/or vagina may occur in virginal victims or in the elderly. Lacerations may also be noted in the area of the urethra, the rectum, and at times through the vaginal vault into the abdominal cavity. In addition, bite marks may be noted in any of these regions. Occasionally, foreign objects are inserted into the vagina, the urethra, or the rectum and may be found.

In recent years, some authorities have advised close inspection with a magnifying glass or colposcope of the vulva and vagina of infants and children suspected to be victims of rape. Muram and Elias, however, in a study of 130 prepubertal girls (mean age 5.5) identified as victims of sexual abuse, could identify evidence of trauma in 96% with unaided inspection. Four additional cases were identified by colposcopy, but the lesions were obvious on repeat unaided examination. Simple visual examination without the aid of a colposcope should be sufficient to detect signs of trauma in children.

Where oral penetration has been effected, injury of the mouth and pharynx should be sought.

INFECTION. Most victims are concerned about possible infections incurred as a result of the rape, but until recently no careful follow-up studies in victims had been performed.

PHYSICIAN'S RESPONSIBILITIES IN CARING FOR RAPE-TRAUMA VICTIM

Medical
  Treat injuries
  Diagnose and treat STD
  Prevent pregnancy
Medical-legal
  Document history carefully
  Examine patient thoroughly and specifically note injuries
  Collect articles of clothing
  Collect vaginal (rectal and pharyngeal) samples for sperm and acid phosphatase
  Comb pubic hair for hair samples
  Collect fingernail scrapings where appropriate
  Collect saliva for secretion substance
  Turn specimens over to forensic authorities and receive receipts for chart
Emotional support
  Discuss degree of injury, probability of infection, and possibility of pregnancy
  Discuss general course that can be predicted
  Consult with rape-trauma counselor
  Arrange follow-up visit for medical and emotional evaluation in 1 to 4 weeks
  Reassure as far as possible

To determine actual risk it is important to know the prevalence of existing sexually transmitted diseases in the victim population. Recently, Jenny et al. examined 204 girls and women within 72 hours of a rape and discovered that 88 (43%) were harboring at least one STD. These included *Neisseria gonorrhoeae* in 13 of 204 (6% of all tested), cytomegalovirus in 13 of 170 (8%), *Chlamydia trachomatis* in 20 of 198 (10.1%), *Trichomonas vaginalis* in 30 of 204 (14.7%), herpes simplex virus in 4 of 170 (2.4%), *Treponema pallidum* in 2 of 199 (1.0%), HIV-I in 1 of 123 (0.8%) and bacterial vaginosis in 70 of 204 (34.3%). In 109 patients (53%) who returned for follow-up (excluding those who were found to be infected on the first visit or who were treated prophylactically), there were 3 of 71 (4%) cases of gonorrhea, 1 of 65 (20%) of chlamydia, 10 of 81 (12%) of trichomoniasis, and 15 of 77 (19%) of bacterial vaginosis. These authors concluded that women who were raped have a higher than average prevalence of preexisting STDs but are also at a substantial risk of acquiring such disease as a result of the assault.

It must be remembered that infection may not be limited to the vagina but may also include the pharynx or the rectum. Specific history to raise a suspicion of this possibility should be sought. Cultures should be performed for *Neisseria gonorrhoeae* and *Chlamydia trachomatis*. In addition, investigation for syphilis, using either dark-field studies and serology at the time the victim is seen and at a follow-up visit or serology alone, should be performed.

Because the victim is also at risk for infection by the herpes virus, hepatitis B virus, cytomegalovirus, HIV, condyloma acuminatum, and a variety of other sexually transmitted diseases, the physician may wish to screen for those that seem appropriate at the time the victim is seen in the acute stage.

Cultures of the cervical mucus for *Neisseria* gonococcus and for *Chlamydia trachomatis* are indicated. In addition, cultures of the rectum and of the oral pharynx are indicated when the history suggests that this would be productive. A wet mount for *Trichomonas vaginalis* and a potassium hydroxide mount for *Candida albicans* are also useful (see box below).

At follow-up visits the patient should again be investigated for signs and symptoms of the sexually transmitted diseases and appropriate repeat cultures and serologies should be obtained.

SEXUALLY TRANSMITTED DISEASES AND TESTS AVAILABLE TO PHYSICIANS CARING FOR A RAPE-TRAUMA VICTIM

Should perform
    Gonorrhea—culture for *Neisseria gonorrhoeae*
    Chlamydia trachomatis—culture
    Syphilis—dark-field microscopy, serology
Could perform
    Herpes simplex—culture lesion or serology
    Hepatitis B—screening serology
    HIV—serology
    Cytomegalovirus—serology
    Condyloma virus—study lesion
    Trichomonas—saline preparation
    Candida—potassium hydroxide preparation

Prophylactic antibiotics are useful in acute rape victim management. The patient should be given a single dose of ceftriaxone 250 mg IM plus doxycycline 100 mg PO two times a day for 7 days. An alternative therapy is spectinomycin 2 g IM (single dose) followed by doxycycline. If the patient is pregnant, erythromycin may be substituted for doxycycline. This should prevent gonorrhea, syphilis, and *Chlamydia* infection but will have no effect on herpes, condylomata, or many of the other problems mentioned.

PREGNANCY. The patient's menstrual history, birth control regimen, and known pregnancy status should be assessed. If the patient is at risk for pregnancy at the time of the assault, an appropriate "morning after" prophylaxis can be offered. This is discussed more fully in Chapter 11. In the experience of most sexual assault centers the chance of pregnancy occurring is quite low. It has been estimated to be approximately 2% to 4% of victims having a single, unprotected coitus. However, if the patient has been exposed at midcycle, the risk will be higher.

Medical-Legal

To be meaningful, medical-legal material must be collected shortly after the assault takes place. Victims should be encouraged to come immediately to a center where they can be evaluated before bathing, urinating, defecating, washing out their mouths, changing clothes, or cleaning their fingernails. In general, evidence for coitus will be present in the vagina for as long as 48 hours after the attack, but in other orifices the evidence may last only up to 6 hours. Appropriate tests should document the patient's physical and emotional condition as judged by her history and physical examination and should include data that document that force was used, evidence for sexual contact, and materials that may help identify the offender. To document that force was used, the physician should carefully describe each injury noted and possibly illustrate with either drawings or photographs. Detail is important, because injuries suffered by sexual assault victims have common patterns.

Documentation of sexual contact must begin with a history of when the patient had intercourse before the attack. If sperm or semen is found in the vagina or cervix of a victim, it must not be confused with such substances deposited during the victim's prior consenting sexual acts. Sexual contact will be verified by analysis of secretions from the vagina or rectum, seeking motile sperm and the presence of acid phosphatase. Nonmotile sperm may be present as well if the attack occurred 12 to 20 hours previously. In some instances, motile sperm will be noted for as long as 2 to 3 days in the endocervix.

It is difficult to ascertain whether ejaculation occurred in the mouth, because residual seminal fluid is rapidly destroyed by bacteria and salivary enzymes, making documentation of such an event difficult after more than a few hours have passed. Seminal fluid may be found staining the skin or the clothing several hours after the attack, and this should be sought. Because acid phosphatase is an enzyme found in high concentrations in seminal fluid, substances removed for analysis should be tested for this enzyme. Table 12-1 demonstrates the survival time of sperm in the pharynx, rectum, and cervix.

In addition to documenting that intercourse has taken place, an attempt should be made to identify the perpetrator. In this regard, all clothing intimately associated with the area of assault should be collected, labeled, and submitted to legal authorities. In addition, smears of vaginal secretions or a Pap smear should be made to permanently document the presence of sperm. Vaginal secretions needed for acid phosphatase reaction and DNA typing should be collected by wet or dry swab and refrigerated until a pathologist can process them. Pubic hair combings should be obtained to attempt to obtain pubic hair of the assaulter. Saliva should be collected from the victim to ascertain whether she secretes an antigen that could differentiate her from substances obtained from the perpetrator. Finally, fingernail scrapings should be obtained for skin or blood if the victim scratched the perpetrator. Specific blood or DNA typing may be conducted to help identify the attacker. All materials collected should be labeled and turned over to the legal authority or pathologist, depending on the system of the unit. A receipt should be obtained, and this should be documented in the patient's chart.

Emotional Support of the Victim

After the physical needs of the patient have been met and after the physician has carefully documented the information concerning the sexual contact, he or she should discuss with the victim the degree of injury, probability of infection or pregnancy, general course that the victim might be expected to follow with respect to these, and how follow-up to aid prevention will be carried out. The physician must allow the victim to give vent to anxieties and to correct misconceptions. The physician should reassure her, insofar as possible, that her well-being will be restored. In doing this the physician may call on other health personnel, such as individuals trained to handle rape-trauma victims, to facilitate counseling and follow-up. The patient should not be released until specific follow-up plans are made and the patient understands what they are. A follow-up visit should be planned within 1 to 4 weeks to reevaluate the patient's medical, infectious disease, pregnancy, and psychological status. At this point, encouragement for continued follow-up counseling should be emphasized. It is important at each visit to emphasize to the patient THAT SHE WAS A VICTIM AND

TABLE 12-1
Survival Time of Sperm

Source	Motile Sperm	Sperm	Acid Phosphatase
Vagina	Up to 8 hr	Up to 7-9 days	Variable (Up to 48 hr)
Pharynx	6 hr	Unknown	100 IU*
Rectum	Undetermined	20 to 24 hr	100 IU*
Cervix	Up to 5 days	Up to 17 days	Similar to vagina

From Anderson S: Sexual assault—medical-legal aspects, an unpublished training packet for pediatric house staff, Harborview Medical Center, Seattle, Wash, 1980.
*Minimum detectable.

HOLDS NO BLAME. At each step she must be allowed to ventilate her feelings and to discuss her current conceptions of the problem.

It is important that the physician realize that some patients will appear to have excellent emotional control when seen immediately after a rape. This is an acute expression of the patient's defense mechanisms and should not be misinterpreted to indicate that the patient is coping with the circumstances. All the recommendations just listed should be followed *regardless* of the patient's apparent condition. Specific plans for follow-up are equally important in such an individual, because it must be anticipated that she will follow the same post-rape emotional process as anyone else.

Finally, it is important to emphasize and re-emphasize that at no time during the management or follow-up care of the rape victim should any comments be made by health care professionals suggesting that the patient was anything other than a victim. These women are sensitive to any accusations and insinuations and may even believe that they may have in some way been responsible for the rape. Their future well-being may be severely affected by creating such an impression.

INCEST

Incest must be placed within the context of child sexual abuse. The actual overall incidence of such abuse is difficult to estimate, although several authorities claim that about 10% of all child abuse cases involve sexual abuse. Sarafino estimates that roughly 336,000 children are sexually abused each year in the United States. Retrospective historical data derived from adults imply that incestual activity may be experienced in as many as 15% to 25% of all women and approximately 12% of all men. These figures seem appropriate for the population in general but vary from group to group, being higher in young prostitutes.

Sexual abuse of children may be divided into two types, the first in which the child is victimized by a stranger and the second in which a family member is the perpetrator. It has been estimated that about 80% of all sexual abuse cases of children involve a family member. Rimsza and Niggemann found that only 18% of 311 children and adolescents who were evaluated for sexual abuse were assaulted by strangers.

In the case of child sexual abuse involving a stranger the act is usually a single episode and is usually reported to the authorities. The child is capable in most instances of clearly stating what happened, and the act may involve any form of sexual activity and may have taken place because of enticement, coercion, or physical force. In such instances the child should be interviewed carefully and allowed to tell what happened. The police or protective services should be notified, and, where appropriate, the techniques used in evaluating a rape victim should be applied. Appropriate prophylaxis against infection should be employed, and counseling should be arranged with a mental health care worker, who should see the child immediately and also take the responsibility for planning long-term follow-up. The molester should be apprehended, and if it is an individual living in the home, he or she should be made to leave. Most communities have sexual abuse crisis intervention centers, and these are appropriate in such circumstances.

In each case the child should be carefully told that HE OR SHE WAS A VICTIM OF A WRONGFUL ACT AND THAT IN NO WAY WAS HE OR SHE TO BLAME. Statements that imply that the child might in some way have enticed the perpetrator into performing the act are inappropriate and may lead to serious compromise in the development of the child's self-esteem in the future. The welfare of siblings must also be considered, and an effort to discover the siblings' status should be made.

About 80% of child sexual abuse involves a parent, guardian, other family member, or mother's significant other. Father-daughter incest accounts for about 75% of reported cases, with mother-son, father-son, mother-daughter, brother-sister, or incest involving another close family member comprising the remaining 25%. Brother-sister incest may be the commonest form but may not be reported often.

Different states define incest in different legal terms. In some, intercourse is required; in others, it is not. Incest is noted to occur in all social groups, including cultures where it is a stated taboo.

Families in which incestual activity is taking place may appear normal, but family members frequently have limited contact with the outside world. Family relationships are often chaotic, including such problems as alcohol and drug abuse and severe mental illness. In father-daughter incestual relationships the father is frequently a passive, introspective person who experiences a weak sexual relationship with the mother. He may therefore turn his attentions to his daughter or daughters out of loneliness, and the sexual activity may be quite affectionate. Frequently the mother is aware of the situation, but both parents agree consciously or subconsciously that the incestuous relationship is more acceptable than an extramarital one. In such situations the daughter may assume more of the role of the wife around the house, fulfilling many homemaker duties.

Children who have been victimized by incest often feel guilty during adolescence. Many may be afraid to withdraw from the relationship out of fear that in so doing they would destroy the family and the security it provides. Such victims frequently feel humiliated and develop a weak ego and self-image. Because of this these women may have difficulty in developing appropriate relationships with members of the opposite sex and may make poor choices in their interpersonal relationships in the future. They frequently choose chaotic family existences after they leave home. Fewer than 10% of children involved in incestuous relationships have normal psychological development at the time of evaluation. Usually they exhibit guilt, anger, behavior problems, unexplained physical complaints, lying, stealing, school failure, running away, and sleep disturbances.

Gynecologists may see such individuals as teenagers or young adults and may note that some or all of these complaints have been fully developed. When such a profile occurs, the gynecologist should seek a history of incest to fully understand the psychopathology of the patient. Appropriate questions like, "Were you physically or sexually abused or raped as a child or adolescent?" should be asked as part of a routine history. Affirmative answers to any of these questions require specific detailed and discreet questioning of the individual involved and the circumstances of the incestuous act. The physician should assess the kinds of counseling the patient may already have experienced. Questioning should be nonjudgmental, clear, and specific. For example, the patient should be questioned about the sexual activity experienced and whether it included touching, genital manipulation, or intercourse. Often the individual is relieved to tell the health profes-sional about her experience, because it may be something that she has never previously discussed. The knowledge that this is a common human experience and that the individual is blameless can be very helpful. The physician must then determine the necessity for an appropriate referral to a mental health worker.

Incest victims as adults frequently choose partners with inadequate personalities who may be capable of physical and sexual violence. This may be their unconscious desire to gravitate to a familiar relationship. It is equally possible that their poor social self-image may prevent them from achieving a stronger and more normal relationship.

Several studies have looked at the long-term follow-up of incest victims. Two separate studies in the 1970s by Lukianowicz and Meiselman found that daughters in father-daughter incestual relationships demonstrated difficulties in sexual adjustment, including promiscuity and homosexuality. In 28 cases, 11 girls became promiscuous, as well as delinquent, and 4 of these became prostitutes. Of the 11, 5 married and had problems with sexual arousal, and 4 demonstrated psychiatric symptoms of depression, anxiety, and suicidal ideology. Six, however, demonstrated no specific ill effects.

In another study by Browning and Boatman a gradual improvement in symptomatology occurred with time, regardless of whether treatment plans were followed. In specific instances of incestual relationships with uncles, however, there was great anxiety over the possibility of repeat incest when the uncles were left at large. In this same study violence was reported, including suicides in fathers and one murder of a mother by her son.

Earlier studies had suggested that the degree of emotional disturbance was greater the closer the relationship of the relative and that the degree was also related to whether genital contact actually took place. In a 1980 study of 796 college students Finkelhor reported that about one third of the incestual activity occurred only once but that in 27% the activity continued with varying frequency for more than a year. Of the involved individuals, 30% considered their experience positive, 30% negative, and the rest did not feel strongly one way or the other. In this series, women students who had sexual incestuous experiences as children were more likely to be sexually active. Experiences with siblings seemed to have a more positive effect on sexual development as long as the overall experience with the sibling was positive. Men who had sibling sexual experiences did not seem to have a higher current level of frequency of intercourse and seemed to have lower self-esteem. Thus it is difficult to predict what overall long-term potential problems may occur in victims of incestuous experiences.

ABUSE

The Battered Woman

Domestic violence and *spouse abuse* are terms referring to violence occurring between partners in an ongoing relationship even if they are not married. A battered woman is defined as any woman over the age of 16 with evidence of physical abuse on at least one occasion at the hands of an intimate male partner. The battered wife syndrome is defined as a symptom complex occurring as a result of violence in which a woman has at any time received deliberate, severe, or repeated (more than three times) physical abuse from her husband or significant male partner in which the minimal injury is bruising. The actual physical abuse may vary from minimal activity, such as verbal abuse or threat of violence, to throwing an object, throwing an object at someone, pushing, slapping, kicking, hitting, beating, threatening with a weapon, or using a weapon. These acts may be spontaneous or intentionally planned. Most such violence is accompanied by mental abuse and intimidation.

It is difficult to ascertain the specific incidence of domestic violence, but it has been estimated that 1.5 million cases of domestic violence occur in the United States each year, and some have stated that at least 50% of family relationships are violent. In a study at Yale University, 3.8% of women who presented to the surgical services and 3.4% to the psychiatric services of the emergency department were victims of battering. In a recent U.S. Department of Justice study, 57% of 450,000 annual acts of family violence were committed by spouses or exspouses, and the wife was a victim in 93% of cases. In at least one fourth of these cases the violent acts had occurred at least three times in the previous 6 months. In addition, of all female homicide victims, one third to one half were murdered by their male partners. Therefore it can be seen that domestic violence and battered women are common in our society today.

The most common sites for injury are the head, neck, chest, abdomen, breast, and upper extremities. The upper extremities may be fractured as the woman attempts to defend herself. In a study from Yale, 84% of the injuries were severe enough to require medical treatment, and in 81% of the cases patients stated that the assailant had beaten them with the fists. In an English study of 100 women brought to a hostel for battered women, 44% suffered from lacerations and 59% stated that they had been kicked repeatedly. All women stated that they had been hit with a clenched fist. Fractures occurred in 32, and 9 of the women had been beaten and taken to the hostel unconscious. Other studies have demonstrated similar findings.

Murder and suicide are frequent components of the domestic violence problem. In a large study from Denver, Walker reported that three quarters of the battered patients felt that the batterer would kill them during the relationship, and almost half felt that they might kill the batterer. Of these victims, 11% stated that they had actually tried to kill the batterer, and 87% believed that they themselves would be the ones to die if someone was killed. One third of these women stated that they seriously considered committing suicide. Walker noted that victims and their attackers frequently are depressed and may move rapidly between suicidal and homicidal intent.

There is a strong relationship between spouse battering and child abuse. In Walker's study, 53% of men who abused their partners were noted also to abuse their children. Another one third had threatened to abuse their children. Interestingly, in the same relationship, 28% of the wives who themselves were abused stated that they had abused their children while living in the violent household, and an additional 6% thought they might abuse their children at the time they were evaluated.

Physical abuse in pregnancy is also quite common. One study identified an incidence of 10.9% among patients attending an antepartum clinic. In the case of the pregnant patient, the battering is frequently directed at the breasts and abdomen.

It is important that physicians increase their ability to recognize the signs of domestic violence and spouse abuse. A study by Hilberman and Monson demonstrated that 25% of women treated for injuries in an emergency room were victims of wife battering. The physicians who were treating these patients made the correct diagnosis originally in only 3% of cases. Viken has listed a profile of the characteristics of the abused wife. These include a history of having been beaten as a child, raised in a single parent home, married as a teenager, and pregnant before marriage. Such women have frequent visits to clinics and emergency rooms with a variety of somatic complaints including headaches, insomnia, choking sensation, hyperventilation, gastrointestinal symptoms, and chest, pelvic, and back pain. Noncompliance with the advice of physicians with respect to these complaints is frequent. (See box.)

In visits to the physician's office or emergency room the patient often appears shy, frightened, embarrassed, evasive, anxious, or passive and often cries. The batterer may accompany the patient on such visits and stay close at hand to monitor what is said to the physician. Thus the woman may be hesitant to provide information about how she was injured, and the explanation given may not fit the injuries observed. Alcohol or other drug abuse is common in such individuals.

Physicians should become comfortable in asking the patient whether she has been physically abused. Such questions as "Has anyone hurt you or tried to injure you?" and "Have you ever been physically abused either recently or in the past?" are very appropriate introductory questions. The physician should follow up on any positive answers in a nonjudgmental manner in an attempt to learn what is happening. Physical examinations should be complete with particular attention to bruises, lacerations, burns, and other signs of injury. If the patient is wearing sunglasses, she should be asked to remove them so the physician can determine whether there are eye injuries. If the patient is pregnant, bruises seen on the breasts or abdomen should always be discussed. Physicians should carefully note evidence for abuse in their patient record.

Battering acts tend to run in cycles consisting of three phases. The first phase is tension building, in which there is a gradual escalation of tension between the couple manifested by discrete acts that cause family friction. Name calling, intimidating remarks, meanness, and mild physical abuse such as pushing are com-

SOMATIC COMPLAINTS IN ABUSED WOMEN

Headaches
Insomnia
Choking sensation
Hyperventilation
Chest, back, or pelvic pain
Other signs and symptoms
    Shyness
    Fright
    Embarrassment
    Evasiveness
    Jumpiness
    Passivity
    Frequent crying
    Often accompanied by male partner
    Drug or alcohol abuse (often overdose)
    Injuries

(From ACOG Technical Bulletin Number 124: The battered woman, Jan, 1989.)

mon. Dissatisfaction and hostility are often expressed by the batterer in a somewhat chronic form. The victim may attempt to placate the batterer in hopes of pleasing him or calming him. She may actually believe at this point that she has the power to avoid aggravating the situation. She may not respond to his hostile actions and may even be successful from time to time in apparently reducing tensions. This of course will reinforce her belief that she can control the situation. As the tension phase builds, the batterer's anger is less controlled, and the victim may withdraw, fearing that she will inadvertently set off explosive behavior.

Often this withdrawal is the signal for the batterer to become more aggressive. Anything may spark the hostile act, and the acute battering then takes place. This is the cycle's second phase and is represented by an uncontrollable discharge of tension that has built up through the first phase. The attack may take the form of both verbal and physical abuse, and the victim is often left injured. In self defense the victim may actually injure or kill the batterer. In approximately two thirds of cases reported by Walker, alcohol abuse was involved. However, the alcohol use may have been the excuse rather than the reason for the battering.

After the abuse has taken place, the third phase generally follows. In this situation, the batterer apologizes, asks forgiveness, and frequently shows kindness and remorse, showering the victim with gifts and promises. This gives the victim hope that the relationship can be saved and that the violence will not recur. Batterers are often charming and manipulative, offering the victim justification for forgiveness.

The cycles, however, do repeat themselves, with the first phase increasing in length and intensity, the battering becoming more severe, and the third phase tending to decrease in both duration and intensity. The batterer learns that he can control the victim without obtaining much forgiveness. The victim becomes more demoralized and loses her ability to leave the situation even if she has the means and opportunity to do so.

Batterers, too, tend to have a specific profile in most cases. They are men who refuse to take responsibility for their behavior, blaming their victims for their violent acts. They often have strong controlling personalities and do not tolerate autonomy in their partners. They have rigid expectations of marriage and sexual behavior and consider their wives or partners as chattel. They wish to be cared for in their most basic needs, frequently make unrealistic demands on their wives, and show low tolerance for stress. Depression and suicidal gestures are often a part of their behavior pattern, but in general they are aggressive and assaultive in most of their behavior, generally using violence to solve their problems. On the other hand, they are often charming and manipulative, especially in their relationships outside the marriage. They often exhibit low self-esteem, feelings of inadequacy, and a sense of helplessness, all of which are generally made worse by the prospects of losing their wives. It is typical behavior for male batterers to exhibit contempt for women in their usual activities. Therapy is usually ineffective and seems to work only when the man can be made to give up violence as his primary means of solving problems.

Physicians should determine community resources available for handling family violence. The acute situation can be helped by the police department, crisis hotline, rape relief centers, domestic violence programs, and legal aid services for abused women. Hospital emergency rooms and shelters for battered women and children are also excellent resources. Counseling and follow-up care can be offered by healthcare workers in these organizations or by private practitioners who specialize in the care of battered women, their spouses, and their children. Such individuals may be social workers, psychologists, psychiatrists, or other mental health workers trained specifically for this purpose. Many community hospitals, mental health departments, and community mental health services have set up counseling programs for such couples, since the problem is so common. The physician's job is to recognize the problem and either offer counseling or get counseling for the patient so that she understands her rights and alternatives and learns to protect herself and her children from future harm.

The victim of abuse very likely will not wish to leave her home because of economic concerns and a fear that the batterer may continue to pursue her. Although she may have the batterer arrested and served with restraining orders, she may be convinced that she and her children cannot be protected from the batterer. She may also believe that there is a possibility of reconciliation and of change in behavior on the part of the batterer. It is therefore reasonable to discuss an exit plan with the victim to be used should the violence recur. This exit plan should include the following:

1. Have a change of clothes packed for her and her children including toilet articles, necessary medications, and an extra set of keys to the house and car. These can be placed in a suitcase and left with a friend or family member.

2. Keep some cash, a checkbook, and a savings account book with the friend or family member.

3. Other identification papers, such as birth certificates, Social Security cards, voter registration cards, utility bills, and drivers license, should be kept available, since children will need to be enrolled in school, and financial assistance may have to be sought.

4. Have something special, such as a toy or book, for each child.

5. Have financial records available, such as mortgage papers, rent receipts, and an automobile title.

6. Determine a plan on exactly where to go regardless of the time of day or night. This may be to a friend or relative's house or to a shelter for battered women and children.

Rehearsing an exit plan as one would conduct a

fire drill makes it possible for the battered woman to respond even under the stress of the battering.

Long-term aid and referral of the patient, her children, and the batterer to the appropriate resource individuals is an important aspect of the care of such patients. The American College of Obstetrics and Gynecology has prepared a patient education brochure that physicians can keep in their offices and give to individuals who suffer from this problem. Making the brochures available in the office waiting room may encourage women with these needs to get help.

These women often suffer from severe psychiatric problems, such as anxiety, depression, and other pathologic conditions, that may require psychotherapy. Group counseling or individual counseling may also help them to rebuild their lives as single individuals or single parents. It is frequently necessary to help them develop a skill that will enable them to be employable. Counseling programs take these things into consideration. Children of victims who may be victims as well also require counseling to avoid behavior patterns that will lead to aggressive behavior in their later lives.

Wife battering is a common problem that affects the family unit in particular and society in general. It can occur in all segments of society and reflects the violence that is a part of life to-day and the behavior of many. Physicians should learn to detect its presence in their patients and offer ways the victim can seek help. The help may include counseling for the victim, batterer, and children or constructing a plan for the woman to exit the relationship and rebuild her life in safety.

The Elderly

The Select Committee on Aging in investigating domestic violence against the elderly held hearings before the Subcommittee of Human Services of the House of Representatives in 1980. The committee noted that approximately 500,000 to 2.5 million cases involving abuse of the elderly occur per year in the United States. The committee documented that abuse of the elderly may be as large a nationwide problem as child abuse. Usually the abused person is a woman past the age of 75, often with a physical impairment. She is generally white, widowed, and living with relatives. The abuser is generally an adult child living within the family. Counseling issues involve the entire family but particularly the individual causing the abuse. Physicians who care for geriatric patients should be alert for signs and symptoms of this type of domestic abuse; when it is found, community resources should be activated.

_____ KEY POINTS _____

- About 200,000 rapes are reported nationwide each year. This figure may represent many fewer rapes than actually occur.

- Sexual assault happens to people of all ages, races, and socioeconomic groups, but the very young, the mentally and physically handicapped, and the very old are particularly susceptible.

- Two phases of the rape-trauma syndrome occur. The first is the immediate or acute phase and lasts hours to days. The second, the reorganization stage, lasts months to years.

- In caring for rape-trauma victims, the physician's responsibilities are medical, medical-legal, and supportive.

- From 12% to 40% of victims who are sexually assaulted have injuries.

- Rape-trauma victims should always be treated as victims. At no time should guilt be implied.

- About 10% of all child abuse cases involve sexual abuse.

- Roughly 336,000 children are sexually abused each year in the United States.

- Incestuous activity may be experienced by as many as 15% to 25% of all women and approximately 12% of all men.

- Approximately 80% of all cases of sexual abuse of children involve a family member.

- Father-daughter incest accounts for about 75% of reported cases; however, brother-sister incest may be the commonest type, although it may not be reported often.

- As many as 25% of women treated for injuries in an emergency room are likely to be victims of wife battering. Diagnosis of this by a physician is rare.

- There are an estimated 1.5 million cases of domestic violence reported in the United States each year.

- In 93% of the cases, the wife is the victim of the violence.

- More than half of the men who abuse their partners also abuse their children.

- About 10% of antepartum clinic patients may be victims of battering.

- Victims of battering demonstrate multiple somatic complaints.

- Two thirds of batterers who carry out violent acts are under the influence of alcohol, but this may be the excuse rather than the reason.

- Between 500,000 and 2.5 million cases of abuse of the elderly reportedly occur in the United States each year.

BIBLIOGRAPHY

American College of Obstetricians and Gynecologists: The Battered Woman (Technical Bulletin Number 124), Washington, DC, ACOG, 1989.

American College of Obstetricians and Gynecologists: The Abused Woman (ACOG Patient Education Pamphlet APO83), Washington, DC, ACOG, 1989.

Bachmann GA, Moeller TP, and Benett J: Childhood sexual abuse and the consequences in adult women, Obstet Gynecol 71:631, 1988.

Barker B: Suicide by patient: criminal charge against physician, JAMA 238(4):305, 1977.

Batten DA: Incest: a review of the literature, Med Sci Law 23:245, 1983.

Behrman S: Hostility to kith and kin, Br Med J 2(5970):538, 1975.

Benward J and Densen-Gerber J: Incest as a causative factor in antisocial behavior: an exploratory study, Contemp Drug Probl 4:322, 1975.

Browning DH, and Boatman B: Incest: children at risk, Am J Psychiatry 134:69, 1977.

Burgess AW and Holmstrom LL: Rape: victims of crisis, Bowie Md, 1974, RJ Brady Co.

Davis LD: Beliefs of service providers about abused women and abusing men, Soc Work 29:2, 1984.

Elbow M: Theoretical considerations of violent marriages, Soc Casework 58(9):515, 1977.

Finkelhor D: Sex among siblings, Arch Sex Behav 9:195, 1981.

Flugel J: Psychoanalytic study of the family, London, 1926, The Hogarth Press.

Frazer M: Domestic violence: a medicolegal review, J Forensic Sci 31(4):1409, 1986.

Galleno H and Oppenheim W: The battered child syndrome revisited, Clin Orthop Rel Res 162:11, 1982.

Gayford JJ: Battered wives: research on battered wives, R Soc Health J 95(6):288, 1975.

Gelles RJ: Violence in the family: a review of research in the seventies, J Marriage Fam 42(4):873, 1980.

Gelles RJ and Cornel CP, editors: International perspectives on family violence, Lexington Mass, 1983, DC Heath and Co, pp. 1-22.

Gentry CE: Incestuous abuse of children: the need for an objective view, Child Welfare 58:355, 1978.

Giordano NH and Giordano JA: Elder abuse: a review of the literature, Soc Work 29:232, 1984.

Goldberg WG and Tomlanovich MC: Domestic violence, victims and emergency departments: new findings, JAMA 251(24):3259, 1984.

Helton A: Battering during pregnancy, Am J Nurs 86(8):910, 1986.

Hilberman E: Overview: the "wife-beaters' wife" reconsidered, Am J Psychiatry 137(11):1336, 1980.

Hilberman E and Monson K: Sixty battered women, Victimatology 2:460, 1977.

Hillard PJ: Physical abuse in pregnancy, Obstet Gynecol 66(2):185, 1985.

Jenny C, Hooton TM, Bowers A, et al: Sexually transmitted diseases in victims of rape, N Engl J Med 322:713, 1990.

Jones JG: Sexual abuse of children, Am J Dis Child 136:142, 1982.

Kahn M and Sexton M: Sexual abuse of young children, Clin Pediatr 22:369, 1983.

Kaplan HS: The evaluation of sexual disorders, New York, 1983, Brunner/Mazel, Inc.

Kempe CH: Sexual abuse: another hidden pediatric problem, The 1977 C Anderson Aldrich lecture, Pediatrics 62:382, 1978.

Kerns DL: Child abuse and neglect: the pediatrician's role, J Contin Educ Pediatr 21:11, 1979.

Klaus PA and Rand MR: Family violence. Washington, DC, US Department of Justice, Bureau of Justice Statistics, 1984.

Lukianowicz N: Incest. I. Paternal. II. Other types, Br J Psychiatry 120:301, 1972.

Meiselman KC: Incest: a psychological study of cases and effects with treatment recommendations, London, 1978, Jossey-Bass, Inc Publishers.

Morgan SM: Conjugal terrorism: a psychological and community treatment model of wife abuse, Palo Alto, Calif, 1982, R&E Research Associates, Inc.

Muram D and Elias S: Child sexual abuse: genital tract findings in prepubertal girls. II. Comparison of colposcopic and unaided examinations, Am J Obstet Gynecol 160:333, 1989.

Nadelson CC, Notman MT, Zackson H, et al: Follow-up study of rape victims, Am J Psychiatry 139:1267, 1982.

Nakashima II and Zakus GE: Incest: review and clinical experience, Pediatrics 60:696, 1977.

Parker B and Schumacher DN: The battered wife syndrome and violence in the nuclear family of origin: a controlled pilot study, Am J Public Health 67(8):760, 1977.

Pedrick-Cornell C and Gelles RJ: Elderly abuse: the status of current knowledge, Fam Rela 31:457, 1982.

Richwald GA and McCluskey TC: Family violence during pregnancy, Adv Int Matern Child Health 5:87, 1985.

Rimsza ME and Niggemann EH: Medical evaluation of sexually abused children: a review of 311 cases, Pediatrics 69:8, 1982.

Rounsaville B and Weissman MM: Battered woman: a medical problem requiring detection, Int J Psychiatry Med 8(2):191, 1977-1978.

Sarafino EP: An estimate of nationwide incidence of sexual offenses against children, Child Welfare 58:127, 1979.

Sarles RM: Incest, Pediatrics 2:51, 1980.

Select Committee on Aging: Domestic violence against the elderly, Hearings before the Subcommittee of Human Services, House of Representatives, April 21, 1980, Washington, DC, 1980, US Government Printing Office.

Sgroi SM: Sexual molestation of children: the last frontier of child abuse, Child Today 4:18, 1975.

Star B: Patterns of family violence, Social Case Work 60:339, 1980.

US Department of Health and Human Services; Public Health Service; Health Resources and Services Administration: Surgeon General's Workshop on Violence and Public Health: Report. DHHS Publication No HRS-D-MC 86-1. Washington DC, 1986, US Government Printing Office.

Viken RM: Family violence: aids to recognition, Postgrad Med 71(5):115, 1982.

Walker LE: The battered woman syndrome, New York, 1984, Springer Publishing Co, Inc.

Breast Diseases

KEY TERMS AND DEFINITIONS

Axillary Tail of Spence. A lateral projection of glandular tissue that extends from the upper, outer portion of the breast toward the axilla.

Cluster. A mammographic finding of five or more calcifications within a volume of a cubic centimeter.

Cooper's Ligaments. Fibrous septa that extend from the skin over the breast to the underlying pectoralis fascia.

Cystosarcoma Phyllodes. Fibroepithelial breast tumors that are rare and may arise from fibroadenomas.

Diaphanography. The technique of transillumination of the breast by which a camera measures the light transmitted through breast tissue.

Digital Radiography. The technique by which x-ray photons are detected after passing through the breast tissue.

Fibroadenomas. Firm, freely mobile, solitary, solid breast masses usually present in adolescents and teenagers.

Fibrocystic Changes. An exaggerated response of breast tissue to the cyclic changes of ovarian hormones.

Intraductal Papilloma. Benign breast mass that is usually microscopic but may grow to 2 to 3 mm in diameter. The predominant symptom of an intraductal papilloma is spontaneous discharge from one nipple.

Lumpectomy. Conservative surgical procedure for breast carcinoma that involves removal of a wide margin of normal breast tissue surrounding a breast carcinoma less than 4 cm in diameter.

Modified Radical Mastectomy. An operation that includes removal of the breast and only the fascia over the pectoralis major muscle.

Myoepithelial Cells. Specialized cells in the lactiferous ducts that are peripheral to epithelial cells, thus forming a double cellular layer in the ductal system. These cells are believed to be involved in the milk letdown phenomenon.

Paget's Disease. Rare breast carcinoma that has an innocent appearance and looks like eczema or dermatitis of the nipple.

Polymastia. More than two breasts.

Polythelia. More than two nipples.

Radical Mastectomy. An operation that includes en bloc removal of the breast, as well as underlying pectoralis major and pectoralis minor muscles.

Simple Mastectomy. An operation that includes removal of the breast without underlying muscle or fascial tissue.

Thermography. Potential technique to diagnose breast disease by directly measuring either cutaneous temperatures of the breast or infrared radiation from the breast by electronic detectors.

Virginal Hypertrophy of the Breasts. Rare condition in which there is massive hypertrophy of the breasts at puberty.

Xeromammography. Mammographic technique in which the image is produced by a photoelectric process on aluminum plates coated with selenium.

The importance of early detection and diagnosis of breast carcinoma cannot be overemphasized. Breast carcinoma is the most common malignancy of women and is one of the two leading causes of all cancer deaths in women. It is the number one cause of death in women in their 40s. One in 9 women (11% of American women) develops carcinoma of the breast during her lifetime. There is no known method of preventing breast carcinoma. Therefore, the major opportunity to alter the natural course of the disease is the opportunity for early discovery and diagnosis.

It is noteworthy that mortality from breast carcinoma has not changed appreciably over the past 50 years. However, recent improvements in mammography and meticulous physical examination have facilitated earlier detection of breast carcinoma and may improve survival rates.

The prognosis for and survival of a woman with breast carcinoma are improved by early discovery. Thus every gynecologist has an obligation to educate patients concerning self-examination of the breast and to develop a routine for carefully screening patients for breast disease. Detailed physical examination of the breast must be an integral step in evaluating every female patient.

Our culture attaches great significance to the female breast. An individual patient may react to the tremendous anxiety of suspected breast disease with behavior that varies from frequent visits to the physician for breast pain to denial of the presence of an obvious mass. The patient's description of her problem and her reactions to diagnoses, benign or malignant, must never be taken out of the context of this anxiety.

The major emphasis of this chapter is the epidemiology, detection, and diagnosis of breast carcinoma. The chapter also includes a brief discussion of benign breast diseases, since the symptoms of benign breast disease present frequently. Galactorrhea is presented in Chapter 37.

ANATOMY

The breasts are large, modified sebaceous glands contained within the superficial fascia of the anterior chest wall. A lateral projection of glandular tissue extends from the upper, outer portion of the breast toward the axilla and is called the *axillary tail of Spence*. The average weight of the adult breast is 200 to 300 g during the menstruating years. The mature breast consists of approximately 20% glandular tissue and 80% fat and connective tissue. The periphery of breast tissue is predominantly fat, while the central area contains more glandular tissue.

The breast is composed of 12 to 20 lobes arranged in radial fashion from the nipple. Each lobe is triangular and has one central excretory duct that opens to the exterior at the nipple. Milk originates in the secretory cells of the alveoli. It is subsequently transported by the branching collecting ducts of the lobules into the lactiferous sinuses and terminally into the excretory ducts of each respective lobe of the breast. Fibrous septa, *Cooper's ligaments*, extend from the skin to the underlying pectoralis fascia (Figure 13-1). Invasion of these ligaments by malignant cells produces skin retraction, which is a sign of advanced breast carcinoma.

The lymphatic distribution of the breast is complex. Approximately 75% of the lymphatic drainage goes to regional nodes in the axilla. The axilla contains a varying number of nodes, usually between 30 and 60. Other metastatic routes include lymphatics adjacent to the internal mammary vessels. After direct spread into the mediastinum, lymphatic drainage may go to the intercostal glands, which are located posteriorly along the vertebral column, and to subpectoral and subdiaphragmatic areas (Figure 13-2). Metastases from one breast across the midline to the other breast or chest wall occur occasionally.

Breast tissue is sensitive to the cyclic changes in hormonal levels. The epithelium of the breast responds to fluctuating levels of estrogen and progesterone similar to other hormonally sensitive tissue. The stroma of the breasts and the myoepithelial cells of the breasts also respond to estrogen and progesterone. Women often experience breast tenderness and fullness during the luteal phase of the cycle. The average increase in volume of the premenstrual breasts is 25 to 30 ml, as measured by water displacement techniques. Premenstrual breast symptoms are produced by an increase in blood flow, vascular engorgement, and water retention. There is a corresponding enlargement in the lumina of ducts and an increase in ductal and acinar cellular secretory activity. During the follicular phase, there is parenchymal proliferation of the ducts. During the luteal phase, there is dilation of the ductal

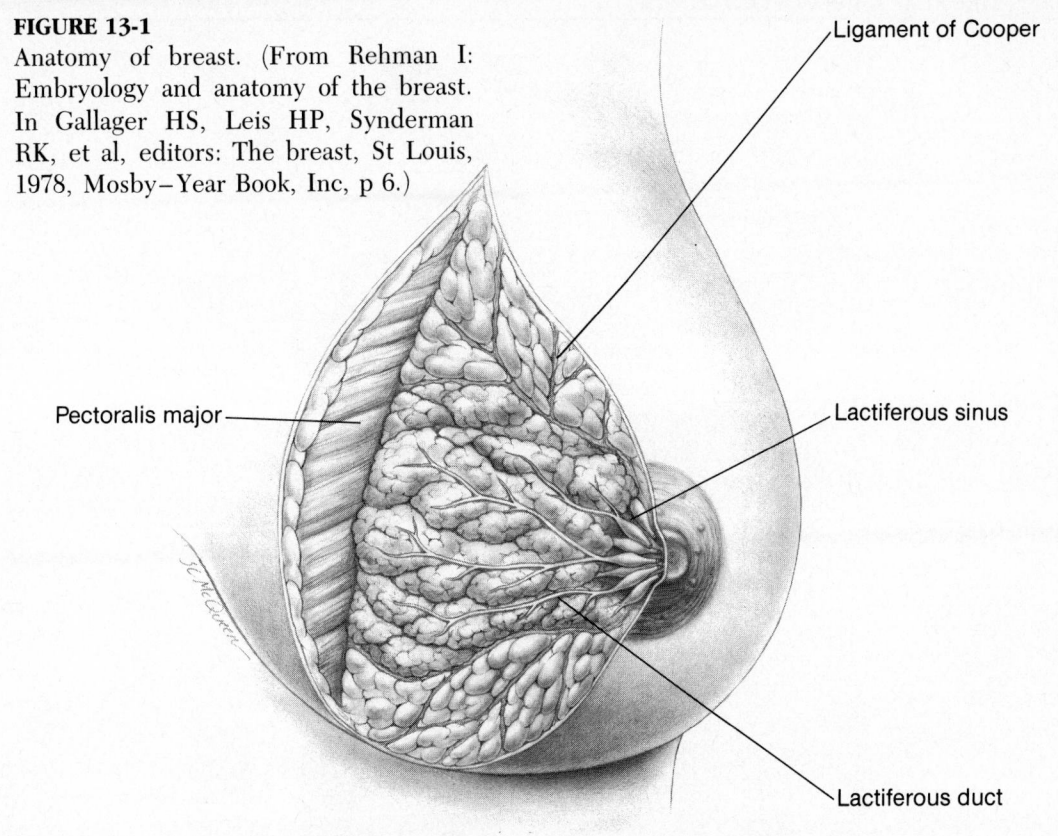

FIGURE 13-1
Anatomy of breast. (From Rehman I: Embryology and anatomy of the breast. In Gallager HS, Leis HP, Synderman RK, et al, editors: The breast, St Louis, 1978, Mosby–Year Book, Inc, p 6.)

Ligament of Cooper

Pectoralis major

Lactiferous sinus

Lactiferous duct

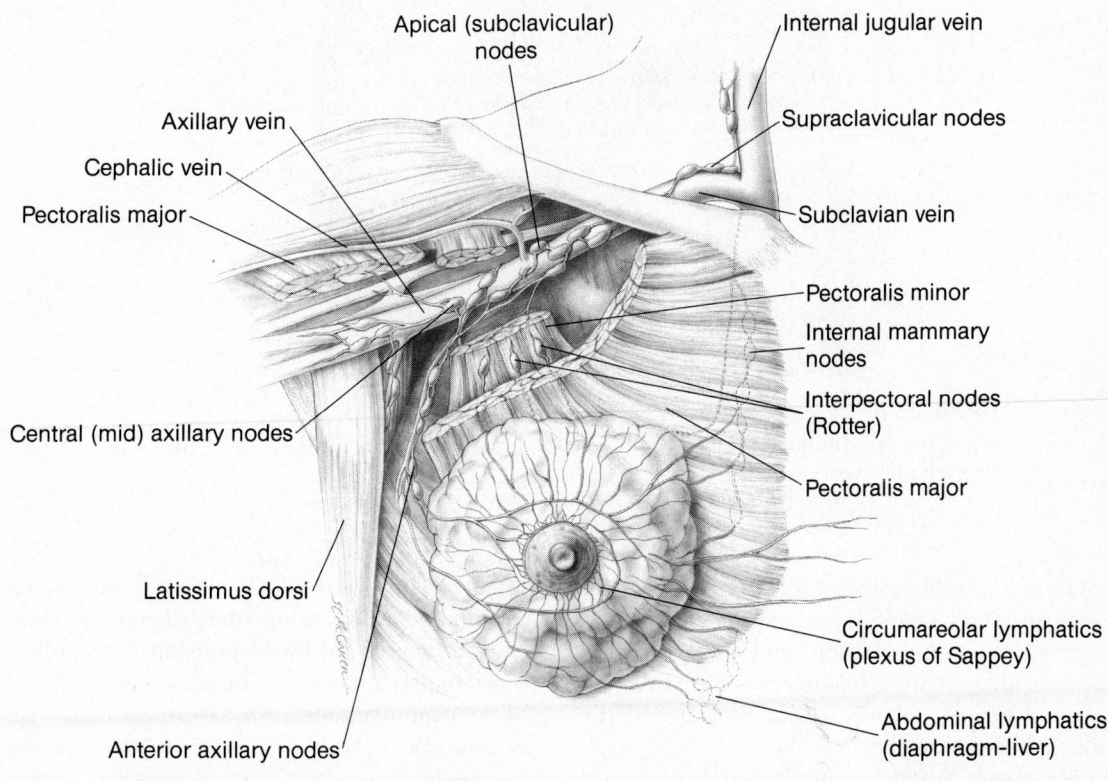

Apical (subclavicular) nodes

Internal jugular vein

Axillary vein

Supraclavicular nodes

Cephalic vein

Subclavian vein

Pectoralis major

Pectoralis minor

Internal mammary nodes

Interpectoral nodes (Rotter)

Central (mid) axillary nodes

Pectoralis major

Latissimus dorsi

Circumareolar lymphatics (plexus of Sappey)

Abdominal lymphatics (diaphragm-liver)

Anterior axillary nodes

FIGURE 13-2
Lymphatics of breast. (From Rehman I: Embryology and anatomy of the breast. In Gallager HS, Leis HP, Synderman RK, et al, editors: The breast, St Louis, 1978, Mosby–Year Book, Inc, p 17.)

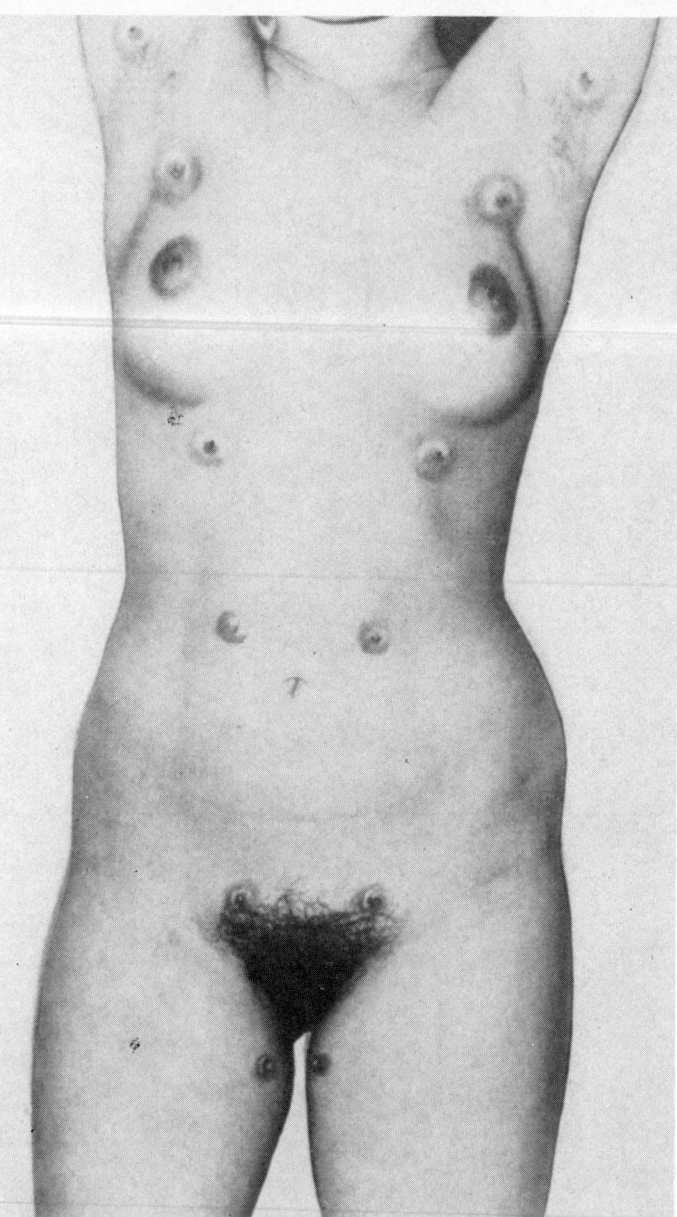

FIGURE 13-3
Extensive polythelia along milk line. (From Degrell I: Atlas of diseases of the mammary gland, Basel, 1976, S Karger AG, p 41.)

system and differentiation of the alveolar cells into secretory cells. The alveolar elements respond to both estrogen and progesterone. When menstruation begins, there is a regression of cellular activity in the alveoli and the ducts become smaller.

Accessory breasts or nipples can occur along the breast lines, which run from the axilla to the groin. Supernumerary nipples (polythelia) or breasts (polymastia) are common anomalies (Figure 13-3), which may be well developed and functional or rudimentary. Underdevelopment of one breast in relationship to the other is a common anomaly. In a recent study of 8408 mammograms, 3% were notable for asymmetric volume reduction relative to the contralateral breast. This asymmetry represented a benign, normal variation unless an associated palpable abnormality was present. Massive hypertrophy of the breasts at puberty

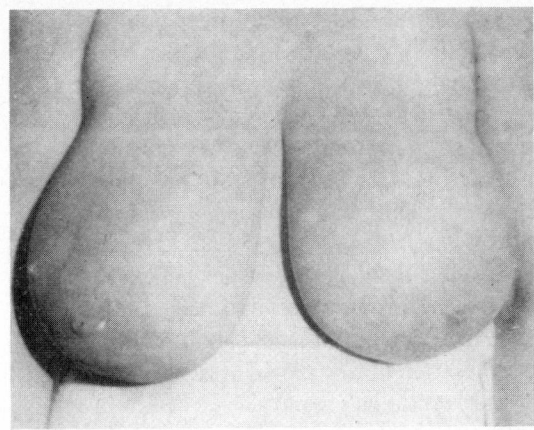

FIGURE 13-4
Virginal hypertrophy, age 13. (From Degrell I: Atlas of diseases of the mammary gland, Basel, 1976, S Karger AG, p 46.)

(virginal hypertrophy) is a rare occurrence that has a deeply disturbing effect on a teenager's self-image (Figure 13-4). This condition is best managed by cosmetic surgery.

BENIGN BREAST DISEASE

The classifications and terminologies of benign breast disease are confusing. Nevertheless, an understanding of these conditions is important. The symptomatology and physical findings of benign disease cause anxiety and fear in the patient, who often thinks the symptoms may be related to breast cancer. The common symptoms of breast disease—pain and tenderness—and the signs—a mass or nipple discharge—may result from either a benign or a malignant process. However, breast pain is a comparatively late symptom in women with breast carcinoma and is the sole presenting symptom in less than 10% of these women.

Numerous epidemiologic studies have found an increased risk of developing breast carcinoma in women with benign breast disease with associated atypical epithelial hyperplasia. This risk varies from twofold to fivefold, depending on the degree of epithelial hyperplasia. The pathophysiology of the association between hyperplasia and subsequent carcinoma is straightforward.

DuPont and Page performed the classic study on the relationship between benign breast disease and subsequent development of carcinoma. They followed more than 3000 women for at least 15 years after benign breast biopsy. The study population was divided into three groups of women according to histology of the original biopsy. The first group consisted of 70% of the women. Their biopsies revealed no proliferative changes, and their diagnoses included adenosis, apocrine metaplasia, duct ectasia, and mild epithelial hyperplasia. During the 15 years of follow-up, only 2% of these women developed breast carcinoma. The second group of women, 26%, had breast biopsies that demonstrated varying degrees of epithelial hyperplasia but without atypia. Of these women, 4% developed breast carcinoma during the 15 years; their relative risk was increased 1.6-fold. The last group consisted of the 4% of women with histology that demonstrated atypical ductal or lobular hyperplasia. Their relative risk was 4 to 5 times greater for developing malignancy; 8% developed carcinoma during the 15-year follow-up.

Fibrocystic Changes

Fibrocystic changes are the most common of all benign breast conditions. This condition has a prolific terminology that includes over 35 different names, with mammary dysplasia and chronic cystic mastitis being the two most common. The exact incidence of fibrocystic changes is difficult to establish. Frantz et al. found histologic evidence of fibrocystic changes in 53% of "normal breasts" examined in a series of 225 autopsies. Clinical evidence of fibrocystic changes is discovered in breast examinations of approximately one in three premenopausal women. It is estimated that 50% of women with the histologic findings of fibrocystic changes experience clinical symptoms serious enough to seek medical therapy.

Fibrocystic changes are an exaggerated response of breast tissue to the cyclic levels of ovarian hormones. The condition is most common in women between the ages of 20 to 50 and unusual after the menopause unless associated with exogenous hormone use. The etiology is believed to be an imbalance of the ratio of estrogen to progesterone. However, Peters et al. have postulated that fibrocystic changes are secondary to increased daily prolactin production.

The classic symptom of fibrocystic changes is cyclic bilateral breast pain. The signs of fibrocystic change include increased engorgement and density of the breasts, excessive nodularity, rapid change and fluctuation in the size of cystic areas, increased tenderness, and occasionally spontaneous nipple discharge. Both signs and symptoms are most disturbing during the premenstrual phase of the cycle. The breast pain is bilateral and it is difficult for the patient to localize. Often the pain radiates to the shoulders and upper arms. Severe localized pain may occur when a simple cyst undergoes rapid expansion . The pathophysiology that produces these symptoms and signs includes cyst formation, epithelial and fibrous proliferation, and varying degrees of fluid retention. The differential diagnosis of breast pain includes referred pain from a dorsal radiculitis or inflammation of the costal chondral junction (Tietze's syndrome). The latter two conditions have symptoms that are not cyclic and are unrelated to the menstrual cycle.

On physical examination the findings of excessive nodularity of fibrocystic changes have been described as similar to palpating the surface of a plateful of peas. Multiple solid areas are described as ill-defined thicknesses or areas of "palpable lumpiness" that are rubbery in consistency and may seem more two dimensional than the three-dimensional mass associated with a carcinoma. During palpation the larger cysts have a consistency similar to a balloon filled with water.

There are three clinical stages, with each stage having predominant histologic findings. Clinically these stages have considerable overlap. The stages are described to allow understanding of the condition's natural history.

The first stage occurs in women in their 20s and is termed *mazoplasia* (mastoplasia). Breast pain is noted primarily in the upper, outer quadrants of the breast. The indurated axillary tail is in the most tender area of the breast. During this phase there is intense proliferation of the stroma.

The second clinical stage of *adenosis* occurs generally in women in their 30s. The breast pain and tenderness are premenstrual but less severe. Multiple small breast nodules vary from 2 to 10 mm in diameter. The histologic picture of adenosis demonstrates marked proliferation and hyperplasia of ducts, ductules, and alveolar cells.

The last stage is termed the *cystic* phase and usually occurs in women in their 40s. There is no severe breast pain unless a cyst increases rapidly in size. In this situation a woman experiences a sudden pain with point tenderness and discovers a lump. Cysts are tender to palpation and vary from microscopic to 5 cm in diameter. The cysts in fibrocystic changes often regress in size. The fluid aspirated from a large cyst is straw colored, dark brown, or green, depending on the chronicity of the cyst.

The histology of fibrocystic changes is characterized by proliferation and hyperplasia of the lobular, ductal, and acinar epithelium. Usually proliferation of fibrous tissue occurs and accompanies epithelial hyperplasia. Many histologic variants of fibrocystic change have been described, including cysts (from microscopic to large, blue, domed cysts), adenosis (florid, blunt duct, sclerosing), fibrosis (periductal and stromal), duct ectasia, apocrine metaplasia, intraductal epithelial hyperplasia, and papillomatosis. Ductal epithelial hyperplasia and atypia and apocrine metaplasia with atypia are the most prominent histologic findings directly associated with the subsequent development of breast carcinoma. If these two conditions are discovered on breast biopsy, the chance of breast carcinoma in the future is fivefold greater than in controls.

The treatment of fibrocystic change depends on the severity of symptoms and varies from mechanical support of the breast to surgical therapy for intractable pain. The vast majority of symptoms can be controlled by medical therapy. If a persistent, dominant three-dimensional mass develops, a tissue biopsy is mandatory. Initial therapy of fibrocystic changes consists of the patient wearing a "support" bra, which provides adequate support for the breasts both night and day. Diuretics during the premenstrual phase occasionally relieve breast discomfort. Minton has advocated advising patients to reduce their consumption of methylxanthines and tobacco. Methylxanthines are commonly found in coffee, tea, cola drinks, chocolate, and many nonprescription medications. Minton studied 106 women with clinical fibrocystic changes and found that in 68% the condition resolved and in another 24% the clinical symptoms improved by decreasing consumption of methylxanthines and nicotine. However, four recent case-control studies have found no association between caffeine or methylxanthine consumption and benign breast disease.

Oral contraceptives or supplemental progestogens during the secretory phase of the cycle have both been used to treat fibrocystic change, but the drug of choice for severe symptoms is danazol. Dosages of 100, 200, and 400 mg daily continuously for 4 to 6 months have been employed. Danazol relieves breast symptoms and decreases nodularity of the breast in approximately 90% of patients. This effect lasts for several months after discontinuation of danazol. Patients who do not respond to danazol should receive a trial of bromocriptine or tamoxifen. Bromocriptine, an inhibitor of prolactin, is given continuously in a dosage of 5 mg daily. Tamoxifen is a synthetic antiestrogen commonly used as a chemotherapeutic agent for breast carcinoma. Tamoxifen competes with estradiol for estrogen receptors in the breast. Small clinical studies have documented a 70% relief of breast symptoms when tamoxifen is prescribed for fibrocystic changes. Women with cyclic breast pain seem to respond better than those with chronic mastalgia.

On rare occasions a woman with severe fibrocystic changes is treated surgically by total mastectomy. Subcutaneous mastectomy produces a better cosmetic result. However, it does not remove all the breast tissue. Thus, if the surgery is being performed prophylactically, the risk of breast cancer remains. Indications for surgery include intractable pain not relieved by medical therapy, a history of multiple breast biopsies, or biopsy evidence of a precancerous lesion.

Fibroadenomas

Fibroadenomas are firm, rubbery, freely mobile, solid, usually solitary breast masses. They are the second most common type of benign breast disease. Fibroadenomas most frequently present in adolescents and women in their 20s. Typically the young woman discovers the painless mass accidentally while bathing. Growth of the mass is usually extremely slow but may be quite rapid. Fibroadenomas do not change in size with the menstrual cycle, and they do not produce breast pain or tenderness.

The average fibroadenoma is 2.5 cm in diameter. Multiple fibroadenomas are discovered in 15% to 20% of patients. After surgical removal, fibroadenomas recur in approximately 20% of women.

Sometimes it is difficult to distinguish a fibroadenoma from a cyst. Mammography is rarely indicated in a woman under age 30.

However, ultrasound is helpful in differentiating a solid from a cystic mass. If the mass cannot be aspirated with a needle, surgical removal is indicated. Only histologic examination of either the aspirate or the biopsy specimen will differentiate this lesion from a medullary or papillary carcinoma. Fibroadenomas can be removed without difficulty under local anesthesia. They are rubbery in consistency, well circumscribed, and easily delineated from surrounding breast tissue.

Cystosarcoma Phyllodes

Cystosarcoma phyllodes are fibroepithelial breast tumors that may arise from fibroadenomas. Cystosarcoma phyllodes are rare in that they represent only 2.5% of fibroepithelial tumors and 1% of breast malignancies. They are the most frequent breast sarcoma. These rapidly growing tumors are most common in the fifth decade of life. One in four of these tumors is malignant, yet only one out of ten metastasizes. If metastatic disease is discovered, it is the stromal tissue that predominates. Treatment of benign cystosarcoma phyllodes is local excision with a wide margin of normal breast tissue. Differentiation of benign from malignant tumors by strict histologic criteria has resulted in poor correlation in some series. Recent studies using flow cytometry have improved on the predictive value in differentiating the biologic nature of the neoplasia.

Intraductal Papilloma

The predominant symptom of an intraductal papilloma is spontaneous discharge from one nipple. This symptom usually appears in a woman in the perimenopausal age group. The discharge from the nipple is *spontaneous* and intermittent. The consistency of the discharge associated with an intraductal papilloma can be watery, serous, or serosanguineous. The amount of discharge varies from a few drops to several milliliters of fluid. During examination of the breast, it is important to circumferentially put pressure on different areas of the areola. This technique helps to identify whether the discharge emanates from a single duct or multiple openings. When the discharge comes from a single duct, the differential diagnosis involves both intraductal papilloma and carcinoma. If multiple ducts are involved, the diagnosis of carcinoma is more likely. Intraductal papillomas are usually microscopic but may grow to 2 to 3 mm in diameter, extending radially from the alveolar margin.

Nipple Discharge

Nipple discharge may be a complaint of women with either benign or malignant breast disease. Leis reported a series of 7588 women with breast operations; 85% had a mass, and 7% had a chief complaint of discharge from the nipple. Of the 560 patients operated on for nipple discharge, 493 findings were benign and 67 malignant.

To be medically significant, discharge from the breast should be spontaneous and persistent in a nonlactating woman. Many normal women can express a few drops of sticky gray, green, or black viscous fluid. The importance of diagnosing the etiology of *spontaneous* nonmilky discharge from the nipple is to rule out carcinoma. The color of the discharge does not differentiate a benign from a malignant process. Malignancies have been associated with clear, serous, or serosanguineous or bloody nipple discharges. Cytology of the discharge is important but often not diagnostic. Most series document a false negative rate of approximately 20%. Therefore a negative cytology should not deter surgical biopsy.

Before excisional biopsy a patient with a persistent discharge of any type should have mammography. In a young woman with a suspected intraductal papilloma, the involved duct, which is usually blue, and a small area of surrounding breast tissue can be removed. Table 13-1 documents that intraductal papillomas and fibrocystic changes are the two most common etiologies of spontaneous nonmilky nipple discharge. In this series, 50 of 432 patients had a carcinoma diagnosed by breast biopsy.

Fat Necrosis

Fat necrosis is rare but important because it is often confused with carcinoma. The patient presents with a firm, tender, indurated, ill-defined mass that may have an area of surrounding ecchymosis. Mammography may demonstrate fine, stippled calcification and stellate contractions. Occasionally there is skin retraction, which further confuses the prebiopsy diagnosis. The usual etiology of fat necrosis is trauma. However, the majority of women do not remember the event that injured the breast. Treatment of fat necrosis is excisional biopsy.

BREAST CARCINOMA

Epidemiology

The etiology of breast carcinoma is poorly understood despite extensive investigation. Epidemiologists have documented some risk factors that provide clues in understanding the pathophysiology of the disease's development in certain high-risk groups of women (Table 13-2). The risk factors can be divided into several categories: heredity, age, hormones, nutrition, demography, radiation, and previous breast disease. Generalizations concerning etiology

---

TABLE 13-1

Relation Between Nipple Discharge and Diagnosis in 432 Operations from New York Medical College, 1960-1975

Discharge	Galactorrhea	Duct Ectasia	Infection	Intraductal Papilloma	Fibrocystic Disease	Cancer
Milky	2	0	0	0	0	0
Multicolored and sticky	0	46	0	0	0	0
Purulent	0	0	14	0	0	0
Watery	0	0	0	3	1	5
Serous	0	5	0	79	52	11
Serosanguineous	0	8	0	59	34	14
Sanguineous	0	6	0	45	28	20
TOTAL	2	65	14	186	115	50

Reprinted with permission from Pilnik S: J Reprod Med 22:286, 1979.

follow similar categories: genetic predisposition, environmental carcinogens, viral agents, and radiation exposure.

Three problems obscure a clear understanding of the risk factors of breast cancer. One is the long latent period before the development of clinically recognizable carcinoma. Second, is the consideration both of the duration and the intensity of factors that may induce or promote cancer. For example, the peak incidence of breast carcinoma in Japanese women after the bombing of Hiroshima and Nagasaki occurred in women who were in the premenarcheal age group at the time of the atomic explosions. Subsequently these teenagers developed breast carcinoma in their mid-30s after the characteristic prolonged latent period. Korenman's estrogen window hypothesis suggests that the radiation (cancer inducer) acted with the background of the unopposed estrogen of adolescents (cancer promoter). Third, epidemiologic studies concentrating on a single risk factor often reach contrary conclusions.

Although there are limits in the clinical applicability of risk factors, selected women at increased risk should be screened at more frequent intervals. Many risk factors are additive. Risk factors are estimates developed by epidemiologists that allow patients and physicians to consider the probability of developing the disease. They have been widely publicized in the lay press. The fact that has not been emphasized is that risk factors identify *only* 25% of women who will eventually develop breast carcinoma.

The United States has one of the highest rates of breast carcinoma in the world. Incidence rates have been increasing gradually over the past 40 years. Presently in the United States, approximately 175,000 new cases of invasive cancer are diagnosed and approximately 44,500 deaths occur yearly from breast carcinoma. The specific risk to an American woman of developing a breast carcinoma is 1 in 9 (11%) during her lifetime. The risk for an American woman without a single risk factor is 1 in 17 (6%). Therefore the message concerning risk should be that every woman in the United States is at risk for breast carcinoma.

TABLE 13-2
Risk Factors for Breast Cancer in Females

Factor	High Risk	Low Risk	Magnitude of Risk Differential*
Age	Old	Young	>>>
Country of birth	North America, Northern Europe	Asia, Africa	>>>
Socioeconomic class	Upper	Lower	>>
Marital status	Never married	Ever married	>
Place of residence	Urban	Rural	>
	Northern U.S.	Southern U.S.	>
Race	White	Black	>
Age at first full-term pregnancy	Older than 30	Younger than 20	>>
Oophorectomy	No	Yes	>>
Body build, postmenopausal	Obese	Thin	>>
Age at menarche	Early	Late	>
Age at menopause	Late	Early	>
Family history of premenopausal bilateral breast cancer	Yes	No	>>>
History of cancer in one breast	Yes	No	>>>
History of fibrocystic disease	Yes	No	>>
Any first-degree relative with breast cancer	Yes	No	>>
History of primary cancer in ovary or endometrium	Yes	No	>>
Radiation to chest	Large doses	Minimal exposure	>>

From Kelsey JL and Berkowitz GS: Cancer Res 48:5615, 1988. Adapted from Kelsey JL: Epidemiol Rev 1:74, 1979. >>>, Relative risk greater than 4.0; >>, relative risk of 2.0 to 4.0; >, relative risk of 1.1 to 1.9.

Berg has made an interesting comparison contrasting breast cancer with another common gynecologic neoplasm, carcinoma of the cervix. In women ages 35 to 39, the rate of breast carcinoma is 55:100,000 women per year. This rate is 3 times greater than the rate for cervical carcinoma in the same age group. The risk of breast carcinoma during a woman's lifetime is similar to the risk of lung cancer in a heavy smoker.

A genetic predisposition to develop breast carcinoma has been recognized in some families. This tendency is not strong enough to develop a specific genetic pattern of inheritance. The basic hypothesis is that women in susceptible families have a genetic predisposition to develop breast carcinoma when exposed to environmental carcinogens. The 2 to 3 times increased risk extends from the mother to first-degree relatives, that is, daughters and sisters. The highest genetic risk (sixfold to ninefold) occurs in first-degree relatives of a premenopausal woman who develops bilateral breast carcinoma.

The frequency of breast carcinoma increases directly with the patient's age (Figure 13-5). Breast carcinoma is almost nonexistent before puberty; the incidence gradually increases during the reproductive years. Eighty-five percent of breast carcinoma occurs after age 40. After menopause the incidence of breast carcinoma increases directly with a woman's age.

The relationship between endogenous ovarian hormones and breast carcinoma has been studied extensively. Several clinical observations support the hypothesis that the risk of breast carcinoma is related to the intensity and duration of exposure to unopposed endogenous estrogen. Breast cancer is most unusual in the prepubertal female. Bilateral oophorectomy before age 35, without hormonal replacement, reduces the risk of breast carcinoma by 70%. Women have an incidence of breast carcinoma 100 times greater than that of men. Coulam et al. have followed 1270 women with chronic anovulation. They discovered a relative risk of 1.45 for the postmenopausal development of breast carcinoma in women with a history of many years of premenopausal unopposed estrogen. Their study is another example of the pro-

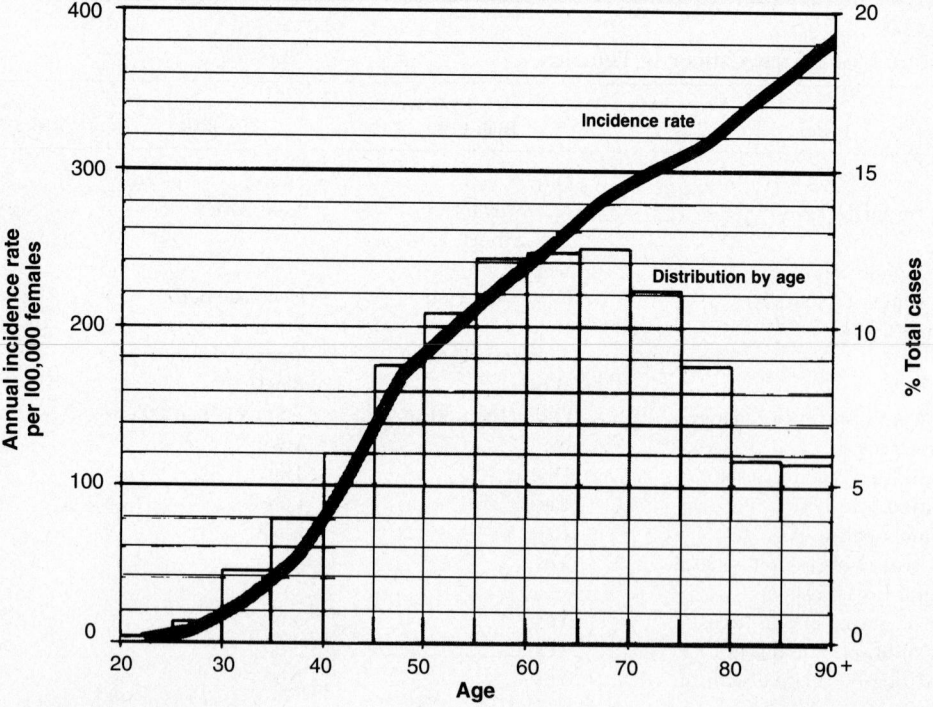

FIGURE 13-5
Incidence in the United States, by age, of female breast cancer. (From Seidman H and Mushinski MH: Breast cancer incidence, mortality, survival, and prognosis. In Feig SA and McLelland R, editors: Breast carcinoma: current diagnosis and treatment, New York, 1983, Masson Publishing USA, Inc. Copyright by American College of Radiology.)

longed latent period between exposure and development of clinical disease.

Obese women are at a higher risk for developing breast carcinoma during the postmenopausal years. The pathophysiology of this tendency is believed to be an increased amount of peripheral conversion of androstenedione to estrone and decreased levels of sex hormone–binding globulin. Marchant described the increased risk associated with prolonged menstrual function. Women with spontaneous menopause before age 45 experience one-half the risk of developing breast carcinoma as do women who are still menstruating at age 54. A similar study documented a twofold increased risk for women who menstruated for 40 years or longer contrasted with that for women who menstruated for 30 years or less.

Demographic data describe significant variations in the incidence of breast carcinoma from country to country. In a descriptive review of the epidemiology of breast carcinoma, De Waard points out that women living in the United States have a much higher rate of breast carcinoma than women living in Africa, Asia, or the Middle East. The age-specific incidence of breast carcinoma in American women is 6 times greater than among women in Japan. Interestingly, studies of Japanese families who moved to the United States demonstrate that their rate of breast carcinoma becomes similar to that of American women after two generations. The demographic data are believed to be due to differences in total dietary fat and obesity. Epidemiologic studies performed within the same culture have demonstrated differences in incidences of breast cancer directly related to the amount of fat in the diet. Several studies have reported a 40% to 50% increase in the risk of developing breast cancer related to alcohol consumption. The possible confounding effects of other dietary factors are difficult to exclude in these studies.

Ionizing radiation is a definite risk factor because of the long-accepted relationship between radiation and malignant transformation. The experience of Japanese women who survived the atomic bomb has been discussed. There are small groups of women who received multiple radiation treatments for postpartum mastitis, irradiation of the thymus in infancy, or multiple fluoroscopic examinations during treatment for tuberculosis who have subsequently developed breast carcinoma at an increased rate. The data concerning relative risk of developing breast carcinoma are most consistent with a linear dose-response relationship.

Previous history of breast disease is an important risk factor. Once the patient has developed carcinoma of one breast, her risk is approximately 1% per year of developing cancer in the other breast. As stated previously, the extent of epithelial hyperplasia and atypia in women with benign breast disease determines the magnitude of risk for developing carcinoma. Women with ovarian, endometrial, or colon carcinoma have a twofold to fourfold greater risk of also developing breast carcinoma.

The age at which a woman delivers her first child is more important as a risk factor than parity. If a woman's first term birth occurs before age 20, she has 50% less risk than a nulliparous woman. If the first term pregnancy occurs after age 35, the risk is 1.5 times greater than for women who have their first baby before age 26. For many years it was believed that nursing an infant offered a protective effect for the future development of breast neoplasia. Subsequent studies have documented that nursing is neither a positive nor a negative risk factor. Reserpine, which elevates prolactin levels, has been shown not to be a risk factor. Rosenberg et al. could find no relationship between cigarette smoking and the incidence of breast cancer.

The vast majority of studies involving exogenous estrogen either in oral contraceptives or given to postmenopausal women have not reported increased incidence of subsequent breast carcinoma. Estrogens are considered tumor promoters in respect to the pathophysiology of breast carcinoma rather than inducers or initiators of carcinoma. Thus any adverse effect should increase with duration of use, and a dose-response curve should be recognized. Some recently reported epidemiologic studies have found an elevated risk for subsets of women under age 45. However, no consistent evidence showed an increase in breast cancer risk through middle age, even in long-term oral contraceptive users or in women with a family history of breast carcinoma (Chapters 11 and 40).

Detection and Diagnosis

Detection of breast carcinoma is defined as the use of screening tests in asymptomatic women at periodic intervals to discover breast malignancies. The advantage of early detection and diagnosis is reduced mortality because of smaller-sized cancers, more localized lesions, and a lower percentage of positive nodes. Established methods of detection include self-examination of the breasts, periodic examination by physicians, and mammography.

Physical examination and mammography are complementary procedures that must be considered together. Breast self-examination (BSE) has the major advantages of no cost to the patient and convenience. Thermography and ultrasound are unproved as methods to detect early breast carcinoma and should be considered experimental. Diagnosis can be established only by biopsy or fine-needle aspiration. A negative mammogram does not rule out breast carcinoma.

The kinetics of growth in breast carcinoma are important for understanding screening and detection. The average breast mass doubles in volume every 100 days and doubles in diameter every 300 days. A breast carcinoma grows for 6 to 8 years before reaching a diameter of 1 cm. In slightly less than another year the carcinoma will reach 2 cm in diameter. The mean diameter of a breast mass discovered by women who perform BSE at monthly intervals is 2 cm.

Greenwald et al. studied the results of BSE and of physician examination on the stage of breast carcinoma at initial diagnosis. Of 293 women with breast carcinoma, cancer was detected in clinical stage I in 54% when the detection method was routine physical examination, in 38% when the detection method was BSE, and in only 27% when the detection of the mass was accidental. In this study, only 50% of women who performed BSE did so on a monthly basis. These authors estimated that the breast cancer mortality might be reduced 19% by BSE and 24% by annual examination of the breasts by physicians.

In another study, Foster and Costanza determined the relationship between BSE and survival of breast cancer patients. Their study group included 1004 newly diagnosed invasive breast carcinoma in Vermont from July 1975 to December 1982. During this time, there was not widespread use of screening mammography in their state. The survival rate at 5 years was 75% for women who examined their own breasts versus 57% for women who did not examine their breasts. The authors concluded that in their population, BSE was responsible for earlier detection, improved survival, smaller tumor size, and fewer axillary node metastases. Their findings persisted after controlling the analysis for the potential bias of confounding variables, such as age, length-biased sampling, and lead-time bias.

Self-Examination of the Breasts

The majority of breast masses are initially discovered by the patient, either accidentally or during BSE. In a group of women having annual mammography and physical examinations by physicians, one of three carcinomas was discovered by the patients in the interval between professional detection methods. Even with widespread national publicity, approximately 50% of women do not perform monthly BSE. However, over 90% of women who regularly practice BSE were instructed in the techniques by their physicians. It is ironic that the group of women who are most eager to perform BSE are between the ages of 18 and 34. This age group has the greatest anxiety concerning breast cancer, yet because of their age they are at the lowest risk. In Foster's and Costanza's study of newly diagnosed carcinomas, 424 women performed BSE and 411 did not. The average size of the breast mass in women who performed BSE monthly was 2.1 cm. For those who performed BSE less than monthly, it was 2.4 cm; for the nonexaminers, 3.2 cm.

The most effective teaching of BSE occurs in a one-to-one relationship. It is ideal to test the patient's ability to palpate masses in manufactured breast models. These models should contain masses with diameters as small as 0.3 to 0.5 cm.

Instructions for the patient concerning the techniques of breast self-palpation should emphasize timing, inspection, and palpation. The few days immediately after a menstrual period are the best time to detect changes in normal lumps or texture of the breasts. Postmenopausal women or women who have had a hysterectomy should be instructed to perform BSE on the same calendar days each month. The patient should inspect her breasts in the mirror, looking for changes in shape and contour of the breasts and changes in the skin or nipples.

Women should be instructed that bilateral soft thickening and nodularity are normal physical findings. Palpation should begin in the shower, since many women have increased tactile sensitivity by using a "wet" technique. After the shower the woman should lie down, initially with one arm at her side and subsequently with the same arm underneath her head. She should be instructed to use the pads of her second, third, and fourth fingers to palpate the contralateral breast. Using the pads of her fingers, in a massaging motion with firm pressure, she should examine the entire breast and surrounding chest wall in a systematic fashion. One of the easier techniques to follow is to palpate the breasts in a clockwise fashion beginning at the nipple and gradually circumscribing larger circles.

Physical Examination

The ability to detect breast lumps varies widely from physician to physician. Fletcher et al. tested the physical examination techniques of 80 different physicians using manufactured breast models. The simulated breasts of the mannequins had a volume of 250 ml and the consistency of the breast tissue of a 50-year-old woman. The ability to detect the mass was directly related to the size of the mass; 87% of 1 cm, 33% of 0.5 cm, and 14% of 0.3 cm masses were discovered. The most disturbing finding was the wide range of detection rates among physicians, from 17% to 83%. In general, physicians with higher discovery rates spent more time performing the examination. The number of masses detected by a physician increased in those who used a consistent geometric pattern of examination with variable pressure exerted by the fingertips.

A thorough breast examination by the physician should take 3 to 5 minutes to complete. This time is also an ideal opportunity to instruct the patient in the technique of BSE. A complete breast examination involves inspecting and palpating the breasts with the patient in the sitting as well as the supine position.

Initially, with a woman sitting on the examining table, the physician inspects the contour, symmetry, and vascular pattern of the breasts and skin for irritation, retraction, or edema. It is important to have the patient place her arms above her head and subsequently place her hands on her hips. This sequence will contract the pectoralis muscles, which may allow the physician to visualize an abnormality. The patient in the sitting position is in the optimal position for the physician to determine the presence of adenopathy in the axilla (Figure 13-6).

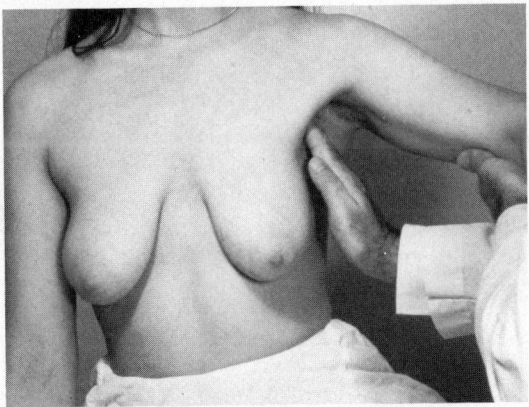

FIGURE 13-6
Examination of axilla in sitting position during breast examination. (From Marchant DJ: Clin Obstet Gynecol 25:361, 1982.)

The patient's breasts should be subsequently examined with the woman in the supine position. It is important to examine both nipples for retraction, skin irritation, or a discharge. The areola should be compressed to identify any discharge. The normal breast has a small depression directly below the nipple. The skin of the breast is again carefully inspected for unusual vascular patterns, edema, erythema, or retraction.

Palpation is performed with the patient's arms at her side and raised above the head and should not be limited to the breast tissue alone. The examiner should palpate the axilla, the supraclavicular areas, and the adjacent chest wall. Palpation should use the pads of the first three fingers placed together, exerting firm but gentle pressure. Each physician determines his or her own systematic approach, the majority preferring concentric circles. It is very important that the physician draw a descriptive picture of any positive finding. This picture should include notations concerning the site, shape, size, consistency, and mobility of the mass. Special notation should be made as to whether the mass is tender and whether it is attached to skin or deep structures (Figure 13-7).

Mammography

Mammography is the only reliable method of detecting breast carcinoma at an early and highly curable stage, ideally occult cancer.

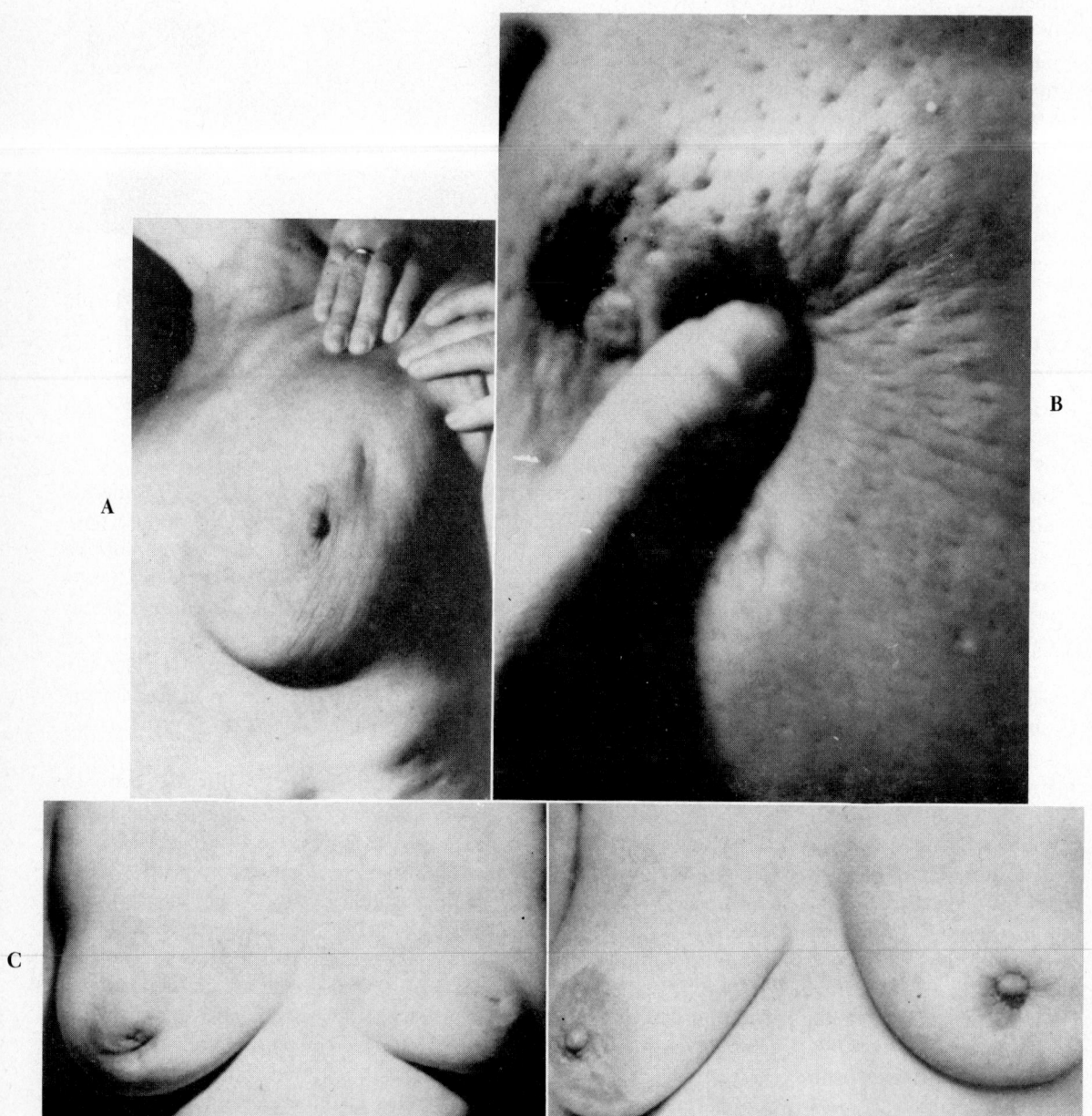

FIGURE 13-7
Signs of breast carcinoma. **A,** Retraction found during physical examination. **B,** Peau d'orange from underlying carcinoma. **C,** Retraction of right nipple. **D,** Retraction of left nipple from carcinoma. (From Degrell I: Atlas of diseases of the mammary gland, Basel, 1976, S Karger AG, p 20.)

Mammography is also the most accurate method of detecting nonpalpable breast carcinoma. The clinical advantages of discovering breast carcinoma during its earliest stage include higher percentage of localized disease, lower incidence of positive regional nodes, and reduced mortality. The 5-year survival of women whose breast cancer is believed to be localized to the breast with negative axillary nodes is 85%. In contrast, the 5-year survival is only 53% when axillary nodes are positive. Ten-year survival statistics in women with negative nodes are approximately 74%, and 39% in women with positive nodes. Therefore, with increasing emphasis on conservative surgery for early carcinomas, mammography will save not only lives but also breasts.

Most physicians are able to consistently palpate breast masses when they are 1 cm in diameter or greater. Mammography may discover fine calcifications in breast neoplasms months to years before the carcinoma enlarges to a size that may be palpated on physical examination. Studying the kinetics of growth of breast cancer helps the clinician to appreciate why breast carcinoma is so often a systemic disease. Breast carcinoma must develop neovascularization to grow beyond 1 to 2 mm in diameter. Neovascularization provides the breast carcinoma the capability of metastasizing via the vascular system. The average breast carcinoma grows for 3 years, to enlarge from 1 mm to 1 cm.

Image quality in mammography has undergone major improvements during the past 15 years. New equipment has decreased the radiation exposure associated with mammography approximately tenfold. Because of these two changes, the guidelines regarding the use of mammography for detection of early breast carcinoma have been expanded. Conservative estimates are that 50 million American women should be screened by mammography each year. This challenge to radiologists has been summarized by McLelland. He believes there are two definite restraints on the optimal use of mammography to identify early breast carcinoma: a lack of properly trained and committed radiologists and the cost of the test. McLelland emphasizes that mammography is a technically demanding procedure that requires an experienced and meticulous interpretation of the films, as well as correlation of the images with a thorough clinical examination.

Historically, two landmark studies laid the foundation for the scientific credibility of mammography as a screening procedure. The first large, randomized control study was undertaken in the early 1960s by the Health Insurance Plan of New York (HIP). The HIP investigation involved yearly screening by both mammography and physical examination for 5 years. The women were followed for 10 to 14 years, and the study demonstrated a 30% reduction in mortality from breast carcinoma in the women who had annual mammography compared with the control group.

The second pivotal study was performed in 29 centers throughout the United States during the late 1970s. This immense undertaking was sponsored by the National Institutes of Health and was named the Breast Cancer Detection Demonstration Project (BCDDP). The BCDDP involved screening 275,000 women, and during the 5 years of the project, 3557 breast carcinomas were found, 42% discovered only by mammography.

The definite improvements in mammographic diagnosis over the 12-year interval between the two studies is documented by comparing their results. Cancer detection was approximately two times more frequent in the BCDDP study. In women ages 40 to 49, mammography found 39% of carcinomas in the HIP investigation, compared with 85% identified in the BCDDP project. Most important, in the detection of carcinoma less than 1 cm, the results were 36% in the BCDDP versus 8% in the HIP. Two more recent studies from the Netherlands have documented a 50% to 70% reduction in number of deaths secondary to breast carcinoma in those women screened by regular mammography.

In the mid-1970s there was an intense controversy over the risks versus benefits of mammography in women under age 50. At that time the benefits of screening premenopausal women were questioned, and the higher sensitivity of the breasts of younger women to the harmful effect of radiation was stressed. However, improved diagnostic techniques and equipment have eliminated the controversy, and the American Cancer Society expanded its recommendations for mammography in 1983 (see box on p. 13-16).

Nemoto et al. surveyed 12,315 new breast carcinomas diagnosed in 1977. Patients initially discovered 73%, physicians found 23%, and only 4% were initially identified by mammography. It is speculated that these percentages

AMERICAN CANCER SOCIETY GUIDELINES FOR MAMMOGRAPHIC SCREENING OF ASYMPTOMATIC WOMEN

1. Baseline mammogram for all women at age 35 to 40 years
2. Mammography at 1- to 2-year intervals from 40 to 49 years
3. Annual mammogram for women 50 years or older

From Kopans DB, Meyer JE, and Sadowsky N: N Engl J Med 310:966, 1984. Reprinted by permission of The New England Journal of Medicine.

will be reversed by the increased use of mammography during the 1990s.

Present recommendations to detect breast cancer include encouraging all women to perform BSE annually. For women ages 35 to 40, it is important to emphasize annual physical examination of the breast for the rest of their lives and to obtain a baseline mammogram. Women ages 40 to 49 should obtain a mammogram approximately every 1 to 2 years. These guidelines were reaffirmed at a consensus conference in Washington, D.C., in June 1989. However, because one third of breast carcinomas occur before age 50, increasing emphasis is being placed on early discovery in young women. Thus we obtain the initial baseline examination at age 35 and advise patients to have mammography every 12 to 18 months between ages 40 and 49. After age 50, every asymptomatic woman should have a mammogram at least yearly. More frequent physical examinations and mammograms may be indicated, depending on individual risk factors and the finding of precursors of breast carcinoma.

Mammography is established as part of the diagnostic workup of women with breast symptoms. Often significant occult disease is identified in another quadrant of the same breast or in the contralateral breast. All patients with breast masses or persistent spontaneous nipple discharge should have mammograms of both breasts before biopsy. Mammography is also indicated in evaluating a breast mass the patient has found but that the physician cannot confirm by palpation. This technique is helpful in difficult clinical problems, such as the evaluation of large breasts or following augmentation mammoplasty. It is important to stress once again that mammography and physical exami-

nation are complementary procedures. One procedure does not replace the necessity of carefully performing the other.

There are two major types of radiologic equipment to obtain mammograms: xeromammography and screen film mammography. Xeromammography is used less often. Although there are minor advantages and disadvantages for each technique, the sensitivity and specificity of mammography depend primarily on the skill of the technician and radiologist and not on the equipment used.

In xeromammography the image is produced by a photoelectric process on aluminum plates coated with selenium. The two definite advantages of xeromammograms are wide recording latitude and edge enhancement. Wide recording latitude emphasizes subtle differences in density of breast tissues. The edge-enhancement phenomenon improves the visualization of microcalcifications and spiculations, especially in dense breasts.

Screen film mammography was developed initially to reduce the radiation exposure from mammography by the use of specialized x-ray equipment. This technique is excellent to delineate soft tissue masses from surrounding tissue. Reduced exposure time causes less distortion of the image by motion. This technique requires firm breast compression to obtain optimal results, including uniform tissue thickness, maximal geometric detail, and increased image contrast.

Optimal identification of early breast carcinoma by mammography depends on a competent technician obtaining excellent images and the radiologist searching for subtle changes. Breast cancer may be detected by visualizing clusters of fine calcifications or spiculations or poorly defined multinodular masses with irregular contours, all characteristic of malignancy.

Isolated clusters of tiny calcifications are the most common and important diagnostic sign of an early carcinoma. Calcifications are often smaller than 0.5 mm in diameter and thus must be identified by a magnifying lens. The presence of five or more calcifications within a volume of 1 cm^3 is termed a *cluster*. Subsequent breast biopsies will find 25% of clusters associated with cancer and 75% with benign disease. Conversely, approximately 68% of occult breast carcinomas and 34% of palpable breast cancers demonstrate calcifications on mammographic examination.

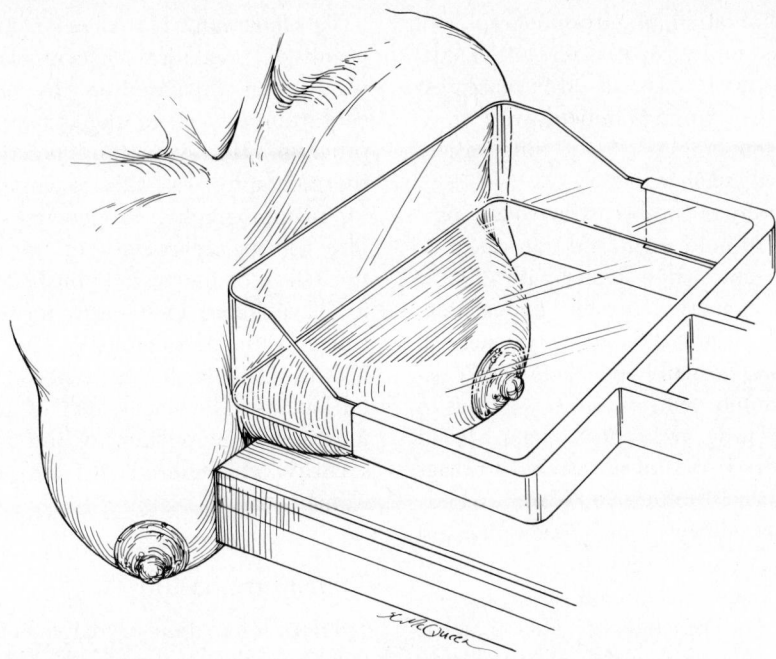

FIGURE 13-8
Mammography being performed with appropriate compression applied. (Redrawn from Wilson OL: Mammographic technique. In Parsons CA, editor: Diagnosis of breast disease: imaging, clinical features, and pathology, London, © 1983, Chapman & Hall Ltd, p 67.)

Sickles emphasized the importance of firm breast compression to spread apart areas of dense tissue within the breast and possibly identify "hidden" carcinoma (Figure 13-8). He further advocated the importance of side-by-side comparison of both breasts and evaluating current films with previous ones. This facilitates identification of the less classic, indirect signs of breast carcinoma, such as a single dilated duct with intraductal carcinoma, asymptomatic architectural distortion in dense breasts, and a developing density.

The relationship between high levels of radiation and increased risk for breast carcinoma raises questions concerning the relative risk of the carcinogenic effect of mammography. The measured radiation dose to the breast by state-of-the-art mammography equipment is approximately 0.1 rad (0.01 Gy) for a two-view examination. Feig and Ehrlich (1990) have estimated the lifetime radiation risk, or numbers of excess breast carcinomas, that could be related to mammography of 1 million women. These rates are related to age at time of exposure. For women ages 40 to 44, the lifetime risk is 5.2 excess cancers versus an annual natural breast cancer incidence of 115 cases. In contrast, for women ages 60 to 64, the numbers would be 0.8 versus 292 spontaneous cancers. Thus the benefits of screening far outweigh any possible radiation risk. This lifetime radiation risk of death, which is approximately between one and two per million, is similar to driving 220 miles by car, riding a bike for 10 miles, or smoking 1.5 cigarettes.

The incidence of breast carcinoma in the United States is 1000 cases per million women per year for women in their early 40s. In summary, the risk of radiation from mammography is negligible compared with the benefits of the discovery of early and potentially curable breast carcinoma.

Ultrasound

Ultrasound has a definite role as a complementary procedure to other imaging techniques in the diagnosis of breast disease, particularly in differentiating cystic from solid masses. The primary advantage of ultrasound is the ability to produce images of breast tissue on multiple occasions without harmful effects.

The greatest limitation of ultrasonography of the breast is the limited spatial resolution. Microcalcifications are not visualized because resolution of less than 2 mm is difficult with ultrasound. Also, sonography cannot differentiate benign from malignant masses.

Ultrasonography of the breast is usually performed by a hand-held, real-time transducer or sometimes by automated water-bath instruments. Breast cancer is usually hypoechoic, and early cancers are difficult to distinguish from surrounding normal hypoechoic breast tissue. The most important use of ultrasound is to differentiate a cystic breast mass from a solid mass. The accuracy rate of ultrasound to diagnose a cystic mass is 96% to 100% and exceeds the combined accuracy of mammography and physical examination. Ultrasound may be used as a guide for needle aspiration and occasionally in localization procedures. This imaging technique also may be useful in diagnosing women with augmentation mammoplasty and in the differential diagnosis of masses in the dense breast tissue of younger women.

Sickles et al. reported a comparison study using state-of-the-art equipment. Mammography detected 62 of 64 (97%) carcinomas, while ultrasound diagnosed only 37 of 64 (58%). Only 8% of carcinomas smaller than 1 cm in diameter were discovered by ultrasound. The majority of breast carcinomas visualized by ultrasound can be palpated clinically. In a small series of 31 proved carcinomas, Egan and Egan found 68% diagnosed by ultrasound versus 77% by mammography.

In summary, ultrasound should not be used as a sole imaging technique for breast disease. It is more time consuming and usually slightly more expensive than mammography. Because of its lack of sensitivity and specificity for early breast carcinoma, it should not be used in an attempt to detect subclinical disease.

Thermography

Thermography is unreliable as a screening technique for breast carcinoma or as a technique to determine women at increased risk for subsequent breast neoplasia. Lawson first described the elevation of skin temperature associated with breast carcinoma in 1956. Although thermography has been used clinically since that time, because of its extremely high false-positive and false-negative rates, it still must be considered experimental.

Thermography is ineffective in detection of occult or preclinical cancers. This technique was initially included in the national multi-center breast cancer detection demonstration program. However, the detection rate with thermography was 42% as compared to 92% for mammography. Proponents of thermography list the advantages of the low cost and the safety of the test. Published clinical studies have found low sensitivity and poor specificity with thermography. Therefore its clinical use should be restricted to experimental studies. The major fault of a normal thermography examination is the false sense of security engendered in the symptom-free woman.

Transillumination

Transillumination, or diaphanography, is the technique that measures the light transmitted through breast tissue. The breast acts as a filter for the light; the hypothesis is that malignant tissue absorbs more infrared light than does benign tissue. Present techniques employ a high-intensity tungsten lamp source and measure transmission by a camera with infrared film. In dense breasts, only 1% of emitted light is transmitted. This technique is definitely experimental and unproved. To date results of research studies using transillumination do not begin to compare with results obtained with mammography.

Computed Tomography

Computed tomography (CT) has limited value when compared with mammography because of higher radiation dose and longer study times. The thickness of cross-sectional slices with CT miss the majority of areas of microcalcification. CT scans have demonstrated some preclinical cancers after injection with radio-contrast media. This imaging technique is excellent for studying the most medial and lateral aspects of the breast. However, the increased expense and radiation exposure virtually eliminate CT scans for screening programs.

Magnetic Resonance Imaging

Research with magnetic resonance imaging (MRI) for the detection of breast carcinoma is in its infancy. Because of higher costs, this imaging technique will not be used in screening but as a diagnostic test. The ability of MRI to differentiate benign from malignant tissue may help to reduce the frequency of breast biopsy. Other potential uses of MRI are to help differentiate solid from cystic masses and to determine preoperative staging. However, MRI probably will not be used in screening programs, since the average examination takes 45 minutes to 1 hour, and MRI cannot identify microcalcifications. Another limitation of MRI is the loss of image quality with respiratory movements.

Digital Radiography

Digital radiography is the technique by which x-ray photons are detected after passing through the breast tissue. This imaging technique potentially may be the screening modality of the future, for it reduces radiation exposure to one tenth of the amount of modern mammographic equipment. However, the high cost per test may make it financially impractical to use digital radiography for screening.

Needle Aspiration

The presence of a dominant breast mass in a woman over age 25 demands investigation to rule out carcinoma. In premenopausal women, approximately one out of three dominant masses is a benign cyst. Breast cancer is rarely cystic. Cysts are usually round, mobile, and rubbery in consistency and may be tender to palpation. In women over age 35, mammography usually should be performed prior to needle aspiration, as hematoma formation may delay obtaining reliable mammograms. The relief of a patient's anxiety produced by successfully aspirating a newly discovered breast mass is most gratifying.

Needle aspiration of a breast cyst can be performed easily and rapidly in the office. Initially the skin is prepared with an iodine solution. Many physicians do not use local anesthesia as the skin over the breast is the only sensitive area. Breast tissue itself has few pain fibers. However, an injection of local anesthesia into a small area of the skin may alleviate the patient's anxiety. The suspected cyst is secured between the thumb and first two fingers of one hand. The other hand introduces a 20-gauge needle (3.8 cm long) attached to a 10 or 20 ml syringe. One feels a "give" or reduced resistance after puncturing the cyst wall. Smaller

cysts can be aspirated using 22- to 25-gauge needles. Technically it is easier to manipulate these smaller needles without the syringe attached. Complete aspiration of all the fluid from the cyst is facilitated by negative pressure from the syringe and firm pressure on the cyst wall. With withdrawal of the fluid the cyst wall collapses, and usually a residual mass cannot be palpated. After withdrawal of the needle, firm pressure is applied for 5 to 10 minutes to reduce the possibility of hematoma formation. Complications of needle aspiration are minimal, with hematoma formation being the only substantial one. Infection is very rare. The theoretical risk of spreading cancer along the needle track has not been substantiated.

The color of the fluid obtained via aspiration varies from clear to grossly bloody. If the aspirated fluid is clear, it is not necessary to submit it for cytologic evaluation. Strawbridge et al. discovered malignant cells in only three samples of clear fluid from 834 aspirated breast cysts. If the aspirated fluid is not clear, it should be placed on a cover slip and sent for cytologic interpretation. The aspirated fluid may be turbid and yellow, brown or green, or bloody. Bloody fluid is usually from a traumatic tap, but the rare cystic carcinoma must be considered.

No further workup is necessary if the aspirated fluid is clear and no residual mass is palpated immediately after the procedure and again 1 month later. However, if the aspirate is bloody or the mass remains, a biopsy should be performed. Obviously, if fluid is not obtained or the mammogram is suspicious, definitive diagnosis by biopsy or fine-needle aspiration cytology is mandatory. Cysts that recur within 2 weeks or necessitate more than one repeat aspiration should be biopsied.

Biopsy

The definitive diagnosis and ultimate foundation for treatment of breast carcinoma depends on histologic diagnosis of biopsy material. The common indications for tissue biopsy include bloody discharge from the nipple, a persistent three-dimensional mass, and/or suspicious mammography. Nipple retraction or elevation and skin changes, such as erythema, induration, or edema, are also indications for breast biopsy. Obviously, the suspicious area must be sampled appropriately. A small biopsy may be appropriate for a large mass. However,

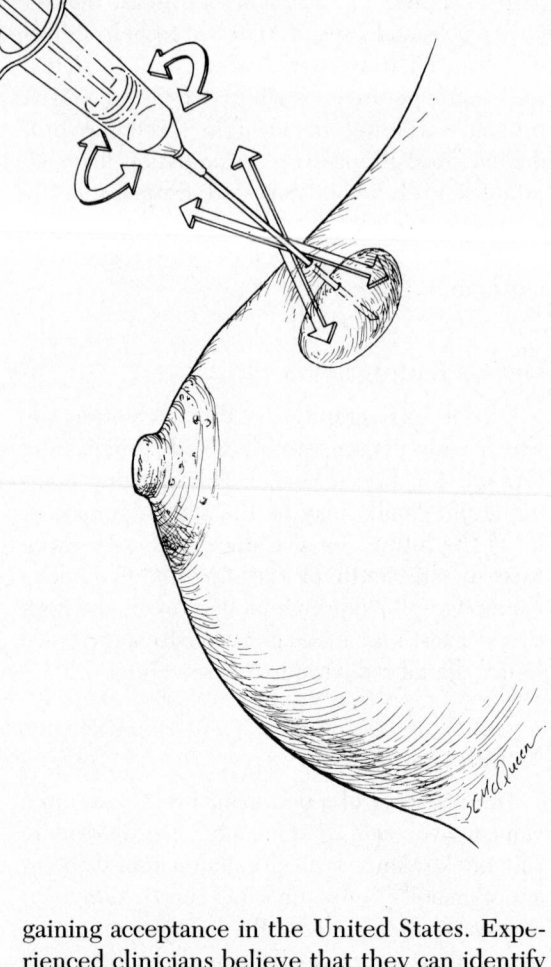

FIGURE 13-9
Needle biopsy and aspiration with negative pressure. Needle is rotated, moved back and forth, and slightly in and out to aspirate representative specimen. (From Vorherr H: Am J Obstet Gynecol 148:128, 1984.)

it is important to obtain a large wedge of breast tissue so as not to miss an occult carcinoma identified by mammography. The technique of excisional biopsy is to obtain a 1 cm margin of normal tissue around the mass.

Today the majority of open breast biopsies are performed under local anesthesia on an outpatient basis. Fifteen years ago, it was common practice to perform a biopsy, frozen section, and definitive surgery during the same operation. The modern two-step approach significantly decreases anxiety for the patient. The 1- to 2-week interval between biopsy and therapy gives the woman a chance to contemplate alternative choices in therapy. The incidence of carcinoma in biopsies corresponds directly with the patient's age. Approximately 20% of breast biopsies in women aged 50 are positive, and this figure increases to 33% in women aged 70 or older.

In performing an outpatient breast biopsy, the primary consideration is appropriate sampling of the suspicious area. Mammography is performed before biopsy to help identify subclinical pathology in both breasts. Radiologic location of suspicious areas facilitates excision of nonpalpable lesions. Cosmetic results are important, and the majority of biopsies can be performed with curvilinear incisions, often in the circumareolar area. It is important to send the laboratory a small sample (1 g of suspicious tissue) to determine the presence or absence of estrogen and progesterone receptors. These receptors are heat labile, and therefore the tissue must be frozen within 30 minutes.

Fine-needle aspiration cytology has been popular in Europe for the past 20 years and is gaining acceptance in the United States. Experienced clinicians believe that they can identify the gritty feeling of a classic breast carcinoma. When the fine-needle aspirate cytology is positive, this technique reduces the incidence of open biopsy. If the aspirate is nondiagnostic, an open biopsy subsequently must be performed. Vorherr suggests a 16-gauge, multiholed needle to obtain both a cytologic and a histologic specimen (Figure 13-9). Others prefer a thin needle that removes a small core of tissue. Fine-needle aspiration cytology is approximately 70% to 90% accurate, with a false negative rate of approximately 20%. Drawbacks of fine-needle aspiration cytology are that it does not differentiate noninvasive from invasive carcinoma and does not delineate the extent of an in situ ductal carcinoma that may be surrounding an invasive carcinoma.

In summary, regardless of the diagnostic accuracy of imaging techniques and needle aspiration, open breast biopsy is the definitive step to establish that a dominant breast mass is not carcinoma.

Classification

Breast cancer is usually asymptomatic before the development of advanced disease. Breast pain is experienced by only 10% of women with early breast carcinoma. The classic sign of a breast carcinoma is a solitary, solid, three-dimensional, dominant breast mass. The borders of the mass are usually indistinct, which makes it difficult to define precisely the size of the mass. Often the mass is not freely mobile. Far-advanced local disease produces changes in the skin and nipples of the breast, including retraction, dimpling, induration, edema (peau d'orange), ulceration, and signs of inflammation.

The prognosis and treatment of breast carcinoma are primarily related to the stage of the disease and extent of spread to regional nodes (Figure 13-10). Variations in histologic types and degree of cellular atypia of breast cancer are of secondary importance. There have been numerous classifications of breast carcinoma

TABLE 13-3
Simplified Classification of Breast Carcinoma

Type of Carcinoma	Percentage of All Cases Diagnosed
Ductal carcinoma	
In situ	5%
Infiltrating	80%
Lobular carcinoma	
In situ	3%
Infiltrating	9%
Inflammatory carcinoma	2%
Paget's disease	1%

that contain mixtures of both clinical and pathologic subgroups. A condensed classification is presented in Table 13-3. Most carcinomas originate in the epithelium of the collecting ducts or terminal lobular ducts. Both in situ and invasive carcinoma have been described, often in the same quadrant of the breast. Bilateral breast carcinoma occurs in approximately 1% of all newly diagnosed cases. The prevalence of bilateral breast cancer is twofold greater in lobular neoplasia.

Intraductal carcinoma in situ is a disease in which the cellular abnormalities are limited to the ductal epithelium. It is most commonly discovered in perimenopausal and postmenopausal women. Intraductal carcinoma in situ is not usually detected by palpation because the disease does not produce a definitive mass. Mammography sometimes demonstrates the fine stippling of microcalcifications. Reviews by Betsill et al. and Page et al. document carcinoma developing in approximately 35% of women with this disease within 10 years of initial diagnosis. If the primary treatment is simple mastectomy, 5% to 10% of women will have a simultaneous invasive carcinoma in the same breast.

Lobular carcinoma in situ has less malignant potential than does intraductal carcinoma in situ. However, it has a much greater tendency to be bilateral and to present as multifocal disease. Three of four patients are in the premenopausal age group. Lobular carcinoma in situ is not detected by palpation, and mammography shows no charcteristic pattern. The latent period is longer than with intraductal carcinoma in situ; often over 20 years will

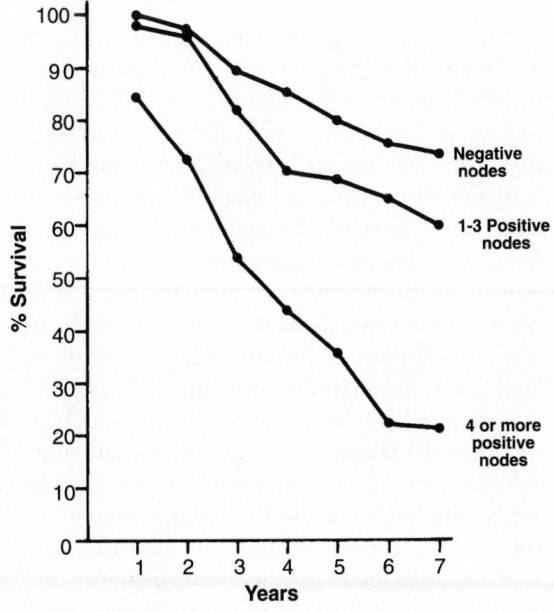

FIGURE 13-10
Survival with breast carcinoma in relation to positive nodes. (From Gambrell RD: Am J Obstet Gynecol 150:122, 1984.)

elapse before infiltrating carcinoma develops. Approximately 20% of women with this disease will develop invasive breast carcinoma during the remainder of their life.

Infiltrating ductal carcinoma is the most common breast malignancy. Histologically, nonuniform malignant epithelial cells of varying sizes and shapes infiltrate the surrounding tissue. The degree of fibrous response to the invading epithelial cells determines the firmness to palpation and texture during biopsy. Approximately 10% of infiltrating ductal carcinomas are of a uniform histologic picture and are classified as medullary, colloid, comedo, tubular, or papillary carcinomas. In general the specialized forms are grossly softer, mobile, and well delineated. They are usually smaller and have a more optimistic prognosis than the more common nonhomogeneous variety. Medullary carcinomas are soft, with extensive stromal infiltration by lymphocytes and plasma cells. Colloid carcinomas have a similar soft consistency, with extensive deposition of extracellular mucin.

Infiltrating lobular carcinomas are characterized by the uniformity of the neoplastic cells. Often the malignant epithelial cells infiltrate the stroma in a single-file fashion. This neoplasia tends to have a multicentric origin in the same breast and tends to involve both breasts more often than infiltrating ductal carcinoma. Histologic subdivisions of infiltrating lobular carcinoma include small cell, round cell, and signet cell carcinomas.

Inflammatory carcinomas comprise approximately 2% of breast cancers. This type is recognized clinically as a rapidly growing, highly malignant carcinoma. Infiltration of malignant cells into the lymphatics of the skin produces a clinical picture that simulates a skin infection. There is not a specific histologic cell type.

Paget's disease is rare, comprising slightly less than 1% of breast carcinomas (Figure 13-11). This lesion has an innocent appearance and looks like eczema or a dermatitis of the nipple. The clinical picture is produced by an infiltrating ductal carcinoma that invades the epidermis. Paget's disease has an excellent prognosis.

Treatment

The treatment of breast carcinoma is complex, with many variables to consider. Proper treatment varies from patient to patient. The four most important variables for treatment selection are the tumor's size; the inherent aggressiveness, as determined by the histology of the initial lesion; the presence of positive nodes; and the receptor status of the tumor. When generalizations are offered concerning the preferred method of therapy, it is important to remember that breast carcinoma is a heterogeneous group of neoplasms. Unfortunately, neither clinical nor pathologic staging of the disease is nearly as precise as one would postulate in a carcinoma involving an external organ. Microscopic metastatic disease occurs early via both hematogenous and lymphatic routes. For example, 30% to 40% of women without gross adenopathy in the axilla will have positive nodes discovered during histologic examination. Approximately two thirds of all women with breast carcinoma eventually develop distant metastatic disease regardless of the type of initial therapy. Women with negative nodes have a 75% 10-year survival (Table 13-4).

It is important to understand the natural history of untreated breast carcinoma. In series of women refusing therapy, 20% will be alive at 5 years and 5% will be alive at 10 years. Breast carcinoma is a systemic disease that may recur many years, sometimes decades, after initial diagnosis.

The major changes in management of breast carcinoma over the past 10 to 20 years have resulted from changing concepts regarding the biology of the disease, with the understanding that many women with breast carcinoma have systemic disease at the time the diagnosis is initially established. The pathophysiology of a developing breast carcinoma results in years of growth of the neoplasia before discovery. Because occult vascular dissemination is likely to occur, treatment of breast carcinoma involves both local and systemic therapy. It is beyond the scope of this book to present the details of treatment of breast carcinoma. Thorough clinical and surgical staging is the cornerstone of any treatment plan. The standard system involves the TNM classification, where the tumor size and characteristics are described (T), regional lymph node involvement is documented (N), and distant metastases are noted (M).

Veronesi et al. have listed the three major objectives of treating breast carcinoma: control of local disease, treatment of distant metastasis, and improved quality of life for women treated

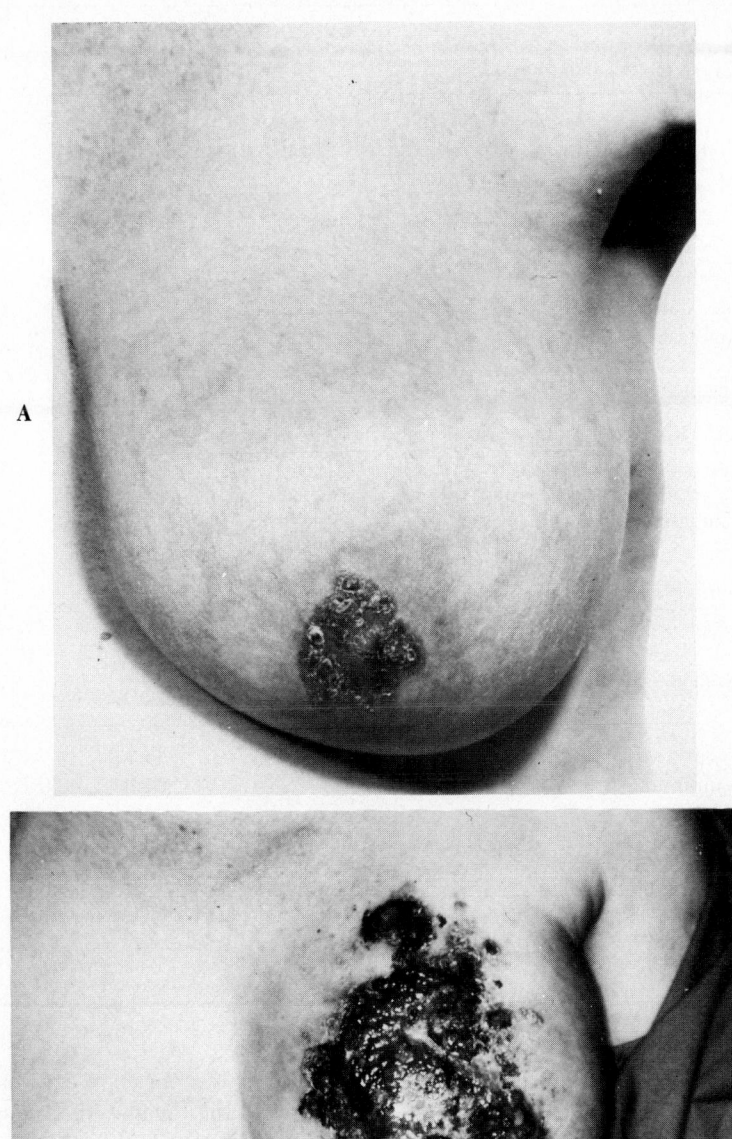

FIGURE 13-11
A, Paget's disease of left nipple. **B,** Extensive Paget's disease involving skin of breast. (From McKinna JA: Clinical features of breast disease. In Parsons CA, editor: Diagnosis of breast disease: imaging, clinical features, and pathology, London, © 1983, Chapman & Hall Ltd, p 38.)

TABLE 13-4
Stages and Survival of Women with Breast Cancer

Clinical Staging (American Joint Committee)	Crude 5-Year Survival (%)	Range of Survival (%)
Stage I	85	82-94
Tumor <2 cm in diameter		
Nodes, if present, not felt to contain metastases		
Without distant metastases		
State II	66	47-74
Tumors <5 cm in diameter		
Nodes, if palpable, not fixed		
Without distant metastases		
Stage III	41	7-80
Tumor >5 cm or,		
Tumor of any size with invasion of skin or attached to chest wall		
Nodes in supraclavicular area		
Without distant metastases		
State IV	10	—
With distant metastases		

Histologic Staging (NSABP*)	Crude Survival (%)		5-Year Disease-Free Survival (%)
	5-Year	10-Year	
All patients	63.5	45.9	60.3
Negative axillary lymph nodes	78.1	64.9	82.3
Positive axillary lymph nodes	46.5	24.9	34.9
1-3 positive axillary lymph nodes	62.2	37.5	50.0
>4 positive axillary lymph nodes	32.0	13.4	21.1

From Henderson IC and Canellos GP: N Engl J Med 302:18, 1980. Reprinted by permission of The New England Journal of Medicine.
*National Surgical Adjuvant Breast Project.

for the disease. There are several methods for controlling local disease. However, no difference in long-term survival rates has been documented, regardless of the extent of surgical therapy or aggressiveness of local radiotherapy. During the past 10 years, revolutionary changes have involved multiple therapeutic options in both local and systemic therapy for breast carcinoma. Women are assuming an increasingly active role in deciding their own treatment regimen. Breast conservation is a frequent choice for the control of local disease. Chemotherapy is used not only for patients with proved metastatic disease but also for women at high risk for recurrent disease. Recent emphasis on conservative surgery (lumpectomy) plus radiation therapy to control multicentric foci of cancer in the same breast and on

reconstructive surgery after mastectomy has improved the quality of life of women with breast carcinoma (Table 13-5).

Surgical Therapy

The decision concerning appropriate therapy and extent of the surgical operation to treat breast carcinoma should be made by the patient in consultation with the surgeon, radiotherapist, and medical oncologist who will treat her. As emphasized, the size of the tumor, the initial extent of disease, virulence of the neoplasms, and presence of estrogen and progesterone receptors are the key medical factors in the decision. Intensive discussions concerning breast reconstruction or external prostheses are important to help the patient and family con-

TABLE 13-5
Ten-Year Disease-Free Survival Rates of
Women with Breast Cancer

	Conservation Surgery and Radiation	Radical or Modified Radical Mastectomy Alone
Minimal breast cancer	92%	95%
Stage I	78%	80%
Stage II	73%	65%

Reprinted with permission from Montague ED: Cancer 53:702, 1984.

template the effects of surgery on body image. Morris et al. have studied the psychological and social adjustments to mastectomy in 160 women. These patients were followed at intervals of 3, 12, and 24 months after surgery. One in four women was still having problems with depression and associated marital and sexual problems 2 years after initial therapy.

Until approximately 20 years ago, radical mastectomy was the standard operation for carcinoma of the breast. Radical mastectomy was designed to control local disease by an extensive en bloc removal of the breast and underlying pectoralis major and pectoralis minor muscles and complete axillary dissection. It is a cosmetically mutilating operation, leaving a major deformity of the chest wall. With an increased understanding that cancer of the breast is often a systemic disease, the therapeutic emphasis has changed to less radical surgery and increased use of radiotherapy and chemotherapy. It has also been recognized that often patients are not cured even with extensive local therapy. Thus protocols have been designed for more conservative approaches to local disease, and less radical operations have grown in popularity. The modified radical mastectomy removes the breast and only the fascia over the pectoralis major muscle. The pectoralis minor muscle may be removed to facilitate the axillary dissection. Simple mastectomy includes removal of the breast without underlying muscle tissue.

The place of radical or modified radical mastectomy in stages I and II breast cancer has been challenged. Veronesi et al. published a controlled study of 701 women with carcinomas measuring less than 2 cm in diameter without palpable axillary lymph nodes. The women were randomized preoperatively into two treatment groups. One group of 349 patients had radical mastectomy. The other group included 352 women who had excision of a quadrant of the breast to control the primary lesion, axillary dissection, and radiotherapy involving both external and interstitial sources. Five-year survival rates were virtually identical—90% in both groups. Five-year disease-free survival rates were similar, 83% and 84%. Fisher et al., in the National Surgical Adjuvant Breast Project, have reported similar findings with breast carcinomas less than 4 cm, if the surgical margins were free of tumor. Three additional randomized prospective studies found no difference in therapeutic results contrasting conservative surgery and postoperative irradiation versus radical surgery for stage I or II breast carcinoma. These studies found local recurrence rates of 5% at 5 years and approximately 10% at 10 years. Radiotherapy was begun 1 to 2 weeks postoperatively and given for approximately 5 weeks. The radiotherapeutic dosage was 180 to 200 cGy per day for a total dose of approximately 5000 cGy.

It is important to offer every woman alternatives in treatment for stages I and II breast carcinoma. The cosmetic result obtained by lumpectomy and radiation therapy depends on the size and shape of the breast and the size of the initial tumor. For some women, mastectomy followed by reconstructive surgery may give a superior cosmetic result.

Medical Therapy

The two major factors in predicting the likelihood of systemic disease in breast carcinoma are the diameter of the primary tumor and the number of positive axillary nodes. Women whose initial tumor is less than 2 cm in diameter and who have negative axillary tumors have excellent disease-free survival, with a 5-year relapse rate of only 11%. Other factors, such as mitotic index, thymidine-labeling index, DNA content, and estrogen and progesterone receptors, are also predictors of extended disease-free survival in women with breast carcinoma.

The presence and concentration of receptors should be obtained at the initial diagnostic surgery, as receptor status may change after radiotherapy or chemotherapy. In general, receptor-positive tumors are usually more well differentiated and exhibit a less aggressive clinical behavior, including a lower risk of recurrence and lower capacity to proliferate. When estrogen receptors are positive, approximately 60% of breast cancers will respond to hormonal therapy; an 80% response is noted when both estrogen and progesterone receptors are present. If estrogen receptors are negative, less than 10% of tumors respond to hormonal manipulation.

Hormonal therapy may include ablative surgery but is usually accomplished by drugs that change endocrine function by blocking receptor sites or blocking synthesis of hormones. In the past the most commonly used ablative surgery was bilateral oophorectomy in a premenopausal woman with breast carcinoma. Hormonal therapy is effective in producing a response in advanced metastatic carcinoma for approximately 1 year. Metastatic disease in soft tissue and bone is the most sensitive to hormonal manipulation. Tamoxifen, an oral antiestrogen, is an alternative to surgical castration and presently is the most frequently prescribed hormonal agent for breast carcinoma. Adrenalectomy or hypophysectomy has largely been replaced by medical adrenalectomy using aminoglutethimide. Oral estrogens, depo-medroxyprogesterone, androgens, danazol, and gonadotrophin hormone–releasing hormone (GH-RH) agonists have also been used to treat breast carcinoma. Two endocrine agents used simultaneously do not produce better results than a single agent. However, Levine and Lippman have combined hormonal therapy and chemotherapy. They believe "synchronization" of the cancer with hormonal therapy improves the cytotoxicity of chemotherapy.

Adjuvant chemotherapy has produced positive responses and an increase in disease-free survival in many clinical studies. Initially, chemotherapy was selected to treat women with positive axillary nodes or remote disease. Chemotherapy has proved effective in shrinking measurable metastatic disease in both premenopausal and postmenopausal women. Recently, chemotherapy has been given in hopes of eradicating occult metastatic disease. Approximately 30% of women who receive local surgery and/or irradiation to the breast with negative axillary nodes will subsequently develop systemic metastatic disease. Recent reports have demonstrated significant prolongation of disease-free survival after treatment with tamoxifen or adjuvant chemotherapy in high-risk patients with operable breast carcinoma and negative axillary nodes. In the treatment of early-stage breast cancer, the rate of local and distal recurrences after local therapy is decreased by adjuvant chemotherapy, either combination cytotoxic drugs or tamoxifen. It is important to note that improvements in disease-free survival have not always been followed by similar improvements in overall survival. The hope for the future is to identify those patients at high risk so as not to expose all women with breast carcinoma to the expense and side effects of chemotherapy.

It is now firmly established that combinations of cytotoxic drugs are superior to a single agent. The chemotherapeutic agents most frequently chosen for breast carcinoma include cyclophosphamide, methotrexate, Adriamycin, 5-fluorouracil, and vinblastine. The average total response rate to combined chemotherapy is 55%. Approximately 10% to 20% of women treated with combination chemotherapy experience a complete remission for about 18 months.

_____ KEY POINTS _____

- One out of 9 women, 11% of American females, develops carcinoma of the breast during her lifetime.

- The breast consists of approximately 20% glandular tissue and 80% fat and connective tissue.

- Skin retraction, a sign of advanced breast carcinoma, is caused by malignant invasion of Cooper's ligaments.

- Lymphatic drainage of the breast is complex, with 75% going to regional axillary nodes; other routes are adjacent to internal mammary vessels, mediastinum, and intercostal glands.

- The classic symptom of fibrocystic changes is cyclic bilateral breast pain. The signs of fibrocystic changes include increased engorgement and density of the breasts, excessive nodularity, rapid change and fluctuation in the size of cystic areas, increased tenderness, and occasionally spontaneous nipple discharge.

- Treatment of the fibrocystic breast changes includes mechanical support, diuretics, avoidance of methylxanthines, danazol, oral contraceptives, and, very rarely, surgery.

- The importance of diagnosing the etiology of *spontaneous* discharge from the nipple is to rule out carcinoma. The color of the nonmilky discharge does not differentiate a benign from a malignant process.

- Intraductal papilloma and fibrocystic changes are the two most common etiologies of spontaneous nonmilky nipple discharge.

- Fat necrosis caused by trauma may present as a firm, indurated, poorly defined mass that has a mammographic appearance of stippled calcifications.

- Risk factors identify only 25% of women who will eventually develop breast carcinoma.

- In the United States there are approximately 175,000 new cases diagnosed and approximately 44,500 deaths yearly from breast carcinoma.

- The frequency of breast carcinoma increases directly with the patient's age; 85% occur after 40 years of age.

- Obesity, dietary fats, alcohol, radiation, and family history of affected first-degree relatives are risk factors for breast carcinoma.

- Once a woman has developed carcinoma of one breast, her risk is approximately 1% per year of developing cancer in the other breast.

Fisher B, Redmond C, Dimitrov NV, et al: A randomized clinical trial evaluating sequential methotrexate and fluorouracil in the treatment of patients with node-negative breast cancer who have estrogen-receptor-negative tumors, N Engl J Med 320:473, 1989.

Fisher B, Redmond C, Fisher ER, et al: Ten-year results of a randomized clinical trial comparing radical mastectomy and total mastectomy with or without radiation, N Engl J Med 312:674, 1985.

Fletcher SW, O'Malley MS, and Bunce LA: Physicians' abilities to detect lumps in silicone breast models, JAMA 253:2224, 1985.

Forbes JF: Breast disease, Clinical Surgery International, New York, 1986, Churchill Livingstone, Inc.

Foster RS and Costanza MC: Breast self-examination practices and breast cancer survival, Cancer 53:999, 1984.

Fowler PA, Casey CE, and Cameron GG: Cyclic changes in composition and volume of the breast during the menstrual cycle, measured by magnetic resonance imaging, Br J Obstet Gynaecol 97:595, 1990.

Frable WJ: Fine-needle aspiration biopsy: a review, Hum Pathol 14:9, 1983.

Frantz VK, Pickren JW, Melcher GW, et al: Incidence of chronic cystic disease in so-called "normal breasts," Cancer 4:762, 1951.

Furnival CM and Porter AJ: Breast cancer again: diagnostic alternatives? Med J Aust 149:397, 1988.

Gautherie M: Thermobiological assessment of benign and malignant breast disease, Am J Obstet Gynecol 147:861, 1983.

Gold RH, Bassett LW, and Kimme-Smith C: Breast imaging: state-of-the-art, Invest Radiol 21:298, 1986.

Goldhirsch A, Stjernsward J, Zava D, et al: Randomized trial of chemo-endocrine therapy, endocrine therapy, and mastectomy alone in postmenopausal patients with operable breast cancer and axillary node metastasis, Lancet 1:1256, 1984.

Goldwyn RM: Breast reconstruction after mastectomy, N Engl J Med 317:1711, 1987.

Golinger RC: Hormones and the pathophysiology of fibrocystic mastopathy, Surg Gynecol Obstet 146:273, 1978.

Greenwald P, Nasca PC, Lawrence CE, et al: Estimated effect of breast self-examination and routine physician examinations on breast-cancer mortality, N Engl J Med 299:271, 1978.

Hare WSC, Tjandra JJ, Russell IS, et al: Comparison of mammary serum antigen assay with mammography in patients with breast cancer, Med J Aust 149:402, 1988.

Harris VJ and Jackson VP: Indications for breast imaging in women under age 35 years, Radiology 172:445, 1989.

Henderson IC: Adjuvant chemotherapy for early breast cancer, Br J Cancer 61:652, 1990.

Henderson IC, Hayes DF, Parker LM, et al: Adjuvant systemic therapy for patients with node-negative tumors, Cancer 65:2132, 1990.

Hicks MJ, Davis JR, Layton JM, et al: Sensitivity of mammography and physical examination of the breast for detecting breast cancer, JAMA 242:2080, 1979.

Hildreth NG, Shore RE, Dvoretsky PM, et al: The risk of breast cancer after irradiation of the thymus in infancy, N Engl J Med 321:1281, 1989.

Hindle WH: Breast disease for gynecologists, Norwalk, CT, 1990, Appleton & Lange.

Howe HL: Proficiency in performing breast self-examination, Patient Counselling and Health Education, fourth quarter, 151, 1980.

Jeffries DO and Adler DD: Mammographic detection of breast cancer in women under the age of 35, Invest Radiol 25:67, 1990.

Jensen RA, Page DL, DuPont WD, et al: Invasive breast cancer risk in women with sclerosing adenosis, Cancer 64:1977, 1989.

Kaufman DW, Miller DR, Rosenberg L, et al: Noncontraceptive estrogen use and the risk of breast cancer, JAMA 252:63, 1984.

Kelsey JL and Berkowitz GS: Breast cancer epidemiology, Cancer Res 48:5615, 1988.

Kopans DB: "Early" breast cancer detection using techniques other than mammography, AJR 143:465, 1984.

Kopans DB, Meyer JE, and Sadowsky N: Breast imaging, N Engl J Med 310:960, 1984.

Kopans DB, Swann CA, White G, et al: Asymmetric breast tissue, Radiology 171:639, 1989.

Korenman SG: Estrogen window hypothesis of the etiology of breast cancer, Lancet 1:700, 1980.

Korenman SG: The endocrinology of breast cancer, Cancer 46:874, 1980.

Lamas AM, Horwitz RI, and Peck D: Usefulness of mammography in the diagnosis and management of breast disease in postmenopausal women, JAMA 252:2999, 1984.

Layde PM, Webster LA, Baughman AL, et al: The independent associations of parity, age at first full-term pregnancy, and duration of breastfeeding with the risk of breast cancer, J Clin Epidemiol 42:963, 1989.

Leis HP and Kwon CS: Fibrocystic disease of the breast, J Reprod Med 22:291, 1979.

Leis HP Jr: The significance of nipple discharge. In Schwartz GF and Marchant D, editors: Breast disease, diagnosis and treatment, New York, 1980, Symposia Specialists, p 111.

Levine RM and Lippman ME: Breast cancer management: recent advances and recommendations, Adv Intern Med 29:215, 1984.

Levinson W and Dunn PM: Nonassociation of caffeine and fibrocystic breast disease, Arch Intern Med 146:1773, 1986.

Levitt SH and Mandel J: Benefits versus risks in conservation surgery with irradiation for breast cancer, Am J Med 77:93, 1984.

London RS, Sundaram GS, and Goldstein PJ: Medical management of mammary dysplasia, Obstet Gynecol 59:519, 1982.

London SJ, Colditz GA, Stampfer MJ, et al: Prospective study of relative weight, height, and risk of breast cancer, JAMA 262:2853, 1989.

Love SM, Gelman RS, and Silen W: Fibrocystic "disease" of the breast—non-disease? N Engl J Med 307:1010, 1982.

Lubin F, Ron E, Wax Y, et al: A case-control study of caffeine and methylxanthines in benign breast disease, JAMA 253:2388, 1985.

Ludwig Breast Study Group: Prolonged disease-free survival after one course of perioperative adjuvant chemotherapy for node-negative breast cancer, N Engl J Med 320:491, 1989.

Mansour EG, Gray R, Shatila AH, et al: Efficacy of adjuvant chemotherapy in high-risk, node-negative breast cancer: an intergroup study, N Engl J Med 320:485, 1989.

Marchant DJ: Epidemiology of breast cancer, Clin Obstet Gynecol 25:387, 1982.

Marchant DJ, Kase NG, and Berkowitz RL, editors: Breast disease, New York, 1986, Churchill Livingstone, Inc, pp 6-7.

McLelland R: Mammography 1984: challenge to radiology, AJR 143:1, 1984.

Meyer JE, Eberlein TJ, Stomper PC, et al: Biopsy of occult breast lesions: analysis of 1261 abnormalities, JAMA 263:2341, 1990.

Miller AB, Howe GR, Sherman GJ, et al: Mortality from breast cancer after irradiation during fluoroscopic examinations in patients being treated for tuberculosis, N Engl J Med 321:1285, 1989.

Minton JP: Methylxanthines in breast disease. In Schwartz GF and Marchant D, editors: Breast disease, diagnosis and treatment, New York, 1980, Symposia Specialists, p 143.

Montague ED: Conservation surgery and radiation therapy in the treatment of operable breast cancer, Cancer 53:700, 1984.

Monyak D and Levitt S: The changing role of radiation therapy in the treatment of primary breast cancer, Invest Radiol 24:483, 1989.

Morris T: Psychological adjustment to mastectomy, Cancer Treat Rev 6:41, 1979.

Morris T, Greer HS, and White P: Psychological and social adjustments to mastectomy, Cancer 40:2381, 1977.

Moskowitz M: Mammography to screen asymptomatic women for breast cancer, AJR 143:457, 1984.

Murad TM, Hines JR, Beal J, et al: Histopathological and clinical correlations of cystosarcoma phyllodes, Arch Pathol Lab Med 112:752, 1988.

NCI Breast Cancer Screening Consortium: Screening mammography: a missed clinical opportunity? JAMA 264:54, 1990.

Nemoto T, Natarajan N, Smart CR, et al: Patterns of breast cancer detection in the United States, J Surg Oncol 21:183, 1982.

NIH Consensus Conference: Treatment of early-stage breast cancer, JAMA 265:391, 1991.

Nyirjesy I and Billingsley FS: Detection of breast carcinoma in a gynecologic practice, Obstet Gynecol 64:747, 1984.

O'Malley MS and Fletcher SW: Screening for breast cancer with breast self-examination: a critical review, JAMA 257:2197, 1987.

Page DL: Cancer risk assessment in benign breast biopsies, Hum Pathol 17:872, 1986.

Page DL, Dupont WD, Rogers LW, et al: Intraductal carcinoma of the breast: follow-up after biopsy only, Cancer 49:751, 1982.

Palmer MD, DeRisi DC, Pelikan A, et al: Treatment options and recurrence potential for cystosarcoma phyllodes, Surg Obstet Gynecol 170:193, 1990.

Paulus DD: Conservative treatment of breast cancer: mammography in patient selection and follow-up, AJR 143:483, 1984.

Peters F, Schuth W, Scheurich B, et al: Serum prolactin levels in patients with fibrocystic breast disease, Obstet Gynecol 64:381, 1984.

Pilnik S: Clinical diagnosis of benign breast disease, J Reprod Med 22:277, 1979.

Redding WH, Monaghan P, Imrie SF, et al: Detection of micrometastases in patients with primary breast cancer, Lancet 2:1271, 1983.

Roberts MM, Jones V, Elton RA, et al: Risk of breast cancer in women with history of benign disease of the breast, Br Med J 288:275, 1984.

Rosen PP, Braun DW, and Kinne DE: The clinical significance of preinvasive breast cancer, Cancer 46:919, 1980.

Rosenberg L, Miller DR, Kaufman DW, et al: Breast cancer and oral contraceptive use, Am J Epidemiol 119:167, 1984.

Rosenberg L, Schwingl PJ, Kaufman DW, et al: Breast cancer and cigarette smoking, N Engl J Med 310:92, 1984.

Schatzkin A, Greenwald P, Byar DP, et al: The dietary fat–breast cancer hypothesis is alive, JAMA 261:3284, 1989.

Schlesselman JJ: Cancer of the breast and reproductive tract in relation to use of oral contraceptives, Contraception 40:1, 1989.

Schnitt SJ, Silen W, Sadowsky NL, et al: Ductal carcinoma in situ (intraductal carcinoma) of the breast, N Engl J Med 318:898, 1988.

Schuh ME, Nemoto T, Penetrante RB, et al: Intraductal carcinoma: analysis of presentation, pathologic findings, and outcome of disease, Arch Surg 121:1303, 1986.

Senie RT, Rosen PP, Lesser ML, et al: Breast self-examination and medical examination related to breast cancer stage, Am J Public Health 71:583, 1981.

Shapiro S: Determining the efficacy of breast cancer screening, Cancer 63:1873, 1989.

Shimizu Y, Schull WJ, and Kato H: Cancer risk among atomic bomb survivors: the RERF life span study, JAMA 264:601, 1990.

Sickles EA: Mammographic features of "early" breast cancer, AJR 143:461, 1984.

Sickles EA: Breast masses: mammographic evaluation, Radiology 173:297, 1989.

Sickles EA, Filly RA, and Callen PW: Breast cancer detection with sonography and mammography: comparison using state-of-the-art equipment, AJR 140:843, 1983.

Sigurdsson H, Baldetorp B, Borg A, et al: Indicators of prognosis in node-negative breast cancer, N Engl J Med 322:1045, 1990.

Sinclair RA: The breast: tissue changes and cancer risk, Med J Aust 149:424, 1988.

Strawbridge HTG, Bassett AA, and Foldes I: Role of cytology in management of lesions of the breast, Surg Gynecol Obstet 152:1, 1981.

Strax P: Control of breast cancer through mass screening: from research to action, Cancer 63:1881, 1989.

Sundaram GS, Manimekalai S, Wenk RE, et al: Estrogen and progesterone receptor assays in human breast cancer: a brief review of the relevant terms, methods, and clinical usefulness, Obstet Gynecol Surv 39:719, 1984.

Sutherland HJ, Lockwood GA, and Boyd NF: Ratings of the importance of quality of life variables: therapeutic implications for patients with metastatic breast cancer, J Clin Epidemiol 43:661, 1990.

Tabar L, Gad A, Akerlund E, et al: Screening for breast cancer in Sweden. In Feig AS and McLelland R, editors: Breast carcinoma: current diagnosis and treatment, New York, 1983, American College of Radiology and Masson Publishing USA, Inc.

VanDeVijver MJ, Peterse JL, Mooi WJ, et al: Neu-protein overexpression in breast cancer: association with comedo-type ductal carcinoma in situ and limited prognostic value in stage II breast cancer, N Engl J Med 319:1239, 1988.

Verbeek ALM, Holland R, Sturmans F, et al: Reduction of breast cancer mortality through mass screening with modern mammography, Lancet 1:1222, 1984.

Veronesi V, Sacozzi R, Del Vecchio M, et al: Comparing radical mastectomy with quadrantectomy, axillary dissection, and radiotherapy in patients with small cancers of the breast, N Engl J Med 305:6, 1981.

Vorherr H: Breast aspiration biopsy, Am J Obstet Gynecol 148:127, 1984.

Wile AG and DiSaia PJ: Hormones and breast cancer, Am J Surg 157:438, 1989.

Wingo PA, Layde PM, Lee NC, et al: The risk of breast cancer in postmenopausal women who have used estrogen replacement therapy, JAMA 257:209, 1987.

Problems of Prenatal DES Exposure

KEY TERMS AND DEFINITIONS

Abnormal Transformation Zone. Area in the vagina or on the cervix that may contain columnar epithelium and squamous metaplasia and that often contains intraepithelial neoplasia that has an abnormal colposcopic pattern.

Adenosis. The presence of glandular (columnar) epithelium in the vagina.

Cervicovaginal Ridge. A structural change in the cervix or upper vagina of DES-exposed females (hood, cockscomb, pseudopolyp, collar).

Clear Cell Adenocarcinoma of the Vagina and Cervix. Rare genital tract malignancy that occurs with increased frequency in DES females.

Colposcope. An instrument used to magnify and examine the epithelium of the transformation zone to identify abnormal areas in the lower genital tract that warrant biopsy.

Diethylstilbestrol (DES). An orally active synthetic nonsteroidal estrogen.

Ectropion. The presence of glandular (columnar) epithelium on the ectocervix (portio of the cervix).

Intraepithelial Neoplasia. Premalignant changes in the surface epithelium. This may also be termed *dysplasia* or *carcinoma in situ*, depending on its severity, and is similar to changes seen in the non-DES-exposed.

Müllerian Ducts. Paired structures in the embryo that in part lead to the formation of the female reproductive tract, primarily the upper vagina, cervix, uterus, and fallopian tubes.

Normal Transformation Zone. Area of columnar epithelium and squamous metaplasia in the vagina or on the cervix that has normal colposcopic patterns.

Squamous Metaplasia. Physiologic process by which squamous epithelium replaces the columnar epithelium of adenosis and ectropion.

Uterine Constriction Ring and T-Shaped Uterus. Types of abnormal shapes of the endometrial cavity diagnosed by hysterosalpingogram in DES females.

Vaginal Epithelial Changes (VECs). Epithelial changes in the vagina of DES-exposed women that consist of adenosis or squamous metaplasia or both.

Diethylstilbestrol (DES) was initially synthesized in 1938 and was the first commercially available, orally active estrogen. It is derived from the stilbene molecule and biologically acts in a fashion similar to steroidal estrogens such as estradiol (Figure 14-1). Because it was relatively inexpensive and is orally active, its use for human therapy became widespread. In the late 1940s, DES treatment was used during pregnancy to prevent complications such as threatened abortion and prematurity. Many initial studies reported beneficial effects for DES pregnancy therapy, but some investigations in the early 1950s did not confirm these initial claims. The popularity of the drug for pregnancy support subsequently waned but continued into the 1960s. Finally, in 1971 it was noted that young women whose mothers

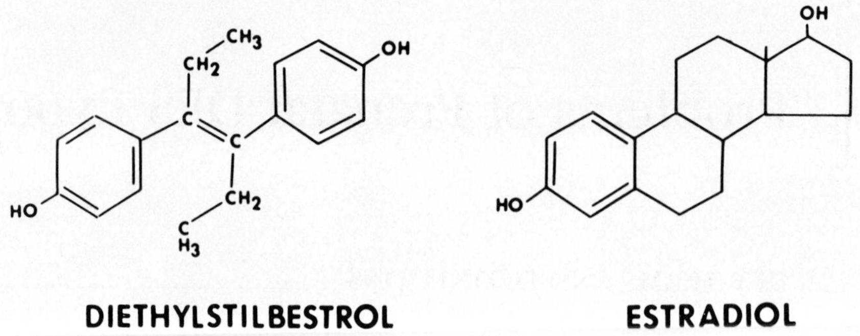

DIETHYLSTILBESTROL   **ESTRADIOL**

FIGURE 14-1
Structures of diethylstilbestrol and estradiol.

took DES during pregnancy were at increased risk to develop a rare malignancy, clear cell adenocarcinoma of the vagina. Soon after this association was established, the use of estrogens for treatment of pregnancy complications in the United States was proscribed by the Food and Drug Administration.

The size of the DES-exposed population is unknown, but it is estimated that in the United States there have been approximately 3 million pregnant women treated with nonsteroidal synthetic estrogens, primarily DES. Soon after the initial association with clear cell adenocarcinoma of the vagina, intrauterine exposure to DES was also associated with clear cell adenocarcinoma of the cervix. Subsequently, a number of nonmalignant epithelial structural abnormalities of the female genital tract were also discovered in this population.

This chapter reviews the various alterations of the genital tract in DES females, including changes that have been observed in their reproductive functions. The histogenesis of DES-associated genital changes is reviewed. In addition, a brief summary is provided of psychologic studies of DES females and the current health status of DES-exposed males and mothers. The management of clear cell adenocarcinoma of the vagina is discussed in Chapter 31.

LOWER GENITAL TRACT (VAGINA AND CERVIX) ABNORMALITIES

Several nonneoplastic abnormalities of the cervix and vagina are found frequently in the genital tract of females exposed to DES in utero. These changes include vaginal adenosis, cervical ectropion, structural abnormalities of the cervix and upper vagina, and alterations in the shape of the endometrial cavity.

Vaginal adenosis (Figure 14-2) consists of glandular (columnar) epithelium or its mucinous products in the vagina; cervical ectropion refers to similar changes on the ectocervix. The columnar epithelium of vaginal adenosis usually contains various cell types. One resembles the epithelium of the endocervix (Figure 14-2, A), and the other contains cells similar to the epithelium of the endometrium and fallopian tubes (so-called tuboendometrial cells) (Figure 14-2, B). It appears that the clear cell adenocarcinomas arise from the tuboendometrial cells.

Squamous metaplasia is frequently seen with adenosis and ectropion and is the physiologic process by which columnar epithelium is replaced by squamous epithelium. This process occurs normally in both DES-exposed and unexposed females.

Structural malformations of the lower genital tract, including transverse ridges, cervical collars, hoods, cockscombs, hypoplasia of the cervix, and pseudopolyps, have been described (Figure 14-3). Upper genital tract abnormalities (changes in the shape of the endometrial cavity) have also been identified on hysterosalpingogram examinations (Figure 14-4).

Frequency

Adenosis has been reported to occur in 30% to 90% of DES-exposed subjects. However, data from case-control studies that are not influenced by the potential bias of self-selection or physician referral suggest the overall prevalence is 30% to 40%. Specific risk factors affect the occurrence of vaginal adenosis in the exposed, including the age of the patient, the

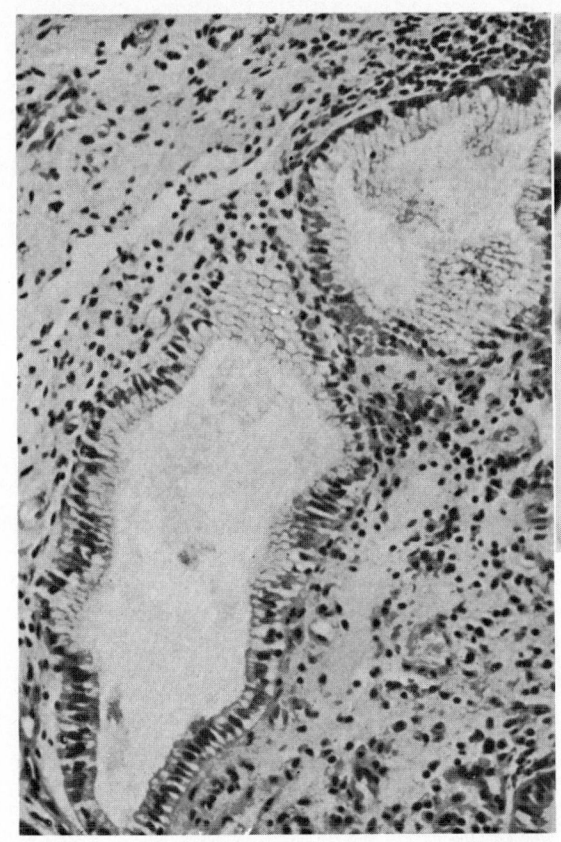

A

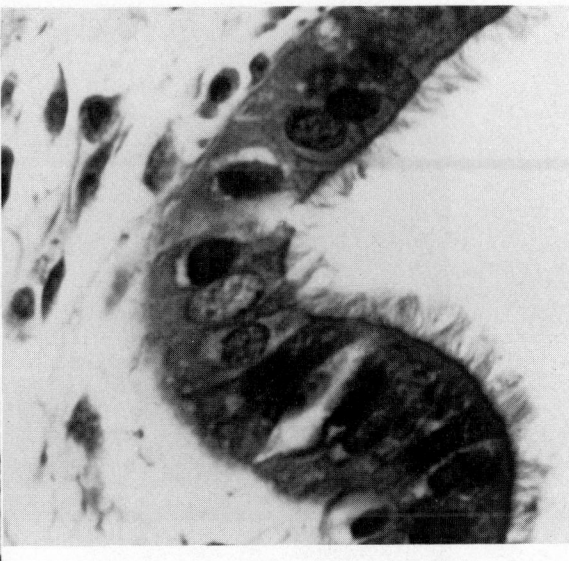

B

FIGURE 14-2
Vaginal adenosis. **A,** Glands are lined by endo-cervical-type epithelium (×200). **B,** Glands are lined by ciliated tuboendometrial cells (×890). (**A** from Herbst AL and Scully RE: Cancer 25:745, 1970. **B** from Herbst AL, editor: Intrauterine exposure to diethylstilbestrol in the human, Washington, DC, 1978, American College of Obstetricians and Gynecologists.)

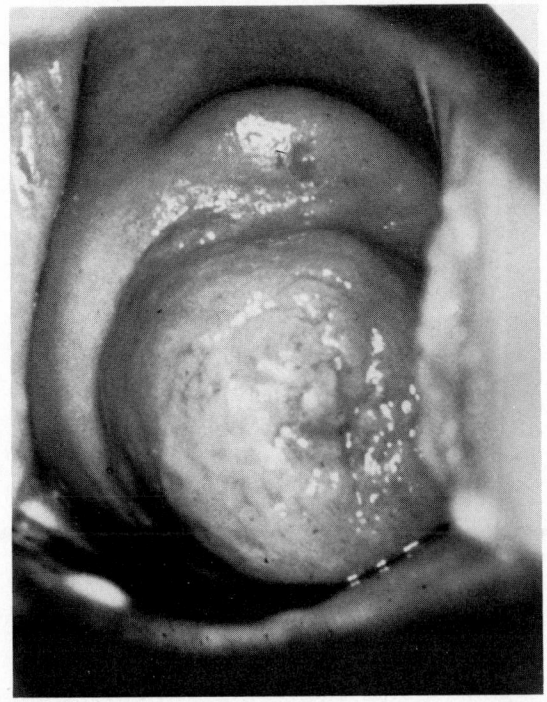

FIGURE 14-3
Vaginal hood. (From Robboy SJ, Scully RE, and Herbst AL: J Reprod Med 15:13, 1975.)

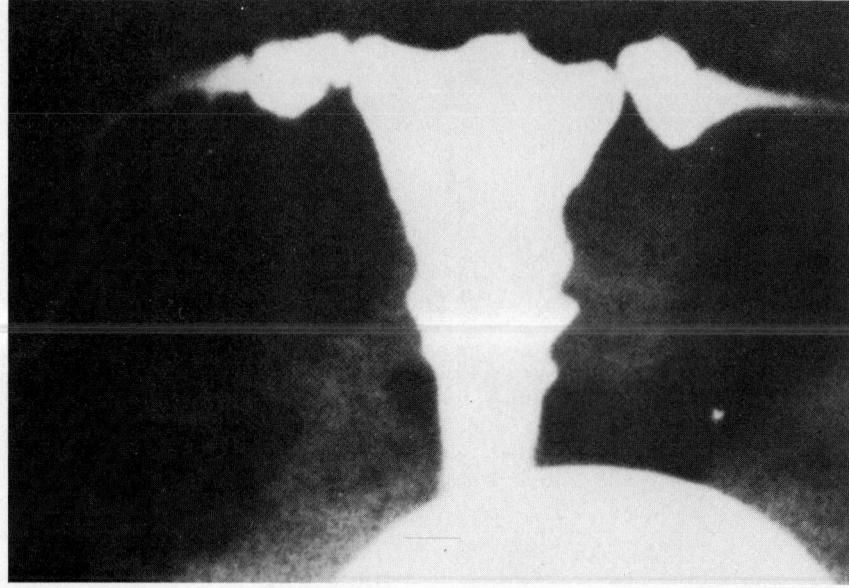

FIGURE 14-4
Hysterosalpingogram. Constrictions are noted in proximal portion of hornlike extension from uterine cavity. Uterine cavity is somewhat irregular. (From Kaufman RH, Adam H, Binder GL, et al: Am J Obstet Gynecol 137:299, 1980.)

total dosage of the drug ingested by the mother, and the time during pregnancy the treatment was begun. The term *vaginal epithelial changes* (VECs) has been used by some investigators to indicate the changes of vaginal adenosis and squamous metaplasia in the vagina.

Biopsy studies have indicated the highest rate of adenosis occurs among those whose mothers began DES in early pregnancy, and changes are rarely observed in subjects whose mothers started treatment after the eighteenth week. A larger dosage of the drug or initiation of treatment early in pregnancy also leads to a greater frequency of adenosis. As subjects grow older, the columnar epithelium is replaced in many instances by squamous metaplasia. Over years the healing process appears to proceed in a high proportion of the DES-exposed subjects, but in some a decrease in the size of the areas of the columnar epithelium does not appear to have occurred (Table 14-1).

The factors that seem to promote the changes of squamous metaplasia are not clearly identified, although some have theorized that a more acid pH of the vagina may accelerate the process. Cervicovaginal structural abnormalities (ridges, hoods, collars etc.) occur in approximately 25% of DES-exposed subjects.

TABLE 14-1
Changes in Lower Genital Tract Abnormalities in DES-Exposed Females

	No Change	Decreased Area or Extent	Disappearance
Cervical ectropion	30	53	38
(N = 121)	(25%)	(44%)	(31%)
Cervicovaginal ridge (N = 123)	58	30	35
	(47%)	(24%)	(29%)

Adapted from Antonioli DA, Burke L, and Friedman EA: Am J Obstet Gynecol 137:847, 1980.

These changes, like those of vaginal adenosis, are more common with higher dosages of maternal medication and initiation of DES treatment early in pregnancy. These structural abnormalities also undergo modification over a period of years and in some subjects disappear entirely. Follow-up studies of DES females for up to 5 years by Antonioli et al. indicated that the epithelial changes of cervical ectropion decreased or disappeared in about three fourths, while cervicovaginal ridges decreased or disappeared in one half.

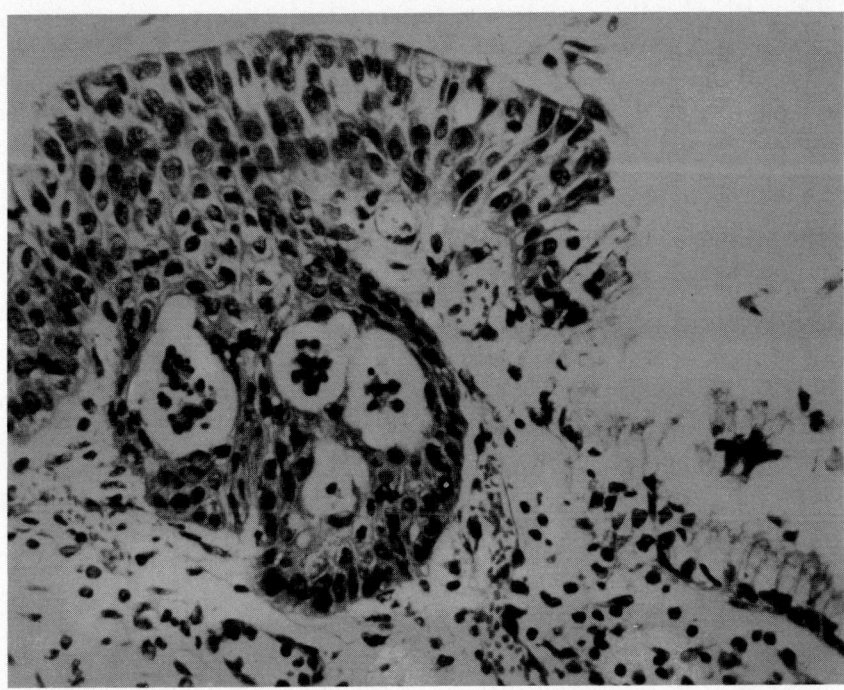

FIGURE 14-5
Squamous metaplasia of surface epithelium and underlying gland (×310). (From Herbst AL, Scully RE, and Robboy SJ: Hosp Pract 10:51, 1975.)

Examination of the DES-Exposed Female

The initial examination of the DES exposed is conducted much like a thorough gynecologic pelvic examination (Chapter 5). One difference is that careful inspection and palpation of the entire vaginal mucosa and cervix are performed first. Surgical lubricants should not be used at this stage in the examination, since they interfere with the interpretation of cytologic specimens (Pap smear). After thorough palpation is completed, an appropriately sized speculum is inserted into the vagina. For very young patients, a special narrow pediatric speculum should be used. The speculum is gently rotated to allow full visualization of the entire vagina and cervix, with care taken not to obscure any small lesion of the anterior or posterior vaginal wall.

Cytologic samples are obtained from the vagina, including the fornices, as well as from the ectocervix and the endocervical canal. These three samples are submitted separately to identify the location of any abnormal cells seen on the smears. Colposcopy (Chapter 26) permits a detailed assessment of the cervicovaginal epithelium (transformation zone).

The appearance of vaginal adenosis is often similar to the "grapelike" appearance of columnar epithelium on the cervix. Squamous metaplasia may give rise to an atypical appearing transformation with areas of "mosaicism" and "punctation," findings that often suggest the presence intraepithelial neoplasia in the unexposed female. However, in DES-exposed offspring such changes often indicate the presence of active squamous metaplasia (Figure 14-5) rather than a dysplastic process. Colposcopy allows for the careful evaluation of the transformation zone in the DES-exposed female and provides a guide for biopsy sites in individuals whose Pap smears indicate intraepithelial neoplasia. However, colposcopy is of limited value in the detection of clear cell adenocarcinomas, which usually do not provide the examiner with any unique colposcopic pattern, unlike squamous cell carcinomas. Biopsies should be performed on any suspicious nodular areas or from the most abnormal parts of the transformation zone if there is an atypical Pap smear.

Following colposcopy, the examination is usually continued by doing an iodine stain of the vagina and cervix with half-strength Lugol's solution. The stain identifies the normal glycogen-containing squamous epithelium and provides the examiner with a useful marker of the boundary between normal squamous epithelium and nonglycogenated areas of metaplasia, adenosis, and ectropion. The technique provides a simple method to detect changes in the size and extent of the non-iodine-staining areas on subsequent examinations. A routine bimanual vaginal and rectal examination completes the evaluation.

The intervals for follow-up examinations depend on the findings as well as the completeness of the initial examination. Yearly intervals are adequate for most individuals. Semiannual examinations are often done for those who have large areas of vaginal adenosis, while the findings of cellular atypia in the vagina or cervical epithelium usually necessitate more frequent follow-up.

Management

The tuboendometrial gland of vaginal adenosis is believed capable of providing the origin of clear cell adenocarcinoma. However, the risk of these tumors developing in an area of adenosis is extremely small. Only about 16 cancers have been identified in the hundreds of thousands of DES-exposed females who have been followed and examined regularly for vaginal adenosis or cervical ectropion in the United States as of 1990. Therefore unless atypia of the columnar epithelium is determined on biopsy or suggested cytologically, therapy for adenosis is not needed.

Because the extensive transformation zone in the DES-exposed female often extends far into the vagina, it has been hypothesized that a higher incidence of dysplasia or intraepithelial neoplasia may occur (Chapter 26). This larger transformation zone would theoretically provide a greater surface area of immature metaplastic epithelium that could be influenced by potential carcinogens. However, current data from case-control studies have not established that intraepithelial neoplasia develops more frequently in DES-exposed subjects in comparison to those not exposed. However, a national collaborative study, the DES Adenosis (DESAD) Project, published by Robboy et al. did show twice the frequency of dysplasia in DES-exposed women. As noted by Bornstein et al. other factors, including increased rates of herpes simplex virus and human *Papillomavi-rus* infections, were observed among the DES exposed in that study, and a clear-cut association was not established. Although abnormal colposcopic findings (white epithelium, punctation, and mosaicism) are found frequently in DES-exposed women, it has been demonstrated that these abnormal colposcopic areas often contain active squamous metaplasia rather than a neoplastic process. It is important that therapy be based on an accurate histologic diagnosis and not be influenced by the issue of DES exposure.

One of the major difficulties in the appropriate management of epithelial changes in the genital tract of the DES-exposed woman is the accurate diagnosis of intraepithelial neoplasia. The histologic changes of active, immature squamous metaplasia may be difficult to distinguish microscopically from the premalignant changes of dysplasia or carcinoma in situ. Additional techniques to identify premalignant epithelium include the determination of the DNA content of the lesion measured in tissue sections. This leads to an estimate of the ploidy level in the cells of the section (Chapter 26). Tissues having a normal diploid (2N) distribution are "euploid" and normal. *Polyploidy* refers to the nuclear DNA measurement being increased by multiples of the diploid amount (4N, 8N, etc.). *Aneuploidy* is the condition in which the DNA content reveals a wide distribution of intermediate modal values that differ from the diploid or polyploid ranges; often a wide range of intermediate values is encountered. Metaplasia usually contains diploid values and occasionally some polyploid values. Tissues showing an aneuploid distribution usually consist of moderate to severe dysplasia or carcinoma in situ. Mild dysplasia, like in some metaplasias, may show a polyploid distribution.

The therapy of intraepithelial neoplasia (dysplasia and carcinoma in situ) of the vagina and cervix in the DES-exposed female involves the same considerations as in those not exposed and is considered in detail in Chapters 26 and 30. Local destruction of the entire area of intraepithelial neoplasia is important. In the vagina this can be accomplished by local surgical excision or laser vaporization. In the cervix, laser treatment can also be utilized and occasionally local surgical therapy in the form of conization is indicated. Although cryotherapy (freezing) has been used successfully to treat intraepithelial neoplasia of the cervix in the unexposed woman, it has been reported to be followed by cervical stenosis and infertility in DES-exposed females. For that reason this modality of therapy should be avoided.

Contraceptive Advice

No data indicate that any contraceptive method, including oral contraceptive steroids, is contraindicated in the DES-exposed female. There has been concern regarding the potential increased risk of endocrine-related tumors, such as endometrial or breast carcinomas, in those subjects who have already been exposed in utero to high doses of exogenous estrogens. Concern involves potential future risks of increasing the lifetime exposure to any estrogen.

Barrier contraceptives and jellies have been frequently prescribed and appear to have the same risks and benefits for the DES-exposed female as for the unexposed population. The intrauterine device has also been used, although there is concern about prescribing it for the use by DES-exposed female because of the abnormal contours of the endometrial cavity that have been demonstrated on hysterosalpingograms in many subjects. It has not yet been demonstrated thus far, however, that the intrauterine device causes excessive risk for the DES-exposed female.

The diaphragm offers an effective method (Chapter 11) without major risk of side effects. For those individuals who prefer not to use a barrier method, oral contraceptives provide an effective and more convenient form of contraception.

DEVELOPMENT OF KIDNEYS AND URETERS

A number of studies have been done comparing the results of X-ray examinations of the kidneys and ureters (intravenous pyelograms) to evaluate the frequency of anatomic changes, such as duplication of a ureter or absence of a kidney. It appears that such changes have been observed in about 5% of the DES-exposed subjects studied, and this is the frequency anticipated in the general population. Thus DES exposure does not appear to cause anatomic abnormalities of the urinary tract.

IMMUNE FUNCTION

There has been some concern based on experimental animal studies that DES-exposed offspring may have an altered immune state and may be subject to an increased frequency of autoimmune diseases. Ways et al. studied eight DES daughters and found their T cell response to the mitogen phytohemagglutinin (PHA) was significantly higher than in nonexposed controls. In addition, Noller et al. studied 1171 DES-exposed females and 922 controls. There was a trend of an increase of autoimmune diseases among the DES females (49 in 1162) compared to controls (15 in 922), with a relative prevalence of 1.8, but the 95% confidence limits overlapped 1.0 (0.99 to 3.1). While not establishing a definitive clinical association, these data raise concern of a possibility of altered immune function in DES females.

REPRODUCTION

Hysterosalpingogram Studies

Various abnormalities in the shape of the endometrial cavity have been identified on hysterosalpingograms (HSGs) performed on DES-exposed females (see Figure 14-4). Irregularities in the shape and size of the endometrial cavity have been observed, characterized as T-shaped uterus, constriction rings near the entrance of the fallopian tube into the uterus, as well as irregular contours of the surface, and a smaller than normal endometrial cavity. HSG abnormalities occur in more than half of DES-exposed subjects. It appears that those who have cervicovaginal structural abnormalities or vaginal epithelial changes also are at greater risk for HSG abnormalities. These associations appear in part to be related to the increased risk for uterine changes in individuals whose mothers began DES treatment in early pregnancy.

Menstrual Patterns

There are conflicting reports regarding menstrual function in the DES-exposed female. In general, it has been reported that menarche in the DES exposed is comparable to that of the general population—about 12 years of age. Some studies have indicated no differences in menstrual histories between the exposed and unexposed. In contrast, others have reported differences, noting primarily oligomenorrhea and a shorter duration of menstrual flow in DES-exposed women. Current data do not allow a definitive conclusion.

Fertility

In the 1980s many DES-exposed females entered their reproductive years. Some studies have suggested decreased fertility among DES-exposed women, while others have not reported such results. Table 14-2 summarizes the findings in four case-control studies that evaluated fertility in this group. Two studies found no differences, while in the other two studies the differences were significant. The follow-up study of Senekjian et al. evaluated the causes of primary infertility and, not surprisingly, noted abnormal HSGs in approximately half the exposed subjects and in none of the controls. While there is no evidence the abnormal HSGs contributed to the primary infertility, the study demonstrated that a "tubal factor" was significantly more likely to occur in the DES-exposed subjects. No differences were found in ovulatory or male factors or in endometriosis; the latter actually occurred more often in the unexposed females. Although not statistically significant, 63% of the infertile DES-exposed females had a cervical factor (stenosis or poor postcoital test) compared with 25% of unexposed women. The tubal factor appeared to be primarily related to adhesions secondary to pelvic inflammatory disease (PID) in the exposed subjects. It has not been established that DES-exposed women are more susceptible to PID, but they should be vigorously treated with appropriate intravenous antibiotics if PID is thought to exist (Chapter 22).

Pregnancy Outcome

Unfavorable pregnancy outcomes, including premature live birth, ectopic pregnancy, and nonviable birth, have been reported more commonly among DES-exposed females. The most reliable source of data to evaluate these outcomes comes from case-control studies that have calculated the outcome of first pregnancies. Table 14-3 summarizes the results of one such study among DES-exposed females and unexposed controls. The incidence of premature birth with first pregnancies was higher in the exposed group. In addition, first-trimester and midtrimester pregnancy loss occurred in a higher proportion among exposed women. Seven percent of exposed women experienced ectopic pregnancy ($P < 0.01$). It also appears that unfavorable outcome may be more frequent among those noted to have cervicovaginal ridges on pelvic examination. However, these ridges are not stable and can disappear with time; their relation to adverse pregnancy outcome is not certain. The Herbst et al. (1989) study also noted that 12 of 30 exposed women who had cervical therapy with cautery or cryosurgery experienced at least one subsequent pregnancy loss compared with only 2 of 17 controls ($P < 0.05$), again suggesting that these modalities should be avoided. Although reproductive performance has been associated with an increased proportion of unfavorable outcomes, over 80% of DES females who desire pregnancy have delivered at least one live-born infant.

Management

Although there may be an increased risk for unfavorable outcome in DES-exposed females with an abnormal hysterosalpingogram, the results of this examination have not been correlated with any individual or specific adverse pregnancy outcome. Therefore routine hysterographic evaluation of DES-exposed females is not warranted. The indications for obtaining HSGs in these individuals are similar to those for unexposed women who are undergoing infertility evaluation.

Careful prenatal care is required for the DES-exposed woman. An early vaginal ultrasound should be performed to confirm intrauterine pregnancy and detect any early ectopic pregnancy. Careful surveillance in the second and third trimesters is needed to treat preterm dilation of the cervix. Michaels et al. studied

TABLE 14-2
Fertility in DES Exposed and Unexposed

| Study | Conception Rate | |
	Exposed	Unexposed
Herbst et al. (1980)	67%	86%
Barnes et al. (1980)	47%	50%
Cousins et al. (1980)	46%	41%
Senekjian et al. (1988)*	82%	95%

*Follow-up of Herbst et al. (1980). Rates of at least one pregnancy.

TABLE 14-3
First Pregnancy Outcome in DES Exposed and Unexposed

Evaluable Pregnancy Outcome	Exposed (*N* = 158)	Unexposed (*N* = 157)
Term birth	85 (54%)	130 (83%)
Premature*	32 (20%)	8 (5%)
Second-trimester loss (weeks 14 to 26)	4 ⎱ (19%)	1 ⎱ (12%)
Spontaneous abortion (≤13 weeks)	26 ⎰	18 ⎰
Ectopic pregnancy	11 (7%)	0

Adapted from Herbst AL, Senekjian EK, and Frey KW: Semin Reprod Endocrinol 7:124, 1989.
*Births were scored as premature if the duration of pregnancy was 26 weeks or more and birth weight was less than 2500 g.
All but one premature baby in each group survived.

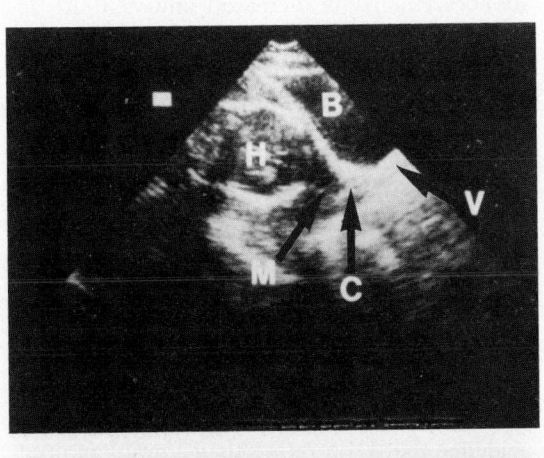

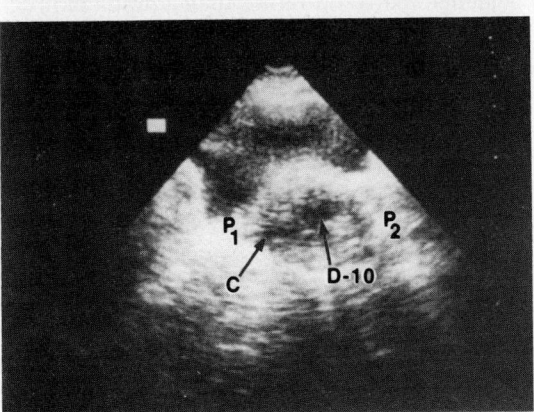

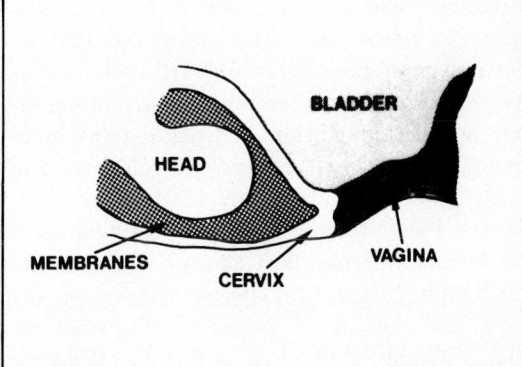

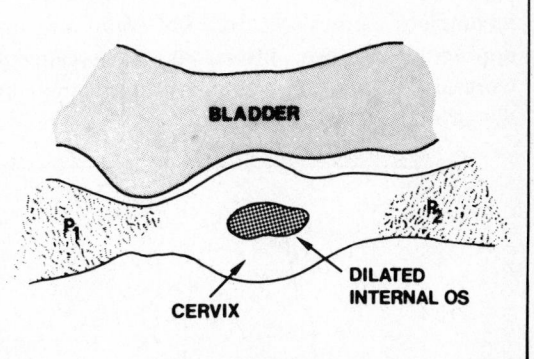

FIGURE 14-6
DES-exposed patient, 21.1 weeks pregnant, with membrane herniation. Internal os dilated to 20 mm, and cervix to 10 mm. **A**, Longitudinal view. **B**, Transverse view. *H*, Head; *M*, membrane herniation; *B*, bladder; *C*, cervix; *V*, vagina; *P1*, right parametrium; *P2*, left parametrium; *D-IO*, dilated internal os. (Reprinted with permission from Michaels WH, Thompson HO, Schreiber FR, et al: Obstet Gynecol 73:230, 1989.)

DES exposed and unexposed during pregnancy to monitor for cervical dilation (Figure 14-6). Cervical cerclage was placed when indicated by their ultrasound findings. Five of 21 DES-exposed patients required cerclage for cervical incompetence. The results were comparable, except control subjects delivered on the average 8 days later. There were no pregnancy losses in the exposed or unexposed due to cervical incompetence, and the technique appears safe and effective.

CLEAR CELL ADENOCARCINOMA OF THE VAGINA AND CERVIX

In 1971 a special registry was established to centralize data on the clinical outcome, histopathology, and epidemiology of clear cell adenocarcinomas of the vagina and cervix that occur in women born after 1940. All such cancers were studied, regardless of a history of maternal hormone ingestion. Through 1990 more than 555 cases of these rare carcinomas had been added. Approximately 65% of the cases reported were associated with a positive maternal history, whereas 25% showed no history of DES-type treatment. The remainder of the cases had therapy for high-risk pregnancy either with unidentified or with non-DES-type drugs. It is likely that some of the so-called negative cases may be due to faulty memory or incomplete medical records, but some are undoubtedly negative, insofar as these cancers were also known to occur in young women in the pre-DES era.

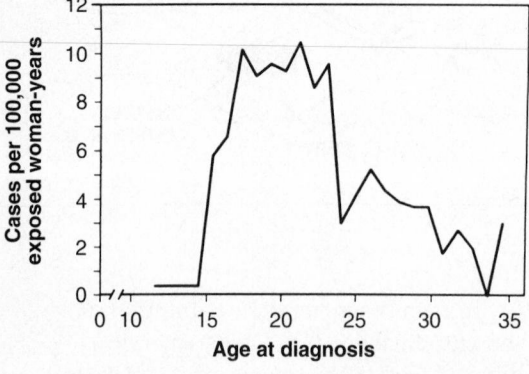

FIGURE 14-7
Incidence rates of clear cell adenocarcinoma, according to age, among white female residents of the United States who were prenatally exposed to diethylstilbestrol. (Reprinted with permission from Melnick S, Cole P, Anderson D, et al: N Engl J Med 316:514, 1987.)

The age of DES patients diagnosed with clear cell adenocarcinoma has varied from 7 to 36 years. Figure 14-7 shows the age-incidence curve for these individuals. It can be seen that the tumors are extraordinarily rare before age 14 and then there is a rapid rise in the age-incidence curve, which plateaus at about age 19, after which there is a drop to lower levels through the 20s and 30s. Similar results for DES history and age distribution were reported by Hanselaar et al. on 55 patients from the Netherlands

These tumors are uncommon, even among DES-exposed females, and the risk of cancer occurring in this population is estimated to be less than 1 cancer per 1000 exposed women. It does appear, however, that the risk of clear cell adenocarcinoma is increased among those females whose mothers began DES treatment in early pregnancy. As noted previously, vaginal adenosis is also more frequent among those whose mothers started DES early in pregnancy. In addition a maternal history of miscarriage, the daughter's birth in the fall, and premature birth also appear to be factors contributing to the development of clear cell adenocarcinoma. However, DES is a primary factor. In addition, a recent study indicates that maternal vaginal bleeding during the index pregnancy *reduces* the risk of clear cell adenocarcinoma and vaginal adenosis, providing further evidence that DES rather than a problem pregnancy is the primary factor in the development of these lesions. Insofar as clear cell adenocarcinomas have developed in DES-exposed females through their 20s and early 30s, these cancers will continue to be diagnosed for a number of years, since DES pregnancy usage is known to have continued, albeit on a limited basis, until 1971. The therapeutic results of treatment of these tumors are considered in Chapter 31.

HISTOGENESIS OF DES-ASSOCIATED ABNORMALITIES

Although there are various interpretations, the development of the human vagina is believed to evolve primarily from the müllerian ducts and the urogenital sinus. The paired müllerian (paramesonephric) ducts arise as invaginations of the celomic epithelium near the urogenital ridge, extend caudally, and then fuse at the urogenital sinus. The müllerian-derived co-

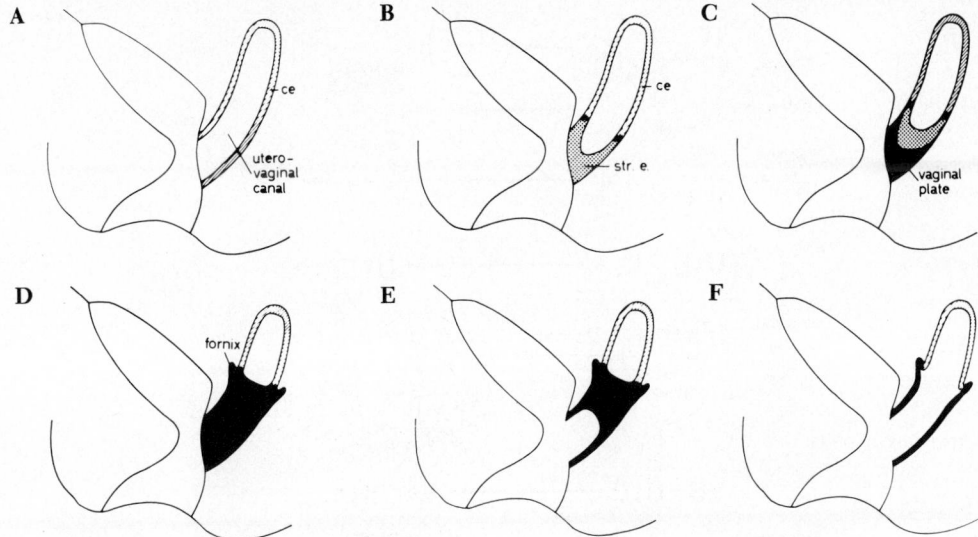

FIGURE 14-8

Diagrams of successive stages in development of human vagina. **A,** Uterovaginal canal is lined with columnar epithelium *(ce),* which later, **B,** undergoes transformation into stratified squamous type *(str e).* Transition between these two epithelial types is indefinite. At same time as transformation takes place, uterovaginal canal is changed into solid structure in same region, **B. C,** Vaginal plate has appeared between dorsal wall of urogenital sinus and region with stratified epithelium in uterovaginal anlage. Vaginal plate grows cranially, stratified epithelium is resorbed, and plate finally is in contact with columnar epithelium, **D.** Lumen formation in solid vaginal plate begins caudally, **E,** and progresses cranially, **F.** (From Forsberg JG and Kalland T: Embryology of the genital tract in humans and in rodents. In Herbst AL and Bern HA, editors: Developmental effects of diethylstilbestrol [DES] in pregnancy, New York, 1981, Thieme-Stratton, Inc.)

lumnar epithelium is then replaced by a solid core of squamous epithelium that arises from the vaginal plate (Figure 14-8). The vaginal plate grows cephalad from the urogenital sinus, and the solid core of squamous epithelium ultimately canalizes to form the permanent lining of the vagina, which consists primarily of squamous epithelium.

The laboratory mouse has been used frequently to study the effects of hormones on the developing genital tract. In the newborn mouse the vagina is immature, and the reproductive tract continues to develop neonatally, similar to the changes that occur in humans during the latter part of intrauterine life. By administering estrogens, such as estradiol or DES, to neonatal mice, it has been found that the squamous transformation of columnar epithelium is arrested, resulting in the persistence of müllerian-type columnar epithelium in the upper vagina and cervix.

In utero exposure to DES in humans may

have a similar effect, that is, a DES-induced persistence of glandular epithelium in the vagina leading to adenosis. The increased risk of clear cell adenocarcinoma in subjects whose mothers began DES treatment in early pregnancy may in part be due to the larger area of ectopic glandular epithelium in the vagina of these patients. Insofar as clear cell adenocarcinomas are related to the tuboendometrial cell of adenosis, increased areas of tuboendometrial-type epithelium in patients exposed to DES in early gestation may provide a greater area for interaction with an unidentified carcinogen. Endogenous estrogens could act as such a promoter insofar as the adenocarcinomas primarily occur after the onset of menstruation. However, not all the factors that lead to the appearance of these tumors are understood at present.

The structural abnormalities of the uterus and cervicovaginal areas may also be associated with anomalous development of the müllerian

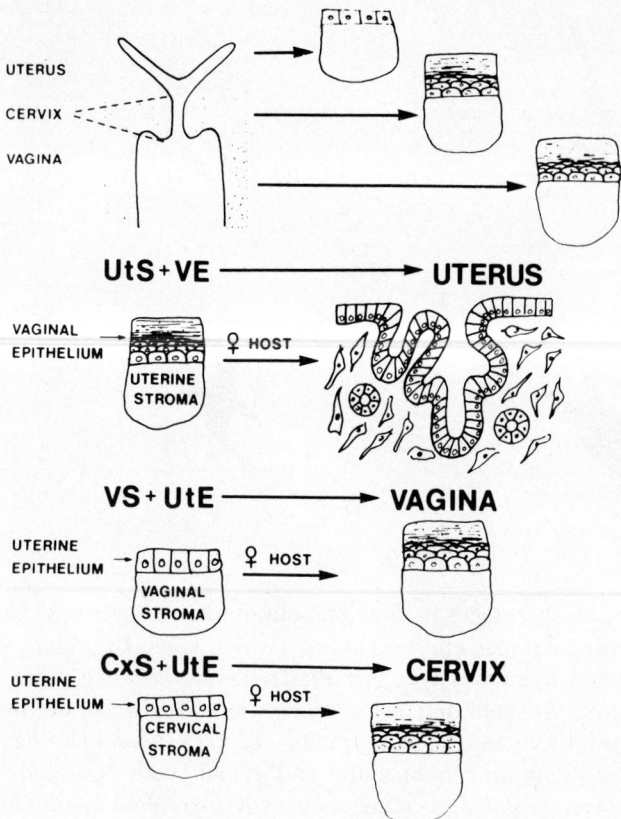

FIGURE 14-9

Summary of recombination experiments between epithelium and stroma from uterus, cervix, and vagina from neonatal mice (1 to 5 days old). Upper portion of figure depicts morphologic organization of epithelium in these organs: uterine epithelium is a simple columnar glandular epithelium, whereas vaginal and cervical epithelium is stratified squamous. Uterine stroma *(UtS)* induces uterine morphogenesis and cytodifferentiation from vaginal epithelium *(VE)*. In reciprocal recombination composed of vaginal stroma *(VS)* plus uterine epithelium *(UtE)*, simple columnar epithelium normally is induced to differentiate as vaginal epithelium. Similarly, cervical stroma *(CxS)* induces development of stratified epithelium from *UtE*. (From Cunha GR and Fujii H: Stromal parenchymal interactions in normal and abnormal development of the genital tract. In Herbst AL and Bern HA, editors: Developmental effects of diethylstilbestrol [DES] in pregnancy, New York, 1981, Thieme-Stratton, Inc.)

ducts. Although the mechanism is not clear, some unfavorable pregnancy outcomes observed in DES-exposed women may be related to the configuration of the endometrial cavity or to anomalies of the cervix. A defect in the development of the myometrium or in cervical-uterine connective tissue is also possible. Recently it has been shown experimentally that the stroma of different parts of the embryonic female genital tract can have inductive effects that determine the histology of the overlying epithelium (Figure 14-9). For example, combining cervical stroma with uterine epithelium leads to cervical differentiation, while combining vaginal stroma with cervical epithelium leads to vaginal epithelial development. These observations suggest a primarily stromal action of DES that could account for both the epithelial and the connective tissue abnormalities often observed. Presumably, DES ingested by the mother crosses the uteroplacental barrier and enters the fetal circulation. It is known that estrogen receptors develop in the fetal genital tract in early intrauterine life. Insofar as DES is a nonsteroidal estrogen, it appears that it may not be metabolized in the fetal tissues in the same manner as steroidal estrogens. This would allow it to have the developmental effects noted in exposed offspring.

The genital abnormalities associated with DES in humans pertain to the ingestion of any stilbene-type estrogen (see Figure 14-1). Ingestion of steroidal estrogens during pregnancy has not been reported to be associated with such changes.

PSYCHOLOGIC STUDIES

There have not been extensive psychologic studies of DES-exposed females compared to those of unexposed females. As might be anticipated, increased anxiety and concern have existed among the exposed population in regard to health risks they encounter as a consequence of intrauterine exposure to DES. A major problem has also been the guilt and anxiety felt by the mothers of these patients because of concern about damage to their daughters. The guilt is present despite the fact that the medication prescribed to help them achieve a better pregnancy outcome. A number of self-help and consumer groups have been formed to deal with some of these issues.

DES-EXPOSED MALES

Abnormalities have been described in DES-exposed males, including cryptorchidism, hypoplasia of the testis, more frequent epididymal cysts, and abnormalities in semen analyses. It should be remembered that the effect of DES on the female genital tract appears to occur primarily on the müllerian ducts. In the male genital tract the müllerian remnants are found in the epididymis of the testis and the utricle of the prostate. An increased risk in development of malignancy in DES-exposed

TABLE 14-4
Breast Cancer Occurrence in DES Exposed and Unexposed

Study	Exposed	Unexposed
Herbst and Bern (1981)	35/655	28/645
Brian et al. (1980)	8/408	9.4*
Greenberg et al. (1984)	118/3033	80/3033
Hadjimichael et al. (1984)	38/1531	24/1405

*Expected number derived from general population statistics.

males has not been demonstrated. The testicular and semen changes observed with increased frequency among DES-exposed males in some studies have not been verified in others. Data regarding fertility rates among DES-exposed men are not sufficient to evaluate adequately the risk of infertility in this group.

DES-EXPOSED MOTHERS

Because of the high doses of estrogen taken during pregnancy by DES mothers, there have been concerns of an increased risk of estrogen-sensitive tumors in this group. In particular, breast cancer and endometrial cancer, as well as other genital tract cancers, have been evaluated in case-control studies. Currently, increased risk has not been conclusively demonstrated. Table 14-4 summarizes the occurrence of breast cancer, citing studies that have evaluated this in DES-exposed women. Only one study showed a slightly increased risk of breast cancer among those exposed who are now over age 60 years. At present the guidelines for breast cancer screening and examination in DES-exposed mothers is the same as for unexposed women (Chapter 13).

_____ KEY POINTS _____

- Vaginal adenosis occurs in about one third of DES-exposed females.

- Cervicovaginal ridges occur in about one fourth of DES-exposed females.

- Vaginal adenosis is more frequent among those whose mothers took DES in early pregnancy, in those whose mothers took DES at a higher dose, and in exposed females who are younger at the time of examination.

- Adenosis and ectropion usually heal by the physiologic process of squamous metaplasia.

- Adenosis, ectropion, and cervicovaginal ridges heal spontaneously in many but not all DES-exposed females.

- Unfavorable pregnancy outcomes, particularly premature birth, midtrimester loss, and ectopic pregnancy, occur in about one half of DES-exposed females.

- Over 80% of DES daughters have a live-born child.

- Routine hysterosalpingogram studies are not indicated for DES-exposed females.

- Vaginal ultrasound is an effective modality for following cervical dilation in DES females through pregnancy to indicate those requiring cerclage.

- Analysis of nuclear DNA content is useful to help distinguish intraepithelial neoplasia from squamous metaplasia.

- Primary infertility is more frequent in DES females, and tubal factors appear to be a contributory cause. An increased frequency of endometriosis has not been demonstrated.

- The risk of development of clear cell adenocarcinoma of the vagina and cervix is increased in DES-exposed females, but these tumors occur in less than 1 per 1000 exposed and have been noted in those 7 to 36 years of age.

- Abnormal development of the müllerian ducts in utero results in reproductive tract alterations in the DES-exposed female.

- Factors that appear to increase the risk of development of clear cell adenocarcinoma, in addition to uterine DES exposure, include history of miscarriage in the mother and the daughter's prematurity and birth in the Fall.

- Current data do not indicate an increased risk of breast cancer in DES mothers.

BIBLIOGRAPHY

Antonioli DA, Burke L, and Friedman EA: Natural history of diethylstilbestrol-associated genital tract lesions: cervical ectopy and cervicovaginal hood, Am J Obstet Gynecol 137:847, 1980.

Barnes AB: Menstrual history of young women exposed in utero to diethylstilbestrol, Fertil Steril 32:148, 1979.

Barnes AB, Colton T, Gundersen J, et al: Fertility and outcome of pregnancy in women exposed in utero to diethylstilbestrol, N Engl J Med 302:609, 1980.

Bibbo M, Gill WB, Azizi F, et al: Follow-up study of male and female offspring of DES-exposed mothers, Obstet Gynecol 49:1, 1977.

Bornstein J, Adam E, Adler-Storthz K, et al: Development of cervical and vaginal squamous cell neoplasia as a late consequence of in utero exposure to diethylstilbestrol, Obstet Gynecol Surv 43:15, 1988.

Brian DD, Tilley BC, Labarthe DR, et al: Breast cancer in DES-exposed mothers: absence of association, Mayo Clin Proc 55:89, 1980.

Cousins L, Karp W, Lacey C, et al: Reproductive outcome of women exposed to diethylstilbestrol in utero, Obstet Gynecol 56:70, 1980.

Cunha G and Fujii H: Stromal-parenchymal interactions in normal and abnormal development of the genital tract. In Herbst AL and Bern HA, editors: Developmental effects of diethylstilbestrol (DES) in pregnancy, New York, 1981, Thieme-Stratton, Inc.

DeCherney AH, Cholst I, and Naftolin A: Structure and function of the fallopian tubes following exposure to diethylstilbestrol (DES) during gestation, Fertil Steril 36:741, 1981.

Dieckmann WE, Davis ME, Rynkiewicz SM, et al: Does the administration of diethylstilbestrol during pregnancy have therapeutic value? Am J Obstet Gynecol 66:1062, 1953.

Dodds EC, Goldberg L, Larson W, et al: Oestrogenic activity of certain synthetic compounds, Nature 141:247, 1938.

Forsberg MD and Kalland T: Embryology of the genital tract in humans and in rodents. In Herbst AL and Bern HA, editors: Developmental effects of diethylstilbestrol (DES) in pregnancy, New York, 1981, Thieme-Stratton, Inc.

Fu Y, Robboy SJ, and Prat J: Nuclear DNA study of vaginal and cervical squamous cell abnormalities in DES-exposed progeny, Obstet Gynecol 52:129, 1978.

Greenberg ER, Barnes AB, Resseguie L, et al: Follow-up study of mothers exposed to diethylstilbestrol in pregnancy, N Engl J Med 311:1393, 1984.

Hadjimichael OC, Meigs JW, Falcier FW, et al: Cancer risk among women exposed to exogenous estrogens during pregnancy, JNCI 73:831, 1984.

Hanselaar AGJM, Van Leusen NDM, DeWilde PCM, and Vooijs GP: Clear cell adenocarcinoma of the vagina and cervix: a report of the Central Netherlands Registry with emphasis on early detection and prognosis, Cancer 67:1971,1991.

Herbst AL, editor: Intrauterine exposure to diethylstilbestrol in the human, Chicago, 1978, American College of Obstetricians and Gynecologists (monograph).

Herbst AL and Anderson D: Recent advances in clear cell adenocarcinoma of the vagina and cervix secondary to intrauterine exposure to DES, Semin Surg Oncol 6:343, 1990.

Herbst AL, Anderson S, Hubby M, et al: Risk factors for the development of DES-associated clear cell adenocarcinoma: a case control study, Am J Obstet Gynecol 154:814, 1986.

Herbst AL and Bern HA, editors: Developmental effects of diethylstilbestrol (DES) in pregnancy, New York, 1981, Thieme-Stratton, Inc.

Herbst AL, Cole P, Colton T, et al: Age-incidence and risk of diethylstilbestrol-related clear cell adenocarcinoma of the vagina and cervix, Am J Obstet Gynecol 128:43, 1977.

Herbst AL, Hubby MM, Azizi F, et al: Reproductive and gynecologic surgical experience in diethylstilbestrol-exposed daughters, Am J Obstet Gynecol 141:1019, 1981.

Herbst AL, Hubby MM, Blough RR, et al: A comparison of pregnancy experience in DES-exposed and DES-unexposed daughters, J Reprod Med 24:62, 1980.

Herbst AL and Scully RE: Adenocarcinoma of the vagina in adolescence: a report of 7 cases including 6 clear cell carcinomas (so-called mesonephromas), Cancer 25:745, 1970.

Herbst AL, Scully RE, and Robboy SJ: Effects of maternal DES ingestion on the female genital tract, Hosp Pract 10:51, 1975.

Herbst AL, Senekjian EK, and Frey KW: Abortion and pregnancy loss among diethylstilbestrol-exposed women, Semin Reprod Endocrinol 7:124, 1989.

Herbst AL, Ulfelder H, and Poskanzer DC: Adenocarcinoma of the vagina: association of maternal stilbestrol therapy with tumor appearance in young women, N Engl J Med 284:878, 1971.

Jeffries JA, Robboy SJ, O'Brien PC, et al: Structural anomalies of the cervix and vagina in women enrolled in the Diethylstilbestrol Adenosis (DESAD) Project, Am J Obstet Gynecol 148:59, 1984.

Kaufman RH, Adam H, Binder GL, et al: Upper genital tract changes and pregnancy outcome in offspring exposed in utero to diethylstilbestrol, Am J Obstet Gynecol 137:299, 1980.

Kaufman RH, Noller KL, Adam E, et al: Upper genital tract abnormalities and pregnancy outcome in diethylstilbestrol-exposed progeny, Am J Obstet Gynecol 148:973, 1984.

Melnick S, Cole P, Anderson D, et al: Rates and risks of diethylstilbestrol-related clear cell adenocarcinoma of the vagina and cervix: an update, N Engl J Med 316:514, 1987.

Michaels WH, Thompson HO, Schreiber FR, et al: Ultrasound surveillance of the cervix during pregnancy in diethylstilbestrol-exposed offspring, Obstet Gynecol 73:230, 1989.

Noller KL, Blair PB, O'Brien PC, et al: Increased occurrence of autoimmune disease among women exposed in utero to diethylstilbestrol, Fertil Steril 49:1080, 1988.

Noller KL, Townsend DE, Kaufman RH, et al: Maturation of vaginal and cervical epithelium in women exposed in utero to diethylstilbestrol (DESAD Project), Am J Obstet Gynecol 146:279, 1983.

Robboy SJ, Noller KL, O'Brien, P, et al: Increased incidence of cervical and vaginal dysplasia in 3980 DES-exposed young women, JAMA 252:2979, 1984.

Robboy SJ, Scully RE, and Herbst AL: Pathology of vaginal and cervical abnormalities associated with prenatal exposure to diethylstilbestrol (DES), J Reprod Med 15:5, 1975.

Robboy SJ, Welch WR, Young RH, et al: Topographic relation of cervical ectropion and vaginal adenosis to clear cell adenocarcinoma, Obstet Gynecol 60:546, 1982.

Senekjian EK, Potkul RK, Frey K, et al: Infertility among daughters either exposed or not exposed to diethylstilbestrol, Am J Obstet Gynecol 158:493, 1988.

Sharp GB and Cole P: Vaginal bleeding and diethylstilbestrol exposure during pregnancy: relationship to genital tract clear cell adenocarcinoma and vaginal adenosis in daughters, Am J Obstet Gynecol 162:994, 1990.

Ways SC, Mortola JF, Zvaifler NJ, et al: Alterations in immune responsiveness in women exposed to diethylstilbestrol in utero, Fertil Steril 48:193, 1987.

Abortion

_____ KEY TERMS AND DEFINITIONS _____

Anembryonic Gestation (Blighted Ovum). Ultrasonic visualization of a gestational sac without a fetus in a pregnancy ≥7.5 weeks' gestation.

Abortion. Termination of pregnancy before 20 weeks' gestation calculated from date of onset of last menses. An alternative definition is delivery of a fetus with a weight of less than 500 g. If abortion occurs before 12 weeks' gestation, it is called *early;* from 12 to 20 weeks it is called *late.*

Aneuploid Abortus. An abortus with the number of chromosomes less or greater than the normal 46.

Cerclage. A circular ligature used to treat the incompetent cervix. The suture is placed beneath the epithelium of the cervix at the level of the internal cervical os.

Complete Abortion. Spontaneous expulsion of all fetal and placental tissue from the uterine cavity before 20 weeks' gestation.

Euploid Abortus. An abortus in which the chromosome complement is normal, 46,XX or 46,XY.

Incompetent Cervix (Cervical Incompetence). Condition whereby the internal cervical canal dilates at 16 weeks of gestation or later, resulting in recurrent premature pregnancy loss.

Incomplete Abortion. Passage of some but not all fetal or placental tissue through the cervix before 20 weeks' gestation.

Induced Abortion. Intentional medical or surgical termination of pregnancy before 20 weeks' gestation. Also called *elective pregnancy termination* if performed for woman's desires or *therapeutic abortion* if performed for reasons of maintaining health of the mother.

Inevitable Abortion. Uterine bleeding from a gestation of less than 20 weeks accompanied by cervical dilation but without expulsion of any placental or fetal tissue through the cervix.

Intrauterine Fetal Death. Ultrasonic visualization of fetus more than 15 mm long, crown-rump length, without fetal heart activity.

Lupus Anticoagulant Activity. Prolongation of activated partial thromboplastic time, usually associated with antiphospholipid antibodies. The presence of this activity and these antibodies is associated with recurrent pregnancy loss caused by thrombosis in the placental circulation.

Metroplasty. A surgical procedure to unify the endometrial cavity of a bicornuate uterus or remove the septum of a septate uterus.

Missed Abortion. Fetal death before 20 weeks' gestation without expulsion of any fetal or maternal tissue for at least 8 weeks thereafter.

Recurrent Spontaneous Abortion. The loss of three or more pregnancies before 20 weeks' gestation. Functionally, however, physicians should do a work up for recurrent spontaneous abortion after two pregnancy losses.

Septic Abortion. Any type of abortion that is accompanied by uterine infection.

Subchorionic Hematoma. An ultrasonographically visible hematoma elevating amniotic membrane.

Threatened Abortion. Any uterine bleeding from a gestation of less than 20 weeks without any cervical dilation or effacement.

Uterine Adhesions. Tissue within the uterine cavity that obliterates part or all of the endometrium.

About 15% to 20% of all known human pregnancies terminate in clinically recognized abortion. However, the incidence of total human embryonic loss is estimated to be much higher. In 1952 Hertig and Rock, using morphologic techniques, reported that about 40% of all human embryos either fail to implant or are aborted before the time of the expected menses. Although several studies using an HCG immunoassay of urine samples of normal women attempting to conceive indicated that the rate of early pregnancy loss after implantation could be as high as 60%, these rates were probably overestimated because of the lack of specificity of the HCG assay. Recently, Wilcox et al. measured HCG in daily urine samples of a group of 221 healthy women attempting to conceive. In this study the HCG assay was extremely sensitive and the antibody used was highly specific and did not cross react with LH. Of the 198 pregnancies that occurred, 22% ended before the pregnancy was clinically recognized and the total pregnancy loss, including clinically recognized abortions, was 31%. Because some fertilized ova do not implant and thus do not secrete detectable HCG and other abnormal pregnancies do not secrete sufficient intact HCG to be detectable by immunoassay, the rate of human pregnancy loss is probably even higher; it has been estimated by Léridon to be as high as 70% (Table 15-1). Therefore the process of human reproduction is inefficient. However, because most early pregnancy losses are the result of chromosomal or genetic abnormalities, the high frequency of abortion, as stated by Austin, is "an important and valuable provision of Nature . . . and . . . is in the best interests of the race," because "disadvantageous features from gene mutation are prevented from being incorporated into the overall hereditary pattern."

About 80% of abortions occur in the first trimester, with the incidence decreasing with increasing gestational age. Harlap et al. reported that the incidence of clinical abortion is relatively stable during each week of gestation before 12 weeks and declines steadily thereafter (Figure 15-1). These investigators also reported that if conception occurs within 3 months after a prior live birth, the incidence of abortion is increased compared with the relatively stable rate if conception occurs later than 3 months.

Obtaining accurate data to determine the true incidence of spontaneous abortion overall, as well as in particular subgroups of women, is difficult because of possible sources of bias produced by the selection process. Retrospective hospital-based studies of pregnant women often

TABLE 15-1

Life Table for Intrauterine Mortality in the Human (Per 100 Ova Exposed to Risk of Fertilization)

Week After Ovulation	Death (Expulsion of Dead Embryos)	Survivors
—	16 (not fertilized)	100
0	15 (failed to cleave)	84 (fertile)
1	27	69 (implanted)
2	5.0	42
6	2.9	37
10	1.7	34.1
14	0.5	32.4
18	0.3	31.9
22	0.1	31.6
26	0.1	31.5
30	0.1	31.4
34	0.1	31.3
38	0.2	31.32
Live births (including birth defects)		31
Natural wastage		69

From Léridon H: Intrauterine mortality. In Léridon H, editor: Human fertility, Chicago, 1977, The University of Chicago Press.

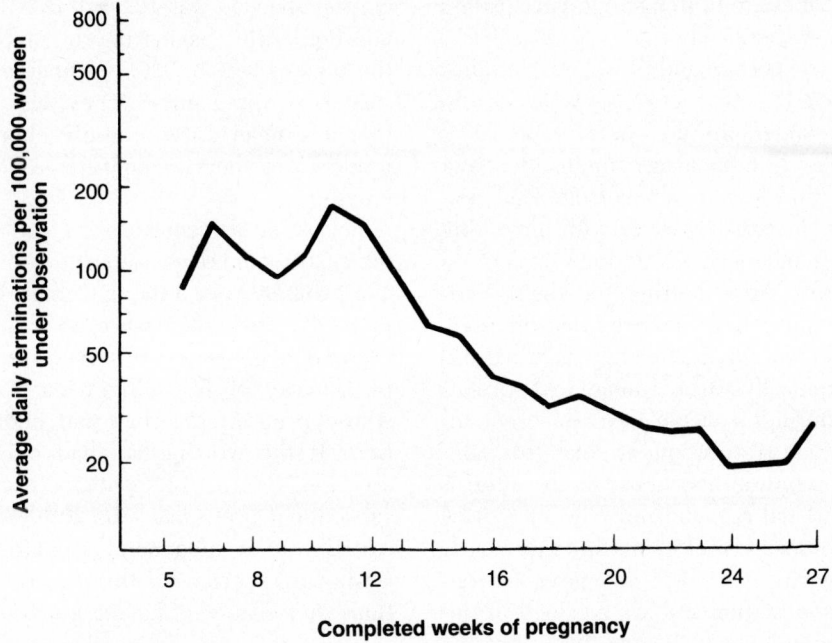

FIGURE 15-1

Spontaneous abortion by week of pregnancy. (From Harlap S, Shiono PH, and Ramcharan S: A life table of spontaneous abortions and the effects of age, parity, and other variables. In Porter IH and Hook, EB, editors: Human embryonic and fetal death, New York, 1980, Academic Press.)

fail to obtain correct information regarding the occurrence of abortion in first pregnancies. In most prospective studies the early pregnancy losses not requiring medical treatment are underrepresented. Probably the most accurate data come from the Cambridge early-pregnancy-loss study reported by Regan et al. In this study 630 women who were contemplating pregnancy were interviewed before conception and examined by ultrasonography as soon as pregnancy was suspected and then serially throughout the first trimester. The overall incidence of spontaneous abortion was 12%, and half had occurred before 8 weeks' gestation. The abortion rate in primigravidas was only 5%, whereas it was 14% in multigravidas (Table 15-2). Women whose last pregnancy was successful also had a low abortion rate (5%), whereas women whose last pregnancy aborted had about a 20% abortion rate. The highest rate of abortion (24%) occurred in that group of women who had been pregnant in the past but all the prior pregnancies terminated in abortion. This study indicates that reproductive history is the most relevant predictive factor for pregnancy outcome in a subsequent pregnancy

TABLE 15-2

Effect of Mother's Reproductive History on Risk of Spontaneous Abortion (n = 407)

History	No. of Patients	No. of Patients Aborting	Percentage
Last pregnancy aborted	214	40	19
Only abortions in the past	98	24	24
Only pregnancy aborted	59	12	20
Last pregnancy successful	95	5	5
All pregnancies successful	73	3	4
Only pregnancy successful	62	3	5
Previous termination of pregnancy	32	2	6
Primigravida	87	4	5
TOTAL	407		

From Regan L et al: Br Med J 299:541, 1989.

and the risk of abortion in primigravidas is less than previously believed.

Several retrospective and prospective studies have reported that if a fetus is viable, as observed ultrasonographically, in a woman less than 12 weeks' gestational age, the incidence of subsequent fetal loss is between 2% and 3%. The loss rate increases slightly with increasing maternal age and becomes as high as 20% in those who also have uterine bleeding. Pedersen and Mantoni have reported that the presence of a subchorionic hematoma, as visualized ultrasonographically, in a woman with threatened abortion and a viable fetus does not increase the risk of subsequent fetal loss. Because most clinical abortions occur after 8 weeks' gestational age and only 3% of fetuses that are viable at 8 weeks subsequently abort, the vast majority of clinical abortuses die before 8 weeks' gestation and are retained in the uterus for several weeks before the symptoms of abortion, uterine bleeding, and cramping occur.

Warburton and Fraser studied the incidence of abortion over a 10-year period in a group of more than 2000 women who had had at least one pregnancy of at least 20 weeks' gestation. The overall incidence of clinical abortion was 14.7%, and the risk of a pregnancy terminating in spontaneous abortion increased with increasing parity, maternal age, and paternal age (Table 15-3). Each of these parameters was an independent risk factor for abortion, and this information has been confirmed in other studies. These investigators also found that in this group of women who before this had delivered at least one live-born infant, the incidence of clinical abortion was 12.3% if they had no prior abortion. After having one or more abortions, there was a 24% to 32% risk of abortion in each successive pregnancy. They also recognized that a woman with multiple abortions has a tendency to abort at about the same gestational length.

Poland et al. reported that the overall incidence of spontaneous abortion in a group of 472 women was 14% and that it increased markedly after they were 35 years old. This group of investigators observed the subsequent pregnancies of 46 multigravida women, all of whose prior pregnancies had ended in abortion. If the woman had had only one prior abortion, the rate of spontaneous abortion in a subsequent pregnancy was 20%, similar to the overall rate in the general population, but after a woman experienced three consecutive abortions, her chance of having a subsequent abor-

TABLE 15-4

Outcome of First Pregnancy After History of Spontaneous Abortion Only

No. of Consecutive Spontaneous Abortions	Outcome		
	Live Birth (%)	Spontaneous Abortion (%)	Total Pregnancies
1*	79	19	145
2	65	35	26
3*	50	47	30
TOTAL			201

From Poland BJ, Miller JR, Jones DC, et al: Am J Obstet Gynecol 127:685, 1977.
*0.005 < P < 0.006 (47% versus 19%).

TABLE 15-3

Relation of Abortion Frequency to Maternal and Paternal Age at Conception

Maternal Age	% Abortion Frequency	Paternal Age	% Abortion Frequency
<20	12.2	<20	12.0
20-24	14.3	20-24	11.8
25-29	13.7	25-29	15.7
30-34	15.5	30-34	13.1
35-39	18.7	35-39	15.8
40-44	25.5	40-44	19.5
		44 +	23.1
MEAN	14.7	MEAN	14.7

From Warburton D and Fraser FC: Am J Hum Genet 16:1, 1964.

tion was nearly 50% (Table 15-4). This figure is similar to the 55% figure reported by James. These figures obtained from clinical studies are much lower than the calculated value of 84% for a similar population reported by Malpas using mathematic assumptions. Thus for women with no live births and a reproductive history of three pregnancies terminating in abortion, the chance of having an abortion in a subsequent pregnancy is about 50%, whereas women with at least one live birth and three spontaneous abortions have only a 30% chance that the next pregnancy will terminate in abortion.

ETIOLOGY

The causes of spontaneous abortion can be divided into two major categories, fetal and maternal, also called *genetic* and *environmental*. By far the major causes of abortion are genetic. There have been several large cytogenetic studies of spontaneous abortion, including the survey of 1500 abortuses by Boué, Boué, and Lazar and the 1980 study by Kajii et al. of 565 abortuses, using chromosomal banding techniques. These and other large studies indicate that the incidence of chromosomal anomalies in abortuses is about 50%. Only about 5% of the abnormal karyotypes are abnormalities in the structure of individual chromosomes, such as translocation. The vast majority are numerical abnormalities as a result of errors occurring during gonadogenesis (chromosomal nondisjunction during meiosis), fertilization (triploidy as a result of digyny or dispermy), or the first division of the fertilized ovum (tetraploidy or mosaicism). Except for monosomy, it is possible to determine the parental origin of the chromosome abnormality. Jacobs and Hassold reported that 26% of all fetal loss is caused by errors of maternal gametogenesis, 5% by errors of paternal gametogenesis, 4% by errors of fertilization and 4% by errors of zygote division (Table 15-5).

In most surveys of chromosomal anomalies of abortuses the relative frequency of the different types of anomalies is similar. The most common type of anomaly is autosomal trisomy, which accounts for about half the abnormal karyotypes (Table 15-6). Trisomies of all autosomes except for autosome 1 have been reported after karyotyping of abortions, with trisomy 16 being the most common. About one third of all autosomal trisomies in abortuses are trisomy 16, with trisomy 13, 15, 21, and 22 being next most common. Many trisomies occurring in abortions have not been reported in live births, probably because the phenotype is incompatible with fetal development.

The second most common chromosome abnormality is monosomy 45,X, which occurs in 15% to 20% of abortuses with abnormal karyotypes. It is estimated that the survival rate of 45,X conceptions is about 1 in 300. About 15% of chromosomal anomalies in abortuses are triploidy, with tetraploidy being less common, about 5% to 10%. To summarize, autosomal trisomy is the most common abnormal karyotype

TABLE 15-5
Chromosome Abnormalities by State at Which Error Occurred

| | Chromosomal Abnormalities (% of All Recognizable Fetal Loss) | | | | | |
| | | Polyploidy | | Structural | | |
Stage	Trisomy	Triploid	Tetraploid	Familial	De Novo	Total
Maternal gametogenesis	23.0	1.6	—	0.67	0.75*	26
Paternal gametogenesis	2.0	2.4	—	0.33	0.25*	5
Fertilization	—	4.0	—	—	—	4
Zygote	—	—	4.0	—	—	4
TOTAL	25.0	8.0	4.0	1.0	1.0	39

From Jacobs PA and Hassold TJ: The origin of chromosome abnormalities in spontaneous abortion. In Porter IH and Hook EB, editors: Human embryonic and fetal death, New York, 1980, Academic Press.
*Based on only four cases.

(~50%), followed in decreasing frequency by monosomy 45,X (~20%), triploidy (15%), tetraploidy (10%), and structural abnormalities (5%). The most common single chromosomal abnormality is monosomy 45,X. Karyotypes of abortuses of women who have had more than one abortion tend to be similar if the first abor-

TABLE 15-6
Chromosome Results of 447 Abortuses

	Karyotyped (Banded)	% of All Known Karyotype
Chromosomally normal		
46,XY	111	24.8
46,XX	95	21.3
TOTAL	206	46.1
Chromosomally abnormal		
45,X	44	9.8
Primary autosomal trisomy	138	30.9
Double trisomy	7	1.7
Triple trisomy	1	0.4
Triploidy	29	6.5
Tetraploidy	8	1.8
Mosaicism	1	0.4
Structural rearrangement	11	2.5
Others (XXY, Monosomy 21)	2	0.8
TOTAL	241	53.9

From Kajii T and Ferrier A: Hum Genet 55:87, 1980.

tus had either a normal karyotype or an autosomal trisomy (Table 15-7).

The various surveys have revealed no seasonal variability in the incidence of any type of chromosomal abnormality in abortions. There is also no effect of paternal age. Maternal age, however, is directly related to the incidence of trisomies, mainly those in the D and G group. Maternal age has no effect on the incidence of the other chromosomal anomalies in abortions, although there is evidence that monosomy 45,X is associated with a younger maternal age than other aneuploid or euploid abortions. Chromosome abnormalities in the parents are an uncommon cause of abortions—more than 95% of couples who have two or more spontaneous abortions are chromosomally normal.

In 1985 Tharapel et al. reviewed the cytogenic results of the 79 published surveys of couples with 2 or more pregnancy losses, comprising a total of 8208 women and 7834 men. The composite prevalence of major chromosome abnormalities in either parent was about 3%, 5 to 6 times higher than the general population. Abnormalities occurred in the female parent about twice as frequently as the male. About half of all chromosomic abnormalities were balanced reciprocal translocations, and one fourth were Robertonian translocations. About 12% were sex chromosomal mosaicism in the female, and the rest were inversions and other

TABLE 15-7
Karyotypes of Abortions in Women with Two Karyotyped Abortions—Combined Series

First Abortion	Second Abortion												Total
	Normal		Monosomy		Trisomy		Triploidy		Tetraploidy		Structural Rearrangements		
	Number	Percentage	Number	Percentage	Number	Percentage	Number	Percentage	Number	Percentage	Number	Percentage	
Normal	69	84.1	2	2.4	6	6.3	5	6.1	0	0	0	0	82
Monosomy	7	58.3	1	8.3	3	25.0	1	8.3	0	0	0	0	12
Trisomy	10	25.0	1	0.3	27	67.5	2	5.0	0	0	0	0	40
Triploidy	6	50.0	1	8.3	3	25.0	2	16.7	0	0	0	0	12
Tetraploidy	1	100.0	0	0	0	0	0	0	0	0	0	0	1
Structural rearrangement	0	0	1	14.7	0	0	0	0	0	0	6	85.7	7

From Warburton D, Stein Z, Kline J, et al: Chromosome abnormalities in spontaneous abortion: data from the New York City study. In Porter IH and Hook EB, editors: Human embryonic and fetal death, New York, 1980, Academic Press.

sporadic abnormalities. Thus both members of couples with 2 or more spontaneous abortions should be karyotyped. If translocation is found in 1 parent, about 80% of their pregnancies will abort. If abortion does not occur in a subsequent pregnancy, fetal cytogenic studies are indicated, because there is about a 3% to 5% incidence of unbalanced fetal karyotype in these gestations (Table 15-7).

Using a definition of gestational age as time from onset of the last menstrual period to time of abortion, Kajii et al. reported that the greatest prevalence of chromosomally abnormal abortions (74%) occurred at 9 weeks of gestation, and gradually decreased thereafter. The lower prevalence of abnormal karyotypes occurring in gestations terminating at less than 9 weeks may be artifactual, because the success of karyotyping by culture is less likely if an embryo is not present, and the frequency of empty gestational sacs is greatest in abortions of 8 weeks or less. However, the lower rate may also be the result of the fact that chromosomally abnormal conceptuses may be retained in utero longer than ones destined to abort that are chromosomally normal.

Abortion of chromosomally normal conceptuses is found to occur later in gestation than abortion of chromosomally abnormal ones. The peak incidence of euploid abortion is about 12 to 13 weeks of gestation; the peak incidence of aneuploid abortions is about 11 weeks. Stein et al. reported that the incidence of chromosomally normal abortions increased markedly after a maternal age of 35, rising to more than 30% of clinically recognized conceptions after age 40 (Figure 15-2). Whether this increase in risk of abortion of euploid conceptions is the result of an increase in genetic abnormalities or abnormalities in the maternal environment has not yet been elucidated, but there is an increased incidence of both first- and second-trimester abortions after age 35, and uterine abnormalities generally are a cause of second-trimester abortion (Figure 15-3).

There are many possible causes for abortion of chromosomally normal conceptions. Simpson has postulated that a common, but yet unproven, cause is a genetic abnormality, most probably a mutation, or polygenic factors. He based this assumption on the fact that about 2% of live births have a disorder involving a single gene mutation or polygenic inheritance, whereas only 0.5% of live births have a chromosomal abnormality. Thus, in humans, genetic abnormalities are more common than

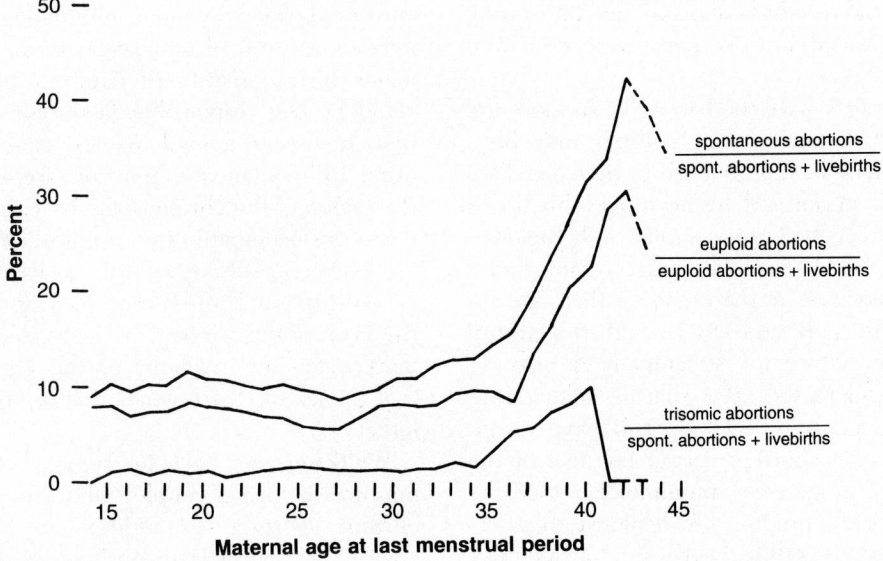

FIGURE 15-2
Estimated rates *(%)* of spontaneous abortion, euploid abortion, and trisomic abortion by maternal age for private and public patients combined. Broken line, denominator less than 25. (From Stein Z, Kline J, Susser E, et al: Maternal age and spontaneous abortion. In Porter IH and Hook EB, editors: Human embryonic and fetal death, New York, 1980, Academic Press.)

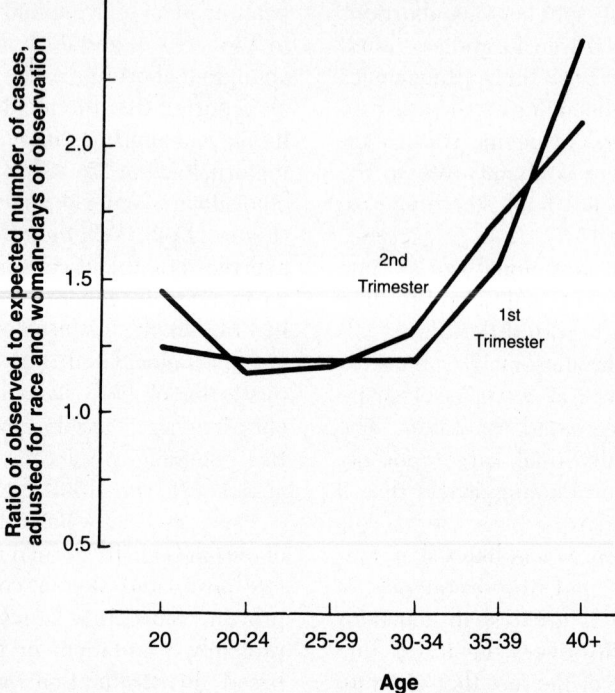

FIGURE 15-3

Spontaneous abortions by age. (From Harlap S, Shiono PH, and Ramcharan S: A life table of spontaneous abortions and the effects of age, parity, and other variables. In Porter IH and Hook EB, editors: Human embryonic and fetal death, New York, 1980, Academic Press.)

chromosomal abnormalities. These genetic disorders could produce abortion by interfering with fetal metabolism or embryonic structural differentiation.

Two reports published in 1985 support the concept that genetic abnormalities may be a cause of spontaneous abortion in humans. Thomas et al. performed histocompatibility locus antigen (HLA) typing in couples with repeated abortion and showed that these couples had a greater frequency of sharing more than one antigen at the A, B, and DR locus than a control population. Other investigators have also reported an increased HLA sharing among couples with recurrent abortion and have postulated that the abortion occurs because of the absence of a maternal immunologic blocking factor normally produced in response to paternal antigens. It is thought that the blocking factor, a circulating IgG antibody, is important in allowing the fetal allograft not to be rejected by the maternal immune system. Thomas et al. and Houwert-de Jong et al. reported that the women who had repeated abortions had a normal maternal lymphocytic immune response to stimulation by paternal lymphocytes. They

therefore concluded that the cause of the recurrent abortions was not immunologic but genetic as a result of homozygosity for recessive major histocompatibility complex genes that could be the responsible factor for the abortion. In several animal species, genes contributing to spontaneous abortion are located in the region of the chromosome that controls the major histocompatibility complex. In humans the histocompatibility complex is located in the HLA locus on chromosome 6. The sharing of the HLA antigens could be just the detectable marker for the segment of the chromosome that carries recessive genes that are potentially lethal.

Weitkamp and Schacter reported that chromosomally normal couples who experience recurrent abortion, in addition to having increased sharing of HLA-A alleles, also have an increased incidence of the transferrin C3 allele and a decreased frequency of the most common transferrin allele, C1. These transferrin alleles are located on chromosome 3. Although transferrin genes have been associated with abortion in several animal species, the effect of transferrin on spontaneous abortion may not be necessarily direct but, as with HLA antigens, could be an effect of genes closely located to the transferrin locus.

Thus these two reports support the concept that the presence of certain recessive genes located on chromosomes 3 and 6 could interfere with normal fetal development and increase the possibility of spontaneous abortion of euploid embryo. Further evidence for a genetic mechanism is the fact that in the gestation after a spontaneous abortion in a primigravida, there is an increased frequency of congenital malformations and perinatal deaths.

Environmental Causes

In contrast to the frequent genetic causes of abortion, maternal or environmental causes are less common. Uterine abnormalities, either congenital or acquired, may not provide the optimal environment for nourishment and survival of the embryo and thus may cause abortion of a genetically normal embryo. Congenital uterine abnormalities can be divided into those brought about by abnormal uterine fusion, those produced by maternal diethylstilbestrol (DES) ingestion, and those caused by abnormal cervical function. The latter condition, the incompetent cervix, can also be acquired after mechanical cervical dilation.

Anomalies of Uterine Development

Anomalies of uterine development are relatively common, with the incidence reported in the literature ranging from about 1:200 to 1:600 women. Overall, about 20% to 25% of women with anomalies of uterine fusion have severe problems with reproduction, recurrent abortion being the most serious. Although it has been stated that the bicornuate and septate uteri are the anomalies most frequently associated with abortion, this belief has arisen from the fact that these anomalies can be corrected surgically and thus are more frequently reported as a cause of abortion before surgical correction. In a study of all 182 women with uterine anomalies detected during an 18-year period at a large Finnish hospital, Heinonen et al. reported that the least common uterine anomaly, the unicornuate uterus, was associated with the greatest incidence of spontaneous abortion, about 50%. This incidence was higher than the 25% to 30% incidence of abortion that occurred in women with either a septate or bi-

cornuate uterus. Buttram and Gibbons also reported that a unicornuate uterus was the uterine developmental anomaly associated with the highest incidence of abortion.

Surgical correction of bicornuate and septate uteri is possible by using one of the transfundal metroplasty techniques described by Strassman, Jones, or Tompkins (Figure 15-4) or by transcervical hysteroscopic resection of the uterine septum. The Strassmann technique of metroplasty is usually used for a bicornuate uterus, whereas the other techniques are used for resection of a uterine septum. In the series of Heinonen et al., about one fifth of the women with bicornuate and septate uteri had a metroplasty performed, and the abortion rate declined from 84% to 12%. Similar results were reported in the series of 43 patients of Rock and Jones and the 21 patients of Musich and Behrman. In both these reports the live birth rate increased from 7% to 8% before metroplasty to 75% to 77% after unification of the uterine cavity. DeCherney et al. reported that of 103 patients with recurrent abortion and a uterine septum, it was possible to perform a hysteroscopic resection in about 70%. Of these patients, 80% had a subsequent successful delivery. In the 30% of patients with a septum greater than 1 cm thick, a metroplasty was not performed.

March and Israel reported that it was possible to incise the septum, even those thicker than 1 cm, of all 82 women with recurrent abortion, using flexible scissors placed transcervically through the hysteroscope. After this treatment the abortion rate declined from 95% to 13%. Because these results are as good as or better than those for an abdominal metroplasty without the need to perform a laparotomy or subsequent cesarean section, hysteroscopic incision should now be the treatment of choice for the septate uterus.

Uterine Anomalies After Diethylstilbestrol (DES)

Comparative studies have shown that women exposed to DES during their fetal life have impaired reproductive function compared with controls. Numerous studies, including the comparative ones of Barnes et al. and Herbst et al., indicate that women exposed to DES who subsequently conceived have a significantly greater incidence of spontaneous abortion than controls (Table 15-8). In 1980

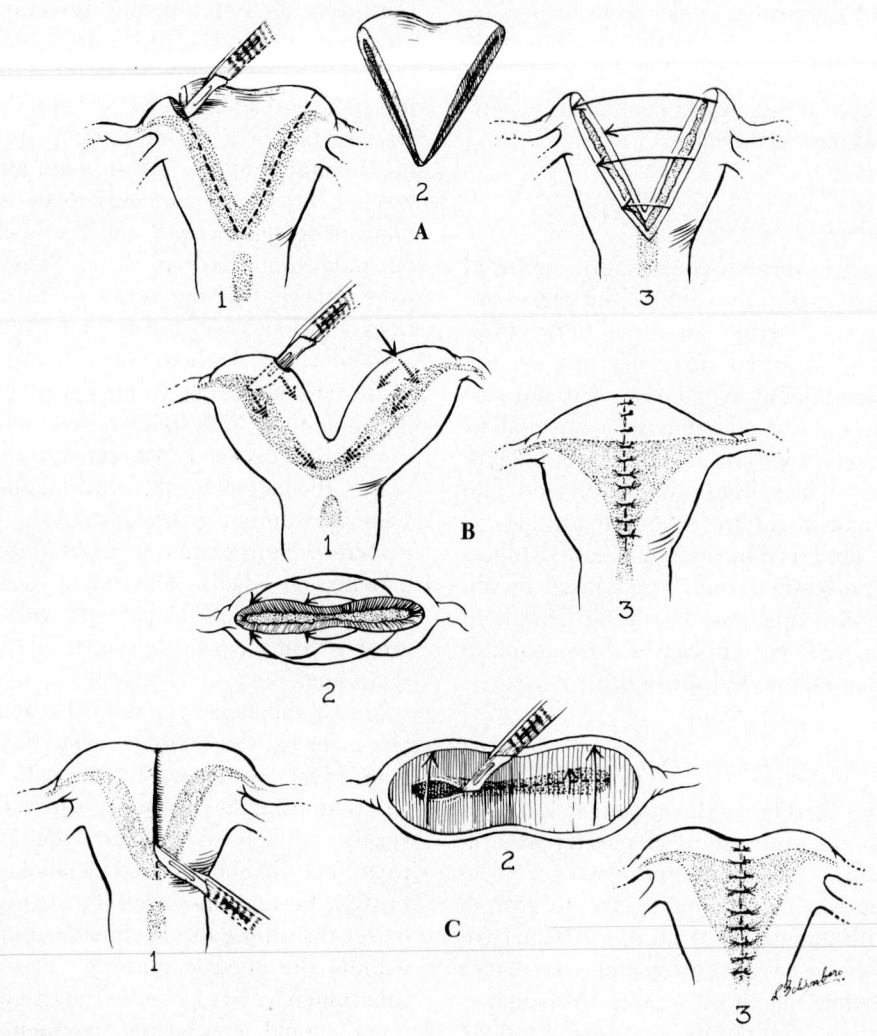

FIGURE 15-4
A, Wedge technique of Jones and Jones. **B,** Transverse fundal incision of Strassmann. **C,** Median bivalving technique of Tompkins. (From Rock JA and Jones HW: Fertil Steril 28:798, 1977. Reproduced with permission of the publisher, The American Fertility Society.)

TABLE 15-8
Numbers and Percentages of Women Exposed to DES and of Control Subjects Who Had Unfavorable Outcomes of Pregnancy, and Relative Risks of Unfavorable Outcomes with DES Exposure

Outcome	Exposed to DES (n = 220)*	Controls (n = 224)*	Relative Risk	P Value	95% Confidence Limits on Relative Risk
Any unfavorable outcome	83 (37.7)	50 (22.3)	1.69	0.001	1.20-2.18
Miscarriage	57 (25.9)	36 (16.1)	1.61	0.008	1.11-2.34
Ectopic pregnancy	8 (3.6)	3 (1.3)	2.77	ns†	0.73-10.46
Premature birth	17 (7.7)	10 (4.5)	1.71	ns	0.80-3.65
Stillbirth	8 (3.6)	3 (1.3)	2.77	ns	0.80-3.65
Never had a full-term live birth	42 (19.1)	11 (4.9)	3.90	0.001	2.06-7.37

From Barnes AB, Colton T, Gundersen J, et al: N Engl J Med 302:609, 1980. Reprinted by permission of The New England Journal of Medicine.
*Figures in parentheses denote percentages in this column.
†Not significant ($P > 0.10$).

Kaufman et al. reported that women exposed to DES who had an abnormal hysterosalpingogram (HSG), mainly a small, T-shaped uterine cavity, had a greater chance of having a spontaneous abortion with a subsequent pregnancy than did DES-exposed women with a normal HSG. However, in a larger series published in 1984 these same investigators reported that the percentage of first or all pregnancies in women exposed to DES that ended in spontaneous abortion was similar regardless of whether their HSG revealed abnormalities in the shape of the cavity or intrauterine defects. Haney et al. reported that the endometrial cavity of women exposed to DES in utero had a significantly smaller surface area than normal, which could perhaps contribute to the increased spontaneous abortion rate in women exposed to DES in utero. No therapy, including routine uterine cerclage, has been shown to be beneficial in lowering the abortion rate in women exposed to DES who have abnormalities of the uterine cavity and recurrent abortion.

Acquired Uterine Defects

LEIOMYOMAS. Leiomyomas are common benign uterine tumors, which are present in about one fourth of women of reproductive age. Uterine leiomyomas, especially if they are submucosal, can be associated with repetitive abortion. Although a causal relationship is difficult to establish, in a review of the literature, Buttram and Reiter reported that when myomectomy was performed for recurrent abortion in a total of 1941 women, the spontaneous abortion rate was reduced from 41% to 19%. These data indicate that, on occasion, uterine leiomyomas are a cause of abortion.

INCOMPETENT CERVIX. Cervical incompetence is characterized by an asymptomatic dilation of the internal cervical os, leading to dilation of the cervical canal and external os during the second trimester of pregnancy. The consequent lack of support of the fetal membranes leads to their spontaneous rupture, which is usually followed by expulsion of the fetus and placenta. The incidence of this problem, which was originally described in 1948, has been estimated to vary from 1 in 57 to 1 in 1730 pregnancies. Mann estimated that about 20% of midtrimester pregnancy losses are caused by cervical incompetence. Although excessive mechanical cervical dilation at the time of dilation and curettage was formerly the most common cause of this problem, since recognition of this syndrome, the use of excessive mechanical cervical dilation is less common. Consequently, as stated in the review by Cousins, the most common cause of cervical incompetence now is a congenital defect in the cervical tissue. The diagnosis of cervical incompetence is best made by a history of second-trimester pregnancy loss accompanied by spontaneous rupture of the fetal membranes without preceding uterine contractions. Cervical incompetence has been found to be associated with uterine anomalies, particularly uterus didelphys, as well as with anomalies produced by fetal DES exposure.

The best treatment of cervical incompetence is placement of a concentric nonabsorbable silk or Mersilene suture at the level of the internal os (cerclage), using either the technique described by Shirodkar or McDonald (Figure 15-5). Because, as reported by Harger, these techniques yield a similar rate of success, with the rate of fetal survival increasing from about 20% before suture placement to 80% after the cerclage procedure, the McDonald procedure is preferable, since this procedure is technically easier and is associated with less morbidity than the Shirodkar technique is. It is recommended that the suture be placed electively between 12 to 14 weeks of gestation after major embryogenesis has been completed and the incidence of spontaneous abortion caused by genetic abnormality has markedly lessened. An ultrasound examination should be performed before cerclage to document a normal gestation. Occasionally if there is a markedly shortened cervix or placement of the McDonald cerclage has failed to maintain the pregnancy, a transabdominal cerclage, as described by Benson and Durfee, should be performed. If the suture is placed externally, it is usually removed at 38 weeks' gestation, and vaginal delivery allowed. However, because of cervical scarring, cesarean section is required in about 15% of pregnancies.

INTRAUTERINE ADHESIONS. Adhesions in the uterine cavity can cause partial or complete obliteration of the endometrium, leading to menstrual abnormalities and amenorrhea, as well as being a cause of abortion. The latter is thought to be the result of insufficient endometrium to support adequate fetal growth. The major cause of adhesions is curettage of the endometrial cavity in association with a pregnancy or in the early puerperium (Table 15-9). In the series of March and Israel the most common antecedent factor was curettage for incomplete abortion. Curettage after a missed abortion or after postpartum hemorrhage had a high incidence of subsequent intrauterine adhesion (IUA) formation. On occasion IUAs develop after a diagnostic curettage, as well as in women with genital tuberculosis. The diagnosis of IUA is usually made by the finding of filling defects

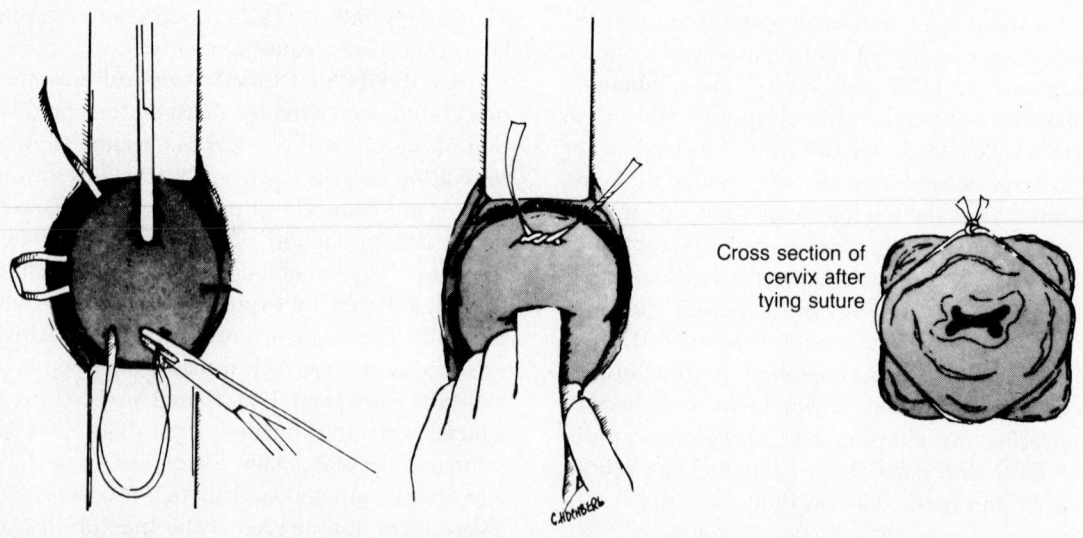

Cross section of
cervix after
tying suture

FIGURE 15-5
Steps in performing McDonald cerclage using Mersilene suture. Index finger is used to ensure closure of internal os. (From March CM: Recurrent abortion. In Mishell DR Jr and Davajan V, editors: Infertility, contraception, and reproductive endocrinology, ed 2, Oradell, NJ, 1986, Medical Economics Books. Reproduced with permission. All rights reserved.)

TABLE 15-9

Definite Causes of IUA in 1856 Cases

	No. of Cases	Percent
Trauma associated with pregnancy		
Curettage after abortion	1237	66.7
Spontaneous	544	
Induced	557	
Unknown	136	
Postpartum curettage	400	21.5
Cesarean section	38	2.0
Evacuation of hydatidi-form mole	11	0.6
Trauma without pregnancy		
Myomectomy	24	1.3
Diagnostic curettage	22	1.2
Cervical manipulation (biopsy, polypectomy, etc.)	10	0.5
Curettage because of menometrorrhagia	8	0.4
Insertion of IUD	3	
Insertion of radium	1	0.3
Without known trauma		
Postpartum; after abortion; others	28	1.5
Genital tuberculosis	74	4.0
TOTAL	1856	100.00

From Schenker JG and Margalioth EJ: Fertil Steril 37:593, 1982. Reproduced with permission of the publisher, The American Fertility Society.

seen at the time of hysterosalpingogram. The defects are typically irregular with sharp contours and homogeneous opacity that persist in a series of films (Figure 15-6). The diagnosis is best confirmed by hysteroscopy.

The recommended treatment for IUA is lysis of the adhesions by miniature scissors during hysteroscopy. After adhesion lysis, either an IUD or small Foley catheter is usually placed in the cavity, and high-dose estrogen (conjugated equine estrogen 2.5 mg bid) is administered for 60 days. Medroxyprogesterone acetate 10 mg per day is added for the last 5 to 10 days, and then the foreign body is removed. March and Israel reported that the abortion rate decreased from 83% to 13% after hysterographic lysis of adhesions. To minimize the chances of development of IUA, curettage of the pregnant or recently pregnant uteri should be gentle and superficial and not extend deep into the mucosa. After curettage for missed abortion or postpartum hemorrhage, consideration should be given to prophylactic high dose estrogen treatment orally for 1 to 2 months to enhance endometrial growth.

Endocrine Causes

Progesterone Deficiency

Maintenance of the endometrium for the first 7 weeks of gestation depends on progesterone produced by the corpus luteum. The function of the latter depends on HCG produced by the trophoblast. When progesterone secretion from the corpus luteum is lower than normal or the endometrium has an inadequate response to normal circulating levels of progesterone, endometrial development may be inadequate to support the implanted blastocyst and may lead to spontaneous abortion. Several investigators have reported that in conception cycles, midluteal peak progesterone levels in the circulation are always greater than 9 ng/ml. Horta et al. measured daily plasma progesterone levels during the luteal phase of a group of normal fertile women, as well as in a group of women whose previous three gestations terminated in spontaneous abortion. In the former group the lowest midluteal peak progesterone level was 9 ng/ml, whereas in the latter group mean progesterone levels reached a peak of 6 ng/ml, significantly lower than the normal fertile group. Hensleigh and Fainstat also reported that five of nine women with recurrent spontaneous abortion had maximum midluteal serum progesterone levels less than 10 ng/ml.

Diagnosis of luteal insufficiency as a cause of infertility has also been made by performing histologic examination of the endometrium and finding a discrepancy of 3 days or more between the expected and actual endometrial dating pattern in at least two menstrual cycles. Several investigators using this method of diagnosis have reported luteal deficiency to occur in as many as one third of women with recurrent abortion, whereas others have reported it to be an uncommon cause of abortion. This discrepancy may have occurred because the precision of endometrial dating by histologic examination varies among different observers.

Several investigators have treated women with recurrent abortion and evidence of luteal deficiency with progesterone vaginal supposito-

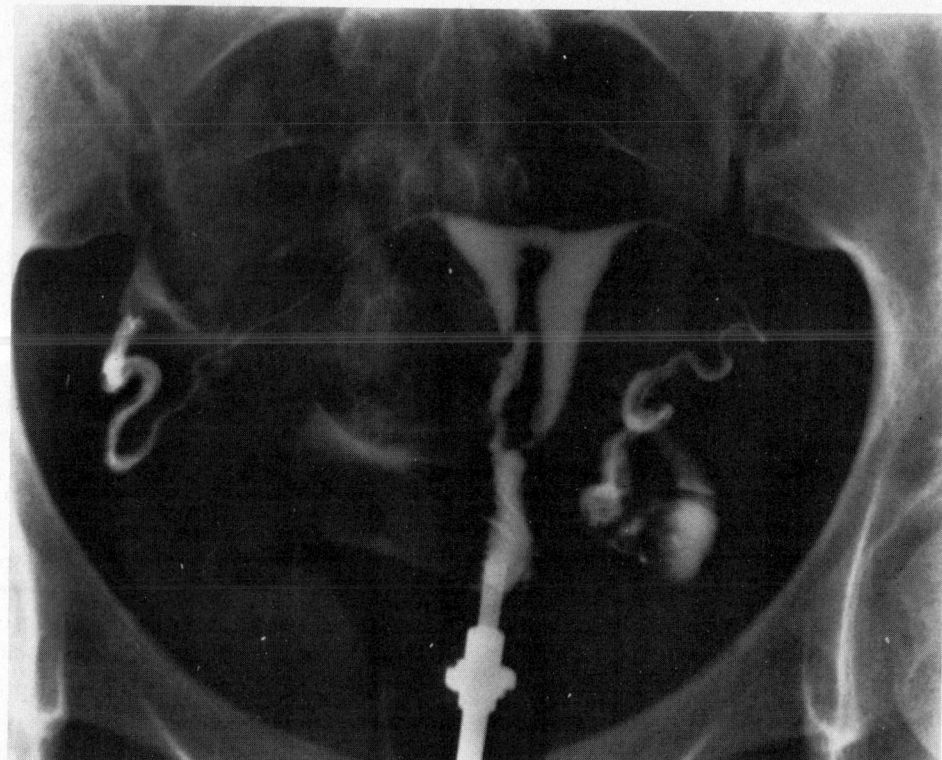

FIGURE 15-6

Endometrial adhesions. The patient was a 23-year-old gravida 5, para 0, spontaneous abortus 4, ectopic 1 (G5 PO SAB4 ECT), with previous left linear salpingostomy, being evaluated for recurrent abortion. Irregular, linear filling defect represents adhesions between anterior and posterior walls of endometrial cavity, extending from internal os to level near fundus. (From Richmond JA: Hysterosalpingography. In Mishell DR Jr and Davajan V, editors: Infertility, contraception, and reproductive endocrinology, ed 2, Oradell NJ, 1986, Medical Economics Books. Reprinted with permission. All rights reserved.)

ries 25 mg twice daily or intramuscular progesterone 12.5 mg/day beginning 3 days after ovulation and continuing throughout the first trimester. With this treatment, term pregnancy rates have been reported to range from 80% to 90%. However, no randomized placebo studies have been reported to verify the effectiveness of progesterone in preventing abortion in women with luteal insufficiency.

There is no evidence that administration of synthetic progestins, which themselves may be luteolytic, are of benefit in reducing the incidence of abortion. There is also no benefit to be derived by initiating progesterone therapy after the expected menstrual period is missed, especially if the women develop symptoms of threatened abortion. Low progesterone levels at this time are a result, not the cause, of the abortion.

Thyroid Disease

Although older studies indicate that hypothyroidism may be a cause of abortion, a study by Montoro et al. reported that no abortions occurred in 11 pregnancies of nine markedly hypothyroid women. In three recent studies of large numbers of women with recurrent abortion, only a few women in one of the studies were found to have abnormal thyroid function.

Stagnaro-Green et al. studied a large group of unselected women in the first trimester of pregnancy with thyroid function tests and assays for thyroid autoantibodies. They found that the spontaneous abortion rate was twice as high, 17% versus 8.4%, among the group of women in whom thyroid autoantibodies were detected. Because only 2 of the 50 women who aborted had significantly abnormal thyroid function, it remains unclear whether the presence of thyroid antibodies (1) is associated with mild subclinical hypothyroidism or (2) reflects a generalized activation of the immune system. This study indicates that the presence of thyroid autoantibodies may be an independent marker for identifying an individual with an increased risk of having an early pregnancy loss. However, there is no definitive evidence that hypothyroidism is a cause of abortion in humans.

Diabetes Mellitus

Although uncontrolled diabetes mellitus has been associated with an increased abortion rate, Crane and Wahl found the incidence of spontaneous abortion was similar in a group of women with either gestational diabetes (12.3%) or frank diabetes (12.2%) and matched control groups (10.9% and 14.5%). In this study the diabetes was controlled with insulin. They also reported that the number of women with multiple spontaneous abortions was similar in the diabetic and control groups. Mills et al. performed a prospective study of insulin-dependent diabetic and non-diabetic women enrolled within 3 weeks of conception. The spontaneous abortion rate in both groups was 16%. However, a small group of diabetic women who were not well controlled and had elevated blood glucose and glycosylated hemoglobulin levels had a significantly increased risk of spontaneous abortion. Thus it appears that diabetes, when controlled by diet or insulin, is not a cause of abortion. However, diabetes without good metabolic control is associated with an increased risk of early pregnancy loss, and a direct correlation exists between the level of hemoglobin A_1 and the rate of abortion.

Immunologic Factors

As mentioned, the foreign antigens produced by the fetus should cause it to be rejected by the mother's immune system. Although some protection from this immunologic effect is offered by progesterone, it has been hypothesized by Rocklin et al. and others that a maternal blocking factor, an IgG antibody, coats the foreign fetal antigens and prevents the fetus from being rejected. These investigators reported that women with recurrent abortion lacked this blocking factor.

Several recent studies could not confirm as a cause of abortion the sharing of major histocompatibility locus antigens (HLA), which, as discussed, may cause the maternal immune system to fail to produce blocking antibodies. Caudle et al. and Houwert-de Jong et al. found no difference in the degree of HLA antigen sharing in couples with recurrent abortion and a control group. Smith and Cowchock likewise found no difference in the incidence of HLA sharing between a group of couples with recurrent spontaneous abortion whose etiology for the condition was determined and another group whose etiology could not be determined. Sargent et al. performed a prospective study of couples with recurrent abortion before and after conception and found no difference in the incidence of HLA sharing among the couples who subsequently had a successful pregnancy and those whose pregnancies aborted. Furthermore, they could not confirm that after pregnancy occurred in these women, as well as in normal controls, there was an increase in production of maternal immunologic factors to fetal (paternal) HLA antigens. However, Mowbray et al. performed a randomized treatment trial in a group of women with recurrent abortion and no detectable antibody against paternal lymphocytes. Women injected with paternal white cells had a significantly greater chance of a subsequent successful pregnancy (78%) than those injected with their own white cells (37%). However, in the study by Smith and Cowchock, after immunization of women with recurrent abortion of unknown etiology with paternal white cells, the rate of successful pregnancy was only 50%, similar to the 62% rate reported by Houwert-de Jong et al., in a group of women with a history of recurrent abortion who received no treatment. Furthermore, in the former study, after immunization the outcome of the pregnancy was not related to the development of blocking antibodies (Table 15-10). Thus the data regarding an immunologic cause of abortion are conflicting, with the majority of the evidence failing to confirm an immunologic etiology. For this reason, at present it is not cost effective or necessary to perform the expensive HLA typing of each member of the couple with a history of recurrent abortion. Immunization of the wife with her husband's white blood cells should be performed only under experimental protocols with informed consent, because the procedure has not been proven to be beneficial.

TABLE 15-10

Pregnancy Outcome with Respect to Development of Lymphocytotoxic Antibody and/or Mixed Lymphocyte Reaction Blocking Factors After Immunization.

| Pregnancy Outcome | Lymphocytotoxic Acetate | | | | Mixed Lymphocyte Reaction Blocking Factors | | | |
| | Neg → Pos | | Neg → Neg | | Neg → Pos | | Neg → Neg | |
	Number	Percentage	Number	Percentage	Number	Percentage	Number	Percentage
Aborted	20/27	74	7/27	26	9/25	36	16/25	64
Delivered	10/21	48	11/21	52	6/18	33	12/18	67

From Smith JB and Cowchock FS: J Reprod Immunol 14:99, 1988.

Lupus Anticoagulant Activity and Antiphospholipid (Anticardiolipin) Antibodies

The presence of lupus anticoagulant activity, as well as elevated levels of certain antiphospholipid antibodies, particularly the anticardiolipin antibody, has been found to be associated with an increased rate of spontaneous abortion and intrauterine fetal death. These antibodies are immunoglobulins of the IgG or IgM class. Although in vitro these immunoglobulins have anticoagulant activity by interfering with activation of the prothrombin activator complex and thus prolonging the partial thromboplastin time, clinically the presence of these antibodies is associated with thrombosis. Although the exact mechanism for an increased incidence of thrombosis is not known, some investigators have shown that when the antibody is present, it inhibits prostacyclin production from endothelial tissues, leading to a relative excess of thromboxane, which could enhance thrombosis. The presence of lupus anticoagulant activity is usually documented by performing an activated partial thromboplastic time (APTT). If the test is prolonged, an equal amount of normal plasma is added to the patient's plasma and the APTT is repeated. If it is still prolonged, the presence of lupus anticoagulant is likely and can be confirmed by correcting the APTT with addition of phospholipid. The antiphospholipid antibodies that are associated with lupus anticoagulant activity bind several phospholipids, including cardiolipin. The majority of patients with lupus anticoagulant activity, but not all, also have anticardiolipin antibodies. The presence of the anticardiolipin antibody, as well as other antiphospholipid antibodies, can be determined by specific solid-phase or enzyme-linked immunoassays.

Deleze et al. reported that about 80% of women with systemic lupus erythromatosus and recurrent fetal loss had antiphospholipid antibodies, whereas they were present in only 15% of women with SLE without fetal loss. These antibodies are found also in women (1) with other immunologic diseases, (2) with subclinical autoimmune disease, and (3) with recurrent abortion, thrombosis, or thrombocytopenia. Several groups have reported that lupus anticoagulant activity is found in about 10% of women with recurrent spontaneous abortion of undetermined etiology, although other investigators report that its prevalence in such women may reach 50%. Anticardiolipin antibody has been reported to occur in 13% to 40% of such individuals. Lockwood et al. reported that the presence of lupus anticoagulant in a normal obstetrical population was only about 0.3%, and about 2% of these women had anticardiolipin antibodies. It thus appears that tests to detect the presence of both lupus anticoagulant activity and anticardiolipin antibody should be performed in individuals with recurrent abortions, since a causal relation apparently exists.

Currently there is no general agreement about therapy for individuals with recurrent abortion and the presence of lupus anticoagulant activity or anticardiolipin antibodies. Different investigators have used corticosteroids, aspirin, heparin, or various combinations of these agents. Corticosteroids suppress the levels of antiphospholipid antibodies, and aspirin inhibits platelet aggregation. According to the recent review by Reece et al., the most widely used therapeutic regimen is daily ingestion of 20 to 60 mg of prednisone with 75 to 80 mg of aspirin. Although the total number of patients treated with this regimen reported in the literature to date is relatively small, (about 100), in their summary Reece et al. found that the overall live birth rate with this therapy was about 80%. Nevertheless, no prospective, randomized, double-blind, placebo controlled trials have been reported to date to document that such therapy is responsible for increasing the live birth rate. Furthermore, serious maternal, as well as fetal, complications have been reported to occur when high-dose corticosteroid therapy is given throughout pregnancy. Therefore such therapy, although shown to be very successful in several small series, must still be regarded as investigational. Precise therapeutic regimens have not been established, but, if used, the least dose of corticosteroid that corrects the APPT should be given, and the dose should be adjusted periodically throughout gestation.

Infections

Numerous infectious agents present in the cervix, uterine cavity, or seminal fluid have been postulated to be etiologic factors for abortion. Although there is evidence that clinical endometritis caused by any infectious agent can produce an abortion, the evidence is unclear as to whether subclinical infections with certain microorganisms or viruses are a cause of spontaneous abortion. The parasite *Toxoplasma gondii* may infect the embryo and cause an abortion. However, it is difficult to document the presence of this organism before abortion because there is a lack of correlation between serologic immunoassays for this organism and its detection in the endometrium by immunofluorescence. Furthermore, Kimball et al. reported that there is a similar incidence of positive immunologic screening tests for this organism in women with a history of none, one, or more than one abortion.

Although *Listeria monocytogenes* produces abortion in several animal species, there is no evidence that it is an abortifacient in women. Rabau and David found no bacteriologic or serologic evidence of *Listeria* infection in 554 women who had aborted, including 74 with recurrent abortions, and Stray-Pedersen et al. were unable to isolate this organism from a group of 48 women with recurrent abortion. *Chlamydia trachomatis* is a common sexually transmitted pathogen, but there is no evidence that it causes abortion in asymptomatic women.

Infection with herpes simplex virus in the genital tract has been reported to cause abortion. Nahmias et al. reported that if genital herpes initially occurs in the first half of pregnancy, the abortion rate is about 34%. Naib et al. reported that if pregnancy occurs within 18 months after initial detection of herpes infection, the abortion rate was 55%. Both these rates were significantly higher than the 11.5% abortion rate in the control population.

Several authors have suggested that T strain mycoplasma, both *Ureaplasma urealyticum* and *Mycoplasma hominis*, can cause abortion. Data indicating the first organism as a cause of abortion are stronger than for the latter. Stray-Pedersen et al. found that although the incidence of cervical colonization of *U. urealyticum* was similar in a group of women with recurrent abortion and controls, the incidence of endometrial colonization was significantly more common (28%) in the group with recurrent abortions than in the control group (7%). In this study the cultures were obtained at least 6 months after the last abortion, and there were no clinical or laboratory signs of infection in any of the women. These investigators could not correlate the presence of *M. hominis* in the uterus with an increased frequency of abortion.

Stray-Pedersen and Stray-Pedersen reported that eradication of *U. urealyticum* in the endometrium by tetracyline treatment for 10 days resulted in a significantly lower subsequent abortion rate (19%). However, there are no randomized placebo controlled treatment studies to prove that these organisms cause abortion and that treatment is effective.

Environmental Factors

Smoking

In a retrospective study Kline et al. reported that women who smoked during pregnancy had a significantly greater chance of having a spontaneous abortion than did a control group (Table 15-11). For women who smoked more than 14 cigarettes per day the risk of having an abortion was 1.7 times greater than for women who did not smoke, but smoking less than this did not result in a significantly greater incidence of abortion. These investigators found that heavy smokers had an increased risk of aborting chromosomally normal embryos only. There was no increased risk of an aneuploid abortion in smokers. These data indicate that smoking acts as a toxic agent to destroy chromosomally normal fetuses.

TABLE 15-11

Frequency (%) of Smoking Among Women Experiencing Spontaneous Abortions (Cases) and Women Delivering at 28 Weeks' Gestation or Later (Controls)

No. of Cigarettes per Day	% Distribution		Adjusted Odds Ratio	95% Confidence Interval
	Cases	Controls		
None	62.0	69.8	1.00	—
1-13	20.5 ⎫ 37.9	20.0 ⎫ 30.2	1.07 ⎫ 1.28	.80-1.42
14-80	17.4 ⎭	10.2 ⎭	1.73 ⎭	1.23-2.43
TOTAL	648	645		

From Kline J, Stein Z, Susser M, et al: Environmental influences on early reproductive loss in a current New York City study. In Porter IH and Hook EB, editors: Human embryonic and fetal death, New York, 1980, Academic Press.

TABLE 15-12

Frequency (%) of Alcohol Consumption among Women Experiencing Spontaneous Abortions (Cases) and Women Delivering at 28 Weeks' Gestation or Later (Controls)

Frequency of Alcohol Consumption During Pregnancy	% Distribution		Adjusted Odds Ratio	95% Confidence Interval
	Cases	Controls		
Never	42.6	43.7	1.00	
Twice a month and less	28.9	38.0	.77	.59-.99
Less than twice a month	10.8	10.4	1.04	.71-1.52
2 to 6 days a week	13.3 ⎫ 17.9	6.5 ⎫ 7.9	1.96 ⎫ 2.36	1.30-2.95
Daily	4.5 ⎭	1.4 ⎭	3.00 ⎭	1.39-6.49
TOTAL	648	645		

From Kline J, Stein Z, Susser M, et al: Environmental influences on early reproductive loss in a current New York City study. In Porter IH and Hook EB, editors: Human embryonic and fetal death, New York, 1980, Academic Press.

Alcohol

Kline et al. also reported that drinking alcohol, acting independently from smoking, was a risk factor for abortion (Table 15-12). Women who drank alcohol at least 2 days a week had about a two fold greater risk of having an abortion than women who did not drink during pregnancy, with the risk increasing to threefold with daily ingestions of alcohol. As with smoking, an increased risk of abortion was confined to chromosomally normal embryos, indicating that drinking alcohol, like smoking, can act as a toxic agent on the normal embryo to cause its death. Harlap and Shiono found that even moderate drinking of alcohol increased the risk of second, but not first, trimester pregnancy loss, confirming the toxic effect of alcohol on the embryo.

Irradiation

Animal studies have shown that ionizing radiation can produce congenital malformation, growth retardation, and embryonic death. These effects are dose related, and there is a threshold dose below which an adverse effect does not occur. Although there is evidence in the human that high-energy radiation exposure is associated with teratogenic effects and growth retardation, there is no conclusive evidence that similar exposure increases the risk of spontaneous abortion.

Extrapolation from animal data indicates that the embryo is most sensitive to the lethal effect of irradiation during the day of implantation and a few days later (Table 15-13). The sensitivity decreases during the period of early embryogenesis, after which the minimum lethal

TABLE 15-13

Estimation of Abortigenic Hazards of
X-Irradiation to Human Embryo from Animal
Experiments

Stage of Human Gestation (Days)	Lethal Dose/50 (Rads)	MLD (Rads)
1	70-100	10
14	140	25
18	150	25
28	220	50
50	260	50
Late fetus to term	300-400	50

From Brent RL: Radiation-induced embryonic and fetal loss from conception to birth. In Porter IH and Hook EB, editors: Human embryonic and fetal death, New York, 1980, Academic Press.

TABLE 15-14

Causes of Vaginal Bleeding Before Twentieth
Week of Pregnancy

Final Diagnosis	No. of Patients	Percentage
Threatened abortion	211	13.6
Inevitable and incomplete abortion	951	61.4
Complete abortion	203	13.1
Septic abortion	67	4.3
Missed abortion	27	1.7
Benign hydatidiform mole	12	0.8
Tubal pregnancy	78	5.1
TOTAL	1549	

From Cavanagh D, Fleisher A, and Ferguson JH: Am J Obstet Gynecol 90:216, 1964.

dose (MLD) remains constant to term gestation. Brent reported that the MLD of irradiation to rats is 5 rads on the day of implantation. These data thus indicate that there is little likelihood that irradiation of less than 5 rads (severalfold greater than the amount used in nearly all diagnostic procedures) will cause an abortion in the human, even if it is administered during the time of implantation.

Environmental Toxins

Little valid information exists concerning the effect of environmental toxins on human abortion. Although some studies have shown an increased risk of abortion among female anesthesiologists, other studies have not found such an effect. Most studies reporting such a relation are retrospective questionnaire studies of marginal validity. A well-done case control study by Axelsson et al. indicated that the incidence of abortion in women exposed to anesthetic gases was not significantly increased.

Information concerning a possible abortifacient effect after increased exposure to other environmental toxins is even less clear. Vianna reported that the entire population of women exposed to toxic chemical wastes in the Love Canal area had no significant excess of spontaneous abortions, although groups of women living in certain areas with a higher exposure may have had an increased risk of abortion.

DIAGNOSIS

Threatened Abortion

It has been estimated that bleeding occurs during the first 20 weeks of pregnancy in about 30% to 40% of human gestations, with about half of these pregnancies ending in spontaneous abortion. The risk of abortion is greater among those women who bleed for 3 or more days (24%) than among those who bleed only 1 or 2 days (7%). There is no evidence that women with gestational bleeding who do not abort have an increased incidence of complications of pregnancy, but they may have a slightly increased incidence of fetal anomalies and preterm birth. To determine the prognosis of the pregnancy in a woman with threatened abortion, ultrasonography, endocrinologic studies, and a combination of both techniques have been used.

The refinement of sonographic technology and the development of the vaginal probe have made it possible for a high-frequency transducer crystal to be placed in the probe in close proximity to the uterus. The images produced by this technique have much greater resolution that those obtained by the transabdominal transducer. With the use of abdominal ultrasonography, Kadar et al. reported that a gestational sac should be seen when the serum HCG level was greater than 6500 mIU/ml. However, with improved technology and use of the vaginal probe, it is now possible to always detect a gestational sac in a normal pregnancy

TABLE 15-15

Relationship of Gestational Age, HCG Levels, and Transvaginal Ultrasound Findings

Ultrasound findings	Days from LMP	β-HCG mIU/ml	
		1st International Reference Preparation (1st IRP)	2nd International Standard (IS)
Sac	34.8 ± 2.2	1398 ± 155	914 ± 106
Fetal pole	40.3 ± 3.4*	113 ± 298*	3783 ± 683
Fetal heart motion	46.9 ± 6.0*	17208 ± 3772*	13178 ± 2898*

From Fossum GT et al: Fertil Steril 49:788, 1988.
*P <0.05 when compared with sac

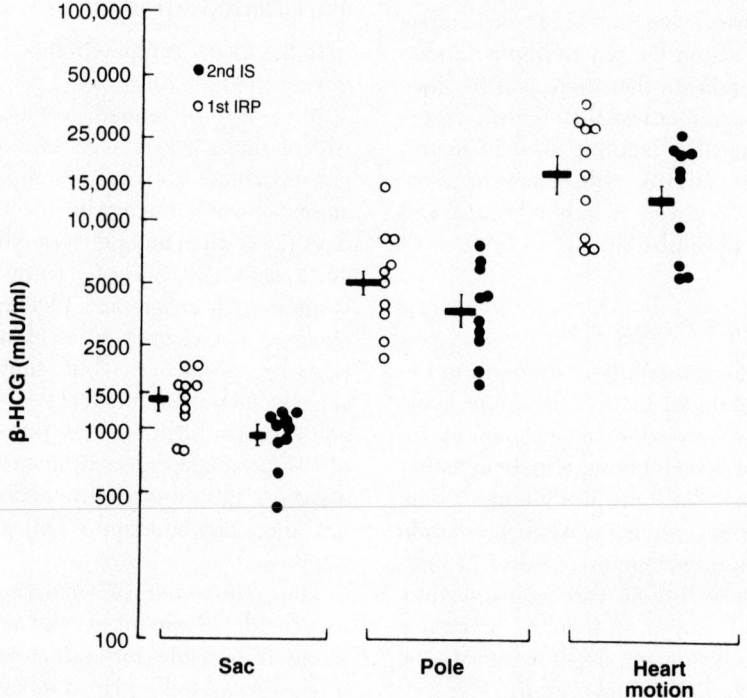

FIGURE 15-7

Relationship between transvaginal ultrasound findings and serum HCG levels (range and mean ± SEM) using two WHO standards: 1st International Reference Preparation (1st IRP) and 2nd International Standard (2nd IS). (From Fossum GT et al: Fertil Steril 49:788, 1988.)

when the HCG level is much lower. Fossum et al. studied a group of women with normal gestations with transvaginal ultrasonography beginning 26 to 36 days after the onset of menses. The mean gestational duration for initial appearance of the fetal sac was 40 days. Fetal heart activity initially appeared at a mean of 47 days after the onset of menses (Table 15-15). A gestational sac was always visualized if the serum HCG was more than 2100 mIU/ml (1st International Reference Preparation [1st IRP]) (Figure 15-7). Cacciatore et al. in a more recent study of similar design reported that a gestational sac was always present when the HCG was more than 1000 mIU/ml 33 days after the last menses. However, it requires great experience to differentiate a true from a false gestational sac at this stage of gestation.

In addition to facilitating visualization of gestational structures much sooner after conception, use of vaginal sonography has also enabled the etiology and prognosis of the symptom of threatened abortion to be established with greater accuracy than had previously been possible with transabdominal ultrasonography. The diagnosis of intrauterine death or anembryonic gestation can be easily established and the contents of the uterus promptly evacuated, avoiding the occurrence of missed abortion. There have been several reports of ultrasonographic studies of groups of women with threatened abortion by Jouppila, Mantoni, and Cashner. About two thirds of such pregnancies have a live fetus present, and about 85% of these fetuses subsequently deliver and survive. The incidence of low birth weight or preterm birth in such pregnancies was increased in one series and not in another. The remaining 15% of the pregnancies abort, usually in the second trimester. Of the one third of women with a threatened abortion who do not have a live fetus present, about half have an anembryonic gestation with the remainder being about equally divided between fetal death and incomplete abortion, with an occasional molar gestation.

Inevitable, Incomplete, and Complete Abortions

In a patient bleeding during the first half of pregnancy the diagnosis of inevitable abortion is strengthened if the bleeding is profuse and associated with uterine cramping pains. Women with threatened abortion who do not abort usually do not have cramps. When bleeding or pain in the first half of pregnancy is severe enough to require hospitalization, the most likely diagnosis is inevitable or incomplete abortion, occurring in more than 60% of women who are hospitalized for vaginal bleeding in the first half of pregnancy (Table 15-14). The diagnosis can be confirmed by examination of the cervical os. If cervical dilation has occurred with or without rupture of membranes, the abortion is inevitable. If only a portion of the products of conception have been expelled and the cervix remains dilated, a diagnosis of incomplete abortion is made. However, if all fetal and placental tissue has been expelled, the cervix is closed, bleeding from the canal is minimal or decreasing, and uterine cramps have ceased, a diagnosis of complete abortion can be made. A complete abortion usually occurs *before* 6 weeks' and *after* 14 weeks' gestation. Abortions occurring *between* 6 weeks' and 14 weeks' gestation are usually incomplete and may be accompanied by profuse uterine bleeding.

Missed Abortion

The diagnosis of missed abortion is suspected clinically when the uterus fails to continue to enlarge with or without uterine bleeding or spotting. Typically after an episode of bleeding subsides, a continuous brown vaginal discharge is noted. When a dead fetus is retained in the uterus beyond 5 weeks after fetal death, consumptive coagulability with resultant hypofibrogenemia may occur. The incidence of this condition is correlated with both the length of gestation and the duration of fetal death: it is uncommon in gestations of less than 14 weeks' duration or duration of fetal death less than 6 weeks. As recently stated by Pridjian and Moawad, with the use of ultrasonography the term *missed abortion* is no longer relevant because the diagnosis of anembryonic gestation or fetal death can be easily determined without delay. The uterus can then be promptly evacuated, avoiding the possibility of the adverse consequences associated with prolonged retention of necrotic fetal tissue.

Septic Abortion

Infection occurs in about 1% to 2% of all spontaneous abortions, with the incidence increasing if the abortion has been induced by a nonsterilized instrument. Any patient with uterine bleeding or spotting during the first half of pregnancy accompanied by clinical signs of infection must be considered to have a septic abortion if no obvious source of infection outside the genital tract is evident.

Septic abortions can be threatened, inevitable, or incomplete. The infection frequently spreads from the endometrium through the myometrium to the parametrium and sometimes to the peritoneum. Thus in addition to endometritis, parametritis and peritonitis frequently occur in women with septic abortions. In addition to an elevated temperature and leukocytosis, lower abdominal tenderness, cervical motion tenderness, and a foul uterine discharge are signs of septic abortion. The cause of the infection is usually polymicrobial, with *Escherichia coli* and other aerobic gram-negative rods frequently involved. Group B betahemolytic streptococci, anaerobic streptococci, *Bacteroides* species, and on occasion *Clostridium perfringens* are other organisms that can cause septic abortion. Because endotoxins can be released from the gram-negative bacilli, endotoxic shock may accompany septic abortion, particularly if it is caused by insertion of nonsterile agents into the uterine cavity.

TREATMENT

Threatened Abortion

Although some physicians recommend that patients with threatened abortion restrict their physical activities or stay at bed rest, there is no evidence that these measures or any active medical therapy improves the prognosis of threatened abortion. Treatment with natural progesterone or synthetic progestins was previously advocated, but there is no evidence that such therapy improves the prognosis. Because such treatment may increase the probability of having a missed abortion, the use of this or any type of hormonal therapy is contraindicated. Nevertheless, staying at home with restriction of physical activities and avoidance of coitus is usually advised until the bleeding ceases. If bleeding increases, especially if it is accompanied by uterine cramps, it is likely that the abortion is becoming inevitable and the patient should be examined in a medical facility. Serial HCG measurements and uterine sonography aid in predicting the outcome. If ultrasonography reveals the presence of an anembryonic

gestation or intrauterine fetal death, it is probably best to evacuate the uterine contents medically with an oxytocic agent or surgically with curettage, depending on the stage of gestation.

Inevitable and Incomplete Abortion

Most abortions that occur between 8 and 14 weeks of pregnancy are incomplete and require surgical evacuation. This procedure can usually be accomplished on an outpatient basis in a hospital or surgical outpatient facility, since bleeding may be profuse and it may be necessary to administer a blood transfusion. Women with an incomplete abortion who do not develop sepsis or hypotension can usually be treated in the emergency room. After measurement of vital signs and placement of an intravenous line with an 18-gauge needle, blood is drawn for a complete blood count, as well as typing and cross matching for possible transfusion. An infusion of 10 to 30 units of oxytocin in 1000 ml of 5% Ringer's lactate is advocated, and an intramuscular analgesic (meperidine 75 mg and diazepam [Valium] 5 mg) is given, followed by placement of a paracervical block at 3 and 9 o'clock with 10 ml of 1% lidocaine (Xylocaine). Approximately 5 to 10 minutes later the uterine contents are evacuated with sponge forceps, and the cavity is curetted gently with a sharp curette. Deep curettage should be avoided to prevent the subsequent development of uterine synechiae. After the procedure the patient's vital signs and amount of vaginal bleeding should be monitored for 4 to 8 hours, after which the patient may be discharged home to remain at bed rest for 24 hours and avoid intercourse for 2 weeks. Oral ergonovine maleate 0.2 mg is administered every 4 to 6 hours for 1 to 2 days. In addition, iron sulfate 200 mg should be administered orally three times a day until hemoglobin levels return to normal and tissue iron stores are replenished. If the mother is Rh negative and the father Rh positive, 50 µg anti-D gamma globulin should be administered intramuscularly. Numerous investigations, including the large series reported by Decenzo and Cavanagh, have shown this management approach to have good results.

Women with a complete abortion, usually before 8 weeks' gestation, need not be hospitalized but can be treated as outpatients with administration of ergonovine maleate as described. However, if patients are already in the hospital and are thought to spontaneously pass all the products of conception, a curettage should be performed as described to be certain that the abortion is not incomplete.

Septic Abortion

Septic abortion is a potentially fatal condition with an estimated fatality rate of 0.4 to 0.6 per 100,000 spontaneous abortions. In the United States between 1975 and 1977, Grimes, et al. reported that 41 women died after having a spontaneous abortion; 15 (37%) of these deaths were the result of sepsis. All patients with the diagnosis of septic abortion should have a complete blood count, urinalysis, chemistry, and electrolyte panel obtained. In addition, a specimen of the uterine discharge should be sent to the laboratory for culture and sensitivity. A Gram stain of the discharge should be performed in the admitting area. If the patient is seriously ill, blood cultures, a chest x-ray examination, and tests of blood coagulability should be obtained. Antibiotics should be administered intravenously and the uterine contents evacuated. It is best to use combination antibiotic therapy including an agent that will be effective against anaerobic bacteria. After adequate blood levels of antibiotics are obtained, usually within 2 hours, the uterus should be evacuated as described previously.

If the uterus is larger than 14 weeks gestation and the cervix is closed (threatened septic abortion), management is more difficult. The uterine cavity needs to be evacuated to provide drainage of the infected material. This can be performed either by curettage, dilation and evacuation, oxytocics, or prostaglandins. Sometimes it is necessary to perform a hysterectomy if the sepsis is severe and the uterus cannot be evacuated through the cervical canal. All patients with septic abortions need to have close monitoring of vital signs and urinary output. If signs of septic shock should develop, a central venous pressure catheter should be placed and additional intravenous fluids administered. Additional therapeutic agents, such as nasal oxygen, vasopressor agents, digitalis, and corticosteroids, may also be used.

Recurrent Abortion

The expected probability of a woman's having three consecutive spontaneous abortions is about 0.3% to 0.4%, but the actual incidence is reported to range from 0.4% to 0.8%, indicating that there is a specific cause for recurrent pregnancy loss in some women.

The abortuses of women who have three or more abortions are more likely to be chromosomally normal (80% to 90%) than those of women with a single spontaneous abortion. Women with recurrent abortions also have a tendency to abort later in gestation, with two thirds of such abortions occurring beyond 12 weeks' gestation, indicating that maternal or environmental factors are a more likely cause of repeated pregnancy loss. Recurrent abortion is also called *habitual abortion*, but this term implies that every pregnancy will end in an abortion. As stated, if a woman has had no live births and three abortions, she has about a 50% chance of having a term gestation in her next pregnancy, and if she has had one live birth, this chance is increased to about 70%. Thus the term habitual abortion should not be used.

Couples with recurrent abortion require careful, sympathetic management by the practitioner, because an abortion is an emotionally traumatic experience that can result in as much grief as intrauterine fetal death in late pregnancy or a neonatal death. With recurrent abortion this emotional trauma is magnified, and the practitioner needs to express sympathy and understanding as counseling is performed and a diagnostic regimen is outlined.

Because the etiology of a second-trimester loss is more likely to be uterine in origin and thus more likely to be able to be diagnosed, a diagnostic evaluation should be performed after a woman has had only one second-trimester spontaneous abortion. There is no need to wait for a woman to have three first-trimester abortions with their accompanying emotional trauma before beginning a diagnostic evaluation. Because one early abortion is relatively common, it is recommended that diagnostic evaluation be initiated only after a woman has two first-trimester abortions.

After a history and physical examination are performed with pertinent questions regarding cervical incompetence, a complete blood count, a serum TSH, and a midluteal serum progesterone measurement should be obtained. A hysterogram should be performed to rule out congenital uterine anomalies, submucous leiomyomas, and intrauterine adhesions. If no abnormalities are found, a karyotype of the husband and wife should be performed to determine if some chromosomal anomaly, such

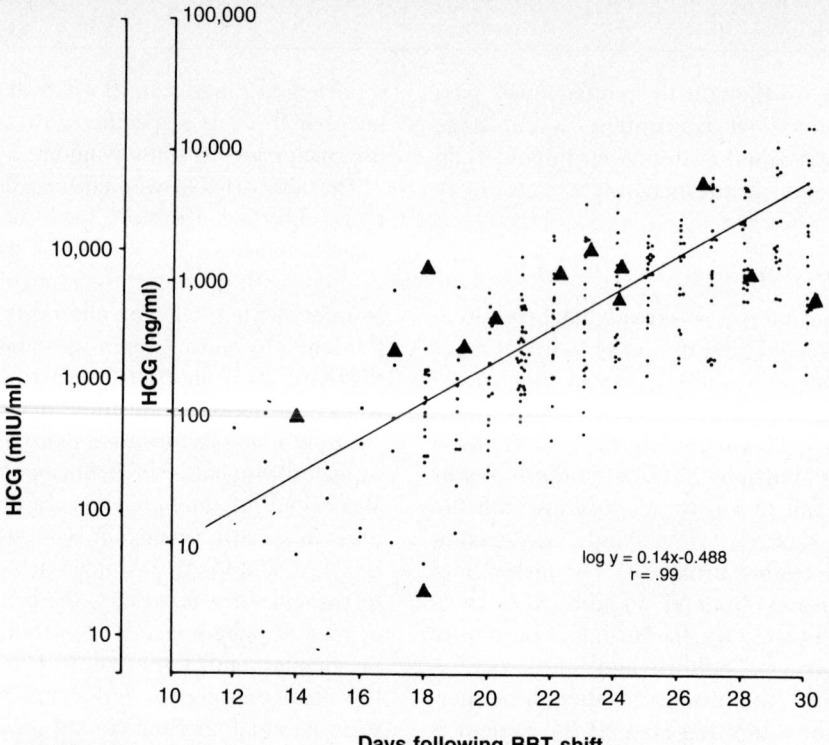

FIGURE 15-8

β-HCG RIA values during first 30 days of successful pregnancies. Each point represents concentration of HCG on specific day from 189 successful pregnancies. ▲, twin gestation. Line represents linear regression of means of data taken by days (5.7 mIU; 1 ng). (From Batzer FR, Schlaff S, Goldfarb AF, et al: Fertil Steril 35:307, 1981. Reproduced with permission of the publisher, The American Fertility Society.)

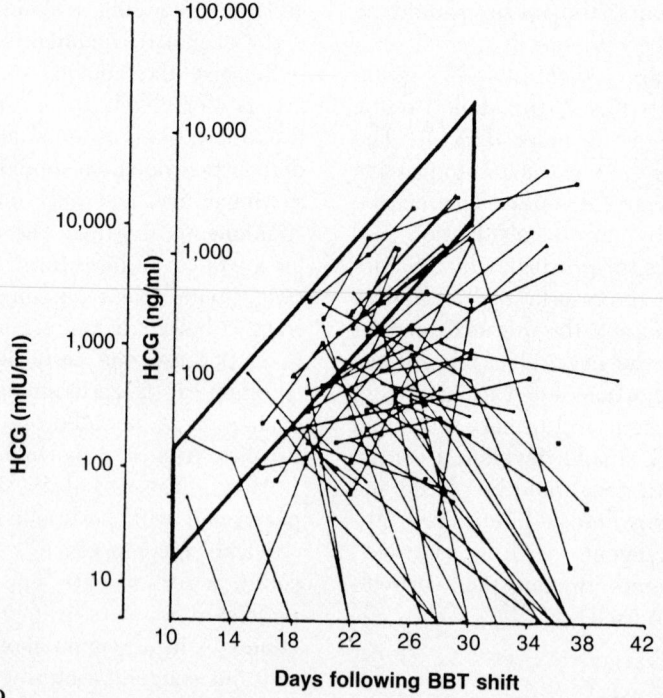

FIGURE 15-9

Serial β-HCG RIA values in 53 patients who aborted spontaneously. Twenty-six patients had a negative slope. Five patients with a normal slope aborted in second trimester. Solid line encloses 95% confidence limits in successful pregnancies. (From Batzer FR, Schlaff S, Goldfarb AF, et al: Fertil Steril 35:307, 1981. Reproduced with permission of the publisher, The American Fertility Society.)

as balanced translocation or 45,X mosaicism, exists. The value of obtaining endometrial bacteriologic cultures and HLA typing of husband and wife is controversial and does not appear to be cost effective. Tests to detect lupus anticoagulant activity and antiphospholipid antibodies should be performed.

If any of these tests reveals an abnormality that can be corrected with appropriate surgical or medical therapy as described, such therapy should be initiated. If a chromosomal abnormality is found, genetic counseling is indicated. There have been three series of large numbers of couples with recurrent abortion who have undergone a comprehensive diagnostic evaluation (Table 15-16). Although different criteria for abnormal diagnostic tests were used by each group of investigators, no specific etiologic factor for the recurrent abortion (all tests normal) was found in 35% to 44% of the couples studied.

If no diagnosis can be obtained, the couple should be counseled regarding the probability of abortion in a subsequent pregnancy. After conception, measurement of HCG levels twice weekly will allow early prognosis of the outcome of the pregnancy. In normal gestations the levels of HCG double about every 2 days, and the rate of increase in a particular patient can be compared with the expected normal rate of increase (Figure 15-8). In most individuals with an early abortion, levels of HCG will rise at a slower rate than normal, plateau, and then decline (Figure 15-9). Batzer et al. found that when β-HCG doubling time in the first month of gestation was normal, it predicted a good outcome 88% of the time, and when abnormal, predicted a poor outcome 76% of the time. If HCG levels are increasing normally, an ultrasound examination should be performed after they reach 2500 mIU/ml, at which time a gestational sac should be found. A repeat ultrasound 2 weeks later should demonstrate a normal fetal heart rate. These findings

are reassuring, both to the mother and to the clinician.

Some individuals recommend that prophylactic antibiotic treatment be given to the husband and wife in the conception cycle or that progesterone supplementation be given to all women with recurrent abortion in the first trimester of pregnancy. Neither of these modalities has been demonstrated to improve the outcome of the pregnancy.

TABLE 15-16

Identification of Etiologic Factors in 195 Couples According to Prior Obstetric History

Etiologic Factor	Total	
	Number	Percentage
Uterine body abnormalities	30	15.4
Müllerian fusion anomaly	19	
Fixed retroversion	5	
Uterine fibroids	4	
Synechiae	2	
Cervical incompetence	25	12.8
Endocrine dysfunction	10	5.1
Luteal insufficiency	6	
Thyroid dysfunction	4	
Endometrial infection	29	14.9
U. urealyticum	22	
T. gondii	7	
Chromosomal abnormalities	5	2.6
Systemic disorders (ulcerative colitis)	2	1.0
Sperm factors	8	4.1
Excessive smoking	1	0.5
Total "known etiology"	110	56.4
"Unknown etiology"	85	43.6
TOTAL	195	100

From Stray-Pedersen B and Stray-Pedersen S: Am J Obstet Gynecol 148:140, 1984.

_____ KEY POINTS _____

- About 15% to 20% of all human pregnancies terminate in clinically recognized abortion.

- In the human the total embryonic loss before 12 weeks' gestation is about 30%.

- About 80% of abortions occur in the first trimester, with the incidence decreasing with increasing gestational age.

- If a fetus is viable, as observed ultrasonographically, in women less than 12 weeks' gestational age, the subsequent fetal loss is between 2% and 3%.

- The risk of a pregnancy terminating in spontaneous abortion increases independently with increasing parity, maternal age, and paternal age.

- Women with multiple abortions have a tendency to abort at about the same gestational age.

- For a woman with a reproductive history of three prior pregnancies terminating in abortion with no live births, her chance of having an abortion in a subsequent pregnancy is about 50%; if she has had at least one live birth and three spontaneous abortions, the chance that her next pregnancy will terminate in abortion is only about 30%.

- The major cause of abortion is genetic, and the incidence of chromosomal anomalies in abortuses is about 50%.

- Only about 5% of the abnormal karyotypes of abortuses are structural abnormalities of the chromosomes, such as translocation.

- Autosomal trisomy is the most common abnormal karyotype (50%), followed in decreasing frequency by monosomy 45,X (20%), triploidy (15%), tetraploidy (10%), and structural abnormalities (5%).

- The most common single chromosomal abnormality is monosomy 45,X.

- It is not cost effective or necessary to perform HLA typing of each member of the couple that has recurrent abortion.

- Lupus anticoagulant activity is found in about 10% of women with recurrent spontaneous abortion of undetermined etiology.

- Karyotypes of abortuses of women who have had more than one abortion tend to be similar if the first abortus had either a normal karyotype or an autosomal trisomy.

- Maternal age is directly related to the incidence of trisomic abortions.

- Monosomy 45,X abortion is associated with a younger maternal age than other aneuploid or euploid abortions.

- Abortion of chromosomally normal conceptuses is found to occur later in gestation than abortion of chromosomally abnormal conceptuses does, with the peak incidence of euploid abortion being about 12 to 13 weeks of gestation; the peak incidence of aneuploid abortions is about 11 weeks.

- The incidence of chromosomally normal abortions increases markedly after a maternal age of 35, rising to more than 30% of clinically recognized conceptions after age 40.

- About 20% to 25% of women with anomalies of uterine fusion have severe problems with reproduction, with recurrent abortion being the most serious.

- The least common uterine anomaly, the unicornuate uterus, is associated with the greatest incidence of spontaneous abortion, about 50%.

- Women with either a septate or bicornuate uterus have a 25% to 30% incidence of spontaneous abortion.

- Women with recurrent abortion as a result of bicornuate and septate uteri have a decline in the abortion rate from about 88% to 15% after surgical correction.

- Women exposed to DES who subsequently conceive have a significantly greater incidence of spontaneous abortion than controls do.

- In women with an incompetent cervix the rate of fetal survival increases from about 20% to 80% after cerclage.

- Spontaneous and induced abortions cause about two thirds of intrauterine adhesions.

- Diabetes, if controlled by diet or insulin, is not a cause of abortion, whereas if uncontrolled, it is a cause.

- In women who smoke more than 14 cigarettes per day the risk of having an abortion is 1.7 times greater than in women who do not smoke.

- Smoking and drinking alcohol introduce toxic agents that can destroy chromosomally normal fetuses.

- Women who drink alcohol at least 2 days a week have about a twofold greater risk of having an abortion.

- Irradiation of less than 5 rads will not cause an abortion in the human.

- Threatened abortion occurs in about 30% to 40% of human gestations, with only about half of these pregnancies ending in spontaneous abortion.

- The prevalence of major chromosomal abnormalities present in either partner of a couple with 2 or more pregnancy losses is about 3%, 5 to 6 times higher than in the general population. Abnormalities occur in the female parent about twice as frequently as the male, with balanced reciprocal translocations occurring in half of these individuals.

- The most widely used therapeutic regimen to treat lupus anticoagulant activity in women with recurrent abortion is 20 to 60 mg of prednisone with 75 to 80 mg of aspirin per day.

- Complete abortion usually occurs *before* 6 weeks' and *after* 14 weeks' gestation. Abortions occurring *between* 6 weeks' and 14 weeks' gestation are usually incomplete.

- When a dead fetus is retained in the uterus beyond 5 weeks after fetal death, consumptive coagulability with resultant hypofibrogenemia may occur.

- About 1% to 2% of all spontaneous abortions become infected.

- The expected probability of a woman's having three consecutive abortions is about 0.3% to 0.4%, but the actual incidence is reported to range from 0.4% to 0.8%.

- The abortuses of women who have three or more abortions are more likely to be chromosomally normal (80% to 90%) than those of women with a single spontaneous abortion.

- Women with recurrent abortions also have a tendency to abort later in gestation, with two thirds of such abortions occurring beyond 12 weeks' gestation, indicating that maternal or environmental factors are a more likely cause of repeated pregnancy loss.

- A diagnostic evaluation should be performed after a woman has had only one second-trimester spontaneous abortion or two first-trimester abortions.

- In most individuals with an early abortion, levels of HCG will rise at a slower rate than normal, plateau, and then decline.

BIBLIOGRAPHY

Austin CR: Pregnancy losses and birth defects. In Austin CR and Short RV, editors: Reproduction in mammals, vol 2, London, 1972, Cambridge University Press.

Axelsson G and Rylander R: Exposure to anaesthetic gases and spontaneous abortion: response bias in a postal questionnaire study, Int J Epidemiol 11:250, 1982.

Balasch J, Font J, Lopez-Soto A, et al: Antiphospholipid antibodies in unselected patients with repeated abortion, Hum Reprod 5:43, 1990.

Barnes AB, Colton T, Gundersen J, et al: Fertility and outcome of pregnancy in women exposed in utero to diethylstilbestrol, N Engl J Med 302:609, 1980.

Batzer FR, Schlaff S, Goldfarb AF, et al: Serial β-subunit human chorionic gonadotropin doubling time as a prognosticator of pregnancy outcome in an infertile population, Fertil Steril 35:307, 1981.

Benson RC and Durfee RB: Transabdominal cervicouterine cerclage during pregnancy for the treatment of cervical incompetency, Obstet Gynecol 25:145, 1965.

Boué J, Boué A, and Lazar P: Retrospective and prospective epidemiological studies of 1500 karyotyped spontaneous human abortions, Teratology 12:11, 1975.

Branch DW, Scott JR, Kochenour NK, and Hershgold E: Obstetric complications associated with the lupus anticoagulant, N Engl J Med 313:1322, 1985.

Brent RL: Radiation-induced embryonic and fetal loss from conception to birth. In Porter IH and Hook EB, editors: Human embryonic and fetal death, New York, 1980, Academic Press.

Buttram VC and Gibbons WE: Müllerian anomalies: a proposed classification (an analysis of 144 cases), Fertil Steril 32:40, 1979.

Buttram VC Jr and Reiter RC: Uterine leiomyomata: etiology, symptomatology, and management, Fertil Steril 36:433, 1981.

Cacciatore B, Tiitinen A, Stenman U-H, and Ylostalo P: Normal early pregnancy: serum HCG levels and vaginal ultrasonographic findings, Br J Obstet Gynecol 97:899, 1990.

Cashner KA, Christopher CR, and Dysert GA: Spontaneous fetal loss after demonstration of a live fetus in the first trimester, Obstet Gynecol 70:827, 1987.

Caudle MR, Rote NS, Scott JR, et al: Histocompatibility in couples with recurrent spontaneous abortion and normal fertility, Fertil Steril 39:793, 1983.

Cavanagh D, Fleisher A, and Ferguson JH: Inevitable and incomplete abortion, Am J Obstet Gynecol 90:216, 1964.

Chartier M, Roger M, Barrat J, et al: Measurement of plasma human chorionic gonadotropin (hCH) and β-hCG activities in the late luteal phase: evidence of the occurrence of spontaneous menstrual abortions in infertile women, Fertil Steril 31:134, 1979.

Cousins L: Cervical incompetence, 1980: a time for reappraisal, Clin Obstet Gynecol 23:467, 1980.

Crane JP and Wahl N: The role of maternal diabetes in repetitive spontaneous abortion, Fertil Steril 36:477, 1981.

Creasy MR, Crolla JA, and Alberman ED: A cytogenetic study of human spontaneous abortions using banding techniques, Hum Genet 31:177, 1976.

Decenzo JA and Cavanagh D: Management of incomplete abortion on an outpatient basis, Am J Obstet Gynecol 97:17, 1967.

DeCherney AH, Russell JB, Graebe RA, et al: Resectoscopic management of Müllerian fusion defects, Fertil Steril 45:726, 1986.

Deleze M, Alarcon-Segovia D, Valdes-Macho E, et al: Relationship between antiphospholipid antibodies and recurrent fetal loss in patients with systemic lupus erythematosus and apparently healthy women, J Rheumatol 16:768, 1989.

Fossum GT, Davajan V, and Kletzky OA: Early detection of pregnancy with transvaginal ultrasound, Fertil Steril 49:788, 1988.

Grimes DA, Cates W Jr, and Selik RM: Fatal septic abortion in the United States, 1975-1977, Obstet Gynecol 57:739, 1981.

Haney AF, Hammond CB, Soules MR, et al: Diethylstilbestrol-induced upper genital tract abnormalities, Fertil Steril 31:142, 1979.

Harger JH: Comparison of success and morbidity in cervical cerclage procedures, Obstet Gynecol 56:543, 1980.

Harger JH, Archer DF, Marchese SG, et al: Etiology of recurrent pregnancy losses and outcome of subsequent pregnancies, Obstet Gynecol 62:574, 1983.

Harlap S, Shiono PH, and Ramcharan S: A life table of spontaneous abortions and the effects of age, parity, and other variables. In Porter IH and Hook EB, editors: Human embryonic and fetal death, New York, 1980, Academic Press.

Harlap S and Shiono PH: Alcohol, smoking, and incidence of spontaneous abortions in the first and second trimester, Lancet 2:173, 1980.

Heinonen PK, Saarikoski S, and Pystynen P: Reproductive performance of women with uterine anomalies, Acta Obstet Gynecol Scand 61:157, 1982.

Hensleigh PA and Fainstat T: Corpus luteum dysfunction: serum progesterone levels in diagnosis and assessment of therapy for recurrent and threatened abortion, Fertil Steril 32:396, 1979.

Herbst AL, Hubby MM, Azizi F, et al: Reproductive and gynecologic surgical experience in diethylstilbestrol-exposed daughters, Am J Obstet Gynecol 141:1019, 1981.

Herbst AL, Hubby MM, Blough RR, et al: A comparison of pregnancy experience in DES-exposed and DES-unexposed daughters, J Reprod Med 24:62, 1980.

Hertig AT, Rock J, Adams EC, et al: Thirty-four fertilized human ova, good, bad and indifferent, recovered from 210 women of known fertility, Pediatrics 23:202, 1959.

Horta JLH, Fernandez JG, Soto de Leon B, et al: Direct

evidence of luteal insufficiency in women with habitual abortion, Obstet Gynecol 49:705, 1977.

Houwert-de Jong MH, Termijtelen A, Eskes TKAB, et al: The natural course of habitual abortion, Eur J Obstet Gynecol Reprod Biol 33:221, 1989.

Howard MA, Firkin BG, Healy DL, and Choong S-CC: Lupus anticoagulant in women with multiple spontaneous miscarriage, Am J Hematol 26:175, 1987.

Jacobs PA and Hassold TJ: The origin of chromosome abnormalities in spontaneous abortion. In Porter IH and Hook EB, editors: Human embryonic and fetal death, New York, 1980, Academic Press.

James WH: On the possibility of segregation in the propensity to spontaneous abortion in the human female, Ann Hum Genet 25:207, 1961.

Jouppila P: Clinical and ultrasonic aspects in the diagnosis and follow-up of patients with early pregnancy failure, Acta Obstet Gynecol Scand 59:405, 1980.

Kadar N, DeVore G, and Romero R: Discriminatory hCG zone: its use in the sonographic evaluation for ectopic pregnancy, Obstet Gynecol 58:156, 1981.

Kajii T, Ferrier A, Niikawa N, et al: Anatomic and chromosomal anomalies in 639 spontaneous abortuses, Hum Genet 55:87, 1980.

Kajii T and Ohama K: Inverse maternal age effect on monosomy X, Hum Genet 51:147, 1979.

Kaufman RH, Adam E, Binder GL, et al: Upper genital tract changes and pregnancy outcome in offspring exposed in utero to diethylstilbestrol, Am J Obstet Gynecol 137:299, 1980.

Kaufman RH, Noller K, Adam E, et al: Upper genital tract abnormalities and pregnancy outcome in diethylstilbestrol-exposed progeny, Am J Obstet Gynecol 148:973, 1984.

Kline J, Shrout P, Stein ZA, et al: Drinking during pregnancy and spontaneous abortion, Lancet 2:176, 1980.

Kline J, Stein Z, Susser M, et al: Environmental influences on early reproductive loss in a current New York City study. In Porter IH and Hood EB, editors: Human embryonic and fetal death, New York, 1980, Academic Press.

Kline J, Stein ZA, Susser M, et al: Smoking: a risk factor for spontaneous abortion, N Engl J Med 297:793, 1977.

Lauritsen JG: Aetiology of spontaneous abortion, Acta Obstet Gynecol Scand (Suppl) 52:3, 1976.

Léridon H: Human fertility, Chicago, 1977, University of Chicago Press.

Lockshin MD, Druzin ML, Goei S, et al: Antibody to cardiolipin as a predictor of fetal distress or death in pregnant patients with systemic lupus erythematosus, N Eng J Med 313:152, 1985.

Lockshin MD, Druzin ML, and Qamar T: Prednisone does not prevent recurrent fetal death in women with antiphospholipid antibody, Am J Obstet Gynecol 160:439, 1989.

Lockwood CJ, Romero R, Feinberg RF, et al: The prevalence and biologic significance of lupus anticoagulant and anticardiolipin antibodies in a general obstetric population, Am J Obstet Gynecol 161:369, 1989.

Lubbe WF and Liggins GC: Lupus anticoagulant and pregnancy, Am J Obstet Gynecol 153:322, 1985.

MacKenzie WE, Holmes DS, and Newton JR: Spontaneous abortion rate in ultrasonographically viable pregnancies, Obstet Gynecol 71:81, 1988.

Malpas P: A study of abortion sequences, Br J Obstet Gynaecol 45:932, 1938.

Mann EC: Habitual abortion, Am J Obstet Gynecol 77:706, 1959.

Mantoni M: Ultrasound signs in threatened abortion and their prognostic significance, Obstet Gynecol 65:471-75, 1985.

March CM and Israel R: Gestational outcome following hysteroscopic lysis of adhesions, Fertil Steril 36:455, 1981.

March CM and Israel R: Hysteroscopic management of recurrent abortion secondary to septate uterus, Am J Obstet Gynecol 156:834, 1987.

Mills JL, Simpson JL, Driscoll SG, et al: Incidence of spontaneous abortion among normal women and insulin-dependent diabetic women whose pregnancies were identified within 21 days of conception, N Engl J Med 319:1618, 1988.

Montoro M, Collea JV, Frasier D, et al: Successful outcome of pregnancy in women with hypothyroidism, Ann Intern Med 94:31, 1981.

Mowbray JF, Gibbings C, Liddell H, et al: Controlled trial of treatment of recurrent spontaneous abortion by immunisation with paternal cells, Lancet 1:941, 1985.

Musich Jr and Behrman SJ: Obstetric outcome before and after metroplasty in women with uterine anomalies, Obstet Gynecol 52:63, 1978.

Nahmias AJ, Josey WE, Naib ZM, et al: Perinatal risk associated with maternal genital herpes simplex virus infection, Am J Obstet Gynecol 110:825, 1971.

Naib ZM, Nahmias AJ, Josey WE, et al: Association of maternal genital herpetic infection with spontaneous abortion, Obstet Gynecol 35:260, 1970.

Naylor AF and Warburton D: Sequential analysis of spontaneous abortion. II. Collaborative study data show that gravidity determines a very substantial rise in risk, Fertil Steril 31:282, 1979.

Ordi J, Barquinero J, Vilardell M, et al: Fetal loss treatment in patients with antiphospholipid antibodies, Ann Rheumat Dis 48:798, 1989.

Pedersen JF and Mantoni M: Prevalence and significance of subchorionic hemorrhage in threatened abortion: a sonographic study, Am J Roentgenol 154:535, 1990.

Poland BJ, Miller JR, Jones DC, et al: Reproductive counseling in patients who have had a spontaneous abortion, Am J Obstet Gynecol 127:685, 1977.

Portnoi M-F, Joye N, Van Den Akker J, et al: Karyotypes of 1142 couples with recurrent abortion, Obstet Gynecol 72:31, 1988.

Pridjian G and Moawad AH: Missed abortion: still appropriate terminology? Am J Obstet Gynecol 161:261, 1989.

Rabau E and David A: Listeria monocytogenes in abortion, J Obstet Gynaecol Br Comm 70:481, 1963.

Reece EA, Gabrielli S, Cullen MT, et al: Recurrent adverse pregnancy outcome and antiphospholipid antibodies, Am J Obstet Gynecol 163:162, 1990.

Regan L, Braude PR, and Trembath PL: Influence of past reproductive performance on risk of spontaneous abortion, Brit Med J 299:541, 1989.

Roberts JM and Laros RK: Hemorrhagic and endotoxic shock: a pathophysiologic approach to diagnosis and management, Am J Obstet Gynecol 110:1041, 1971.

Rock JA and Jones HW: The clinical management of the double uterus, Fertil Steril 28:798, 1977.

Rock JA and Zacur HA: The clinical management of repeated early pregnancy wastage, Fertil Steril 39:123, 1983.

Rocklin RE, Kitzmiller JL, Carpenter CB, et al: Maternal-fetal relation: absence of an immunologic blocking factor from the serum of women with chronic abortions, N Engl J Med 295:1209, 1976.

Sachs ES, Jahoda MGJ, Van Hemel JO, et al: Chromosome studies of 500 couples with two or more abortions, Obstet Gynecol 65:375, 1985.

Sargent IL, Wilkins T, and Redman CWG: Maternal immune responses to the fetus in early pregnancy and recurrent miscarriage, Lancet 2:1099, 1988.

Schenker JG and Margalioth EJ: Intrauterine adhesions: an updated appraisal, Fertil Steril 37:593, 1982.

Sider D, Wilson WG, Sudduth K, et al: Cytogenetic studies in couples with recurrent pregnancy loss, Southern Med J 81:1521, 1988.

Simpson JL, Mills JL, Holmes LB, et al: Low fetal loss rates after ultrasound-proved viability in early pregnancy, JAMA 258:2555, 1987.

Simpson JL: Genes, chromosomes, and reproductive failure, Fertil Steril 33:107, 1980.

Smith A and Gaha TJ: Data on families of chromosome translocation carriers ascertained because of habitual spontaneous abortion, Aust NZ J Obstet Gynaecol 30:57, 1990.

Smith JB and Cowchock FS: Immunological studies in recurrent spontaneous abortion: effects of immunization of women with paternal mononuclear cells on lymphocytotoxic and mixed lymphocyte reaction blocking antibodies and correlation with sharing of HLA and pregnancy outcome, J Reprod Immunol 14:99, 1988.

Stabile I, Campbell S, and Grudzinskas JG: Ultrasonic assessment of complications during first trimester of pregnancy, Lancet 2:1237, 1987.

Stagnaro-Green A, Roman SH, Cobin RH, et al: Detection of at-risk pregnancy by means of highly sensitive assays for thyroid autoantibodies, JAMA 264:1422, 1990.

Stein Z, Kline J, Susser E, et al: Maternal age and spontaneous abortion. In Porter IH and Hook EB, editors: Human embryonic and fetal death, New York, 1980, Academic Press.

Stillman RJ: In utero exposure to diethylstilbestrol: adverse effects on the reproductive tract and reproductive performance in male and female offspring, Am J Obstet Gynecol 142:905, 1982.

Stray-Pedersen B, Eng J, and Reikvam TM: Uterine T-mycoplasma colonization in reproductive failure, Am J Obstet Gynecol 130:307, 1978.

Stray-Pedersen B and Stray-Pedersen S: Etiologic factors and subsequent reproductive performance in 195 couples with a prior history of habitual abortion, Am J Obstet Gynecol 148:140, 1984.

Strobino BA and Pantel-Silverman J: First-trimester vaginal bleeding and the loss of chromosomally normal and abnormal conceptions, Am J Obstet Gynecol 157:1150, 1987.

Tharapel AT, Tharapel SA, and Bannerman RM: Recurrent pregnancy losses and parental chromosome abnormalities: a review, Br J Obstet Gynaecol 92:899, 1985.

Tho PT, Byrd TR, and McDonough PG: Etiologies and subsequent reproductive performance of 100 couples with recurrent abortion, Fertil Steril 32:389, 1979.

Thomas ML, Harger JH, Wagener DK, et al: HLA sharing and spontaneous abortion in humans, Am J Obstet Gynecol 151:1053, 1985.

Triplett DA, Brandt JT, Musgrave KA, and Orr CA: The relationship between lupus anticoagulants and antibodies to phospholipid, JAMA 259:550, 1988.

Warburton D, Stein Z, Kline J, et al: Chromosome abnormalities in spontaneous abortion: data from the New York City study. In Porter IH and Hook EB, editors: Human embryonic and fetal death, New York, 1980, Academic Press.

Warburton D: Monosomy X: a chromosomal anomaly associated with young maternal age, Lancet 1:167, 1980.

Warburton D and Fraser FC: Spontaneous abortion risks in man: data from reproductive histories collected in a medical genetics unit, Am J Hum Genet 16:1, 1964.

Weitkamp LR and Schacter BZ: Transferrin and HLA: spontaneous abortion, neural tube defects, and natural selection, N Engl J Med 313:925, 1985.

Wilcox AJ, Weinberg CR, O'Connor JF, et al: Incidence of early loss of pregnancy, N Engl J Med 319:189, 1988.

Wilson RD, Kendrick V, Wittmann BK, and McGillivray B: Spontaneous abortion and pregnancy outcome after normal first-trimester ultrasound examination, Obstet Gynecol 67:352, 1986.

Ectopic Pregnancy

KEY TERMS AND DEFINITIONS

Abdominal Pregnancy. Pregnancy that develops in any portion of the peritoneal cavity. It usually occurs after a secondary implantation of the trophoblast after tubal abortion (secondary abdominal pregnancy). A primary abdominal pregnancy is one that implants directly into the peritoneal cavity.

Arias-Stella Reaction. Hypersecretory appearance of endometrial glands. The cells demonstrate hyperchromatism, pleomorphism, increased mitotic activity, and hypertrophy.

Cervical Pregnancy. Pregnancy developing in the cervical canal below the level of the internal os.

Chronic Ectopic Pregnancy. Ectopic gestational tissue in the peritoneal cavity after tubal abortion or rupture. It produces chronic symptoms of lower abdominal pain and usually forms adhesions to bowel and peritoneum.

Cornual Pregnancy. Pregnancy developing in one horn of a bicornuate uterus.

Culdocentesis. Aspiration of fluid in cul-de-sac (pouch) of Douglas via a needle placed through the vagina.

Decidual Cast. Sloughing of nearly all of the decidua lining the endometrial cavity.

Ectopic Pregnancy. Pregnancy that develops after implantation of the blastocyst anywhere other than the endometrium lining the uterine cavity.

Hemoperitoneum. Blood in the peritoneal cavity. The blood from a ruptured ectopic pregnancy initially clots and then lyses so that hemoperitoneum is a combination of blood clots and hemorrhagic fluid that will not clot.

Heterotopic Pregnancy. Combined intrauterine and extrauterine pregnancy.

Interstitial Pregnancy. Pregnancy developing in the interstitial portion of the oviduct.

Ovarian Pregnancy. Pregnancy developing in the ovary. For the diagnosis to be made, the following four characteristics must be fulfilled: (1) the tube on the affected side should be intact, (2) the gestational site must occupy the normal position of the ovary, (3) the gestational site must be connected to the uterus by the ovarian ligament, and (4) histologically identified ovarian tissue must be present in the sac wall.

Persistent Ectopic Pregnancy. Continued growth of viable trophoblastic tissue after conservative treatment of an unruptured ectopic pregnancy; manifestations include HCG titers that do not fall and/or low pelvic pain.

Ruptured Ectopic Pregnancy. Ectopic pregnancy that has eroded through the tissue in which it has implanted, producing hemorrhage from exposed vessels.

Salpingitis Isthmica Nodosa. (Tubal Diverticulum). Direct invasion of the tubal muscularis by the tubal epithelium for varying distances between the lumen and the serosa.

Salpingostomy. Operative opening made in the oviduct and used to remove an unruptured tubal pregnancy for the purpose of retaining the oviduct.

Salpingotomy. Operative opening made in the oviduct, followed by removal of an ectopic pregnancy and closure of the incision in the oviduct.

Tubal Abortion. Tubal pregnancy that is extruded out of the fimbrial end of the oviduct.

Tubal Pregnancy. Pregnancy occurring in the oviduct in the ampulla, fimbria, or isthmus. This is the most common site of ectopic pregnancy.

Unruptured Tubal Gestation. Tubal pregnancy that has not yet eroded through the wall of the oviduct.

Ectopic pregnancy was probably first described in AD 963 by Albucasis, an Arab writer. In 1876, before the initiation of surgical therapy, the mortality from ectopic pregnancy was estimated to be 60%. The first successful operative treatment of ectopic pregnancy was performed in 1883 by Lawson Tait in England. In 1887 he reported that he had performed salpingectomy on four women with ectopic pregnancy and that they all survived.

EPIDEMIOLOGY

The incidence of ectopic pregnancy is expressed in different ways in the literature, with the most common denominator being number of recognized conceptions (number of ectopic pregnancies per 1000 conceptions). Other denominators include the number of women of reproductive age (number of ectopic pregnancies per 10,000 women aged 14 to 44) and number of total births (number of ectopic pregnancies per 1000 births).

It would be best to be able to calculate the incidence of ectopic pregnancies per 1000 total conceptions; however, since most spontaneous abortions and many elective abortions are not reported, the denominator is always smaller than the actual number, yielding a spuriously increased incidence. Nevertheless, since an unknown number of ectopic pregnancies remain asymptomatic and thus are not reported, the numerator is also lower. Thus the true inci-

dence of ectopic pregnancies per 1000 total conceptions can never be accurately calculated, but the incidences reported are good approximations and, since the same methodology is used, can be validly compared.

The incidence of ectopic pregnancy varies among different countries, with rates as high as 1 in 28 and 1 in 40 deliveries reported in Jamaica and Vietnam. In the United States the incidence per live births in different series has varied from 1 in 64 to 1 in 241. The annual ectopic pregnancy rate in the United States in 1987 was 1.52 per 1000 women aged 15 to 44 and 1.87 per 1000 women at risk for pregnancy.

During the past 30 years the incidence of ectopic pregnancy has been steadily increasing in the United States, as well as in several European countries (Table 16-1). Weström et al. reported that in 20 years the rate of ectopic pregnancy doubled in Sweden, increasing from 5.8 per 1000 diagnosed conceptions between 1960 and 1964 to 11.1 between 1975 and 1979. The Centers for Disease Control reported a similar marked increase in the United States. Between 1970 and 1987 there was a fivefold increase in the annual number of women hospitalized for ectopic pregnancies (from 17,800 to 88,000), and there was a tripling of the rate per 1000 pregnancies (from 4.5 to 16.8) (Table 16-2). Thus in the United States in 1987 nearly 2 of every 100 women who were known to conceive were hospitalized for ectopic gestation. This increased incidence of ectopic pregnancy is thought to be mainly the result of increased incidence of salpingitis, a major risk factor for ectopic pregnancy, as well as improved diagnostic techniques.

In both the Swedish and United States studies there was also a marked increase in the rate of ectopic pregnancy with increasing age when calculated as incidence per 1000 reported conceptions. In the United States the rate increased from 6.3 in women aged 15 to 24 years to 20.5 in those aged 35 to 44 years. However, when the number was calculated per 10,000 women aged 15 to 44, the rate of ectopic pregnancy was lowest in the older group, reflecting the lower total number of pregnancies in this group. These data indicate that the incidence rate of ectopic pregnancy should be calculated using total pregnancies as the denominator to determine the actual risk for a woman exposed to pregnancy. Because of the lower pregnancy

TABLE 16-1

Increases in Incidence of Ectopic Pregnancy as Reported in Different Regions

Geographic Area	Period	Increase Factor
Czechoslovakia, Prague	1955-1966	1.7
England and Wales	1966-1976	1.6
Finland		
Helsinki	1968-1976	1.9
Turku	1966-1975	1.8
Scotland (unpublished observations)	1964-1974	1.7
Sweden		
Lund	1960-1979	1.9
Uppsala	1960-1975	2.5
United States	1965-1977	2.7

From Weström L, Bengtsson LPH, and Mårdh P-A: Br Med J 282:15, 1981.

TABLE 16-3
Misdiagnose:

Gastrointestin
Intrauterine p
Pelvic inflamr
Psychiatric di:
Spontaneous :
Sequelae of r(
Urinary tract
Adnexal cyst
Dysfunctional
Fetal death ir
Placental abn(

   TOTAL

From Dorfman
American Colle
*Based on all r(
†These percent

levels of eit
interfere wi
creased rate
reported in
logically an(
of progestin
duced loca
IUD, as w
only oral co
ically incre:
terone occu
ther clomip
otrophins,
pregnancie:
ceiving afte
ties.

   Another
of embryon
44 human (
by microdi:
found that :
half had gr
types of abr
mal tubal
have not b(
pregnancy,
creased inc
that the ch
gestations :
gestations.

rate in older women, overall only about 11% of ectopic pregnancies in the United States occur in women aged 35 to 44, whereas more than half (58%) occur in women aged 25 to 34.

Most ectopic pregnancies occur in multigravid women. Only 10% to 15% of ectopic pregnancies occur in nulligravid women, whereas more than half occur in women who have been pregnant three or more times.

In the United States the rates of ectopic pregnancy were similar in each section of the country, but the rates were about twice as high for nonwhite as for white women (Figure 16-1). About 2.6% of all reported pregnancies in nonwhite women aged 35 to 44 in the United States were ectopic.

TABLE 16-2
Numbers and Rates of Ectopic Pregnancies by Year (United States, 1970-1987)

Year	Number*	Rate†
1970	17,800	4.5
1971	19,300	4.8
1972	24,500	6.3
1973	25,600	6.8
1974	26,400	6.7
1975	30,500	7.6
1976	34,600	8.3
1977	40,700	9.2
1978	42,400	9.4
1979	49,900	10.4
1980	52,200	10.5
1981	68,000	13.6
1982	61,800	12.3
1983	60,600	14.0
1984	75,400	14.9
1985	78,400	15.2
1986	73,700	14.3
1987	88,000	16.8
TOTAL	877,400‡	10.7

From Centers for Disease Control: Ectopic pregnancies—United States, 1979-1987, vol 39, no SS-4, p 9.
*Rounded to nearest hundred.
†Rate per 1000 pregnancies (live births, legally induced abortions, and ectopic pregnancies).
‡Because of rounding, the total differs from the sum of the numbers.

MORTALITY

Even with the increased use of surgery and blood transfusions and earlier diagnosis, ectopic pregnancy remains a major cause of maternal death in the United States today. About 40 to 50 deaths from ectopic pregnancy occur annually. Ectopic pregnancy is the most common cause of maternal death in the first half of pregnancy. Although the percentage of all maternal deaths in the United States that are the result of ectopic pregnancy increased from 8% in 1970 to 14% in 1980, the percentage of ectopic pregnancies that become fatal has decreased. The overall death-to-case rate of ectopic pregnancy has decreased sevenfold from 3.5 per 1000 women with ectopic pregnancy in 1970 to 0.5 in 1987 (Figure 16-2). The death-to-case rate is similar in all age groups but is about 3 times higher in black women. Because the incidence of ectopic pregnancy is also higher in blacks in the United States, a pregnant black woman is about 5 times more likely to die of ectopic pregnancy than a white woman. Ectopic pregnancy is the most common single cause of all maternal deaths among

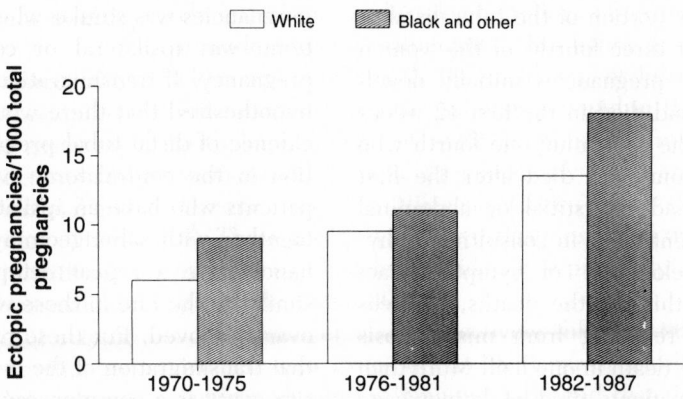

FIGURE 16-1
Ectopic pregnancy rate by race and selected periods, United States, 1970-1987. (From Nederlof KP et al: MMWR 39[SS-4]: 9, 1990.)

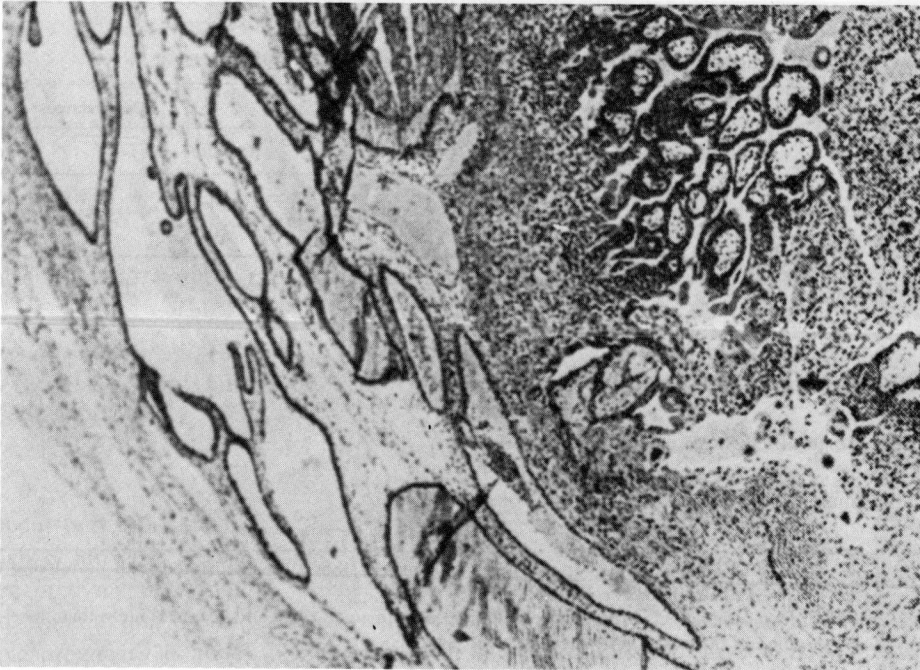

FIGURE 16-3
Tubal pregnancy with placental villi and trophoblastic cells to the right and wall of the tube to the left showing marked degree of follicular salpingitis. (Original magnification, ×70.) (From Bone NL and Greene RR: Am J Obstet Gynecol 82:1166, 1961.)

compared with a group of women without prior clinical evidence of salpingitis. The risk that the first pregnancy after acute salpingitis would be ectopic increased both with the number of episodes of infection and with the increasing age of the women at the time of infection.

In two histopathology studies of oviducts removed from women with ectopic pregnancy, Majmudar et al. and Green and Kott found that about half contained lesions of salpingitis isthmica nodosa (SIN) when numerous sections of the tube were examined. In their control groups only 5% of oviducts had SIN. SIN was defined as the microscopic presence of tubal epithelium within the myosalpinx or beneath the tubal serosa (Figure 16-4). With serial sectioning it has been determined that SIN is actually a diverticulum or intrauterine extension of the tubal lumen (Figure 16-5). Associated histologic evidence of chronic salpingitis was seen in only 6% of these oviducts in the first series, indicating that SIN was not necessarily the result of infection. These findings agreed with those of Persaud, who observed tubal diverticula (histologically similar to SIN) in the isthmus and proximal ampulla of half of the oviducts removed for tubal pregnancy. In both these series the tubal pregnancy usually implanted at a portion of the tube distal to the SIN, indicating that mechanical entrapment of the blastocyst is not the mechanism whereby SIN causes tubal gestation. These investigators postulated that SIN itself or associated tubal anomalies may be responsible for dysfunction of the tubal transport mechanism without anatomic obstruction.

It is likely that adhesions between the tubal serosa and bowel or peritoneum may interfere with normal tubal motility and cause ectopic pregnancy because as reported by Brenner et al. and DeCherney, respectively, 17% to 27% of patients with ectopic pregnancy have had previous abdominal surgical procedures not involving the oviduct. On the other hand, neither endometriosis nor a congenital anomaly of the tube has been associated with an increased incidence of ectopic pregnancy.

An operative procedure on the oviduct itself is a cause of ectopic pregnancy whether the oviduct is morphologically normal, as occurs

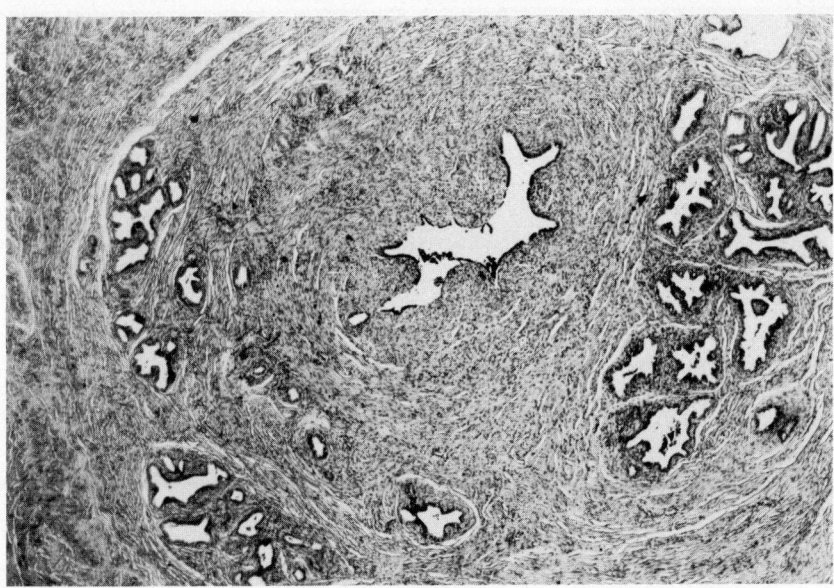

FIGURE 16-4
Microscopic section of fallopian tube showing typical lesion of salpingitis isthmica no-dosa. Multiple glandular inclusions of tubal mucosa are seen in myosalpinx without continuity with luminal epithelium. (H&E, ×12.) (From Majmudar B, Henderson PH III, and Semple E: Obstet Gynecol 62:73, 1983. Reprinted with permission from The American College of Obstetricians and Gynecologists.)

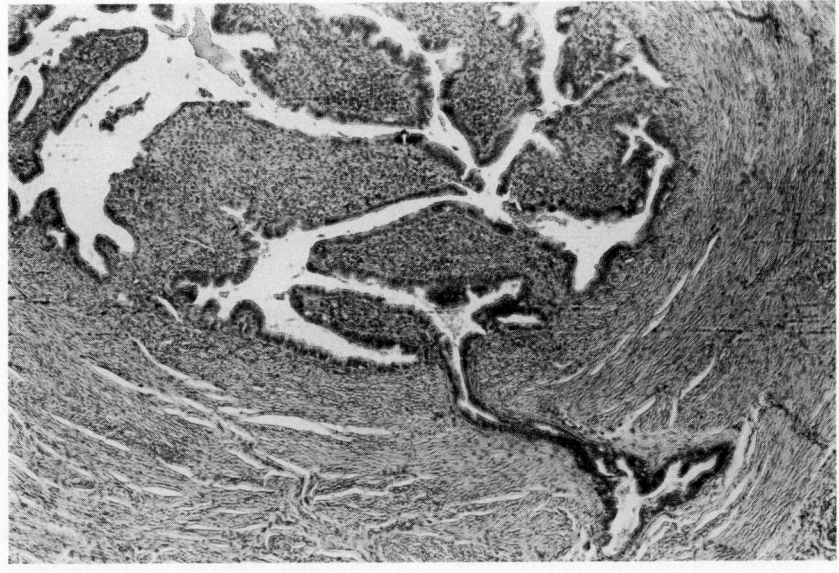

FIGURE 16-5
Tubal mucosa showing its actual extension into myosalpinx. (H&E, ×12.) (From Majmudar B, Henderson PH III, and Semple E: Obstet Gynecol 62:73, 1983. Reprinted with permission from The American College of Obstetricians and Gynecologists.)

TABLE 16-4

Ectopic Pregnancies as Percentage of Pregnancies Associated with Tubal Sterilization

Route of Operation	Number of Women	Total Pregnancies	
		Number	% Ectopic
Transabdominal (laparotomy)	9092	65	20.0
Transvaginal	8190	35	2.9
Transabdominal or transvaginal	1290	7	0.0
Laparoscopic			
Coagulation-transection	12,806	55	14.5
Coagulation only	5724	14	42.9
TOTAL	37,102	176	15.9
Laparoscopic spring-loaded clip	977	22	0.0
Laparoscopic Falope-Ring	3876	15	60.0

From Tatum HJ and Schmidt FH: Fertil Steril 28:407, 1977. Reproduced with permission of the publisher, The American Fertility Society.

with sterilization procedures, or abnormal, as occurs with postsalpingitis reconstructive surgery. The incidence of ectopic pregnancy in pregnancies occurring after salpingoplasty or salpingostomy procedures for distal tubal disease ranges from 15% to 25%, probably because the damage to the endosalpinx remains. The rate of ectopic pregnancy in pregnancies after reversal of sterilization procedures is lower, about 4%, because the tubes have not been damaged by infection.

Tatum and Schmidt reported that when women conceive after a tubal sterilization has been performed, the overall incidence of ectopic pregnancy is about 16% (Table 16-4). In their review as well as that of McCausland, it was reported that if pregnancy occurred after tubal sterilization by laparoscopic fulguration without concomitant transection, the ectopic pregnancy rate was about 50%. McCausland hypothesized that with the extensive tissue destruction caused by electrocoagulation, a uteroperitoneal fistula could develop that would allow sperm to pass into the distal segment of the oviduct and fertilize the egg (Figure 16-6). Such fistulas were demonstrated radiographically by Shah et al. in 11% of 150 women after laparoscopic electrocoagulation and demonstrated histologically by McCausland, who called the process endosalpingosis or endosalpingoblastosis. McCann and Kessel also reported a 50% ectopic pregnancy rate after failure of laparoscopic electrocoagulation but only

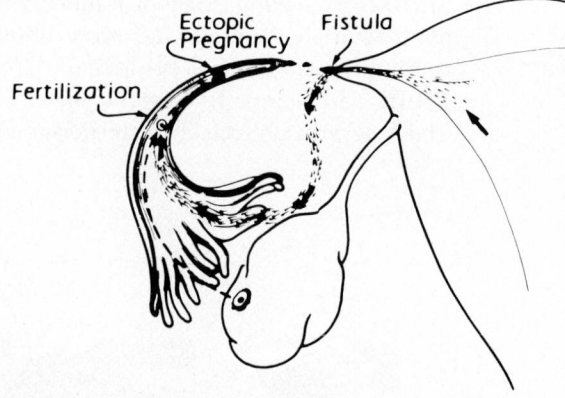

FIGURE 16-6

Mechanism of ectopic pregnancy after sterilization. (From Corson SL and Batzer FR: J Reprod Med 31:78, 1986.)

a rare ectopic pregnancy occurred after failure of sterilization with metal clips or silicone rings.

With the marked increase in use of female sterilization techniques, failure of sterilization is becoming a more common cause of ectopic pregnancy. In contrast to a large series of ectopic pregnancies in the United States in the 1950s and 1960s reported by Breen, in which only 0.6% of women with ectopic pregnancy had had tubal sterilization, Brenner et al. reported that 3% of 300 ectopic pregnancies occurring in 1976 to 1977 were the result of tubal sterilization failure.

TABLE 16-5
Percent Distribution of Current Contraceptive Methods and Relationship with Ectopic Pregnancy

Current Method	Women with Ectopic Pregnancy (No. = 475)	Control Subjects (No. = 2923)	Relative Risk (95% Confidence Interval)
IUD	14.1	17.0	0.4 (0.3-0.6)
Traditional methods	12.0	19.6	0.4 (0.3-0.5)
Oral contraceptives	6.7	26.5	0.1 (0.1-0.2)
None	67.2	36.9	1.0 (Referent)
TOTAL	100.0	100.0	

From Ory HW, The Women's Health Study: Obstet Gynecol 57:137, 1981. Reprinted with permission from The American College of Obstetricians and Gynecologists.

Women who have had a prior ectopic pregnancy, even if treated by unilateral salpingectomy, are at increased risk for having a subsequent ectopic pregnancy. Of women who conceive after having one ectopic pregnancy, about 15% of subsequent pregnancies are ectopic. In the series of Brenner et al. and Breen, 7% of the women with ectopic pregnancy had a prior ectopic pregnancy.

Contraceptive Failures

As summarized by Tatum and Schmidt, pregnancies occurring as a result of a failure of certain contraceptive methods have a greater chance of being ectopic. Although women who become pregnant while using diaphragms or combination oral contraceptives do not have an increased chance of having an ectopic pregnancy, women who become pregnant while using IUDs or progestin-only oral contraceptives have about a 5% chance of having an ectopic pregnancy. The incidence of ectopic pregnancy in women who become pregnant with the progesterone-releasing IUD is even higher, about 15%. Women using these methods of contraception who elect to have their pregnancies terminated should have a histologic examination of the uterine cavity to be sure the pregnancy was intrauterine.

Women using any type of contraception have a significantly decreased chance of having an ectopic pregnancy as compared with sexually active, noncontraceptive users (Table 16-5). Oral contraceptives prevent ectopic pregnancy to a greater extent than barrier methods or IUDs, but women using the latter methods have less than half the chance of having an ectopic pregnancy than women using no method have. Ory as well as Tatum and Schmidt have reported that the chance of a pregnancy being ectopic in a woman using an IUD is increased if the IUD has been in place for 2 years or more. This increase with longer duration of IUD use is most likely due to the fact that the intrauterine pregnancy rate with IUDs is highest in the first year of use and declines steadily thereafter. Thus the IUD prevents both tubal and uterine pregnancies but is more effective in preventing intrauterine pregnancies. After discontinuation of any method of contraception, including the IUD, the ectopic pregnancy rate is not increased. An exception is women who were using the shield-type of IUD with its multifilament tailstring, which enhanced the development of salpingitis. As reported by Chow et al., women discontinuing use of the shield IUD have a 2.4 times increased risk of having an ectopic gestation.

Herbst et al. as well as others have shown that the incidence of ectopic gestation is significantly greater (4 to 5 times) in women who have been exposed to diethylstilbestrol (DES) in utero than in a control group. In various series the ectopic pregnancy rate in such individuals is about 4% to 5%. Kaufman et al. reported that among women exposed to DES whose hysterosalpingograms demonstrated abnormalities in the uterine cavity, the ectopic pregnancy rate was 13%.

Hormonal Alterations

As occurs with exogenous progesterone administration, if increased levels of exogenous or endogenous estrogens are present shortly after the time of ovulation, the incidence of ectopic pregnancy is increased. Morris and Van Wagenen reported that 3 of 30 pregnancies were ectopic in women receiving postovulatory high-dose estrogen to prevent pregnancy. Several investigators have reported that the ectopic pregnancy rate is about 1.5% for conceptions occurring after ovulation has been induced with clomiphene citrate. McBain et al. as well as Gemzell reported the ectopic rate in pregnancies occurring after human menopausal gonadotrophin–induced ovulation to be about 3% to 4%. McBain et al. reported that if the urinary estrogen excretion during human menopausal gonadotrophin therapy exceeded 200 μg per day, the ectopic rate was 12.5%. These reports indicate that increased levels of estrogen as well as of progesterone interfere with tubal motility and increase the chance of ectopic gestation. Ectopic gestation has also been reported to occur after in vitro fertilization and embryonic transfer. The mechanism remains obscure but may be related to altered sex steroid hormone levels, proximal tubal disease, or both.

Previous Abortion

Although some studies have suggested that a prior induced abortion increases the risk of ectopic pregnancy, Levin et al. showed that when statistical techniques were used to control the effects of other risk factors, the history of one prior induced abortion did not significantly increase the risk of ectopic pregnancy (Table 16-6). In this study, the risk for ectopic pregnancy doubled if a woman had had two or more prior induced abortions, which (although not significant) indicates a possible association between multiple induced abortions and subsequent ectopic gestation, probably related to postabortal infection. A more recent study by Holt et al., using a different type of control group, reported no significantly increased incidence of ectopic pregnancy in women having one prior abortion (RR = 0.9) and women having two or more prior abortions (RR = 1.2).

PATHOLOGY

Most ectopic pregnancies occur in the oviduct. In Breen's series 97.7% of the ectopic pregnancies were tubal, 1.4% were abdominal, and less than 1% were ovarian or cervical (Figure 16-7). The majority of tubal gestations,

TABLE 16-6

Standardized* Relative Risks of Ectopic Pregnancy and 95% Confidence Intervals According to Selected Characteristics

History Characteristic	Relative Risk	95% Confidence Interval
One induced abortion	1.3	0.6-2.7
Two or more induced abortions	2.6	0.9-7.4
Ectopic pregnancy	7.7	1.9-31.5
Pelvic infection	7.5	3.5-16.0
Pelvic operation	2.6	1.4-4.6

From Levin AA, Schoenbaum SC, Stubbfield PG, et al: Am J Public Health 72:253, 1982.
*Standardized using the multiple logistic regression model.

81%, were located in the ampullary portion of the oviduct, being about equally divided between the distal and middle third of the tube. About 12% of tubal gestations occur in the isthmus and 5% in the fimbrial region. Although Breen considered pregnancies located in the cornual area of the uterus to be uterine in origin, they are in fact pregnancies implanted in the interstitial portion of the oviduct. About 2% of all ectopic pregnancies are interstitial and are associated with severe morbidity, because they become symptomatic later in gestation than other tubal pregnancies, are difficult to diagnose, and frequently produce massive hemorrhage when they rupture (Figure 16-8). A true cornual pregnancy is one located in the rudimentary horn of a bicornuate uterus, and this is quite rare. In a review of 240 true cornual pregnancies reported by O'Leary and O'Leary, about 90% of them ruptured with massive hemorrhage.

About 1 in 200 ectopic pregnancies are true ovarian pregnancies that fulfill the four criteria originally described by Spiegelberg. In IUD users the incidence increases to 1 in 15. Many patients with ovarian pregnancies are believed clinically to have a ruptured corpus luteum cyst. In Hallatt's series of 25 primary ovarian pregnancies, correct diagnosis was made during the surgical procedure for only 28%. In his series the hemorrhagic mass was always located adjacent to the corpus luteum, never within it. Ovarian pregnancy is also associated with profuse hemorrhage, with 81% of Hallatt's cases having a hemoperitoneum greater than 500 ml. Nevertheless, most can be successfully treated

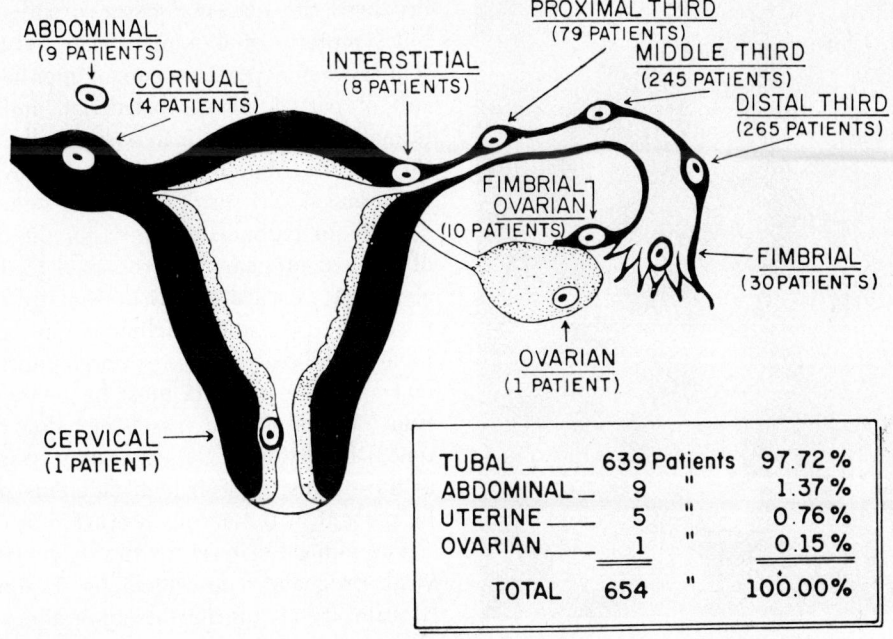

FIGURE 16-7
Anatomic site of ectopic pregnancy. (From Breen JL: Am J Obstet Gynecol 106:1004, 1970.)

by ovarian resection and not oophorectomy.

Most abdominal pregnancies occur secondary to tubal abortion with secondary implantation into the peritoneal cavity (Figure 16-9). On rare occasions a primary abdominal pregnancy may occur. For the latter diagnosis to be made the following three criteria originally set forth by Studdiford must be present: (1) the tubes and ovaries must be normal with no evidence of recent or past injury; (2) there must be no evidence of a uteroplacental fistula; and (3) the pregnancy must be related only to the peritoneal surface and early enough in gestation to eliminate the possibility of secondary implantation after primary tubal nidation. An unusual type of primary abdominal pregnancy may implant in the spleen or liver and produce massive intraperitoneal hemorrhage.

The prognosis for fetal survival in abdominal pregnancy is poor, found to be 11% by Clark and Guy. Diagnosis is difficult but has become easier with the use of ultrasonography. Once the diagnosis is established, a laparotomy with removal of the fetus should be performed immediately to prevent a possible fatal hemorrhage. On occasion, when the placenta is tightly adherent to bowel and blood vessels, it should be left in the abdominal cavity. In such

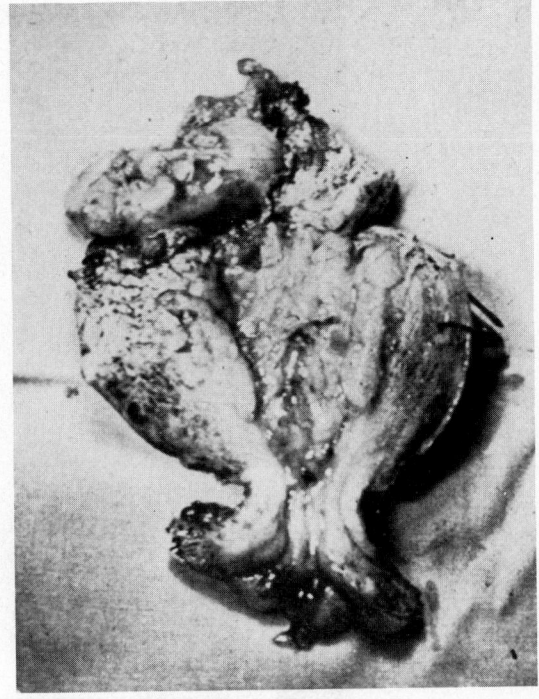

FIGURE 16-8
Anterior view of uterus that has been opened with an anterior Y incision, showing conceptus replaced in site it had formerly occupied in cornual bed. (From Kalchman GG and Meltzer RM: Am J Obstet Gynecol 96:1139, 1966.)

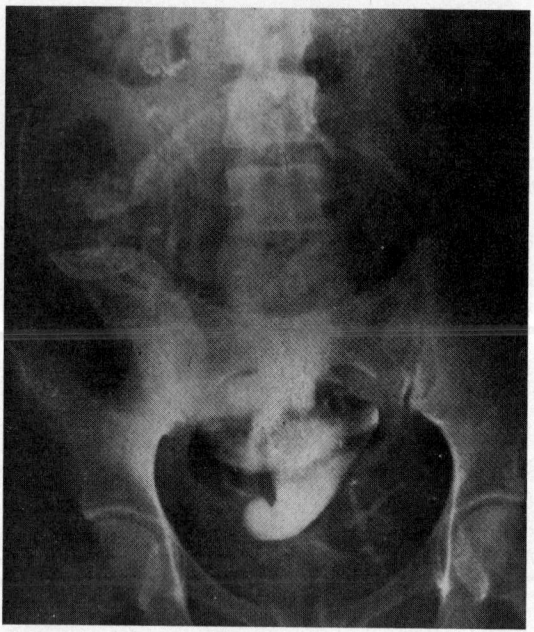

FIGURE 16-9
Hysterosalpingography demonstrating size of uterus and fetus, which is located outside of uterus. (From Clark JF and Guy RS: Am J Obstet Gynecol 96:511, 1966.)

instances the placental tissue usually resorbs, but symptoms of abdominal pain and intermittent fever may persist for many months as a result of partial bowel obstruction and abscess formation. Thus when it is surgically feasible, the placenta should be entirely removed. Partial removal may result in massive hemorrhage.

The four pathologic criteria for the diagnosis of cervical pregnancy as reported by Rubin et al. are (1) cervical glands must be present opposite the placental attachment, (2) the attachment of the placenta to the cervix must be intimate, (3) the placenta must be below the entrance of the uterine vessels or below the peritoneal reflection of the anteroposterior surface of the uterus, and (4) fetal elements must not be present in the corpus uteri (Figure 16-10).

The clinical criteria for the diagnosis of cervical pregnancy described by Paalman and McElin are (1) uterine bleeding after amenorrhea without cramping pain, (2) a softened cervix that is disproportionately enlarged to a size equal to or larger than the corpus, (3) complete confinement and firm attachment of the prod-

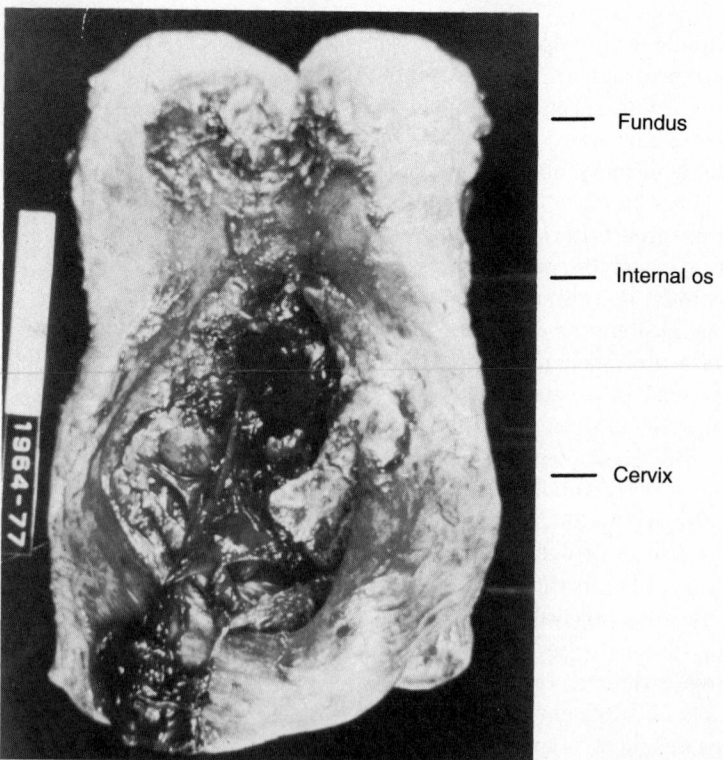

Fundus

Internal os

Cervix

FIGURE 16-10
Cervical pregnancy, 10 weeks' gestation. (From Parente JT, Ou C-S, and Levy J: Obstet Gynecol 62:79, 1983. Reprinted with permission from The American College of Obstetricians and Gynecologists.)

ucts of conception to the endocervix, and (4) a snug internal os.

Most cervical pregnancies occur after a previous sharp uterine curettage. The differential diagnosis is difficult and includes incomplete abortion, placenta previa, carcinoma of the cervix, and degenerative leiomyoma. Although this entity was primarily associated with a high mortality because of massive hemorrhage, currently, with better methods of diagnosis and modern techniques of treatment, death is rare. More than half of the patients with cervical pregnancy require a hysterectomy for treatment, and it is nearly always necessary if the pregnancy has advanced more than 18 weeks in gestational age. Even if a hysterectomy is not performed, the prognosis for future fertility is poor.

Recently there have been case reports in which cervical pregnancy was successfully treated by systemic methotrexate. Other case reports have indicated that angiographic uterine artery embolization allowed evacuation of this pregnancy to be easily performed transcervically with minimal blood loss.

Another uncommon form of ectopic gestation is combined intrauterine and extrauterine pregnancy (94% tubal and 6% ovarian). With the use of mathematic calculation the incidence of this entity has previously been estimated to be either 1 in 16,000 or 1 in 30,000 pregnancies. However, a review of the recent experience at one institution by Reece et al. revealed that 1 of 8000 pregnancies was combined intrauterine and extrauterine and 1 of 70 ectopic pregnancies was associated with an intrauterine pregnancy. Bello et al. estimated that the incidence of heterotopic pregnancy may be as high as 1 of 4000 pregnancies. Combined intrauterine and extrauterine pregnancy may be more common after pharmacologic ovulation induction with the subsequent increase in multiple ovulation. With the increased use of these agents as well as increased incidence of salpingitis, combined intrauterine and extrauterine pregnancy may occur more frequently than previously estimated and should be suspected when any of the following clinical criteria are present: (1) a fundus compatible with gestational age estimated by date of onset of last menses in a patient believed to have an ectopic gestation; (2) two corpora lutea at laparotomy or laparoscopy and an enlarged, soft, and globular uterus; (3) the absence of withdrawal bleeding and the presence of pregnancy symptoms after excision of an ectopic pregnancy; (4) hemoperitoneum after the termination of an intrauterine pregnancy; and (5) the combination of abdominal pain, adnexal mass with pain and tenderness, peritoneal irritation, and a uterus enlarged more than 8 weeks' gestational age.

A chronic ectopic pregnancy occurs when the intraperitoneal hemorrhage associated with tubal abortion or rupture is relatively minor and ceases spontaneously, but the ectopic gestation neither resolves completely nor implants and continues to develop as an abdominal pregnancy. The trophoblast continues to secrete human chorionic gonadotrophin (HCG) in small amounts, with the circulating levels less than 1000 mIU/ml in 50% and less than 100 mIU/ml in 20%. In the series of Cole and Corlett about 6% of all surgically treated ectopic pregnancies in one institution were classified as chronic. The most common (72%) gross pathologic finding was dense adhesions produced by the inflammatory response to the trophoblast. These adhesions attach omentum and bowel to the site of the ectopic pregnancy. In one third of the cases a collection of clotted blood or old hematoma was present. Cole and Corlett reported that because of the extensive disease it is necessary to perform a hysterectomy in 25% and an oophorectomy in 60% of patients with a chronic ovarian ectopic pregnancy.

HISTOPATHOLOGY

When the blastocyst implants in the tube, it does not grow mainly in the tubal lumen as has been assumed for many years. In a recent review of the pathology of tubal gestation, Budowick et al. found that after implanting on the mucosa of the endosalpinx, the trophoblast invades the lamina propria and then the muscularis of the oviduct and grows mainly between the lumen of the tube and its peritoneal covering (Figure 16-11). Growth occurs both parallel to the long axis of the tube and circumferentially around it. As the trophoblast invades vessels, retroperitoneal tubal hemorrhage occurs that is mainly extraluminal but may extrude from the fimbriated end and create a hemoperitoneum before tubal rupture (Figure 16-12).

The stretching of the peritoneum covered by this hemorrhage results in episodic pain before the final perforation into the peritoneal cavity. Rupture occurs when the serosa is maximally

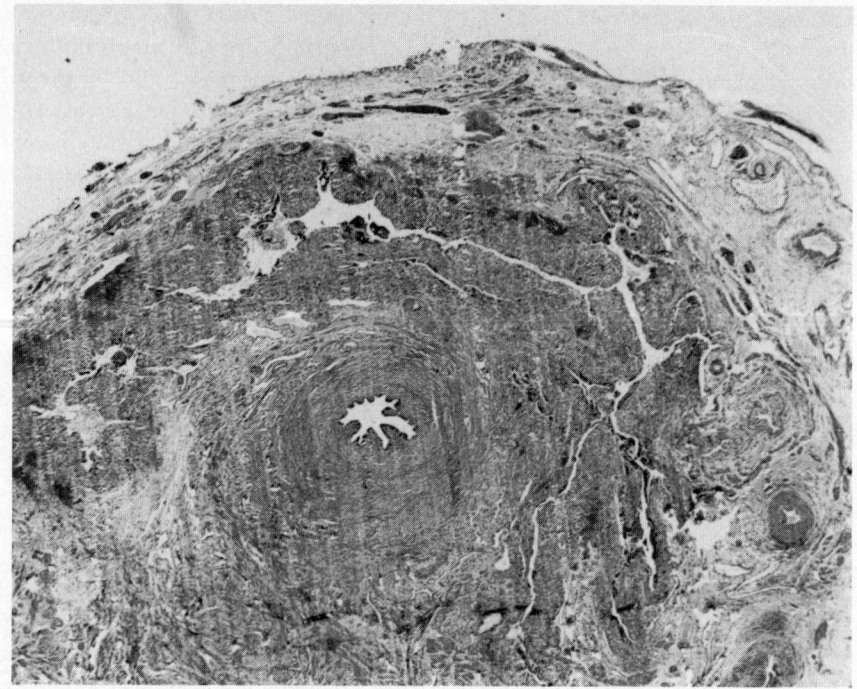

FIGURE 16-11

Low-power photograph showing tube almost completely surrounded by cleftlike space. Closer inspection revealed that cleft was produced by trophoblast that had implanted elsewhere, perforated wall of tube, and was dissecting along broad ligament between tube and peritoneum. (From Budowick M, Johnson TRB, Genadry R, et al: Fertil Steril 34:169, 1980. Reproduced with permission of the publisher, The American Fertility Society.)

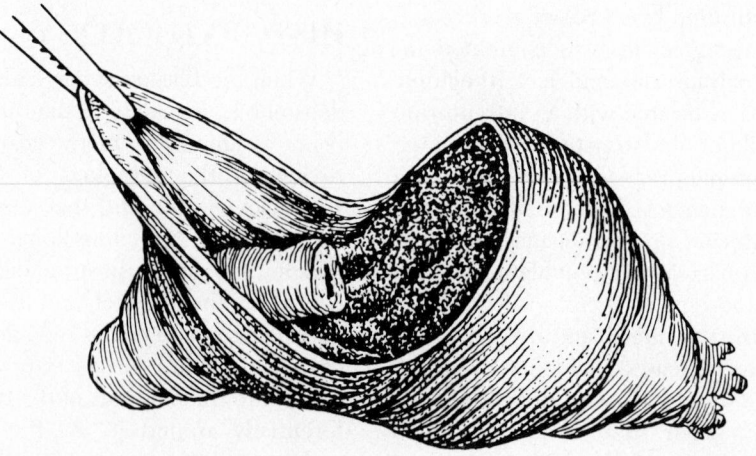

FIGURE 16-12

Artist's rendition of dissected ampullary ectopic pregnancy showing space between tube and peritoneum, revealed when blood clots and placenta were removed. Toward fimbriated end, no dissection was performed and external appearance is that of dilated tube. (From Budowick M, Johnson TRB, Genadry R, et al: Fertil Steril 34:169, 1980. Reproduced with permission of the publisher, The American Fertility Society.)

stretched, producing necrosis secondary to an inadequate blood supply.

Hemoperitoneum is nearly always found in ectopic pregnancy other than that which is cervical in origin. Usually there is a combination of clotted and unclotted blood in the peritoneal cavity. The unclotted blood has not clotted because it results from lysis of blood that has previously coagulated, similar to what occurs during menstrual bleeding. The hematocrit value of this nonclotting blood is nearly always greater than 15%, such a finding being reported in 98% of specimens obtained by culdocentesis in the series of ectopic pregnancies reported by Brenner et al. At the time of laparotomy for a ruptured ectopic pregnancy, about half of the patients have less than 500 ml of hemoperitoneum, one quarter between 500 and 1000 ml, and one fifth more than 1000 ml.

When the oviduct is removed and examined histologically, inflammatory cells are nearly always seen. These include plasma cells, lymphocytes, and histiocytes. Chorionic villi, which are frequently degenerated or hyalinized, as well as nucleated red cells are diagnostic of ectopic pregnancy. Decidual reaction in the tube is uncommon.

Because of limited space or inadequate nourishment, the trophoblastic tissue of most ectopic pregnancies does not grow as rapidly as that of pregnancies within the uterine cavity. As a result, HCG production does not increase as rapidly as in a normal pregnancy, and although steroid production of the corpus luteum is initiated, elevated progesterone levels cannot be maintained. Thus initially the endometrium becomes decidualized because of continued progesterone production by the corpus luteum. Sometimes the secretory cells of the endometrial glands become hypertrophied with hyperchromatism, pleomorphism, and increased mitotic activity, as originally described by Arias-Stella (Figure 16-13). The Arias-Stella reaction can be confused with neoplasia, but it is not unique for ectopic pregnancy, because it can occur with intrauterine pregnancy, as well as after stimulation with clomiphene. In a histologic study of the endometrium in 84 women with ectopic pregnancies, Ollendorff et al. found that about 40% had secretory endometrium with the remaining number about equally diveded among proliferative endometrium, decidual reaction, and Arias-Stella reaction. When progesterone levels fall as a result of insufficient daily increase of HCG, the endometrium is no longer maintained, and it

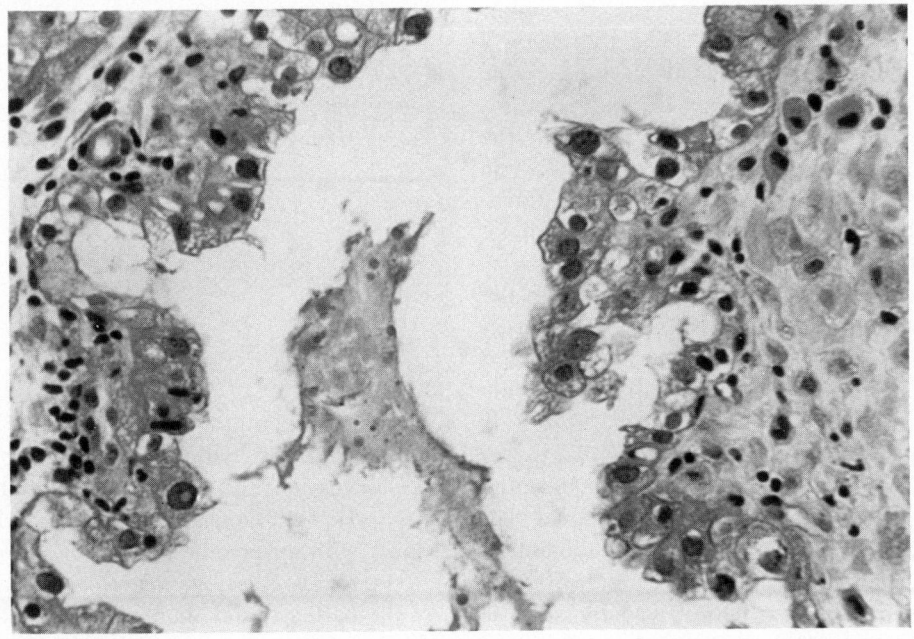

FIGURE 16-13
Arias-Stella reaction. (From DeCherney AH and Maheux R: Curr Probl Obstet Gynecol 6:2, 1983. Reproduced with permission.)

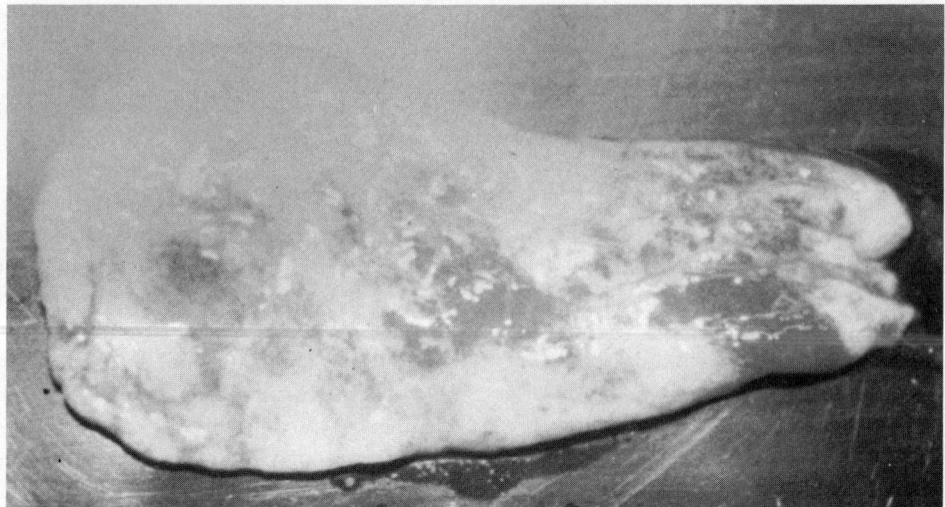

FIGURE 16-14
Decidual cast. (From DeCherney AH and Maheux R: Curr Probl Obstet Gynecol 6:2, 1983. Reproduced with permission.)

sloughs, producing uterine bleeding. Sometimes nearly all the decidua is passed through the cervix intact, producing a decidual cast that may be clinically confused with a spontaneous abortion (Figure 16-14).

SYMPTOMS

The most common symptoms of ectopic pregnancy are abdominal pain, absence of menses, and irregular vaginal bleeding (Table 16-7). Pain is nearly a universal symptom but is not type specific. Before rupture occurs, the pain may be only a vague soreness or colicky in nature. Its location may be generalized, unilateral, or bilateral. Shoulder pain occurs in about one fourth of patients with ectopic pregnancy as a result of diaphragmatic irritation from the hemoperitoneum. During rupture of the pregnancy the pain usually becomes intense, and syncope occurs in about one third of patients with tubal rupture.

The majority of patients with ectopic pregnancy fail to have menses at the expected time but have one or more episodes of irregular vaginal bleeding when the decidual endometrial tissue is sloughed. The interval of amenorrhea is usually 6 weeks or more. The bleeding is usually characterized as spotting but may simulate menstrual bleeding. It is rarely as heavy as that which occurs in spontaneous abortion. Other symptoms include dizziness, an urge to defecate, breast tenderness, and nausea. About

TABLE 16-7
Symptoms of Ectopic Pregnancy

Symptoms	% Patients with Symptom
Abdominal pain	90-100
Amenorrhea	75-95
Vaginal bleeding	50-80
Dizziness, fainting	20-35
Urge to defecate	5-15
Pregnancy symptoms	10-25
Passage of tissue	5-10

From Weckstein LN: Obstet Gynecol Surv 40:259, 1985.

5% to 10% of women will note passage of a decidual cast.

SIGNS

The most common presenting sign is abdominal tenderness, which, together with adnexal tenderness elicited at the time of the bimanual pelvic examination, is present in nearly all patients with an ectopic pregnancy (Table 16-8). It is possible to palpate an adnexal mass in half of the patients, and about one third have some degree of uterine enlargement that is nearly always smaller than a normal 8-week gestation except when interstitial gestation is present. Tachycardia and hypotension can occur after rupture if blood loss is profuse, but tempera-

TABLE 16-8
Signs of Ectopic Pregnancy

Sign	% Patients with Sign
Adnexal tenderness	75-90
Abdominal tenderness	80-95
Adnexal mass*	50
Uterine enlargement	20-30
Orthostatic changes	10-15
Fever	5-10

From Weckstein LN: Obstet Gynecol Surv 40:259, 1985.
*20% present on the side opposite the ectopic pregnancy.

ture elevation is an uncommon finding, being present in only about 5% to 10% of patients, and is rarely greater than 38° C.

DIAGNOSIS

Laboratory Tests

At the time of rupture a hematocrit of less than 30% is found in about one fourth of patients. About half of the patients have a normal leukocyte count, with a mild elevation of 10,000 to 15,000/mm^3 in one third and a greater elevation in one fifth.

HCG is present in the circulation of nearly every patient with an ectopic gestation, but the levels are lower than 3000 mIU/ml in about half. The incidence of positive qualitative pregnancy tests depends on the sensitivity of the assay. With use of the sensitive enzyme-linked immunosorbent assays (ELISA), more than 90% of patients with an ectopic pregnancy will have a positive pregnancy test. This incidence increases to nearly 100% if a radioimmunoassay for HCG is used.

Differential Diagnosis

The diagnosis is usually obvious for patients with the classic symptoms of ruptured ectopic pregnancy: a history of irregular bleeding followed by sudden onset of pain and syncope accompanied by signs of peritoneal irritation. However, before rupture the symptoms and signs are nonspecific and also occur with other gynecologic disorders. Entities frequently confused with ectopic pregnancy include salpingitis, threatened or incomplete abortion, ruptured corpus luteum, appendicitis, dysfunctional uterine bleeding, adnexal torsion, degenerative uterine leiomyoma, and endometriosis.

In the series of Brenner et al., about 50% of the patients with ruptured ectopic pregnancy had at least one medical consultation without the correct diagnosis having been made before the admission when the diagnosis was established. About 33% were seen once, 11% twice, and the remainder three to five times before the diagnosis was made. Other studies have confirmed this high frequency of misdiagnosis and physician delay in determining that an ectopic pregnancy is present. Because of the possibility of a fatal outcome from undiagnosed ruptured ectopic pregnancy, it is essential that the diagnosis of ectopic pregnancy be considered in any woman of childbearing age with abdominal pain and irregular menstrual bleeding even if she has had a previous tubal sterilization procedure or is wearing an IUD.

Establishment of Diagnosis

Ectopic pregnancy should be suspected in any patient who develops the symptoms just listed, particularly if she has previously had a pelvic operation, especially tubal operation, whether it was a tubal reconstructive procedure or a sterilization procedure. Other risk factors include one or more episodes of salpingitis, a previous ectopic gestation, current use of an IUD, use of a progestin-only oral contraceptive, use of pharmacologic methods of ovulation induction, as well as a prior history of infertility. In any patient with the symptoms of ectopic gestation the diagnosis is facilitated by a sensitive assay for HCG and pelvic ultrasonography and can be established by laparoscopy or laparotomy. Culdocentesis and measurement of serum progesterone levels may also be of assistance.

Culdocentesis

The finding of nonclotting blood, especially if the hematocrit is above 15%, is of great diagnostic assistance in establishing the diagnosis of ectopic pregnancy. In the literature review of Cartwright et al. of nearly 5000 ectopic pregnancies, a positive finding at culdocentesis was reported to be present between 70% and 97% of the time, with most series reporting a positive finding at culdocentesis in more than 90% of ectopic pregnancies. A positive finding at culdocentesis indicates hemoperitoneum. This may be caused by other pathologic conditions, most frequently a hemorrhagic corpus luteum or upper abdominal pathology. However, about 85% of patients with hemoperitoneum suspected of having an ectopic pregnancy do have one. The finding of nonclotting blood at the time of culdocentesis does not always indicate that rupture of the ectopic pregnancy has occurred, as mentioned previously. Finally, hemoperitoneum can occur without causing symptoms or signs of peritoneal irritation.

Human Chorionic Gonadotrophin

Although a negative qualitative urine test for HCG does not rule out ectopic pregnancy, if a sensitive ELISA is negative, the diagnosis is unlikely. If β-HCG is not detected with use of radioimmunoassay of serum, the diagnosis of ectopic pregnancy can, with a rare exception, be ruled out. Although about 85% of women with ectopic pregnancy have serum HCG levels lower than those seen in normal pregnancy at a similar gestational age, a single quantitative HCG assay usually cannot be used to diagnose ectopic pregnancy because the actual dates of ovulation and conception are not known for most women. Even if the date of ovulation is known, 10% of women with normal gestations will have HCG levels lower than the normal 90% confidence limits. Furthermore, low HCG levels are found also in women with various stages of spontaneous abortion, conditions which must be considered in the differential diagnosis.

In normal pregnancies in early gestation the levels of circulating HCG double about every 2 days. In abnormal pregnancies (ectopic gestations and those destined to abort), HCG levels usually do not increase at the same rate. Kadar et al. reported that if the percentage increase in HCG during a 2-day period is less than 66%, the chance that the patient has an abnormal pregnancy is high (Table 16-9). In their series only 15% of normal pregnancies failed to have this amount of increase and only 13% of ectopic pregnancies had this normal rate of increase.

Cartwright and DiPietro reported that of 25 patients with surgically treated ectopic pregnancies and serial HCG levels, 20 showed a plateau or decrease in HCG levels over a 48-hour period or longer before surgical excision (Figure 16-15).

Romero et al. reported that 90% of patients with ectopic pregnancies had one of two main patterns of serial HCG values. About half had

TABLE 16-9
Lower Normal Limits of Percentage Increase of Serum HCG during Early Pregnancy

Sampling Interval (Days)	Increase in HCG (%)
1	29
2	66
3	114
4	175
5	255

From Kadar N, Caldwell BV, and Romero R: Obstet Gynecol 58:162, 1981. Reprinted with permission from The American College of Obstetricians and Gynecologists.

falling HCG levels and the other half had a subnormal rate of increase with a slope of less than 0.11 (correspondingly to a 66% increase in 48 hours and a 114% increase in 3 days). Thus the sensitivity of measuring serial HCG levels to diagnose ectopic pregnancy compared with an intrauterine pregnancy is 90%. However, the false positive rate of intrauterine pregnancies with a subnormal slope was 12.5%. Kratzer and Taylor reported similar results when comparing the rates of HCG increase in ectopic and intrauterine pregnancies, but no differentiation between ectopic pregnancies and spontaneous abortion could be made with this technique (Figure 16-16). Lindblom et al. reported a refinement of this technique that increased the positive predictive value of diagnosing ectopic pregnancy to 95%. In their series of patients presenting with symptoms or a history suspicious of ectopic pregnancy, all women with subsequent falling HCG titers were excluded. Only those whose initial HCG titers were between 10 and 4000 mIU/ml were included as about 4000 mIU/ml ultrasonography aids in the diagnosis. An HCG score was calculated for each patient by plotting the slope of the rise of HCG against the initial level (Figure 16-17). With this modified technique, 18 of 19 ectopic pregnancies and 21 of 22 intrauterine pregnancies were currently identified prospectively, reflecting a high degree of accuracy. Thus serial HCG measurements aid in the early diagnosis of unruptured ectopic gestation.

PROGESTERONE

Since a single HCG determination does not provide sufficient information to diagnose ec-

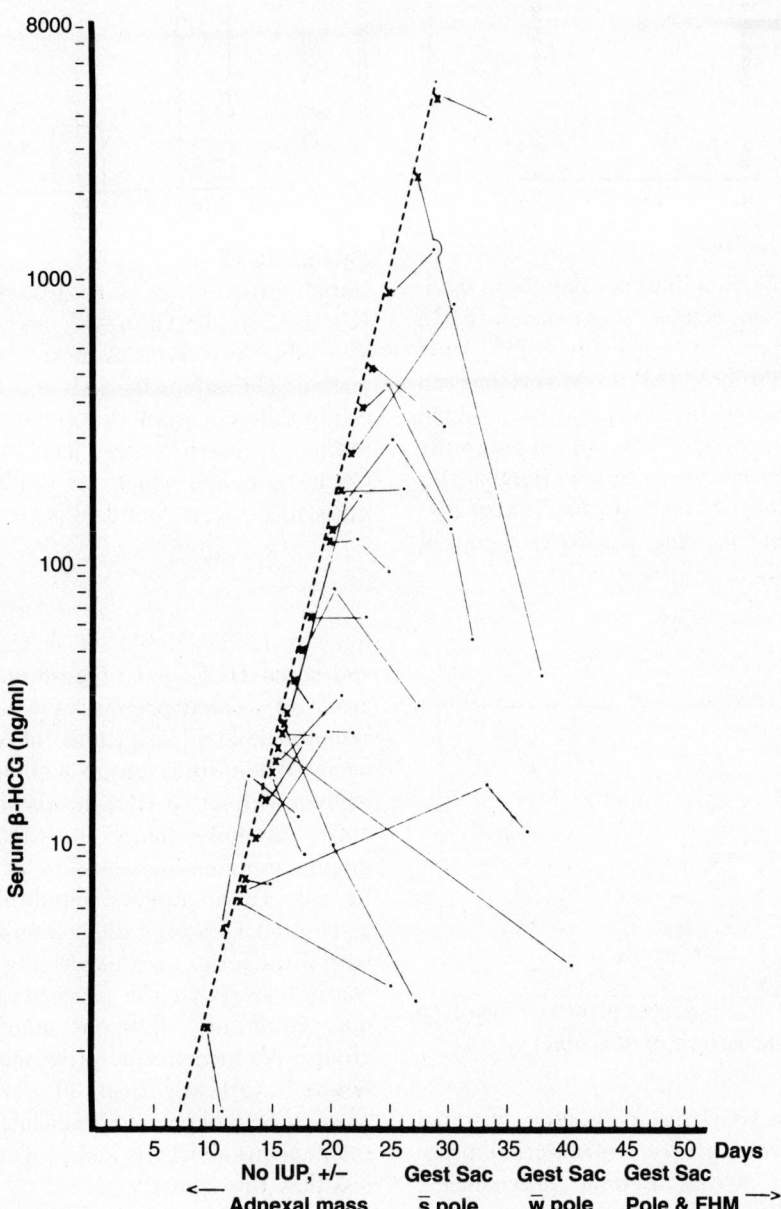

FIGURE 16-15

Serial quantitated serum β-HCG levels for 25 patients with ectopic pregnancy. Broken line represents average HCG progression for first 30 days of normal pregnancy, with corresponding sonographic findings below. Each patient's first determined value is arbitrarily placed on standard line. (From Cartwright PS and DiPietro DL: Obstet Gynecol 63:76, 1984. Reprinted with permission from The American College of Obstetricians and Gynecologists.)

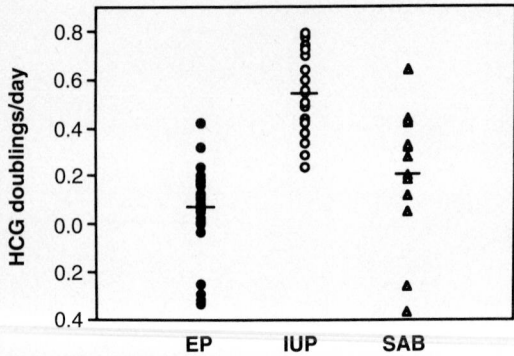

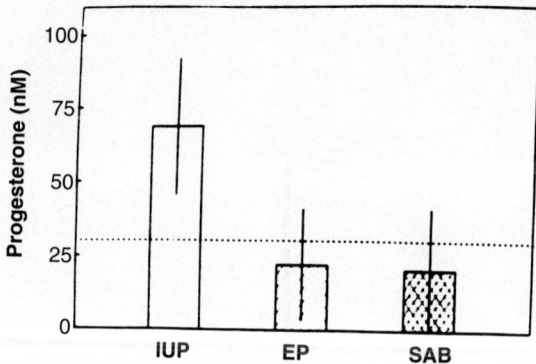

FIGURE 16-16
Number of HCG doublings per day for individual samples from ectopic pregnancies (EP●), normal intrauterine pregnancies (IUP⁰), and spontaneous abortions (SAB Δ). Means for each group are indicated by horizontal bars. Mean rate for ectopic pregnancies was significantly less than that for intrauterine pregnancies ($p<0.05$, by Student t test). (From Kratzer PG, Taylor RN, et al: Am J Obstet Gynecol 163:1497, 1990.)

FIGURE 16-18
Initial serum level of progesterone in viable IUP (n=24), in SAB (n=37), and in EP (n=97). The values are given as means ± standard deviation. The values for SAB and EP are significantly different from IUP ($P<0.001$). The dotted line is discriminatory level of progesterone (30 nM), below which no viable intrauterine pregnancies were found.

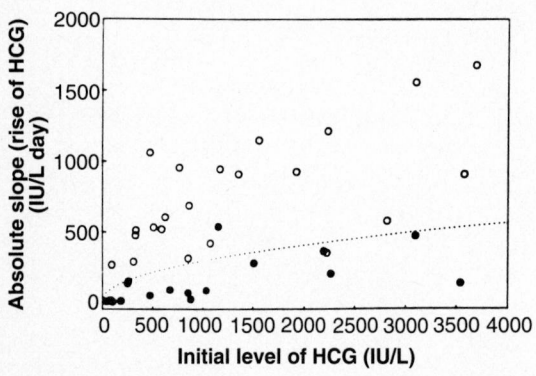

FIGURE 16-17
Slope of serum HCG rise as function of initial HCG level. *Open circles*, Intrauterine pregnancies. *Filled circles*, Ectopic pregnancies. *Dotted line*, Discriminatory function (see text). (From Lindblom B, Hahlin M, Sjoblom P, et al: Am J Obstet Gynecol 161: 397, 1989.)

topic pregnancy because of the inability to determine gestational age with precision, and serial determinations require a 2- to 3-day delay, several investigators have reported that measurement of a single serum progesterone value is of help in establishing the diagnosis of ec-

topic gestation. Hahlin et al. measured initial and serial HCG and progesterone levels in a group of women presenting with a history of symptomatology suspicious of ectopic pregnancy. Their study group included only those women with initial HCG levels between 20 and 4000 mIU/ml—those in whom ultrasonographic examination would be of least diagnostic aid. These authors found that the initial level of HCG did not differ from that of women with intrauterine pregnancy (Figure 16-18). In contrast to HCG, the progesterone slope was not significantly different among the three groups. No intrauterine pregnancy had progesterone levels less than 30 nM/L (10ng/ml), whereas 88% of ectopic pregnancies and 83% of spontaneous abortions had progesterone values less than this amount.

Sauer et al. found that measurement of pregnanediol glucuronide in a single random urine specimen by a rapid enzyme immunoassay was also very useful to differentiate ectopic from intrauterine pregnancy when a level of 9 ug/ml was used to discriminate the two entities. In their study, this single rapid assay was as effective as measurement of serum progesterone in distinguishing ectopic from intrauterine pregnancies between 5 and 8 weeks from the onset of the last menses (Table 16-10).

TABLE 16-10

Applicability of a Single Random Test for Detecting Ectopic Gestations Based on Normal Pregnancies Representing Positive Pregnancy Tests*

		Serum β-hCG (%)	Serum progesterone (%)	Urinary pregnanediol-3α-glucuronide (%)
Sensitivity	(TP/TP + FN)	100	94	100
Specificity	(TN/TN + FP)	93	68	75
Predictive value	(+) test (TP/TP + FP)	87	63	69
Predictive value	(−) test (TN/TN + FN)	100	95	100
Efficiency	(TP+TN) TOTAL	96	78	84

From Sauer MV et al: Am J Obstet Gynecol 159:1531, 1988.
TP, True positive; *TN*, true negative; *FP*, false positive; *FN*, false negative.
*Serum progesterone ≥10 ng/ml; urinary pregnanediol-3α-glucuronide ≥9 μg/ml; and serum HCG within the 95% confidence interval of normal value for a specific gestational age)

ULTRASONOGRAPHY

With the use of abdominal ultrasonography, Kadar et al. reported in 1981 that if the HCG level was greater than 6500 mIU/ml and no gestational sac was seen in the uterus, nearly all the patients had an ectopic pregnancy. However, this technique was not clinically useful, because about 90% of women with ectopic pregnancies had HCG levels below this threshold.

Development of the transvaginal transducer probes with 5.0 to 7.0 MHz scanning frequency has enabled more precise imaging of the pelvic organs in the early pregnancy than is possible with transabdominal ultrasonography. With these probes it is nearly always possible to identify a gestational sac in the uterus before the HCG level reaches 2500 mIU/ml (1st International Reference Preparation [1st IRP]), about 5 to 6 weeks after the last menses. Because combined extrauterine and intrauterine pregnancy is a rare event, the finding of an intrauterine gestational sac should nearly always exclude the presence of an ectopic pregnancy. When a gestational sac is not present and the HCG level is more than 2500 mIU/ml, a pathologic pregnancy—either an ectopic or a blighted ovum—should be suspected. Usually an adnexal mass and/or a gestational saclike structure can be identified in the oviduct when an ectopic pregnancy that produces levels of HCG above 2500 mIU/ml is present (Figure 16-19).

Kivitoski and Martin evaluated a series of pa-

tients with suspected ectopic pregnancy by both transabdominal and transvaginal ultrasonography and found that the latter technique was significantly more accurate in identifying an adnexal gestational sac—64% for transvaginal and 33% for transabdominal—when an early ectopic pregnancy was present. Shapiro et al. reported rates of identifying an adnexal mass to be 91% and 50% respectively with the two techniques.

Thus diagnostic criteria for the ultrasonographic diagnosis of ectopic pregnancy include the detection of an adnexal mass and/or the absence of a gestational sac with use of currently available vaginal transducers, when the HCG level is above a certain threshold, about 2500 mIU/ml.

Both Timor-Tritsch and Cacciatore et al. have reported the diagnosis of ectopic pregnancy with this technique has an excellent sensitivity and specificity—more than 97%—with a positive and negative predictive value of more than 98%. About two thirds of women presenting with symptoms of ectopic pregnancy have HCG levels above 2500 mIU/ml, and the diagnosis can usually be reliably made with ultrasonography. For the other one third with lower HCG levels, unless a gestational sac is evident on ultrasonography, other diagnostic techniques, such as serial HCG determination, should be performed. Repeat ultrasonographic examinations at 3- to 5-day intervals are often helpful in establishing a correct diagnosis.

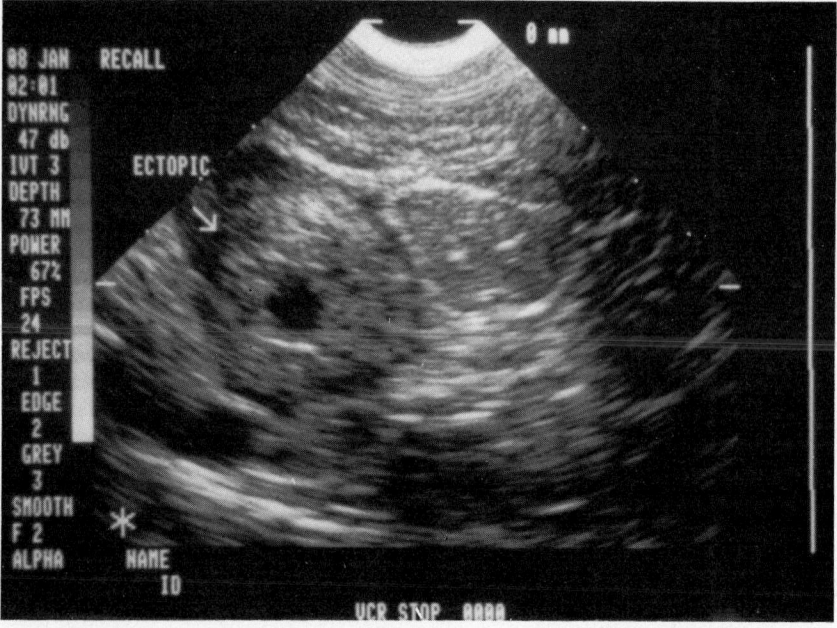

FIGURE 16-19
Ultrasound of ectopic pregnancy. (Photo Courtesy Advanced Technology Laboratories, Bothell, Washington, 1991.)

Dilation and Curettage

If the gestational age is known to exceed 5 weeks and HCG is present and no intrauterine gestational sac is seen with ultrasonography, a curettage with histologic examination of the scrapings, by frozen section if desired, can be undertaken to determine if any products of gestation are present in the uterus. If no chorionic villi are visualized in the scrapings, laparoscopy should be performed to establish the diagnosis of ectopic pregnancy. The finding of a decidual reaction or the Arias-Stella reaction in the scrapings cannot establish the diagnosis of ectopic pregnancy, because these findings can also appear with intrauterine gestation and have been reported to occur in only about half of the patients with ectopic gestation.

Laparoscopy

A definitive diagnosis of ectopic pregnancy can nearly always be made by direct visualization of the pelvis with laparoscopy. However, sometimes because of hemoperitoneum, adhesions, or obesity, it is difficult to visualize the pelvic organs. In a study by Samuellson and Sjovall, 4 of 166 ectopic pregnancies were not visualized by the laparoscopist, and 6 of 120 patients with an intrauterine pregnancy were

thought to have ectopic pregnancies. Thus there is a 2% to 5% chance of a false positive or false negative diagnosis with laparoscopy. If sufficient hemoperitoneum is present to prevent adequate laparoscopic visualization, exploratory laparotomy should be performed.

Clinical Evaluation of Patients with Suspected Ectopic Pregnancy

Flow sheets have been developed by several authors to aid the clinician in the diagnosis of the patient with ectopic pregnancy who is not hypotensive and requires immediate laparotomy. They involve the use of ultrasonography and serial quantitative HCG assays. These diagnostic aids are of particular use in following an asymptomatic patient, beginning shortly after conception if the patient is at high risk for ectopic pregnancy, such as when she has had a prior ectopic pregnancy or distal tubal infertility surgery. Performing a quantitative HCG assay twice weekly and calculating the rate of increase, as well as performing ultrasonography beginning 3 weeks after ovulation, will help to establish the diagnosis of ectopic pregnancy before tubal rupture. The combination of these two techniques is particularly applicable to stable patients treated in institutions with adequate facilities for ultrasound and serial quantitative Beta HCG assays.

However, when ultrasonography is not immediately available for the patient who develops symptoms of an ectopic pregnancy that are of sufficient magnitude to require emergency care, a sensitive qualitative pregnancy test and culdocentesis are usually all the diagnostic aids necessary to establish the diagnosis. If both these tests are positive, it is most likely that an ectopic pregnancy is present, and laparoscopy or laparotomy or both should be performed, depending on the findings of the physical examination. For the patient with a positive finding at culdocentesis and a negative quantitative HCG assay, the diagnosis of ruptured corpus luteum is likely, and the patient should have either a laparoscopy or radioimmunoassay for HCG, depending on her clinical condition.

The patient with a negative finding at culdocentesis and a positive qualitative HCG assay will benefit most from ultrasound and serial quantitative HCG assays. If an ectopic pregnancy is not diagnosed by ultrasound, she must still be warned that she may have an ectopic pregnancy and be prepared to enter the hospital quickly if her symptoms suddenly worsen.

MANAGEMENT

Surgical Therapy

The treatment of ectopic gestations in uncommon locations other than the oviduct was discussed earlier in the chapter (see "Pathology"). An interstitial pregnancy, because it usually becomes symptomatic at a late gestational age, is usually large and may require hysterectomy. Otherwise a resection of the cornual region of the uterus may be sufficient. On occasion, tubal gestations abort through the fimbriated end of the oviduct or regress spontaneously without symptoms; however, the vast majority require surgical treatment, which can be either a radical or a conservative procedure. If the pregnancy has produced rupture of the oviduct and has involved the entire oviduct or if no further pregnancies are desired, radical tubal operation is usually performed. Radical operation consists of salpingectomy with or without accompanying oophorectomy or hysterectomy. It was previously advocated that an elective ipsilateral oophorectomy be performed in a woman wishing future fertility, theoreti-

cally to increase the chance of conception and reduce the chance of another ectopic pregnancy by having ovulation occur each month from the ovary proximal to the remaining tube. Results from various studies yield conflicting data. Some studies report similar conception rates in women treated with salpingectomy and salpingo-oophorectomy, whereas others report higher pregnancy rates in women having the ovary removed, and still others report lower subsequent pregnancy rates in women having the ovary removed. Because the subsequent ectopic pregnancy rate in these studies was not decreased when oophorectomy was performed and because the number of eggs available for the in vitro fertilization procedure is greater with two ovaries, it is best not to remove the ipsilateral ovary unless its involvement in the pathologic process technically necessitates its removal.

Removal of the uterus may sometimes be indicated if another disease, such as leiomyoma, is present. On occasion a hysterectomy can be performed if the woman has undergone a prior tubal sterilization and develops a tubal pregnancy. However, because of the increased operating time and morbidity associated with hysterectomy, as well as the need for extensive preoperative counseling, elective hysterectomy should usually not be performed at the time of laparotomy for ectopic pregnancy.

Resection of the distal portion of the interstitial oviduct, commonly called a cornual resection, is frequently performed at the time of salpingectomy, but the procedure is unnecessary because it does not prevent a subsequent interstitial pregnancy. Of the 75 cases of interstitial pregnancy after homolateral salpingectomy reported by Kalchman and Meltzer, 20% had been preceded by a cornual resection. In Hallatt's series of repeat ectopic pregnancies, 8 of 10 ruptured homolateral interstitial pregnancies were preceded by deep cornual resection. Thus cornual resection does not prevent a subsequent interstitial pregnancy, and if it is performed, it should be only superficial.

Although a colpotomy incision has been used to perform salpingectomy in an unruptured tubal pregnancy, as well as to aid in establishing the diagnosis, because of the extensive use of laparoscopy for diagnosis, this incision is used infrequently.

Conservative treatment (not removing the oviduct) for an unruptured ectopic pregnancy is being used with increasing frequency for women who desire future fertility. When conservative surgery is correctly performed for an unruptured ectopic pregnancy, the repeat ectopic pregnancy rate is not increased compared with that of salpingectomy, whereas the subsequent live birth rate is increased. The techniques used include salpingotomy, salpingostomy, fimbrial evacuation, and partial salpingectomy, also called *segmental resection* of the portion of the oviduct containing the ectopic pregnancy. Fimbrial evacuation of the gestational products by digital expression or blunt curettage traumatizes the endosalpinx and has a high rate of recurrent ectopic pregnancy (24%), about twice as high as the rate after salpingectomy. In addition, this procedure may not remove the tubal gestation, and another operative procedure may be required a few days later. The best results of conservative operation occur after salpingotomy or salpingostomy. The latter technique is used more frequently in the United States (Figure 16-20).

These techniques can be performed for the vast majority of unruptured tubal pregnancies not located in the isthmic portion of the oviduct. It is best to use microsurgical principles when performing salpingostomy, and when the unruptured pregnancy is small (less than 5 cm), it is possible to perform the salpingostomy with a laparoscopic procedure. Results of a prospective randomized trial of treatment of unruptured ectopic gestation by linear salpingostomy performed by either laparoscopy or laparotomy was reported by Vermesh et al. Treatment with either of these techniques was similarly safe and effective, but the estimated blood loss and length of hospital stay were both significantly less in the group treated by laparoscopy. After salpingostomy, because persistence of trophoblast tissue has been reported in a small percentage of women treated in this manner, serial quantitative HCG assays should be performed postoperatively. If hemostasis cannot be maintained after a salpingostomy, which frequently occurs for those unruptured pregnancies located in the isthmus, a segmental resection of the oviduct can be performed and a reanastomosis done a few months later. Timonen and Nieminen reported that women who had a

FIGURE 16-20
A, Incision is made into the antimesenteric border of the fallopian tube. **B**, Ectopic pregnancy is gently removed from within the fallopian tube. **C**, Salpingostomy site is allowed to heal by secondary intention. **D**, Salpingotomy is completed by primary closure. (From Leach RE and Ory SJ: J Reprod Med 34:325, 1989.)

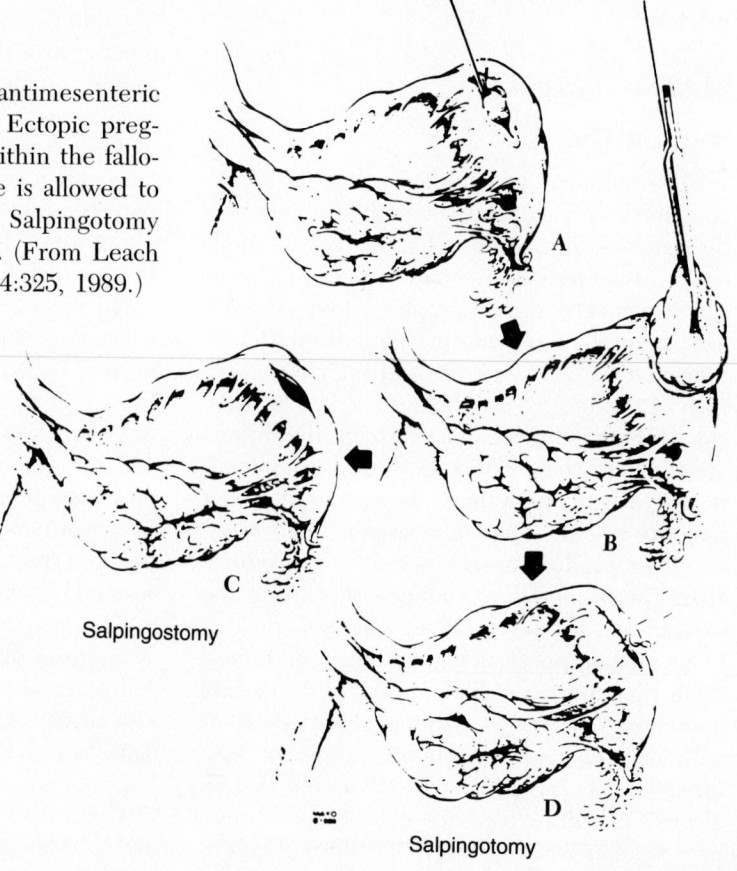

Salpingostomy

Salpingotomy

segmental resection had a lower subsequent term pregnancy rate (17%) than women who had salpingectomy (29%). Therefore DeCherney and Maheux recommended that a partial salpingectomy be performed only if salpingostomy is impossible and the contralateral oviduct is absent or irrevocably damaged.

In his review of the conservative management of ectopic gestation, Vermesh presented a useful flow sheet developed to guide the clinician (Figure 16-21).

Medical Therapy

In 1982 Tanaka et al. reported the successful use of methotrexate in a patient with an unruptured interstitial pregnancy. In 1987 Ichinoe et al. reported the use of methotrexate in 23 patients with unruptured tubal pregnancies. Methotrexate was given in 5-day courses every other week until the HCG titer fell to 20 mIU/ml. The total dosage ranged from 60 to 300 mg. Of the 23, only 1 required subsequent laparotomy, and tubal patency was observed in 10 of 19 who had a subsequent hysterosalpingogram and/or laparoscopy. Several other investigators

have been using this technique with a careful research protocol involving the use of systemic methotrexate in combination with citrovorum factor. As summarized by Leach and Ory, of 83 patients who were treated with methotrexate for tubal gestation, 7% required subsequent surgical intervention and about 25% had some degree of toxicity. Patency rates of the affected tube after surgery were 70%. Stovall et al. used an individualized reduced dose of methotrexate and citrovorum factor after establishing the diagnosis of unruptured ectopic pregnancy at the time of laparoscopy. Of 36 patients who were treated, 2 required a subsequent laparotomy and 3 experienced toxic side effects. The major disadvantage with this therapy was a prolonged response time. Results of subsequent fertility rates and data regarding fetal wastage or abnormal subsequent pregnancies have not bee reported to date. For these reasons the use of systemic methotrexate must still be regarded as experimental.

To avoid high doses and prolonged courses of systemic administration of methotrexate, some investigators have been injecting from 12.5 to 100 mg of methotrexate diluted in 2 to 4 ml of

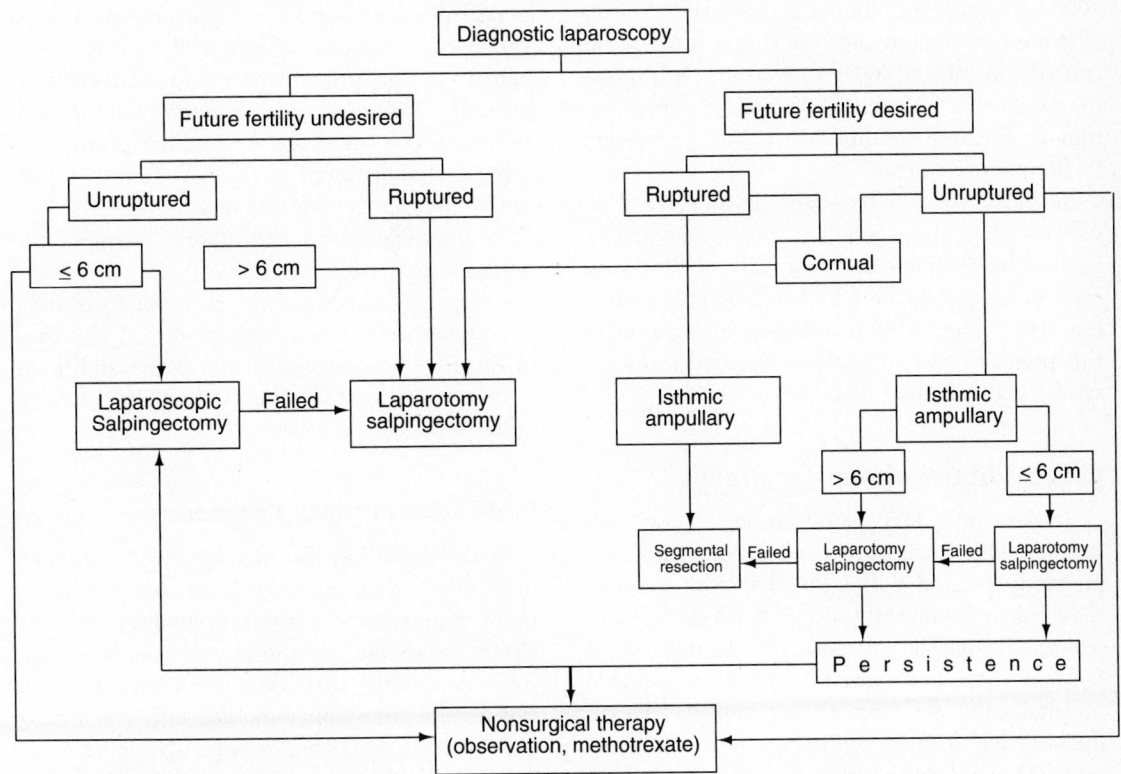

FIGURE 16-21
Conservative management of ectopic gestation. (From Vermesh M: Fertil Steril 51:559, 1989.)

saline directly into the ectopic gestational sac at the time of laparoscopy. In a series of 27 patients receiving such treatment reported by Pansky et al. only 3 required subsequent laparoscopy because of rising HCG levels. The HCG titers declined normally in the other 21, but the decline was slow in some, taking 5 weeks to drop 10 mIU/ml. Kooi and Kock reported similar good results with rapidly falling HCG titers in 17 of 24 patients. One had a tubal rupture 3 days after laparoscopy. The remaining 7 had plateauing HCG levels after the procedure and received systemic methotrexate, after which their titers fell. Of 14 patients who wished to subsequently conceive and were followed, 9 had intrauterine gestations and none had repeat ectopic pregnancies. To avoid any toxic effects of methotrexate, Lingblom et al. and others had injected small amounts of prostaglandin $F_2\alpha$ diluted in 3 to 10 ml of saline into small, unruptured ectopic gestations at the time of diagnostic laparoscopy. In nearly all patients so treated, HCG titers fell rapidly and there were no reports of tubal rupture. Best results with this technique were obtained when the diameter of the tubal gestation was less than 2 cm and the HCG titer was less than 1000 mIU/ml. Lindblom et al. followed a group of women so treated and reported a subsequent conception rate of 90%, with a 60% intrauterine pregnancy rate and a 30% rate of repeat ectopics. Further studies with this promising technique are warranted.

Recently there have been case reports in which cervical pregnancy was successfully treated by systemic methotrexate. Other case reports have indicated that angiographic uterine artery embolization allowed evacuation of this pregnancy to be easily performed transcervically with minimal blood loss.

Observation without Treatment

As late as 1955 Lund reported on 119 women with unruptured tubal pregnancy expectantly treated with only bed rest and frequent observation. Of these 119, 68 (57%) were eventually discharged from the hospital without operation, but about 60% of them required hospitalization for more than 1 month. The remainder had a tubal rupture or required operative intervention for other reasons. The subsequent fertility rates were similar in the group treated surgically and those requiring no fur-

ther operation. In 1982 Mashiach et al. reported that if at the time of the initial laparoscopy a small unruptured tubal pregnancy was found and that if serial HCG levels subsequently fell, it was possible to avoid surgical therapy, although they performed a repeat laparoscopy before discharge.

In 1987 Garcia et al. followed a group of 13 women with suspected ectopic pregnancy who were clinically stable, had elevated but falling HCG levels, and had a cyanotic intact tubal mass less than 4 cm in diameter visualized at the time of laparoscopy. The women were hospitalized for a minimum of 5 days, and daily ultrasonography and serum HCG measurements were obtained. Of the 13, 9 had steadily falling HCG levels and were discharged 5 days after laparoscopy. Of the remaining 4, 3 remained asymptomatic but their HCG titers remained level for as long as 3 weeks and then declined; the fourth woman, whose HCG also plateaued, developed increased abdominal pain 9 days after laparoscopy and had a salpingectomy performed. The majority of these women had a subsequent normal hysterosalpingogram or visualization of grossly normal oviducts at the time of a second laparoscopy 6 months later. Fernandez and Rainhorn reported that 4 of 14 women with small, unruptured ectopic pregnancies at the time of laparoscopy observed expectedly required subsequent reoperation. Whether this rigid and expensive protocol of ectopic management results in better subsequent pregnancy rates than removing the ectopic pregnancy by a laparoscopic linear salpingoplasty awaits further study.

At present it is considered better to remove the unruptured ectopic pregnancy at the time of the first laparoscopy to avoid the additional expense of hospitalization, serial HCG assays, and a second laparoscopy.

Persistent Ectopic Pregnancy

With increasing use of conservative modalities rather than salpingectomy for the treatment of unwanted ectopic pregnancy, the entity of persistent ectopic gestation is becoming more commonly seen. Manifestations of persistent ectopic pregnancy include either acute abdominal symptoms and/or a persistent or rising HCG titer after conservative treatment of an unruptured ectopic gestation. In several reports the incidence of persistent ectopic preg-

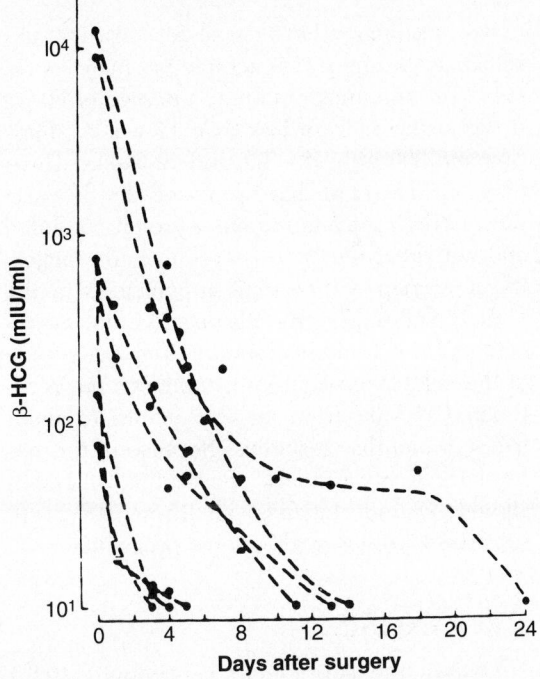

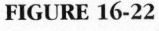

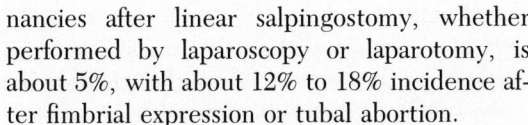

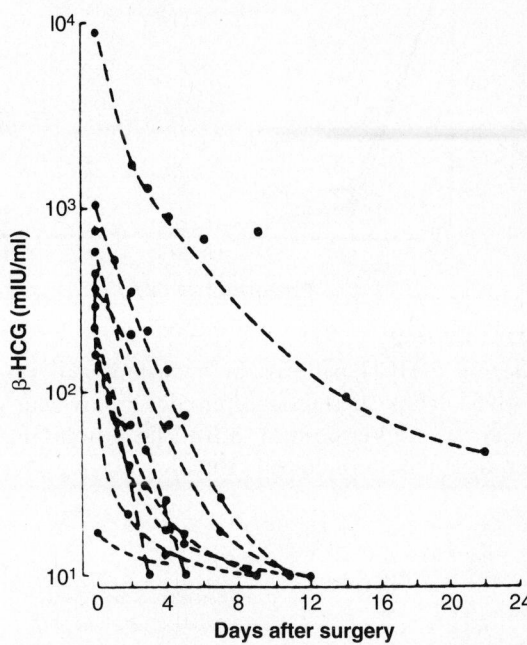

FIGURE 16-22
Serial serum levels of β-HCG in the postoperative period in patients treated with either salpingectomy or partial resection of the fallopian tube. (From Kamrava MM, Taymor M, et al: Obstet Gynecol 62:486, 1983.)

FIGURE 16-23
Serial serum levels of β-HCG in the postoperative period in patients treated with either linear salpingostomy or fimbrial expression. (From Kamrava MM, Taymor M, Berger MJ, et al: Obstet Gynecol 62:486, 1983.)

nancies after linear salpingostomy, whether performed by laparoscopy or laparotomy, is about 5%, with about 12% to 18% incidence after fimbrial expression or tubal abortion.

Stock reviewed the histologic finding of five women with persistent ectopic gestation treated by subsequent salpingectomy. He observed that in all five instances the implantation sites in the oviduct were medial to the previous surgical incision site, indicating the site of the previous surgical incision was medial to the maximally dilated area of the tube where the salpingostomy incision was made.

Kamrava et al. studied the disappearance rate of HCG in 2 patients with ectopic pregnancy treated by salpingectomy or partial resection (Figure 16-22) compared with 9 patients treated by linear salpingostomy or fimbrial expression (Figure 16-23). With one exception, in each group the disappearance curve of HCG was similar to that reported after other pregnancy terminations: an initial rapid component followed by a slow component. The dura-

tion of detectable HCG in serum is directly related to the initial titer and can remain detectable for as long as 1 month.

Lundorff et al. reported that risk factors for persistent ectopic gestation include a preoperative HCG level above 3000 mIU/ml and/or an HCG level above 1000 mIU/ml 7 days after surgery. Vermesh et al. measured both HCG and progesterone preoperatively and every 3 days after conservative tubal surgery for an unruptured ectopic gestation in a group of 114 women. Of these 114, 6 (5.3%) had persistent ectopic gestation. All 6 had an initial sharp drop in HCG levels to 25% of pretreatment 6 days after surgery, similar to the remainder of the group who did not have persistent ectopic gestation. After 6 days, titers of the former group plateaued or rose slightly (Figure 16-24). Progesterone levels showed the same type of pattern (Figure 16-25).

Based on these data, persistent ectopic gestation is likely if a day 12 serum HCG is more than 10% of the initial level and/or a day 9 se-

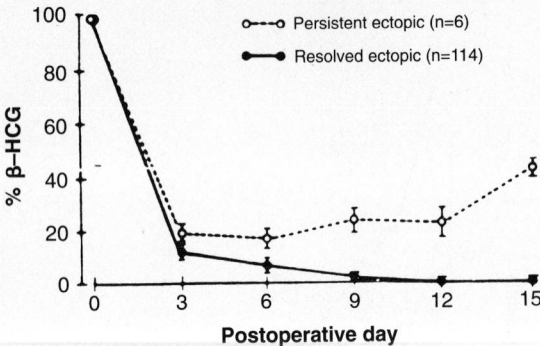

FIGURE 16-24

Serum β-HCG patterns in persistent and resolved ectopic gestations after conservative surgery. (From Vermesh M, Silva PD, Rosen GF, et al: Fertil Steril 50:584, 1988.)

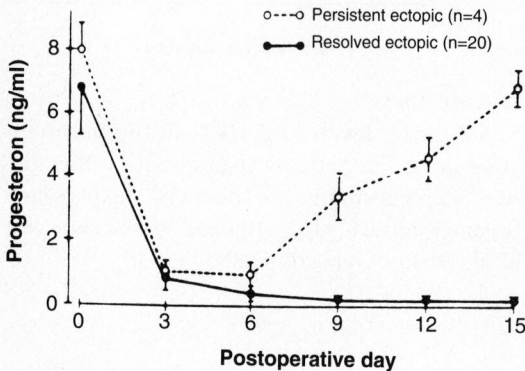

FIGURE 16-25

Serum progesterone patterns in persistent and resolved ectopic gestations after conservative surgery. (From Vermesh M, Silva PD, Rosen GF, et al: Fertil Steril 50:584, 1988.)

rum progesterone is higher than 1.5 μg/ml. They recommended that HCG or progesterone be measured initially on day 6 postoperatively and at 3-day intervals thereafter. Increasing levels of these hormones beyond day 6 are suggestive of persistent ectopic gestation.

Methods used to treat this condition include salpingectomy, salpingostomy, methotrexate, or expectant management. Expectant management is usually reserved for the asymptomatic patient whose titers do not rise. Surgical management, either by laparoscopy or laparotomy, is reserved for those patients who become symptomatic and/or whose HCG titers rise.

Rh Factor

It is recommended that all Rh-negative, unsensitized women with ectopic pregnancies receive Rh immunoglobulin at a dosage of 50 μg if the gestation is of less than 12 weeks' duration and 300 μg if it is beyond 12 weeks. However, Grimes et al. have reported that because most of their hospitalizations were unscheduled and not preceded by Rh screening, the majority of women with ectopic pregnancies in the United States who are Rh negative do not receive Rh(D) immunoglobulin. The magnitude of the risk of sensitization is unknown but is estimated to vary from nil at 1 month to about 9% at 3 months' gestation. Because of the potential benefits and lack of risk, this treatment should be undertaken in all Rh-negative, unsensitized women with ectopic pregnancy.

PROGNOSIS

Overall the subsequent conception rate in women with an ectopic pregnancy is about 60%. A little less than half of these pregnancies terminate in another ectopic pregnancy or spontaneous abortion, so only about one third of women with an ectopic pregnancy have a subsequent live birth. However, these general figures are modified by several factors, particularly age, parity, evidence of contralateral tubal disease, whether the ectopic material is ruptured, and use of an IUD (Table 16-11). Makinen et al. reported that if a woman was using an IUD at the time of ectopic pregnancy, her subsequent fertility rate was normal and she had no increased risk of a subsequent ectopic pregnancy. The subsequent fertility rate is significantly higher in parous women under the age of 30. However, if the ectopic pregnancy occurs in a woman's first pregnancy, her subsequent conception rate is only about 35%. On the other hand, women with high parity (more than three deliveries) who develop an ectopic pregnancy have a relatively high rate of conception (≈80%). The subsequent conception rate is lower in women who have had a history of salpingitis as well as in those who have gross evidence of damage to the opposite oviduct as a result of previous salpingitis. Future fertility is significantly higher in women who have an unruptured tubal pregnancy than in those with a ruptured ectopic pregnancy so that early diagnosis with serial HCG and ultrasound is desirable. In the report of Sherman et al., whereas only 65% of patients with a ruptured

TABLE 16-11
Factors Significantly Associated with Postoperative Fertility of 151 Patients with Primary Ectopic Pregnancy

Factor	Fertile Patients b (No. = 114)	Infertile Patients c (No. = 37)	Significant Difference (P)
Mean age (years ± SD)	26.2 ± 4.7	28.0 ± 4.4	<0.05
History of sterility	17 (15%)	15 (41%)	<0.003
Adhesions or tubal disease or both	20 (18%)	19 (51%)	<0.001
Unruptured ectopic pregnancy	77 (68%)	17 (46%)	<0.03

From Sherman D, Langer R, Sadovsky G, et al: Fertil Steril 37:497, 1982. Reproduced with permission of the publisher, The American Fertility Society.
b, Subsequent intrauterine pregnancies.
c, Subsequent sterility or repeat ectopic pregnancy only.

ectopic pregnancy subsequently conceived, the conception rate in women with an unruptured tubal pregnancy was 82%.

The rate of repeat ectopic pregnancies after a single ectopic pregnancy ranges from 8% to 20% with a mean of about 15%. Thus about one of four conceptions after an ectopic pregnancy is a repeat ectopic pregnancy. Only about one of three nulliparous women who have an ectopic pregnancy ever conceives again (35%), and about one third of them have another ectopic pregnancy (13%). With two ectopic pregnancies the subsequent fertility is decreased even further, with infertility rates as high as 90% being reported.

In two large groups of patients with unruptured ectopic pregnancy treated by conservative surgery, Langer et al. and Pouly et al. reported a high incidence of subsequent fertility (80% to 86%) and a low incidence of subsequent ectopic pregnancy (11% to 22%). The intrauterine pregnancy rates were 64% to 70%. In both series the intrauterine pregnancy rates were highest (82% to 86%) in patients with no history of infertility or gross evidence of prior salpingitis. The intrauterine pregnancy rates were significantly lower (41% to 56%) in women with these problems. Sherman et al. and Toumivaara and Kauppila reported that in patients with a normal contralateral tube and no history of infertility, pregnancy rates were similar whether the patients were treated with salpingectomy or salpingostomy. However, in the group of women with evidence of prior tubal infection and/or a history of infertility, subsequent intrauterine conception rates were higher when they were treated with salpingostomy (73% to 76%) than with salpingectomy

(43% to 44%). Most studies in the literature indicate that the overall subsequent ectopic pregnancy rate is similar among women treated radically or conservatively, and these two studies indicate that conservative surgery is most beneficial in women with evidence of contralateral tubal damage or peritubal adhesions, and/or history of infertility.

To compare the results of conservative tubal surgery using salpingotomy and salpingostomy, Tulandi and Guralnick performed a randomized study of these two techniques in women in a group of 34 women with unruptured ampullary ectopic pregnancies. They compared the results of subsequent fertility with these two techniques, as well as with a historical control group treated by salpingectomy. The data, unlike other studies, were analyzed by life table analysis. In this study they found the cumulative probability of intrauterine pregnancy was higher after both conservative treatments than after salpingotomy. At 6 and 12 months after surgery the cumulative probability of the incidence of intrauterine pregnancy was greater with patients treated by salpingostomy than after salpingectomy, but by 18 months the pregnancy rates were similar with the two techniques (Figure 16-26). These findings suggest that intrauterine pregnancy occurs earlier after salpingostomy than after salpingotomy, indicating that tubal suturing delays the return of tubal function but does not alter the ultimate rate of intrauterine pregnancy. These authors also reported that ectopic pregnancy rates were higher with the two conservative methods of treatment compared with salpingectomy, in contrast to most other studies.

There have been several reports of the use of

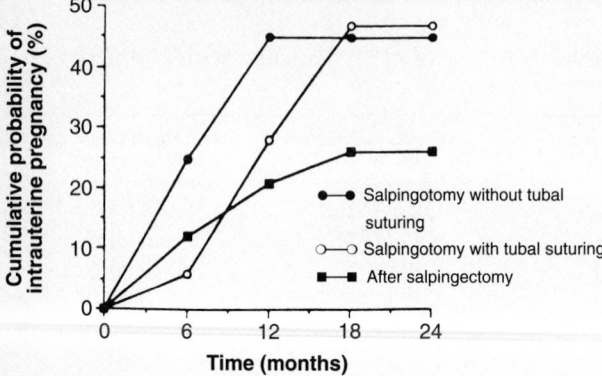

FIGURE 16-26

Cumulative probability of IUP after conservative surgical treatment of tubal EP by salpingotomy without tubal suturing; salpingotomy with tubal suturing; and after salpingectomy. (From Tulandi T and Guralnick M: Fertil Steril 55:53, 1991.)

conservative microsurgery, either salpingostomy or salpingotomy, in women with an unruptured tubal pregnancy in the only remaining oviduct. In the great majority of the subjects the other oviduct had been previously removed for another ectopic gestation. In the total of 90 patients so treated in six different centers, the conception rate was 81% with an intrauterine pregnancy rate of 57% (Table 16-12). About one fourth of the women had a subsequent ectopic gestation. Because this intrauterine pregnancy rate is higher than that achieved by in vitro fertilization and embryo transfer, it is now recommended that all women with an unruptured tubal pregnancy have a salpingostomy performed even if they have had two ectopic pregnancies and have only one oviduct remaining.

TABLE 16-12

Results of Conservative Surgery for Tubal Pregnancy in Women with a Solitary Tube

Author	Year	No. of patients desiring pregnancy	IUP	EUP
Henri-Suchet et al.	1979	14	8	2
DeCherney et al.	1982	12	6	2
Langer et al.	1982	8	5	2
Valle and Lifchez	1983	11	11	0
Oelsner et al.	1986	21	10	9
Pouly et al.	1986	24	11	7
TOTAL		90	51(57%)	22(24%)

From Vermesh M: Fertil Steril 51:559, 1989.

_____ KEY POINTS _____

- Diagnostic criteria for the ultrasonographic diagnosis of ectopic pregnancy include the detection, with use of currently available vaginal transducers, of an adnexal mass and/or the absence of a gestational sac when the HCG level is above a certain threshold, about 2500 mIU/ml.

- The annual ectopic pregnancy rates in the United States are about 1.5 per 1000 women aged 15 to 44 and 1.9 per 1000 women at risk for pregnancy.

- Between 1970 and 1987 there was nearly a fivefold increase in the annual number of women hospitalized for ectopic pregnancies in the United States (from 17,800 to 88,000) and tripling of the rate per 1000 live births (from 4.8 to 14.5) and a doubling of the rate per reported pregnancies (from 4.5 to 16.8).

- In the United States in 1987 nearly 2 of every 100 women who were known to conceive were hospitalized for ectopic gestation.

- In the United States the rate of ectopic pregnancy increased from 6.3 per 1000 conceptions in women aged 15 to 24 to 20.5 per 1000 conceptions in those aged 25 to 34.

- Only 10% to 15% of ectopic pregnancies occur in nulligravid women, and more than half of the ectopic pregnancies occur in women who have been pregnant three or more times.

- Most series report that nonclotting blood is obtained by culdocentesis in more than 90% of ectopic pregnancies.

- About 85% of women with an ectopic pregnancy have serum HCG levels lower than those seen in normal pregnancy at a similar gestational age.

- In women with an ectopic gestation, about 90% have an abnormal pattern of serial HCG levels. Half of these have falling levels and half have a subnormal increase.

- Laparoscopy has a 2% to 5% misdiagnosis rate (false positive or false negative) for ectopic pregnancy.

- Ultrasonography with a vaginal probe allows visualization of an intrauterine gestation when the HCG level is more than 2000 mIU/ml.

- If the pregnancy has produced rupture of the oviduct or has involved the entire oviduct or if no further pregnancies are desired, salpingectomy is the treatment of choice.

- About two thirds of women with symptomatic ectopic pregnancy have HCG levels above 2500 mIU/ml, and this can be reliably diagnosed by ultrasonography.

- Similar subsequent conception rates and ectopic pregnancy rates occur in women treated with salpingectomy or salpingo-oophorectomy.

- Cornual resection does not prevent a subsequent interstitial pregnancy.

- Most series report that when an unruptured ectopic pregnancy is present, the repeat ectopic pregnancy rate with salpingostomy is not increased as compared with salpingectomy, whereas the subsequent live birth rate is increased if the other tube is grossly abnormal.

- Fimbrial evacuation of the gestational products by digital expression has about twice the rate of recurrent ectopic pregnancy as salpingectomy.

- It is recommended that all Rh-negative unsensitized women with ectopic pregnancies receive Rh immunoglobulin.

- Overall the subsequent conception rate in women with an ectopic pregnancy is about 60%. A little less than half of these pregnancies terminate in another ectopic pregnancy or spontaneous abortion, so only about one third of women with an ectopic pregnancy have a subsequent live birth.

- If the ectopic pregnancy occurs in a woman's first pregnancy, her chance of subsequent conception is only about 35%.

- The subsequent conception rate is lower in women who have had a history of salpingitis, as well as in those who have gross evidence of damage in the opposite oviduct caused by previous salpingitis.

- Future fertility is significantly higher in women who have an unruptured tubal pregnancy than in those with a ruptured ectopic pregnancy.

- Conservative tubal surgery is most beneficial in women with evidence of contralateral tubal damage or peritubal adhesions or a history of infertility.

- About one of four conceptions after an ectopic pregnancy is a repeat ectopic pregnancy.

- About one third of nulliparous women with an ectopic pregnancy have a subsequent ectopic pregnancy.

- In women with one remaining oviduct where unruptured ectopic pregnancy is treated by salpingostomy, the conception rate is 81%, with an intrauterine pregnancy rate of 56% and a subsequent ectopic gestation rate of 24%.

BIBLIOGRAPHY

Atrash HK, Friede A, et al: Ectopic pregnancy mortality in the United States, 1970-1983, Obstet Gynecol 70:817, 1987.

Barnes AB, Wennberg CN, and Barnes BA: Ectopic pregnancy: incidence and review of determinant factors, Obstet Gynecol Surv 38:345, 1983.

Bick MB, Joubert SM, Norman RJ, et al: Serum progesterone in the uterine tubes with tubal pregnancy, Fertil Steril 50:752-755, 1988.

Braunstein GD and Asch RH: Predictive value analysis of measurements of human chorionic gonadotropin, pregnancy specific β_1-glycoprotein, placental lactogen, and cystine aminopeptidase for the diagnosis of ectopic pregnancy, Fertil Steril 39:62, 1983.

Breen JL: A 21-year survey of 654 ectopic pregnancies. Am J Obstet Gynecol 106:1004, 1970.

Brenner PF, Roy S, and Mishell DR Jr: Ectopic pregnancy: a study of 300 consecutive surgically treated cases, JAMA 243:673, 1980.

Budowick M, Johnson TRB, Genadry R, et al: The histopathology of the developing tubal ectopic pregnancy, Fertil Steril 34:169, 1980.

Cacciatore B, Stenman U-H, et al: Diagnosis of ectopic pregnancy by vaginal ultrasonography in combination with a discriminatory serum HCG level of 1000 (IU/ICIRP), BGOB 97:904, 1990.

Cartwright PS and DiPietro DL: Ectopic pregnancy: changes in serum human chorionic gonadotropin concentration, Obstet Gynecol 63:76, 1984.

Cartwright PS, Vaughn B, and Tuttle D: Culdocentesis and ectopic pregnancy, J Reprod Med 29:88, 1984.

Centers for Disease Control: Ectopic pregnancies—United States, MMWR 39, NO. SS, 1988.

Chavkin W: The rise in ectopic pregnancy—exploration of possible reasons, Int J Gynaecol 20:342, 1982.

Chow W-H, Daling JR, Weiss NS, et al: IUD use and subsequent tubal ectopic pregnancy, Am J Public Health 76:536, 1986.

Clark JF and Guy RS: Abdominal pregnancy, Am J Obstet Gynecol 96:511, 1966.

Cole T and Corlett R Jr: Chronic ectopic pregnancy, Obstet Gynecol 59:63, 1982.

Corson SL and Batzer FR: Ectopic pregnancy: a review of the etiologic factors, J Reprod Med 31:78, 1986.

DeCherney AH and Kase N: The conservative surgical management of unruptured ectopic pregnancy, Obstet Gynecol 54:451, 1979.

DeCherney AH and Maheux R: Modern management of tubal pregnancy, Curr Probl Obstet Gynecol 6:1, 1983.

DeCherney AH, Romero R, and Naftolin F: Surgical management of unruptured ectopic pregnancy, Fertil Steril 35:21, 1981.

Delke I, Veridiano NP, and Tancer ML: Abdominal pregnancy: review of current management and addition of 10 cases, Obstet Gynecol 60:200, 1982.

Di March JM, Kosasa Ts, et al: Persistent ectopic pregnancy, Obstet Gynecol &):555, 1987.

Dorfman SF: Deaths from ectopic pregnancy—United States, 1979 to 1980, Obstet Gynecol 62:334, 1983.

Dorfman SF: Epidemiology of ectopic pregnancy, Clin Obstet Gynecol 30:174, 1987.

Dorfman SF, Grimes DA, Cates W Jr, et al: Ectopic pregnancy mortality—United States, 1979 to 1980: clinical aspects, Obstet Gynecol 64:386, 1984.

Elias S, LeBeau M, Simpson JL, et al: Chromosome analysis of ectopic human conceptuses, Am J Obstet Gynecol 141:698, 1981.

Fernandez H and Rainhorn JD: Spontaneous resolution of ectopic pregnancy, Obstet Gynecol 71:171, 1988.

Gaetano V and Henno D: Combined pregnancy: The Mount Sinai experience, Obstet Gynecol Surv 41:603, 1986.

Garcia AJ, Aubert JM, Sama J, and Josimovich JB: Expectant management of presumed ectopic pregnancies, Fertil Steril 48:395, 1987.

Green LK and Kott ML: Histopathologic findings in ectopic tubal pregnancy, Int J Gynecol Pathol 8:255, 1989.

Grimes DA, Geary FH Jr, and Hatcher RA: Rh immunoglobulin utilization after ectopic pregnancy, Am J Obstet Gynecol 140:246, 1981.

Hahlin M, Wallin A, Sjoblom P, and Lindblom B: Single progesterone assay for early recognition of abnormal pregnancy, Hum Reprod 5:662, 1990.

Hallatt JG: Primary ovarian pregnancy: a report of twenty-five cases, Am J Obstet Gynecol 143:55, 1982.

Holt VL, Daling JR, Voigt LF, et al: Induced abortion and the risk of subsequent ectopic pregnancy, Am J Public Health 70: 1234, 1989.

Ichinoe K, Wake H, Shinkai N, et al: Nonsurgical therapy to preserve oviduct function in patients with tubal pregnancies, Am J Obstet Gynecol 156:484, 1987.

Kadar N, Caldwell BV, and Romero R: A method of screening for ectopic pregnancy and its indications, Obstet Gynecol 58:162, 1981.

Kalchman GG and Meltzer RM: Interstitial pregnancy following homolateral salpingectomy, Am J Obstet Gynecol 196:1139, 1966.

Kamrava MM, Taymor M, Berger MJ, et al: Disappearance of human chorionic gonadotropin following removal of ectopic pregnancy, Obstet Gynecol 62:486, 1983.

Kaufman RH, Noller K, Adam E, et al: Upper genital tract abnormalities and pregnancy outcome in diethylstilbestrol-exposed progeny, Am J Obstet Gynecol 148:973, 1984.

Kivitoski AI and Martin CM: Transabdominal and transvaginal ultrasonography in the diagnosis of ectopic pregnancy: a comparative study, Am J Obstet Gynecol 163:123, 1990.

Kooi S and Kock H: Treatment of tubal pregnancy by local injection of methotrexate after adrenaline injection into the mesosalpinx: a report of 25 patients, Fertil Steril 54:580, 1990.

Kratzer PG and Taylor RN: Corpus luteum function in early pregnancies is primarily determined by the rate of change of human chorionic gonadotropin levels, Am J Obstet Gynecol 163:1497, 1990.

Langer R, Raszier A, Ron-El R, et al: reproductive outcome after conservative surgery for unruptured tubal pregnancy: a 15-year experience, Fertil Steril 53:227, 1990.

Leach RE and Ory SJ: Modern management of ectopic pregnancy, J Reprod Med 34:325, 1989.

Leeton JK, and Davison G: Nonsurgical management of unruptured tubal pregnancy with intra-amniotic methotrexate: preliminary report of two cases, Fertil Steril 50:167, 1988.

Levin AA, Schoenbaum SC, Stubblefield PG, et al: Ectopic pregnancy and prior induced abortion, Am J Public Health 72:253, 1982.

Lindblom B, Hahlin M, et al: Serial human chorionic gonadotropin determinations by fluoroimmunoassay for differentiation between intrauterine and ectopic gestation, Am J Obstet Gynecol 161:397, 1989

Lindblom B, Hahlin M, Lundorf P, and Thorburn J: Treatment of tubal pregnancy by laparoscopy-guided injection of prostaglandin $F\alpha_2$, Fertil Steril 54:404, 1990.

Lund J: Early ectopic pregnancy, J Obstet Gynaecol Br Emp 62:70, 1955.

Lundorff P, Hahlin M, Sjoblom P, and Lindblom B: Persistent trophoblast after conservative treatment of tubal pregnancy: prediction and detection, Obstet Gynecol 77:129, 1991.

Majmudar B, Henderson PH III, and Semple E: Salpingitis isthmica nodosa: a high-risk factor for tubal pregnancy, Obstet Gynecol 62:73, 1983.

Makinen JI, Salmi TA, Nikkanen VPJ, and Koskineew EYJ: Encouraging rates of fertility after ectopic pregnancy, Int J Fertil 34:46, 1989.

Mangan CE, Borow L, Burtnett-Rubin MM, et al: Pregnancy outcome in 98 women exposed to diethylstil bestrol in utero, their mothers, and their unexposed siblings, Obstet Gynecol 59:315, 1982.

Marchbanks PA and Annegers JF: Risk factors for ectopic pregnancy: population based study, JAMA 259:1823, 1988.

Matthews CP, Coulson P, and Wild RA: Serum progesterone levels as an aid in the diagnosis of ectopic pregnancy, Obstet Gynecol 68:390, 1986.

McBain JC, Evans JH, Pepperell RJ, et al: An unexpectedly high rate of ectopic pregnancy following the induction of ovulation with human pituitary and chorionic gonadotrophin, Br J Obstet Gynaecol 87:5, 1980.

McCann MF and Kessel E: International experience with laparoscopic sterilization: follow-up of 8500 women, Adv Planned Parent 12:199, 1978.

McCausland A: High rate of ectopic pregnancy following laparoscopic tubal coagulation failures, Am J Obstet Gynecol 136:97, 1980.

McCausland A: Endosalpingosis ("endosalpingoblastosis") following laparoscopic tubal coagulation as an etiologic factor of ectopic pregnancy, Am J Obstet Gynecol 143:12, 1982.

Morris JM and Van Wagenen G: Interception: the use of postovulatory estrogens to prevent implantation, Am J Obstet Gynecol 115:101, 1973.

Nagamani M, London S, and St Amand P: Factors influencing fertility after ectopic pregnancy, Am J Obstet Gynecol 149:533, 1984.

Nederlof KP, Lawson HW, Saftlas AF, et al: Ectopic pregnancy Surveillance: United States, 1970-1987, NNWR 39 (55-4):9, 1990.

Niles JH and Clark JJ: Pathogenesis of tubal pregnancy, Am J Obstet Gynecol 105:1230, 1969.

Nyberg DA, Mack A, Laing FC, et al: Early pregnancy complications: endovaginal sonographic findings correlated with human chorionic gonadotropin levels, Radiology 167:619, 1988.

Oelsner G, Rabinovitch O, Morad J, et al: Reproductive outcome after microsurgical treatment of tubal pregnancy in women with a single fallopian tube, J Reprod Med 31:483, 1986.

O'Leary JL and O'Leary JA: Rudimentary horn pregnancy, Obstet Gynecol 22:371, 1963.

Ollendorff BA and Felgin MD: The value of curettage in the diagnosis of ectopic pregnancy, Am J Obstet Gynecol 157:71, 1987.

Ory HW, The Women's Health Study: Ectopic pregnancy and intrauterine contraceptive devices: new perspectives, Obstet Gynecol 57:137, 1981.

Paalman RJ and McElin TW: Cervical pregnancy, Am J Obstet Gynecol 77:1261, 1959.

Pansky M, Bukovsky I, Golan A, et al: Local methotrexate injection: a nonsurgical treatment of ectopic pregnancy, Am J Obstet Gynecol 161:393, 1989.

Parente JT, Ou C-S, and Levy J: Cervical pregnancy analysis: a review and report of five cases, Obstet Gynecol 62:79, 1983.

Persaud V: Etiology of tubal ectopic pregnancy, Obstet Gynecol 36:257, 1970.

Peterson HB: Extratubal ectopic pregnancies, J Reprod Med 31:108, 1986.

Pouly JL, Mahnes H, Mage G, et al: Conservative laparoscopic treatment of 321 ectopic pregnancies, Fertil Steril 46:1093, 1986.

Reece EA, Petrie RH, Sirmans MF, et al: Combined intrauterine and extrauterine gestations: a review, Am J Obstet Gynecol 146:323, 1983.

Romero R, Kadar H, Castro D, et al: The value of serial human chorionic gonadotropin testing as a dignostic tool in ectopic pregnancy, Am J Obstet Gynecol 155:392, 1986.

Rubin GL, Peterson HB, Dorfman SF, et al: Ectopic pregnancy in the United States 1970 through 1978, JAMA 249:1725, 1983.

Saito M, Koyama T, Yaoi Y, et al: Site of ovulation and ectopic pregnancy, Acta Obstet Gynecol Scand 54:227, 1975.

Sauer MV, Vermesh M, Anderson R, et al: Rapid measurement of urinary pregnanediol glucuronide to diagnose ectopic pregnancy, Am J Obstet Gynecol 159:1531, 1988.

Schenker JG and Evron S: New concepts in the surgical management of tubal pregnancy and the consequent postoperative results, Fertil Steril 40:709, 1983.

Schoen JA and Nowak RJ: Repeat ectopic pregnancy: a 16-year clinical survey, Obstet Gynecol 45:542, 1975.

Shapiro BS and Cullen M: Transvaginal ultrasonography for the diagnosis of ectopic pregnancy, Fertil Steril 50:425, 1988.

Shaw A, Courey NG, and Cunanan RG: Pregnancy following laparoscopic tubal electrocoagulation and division, Am J Obstet Gynecol 192: 459, 1977.

Sherman D, Langer R, Sadovsky G, et al: Improved fertility following ectopic pregnancy, Fertil Steril 37:497, 1982.

Siegler AM, Wang CF, and Westoff C: Management of unruptured tubal pregnancy, Obstet Gynecol Surv 36:599, 1981.

Sivin I: Copper T IUD use and ectopic pregnancy rates in the United States, Contraception 19:151, 1979.

Stock RJ: Persistent tubal pregnancy, Obstet Gynecol 77:267, 1991.

Stovall TG, Ling F, Kellerman AL, and Buster JE: Outpatient chemotherapy of unruptured ectopic pregnancy, Fertil Steril 51:435, 1989.

Stratford B: Abnormalities of early human development, Am J Obstet Gynecol 107:1223, 1970.

Tanaka T, Hayashi H, Kutsuzawa T, et al: Treatment of interstitial ectopic pregnancy with methotrexate: report of a successful case, Fertil Steril 37:851, 1982.

Tatum HJ and Schmidt FH: Contraceptive and sterilization practices and extrauterine pregnancy: a realistic perspective, Fertil Steril 28:407, 1977.

Timonen S and Nieminen U: Tubal pregnancy, choice of operative method of treatment, Acta Obstet Gynecol Scand 46:327, 1967.

Timor-Tritsch IE, Yeh MN, Peisner DB, et al: The use of transvaginal ultrasonography in the diagnosis of ectopic pregnancy, Am J Obstet Gynecol 161:157, 1989.

Tulandi T and Guralnick M: Treatment of tubal ectopic pregnancy by salpingotomy with or without tubal suturing and salpingectomy, Fertil Steril 55:53, 1991.

Tuomivaara L and Kauppila A: Radical or conservative surgery for ectopic pregnancy? A follow-up study of fertility of 323 patients, Fertil Steril 50:580, 1988.

Vermesh M, Silva PD, Rosen GF, et al: Persistent tubal ectopic gestation: patters of circulation β-human chorionic gonadotropin and progesterone, and management options, Fertil Steril 50:584, 1988.

Vermesh M, Silva PD, et al: Management of unruptured ectopic gestation by linear salpingostomy: a prospective, randomized clinical trial of laparoscopy versus laparotomy, Obstet Gynecol 73:400, 1989.

Vermesh M: Conservative management of ectopic gestation, Fertil Steril 51:559, 1989.

Weckstein LN: Current perspective on ectopic pregnancy, Obstet Gynecol Surv 40:259, 1985.

Weckstein LN, Boucher AR, Tucker H, et al: Accurate diagnosis of early ectopic pregnancy, Obstet Gynecol 65:393, 1985.

Weström L, Bengtsson LPH, and Mårdh P-A: Incidence, trends and risks of ectopic pregnancy in a population of women, Br Med J 282:15, 1981.

Yeko TR, Gorrill MJ, Hughes LH, et al: Timely diagnosis of early ectopic pregnancy using a single blood progesterone measurement, Fertil Steril 48:10, 1987.

Benign Gynecologic Lesions

———————— KEY TERMS AND DEFINITIONS ————————

Brenner Tumor. A small, smooth, solid fibroepithelial tumor of the ovary. It may be benign or malignant.

Degeneration of a Myoma. The process by which a myoma outgrows its blood supply and begins to necrose centrally. Forms of degeneration include hyaline, myxomatous, calcific, cystic, fat, and red degeneration.

Dermoid (Benign Cystic Teratoma). A benign germ cell tumor that may contain elements of all three germ cell layers.

Dysontogenetic Cysts. Thin-walled cysts of embryonic origin.

Endometrial Polyp. A localized outgrowth of endometrial glands and stroma projecting beyond the surface of the endometrium and including a vascular stalk.

Follicular Hematoma. Follicular cysts filled with blood, usually from hemorrhage in the vascular theca zone.

Gartner's Duct Cysts. Cysts primarily of mesonephric origin found laterally in the vagina.

Hematometra. A uterus distended with blood, secondary to partial or complete obstruction of any portion of the lower genital tract.

Hidradenitis Suppurativa. A chronic infection involving skin, subcutaneous tissue, and apocrine glands.

Hidradenoma. A rare, small, benign vulvar tumor originating from apocrine sweat glands.

Hydatid Cysts of Morgagni. Pedunculated paratubal cysts found near the fimbria of the oviduct.

Hydrometra. A collection of clear fluid in the uterine cavity.

Hyperreactio Luteinalis. Multiple theca lutein cysts causing bilateral ovarian enlargement during pregnancy.

Intravenous Leiomyomatosis. An extremely rare condition in which benign smooth muscle fibers invade and slowly grow into the venous channels of the pelvis.

Itch-Scratch Cycle. The cycle of itching leading to scratching. The scratching leads to excoriation, irritation, and healing, with subsequent irritation and itching.

Leiomyoma (Myoma or Fibroid). A benign tumor of muscle cell origin found in any tissue that contains smooth muscle.

Leiomyomatosis Peritonealis Disseminata. A benign disease with multiple small nodules over the surface of the pelvis and abdominal peritoneum, grossly mimicking disseminated carcinoma.

Lichenification. Changes in the skin from chronic irritation, characterized by whiteness, thickening, and leathery appearance.

Luteoma of Pregnancy. A rare, specific, benign, hyperplastic reaction of ovarian theca lutein cells during pregnancy.

Meigs' Syndrome. The constellation of symptoms of ascites and hydrothorax associated with a benign ovarian fibroma, resolving after the removal of the tumor.

Nabothian Cysts. Cervical retention cysts lined by endocervical-type columnar cells.

Parasitic Myoma. A myoma that outgrows its uterine blood supply and obtains a secondary blood supply from another organ, such as the omentum.

Prominence or **Tubercle of Rokitansky.** The protrusion of solid elements of a dermoid into the cyst cavity.

Pruritus. A symptom of intense itching with an associated desire to scratch.

Pyometra. A collection of pus in the uterine cavity.

Struma Ovarii. A specialized ovarian teratoma that consists of thyroid tissue as a major or exclusive component. It may rarely produce sufficient thyroid hormone to induce hyperthyroidism.

Submucosal Myoma. A myoma located immediately below the endometrial lining.

Subserosal Myoma. A myoma found just beneath the serosa of the uterus.

Syringoma. A benign tumor of the eccrine sweat glands.

Vulvodynia. A term describing chronic vulvar discomfort.

This book is divided primarily into chapters dealing with benign diseases and chapters dealing with malignant ones. For the clinician, however, the difference is not always clear. As in all areas of medicine, gynecologic problems do not fall into definitive categories, and those that include malignant disease often overlap with those that include benign disease. When the diagnosis from the history, physical examination, and laboratory tests is clear, management is usually self-evident. When a specific diagnosis is unclear, tissue biopsy is appropriate. This chapter deals primarily with benign lesions; however, the symptoms and differential diagnoses of these lesions have tremendous overlap with those of malignant disease.

The discussions in this chapter are arranged anatomically, beginning with the vulva and then covering the vagina, cervix, uterus, oviducts, and ovaries. This chapter does not attempt to be encyclopedic; rather, lesions have been selected based on their clinical importance and incidence. Therefore, lesions such as glomus tumors of the vulva or papillomas of the cervix have been omitted. Because several nonneoplastic abnormalities and lesions present in ways similar to those of benign tumors, this chapter also discusses entities that are not specifically abnormal growths. Lesions such as torsion of the ovary, lacerations of the vagina, and hematomas of the vulva are examples of these common clinical problems.

The successful clinician must use deductive as well as inductive reasoning in solving a problem. To have mastered both these techniques, he or she not only must be adept at physical examination and history taking but also must be able to form a complete list of possible lesions that may be involved in the patient's complaint. An understanding of the entities of this chapter will be helpful toward that goal.

VULVA

Urethral Caruncle

A urethral caruncle is a small, fleshy outgrowth of the edge of the urethra. The tissue of the caruncle is soft, smooth, friable, and bright red and initially appears as an eversion of the urethra (Figure 17-1). Urethral caruncles are generally small, single, and sessile but may be pedunculated and grow to be 1 to 2 cm in diameter. They occur most frequently in postmenopausal women and must be differentiated from urethral carcinomas. If a urethral caruncle is diagnosed in a child, most likely the correct diagnosis is urethral prolapse. Urethral caruncles are believed to arise from an ectropion of the posterior urethral wall secondary to retraction and atrophy of the postmenopausal vagina. The growth of the caruncle is secondary to chronic irritation or infection. Histologically the caruncle is composed of transitional and stratified squamous epithelium with a loose connective tissue (Figure 17-2). Caruncles are frequently subdivided into papillomatous, granulomatous, and angiomatous varieties. They are often secondarily infected, producing ulceration and bleeding.

The symptoms associated with urethral caruncles are variable. Many women are asymptomatic, whereas others experience dysuria, frequency, and urgency. Sometimes the caruncle produces point tenderness after contact with undergarments or during intercourse. Ulcerative lesions usually produce spotting on contact more commonly than hematuria.

The differential diagnosis of urethral caruncles includes primary carcinoma of the urethra and prolapse of the urethral mucosa. Although urethral caruncles are not a precursor for urethral carcinoma, grossly the two are often confused. Both diseases are most common in post-

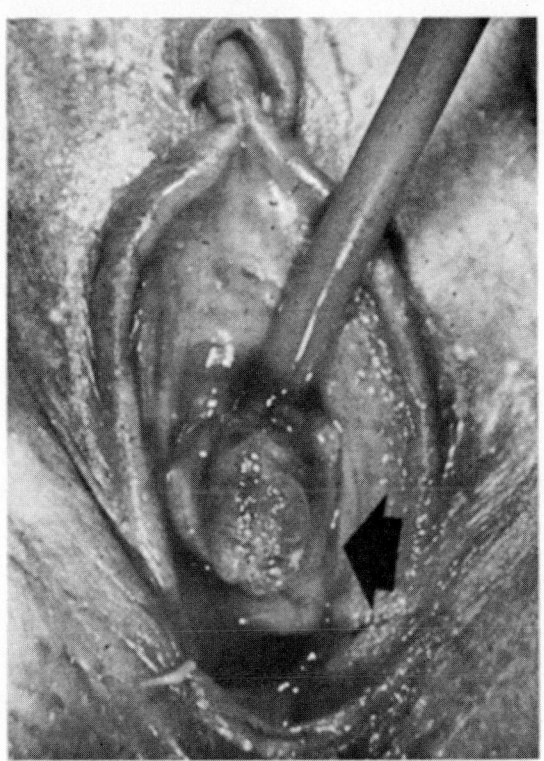

FIGURE 17-1
Large benign urethral caruncle, thought clinically to be urethral carcinoma because of its size *(arrow)*. (From Marshall FC, Uson AC, and Melicow MM: Surg Gynecol Obstet 110:724, 1960. By permission of Surgery, Gynecology & Obstetrics.)

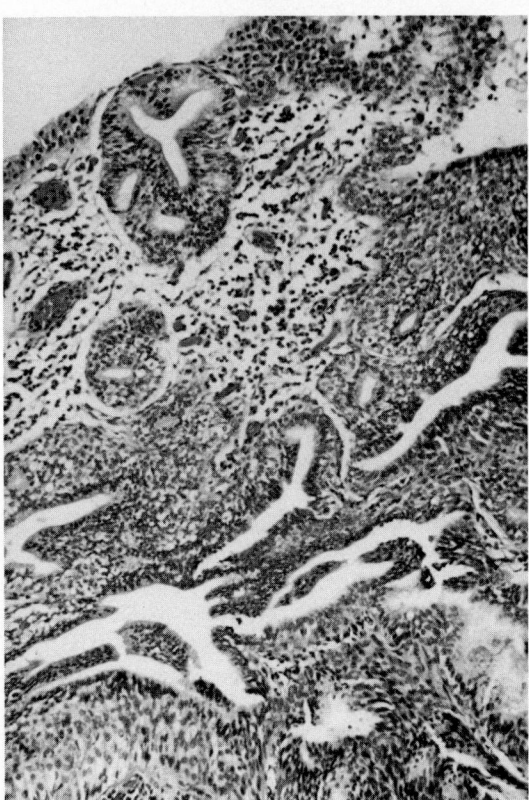

FIGURE 17-2
Urethral caruncle. Hyperemia, inflammation, and some infolding of transitional epithelium. (H&E stain). (From Kaufman RH: Solid tumors. In Gardner HL and Kaufman RH, editors: Benign diseases of the vulva and vagina, ed 2, Boston, 1981, GK Hall & Co, p 88. Reproduced with permission.)

menopausal women. Marshall et al. reported a series of 394 urethral tumors. A clinical diagnosis of urethral caruncle was made in 376 of these women. Histologic examination of biopsy material demonstrated urethral carcinoma in nine patients in their series. Thus, approximately 1 out of 40 women with a clinical diagnosis of urethral caruncle has a malignant urethral neoplasm. Urethral carcinoma is primarily a disease of postmenopausal women. The symptoms of a urethral carcinoma include bleeding, urinary frequency, and dysuria, and the signs include a mass protruding from the urethra with associated tenderness and induration of the urethra.

The diagnosis of a urethral caruncle is established by biopsy under local anesthesia. Small asymptomatic urethral caruncles do not need

treatment. Initial therapy is oral or topical estrogen and avoidance of irritation. If the caruncle does not regress or is symptomatic, it may be destroyed by cryosurgery, laser therapy, fulguration, or operative excision. Following operative destruction, a Foley catheter should be left in place for 48 to 72 hours. Follow-up is necessary to ensure that the patient does not develop urethral stenosis.

Urethral prolapse is predominantly a disease of the premenarchal female (Figure 17-3), although it does occur in postmenopausal women. The annular rosette of friable, edematous prolapsed mucosa does not have the bright-red color of a caruncle and is not as circumscribed in gross configuration. It may be ulcerated with necrosis or grossly edematous. Therapy of a prolapsed urethra is hot sitz baths

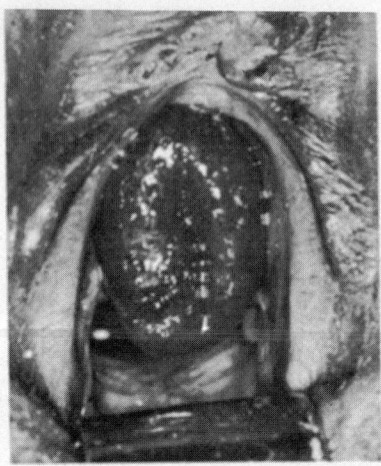

FIGURE 17-3
Prolapse of urethral mucosa in 7-year-old child. Edematous red collar of tissue surrounds urethral meatus. (From Kaufman RH: Solid tumors. In Gardner HL and Kaufman RH, editors: Benign diseases of the vulva and vagina, ed 2, Boston, 1981, GK Hall & Co, 1981, p 89. Reproduced with permission.)

and antibiotics to reduce inflammation and infection. In rare cases it may be necessary to excise the redundant mucosa.

Cysts

The most common large cyst of the vulva is a cystic dilation of an obstructed Bartholin's duct. Approximately 2% of new gynecologic patients present with an asymptomatic Bartholin's duct cyst. Treatment is not necessary in women younger than 40 unless the cyst becomes infected or enlarges enough to produce symptoms. A more complete discussion of Bartholin's duct cysts and abscesses is included in Chapter 21. Occasionally the ducts of mucous glands of the vestibule are occluded. The resulting cysts may be clear, yellow, or blue. Similar small mucous cysts occur in the periurethral region. Wolffian duct cysts or mesonephric cysts are rare, but when they do occur, they are found near the clitoris and lateral to the hymeneal ring.

The most common small vulvar cysts are epidermal inclusion cysts or sebaceous cysts. Because these cysts cannot be differentiated grossly and since a continuing controversy exists with respect to their histogenesis, these two cysts are discussed together in this chapter. However, numerically, many more epithelial cysts are discovered, sebaceous cysts of the vulva being a rarity. These cysts are located immediately beneath the epidermis. Most commonly they are discovered on the anterior half of the labia majora. These cysts are usually multiple, freely movable, round, slow growing, and nontender. They are firm to shotty in consistency, and their contents are usually under pressure. Grossly, they are white or yellow, and the contents are caseous, like a thick cheese.

An inclusion cyst may develop following trauma when an infolding of squamous epithelium has occurred beneath the epidermis in the site of an episiotomy or obstetric laceration. Most inclusion cysts of the vagina are directly related to previous trauma, while most inclusion cysts of the vulva are not related to trauma. Alternative theories of histogenesis include embryonic remnants and occlusion of pilosebaceous ducts of sweat glands. The histology of these cysts is characterized by an epithelial lining of keratinized, stratified squamous epithelium with a center of cellular debris that grossly resembles sebaceous material. Most vulvar epidermal cysts do not have sebaceous cells or sebaceous material identified on microscopic examination. These cysts are asymptomatic unless they are secondarily infected. Large epidermal cysts may be confused with fibromas, lipomas, and hidradenomas.

Most of these cysts require no treatment. If the cyst becomes infected, treatment consists of heat applied locally and incision and drainage. Cysts that become recurrently infected or produce pain should be excised when the acute inflammation has subsided.

Nevus

A nevus, commonly referred to as a *mole*, is a localized nest or cluster of melanocytes. These undifferentiated cells arise from the embryonic neural crest and are present from birth. Many nevi are not recognized until they become pigmented at the time of puberty. Vulvar nevi are one of the most common benign neoplasms in females. As with nevi in other parts of the body, they exhibit a wide range in depth of color, from blue to dark brown to black, and some may be amelanotic. The diameter of most nevi ranges from a few millimeters to 2 cm. Grossly, a benign nevus may be flat,

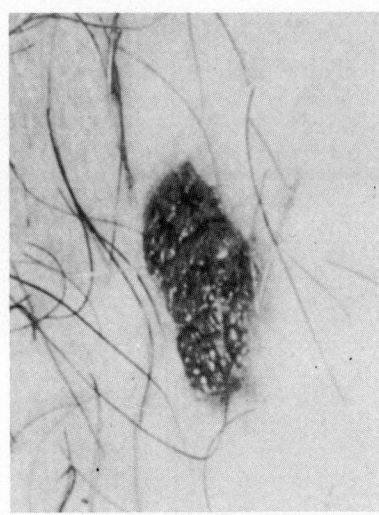

FIGURE 17-4
Compound nevus, usually a slightly elevated pigmented lesion. (From Kaufman RH: Solid tumors. In Gardner HL and Kaufman RH, editors: Benign diseases of the vulva and vagina, ed 2, Boston, 1981, GK Hall & Co, p 64. Reproduced with permission.)

elevated, or pedunculated. Other pigmented lesions in the differential diagnosis include hemangiomas, endometriosis, malignant melanoma, vulvar intraepithelial neoplasia, and seborrheic keratosis.

Vulvar nevi are generally asymptomatic. Most women do not closely inspect their vulvar skin and are unaware of biologic changes in gross appearance of these lesions. Histologically, the lesions are subdivided into three major groups: junctional, compound (Figure 17-4), and intradermal nevi.

Although the vulvar area contains approximately 1% of the skin surface of the body, 5% to 10% of all malignant melanomas in women arise from this region. The biologic reasons for this discrepancy are unknown. Speculation includes the hypothesis that junctional activity is common in vulvar nevi, and the many irritants to which vulvar skin is exposed may lead to malignancy. It is estimated that 30% of malignant melanomas arise from a preexisting nevus. The majority of women who develop melanomas are in their 50s.

Ideally, all flat vulvar nevi should be excised and examined histologically. This may be accomplished with local anesthesia or coincidentally with obstetric delivery or gynecologic sur-

gery. Proper excisional biopsy should be three dimensional and adequate in width and depth. Approximately 5 to 10 mm of normal skin surrounding the nevus should be included, and the biopsy should include the underlying dermis as well. Some patients are reluctant to have a "normal"-appearing nevus removed. Recent changes in growth or color, ulceration, bleeding, pain, or the development of satellite lesions mandates biopsy. Friedman et al. (1985) listed the characteristic clinical features of an early malignant melanoma, which may be remembered by thinking ABCD: *asymmetry*, *border* irregularity, *color* variegation, and a *diameter* usually greater than 6 mm.

Hemangioma

Hemangiomas are rare malformations of blood vessels rather than true neoplasms. Vulvar hemangiomas frequently are discovered first in children. They are usually single, 1 to 2 cm in diameter, flat, and soft, and they range from brown to red or purple. Histologically the multiple channels of hemangiomas are predominantly thin-walled capillaries arranged randomly and separated by thin connective tissue septa. These tumors change in size and compression and are not encapsulated. Most hemangiomas are asymptomatic; occasionally they may become ulcerated and bleed.

There are four different types of vulvar hemangiomas. The strawberry or cavernous hemangioma is a congenital defect discovered in young children. It is usually bright red to dark red, is elevated, and rarely increases in size after age 2. Approximately 60% of vulvar hemangiomas discovered during the first year of life spontaneously regress in size. Senile or cherry angiomas are common small lesions that arise on the labia majora of postmenopausal women. They are most often less than 3 mm in diameter, multiple, and red-brown to dark blue. Angiokeratomas are approximately twice the size of cherry angiomas, are purple, and occur in women between the ages of 30 and 50. They are noted for their rapid growth and tendency to bleed during strenuous exercise. In the differential diagnosis of an angiokeratoma is Kaposi's sarcoma and angiosarcoma. Pyogenic granulomas are an overgrowth of inflamed granulation tissue. These lesions grow under the hormonal influence of pregnancy, with similarities to lesions in the oral cavity. Pyogenic granulomas are usually approximately 1 cm in diameter and may be mistaken clinically for malignant melanomas, basal cell carcinomas, vulvar condylomas, or nevi.

The diagnosis is usually established by gross inspection of the vascular lesion. Asymptomatic hemangiomas and hemangiomas in children rarely require therapy. When the differential diagnosis is questionable, excisional biopsy should be performed. A hemangioma that is associated with troublesome bleeding may be destroyed by cryosurgery or use of a laser. Obviously, if the histologic diagnosis is questionable, any bleeding vulvar mass should be treated by excisional biopsy so that the definitive pathologic diagnosis can be established. Surgical removal of a large, cavernous hemangioma may be technically quite difficult. Lymphangiomas of the vulva do exist but are extremely rare.

Fibroma

Fibromas are the most common benign solid tumors of the vulva. They are more frequent than lipomas, the other common benign tumors of mesenchymal origin. Fibromas occur in all age groups and most commonly are found in the labia majora (Figure 17-5). However, they actually arise from deeper connective tissue. They grow slowly and vary from a few centimeters to one gigantic vulvar fibroma reported to weigh more than 250 pounds. The smaller fibromas are discovered as subcutaneous nodules. As they increase in size and weight, they become pedunculated. Smaller fibromas are firm; however, larger tumors often become cystic after undergoing myxomatous degeneration.

Fibromas have a smooth surface and a distinct contour. On cut surface the tissue is gray-white. Fat or muscle cells microscopically may be associated with the interlacing fibroblasts. Fibromas have a low-grade potential for becoming malignant. Smaller fibromas are asymptomatic; larger tumors may produce acute pain when they degenerate or chronic pressure symptoms. Treatment is operative removal if the fibromas are symptomatic and/or continue to grow. Occasionally they are removed for cosmetic reasons.

Lipoma

Lipomas are benign, slow-growing, circumscribed tumors of fat cells arising from the sub-

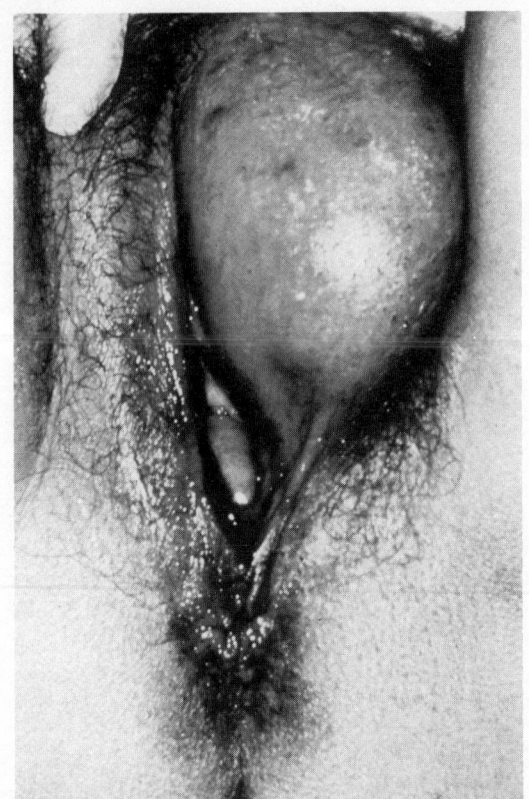

FIGURE 17-5
Vulvar fibroma, which is the most common benign solid tumor of the vulva. (From Friedrick EG, editor: Vulval disease, ed 2, Philadelphia, 1983, WB Saunders Co, p 283.)

cutaneous tissue of the vulva (Figure 17-6). Lipomas of the vulva are similar to lipomas of other parts of the body. When discovered they are softer and usually larger than fibromas. The largest vulvar lipoma reported in the literature weighed 44 pounds. Lipomas are the second most frequent benign vulvar mesenchymal tumor. Because of the fat distribution of the vulva, most lipomas are discovered in the labia majora and are superficial in location. They are slow growing, and their malignant potential is low.

When a lipoma is cut, the substance is soft, yellow, and lobulated. Histologically, lipomas are usually more homogeneous than fibromas. Occasionally associated with the adipose cells of a true lipoma are prominent areas of connective tissue. Unless extremely large, lipomas do not produce symptoms. Excision is usually performed to establish the diagnosis, although smaller tumors may be followed conservatively.

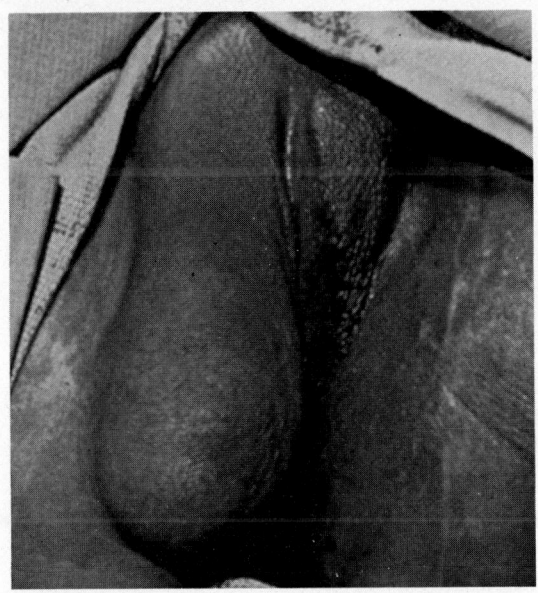

FIGURE 17-6
Lipoma. (From Friedrich EG, editor: Vulvar disease, ed 2, Philadelphia, 1983, WB Saunders Co, p 233.)

Hidradenoma

The hidradenoma is a rare, small, benign vulvar tumor that originates from apocrine sweat glands of the inner surface of the labia majora and nearby perineum. The majority of hidradenomas are cystic. For unknown reasons, they are discovered exclusively in white women between the ages of 30 and 70, most commonly in the fourth decade of life. These tumors have not been reported prior to puberty. Hidradenomas may be cystic or solid. In a review by Woodworth et al., 55% were cystic. While 38% originated from the labia majora, 26% arose from the labia minora.

These tumors are well defined and usually sessile, pinkish-gray nodules not larger than 2 cm in diameter. In most cases the surface epithelium is white, but occasionally necrosis of a central indented area occurs with a protrusion of reddish-brown granulation tissue. These latter lesions may be confused with pyogenic granulomas.

These tumors have well-defined capsules. Histologically, because of its hyperplastic, adenomatous pattern, a hidradenoma may be mistaken at first glance for an adenocarcinoma. On close inspection, however, although there is glandular hyperplasia with numerous tubular ducts, there is a paucity of mitotic figures and a lack of significant cellular and nuclear pleomorphism (Figure 17-7). Hidradenomas are generally asymptomatic. However, they may cause pruritus or bleeding if the tumor undergoes necrosis. Excisional biopsy is the treatment of choice.

Syringoma

The syringoma is a very rare, cystic, asymptomatic, benign tumor, which is an adenoma of the eccrine sweat glands. It appears as small subcutaneous papules that are either skin colored or yellow and that may coalesce to form cords of firm tissue. Identical tumors are often found in the eccrine glands of the eyelids. This tumor is usually treated by excisional biopsy. The most common differential diagnosis is Fox-Fordyce disease, a condition of multiple retention cysts of apocrine glands accompanied by inflammation of the skin. The latter disease often produces intense pruritus, while syringoma is generally asymptomatic. Fox-Fordyce disease is treated by oral or topical estrogens and topical retinoic acid.

Endometriosis

Endometriosis of the vulva is rare. Only 1 in 500 women with endometriosis will present with vulvar lesions. The firm, small nodule or nodules may be cystic or solid and vary from a few millimeters to several centimeters. The subcutaneous lesions are blue, red, or purple, depending on their size, activity, and closeness to the surface of the skin. The gross and microscopic pathologic picture of vulvar endometriosis is similar to endometriosis of the pelvis (Chapter 18).

Endometriosis of the vulva is usually found at the site of an old, healed obstetric laceration, episiotomy site, or area of operative removal of a Bartholin's duct cyst. The pathophysiology of development of vulvar endometriosis may be secondary to metaplasia, retrograde lymphatic spread, or potential implantation of endometrial tissue during operation. Paull and Tedeschi documented 15 cases of vulvar endometriosis they believed were associated with prophylactic postpartum curettage of the uterus to prevent postpartum bleeding. In their series there was not a single case of vulvar endometriosis in 13,800 deliveries without curettage, but 15 cases of vulvar endometriosis were

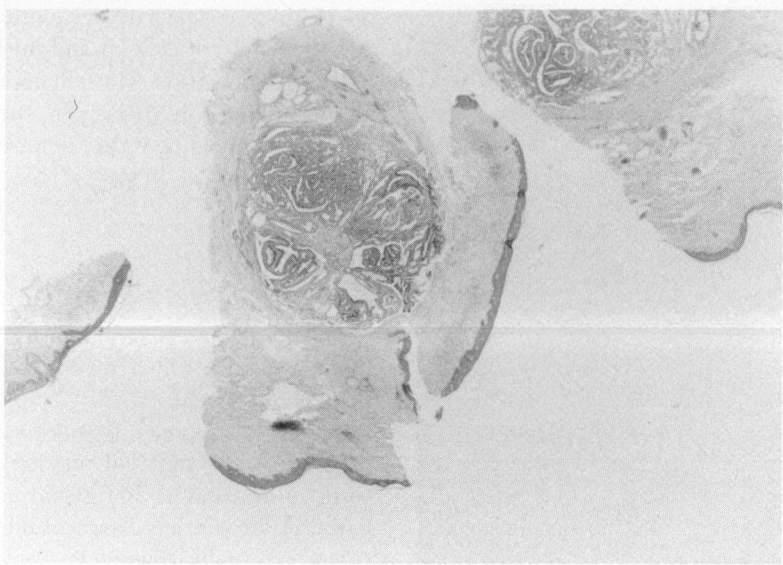

FIGURE 17-7
Hidradenoma. Numerous acini. Distinct apocrine gland–type epithelium is present on left. (H&E stain.) (From Kaufman RH: Cystic tumors. In Gardner HL and Kaufman RH, editors: Benign diseases of the vulva and vagina, ed 2, Boston, 1981, GK Hall & Co, p 101. Reproduced with permission.)

associated with 2028 deliveries with prophylactic curettage.

The most common symptoms of endometriosis of the vulva are pain and introital dyspareunia. The classic history is cyclic discomfort and an enlargement of the mass associated with menstrual periods. Treatment of vulvar endometriosis is by excision or laser vaporization.

Granular Cell Myoblastoma

Granular cell myoblastoma is a rare, slow-growing, solid vulvar tumor. The tumor originates from neural sheath (Schwann) cells and is sometimes called a *schwannoma*. These tumors are found in connective tissues throughout the body, most commonly in the tongue, and occur in any age group. Approximately 7% of solitary granular cell myoblastomas are found in the subcutaneous tissue of the vulva. Twenty percent of multiple granular cell myoblastomas are located in the vulva.

These tumors are subcutaneous nodules, usually 1 to 5 cm in diameter. They are benign but characteristically infiltrate the surrounding local tissue. As they grow, they may also cause ulcerations in the skin. The overlying skin often has hyperplastic changes that may look sim-

ilar to invasive squamous cell carcinoma. Grossly, these tumors are not encapsulated. The cut surface of the tumor is yellow. Histologically, there are irregularly arranged bundles of large, round cells with indistinct borders and pink-staining cytoplasm. Initially the cell of origin was believed to be striated muscle; however, electron microscopic studies have demonstrated that this tumor is from cells of the neural sheath.

The tumor nodules are painless. Treatment involves wide excision to remove the filamentous projections into the surrounding tissue. If the initial excisional biopsy is not adequate and aggressive enough, these benign tumors tend to recur.

von Recklinghausen's Disease

The vulva is sometimes involved with the benign neural sheath tumors of von Recklinghausen's disease (generalized neurofibromatous and café-au-lait spots). The vulvar lesions of this disease are fleshy, brownish red, polypoid tumors. Approximately 18% of women with von Recklinghausen's disease have vulvar involvement. Excision is the treatment of choice for symptomatic tumors.

Other Abnormal Tissue

Other examples of diseases or aberrant tissue presenting as vulvar masses include leiomyomas, myomas, squamous papillomas, sebaceous adenomas, dermoids, accessory breast tissue and müllerian or wolffian duct remnants, epidermal inclusion cysts, sebaceous cysts, mucous cysts, and skin diseases such as seborrheic keratosis, condyloma acuminata, and molluscum contagiosum. Some of these diseases are discussed in this chapter, others in Chapter 21.

Hematomas

Hematomas of the vulva are usually secondary to blunt trauma such as a straddle injury from a fall, an automobile accident, or a physical assault. Traumatic injuries producing vulvar hematoma have been reported secondary to a wide range of recreational activities, including bicycle and motorcycle riding, sledding, water skiing, cross-country skiing, riding go-carts, and amusement park rides (Figure 17-8). Spon-

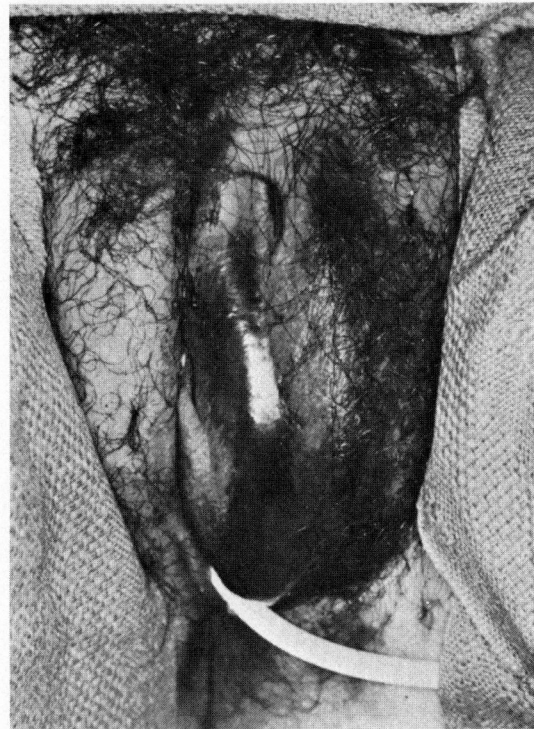

FIGURE 17-8
Vulva hematoma from straddle injury that produced urethral obstruction. (From Naumann RO and Droegemueller W: Am J Obstet Gynecol 142:358, 1982.)

taneous hematomas are rare and usually occur from rupture of a varicose vein during pregnancy or the postpartum period.

The management of vulvar hematomas is usually conservative unless the hematoma is rapidly expanding. The bleeding that produces a vulvar hematoma is usually venous in origin. Therefore it may be controlled by direct pressure. Compression and application of an ice pack to the area are appropriate therapy. Operative therapy is indicated in an attempt to identify and ligate the damaged vessel only if the hematoma continues to expand. Obvious bleeding vessels are ligated and a pack placed to promote hemostasis.

The majority of hematomas regress with time. However, Reid et al. have emphasized the problems associated with a chronic expanding hematoma. The most familiar clinical example of this problem is the chronic subdural hematoma, but a similar situation may accompany vulvar hematomas. The underlying pathophysiology is the repetitive episodes of bleeding from capillaries in the granulation tissue of the hematoma, which result in a chronic, slowly expanding vulvar mass. Treatment of a chronic expanding hematoma is drainage and debridement.

DERMATOLOGIC DISEASES

The skin of the vulva is similar to the skin over any surface of the body and is therefore susceptible to any generalized skin disease or involvement by systemic disease. The most common generalized skin diseases involving the vulva include contact dermatitis, neurodermatitis, psoriasis, seborrheic dermatitis, cutaneous candidiasis, and lichen planus. The diagnosis and treatment of these lesions are often obscured or modified by the environment of the vulva. The moisture and heat of the intertriginous areas may produce irritation, maceration, and a wet weeping surface. Therefore it is important that the gynecologist examine the skin of the entire body, as the patient may have more classic lesions of the dermatologic disease in another location. The skin of the vulva is susceptible to acute infections produced by streptococcus or staphylococcus, such as folliculitis, furunculitis, impetigo, and a special chronic infection, hidradenitis suppurativa.

The nonspecific symptom complex of vulvar pruritus and burning is presented next as an introduction to the discussion of dermatologic diseases of the vulva.

Pruritus and Vulvodynia

Pruritus is a symptom of intense itching with an associated desire to scratch and rub the affected area. In some women pruritus becomes an almost unrelenting symptom with the development of an "itch-scratch" cycle. The itch-scratch cycle is a complex of itching leading to scratching, producing excoriation and then healing. The healing skin itches, leading to further scratching. *Vulvodynia* is a term recently developed to describe chronic vulvar discomfort, including burning, stinging, and "rawness." Patients with persistent vulvodynia in which a physical cause has not been identified are often grouped under the semantic term *burning vulvar syndrome.* Pruritus and vulvodynia are nonspecific symptoms, and their differential diagnosis includes a wide range of vulvar diseases, including skin infections, sexually transmitted diseases, specific dermatosis, vulvar dystrophies, lichen sclerosis, premalignant and malignant disease, contact dermatitis, neurodermatitis, atrophy, diabetes, drug allergies, vitamin deficiencies, pediculosis, scabies, psychologic causes, and systemic diseases such as leukemia and uremia. The differential diagnosis of vulvodynia also includes neurologic diseases, especially of the nerve roots; herpes simplex infection; vulvar vestibulitis; contact dermatitis; and psychogenic causes.

The management of pruritus and vulvodynia involves establishing a diagnosis, treating of the offending cause, and improving local hygiene. For successful treatment the itch-scratch cycle must be interrupted before the condition becomes chronic, resulting in *lichenification* of the skin. During the latter process the skin becomes white, thickened, and "leathery." The resulting dry, scaly skin frequently cracks, forms fissures, and becomes secondarily infected, thus complicating the treatment. Chapter 30 discusses vulvar dystrophies.

Vulvar vestibulitis, also known as *vestibular adenitis*, is a rare syndrome of unknown etiology. Patients experience vulvar burning and pain at the introitus, particularly the area of the vulvar vestibule. Signs of this syndrome include focal ulceration and inflammation of the mucosa of the vestibule. Grossly, there are small areas of erythematous epithelium that are punctate and 3 to 10 mm in diameter, and sometimes there are associated small ulcerations. The patient is able to identify these small foci of pain when tested by repetitively touching the area with a cotton-tipped applicator. Classically, most patients have one to 10 lesions, with 75% being located in the skin between the two Bartholin's glands. Vulvar vestibulitis is similar to interstitial cystitis, another condition in which tissue that arose from the urogenital sinus produces a chronic pain syndrome without a recognized etiology. Vulvar vestibulitis has a spontaneous remission in approximately one of three patients. It may be treated medically with topical anesthetics such as viscous xylocaine. However, refractory cases are treated either by the laser or by surgical removal of the involved skin.

Contact Dermatitis

The vulvar skin, especially the intertriginous areas, is a frequent site of contact dermatitis. Contact dermatitis may be one of two basic pathophysiologic processes: a primary irritant (nonimmunologic) or a truly allergic (immunologic) etiology. Commonly, biologic fluids such as urine and feces cause irritation of the vulvar skin. Rarely, some women will be allergic to semen. The majority of chemicals that produce hypersensitivity of the vulvar skin are cosmetic or therapeutic agents, including vaginal contraceptives, lubricants, sprays, perfumes, douches, fabric dyes, fabric softeners, synthetic fibers, bleaches, soaps, chlorine, dyes in toilet tissues, and local anesthetic creams. Some of the most severe cases of contact dermatitis involve lesions of the vulvar skin secondary to poison ivy or poison oak.

Acute contact dermatitis results in a red, edematous inflamed skin. The skin may become weeping and eczematoid. The most severe skin reactions form vesicles, and any stage may become secondarily infected. The common symptoms of contact dermatitis include vulvar tenderness, burning, and pruritus.

The foundation of treatment of contact dermatitis is to withdraw the offending substance. Sometimes the distribution of the vulvar erythema helps to delineate the irritant. For example, localized erythema often results from vaginal medication, while generalized erythema of the vulva is secondary to an allergen in clothing. It is possible to use a vulvar chemical innocuously for many months or years before the topical vulvar "allergy" develops. Initial treatment of severe lesions is with wet compresses of Burow's solution (diluted 1 to 20) for 30 minutes several times a day. This is followed by drying the vulva with cool air from a hair dryer. The vulvar skin should remain clean and dry. Cotton undergarments that allow the vulvar skin to aerate should be worn, and constrictive, occlusive, or tight-fitting clothing such as pantyhose should be avoided. Vulvar dryness may be facilitated by using a nonmedicated baby powder. Hydrocortisone (0.5% to 1%) and fluorinated corticosteroids (Valisone, 0.1%, or Synalar, 0.01%) as lotions or creams may be rubbed into the skin two to three times a day for a few days to control symptoms. Synthetic systemic corticosteroids (prednisone, 50 mg a day for 7 to 10 days) are sometimes necessary for treatment of poison ivy and poison oak. Antipruritic medications, such as antihistamines, are not of great therapeutic benefit except as soporific agents.

Psoriasis

Psoriasis is a common, generalized skin disease of unknown etiology. Susceptibility to develop psoriasis is believed to be multifactorial inheritance. Generally, women develop psoriasis during their teenage years, with approximately 3% of adult women being affected. The disease is chronic with an extremely variable and unpredictable course marked by spontaneous remissions and exacerbations. Twenty-five percent of women have a family history of the disease. Common areas of involvement are the scalp and fingernails.

Vulvar psoriasis usually affects intertriginous areas and is manifested by red to red-yellow papules. These papules tend to enlarge, becoming well-circumscribed, dull-red plaques. The classic silver scales and bleeding on gentle scraping of the plaque help to establish the diagnosis. In the vulvar region the amount of scales is extremely variable. Under the influence of the moisture and heat of the vulva, vulvar psoriasis may look similar to candidiasis. Initial treatment is a topical fluorinated corticosteroid preparation. If this treatment is not successful, a dermatologist should be consulted.

Seborrheic Dermatitis

Seborrheic dermatitis is a common chronic skin disease of unknown etiology that classically affects the face, scalp, sternum, and the area behind the ears. Rarely, the mons pubis and vulvar areas may be involved. Vulvar lesions are pale to yellow-red, erythematous, and edematous, and they are covered by a fine nonadherent scale, which is usually oily. Excessive sweating and emotional tension precipitate attacks. The pruritus associated with seborrheic dermatitis varies from mild to severe. Treatment is similar to that for contact dermatitis, with hydrocortisone cream being the most effective medication. The differential diagnosis of seborrheic dermatitis includes psoriasis, cutaneous candidiasis, and contact dermatitis.

Lichen Planus

Lichen planus is a unique, chronic eruption of violaceous papules. These tiny flat papules appear in women over 30 years of age on flexor surfaces, mucous membranes, and vulvar skin. Papules often develop in linear scratch marks. The lesions are intensely pruritic and sometimes painful, and the initial onset usually follows a time of intense emotional stress. The etiology of this disease is believed to be related to an autoimmune cell-mediated response. Some women also develop an erosive desquamative vaginitis even though they have normal circulating levels of estrogen. This vaginitis may be mistakenly treated as atrophic vaginitis. Treatment of local lesions is use of a topical steroid cream. If the patient is intensely symptomatic, oral steroids may be necessary.

Hidradenitis Suppurativa

Hidradenitis suppurativa is a chronic, unrelenting, refractory infection of the skin and subcutaneous tissue. Initially it develops from one or more subcutaneous nodules. Subsequently, deep scars and pits are formed. The patient undergoes great emotional distress as this condition is both painful and associated with a foul-smelling discharge. If treatment is unsuccessful with antibiotics and topical steroids, other medical therapies of the early stages of the disease include antiandrogens and isotretinoin. Gradually a deep-seated chronic infection of apocrine glands develops, with occlusion of dilated ducts with inspissated keratin material. In the advanced stages, hidradenitis suppurativa progresses to multiple draining abscesses and sinuses. Bhatia et al. recommend that the diagnosis be confirmed by biopsy. The treatment of choice is early, aggressive, wide operative excision of the infected skin. The differential diagnosis of hidradenitis suppurativa includes Crohn's disease of the vulva and granulomatous sexually transmitted diseases.

Edema

Edema of the vulva may be a symptom of either local or generalized disease. Two of the most common causes of edema of the vulva are secondary reactions to inflammation or to lymphatic blockage. Vulvar edema is often noted before edema in other areas of the female body is noted. The loose connective tissue of the vulva and its dependent position predispose to early development of pitting edema. Systemic causes of vulvar edema include circulatory and renal failure, ascites, and hypoproteinemia. Vulvar edema also may occur after intraperitoneal dextran is given to prevent adhesions following infertility operations. Local causes of vulvar edema include allergy, neurodermatitis, inflammation, trauma, and lymphatic obstruction due to carcinoma or infection. Infectious diseases that are associated with vulvar edema include tuberculosis, syphilis, filariasis, and lymphogranuloma venereum.

VAGINA

Urethral Diverticulum

A urethral diverticulum is a permanent, epithelialized, saclike projection that arises from the posterior urethra. It is a common problem, being discovered in approximately 3% of women. The majority of cases are initially diagnosed in reproductive-age females, with the peak incidence in the fourth decade of life. The symptoms of a urethral diverticulum are nonspecific and are identical to the general symptoms of a lower urinary tract infection. To diagnose this elusive condition, one should suspect urethral diverticulum in any woman with chronic or recurrent lower urinary tract symptoms. The urologic aspects of this condition are discussed in Chapter 20. Histologically the diverticulum is lined by epithelium; however, there is a lack of muscle in the saclike pocket.

Urethral diverticula may be congenital or acquired. Few urethral diverticula present in children; therefore it is assumed that most diverticula are not congenital. Huffman made the analogy that anatomically the urethra is similar to a tree with many stunted branches that rep-

TABLE 17-1

Location of the Ostium in 108 Female Patients with Diverticulum of the Urethra

Site	No. of Patients
Distal (external) third of the urethra	11
Middle third of the urethra	55
Proximal (inner) third of the urethra (including vesical neck)	18
Multiple sites	18
Unknown	6

From Lee RA: Clin Obstet Gynecol 27:491, 1984.

resent the periurethral ducts and glands. It is assumed that the majority of urethral diverticula result from repetitive or chronic infections of the periurethral glands. The suburethral infection may cause obstruction of the ducts and glands, with subsequent production of cystic enlargement and retention cysts. These cysts may rupture into the urethral lumen and produce a suburethral diverticulum. Occasionally a suburethral diverticulum has associated stone formation in the dilated retention cyst. Urethral diverticula are small, from 3 mm to 3 cm in diameter. The majority of urethral diverticula open into the midportion of the urethra (Table 17-1). Occasionally, multiple suburethral diverticula occur in the same woman.

The most common symptoms associated with urethral diverticula are urinary urgency, frequency, and dysuria. Ginsburg and Genadry discovered that 90% of their patients had symptoms of chronic lower urinary tract infection as the presenting complaint. Other authors have stressed the three Ds associated with a diverticula: *dysuria, dyspareunia,* and *dribbling* of the urine. Although for years postvoiding dribbling has been termed a classic symptom of urethral diverticulum, it is reported by fewer than 10% of women with this condition. In Lee's series a palpable, tender mass was felt in 56 of 108 patients. Ginsburg and Genadry found a palpable mass in 46 of 70 women with a urethral diverticulum. It is interesting that in most large series, approximately 20% of the women are asymptomatic. A classic sign of a suburethral diverticulum is the expression of purulent material from the urethra after compressing the suburethral area during a pelvic examination.

The foundation of diagnosing urethral diver-

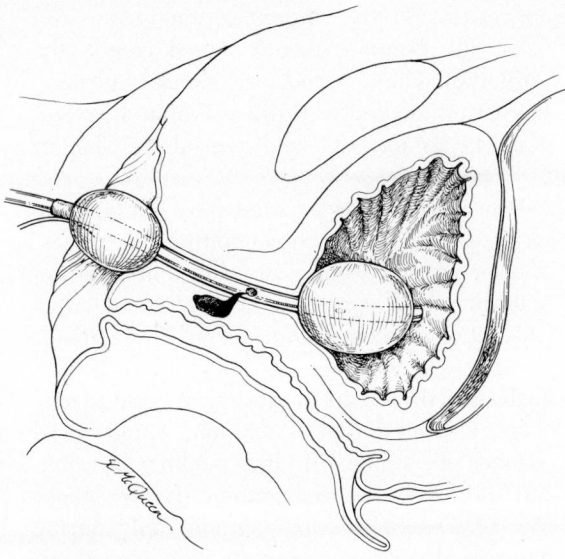

FIGURE 17-9
Double-balloon catheter in use for positive-pressure urethrography. (From Mattingly RF and Thompson JD, editors: TeLinde's operative gynecology, ed 6, Philadelphia, 1985, JB Lippincott Co, p 751.)

ticulum is the physician's awareness of the possibility of this defect occurring in women with chronic symptoms of lower urinary tract infection. Subsequently it is important to appreciate that a single diagnostic procedure may not identify the diverticulum. The two most common methods of diagnosing urethral diverticulum are voiding cystourethrography and cystourethroscopy. Approximately 70% of urethral diverticula will be filled by contrast material on a postvoiding x-ray film with a lateral view. Cystourethroscopy will demonstrate the urethral opening of the urethral diverticulum in approximately 6 of 10 cases. Other diagnostic tests used to identify urethral diverticula include urethral pressure profile recordings and a positive-pressure urethrography. The latter test is done with a special double-balloon urethral catheter (Davis catheter) (Figure 17-9). Ultrasound has been used to diagnose urethral diverticulum but is of limited diagnostic benefit. The differential diagnosis includes Gartner's duct cyst, an ectopic ureter that empties into the urethra, and Skene's glands cysts.

Several different operations can correct urethral diverticula. Excisional surgery should be scheduled when the diverticulum is not acutely infected. Operative techniques can be divided into transurethral and transvaginal approaches, with most gynecologists preferring the transvaginal approach as described by Lee. The vast majority of diverticula enter into the posterior aspect of the urethra. Diverticula of the distal one-third may be treated by simple marsupialization. Following operations, approximately 80% of patients obtain complete relief from symptoms. Some diverticula have multiple openings into the urethra. Complete excision of this network of fistulous connections is important. The recurrence rate varies between 10% and 20%, and many failures are due to incomplete surgical resection. The most serious consequences of surgical repair of urethral diverticula are urinary incontinence and urethrovaginal fistula. Postoperative incontinence usually follows operative repairs of large diverticula that are near the bladder neck. This incontinence is secondary to damage to the urethral sphincter. The incidence of each of these complications is approximately 1% to 2%.

Inclusion Cysts

Inclusion cysts are the most common cystic structures of the vagina. In Deppisch's series of 64 women with cystic masses of the vagina, 34 had inclusion cysts. The cysts are usually discovered in the posterior or lateral walls of the lower third of the vagina. Inclusion cysts vary from 1 mm to 3 cm. Deppisch reported a mean diameter of 1.6 cm. Similar to inclusion cysts of the vulva, inclusion cysts of the vagina are more common in parous women. Inclusion cysts usually result from birth trauma or gynecologic surgery. Often they are discovered in the site of a previous episiotomy or at the apex of the vagina following hysterectomy.

Histologically, inclusion cysts are lined by stratified squamous epithelium. These cysts contain a thick, pale-yellow substance that is oily and formed by degenerating epithelial cells. Often these cysts are erroneously called sebaceous cysts in the misbelief that the central material is sebaceous. Similar to vulvar inclusion cysts, the etiology is either a small tag of vaginal epithelium buried beneath the surface following a gynecologic or obstetric procedure or a misplaced island of embryonic remnant that was destined to form epithelium.

The majority of inclusion cysts are asymptomatic. If the cyst produces dyspareunia or pain, excisional biopsy is appropriate.

Dysontogenetic Cysts

Dysontogenetic cysts of the vagina are thin-walled, soft cysts of embryonic origin. Whether the cysts arise from the mesonephros (Gartner's duct cyst), the perimesonephrium (müllerian cyst), or the urogenital sinus (vestibular cyst) is predominantly of academic rather than clinical importance. The cysts may be differentiated histologically by the epithelial lining. Most mesonephric cysts have cuboidal, nonciliated epithelium. Most perimesonephric cysts have columnar, endocervical-like epithelium. Although most commonly single, dysontogenetic cysts may be multiple. The cysts are usually 1 to 5 cm in diameter and are usually discovered in the upper one half of the vagina. Sometimes multiple small cysts may present like a string of large, soft beads. A large cyst presenting at the introitus may be mistaken for a cystocele, anterior enterocele, or obstructed aberrant ureter. Approximately 1 in 200 females develop these cysts.

Embryonic cysts of the vagina, especially those on the anterior lateral wall, are usually Gartner's duct cysts. The distal portion of the mesonephric duct runs parallel with the vagina. It is assumed that a segment of this embryonic structure fails to regress, and the obstructed vestigial remnant becomes cystic.

Most of these benign cysts are asymptomatic, sausage-shaped tumors that are discovered only incidentally during pelvic examination. Small asymptomatic Gartner's duct cysts may be followed conservatively. Deppisch, in a series of 25 women undergoing operations for symptomatic dysontogenetic cysts, reported a wide range of symptoms, including dyspareunia, vaginal pain, urinary symptoms, and a palpable mass. Sometimes large cysts interfere with the use of tampons.

Operative excision is indicated for chronic mechanical symptoms. Rarely one of these cysts becomes infected, and if operated on during the acute phase, marsupialization of the cyst is preferred. Occasionally, excision of the vaginal cyst is a much more formidable operation than anticipated. The cystic structure may extend up into the broad ligament and anatomically be in proximity to the distal course of the ureter.

Tampon Problems

The vaginal tampon has achieved immense popularity and ubiquitous use by women. It is not surprising that there are rare associated risks with tampon usage: vaginal ulcers, the "forgotten" tampon, and toxic shock syndrome. The latter, related to toxins elaborated by *Staphylococcus aureus*, is discussed in Chapter 21.

Wearing tampons for a few days has been associated with microscopic epithelial changes. The majority of women develop epithelial dehydration and epithelial layering, and some will develop microscopic ulcers. These minor changes take between 48 hours to 7 days to heal. Friedrich, in a study of colposcopic changes related to the tampon, found serial changes of epithelial drying, peeling, layering, and ultimately microulceration. In his study, 15% of women wearing tampons only during the time of normal menstruation developed microulcerations.

Barrett et al. were the first to describe large macroscopic ulcers of the vaginal fornix in four women who were tampon "abusers." Each of these young women wore vaginal tampons for prolonged lengths of time for persistent vaginal discharge or spotting, changing the individual tampon several times per day. The ulcers had a base of clean granulation tissue with smooth, rolled edges. Jimmerson and Becker found birefractal foreign body fragments in biopsy specimens (fibers from tampons) in the vaginal ulcers of 4 of 10 women. The pathophysiology of the ulcer is believed to be secondary to drying and pressure necrosis induced by the tampon. Obviously, many of these young women use tampons for the identical symptoms that are associated with a vaginal ulcer, that is, spotting and vaginal discharge. Often the intermenstrual spotting is believed to be breakthrough bleeding from oral contraceptives, and the possibility of a vaginal ulcer from chronic tampon usage is overlooked.

Vaginal ulcers are not uncommon secondary to several types of foreign objects, including diaphragms, pessaries, and medicated silicon rings. Management is conservative, as the ulcers heal spontaneously when the foreign object is removed. Any persistent ulcer should be biopsied to rule out carcinoma.

A woman with a "lost" or "forgotten" tampon presents with a classic foul vaginal discharge and occasionally spotting. The tampon is usually found high in the vagina. The odor from a forgotten tampon is overwhelming. The woman should be treated with an antibiotic vaginal cream (Sultrin) for the next 5 to 7 days.

Local Trauma

The most frequent etiology of trauma to the lower genital tract of adult females is coitus. Approximately 80% of vaginal lacerations occur secondary to sexual intercourse. Other causes of vaginal trauma are straddle injuries, penetration injuries by foreign objects, sexual assault, vaginismus, and water skiing accidents. The management of vulvar and vaginal trauma in children is discussed in Chapter 10.

The predisposing factors believed to be related to coital injury include virginity, the postpartum and postmenopausal vaginal epithelium, pregnancy, intercourse after a prolonged period of abstinence, hysterectomy, and inebriation. Smith et al. reviewed 19 injuries from normal coitus; 12 of the women in his series were between the ages of 16 and 25 and 5 were over age 45. The most common injury is a transverse tear of the posterior fornix. Similar linear lacerations often occur in the right or left vaginal fornices. The location of the coital injury is believed to be related to the poor support of the upper vagina, which is supported only by a thin layer of connective tissue. The most prominent symptom of a coital vaginal laceration is profuse or prolonged vaginal bleeding. Many women experienced sharp pain during intercourse, and 25% noted persistent abdominal pain. The most troublesome but extremely rare complication of vaginal laceration is vaginal evisceration.

Often the history of the coital injury is not obtained, and the patient may even give misleading information. However, coital injury to the vagina should be considered in any woman with profuse or prolonged abnormal vaginal bleeding.

Management of coital lacerations involves prompt suturing under adequate anesthesia. There is no place for conservative management. Secondary injury to the urinary and gastrointestinal tracts should be ruled out.

CERVIX

Endocervical and Cervical Polyps

Endocervical and cervical polyps are the most common benign neoplastic growths of the cervix. In an extensive series Farrar and Nedoss reported an incidence of endocervical polyps in 4% of all gynecologic patients. Endocervical polyps are most common in multiparous women in their 40s and 50s. The majority are smooth, soft, reddish-purple to cherry red, and fragile. They readily bleed when touched. Endocervical polyps may be single or multiple and are a few millimeters to 4 cm in diameter. The stalk of the polyp is of variable length and width (Fig. 17-10). Polyps may arise from either the endocervical canal (endocervical polyp) or ectocervix (cervical polyp). Endocervical polyps are more common than cervical polyps. The terms *endocervical* and *cervical* polyps are used to describe the same abnormality because they are treated in a similar fashion. Polyps whose base is in the endocervix usually have a narrow, long pedicle and occur during the reproductive years, while polyps that arise from the ectocervix have a short, broad base and usually occur in postmenopausal women.

The general hypothesis of the origin of endocervical polyps is that they are usually secondary to inflammation. Focal hyperplasia and localized proliferation are the response of the cervix to local inflammation. The color of the polyp depends in part on its origin, with most endocervical polyps being cherry red and most cervical polyps grayish-white.

The classic symptoms of an endocervical polyp are intermenstrual bleeding, especially following contact such as coitus or an examination. Sometimes an associated leukorrhea emanates from the infected cervix. A large polyp may dilate the cervix as its dependent portion protrudes into the vagina. Many endocervical polyps are asymptomatic and recognized for the first time during a routine speculum examination. Often the polyp seen on inspection is difficult to palpate because of its soft consistency.

Histologically the surface epithelium of the polyp is columnar or squamous epithelium, depending on the site of origin and the degree of squamous metaplasia (Figure 17-11). The stalk is composed of an edematous, inflamed, loose, and richly vascular connective tissue. During pregnancy, focal areas of decidual changes may develop in the stroma. Often there is ulceration of the stalk's most dependent portion, which explains the symptom of contact bleeding. Malignant degeneration of an endocervical polyp is extremely rare. Considerations in the differential diagnosis include endometrial polyps, small prolapsed myomas, retained products of conception, squamous papilloma, sarcoma, and cervical malignancy. Microglandular endocervical hyperplasia sometimes presents as a 1 to 2 cm polyp. This is an exaggerated

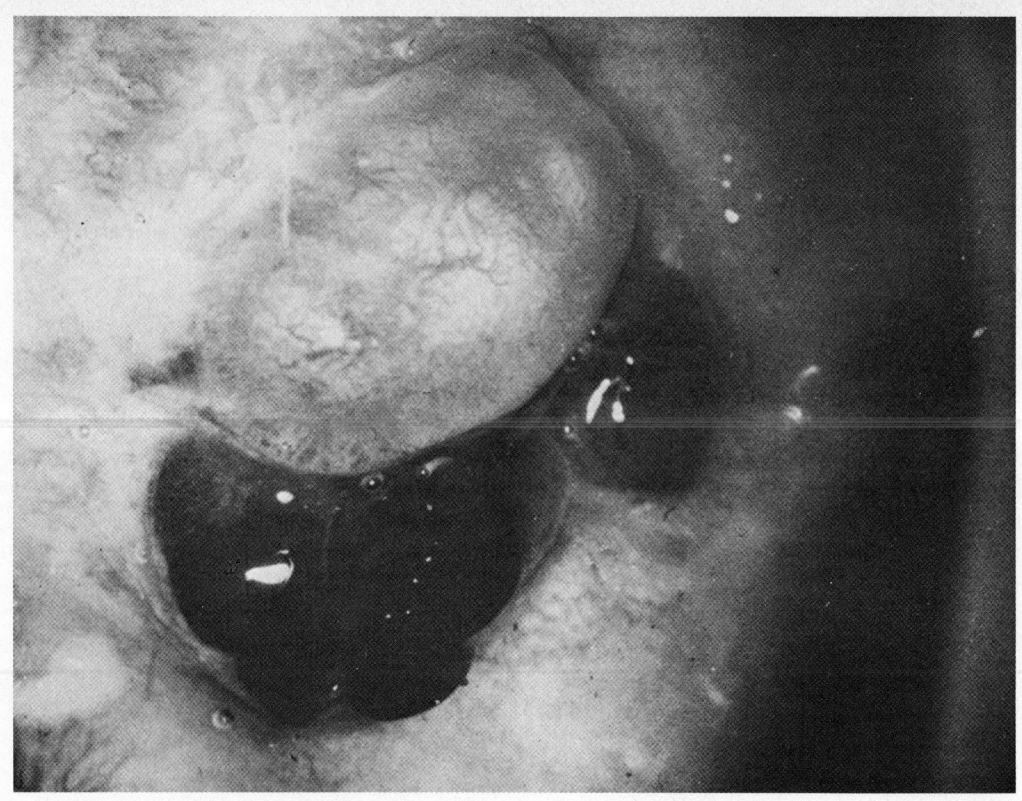

FIGURE 17-10
Endocervical polyp: clinical appearance. (From Gompel C and Silverberg SG, editors: Pathology in gynecology and obstetrics, ed 2, Philadelphia, 1977, JB Lippincott Co, p 74.)

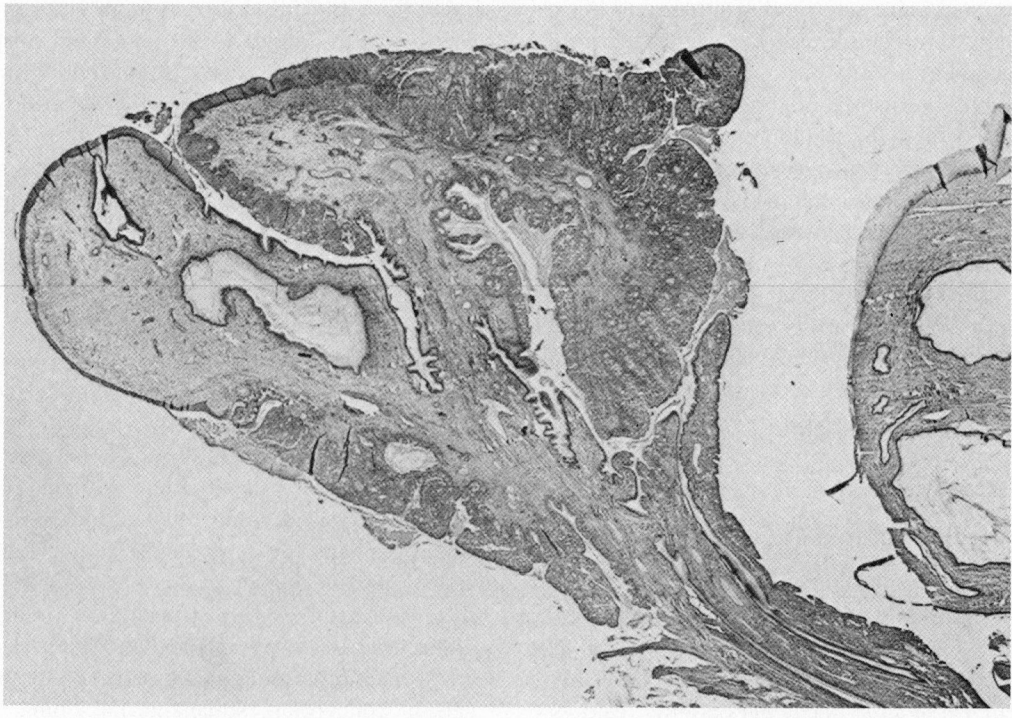

FIGURE 17-11
Endocervical polyp with zones of squamous metaplasia. (From Gompel C and Silverberg SG, editors: Pathology in gynecology and obstetrics, ed 2, Philadelphia, 1977, JB Lippincott Co, p 74.)

histologic response, usually to oral contraceptives.

Most endocervical polyps may be managed in the office by grasping the base of the polyp with an appropriately sized clamp. The polyp is avulsed with a twisting motion and sent to the pathology laboratory for microscopic evaluation. If the base is broad or bleeding ensues, the base may be treated with chemical cautery, electrocautery, or cryocautery. If abnormal bleeding continues after the polyp is removed, endometrial sampling should be performed to diagnose an unrelated endometrial hyperplasia or carcinoma that might have produced symptoms identical to those of the polyp.

Nabothian Cysts

Nabothian cysts are retention cysts of endocervical columnar cells occurring where a tunnel or cleft has been covered by squamous metaplasia. These cysts are so common that they are considered a normal feature of the adult cervix. Many women have multiple cysts. Grossly, these cysts may be translucent or opaque whitish blobs. Nabothian cysts vary from microscopic to macroscopic size, with the majority between 3 mm and 3 cm in diameter. Rarely, a woman with several large nabothian cysts may develop gross enlargement of the cervix. These mucous retention cysts are produced by the spontaneous healing process of the cervix. The cervix is in an almost constant process of repair, and squamous cells block the cleft of a gland orifice. The endocervical columnar cells continue to secrete, and thus a mucous retention cyst is formed. Nabothian cysts are asymptomatic, and no treatment is necessary.

Lacerations

Cervical lacerations frequently occur with both normal and abnormal deliveries. Lacerations may occur in nonpregnant women with mechanical dilation of the cervix. Obstetric lacerations vary from minor superficial tears to extensive full-thickness lacerations at 3 and 9 o'clock, respectively, which may extend into the broad ligament. In gynecology the atrophic cervix of the postmenopausal woman predisposes to the complication of cervical laceration when the cervix is mechanically dilated for a diagnostic dilation and curettage.

Acute cervical lacerations bleed and should be sutured. Cervical lacerations that are not repaired may give the external os of the cervix a fish-mouthed appearance; however, they are usually asymptomatic. Extensive cervical lacerations may lead to incompetence of the cervix during pregnancy. The use of laminaria tents to slowly soften and dilate the cervix before mechanical instrumentation of the endometrial cavity has reduced the magnitude of iatrogenic cervical lacerations. Furthermore, the practice of routine inspection of the cervix, stabilized with one or more ring forceps, following every second- or third-trimester delivery has enabled physicians to discover and repair extensive cervical lacerations.

Cervical Myomas

Cervical myomas are smooth, firm masses that are usually solitary and are similar to myomas of the fundus (Figures 17-12 and 17-13). Depending on the series, 3% to 8% of myomas are categorized as cervical myomas. In fact, because of the relative paucity of smooth muscle fibers in the cervical stroma, the majority of myomas that appear to be cervical actually arise from the isthmus of the uterus.

Most cervical myomas are small and asymptomatic. When symptoms do occur, they are dependent on the direction in which the enlarging myoma expands. Cervical myomas may

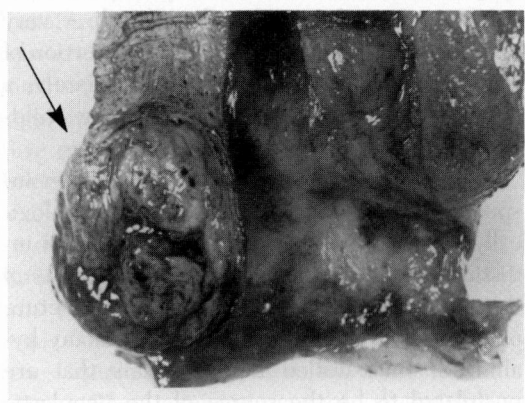

FIGURE 17-12
Leiomyoma, originating in cervix and dilating endocervical canal. It is soft, showing degenerative changes. (From Janovski NA, editor: *Color atlas of gross gynecologic and obstetric pathology*, New York, 1969, McGraw-Hill Book Co, p 71.)

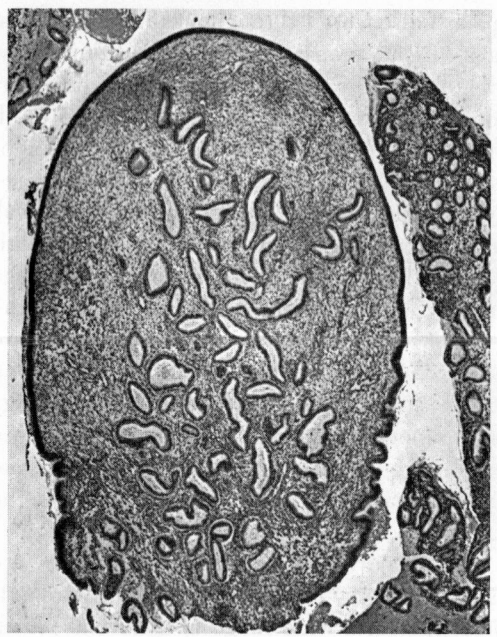

FIGURE 17-14
Typical small endometrial polyp. (From Novak ER and Woodruff JD, editors: Novak's gynecologic and obstetric pathology, ed 6, Philadelphia, 1967, WB Saunders Co, p 206.)

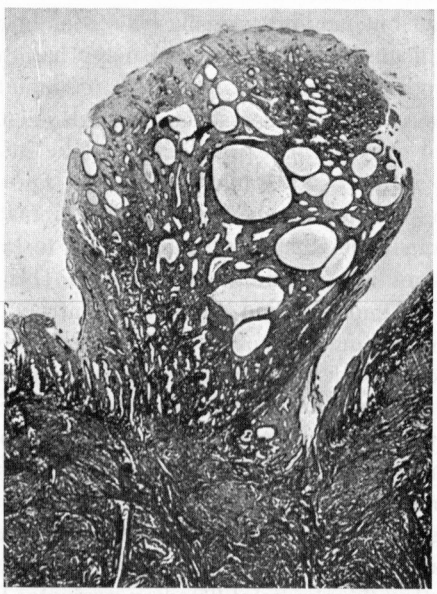

FIGURE 17-15
Endometrial polyp showing hyperplastic, nonfunctioning structure. This is much more common than the functioning type. (From Novak ER and Woodruff JD, editors: Novak's gynecologic and obstetric pathology, ed 6, Philadelphia, 1967, WB Saunders Co, p 207.)

polyp has been estimated to be as high as 0.5%. However, an epidemiologic, population-based, case-control study from Sweden by Pettersson et al. estimates that the increased risk of subsequent endometrial carcinoma in women with endometrial polyps is only twofold. This study provides a more realistic appraisal of the risk. Malignant change, when found in an endometrial polyp, is usually curable, and the endometrial carcinoma is most often of a low stage and grade. It is interesting that benign polyps have been found in approximately 20% of uteri removed for endometrial carcinoma.

As most endometrial polyps are asymptomatic, the diagnosis is not usually established until the uterus is opened following hysterectomy for other reasons. Endometrial polyps have been discovered by hysteroscopy and hysterosalpingography during the diagnostic workup of a woman with a refractory case of abnormal uterine bleeding.

The management of endometrial polyps is removal by curettage or via the hysteroscope. Because of the frequent association of endometrial polyps and other endometrial pathology, it is important to examine histologically both the polyp and the associated endometrial lining. Polyps, because of their mobility, often tend to elude the curette. Postcurettage hysteroscopic studies have demonstrated that routine use of a long, narrow polyp forceps at the time of curettage at best results in discovery and removal of only approximately one in four endometrial polyps.

Hematometra

A hematometra is a uterus distended with blood and is secondary to gynatresia, which is partial or complete obstruction of any portion of the lower genital tract. Obstruction of the isthmus of the uterus, cervix, or vagina may be congenital or acquired. The two most common congenital causes of hematometra are an imperforate hymen and a transverse vaginal septum. Among the leading causes of acquired lower tract stenosis are senile atrophy of the endocervical canal and endometrium, scarring of the isthmus by synechiae, cervical stenosis associated with surgery, radiation therapy, cryocautery or electrocautery, malignant disease of the endocervical canal, and cervical obstruction by tissue following suction curettage.

The symptoms of hematometra depend on

the age of the patient, her menstrual history and the rapidity of the accumulation of blood in the uterine cavity, and the possibility of secondary infection producing pyometra. Thus common symptoms of hematometra include primary or secondary amenorrhea and possibly cyclic lower abdominal pain. During the early teenage years the combination of primary amenorrhea and cyclic episodic cramping lower abdominal pains suggests the possibility of a developing hematometra. Occasionally the obstruction is incomplete, and there is associated spotting of dark-brown blood. Hematometra in postmenopausal women may be entirely asymptomatic. On pelvic examination a mildly tender, globular uterus is usually palpated.

The diagnosis of hematometra is generally suspected by the history of amenorrhea and cyclic abdominal pain. The diagnosis is usually confirmed by probing the cervix with a narrow metal dilator with release of dark brownish-black blood from the endocervical canal. Often the blood retained inside the uterus becomes secondarily infected and has a foul odor.

Management of hematometra is dependent on operative relief of the lower tract obstruction. Treatment of congenital obstruction is discussed in Chapter 9. Appropriate biopsy specimens of the endocervical canal and endometrium should be obtained to rule out malignancy when the cause of hematometra is not obvious. If the uterus is significantly enlarged or if there is any suspicion that the retained fluid is infected, drainage should be accomplished first. Biopsy should be postponed for approximately 1 month to diminish the chances of infection or uterine perforation. Hematometra following operations or cryocautery usually resolves with cervical dilation. Hematometra following a first-trimester abortion is treated by repeat suction aspiration of the products of conception that are blocking the internal os.

Leiomyomas

Leiomyomas, also called *myomas*, are benign tumors of muscle cell origin. These tumors are often referred to by their popular names, *fibroids* or *fibromyomas*, but both terms are semantic misnomers if one is referring to the cell of origin. Most leiomyomas contain varying amounts of fibrous tissue, which is believed to be secondary to degeneration of some of the smooth muscle cells.

Leiomyomas are the most frequent pelvic tumors, with the highest incidence occurring during the fifth decade of a woman's life. Although leiomyomas arise throughout the body in any structure containing smooth muscle, in the pelvis the majority are found in the corpus of the uterus. Occasionally, leiomyomas may be found in the fallopian tube or the round ligament, and approximately 5% of uterine myomas originate from the cervix. Myomas may be single but most often are multiple. Myomas are discovered in one of four white women and one of two black women. They vary greatly in size from microscopic to large, multinodular uterine tumors that may weigh more than 50 pounds and literally fill the patient's abdomen. Myomas are more prone to grow and become symptomatic in nulliparous women and women with earlier menarche. The question as to why some women develop myomas while others do not is unanswered.

All myomas initially develop from the myometrium, beginning as intramural myomas. As they grow, they remain attached to the myometrium with a pedicle of varying width and thickness. Myomas are classed into subgroups by their relative anatomic relationship and position to the layers of the uterus (Figure 17-16). The three most common types of myomas are intramural (Figures 17-17 and 17-18), subserous, and submucous, with special nomenclature for broad ligament and parasitic myomas. Continued growth in one direction determines which myomas will be located just below the endometrium, submucosal, and which will be found just beneath the serosa, subserosal (Figure 17-19). Although only 5% to 10% of myomas become submucosal, they usually are the most troublesome clinically. These submucosal tumors may be associated with abnormal vaginal bleeding or distortion of the uterine cavity that may produce infertility or abortion. Rarely, a submucosal myoma enlarges and becomes pedunculated. The uterus will try to expel it, and the prolapsed myoma may protrude through the external cervical os. Subserosal myomas give the uterus its knobby contour during pelvic examination.

Further growth of a subserosal myoma may lead to a pedunculated myoma wandering into the peritoneal cavity. This myoma may outgrow its uterine blood supply and obtain a secondary blood supply from another organ, such as the omentum, and become a parasitic myoma. Growth of a myoma in a lateral direction

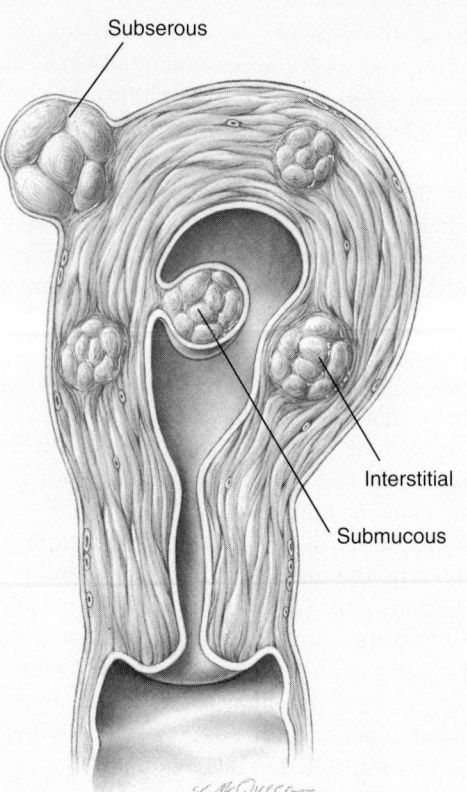

FIGURE 17-16

Drawing of cut surface of uterus showing characteristic whorl-like appearance and varying locations of leiomyomas. (From Novak ER and Woodruff JD, editors: Novak's gynecologic and obstetric pathology, ed 6, Philadelphia, 1967, WB Saunders Co, p 215.)

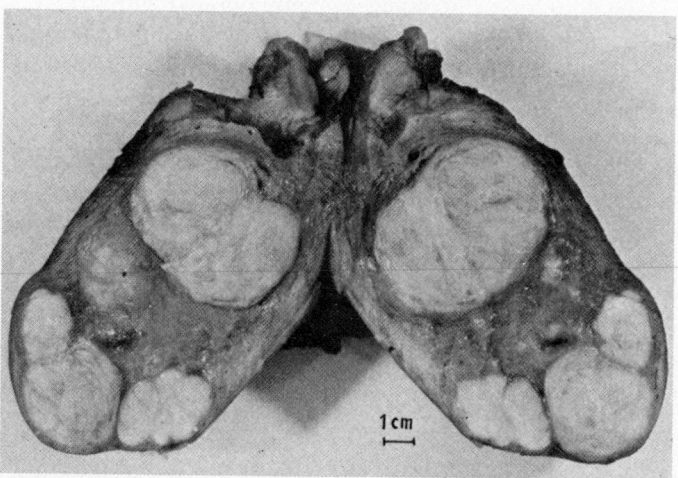

FIGURE 17-17

Intramural leiomyomata. (From Gompel C and Silverberg SG, editors: Pathology in gynecology and obstetrics, ed 2, Philadelphia, 1977, JB Lippincott Co, p 186.)

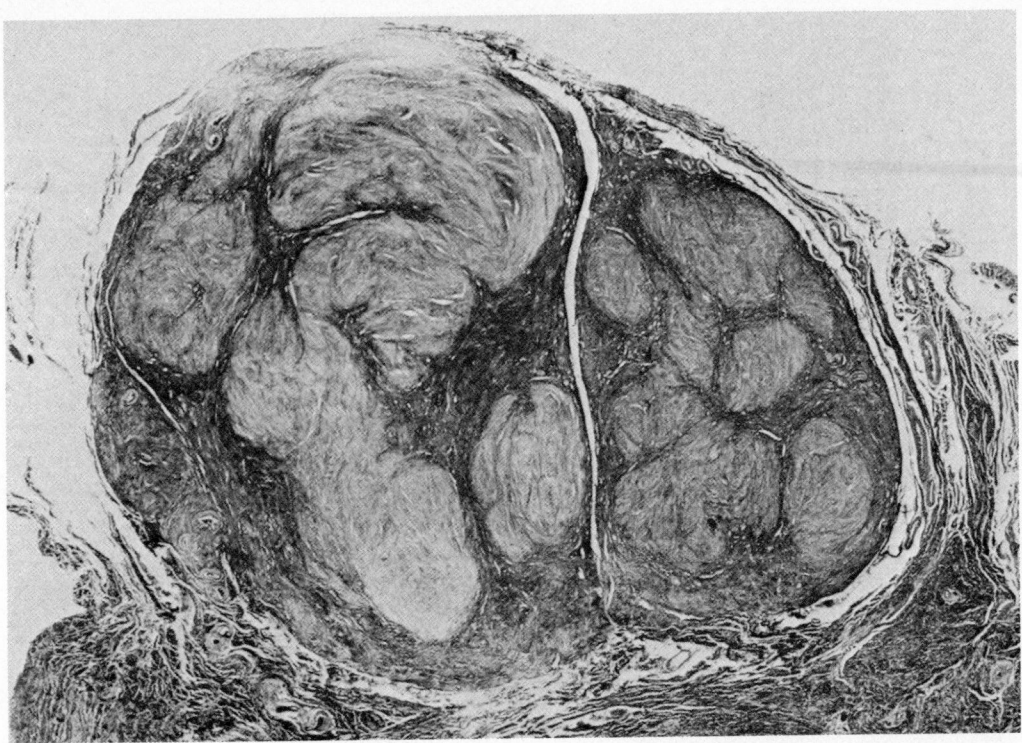

FIGURE 17-18
Intramural leiomyoma. (From Gompel C and Silverberg SG, editors: Pathology in gynecology and obstetrics, ed 2, Philadelphia, 1977, JB Lippincott Co, p 187.)

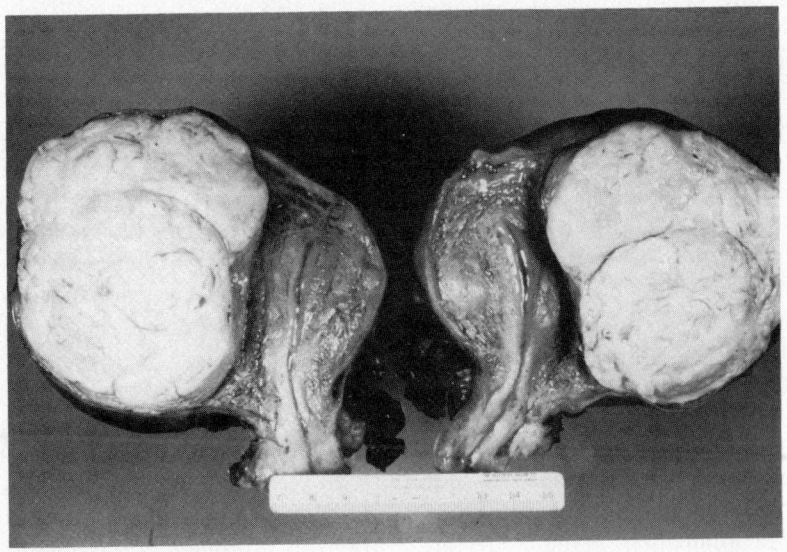

FIGURE 17-19
Large subserosal myoma. (Courtesy William Droegemueller and Vern L. Katz.)

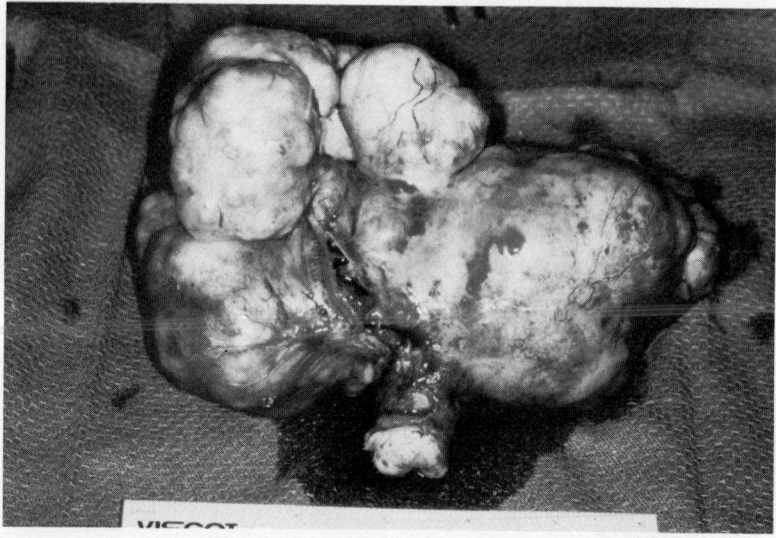

FIGURE 17-20
Hysterectomy specimen of myomatous uterus. (Courtesy Vern L. Katz and William Droegemueller.)

may result in a broad ligament myoma (Figure 17-20). The clinical significance of broad ligament myomas is that they are difficult to differentiate on pelvic examination from a solid ovarian tumor. Broad ligament myomas often produce a hydroureter as they enlarge.

Small myomas are round, firm, solid tumors. With continued growth the myometrium at the edge of the tumor is compressed and forms a pseudocapsule. Although myomas do not have a true capsule, this pseudocapsule is a valuable surgical plane during a myomectomy.

The etiology of uterine leiomyomas is incompletely understood. It is known that each tumor results from an original single muscle cell. Each uterine myoma is monoclonal in that all cells have identical electrophoretic variance of glucose-6-phosphate dehydrogenase. Pathologists have two different theories as to the cell of origin of this smooth muscle tumor. One hypothesis proposes that the cell of origin is from persistent, small, embryonic cell rests, whereas the other theory proposes that myomas originate from the smooth muscle of blood vessels.

The stimulus for growth of myomas is similarly unclear; however, the growth may be related to estrogen stimulation. Myomas are rare before menarche, and most myomas diminish in size following menopause or castration, with the reduction of a significant amount of circu-

lating estrogen. Myomas often enlarge during pregnancy and occasionally enlarge secondary to oral contraceptive therapy with relatively high levels of estrogens. Medically induced hypoestrogenic states produce reductions in the size of myomas. Soules and McCarty studied the steroid receptor content of leiomyomas. Estrogen receptors are found in higher concentrations in myomas than in the surrounding myometrium. Women who smoke cigarettes and are thus relatively estrogen deficient have a lower incidence of myomas. Many women, though, have small myomas that do not grow under the influence of high circulating estrogen levels. Thus the relationship between estrogen and myoma growth is complex. Cramer et al. are studying the growth potential of uterine leiomyomas in vitro and have found heterogeneity in hormonal responsiveness. Other investigators have suggested that growth hormone may also influence the growth of these tumors.

Grossly, a myoma has a lighter color than the normal myometrium. On cut surface the tumor has a glistening, pearl-white appearance, with the smooth muscle arranged in a trabeculated or whorled configuration. Histologically, there is a proliferation of mature smooth muscle cells. The nonstriated muscle fibers are arranged in interlacing bundles. Between bundles of smooth muscle cells are variable

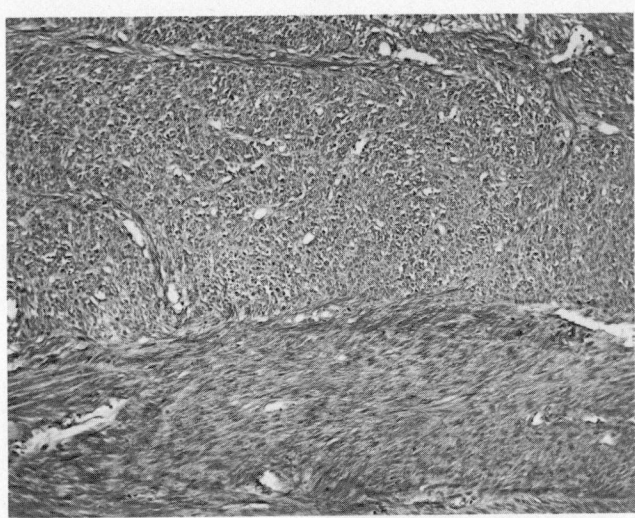

FIGURE 17-21
Histologic section of leiomyoma. (Courtesy Daniel R. Mishell, Jr., M.D.)

amounts of fibrous connective tissue, especially toward the center of any large tumor (Figures 17-21, 17-22, and 17-23). The amount of fibrous tissue is proportional to the extent of atrophy and degeneration that has occurred over time.

The eventual fate of most myomas is determined by their relatively poor vascular supply. This supply is found in one or two major arteries at the base or pedicle of the myoma. The arterial supply of myomas is significantly less than that of a similar-sized area of normal myometrium. Thus, with continued growth, degeneration occurs because the tumor outgrows its blood supply. The severity of the discrepancy between the myoma's growth and its blood supply determines the extent of degeneration: hyaline, myxomatous, calcific, cystic, fatty, or red degeneration and necrosis. The mildest form of degeneration of a myoma is hyaline degeneration. Grossly, in this condition the surface of the myoma is homogeneous with loss of the whorled pattern. Histologically with hyaline degeneration, cellular detail is lost as the smooth muscle cells are replaced by fibrous connective tissue.

The most acute form of degeneration is red or carneous infarction. This acute muscular infarction causes severe pain and localized peritoneal irritation. This form of degeneration occurs during pregnancy in approximately 5% to 10% of gravid women with myomas. The ultra-

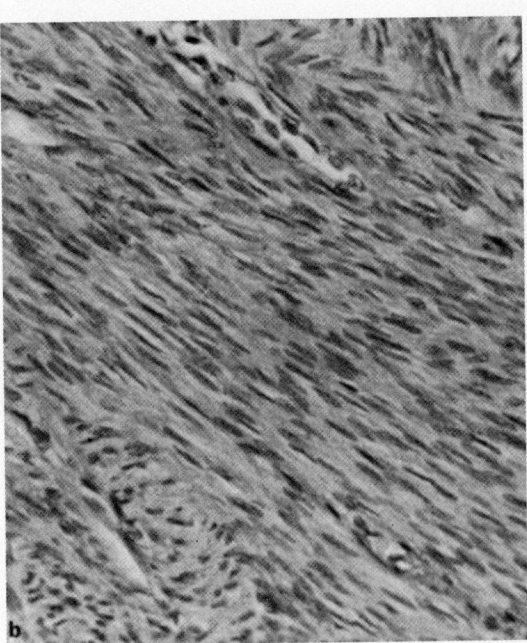

FIGURE 17-22
Leiomyoma showing interlacing bundles of smooth muscles with spindle nuclei without degeneration. (From Demopoulos RI: Benign lesions of the myometrium. In Blaustein A, editor: Pathology of the female genital tract, New York, 1977, Springer-Verlag New York, Inc, p 302.)

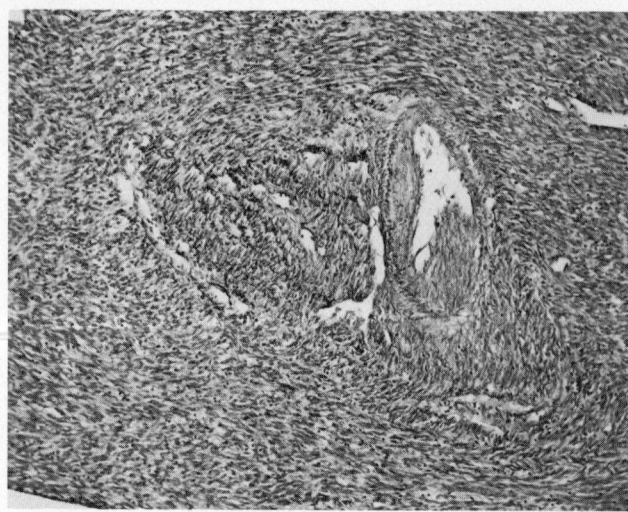

FIGURE 17-23
Leiomyoma histologic section of a cellular myoma. (Courtesy Daniel R. Mishell, Jr., M.D.)

sound appearance of painful myomas is one of mixed echodense and echolucent areas. Serial ultrasound examinations have also demonstrated that most (80%) myomas do not change size during pregnancy; if a change in size does occur, it is usually not associated with painful symptomatology. During pregnancy this complication should be treated medically, for attempts at operative removal result in profuse blood loss. If the patient is not pregnant, acute degeneration is not a contraindication to myomectomy. Obviously the more advanced forms of degenerating myomas may become secondarily infected, especially when large necrotic areas exist. The histologic changes of degeneration are found more commonly in larger myomas. However, two thirds of all myomas show some degree of degeneration, with the three most common types being hyaline degeneration (65%), myxomatous degeneration (15%), and calcific degeneration (10%).

The literature emphasizes that the incidence of malignant degeneration is estimated to be between 0.3% and 0.7%. The term *malignant degeneration* is ambiguous. It is unknown as to whether myomas degenerate into sarcomas or if sarcomas arise spontaneously in myomatous uteri. In a recent series of 1429 hysterectomies in patients with a preoperative diagnosis of symptoms related to myomas, leiomyosarcomas were found histologically in 0.49%.

The symptoms related to myomas are related to primarily pressure from an enlarging pelvic mass, pain including dysmenorrhea, abnormal uterine bleeding, infertility, and pregnancy complications, including abortion, premature labor, and dystocia. The severity of symptoms is often directly related to the number, location, and size of the myomas. However, the majority of women with uterine myomas are asymptomatic.

One of three women with myomas experiences pelvic pain. Acquired dysmenorrhea is the most frequent complaint, with a study by Iosif and Akerlund from Sweden documenting an associated increase in myometrial activity. Various forms of vascular compromise, either acute degeneration or torsion of the pedicle, produce severe pelvic pain. Milder pelvic discomfort is described as pelvic heaviness or a dull aching sensation that may be secondary to edematous swelling in the myoma.

An enlarged myoma or myomas often produce pressure symptoms similar to those of an enlarging pregnant uterus. Sometimes a woman will notice that her abdominal girth is increasing without appreciable change in weight. Alternately, an anterior myoma pressing on the bladder may produce urinary frequency and urgency. In general, urinary symptoms are more common than rectal symptoms. Bilateral hydroureter from partial obstruction is a frequent finding with larger masses. Abnormal bleeding is experienced by 30% of women with myomas. The most common symptom is menorrhagia, but intermenstrual spotting and disruption of a normal pattern are other frequent complaints. The exact cause-and-effect relationship between myomas and abnormal bleeding is difficult to determine and is poorly understood. The explanation is straightforward when there are areas of ulceration over submucous myomas. However, ulceration is a clinical rarity. The most popular theory is that myomas result in an abnormal venous pattern with stasis and a change in venous drainage. The theory that the amount of menorrhagia is directly related to an increase of endometrial surface area has been disproved. One of three women with abnormal bleeding and myomas also has endometrial hyperplasia, which may be the cause of the symptom and related to a submucous myoma.

Occasionally, myomas are the only identifiable abnormality after a detailed infertility investigation. Myomectomy is indicated in longstanding infertility and recurrent abortion after all other potential factors have been investigated and treated. Successful term pregnancy rates of 40% to 50% have been reported following a myomectomy. The success of an operation is most dependent on the age of the patient, the size of the myomas, and most important, the number of compounding factors that affect the couple's fertility.

Growth of a uterine myoma after menopause is a disturbing symptom. This is the classic symptom of a leiomyosarcoma, and thus the patient should have a total abdominal hysterectomy so that the tissue may be examined histologically.

Rarely, a secondary polycythemia is noted in women with uterine myomas. The mechanism is unclear; however, the polycythemia diminishes following removal of the uterus.

The diagnosis of uterine myomas is usually confirmed by palpating an enlarged, firm, irregular uterus during pelvic examination. The three conditions that commonly enter into the differential diagnosis include pregnancy, adenomyosis, and an ovarian neoplasm. The discrimination between large ovarian tumors and myomatous uteri may be difficult. Extension of myomas laterally may make palpation of normal ovaries impossible during the pelvic examination. Degeneration of myomas may cause a change of consistency from firm to soft, and some may become cystic. Often, if pregnancy has been excluded, placing a metal sound in the uterine cavity will help to establish the clinical diagnosis. The uterine cavity is generally enlarged and often irregular with myomas, while an ovarian tumor is usually associated with a normal-sized uterus. The mobility of the pelvic mass and whether the mass moves independently or as part of the uterus may be helpful diagnostically. Submucosal myomas may be diagnosed by direct observation during hysteroscopy or indirectly as a filling defect on hysterosalpingography.

Although the majority of uterine myomas may be diagnosed by pelvic examination, difficult cases will benefit from ultrasound examination or a search for concentric calcifications on an abdominal x-ray film. There are several recent reports of computed tomography (CT) and magnetic resonance imaging (MRI) studies of uterine myomas. However, these imaging techniques are more expensive than ultrasound. Until CT and MRI can distinguish between benign and malignant myomas, they will rarely be ordered in routine clinical management of myomas. Serial ultrasound and MRI examinations have been used to evaluate progression in size or response to therapy of myomas.

The management of a woman with small, asymptomatic myomas is judicious observation. When the tumor is first discovered, it is appropriate to perform a pelvic examination at 4- to 6-month intervals to determine the rate of growth. The majority of women will not need an operation, especially those women in the perimenopausal period, where the condition usually improves with diminishing levels of circulating estrogens.

Women with symptomatic leiomyomas should be investigated thoroughly for concurrent problems such as endometrial hyperplasia. If their symptoms do not improve with conservative management, operative therapy may be considered. The choice between a myomectomy and hysterectomy is usually determined by the patient's age, parity, and most important, future reproductive plans.

Classic indications for a myomectomy include a rapidly expanding pelvic mass, persistent abnormal bleeding, pain or pressure, previous repetitive abortion, longstanding infertility, or enlargement of an asymptomatic myoma to more than 8 cm in a woman who has not completed childbearing. Contraindications to a myomectomy include pregnancy, advanced adnexal disease, malignancy, and the situation in which enucleation of the myoma would result in a severe reduction of endometrial surface so that the uterus would not be functional. The choice between the two operations is not always an easy one. To quote Richard TeLinde, "All indications and contraindications in medicine are relative, a fact that is especially true when one considers hysterectomy versus myomectomy."

Within 20 years of the myomectomy procedure, one in four women subsequently has a hysterectomy performed, the majority for recurrent leiomyomas. Submucous myomas may be resected via the cervical canal using the hysteroscope. Although preliminary studies using laser surgery have been reported, most investigators advocate using a urologic resectoscope. Though the majority of women have relief of symptoms with hysteroscopic surgery, large numbers and long-term follow-up are pending.

The indications for hysterectomy for myomas are similar to indications for myomectomy, with a few additions. Many gynecologists selectively perform a hysterectomy for asymptomatic myomas when the uterus has reached the size of a 12- to 14-week gestation. The hypothesis is that most myomas of this size will eventually produce symptoms. Another previously mentioned indication for hysterectomy is growth of a myoma after the menopause. Prolapse of a myoma through the cervix is optimally treated by vaginal removal and ligation of the base of the myoma with antibiotic coverage. If hysterectomy is indicated, usually it is postponed for several weeks after removal of the prolapsed myoma, until the concurrent endometritis is resolved. Hysteroscopic resection has greatly aided transvaginal removal of prolapsed myoma. Finally, the lateral growth of myomas may make it impossible to evaluate the adnexa during pelvic examination.

It is possible to treat leiomyomas medically by reducing the circulating level of estrogen. Medroxyprogesterone acetate (Depo-Provera), danazol, and GnRH analogues have undergone clinical trials. Several studies in the past 5 years have reported the use of GnRH agonists to treat myomas. A variety of GnRH agonists given as a depot intramuscular injection, subcutaneously, and intranasally have been inves-

tigated. Reduction in uterine volume and myoma size by 40% to 90% has been documented in 80% to 100% of patients. Seventy-five percent of the reduction occurs within the first 2 to 4 months, with maximal reduction occurring by 8 months. After cessation of therapy, myomas gradually resume their pretreatment size. By 6 months after treatment, most myomas will have returned to the full pretreatment size. During treatment, Doppler flow studies have demonstrated increased resistance in the uterine arteries and in the smaller arteries feeding the myoma. Also during treatment, binding of epidermal growth factor is reduced in myomas. These two effects are concomitant with reduction of size in the myomas. Estrogen receptors, however, increase in amount during GnRH therapy. Several investigators have advocated preoperative treatment of myomas with GnRH agonists. Reduction in blood loss at the time of hysterectomy or myomectomy is an important advantage to such therapy. Medical therapy is useful perimenopausally to avoid hysterectomy.

Two associated but rare diseases should be noted: intravenous leiomyomatosis and leiomyomatosis peritonealis disseminata. *Intravenous leiomyomatosis* is a rare condition in which benign smooth muscle fibers invade and slowly grow into the venous channels of the pelvis. The tumor grows by direct extension and grossly appears like a "spaghetti" tumor. Only 25% of tumors extend beyond the broad ligament, yet case reports exist of tumor growth into the vena cava and right heart.

Leiomyomatosis peritonealis disseminata (LPD) is a benign disease with multiple small nodules over the surface of the pelvis and abdominal peritoneum. Grossly, LPD mimics disseminated carcinoma (Figure 17-24). However, histologic examination demonstrates benign-appearing myomas. This disorder is usually associated with a recent pregnancy.

OVIDUCT

Leiomyomas

Both benign and malignant tumors of the oviduct are uncommon compared with other gynecologic neoplasms. Although these tumors are underreported, fewer than 100 women with myomas or leiomyomas of the oviduct are described in the literature. Tubal leiomyomas may be single or multiple and usually are dis-

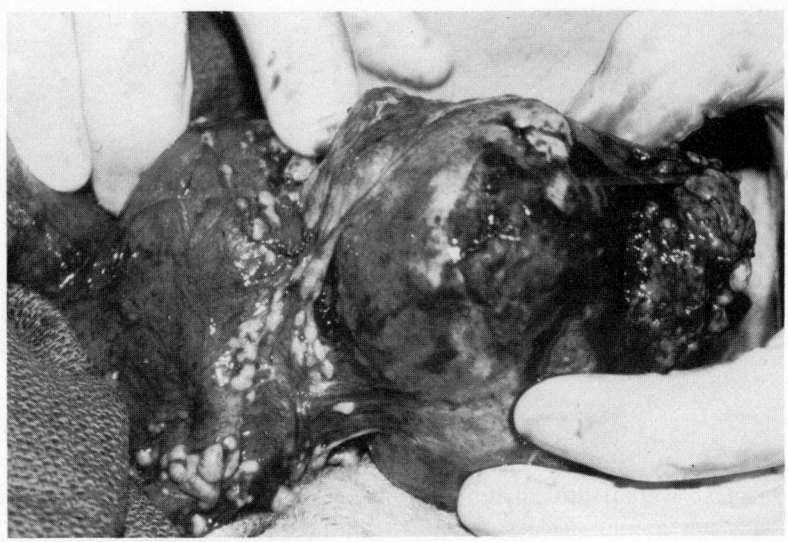

FIGURE 17-24
Photograph of leiomyomata peritonealis disseminata. (Courtesy William Droege-mueller and Vern L. Katz.)

covered in the interstitial portion of the tubes. They usually coexist with the more common uterine leiomyomas. Myomas may originate from muscle cells in the walls of the tube or blood vessels or from smooth muscle in the broad ligament.

Leiomyomas of the tube present as smooth, firm, mobile, usually nontender masses that may be palpated during the bimanual examination. Similar to uterine myomas, they may be subserosal, interstitial, or submucosal. During laparoscopy the myomas appear as a spherical mass that protrudes from beneath the peritoneal surface. They vary from a few millimeters to 15 cm in diameter. Histologically they are identical to uterine leiomyomas.

The majority of the myomas of the oviduct are asymptomatic. Rarely, they may undergo acute degeneration or be associated with unilateral tubal obstruction or torsion. Treatment of a symptomatic tubal leiomyoma is excision.

Another benign tumor of the oviduct is the *angiomyoma* or *adenomatoid tumor*. They are small, gray-white, circumscribed nodules, 1 to 2 cm in diameter. These benign tumors are found below the serosa of the fundus of the uterus and the broad ligament. Microscopically they are composed of small tubules lined by a low cuboidal or flat epithelium. Histologic studies have established that the thin-walled

channels that comprise these tumors are of mesothelial origin. These tumors do not become malignant; however, they may be mistaken for a low-grade neoplasm when initially viewed during a frozen section evaluation.

Paratubal Cysts

Paratubal cysts are frequently incidental discoveries during gynecologic operations for other abnormalities. They are often multiple and may vary from 0.5 cm to more than 20 cm in diameter. The majority of cysts are asymptomatic and slow growing and are discovered during the third and fourth decade of life. When paratubal cysts are pedunculated and near the fimbrial end of the oviduct, they are called *hydatid cysts of Morgagni* (Figure 17-25). Cysts near the oviduct may be of mesonephric, mesothelial, or paramesonephric origin.

The histogenesis of the majority of paratubal cysts had been believed to be from the mesonephric duct, with the cysts arising from the main duct or accessory tubules. These latter cysts often develop between the leaves of the broad ligament in the mesosalpinx, with the ovary being separate. However, a recent histologic study of 79 paratubal cysts by Samaha and Woodruff has documented that 60 of the cysts were of tubal origin. Thus the majority of

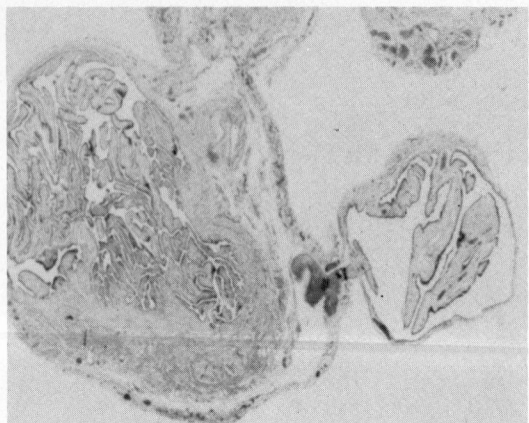

FIGURE 17-25
Normal tube to right with pedunculated hydatid cyst of Morgagni to right (accessory lumen with papillary fronds, really mucosal folds of tube). (From Samaha M and Woodruff JD: Obstet Gynecol 65:692, 1985. Reprinted with permission from The American College of Obstetricians and Gynecologists.)

grossly identified "paratubal cysts" are in reality accessory lumina of the fallopian tubes. The remaining 19 cysts in Samaha and Woodruff's series were of mesothelial origin. Paratubal cysts are thin walled and smooth and contain clear fluid. Often there are multiple small cysts. These cysts are thin-walled and are filled with clear fluid. Occasionally there is a papillomatous proliferation on the internal wall of these cysts.

The majority of paratubal cysts are asymptomatic and are usually discovered incidentally during gynecologic operations. When paratubal cysts are symptomatic, they generally produce a dull pain. Often during pelvic examination it is difficult to distinguish a paratubal cyst from an ovarian mass. At operation the oviduct is often found stretched over a large paratubal cyst. The oviduct should not be removed in these cases, as it will return to normal size after the paratubal cyst is excised. Stein et al. recently reported a retrospective 10-year review of 168 women with parovarian tumors. Three low-grade malignant neoplasms were found in this series. These malignancies were in women of reproductive age who had cysts greater than 5 cm in diameter with internal papillary projections. The authors cautioned that the differentiation between benign and malignant parovarian masses cannot be made by external examination of the cyst. Therefore they expressed

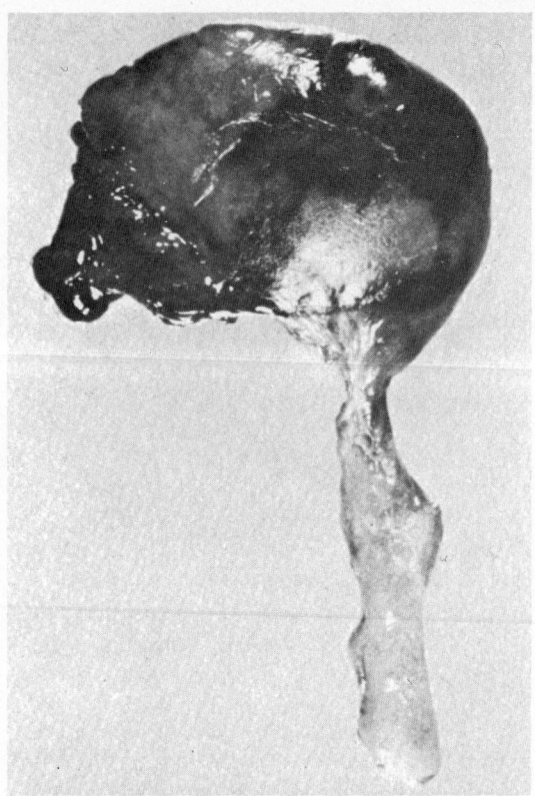

FIGURE 17-26
Right fallopian tube showing hemorrhage, edema, and infarction secondary to torsion. (From Chambers JT, Thiagarajah S, and Kitchin JD: Obstet Gynecol 54:488, 1979. Reprinted with permission from The American College of Obstetricians and Gynecologists.)

concern about the practice of aspirating cysts via the laparoscope because of the potential hazard of missing or disseminating a malignant disease.

Paratubal cysts may grow rapidly during pregnancy, and most of the cases of torsion of these cysts have been reported during pregnancy or the puerperium. Treatment is simple excision.

Torsion

Acute torsion of the oviduct is a rare event; however, it has been reported with both normal and pathologic fallopian tubes. Pregnancy predisposes to this problem. Tubal torsion usually accompanies torsion of the ovary, as they have a common vascular pedicle. (See discussion of ovarian torsion later in this chapter.) Torsion of the fallopian tube is secondary to an ovarian mass in approximately 50% to 60% of patients. The right tube is involved more frequently than the left (Figure 17-26). The degree of tubal torsion varies from less than one turn to four complete rotations. Torsion of the oviduct is usually seen in women of reproductive age. However, it occurs also in preadolescent children, especially when part of the tube in enclosed in the sac of a femoral or inguinal hernia.

Youssef et al. have subdivided the pathophysiology and etiology of tubal torsion into intrinsic and extrinsic causes. Prominent intrinsic causes include congenital abnormalities such as increased tortuosity due to excessive length of the tube, and pathologic processes, such as hydrosalpinx, hematosalpinx, tubal neoplasms, and previous operation, especially tubal ligation. Torsion of the fallopian tube following tubal ligation is usually of the distal end. Extrinsic causes of tubal torsion are ovarian and peritubal tumors, adhesions, trauma, and pregnancy.

The most important symptom of tubal torsion is acute lower abdominal and pelvic pain. The onset of this pain may be gradual or sudden, and the pain is usually located in the iliac fossa with radiation to the thigh and flank. The duration of pain is generally less than 48 hours, and it is associated with nausea and vomiting in two thirds of the cases. Unless there is associated torsion of the ovary, a specific mass is usually not palpable on pelvic examination.

The preoperative diagnosis of tubal torsion is made in less than 20% of reported cases. However, the number of cases diagnosed preoperatively has increased dramatically with the use of vaginal ultrasonography. Because of the severity of the pain a wide differential diagnosis of abdominal and pelvic pathology must be considered. The differential diagnosis includes acute appendicitis, ectopic pregnancy, pelvic inflammatory disease, and rupture or torsion of an ovarian cyst.

Exploratory operation determines the extent of hypoxia and the choice of operative techniques. With tubal torsion, usually the tubes are gangrenous and must be excised. The twisted tube is usually filled with a bloody or serous fluid. Occasionally, with a minor degree of torsion, it is possible to restore normal circulation to the tube and salvage it. The tube is usually sutured into a secure position to prevent recurrence.

OVARY

Functional Cysts

Follicular Cysts

Follicular cysts are by far the most frequent cystic structures in normal ovaries. The cysts are frequently multiple and may vary from a few millimeters to as large as 15 cm in diameter. Physiologically, however, a normal follicle may become cystic, and therefore it is important to have a minimal diameter for a follicular cyst. Throughout the literature this diameter is generally between 2.5 and 3 cm. Follicular cysts are not neoplastic and are believed to be dependent on gonadotrophins for growth. They arise from a temporary pathologic variation of a normal physiologic process. Clinically, they may present with the signs and symptoms of ovarian enlargement and therefore must be differentiated from a true ovarian neoplasm. Functional cysts may be solitary or multiple. Solitary cysts occur during the fetal and neonatal periods and rarely during childhood, but there is an increase in frequency during the perimenarchal period. These cysts are found most commonly in young, menstruating women. Large solitary follicular cysts in which the lining is luteinized are occasionally seen during pregnancy and the puerperium. Multiple follicular cysts in which the lining is luteinized are associated with either intrinsic or extrinsic elevated levels of gonadotrophins.

Follicular cysts are translucent, thin walled, and are filled with a watery, clear to straw-colored fluid. If a small opening in the capsule of the cyst suddenly develops, the cyst fluid will squirt out under pressure. These cysts are situated in the ovarian cortex, and sometimes they appear as translucent domes on the surface of the ovary. Histologically, the lining of the cyst is usually composed of a closely packed layer of round, plump granulosa cells with the spindle-shaped cells of the theca interna deeper in the stroma. In many cysts the lining of granulosa cells is difficult to distinguish, having undergone pressure atrophy. All that remains is a hyalinized connective tissue lining.

The temporary disturbance in follicular function that produces the clinical picture of a follicular cyst is poorly understood. Follicular cysts may result from either the dominant mature follicle's failing to rupture (persistent follicle) or an immature follicle's failing to undergo the normal process of atresia. In the latter circumstance the incompletely developed follicle fails to reabsorb follicular fluid. Some follicular cysts lose their ability to produce estrogen, while in others the granulosa cells remain productive with prolonged secretion of estrogens. Occasionally, follicular cysts are better termed *follicular hematomas*, as blood from the vascular theca zone fills the cavity of the cyst.

The majority of follicular cysts are asymptomatic and are discovered only during a routine pelvic examination. Because of their thin walls, these cysts often are ruptured during examination. The patient experiences a transient tenderness or no pain whatsoever. Only rarely is there significant intraperitoneal bleeding associated with the rupture of a follicular cyst. Women who are chronically anticoagulated may bleed, not infrequently, from either a follicular or corpus luteum cyst. Occasionally, menstrual irregularities and abnormal uterine bleeding may be associated with follicular cysts, which produce prolonged elevated blood estrogen levels. The syndrome associated with such follicular cysts is of a regular cycle with a prolonged intermenstrual interval, followed by episodes of menorrhagia. Some women with larger follicular cysts notice a vague, dull sensation or a heaviness in the pelvis.

The initial management of a suspected follicular cyst is conservative observation. The majority of follicular cysts disappear spontaneously by either reabsorption of the cyst fluid or silent rupture within 4 to 8 weeks of initial diagnosis. However, a persistent ovarian mass necessitates operative intervention to differentiate a physiologic cyst from a true neoplasm of the ovary. There is no way to make the differentiation on the basis of signs, symptoms, or the initial growth pattern during early development of either process. Vaginal ultrasound examination may help to differentiate simple from complex cysts and also may help during conservative management by providing dimensions to determine if the cyst is increasing in size. Spanos suggested prescribing oral contraceptives for 4 to 6 weeks for young women with adnexal masses. This therapy removes any influence that pituitary gonadotrophins may have on the persistence of the ovarian cyst. It also allows for several weeks of observation. In Spanos's series, 80% of cystic masses 4 to 6 cm in size disappeared during the time the patient was taking oral contraceptives. Steinkampf et al. performed a randomized prospective controlled study of the effect of oral contraceptives on functional ovarian masses in women of reproductive age. Their study group consisted of infertility patients who had recently been treated by ovulation induction. In their series there was no difference in the rate of disappearance of functional ovarian cysts between the group that received oral contraceptives and the control group.

Indications for immediate operation include the presence of any adnexal mass after the menopause or before puberty, a solid adnexal mass at any age, a cystic mass larger than 8 cm, or a cystic mass from 5 to 8 cm that has been observed for longer than 8 weeks in a menstruating woman. Operative management is cystectomy, not oophorectomy. There is increasing enthusiasm for managing simple cysts in young women via the laparoscope. However, this procedure has an accompanying risk of spilling malignant cells into the peritoneal cavity if the cyst is an early carcinoma. Therefore strict criteria are important concerning the patient's age, size of the mass, ultrasonic characteristics, and in ensuring that the cyst is nonadherent, has no papillae, and is smooth and thin walled. DeWilde et al., in a series of follicular cysts averaging 6 cm in diameter, found that the recurrence rate following laparoscopic fenestration was approximately 2%.

Corpus Luteum Cysts

Corpus luteum cysts are less common than follicular cysts, but clinically they are more important. This discussion collectively groups corpus luteum cysts and persistently functioning mature corpora lutea (Figure 17-27). Pathologists are sometimes able to make a distinction between a hemorrhagic cystic corpus luteum and a corpus luteum cyst, but at other times this difference cannot be established. All corpora lutea are cystic with gradual reabsorption of a limited amount of hemorrhage, which may form a cavity. Clinically, corpora lutea are not termed *corpus luteum cysts* unless they are a minimum of 3 cm in diameter. Corpus luteum cysts may be associated with either normal endocrine function or prolonged secretion of progesterone.

Corpora lutea develop from mature graafian follicles. Intrafollicular bleeding does not occur during ovulation. However, 2 to 4 days later, during the stage of vascularization, thin-walled capillaries invade the granulosa cells from the theca interna. Spontaneous but limited bleeding fills the central cavity of the maturing corpus luteum with blood. Subsequently this blood is absorbed, forming a small cystic space. When the hemorrhage is excessive, the cystic space enlarges. If the hemorrhage into the central cavity is brisk, intracystic pressure increases and rupture of the corpus luteum is a possibility. If rupture does not occur, the size of the resulting corpus luteum cyst usually varies between 3 and 10 cm. Occasionally a cyst may be 11 to 15 cm in diameter. If a cystic central cavity persists, blood is replaced by clear fluid, and the result is a hormonally inactive corpus albicans cyst (Figure 17-28). A corpus luteum of pregnancy is normally 3 to 5 cm in diameter with a central cystic structure, occupying at least 50% of the ovarian mass.

Most corpus luteum cysts are small, the average diameter being 4 cm. Grossly, they have a smooth surface and, depending on whether the cyst represents acute or chronic hemorrhage, are purplish red to brown (Figure 17-29). When a corpus luteum is cut, the convoluted lining is yellowish-orange, and the center contains an organizing blood clot. Both the granulosa and the theca cells undergo luteinization. In chronic corpus luteum cysts the wall becomes gray-white, and the polygonal luteinized cells usually undergo pressure atrophy. Hallatt et al. reviewed 173 ruptured corpora lutea with hemoperitoneum. In their institution the frequency of serious bleeding from a

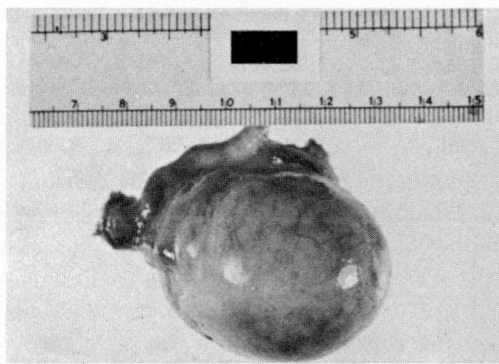

FIGURE 17-27
Corpus luteum cyst, 3 to 4 cm in diameter, externally smooth. (From Janovski NA, editor: Color atlas of gross gynecologic and obstetric pathology, New York, 1969, McGraw-Hill Book Co, p 155.)

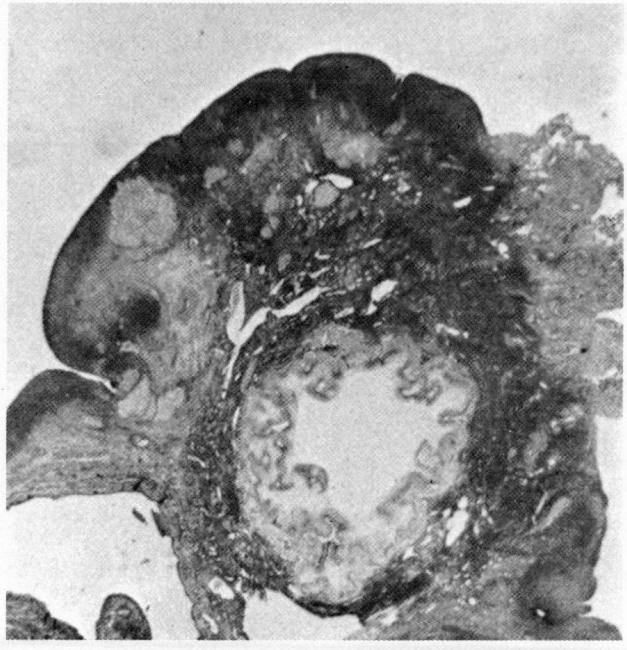

FIGURE 17-28
Corpus albicans cyst. Lining of cyst is composed of hyalinized connective tissue. (From Blaustein A: Nonneoplastic cysts of the ovary. In Blaustein A, editor: Pathology of the female genital tract, New York, 1977, Springer-Verlag New York, Inc, p 396.)

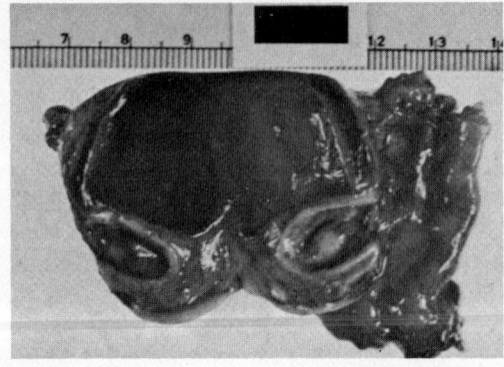

FIGURE 17-29
Corpus luteum cyst with thickened cyst wall and definite lutein cell lining recognized by its color. Cyst is filled with hemorrhagic gelatinous material. (From Janovski NA, editor: Color atlas of gross gynecologic and obstetric pathology, New York, 1969, McGraw-Hill Book Co, p 157.)

corpus luteum cyst compared with ectopic pregnancy was one in four.

Corpus luteum cysts vary from being asymptomatic masses to those causing catastrophic and massive intraperitoneal bleeding associated with rupture. Many corpus luteum cysts produce dull, unilateral, lower abdominal and pelvic pain. The enlarged ovary is moderately tender on pelvic examination. Depending on the amount of progesterone secretion associated with cysts, the menstrual bleeding may be normal or delayed several days to weeks with subsequent menorrhagia. Halban in 1915 described a syndrome of a persistently functioning corpus luteum cyst that has clinical features similar to an unruptured ectopic pregnancy. Halban's classic triad was a delay in a normal period followed by spotting, unilateral pelvic pain, and a small, tender adnexal mass. This triad of symptomatology is very similar to the classic triad of an anomalous period or delay in a normal period, spotting, and unilateral pelvic pain that is exhibited by the classic ectopic pregnancy. The differential diagnosis between these two conditions without a sensitive pregnancy test is difficult.

Corpus luteum cysts may cause intraperitoneal bleeding. The amount of bleeding varies from slight to significant hemorrhage, necessitating blood transfusion. Internal bleeding often follows coitus, exercise, trauma, or a pelvic examination. However, episodes of bleeding usually do not recur, which differs from an ec-

topic pregnancy. Women undergoing chronic warfarin (Coumadin) therapy are especially prone to develop ovarian hemorrhage from a corpus luteum cyst. Bleeding occurs usually between days 20 to 26 of their cycle, and these women have a 31% chance for subsequent hemorrhage from a recurrent corpus luteum cyst. Oral contraceptives are commonly used to suppress ovulation and avoid recurrent hemorrhage.

Hallatt et al. reported that sudden, severe, lower abdominal pain was a prominent symptom in all patients with hemoperitoneum caused by a ruptured corpus luteum cyst (Table 17-2). One of three women also noted unilateral cramping and lower abdominal pain for 1 to 2 weeks before overt rupture. The right ovary was the source of hemorrhage in 66% of their series. Tang et al. have also reported a right-sided predominance in the incidence of hemorrhage from corpus luteum cysts. They postulated that the difference is related to a higher intraluminal pressure on the right side because of the differences in ovarian vein architecture. Most ruptures occur between days 20 and 26 of the cycle, although in the series of Hallatt et al. 28% of the women had a delay in menses not explained by pregnancy or history (Table 17-3).

The differential diagnosis of a woman with acute pain and suspected ruptured corpus lu-

TABLE 17-2
Symptoms of 173 Women with Ruptured Corpus Luteum

	Number	Percent
Location		
Right ovary	114	66
Left ovary	56	32
Unknown	3	2
Abdominal pain	173	100
Onset with intercourse	29	17
Right ovary	21	72
Left ovary	8	28
Duration		
Less than 24 hours	94	54
1 to 7 days	40	23
Over 7 days	14	8
Unknown	25	15
Nausea or vomiting or diarrhea	60	35

From Hallatt JG, Steele CH, and Snyder M: Am J Obstet Gynecol 149:6, 1984.

TABLE 17-3
Menstrual History in 173 Women with
Ruptured Corpus Luteum

	Number	No.
Last menstrual period to operation		
Under 14 days		5
14 to 31 days (pregnant = 2)		77
31 to 60 days (pregnant = 15)		56
Over 60 days (pregnant = 10)		18
No menstrual period		14
Hysterectomy	5	
Amenorrhea after oral contraceptives	5	
Secondary amenorrhea	2	
Menarche	1	
Menopause	1	
History of irregular menses		14
Unknown		3

From Hallatt JG, Steele CH, and Snyder M: Am J Obstet
Gynecol 149:6, 1984.

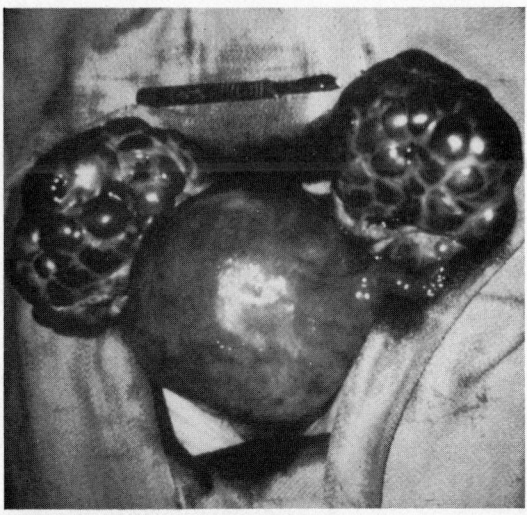

FIGURE 17-30
Bilateral theca lutein cysts. (Courtesy Daniel
R. Mishell, Jr., M.D.)

teum cyst includes ectopic pregnancy, ruptured endometrioma, and adnexal torsion. A sensitive serum or urinary assay for human chorionic gonadotrophin (HCG) may help to differentiate a bleeding corpus luteum from ectopic pregnancy (Chapter 16). Vaginal ultrasound is occasionally useful in establishing a preoperative diagnosis. Culdocentesis is helpful in establishing the rapidity and severity of the hemorrhage. If the hematocrit of the fluid obtained from the posterior cul-de-sac is greater than 15%, operative therapy becomes a necessity. Cystectomy is the operative treatment of choice, with preservation of the remaining portion of the ovary. In the series of DeWilde et al. of persistent corpus luteum cysts treated by fenestration via the laparoscope, 6 of 44 (14%) recurred. Obviously, it was impossible for the authors to distinguish between a recurrent corpus luteum cyst and the development of a new corpus luteum. Unruptured corpus luteum cysts may be followed conservatively.

Theca Lutein Cysts

Theca lutein cysts are by far the least common of the three types of physiologic ovarian cysts (Figure 17-30). Unlike corpus luteum cysts, theca lutein cysts are almost always bilat-

eral and produce moderate to massive enlargement of the ovaries. These cysts arise from either prolonged or excessive stimulation of the ovaries by endogenous or exogenous gonadotrophins or increased ovarian sensitivity to gonadotrophins. Approximately 50% of molar pregnancies and 10% of choriocarcinomas have associated bilateral theca lutein cysts (Chapter 29). In these patients the HCG from the trophoblast produces luteinization of the cells in immature, mature, and atretic follicles. The cysts are also discovered in the latter months of pregnancies with conditions that produce a large placenta, such as twins, diabetes, and Rh sensitization. It is not uncommon to iatrogenically produce theca lutein cysts in women receiving drugs to induce ovulation. Theca lutein cysts are occasionally discovered in association with normal pregnancy and in newborn infants secondary to transplacental effects of maternal gonadotrophins. Rarely, these cysts are found in young girls with junvenile hypothyroidism.

Grossly the total ovarian size may be voluminous, 20 to 30 cm in diameter, with multiple theca lutein cysts. This condition of bilateral ovarian enlargement of gray to bluish tinged cysts is also called *hyperreactio luteinalis*. The bilateral enlargement is secondary to hundreds of thin-walled locules or cysts producing a honeycombed appearance. Grossly the external surface of the ovary appears lobulated. The small cysts contain a clear to straw-colored

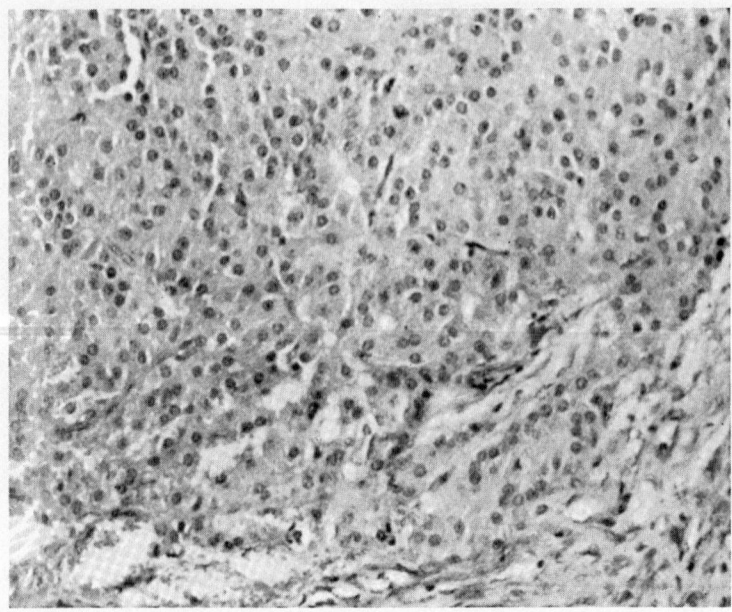

FIGURE 17-31
Luteoma. Solid mass of uniform polygonal "luteinized" cells with spherical nuclei. (H&E stain; ×220.) (From Dische FE and Ritchie JM: J Pathol 100:Plate XXXVI, 1970.)

fluid. Histologically the lining of the cyst is composed of theca lutein cells (paralutein cells), believed to originate from ovarian connective tissue. Occasionally there is also luteinization of granulosa cells. These voluminous and congested ovaries are slow growing. Generally only the larger cysts produce vague symptoms, such as a sense of pressure in the pelvis. Ascites and increasing abdominal girth have been reported with hyperstimulation from exogenous gonadotrophins. Rarely, associated adnexal torsion may occur. Montz et al., in reviewing the natural history of 102 theca lutein cysts, found that approximately 1% of patients experienced acute complications of either torsion or intraperitoneal bleeding. They also discovered that theca lutein cysts persisted in some patients for weeks after HCG levels were nondetectable.

The presence of theca lutein cysts is established by palpation and often confirmed by ultrasound examination. Treatment is conservative because these cysts gradually regress. If these cysts are discovered incidentally at cesarean delivery, they should be handled delicately. No attempt should be made to drain or puncture the multiple cysts because of the possibility of hemorrhage. Bleeding is difficult to control in these cases because of the thin walls that comprise the cysts.

A condition related to theca lutein cysts is the *luteoma* of pregnancy. The condition is rare and not a true neoplasm, but rather a specific, benign, hyperplastic reaction of ovarian theca lutein cells (Figure 17-31). These nodules do not arise from the corpus luteum of pregnancy. Fifty percent of luteomas are multiple, and approximately 30% of those reported have bilateral nodules. In appearance they are discrete and brown to reddish brown and may be solid or cystic.

The majority of patients with luteomas are asymptomatic, and the nodules are discovered incidentally at cesarean delivery or postpartum tubal ligation. Most reported cases are in multiparous black women. Masculinization of the mother occurs in 30% of cases, and masculinization of the external genitalia of the female fetus may sometimes occur. These tumors regress spontaneously following completion of the pregnancy.

Benign Neoplasms of the Ovary

Benign Cystic Teratoma (Dermoid Cyst, Mature Teratoma)

Benign ovarian teratomas are usually cystic structures that on histologic examination contain elements from all three germ cell layers.

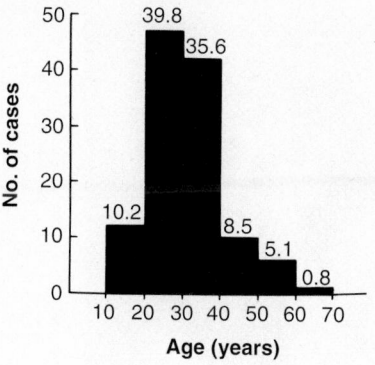

FIGURE 17-32
Age distribution of cystic teratomas. (From Lakkis WG, Martin MC, and Gelfand MM: Originally published in Canadian Journal of Surgery 28:444, 1985.)

The word *teratoma* was first advanced by Virchow and translated literally means "monstrous growth." Teratomas of the ovary may be benign or malignant. Although *dermoid* is a misnomer, it is the most common term used to describe the benign cystic tumor, composed of mature cells, whereas the malignant variety is composed of immature cells (immature teratoma). *Dermoid* is a descriptive term in that it emphasizes the preponderance of ectodermal tissue with some mesodermal and rare endodermal derivatives. Malignant teratomas that are immature are usually solid with some cystic areas and histologically contain immature or embryonic-appearing tissue. (See Chapter 29 for further discussion of malignant teratomas.) Benign teratomas may undergo malignant transformation. This occurs in approximately 1% to 2% of dermoids, usually in women over age 40. The malignant component is generally a squamous carcinoma. Nonovarian teratomas may arise in midline structures of the body where the germ cell has resided during embryonic life.

Benign teratomas are among the most common ovarian neoplasms. These slow-growing tumors occur from infancy to the postmenopausal years. Depending on the series, dermoids represent 20% to 25% of all ovarian neoplasms and approximately 33% of all benign tumors, if follicular and corpus luteum cysts are excluded. Dermoids are the most common ovarian neoplasm in prepubertal females and are also common in teenagers. However, more than 50% of benign teratomas are discovered in women between the ages of 25 and 50 years. In the series of Lakkis et al. of 118 patients with dermoids, 86% of the patients were less than 40 years of age, and 3.4% had recurrences (Figure 17-32). In most large series of benign tumors in postmenopausal women, dermoids account for approximately 20% of the neoplasms.

Dermoids vary from a few millimeters to 25 cm in diameter. However, 80% are less than 10 cm. These tumors may be single or multiple, with as many as nine individual dermoids having been reported in the same ovary. Benign teratomas occur bilaterally 10% to 15% of the time. Often, dermoid cysts are pedunculated. These cysts make the ovary heavier than normal, and thus they are usually discovered either in the cul-de-sac or anterior to the broad ligament. Grossly, the cysts are smooth and pearly gray. On palpation these tumors, which have both cystic and solid components, have a doughy consistency (Figure 17-33).

The cysts are usually unilocular. When they are opened, thick sebaceous fluid, often with tangled masses of hair and firm areas of cartilage and teeth, pours from the cyst (Figure 17-34). The sebaceous material is a thick fluid at body temperature but solidifies when it cools in room air.

Benign teratomas are believed to arise from a single germ cell after the first meiotic division. Therefore they develop from totipotential stem cells, and they are neoplastic sequelae from a transformed germ cell. Dermoids have a chromosomal makeup of 46,XX. Linder et al.,

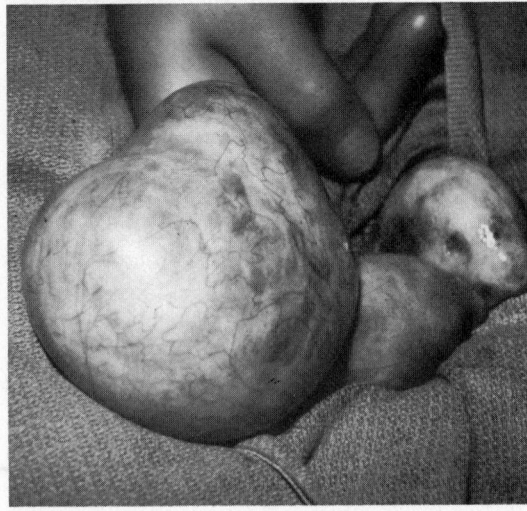

FIGURE 17-33
Gross appearance of bilateral dermoid cysts of the ovary. (Courtesy Daniel Mishell, M.D.)

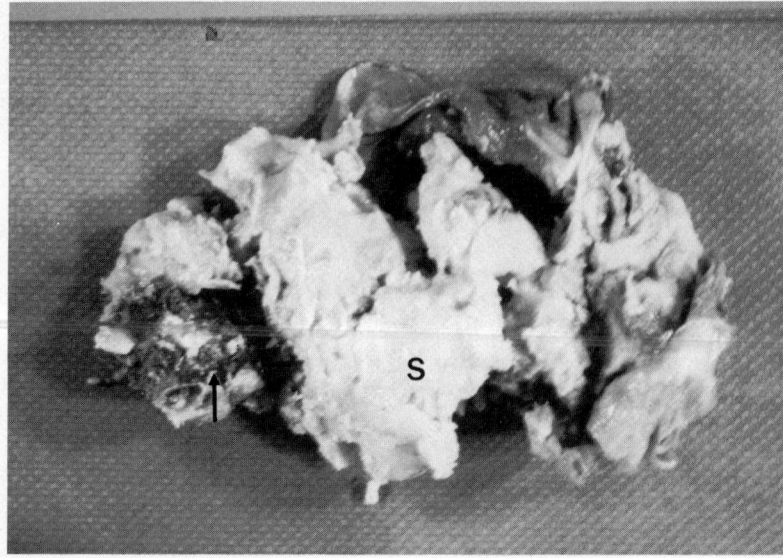

FIGURE 17-34
Benign cystic teratoma. This section from the tumor demonstrates areas of hair (*dark arrows*) and solid sebaceous material (*S*). (Courtesy Deborah Jean Dotters, M.D.)

in a series of experiments using chromosome banding techniques and electrophoretic variance, discovered that the chromosomes of dermoids were different from the chromosomes of the host. They postulated that dermoids began by parthenogenesis from secondary oocytes. An alternative hypothesis was that the dermoid resulted from fusion of the second polar body with the oocyte. The studies by Linder et al. ruled out the possibility that dermoids arise from somatic cells or from an oogonium before the first stage of meiosis. The first meiotic division occurs at approximately 13 weeks of gestation. Thus dermoids begin in fetal life sometime after this point.

Histologically, benign teratomas are comprised of mature cells, usually from all three germ layers (Figure 17-35). A combination of skin and skin appendages, including sebaceous glands, sweat glands, hair follicles, muscle fibers, cartilage, bone, teeth, glial cells, and epithelium of the respiratory and gastrointestinal tracts, may be visualized. Teeth are predominantly premolar and molar forms. The fluid in dermoid cysts is usually sebaceous. Most solid elements arise and are contained in a protrusion or nipple (mamilla) in the cyst wall termed the *prominence* or *tubercle of Rokitansky*. The wall of the cyst will often contain granulation

tissue, giant cells, and pseudoxanthoma cells.

Approximately 50% of dermoids are asymptomatic and are discovered incidentally by pelvic examination or coincidentally visualized by an abdominal x-ray or ultrasound examination. Specific complications of dermoid cysts include torsion, rupture, infection, hemorrhage, and malignant degeneration. Three medical diseases also may be associated with dermoid cysts: thyrotoxicosis, carcinoid syndrome, and autoimmune hemolytic anemia. Torsion of a dermoid is the most frequent complication, occurring in 11% of the series by Pantoja et al. of 253 tumors. Because of its weight, the benign teratoma is often pedunculated, which may predispose to torsion. Torsion is more common in younger women (Figure 17-36).

Rupture or perforation of the contents of a dermoid into the peritoneal cavity or an adjacent organ is a most serious complication. The incidence varies between 0.7% and 4.6%. However, most series report less than 1%. Rupture is more common in pregnancy. Rupture may occur either catastrophically, which produces an acute abdomen, or by a slow leak of the sebaceous material. The latter is clinically more common, with the sebaceous material producing a severe chemical granulomatous peritonitis. Waxman and Boyce warn that this

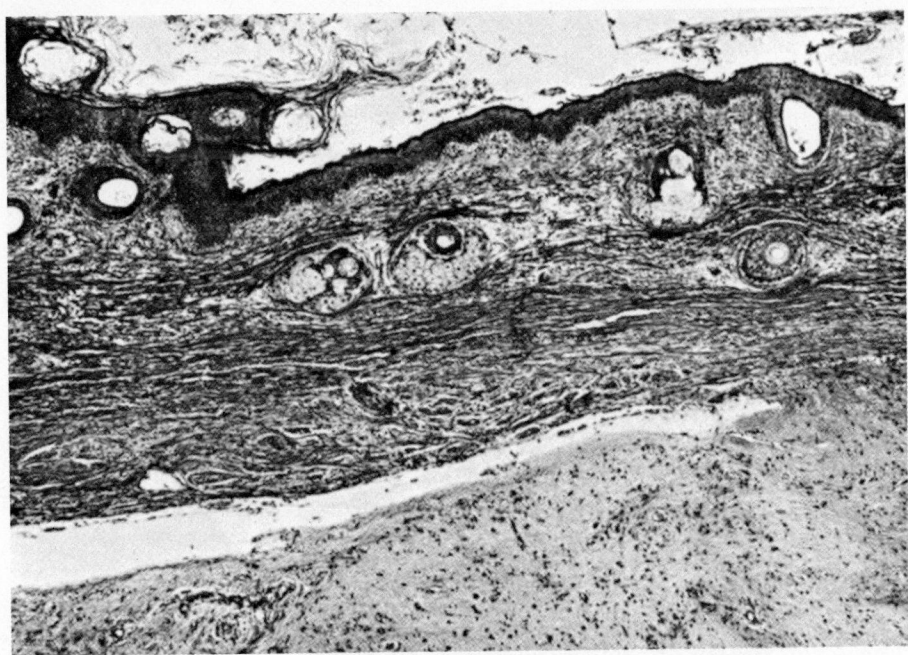

FIGURE 17-35
Mature cystic teratoma. Lining of cyst is composed of skin with its appendages. Mature neural tissue is seen beneath the cutaneous structures. (H&E stain; ×61.) (Reprinted by permission from Talerman A: Germ cell tumors of the ovary. In Blaustein A, editor: Pathology of the female genital tract, New York, 1977, Springer-Verlag New York, Inc, p 559.)

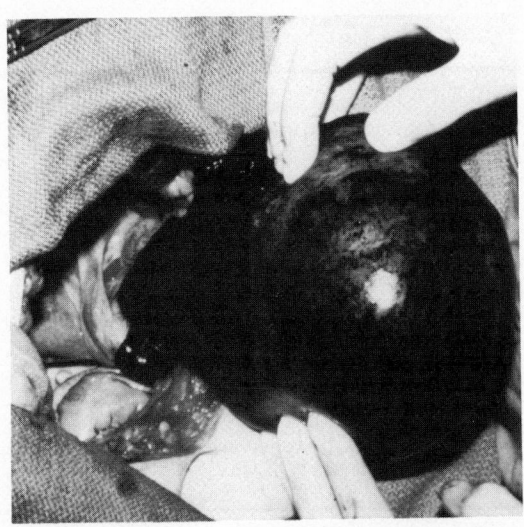

FIGURE 17-36
Torsion of the ovary. (Courtesy Daniel Mishell, M.D.)

possibility should be considered and a frozen section obtained so that the true diagnosis is established. Thus a young woman will not be mistakenly treated for suspected ovarian carcinoma with metastasis because of the identical gross appearance of a slow-leaking dermoid cyst.

Infection, hemorrhage, and malignant degeneration are all unusual complications of dermoids, occurring in less than 1% of patients.

Adult thyroid tissue is discovered microscopically in approximately 12% of benign teratomas. *Struma ovarii* is a teratoma in which the thyroid tissue has overgrown other elements and is the predominant tissue (Figure 17-37) Strumae ovarii comprise 2% to 3% of ovarian teratomas. These tumors are usually unilateral and measure less than 10 cm in diameter. Less than 5% of women with struma ovarii develop thyrotoxicosis, which may be secondary to the production of increased thyroid hormone by either the ovarian or the thyroid gland.

Another rare finding with dermoids is the presence of a primary carcinoid tumor from the gastrointestinal or respiratory tract epithelium contained in the dermoid. One of three of these tumors is associated with the typical car-

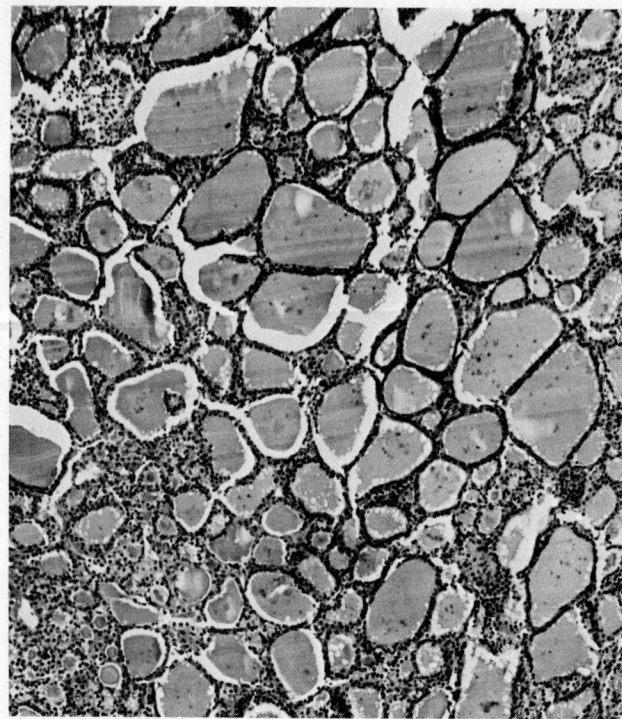

FIGURE 17-37
Struma ovarii. Tumor is composed of normal thyroid tissue. (H&E stain; ×76.) (Reprinted by permission from Talerman A: Germ cell tumors of the ovary. In Blaustein A, editor: Pathology of the female genital tract, New York, 1977, Springer-Verlag New York, Inc, p 563.)

cinoid syndrome even without metastatic spread. If the carcinoid is functioning, it may be diagnosed by measuring serum serotonin levels or urinary levels of 5-hydroxyindoleacetic acid. The autoimmune hemolytic anemia associated with dermoids is the rarest of the three medical complications.

The diagnosis of a dermoid cyst is often established when a semisolid mass is palpated anterior to the broad ligament. Approximately 50% of dermoids have pelvic calcifications on x-ray examination. Often an ovarian teratoma is an incidental finding during radiologic investigation of the genitourinary or gastrointestinal tract. There is an ongoing debate as to whether dermoids have a typical ultrasound picture. Early reports have emphasized an echogenic focus with acoustic shadowing situated within a predominantly cystic mass as classic for dermoid cysts. Laing et al. have found that only one of three dermoids have this "typical picture." In their series of 45 patients with 51 biopsy-proven dermoid cysts, 24% of the dermoid cysts were predominantly solid, 20%

TABLE 17-4
Ultrasonographic Appearance of Dermoid Cysts

Appearance	No. of Dermoids	Percent
Cystic	10	20.0
Solid	12	23.5
Cystic and solid	17	33.0
Not visualized	12	23.5
TOTAL	51	100.0

From Laing FC, Van Dalsem VF, Marks WM, et al: Obstet Gynecol 57:103, 1981. Reprinted with permission from The American College of Obstetricians and Gynecologists.

were almost entirely cystic, and 24% were not visible (Table 17-4). Treatment of benign cystic teratomas is cystectomy and is discussed in Chapter 29.

Endometriomas

Endometriosis of the ovary is often associated with endometriosis in other areas of the

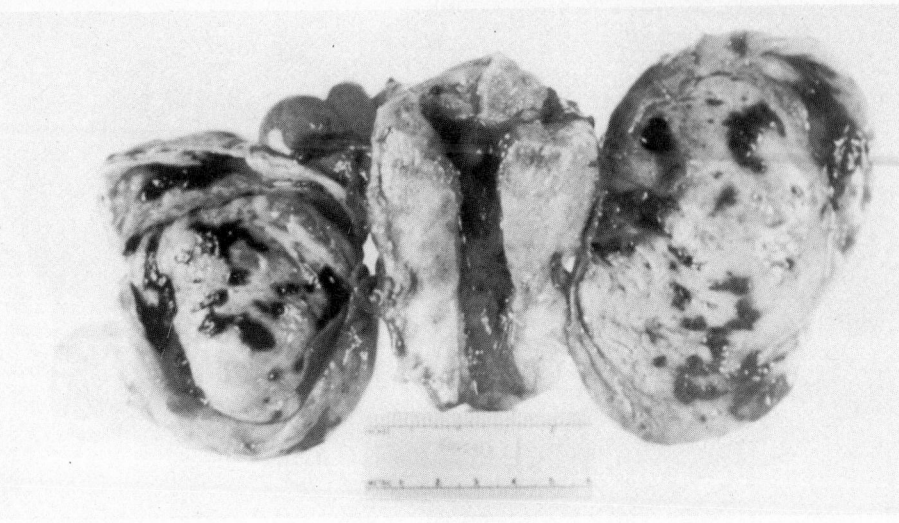

FIGURE 17-38
Endometriosis of ovaries. Wall of endometriotic cyst is thickened and fibrotic. Inner surface shows areas of dark-brown discoloration. (From Janovski NA, editor: Color atlas of gross gynecologic and obstetric pathology, New York, 1969, McGraw-Hill Book Co, p 159.)

pelvic cavity. Approximately two out of three women with endometriosis have ovarian involvement. Interestingly, only 5% of these women have enlargement of the ovaries that is detectable by pelvic examination. However, because of the frequency of the disease, endometriosis is one of the most common causes of enlargement of the ovary. Because most authors do not classify endometriosis as a neoplastic disease, often the diagnosis of endometriosis is not given due consideration in the differential diagnosis of an adnexal mass. Ovarian endometriosis is similar to endometriosis elsewhere and is described in greater detail in Chapter 18.

The size of ovarian endometriomas varies from small, superficial, blue-black implants that are 1 to 5 mm in diameter to large, multiloculated, hemorrhagic cysts that may be 5 to 10 cm in diameter (Figure 17-38). Semantically, areas of ovarian endometriosis that become cystic are termed *endometriomas*. Rarely, large chocolate cysts of the ovary may reach 15 to 20 cm (Figure 17-39), and they are frequently bilateral. The surface of an ovary with endometriosis is often irregular, puckered, and scarred.

Although most patients with endometriomas are asymptomatic, the most prominent symptoms of ovarian endometriosis are pelvic pain, dyspareunia, and infertility. Approximately 10% of the operations for endometriosis are for acute symptoms, usually related to a ruptured ovarian endometrioma that was previously asymptomatic. Smaller cysts generally have thinner cyst walls, and thus perforation occurs commonly secondary to cyclic hemorrhage into the cystic cavity.

On pelvic examination the ovaries are usually tender and immobile, secondary to associated inflammation and adhesions. Most commonly the ovaries are densely adherent to surrounding structures, including the peritoneum of the pelvic sidewall, the oviduct, the broad ligament, and sometimes the small or large bowel. Histologically, endometrial glands, endometrial stroma, and large phagocytic cells containing hemosiderin may be identified (Figure 17-40). Pressure atrophy may lead to the loss of architecture of the endometrial glands.

The choice between medical and operative management depends on several factors, including the patient's age, future reproductive plans, and severity of symptoms. In general, medical therapy is not successful in treating ovarian endometriosis if the disease has produced ovarian enlargement.

On pathologic examination it is important to distinguish endometriosis from benign endometrial tumors, which are usually adenofibromas.

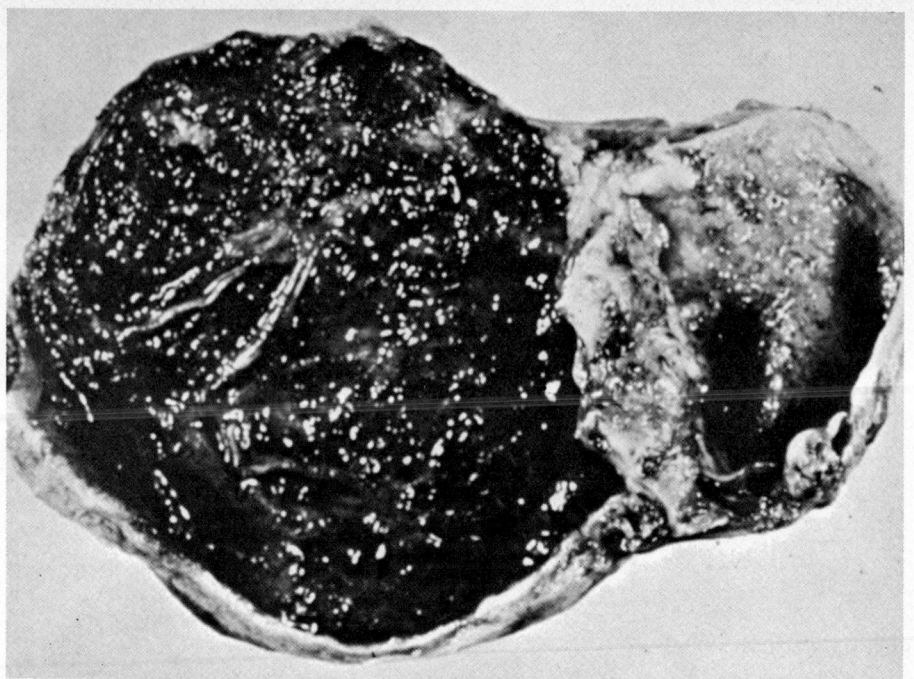

FIGURE 17-39
Opened endometrioma showing large cyst lined by hemorrhagic tissue. (From Czernobilsky B: Primary epithelial tumors of the ovary. In Blaustein A, editor: Pathology of the female genital tract, New York, 1977, Springer-Verlag New York, Inc, p 476.)

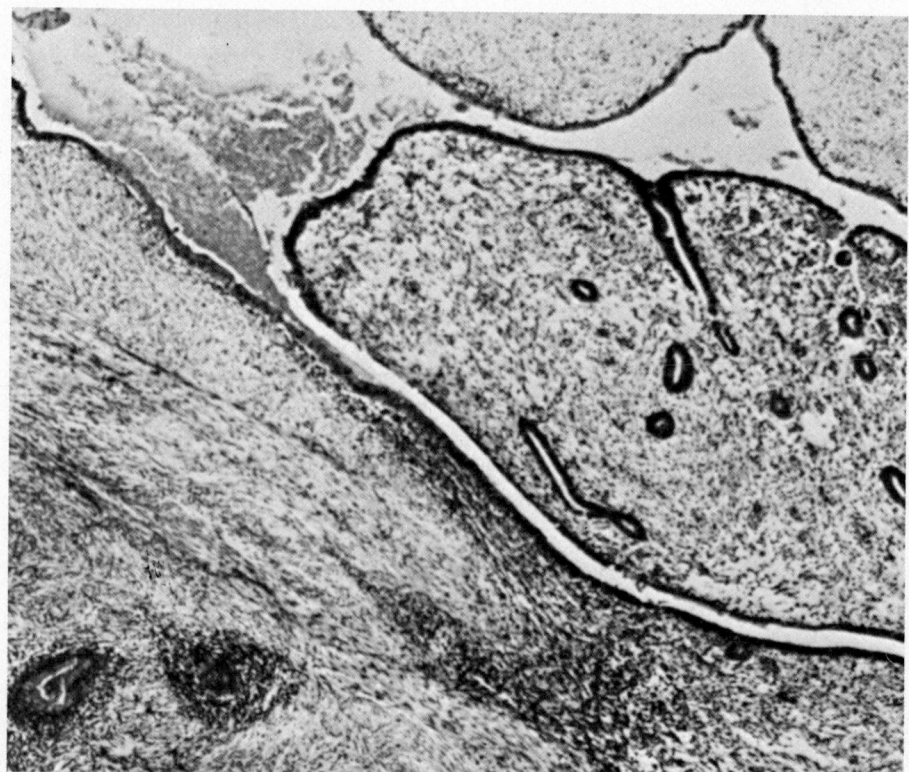

FIGURE 17-40
Wall of endometrioma lined by endometrial-type epithelium with underlying endometrial stroma. Note polypoid projections of endometrial tissue projecting into cyst lumen. (H&E stain; ×40.) (From Czernobilsky B: Primary epithelial tumors of the ovary. In Blaustein A, editor: Pathology of the female genital tract, New York, 1977, Springer-Verlag New York, Inc, p 476.)

The latter tumor is a true neoplasm, and there is a malignant counterpart.

Fibroma

Fibromas are the most common benign, solid neoplasms of the ovary. Their malignant potential is low, less than 1%. These tumors comprise approximately 5% of benign ovarian neoplasms and approximately 20% of all solid tumors of the ovary.

Fibromas vary in size from small nodules to huge pelvic tumors weighing 50 pounds. One of the predominant characteristics of fibromas is that they are extremely slow-growing tumors. The average diameter of a fibroma is approximately 6 cm; however, larger tumors have reached 30 cm in diameter. In most series, less than 5% of fibromas are greater than 20 cm in diameter. The diameter of a fibroma is important clinically, because the incidence of associated ascites is directly proportional to the size of the tumor. Ninety percent of fibromas are unilateral; however, multiple fibromas are found in the same ovary in 10% to 15% of cases. The average age of a woman with an ovarian fibroma is 48. Thus this tumor often presents in a postmenopausal woman. The tumor arises from the undifferentiated fibrous stroma of the ovary.

The pelvic symptoms that develop with growth of fibromas include pressure and abdominal enlargement, which may be secondary to the size of the tumor and ascites. Smaller tumors are asymptomatic; because these tumors do not elaborate hormones, there is no change in the pattern of menstrual flow. Fibromas may be pedunculated and thus easily easily palpable during one examination yet difficult to palpate during a subsequent pelvic examination. Sometimes on pelvic examination the fibromas appear to be softer than a solid ovarian tumor because of the edema and/or occasional cystic degeneration. *Meigs' syndrome* is the association of an ovarian fibroma, ascites, and hydrothorax. Both the ascites and the hydrothorax resolve after removal of the ovarian tumor.

The ascites is caused by transudation of fluid from the ovarian fibroma. Samanth and Black reported that the incidence of ascites was directly related to the size of the fibroma. Fifty percent of patients have ascites if the tumor is greater than 6 cm. However, true Meigs' syndrome is rare, occurring in less than 5% of fibromas. The hydrothorax develops secondary to a flow of ascitic fluid into the pleural space via the lymphatics of the diaphragm. Statistically the right pleural space is involved in 75% of reported cases, the left in 10%, and both sides in 15%. The clinical features of Meigs' syndrome are not unique to fibromas, and a similar clinical picture is found with many other ovarian tumors.

Grossly, fibromas are heavy, solid, well encapsulated, and grayish-white. The cut surface usually demonstrates a homogeneous white or yellowish white solid tissue with a trabeculated or whorled appearance similar to that of myomas. The vast majority of fibromas are grossly edematous (Figure 17-41). Less than 10% of fibromas have calcifications or small areas of hyaline or cystic degeneration. Histologically, fibromas are composed of connective tissue, stromal cells, and varying amounts of collagen interposed between the cells. The connective tissue cells are spindle-shaped, mature fibroblasts. They are arranged in an imperfect pattern. A few smooth muscle fibers may be occasionally identified. It is sometimes difficult to distinguish fibromas from nonneoplastic thecomas. Histologically the pathologist must differentiate fibromas from fibrosarcomas and also look for epithelial elements of an associated Brenner tumor.

The management of fibromas is straightforward; any woman with a solid ovarian neoplasm

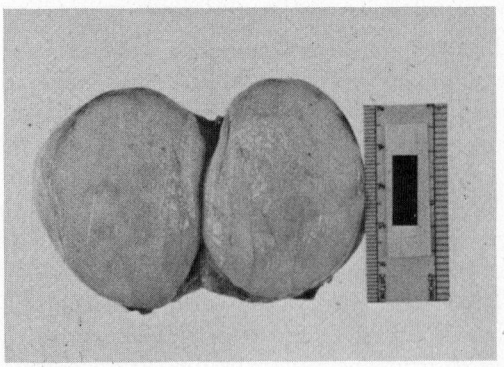

FIGURE 17-41
Fibroma of ovary. Cut surface shows somewhat edematous, interlacing bundles of connective tissue. (From Janovski NA, editor: Color atlas of gross gynecologic and obstetric pathology, New York, 1969, McGraw-Hill Book Co, p 163.)

should have an exploratory operation soon after the tumor is discovered. Simple excision of the tumor is all that is necessary. Following excision of the tumor, there is resolution of all symptoms, including ascites. Because these tumors are frequently discovered in postmenopausal women, often a bilateral salpingo-oophorectomy and total abdominal hysterectomy are performed. Conversely, it is important to note that most women who preoperatively have a solid ovarian tumor and ascites subsequently are found to have ovarian carcinoma.

Brenner Tumors

Brenner tumors are rare, small, smooth, solid, fibroepithelial ovarian tumors that are generally asymptomatic. The benign proliferative and malignant forms together comprise approximately 2% of ovarian tumors, and they usually occur in women aged 40 to 60 years. Approximately 30% of Brenner tumors are discovered as small, solid tumors in association with a concurrent serous cystic neoplasia, such as serous or mucinous cystadenomas of the ipsilateral ovary. Some are microscopic, with the entire tumor contained in a single low-powered microscopic field, and others may reach a diameter of 20 cm; the majority are less than 5 cm in diameter. The tumor is usually unilateral, with bilateral Brenner tumors being reported in only 5% to 15% of the women in large series.

The Brenner tumor was first described in 1898. Robert Meyer established that it was a distinct independent neoplasm from granulosa cell tumors in 1932. Since that time there has been a continuing controversy in the gynecologic pathology literature as to the histogenesis of the neoplasm. Most authorities accept the theory that the tumor results from metaplasia of coelomic epithelium into uroepithelium. Detailed three-dimensional histologic studies have demonstrated a downward growth in a cordlike fashion of epithelium from the surface of the ovary to deeper areas in the ovarian cortex. Others have postulated that the solid nests of epithelial cells of the tumor originate from the rete ovarii or Walthard rests. Shevchuk et al., in an electron microscopy study, confirmed the histologic and ultrastructural similarity between epithelium in Brenner tumors and transitional epithelium. These authors argue that because of the histogenesis from coelomic in-

clusion cysts and also the mixture of müllerian-type epithelium in 30% of Brenner tumors, it might be appropriate to classify Brenner tumors in the epithelial group of ovarian neoplasms.

Approximately 90% of these small neoplasms are discovered incidentally during a gynecologic operation, although large tumors may produce unilateral pelvic discomfort. Postmenopausal bleeding is sometimes associated with Brenner tumors, as endometrial hyperplasia is a coexisting abnormality in 10% to 16% of cases. It is postulated that luteinization of the stroma produces estrogen with resulting hyperplasia. Similar to fibromas, Brenner tumors are slow growing.

Grossly, Brenner tumors are smooth, firm, gray-white, solid tumors that grossly resemble fibromas. Upon sectioning, the tumor usually appears gray; however, occasionally there is a yellowish tinge with small cystic spaces (Figure 17-42). Approximately 1% to 2% of these tumors undergo malignant change (Chapter 29). Histologically, Brenner tumors have two principal components: solid masses or nests of epithelial cells and a surrounding fibrous stroma. The epithelial cells are uniform and do not appear anaplastic (Figure 17-43). The histology and ultrastructure of the epithelial cells of a Brenner tumor are similar to transitional epithelium of the urinary bladder. The pale epithelial cells have a "coffee bean"–appearing nucleus, which is also described as a longitudinal groove in the cell's nucleus. Electron microscopy has demonstrated that the longitudinal groove during routine microscopy is produced by prominent indentation of the nuclear membrane. An additional ovarian neoplasm is frequently found associated with Brenner tumors. Balasa et al., in a review of 302 tumors, reported 100 other concurrent neoplasms, with the majority being serous and mucinous cystadenomas or teratomas.

Management of Brenner tumors is operative with simple excision being the procedure of choice. However, as with ovarian fibromas, the patient's age often is the principal factor in deciding the extent of the operation.

Adenofibroma and Cystadenofibroma

Adenofibromas and cystadenofibromas are closely related. Both of these benign firm tumors are rare solid variations of serous cystadenomas. They differ from benign epithelial cys-

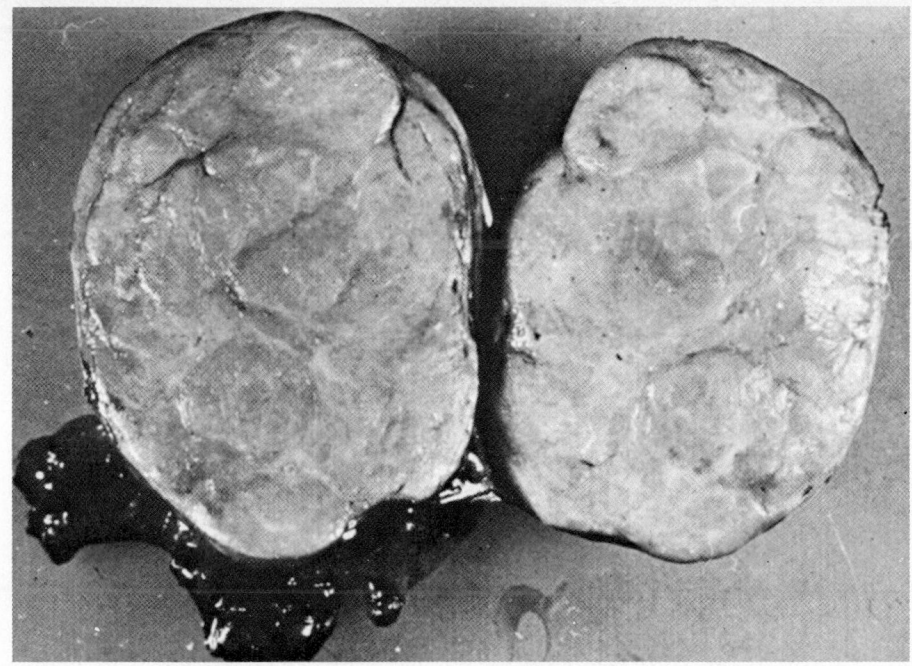

FIGURE 17-42
Cut section of solid, nodular Brenner tumor. (From Czernobilsky B: Primary epithelial tumors of the ovary. In Blaustein A, editor: Pathology of the female genital tract, New York, 1977, Springer-Verlag New York, Inc, p 489.)

A

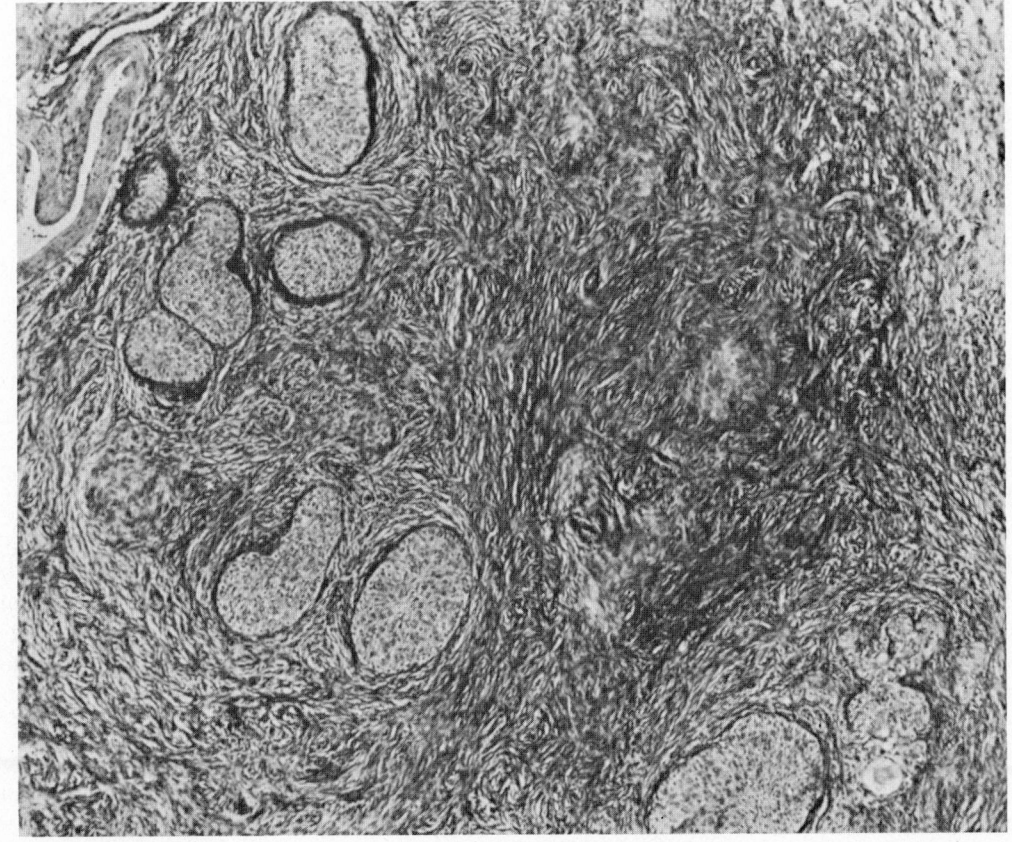

FIGURE 17-43
A, Brenner tumor of ovary that measured 3 mm in diameter; shows characteristic nests of epithelium in dense fibrous stroma. Tumor was an incidental microscopic finding. (H&E stain; ×25.)

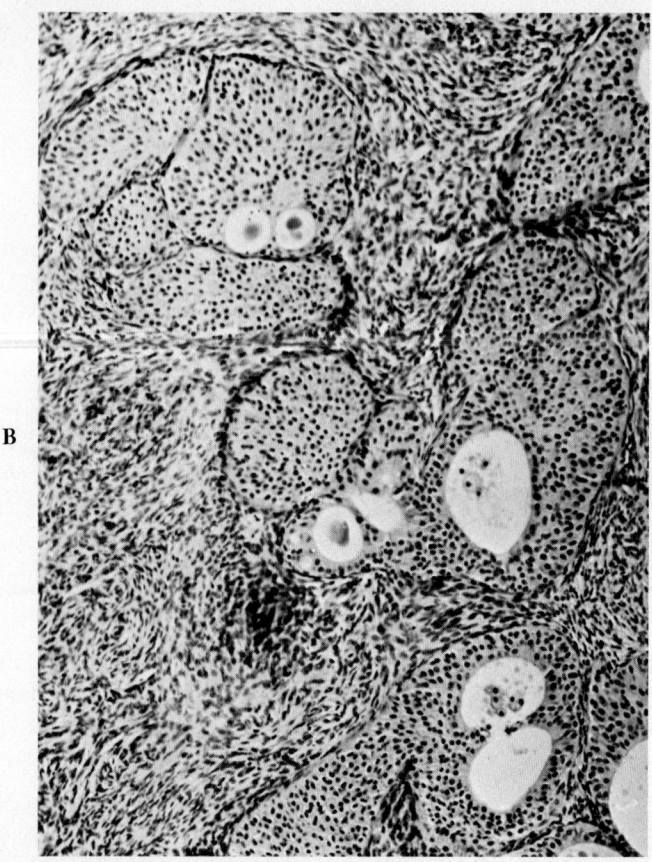

FIGURE 17-43, cont'd

B, Brenner tumor showing solid and partly cystic epithelial nest in dense fibrous stroma. (H&E stain; ×113.) (**A** from Balasa RW, Adcock LL, Prem KA, et al: Obstet Gynecol 50:121, 1977; **B** from Czernobilsky B: Primary epithelial tumors of the ovary. In Blaustein A, editor: Pathology of the female genital tract, New York, 1977, Springer-Verlag New York, Inc, p 490.)

tadenomas in that there is a preponderance of connective tissue. Most pathologists emphasize that at least 25% of the fibroma consists of fibrous connective tissue. Obviously, cystadenofibromas have microscopic or occasional macroscopic areas that are cystic. The varying degree of fibrous stroma and epithelial elements produces a spectrum of tumors, which have resulted in a confusing nomenclature with terms such as *papillomas, fibropapillomas,* and *fibroadenomas.*

Adenofibromas are usually small fibrous tumors that arise from the surface of the ovary. They are bilateral in 20% to 25% of women. They usually occur in postmenopausal women and are 1 to 15 cm in diameter. Grossly, they are gray or white tumors, and it is difficult to distinguish them from fibromas. Papillary ade-

nofibromas, which project from the surface of the ovary, may at first glance appear to be external excrescences of a malignant tumor. Histologically, small precursors of adenofibromas are identified in many normal ovaries. Under the microscope, true cystic gland spaces lined by cuboidal epithelium are characteristic. However, differing from serous cystadenomas, the fibrous connective tissue surrounding the cystic spaces is abundant and is the predominant tissue of the tumor.

Smaller tumors are asymptomatic and are only discovered incidentally during abdominal or pelvic operations. Large tumors may cause pressure symptoms or rarely undergo adnexal torsion.

Because adenofibromas are usually discovered in postmenopausal women, the treatment of choice is bilateral salpingo-oophorectomy and total abdominal hysterectomy. As these tumors are benign and as malignant transformation is rare, simple excision of the tumor and inspection of the contralateral ovary is appropriate in younger women.

Torsion

Torsion of the ovary or both the oviduct and the ovary (adnexal torsion) is an unusual but important cause of acute lower abdominal and pelvic pain. Torsion of the ovary may occur separately from torsion of the fallopian tube, but most commonly the two adnexal structures are affected together. In Hibbard's review of 128 cases of adnexal torsion, this syndrome accounted for approximately 3% of gynecologic operative emergencies at the University of Southern California Medical Center.

Adnexal torsion occurs most commonly during the reproductive years, with the average patient being in her mid-20s. Nevertheless, adnexal torsion is also a complication of benign ovarian tumors in the postmenopausal woman. Pregnancy appears to predispose women to adnexal torsion, with approximately one in five women being pregnant when the condition is diagnosed. Most susceptible are ovaries that are enlarged secondary to ovulation induction during early pregnancy. One series reported four cases of adnexal torsion out of 648 pregnancies resulting from ovulation induction. The most common etiology of adnexal torsion is ovarian enlargement by an 8 to 12 cm benign mass of the ovary. Ovarian tumors are discovered in 50% to 60% of women with adnexal torsion. Torsion of a normal ovary or adnexum is also possible and occurs more frequently in children. Hibbard reports that because of their relative prevalence, dermoids are the tumor most frequently reported in a series of women with adnexal torsion. However, the relative risk of adnexal torsion is higher with parovarian cysts, solid benign tumors, and serous cysts of the ovary. The right ovary has a greater tendency to twist (3 to 2) than does the left ovary. Torsion of a malignant ovarian tumor is comparatively rare (2.5% in Hibbard's report).

Patients with adnexal torsion present with acute, severe, unilateral, lower abdominal and pelvic pain. Often the patient relates the onset of the severe pain to an abrupt change of position. A unilateral palpable adnexal mass is found in over 90% of patients. Approximately two thirds of patients have associated nausea and vomiting. These associated gastrointestinal symptoms sometimes lead to a preoperative diagnosis of acute appendicitis or small intestinal obstruction. Many patients have noted intermittent previous episodes of similar pain for several days to several weeks. The hypothesis is that previous episodes of pain were secondary to partial torsion, with spontaneous reversal without significant vascular compromise. With progressive torsion, initially venous and lymphatic obstruction occurs. This produces a cyanotic, edematous ovary, which on pelvic examination presents as a unilateral, tender adnexal mass. Further progression of the torsion interrupts the major arterial supply to the ovary, resulting in hypoxia, adnexal necrosis, and a concomitant low-grade fever and leukocystosis. Approximately 10% of women with adnexal torsion have a repetitive episode affecting the contralateral adnexum.

Most patients with adnexal torsion present with symptoms and signs severe enough to demand operative intervention. If the diagnosis is questionable, laparoscopy may be appropriate. Increasingly, women with ovarian torsion are being treated via laparoscopic surgery. The most common gynecologic conditions that may be confused with adnexal torsion are a ruptured corpus luteum or an adnexal abscess. In recent series emphasizing the early diagnosis of adnexal torsion, conservative management has been possible in 75% of cases.

Because the majority of cases of adnexal torsion occur in young women, a conservative operation is ideal. The clinician should maintain a high index of suspicion for adnexal torsion so that early and conservative surgery is possible. However, it is often difficult to grossly differentiate between partial torsion and complete torsion. If partial torsion is confirmed, it is acceptable to untwist the pedicle, perform a cystectomy, and stabilize the ovary with sutures so as to prevent recurrence. Conservative operation has the risk of releasing venous thrombi into the general circulation if the degree of torsion is underestimated. Thus with vascular compromise the proper operation is unilateral salpingo-oophorectomy. The vascular pedicle should be clamped with care so as not to injure the ureter, which may be tented up by the torsion, yet sufficiently distant from the ovary so as to include all areas of vascular thrombosis.

—————————— **KEY POINTS** ——————————

- Symptoms of urethral caruncles are variable. Some urethral caruncles are asymptomatic; others cause dysuria, frequency, and urgency. They must be differentiated from urethral carcinoma by biopsy. Treatment of urethral caruncles is topical or oral estrogen therapy.

- The vulva contains 1% of the skin surface of the body, but 5% to 10% of all malignant melanomas in women arise from this region. All vulvar nevi should be excised and examined histologically.

- Symptoms of an early malignant melanoma include *asymmetry*, *border* irregularity, *color* variegation, and a *diameter* usually greater than 6 mm (ABCD).

- Hidradenomas are asymptomatic vulvar tumors originating from apocrine glands and are found in white women between 30 and 70 years of age.

- Endometriosis of the vulva is rare, with only 1 in 500 patients with endometriosis having vulvar involvement.

- Treatment of vulvar hematomas is conservative unless they are expanding.

- The most common causes of vulvar contact dermatitis are cosmetic and local therapeutic agents.

- Vulvar psoriasis usually involves intertriginous areas and is manifested by red to red-yellow papules. These lesions enlarge, becoming dull-red plaques.

- The treatment of hidradenitis suppurativa is wide operative excision.

- Urethral diverticula occur in approximately 3% of women, and the diagnosis should be suspected in any woman with chronic or recurrent lower urinary tract symptoms.

- Of women with urethral diverticula, 20% are asymptomatic, while tender masses may be palpated in more than half of the patients.

- Prolonged tampon use may be associated with ulcerations of the vagina, discharge, and bleeding.

- Biopsy examination of any persistent vaginal ulcer should be done to rule out carcinoma.

- Endocervical polyps are smooth, soft, red, fragile masses. They are found most commonly in multiparous women in their 40s and 50s.

- Approximately 1 in 4 women with abnormal bleeding will have an endometrial polyp.

- Malignant transformation of endometrial polyps has been estimated to occur in 0.5% of cases and is most often an endometrial carcinoma of low grade and stage.

- Leiomyomas of the uterus are the most frequent pelvic tumors and occur most commonly in the fifth decade of life.

- Five to ten percent of myomas are submucosal, often presenting with symptoms of abnormal vaginal bleeding and distortion of the uterine cavity that may lead to infertility or abortion.

- Broad ligament leiomyomas may produce hydroureters as they enlarge.

- Each individual uterine myoma is monoclonal, arising from a single muscle cell.

- The stimulus for growth of myomas is unclear; however, it is partially related to estrogen levels.

- Acute muscular infarction, as is seen with red degeneration of a myoma, causes severe pain and localized peritoneal irritation.

- The malignant transformation of a fibroid is rare, probably occurring in less than 0.3% of cases.

- The majority of women with uterine myomas are asymptomatic, but one of three will experience pelvic pain, with dysmenorrhea being the most frequent complaint.

- Abnormal bleeding is experienced by 30% of women with myomas, with the most common symptom being menorrhagia, but intermenstrual spotting and disruption of the normal pattern are other frequent complaints.

- The management of women with small, asymptomatic myomas is conservative, and the majority of women will not need operations.

- Prolapse of a myoma through the cervix is optimally treated by vaginal removal and ligation of the base of the myoma.

- Gonadotrophin-releasing hormone (GnRH) agonists will reduce the size of myomas by 40% to 90% in 80% of patients. However, within 6 months after treatment, the myoma will return to pretreatment size.

- Women with symptomatic leiomyomas should be investigated thoroughly for concurrent problems, such as endometrial hyperplasia. If their symptoms do not improve with conservative management, operative therapy is indicated.

- Classic indications for myomectomy include rapidly expanding pelvic mass, persistent abnormal bleeding, pain or pressure, previous repetitive abortion, or longstanding infertility.

- Hematometra in postmenopausal women is often asymptomatic.

- The main symptom of torsion of the tube is pain, usually located in the iliac fossa with radiation to the thigh and flank. In two thirds of cases the pain is associated with nausea and vomiting.

- Follicular cysts are the most common cystic structures in normal ovaries.

- Indications for operation on a cyst in the ovary include a mass after the menopause or before puberty, a solid tumor at any age, a cystic mass greater than 8 cm, or a cystic mass 5 to 8 cm in size that has been observed for more than 8 weeks.

- Women taking warfarin (Coumadin) are especially prone to develop hemorrhage from rupture of a corpus luteum cyst.

- The treatment of unruptured corpus luteum cysts is conservative. However, if the cyst persists or intraperitoneal bleeding occurs, necessitating operation, the treatment is cystectomy.

- Benign ovarian teratomas comprise 15% to 25% of all ovarian neoplasms.

- Benign ovarian teratomas vary from a few millimeters to 25 cm, may be single or multiple, and are bilateral 10% to 15% of the time.

- Dermoids are believed to arise during fetal life from a single germ cell. They are 46,XX in karyotype.

- Although most dermoids are asymptomatic, torsion and rupture are two important complications.

- Fifty percent of dermoids have calcifications visible on a pelvic x-ray film.

- The most prominent symptoms of ovarian endometriosis are pelvic pain, dyspareunia, and infertility.

- Histologically, ovarian endometriosis usually demonstrates endometrial stroma, large phagocytic cells, and endometrial glands. However, pressure atrophy may lead to loss of architecture of the endometrial glands.

- Fibromas are the most common, benign, solid neoplasms of the ovary. They have a low malignant potential.

- Fibromas vary in size from small nodules to huge pelvic tumors weighing as much as 50 pounds. Ninety percent of fibromas are unilateral, and most have an average diameter of 6 cm.

- Fifty percent of patients with an ovarian fibroma will have ascites if the tumor is greater than 6 cm.

- Brenner tumors are smooth, solid, fibroepithelial tumors of the ovary. They usually occur in women between the ages of 40 and 60 years and are predominantly unilateral.

- Adnexal torsion occurs most commonly in the reproductive years, with the average age of patients being mid-20s. Pregnancy predisposes to adnexal torsion.

- Ovarian tumors are discovered in 50% to 60% of women with adnexal torsion.

BIBLIOGRAPHY

Aharoni A, Reiter A, Golan D, et al: Patterns of growth of uterine leiomyomas during pregnancy: a prospective longitudinal study, Br J Obstet Gynaecol 95:510, 1988.

Ahnaimugan S and Asuen MI: Coital laceration of the vagina, Aust NZ J Obstet Gynaecol 20:180, 1980.

Axe S, Parmley T, Woodruff JD, et al: Adenomas in minor vestibular glands, Obstet Gynecol 68:16, 1986.

Baggish MS and Baltoyannis P: Carbon dioxide laser treatment of cervical stenosis, Fertil Steril 48:24, 1987.

Balasa RW, Adcock LL, Prem KA, et al: The Brenner tumor, Obstet Gynecol 50:120, 1977.

Baron JA, LaVecchia C, and Levi F: The antiestrogenic effect of cigarette smoking in women, Am J Obstet Gynecol 162:502, 1990.

Barrett KF, Bledsoe S, Greer BE, et al: Tampon-induced vaginal or cervical ulceration, Am J Obstet Gynecol 127:332, 1977.

Bernardus RE, Van Der Slikke JW, Roex AJM, et al: Torsion of the fallopian tube: some considerations on its etiology, Obstet Gynecol 64:675, 1984.

Bhatia NN, Bergman A, and Broen EM: Advanced hidradenitis suppurativa of the vulva, J Reprod Med 29:436, 1984.

Birch HW and Sondag DR: Granular-cell myoblastoma of the vulva, Obstet Gynecol 18:443, 1961.

Blaustein A, editor: Pathology of the female genital tract, ed 3, New York, 1987, Springer-Verlag, New York, Inc.

Brown JV and Stenchever MA: Cavernous lymphangioma of the vulva, Obstet Gynecol 73:877, 1989.

Burton CA, Grimes DA, and March CM: Surgical management of leiomyomata during pregnancy, Obstet Gynecol 74:707, 1989.

Buttram VC and Reiter RC: Uterine leiomyomata: etiology, symptomatology, and management, Fertil Steril 36:433, 1981.

Carneiro SJC, Gardner HL, and Knox JM: Syringoma: three cases with vulvar involvement, Obstet Gynecol 39:95, 1972.

Chambers JT, Thiagarajah S, and Kitchin JD: Torsion of the normal fallopian tube in pregnancy, Obstet Gynecol 54:487, 1979.

Choo YC, Mak KC, Hsu C, et al: Postmenopausal uterine bleeding of nonorganic cause, Obstet Gynecol 66:225, 1985.

Coates JB and Hales JS: Granular cell myoblastoma of the vulva, Obstet Gynecol 41:796, 1973.

Coutinho EM and Goncalves MT: Long-term treatment of leiomyomas with gestrinone, Fertil Steril 51:939, 1989.

Cramer SF, Robertson AL, Ziats NP, et al: Growth potential of human uterine leiomyomas: some in vitro observations and their implications, Obstet Gynecol 66:36, 1985.

David GD: The management of vulvar vestibulitis syndrome with the carbon dioxide laser, J Gynecol Surg 5:87, 1989.

DeCrespigny LC, Robinson HP, Davoren RAM, et al: The 'simple' ovarian cyst: aspirate or operate? Br J Obstet Gynaecol 96:1035, 1989.

Deppisch LM: Cysts of the vagina, Obstet Gynecol 45:623, 1975.

DeWilde R, Bordt J, Hesseling M, et al: Ovarian cystostomy, Acta Obstet Gynecol Scand 68:363, 1989.

Dick HM and Honore LH: Dental structures in benign ovarian cystic teratomas (dermoid cysts), Oral Surg Oral Med Oral Pathol 60:299, 1985.

Dische FE and Ritche JM: Luteoma of pregnancy, J Pathol 100:77, 1970.

Donnez J, Schrurs B, Gillerot S, et al: Treatment of uterine fibroids with implants of gonadotropin-releasing hormone agonist: assessment by hysterography, Fertil Steril 51:947, 1989.

Dreyer L, Simson IW, Sevenster CBO, et al: Leiomyomatosis peritonealis disseminata: a report of two cases and a review of the literature, Br J Obstet Gynaecol 92:856, 1985.

Duckman S, Suarez JR, and Sese LQ: Giant cervical polyp, Am J Obstet Gynecol 159:852, 1988.

Dunnihoo DR and Wolff J: Bilateral torsion of the adnexa: a case report and a review of the world literature, Obstet Gynecol 64:55S, 1984.

Evans AT, Symmonds RE, and Gaffey TA: Recurrent pelvic intravenous leiomyomatosis, Obstet Gynecol 57:260, 1981.

Farrar HK and Nedoss BR: Benign tumors of the uterine cervix, Am J Obstet Gynecol 81:124, 1961.

Fedele L, Vercellini P, Bianchi S, et al: Treatment with GnRH agonists before myomectomy and the risk of short-term myoma recurrence, Br J Obstet Gynaecol 97:393, 1990.

Friedel W and Kaiser IH: Vaginal evisceration, Obstet Gynecol 45:315, 1975.

Friedman AJ, Barbieri RL, Benacerraf BR, et al: Treatment of leiomyomata with intranasal or subcutaneous leuprolide, a gonadotropin-releasing hormone agonist, Fertil Steril 48:560, 1987.

Friedman AJ, Harrison-Atlas D, Barbieri RL, et al: A randomized, placebo-controlled, double-blind study evaluating the efficacy of leuprolide acetate depot in the treatment of uterine leiomyomata, Fertil Steril 51:251, 1989.

Friedman AJ, Hoffman DI, Comite F, et al: Treatment of leiomyomata uteri with leuprolide acetate depot: a double-blind, placebo-controlled, multicenter study, Obstet Gynecol 77:720, 1991.

Friedman AJ, Rein MS, Harrison-Atlas D, et al: A randomized, placebo-controlled, double-blind study evaluating leuprolide acetate depot treatment before myomectomy, Fertil Steril 52:728, 1989.

Friedman RJ, Rigel DS, and Kopf AW: Early detection of malignant melanoma: the role of physician examination and self-examination of the skin, CA 35:130, 1985.

Friedrich EG: Tampon effects on vaginal health, Clin Obstet Gynecol 24:395, 1981.

Friedrich EG: The vulvar vestibule, J Reprod Med 28:773, 1983.

Friedrich EG: Vulvar disease, ed 2, Philadelphia, 1983, WB Saunders Co.

Friedrich EG and Wilkinson EJ: Vulvar surgery for neurofibromatosis, Obstet Gynecol 65:135, 1985.

Gardner HL and Kaufman RH: Benign diseases of the vulva and vagina, ed 2, Boston, 1981, GK Hall & Co.

George M, Lhomme C, Lefort J, et al: Long-term use of an LH-RH agonist in the management of uterine leiomyomas: a study of 17 cases, Int J Fertil 34:19, 1989.

Ginsburg D and Genadry R: Suburethral diverticulum: classification and therapeutic considerations, Obstet Gynecol 61:685, 1983.

Goldstein SR, Subramanyam B, Snyder JR, et al: The postmenopausal cystic adnexal mass: the potential role of ultrasound in conservative managment, Obstet Gynecol 73:8, 1989.

Gompel C and Silverberg SG: Pathology in gynecology and obstetrics, ed 3, Philadelphia, 1985, JB Lippincott Co.

Grimes DA and Hughs JM: Use of multiphasic oral contraceptives and hospitalizations of women with functional ovarian cysts in the United States, Obstet Gynecol 73:1037, 1989.

Hallatt JG, Steele CH, and Snyder M: Ruptured corpus luteum with hemoperitoneum: a study of 173 surgical cases, Am J Obstet Gynecol 149:5, 1984.

Hamlin DJ, Pettersson H, Fitzsimmons J, et al: MR imaging of uterine leiomyomas and their complications, J Comput Assist Tomogr 9:902, 1985.

Hart WR: Paramesonephric mucinous cysts of the vulva, Am J Obstet Gynecol 107:1079, 1980.

Herndon JH: Itching: the pathophysiology of pruritus, Int J Dermatol 14:465, 1975.

Hibbard LT: Adnexal torsion, Am J Obstet Gynecol 152:456, 1985.

Hricak H, Tschalakoff D, Heinrichs L, et al: Uterine leiomyomas: correlation of MR, histopathologic findings, and symptoms, Radiology 158:385, 1986.

Huddock JJ, Dupayne N, and McGeary JA: Traumatic vulvar hematomas, Am J Obstet Gynecol 70:1064, 1955.

Huffman JW: The detailed anatomy of the paraurethral ducts in the adult human female, Am J Obstet Gynecol 55:86, 1948.

Hunter DJS: Management of a massive ovarian cyst, Obstet Gynecol 56:254, 1980.

Imperial R and Helwig EB: Angiokeratoma of the vulva, Obstet Gynecol 29:307, 1967.

Iosif CS and Akerlund M: Fibromyomas and uterine activity, Acta Obstet Gynecol Scand 62:165, 1983.

Israel SL: The clinical similarity of corpus luteum cyst and ectopic pregnancy, Am J Obstet Gynecol 44:22, 1942.

Janovski NA: Dysontogenetic cyst of the vulva, Obstet Gynecol 20:227, 1962.

Janovski NA: Color atlas of gross gynecologic and obstetric pathology, New York, 1969, McGraw-Hill Book Co.

Jimmerson SD and Becker JD: Vaginal ulcers associated with tampon usage, Obstet Gynecol 56:97, 1980.

Junaid TA and Thomas SM: Cysts of the vulva and vagina: a comparative study, Int J Gynaecol Obstet 19:239, 1981.

Katz VL, Dotters DJ, and Droegemueller W: Complications of uterine leiomyomas in pregnancy, Obstet Gynecol 73:593, 1989.

Kemmann E, Ghazi DM, and Corsan GH: Adnexal torsion in menotropin-induced pregnancies, Obstet Gynecol 76:403, 1990.

Kessel B, Liu J, Mortola J, et al: Treatment of uterine fibroids with agonist analogs of gonadotropin-releasing hormone, Fertil Steril 49:538, 1988.

Klein HZ and Smith RL: Fibromyoma of the uterine tube, Obstet Gynecol 26:515, 1965.

Knox JM: Cutaneous inflammations and infections, Clin Obstet Gynecol 21:991, 1978.

Kolstad P and Stafl A: Atlas of colposcopy, ed 2, Baltimore, 1977, University Park Press.

Koonings PP and Grimes DA: Adnexal torsion in postmenopausal women, Obstet Gynecol 73:11, 1989.

Laing FC, Van Dalsem VF, Marks WM, et al: Dermoid cysts of the ovary: their ultrasonographic appearances, Obstet Gynecol 57:99, 1981.

Lakkis WG, Martin MC, and Gelfand MM: Benign cystic teratoma of the ovary: a 6-year review, Can J Surg 28:444, 1985.

Lambert B, and De Brux J: Theca lutein cysts of pregnancy without mole or chorioepithelioma, Obstet Gynecol 22:643, 1963.

Leach GE and Bavendam TG: Female urethral diverticula, Urology 30:407, 1987.

Lee RA: Diverticulum of the female urethra: postoperative complications and results, Obstet Gynecol 61:52, 1983.

Lee RA: Diverticulum of the urethra: clinical presentation, diagnosis, and management, Clin Obstet Gynecol 27:490, 1984.

Leibsohn S, d'Ablaing G, Mishell DR Jr, et al: Leiomyosarcoma in a series of hysterectomies performed for presumed uterine leiomyomas, Am J Obstet Gynecol 162:968, 1990.

Letterie GS, Coddington CC, Winkel CA: et al: Efficacy of a gonadotropin-releasing hormone agonist in the treatment of uterine leiomata: long-term follow-up, Fertil Steril 51:951, 1989.

Linder D, McCau BK, and Hecht F: Parthenogenic origin of benign ovarian teratomas, N Engl J Med 292:63, 1975.

Loffer FD: Removal of large symptomatic intrauterine growths by the hysteroscopic resectoscope, Obstet Gynecol 76:836, 1990.

Lucente V and Benson JT: Vaginal mullerian cyst presenting as an anterior enterocele: a case report, Obstet Gynecol 76:906, 1990.

Luesley DM, Williams DR, Gee H, et al: Management of postconization cervical stenosis by laser vaporization, Obstet Gynecol 67:126, 1986.

Lumsden MA, West CP, Bramley T, et al: The binding of epidermal growth factor to the human uterus and leiomyomata in women rendered hypo-oestrogenic by continuous administration of an LHRH agonist, Br J Obstet Gynaecol 95:1299, 1988.

Luxman D, Bergman A, Sagi J, and David MP: The postmenopausal adnexal mass: correlation between ultrasonic and pathologic findings, Obstet Gynecol 77:726, 1991.

Lynch PJ: Vulvodynia: a syndrome of unexplained vulvar pain, psychologic disability and sexual dysfunction, J Reprod Med 31:773, 1986.

MacKay B, Bennington JL, and Skoglund RW: The adenomatoid tumor: fine structural evidence for a mesothelial origin, Cancer 27:109, 1971.

Maheux R, Guilloteau C, Lemay A, et al: Luteinizing hormone–releasing hormone agonist and uterine leiomyoma: a pilot study, Am J Obstet Gynecol 152:1034, 1985.

Maiman M, Seltzer V, and Boyce J: Laparoscopic excision of ovarian neoplasms subsequently found to be malignant, Obstet Gynecol 77:563, 1991.

Maloney ME: Exploring the common vulvar dermatoses, Contemp Ob/Gyn, 29:91, 1988.

Marshall FC, Uson AC, and Melicow MM: Neoplasms and caruncles of the female urethra, Surg Gynecol Obstet 110:723, 1960.

Mathias CGT and Maibach HI: Dermatotoxicology monographs. I. Cutaneous irritation: factors influencing the response to irritants, Clin Toxicol 13:333, 1978.

Matta WHM, Shaw RW, and Nye M: Long-term follow-up of patients with uterine fibroids after treatment with the LHRH agonist buserelin, Br J Obstet Gynaecol 96:200, 1989.

Matta WHM, Stabile I, Shaw RW, et al: Doppler assessment of uterine blood flow changes in patients with fibroids receiving the gonadotropin-releasing hormone agonist buserelin, Fertil Steril 49:1083, 1988.

Mattingly RF and Thompson JD, editors: TeLinde's operative gynecology, ed 6, Philadelphia, 1985, JB Lippincott Co.

McKay M: Vulvodynia versus pruritus vulvae, Clin Obstet Gynecol 28:123, 1985.

Meigs JV, Armstrong SH, and Hamilton HH: A further contribution to the syndrome of fibroma of the ovary with fluid in the abdomen and chest, Meigs' syndrome, Am J Obstet Gynecol 46:19, 1943.

Melody GF: Obstructed cervix, Obstet Gynecol 10:190, 1957.

Montz FJ, Schlaerth JB, and Morrow CP: The natural history of theca lutein cysts, Obstet Gynecol 72:247, 1988.

Mostafa SAM, Bargeron CB, Flower RW, et al: Foreign body granulomas in normal ovaries, Obstet Gynecol 66:701, 1985.

Mutter GL: Teratoma genetics and stem cells: a review, Obstet Gynecol Surv 42:661, 1987.

Naumann RO and Droegemueller W: Unusual etiology of vulvar hematomas, Am J Obstet Gynecol 142:357, 1982.

Neuwirth RS: Urethral prolapse—a cause of vaginal bleeding in young girls, Obstet Gynecol 22:290, 1963.

Neuwirth RS: Hysteroscopic management of symptomatic submucous fibroids, Obstet Gynecol 62:509, 1983.

Nichols DH and Julian PJ: Torsion of the adnexa, Clin Obstet Gynecol 28:375, 1985.

Novak ER and Woodruff JD, editors: Novak's gynecologic and obstetric pathology with clinical and endocrine relations, ed 8, Philadelphia, 1979, WB Saunders Co.

Ong HC and Chan WF: Mucinous cystadenoma, serous cystadenoma and benign cystic teratoma of the ovary, Cancer 41:1538, 1978.

Pantoja E, Rodriguez-Ibanez I, Axtmayer RW, et al: Complications of dermoid tumors of the ovary, Obstet Gynecol 45:89, 1975.

Papadaki L and Beilby JOW: Ovarian cystadenofibroma: a consideration of the role of estrogen in its pathogenesis, Am J Obstet Gynecol 121:501, 1975.

Parazzini F, LaVecchia C, Negri E, et al: Epidemiologic characteristics of women with uterine fibroids: a case-controlled study, Obstet Gynecol 72:853, 1988.

Parker WH and Berek JS: Management of selected cystic adnexal masses in postmenopausal women by operative laparoscopy: a pilot study, Am J Obstet Gynecol 163:1574, 1990.

Pauerstein CJ: The fallopian tube: a reappraisal, Philadelphia, 1974, Lea & Febiger.

Paull T and Tedeschi LG: Perineal endometriosis at the site of episiotomy scar, Obstet Gynecol 40:28, 1972.

Peckham EM, Maki DG, Patterson JJ, et al: Focal vulvitis: a characteristic syndrome and cause of dyspareunia, Am J Obstet Gynecol 154:855, 1986.

Perl V, Marquez J, Comaru-Schally AM, et al: Treatment of leiomyomata uteri with D-Trp6-luteinizing hormone–releasing hormone, Fertil Steril 48:383, 1987.

Peters WA, Thiagarajah S, and Thornton WN: Ovarian hemorrhage in patients receiving anticoagulant therapy, J Reprod Med 22:82, 1979.

Peterson WF and Novak ER: Endometrial polyps, Obstet Gynecol 8:40, 1956.

Pettersson B, Adami H-O, Lindgren A, et al: Endometrial polyps and hyperplasia as risk factors for endometrial carcinoma, Acta Obstet Gynecol Scand 64:653, 1985.

Price FV, Edwards R, and Buchsbaum HJ: Ovarian remnant syndrome: difficulties in diagnosis and management, Obstet Gynecol Surv 45:151, 1990.

Radisavljevic SV: The pathogenesis of ovarian inclusion cysts and cystomas, Obstet Gynecol 49:424, 1977.

Rafla N: Vaginismus and vaginal tears, Am J Obstet Gynecol 158:1043, 1988.

Reid JD, Kommareddi S, Lankerani M, et al: Chronic expanding hematomas, JAMA 244:2441, 1980.

Rein MS, Friedman AJ, Stuart JM, et al: Fibroid and myometrial steroid receptors in women treated with gonadotropin-releasing hormone agonist leuprolide acetate, Fertil Steril 53:1018, 1990.

Rice JP, Kay HH, and Mahony BS: The clinical significance of uterine leiomyomas in pregnancy, Am J Obstet Gynecol 160:1212, 1989.

Richardson DA, Hajj SN, and Herbst AL: Medical treatment of urethral prolapse in children, Obstet Gynecol 59:69, 1982.

Robboy SJ, Ross JS, Prat J, et al: Urogenital sinus origin of mucinous and ciliated cysts of the vulva, Obstet Gynecol 51:347, 1978.

Roberts CL and Marshall HK: Fibromyoma of the fallopian tube, Am J Obstet Gynecol 82:364, 1961.

Roberts DB: Necrotizing fasciitis of the vulva, Am J Obstet Gynecol 157:568, 1987.

Roehrborn CG: Long-term follow-up study of the marsupilization technique for urethral diverticula in women, Surg Gynecol Obstet 167:191, 1988.

Rulin MC and Preston AL: Adnexal masses in postmenopausal women, Obstet Gynecol 70:578, 1987.

Samaha M and Woodruff JD: Paratubal cysts: frequency, histogenesis, and associated clinical features, Obstet Gynecol 65:691, 1985.

Samanth KK and Black WC: Benign ovarian stromal tumors associated with free peritoneal fluid, Am J Obstet Gynecol 107:538, 1970.

Sauer M, Rodi I, and Bustillo M: Unilateral vulvar edema after intraperitoneal Hyskon administration, Fertil Steril 44:546, 1985.

Schlaff WD, Zerhouni EA, Huth JAM, et al: A placebo-controlled trial of a depot gonadotropin-releasing hormone analogue (leuprolide) in the treatment of uterine leiomyomata, Obstet Gynecol 74:856, 1989.

Shevchuk MM, Fenoglio CM, and Richart RM: Histogenesis of Brenner tumors. I. Histology and structure, Cancer 46:2607, 1980.

Silvers DN and Halperin AJ: Cutaneous and vulvar melanoma: an update, Clin Obstet Gynecol 21:1117, 1978.

Smith NC, Van Coeverden de Groot HA, and Gunston KD: Coital injuries of the vagina in nonvirginal patients, S Afr Med J 64:746, 1983.

Soper DE, Patterson JW, Hurt WG, et al: Lichen planus of the vulva, Obstet Gynecol 72:74, 1988.

Soules MR and McCarty KS: Leiomyomas: steroid receptor content, Am J Obstet Gynecol 143:6, 1982.

Spanos WJ: Preoperative hormonal therapy of cystic adnexal masses, Am J Obstet Gynecol 116:551, 1973.

Stein AL, Koonings PP, Schlaerth JB, et al: Relative frequency of malignant parovarian tumors: should parovarian tumors be aspirated? Obstet Gynecol 75:1029, 1990.

Steinkampf MP, Hammond KR, and Blackwell RE: Hormonal treatment of functional ovarian cysts: a randomized prospective study, Fertil Steril 54:775, 1990.

Stern JL, Buschema J, Rosenshein NB, et al: Spontaneous rupture of benign cystic teratomas, Obstet Gynecol 57:363, 1981.

Sutherland JA, Wilson EA, Edger DE, et al: Ultrastructure and steroid-binding studies in leiomyomatosis peritonealis disseminata, Am J Obstet Gynecol 136:992, 1980.

Tang LCH, Cho HKM, Chan SYW, et al: Dextropreponderance of corpus luteum rupture, J Reprod Med 30:764, 1985.

Thomas R, Barnhill D, Bibro M, et al: Hidradenitis suppurativa: a case presentation and review of the literature, Obstet Gynecol 66:592, 1985.

Thorp JM Jr, Wells SR, and Droegemueller W: Ovarian suspension in massive ovarian edema, Obstet Gynecol 76:912, 1990.

Valente PT: Leiomyomatosis peritonealis disseminata, Arch Pathol Lab Med 108:669, 1984.

Van Bogaert LJ: Clinicopathologic findings in endometrial polyps, Obstet Gynecol 71:771, 1988.

Venter PF, Rohm GF, and Slabber CG: Giant neurofibromas of the labia, Obstet Gynecol 57:128, 1981.

Vollenhoven BJ, Shekleton P, McDonald J, et al: Clinical predictors for buserelin acetate treatment of uterine fibroids: a prospective study of 40 women, Fertil Steril 54:1032, 1990.

Waxman M and Boyce JG: Intraperitoneal rupture of benign cystic ovarian teratoma, Obstet Gynecol 48:95, 1976.

Weissberg SM and Dodson MG: Recurrent vaginal and cervical ulcers associated with tampon use, JAMA 250:1430, 1983.

West CP, Lumsden MA, Lawson S, et al: Shrinkage of uterine fibroids during therapy with goserelin (Zoladex): a luteinizing hormone–releasing hormone agonist administered as a monthly subcutaneous depot, Fertil Steril 48:45, 1987.

Westhoff CL and Beral V: Patterns of ovarian cyst hospital discharge rates in England and Wales, 1962-79, Br Med J 289:1348, 1984.

Wolfe SA and Mackles A: Malignant lesions arising from benign endometrial polyps, Obstet Gynecol 20:542, 1962.

Woodworth H, Dockerty MB, Wilson RB, et al: Papillary hidradenoma of the vulva: a clinicopathologic study of 69 cases, Am J Obstet Gynecol 110:501, 1971.

Youssef AF, Fayad MM, and Shafeek MA: Torsion of the fallopian tube, Acta Obstet Gynecol Scand 41:291, 1962.

Endometriosis and Adenomyosis

KEY TERMS AND DEFINITIONS

Adenomyoma. An isolated area of endometrial glands and stroma in the uterine musculature that can be identified grossly.

Adenomyosis. The growth of endometrial glands and stroma in the uterine myometrium at a depth of at least 2.5 mm from the basalis layer of the endometrium.

Chocolate Cyst. A cystic area of endometriosis in the ovary.

Coelomic Metaplasia. The potential ability of coelomic epithelium to develop into several different histologic cell types.

Danazol. A synthetic steroid, an attenuated androgen, that is active when taken orally.

Dyschezia. Difficult or painful evacuation of feces from the rectum.

Endometrioma. A small area of endometriosis that can be identified macroscopically.

Endometriosis. The presence and growth of glands and stroma identical to the lining of the uterus in an aberrant location.

Retrograde Menstruation. The flow of menstrual blood, endometrial cells, and debris via the fallopian tubes into the peritoneal cavity.

ENDOMETRIOSIS

Endometriosis is a benign, but in many women, a progressive disease. The wide spectrum of clinical problems that occur with endometriosis has frustrated gynecologists, fascinated pathologists, and burdened patients for years. Though the first histologic description of aberrant endometrial glands and stroma was published in 1860, the classic studies of Sampson in the 1920s were the first to emphasize the clinical and pathologic correlations of endometriosis. Even today, many aspects of the disease remain enigmatic.

By definition, endometriosis is the presence and growth of the glands and stroma of the lining of the uterus in an aberrant or heterotopic location. Adenomyosis is the growth of endometrial glands and stroma in the uterine myometrium at a depth of at least 2.5 mm from the basalis layer of the endometrium. Adenomyosis is sometimes termed *internal endometriosis;* however, this is a semantic misnomer because clinically they are separate diseases.

It is generally believed that the incidence of endometriosis has been increasing over the past 25 years. This "opinion" is secondary to an enlightened awareness of mild to moderate endometriosis as diagnosed by the increasing use of laparoscopy. Some speculate the "epidemic of endometriosis" is secondary to changes in society that have resulted in delayed childbearing for many women. The age-specific incidence or prevalence of endometriosis is unknown. Any statements concerning the incidence or prevalence of endometriosis are approximations. Many patients are diagnosed incidentally during laparoscopy or exploratory celiotomy for a variety of other indications. Conservative estimates find that endometriosis is present in 5% to 15% of laparotomies performed on reproductive-age females. If the women are infertile, the incidence of endometriosis is 30% to 45%.

The etiology of endometriosis is uncertain and may involve retrograde menstruation, vascular dissemination, metaplasia, genetic predisposition, immunologic defects, and hormonal influences. Visualization in the vast majority of endometriosis cases necessitates either laparoscopy or celiotomy. Because few patients have these procedures performed repetitively, the natural history of the disease remains a mystery. Clinically, it is most difficult to predict the natural course of endometriosis in any one individual. For example, the clinician is uncertain as to which patient with mild disease in her 20s will progress to severe disease at a later age.

The typical patient with endometriosis is in her mid-30s, is nulliparous and involuntarily infertile, and has symptoms of secondary dysmenorrhea and pelvic pain. However, in clinical practice the majority of cases are not "classic." Aberrant endometrial tissue grows under the cyclic influence of ovarian hormones; therefore the disease is most commonly found during the reproductive years. Approximately 5% of women with endometriosis are diagnosed following menopause. Postmenopausal endometriosis is usually stimulated by exogenous estrogen. Teenagers with endometriosis should be investigated for obstructive anatomic abnormalities that increase the amount of retrograde menstruation.

Endometriosis is a disease not only of great individual variability, but also of contrasting pathophysiologic processes (Table 18-1). It is a benign disease, yet it has the characteristics of a malignancy—locally infiltrative, invasive, and widely disseminating. Although the growth of ectopic endometrium is stimulated by physiologic levels of estrogen and progesterone, both low ("pseudomenopause") and high ("pseudopregnancy") levels of these hormones are usually therapeutic. Another contrast often noted is the inverse relationship between the extent of pelvic endometriosis and the severity of pelvic pain. Women with extensive endometriosis may be asymptomatic, whereas other patients with minimal implants may have incapacitating pelvic pain. Finally, there is only speculation as to the underlying pathophysiology that produces infertility in women with endometriosis. Infertility associated with endometriosis is discussed in Chapter 39.

Until the natural history of endometriosis is understood, the clinician will have more questions than answers concerning this benign, usu-

TABLE 18-1
Endometriosis: A Disease of Clinical Contrasts

Characteristics	Contrasts
Benign disease	Locally invasive
	Widespread disseminated foci
	Proliferates in pelvic lymph nodes
Minimal disease	Severe pain
Many large endometriomas	Asymptomatic patient
Cyclic hormones cause growth	Continuous hormones reverse the growth pattern

ally progressive, and sometimes recurrent disease. These questions are a stimulating challenge to future investigators.

Etiology

There are several theories to explain the histogenesis of endometriosis. However, no single theory adequately explains the protean manifestations of the disease. Most important, there is only vague speculation as to why some women develop endometriosis, while others do not. Our ignorance surrounding the exact pathogenesis of the disease detracts from discovering a clinical means of prevention.

Retrograde Menstruation

The most popular theory is that endometriosis results from retrograde menstruation. Sampson suggested that pelvic endometriosis was secondary to implantation of endometrial cells shed during menstruation. These cells attach to the pelvic peritoneum and under hormonal influence grow as homologous grafts. Endometriosis is most often discovered in areas immediately adjacent to the tubal ostia or in the dependent areas of the pelvis.

A number of experiments in monkeys and clinical observations in humans support this hypothesis. Monkeys developed classic endometriosis when the cervix was sutured to prevent the normal egress of menstrual blood. In these experiments the development of endometriosis was dependent on repetitive "seeding" of the peritoneal cavity. Retrograde menstruation is the rule rather than the exception in all women.

This fact has been noted at laparoscopy during the first days of menstrual flow. Studies by Blumenkrantz et al. observed bloody dialysate fluid 24 to 48 hours before menstruation in the majority of women being treated with peritoneal dialysis. This bloody peritoneal fluid contained viable endometrial cells. Epidemiologic studies have discovered that women with histories of menstrual flow lasting longer than 7 days have more than 2 times the prevalence of endometriosis than women with shorter menstrual periods. Endometriosis is frequently found in women with outflow obstruction of the genital tract.

Metaplasia

In contrast to the theory of seeding from retrograde menstruation is the theory of metaplasia from the coelomic (celomic) epithelium. The müllerian ducts and nearby mesenchymal tissue form the majority of the female reproductive tract. The müllerian duct is derived from the coelomic epithelium during fetal development. The metaplasia hypothesis postulates that the coelomic epithelium retains the ability for multipotential development. It is well known that the surface epithelium of the ovary can differentiate into several different histologic cell types. The decidual reaction of isolated areas of peritoneum during pregnancy is an example of this process.

Metaplasia occurs after an "induction phenomenon" has stimulated the multipotential cell. The induction substance may be a combination of menstrual debris and the influence of estrogen and progesterone. Recently, Batt and Smith have hypothesized that the histogenesis of endometriosis in peritoneal pockets of the posterior pelvis results from a congenital anomaly involving rudimentary duplication of the müllerian system. The peritoneal pockets that they describe are found in the posterior pelvis, the posterior aspects of the broad ligament, and the cul-de-sac of Douglas. The endometriosis in these pockets contains both endometrial glands and stroma in more than 90% of affected women. The pockets may be either unilateral or bilateral. To confirm this hypothesis, peritoneal pockets and associated endometriosis must be identified in premenarcheal females.

Lymphatic and Vascular Metastasis

The theory of endometrium being transplanted via lymphatic channels and the vascular system helps to explain rare and remote sites of endometriosis, such as the spinal column and nose. Endometriosis has been observed in the pelvic lymph nodes of approximately 30% of women with the disease. Hematogenous dissemination of endometrium is the best theory to explain endometriosis of the forearm and thigh, as well as multiple lesions in the lung.

Iatrogenic Dissemination

Endometriosis of the anterior abdominal wall is sometimes discovered in women after a cesarean operation. The hypothesis is that endometrial glands and stroma are displaced during the procedure. The aberrant tissue is found subcutaneously at the abdominal incision. Rarely, iatrogenic endometriosis may be discovered in an episiotomy scar.

Immunologic Defects

Recent investigations have suggested that changes in the immune system are related to the pathogenesis of endometriosis. Whether endometriosis is an autoimmune disease has been intensely debated the past 5 years. Studies have demonstrated abnormalities in cell-mediated and humoral components of the immune system in both peripheral blood and peritoneal fluid. However, these studies have been inconsistent in their findings. Similarly, antiendometrial antibodies have been identified in the serum and peritoneal fluid of women with endometriosis. Studies by Dmowski et al. suggest a specific defect in local cell-mediated immunity in women with endometriosis. It is well known that a defect in host response is necessary before antibodies will be developed. The primary defect probably involves a change in function of the peritoneal macrophages so prevalent in the peritoneal fluid of patients with endometriosis. Halme et al. hypothesize that normal women who do not develop endometriosis have monocytic-type macrophages in their peritoneal fluid that have a short life span and limited function. Conversely, women who develop endometriosis have more peritoneal macrophages that are larger and more aggressive and secrete such substances as prostaglandins, fibronectin, and other growth factors that enhance the development of endometriosis. Combining the immunologic etiology with other theories helps partly to explain why

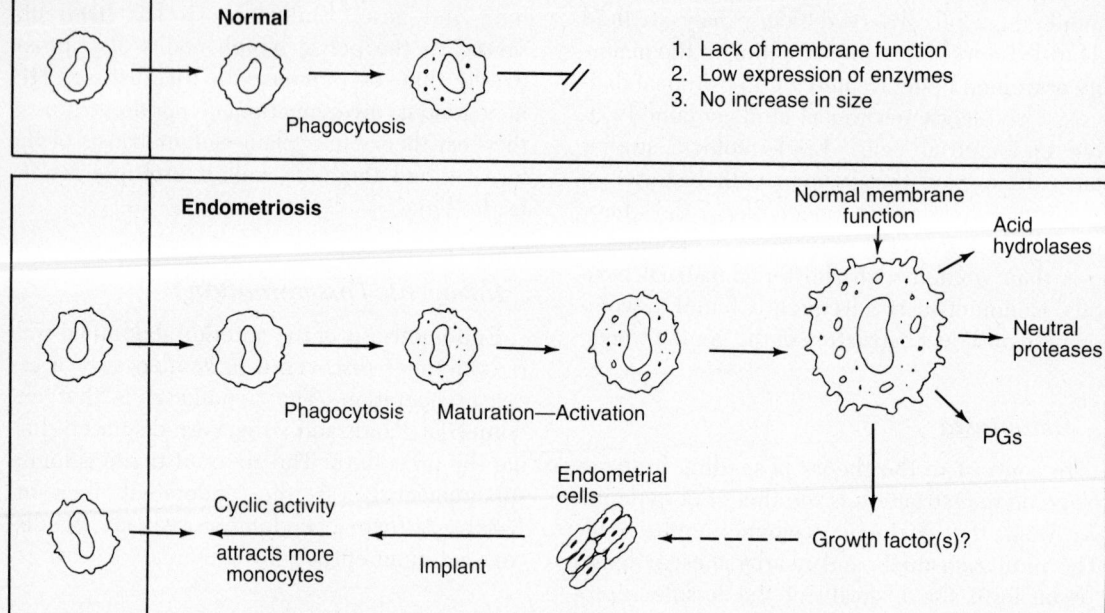

FIGURE 18-1

Hypothesis regarding pathophysiologic characteristics of human peritoneal macrophages in endometriosis. The presence of higher numbers and larger, more mature macrophages in endometriosis may lead to secretion of putative growth factors facilitating implantation and growth of endometrial cells. (Redrawn from Halme J et al: Am J Obstet Gynecol 156:787, 1987.)

some women develop endometriosis while others do not. In summary, it is not yet established whether endometriosis is related to a systemic or local immunologic problem (Figure 18-1).

Genetic Predisposition

Several studies have documented a familial predisposition to endometriosis with grouping of cases of endometriosis in mothers and their daughters. An investigation by Simpson et al. of the disease demonstrated a sevenfold increase in the incidence of endometriosis in relatives of women with the disease as compared to controls. One out of 10 women with severe endometriosis will have a sister or mother with clinical manifestations of the disease. Women who have a family history of endometriosis are likely to develop the disease earlier in life and to have more advanced disease than women whose first-degree relatives are free of the disease. Researchers speculate that the predisposition to develop endometriosis is transmitted via polygenic or multifactorial inheritance patterns. The expression of this genetic tendency

may depend on an interaction with environmental factors.

In summary, most authorities believe that several factors are probably involved in the etiology of endometriosis, including transport of endometrium, a genetic predisposition, and a local immunologic defect. Each factor may contribute to the development of this enigmatic disease (see box below).

Pathology

The majority of endometrial implants are located in the dependent portions of the female pelvis (Figure 18-2). The ovaries are the most

---

ETIOLOGY OF ENDOMETRIOSIS

Retrograde menstruation
Metaplasia
Lymphatic and vascular metastases
Immunologic defect
Genetic predisposition
Iatrogenic dissemination

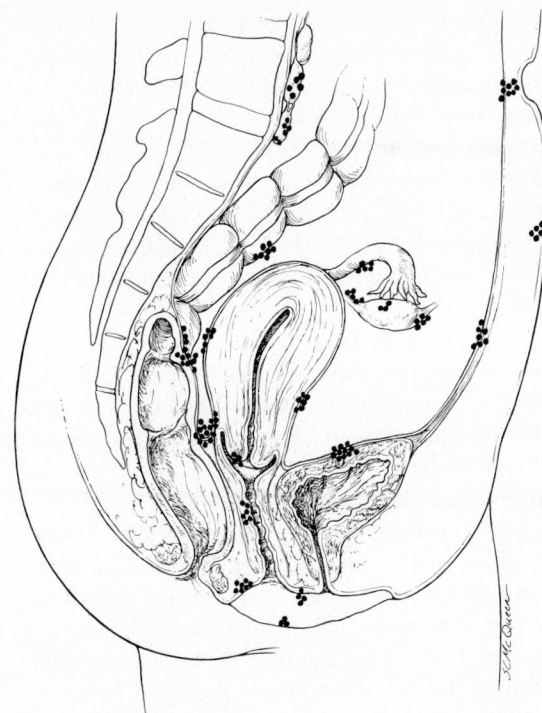

FIGURE 18-2
Common pelvic sites of endometriosis.

common site, being involved in two of three patients with endometriosis. In most of these patients the involvement is bilateral. The pelvic peritoneum over the uterus, the anterior and posterior cul-de-sac, and the uterosacral, round, and broad ligaments are also common sites where endometriosis develops. Pelvic lymph nodes are involved in 30% of cases (Figure 18-3). The cervix, vagina, and vulva are other possible pelvic locations.

Approximately 10% to 15% of cases involve the rectosigmoid. Depending on the amount of associated scarring, endometriosis of the bowel may be difficult to differentiate grossly from a primary neoplasm of the large intestine.

Rare sites of endometriosis include the umbilicus, areas of previous surgical incisions of the anterior abdominal wall or perineum, the bladder, kidney, lung, arms, legs, and even the male urinary tract (Table 18-2).

Gross pathologic changes of endometriosis exhibit wide variability in color, shape, size, and associated inflammatory and fibrotic changes. The visual manifestations of endometriosis in the female pelvis are protean and have many appearances. Recently, increased

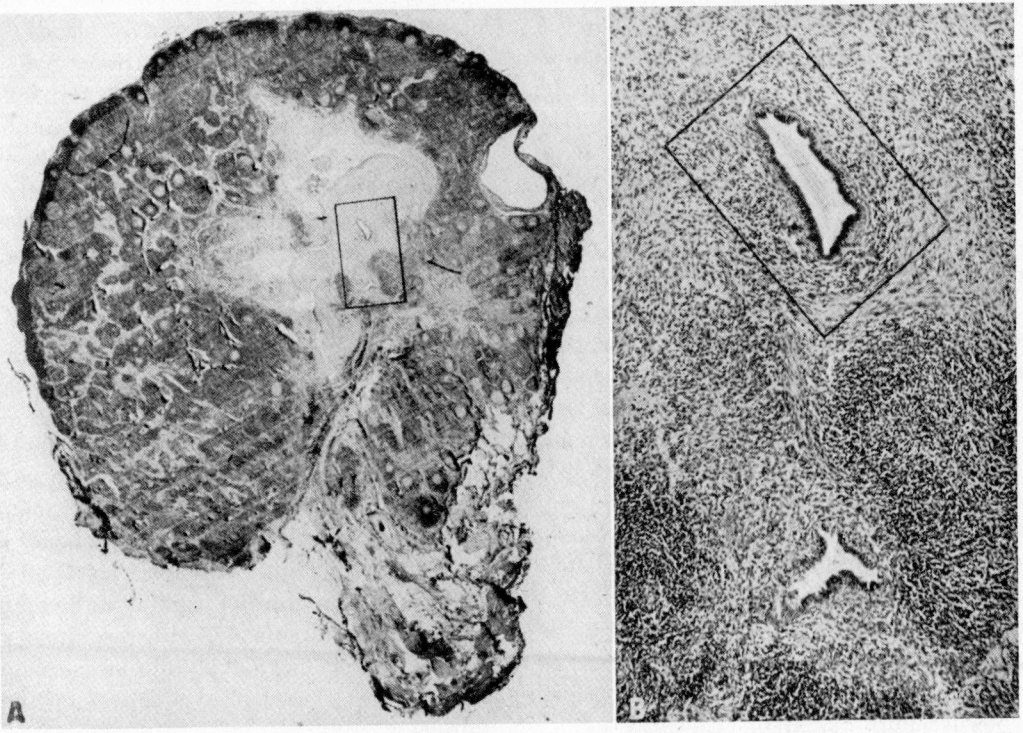

FIGURE 18-3
Endometriosis in right ureteral lymph node. **A,** Low-power view. **B,** Higher-power view showing two glands and surrounding stroma. (From Javert CT: Cancer 2:403, 1949.)

TABLE 18-2
Anatomic Distribution of Endometriosis

Common Sites	Rare Sites
Ovaries	Umbilicus
Pelvic peritoneum	Episiotomy scar
Ligaments of the uterus	Bladder
Sigmoid colon	Kidney
Appendix	Lungs
Pelvic lymph nodes	Arms
Cervix	Legs
Vagina	Nasal mucosa
Fallopian tubes	Spinal column

awareness and anticipation have focused on the subtle lesions of endometriosis. During the past 5 years clinicians have closely inspected the pelvic peritoneum to identify abnormal areas and small, nonhemorrhagic lesions. Clinically, more emphasis has been placed on biopsy confirmation of endometriosis because of increasing awareness of its subtle lesions. The gross appearance of the implant depends on the site, activity, relationship to day of menstrual cycle, and chronicity of the area involved. The color of the lesion varies widely and may be red, brown, black, white, or yellow or a pink, clear, or red vesicle. The predominant color depends on the blood supply, the amount of hemorrhage, and fibrosis. The color also appears related to the size of the lesion, degree of edema, and the amount of inspissated material. Other peritoneal lesions that grossly appear similar to endometriosis, but on histologic examination are not, include necrotic areas of ectopic pregnancy, fibrotic reactions to suture, hemangiomas, adrenal rest, Walthard's rest, breast cancer, ovarian cancer, epithelial inclusions, residual carbon from laser surgery, peritoneal inflammation, psammoma bodies, peritoneal reactions to oil-based hysterosalpingogram dye, and splenosis.

New lesions are small, sometimes blood-filled cysts that are less than 1 cm in diameter. Initially these areas are raised above the surrounding tissues. With time the areas of endometriosis become larger and assume a light or dark brown color, and they may be described as "powder burn" areas or "chocolate cysts." The older lesions have more intense scarring and are usually puckered or retracted from the surrounding tissue.

The pattern of ovarian endometriosis is also variable (Figure 18-4). Individual areas range from 1 mm to large chocolate cysts 8 to 14 cm in diameter. The associated adhesions may be filmy or dense. Larger cysts are usually densely adherent to the surrounding pelvic sidewalls or broad ligament. The pathophysiology of this adhesive process is believed to be repetitive episodes of bloody fluid leaking from the cyst, producing an intense inflammatory response.

The three cardinal histologic features of endometriosis are ectopic endometrial glands, ectopic endometrial stroma, and hemorrhage into the adjacent tissue (Figures 18-5 and 18-6). Previous hemorrhage can be discovered by identifying large macrophages filled with hemosiderin near the periphery of the lesion. In the majority of cases the aberrant endometrial glands and stroma respond in cyclic fashion to estrogen and progesterone. Depending on the local blood supply, these changes may or may not be in synchrony with the endometrial lining of the uterus. The ectopic endometrial stroma will undergo classic decidual changes similar to pregnancy when exposed to physiologic or pharmacologic levels of progesterone.

In approximately 25% of the cases of endometriosis, viable endometrial glands and stroma cannot be identified. Repetitive episodes of hemorrhage may lead to severe inflammatory changes and result in the glands and stroma undergoing necrobiosis secondary to pressure atrophy or lack of blood supply. In these cases a presumptive diagnosis of endometriosis is made by visualizing the intense inflammatory reaction and the large macrophages filled with blood pigment.

Clinical Diagnosis

Symptoms

The classic symptoms of endometriosis are cyclic pelvic pain and infertility. The chronic pelvic pain usually presents as secondary dysmenorrhea and/or dyspareunia. However, approximately one third of patients with endometriosis are asymptomatic, with the disease being discovered incidentally during an abdominal operation or visualized at laparoscopy for an unrelated problem.

Clinicians have appreciated the paradox that the extent of pelvic pain is often inversely related to the amount of endometriosis in the female pelvis. Women with large, fixed adnexal

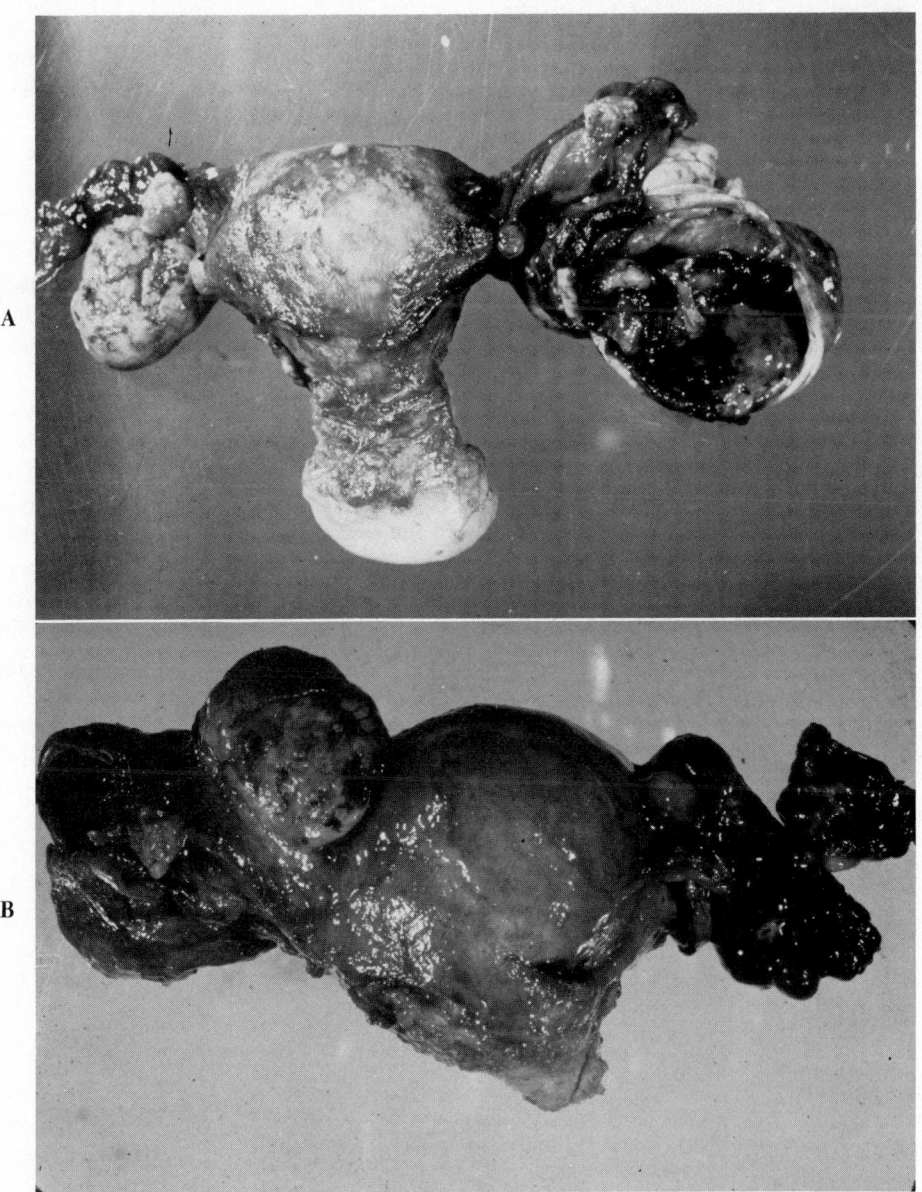

FIGURE 18-4
A, Total hysterectomy specimen from woman with endometriosis. Right ovary was partially destroyed by endometrioma. **B,** Anterior view of same specimen. Note small endometrial implants on surface of right ovary. (Courtesy Fred Askin, M.D.)

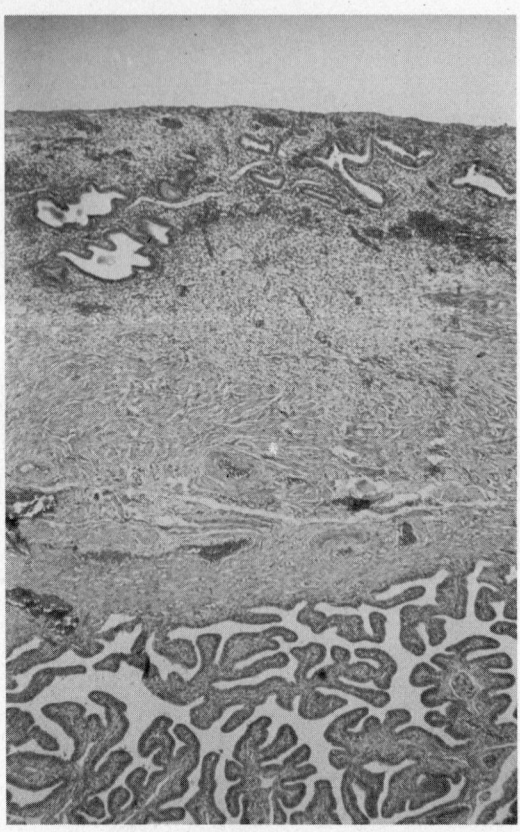

FIGURE 18-5
Endometriosis on fallopian tube. Serosa of tube is being invaded by glands and stroma. (Courtesy Fred Askin, M.D.)

masses sometimes have minor symptoms, while other patients with only a few small foci of peritoneal implants may experience moderate to severe chronic pain. Recently, Fedele et al. could find no correlation between the anatomic stage of the disease and the patient's perception of severity of pelvic pain. In their study, 124 women were staged according to the revised scoring system of the American Fertility Society. No relationship was found between stage of the disease and frequency or severity of pain symptoms.

The cyclic pelvic pain is related to the sequential swelling and the extravasation of blood and menstrual debris into the surrounding tissue. The chemical mediator of this intense sterile inflammation and pain is believed to be prostaglandins.

The secondary dysmenorrhea is constant, beginning 24 to 48 hours before menstruation. It varies from a dull ache to severe pelvic pain. It may be unilateral or bilateral and may radiate to the lower back, legs, and groin. Patients often complain of pelvic heaviness or a perception of their internal organs being swollen. Unlike primary dysmenorrhea, the pain may last for several days, including the entire duration of menstrual flow.

The dyspareunia associated with endometriosis is described as pain deep in the pelvis. The etiology of this symptom seems to be immobility of the pelvic organs during coital activity or

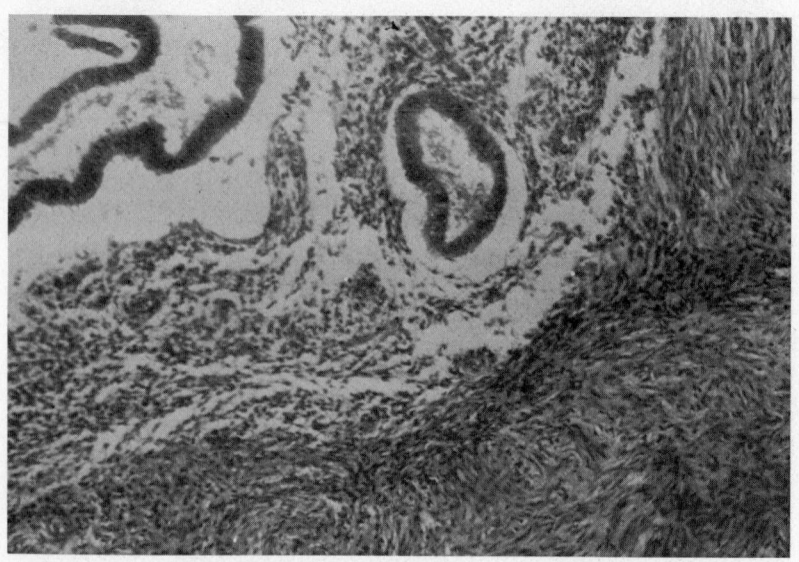

FIGURE 18-6
High-power view of endometrial glands in ovarian stroma. (Courtesy Fred Askin, M.D.)

direct pressure on areas of endometriosis in the uterosacral ligaments or the cul-de-sac of Douglas. Sometimes patients describe areas of point tenderness. The pain, besides being experienced during deep penetration, may continue for several hours following intercourse.

Abnormal bleeding is a symptom noted by 15% to 20% of women with endometriosis. The most frequent complaints are premenstrual spotting and menorrhagia. Usually this abnormal bleeding is not associated with an anovulatory pattern. On the other hand, patients with endometriosis frequently have ovulatory dysfunction. Approximately 15% of women with endometriosis have coincidental anovulation.

An increased incidence of first-trimester abortion in women with untreated endometriosis has been reported. Recent epidemiologic studies, however, question a true increased incidence and, if there is, raise serious doubt as to a cause-and-effect relationship.

Less common yet troublesome are the symptoms resulting from endometriosis influencing the gastrointestinal and urinary tracts. Cyclic abdominal pain, intermittent constipation, diarrhea, dyschezia, urinary frequency, dysuria, and hematuria are all possible symptoms. Bowel obstruction and hydronephrosis may occur. One rare clinical manifestation of endometriosis is catamenial hemothorax, bloody pleural fluid occurring during menses.

Signs

The most prominent pelvic finding of endometriosis is a fixed retroverted uterus with scarring and tenderness posterior to the uterus. The characteristic nodularity of the uterosacral ligaments and cul-de-sac of Douglas may be palpated on rectovaginal examination. Advanced cases have extensive scarring and narrowing of the posterior vaginal fornix. The ovaries may be enlarged and tender and are often fixed to the broad ligament or lateral pelvic sidewall. The adnexal enlargement is rarely symmetric, as one might expect in some benign pelvic conditions.

Endometriosis is a disease that produces tenderness of the pelvic structures and scarring that restricts movement of the pelvic organs. Occasionally the physician discovers endometriosis in a an old surgical incision or a site of a previous amniocentesis. Speculum examination may demonstrate a small area of endometriosis

on the cervix or upper vagina. If a patient presents with secondary dysmenorrhea, deep dyspareunia, and infertility and if on pelvic examination the physician discovers bilateral adnexal tenderness, a fixed posterior uterus, and beading of the uterosacral ligaments, the diagnosis is straightforward. If the diagnosis of endometriosis is in doubt, an experienced clinician will instruct the patient to return for a pelvic examination on the first day of her menstrual flow. This is the time of maximum swelling and tenderness of the areas of endometriosis. The diagnosis can be confirmed in most cases by direct laparoscopic visualization of endometriosis with its associated scarring and adhesion formation. In many patients it is discovered for the first time during an infertility investigation. Biopsy of selected implants gives confirmation of the diagnosis. However, sometimes the pathologist may be unable to find glandular elements and endometrial stroma in the biopsy specimens.

When laparoscopy is undertaken to establish the diagnosis of endometriosis, it is important to describe systematically the extent of the pathology (Figures 18-7 to 18-9). This will help to establish a starting point to measure the results of future therapy. Several systems have been devised to quantitate the extent of the endometriosis. The American Fertility Society classification of endometriosis is useful for patients with infertility or with pelvic pain (Chapter 39). For patients with pelvic pain the staging system depicted in Table 18-3 is an alternative model to follow to establish the success or failure of therapy.

A promising method is being developed in experimental animals to help improve laparoscopic diagnosis of endometriosis. This technique will potentially become a new form of therapy. Animals are treated with drugs such as tamoxifen or clomiphene citrate; after these drugs are absorbed by the cell, fluorescence is induced with an argon laser. In experimental photodynamic therapy, endometriosis tissue is destroyed by an interaction between the retained photosensitizing drug and the absorbed laser light.

Unfortunately, ultrasound examination shows no specific pattern for pelvic endometriosis. Ultrasound is helpful in differentiating solid from cystic lesions but cannot distinguish an endometrioma from a hemorrhagic ovarian cyst. Therefore pelvic ultrasound may give additional and confirmatory information, but can-

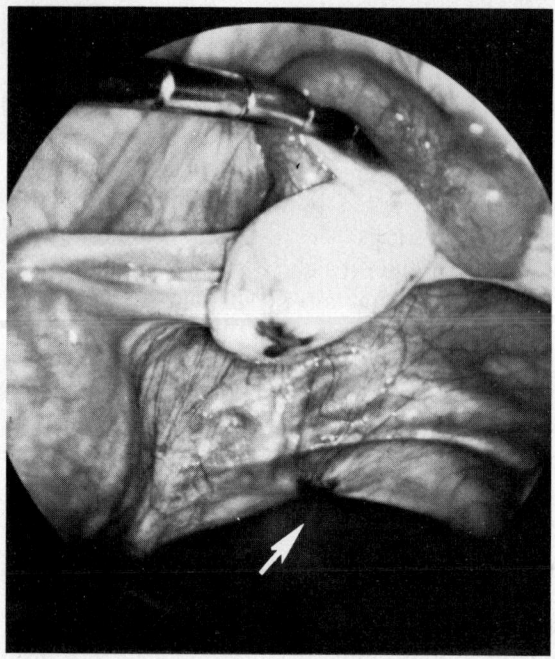

FIGURE 18-7
Laparoscopic view of ovarian and pelvic endometriosis. Tube is being elevated by a probe. Note retracted area of broad ligament around endometriosis *(arrow)*. (Courtesy Jaroslav Hulka, M.D.)

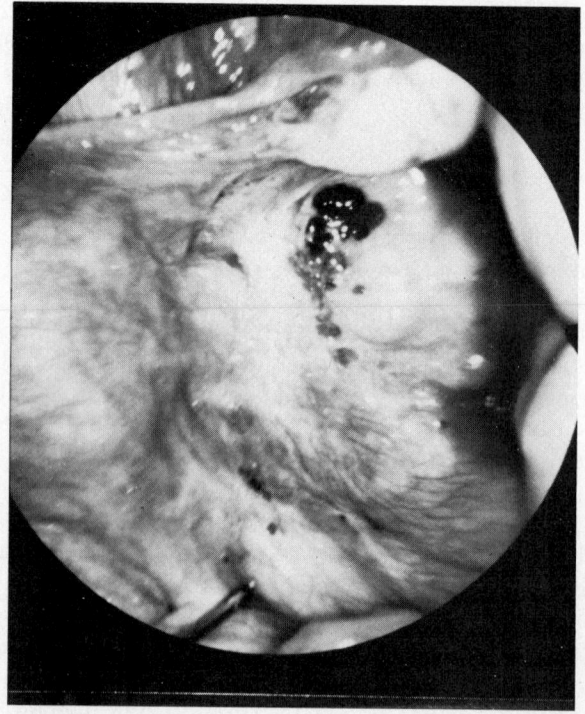

FIGURE 18-8
Laparoscopic view of endometriosis on posterior leaf of broad ligament and cul-de-sac. Note the many adhesions. (Courtesy Jaroslav Hulka, M.D.)

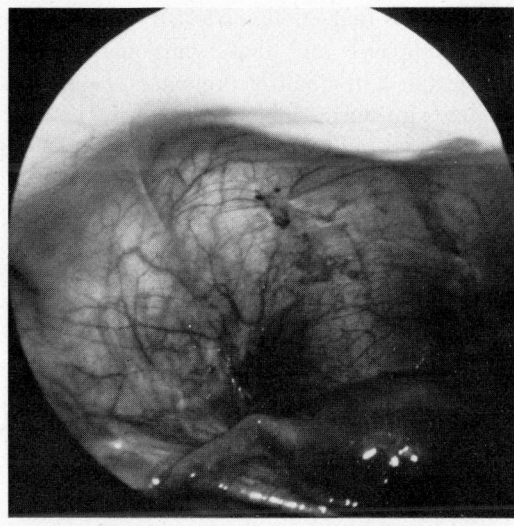

FIGURE 18-9
Laparoscopic view of endometrial implants on sigmoid colon. (Courtesy Jouko Halme, M.D., Ph.D.)

TABLE 18-3
Classification of Endometriosis

Extent of Disease	Findings
Mild	1. Scattered, superficial implants on structures other than uterus, tubes, or ovaries; no scarring
	2. Rare, superficial implants on ovaries
	3. No significant adhesions
Moderate	1. Involvement of one or both ovaries with multiple implants or small endometriomas (≤2 cm)
	2. Minimal peritubular or periovarian adhesions
	3. Scattered, scarred implants on other structures
Severe	1. Large ovarian endometriomas (≥2 cm)
	2. Significant tubal or ovarian adhesions
	3. Tubal obstruction
	4. Obliteration of cul-de-sac, major uterosacral involvement
	5. Significant bowel or urinary tract disease

From Puleo JG and Hammond CB: Fertil Steril 40:165, 1983. Reproduced with permission of the publisher, The American Fertility Society.

not be used for primary screening. Similarly, endometriosis has a variable appearance on magnetic resonance imaging (MRI), with considerable overlap with other pelvic conditions. The sensitivity and specificity of MRI in diagnosing endometriosis is approximately 60%. Thus MRI also has limited value as a primary modality in detecting or staging the disease.

Although a benign disease, endometriosis exhibits characteristics of both malignancy and sterile inflammation. Therefore the common considerations in the differential diagnosis include chronic pelvic inflammatory disease, ovarian malignancy, degeneration of myomas, hemorrhage or torsion of ovarian cysts, adenomyosis, primary dysmenorrhea, and functional bowel disease.

Occasionally a large endometrioma of the ovary may rupture into the peritoneal cavity. This results in an acute surgical abdomen and brings into the differential diagnosis conditions such as ectopic pregnancy, appendicitis, diverticulitis, and a bleeding corpus luteum cyst. Studies have not demonstrated any temporal relationship between the timing of an endometrioma's acute rupture and the day of the menstrual cycle.

Natural History

Endometriosis is a chronic and sometimes progressive disease. The rate of progression of the disease varies widely from one patient to another. Serial pelvic examinations are a poor indicator of progression of the disease. Therefore the natural history of the disease is largely speculation. In some centers, second-look or reassessment laparoscopy is performed routinely. These limited studies have given insight into the success of therapy. During the past few years interest has centered on measuring serum levels of cancer antigen-125 (CA-125) as a chemical marker and noninvasive test for endometriosis. CA-125 levels are elevated in most patients with endometriosis and increase incrementally with advanced stages. However, assays for serum levels of CA-125 have a low specificity because they also increase with other pelvic diseases. Therefore it is unlikely that this assay will become a screening or diagnostic test. However, physicians may be able to follow the course of persistent or recurrent disease or predict the success of therapy by measuring serial CA-125 levels.

It would be optimal to identify women who are going to develop endometriosis. Clinicians should note the genetic factors in endometriosis and identify family members at risk. The optimal preventive therapy for a young teenagers not desirous of pregnancy until her late 20s is unknown. Clinical options include no treatment, continuous use of oral contraceptives, or cyclic oral contraceptive therapy. Controlled prospective studies are needed to answer the difficult clinical question of the best method to inhibit progression of the disease.

Approximately 10% of teenagers who develop endometriosis have associated congenital outflow obstruction. Therefore teenagers with pelvic pain should be examined for this rare possibility.

Until 25 years ago there was a general belief that pregnancy improved endometriosis. A careful study by McArthur and Ulfelder of external endometriosis, which could be observed throughout the pregnancy, discovered that this generalization was not invariably true. In some cases endometriomas rapidly increase in size during the first few weeks of pregnancy. In general, during the third trimester, symptoms are less severe and the size of the external lesions decreases.

Endometriosis is dependent on ovarian hormones to stimulate growth. With a natural menopause, there is a gradual relief of symptoms. Following surgical menopause, areas of endometriosis rapidly disappear. However, it is important to note that 5% of symptomatic cases of endometriosis present after menopause. The vast majority of the cases in women in their late 50s or early 60s are related to the use of exogenous estrogen.

Management

The appropriate treatment for endometriosis varies widely because of the spectrum of clinical symptoms and vast differences in extent of the disease from one patient to another. Therefore the treatment plan must be individualized. Choice of therapy depends on multiple variables, including the patient's age, her future reproductive plans, the location and extent of her disease, her symptoms, and associated pelvic pathology. Most patients should undergo a diagnostic laparoscopy to establish the nature and extent of endometriosis before therapy.

Treatment of endometriosis can be medical, surgical, or a combination of both. The clinical observations that endometriosis regresses after the menopause and that symptoms improve during the latter half of pregnancy have been the basis for hormonal palliation of the disease. The glands and stroma contained in areas of endometriosis and the endometrial glands and stroma of the uterus usually react to hormones in a similar fashion. Most of the sex steroids, alone or in combination, have been tried in clinical studies to suppress the growth of endometriosis. Optimal regression secondary to treatment is observed in small endometriomas that are less than 1 to 2 cm in diameter. Response in larger areas of endometriosis may be minimal with steroid therapy. This poor therapeutic result may be governed by the reduction of blood supply to the mass caused by surrounding scar tissue.

Surgical therapy is divided into conservative and definitive operations. Conservative surgery involves the resection or destruction of endometrial implants, lysis of adhesions, and attempts to restore normal pelvic anatomy. Definitive surgery involves surgical castration with the removal of both ovaries, the uterus, and all visible ectopic foci of endometriosis.

Medical Therapy

The primary goal of the hormonal treatment of endometriosis is induction of amenorrhea. It is hoped that hormonal treatment will create an environment that will inhibit growth and promote regression of the disease. The endometrium within the uterine cavity is dissimilar to ectopic endometrium in receptor content. The two types of endometrium do not always respond the same to the levels of circulating hormones. Amenorrhea is the best clinical marker available to assess clinical response. Both clinical symptomatology and findings on second-look laparoscopy have demonstrated that clinical improvement directly correlates with establishment of amenorrhea. To date no hormonal therapy has been able to produce long-lasting cures with ablation of all foci of endometriosis after discontinuation of hormonal management.

DANAZOL. Since its approval by the Food and Drug Administration in the mid 1970s, danazol has been a popular drug for the treatment of endometriosis. Danazol also may be prescribed for women with benign cystic mastitis, menorrhagia, and hereditary angioneurotic edema. Danazol is an attenuated androgen that is active when given orally. Chemically it is a

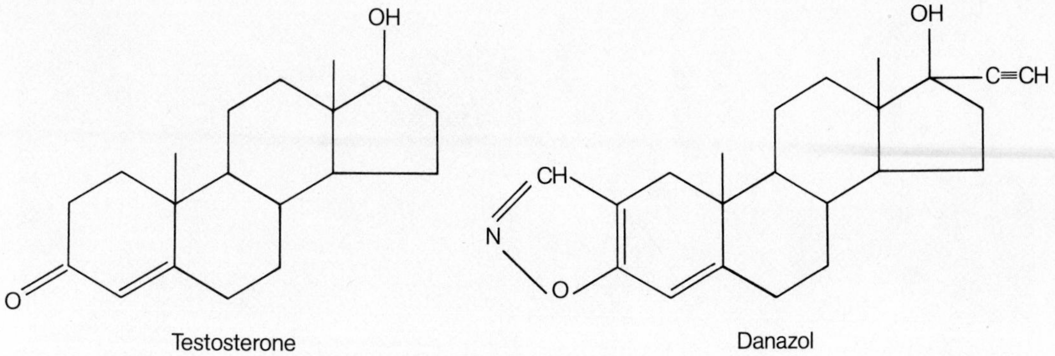

FIGURE 18-10
Chemical structures of danazol and testosterone.

synthetic steroid that is the isoxazole derivative of ethisterone (17-alpha-ethinyltestosterone) (Figure 18-10). The drug is mildly androgenic and anabolic. Many of danazol's side effects are directly related to these two properties. Dmowski et al. determined that the androgenic effects of testosterone are approximately 200 times greater than those of danazol.

Danazol was initially prescribed for its "pseudomenopausal effect." The drug significantly decreases follicle-stimulating hormone (FSH) and luteinizing hormone (LH) levels in castrated females. However, in premenopausal women, basal levels of gonadotrophins are not influenced. The midcycle surge of FSH and LH is eliminated by a dose of 800 mg a day. The term *pseudomenopause* is a misnomer because during the physiologic menopause, gonadotrophins are elevated.

Danazol binds to androgen and progesterone receptors and also binds to sex hormone–binding globulin. The latter effect results in a threefold increase in endogenous free testosterone levels. Danazol directly inhibits several steroidogenic enzymes in both the ovary and the adrenal gland, thus reducing circulating steroid levels. In vitro and in vivo studies have shown that danazol may also modulate immunologic functions through an effect on macrophages and/or T lymphocytes. Until the basic mechanisms are further elucidated, the student can remember the misnomer pseudomenopause, which helps to describe danazol's effects at the target organs. For clinicians the effect on the target organ is the desired goal.

The explanations of the exact mechanism of action and underlying pharmacologic properties of danazol are controversial and speculative. Dosages of 800 mg daily produce amenorrhea and inhibition of ovulation within 4 to 6

weeks after the onset of therapy. Danazol definitely produces a hypoestrogenic, hypoprogestational effect on steroid-sensitive end organs. Luciano has found that plasma levels of estrogen and progesterone remain in the early follicular range. Danazol induces atrophic changes in the endometrium of the uterus and similar changes in endometrial implants (Figure 18-11). An endometrial biopsy performed after several weeks of therapy shows endometrial atrophy with few glands and an inactive stroma. It would be difficult to differentiate the biopsy of a young woman taking danazol from the biopsy of a postmenopausal woman.

The standard prescribed dosage of danazol is 400 to 800 mg a day for approximately 6 to 9 months. The half-life of this oral drug is between 4 and 5 hours. Therefore, for the 800 mg dosage regimen, it is best to recommend one tablet four times a day rather than two tablets in the morning and two at night. Prescribing danazol 200 mg every 6 hours results in mean serum estradiol concentrations that are 40% lower than with the alternative regimen, 400 mg twice a day. The drug is started on the fifth day after the onset of menses. The length of therapy of oral danazol should be individualized, depending partly on the stage of endometriosis. Women should use mechanical contraceptives for the first month, as danazol has produced female pseudohermaphroditism in a developing fetus. If one is certain the patient is not pregnant, danazol is begun on the first day of the menstrual bleeding. By starting the hormone earlier in the cycle, the patient will experience less breakthrough bleeding during the first 4 to 6 weeks.

A major drawback of the medication is its expense. A 200 mg tablet costs approximately $1.00 to $1.50, resulting in a total cost of $120

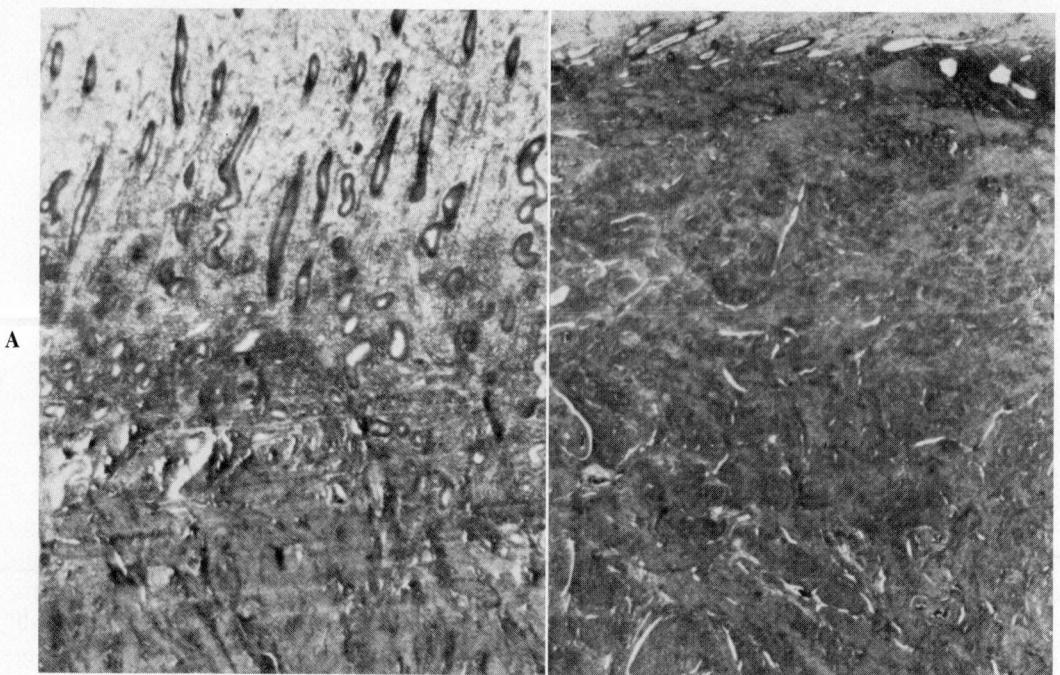

FIGURE 18-11
A, Untreated endometrium. **B,** Endometrium after 4 months of treatment with danazol. (From Greenblatt RP, Dmowski WP, Mahesh VB, and Scholer HFL: Fertil Steril 22:108, 1971. Reproduced with permission of the publisher, American Fertility Society.)

to $180 per month. Because of this factor, many investigators have reduced the total daily dosage of the drug. Dmowski et al. and Low et al. compared 600, 400, 200, and even 100 mg of danazol daily. The relief of the symptoms of endometriosis was directly related to the incidence of amenorrhea. The lower dosages of danazol are not as effective at producing amenorrhea and anovulation. The clinical success rates using lower dosages are slightly less with advanced disease than when 400 to 800 mg daily is used. A woman with an atrophic endometrium may occasionally experience breakthrough bleeding.

Side effects of the hormonal pseudomenopause are encountered by 80% of patients taking danazol. Approximately 10% to 20% of women discontinue the drug because of the side effects. Virtually all of the symptoms disappear on cessation of drug therapy. However, there are scattered reports of deepening of the voice that did not resolve after discontinuing the drug. Symptoms that have been related to danazol therapy include menopausal hot flushes, atrophic vaginitis, emotional lability,

weight gain averaging 8 to 10 pounds, fluid retention, migraine headaches, dizziness, fatigue, depression, oily skin, facial hair, and deepening of the voice (Table 18-4). Recent studies have demonstrated that danazol decreases high-density lipoprotein (HDL) levels and elevates low-density lipoprotein (LDL) levels. With increasing emphasis on the prevention of atherosclerotic disease, this finding should not be ignored. However, the clinical impact of these changes occuring for a few months in young women is not known.

Danazol is metabolized in the liver with cleavage of the isoxazol ring. The biologic effects of danazol are believed to be from the parent compound and not the metabolites. Holt and Keller reported a mild elevation in serum liver enzyme levels in six of seven women treated for endometriosis. Alkaline phosphatase levels were not changed. Clinicians should be alert to these changes, and women who take danazol for longer than 6 months should have serum liver enzyme determinations.

The standard length of treatment with dana-

TABLE 18-4
Adverse Reactions to Danazol (800 mg/day)

Androgenic action

Acne	17%
Edema	6%
Weight gain	5%
Hirsutism	6%
Voice changes	3%

Antiestrogenic action

Flushes and sweats	15%
Uterine spotting	10%
Decrease in breast size	5%
Change in libido	3% to 5%
Atrophic vaginitis	3%

Idiopathic drug reactions

GI disturbances	8%
Weakness, dizziness	8%
Muscle cramps	4%
Skin rashes	3%
Headaches	2%
Sleep disturbances	Uncommon

From Luciano AA: Contemp OB/GYN 19:228, 1982. Modified from Greenblatt R, editor: Recent advances in endometriosis: proceedings of a symposium, Augusta, GA, March 5-6, 1975. Excerpta Medica, 1976, p 368.

zol is 6 to 9 months. Approximately three of four patients note significant improvement in their symptoms, and about 90% have objective improvement discovered at second-look laparoscopy. The uncorrected fertility rate following danazol therapy is approximately 40%. Unfortunately, 15% to 30% of patients will have recurrence of symptoms within 2 years following therapy.

Several randomized, double-blind clinical studies have compared the therapeutic effectiveness of danazol with gonadotrophin-releasing hormone (GnRH) agonists. The results do not show significant differences between the efficacies of these two drugs. Danazol was found superior to continuous oral contraceptives in a comparison study. Noble and Letchworth found greater subjective relief of symptoms and more objective regression of endometriosis during second-look laparoscopy in the danazol group. Fewer patients discontinued danazol because of side effects.

GnRH AGONISTS. In 1971 Schally and Guellemin first characterized and sequenced the structure of the native decapeptide, gonadotrophin-releasing hormone (GnRH). This discovery led to their winning the Nobel prize and also to the development of GnRH agonists, which are 10 to 200 times more potent and have much longer half-lives than the natural hormone. With chronic administration of GnRH analogues, specific suppression of gonadotrophin secretion occurs, with secondary diminution of ovarian steroidogenesis. The GnRH analogues bind with receptors for a prolonged time and induce protracted periods of downward regulation.

Multiple GnRH agonists have been developed and are in various stages of investigation and approval by the Federal Food and Drug Administration. These agonists may be administered by intravenous, intramuscular, subcutaneous, intravaginal, or intranasal routes. The oral route is not practical because the hormone is inactivated by enzymes in the gastrointestinal tract. Currently the three routes used most frequently in clinical practice include monthly intramuscular injection, daily subcutaneous injections, and topical absorption by self-administered nasal spray. At present the two most widely used agonists are leuprolide acetate (Lupron, injectable) and nafarelin acetate (Synarel, intranasal). The usual dose of leuprolide acetate is 3.75 to 7.5 mg intramuscularly once per month or 0.5 mg daily subcutaneously. Nafarelin acetate nasal spray is given in a dose of one spray (200 µg) in one nostril in the morning and one spray (200 µg) in the other nostril in the evening.

Preliminary studies determined the dose-response curve of the GnRH agonists, establishing the optimal dose to produce amenorrhea and sufficient down regulation to produce extremely low levels of circulating estrogen. Chronic use of GnRH agonists produces a "medical oophorectomy." A dramatic reduction occurs in serum estrone, estradiol, testosterone, and androstenedione levels similar to the hormonal levels in castrated women. The total serum estrone and estradiol levels and the free serum estradiol concentration are 25% to 50% of those measured in women taking danazol chronically for endometriosis (Figure 18-12).

Most important, GnRH agonists have no effect on sex hormone–binding globulin. Thus the androgenic side effects from danazol caused

GnRH AGONISTS IN ENDOMETRIOSIS

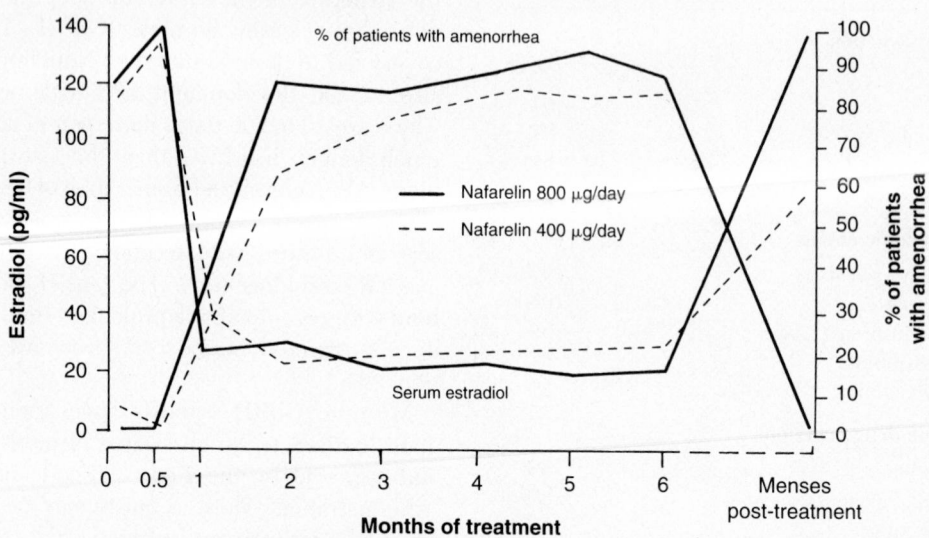

FIGURE 18-12

Decrease in serum estradiol levels and the development of amenorrhea in patients receiving nafarelin. (Redrawn from Henzl MR: Clin Obstet Gynecol 31:847, 1989.)

by the increase in free serum testosterone are not observed. Similarly, no significant changes occur in total serum cholesterol, HDLs, or LDLs during therapeutic periods of as long as 6 months. Endometrial samples obtained after several months of chronic agonist therapy demonstrated either atrophic or early proliferative endometrium.

The side effects associated with GnRH agonist therapy are primarily those associated with estrogen deprivation, similar to menopause. The three most common symptoms are hot flushes, vaginal dryness, and insomnia. Bone mineral content has been studied during agonist therapy with conflicting results. Some quantitative computed tomography studies have demonstrated a decrease in trabecular bone of the spine without changes in the compact bone of the distal radius. Other studies have not demonstrated any changes in bone mineral content. However, it is believed that the decrease in bone density is partially or completely reversible after discontinuing therapy.

The clinical response to agonist therapy depends on when the therapy is initiated in regard to the menstrual cycle. If agonist therapy is begun during the follicular phase, an initial rapid rise in FSH and E_2 levels occurs for ap-

proximately 3 weeks. FSH levels fall to basal levels by the third to fourth week of therapy. E_2 levels rapidly decline after 21 days of therapy. The expected LH surge does not occur, and serum progesterone levels do not become elevated. Amenorrhea is induced within 6 to 8 weeks. In contrast, beginning agonist therapy during the luteal phase diminishes the length of the initial response. LH levels are elevated for approximately 1 week, and serum estradiol levels are suppressed to those of a castrated female within 2 weeks. Amenorrhea is induced in 4 to 5 weeks. However, when beginning GnRH therapy during the luteal phase, it is important to ensure that the patient is not pregnant.

GnRH agonist therapy results in amelioration of symptomatology in 75% to 90% of patients with endometriosis, depending on the extent of the disease in the study group. The greatest therapeutic effects are seen in patients whose areas of endometriosis are less than 1 cm in diameter. In comparison studies the results of GnRH agonist therapy are directly comparable with those obtained with danazol. Growth of endometriosis is either arrested, diminished, or eliminated.

Henzl et al. performed a multicenter, double-blind, double-placebo randomized study of GnRH agonist and danazol therapy in which neither physicians nor patients were aware of their group's status. The 235 patients received laparoscopy both before and after 6 months of treatment and were assigned to three different protocols. One group received 400 μg of intranasal nafarelin acetate per day; the second, 800 μg of intranasal nafarelin per day; and the third, 800 mg of oral danazol per day. This large investigation demonstrated that the therapeutic response to the two drugs was similar. More than 80% of patients had a reduction in the extent of endometriosis, according to the American Fertility Society classification. Before therapy, 46% had stage III or IV disease; after therapy, 26% had stage III or IV disease. Interestingly, endometriosis was progressive in 4% to 8% of patients throughout the study.

After 6 months of GnRH agonist therapy, ovarian function will return to normal in 6 to 12 weeks. Endometriomas and severe adhesive disease have not responded to hormonal therapy. The primary advantage of GnRH agonists over danazol is better patient compliance. Most patients find the side effects of GnRH agonists more tolerable. In current studies, norethindrone or very low doses of estrogen are "added back" and combined with chronic GnRH agonist therapy. It is hoped that the addition of norethindrone or low-dose estrogen will make the side effects less bothersome without compromising the agonist's therapeutic effect. The greatest advantage of GnRH agonists is their production of a pseudomenopause or medical castration without the androgenic side effects of danazol on other steroid-sensitive organs.

ORAL CONTRACEPTIVES. Kistner was the first to popularize the continuous use of high-dosage, combination oral contraceptives for endometriosis. In the late 1950s up to 40 mg of norethynodrel with mestranol (Enovid) daily were given to produce amenorrhea and a "pseudopregnancy." Most of the published studies involved the first-generation, high-estrogen-content oral contraceptives. However, more recent reports have established that the present low-estrogen combination pills, specifically the ones with a relatively high progestin potency, are equally effective.

The regimen is started by a single daily oral contraceptive tablet beginning on the third day of the patient's period. The pills are taken continuously until breakthrough bleeding occurs, and then the daily dosage is doubled to relieve breakthrough bleeding. After 5 days of a double dose, the majority of patients can return to one to two pills a day, thereby maintaining their amenorrhea on a comparatively low dosage of steroids. As in other hormonal regimens for endometriosis, amenorrhea is the desired endpoint. The optimal regimen is the lowest daily dose of steroids that will produce amenorrhea in the individual patient. Most patients are able to maintain the amenorrhea for 6 to 9 months, using at most three to four contraceptive tablets a day. It is important to emphasize to the patient the goal of continuous rather than intermittent oral contraceptive therapy.

The initial histologic response is similar to that of normal pregnancy, with an increase in vascularity and edema in the endometrial implants. This transient growth phase may cause an acute exacerbation of the clinical symptoms. Occasionally, large ovarian endometriomas rupture, resulting in an acute surgical abdomen during the first 6 weeks of oral contraceptive therapy. During prolonged therapy the endometrial glands atrophy and the stroma undergoes a marked decidual reaction. Subsequently, in most smaller endometriomas that are less than 1 to 2 cm, there is necrobiosis and absorption.

The many side effects of inducing amenorrhea with oral contraceptives include weight gain, breast tenderness, nausea, chloasma, an increase in appetite, irritability, depression, edema, hypertension, and vaginal discharge. Approximately one of three women discontinue this therapy because of the side effects.

The results of continuous oral contraceptive therapy include a decrease in symptomatology in approximately 80% of patients during therapy and an uncorrected pregnancy rate of about 30% after therapy.

OTHER HORMONAL TREATMENTS. For women who cannot tolerate the high dosage of estrogen in the pseudopregnancy regimen or who have a contraindication to estrogen therapy, treatment with progestins only has been successful. Medroxyprogesterone (Depo-Provera), if given in a dosage of 100 mg intramuscularly every 2 weeks for four doses and then 200 mg every month for four doses, will produce a prolonged amenorrhea. The medication is acceptable for the older woman who has completed childbearing. The time of resumption of ovulation following discontinuation of injectable medroxyprogesterone is prolonged and extremely variable. Some women will not ovulate for more than a year after their last injection. Therefore this form of therapy should not be prescribed for a young woman who is contemplating pregnancy in the near future. Oral medroxyprogesterone in a dosage of 30 to 50 mg a day is an alternative mode of therapy but is more expensive.

The most persistent side effects while taking medroxyprogesterone are breakthrough spotting or bleeding. Approximately 40% of patients develop abnormal bleeding associated with high-dose progestin therapy. If there is no contraindication to estrogen, this symptom can be alleviated by small doses of oral estrogen. Many women find unacceptable the changes in mood, depression, and irritability produced by high-dose progestins. Gestrinone is a progestin originally developed as a once-a-week oral contraceptive. Recently, this drug has undergone clinical trials for endometriosis. The dosage ranges from 2.5 to 7.5 mg per week. Gestrinone acts as an agonist-antagonist of progesterone receptors and an agonist of androgen receptors and also binds weakly to estrogen receptors both in vitro and in vivo. Alternative routes of giving the drug include implants and vaginal suppositories.

Clinical results with progestin-only therapy are similar to those with continuous oral contraceptives. Some pathologists postulate that suppression of growth of endometriosis by progestins equals the suppression by oral contraceptives, but there is less necrobiosis and absorption. Progestins used in combination with GnRH agonists may ameliorate the side effects associated with the hypoestrogenic state produced by the agonists alone. Preliminary studies have found that progestins diminish hot flushes and produce a bone-sparing effect during the months of GnRH agonist therapy.

For historical interest, it is important to mention two other hormonal regimens, methyltestosterone and stilbestrol. Both therapies enjoyed initial enthusiasm but are rarely prescribed today.

Surgical Therapy

The choice between medical treatment to suppress endometriosis and surgical therapy to remove it depends on the patient's age, symptomatology, and reproductive desires. Because endometriosis is a puzzling disease, with great individual variation in its natural course, many therapeutic regimens exist. Thus, the time-honored admonition that each patient must have individualized treatment still holds (Table 18-5).

Surgery has been the foundation of treatment for women with moderate or severe en-

TABLE 18-5
Endometriosis Treatment Algorithm

| Chief Complaint | Desires Childbearing | | Childbearing Complete |
	Infertility	Pelvic Pain	Pelvic Pain
Stages I and II	1. Expectant Rx 2. Laparoscopic Rx 2. Medical Rx 3. CSEL ± PSN 3. IVF/ET	1. Laparoscopic Rx 2. Medical Rx 3. CSEL + PSN	1. Laparoscopic Rx 2. Medical Rx 3. TAH ± BSO 3. CSEL ± PSN
Stage III	1. Laparoscopic Rx 1. CSEL ± PSN 2. Medical Rx 3. IVF/ET	1. Laparoscopic Rx 2. CSEL + PSN 3. Medical Rx	1. Laparoscopic Rx 2. Medical Rx 3. TAH ± BSO 3. CSEL + PSN
Stage IV	1. CSEL + perioperative medical Rx 2. CSEL alone 3. Laparoscopic Rx + postoperative medical Rx 4. IVF/ET	1. CSEL + PSN + perioperative medical Rx 2. Medical Rx 3. Laparoscopic Rx + medical Rx	1. TAH ± BSO 1. CSEL + PSN + medical Rx 2. Laparoscopic Rx + medical Rx

From Wheeler JM and Malinak LR: Obstet Gynecol Clin N Am 31:150, 1989.
Rx, Treatment; *CSEL*, Conservative surgery for endometriosis at laparotomy; *PSN*, Presacral neurectomy, *TAH*, Total abdominal hysterectomy; *BSO*, Bilateral salpingo-oophorectomy; *IVF/ET*, In vitro fertilization/embryo transfer; ±, Indicates adjunctive treatment option based on individual patient findings.

dometriosis when the disease involves organs other than the pelvic genital tract. A surgical approach is mandatory in cases involving acute rupture of large endometriomas, ureteral obstruction, compromise in the large bowel's function, or adnexal enlargements with a diameter of 8 cm or larger. During the past 10 years, clinicians have increasingly emphasized laparoscopic treatment of endometriosis. Surgical techniques using the laparoscope have been marketed with descriptive names such as "pelviscopy" or "video laseroscopy." Wheeler and Malinak use the term "manage" rather than "treat" endometriosis. Their rationale is that the diagnosed recurrence rate of endometriosis is approximately one in three patients after 5 years, and since many patients do not have second-look laparoscopy, the actual recurrence rate is probably higher. This recurrence rate reflects both persistence and proliferation of initially microscopic disease.

Laparoscopy is employed frequently for diagnostic reasons and can also be used therapeutically. The major advantage of treating endometriosis with the laparoscope, using either the laser or electrocautery, is that patients may be treated at the time of diagnosis. Presently, four types of lasers have been directed toward areas of endometriosis via the laparoscope: the carbon dioxide (CO_2), the argon, the potassium-titanyl-phosphate (KTP), and the neodymium:yttrium-aluminum-garnet (Nd:YAG) lasers. Recently a sapphire probe has been added to the Nd:YAG laser that results in more precise destruction. Depending on the laser chosen, endometriosis is coagulated and/or vaporized.

Laser therapy is a precise and almost bloodless technique resulting in a short patient stay with few complications. Other advantages include the speed of the surgical procedure, accuracy, control, and minimal tissue damage to the surrounding areas. (One must emphasize, however, that these are impressions; in general, truly randomized and carefully controlled series are lacking.) Also, most of the tissue debris after laser therapy is evacuated. Therefore minimal fibrosis or scarring occurs in surrounding areas. It is possible to lyse adhesions, obtain tissue for biopsy, remove small implants, and cauterize (using electrocautery) other implants via the laparoscope.

Adhesions in the pelvis have varying characteristics. They may be minimal or extensive, filmy or dense, and avascular or vascular. De-

pending on the laser used, the surgeon must adjust spot size, power setting (watts), and time of application to control depth of penetration. The laser is preferable to electrocautery when endometriosis is adjacent to the ureter, bladder, or bowel because the depth of penetration can be controlled. Follow-up studies have documented pain improvement in 70% to 80% of patients treated by laser therapy via the laparoscope.

The surgical techniques for invasive carcinoma and for endometriosis are similar. The infiltrative nature of both disease processes and the associated scarring from endometriosis result in a loss of cleavage planes and tedious, difficult dissections. Technically it is easier to palpate rather than visualize the extent of the infiltrative process of endometriosis. Special care must be taken not to injure the bladder or bowel during excision of areas impinging on these structures.

Conservative surgery has as its goal the removal of all macroscopic, visible areas of endometriosis with preservation of ovarian function. Conservative operations include removal or destruction of implants, lysis of adhesions, appendectomy, and sometimes an anterior uterine suspension and/or presacral neurectomy. Throughout these procedures the surgeon observes the principles of microsurgery and plastic surgery, including minimal and gentle handling of tissues, avoiding hypoxia of the peritoneum, and attempting to restore the pelvic anatomy to normal. In selecting a microsurgical approach, it is current practice to use a fine suture of Dexon or Vicryl and almost constant irrigation with lactated Ringer's solution containing heparin and/or corticosteriods. At the completion of the operation, most surgeons perform a simple anterior suspension of the uterus by suturing the round ligaments to the anterior rectus fascia. In theory this prevents the adnexa from adhering to raw areas in the posterior cul-de-sac, but the efficacy has not been established. Approximately one in four women will have a second operation for a recurrence of endometriosis.

It is a time-honored tradition to perform a dilation and curettage (D&C) in hopes of decreasing the amount of retrograde menstruation. There are no control studies to document the benefits of either D&C or uterine suspension. If the patient has midline pain, such as dysmenorrhea or dyspareunia, occasionally a pre-sacral neurectomy or resection of the uterosacral ligaments may be performed.

Somewhere between conservative and definitive surgery for endometriosis there is a place for total abdominal hysterectomy with ovarian preservation. This operation is selected for women who have completed childbearing but are in their late 20s or early 30s. It is interesting that without repetitive episodes of retrograde menstruation, the endometriosis remains quiescent in the majority of these patients. In approximately 5% to 10% of women the disease is progressive, and they subsequently have a second operation involving oophorectomy.

Definitive surgical treatment is reserved for patients with far-advanced disease and for whom future fertility is not a consideration. Patients with pain that continues after medical and conservative surgery are treated by definitive surgery, which involves castration. Definitive surgery involves total abdominal hysterectomy, bilateral salpingo-oophorectomy, and the removal of all visible endometriosis. If the surgeon believes that it is not possible to surgically remove all the areas of endometriosis, it is best to treat a premenopausal woman with medroxyprogesterone or continuous oral contraceptive therapy for approximately 1 year to relieve menopausal symptoms before beginning cyclic exogenous estrogen therapy.

Medical therapy and surgical therapy are often performed in combination for advanced stages of the disease. Clinicians debate the advantages of either preoperative or postoperative medical therapy. Presently the majority favor preoperative medical treatment followed by surgery. In the future, photodynamic therapy for endometriosis may become a clinical reality. This procedure would involve intravenous injection of a special dye that would be concentrated in areas of endometriosis. Then a laser light would produce a photochemical reaction to destroy the areas.

If a patient has recurrent symptoms following definitive surgery for endometriosis and has not been taking exogenous estrogen, it is possible that she has a remnant of residual ovary, which can be diagnosed by measuring serum gonadotrophin levels. If the FSH and LH levels are not in menopausal range, some viable ovarian tissue remains, usually in the retroperitoneal space.

Most surgeons routinely remove the appendix when performing surgery for endometriosis not related to infertility. Pittaway published a series of more than 100 consecutive patients with endometriosis; 13% had histologic evidence of endometriosis in the appendix. This involvement could be discovered by gross examination in only 60% of patients. Appendectomy is generally contraindicated in infertility surgery because of the remote potential of infection, leakage from the stump, or adhesion formation.

The efficacy of oral contraceptives or danazol immediately before or following surgery for endometriosis is unresolved in clinical practice. Those who advocate hormones before surgery believe that it makes the dissection easier, but most surgeons do not use hormones preoperatively. Oral contraceptives carry the additional hazard of producing a hypercoagulable state during the perioperative period. Oral contraceptives and danazol may help eradicate microscopic endometriosis postoperatively. Obviously, they would not be prescribed for a prolonged period of time if fertility was the primary concern.

Gastrointestinal Tract Endometriosis

The frequency of gastrointestinal tract involvement in series of women with histologically proven endometriosis varies from 3% to 34%. Most large series document a frequency of approximately 5% (Figure 18-13). The severity and extent of involvement of the bowel by ectopic endometrium varies from the incidental finding of a spot on the serosa of the bowel to obstruction of the rectosigmoid. Most cases are insignificant and do not produce clinical symptoms. In the majority of cases, endometriosis of the gastrointestinal tract involves the sigmoid colon and the anterior wall of the rectum (Figure 8-14).

Endometriosis of the appendix is fairly common. The incidence in patients with pelvic endometriosis is reported between 1% and 13% (Figure 18-15). Endometriosis of the appendix is usually an incidental pathologic finding. It is not clinically important because pathophysiologically the aberrant endometrium in the appendix wall does not produce symptoms.

Endometriosis of the small bowel is rare. Approximately 200 cases of endometriosis of the ileum have been reported in the literature. This is a troublesome process because of the high incidence of associated small bowel obstruction.

Classic symptoms of endometriosis of the

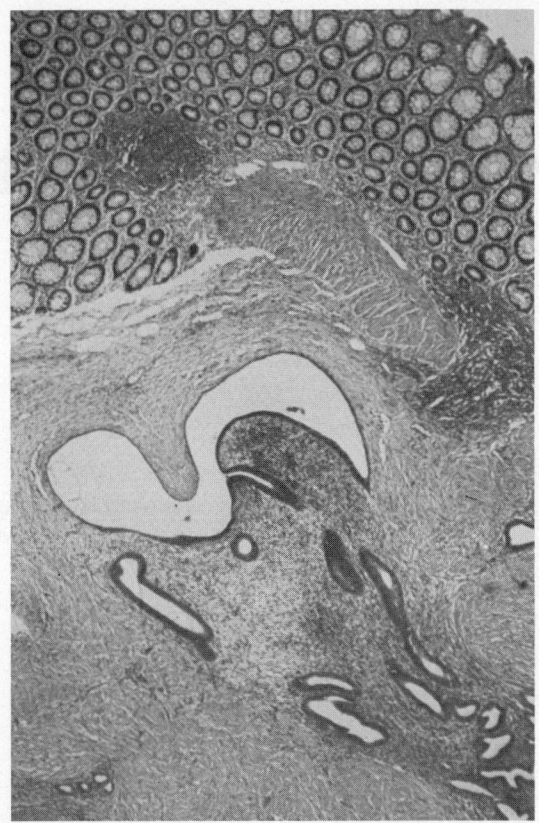

FIGURE 18-13
Endometriosis in bowel wall. (Courtesy Fred Askin, M.D.)

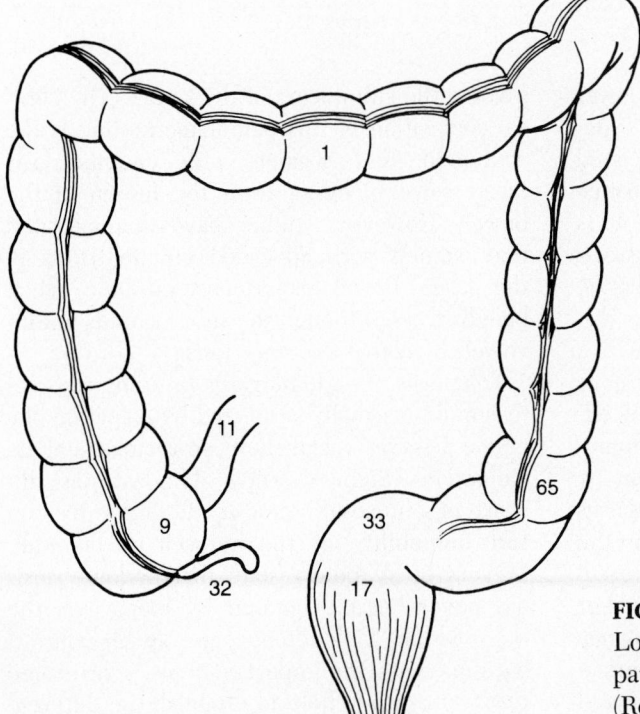

FIGURE 18-14
Locations of 168 bowel lesions found in 163 patients with endometriosis of the bowel. (Redrawn from Weed JC and Ray JE: Obstet Gynecol 69:727, 1987.)

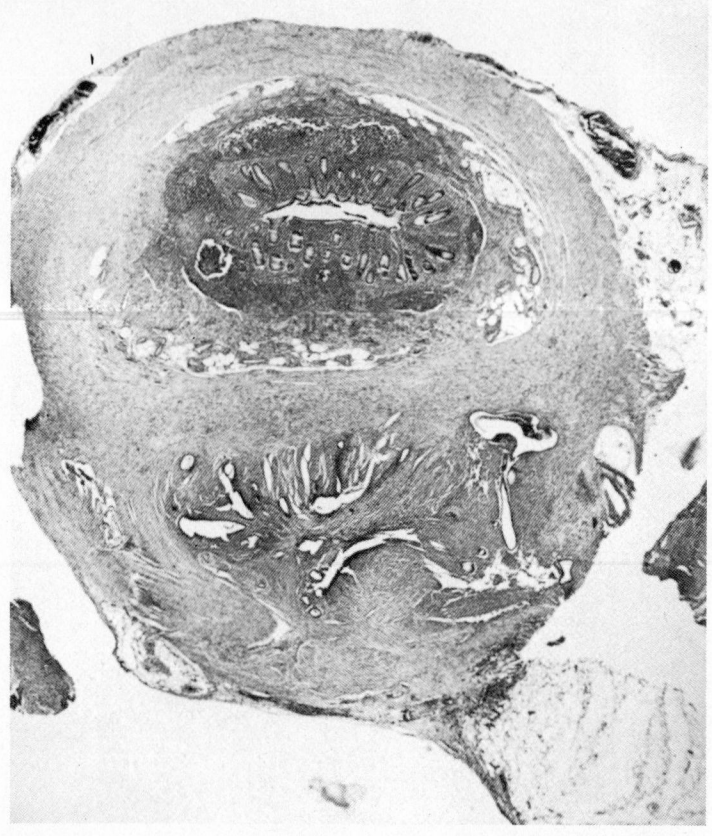

FIGURE 18-15
Cross section of appendix showing lumen of bowel and island of endometriosis.
(From Dougherty CM: Surgical pathology of gynecologic disease, New York, 1968,
Harper & Row, Publishers, Inc, p 636.)

large bowel include cyclic cramping and lower abdominal pain and pain with defecation, especially during the menstrual period. Associated with the abdominal and pelvic pain is a change in bowel function, usually constipation. It is difficult to differentiate the symptoms associated with endometriosis from the constellation of symptoms associated with inflammatory disease of the colon or malignancy. Women with a gastrointestinal malignancy usually experience intermittent rather than cyclic intestinal bleeding. Early diagnosis of gastrointestinal endometriosis demands a high index of suspicion by the physician. The initial clue to the diagnosis of the patient with multiple symptoms is the cyclic nature of these symptoms. Bowel resection is indicated for obstruction of the bowel or with extensive lesions in which malignancy may not be ruled out. On pathologic examination the aberrant endometrial glands and stroma penetrate the serosa of the bowel and muscularis. It is unusual for endometriosis to involve the submucosa of the bowel. The clinical correlation of this pathologic finding is the statement that women with endometriosis rarely have bleeding from the lumen of the bowel. However, studies have demonstrated that women with advanced endometriosis of the large bowel experience episodic rectal bleeding, even though the submucosa is not involved by active endometriosis.

Diagnosis of endometriosis invading the rectosigmoid is usually suspected by palpation of a pelvic mass or "rectal shelf" on rectovaginal examination. Sigmoidoscopy demonstrates absence of a mucosal lesion in addition to fixation and immobility of the anterior rectal wall. Meyers et al. boldly state that endometriosis has never been diagnosed by biopsy via the colonoscope. Colonoscopy and an air-contrast barium enema are important steps in suspected cases, since they help to establish the differential diagnosis and the degree of obstruction. There is no specific radiologic appearance for endometriosis. However, a filling defect and absence of a mucosal lesion with the presence of extramucosal involvement are usually demonstrated. The definitive diagnosis and differentiation of endometriosis from carcinoma of the bowel may be delayed until a frozen section is obtained during exploratory surgery.

The treatment of endometriosis of the gastrointestinal tract is dependent on the extent and severity of symptoms. Endocrine therapy is not recommended for advanced cases. The importance of preoperative preparation of the bowel in difficult cases should not be forgotten. Surgical procedures vary from superficial excision of the endometriosis to bowel resection with anastomosis. Superficial excision involves delicate, tedious surgery to ensure that the lumen of the bowel is not entered.

Urinary Tract Endometriosis

Endometriosis in the female pelvis occasionally produces dysfunction in adjacent pelvic organs. Approximately 10% of women with endometriosis have involvement of the urinary tract by implants of endometriosis and associated retroperitoneal fibrosis. In most cases an incidental finding of aberrant endometrial glands and stroma is discovered on the bladder peritoneum and anterior cul-de-sac. The most serious consequence of urinary tract involvement is ureteral obstruction, which occurs in about 1% of women with moderate or severe pelvic endometriosis.

Patients with endometriosis involving the urinary tract have nonspecific clinical presentations. Hematuria and flank pain are experienced by less than 25% of women. One of three women with documented complete ureteral obstruction secondary to endometriosis has no pelvic symptoms whatsoever. The clinical challenge is to diagnose ureteral obstruction at an early stage, before loss of renal function. The obstruction is always in the distal one third of the course of the ureter. The importance of an intravenous pyelogram in all women with retroperitoneal endometriosis cannot be overemphasized.

Treatment of endometriosis of the peritoneum over the bladder can be accomplished by medical or surgical means. Ureteral obstruction may be intrinsic, from active endometriosis, or extrinsic, from longstanding fibrotic reactions to retroperitoneal inflammation. There are few reports of intrinsic endometriosis of the ureter responding to danazol or GnRH agonists. However, long-term follow-up with serial intravenous pyelograms must be undertaken to ensure that the disease process does not recur.

Surgical therapy is preferred for ureteral obstruction secondary to endometriosis. Because the operations are rare, they must be individualized. However, surgical castration and the relief of urinary obstruction by ureterolysis or by ureteroneocystostomy are the usual alternatives. If ureterolysis is the operation of choice, peristalsis in the involved segment of the ureter should be observed, along with adequate resection of the endometriosis and surrounding inflammation in the retroperitoneal space. Ureteroneocystostomy has the advantage of bypassing the urinary obstruction and making it technically easier to resect the area of endometriosis.

ADENOMYOSIS

Adenomyosis is frequently referred to as *endometriosis interna*. This term is misleading because endometriosis and adenomyosis are discovered in the same patient in less than 20% of women. More important, endometriosis and adenomyosis are two clinically different diseases. The only common feature is the presence of ectopic endometrial glands and stroma. Adenomyosis is derived from aberrant glands of the basalis layer of the endometrium. Therefore these glands do not usually undergo the traditional cyclic proliferative and secretory changes that are associated with differing levels of ovarian hormone production.

Adenomyosis is usually diagnosed incidentally by the pathologist examining histologic sections of surgical specimens. The frequency of the histologic diagnosis is directly related to how meticulously the pathologist searches for the disease. If multiple serial sections of the uterus are obtained, the incidence may exceed 60% in women 40 to 50 years of age. Adenomyosis is also a common incidental finding during autopsy. Serial histologic slides confirm the continuity of downward growth of the basalis layer of the endometrium. Thus the histogenesis of adenomyosis is direct extension from the endometrial lining.

The pathogenesis of adenomyosis remains unknown. The current theory is that high levels of estrogen stimulate hyperplasia of the basalis layer of the endometrium. For an unknown reason the barrier between the endometrium and myometrium is broken. Because adenomyosis is discovered most often in parous women, one hypothesis is that chronic postpartum endometritis may cause the initial break in the barrier. Initially the stroma and subsequently the glands begin to invade the myometrium along the path of least resistance. In most instances this growth is adjacent to lymphatic and vascular channels.

Pathology

There are two distinctly different pathologic presentations of adenomyosis. Most common is a diffuse involvement of both anterior and posterior walls of the uterus. The posterior wall is usually involved more than the anterior wall. The individual areas of adenomyosis are not encapsulated. The second presentation is a focal area or adenomyoma. This results in an asymmetric uterus, and this special area of adenomyosis may have a pseudocapsule.

In the more common, diffuse type of adenomyosis the uterus is uniformly enlarged, usually 2 to 3 times normal size. Sometimes it is difficult to distinguish grossly from uterine lei-

omyomas. When the myometrium is transected by a knife, the cut surface protrudes convexly and has a spongy appearance. The cut surface of a uterus with adenomyosis is darker than the white surface of a myoma. Sometimes there are discrete areas of adenomyosis that are not densely encapsulated and contain small, dark cystic spaces. There is no distinct cleavage plane around focal adenomyomas as there is with uterine myomas.

Benign endometrial glands and stroma are seen within the myometrium. These glands rarely undergo the same cyclic changes as the normal uterine endometrium. Studies have demonstrated a lack of progesterone receptors in tissue from adenomyosis. There are also fewer estrogen receptors than in normal endometrium. This deficiency of receptors helps to explain the lack of responsiveness of adenomyosis to hormonal therapy.

The standard criterion used in diagnosis of adenomyosis is the finding of endometrial glands and stromas more than one low-powered field (2.5 mm) from the basalis layer of the endometrium (Figure 18-16). The small areas of adenomyosis have the same general appearance as the basalis layers of the endometrium.

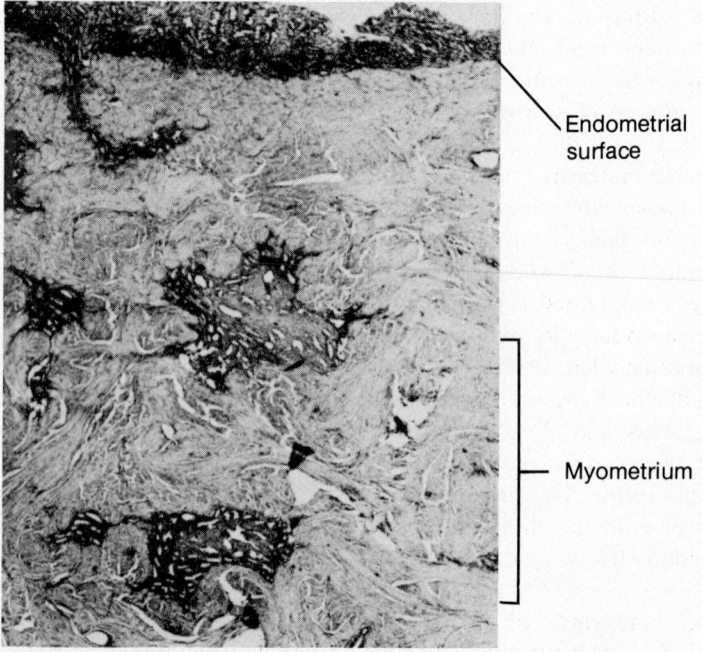

FIGURE 18-16
Adenomyosis. Note islands of endometrial tissue deep within myometrium. (From Janovski NA and Dubrauszky V: Atlas of gynecologic and obstetric diagnostic histopathology, New York, 1967, McGraw-Hill Book Co, p 217.)

Histologically the glands exhibit an inactive or proliferative pattern. Occasionally one sees cystic hyperplasia and rarely a secretory pattern. Although the areas do not undergo full menstrual-type changes, bleeding may occur in these ectopic areas, as evidenced by both gross and microscopic findings. It is not unusual to see histologic variability in several different fossae deep in the walls of the myometrium from the same uterus. Some fossae of adenomyosis undergo decidual changes either during pregnancy or during estrogen-progestin therapy for endometriosis. The reaction of the myometrium to the ectopic endometrium is hyperplasia and hypertrophy of individual muscle fibers (Figure 18-17). Surrounding most foci of glands and stroma are localized areas of hyperplasia of the smooth muscle of the uterus. This change in the myometrium produces the globular enlargement of the uterus.

Clinical Diagnosis

The majority of women with adenomyosis are asymptomatic or have minor symptoms that do not annoy them enough to seek medical care. They attribute the increase in dysmenorrhea or menstrual bleeding to the aging process and tolerate the symptoms. Symptomatic adenomyosis usually presents in women between the ages of 35 and 50. Unlike those with endometriosis, the majority of women women with symptomatic adenomyosis are parous and frequently have had several children.

The classic symptoms of adenomyosis are secondary dysmenorrhea and menorrhagia. The acquired dysmenorrhea becomes increasingly more severe as the disease progresses. Occasionally the patient complains of dyspareunia, which is midline in location and deep in the pelvis. On pelvic examination the uterus is diffusely enlarged, usually 2 to 3 times normal size. It is most unusual for the uterine enlargement associated with adenomyosis to be greater than 14 week size gestation unless the patient also has uterine myomas. The uterus is globular and tender immediately before and during menstruation (Figure 18-18). There are often differences in tenderness and consistency of the uterus from one pelvic examination to another. This depends on the time of the pelvic examination in relation to the patient's menstrual cycle.

The diagnosis of adenomyosis is confirmed only following histologic examination of the hysterectomy specimen. Frequently the clinical diagnosis is inaccurately assigned to the patient who has chronic pelvic pain. Traditionally the patient will have endometrial sampling to rule out other organic causes of abnormal bleeding. Many times adenomyosis is diagnosed retrospectively following a hysterectomy for other indications. Adenomyosis may coexist with both endometrial hyperplasia and endometrial carcinoma. Approximately two out of three women with adenomyosis have coexistent pelvic pathology, most commonly myomas but also endometriosis, endometrial hyperplasia, and salpingitis isthmica nodosa. Emge has speculated that unopposed estrogen is a potential cause of adenomyosis. The two most common conditions in the differential diagnosis of adenomyosis are small uterine myomas and dysfunctional uterine bleeding in the slightly enlarged uterus of a multiparous woman. Ultrasound and magnetic resonance imaging have been used to help differentiate between adenomyosis and uterine myomas in a young woman desiring future childbearing.

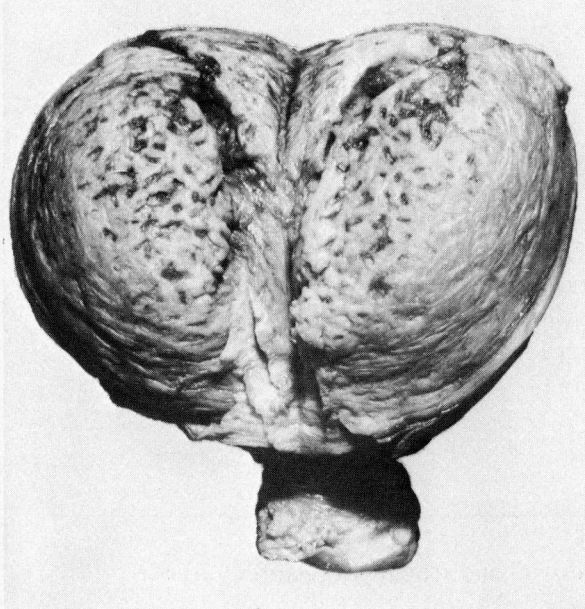

FIGURE 18-17
Adenomyosis. This hysterectomy specimen from a 32-year-old woman has been bisected to demonstrate the hypertrophied myometrium. (From Jeffcoate TNA: Principles of gynaecology, ed 4, London, Butterworths, 1975, p 353.)

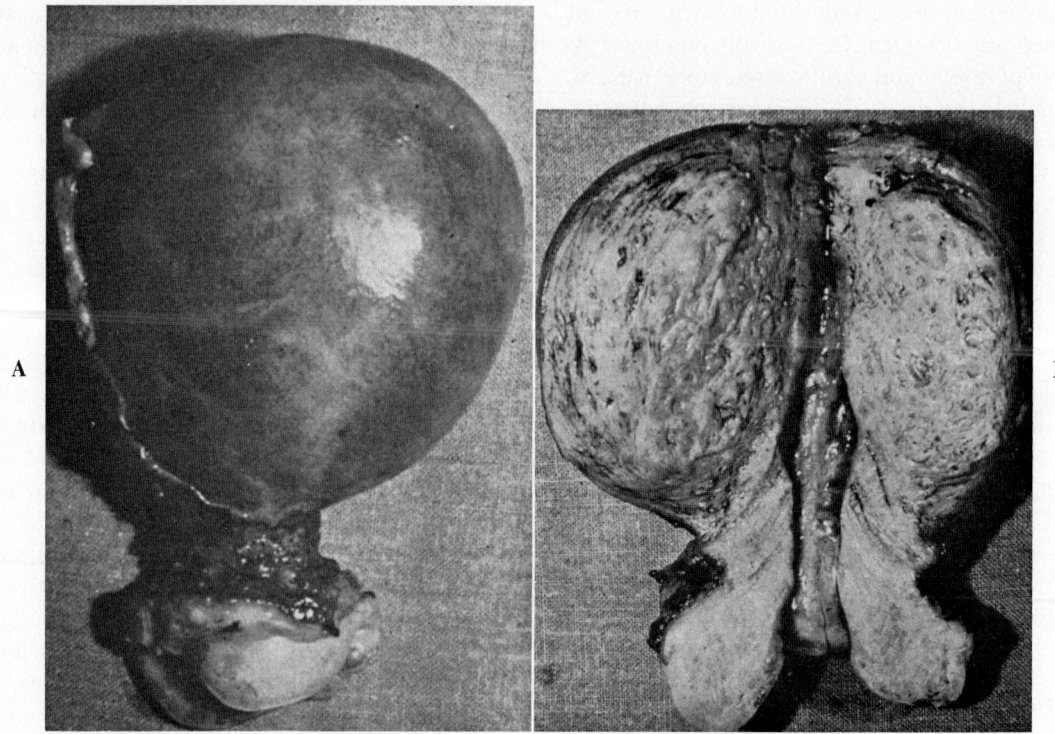

FIGURE 18-18
A, Hysterectomy specimen from 37-year-old woman showing adenomyosis. Note globular appearance of uterus. **B,** Bisection of posterior wall of uterus. (From Emge LA: Am J Obstet Gynecol 83:1551, 1962.)

Management

There is no satisfactory medical treatment for adenomyosis. Occasionally, patients with adenomyosis are treated with cyclic hormones or prostaglandin synthetase inhibitors for their abnormal bleeding and pain. Hysterectomy is the definitive treatment if this therapy is appropriate for the woman's age, parity, and plans for future reproduction. Before hysterectomy, endometrial sampling should be performed to rule out endometrial malignancy. Size of the uterus, degree of prolapse, and presence of associated pelvic pathology determine the choice of abdominal or vaginal route for the hysterectomy. For the woman in her late 40s, the ovaries are often removed as a prophylactic measure against ovarian carcinoma, regardless of whether the woman has an abdominal or vaginal hysterectomy.

_____ KEY POINTS _____

- Endometriosis is a benign, usually progressive, and sometimes recurrent disease that invades locally and disseminates widely.

- Endometriosis is present in 5% to 15% of celiotomies performed on women of reproductive age.

- The incidence of endometriosis is 30% to 45% in women with infertility.

- Approximately 5% of women with endometriosis are diagnosed following menopause. Postmenopausal endometriosis is usually secondary to the use of exogenous estrogen.

- The clinical course of endometriosis differs for each patient, and treatment must be individualized.

- Possible etiologic factors of endometriosis include retrograde menstruation, metaplasia, vascular metastasis, immunologic defects, iatrogenic dissemination, and a genetic predisposition.

- The ovaries and the pelvic peritoneum are the most frequent sites for endometriosis. Pelvic lymph nodes are involved in 30% of cases. Approximately 10% to 15% of women with endometriosis have involvement of the rectosigmoid.

- Visually, endometriosis may appear in many forms, including red, brown, black, white, yellow, pink, or clear vesicles and lesions. Biopsy is essential for diagnosis.

- Three cardinal features of microscopic endometriosis are ectopic endometrial glands, ectopic endometrial stroma, and hemorrhage into the adjacent tissue.

- Classic symptoms of endometriosis are cyclic pelvic pain and infertility. However, approximately one third of patients with endometriosis are asymptomatic.

- The severity of endometriosis is not related to the severity of pain symptoms.

- The most prominent pelvic sign of endometriosis is a fixed, retroverted uterus with scarring and tenderness posterior to the uterus. The classic sign of endometriosis is tender nodularity of the uterosacral ligaments.

- Viable endometrial glands and stroma cannot be identified on pathologic examination in approximately 25% of cases of endometriosis.

- Neither ultrasound nor magnetic resonance imaging is useful as a primary modality in detecting or staging endometriosis.

- Approximately 10% of teenagers who develop endometriosis have associated congenital outflow obstruction.

- The primary goal of the hormonal treatment of endometriosis is induction of amenorrhea.

- The side effects of danazol are related to its androgenic and anabolic properties, as well as to the pseudomenopause produced by the drug.

- Danazol acts as a mild androgen and leads to substantial reduction in estradiol levels.

- Danazol decreases high-density lipoprotein levels and increases low-density lipoprotein levels.

- Approximately three of four women note significant improvement in symptoms following danazol therapy. One in four will have a recurrence of symptoms within 2 years following completion of medical therapy.

- GnRH agonists produce a "medical castration" without the side effects of danazol on steroid-sensitive target organs.

- Approximately 40% of women treated with progestin therapy for endometriosis develop abnormal bleeding.

- Gonadotrophin-releasing hormone (GnRH) agonists and progestins, given together, diminish the side effects caused by GnRH agonists given alone.

- GnRH agonists work by suppressing gonadotrophin secretion, leading to decreased ovarian steroidogenesis.

- GnRH agonists may be given by intranasal, intramuscular, subcutaneous, intravenous, or intravaginal routes, but not via the gastrointestinal tract.

- Initial clinical response to GnRH agonist therapy depends on when the therapy is begun in relation to the menstrual cycle.

- The goals of conservative surgery include removal of macroscopic endometriosis, lysis of adhesions, and restoration of normal anatomy.

- Laparoscopic management of endometriosis includes the use of laser vaporization/coagulation. Advantages of this modality include speed, precision, and minimal tissue damage to surrounding areas.

- The principles of microsurgery are essential to the surgical treatment of endometriosis: minimal and gentle handling of tissue, avoiding hypoxia of the peritoneum, and attempting to restore normal pelvic anatomy.

- Approximately 5% of women with endometriosis will have involvement of the gastrointestinal tract.

- Adenomyosis rarely causes uterine enlargement greater than a size at 14 weeks' gestation unless there is concomitant uterine pathology.

- Adenomyosis is discovered microscopically in one of three hysterectomy specimens and is frequently asymptomatic.

- Symptomatic adenomyosis primarily occurs in parous women over age 35. The classic symptoms are secondary dysmenorrhea and menorrhagia. The most common physical sign is a diffusely enlarged uterus, usually 2 to 3 times normal size.

BIBLIOGRAPHY

Adamson GD: Diagnosis and clinical presentation of endometriosis, Am J Obstet Gynecol 162:568, 1990.

Adamson GD, Lu J, and Subak LL: Laparascopic CO_2 laser vaporization of endometriosis compared with traditional treatments, Fertil Steril 50:704, 1988.

Andrews WC: Medical versus surgical treatment of endometriosis, Clin Obstet Gynecol 23:917, 1980.

Arrivé L, Hricak H, and Martin MC: Pelvic endometriosis: MR imaging, Radiology 171:687, 1989.

Athey PA and Diment DD: The spectrum of sonographic findings in endometriosis, J Ultrasound Med 8:487, 1989.

Azziz R: Adenomyosis: current perspectives, Obstet Gynecol Clin North Am 16:221, 1989.

Barbieri RL: Comparison of the pharmacology of nafarelin and danazol, Am J Obstet Gynecol 162:581, 1990.

Barbieri RL: Etiology and epidemiology of endometriosis, Am J Obstet Gynecol 162:565, 1990.

Barbieri RL and Ryan KJ: Danazol: endocrine pharmacology and therapeutic applications, Am J Obstet Gynecol 141:453, 1981.

Batt RE and Smith RA: Embryologic theory of histogenesis of endometriosis in peritoneal pockets, Obstet Gynecol Clin North Am 16:15, 1989.

Bird CC, McElin TW, and Manalo-Estrella P: The elusive adenomyosis of the uterus—revisited, Am J Obstet Gynecol 112:583, 1972.

Blumenkrantz MJ, Gallagher N, Bashore RA, et al: Retrograde menstruation in women undergoing chronic peritoneal dialysis, Obstet Gynecol 57:667, 1981.

Burry KA, Patton PE, and Illingworth DR: Metabolic changes during medical treatment of endometriosis: nafarelin acetate versus danazol, Am J Obstet Gynecol 160:1454, 1989.

Buttram VC: Evolution of the revised American Fertility Society classification of endometriosis, Fertil Steril 43:347, 1985.

Buttram VC, Reiter RC, and Ward S: Treatment of endometriosis with danazol: report of a 6-year prospective study, Fertil Steril 43:353, 1985.

Candini GB, Fedele L, Vercellini P, et al: Repetitive conservative surgery for recurrence of endometriosis, Obstet Gynecol 77: 421, 1991.

Cedars MI, Lu JKH, Meldrum DR, et al: Treatment of endometriosis with a long-acting gonadotropin-releasing hormone agonist plus medroxyprogesterone acetate, Obstet Gynecol 75:641, 1990.

Confino E, Harlow L, and Gleicher N: Peritoneal fluid and serum autoantibody levels in patients with endometriosis, Fertil Steril 53:242, 1990.

Cornillie FJ, Oosterlynck D, Lauweryns JM, et al: Deeply infiltrating pelvic endometriosis: histology and clinical significance, Fertil Steril 53:978, 1990.

Coronado C, Franklin RR, Lotze EC, et al: Surgical treatment of symptomatic colorectal endometriosis, Fertil Steril 53:411, 1990.

Corson SL, Unger M, Kwa D, et al: Laparoscopic laser treatment of endometriosis with the ND:YAG sapphire probe, Am J Obstet Gynecol 160:718, 1989.

Dawood MY, Lewis V, and Ramos J: Cortical and trabecular bone mineral content in women with endometriosis: effect of gonadotropin-releasing hormone agonist and danazol, Fertil Steril 52:21, 1989.

Dickey RP, Taylor SN, and Curole DN: Serum estradiol and danazol. I. Endometriosis response, side effects, administration interval, concurrent spironolactone and dexamethasone, Fertil Steril 42:709, 1984.

Dlugi AM, Miller JD, Knittle J, et al: Lupron depot (leuprolide acetate for depot suspension) in the treatment of endometriosis: a randomized, placebo-controlled, double-blind study, Fertil Steril 54:419, 1990

Dlugi AM, Rufo S, D'Amico JF, et al: A comparison of the effects of buserelin versus danazol on plasma lipoproteins during treatment of pelvic endometriosis, Fertil Steril 49:913, 1988.

Dmowski WP: Danazol-induced pseudomenopause in the management of endometriosis, Clin Obstet Gynecol 31:829, 1989.

Dmowski WP, Kapetanakis E, and Scommegna A: Variable effects of danazol on endometriosis at 4 low-dose levels, Obstet Gynecol 59:408, 1982.

Dmowski WP and Radwanska E: Current concepts on pathology, histogenesis and etiology of endometriosis, Acta Obstet Gynecol Scand Suppl 123:29, 1984.

Dmowski WP, Steele RW, and Baker GF: Deficient cellular immunity in endometriosis, Am J Obstet Gynecol 141:377, 1981.

Dodin S, Lemay A, Maheux R, et al: Bone mass in endometriosis patients treated with GnRH agonist implant or danazol, Obstet Gynecol 77:410, 1991.

Dougherty CM: Surgical pathology of gynecologic disease, New York, 1968, Harper & Row, Publishers, Inc.

Eisermann J, Gast MJ, Pineda J, et al: Tumor necrosis factor in peritoneal fluid of women undergoing laparoscopic surgery, Fertil Steril 50:573, 1988.

El-Roeiy A, Dmowski WP, Gleicher N, et al: Danazol but not gonadotropin-releasing hormone agonists suppresses autoantibodies in endometriosis, Fertil Steril 50:864, 1988.

Emge LA: The elusive adenomyosis of the uterus, Am J Obstet Gynecol 83:1541, 1962.

Erickson LS and Ory SJ: GnRH analogues in the treatment of endometriosis, Obstet Gynecol Clin North Am 16:123, 1989.

Falk RJ and Mullin BR: Exacerbation of adenomyosis symptomatology by estrogen-progestin therapy: a case report and histopathological observations, Int J Fertil 34:386, 1989.

Fedele L, Bianchi S, Viezzoli T, et al: Gestrinone versus danazol in the treatment of endometriosis, Fertil Steril 51:781, 1989.

Fedele L, Arcaini L, Vercellini P, et al: Serum CA-125 measurements in the diagnosis of endometriosis recurrence, Obstet Gynecol 72:19, 1988.

Fedele L, Parazzini F, Bianchi S, et al: Stage and localization of pelvic endometriosis and pain, Fertil Steril 53:155, 1990.

Fedele L, Marchini M, Bianchi S, et al: Endometrial patterns during danazol and buserelin therapy for endometriosis: comparative structural and ultrastructural study, Obstet Gynecol 76:79, 1990.

Forsgren H, Lindhagen J, Melander S, et al: Colorectal endometriosis, Acta Chir Scand 149:431, 1983.

Gehr TWB and Sica DA: Case report and review of the literature: ureteral endometriosis, Am J Med Sci 294:346, 1987.

Gerbie AB and Merrill JA: Pathology of endometriosis, Clin Obstet Gynecol 31:779, 1989.

Ginsburg KA, Quereshi F, Thomas M, et al: Intramural ectopic pregnancy implanting in adenomyosis, Fertil Steril 51:354, 1989.

Gleicher N, El-Roeiy A, Confino E, et al: Is endometriosis an autoimmune disease? Obstet Gynecol 70:115, 1987.

Gorell HA, Cyr DR, Wang KY, et al: Rectosigmoid endometriosis: diagnosis using endovaginal sonography, J Ultrasound Med 8:459, 1989.

Graham B and Mazier WP: Diagnosis and management of endometriosis of the colon and rectum, Dis Colon Rectum 31:952, 1988.

Greenblatt RP, Dmowski WP, Mahesh VB, et al: Clinical studies with antigonadotropin—danazol, Fertil Steril 22:102, 1971.

Halme J, Becker S, and Haskill S: Altered maturation and function of peritoneal macrophages: possible role in pathogenesis of endometriosis, Am J Obstet Gynecol 156:783, 1987.

Halme J, White C, et al: Peritoneal marcophages from patients with endometriosis release growth factor activity in vitro, J Clin Endocrinol Metab 66:1044, 1988.

Haney AF and Weinberg JB: Reduction of the intraperitoneal inflammation associated with endometriosis by treatment with medroxyprogesterone acetate, Am J Obstet Gynecol 159:450, 1988.

Henzl MR: Gonadotropin-releasing hormone (GnRH) agonists in the management of endometriosis: a review, Clin Obstet Gynecol 31:840, 1988.

Henzl MR, Corson SL, Moghissi K, et al: Administration of nasal nafarelin as compared with oral danazol for endometriosis: a multicenter double-blind comparative clinical trial, N Engl J Med 318:485, 1988.

Holt JP Jr and Keller D: Danazol treatment increases serum enzyme levels, Fertil Steril 41:70, 1984.

Hornstein MD, Gleason RE, and Barbieri RL: A randomized double-blind prospective trial of two doses of gestrinone in the treatment of endometriosis, Fertil Steril 53:237, 1990.

Israel R: Pelvic endometriosis. In Mishell DR, Davajan V, and Lobo RA, editors: Infertility, contraception, and reproductive endocrinology, ed 3, Oradell, NJ, 1990, Medical Economics Books.

Iwasaka T, Okuma Y, Yoshimura T, et al: Endometriosis associated with ascites, Obstet Gynecol 66:72S, 1985.

Jager W, Meier C, Wildt L, et al: CA-125 serum concentrations during the menstrual cycle, Fertil Steril 50:223, 1988.

Janovski NA and Dubrauszky V: Atlas of gynecologic and obstetric diagnostic histopathology, New York, 1967, McGraw-Hill Book Co.

Javert CT: Pathogenesis of endometriosis based on endometrial homeoplasia, direct extension exfoliation and implantation, lymphatic and hematogenous metastasism, Cancer 2:399, 1949.

Johnson WM and Tyndal CM: Pulmonary endometriosis: treatment with danazol, Obstet Gynecol 69:506, 1987.

Kane C and Drouin P: Obstructive uropathy associated with endometriosis, Am J Obstet Gynecol 151:207, 1985.

Kauma S, Clark MR, White C, et al: Production of fibronectin by peritoneal macrophages and concentrations of fibronectin in peritoneal fluid from patients with or without endometriosis, Obstet Gynecol 72:13, 1988.

Kennedy SH, Williams IA, Brodribb J, et al: A comparison of nafarelin acetate and danazol in the treatment of endometriosis, Fertil Steril 53:998, 1990.

Kennedy SH, Mojiminiyi OA, Soper ND, et al: Immunioscrintigraphy of endometriosis, Br J Obstet Gynaecol 97:667, 1990.

Kennedy SH, Sargent IL, Starkey PM, et al: Localization of anti-endometrial antibody binding in women with endometriosis using a double-labelling immunohistochemical method, Br J Obstet Gynaecol 97:671, 1990.

Kennedy SH, Starkey PM, Sargent IL, et al: Antiendometrial antibodies in endometriosis measured by an enzyme-linked immunosorbent assay before and after treatment with danazol and nafarelin, Obstet Gynaecol 75:914, 1990.

Keye WR Jr and Dixon J: Photocoagulation of endometriosis by the argon laser through the laparoscope, Obstet Gynecol 62:383, 1983.

Kirshon B and Poindexter AN III: Contraception: a risk factor for endometriosis, Obstet Gynecol 71:829, 1988.

Klein RS and Cattolica EV: Ureteral endometriosis, Urology 13:477, 1979.

Lemay A, Maheux R, Huot C, et al: Efficacy of intranasal or subcutaneous luteinizing hormone–releasing hormone agonist inhibition of ovarian function in the treatment of endometriosis, Am J Obstet Gynecol 158:233, 1988.

Lemay A and Quesnel G: Potential new treatment of endometriosis: reversible inhibition of pituitary-ovarian function by chronic intranasal administration of a luteinizing hormone–releasing hormone (LH-RH) agonist, Fertil Steril 38:376, 1982.

Low RAL, Roberts DGR, and Lees DAR: A comparative study of various dosages of danazol in the treatment of endometriosis, Br J Obstet Gynaecol 91:167, 1984.

Luciano AA: A guide to managing endometriosis, Contemp OB/GYN 19:211, 1982.

Luciano AA, Turksoy RN, and Carleo J: Evaluation of oral medroxyprogesterone acetate in the treatment of endometriosis, Obstet Gynecol 72:323, 1988.

Mahmood TA and Templeton A: Pathophysiology of mild endometriosis: review of literature, Hum Reprod 5:765, 1990.

Malinak LR: Infertility and endometriosis: operative technique, clinical staging, and prognosis, Clin Obstet Gynecol 23:925, 1980.

Manyak MJ, Nelson LM, Solomon D, et al: Photodynamic therapy of rabbit endometrial transplants: a model for treatment of endometriosis, Fertil Steril 52:140, 1989.

Marana R, Muzii L, Muscatello P, et al: Gonadotrophin-releasing hormone agonist (buserelin) in the treatment of endometriosis: changes in the extent of the disease in CA-125 serum levels after 6-month therapy, Br J Obstet Gynaecol 97: 1016, 1990.

Martin DC, Hubert GD, Zwaag RV, et al: Laparoscopic appearances of peritoneal endometriosis, Fertil Steril 51:63, 1989.

Masahashi T, Matsuzawa K, Onsawa M, et al: Serum CA-125 levels in patients with endometriosis: changes in CA-125 levels during menstruation, Obstet Gynecol 72:328, 1988.

McArthur JW and Ulfelder H: The effect of pregnancy upon endometriosis, Obstet Gynecol Surv 20:709, 1965.

McCarthy S: MR imaging of the uterus, Radiology 171:321, 1989.

Meek SC, Hodge DD, and Musich JR: Autoimmunity in infertile patients with endometriosis, Am J Obstet Gynecol 158:1365, 1988.

Meldrum DR, Pardridge WM, Karow WG, et al: Hormonal effects of danazol and medical oophorectomy in endometriosis, Obstet Gynecol 62:480, 1983.

Metzger DA and Luciano AA: Hormonal therapy of endometriosis, Obstet Gynecol Clin North Am 16:105, 1989.

Meyers WC, Kelvin FM, and Jones RS: Diagnosis and surgical treatment of colonic endometriosis, Arch Surg 114:169, 1979.

Moghissi KS: Gonadotropin-releasing hormones: clinical applications in gynecology, J Reprod Med 35:1097, 1990.

Moghissi KS: Treatment of endometriosis with estrogen-progestin combination and progestogens alone, Clin Obstet Gynecol 31:823, 1989.

Moloney MD, Thornton JG, and Cooper EH: Serum CA-125 antigen levels and disease severity in patients with endometriosis, Obstet Gynecol 73:767, 1989.

Moore JG, Binstock MA, and Growdon WA: The clinical implications of retroperitoneal endometriosis, Am J Obstet Gynecol 158:1291, 1988.

Moore JG, Hibbard LT, Growdon WA, et al: Urinary tract endometriosis: enigmas in diagnosis and management, Am J Obstet Gynecol 134:162, 1979.

Moretuzzo RW, DiLauro S, Jenison E, et al: Serum and peritoneal lavage fluid CA-125 levels in endometriosis, Fertil Steril 50:430, 1988.

Myers WC, Kelvin FM, and Jones RS: Diagnosis and surgical treatment of colonic endometriosis, Arch Surg 114:169, 1979.

Nisolle-Pochet M, Casanas-Roux F, and Donnez J: Histologic study of ovarian endometriosis after hormonal therapy, Fertil Steril 49:423, 1988.

Noble AD and Lechtworth AT: Medical treatment of endometriosis: a comparative trial, Postgrad Med J 55(suppl 5):37, 1979.

Olive DL and Henderson DY: Endometriosis and müllerian anomalies, Obstet Gynecol 69:412, 1987.

Ory SJ: Clinical uses of luteinizing hormone–releasing hormone, Fertil Steril 39:577, 1983.

Pittaway DE: Appendectomy in the surgical treatment of endometriosis, Obstet Gynecol 61:421, 1983.

Pittaway DE and Douglas JW: Serum CA-125 in women with endometriosis and chronic pelvic pain, Fertil Steril 51:68, 1989.

Pittaway DE, Ellington CP, and Klimek M: Preclinical abortions and endometriosis, Fertil Steril 49:221, 1988.

Pittaway DE, Vernon C, and Fayez JA: Spontaneous abortions in women with endometriosis, Fertil Steril 50:711, 1988.

Pratt JH and Williams TJ: Indications for complete pelvic operations and more radical procedures in the treatment of severe or extensive endometriosis, Clin Obstet Gynecol 23:937, 1980.

Prystowsky JB, Stryker SJ, Ujiki GT, et al: Gastrointestinal endometriosis, Arch Surg 123:855, 1988.

Puleo JG and Hammond CB: Conservative treatment of endometriosis externa: the effects of danazol therapy, Fertil Steril 40:164, 1983.

Redwine DB: Age-related evolution in color appearance of endometriosis, Fertil Steril 48:1062, 1987.

Redwine DB: Is "microscopic" peritoneal endometriosis invisible? Fertil Steril 50:665, 1988.

Redwine DB: Peritoneal pockets and endometriosis: confirmation of an important relationship, with further observations, J Reprod Med 34:270, 1989.

Reimnitz C, Brand E, Nieberg RK, et al: Malignancy arising in endometriosis associated with unopposed estrogen replacement, Obstet Gynecol 71:444, 1988.

Riis BJ, Christiansen C, Johansen JS, et al: Is it possible to prevent bone loss in young women treated with luteinizing hormone–releasing hormone agonists? J Clin Endocrinol Metab 70:920, 1990.

Rivlin ME, Krueger RP, and Wiser WL: Danazol in the management of ureteral obstruction secondary to endometriosis, Fertil Steril 44:274, 1985.

Rivlin ME, Miller JD, Krueger RP, et al: Leuprolide acetate in the management of ureteral obstruction caused by endometriosis, Obstet Gynecol 75:532, 1990.

Rolland R and van der Heijden PFM: Nafarelin versus danazol in the treatment of endometriosis, Am J Obstet Gynecol 162:586, 1990.

Rorkelson SJ, Lee RA, and Hildahl DB: Endometriosis of the sciatic nerve: a report of two cases and a review of the literature, Obstet Gynecol 71:473, 1988.

Rossman F, D'Ablaing G III, and Marrs RP: Pregnancy complicated by ruptured endometrioma, Obstet Gynecol 62:519, 1983.

Rovati V, Faleschini E, Vercellini P, et al: Endometrioma of the liver, Am J Obstet Gynecol 163:1490, 1990

Ruponen S and Taina E: Operative treatment of rectal endometriosis, Acta Obstet Gynecol Scand 57:277, 1978.

Sakata M, Terakawa N, Mizutani T, et al: Effects of danazol, gonadotropin-releasing hormone agonist, and a combination of danazol and gonadotropin-releasing hormone agonist on experimental endometriosis, Am J Obstet Gynecol 163:1679, 1990.

Sampson JA: Peritoneal endometriosis due to menstrual dissemination of endometrial tissue into peritoneal cavity, Am J Obstet Gynecol 14:422, 1927.

Sanfilippo JS, Wakim NG, Schikler KN, et al: Endometriosis in association with uterine anomaly, Am J Obstet Gynecol 154:39, 1986.

Schenken RS: Gonadotropin-releasing hormone analogs in the treatment of endometriosis, Am J Obstet Gynecol 162:579, 1990.

Schlaff WD, Dugoff L, Damewood MD, et al: Megestrol acetate for treatment of endometriosis, Obstet Gynecol 75:646, 1990.

Schmidt CL: Endometriosis: a reappraisal of pathogenesis and treatment, Fertil Steril 44:157, 1985.

Schriock E, Monroe SE, Henzl M, et al: Treatment of endometriosis with a potent agonist of gonadotropin-releasing hormone (nafarelin), Fertil Steril 44:583, 1985.

Schweppe K-W and Wynn RM: Endocrine dependency of endometriosis: an ultrastructural study, Eur J Obstet Gynecol Reprod Biol 17:193, 1984.

Seibel MM, Berger MJ, Weinstein FG, et al: The effectiveness of danazol on subsequent fertility in minimal endometriosis, Fertil Steril 38:534, 1982.

Seltzer VL and Benjamin F: Treatment of pulmonary endometriosis with a long-acting GnRH agonist, Obstet Gynecol 76:929, 1990.

Shaw RW: Nafarelin in the treatment of pelvic pain caused by endometriosis, Am J Obstet Gynecol 162:574, 1990.

Shirk GJ: Use of the Nd:YAG laser for the treatment of endometriosis, Am J Obstet Gynecol 160:1344, 1989.

Simpson JL, Elias S, Malinak LR, et al: Heritable aspects of endometriosis, Am J Obstet Gynecol 137:327, 1980.

Stahl C and Grimes EM: Endometriosis of the small bowel: case reports and review of the literature, Obstet Gynecol Surv 42:131, 1987.

Stripling MC, Martin DC, Chatman DL, et al: Subtle appearance of pelvic endometriosis, Fertil Steril 49:427, 1988.

Suginami H, Hamada K, and Yano K: A case of endometriosis of the lung treated with danazol, Obstet Gynecol 66:68S, 1985.

Surrey ES, Gambone JC, Lu JKH, et al: The effects of combining norethindrone with a gonadotropin-releasing hormone agonist in the treatment of symptomatic endometriosis, Fertil Steril 53:620, 1990.

Sutton C and Hill D: Laser laparoscopy in the treatment of endometriosis: a 5-year study, Br J Obstet Gynaecol 97:181, 1990.

Syrop CH and Halme J: Peritoneal fluid environment and infertility, Fertil Steril 48:1, 1987.

Takahashi K, Yoshinok, Nagata H, et al: CA-125 is an effective marker for patients with external endometriosis and on danazol: case reports, Fertil Steril 50:173, 1988.

Takahashi K, Nagata H, Musa AA, et al: Clinical usefulness of CA-125 levels in the menstrual discharge in patients with endometriosis, Fertil Steril 54:360, 1990.

Telimaa S, Kauppila A, Rönnberg L, et al: Elevated serum levels of endometrial secretory protein PP14 in patients with advanced endometriosis, Am J Obstet Gynecol 161:866, 1989.

Torkelson SJ, Lee RA, and Hidahl DB: Endometriosis of the sciatic nerve: a report of two cases and a review of the literature, Obstet Gynecol 71:473, 1988.

Vancillie TG, Hill RH, Riehl RM, et al: Laser-induced fluorescence of ectopic endometrium in rabbits, Obstet Gynecol 74:225, 1989.

Vasquez G, Cornillie F, and Brosens IA: Peritoneal endometriosis: scanning electron microscopy and histology of minimal pelvic endometriotic lesions, Fertil Steril 42:696, 1984.

Weed JC and Ray JE: Endometriosis of the bowel, Obstet Gynecol 69:727, 1987.

West CP: Endometriosis: large scale studies needed to decide on definitive treatment, Br Med J 301:189, 1990.

Wheeler JM and Malinak LR: Recurrent endometriosis: incidence, management, and prognosis, Am J Obstet Gynecol 146:247, 1983.

Wheeler JM and Malinak LR: The surgical management of endometriosis, Obstet Gynecol Clin North Am 16:147, 1989.

Wild RA, Hirisave V, Bianco A, et al: Endometrial antibodies versus CA-125 for the detection of endometriosis, Fertil Steril 55:90, 1991.

Williams TJ and Pratt JH: Endometriosis in 1000 conservative celiotomies: incidence and management, Am J Obstet Gynecol 129:245, 1977.

Wolf GC and Singh KB: Cesarean scar endometriosis: a review, Obstet Gynecol Surv 44:89, 1989.

Yen SSC: Clinical applications of gonadotropin-releasing hormone and gonadotropin-releasing hormone analogs, Fertil Steril 39:257, 1983.

Zawin M, McCarthy S, Scoutt L, et al: Endometriosis: appearance and detection at MR imaging, Radiology 171:693, 1989.

Zorn JR, Mathieson J, Risquez F, et al: Treatment of endometriosis with a delayed release preparation of the agonist d-Trp[6]-luteinizing hormone-releasing hormone: long-term follow-up in a series of 50 patients, Fertil Steril 53:401, 1990.

Disorders of Abdominal Wall and Pelvic Support

Abdominal Wall Hernia. An outpouching of peritoneum, with or without intraabdominal contents, through weak areas of the abdominal wall.

Cystocele. Protrusion of the bladder into the vagina, signifying the relaxation of fascial supports of the bladder.

Descensus of Cervix and Uterus (Prolapse, Procidentia). Protrusion of the cervix and uterus into the barrel of the vagina.

First Degree. Prolapse into the upper vagina.

Second Degree. Prolapse to or near the introitus.

Third Degree (Complete). Prolapse through the introitus.

Enterocele. Herniation of the pouch of Douglas (cul-de-sac) between the uterosacral ligaments into the rectovaginal septum; usually contains small bowel.

Femoral Hernia. A hernia that occurs through the femoral triangle. The hernia sac passes beneath the inguinal ligament through Hesselbach's triangle (an area bounded laterally by the inferior epigastric artery, inferiorly by the inguinal ligament, and medially by the lateral margin of the rectus sheath).

Incarcerated Hernia. A hernia whose contents cannot be reduced readily.

Incisional Hernia. A hernia that occurs in a surgical incision.

Inguinal Hernia. A hernia that occurs through the inguinal canal.

Pessary. A prosthesis inserted into the vagina to help support pelvic structures.

Rectocele. Protrusion of the rectum into the vagina, signifying a relaxation of rectal supports.

Reducible Hernia. A hernia whose contents can be reduced from the sac.

Sliding Hernia. A hernia in which the organ protruding makes up a portion of the wall of the hernia sac.

Spigelian Hernia. A rare hernia at a point where the vertical linea semilunaris joins the lateral border of the rectus muscle.

Strangulated Hernia. A hernia whose contents are incarcerated and whose blood supply to the content's structures is compromised.

Umbilical Hernia. A hernia protruding through the umbilicus.

Urethrocele. Protrusion of the urethra into the vagina, signifying loss of fascial supports of the urethra.

The structural supports of the abdomen and pelvis are susceptible to a number of stresses. In the female these supports are affected by congenital anatomic weaknesses, the stresses of childbearing, injury, surgical damage, and straining. In addition, a combination of chronic stresses, such as lifting heavy objects, straining at stool, or activities that require frequent stretching, plus the aging process, may make older women more susceptible to such abnormalities. This chapter considers hernias of the abdominal wall and pelvic region, as well as conditions that are a result of the loss of pelvic supports.

ABDOMINAL WALL HERNIAS

The abdominal wall is made up of the following structures beginning externally: skin; subcutaneous connective tissue; external oblique, internal oblique, and transversus abdominis muscles with their investing fascia; and parietal peritoneum. The rectus abdominis muscles run longitudinally in the midline from the xiphoid to the pubic symphysis. The investing fasciae of the external oblique, internal oblique, and transversus abdominis muscles completely encase the rectus abdominis muscles cephalic to the semilunar line. Caudally from the semilunar line the muscle is completely behind the aponeurosis of the fasciae of these muscles and lies directly on the peritoneum (Figure 19-1). Normally the investing fasciae join in the midline after surrounding the rectus abdominis muscles.

In the male the descent of the testes from their original retroperitoneal site to the scrotum necessitates passing through the abdominal wall to the inguinal region. At the level of the transversalis fascia where the descent begins, the internal inguinal ring is formed. The medial margin of this ring is defined by the inferior epigastric artery as it courses from the external iliac artery medially and superiorly into the rectus sheath. The inguinal canal runs from the internal inguinal ring obliquely downward, emerging through the external inguinal ring and opening in the external oblique aponeurosis just above the pubic spine and then continuing into the scrotum. This allows for passage of the testes and for the presence of part of the spermatic cord.

In the female the round ligament courses in the same direction but ends short of the labia. An inguinal hernia, that is, a bulge of peritoneum through the internal inguinal ring and into the inguinal canal, is less common in the female than in the male and is frequently identified after stretching of the abdominal wall during or after pregnancy. It may be related to a congenital weakness of this area. Occasionally a femoral-type groin hernia may develop. In this case the defect in the transversalis fascia occurs in Hesselbach's triangle, which is an area bounded laterally by the inferior epigastric artery, inferiorly by the inguinal ligament, and medially by the lateral margin of the rectus sheath (Figure 19-2). The hernia sac passes under the inguinal ligament into the femoral triangle rather than coursing through the inguinal

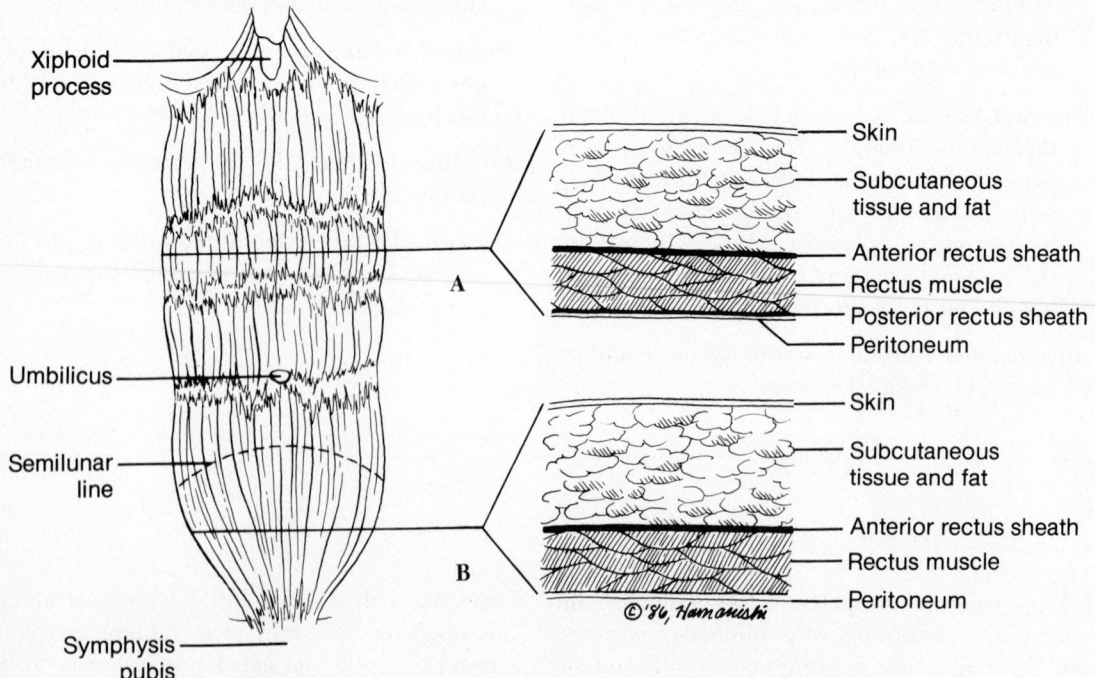

Xiphoid process

Skin

Subcutaneous tissue and fat

Anterior rectus sheath
Rectus muscle
Posterior rectus sheath
Peritoneum

A

Umbilicus

Skin

Subcutaneous tissue and fat

Semilunar line

Anterior rectus sheath
Rectus muscle
Peritoneum

B

©'86, Hamanishi

Symphysis pubis

FIGURE 19-1
Graphic representation of layers of the abdominal wall. **A,** Above semilunar line. **B,** Below semilunar line.

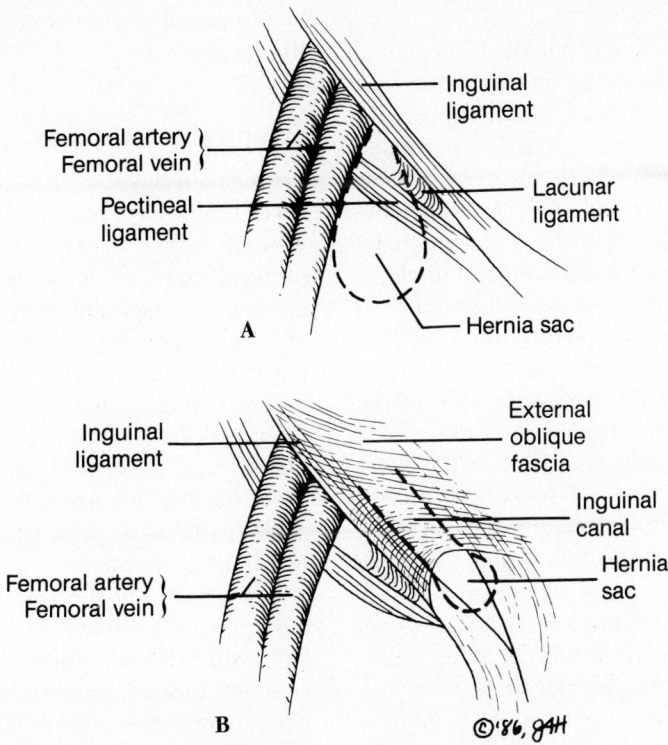

FIGURE 19-2
Graphic representation of right femoral (**A**) and right inguinal (**B**) hernias in the female.

canal. Femoral hernias are more common in females than in males.

The hernia is said to be *reducible* if the contents can be returned to the abdominal cavity. If the contents cannot be reduced, the hernia is said to be incarcerated. An incarcerated hernia may be acute, accompanied by pain, or may be longstanding and asymptomatic. If the blood supply to the incarcerated structure is compromised, the hernia is said to be *strangulated*. Because the hernia sac is primarily prolapsed peritoneum, the hernia itself is not strangulated but only its contents.

On rare occasions a portion of the wall of the hernia sac is composed of an organ such as the sigmoid colon or the cecum. In these instances the hernia is called a *sliding hernia*.

A ventral hernia occurs in the abdominal wall away from the groin. Examples include umbilical hernias, which are caused by congenital relaxation of the umbilical ring, and incisional hernias, which are herniations through separation of fascial planes after operative incision. Two special ventral hernias include the epigastric hernia, which occurs in a defect of the linea alba above the umbilicus, and the

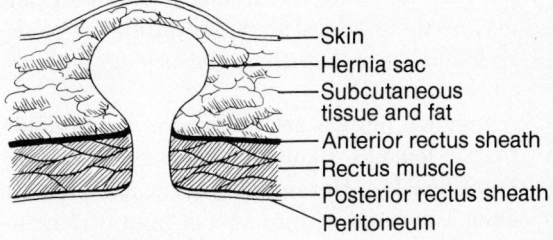

FIGURE 19-3
Graphic representation of umbilical hernia.

rare spigelian hernia, which is a herniation at a point where the vertical linea semilunaris joins the lateral border of the rectus muscle.

Incisional hernias generally involve the separation of the fascia of the abdominal wall with the hernia sac palpated beneath the skin and subcutaneous tissue. The sac wall is composed of peritoneum.

Because the umbilicus consists of a fusion of skin, fascia, and peritoneum, an umbilical hernia generally occurs because the fascial ring is grossly separated, allowing the hernia sac to protrude. This occurs most frequently in obese women. The hernia sac itself is made up of peritoneum and subcutaneous tissue beneath the skin (Figure 19-3).

Etiology

Hernias may be the result of a congenital malformation. The umbilical hernia is the best example. Before 10 weeks' gestation the abdominal contents are partially herniated through the umbilicus into the extra embryonic coelomic cavity. However, after 10 weeks the viscera normally return to the abdominal cavity, and the defect in the abdominal wall closes during subsequent fetal growth. Generally at birth only the space occupied by the umbilical cord remains patent. Following the cutting of the cord the area heals so that the skin in the area of the umbilicus fuses above the closed fascial layer. Some infants at birth will show a small umbilical hernia, but in most instances the fascial defect closes during the first 3 years of life. If it does not close, an umbilical hernia will form. In rare cases the abdominal wall closure process is less complete, leading to an omphalocele, which is a hernia sac at the umbilicus covered only by peritoneum and including bowel and other abdominal contents. Omphaloceles are usually seen in infants with other malformations and possibly chromosome anomalies, such as trisomy 13.

Black infants have umbilical hernias more often than do white. Occasionally umbilical hernias occur in adults after the distention of the abdominal cavity with pregnancy or with ascites.

Inguinal hernias are more common in males than in females. Femoral hernias occur primarily in females. Hernias that occur in adults are often associated with trauma or injury. In many instances the hernia bulge develops slowly after years of heavy labor. It is likely that a congenital anatomic defect was always present but became exaggerated over time, leading to the development of a hernia. Zimmerman and Anson thought that such lesions resulted from inadequate muscle support at the lower area of the inguinal canal, primarily caused by a defect in the internal oblique muscle. Stretching of this area in pregnancy may initiate a hernia, but other factors, such as chronic cough caused by smoking or chronic respiratory disease, may be responsible.

Incisional hernias generally occur because of poor healing of the fascia. This may be secondary to poor nutrition, infection, or necrosis of the fascia secondary to suturing. It may also occur because absorbable suture loses its tensile strength before healing is complete. Stress and strain secondary to chronic cough or retching in the postoperative period may contribute to the process.

Symptoms and Signs

Bulges in the abdominal wall lead to the discovery of most ventral or groin hernias in women, either by a physician at the time of physical examination or by the patient. These hernias are generally symptom free. Occasionally, excessive straining or trauma will be implicated, and the patient may experience a feeling of tearing of tissue. Frequently the bulges are noted during an increase in intraabdominal pressure, such as with pregnancy or ascites. Most hernias are asymptomatic, but in some cases, particularly with larger ones, there may be aching or discomfort. Should intraabdominal organs move into the sac, the patient may experience some discomfort. Organs that strangulate within the sac cause acute pain and discomfort. Incarcerated organs may give nonspecific visceral pain, which is most likely the result of mesenteric stretching.

In cases where a hernia exists but no contents are within the sac, physical examination reveals a weakening at the site of the hernia. It is often possible to feel the "ring" of the hernia as one palpates the defect through the skin and subcutaneous tissue. The patient's straining will generally accentuate the hernia, making it more palpable and visible. In the case of inguinal and femoral hernias it may be necessary for the patient to be standing for one to palpate the hernia.

When there are intraabdominal contents within the hernia sac, the hernia is more easily palpated. The physician should then decide, based on his or her attempts to gently milk the contents from the sac back through the defect ring, whether the contents are reducible. For a hernia that does not reduce easily but in which there is no evidence of vascular compromise it is sometimes useful to apply ice packs to the abdomen in the area of the incarcerated hernia before additional attempts are made to reduce it. In cases of strangulated hernia, evidence of devitalization of an organ, such as fever, leukocytosis, and evidence for an acute abdomen, may be noted.

Management

Nonoperative management of hernias of the ventral wall and groin in women is often feasible. Umbilical hernias in little girls will generally close by age 3 or 4 years and rarely become incarcerated. An incisional hernia, if not too large, can frequently be managed by a corset, which prevents it from becoming incarcerated. Unincarcerated groin hernias are often small and become uncomfortable only with an increase in intraabdominal pressure, such as occurs with pregnancy. Many authors advocate repair, however, because the small neck of these hernias may make incarceration more likely. With pregnancy the opportunity for incarceration is reduced because the increasing size of the uterus pushes bowel contents away from the area of the herniation. Trusses and other supports are generally difficult to fit and are of little value in women.

Larger hernias, hernias that continuously contain intraabdominal contents, hernias that cause continuing discomfort, and those that have been incarcerated should be repaired. Some general principles of operative repair can be stated. The first principle involves the anatomy of the hernia. The hernia almost always consists of a sac of peritoneum with a narrow neck and a fascial defect of some sort. In rare instances, if a peritoneal sac is broad based, it may be possible to simply reduce the sac through the fascial defect without opening it and then to repair the fascial defect. However, if a narrow-necked sac exists, it must be dissected free of the fascial defect, emptied of its contents, and then excised and sutured at the neck (base). The fascial defect is then mobilized completely to remove stress and scarring, and

it is closed with permanent suture. In rare cases the fascial defect may be large and the degree of mobilization that is required may be impossible. In such instances, patching with inert material, such as Mersilene mesh, may be necessary. This is rarely required in women except in the presence of large incisional hernias.

The second principle involves management of the contents of the hernia sac. Usually the hernia sac reduces with ease, but if intraabdominal contents are fixed to the sac wall by adhesions, the sac must be opened and the adhesions carefully separated. Care must be taken not to damage the organs or their blood supply. When these organs are reduced from the sac, the sac may be handled in the usual fashion. When incarceration has occurred, the organs must be inspected for viability before replacement.

Umbilical Hernia

A curved incision is made at the inferior margin of the umbilicus (Figure 19-4). The umbilicus is dissected free of the sac and reflected upward. The sac is then dissected free of the fascial defect and either reduced or excised, depending on the circumstances. The fascial edges are freshened and either closed by direct approximation anterior to posterior using nonabsorbable sutures or mobilized and closed in a "vest over pants" manner, suturing the anterior edge to the posterior edge in an overlapping fashion. Studies have not shown that either of these closures is superior to the other, and the

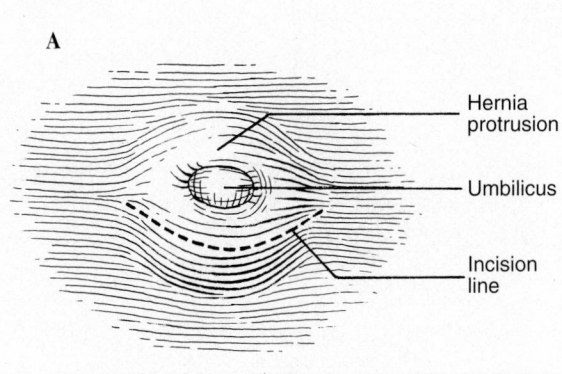

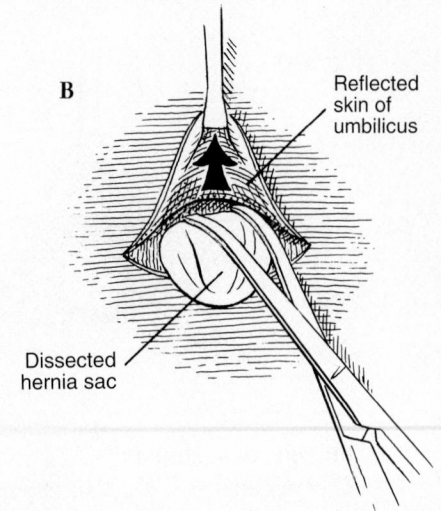

FIGURE 19-4
Repair of umbilical hernia. **A,** Site of incision. **B,** Umbilicus dissected free of sac and reflected upward.　　　　　　　　　　　　　　*Continued.*

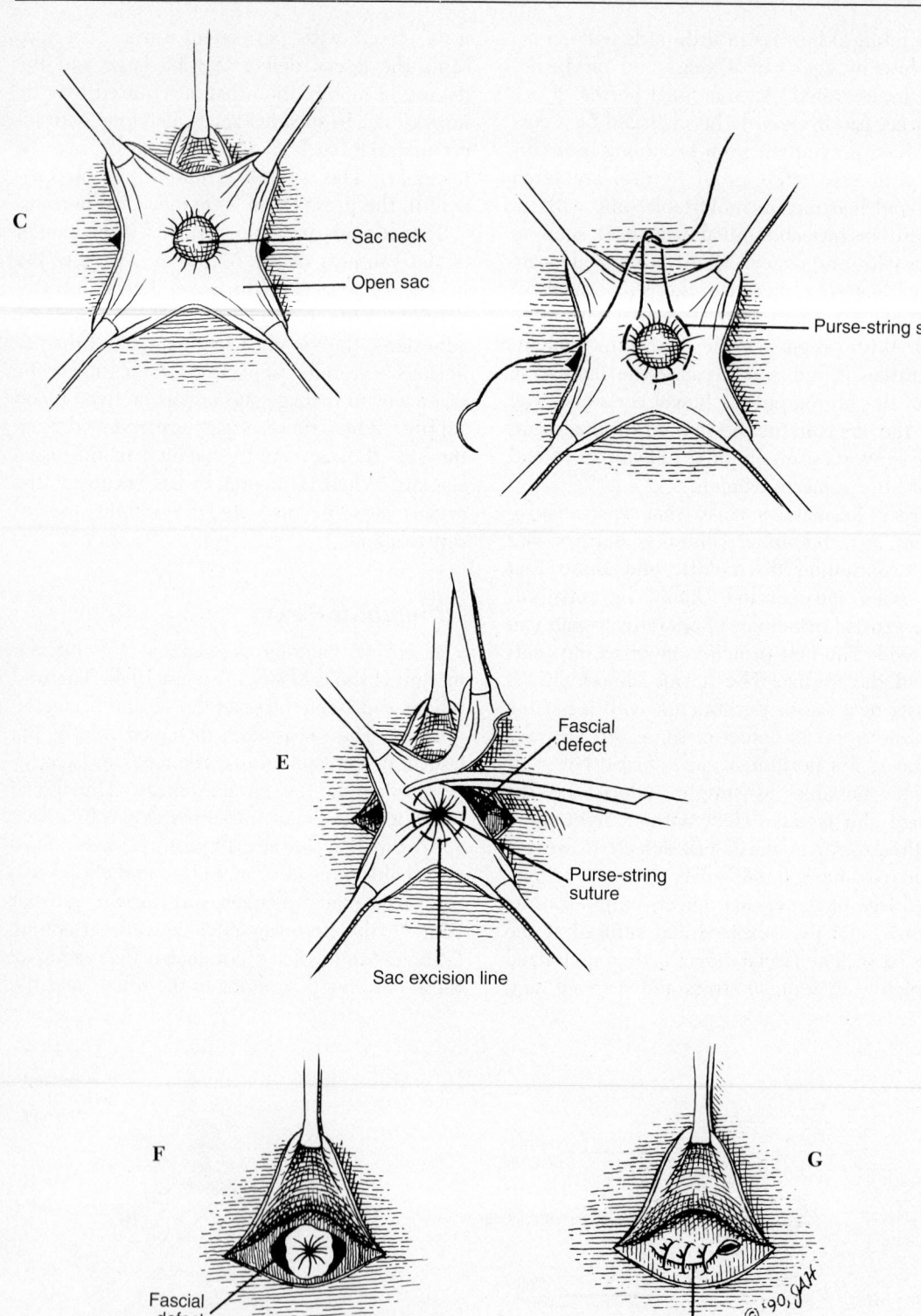

FIGURE 19-4, cont'd
C, Appearance of sac that is cut open. **D,** Placement of purse-string suture at neck of sac. **E,** Sac dissected free of fascial defect after suture is tied. **F,** Appearance of fascial defect after sac excised. **G,** Fascial defect closed; umbilicus will be tacked to it.

approach taken generally is the one that best fits the circumstances. The umbilicus is then tacked to the fascial defect and the skin margin approximated.

Incisional Hernia

Repair of an incisional hernia can be accomplished by incising the skin through the old scar or via a parallel incision and dissecting through the subcutaneous tissue to identify both margins of the separated fascial defect. The peritoneum of the hernia sac is then isolated, dissected free of the margins, and reduced in the most appropriate fashion, with the surgeon exercising care not to damage any organs that may be fixed in the sac by adhesions. The fascial edges are then mobilized completely and closed side to side with interrupted nonabsorbable suture. Rarely the defect is so large that a patch has to be sutured over the defect. With care, however, it is generally possible to mobilize the fascia so that this is not necessary.

Groin Hernia

To repair an inguinal or femoral hernia, an incision is made above the inguinal ligament, usually parallel to its medial portion. Subcutaneous tissue is separated, and the aponeurosis of the external oblique muscle is exposed. The external oblique is then incised from above down through the external inguinal ring, with the surgeon taking care to avoid the ilioinguinal nerve, which is frequently adherent to the external ring. The sac is identified and by careful dissection excised down to its emergence through the transversalis fascia. The sac is opened, and the intraperitoneal contents are reduced. The surgeon should place his or her finger through the sac neck into the peritoneal cavity and palpate the structures immediately within to be sure that there are no other hernia sacs protruding, particularly into the femoral canal. The sac neck is then ligated and transfixed away from the ring, often to Cooper's ligament. The transversalis fascia is approximated with nonabsorbable suture. The external oblique aponeurosis is then closed with nonabsorbable suture, and the skin and subcutaneous tissue are closed. Occasionally on opening the external oblique aponeurosis, only a mass of fat is found. In such instances the diagnosis of a

hernia was made in error and no sac is present. Often, however, there is both fat and a sac, and the surgeon must be careful to determine the contents of the inguinal canal.

Femoral Hernia

When the sac is protruding beneath the inguinal ligament and through the femoral canal, an attempt may be made to reduce it from above. Frequently it is necessary to incise the inguinal ligament to free up the sac neck. In either case the sac should be ligated at its base, with the surgeon making sure that its contents are not damaged and that they are reduced. The sac, as in all cases, is generally handled by excision of excess peritoneum and placing a purse-string suture of absorbable material about the base. Although it is probably not necessary to repair the inguinal ligament, most surgeons will do so. To prevent recurrent hernia in the transversalis fascia, the sac neck is sutured to Cooper's ligament beneath the inguinal ligament. To support the transversalis fascia repair, the external oblique aponeurosis is sutured over the transversalis fascia for extra support, all with interrupted, nonabsorbable suture material.

DISORDERS OF PELVIC SUPPORT

Pelvic support structures are often weakened by childbirth, other pelvic trauma, stress and strain, and the aging process. Abnormalities that result from these relaxation problems include urethrocele, cystocele, rectocele, enterocele, and uterine prolapse (descensus of the cervix and uterus). If a hysterectomy has been performed, prolapse of the vagina may also be a problem. It is unusual to have only one of these conditions. In most cases the relaxation affects all the support structures of the pelvis. Frequently relaxation of the urethra, the bladder neck, and the bladder (urethrocele, cystocele) is associated with urinary incontinence, which is discussed in Chapter 20.

Urethrocele and Cystocele

Attenuation or rupture of the pubovesicle cervical fascia for any reason may allow the descent of the urethra (urethrocele), bladder neck, or bladder (cystocele) into the vaginal ca-

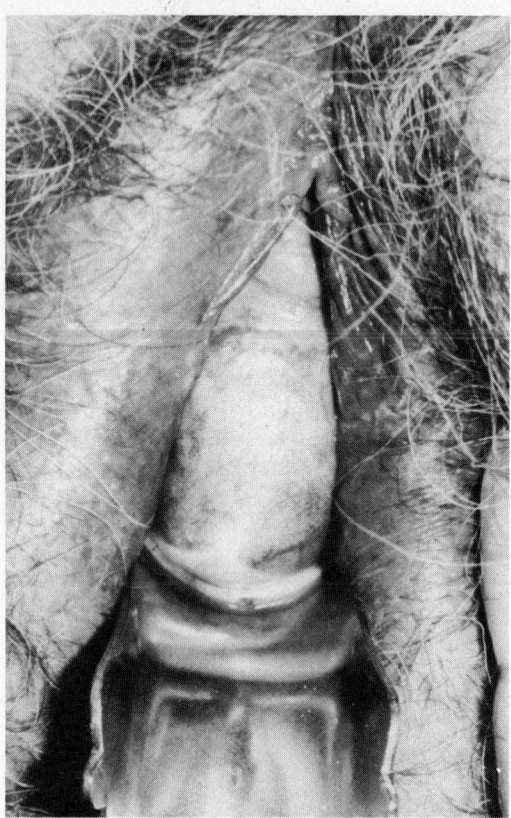

FIGURE 19-5
Cystocele.

nal. Often only a cystocele is present (Figure 19-5), and generally in these cases the patient is continent. When a urethrocele is present as well, the woman usually suffers from stress incontinence. Urethroceles seem to be more common in women with wide subpubic arches (gynecoid type), which allow the full force of the fetal head against this area during descent in labor. Narrower arches, such as those associated with the android or anthropoid pelvic types, seem to protect this region from the descent of the fetal head.

Symptoms and Signs

Symptoms and signs of urethrocele and cystocele consist of a sensation of fullness or pressure and at times a feeling that organs are falling out, stress incontinence, occasional urgency, and often a feeling of incomplete emptying with voiding. The patient and the physician note a soft bulging mass of the anterior vaginal wall. In some patients this must be replaced manually before the patient can void.

Strain or cough accentuates the bulge. The mass may descend to or beyond the introitus. Although urethroceles and cystoceles almost always occur in parous women, they have been noted in nulliparous women who have poor structural supports. This is particularly true in women who have congenital malformations or weaknesses of the endopelvic connective tissue and musculature of the pelvic floor. Most parous women demonstrate some degree of cystocele, and when asymptomatic, they do not require therapy.

Diagnosis

The urethrocele and the cystocele are best demonstrated with a patient in the lithotomy position. A retractor or posterior wall blade of a Graves speculum is used to depress the posterior wall. The patient is then asked to strain, and the degree of the cystocele or urethrocele is noted. The physician should palpate the bladder neck and note whether it is well supported. Generally, if the supports of the bladder neck are adequate, the urethra is adequately supported. If a cystocele and a urethrocele are present, it invariably follows that the bladder neck is not supported. The examination for cystocele and urethrocele is best performed with the bladder at least partially filled (100 to 250 ml).

Urethroceles must be differentiated from inflamed and enlarged Skene's glands and urethral diverticula. Cystoceles must be differentiated from bladder tumors and bladder diverticula, both of which are rare but may occur. Urethroceles and cystoceles are generally soft, pliable, and nontender. Although diverticula may be reducible, a sensation of a mass is usually present. Inflamed Skene's glands are generally tender, and it may be possible to express pus from the urethra when they are palpated. Pus may be expressed also in the presence of a diverticulum of the urethra. In such cases gonococcal and chlamydial infections should be considered.

Management

Treatment of urethroceles and cystoceles may be nonoperative or operative. Nonoperative treatment consists of supporting the herniation of the bladder into the vagina with the use of Smith-Hodge or inflatable pessary (see

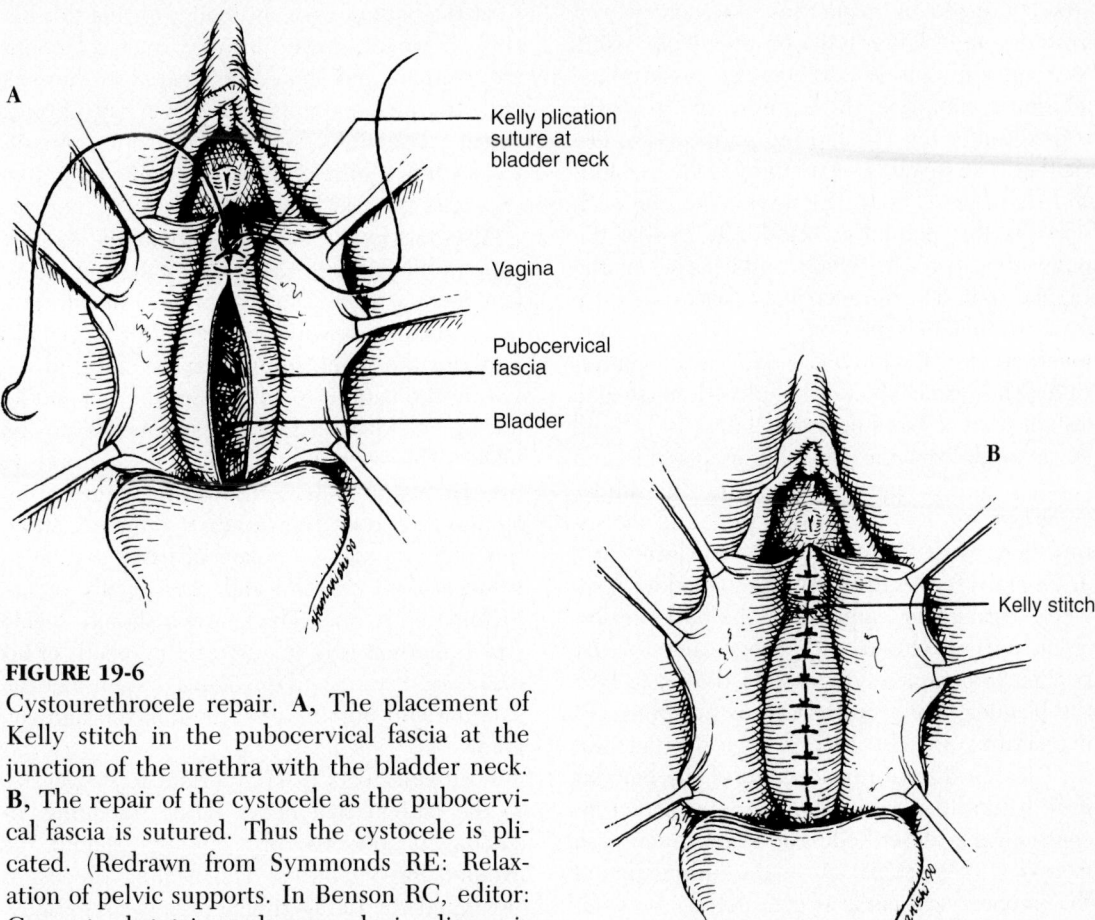

FIGURE 19-6

Cystourethrocele repair. **A,** The placement of Kelly stitch in the pubocervical fascia at the junction of the urethra with the bladder neck. **B,** The repair of the cystocele as the pubocervical fascia is sutured. Thus the cystocele is plicated. (Redrawn from Symmonds RE: Relaxation of pelvic supports. In Benson RC, editor: Current obstetric and gynecologic diagnosis and treatment, ed 5, Los Altos, Calif, 1984, Lange Medical Publications.)

Figure 19-12) or even with the intermittent use of a large tampon. Kegel exercises (see Chapter 20) help to strengthen the pelvic floor musculature and thereby may relieve some of the pressure symptoms produced by the cystocele. In an older woman the use of estrogen systemically or in a vaginal cream may improve both the tone of the pelvic support structures and the vascular supply of these tissues.

A younger woman with a large cystocele should be encouraged to avoid operative repair until she has completed her family. Occasionally the abnormality is so uncomfortable that repair must be performed before childbearing is complete. If this is the case, cesarean delivery should be considered for subsequent pregnancies.

Operative repair of a cystocele is generally performed in conjunction with the repair of a rectocele. It is unusual for anterior supports of the vagina to relax without an accompanying

relaxation of the posterior wall. Repair, therefore, usually consists of an anterior and posterior colporrhaphy. If uterine descensus is noted, this must also be treated. Frequently an enterocele accompanies a cystocele and rectocele and where present must be excised. These problems are discussed later in this chapter.

Anterior wall repair (colporrhaphy) is performed by incising the vaginal epithelium transversely just above the anterior lip of the cervix in the region of the bladder reflection (Figure 19-6). If the woman has undergone a hysterectomy in the past, the incision may be made approximately 1 to 1.5 cm anterior to the vaginal scar. The vagina is then incised longitudinally from the transverse incision to the level of the bladder neck. If no urethrocele is present, this incision is sufficient. If a urethrocele is present, the incision must be continued under the urethra as well. The longitudinal incision is made by separating the vaginal wall from the underlying tissue progressively, using Metzenbaum scissors. When the longitudinal incision is complete, the cut edge of the vagina is held under tension and the pubocervical fascia that is attached is separated from it by blunt and sharp dissection. This is repeated on each side. At this point the bladder is free of the pubocervical fascia, which is itself free of the vaginal wall. The surgeon then places a suture over the bladder neck (Kelly stitch), bringing together the pubocervical fasciae on either side. The stitch should be placed in such a fashion that the pubocervical fascia is sutured as far away from the cut edge as possible and parallel to the previous incision. A similar stitch is taken on the opposite side, and the suture tied. Most appropriate for this closure is 0 or 2-0 polyglycol suture. With the bladder neck well identified and supported, the pubocervical fascia is then closed with progressive similar stitches to completely imbricate the fascia over the bladder. If the urethrocele is present, similar sutures are also placed over the urethra. (In Chapter 20 the replacement of the bladder neck behind the pubic symphysis to correct incontinence is described. The reader may wish to review these steps.) After the imbrication of the pubocervical fascia is completed, the vaginal edges are trimmed and the vagina closed with a row of interrupted 2-0 polyglycol or catgut sutures.

Postoperatively the bladder should be drained for about 5 days. There are several ways to accomplish this. The first is to leave a No. 16 Foley catheter in place for 5 days, remove the catheter on the fifth day, and allow the patient to try to void. After voiding of at least 100 to 200 ml the patient should be catheterized for the presence of residual urine. If residual urine is found in a quantity of more than 150 ml on two successive voidings or if the amount voided is less than 100 ml, the physician should consider replacing the catheter for 24 to 48 hours. If residual urine amounts are less than 150 ml on two consecutive voidings, no further steps are necessary. Occasionally, after an anterior repair, voiding does not occur after 5 days of bladder drainage. At that point the patient may require catheterization for 24 to 48 hours longer, or she may be discharged with a Foley catheter in place for continuous drainage for a week, to be rechecked for voiding and residual urine as an outpatient in 1 week. It is rarely necessary to treat the patient with antibiotics during this period; however, lower urinary tract infections are common and should be treated as they occur. In some patients who have had chronic urinary tract infections, prophylactic antibiotics, such as a sulfa preparation or nitrofurantoin (Furadantin), can be administered.

Alternatives to the above regimen include suprapubic catheter drainage or placing an infant feeding tube (No. 5) through the urethra and attaching it with a labial suture. In both methods the drainage tube can be clamped, allowing the patient to void when she can and allowing residual urine measurements to be taken. The suprapubic technique is simple to use and seems to have a lower incidence of infection than does transurethral catheterization, but patients may complain of extravasation of urine around the site and occasionally of hematoma formation. The surgeon should decide which method is best suited to the needs of his or her institution and develop a system that the surgeon and nursing team understand and can follow.

Postoperatively it is important to emphasize to the patient that heavy lifting, straining, or prolonged periods of standing should be avoided for 3 months. The healing process is slow, and the tissue is generally weak initially. Complete healing should be ensured before the tissue is stressed by normal activities.

Rectocele

Symptoms and Signs

The patient with a rectocele often complains of a heavy or "falling out" feeling in the vagina. She may complain of constipation and occasionally may need to splint the vagina with her fingers to effect a bowel movement. She may also have a feeling of incomplete emptying of the rectum at the time of the bowel movement.

Diagnosis

A rectocele may be identified by retracting the anterior vaginal wall upward and again having the patient strain. The rectum will bulge into the vagina, and this bulge may protrude through the introitus (Figure 19-7). The physician should then place one finger in the rectum and one in the vagina and palpate the hernia. Often the rectovaginal septum is paper thin, and the rectocele can be palpated to its upper margin. If an enterocele is present, it may be

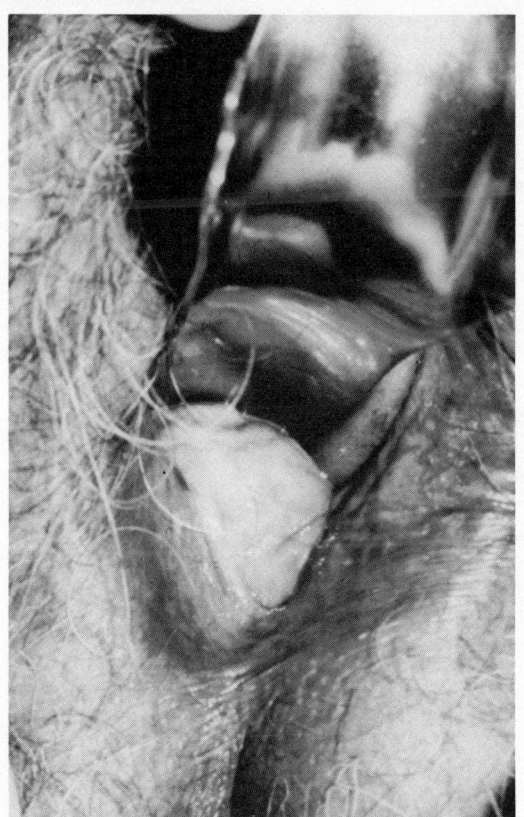

FIGURE 19-7
Rectocele.

possible to differentiate it from the rectocele by having the patient strain. Frequently, however, the diagnosis of a small enterocele is established only at the time of operation.

Management

Nonoperative management of a rectocele is similar to that mentioned for a cystocele. Pessaries, Kegel exercises, and estrogen may be useful in the appropriate situations.

Operative management of a rectocele (posterior colporrhaphy) is generally performed at the time of an anterior colporrhaphy with or without enterocele repair or operation for descensus. Most women with rectoceles also have gaping vaginas and weakness in their perineal body. Therefore as part of a rectocele repair a perineorrhaphy is performed as well. The surgeon should estimate at the time of starting the posterior repair what degree of perineorrhaphy he or she wishes to perform. The margins of the perineum to be narrowed are generally marked by placing Allis clamps at their extreme at the introital opening (Figure 19-8).

The tissue of the introitus is then incised between these clamps, and the vaginal wall is separated from the underlying tissue and rectum in a progressive manner longitudinally in the midline, beginning at the introital incision and being carried forward to the apex of the vagina above the limit of the rectocele. This is done by progressive separation and incision using the Metzenbaum scissors in a fashion similar to that described for cystocele repair.

When the vaginal wall is completely incised, the edges are grasped and placed under tension, and the perirectal connective tissue is separated from the vaginal mucosa by blunt and sharp (if necessary) dissection. This is carried out bilaterally until it is possible for the operator to palpate the perirectal space on each side. The operator then places a finger of his nondominant hand into the rectum using a double-glove technique while an assistant picks up perirectal tissue on either side. The operator then places an 0 nonabsorbable suture (silk or dermalon) into the perirectal tissue on either side. Approximately three to five of these stitches are placed, and these are held without tying. The operator should use his or her finger in the rectum to ensure that no suture is placed into the rectum. The perirectal tissue usually includes portions of the levator ani muscles. When the sutures are tied, these tissues are interposed between rectum and vagina, thereby reducing the rectocele. These sutures also serve to tack the vagina to the levator ani area, thereby, it is hoped, avoiding future vaginal prolapse if a hysterectomy has also been performed. The vaginal edges are then trimmed and the vagina closed with a row of either continuous or interrupted catgut suture.

Attention is then turned to the perineorrhaphy, which is closed in the following fashion. Polyglycol sutures are placed in the lateral margins of the transverse incision, essentially bringing bulbocavernosal muscles together from either side to the midline. The operator should be sure that the bulbocavernosal muscle insertions are included in the sutures by pulling on the suture and noting whether the tension identifies the muscle bundles. The remainder of the perineal incision is then closed with a row of 2-0 polyglycol sutures to the deep tissue, and the skin of the perineum is closed with either interrupted or continuous subcuticular suture of 3-0 chromic catgut or polyglycol.

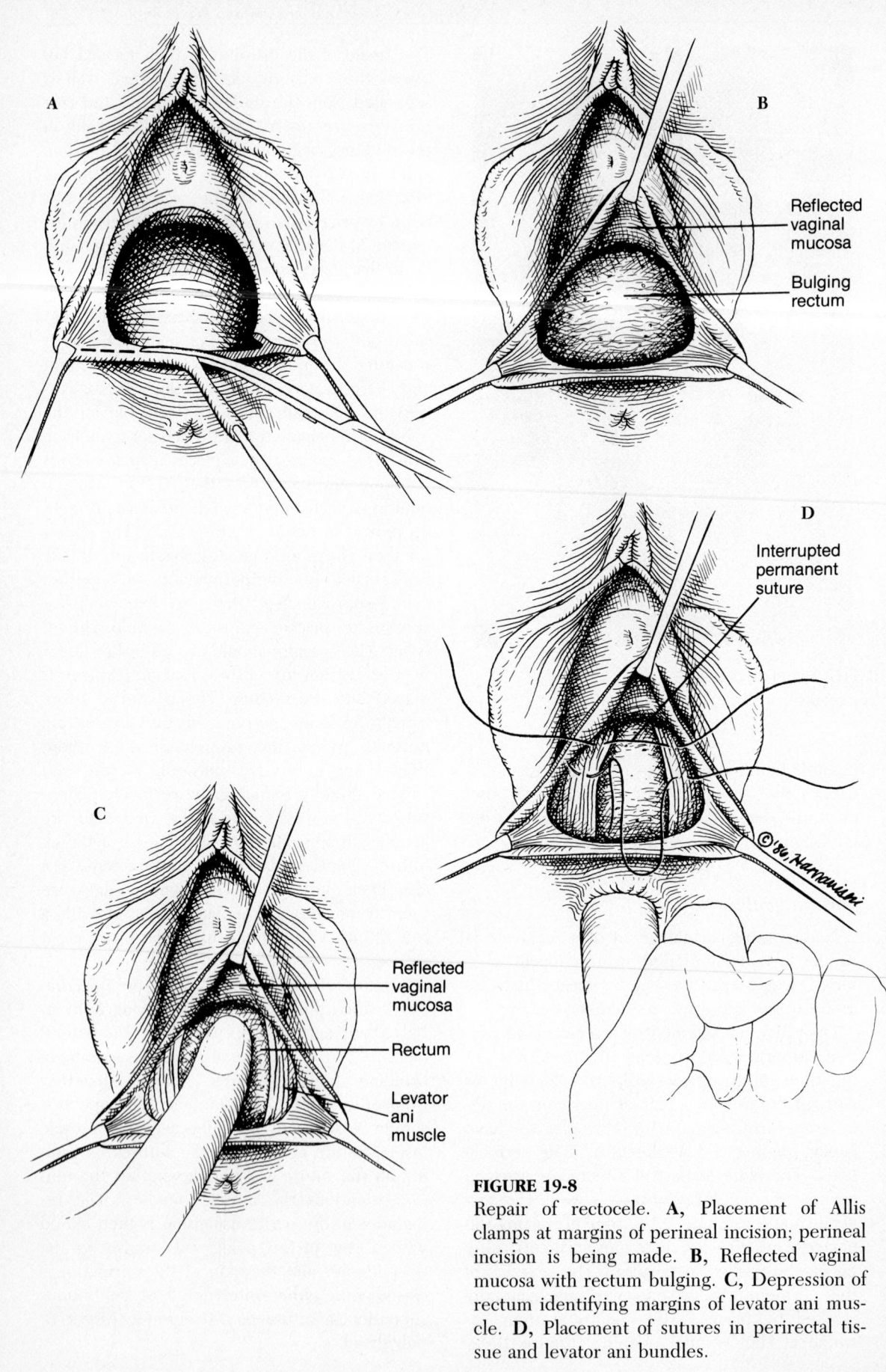

FIGURE 19-8
Repair of rectocele. **A,** Placement of Allis clamps at margins of perineal incision; perineal incision is being made. **B,** Reflected vaginal mucosa with rectum bulging. **C,** Depression of rectum identifying margins of levator ani muscle. **D,** Placement of sutures in perirectal tissue and levator ani bundles.

Enterocele

Enteroceles frequently occur after an abdominal or vaginal hysterectomy and generally are the result of a weakened support for the pouch of Douglas. In the prevention of enteroceles, the uterosacral and cardinal ligaments are the most important support structures and should be incorporated into the vault repair at the time of a hysterectomy and the ligaments from each side joined together.

Diagnosis

An enterocele is not always easy to diagnose. It is a true hernia of the peritoneal cavity emanating from the pouch of Douglas between the uterosacral ligaments and into the rectovaginal septum (Figure 19-9). It may be noticed as a separate bulge above the rectocele, and at times it may be large enough to prolapse through the vagina (Figure 19-10). If such is the case, it may be possible to make the specific diagnosis of enterocele by transilluminating the bulge and seeing small bowel shadows within the sac. It may also be possible to differentiate the enterocele from a rectocele by rectovaginal examination. The contents of an enterocele are always small bowel and may also include omentum. The contents may be easily reducible or may be fixed to the peritoneum of the sac by adhesions.

Management

Enteroceles may be reduced transabdominally as a primary procedure or at the time of other abdominal procedures. In the primary procedure the sac should be reduced upward if possible, and if the uterosacral ligaments are present, these may be brought together in the midline. If the uterosacral ligaments cannot be identified, as with large enteroceles after previously performed hysterectomy, the cul-de-sac may be obliterated by concentric purse-string sutures in the endopelvic fascia. Care must be taken to avoid damaging the ureters, rectum, and sigmoid colon. It is best to perform this procedure with permanent suture. The enterocele has probably occurred because of weakening of pelvic floor structures. Therefore, for optimum results, repair of the lower pelvis using a vaginal approach is probably indicated, even though the enterocele is obliterated abdominally.

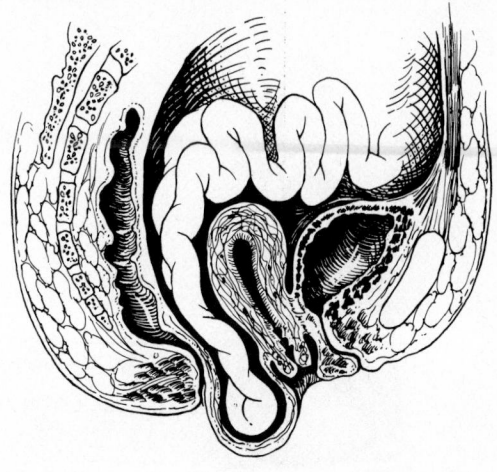

FIGURE 19-9
Enterocele and uterine prolapse. (Reproduced, with permission, from Symmonds RE: Relaxation of pelvic supports. In Benson RC, editor: Current obstetric and gynecologic diagnosis and treatment, ed 5, Copyright 1984, Lange Medical Publications, Los Altos, Calif.)

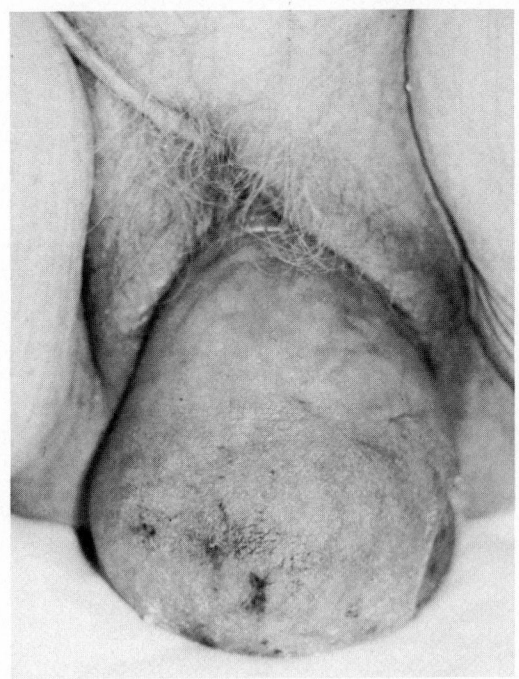

FIGURE 19-10
Elderly patient with vaginal prolapse who proved to have large enterocele with ulcers on the vagina.

Repair of the enterocele can be carried out at the time of the posterior colporrhaphy. The sac will be visualized as the vagina is separated from the rectum. The sac must then be dis-

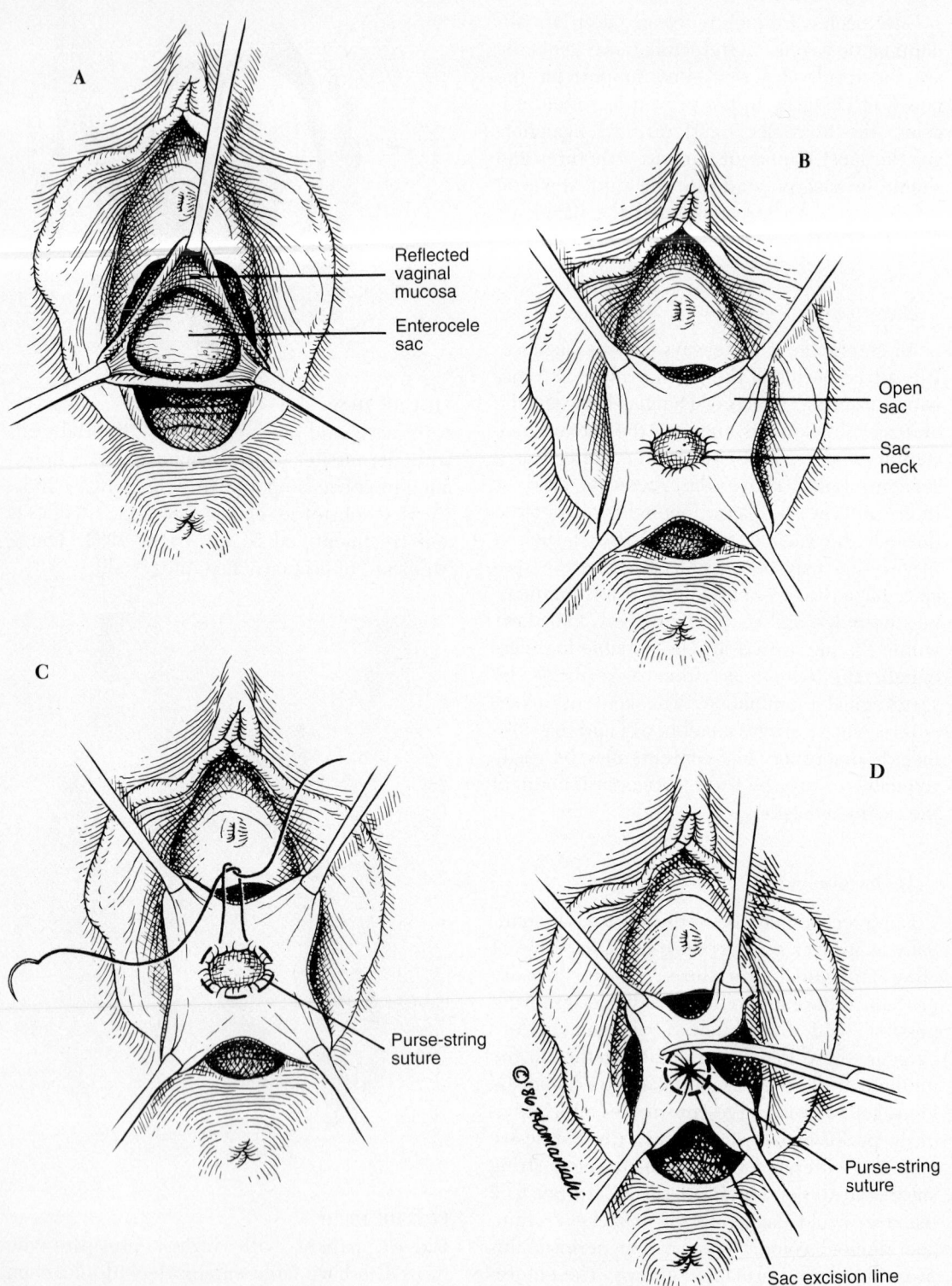

FIGURE 19-11
Repair of enterocele. **A,** Appearance of enterocele sac with vaginal wall reflected.
B, Appearance of open enterocele sac with sac neck identified. **C,** Placing of purse-
string suture at the neck of the enterocele sac. **D,** Excision of enterocele sac.

sected free of underlying tissue and isolated at its neck. It should be opened to ensure that all contents are replaced. The neck of the hernia is then sutured with a purse-string 0-chromic or polyglycol suture ligature and the sac excised (Figure 19-11).

It is important to support the neck of the enterocele sac as much as possible. If uterosacral ligaments can be identified or if they are present when a vaginal hysterectomy has been performed in association with an enterocele repair, they should be used in the repair. This can be accomplished by fixing the uterosacral ligaments to the peritoneum of the sac and the vaginal vault using a suture of 0 polyglycol, beginning on one side of the vagina and continuing through the uterosacral ligament of that side, the peritoneum of the sac, and the uterosacral ligament and vagina of the opposite side. Multiple sutures can be placed if space allows. This technique was described by McCall and is often called the *McCall stitch*. It effectively shortens the cul-de-sac and supports the enterocele neck. If uterosacral ligaments cannot be identified, as is often the case if the uterus has been previously removed, the rectocele repair should be continued to the area of the enterocele sac neck to reinforce this area and support the cul-de-sac as high as possible.

Correctly repaired enteroceles usually will not recur. Enteroceles repaired without proper attention to ligation of the neck of the sac and without appropriate rectocele repair may recur. In such cases a subsequent operation with special attention to these surgical principles is indicated.

Uterine Prolapse (Descensus, Procidentia)

Descensus of the uterus and cervix into or through the barrel of the vagina is associated with injuries of the endopelvic fascia, including the cardinal and uterosacral ligaments, as well as injury to or relaxation of the pelvic floor muscles, particularly the levator ani muscles. Occasionally prolapse is the result of increased intraabdominal pressure, such as with ascites or large pelvic or intraabdominal tumors superimposed on poor pelvic supports. In some instances, sacral nerve disorders, especially injuries to S1 to S4, or diabetic neuropathy may be responsible. Associated factors that increase tension on pelvic floor musculature, such as chronic respiratory disease including chronic bronchitis, asthma, and bronchiectasis, or severe obesity, may be associated. Congenitally damaged or relaxed pelvic floor supports may cause prolapse in young, nulliparous women. Most of the time, however, the patients are multiparous, with the prolapse being at least in part a result of childbirth trauma. Descensus is almost always associated with rectocele and cystocele and, at times, enterocele, supporting the concept of overall relaxation of the pelvic support structures.

A prolapse into the upper barrel of the vagina is called *first degree*. If the prolapse is through the vaginal barrel to the region of the introitus, it is *second degree*. If the cervix and uterus prolapse out through the introitus, it is called *third degree* or *total*. In total prolapse the vagina is everted around the uterus and cervix and completely exteriorized. When this occurs, the patient is in danger of developing dryness, thickening, and chronic inflammation of the vaginal epithelium. Stasis ulcers may result as edema and interference with blood supply to the vaginal wall occur. These ulcers rarely become cancerous, but biopsies should always be taken to ensure that they are not. In almost every case of acquired prolapse, the perineal supports are poor and the perineal body is damaged.

Symptoms and Signs

Major symptoms noted by patients with descensus are a feeling of heaviness, fullness, or "falling out" in the perineal area. In cases where the cervix and uterus are low in the vaginal canal, the cervix may be seen protruding from the introitus, giving the patient the impression that a tumor is bulging out of her vagina. Where total descensus has occurred, the patient is aware that a mass has actually prolapsed out of the introitus. Because prolapse almost always is related to anterior and posterior vaginal wall relaxation, symptoms that were reported earlier for cystocele and rectocele may be present as well.

It is not uncommon for the cervix or vaginal epithelium to become damaged or ulcerated, in which case the patient may report pain or vaginal bleeding. There is often discharge from the cervix and vagina when secondary infection occurs.

Management

Minimum prolapse does not require therapy unless the patient is very uncomfortable. Degrees of prolapse that place the cervix at or through the introitus probably cause greater discomfort and are usually more bothersome to the patient. Medical management of such conditions involves the use of a pessary, usually of the Smith-Hodge, donut, cube, or inflatable variety (Figure 19-12). These require the replacement of the uterus and cervix to their usual position in the pelvis and then the institution of support using one of these devices. Pessaries are available in varying sizes and should be properly fitted to the patient. In general the perineum must be capable of holding the pessary in place, or the pessary will frequently fall out. If the patient is a young woman and pregnant, it is important to replace the uterus before it enlarges and becomes trapped in the lower pelvis or vagina. If this happens, edema may cause incarceration and even loss of blood supply to the uterus. In a postmenopausal woman, estrogen replacement for at least 30 days in the form of systemic estrogen or vaginal estrogen cream may help improve the vitality of the vaginal epithelium, the cervix, and the vasculature of these organs, making the operative procedure and the healing process more efficient. The patient should not undergo operation until all ulcers of the vagina and cervix are healed, because to do otherwise is to risk infection and breakdown of the repair.

Operative repair for prolapse of the uterus and cervix generally involves a vaginal hysterectomy with anterior and posterior colporrhaphy. The hysterectomy is performed carefully, isolating the uterosacral and cardinal ligaments so that they may be used in the support of the vaginal vault. The uterosacral ligaments should be sutured together so that the cul-de-sac is shortened or obliterated and the risk of a subsequent enterocele is lessened.

In some cases a vaginal hysterectomy is not advisable. These circumstances include previous intraabdominal operation for an inflammatory process, such as endometriosis or pelvic inflammatory disease. Where such is the case an abdominal hysterectomy may be performed, followed by a vaginal anterior and posterior colporrhaphy. Under these circumstances the cardinal and uterosacral ligaments should be treated as noted earlier.

In some women the cervix is hypertrophied and elongated to the area of the introitus, but the supports of the uterus itself are good. A cystocele and rectocele may be present, and operative repair can consist of a Manchester-Fothergill operation. This operation combines an anterior and posterior colporrhaphy with the amputation of the cervix and the use of the cardinal ligaments to support the anterior vaginal wall and bladder. Although it was suggested for repair in young women who wish to maintain their reproductive abilities, the loss of the cervix may interfere with fertility or lead to incompetence of the internal cervical os. The op-

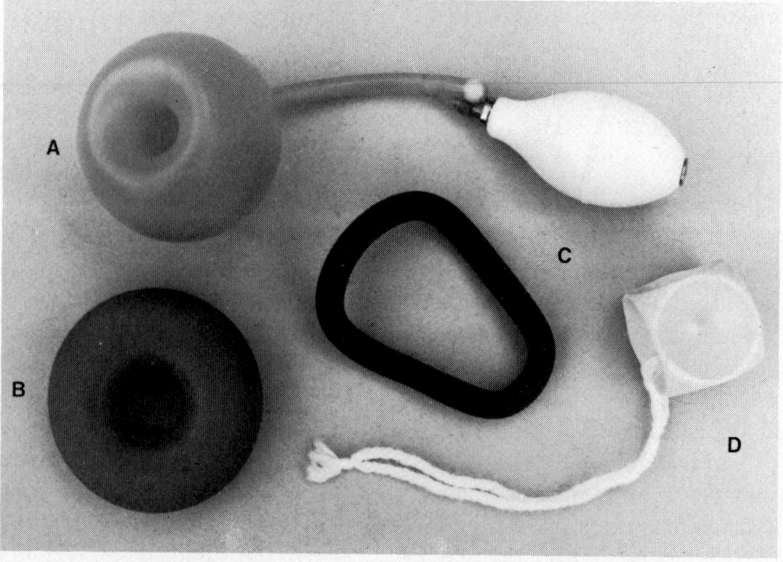

FIGURE 19-12
Examples of pessaries (*A*, Inflatable; *B*, donut; *C*, Smith-Hodge; *D*, cube type.)

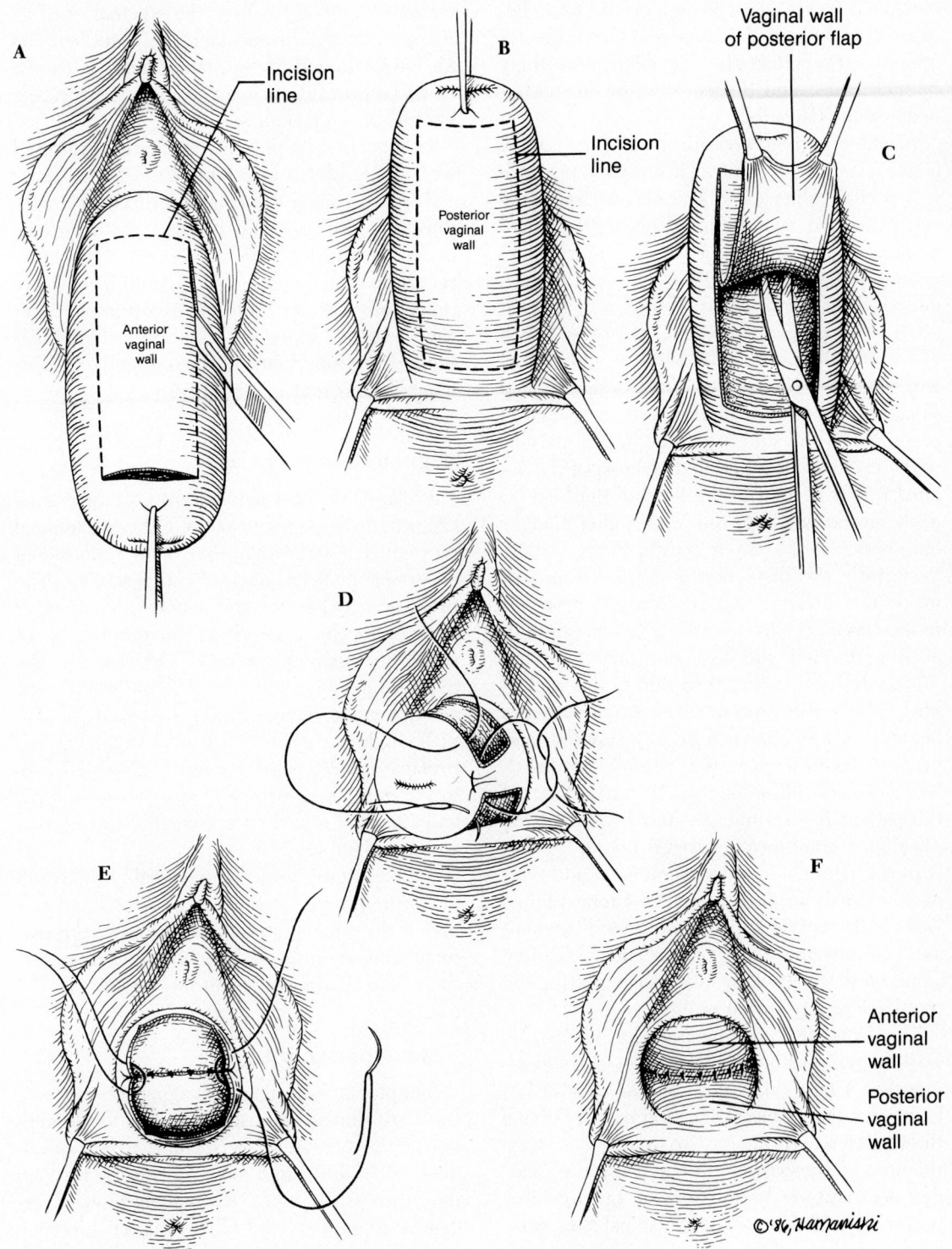

FIGURE 19-13

Le Fort procedure. **A,** Incision of anterior vaginal wall strip. **B,** Incision of posterior wall strip. **C,** Removal of vaginal strip. **D,** and **E,** Placement of sutures. **F,** Appearance of vagina after procedure is completed but before perineorrhaphy is performed.

eration has value in older women who have an elongated cervix and well-supported uterus because it is technically easier and has a shorter operative time than the vaginal hysterectomy in such cases, and the entering of the peritoneal cavity is avoided.

In older women who are no longer sexually active a simple procedure for reducing prolapse is a partial colpocleisis. The classic procedure was described by Le Fort (Figure 19-13) and involves the removal of a strip of anterior and posterior vaginal wall, with closure of the margins of the anterior and posterior wall to each other. This procedure may be performed with or without the presence of a uterus and cervix, and when it is completed, a small vaginal canal exists on either side of the septum, which is produced by the suturing of the lateral margins of the excision. The line of dissection of the vaginal wall is carried to the level of the bladder neck anteriorly and to the reflection of bladder onto cervix at the upper margin of the vagina. Posteriorly the dissection is carried from just inside the introitus to a position just posterior to the cervix. If a hysterectomy has been previously performed, the dissection may begin approximately 1 cm on either side of the vaginal scar. When the procedure is completed, the bladder neck is spared from any scarring, and urinary incontinence is generally avoided. Bladder neck plication may be carried out if the patient is incontinent. After healing of the plication a small introital area is noted; this has cosmetic benefits in older women. In addition, narrow canals are noted on each lateral vaginal wall. If the cervix and uterus are still present and intrauterine pathology occurs, bleeding along these canals could take place, alerting the physician to a potential problem.

The Goodall-Power modification of the Le Fort operation (Figure 19-14) allows for the removal of a triangular piece of vaginal wall beginning at the cervical reflection or 1 cm above the vaginal scar at the base of the triangle, with the apex of the triangle just beneath the bladder neck anteriorly and just at the introitus posteriorly. The cut edge of vaginal wall making up the base of the triangle anteriorly is sutured to the similar wall posteriorly, and the vaginal incision is then closed with a row of interrupted sutures beginning beneath the bladder neck and carried side to side to the area of the introitus. This procedure works well for relatively small prolapses, whereas the Le Fort is best for larger ones.

When a colpocleisis is performed, if an enterocele is found when the vaginal wall is stripped away, the sac must be identified, its neck ligated, and the peritoneum of the sac excised to prevent recurrence of the enterocele behind the colpocleisis.

In most cases a perineorrhaphy is performed with a colpocleisis to reinforce the introitus.

Prognosis for a colpocleisis procedure to reduce the prolapse and prevent recurrence is generally excellent. Ridley reports no prolapse recurrences in 58 patients unless an incomplete procedure was performed in an attempt to salvage vaginal depth and function. Three patients developed stress incontinence where none was present preoperatively.

Vaginal Stump Prolapse

Prolapse of the vaginal stump at some time remote to the performance of either abdominal or vaginal hysterectomy has been reported as occurring in 0.1% to 18.2% of patients. The prolapse may be total and may be accompanied by a cystocele, a rectocele, an enterocele, or some combination thereof. Occasionally the prolapse involves only one of those entities and not the entire vaginal stump. In a study in Munich, Richter reported that of 97 vaginal stump prolapses, 6.2% were cystocele only, 5.1% rectocele only, 9.3% primarily an enterocele type, and 72.2% of mixed type. Specific classification was not given for 7.2%.

Vaginal stump prolapse is probably the result of continuing pelvic support weakness and failure of the vaginal structures, namely, the cardinal and uterosacral ligaments, to maintain their tone or attachment to the vagina.

Symptoms and Signs

Symptoms and signs of vaginal stump prolapse are similar to those delineated for descensus of the uterus. They include pelvic heaviness, backache, and a mass protruding through the introitus. At times, stress incontinence, urgency, frequency, dribbling, vaginal bleeding or discharge (if there is an ulcer), and, depending on the size of the mass, difficulty with sitting or walking may occur.

Diagnosis

Examination may help determine the contents of the herniation depending on where the

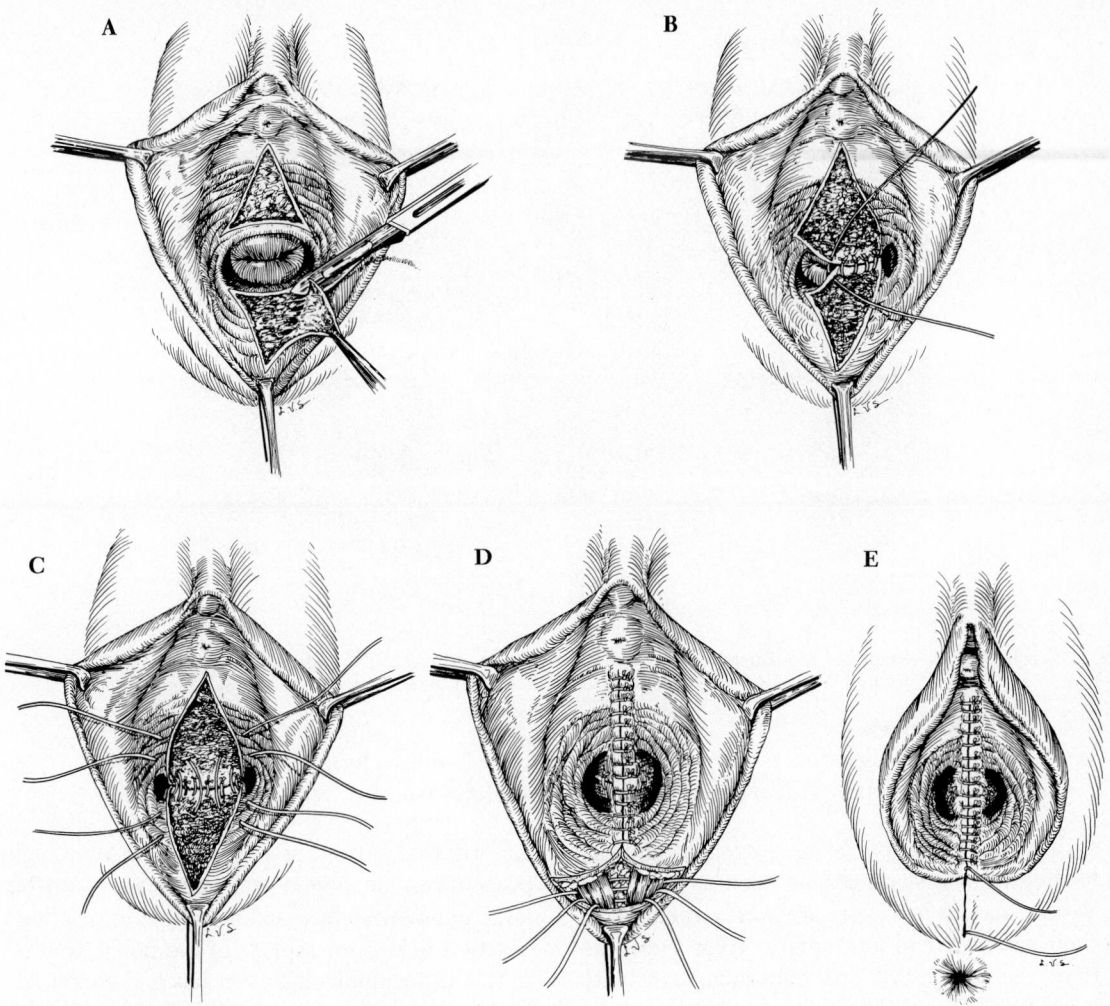

FIGURE 19-14
Goodall-Power modification of Le Fort operation. **A,** Representation of vaginal incision on anterior and posterior wall. **B,** Early placement of sutures. **C,** Later placement of suture. **D,** Vaginal incision completely closed; perineorrhaphy being performed. **E,** Appearance at completion of procedure. (Reprinted, with permission,
from Symmonds RE: Relaxation of pelvic supports. In Benson RC, editor: Current
obstetric and gynecologic diagnosis and treatment, ed 5, Copyright 1984, Lange
Medical Publications, Los Altos, Calif.)

vaginal scar is located in relation to the protruding mass and the extent to which the supports of the pelvis are lost. Rectovaginal examination is often helpful in delineating an enterocele from a rectocele.

Management

Although the management of descensus with
the uterus present is uniformly agreed to be
vaginal hysterectomy with anterior and posterior colporrhaphy, there is much controversy
over the appropriate procedure for vaginal

stump prolapse. Nevertheless, certain principles and facts are important. The first is that
the normal position of the vagina in the standing position is against the rectum and no more
than 30 degrees from the horizontal (Figure 19-
15). The second principle is that pelvic relaxation is a part of the problem and dictates that
an existing cystocele, rectocele, or enterocele
must be repaired as part of the procedure. The
third principle acknowledges that the perineal
body is almost always severely weakened in
such patients and must therefore be recon-
structed as well. Nonsurgical management,

Symphysis pubis   Bladder

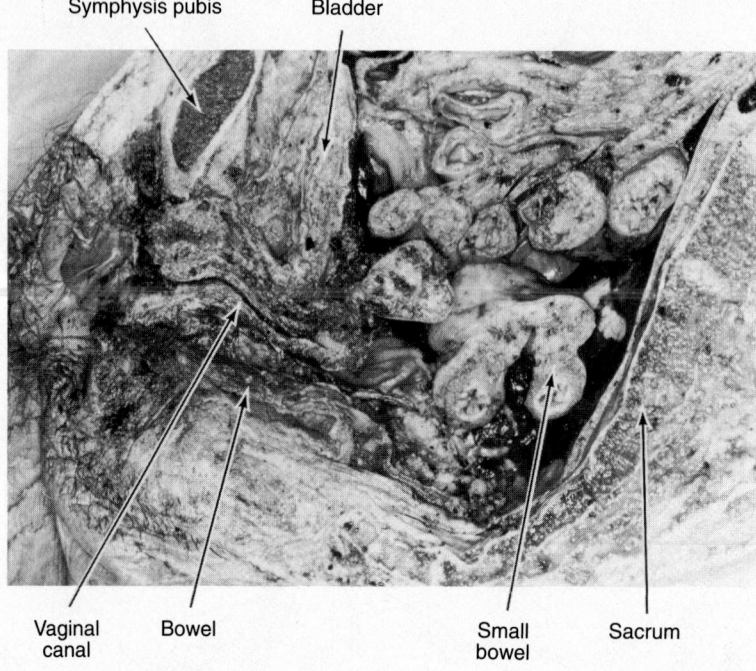

Vaginal   Bowel   Small   Sacrum
canal   bowel

FIGURE 19-15
Pelvis of a dissected cadaver in supine position demonstrating vaginal canal orientation in the pelvis. (Courtesy of Dr. Richard Hebertson.)

such as the use of pessaries, estrogen, and the healing of ulcers, should be used as appropriate. Pessaries, however, are rarely retained in such patients, and attempts to treat these patients nonsurgically are generally met with frustration.

The choices of operative procedures are many. These include those that use the abdominal route, the vaginal route, or some combination thereof. For the abdominal approach a variety of procedures have been tried. These include fixation of the vaginal vault to the anterior abdominal wall, to the lumbar spine, to the sacral promontory, to various tendonous lines in the musculature of the true pelvis, and to the sacrospinous ligament. The anterior abdominal wall fixation increases the diameters of the pouch of Douglas and frequently adds to the risk of subsequent enterocele development, often creating a recurrence in short order. Fixation to the lumbar spine or the sacral promontory is often difficult to achieve directly and frequently requires the interposition of a different material. In the past, ox fascia lata, fascial aponeurosis from the patient, or inert materials such as Mersilene have been used. In such procedures it is important to cover the stent with peritoneum, thereby rendering it retroperitoneal to avoid troublesome adhesions

and internal hernias at a future data. After such procedures the pouch of Douglas may still be large enough to allow an enterocele to develop. Fixation to various aspects of the pelvic wall or to the sacrospinous ligament has had encouraging degrees of success, the latter being the most successful. Using the sacrospinous ligament can frequently be accomplished vaginally. Randall and Nichols report excellent success with both abdominal and vaginal approaches. In 18 patients treated with fixation of the vaginal vault to the sacrospinous ligament via the vaginal route, all had successful outcomes.

Recently Morley and DeLancey reported the results of 100 patients treated at the University of Michigan for vaginal vault prolapse or posthysterectomy enterocele with sacrospinous ligament suspension of the vaginal vault. Of 71 patients who were followed for 1 year or more, 64 (90%) had complete symptomatic relief, 10 had some asymptomatic relaxation of the vaginal walls, and 9 had either vaginal stenosis or stress incontinence. In addition, 4 patients developed cystoceles, and 3 had recurrent prolapse of the vagina. Figure 19-16 depicts the fixation of the vaginal vault to the sacrospinous ligament and the direction of the vagina after the procedure. Miyazaki reports the use of an

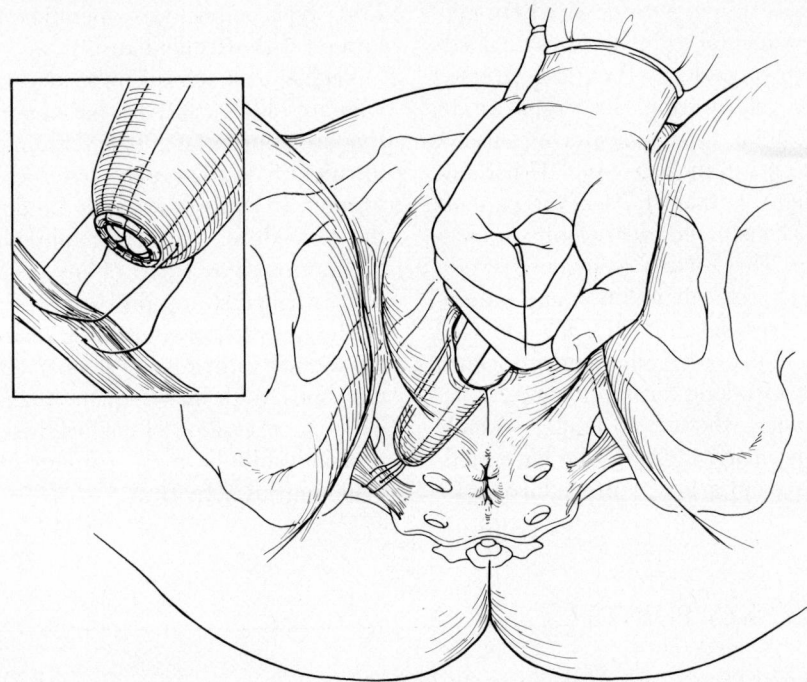

FIGURE 19-16
Sutures tied to bring the new vaginal apex into contact with the ligament and over-lying muscle. Vaginal wall is advanced toward the sacrospinous ligament while tying sutures. A "suture bridge" is to be avoided. (Redrawn from Morley GW and DeLancey JO: Am J Obstet Gynecol 158:872, 1988.)

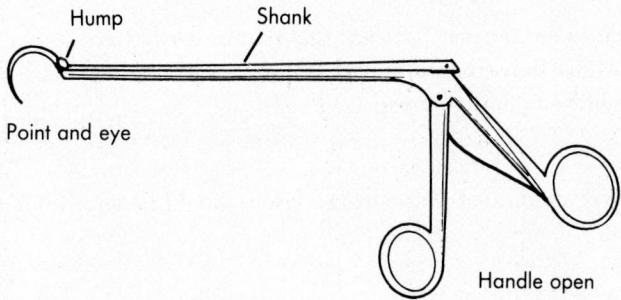

FIGURE 19-17
The Miya hook ligature carrier. (From Miyazaki FS: Obstet Gynecol 70:286, 1987.)

instrument, the Miya hook ligature carrier, to lessen the difficulty of placing a suture into the sacrospinous ligament. This is depicted in Figure 19-17. Some surgeons favor the use of this instrument in the performance of this procedure.

A variety of vaginal procedures have been designed. The best success, however, occurs in procedures in which adequate vaginal length is maintained and the vagina is positioned against the rectum nearly parallel to the horizontal. Recently, Thornton reported on 41 women who underwent repair of vaginal stumps, in which the vaginal approach was used with good lasting success. Of these patients, 20 required a repair of an enterocele and a posterior repair, which especially detailed the attachment of the posterior wall of the vagina to the perirectal fascia and levator ani muscles. In addition, 21 patients underwent a repair of an enterocele with both an anterior and a posterior repair because a cystocele was believed to be a major part of their prolapse problem. Long-term follow-ups were effected, and the success rate was said to be excellent.

Richter and Albrich combined the repair of

cystocele, rectocele, and enterocele where necessary with a unilateral or bilateral vaginal sacrospinal fixation procedure. They also stressed the importance of suturing the vagina in its physiologic position to the perirectal support tissue. The success in their group of 97 patients was also excellent, in that 61.7% of the patients had what were considered ideal results in long-term follow-up. There was a recurrence of cystocele in 14.8%, rectocele in 8.6%, and enterocele in 3.7%. Stress incontinence was reported in 3.7% of their patients and urgency incontinence in 2.5% with long-term follow-up.

In older women who are no longer sexually active, and particularly in those who have medical reasons to avoid a longer procedure, a Le Fort–type colpocleisis operation may be performed with excellent results.

Vaginal colpocleisis procedures for women who are elderly and are no longer sexually active are appropriate. It is extremely important to identify and repair enteroceles in such women, but this can readily be done as part of the procedure. Perineorrhaphy should always be performed as a part of any procedure to repair a vaginal stump prolapse.

The question of continuing sexual activity after vaginal vault repairs is obviously an important one. With an adequate vaginal operation (with the exception of colpocleisis), intercourse is achievable in most patients who wish to maintain this activity.

_____ KEY POINTS _____

- Femoral hernias are more common in females than in males, whereas inguinal hernias are more common in males.

- Congenital fascial defects at the umbilicus generally close within the first 3 years of life.

- In the female, large hernias, hernias that continuously have intraabdominal contents, hernias that cause continuing discomfort, and hernias that have been incarcerated should be operatively repaired.

- In the repair of abdominal wall hernias, fascia should be sutured with nonabsorbable material.

- Urethroceles and cystoceles are more common in women with a gynecoid pelvis than in those with android or anthropoid types.

- Urinary incontinence is usually noted with loss of support of the urethra and bladder neck.

- After cystocele repair, bladder drainage for about 5 days is generally necessary before normal voiding can be anticipated.

- Bladder drainage after cystocele repair may be with a transurethral or suprapubic catheter.

- When an enterocele is present, the sac must be dissected free and ligated at its neck to prevent recurrence.

- Descensus of the uterus and cervix is graded as first degree (prolapse into the upper vagina), second degree (prolapse to or near the introitus), and third degree, or complete, (prolapse through the introitus).

- Prolapse of the vaginal stump at some time after hysterectomy has been reported in 0.1% to 18.2% of patients.

- Vaginal prolapse after hysterectomy includes a mixture of cystocele, rectocele, and enterocele in 72% of cases.

- Vaginal vault prolapse can be repaired abdominally or vaginally.

- Vaginal vault prolapse repair using fixation to the sacrospinous ligament will have a success rate approaching 100%.

BIBLIOGRAPHY

Beecham CT: Classification of vaginal relaxation, Am J Obstet Gynecol 136:957, 1980.

Beecham CT and Beecham JB: Correction of prolapsed vagina or enterocele with fascia, Obstet Gynecol 42:542, 1973.

Glassow F: Inguinal and femoral hernia in women, Int Surg 57:34, 1972.

Halverson K and McVay CB: Inguinal and femoral hernioplasty: a 22 year study of author's methods, Arch Surg 101:127, 1970.

Kuhn RJ and Hollyock VE: Observations on the anatomy of the recto-vaginal pouch and septum, Obstet Gynecol 59:445, 1982.

McCall ML: Posterior culdeplasty—surgical correction of enterocele during vaginal hysterectomy: a preliminary report, Obstet Gynecol 10:595, 1957.

Miyazaki FS: Miya hook ligature carrier for sacrospinous ligament suspension, Obstet Gynecol 70:286, 1987.

Morley GW and DeLancey JO: Sacrospinous ligament fixation for eversion of the vagina, Am J Obstet Gynecol 158:872, 1988.

Nichols DH: Transvaginal sacrospinous fixation, Pelvic Surg 1:10, 1981.

Randall CI and Nichols DH: Surgical treatment of vaginal inversion, Obstet Gynecol 38:327, 1971.

Richter K: Massive eversion of the vagina: pathogenesis, diagnosis and therapy of the "true" prolapse of the vaginal stump, Clin Obstet Gynecol 25:897, 1982.

Richter K and Albrich W: Long-term results following fixation of the vagina on the sacrospinal ligament by the vaginal root (vaginae fixatio sacrospinalis vaginalis), Am J Obstet Gynecol 141:811, 1981.

Ridley JH: Evaluation of the colpocleisis operation: a report of 58 cases, Am J Obstet Gynecol 113:1114, 1972.

Schwartz SI, Shires GT, Spencer FC, and Storer EH: Principles of surgery, ed 4, New York, 1984, McGraw-Hill Book Co.

Seigworth GR: Vaginal vault prolapse with eversion, Obstet Gynecol 54:255, 1979.

Symmonds RE: Relaxation of pelvic supports. In Benson RC, editor: Current obstetric and gynecologic diagnosis and treatment, ed 5, Los Altos, Calif, 1984, Lange Medical Publications.

Symmonds RE, Williams TJ, Lee RA, and Webb MJ: Posthysterectomy, enterocele and vaginal vault prolapse, Am J Obstet Gynecol 140:852, 1981.

Thornton WN Jr and Peters WA: Repair of vaginal prolapse after hysterectomy, Am J Obstet Gynecol 147:140, 1983.

Zacharin RF: Pulsion enterocele: review of functional anatomy of the pelvic floor, Obstet Gynecol 55:135, 1980.

Zimmerman LM and Anson BJ: The anatomy of surgery of hernia, Baltimore, 1953, The Williams & Wilkins Co.

Gynecologic Urology

KEY TERMS AND DEFINITIONS

Cystometry. Method for measuring pressure–volume relationships of the bladder.

Detrusor Dyssynergia. Involuntary contraction of the bladder during distention with urine or other fluids.

Detrusor Pressure. Component of intravesical pressure created by forces in the bladder wall.

Extraurethral Incontinence. The loss of urine through channels other than the urethra.

Flow Rate. Volume of urine expelled via the urethra per unit time expressed in milliliters.

Genuine Stress Incontinence. Condition of immediate involuntary loss of urine when intravesical pressure exceeds the maximum urethral pressure in the absence of detrusor activity.

Incontinence. A condition in which involuntary loss of urine is a social or hygienic problem and one that can be objectively demonstrated.

Intraabdominal Pressure. Pressure surrounding the bladder.

Intravesical Pressure. Pressure within the bladder.

Kegel Exercises. Isometric contractions of the pubococcygeus muscles to improve control of continence.

Osteitis Pubis. An inflammation of the periosteum of the pubic bone, often occurring after suprapubic urethral suspension procedures.

Osteomyelitis Pubis. An infection of the pubic bone, which may occur after pelvic operations.

Overflow Incontinence. Involuntary loss of urine when intravesical pressure exceeds the maximum urethral pressure secondary to an elevation of intravesical pressure associated with bladder distention but in the absence of detrusor activity.

Posterior Urethral Angle (PUV). The angle formed by the posterior aspect of the urethra and the bladder. It is generally less than 120 degrees in continent women.

Reflex Incontinence. The involuntary loss of urine caused by abnormal reflex activity in the spinal cord in the absence of the sensation that is usually associated with the desire to micturate.

Residual Urine. Volume of urine remaining in the bladder immediately after completion of micturition.

Trigone (Bladder). The area of the floor of the urinary bladder that forms a triangle with the urethral opening at the apex and the ureteral openings at the ends of the base.

Trigonitis. Inflammation of the trigone.

Urethral Closure Pressure Profile. Intraluminal pressure along the length of the urethra with the bladder at rest.

Urethral Syndrome. An inflammatory condition of the urethra in which bacterial cultures are found to be negative. In many cases *Chlamydia* can now be cultured.

Urge Incontinence. The involuntary loss of urine associated with a strong desire to void. This may be divided into motor urge incontinence, which is associated with uninhibited detrusor contractions, and sensory urge incontinence, which is not caused by uninhibited detrusor contractions.

The gynecologist frequently consults on and treats urologic problems in the female patient. Perhaps the most commonly seen of these problems involves infection and inflammation of the lower tract (urethritis, trigonitis, and cystitis). However, many women suffer from some degree of urinary incontinence. In a telephone interview study of 851 women ages 18 and older selected at random in Australia, 267 (31%) stated that they had noted some degree of incontinence during the preceding 12 months, and 142 (12%) suffered two or more regular episodes of leakage per month. Daily incontinence was reported by 5%, and 2.3% were incontinent often or continuously.

This condition increases in incidence with age, and because the number of older women in our population is growing, it is likely that this problem will grow in magnitude with time. At a conference of the National Association of Retired People, Teasdale et al. learned (by questionnaire) that 33% of the total responders experienced some form of urinary incontinence. Women accounted for 75% of the respondents, representing 168 individuals. Of these, 118 complained of dribbling, 13 of spontaneous large losses of urine, and 37 of both dribbling and large losses. The older the woman, the higher the incidence of incontinence.

Continence depends on a number of factors, including the neurologic control of micturition, the anatomic relationships of the urinary tract, and the specific effects of a number of systemic, infectious, and neoplastic conditions. This chapter considers the physiology of micturition and the diagnosis and treatment of pathologic entities that affect the female urologic system, and it offers suggestions on diagnosis and management of urinary incontinence.

PHYSIOLOGY OF MICTURITION

A number of factors are in play to maintain continence. Basically these involve those that maintain a urethral closure mechanism and those that affect detrusor function. In the final analysis it is the balance between urethral closure and detrusor function that determines whether micturition occurs or continence is maintained.

The factors affecting the urethral closure mechanism primarily involve urethral tone and include the basic elasticity of the urethra, the presence of smooth and voluntary (striated) muscle, the vascular component supplying the urethra, and the presence of alpha receptors from the sympathetic nervous system, which when stimulated cause contraction of the urethral sphincter.

Bladder detrusor contractility is stimulated by the activity of the parasympathetic nervous system mediated through the neurotransmitter acetylcholine. This stimulates receptors in the bladder wall, which then activate detrusor contraction. Sympathetic nervous system beta receptors within the bladder cause bladder relaxation when stimulated. Bladder contraction may also be affected by irritation and inflammation of the bladder wall, causing uncoordinated contractions.

The act of voiding is under the control of four basic autonomic and somatic nervous system feedback loops. The first loop (loop I) involves a circuit from the cerebral cortex to the brainstem, which inhibits micturition by modifying sensory stimuli emanating from loop II. Loop II, which originates in the sacral micturition (S2 through S4) center and the detrusor muscle wall itself, represents sensory fibers to the brainstem, where modulation of the stimuli by loop I takes place. If cerebral inhibition is not imposed (loop I), the stimuli are returned to the sacral micturition center as a response to the bladder filling, allowing activation of loop III. Loop III involves sensory flow from the bladder wall to the sacral micturition center with returning motor fibers to the urethral sphincter striated muscle, which allows the voluntary relaxation of the urethral sphincter as the detrusor contracts. Loop IV originates in the frontal lobe of the cerebral cortex and runs to the sacral micturition center and then to the urethral striated muscle, allowing urethral voluntary muscles to relax and thus leading to the initiation of voiding. Figure 20-1 demonstrates these four loops as visualized by Williams and Fitzhugh. Table 20-1 summarizes the important aspects of each loop as reviewed by Ostergard.

Both the parasympathetic and sympathetic nervous systems function with the central nervous system in these feedback loops. Basically, the parasympathetic system is involved in the act of voiding via nuclei in S2 through S4 (micturition center). Contraction of the detrusor muscle puts pressure on the bladder neck and the proximal urethra, contributing to the relax-

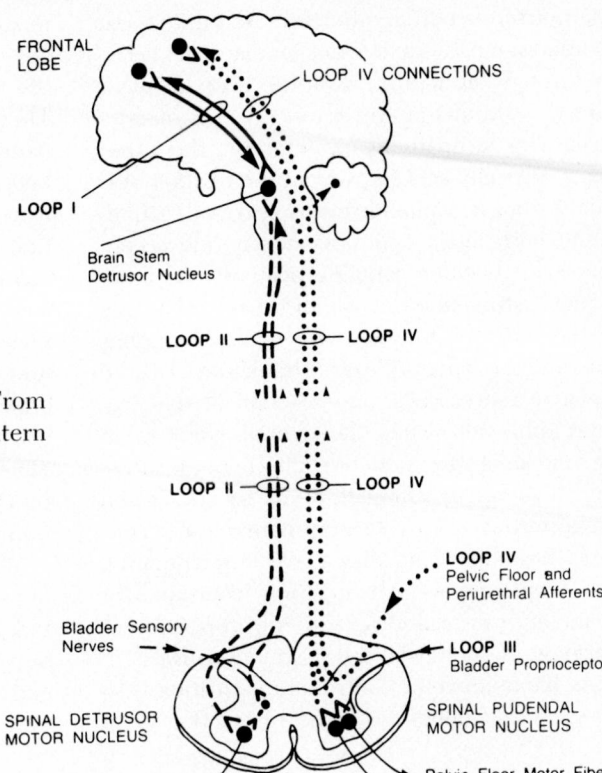

FIGURE 20-1

Central nervous system feedback loops. (From Williams ME and Fitzhugh CP: Ann Intern Med 97:895, 1982.)

TABLE 20-1

Neurologic Control of Micturition: Clinical Considerations on Central Nervous System Reflex Loops

Loop	Origin	Termination	Function	Associated Conditions
I	Frontal lobe	Brainstem	Coordinates volitional control of micturition	Parkinson's disease, brain tumors, trauma, cerebrovascular disease, MS, lower urinary tract disease
II	A. Brainstem B. Bladder wall	Sacral micturition center Brainstem	Detrusor muscle contraction to empty bladder	Spinal cord trauma, MS, spinal cord tumors
III	Sensory afferents of detrusor muscle	Striated muscle of urethral sphincter via pudendal motor nervous and micturition center	Allows relaxation of urethral sphincter in synchrony with detrusor contraction	MS, spinal cord trauma or tumors, diabetic neuropathy, local urinary tract disease
IV	Frontal lobe	Pudendal nucleus	Volitional control of striated external urethral sphincter	Cerebral or spinal trauma or tumor, MS, cerebrovascular disease, lower urinary tract disease

Adapted from Ostergard DR: Obstet Gynecol Surv 34:417, 1979.

ation of the urethral sphincter. As mentioned, the parasympathetic system mediates its activity through the neurotransmitter acetylcholine, directly stimulating receptors in the bladder wall. The sympathetic system, on the other hand, basically acts to prevent micturition. Via this system norepinephrine is secreted, stimulating both alpha and beta adrenergic receptors. The bladder contains primarily beta receptors, stimulation of which causes relaxation of the detrusor muscle. The urethra contains primarily alpha receptors. Stimulation of these alpha receptors causes contraction of the urethral sphincter. Thus the overall effect is to prevent micturition (Figure 20-2). Because estrogen seems to stimulate alpha receptors and progesterone seems to stimulate beta receptors, these hormones play a role in maintaining continence in women in their reproductive years and in women receiving replacement hormone therapy who are postmenopausal.

As the neurogenic control of micturition is so complex and depends on the interaction of so many factors, it is understandable that a host of general systemic diseases or diseases involving the nervous system may affect bladder control. These include, but are not limited to, demyelinating diseases (such as multiple sclerosis), diabetes mellitus, vascular diseases, and central nervous system trauma and tumors. In addition, medications that have an effect on the central or autonomic nervous systems may affect bladder control. Compounds with atropine-like effects may interfere with the initiation of micturition, whereas those with cholinergic effects may cause bladder irritability (Table 20-2). An appendix to this chapter (pp. 629-632) contains an exhaustive list developed by Ostergard of agents that affect bladder function.

With the neurologic principles of micturition in mind, it is appropriate to assess other factors that may influence continence. Recently, Asmussen and Ulmsten noted that the bladder and the urethra are essentially a functional unit, with the bladder's subfunction to store

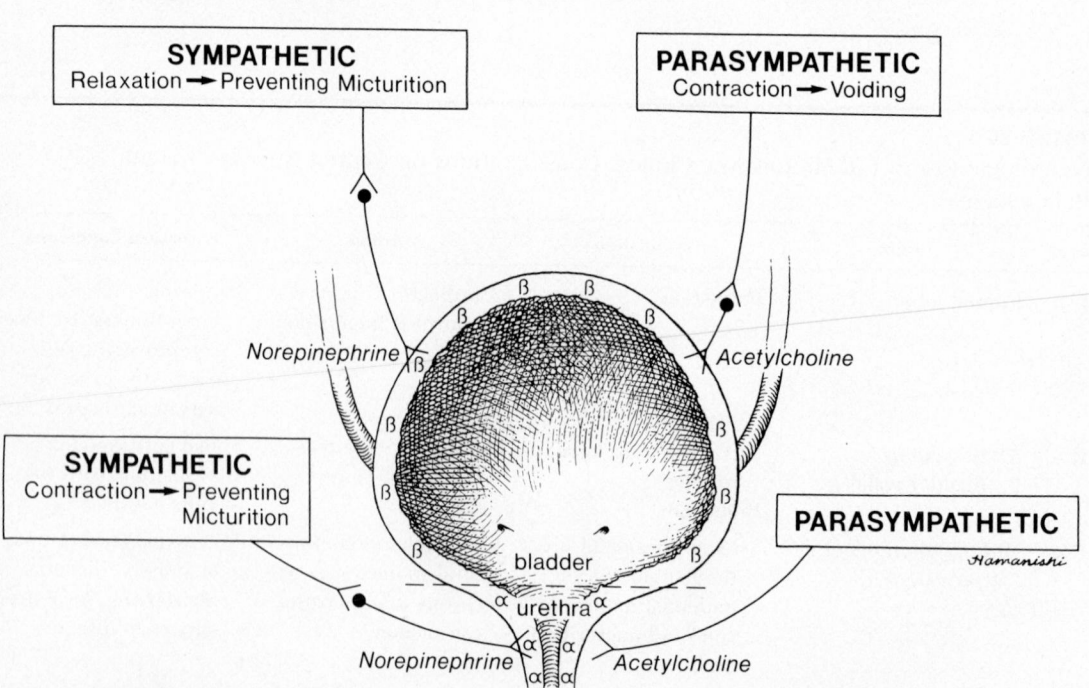

FIGURE 20-2
The innervation of the bladder and urethra. Parasympathetic fibers arising in S2 through S4 have long preganglionic fibers and pelvic ganglia close to the bladder and urethra. These parasympathetic fibers excrete acetylcholine. Sympathetic fibers that have long postganglionic fibers discharge norepinephrine to beta receptors, primarily in the bladder, and alpha receptors, primarily in the urethra. (Redrawn and modified from Raz S: Urol Clin North Am 5:323, 1978.)

TABLE 20-2
Some Common Drugs That Affect Continence and Micturition (See Appendix for Additional Information)

Sympathetic (relaxes bladder; controls urethral sphincter)

Drug	Action
Dopamine	Alpha adrenergic stimulator
Ethylphenylephrine	"
Methamphetamine	"
Norepinephrine	"
Phenylephrine	"
Albuterol	Beta adrenergic stimulator
Ethylnorepinephrine	"
Isoproterenol	"
Methoxyphenamine	"
Terbutaline	"

Parasympathetic (stimulates bladder contraction; relaxes urethral sphincter)

Drug	Action
Pilocarpine	Stimulates acetylcholine
Pralidoxime	"
Pyridostigmine	"

Sympathetic blockers

Drug	Action
Guanethidine	Adrenergic blocker
Hydralazine	"
Methyldopa	"
Reserpine	"

Parasympathetic blockers

Drug	Action
Anisotropine	Parasympathetic inhibitor
Atropine	"
Clidinium	"
Homatropine	"
Papaverine	"
Scopolamine	"

urine and the urethra's to allow it to pass. For urine to pass through the urethra, the maximum urethral pressure must be lower than the intravesical pressure. Intravesical pressure depends on (1) the volume of fluid in the bladder, (2) the part of the intraabdominal pressure transmitted to the bladder, and (3) the tension in the bladder wall related to muscular and nervous system activity. The resting pressure in the bladder is between 20 and 30 cm H_2O.

The intraurethral pressure depends on (1) the striated muscle fibers of the urethral wall, (2) smooth muscle fibers of the urethral wall, (3) the vascular content of the urethral submucosal cavernous plexus, (4) the passive elasticity of the urethral wall, and (5) the part of the intraabdominal pressure transmitted to the urethra.

Anatomically the exact border between the bladder and urethra is difficult to determine. The functional length of the urethra, however, is that part in which the urethral pressure exceeds the bladder pressure. Asmussen and Ulmsten have noted that the urethral closure pressure (UCP) is defined as the maximum urethral pressure minus the bladder pressure. For continence to be present the UCP must be greater than the bladder pressure. Urethral pressure varies with age, increasing up to the age of 20 and then gradually decreasing until menopause. However, after menopause the fall of this pressure is more rapid. Asmussen, Ulmsten, and Henrikksson have demonstrated that the highest pressure zone in the urethra is about midpoint in the functional urethral length, and Westby et al. have located this zone at about 0.5 cm proximal to the urogenital diaphragm. Most of the functional urethral length is, indeed, above the urogenital diaphragm (Figure 20-3). Ulmsten et al. and Gossling et al. have pointed out that the submucosal cavernous plexus of vessels, the bulk of the smooth and striated muscle, and the bulk of the autonomic nerve supply are most prominent in the area in which they record the maximum urethral pressure. Because the urethral pressure displays high pressure zone oscillations that are synchronous with the heartbeat, the submucosal cavernous plexus is probably important in helping to maintain continence (Figure 20-4). Indeed, this structure is under the control of estrogen. Enhorning and also Asmussen and Ulmsten have demonstrated that urethral pressure can oscillate as much as 25 cm H_2O in young women but seldom more than 5 cm H_2O in postmenopausal women. The cavernous plexus is thicker walled and less elastic in older women. Thus not only are the epithelium of the bladder and the bladder neck dependent on hormone stimulation, but so probably is the vascular system of these areas.

Because the maximum urethral pressure area under normal circumstances lies above the urogenital diaphragm and because intraabdominal pressure likely affects both the bladder and this

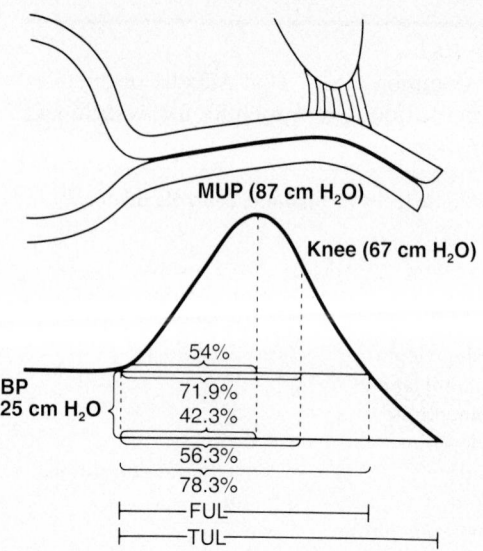

FIGURE 20-3

The location of maximum urethral pressure in relation to the urogenital diaphragm (average value of 25 normal women). KNEE indicates the location of the urogenital diaphragm seen on x-ray film and transformed to the pressure curve. (From Asmussen M and Ulmsten U: On the physiology of continence and pathophysiology of stress incontinence in the female. In Controversies in gynecology and obstetrics, vol 10, Basel, 1983, Karger, S, AG, pp 32-50.)

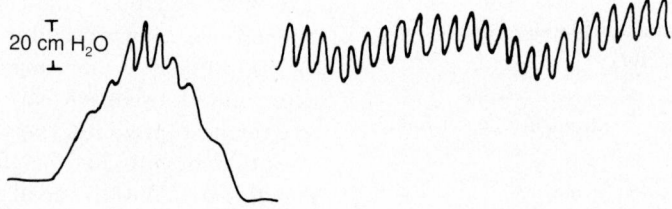

FIGURE 20-4

The maximum urethral pressure shows great variation synchronously with the heartbeat. Variations of 20 cm H_2O as shown in the curve are not uncommon. (From Asmussen M and Ulmsten U: On the physiology of continence and pathophysiology of stress incontinence in the female. In Controversies in gynecology and obstetrics, vol 10, Basel, 1983, Karger, S, AG, pp 32-50.)

area of the urethra equally, if normal anatomic relationships are maintained, a sudden intraabdominal pressure should not, under normal circumstances, cause incontinence. On the other hand, if the functional urethra is displaced from its usual anatomic relationships, it may be excluded from the effect of increased intraabdominal pressure and therefore be susceptible to it. This problem will be addressed further in the discussion of stress incontinence.

DeLancey made some interesting observations on functioning periurethral anatomy by studying serial histologic sections of intact pelvic viscera and surrounding tissue, as well as dissecting 22 fresh and embalmed cadavers. Because the length of the urethra varies from woman to woman, topography of urethral and periurethral structures was expressed in terms of the location along the urethra using percentages of the total urethra. DeLancey considered the zero location as that point in which the

urethra leaves the bladder lumen and the 100th percentile as that point in which the urethra terminates on the perineum. From the standpoint of functional anatomy there is excellent agreement among the measurements made from each of his specimens when percentiles were used. Table 20-3 depicts these anatomic relationships. It can be seen that the intramural urethra represents approximately 20% of the length of the urethra. The portion of the urethra encircled by striated urethral sphincter muscle and associated with the pubourethral ligament and vaginal levator attachment concerns the midurethra, that is, that portion which is from the 20th to 60th percentile along the total length. The 60th to 80th percentile of the urethral length passes through the urogenital diaphragm and is under the influence of the urethrovaginal sphincter muscles. Finally, the last 20%, or distal urethra, traverses the bulbocavernosus muscles. These ure-

TABLE 20-3

Topography of Urethral and Paraurethral Structures*

Approximate Location†	Region of the Urethra	Paraurethral Structures
0-20	Intramural urethra	Urethral lumen traverses the bladder wall
20-60	Midurethra	Striated urethral sphincter muscle
		Pubourethral ligament
		Vaginolevator attachment
60-80	Urogenital diaphragm	Compressor urethrae muscle
		Urethrovaginal sphincter muscle
80-100	Distal urethra	Bulbocavernosus muscle

From DeLancey JO: Obstet Gynecol 68:91, 1986. Reprinted with permission from The American College of Obstetricians and Gynecologists.
*Smooth muscle of the urethra was not considered.
†Expressed as a percentile of total urethral length.

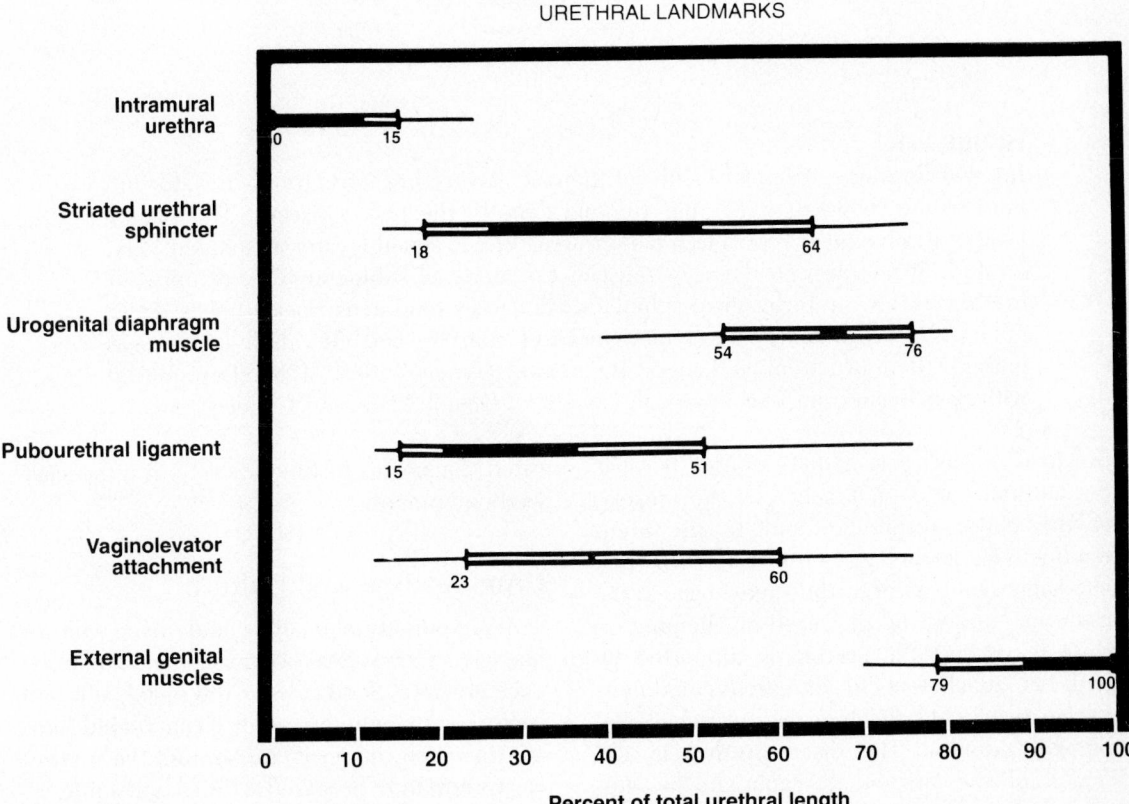

URETHRAL LANDMARKS

Percent of total urethral length

FIGURE 20-5

Average spatial distribution of periurethral structures, as well as the range of values found. Urogenital diaphragm muscles are the compressor urethrae and urethrovaginal sphincter. (From DeLancey JO: Obstet Gynecol 68:91, 1986. Reprinted with permission from The American College of Obstetricians and Gynecologists.)

thral landmarks are depicted in Figure 20-5, which highlights the actual ranges and values found in DeLancey's study. The actual anatomic relationships are depicted in Figure 20-6. DeLancey's observations help to correlate the anatomic relationships to the physiologic observations that others have made.

In a subsequent paper, DeLancey pointed out that additional anatomic factors may influence continence. Using serial histologic sections from 8 female cadavers and the dissections of 34 other cadavers, he noted that the

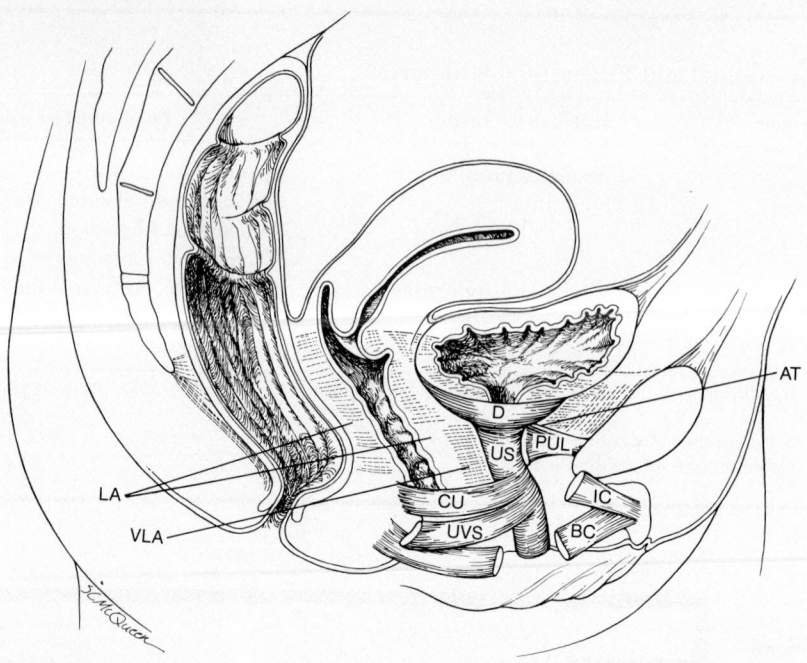

FIGURE 20-6

Interrelationships of approximate location of periurethral structures. Levator ani muscles are shown as light lines running deep to the pelvic viscera. The vaginal levator attachment is shown as a darker area. *VLA*, vaginal levator attachment; *LA*, levator ani muscles; *D*, detrusor muscle; *US*, urethral sphincter; *CU*, compressor urethrae; *UVS*, urethrovaginal sphincter; *AT*, arcus tendineus fasciae pelvis; *PUL*, pubourethral ligament; *IC*, ischiocavernosus muscle; and *BC*, bulbocavernosus muscle. (Redrawn from DeLancey JO: Obstet Gynecol 68:91, 1986. Reproduced with permission from The American College of Obstetricians and Gynecologists.)

proximal urethra gets added support because the anterior vagina is attached to the muscles of the pelvic diaphragm and to the arcus tendineus fasciae pelvis. Contraction of the pelvic diaphragm thus pulls the vagina against the posterior surface of the urethra, helping to close it. At rest the urethra is supported by both its attachment to the arcus tendineus fasciae pelvis and the tone of the pelvic diaphragm muscles. The distal urethra in the region of the urogenital diaphragm is supported by two striated muscle arches, the compressor urethrae and urethrovaginal sphincter. These muscles help to compress the distal urethra, helping to maintain continence during a cough.

DIAGNOSTIC PROCEDURES

Useful testing can be done in the gynecologist's office without the use of sophisticated equipment. These procedures are described next and their benefits noted. Their description is followed by a discussion of more sophisti-

cated diagnostic techniques requiring specialized equipment.

Urine Analysis and Culture

A simple urine analysis and urine culture may give a great deal of information. The presence of white blood cells or red blood cells and bacteria in a catheterized or clean voided sample (in which the perineum around the urethra is appropriately prepared with an antiseptic solution) may suggest urethritis, a diverticulum that is infected, trigonitis, or cystitis. Their presence may also suggest an infection in the upper urinary tract, such as pyelonephritis. Chronic infection in the lower tract may be associated with urgency, frequency, dysuria, and even incontinence. In such instances the urine analysis and urine culture may be diagnostic.

Test for Residual Urine

This simple procedure can be extremely helpful in the evaluation of a patient with cystocele or overflow incontinence. The patient is asked to void, and a catheter is inserted within 10 to 15 minutes thereafter. The urine remaining in the bladder is measured and may be sent for analysis and culture. Under normal circumstances the amount of residual urine should be less than 50 ml after the patient has voided at least 100 to 150 ml. Large amounts of residual urine suggest overflow incontinence resulting from inadequate bladder emptying.

Office Cystometrics

Bladder capacity and bladder function may be measured with sophisticated tools, which are discussed later. Nevertheless it is possible to gain a great deal of information about bladder capacity and bladder function with a relatively simple apparatus. If after a catheter is inserted to check for residual urine, the catheter is left in place and attached to a graduated Asepto syringe without bulb, it is possible to pour sterile saline into the syringe and measure the amount of saline that first causes the patient to have the urge to void. This urge should normally occur after 150 to 200 ml of saline have been infused. However, normal women should be able to continue to maintain continence at that level, with a strong, normally uncontrollable urge to void usually occurring when 400 to 500 ml have been instilled. Thus a normal bladder first transmits an urge to void at 150 to 200 ml, and functional capacity is reached at 400 to 500 ml. Most women can maintain continence with larger volumes, but this is usually accomplished with a great deal of conscious effort.

Stress (Bonney) Test

If a bladder has been previously filled to measure capacity, it should then be emptied to about 250 ml of saline, or if the bladder is empty, 250 ml of saline should be instilled. The catheter is then removed, and the patient is asked to cough while in the recumbent position. If urine spurts from the urethral meatus, stress incontinence may be present. The bladder neck should be gently elevated with the finger or an instrument such as a Kelly clamp, and the patient should be asked to cough once again. Care should be taken not to compress the urethra, thereby mechanically occluding it. If urine no longer spurts from the urethra when the bladder neck is supported,

this suggests that the bladder neck separation from the pubic symphysis may be responsible for the incontinence, and an appropriate operative repair could be expected to produce continence.

Recently Migliorini and Glenning questioned the value of this test because they noted that a group of women with urethral sphincter weakness demonstrated by urodynamic studies were still incontinent even when the bladder neck was elevated (Bonney test). Bhatia and Bergman had previously reached a similar conclusion, stating that they believed the test restored continence by obstructing the urethra and urethrovesicle junction. But it is often noted that patients who have had successful operations to elevate the bladder neck for the treatment of stress incontinence will show obstructive patterns on postoperative urodynamic studies. For the practitioner who is trying to judge clinically whether the replacement of the urethrovesicle junction behind the pubic symphysis will aid continence, the test may still be useful.

Because urine loss with cough should be immediate if stress incontinence is the problem, it may be possible to detect evidence of detrusor instability by observing the time of the spurt of urine in the Bonney test. Classically the detrusor reacts a few seconds after the stimulus; therefore a spurt that occurs after a delay after a cough suggests the presence of a detrusor instability.

After the Bonney test is performed in a recumbent patient, it should be repeated with the patient standing. Frequently the patient will appear to be continent with stress while lying down but may demonstrate incontinence when the influence of gravity on the pelvic organs is brought into play in the standing position.

• • •

Thus with the urine analysis, urine culture, tests for residual urine, information about the amount of urine required to cause the first urge to void, information concerning general bladder capacity, and the Bonney test in both the recumbent and the standing positions, the physician will have a great deal of information concerning the etiology of the patient's urinary problem. More sophisticated urodynamic evaluations using specific and often costly equipment should be performed by individuals who are trained and experienced in these tests. A short discussion of these procedures and the equipment involved follows.

Urethroscopy

Urethroscopy is excellent for visualizing the urethra and therefore offers information about inflammatory processes within the urethra, urethral diverticula, other anatomic defects, and estrogenic effects and permits some estimate of urethral tone. The use of a gas medium such as carbon dioxide is appropriate for these studies. Although the equipment used for performing gas urethroscopy makes it possible to measure pressures within the urethra and the bladder, caution must be exercised because a rapid instillation of carbon dioxide into the lower urinary tract may stimulate detrusor contraction, which may in itself lead to reflex opening of the vesical neck, thus giving false information about the bladder neck and the urethral sphincter.

A variety of equipment is available for this procedure. Relatively inexpensive apparatuses can be used for urethroscopy, as well as for cystometry and uroflowmetry.

Cystoscopy and Cystometry

Cystoscopy may be performed using a water system or a carbon dioxide gas system. The water system is probably best used for diagnosis of detrusor hyperactivity because it does not cause the reflex irritability of the detrusor muscle that has been observed with the gas system. In either case the bladder may be visualized and the presence of inflammation or benign or malignant processes noted.

In attempting to understand the basis of anatomic urinary stress incontinence, the practitioner must realize that what must be determined is the relationship between the simultaneous intraurethral and intravesical pressures (Figure 20-7). For greatest accuracy these must be measured with the patient in the standing and reclining positions, at rest and with straining. The ideal means of evaluating a patient for stress incontinence is to use a multichannel recorder that permits pressure determinations at two points within the urethra (proximal and midpoint to distal), one within the bladder and one intraabdominally as recorded by an intrarectal sensor or by a sensor within the vagina if the vagina is in a relatively normal position (not prolapsed). Should intraabdominal

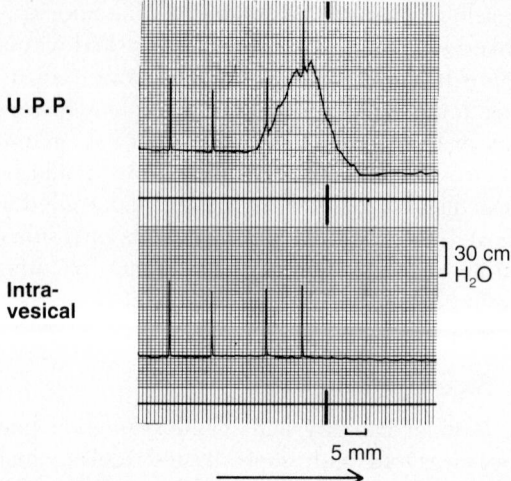

FIGURE 20-7
Simultaneous recordings of urethra and intravesical pressures during coughing. Stress produces a parallel increase of bladder and urethral pressure because the intraabdominal position of the bladder and proximal two thirds of the urethra are displayed. (From Raz S: Urol Clin North Am 5:323, 1978.)

stress be transmitted equally to the bladder and the urethra and should the intravesical pressure be less than the urethral closing pressure, one would expect closing pressure to be overcome and stress incontinence to be demonstrated if an intraabdominal pressure increase is transmitted to the bladder but not to the urethra.

Multiple channel devices involve more expensive equipment and require continuous maintenance. It is possible to add a video urodynamic system to the multichannel recorders, making it possible to identify reflux into the ureters under pressure situations. The video system also makes it possible to actually observe the act of micturition and the effect of stress. Because the data obtained by multichannel pressure recordings plus the ability to actually visualize the patient micturate offer the most accurate diagnostic information that the clinician can obtain, this technique is considered the standard against which other tests are measured.

INFECTIONS OF THE LOWER URINARY TRACT

Infections of the urethra and bladder are almost always associated with some combination of the following: frequency, urgency, dysuria, pyuria, hematuria, acute or chronic pelvic pain, backache, and at times fever. As many as 20% of all women develop urinary tract infections at some time during their life, and by age 70 as many as 10% of women will have chronic urinary tract infections. At times incontinence is associated with acute and chronic infections. Although *Escherichia coli* is the cause of most of the infections, a myriad of organisms including *Enterobacter, Klebsiella, Pseudomonas, Proteus, Streptococcus faecalis, Morganella, Staphylococcus,* and *Chlamydia* are often found. The presence of bacteria in the urine (bacteriuria) does not necessarily prove clinical infection. Bacteriuria is fairly common in women, especially older women. For instance, cumulative data from several studies suggest that 20% of women over 65 years of age will demonstrate bacteriuria, but the percentage increases from about 15% in the 65-to-70-year group to 20% to 50% for women over 80.

The presence of at least 100,000 organisms per milliliter of urine is generally accepted as evidence for a clinical infection. In cases of urethritis and trigonitis the presence of as few as 100 organisms per milliliter may indicate an infection because of the dilution of bladder urine. White blood cells are always seen in the urine (pyuria) when urinary tract infection occurs, and red blood cells may be present in microscopic or macroscopic numbers. Hematuria is common in acute infections.

Many explanations have been offered as to why the female urinary tract is vulnerable to infection. These include the fact that the female urethra is short, thereby allowing easier access of bacteria to the bladder; the proximity of vulva, vagina, and rectum to the opening of the urethra; poor hygiene, including the habit in some women of wiping toward the urethra after a bowel movement; the effects of sexual intercourse on the entrance of bacteria into the urethra and the lower urinary tract; and the effect of loss of estrogen on the reproductive tract of elderly women. To this list it is probably appropriate to add personal immunologic variations that may make one woman more susceptible to certain bacteria than other women. This is particularly true for older women, since immunologic competency diminishes with age.

Additional circumstances that may be responsible for infections in women include the dilation of the urinary tract in pregnancy, urinary tract obstruction, ureteral reflux, and situations of urinary tract relaxation. Other causes of urinary tract infections in both men and women are the need for frequent catheterization, instrumentation, the loss of resistance that occurs in general systemic disease, and overdistention of the bladder in neurogenic conditions where stasis becomes a problem.

Urethritis

Patients with urethritis generally have the typical findings of lower urinary tract infection, which include dysuria, frequency, and urgency. They often have a urethra that is tender to palpation. Under certain circumstances it may be possible to express pus from the urethra; this is particularly common in acute infections with the gonococcus or *Chlamydia*. In these situations the infection involves not only the urethra but the periurethral glands as well. Frequently, significant pyuria is noted in a clean-catch urine sample, particularly that taken early in the voiding. The urine should be inspected, since *Trichomonas* infestation is frequently noted in such instances.

Pus expressed from the urethra should be submitted for culture and for smear with Gram's stain. Intracellular diplococci are suggestive of gonorrhea. *Neisseria Gonorrhoeae* or *Chlamydia* is usually cultured in such situations. Urine obtained by the clean-catch method should also be cultured.

If no specific organism is identified on smear, a broad-spectrum coverage such as a sulfa preparation or nitrofurantoin (Macrodantin), 50 or 100 mg three or four times a day, should be prescribed for 10 days. If *Chlamydia* is suspected, tetracycline should be prescribed for at least 10 days. If gonorrhea is diagnosed, the current recommended treatment consists of ceftriaxone 250 mg IM (single dose) plus doxycycline 100 mg PO two times a day for 7 days. An alternative therapy is spectinomycin 2 gm IM (single dose) followed by doxycycline. Penicillin is no longer the drug of choice because of the many penicillin-resistant strains of gonococcus now present.

Urethral Syndrome

The so-called *urethral syndrome* is characterized by the same symptoms of dysuria, frequency, urgency, and pain that are seen with urethritis, but generally the symptoms are of long standing, and no specific organism can be identified. Classically, urethroscopy has revealed a reddened, chronically inflamed urethra with spasm at the bladder neck. This condition is quite common and may affect as many as 20% to 30% of all women at one time or another. The etiology is unknown, but there are many theories, including allergic, immunologic, infectious, neurologic, atrophic, and psychogenic causes. Some feel the problem resides in the paraurethral glands and that infection with such organisms as mycoplasma, uroplasma, or *Chlamydia* might be responsible. The incidence of these infections, however, has been about the same as in populations of women without the syndrome. Nevertheless, such organisms should be sought and eradicated with appropriate antibiotic therapy when they are found, since this may alleviate symptoms in such cases.

Because the etiology in most cases is unknown, various therapies have been devised with varying success. These include dilation of the urethra with progressive dilators, antispasmodics, estrogen (in postmenopausal women) and more recently, cryosurgery. Sand et al., in a randomized cross-over trial, compared cryosurgery using a specially designed cryoprobe with dilation and massage of the urethra in 24 patients diagnosed as having the urethral syndrome. Of the patients first treated with cryosurgery, 91% achieved relief of their symptoms, compared with 33% of patients first treated with dilation and massage. When crossover of the failures occurred, 75% of women treated with cryosurgery were relieved of symptoms, compared with none of the cryotherapy failures who were then treated with dilation and massage.

Patients diagnosed as having the urethral syndrome deserve a careful evaluation before specific therapy is determined.

Cystitis

Cystitis is perhaps the most common of the urinary tract infections. It is diagnosed when a clean-catch urine sample or catheterized specimen has a bacteria concentration of 100,000 or more per milliliter of urine and when the patient suffers the symptoms of dysuria, frequency, urgency, and pain. White blood cells are almost always seen in large numbers in the urine, as are bacteria. Red blood cells are frequently present in microscopic numbers, but gross hematuria may occur as a result of extravasation of blood across dilated and inflamed capillaries. If the bladder is visualized, it is noted to be uniformly reddened and inflamed. Treatment involves obtaining a culture and beginning the patient on a general antibiotic regimen of sulfa or nitrofurantoin, although a variety of other antibiotics could be used as substitutes for general therapy. These include tetracycline, ampicillin, cephalosporin, nalidixic acid (NegGram), or norfloxacin. When results of the culture are reported, the antibiotic may be changed if the organisms noted are not sensitive to the antibiotic in use. Treatment should be continued for 10 days, although shorter periods are appropriate for certain antibiotics, and the patient should remain well hydrated and should be encouraged to continue treatment even though symptoms generally disappear within 48 hours. Infections frequently recur and become chronic because they are not adequately eradicated. This may result from physician error (treating with too low a dose of antibiotic or for too short a period of time) or patient error (not taking the medication as prescribed). The latter occurrence is generally suspected when the same organism is continuously cultured.

Recurrent infections of different organisms should alert the physician to the need for a more complete evaluation of the urinary tract, including intravenous pyelogram (seeking structural abnormalities of the bladder). Occasionally continuous antibiotic therapy at lower doses for more prolonged periods is necessary to ensure that the patient is no longer infected.

Frequent catheterizations or manipulation of the lower urinary tract often causes urinary tract infections. An indwelling catheter for 24 hours leads to bacteriuria in as many as 50% of patients. When left in place for 96 hours, an indwelling catheter causes bacteriuria in nearly 100% of patients. Many physicians suggest prophylactic antibiotics in patients who must continue catheter use, but no good evidence supports this thesis. Certainly a patient with an indwelling catheter should be monitored for the possibility of bacteriuria and urinary tract infections, be kept well hydrated, and have a urine culture when the catheter is removed. Postoperative and debilitated patients are at greatest risk.

Physicians can counsel their patients about preventive measures by instructing them on proper hygiene. This consists of cleansing the vulvar region at least daily, wiping the rectum away from the urethra, and encouraging good hygiene with respect to coitus. In women who develop frequent urinary tract infections secondary to coitus, one technique is to encourage voiding immediately after intercourse. This tends to wash out bacteria that have entered the urethra before they can cause an infection. Elderly, sexually active women may benefit from either external or systemic estrogen therapy.

Urethral Diverticulum

Etiology

Urethral diverticula occur in perhaps as many as 3% to 4% of all women sometime during their lifetime. Age distribution in published reports ranges from 19 to 76 years, but the majority of diverticula seem to occur between the ages of 30 and 50. Andersen has suggested that the disease occurs more frequently in blacks, with a ratio perhaps as high as 6 to 1.

A variety of etiologies have been suggested, including congenital, acute and chronic inflammatory, and traumatic. The congenital theory stems from the fact that cases have been reported in children and neonates. Evidence for acute and chronic infection stems from the fact that several observers have noted infection and obstruction of periurethral glands, which result in the formation of retention cysts that, when repeatedly infected, may rupture into the lumen of the urethra, giving rise to the diverticulum. Several authors have suggested that the gonococcus is the cause of this, but *E. coli* and other organisms have been found in such processes. Urethral trauma from multiple catheterizations or from childbirth has also been suggested as an etiologic factor. However, many women with diverticula have neither been catheterized nor given birth. The infectious etiology is probably the most common.

Signs and Symptoms

The usual symptoms and signs of a patient with diverticulitis include urgency, frequency, dysuria, and dyspareunia. Frequently a history of recurrent urinary tract infection, dribbling, and incontinence is noted. Occasionally hematuria occurs. In a series reported from the Mayo Clinic, Lee noted that a palpable, tender suburethral mass was present in 51 of 85 pa-

tients (60%) and that protrusion of the diverticulum from the vaginal introitus occurred in 4 patients. Occasionally patients have urinary stones within the diverticula.

Diagnosis

Diagnosis is generally suspected by physical examination and confirmed by cystourethroscopy or voiding cystourethrogram. At times it may be necessary to use a double-catheter balloon technique that essentially closes the urethra at each end and forces contrast medium into the diverticulum under pressure during cystogram.

Management

A variety of procedures have been suggested for the management of urethral diverticula. Lapides has suggested a technique for transurethral marsupialization that involves the resection of the roof of the diverticulum, using transurethral electrocautery. Essentially this technique enlarges the orifice of the diverticulum by incising its roof. Spence and Duckett reported a marsupialization technique in which the diverticulum was opened and sutured to the vaginal epithelial surface. Generally this leads to a fistula and requires secondary closure, making this technique useful in only rare circumstances.

A classic operative approach uses urethroscopy to identify the location of the diverticulum. It is important at this point to note the presence of multiple diverticula. In Lee's report from the Mayo Clinic the diverticulum was noted coming from the distal third of the urethra in only 10 of the 85 patients, whereas 38 patients demonstrated an origin from the middle third, and 13 from the proximal third including the bladder neck. Lee noted multiple diverticula in 18 of his 85 patients.

After the diverticulum is identified and evaluated, an incision is made in the anterior vaginal wall and the diverticulum is dissected free of the pubocervical fascia. The diverticulum's attachment to the urethra is noted, it is excised by sharp dissection, and the urethral wall is closed with a row of interrupted 4-0 catgut sutures. The closure line is generally in the longitudinal axis. Occasionally, however, a transverse closure is necessary because of the nature of the attachment. The pubocervical fascia is

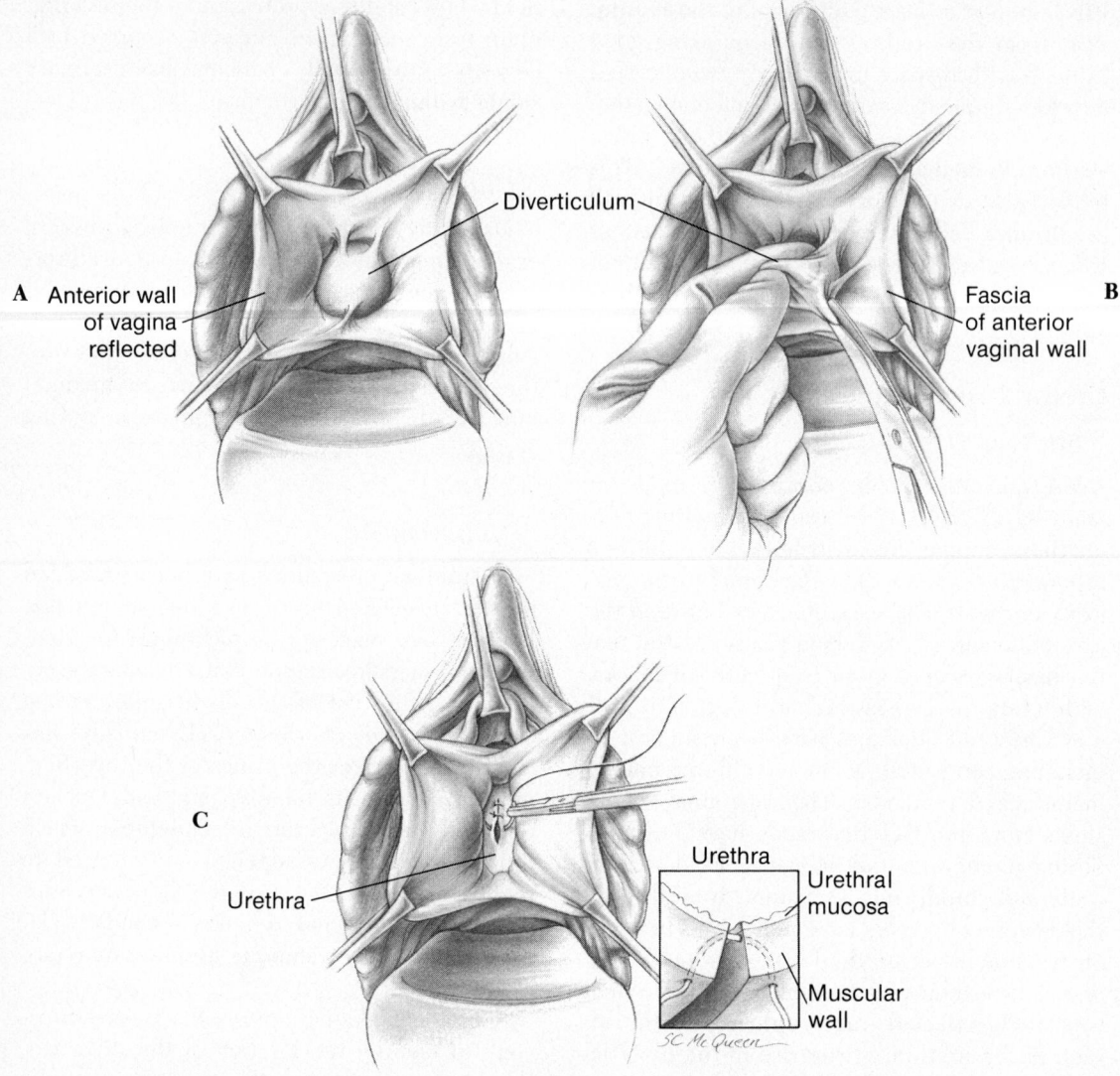

FIGURE 20-8

Resection of urethral diverticulum. **A,** Diverticulum exposed with vaginal lining and endopelvic fascia retracted. **B,** Fingers hold diverticulum on traction, which aids in dissection and identification of ostium. **C,** After complete resection of diverticulum, urethra is closed with fine uninterrupted extramucosal sutures. (Redrawn from Lee RA: Obstet Gynecol 61:52, 1983. Reprinted with permission from The American College of Obstetricians and Gynecologists.)

then reinforced with a row of 3-0 polyglycol reabsorbable interrupted sutures. Hemostasis is scrupulously secured with electrocautery, and the vaginal incision is closed with polyglycol sutures (Figure 20-8).

Most diverticula emanate from the ventral wall of the urethra. Occasionally, however, the diverticulum is noted to be arising from the lateral wall of the urethra or even from the anterior wall. In such cases the dissection must be

carefully carried to the base of the diverticulum and the procedure carried out as stated. In cases of diverticula arising from the dorsal wall of the urethra, it is appropriate to simply excise the diverticulum at its neck and allow the tissue of the urethra to retract. In all cases a No. 16 or 18 Foley catheter is left in place for 6 or 7 days.

Several nuances have been offered to make dissection and subsequent repair easier. One of these is placing a ureteral catheter into the diverticulum and allowing it to coil so that the diverticulum is more easily observable during dissection. Other surgeons have attempted to dilate the neck of the diverticulum before beginning the excision and occasionally have even tried to pack foreign substances such as gauze through the neck to make the dissection easier.

Complications

Major complications of this procedure include urethrovaginal fistula formation, recurrence of the diverticulum, and stricture of the urethra.

In a study from the Mayo Clinic, MacKinnon et al. reported on 140 patients treated operatively, 7 of whom (5%) developed urethrovaginal fistulas. In Lee's report of a later study from the Mayo Clinic, only 1 patient developed a fistula. In another series, Spraitz and Welch, reporting on 94 patients repaired, found 4 with urethrovaginal fistulas.

Recurrence of diverticula is reported in about 5% to 10% of patients in various series. If the diverticulum recurs within the first few months after operation, it may represent a second diverticulum that was overlooked or an inappropriate repair of the diagnosed diverticulum. If the diverticulum occurs after 1 year, it is probably a new lesion.

Stricture of the urethra has rarely been reported in any of the operative series. It is a theoretic possibility.

Other complications involve stress incontinence, which may be related to the dissection of the bladder neck away from its usual location, and the development of the urethral syndrome, probably caused by continuing inflammation and irritation. These conditions generally respond to appropriate specific therapy.

Urolithiasis

Urinary tract stones may occur in patients of either sex and at any age. They may be related to metabolic abnormalities, such as gout or errors of calcium metabolism, but usually they relate to chronic infection and stasis of urine. Risk factors for calculi in women include pregnancy, during which time the urinary tract becomes dilated and stasis is more common; large cystoceles; and obstruction of outflow secondary to anatomic variations or external pressure from other organs.

A variety of management techniques are available, including observation awaiting spontaneous passage, endoscopic removal, surgical removal, and the destruction of the stone with the lithotriptor. The principal consideration, however, should be the correction of the basic problem that caused the stone.

GENUINE STRESS INCONTINENCE

Genuine stress incontinence occurs when increased intraabdominal pressure is not transmitted equally to the bladder and the functional urethra. If intraabdominal pressure plus bladder pressure is sufficient to overcome urethral closing pressure, incontinence will occur. The real problem is the fact that the bladder neck, the base of the bladder, and the proximal urethra are no longer adequately supported. This may result from a separation of the supports that hold the upper vagina and urethra to the pubic symphysis, from a relaxation of pelvic fascia and musculature secondary to childbearing or the aging process, or from some sort of trauma. Because the proximal two thirds of the urethra normally is an intraabdominal structure, an increased intraabdominal pressure would normally be exerted against it as well as the bladder. However, with a change in the anatomic relationships of this portion of the urethra, its intraabdominal position may be lost, thereby making it bear the brunt of such pressure rather than allowing it this degree of protection.

Over the years urethral length has been implicated as a related factor in stress incontinence. Lapides et al. measured urethral length using calibrated intraurethral catheters before and after operative correction of stress incontinence and found the urethra was shorter in cases of incontinence. However, during their procedure, downward traction was exerted to give the most meaningful measurement. Because the bladder neck in such women frequently funnels, accuracy of the measurements by Lapides et al. has been considered suspect. Other studies by multiple investigators using bead-chain urethrocystography have failed to show any change in urethral length before or after standard repair procedures. Thus it seems that, except for the most unusual circumstances, anatomic urethral length is not a major factor in stress incontinence.

The importance of a posterior urethrovesical angle in maintaining continence was first discussed by Jeffcoate and Roberts using urethrocystographic techniques in both continent and incontinent women. They concluded that a normal posterior urethrovesical angle (PUV) of less than 120 degrees was an important aspect of the continence mechanism, because such an angle was characteristically greater than 120 degrees in patients suffering from stress incontinence. This point has been verified by several authors since then. It has been noted that the relationship of the bladder neck and urethra to the pubic symphysis is not the major anatomic feature of the etiology of stress incontinence, because many patients with bladder descent but with a normal PUV angle were continent, whereas some incontinent women had bladders and urethras appropriately positioned to the pubic symphysis but had lost their PUV. Normal continent women demonstrate a bladder base nearly parallel to the horizontal in a standing position and have a sharply defined PUV angle of 90 to 100 degrees. When such bladders are visualized by cystourethrography, it is noted that the angle is maintained even with cough, and funneling does not occur. Most women with stress incontinence usually demonstrate near complete loss of the PUV angle and funneling and posterior descent of the vesical neck.

In the past Green and others have attempted to grade the severity of stress incontinence by the amount of loss of PUV angle. They defined type I loss as showing complete or almost complete loss of PUV angle but with the angle of inclination to the vertical of the urethral axis as being normal (10 to 30 degrees) or at least 45 degrees in the lateral standing–straining configuration, as measured by urethrocystogram. They define a type II defect as representing loss of the PUV angle, with an abnormal angle of inclination to the vertical of the urethral axis generally of 45 to 90 degrees. In 1971 the concept of a saline-moistened Q-tip test was introduced to differentiate these two types of defects. This test involved placing a Q-tip into the urethra and observing the angle the urethra made with the horizontal in the relaxed and voiding positions. Recently Montz and Stanton reevaluated the Q-tip test and discovered that 32% of patients with a positive Q-tip test had either pure detrusor instability or pure sensory urgency after a complete urologic workup. Further, 29% of the patients who had a negative Q-tip test were finally diagnosed as pure genuine stress incontinence. Although these authors noted that the Q-tip test was more likely to be positive in younger patients with a cystourethrocele who had undergone minimal bladder neck repair, they believed that the Q-tip test was not sensitive enough to differentiate stress incontinence from other forms of incontinence and recommended that more sensitive and specific urodynamic investigations be carried out in incontinent women.

Other investigators have noted similar findings and have concluded that the Q-tip test suggests defects in the anterior vaginal wall supports, but not a specific urological diagnosis. The test also quantifies the mobility of the bladder neck and proximal urethra in both continent and incontinent women with and without pelvic support relaxation, but offers no additional information about incontinence to that noted by history or physical examination.

A second test developed to help identify abnormalities of the bladder neck was the bead-chain cystourethrogram. This involved placing a sterile bead chain through the urethra into the bladder and x-raying the patient during the resting stage and during voiding. Recently, however, Fantl et al. demonstrated that 83 cystourethrograms interpreted by three radiologists using five specific radiologic landmarks failed to identify any agreement in interpretation, with a variation in interpretation of from 19.3% to 54.2%. Further, Fantl's group could find no statistically significant difference in the distribution of radiographic characteristics between patients with stress incontinence and detrusor instability.

It is well accepted today that the degree of loss of PUV angle is not as critical as the position of the bladder neck within the abdominal cavity, and Green's classification is no longer used in most centers.

Confusion in diagnosis is commonly caused by the presence of a cystocele. A cystocele is a herniation of the bladder into the vagina and is visualized with the patient in the lithotomy position as a bulge of the anterior vaginal wall. Most patients with cystoceles, however, have well-supported bladder necks and are continent. At times the anatomic defect involves the urethra and the bladder neck as well, forming a cystourethrocele. In such cases, in addition to the presence of the cystocele, the bladder neck is displaced also. Whereas the patient with a cystocele rarely has stress incontinence, the patient with the cystourethrocele frequently has stress incontinence.

Management

Before considering the operative approaches to the treatment of stress incontinence, it is reasonable to discuss other means of management. The first of these is directed toward the strengthening of the levator ani and pubococcygeal muscles. This can be effected by isometric exercises as described by Kegel. Although a number of modifications of these exercises exist, one useful application is to teach the patient to contract these muscles for the count of 10, 5 to 10 times, and to repeat this series several times a day. Interestingly, Kegel in 1956 suggested that the patient contract her pubococcygeal muscles 5 times on waking, 5 times on rising, and 5 times every half hour throughout the day. The patient can be instructed on how to contract these muscles by being told to attempt to stop the urinary stream while she is voiding. After she learns which muscles to contract, she may perform the exercises at any time without any relationship to voiding. These exercises improve the muscular supports of the bladder neck, and in some cases this may be enough to overcome the anatomic weakness that led to the stress incontinence.

Several studies have been performed to demonstrate the ability of patients to overcome stress incontinence by performing pelvic floor exercises. Henalla et al. used a form of pelvic floor exercise under the direction of physical therapists in two different hospitals. Using a perineal pad weighing test to assess the quantity of urine lost during exercise before and after 3 months of therapy, they found that 67% of patients achieved either complete continence or a significant improvement of symptoms. Although the severity of the symptoms before therapy and the patient's age had no effect on outcome, the treatment was noted to be more effective when the symptoms were present for less than a year. Tchou et al. performed urodynamic evaluations on 14 patients before and after pelvic floor exercise therapy. Of these, 9 experienced a reversion of their urinary stress test to negative, and all subjects reported an improvement in symptoms. Henalla et al. in a different study divided 104 patients with stress incontinence into four groups. The first group ($N = 26$) was treated with pelvic floor exercises; the second group ($N = 25$) was treated with a course of 10 interferential (electric current) treatments over a 10-week period (one per week); the third group ($N = 24$) was treated with vaginal conjugated estrogen cream, 2 gm per night for 12 weeks (1.25 mg conjugated estrogen/2 gm dose); and the fourth group ($N = 25$) was given no treatment and served as a control group. The groups were evaluated before and after therapy (after 3 months) with a perineal pad weighing test, and all 100 were available for questionnaire evaluation 9 months after therapy. A total of 65% (17) of the pelvic floor exercise group, 32% (8) of the interferential group, 12% (3) of the estrogen treated group, and none of the controls were found either cured or improved.

In postmenopausal women, estrogen therapy may increase the vasculature and the tone of the bladder neck, thereby increasing urethral closing pressure and again overcoming the effects that have led to mild degrees of stress incontinence. Estrogen also has a positive effect on pelvic supports in many women, and the combination of estrogen and Kegel exercises may occasionally be all that some women require to overcome their stress incontinence.

Other drugs and combinations of drugs have been studied to determine whether nonoperative therapy could aid stress incontinent women. In a study of 30 stress incontinent women using clinical and urodynamic assessment, Kiesswetter et al. compared continence profiles after treatment with an alpha adrenergic stimulant, midodrine; a cholinesterase inhibitor, distigmine bromide; a tricyclic antidepressant, imipramine; or an estriol, triodurin. In each case the patients were treated for 4 weeks and reevaluated. Finally, a suspensory sling operation was performed. After a successful sling operation the profile for continence as outlined by the authors increased 45% compared with an increase of 9% for midodrine, 8.9% for imipramine, and 7.9% for the combination of estriol and distigmine bromide. The urethral pressures showed an increase of mean value of 8.1% after operation, 8.3% after midodrine, 7.9% after imipramine, 3.5% after estriol, and 3.5% after distigmine bromide. The authors believed that estriol plus midodrine

TABLE 20-4

Drugs With Possible Effects on the Lower Urinary Tract

Class	Possible Side Effects	Drug and Usual Indication	Action
Antihypertensives	Incontinence	Reserpine—hypertension Methyldopa—hypertension	Pharmacologic sympathectomy by depleting catecholamines
Dopaminergic agonists	Bladder neck obstruction	Bromocriptine—galactorrhea Levodopa—Parkinson's disease	Increased urethral resistance and decreased detrusor contractions
Cholinergic agonists	Decreased bladder capacity and increased intravesical pressure	Digitalis—cardiotropic	Increased bladder wall tension
Neuroleptics	Incontinence	Major tranquilizers: prochlorperazine, promethazine, trifluoperazine, chlorpromazine, haloperidol	Dopamine receptor blockade, with internal sphincter relaxation
β-Adrenergic agents	Urinary retention	Isoxsuprine—vasodilator Terbutaline—bronchodilator Ritodrine—tocolytic agent	Inhibited bladder muscle contractility
Xanthines	Incontinence	Caffeine	Decreased urethral closure pressure

From Corlett RC: Female Patient 10:20, 1985.

and estriol plus imipramine were favored subjectively by the patients over single-drug therapy, but little difference was noted in urodynamic assessment to show the advantage of one drug or combination over another. Although imipramine is a tricyclic antidepressant, it has alpha-adrenergic enhancement characteristics. Table 20-4 is a summary by Corlett of classes of other agents that may affect urinary function or therapy.

Before the 1950s the operative approach to treat stress incontinence primarily involved vaginal procedures, which included plication of the bladder neck (Kelly procedure) with anterior colporrhaphy to reduce a cystocele. However, after Green attempted to grade the degree of PUV angle loss in such patients, it was demonstrated by Bailey and others that the success rate using the vaginal approach varied according to the etiology. Patients showing an almost complete loss of PUV angle had a 90% success rate when followed for 5 to 10 years after a bladder neck plication and anterior colporrhaphy, but only 50% of patients with lesser PUV angle loss remained continent over that

period. However, after the introduction of suprapubic urethrovesical suspension operations, the 5-year cure rate for these latter patients surpassed 90% in most series. It thus seemed important to determine the type of anatomic defect the patient had and to design appropriate operative management.

For the patient with a definite relaxation of the anterior vaginal wall and a bladder neck that is displaced into the lower pelvis, an anterior colporrhaphy with bladder neck plication is appropriate. This is frequently performed in conjunction with a vaginal hysterectomy if there is evidence for uterine prolapse and a posterior colporrhaphy, because such patients frequently have relaxation of the support structures of both anterior and posterior vaginal walls. The decision of whether to perform a vaginal hysterectomy and posterior wall repair depends on the circumstances of the patient and does not modify the success rate of the anterior colporrhaphy and bladder neck plication in treating stress incontinence.

The anterior colporrhaphy is carried out by incising the vaginal mucosa in the midline and

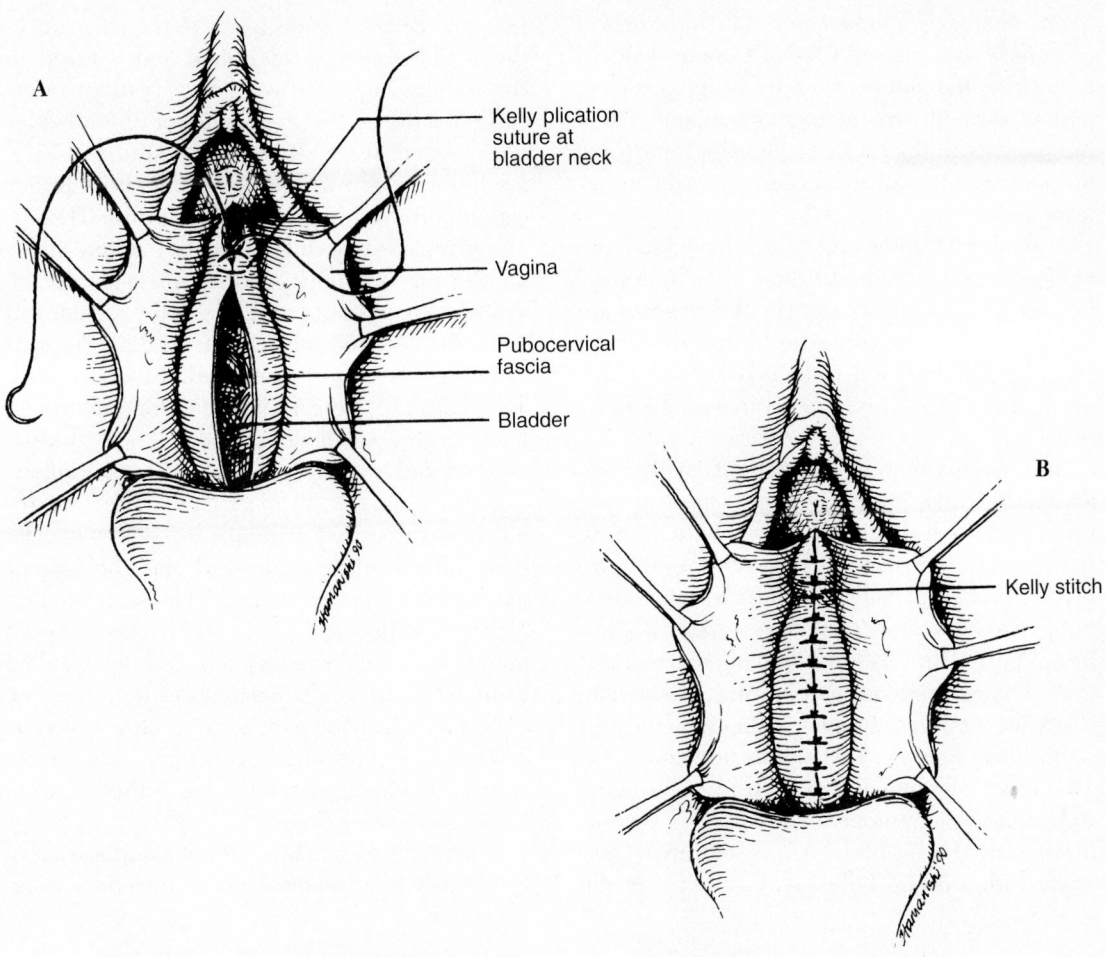

FIGURE 20-9
Cystourethrocele repair. **A,** Appearance of cystourethrocele after plication of bladder neck and repair of cystocele; cut edge of vagina is held apart above repair. **B,** Repair of vagina over cystocele is noted. (Redrawn from Symmonds RE: Relaxation of pelvic supports. In Benson RC, editor: Current obstetric and gynecologic diagnosis and treatment, ed 5, Los Altos, Calif, 1984, Lange Medical Publications.)

separating the pubocervical fascia from the vaginal mucosa by blunt and sharp dissection. The dissection is carried to the area of the bladder neck, and the first plication suture is placed on either side of the bladder neck using a 0 or 2-0 polyglycol suture. The slowly absorbable suture is ideal for this type of repair. Bladder plication is then continued from the area of the bladder neck to reduce an existing cystocele (Figure 20-9). In a patient with a displaced bladder neck and a cystourethrocele, it is often useful to place sutures in paravaginal tissue lateral to the bladder neck and fix this area to the pubic symphysis during the vaginal procedure. The vaginal tissue parallel to the bladder neck is identified and sutured with a polyglycol suture that is placed into the pubic symphysis. One suture on each side frequently suffices; the procedure requires a certain amount of dexterity, but the operator can quickly achieve this with practice.

Modifications of this procedure have been described. Special needles have been developed by Pereyra that can be used to guide sutures from the paravaginal tissue through the space of Retzius. Nonabsorbable material is used, and the suture is tied over the rectus fascia just above the bladder neck. This is carried out through a small suprapubic incision. It is appropriate to follow the steps of this procedure under direct urethrocystoscopy to avoid injuring the bladder neck during the needle placement. Stamey's modification of the Pereyra procedure uses a small tube of Dacron material to buttress the suture, thereby keeping it from pulling through. Stamey reports about 3% of the patients in his series required a removal of the suprapubic suture because of pain or infection.

A number of other procedures have been developed to support the bladder neck by repairing the endopelvic fascia via the vaginal approach. One such procedure recently developed by Raz is being evaluated by some surgeons and seems to be as effective as the Kelly plication.

Appropriate therapy for patients with bladder neck displacement, without significant anterior vaginal wall relaxation but with incontinence, in most instances is by a suprapubic approach. The Marshall-Marchetti-Krantz suprapubic urethrovesical suspension operation was first reported in 1949 and has been the mainstay of most surgeons attempting to alleviate stress incontinence in such patients. The procedure may be done by itself or in conjunction with other abdominal procedures, such as an abdominal hysterectomy. The space of Retzius is entered, the bladder neck is identified generally with a 30 ml bulb Foley catheter in the bladder, and the paravaginal tissue adjacent to the bladder neck is identified and sutured to the pubic symphysis using two or three interrupted sutures on each side of the bladder neck. Again, 0 or 2-0 polyglycol suture is ideal for this procedure, but some operators prefer catgut and even nonabsorbable suture. The operator must be careful not to place undue stress on the bladder neck. Stress can generally be assessed by placing one hand in the vagina and palpating the tension on the bladder neck at the time the sutures are tied (Figure 20-10). The space of Retzius is then drained for 48 hours with a small Penrose drain, and the patient is followed for 5 days with continuous catheter drainage. In most cases, after the removal of the catheter the patient will void. Occasionally, voiding is delayed and the patient may need to be discharged with an indwelling catheter in the bladder to be checked 1 week hence. It is usual to check a patient for residual urine after she voids; residuals of less than 100 to 150 ml, after the patient voids at least 100 to 200 ml, are considered acceptable. Larger residuals should signal continuing catheterization for 48 to 72 hours.

A rare (1% to 2%) but painful complication of the Marshall-Marchetti-Krantz procedure is os-

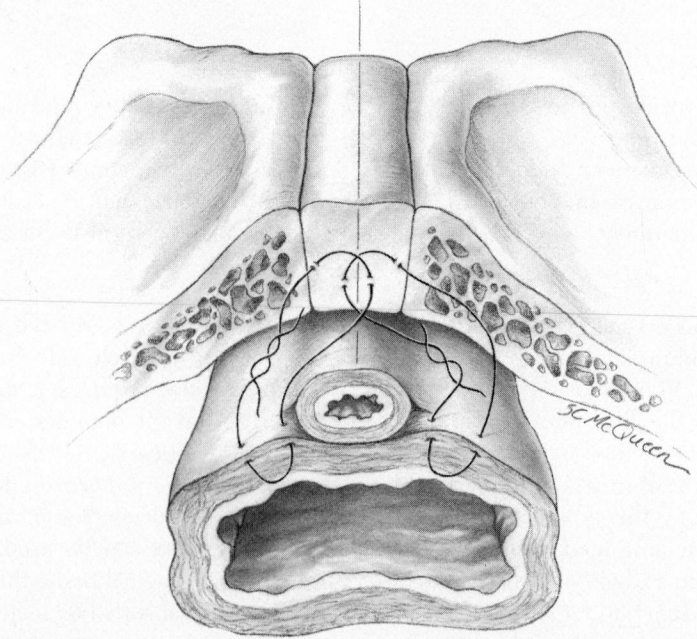

FIGURE 20-10
Demonstration of the relative position of a pair of sutures adjacent to the urethra securely placed into the pubic symphysis. (Redrawn from Buchsbaum HJ and Schmidt JD, editors: Gynecologic and obstetric urology. Reprinted with permission from WB Saunders Co, Philadelphia, 1982.)

teitis pubis. This condition is an inflammatory reaction in the periosteum of the pubic bone more often associated with permanent suture material. This complication after suprapubic cystotomy was first reported in 1923 by Legueu and Rochet. The next year Beer described six patients with pubic symphysis periostitis after suprapubic procedures. It is important to differentiate this condition from true osteomyelitis. The latter condition, seen occasionally after radical pelvic operations and other pelvic procedures, involves infection of the bone and is often associated with positive blood cultures. Hoyme et al. reviewed this subject in relation to radical gynecologic operations. Treatment of osteomyelitis often involves prolonged antibiotic therapy and surgical debridement. Treatment of osteitis pubis includes antibiotics and analgesics and may require the removal of permanent sutures.

In 1961 Burch advocated a modification of the suprapubic bladder neck suspension by suspending the vaginal wall to Cooper's ligament (Figure 20-11). The original description uses 2-0 chromic catgut suture, but polyglycol sutures are probably more appropriate now.

Postoperative care similar to that described for the Marshall-Marchetti-Krantz operation is appropriate. At times patients have difficulty voiding for prolonged periods, and the occasional patient may report that she needs to rise off the commode to a semistanding position to void.

Both the Marshall-Marchetti-Krantz and Burch procedures have their advocates. When properly performed, each procedure cures patients with stress incontinence in 90% to 95% of cases. Frequently failures can be resolved by performing the same procedure again, indicating that the problem was technical performance of the procedure rather than a failure of the type of procedure.

Sand et al. offered some insight into why at least some retropubic urethropexy procedures fail. In a study of 86 patients who were evaluated preoperatively and postoperatively with urodynamic studies, they noted that in women under 50 years of age there was a significant risk of failure if the preoperative urethral closure pressure was less than 20 cm H_2O. Although low urethral closure pressure was found to be an independent risk factor in women un-

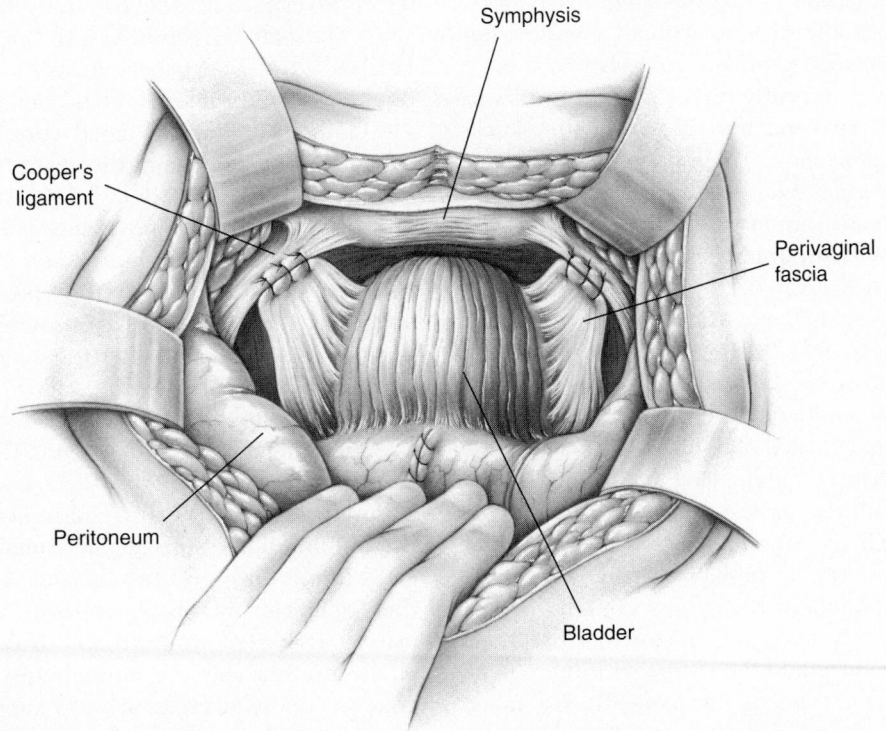

FIGURE 20-11
Burch procedure. The lateral edges of the vagina have been sutured to Cooper's ligament. (Redrawn from Burch JC: Am J Obstet Gynecol 81:281, 1961.)

der 50, it was not found to be so in women over 50. Thus in younger women, the urethral closure pressure preoperatively may help predict success.

In situations where the Marshall-Marchetti-Krantz or Burch operations fail and the operator does not wish to attempt a similar suspension, a fascial sling procedure may be considered. This procedure, which mobilizes the bladder neck completely using a vaginal and abdominal approach, allows for the imposition of a strip of anterior rectus fascia still attached surrounding the bladder neck and then reattached to the anterior rectus fascia on the opposite side. This creates a pulley effect, and with intraabdominal stress, contraction of the abdominal wall muscles allows for a "pulling up" effect on the bladder neck. This procedure is generally effective in creating continence.

The surgeon must exercise care in determining the tension to be applied on the bladder neck when the fascia is fixed. Making the sling too tight may interfere with voiding and may actually damage the bladder neck; making it too loose will abrogate its effectiveness. Generally with a No. 16 or 18 Foley catheter in the urethra it should be possible for the surgeon to judge the tension so that the sling fits comfortably against the urethra without compressing it. Concomitant cystoscopy may also be used.

Beck et al. recently reported their results in treating 170 patients over 22 years with a fascia lata sling procedure. These patients had undergone one or more unsuccessful attempts to correct their stress urinary incontinence. In all patients an intraurethral pressure of 80 to 90 cm of water was created at the site of the sling. Their success rate in curing the stress urinary incontinence was 98.2%, with 100% success noted in their last 148 cases. The most troublesome postoperative problem was delayed voiding, which averaged 59.6 days. Others, including the chapter author, have had similar experiences with this procedure.

Although an anterior rectus sheath fascial sling procedure is probably as effective as a Marshall-Marchetti-Krantz or Burch procedure, it involves a greater degree of dissection, as well as entry into the vagina with the potential risk of ascending infection. It is a more complicated procedure than necessary in most cases.

Other types of sling procedures have been advocated over the years, including using inert materials, such as Mersilene and polypropylene (Marlex), and a variety of human and nonhuman fascial strips. These slings have been fashioned to encircle the urethra and to be put in place by vaginal, abdominal, or combined procedures. In many cases the inert material or nonhuman fascial strips have been rejected or, in the case of the latter, reabsorbed. Risk of morbidity, especially by infection, has been considerable. The anterior rectus sheath sling operation is the safest and most successful, but it should be used only after a Marshall-Marchetti-Krantz or Burch procedure failure.

Some surgeons have suggested that the symptoms of stress urinary incontinence could be relieved by the periurethral injection of Teflon. This procedure was thought to increase urethral resistance by compressing the urethral lumen. Although some success has been reported in women with normal pelvic floor anatomy, the success rate in others has been unpredictable.

Urodynamic Studies After Retropubic Urethropexy for Stress Incontinence

In a study of 29 women with stress incontinence investigated urodynamically before and after Marshall-Marchetti-Krantz operation by Beisland et al., no major changes in the urethral pressure profile could be demonstrated. The authors did note a good correlation between clinical results and the changes in transmission of increased abdominal pressure to the urethra. The operative procedure did not seem to increase the urethral pressure. Those patients with low maximal urethral pressure preoperatively continued to have insufficient urethral sphincter function after the operation. Indeed the operation in some cases may have caused injury to the sphincter because of excessive dissection around the urethra. The authors pointed out that patients with a low urethral closure pressure but with good transmission to the urethra of pressure are not suitable candidates for urethropexy. Insufficiency of the urethral sphincter in postmenopausal women is usually associated with atrophy of the mucosa of the urethra and the epithelium of the vagina, as well as decreased blood supply in the periurethral tissue. The authors suggested such patients should be treated with a combination of alpha-receptor stimulating drugs and estrogen and not by operation.

In a study of 25 women after Burch colposuspension in which 88% had objective evidence of cure, an increase in voiding difficulty and urodynamic evidence of outflow obstruction was seen 6 months after the procedure. Beisland et al. also noted that the Burch procedure, like the Marshall-Marchetti-Krantz operation, does not induce any significant change in resting urethral profile; they believed the changes noted were probably a mechanical obstruction of the bladder neck.

Recently, van Geelen et al. investigated the urodynamic effects of both anterior vaginal wall and Burch procedures. There were no changes in resting urethral pressure profiles in either group of patients after surgery. Pressure transmission rates in the proximal urethra were increased in women treated successfully with the Burch procedure in supine, sitting, and standing positions, but in women unsuccessfully relieved of their incontinence, no significant increase in pressure transmission could be noted. In those women treated successfully with an anterior repair, a significant increase in pressure was observed in the midurethra in the sitting position and in the proximal urethra in the standing position. The authors concluded that the Burch procedure was more effective than an anterior repair in correcting genuine stress incontinence.

Some authors have suggested that the chance of curing genuine stress incontinence with a surgical procedure was increased by performing a hysterectomy as well. Van Geelen et al. did not note this in their study, and in a recent report by Langer et al. no differences were found in the cure rate of 45 patients of whom 22 underwent a Burch procedure without hysterectomy and 23 underwent a Burch procedure with hysterectomy.

It is difficult to compare the results obtained in curing stress incontinence with different procedures. Differences in techniques and skills of different operators and differences in patient selection methods make different procedures difficult to compare. In a large study of 680 surgically treated patients reported by Park and Miller, the Marshall-Marchetti-Krantz procedure and Kelly plication were noted to be equally successful in correcting stress incontinence after 3 years (69% and 66% respectively). Patients who underwent the Pereyra procedure as their primary repair had a 41% success rate after 3 years. Still, the reader must remember that differences in the groups and in the skills of the surgeons involved may have played a role in the outcomes.

DETRUSOR DYSSYNERGIA

Walter and Olesen studied 303 patients complaining of urinary incontinence and discovered that 43% had stress incontinence, 21% urge incontinence, and 36% both urge and stress incontinence. Most patients with urge incontinence suffer from detrusor dyssynergia. This condition is generally chronic and is associated with an urgency-frequency problem often accompanied by painless urine loss. Generally a large volume of urine is lost; leakage may occur in any position and often with a change in position. Stress secondary to running, walking, coughing, sneezing, or laughing may trigger this type of incontinence, but it is generally delayed until several seconds after the stress has occurred. Stress incontinence frequently disappears during the night but urge incontinence continues, often with nocturia. Patients are often unable to stop their stream during the act of voiding, whereas women with stress incontinence can accomplish this.

Detrusor dyssynergia is the result of sudden, spontaneous detrusor muscle activity and has previously been termed *detrusor instability* or *detrusor irritability*. Some 50% to 80% of patients have an underlying functional or psychosomatic component. Patients, however, may suffer from generalized diseases affecting the bladder or its innervation.

The loss of urine is probably triggered by sudden, uninhibited stimulation of receptors in the bladder wall. These may be hyperreactive for emotional reasons or may be a result of chronic irritation. The problem may also be caused by the breakdown of normal neurologic and inhibitory reflexes. Frequently such patients demonstrate symptoms of chronic anxiety.

Recently a study of 86 women with genuine stress incontinence was reported by Sands et al. Of these, 20 (23.3%) also had unstable detrusor function preoperatively. Of these 20, 11 (55%) had stable detrusor function after retropubic urethropexy, whereas 5 of the 66 (7.6%) patients who had stable detrusor function preoperatively developed unstable detrusors postoperatively. Overall, women with both stress incontinence and unstable detrusors experienced a cure rate of only 30% with surgery. No relationship could be found in preoperative symptoms, age, history of previous procedures, and cystometric parameters between those who were cured and those who were not. In addition, none of these criteria could predict which patient who was detrusor stable before surgery would develop instability after surgery. Risks of developing detrusor instability after surgery must be recognized and may require further medical therapy.

Diagnosis

Electronic urethrocystometry and fluid cystometrographic techniques allow the detection of spontaneous involuntary pressure changes within the bladder, which are noted as the bladder fills. These techniques are also useful in detecting patients with true stress incontinence who have an urgency incontinence (detrusor dyssynergic) component to their incontinence. It is important that in such cases both problems be treated, or it is not likely that incontinence will be cured.

Management

Operative procedures are useless in treating urgency incontinence. In fact, they can be expected to have no influence on the problem at all. In those patients who have stress incontinence and detrusor dyssynergia, an operation may have a place in the specific therapy. However, if the major part of the problem seems to be detrusor dyssynergia, this should be treated first, as an operative procedure frequently may not be necessary. Likewise, patients who have undergone an operation for stress urinary incontinence and continue to be incontinent should be evaluated for detrusor dyssynergia. Bates et al. demonstrated that a high percentage of such failures will be found on urethrocystometric studies to have detrusor dyssynergia.

Because the majority of patients with detrusor dyssynergia have psychosomatic problems, retraining or bladder drills may be of use. This should take the form of bladder retraining, which involves a programmed progressive lengthening of the period between voiding with or without the addition of biofeedback techniques. In a study Millard and Oldenburg demonstrated improvement in 74% of women with detrusor dyssynergia using such techniques. Cystometric studies performed on these patients revealed a reversion to stable bladder function.

Postmenopausal women may benefit from estrogen therapy; estrogen not only improves the vasculature of the bladder neck and the mucosa of the urethra and trigone, but also has an alpha-adrenergic stimulating capacity that may help overall urinary control.

Anticholinergic drugs or beta-adrenergic stimulation that will relax the detrusor muscle may be useful. The following may be tried: propantheline (Pro-Banthine) at doses of 15 to 30 mg 4 times a day, oxybutynin chloride (Ditropan) 5 mg every 8 to 12 hours, flavoxate (Urispas) 200 mg every 6 hours, imipramine (Tofranil) 50 mg every 8 hours, or ephedrine sulfate 25 mg every 6 hours. At times these medications in conjunction with bladder retraining have greater efficacy than either alone.

TRUE INCONTINENCE

True incontinence is a loss of urine without abnormal bladder function. This is generally caused by fistulas or by other damage to the urinary tract. Such damage may occur congenitally or secondary to trauma.

OVERFLOW INCONTINENCE

Overflow incontinence occurs when a bladder is overdistended because of its inability to empty. The problem may be caused by a neurologic disorder that interferes with normal bladder reflexes or by partial obstruction of the urethra. Typically the patient complains of voiding small amounts and still having the feeling that there is urine in the bladder. In addition, the patient frequently loses small amounts of urine without any control. This condition is commonly seen in patients with multiple sclerosis, diabetic neuropathy, and trauma or tumors of the central nervous system. A complete general medical and urologic workup is necessary to clarify the patient's condition. Therapy directed at the primary cause may be beneficial. Often the patient must be trained in techniques of intermittent self-catheterization.

_____ **KEY POINTS** _____

- As many as 30% of all women may suffer from some degree of urinary incontinence during their lifetime.

- Continence is determined by the balance between those forces that maintain urethral closure and those that affect detrusor function.

- Parasympathetic nervous system activity via the neurotransmitter acetylcholine stimulates receptors in the bladder wall to activate detrusor contraction.

- Anticholinergic agents decrease detrusor activity.

- Sympathetic nervous system receptors in the bladder are mostly beta receptors and when stimulated cause relaxation.

- Sympathetic nervous system receptors in the urethra are basically alpha receptors. Stimulation causes contraction.

- The highest pressure zone in the urethra is about midpoint in the functional urethra, which is roughly 0.5 cm proximal to the urogenital diaphragm.

- Resting pressure within the bladder is between 20 and 30 cm H_2O.

- A normal bladder transmits a voiding urge at 150 to 200 ml volume, and functional capacity is generally 400 to 500 ml.

- About 20% of all women will develop urinary infections at some time in their life, and by age 70 as many as 10% of women will have chronic urinary tract infections.

- Bacterial counts of 100,000 or greater per milliliter of urine usually indicate a urinary tract infection. *Escherichia coli* is the most common organism seen.

- Bacterial counts of 100 per milliliter may be seen in patients with urethritis.

- Some 3% to 4% of all women will suffer from urethral diverticula, with the majority of cases occurring between the ages of 30 and 50. Most urethral diverticula originate in the middle third of the urethra, but diverticula may occur from any area of the urethra and may be multiple.

- Urethral syndrome can occur in as many as 20% to 30% of women and should not be diagnosed until all infectious organisms have been discounted.

- Some 75% to 80% of women with urinary incontinence suffer from stress incontinence.

- The cure rate for Marshall-Marchetti-Krantz and Burch procedures is usually 90% to 95%.

- Osteitis pubis occurs in 1% to 2% of suprapubic suspension operations.

- Long-term (over 3 years) follow-up of patients who underwent Kelly plication of the bladder neck and those who underwent retropubic urethropexy showed the two procedures had about the same success rate.

- About 20% of women with urinary incontinence suffer from detrusor dyssynergia.

- Some 50% to 80% of patients with detrusor dyssynergia have an underlying functional or psychosomatic component.

- Operative procedures are of no value in treating detrusor dyssynergia unless there is a stress incontinence component as well.

- An indwelling catheter for more than 24 hours leads to urinary tract infection in about 50% of cases and in nearly 100% after 96 hours.

BIBLIOGRAPHY

Andersen MTF: The incidence of diverticula in the female urethra, J Urol 98:96, 1967.

Arnold EP, Webster JR, Loose H, et al: Urodynamics of female incontinence: factors influencing the results of surgery, Am J Obstet Gynecol 117:805, 1973.

Asmussen M and Ulmsten U: A new technique for measurement of the urethra pressure profile, Acta Obstet Gynecol Scand 55:167, 1976.

Asmussen M and Ulmsten U: Simultaneous urethrocystommetry with a new technique, Scand J Urol Nephrol 10:7, 1976.

Asmussen M and Ulmsten U: On the physiology of continence and pathophysiology of stress incontinence in the female. In Controversies in gynecology and obstetrics, vol 10, Basel, 1983, Karger, S, AG.

Bailey KV: A clinical investigation into uterine prolapse with stress incontinence. Treatment by modified Manchester colporrhaphy, J Obstet Gynaecol Br Comm Part I, 61:291, 1954; Part II, 63:663, 1956; Part III, 70:947, 1963.

Barnett RM: The modern Kelly plication, Obstet Gynecol 34:667, 1969.

Bates CP, Bradley W, Glen E, et al: First report of the standardization of terminology of lower urinary tract function, J Urol 48:39, 1976.

Bates P, Bradley WE, Glen E, et al: The standardization of terminology of lower urinary tract function, J Urol 121:551, 1979.

Bates CP, Loose H, and Stanton SLR: The objective study of incontinence after repair operations, Surg Gynecol Obstet 136:17, 1973.

Beck RP and Maughan GB: Simultaneous intraurethral and intravesical pressure studies in normal women and those with stress incontinence, Am J Obstet Gynecol 89:746, 1964.

Beck RP, McCormick S, and Nordstrom L: The fascia lata sling procedure for treating recurrent genuine stress incontinence of urine, Obstet Gynecol 72:699, 1988.

Beer E: Periostitis of the symphysis and descending rami of the pubes following suprapubic operations, Int J Med 37:224, 1924.

Beisland HO, Fossberg E, and Sander S: Urodynamic studies before and after retropubic urethropexy for stress incontinence in females, Surg Gynecol Obstet 155:333, 1982.

Bhatia NN and Bergman A: Urodynamic appraisal of the Bonney test in women with stress urinary incontinence, Obstet Gynecol 62:696, 1983.

Bhatia NN and Ostergard DR: Urodynamics in women with stress urinary incontinence, Obstet Gynecol 60:552, 1982.

Buchsbaum HJ and Schmidt JD, editors: Gynecologic and obstetric urology. Philadelphia, 1982, WB Saunders Co.

Burch JC: Cooper's ligament urethrovesical suspension for stress incontinence, Am J Obstet Gynecol 100:764, 1968.

Cherney C and Boscia JA: Asymptomatic bacteriuria in the elderly, Geriatric Medicine 7:46, 1988.

Corlett RC: Gynecologic urology. I. Urinary incontinence, Female Patient 10:20, 1985.

DeLancey JO: Correlative study of periurethral anatomy, Obstet Gynecol 68:91, 1986.

DeLancey JO: Structural aspects of the extrinsic continence mechanism, Obstet Gynecol 72:296, 1988.

Enhorning G: Simultaneous recording of intravesical and intraurethral pressure, Acta Chir Scand Suppl 276:1, 1971.

Fantl JA, Beachley MC, Bosch HA, et al: Bead-chain cystourethrogram: an evaluation, Obstet Gynecol 58:237, 1981.

Fernie GR, Jewett MAS, Halsall P, et al: Urodynamic characterization of incontinence in the elderly by bladder volume, J Urol 129:772, 1983.

Fossberg E, Veisland HO, and Lundgren RA: Stress incontinence in females: treatment with phenylpropanolamine: a urodynamic and pharmacological evaluation, Urol Int 38:293, 1983.

Frewen WK: Urgency incontinence, J Obstet Gynaecol Br Comm 79:77, 1972.

Gillespie WA, Henderson EP, Linton KB, and Smith PJB: Microbiology of the urethral (frequency and dysuria) syndrome: a controlled study with a 5-year review, Br J Urology 64:270, 1989.

Gossling JA, Dixon JS, Critchley, et al: Comparative studies of the human external sphincter and periurethral levator ani muscles, Br J Urol 53:35, 1981.

Green TH Jr: Development of a plan for diagnosis and treatment of urinary stress incontinence, Am J Obstet Gynecol 83:632, 1962.

Green TH Jr: The problem of urinary stress incontinence in the female: an appraisal of its current status, Obstet Gynecol Surv 23:603, 1968.

Green TH Jr: Urinary stress incontinence differential diagnosis pathophysiology and management, Am J Obstet Gynecol 122:368, 1975.

Hajj SN: Female urinary incontinence: a dynamic evaluation, J Reprod Med 23:33, 1979.

Henalla SM, Hutchins CJ, Robinson P, and MacVicar J: Nonoperative methods in the treatment of female genuine stress incontinence of urine, Br J Obstet Gynaecol 9:222, 1989.

Henalla SM, Kirwan P, Castleden CM, et al: The effect of pelvic floor exercises in the treatment of genuine urinary stress incontinence in women at two hospitals, Br J Obstet Gynaecol 95:602, 1988.

Henriksson L and Ulmsten U: Urodynamic evaluation of the effects of abdominal urethrocystopexy and vaginal sling urethroplasty in women with stress incontinence, Am J Obstet Gynecol 131:77, 1978.

Hilton P and Stanton SL: A clinical and urodynamic assessment of the Burch colposuspension for genuine stress incontinence, Br J Obstet Gynaecol 90:934, 1983.

Hilton P and Stanton SL: Urethral pressure measurements by microtransducer: the results of symptom-free women and in those with genuine stress incontinence, Br J Obstet Gynaecol 90:919, 1983.

Hilton P and Stanton SL: Use of intravaginal oestrogen cream in genuine stress incontinence, Br J Obstet Gynaecol 90:940, 1983.

Hodgkinson CP: Relationships of the female urethra and bladder in urinary stress incontinence, Am J Obstet Gynecol 65:506, 1953.

Hodgkinson CP and Cobert N: Direct urethrocystommetry, Am J Obstet Gynecol 79:648, 1960.

Hodgkinson CP, Ayers MA, and Drukker BH: Dyssynergic detrusor dysfunction in the apparently normal female, Am J Obstet Gynecol 87:717, 1963.

Hodgkinson CP, Drukker BH, and Hershey GJG: Stress urinary incontinence in the female. VIII. Etiology significance of the short urethra, Am J Obstet Gynecol 86:16, 1963.

Holst K and Wilson PD: The prevalence of female urinary incontinence and reasons for not seeking treatment, NZ Med J 101:758, 1988.

Hoyme UB, Tamimi HK, Eschenbach DA, et al: Osteomyelitis pubis after radical gynecologic operations, Obstet Gynecol 63:47S, 1984.

Jeffcoate TNA and Roberts H: Observations of stress incontinence of urine, Am J Obstet Gynecol 64:721, 1952.

Karram MM and Bhatia NN: The Q-tip test: standardization of the technique and its interpretation in women with urinary incontinence, Obstet Gynecol 71:807, 1988.

Kegel AH: Stress incontinence of urine in women: physiologic treatment, J Int Coll Surg 25:487, 1956.

Kiesswetter H, Hennrich F, and Englisch M: Clinical and urodynamic assessment of pharmacologic therapy of stress incontinence, Urol Int 38:58, 1983.

Kujansuu E: The effect of pelvic floor exercises on urethral function in female stress incontinence and urodynamic study, Ann Chir Gynaecol 72:28, 1983.

Langer R, Ron-El R, Neuman M, et al: The value of simultaneous hysterectomy during Burch colposuspension for urinary stress incontinence, Obstet Gynecol 72:866, 1988.

Lapides J: Transurethral treatment of urethral diverticula in women, Trans Am Assoc Genitourin Surg 70:135, 1978.

Lapides J, Ajemian EP, Stewart BH, et al: Physiopathology of stress incontinence, Surg Gynecol Obstet 111:224, 1960.

Lee RA: Diverticulum of the female urethra: postoperative complications and results, Obstet Gynecol 61:52, 1983.

Legueu and Rochet: Les cellulites perivesicales et pelviennes, J Urol Med Chir 15:1, 1923.

Low JA: Clinical characteristics of patients with demonstrable urinary incontinence, Am J Obstet Gynecol 88:322, 1964.

MacKinnon M, Pratt JH, and Pool TL: Diverticulum of the female urethra, Surg Clin North Am 39:953, 1959.

Marchetti AA, Marshall VF, and Shultis LD: Simple vesicourethral suspension for stress incontinence of urine, Am J Obstet Gynecol 74:57, 1957.

Migliorini GR and Glenning PP: Bonney's test—fact or fiction? Br J Obstet Gynaecol 94:157, 1987.

Millard RJ, and Oldenburg BF: The symptomatic urodynamic and psychodynamic results of bladder reeducation programs, J Urol 130:715, 1983.

Mohr JA, Rogers J Jr, Brown TN, et al: Stress urinary incontinence. The simple and practical approach to diagnosis and treatment, J Am Geriatr Soc 31:476, 1983.

Montz FJ and Stanton SL: Q-tip test in female urinary incontinence, Obstet Gynecol 67:258, 1986.

Muellner SR and Fleischner FG: Normal and abnormal micturition study of the bladder behavior by means of fluoroscopy, J Urol 61:233, 1949.

Nichols DH: A Mersilene mesh gauze hammock for severe urinary stress incontinence, Obstet Gynecol 41:88, 1973.

Ostergard DR: The effect of drugs on the lower urinary tract, Obstet Gynecol Surv 34:424, 1979.

Ostergard DR: The neurologic control of micturition and integral voiding reflexes, Obstet Gynecol Surv 34:417, 1979.

Park GS and Miller EJ Jr: Surgical treatment of stress urinary incontinence: a comparison of the Kelly plication, Marshall-Marchetti-Krantz, and Pereyra procedures, Obstet Gynecol 71:575, 1988.

Pereyra AJ: A simplified surgical procedure for the correction of stress incontinence in women, West J Surg 67:223, 1959.

Pereyra AJ and Lebherz TB: Combined urethrovesical suspension and vaginal urethroplasty for correction of stress incontinence, Obstet Gynecol 30:537, 1967.

Rudd T: Urethral pressure profile in continent women from childhood to old age, Acta Obstet Gynecol Scand 59:331, 1979.

Sand PK, Bowen LW, Panganiban R, and Ostergard DR: The low pressure urethra as a factor in failed retropubic urethropexy, Obstet Gynecol 69:399, 1987.

Sand PK, Bowen LW, Ostergard DR, et al: The effect of retropubic urethropexy on detrusor stability, Obstet Gynecol 71:818, 1988.

Sand PK, Bowen LW, Ostergard DR, et al: Cryosurgery versus dilation and massage for the treatment of recurrent urethral syndrome, J Repro Med 34:499, 1989.

Sjoberg B and Nyman CR: Hydrodynamics of micturition in stress incontinent women: comparisons of pressure and flow at different micturition volumes in stress incontinent and continent women, Scand J Urol Nephrol 16:1, 1982.

Spence HM and Duckett JW Jr: Diverticulum of the female urethra: clinical aspects and presentation of a simple operative technique for cure, J Urol 104:432, 1970.

Spraitz AF Jr and Welch JS: Diverticulum of the female urethra, Am J Obstet Gynecol 91:1013, 1965.

Stamey TA: Endoscopic suspension of the vesical neck for urinary incontinence in females: report of 203 consecutive cases, Ann Surg 192:465, 1980.

Tchou DCH, Adams C, Varner RE, and Denton B: Pelvic-floor musculature exercises in treatment of anatomical urinary stress incontinence, Physical Therapy 68:652, 1988.

Teasdale TA, Taffet GE, Luchi RJ, and Adam E: Urinary incontinence in a community-residing elderly population, J Am Geriatr Soc 36:600, 1988.

Te Linde RW: Urethral sling operation, Clin Obstet Gynecol 6:206, 1963.

Van Geelen JM, Theeuwes AGM, Eskes TKAB, and Martin CB Jr: The clinical and urodynamic effects of anterior vaginal repair and Burch colposuspension, Am J Obstet Gynecol 159:137, 1988.

Vesey SG, Rivett A, and O'Boyle PJ: Teflon injection in female stress incontinence: effect on urethral pressure profile and flow rate, B J Urology 62:39, 1988.

Walter S and Olesen KP: Urinary incontinence in genital prolapse in the female: clinical urodynamic and radiologic examinations, Br J Obstet Gynaecol 89:393, 1982.

Walters MD and Diaz K: Q-tip test: a study of continent and incontinent women, Obstet Gynecol 70:208, 1987.

Walters MD and Shields LE: The diagnostic value of history, physical examination, and the Q-tip cotton swab test in women with urinary incontinence, Am J Obstet Gynecol 159:145, 1988.

Westby M, Asmussen M, and Ulmsten U: Localization of maximum intraurethral pressure related to urogenital diaphragm in the female subject as studied by simultaneous urethrocystommetry and voiding urethrocystography, Am J Obstet Gynecol 144:408, 1982.

Williams ME and Fitzhugh CP: Urinary incontinence in the elderly, Ann Intern Med 97:895, 1982.

APPENDIX

Drugs That Affect Bladder Functions

Generic Name	Trade Name	Generic Name	Trade Name
Drugs affecting sympathetic nervous system		**General adrenergic stimulators—cont'd**	
Alpha-adrenergic blockers		Levamphetamine	Ad-Nil, Amodril, Cydril, Maigret
Azapetine	Ilidar	Mazindol	Sanorex
Dihydroergotoxine	Hydergine	Mephentermine	Wyamine
Ergot alkaloids	—	Methamphetamine	Dexoxyn
Phenothiazines	(Various; see below: Drugs Affecting Autonomic Nervous System—Causing Retention)	Methylaminoheptane	Oenethyl
		Methylhexamine	Forthane
		Naphazoline	Privine
		Oxymetazoline	Afrin
Phentolamine	Regitine	Phedrazine*	—
Piperoxan	Benodaine	Phendimetrazine	Dietrol, Plegine
Tolazoline	Priscoline	Phenmetrazine	Preludin
		Phentermine	Ionamin, Wilpo
Beta-adrenergic blockers		Pholedrine	Paredrinal
Alprenolol	—	Propylhexedrine	Benzedrex
Butidrine	—	Pseudoephedrine	Sudafed, Ro-Fedrin
Butoxamine	—	Racephedrine	—
Dichloroisoproterenol	Alderlin, Nethalide, Pronethalol	Synephrine*	—
		Tenaphtoxaline*	—
Isopropylmethoxamine	—	Tetrahydrozoline	Tyzine
Ko692	—	Tramazoline	—
LB-46	Prinololol	Tuaminoheptane	Taumine
M 1999	Sotalol	Tymazoline*	Pernazene
Oxprenolol	—	Xylometazoline	Otrivin
Practolol	Eraldin	***Alpha-adrenergic stimulators***	
General adrenergic stimulators		Amidephrine	—
Adrenalone	Kephrine	Cyclopentamine	Clopane
Aminorex*	—	Dopamine	Intropin
—	Aranthol	Etafedrine	—
Benzphetamine	Didrex	Ethylphenylephrine	Effortil
Chlorphentermine	Pre-Sate	Hydroxyamphetamine	Paredrine
Clortemine	Voranil	Metaraminol	Aramine
Cyclopantamine	Clopane	Methamphetamine	Desoxyn; Efroxine, Methedrine, Norodin, Synodroy
Deoxyepinephrine	Epinine		
Dextroamphetamine	Dexedrine		
Diethylpropion	Tenuate, Tepanil	Methoxamine	Vasoxyl
Epinephrine	—	Methylhexaneamine	Forthane
Ethylnorepinephrine	Bronkephrine	Nordefrin	Cobefrin
Fenfluramine	Pondimin	Norepinephrine	Levarterenol
Hydroxyamphetamine	Paredrine	Novadral	—
H1032*	—	Phenylephrine	Neo-Synephrine, Isophrin, Synasal, Alconefrin Biomydrin, Isohalent Improved
Isometheptene	Octin		

*Not available in the United States.

Continued.

Drugs That Affect Bladder Functions—cont'd

Generic Name	Trade Name	Generic Name	Trade Name
Alpha-adrenergic stimulators—cont'd		**Drugs affecting parasympathetic nervous system**	
Phenylpropylmethylamine	Vonedrine	***Stimulators***	
Propylhexedrine	Benzedrex	Ambenonium	Mytelase
Tyramine	—	Carbachol	Carcholin, Isopto Carbachol
Beta-adrenergic stimulators		Echothiophate	Phospholine
Albuterol	Proventil, Ventolin	Demecarium	Humorsol
Bamethan*	—	Edrophonium	Tensilon
Chlorprenaline	—	Isoflurophate	Floropryl
Dioxethedrine	—	Methacholine	Mecholyl
Etafedrine	—	Pilocarpine	Pilocar
Ethylnorepinephrine	Butanefrine, Bronkephrine	Pralidoxime	Protopam
Hydroxyephedrine	—	Pyridostigmine	Mestinon
Isoethamine	—	***Inhibitors***	
Isoproterenol	Aludrine, Isuprel, Norisodrine	Adiphenine	Trasentine
		Alverine	Prafenil, Spacolin
Methoxyphenamine	Orthoxine	Anisotropine	Valpin
Nylidrin	Arlidin	Atropine	—
Protokylol	Caytine	Belladonna extract	—
Salbutanal	—	Carbofluorene	Pavatrine
Soterenol	—	Clidinium	Librax, Quarzan
Terbutaline	Bricamyl	Cyclopentolate	Cyclogyl
Adrenergic neuron blockers		Diphemanil	Prantal
Alseroxylon	Rautensin, Rauwiloid	Ethaverine	Ethaquin, Laverin, Neopavrin
Bethanidine	Esbatal		
Bretylium	Darenthin	Eucatropine	Euphthalmine
Debrisoquin	Declinax	Glycopyrrolate	Robinul
Deserpidine	Harmonyl	Hexocyclium	Tral
Guanadrel	—	Homatropine hydrobromide	—
Guanethidine	Ismelin		
Guanoclor	Vatensol	Homatropine methylbromide	Homapin, Malcotran, Mesopin, Novatrin
Guanoxan	Envacar		
Hydralazine	Apresoline	Hyoscyamine sulfate	Levsin
Methyldopa	Aldomet	Isometheptene	Isometene, Octin
Methyldopate	Aldomet Ester	Mepenzolate	Cantil
Nialamide	—	Methixene	Trest
Pargyline	Eutonyl	Methscopolamine bromide	Pamine
Rauwolfia	Hyperloid, Raudixin, Rauja, Raulfin, Rautina, Rauval, Venibar	Methylatropine nitrate (atropine methylnitrate)	Metropine
Rescinnamine	Cinatabs, Moderil	Oxyphenonium	Antrenyl
Reserpine	Lemiserp, Rau-Sed, Resercen, Reserpoid, Rolserp, Sandril, Serpasil, Sertina, Vio-Serpine	Papaverine	Cerespan, Pap-Kaps, Pavabid, Pavacap, Pavacen, Pavarine, Pavatest, Paveril, Vasal, Vasospan
Syrosingopine	Singoserp	Pentapiperium	Quilene
Tranylcypromine	—	Penthienate	Monodral
Veratrum alkaloids	Unitensin, Veralba, Veriloid, Vertairs	Pipenzolate	Piptal
		Piperidolate	Dactil
		Poldine	Nacton
		Scopolamine	—

Drugs That Affect Bladder Functions—cont'd

Generic Name	Trade Name	Generic Name	Trade Name
Inhibitors—cont'd		**Causing retention—cont'd**	
Thihexinol	Sorboquel	Isocarboxazid	Marplan
Thiphenamil	Trocinate	Mepazine	—
Tincture of belladonna	—	Mesoridazine	Serentil
Tricyclamol	Elorine	Metaxalone	Skelaxin
Tridihexethyl	Pathilon	Methapyrilene	Histadyl
Tropicamide	Mydriacyl	Methdilazine	Tacaryl
Valethamate	Murel	Methylphenidate	Ritalin
		Methysergide	Sansert
Drugs affecting sympathetic and parasympathetic nervous system—ganglionic blockers		Molindone	Moban
		Nortriptyline	Aventyl
Azamethonium	Pendiomid	Orphenadrine	Norflex
Chlorisondamine	Ecolid	Perphenazine	Trilafon
Hexamethonium	—	Phenelzine	Nardil
Mecamylamine	Inversine	Phenindamine	Thephorin
Methaphan	Arfonad	Piperacetazine	Quide
Pentolinium	Ansolysen	Pipradrol	Meratran
Sparteine	Spartocin, Tocosamine	Prochlorperazine	Compazine
Trimethidinium	Ostensin	Procyclidine	Kemadrin
		Promazine	Sparine
Drugs affecting autonomic nervous system		Promethazine	Phenergan
Causing retention		Protriptyline	Vivactil
Acetophenazine	Tindal	Pyrilamine	—
Amitriptyline	Elavil	Rotoxamine	Turiston
Amphotericin B	Fungizone	Thiopropazate	Dartal
Benztropine	Cogentin	Thioridazine	Mellaril
Biperiden	Akineton	Thiothixene	Navane
Bromodiphenhydramine	Ambodryl	Tranylcypromine	Parnate
Brompheniramine	Dimetane	Trifluoperazine	Stelazine
Butaperazine	Repoise	Triflupromazine	Vesprin
Carbinoxamine	Clistin	Trihexyphenidyl	Artane, Pipanol, Tremin
Carphenazine	Proketazine	Trimeprazine	Temaril
Chlorpheniramine	Chlor-Trimeton, Histaspan, Teldrin	Tripelennamine	Pyribenzamine
		Triprolidine	Actidil
Chlorphenoxamine	Systral, Phenoxene		
Chlorpromazine	Thorazine	**Causing miscellaneous urologic symptoms**	
Chlorprothixene	Taractan	**Frequency**	
Cycrimine	Pagitane	Dantrolene	Dantrium Triavil (mixture)
Deanol	Deaner		
Desipramine	Norpramin, Pertofrane	Iron Sorbitex	Jectofer Etrafon (mixture)
Dexbrompheniramine	Disomer		
Dexchlorpheniramine	Polaramine	**Incontinence**	
Dimethindene	Forhistal, Triten	Estrogens	—
Diphenhydramine	Benadryl	Hydroxystilbamidine	—
Diphenylpyraline	Diafen, Hispril		
Doxepin	Adapin, Sinequan	**Urgency**	
Doxylamine	Decapryn	Disodium Edetate	Endrate
Droperidol	Inapsine		
Ethopropazine	Parsidol	**Frequency, retention, and incontinence**	
Fluphenazine	Prolixin, Permitil	Levodopa	Bendopa, Dopar, Larodopa, Levodopa
Haloperidol	Haldol		
Imipramine	Tofranil, Presamine	Levopropoxyphene	Novrad

Continued.

Combined Preparation Drugs

Drugs affecting sympathetic nervous system

Actifed-C Expectorant
Acutuss
Acutuss Expectorant with
　Codeine
Aerolone Compound
Amesec
Amodrine
Asbron
Ayrcap
AyrLiquid
Bihisdin
Brondilate
Bronkometer
Bronkosol
Bronkotabs
Calcidrine Syrup
Cerose Expectorant
Chlor-Trimeton Expecto-
　rant with Codeine
Citra
Colrex Compound
Copavin
Copavin Compound
Coricidin Nasal Mist
Co-Xan
Dainite
Dainite-Kl
Deltasmyl
Duo-Medihaler
Duovent
Dylephrine

Ephed-Organidin
Ephedrine and Chlorcy-
　clizine
Ephedrine and Nembutal
Ephedrine and Seconal
　Sodium
Ephoxamine
Glynazan/EP
Hyadrine
Hydryllin with Racephe-
　drine Hydrochloride
Iso-Tabs
Isuprel Compound
Lufyllin-EP
Marax
Neo-Vadrin
Norisodrine with Cal-
　cium Iodide
Novalene
NTZ
Numa
Orthoxine and Amino-
　phylline
Pyracort
Quadrinal
Tedral
Tedral-25
Tedral Anti-H
Thalfed
Triaminicin

Drugs inhibiting sympathetic nervous system

Aldoclor
Aldoril
Butiserpazide
Diupres
Diutensen
Enduronyl
Esimil
Eutron
Exna-R
Hydromox-R
Hydropres
Maxitate with Rauwolfia
Metatensin
Naquival

Nyomin
Oreticyl
Protalba-R
Rautrax
Rawiloid + Veriloid
Regroton
Renese-R
Salutensin
Sandril with Pyronil
Serpasil-Esidrix
Singoserp-Esidrix

Drugs inhibiting parasympathetic nervous system

Belbarb
Belladenal
Bellergal
Butibel
Cantil with Phenobar-
　bital
Chardonna
Combid
Daricon-PB
Donnatal
Donphen
Enarax
Histalet
Hybephen
Kinesed
Kolantyl

Levsin with Phenobar-
　bital
Milpath
Nolamine
Pamine
Pathibamate
Pathilon with Phenobar-
　bital
Phenobarbital and Bella-
　donna
Probanthine with Dartal
Probanthine with Phe-
　nobarbital
Robinul-PH
Sidonna
Trasentine-phenobarbital
Valpin-PB

From Ostergard DR: Obstet Gynecol Surv 34:424, 1979.

CHAPTER 21

Infections of the Lower Genital Tract

KEY TERMS AND DEFINITIONS

Acyclovir. An antiviral agent, a purine nucleoside analogue used in the treatment of herpes. This agent comes in oral, topical, and intravenous preparations.

Calymmatobacterium Granulomatis. The gram-negative, nonmotile rod that causes granuloma inguinale.

Clue Cells. Epithelial cells with clusters of bacteria adherent to their external surfaces, obscuring their normal, fine border. They have a granular or stippled appearance and are associated with bacterial vaginosis.

Condyloma Acuminatum. A sexually transmitted viral disease of the vulva, vagina, and cervix caused by the human papillomavirus.

Condyloma Latum. The large, raised, flattened, grayish white lesions of secondary syphilis, most often found on the vulva.

Dark-Field Microscopy. A technique used to identify the spirochetes of syphilis, *Treponema pallidum.*

Donovan Bodies. The pathognomonic clusters of dark-staining bacteria (bipolar in appearance) found in the cytoplasm of large mononuclear cells in patients with granuloma inguinale.

Forme Fruste. A mild form of a disease.

Groove Sign. A depression between groups of inflamed nodes producing a double genitocrural fold in patients with lymphogranuloma venereum.

Gumma. An infectious granuloma characteristic of late or tertiary syphilis.

HIV. The human immunodeficiency virus, responsible for acquired immune deficiency syndrome (AIDS). It is an RNA virus of the retrovirus family.

Koilocystosis. The histologic appearance of cells with perinuclear halos consistent with HPV infection.

Mucopurulent Cervicitis. The counterpart to urethritis in men, diagnosed by gross visualization of yellow mucopurulent material or the presence of 10 or more polymorphonucleocytes per high-powered field on Gram stain of the endocervix.

Nit. The egg of the crab louse.

Podophyllin. A topical resin mixed with benzoin and alcohol used to treat the lesions of condyloma acuminatum.

Sexually Transmitted Disease (STD). A term used to describe an infection acquired primarily through sexual contact; venereal disease.

Toxin 1. The toxin involved in producing the signs and symptoms of toxic shock syndrome. It is a small protein with a molecular weight of 22,000. Its primary effects are the production of increased vascular permeability and profuse leaking of fluid from the intravascular space to the extravascular space.

Western Blot Test. A technique to a identify antibodies to a protein of a specific molecular weight. This test is more specific than the ELISA test for AIDS.

Whiff Test. A test used clinically. The smell of vaginal discharge after the addition of 10% potassium hydroxide. A positive sample associated with either bacterial vaginosis or *Trichomonas* infections will give off a fishy or aminelike smell.

Word Catheter. A short catheter with an inflatable Foley balloon used to help develop a fistulous tract from a Bartholin's duct to the vestibule.

Zidovudine (ZDV). An antiviral agent used against the HIV. It inhibits the reverse transcriptase enzyme.

The discussion of infectious diseases of the female genital tract is divided into two chapters. Infections involving the vulva, vagina, and cervix are discussed in this chapter, and infections involving the uterus, oviducts, and ovaries are discussed in Chapter 22. This separation has been made only to be similar to other chapters of the book and for clarity of presentation. The female genital tract has anatomic and physiologic continuity. Thus infectious agents that colonize and involve one organ often infect adjacent organs. To understand the pathophysiology and natural history of infectious diseases of the genital tract, one must always keep this continuity in mind.

This chapter will focus on infections of the lower genital tract. The symptoms caused by infections in this area produce the most common conditions seen by gynecologists. Therefore the focus of this chapter is on clinical presentation and differential diagnosis of vulvitis, vaginitis, and cervicitis. For more detailed discussions of microbiology and pharmacology, the reader is directed to the bibliography.

Toxic shock syndrome, acquired immune deficiency syndrome (AIDS), and syphilis are discussed in this chapter. Although the most devastating pathologic processes from these diseases occur in sites other than the genital tract, often they obtain entry into the body through the vaginal epithelium.

Many of the infections discussed in this chapter may be acquired through sexual contact and are termed sexually transmitted diseases (STDs). These often coexist—for example, herpes and condyloma or infections of *Chlamydia trachomatis* and *Neisseria gonorrhoeae*. When one disease is suspected, appropriate diagnostic methods must be used to detect other infections. This principle cannot be overemphasized.

INFECTIONS OF THE VULVA

The skin of the vulva is composed of a stratified squamous epithelium containing hair follicles and sebaceous, sweat, and apocrine glands. The subcutaneous tissue of the vulva also contains specialized structures such as the Bartholin glands. Similar to skin elsewhere on the body, the vulvar area is subject to both primary and secondary infections. The three most prevalent primary viral infections of the vulva are herpes genitalis, condyloma acuminatum, and molluscum contagiosum. However, symp-

toms from secondary infections of the vulva caused by organisms that produce vulvovaginitis are among the most common of all gynecologic conditions. To understand the differential diagnosis of vulvar infections, one must consider that vulvar skin is also sensitive to hormonal, metabolic, and allergic influences.

Vulvar itching or burning of acute onset and short duration suggests infection or a contact dermatitis. Approximately 10% of outpatient visits to gynecologists are for vulvar pruritus. The signs of erythema, edema, and superficial skin ulcers of the vulva also suggest infection. Skin fissures and excoriation may be signs of primary infection or may be caused by the patient's scratching as a result of irritation from a vaginal discharge.

Acute Urethral Syndrome and Acute Bacterial Cystitis

Dysuria, urinary frequency, and urinary urgency are the classic symptoms of infections of the lower urinary tract. It is estimated that 10% to 20% of adult women experience these symptoms each year. Women are prone to ascending infections because of the shortness of the female urethra and the fact that the distal one third of the urethra is constantly colonized by bacteria from the vulvar vestibule.

A woman with urinary frequency and dysuria who does not have significant bacterial growth in the urine (less than 10^2 organisms per milliliter) has acute urethral syndrome. Another name for this condition when associated with pyuria is dysuria–sterile pyuria syndrome. The diagnosis of acute urethral syndrome is made by exclusion of other diseases, primarily acute bacterial cystitis and vulvovaginitis. Acute bacterial cystitis is characterized by dysuria and the presence of more than 100 uropathogens per milliliter of urine. Superpubic tenderness is a specific sign for acute bacterial cystitis. However, it is only present in approximately 10% of women. Vulvovaginitis also produces a similar symptom complex and must be excluded from the diagnosis during the physical examination. Table 21-1 lists characteristic features that help to differentiate the three most common causes of dysuria in women.

The most common cause of acute bacterial cystitis is ascending infection from the introitus and distal urethra. The most frequent pathogens involved in premenopausal women are *Escherichia coli* and *Staphylococcus sapro-*

TABLE 21-1
Characteristic Features Which Differ in the Three Major Causes of Dysuria in Women

	Acute Bacterial Cystitis	Urethritis	Vulvitis
Predisposing factors	Previous cystitis Diaphragm use Onset of symptoms within 24 hours after intercourse	New sex partner	History of genital herpes Partner with genital herpes Antibiotic use History of recurrent vulvovaginal candidiasis
Symptoms	Internal dysuria Duration of symptoms ≤4 days Frequency and urgency Gross hematuria	Internal dysuria Duration of symptoms often ≥7 days with chlamydial urethritis	External dysuria Vaginal discharge Vulvar irritation, burning, pruritus, or lesions
Signs	Suprapubic tenderness	Mucopurulent cervicitis Vulvar lesions	Vulvar lesions Vulvitis Curdlike vaginal exudate
Laboratory	Pyuria Microscopic hematuria Rapid nitrite test Urine Gram stain Urine culture	Pyuria Urethral discharge or bartholinitis Endocervical exudate Cervical and urethral tests for *C. trachomatis* and *N. gonorrhoeae* Test lesion for HSV	No pyuria Test lesion for HSV Test vaginal discharge for *C. albicans*

From Holmes KK, Mårdh PH, Sparling PF, et al, editors: Sexually transmitted diseases, ed 2, New York, 1990, McGraw-Hill Book Co.

phyticus. The most common causes of acute urethral syndrome are *C. trachomatis* and *N. gonorrhoeae.* Postmenopausal women often experience similar symptoms related to estrogen deficiency without significant bacterial colonization of the bladder.

The diagnosis of acute urethral syndrome is established primarily by excluding the possibility that the symptom complex is secondary to cervicitis, vulvovaginitis, or cystitis. The patient's perception of the anatomic site of the dysuria may be helpful. Vulvovaginitis tends to produce "external" dysuria in contrast to a deeper, "internal" dysuria associated with cystitis. Rarer causes of similar symptomatology include urethral diverticulum, hypoestrogenism, allergy, vitamin deficiency, urethral spasm and/or stenosis, and psychologic, neurologic, or traumatic causes.

There are two basic diagnostic steps in the workup of a woman with dysuria and urinary frequency. Initially, pelvic examination is performed to discover whether the patient has an associated vaginal or cervical infection. Secondly, a clean-catch, midstream urine speci-

men is obtained. The urine should be examined for both white cells and bacteria. A urine culture is obtained if bacteria are present and the patient has been treated for similar symptoms in the past. Absolute indications for urine culture include patients with complicated histories, previous urinary tract infection within the past month, urinary symptomatology that has been present more than 7 days, pregnancy or intercurrent diseases such as diabetes mellitus or immunosuppression. To obtain accurate estimates of the number of bacteria per milliliter, it is important to culture the urine within 2 hours or refrigerate the specimen until it is sent to the laboratory. The "gold standard" of more than 10^5 uropathogens per milliliter had been the criterion used to make the diagnosis of significant bacteriuria. However, recently bacterial concentrations of as few as 10^2 per milliliter are accepted as bacteriologic confirmation of cystitis. Approximately one out of three women with acute bacterial cystitis will have positive cultures with a single organism in a concentration between 10^2 and 10^5 uropathogens per milliliter. In large series, 50% of women with dysuria and frequency did not have significant bacteriuria. Women, especially in the age group of 15 to 25, with pyuria and a sterile urine culture often have urethral infection by *Chlamydia* or gonorrhea. In general, women with urethral syndrome secondary to *Chlamydia* have more chronic symptoms with a gradual onset and less urgency than women with acute bacterial cystitis.

The initial treatment of choice for women with acute bacterial cystitis is a single-dose regimen of trimethoprim-sulfamethoxazole (two tablets of double strength, 320 mg of trimethoprim and 1600 mg of sulfamethoxazole). Other antibiotic choices for single-dose therapy for uncomplicated acute bacterial cystitis are listed in Table 21-2. The advantages of single-dose therapy are simplicity, better patient compliance, lower cost, and reduction of side effects such as diarrhea and vaginitis. Contraindications to single-dose therapy include chronic infections, systemic manifestations of infection, renal disease, anatomic abnormalities of the urinary tract, pregnancy, or diabetes mellitus. Patients should be seen 2 to 4 weeks after completing initial therapy to rule out reinfection or a relapse.

An alternative to single-dose therapy is short-course therapy of 3 days of certain antibiotics. Multidose regimens of oral therapy for acute cystitis are listed in Table 21-3. If there are complicating factors in a woman who has acute bacterial cystitis, oral therapy should be continued for a minimum of 7 to 14 days. If bacteriuria is not present, the patient should be treated with tetracycline (500 mg every 6 hours) for 7 days to treat a presumptive diagnosis of *Chlamydia* infection. Failure to respond necessitates quantitative cultures of the urine for bacteria and culture of the endocervix for *Chlamydia* and gonorrhea organisms. It is important to stress that uncomplicated lower urinary tract infection is not a threat to renal function in an ambulatory adult woman. Approximately 75% of episodes of acute bacterial infection in women with recurrent cystitis occur within 24 hours of coitus. The incidence of acute infection in these women is reduced dramatically by prescribing postcoital antibiotic prophylaxis.

Chronic urethral syndrome has many causes, including estrogen deficiency, trauma (espe-

TABLE 21-2

Single-Dose Therapy for Uncomplicated Acute Cystitis*

Medication	Dose	Cost/Dose ($)†
Trimethoprim‡	400 mg	1.84
Trimethoprim-sulfamethoxazole‡	320 and 1600 mg	1.42
Nitrofurantoin‡	200 mg	0.28
Amoxicillin	3 g	3.09
Amoxicillin plus clavulanate	500 mg	1.71
Ampicillin	3.5 g	1.12
First-generation cephalosporin	2 g	6.43
Sulfisoxazole	2 g	0.57
Ciprofloxacin	250 mg	3.12
Norfloxacin	400 mg	3.64

From Johnson JR and Stamm WE: Ann Intern Med 111:906, 1989.
*Single-dose therapy should be reserved for patients without complicating factors.
†Costs are based on manufacturer's average wholesale price.
‡Preferred antimicrobial agents.

TABLE 21-3

Multidose Regimens for Oral Therapy for Acute Cystitis

Medication*	Dose (mg)	Interval (Hours)†	Cost/Day ($)‡
Trimethoprim§	100 (200)	12 (24)	0.92
Trimethoprim-sulfamethoxazole§	160 and 800	12	1.42
Nitrofurantoin§	100	6	0.76
Amoxicillin	500	8	1.53
Amoxicillin plus clavulanate	500	8	5.13
First-generation cephalosporin	500	6	6.44
Ciprofloxacin	250	12	3.12
Norfloxacin	400	12	3.64
Sulfisoxazole	500	6	0.56
Tetracycline	500	6	0.36

From Johnson JR and Stamm WE: Ann Intern Med 111:906, 1989.
*Susceptibility of pathogen to selected antibodies should be confirmed with in vitro susceptibility testing in patients with complicating factors.
†Twice-daily dosing can probably be used for all medications listed when there are no complicating factors. Patients without complicating factors can be treated for 3 days. In the presence of complicating factors, therapy should be continued for at least 7 days.
‡Costs are based on manufacturers' average wholesale price (1989 statistics).
§Preferred antimicrobial agents.

cially during intercourse), chronic infection (most commonly with genital *Mycoplasma*), anatomic obstruction, allergy, and neurologic and psychogenic conditions. Chronic urethral syndrome is discussed in detail in Chapter 20.

Infections of Bartholin's glands

Bartholin's glands normally are two rounded, pea-sized glands deep in the perineum. They are located at the entrance of the vagina at 5 and 7 o'clock. A normal Bartholin's gland cannot be palpated. Approximately 2% of adult women develop enlargements of one or both glands, of which there are three common causes. The most common cause is cystic dilation of Bartholin's duct. Secondly, symptomatic enlargement of Bartholin's glands may be related to adenitis or abscess formation (Figure 21-1). Mechanical obstruction of the duct usually precedes overt infection. The most serious sequela of infection is a polymicrobial necrotizing subcutaneous infection, especially in diabetics. Thirdly, in women over the age of 40, enlargement may be caused by the rare adenocarcinoma of Bartholin's glands. More than 85% of women who develop enlargement of the Bartholin's glands do so during their reproductive years. The mean age of discovery of a Bartholin's gland carcinoma is approximately age 50.

The etiology of a Bartholin's duct cyst is obstruction of the duct secondary to nonspecific inflammation or trauma. Histologically, the Bartholin's ducts are lined by transitional epithelium. These ducts are easily obstructed, usually near the distal orifice. Following obstruction, there is continued secretion of glandular fluid, which results in the cystic dilation. Twenty years ago bilateral enlargement of Bartholin's glands was believed to be a pathognomonic sign of gonococcal infection. This is no longer true. Unilateral or bilateral Bartholin's gland infection in the majority of cases is not caused by a sexually transmitted disease. Lee et al. obtained bacterial cultures of fluid from Bartholin's duct cysts and abscesses. More than 80% of cultures from cysts were sterile, as were one in three cultures from Bartholin's abscesses. Brook recently reported positive cultures from 26 of 28 patients. He reported a total of 67 bacterial isolates, 43 of which were anaerobic and 24 of which were aerobic and facultative anaerobic organisms. In summary, positive cultures from Bartholin's gland ab-

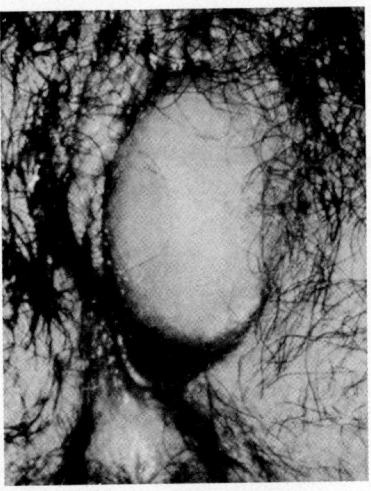

FIGURE 21-1
Bartholin's abscess. Mass is tender and fluctuant and is situated on lower lateral aspect of labium minus at 5 o'clock. (From Kaufman RH: Cystic tumors. In Gardner HL and Kaufman RH, editors: Benign diseases of the vulva and vagina, ed 2, Chicago, 1981, Mosby–Year Book, Inc.)

scesses are often polymicrobial and contain a wide range of bacteria similar to the natural flora of the vagina.

The differential diagnosis of Bartholin's gland cysts includes mesonephric cysts of the vagina and epithelial inclusion cysts. Mesonephric cysts are generally more cephalad in the vagina, and epithelial inclusion cysts are more superficial. Rarely, a lipoma, fibroma, hernia, or hydrocele may be confused with a Bartholin's duct cyst. Bartholin's duct cysts are found in the labia majora, whereas Bartholin's glands are at the base of the labia minora. If one draws a line in an anteroposterior direction from the base of the labia minora, it will approximately bisect the Bartholin's duct cyst.

Most women with Bartholin's duct cysts are asymptomatic. The cysts may vary from 1 to 8 cm in diameter, and they are usually unilateral, tense, and nonpainful. The majority of cysts are unilocular. However, occasionally in chronic or recurrent cysts there are multiple compartments. An abscess of a Bartholin's gland tends to develop rapidly over 2 to 4 days. Symptoms include acute vulvar pain, dyspareunia, and pain during walking. Local symptoms of acute pain and tenderness are secondary to rapid enlargement, hemorrhage, or secondary infection. The signs are those of a classic abscess:

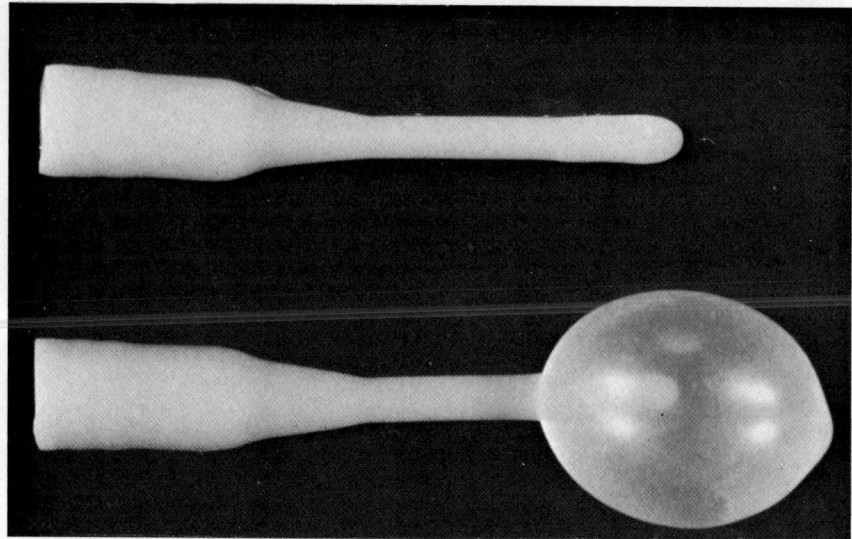

FIGURE 21-2
Word catheters before and after inflation. They are used to develop a fistula from Bartholin's cyst or abscess to vestibule. (From Friedrich EG: Vulvar disease, ed 2, Philadelphia, 1983, WB Saunders Co.

erythema, acute tenderness, edema, and occasionally cellulitis of the surrounding subcutaneous tissue. Without therapy, most abscesses tend to rupture spontaneously by the third or fourth day.

The treatment of infections or enlargement of Bartholin's glands depends on their symptomatology. Asymptomatic cysts in women under the age of 40 do not need treatment. The therapy for acute adenitis without abscess formation is broad-spectrum antibiotics and frequent hot sitz baths.

The treatment of choice for a symptomatic cyst or abscess is the development of a fistulous tract from the dilated duct to the vestibule. Simple incision and drainage of a Bartholin's gland abscess are complicated by a tendency for the abscess to recur. The classic surgical treatment is to develop a fistulous tract to "marsupialize" the duct. After an elliptical wedge of tissue has been removed, the remaining edges of the duct or abscess are everted and sutured to the surrounding skin with interrupted sutures. This forms an epithelialized pouch that provides drainage for the gland. The recurrence rate following marsupialization is approximately 5% to 10%. An alternate surgical approach is to insert a Word catheter (a short catheter with an inflatable Foley balloon) through a stab incision into the duct or abscess

and leave it in place for 4 to 6 weeks (Figure 21-2). During this period a tract of epithelium will form. Davis has described a procedure using a carbon dioxide laser to produce a neostoma in a Bartholin's duct cyst. Recently, Cho et al. described a window operation performed with the patient under local anesthesia. They reported 25 cysts and 22 abscesses without a recurrence. All of the previously mentioned operations may be performed with local anesthesia. Antibiotics are not necessary unless there is an associated cellulitis surrounding the Bartholin's gland abscess.

Excision of a Bartholin's duct and gland is indicated for persistent deep infection, multiple recurrences of abscesses, or enlargement of the gland in women over the age of 40. Excision for gland enlargement in women over 40 is performed to diagnose adenocarcinoma of Bartholin's gland. Because of the richness of the vascular supply to the region, including the vestibular bulbs directly below Bartholin's gland, excision is a more formidable task than one would expect. It is best to have either regional block or general anesthesia for excision. Removal of a Bartholin's gland is often accompanied by morbidity, including intraoperative hemorrhage, hematoma formation, postoperative scarring, and associated dyspareunia. Bartholin's gland secretions are not important for providing lubrication during sexual intercourse. Mucinous secretions from Bartholin's glands do provide moisture for the epithelium of the vestibule but are not important for vaginal lubrication.

Pediculosis Pubis and Scabies

The skin of the vulva is a frequent site of infestation by animal parasites, the two most common being the crab louse and the itch mite. Ideally, early diagnosis and treatment are of the utmost importance to control parasitic infection. However, because many women experience embarrassment, guilt, and anxiety over the potential diagnosis of this infection, delay in diagnosis often interferes with ideal treatment.

Pediculosis pubis is an infestation by the crab louse, *Phthirus pubis.* The crab louse is also called the pubic louse and is a different species than the body or head louse. The louse is transmitted usually by close contact, although it may be acquired from towels or bedding. Lice in the pubic hair are the most contagious of all sexually transmitted diseases. It is estimated that over 90% of sexual partners are infected following a single exposure. *P. pubis* is generally confined to the hairy areas of the vulva. It may occasionally be found in other areas such as the eyelids. The major nourishment of the louse is human blood.

There are three stages in the louse's life cycle: egg (nit), nymph, and adult. The entire life cycle is spent on the host. Eggs are deposited at the base of hair follicles. The adult parasite is approximately 1 mm long and dark gray when its alimentary tract is not filled with blood (Figure 21-3). Of clinical importance for diagnosis is the fact that the louse moves slowly.

Scabies is a parasitic infection of the itch mite, *Sarcoptes scabiei.* Similar to the crab louse, it is transmitted by close contact. Unlike louse infestation, scabies is an infection that is widespread over the body without a predilection for hairy areas. The adult female itch mite digs a burrow just beneath the skin. She lays eggs in this home during her life span of approximately 1 month. The adult itch mite is usually less than 0.5 mm long. Unlike the crab louse, an itch mite travels rapidly over skin and may move up to 2.5 cm in 1 minute.

The predominant clinical symptom of louse

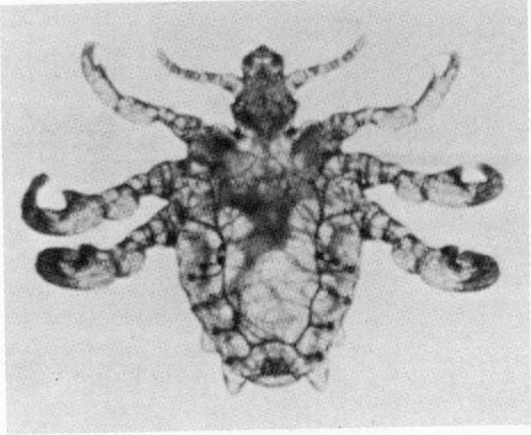

FIGURE 21-3
Pubic louse, *Phthirus pubis,* after blood meal. (From Billstein S: Human lice. In Holmes KK, Mårdh PA, Sparling PF, et al, editors: Sexually transmitted diseases, New York, 1984, McGraw-Hill Book Co.

infestation is constant itching in the pubic area, which is secondary to allergic sensitization. It is estimated that it takes a minimum of 5 days following initial infection to develop allergic sensitization. Examination of the vulvar area without magnification demonstrates eggs and adult lice (Figure 21-4). The tiny rough spots visualized with the naked eye are the alimentary tracts of lice filled with human blood. The vulvar skin may become secondarily irritated or infected by constant scratching. For definitive diagnosis one can make a microscopic slide by scratching the skin papule with a needle and placing the crust under a drop of mineral oil. The louse's body looks like that of a miniature crab with six legs that have claws on them.

The predominant clinical symptom of scabies is severe but intermittent itching. Generally, more intense pruritus occurs at night when the skin is warmer and the mites are more active. Scabies may present as papules, vesicles, or burrows. Any area of the skin may be infected, with the hands, wrists, breasts, vulva, and buttocks being most commonly involved. Scabies has been termed the *great dermatologic imitator,* and the differential diagnosis includes virtually all dermatologic diseases that cause pruritus. A hand-held magnifying lens is helpful for examining suspicious areas. Microscopic slides may be made by use of mineral oil and a scratch technique (Figure 21-5). Mites lack lat-

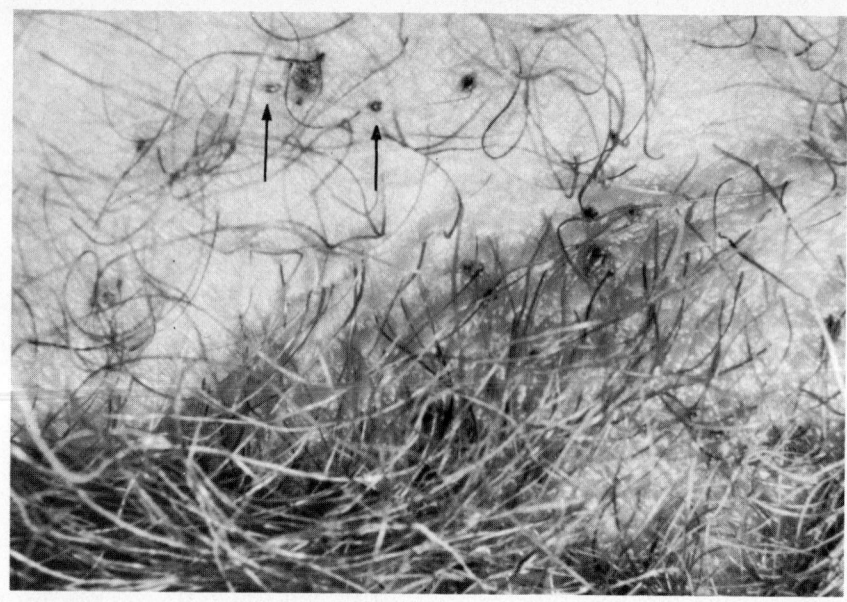

FIGURE 21-4
Crab lice and nits of pediculosis pubis *(arrows.)* (From Gardner HL: Miscellaneous conditions. In Gardner HL and Kaufman RH, editors: Benign diseases of the vulva and vagina, ed 2, Chicago, 1981, Mosby–Year Book, Inc.)

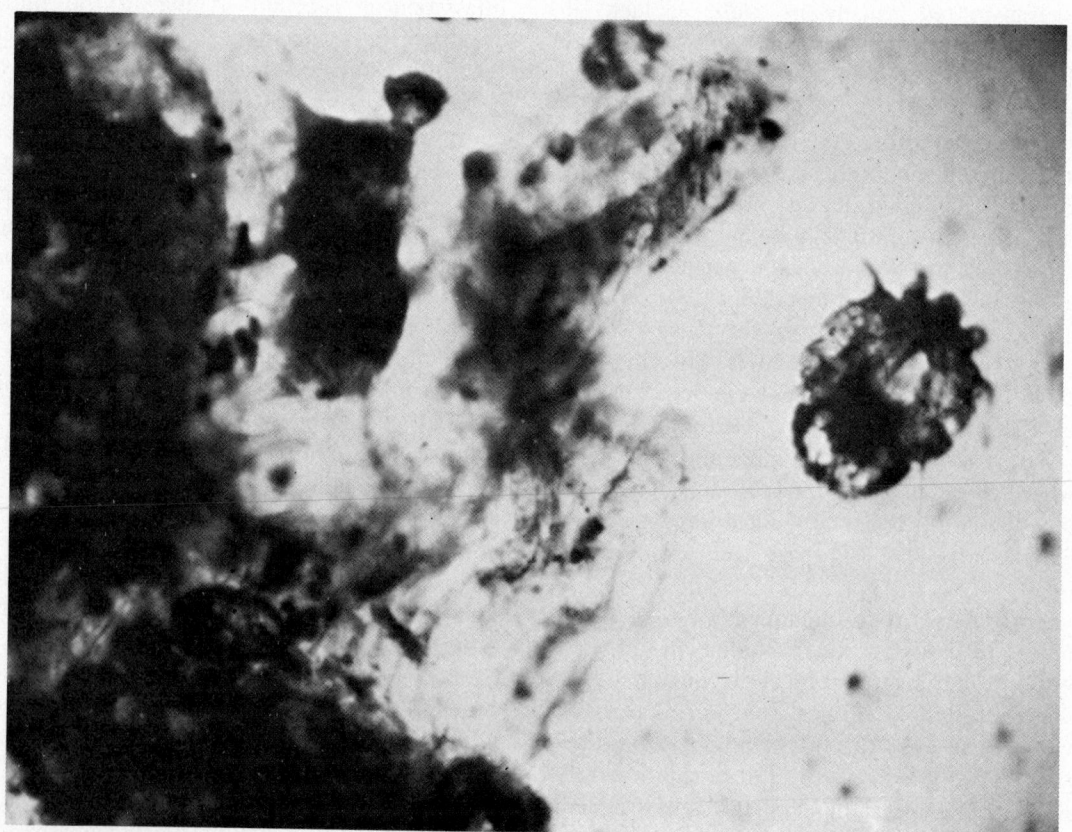

FIGURE 21-5
Skin scrapings of unexcoriated papules fortuitously disclose adults, larve, eggs, and fecal pellets, any of which would be diagnostic of scabies. (From Orkin M and Howard IM: Scabies. In Holmes KK, Mårdh PA, Sparling PF, et al, editors: Sexually transmitted diseases, New York, 1984, McGraw-Hill Book Co.)

eral claw legs but have two anterior triangular hairy buds.

The treatment of pediculosis pubis and scabies involves an agent that kills both the adult parasite and eggs. The current therapy is 5% permethrin (Nix Cream), which was approved by the FDA in 1986. To ensure maximal therapeutic efficacy, a second application for 10 minutes should be applied 10 days later to kill any eggs that have hatched recently. The medication should be used for 10 minutes twice a day for 48 hours when treating scabies. Lindane, which is a 1% gamma-benzene hexachloride preparation (Kwell), is available as a cream, lotion, and shampoo. The infected individual should take a shower and then apply Kwell to the infested areas of the body for 12 hours on 2 successive days. Lindane must remain in direct contact for at least 1 hour to kill eggs. Lindane is contraindicated during pregnancy and in women who are breast-feeding. For scabies, approximately 30 ml of lotion covers the entire skin surface of an adult patient. Patients with scabies have intense pruritus that may persist for several days following effective therapy. An antihistamine will help to alleviate this symptom. The treatment of other family members should be prescribed to avoid reinfection. Obviously, clothes, bedding, and the home environment must be disinfected.

Molluscum Contagiosum

Molluscum contagiosum in adults is an asymptomatic viral disease of the vulvar skin. In contrast, molluscum contagiosum in children may present over the entire body. This benign skin disease is caused by the poxvirus. Poxvirus does not grow on mucous membranes and is spread by close contact. Unlike most sexually transmitted diseases, poxvirus is only mildly contagious. The disease is also acquired via nonsexual contact. The prevalence of the disease has increased rapidly over the past 20 years. The incubation period is several weeks to many months, and many of the skin lesions result from autoinoculation.

The small nodules or domed papules of molluscum contagiosum are usually 1 to 5 mm in diameter (Figure 21-6). A descriptive name for the small nodule is the "water wart." Close inspection reveals that many of the more mature nodules have an umbilicated center. Characteristically, an infected woman will have 1 to 20

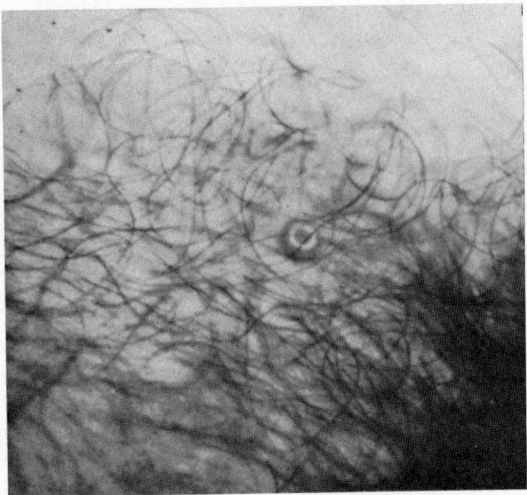

FIGURE 21-6
Papule of molluscum contagiosum with umbilicated center. (From Brown ST: Molluscum contagiosum. In Holmes KK, Mårdh PA, Sparling PF, et al, editors: Sexually transmitted diseases, New York, 1984, McGraw-Hill Book Co.)

solitary lesions randomly distributed over the vulvar skin. A crop of new nodules will persist from several months to years. If the diagnosis cannot be made by simple inspection, the white, waxy material from inside the nodule should be expressed on a microscopic slide. The finding of intracytoplasmic molluscum bodies with Wright's or Giemsa stain confirms the diagnosis (Figure 21-7). The major complication of molluscum contagiosum is bacterial superinfection.

Treatment of individual papules is initiated with injection of a local anesthetic with a small subdermal wheal of 1% lidocaine (Xylocaine). The caseous material is then evacuated and the nodule excised with a sharp dermal curet. The base of the papule is subsequently chemically treated with either ferric subsulfate (Monsel's solution) or 85% trichloroacetic acid. As an alternative the base of the papule may be treated with cryosurgery, electrocautery, or laser therapy.

Condyloma Acuminatum

Condyloma acuminatum is a sexually transmitted viral disease of the vulva, vagina, and cervix caused by the human papillomavirus (HPV). Synonyms for vulvar condylomata acu-

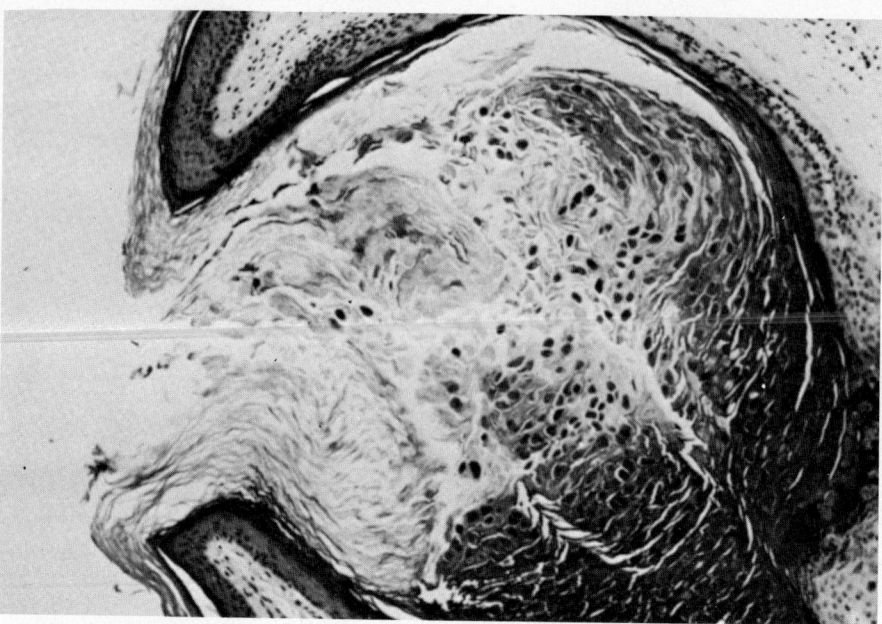

FIGURE 21-7
Papule of molluscum contagiosum with plug of acanthotic and hyperkeratolytic epidermis containing numerous intracytoplasmic inclusions opening to the surface through an apical hole. (H&E stain; ×75.) (From Brown ST: Molluscum contagiosum. In Holmes KK, Mårdh PA, Sparling PF, et al, editors: Sexually transmitted diseases, New York, 1984, McGraw-Hill Book Co.)

minata include genital, venereal, or anogenital warts. In the past few years this disease has reached epidemic levels. HPV is the most common viral sexually transmitted disease. Recent advances in DNA hybridization have demonstrated that the majority of HPV infections are subclinical. Thus the prevalence of the disease depends on the sophistication of the technique used to diagnose subclinical infection, such as cytology, colposcopy, or molecular probes of biopsy material. In a comparison study, Schneider et al. found colposcopy to be far superior to cytology for the detection of early genital human papillomavirus infection. In their study of 214 women, colposcopy was positive for HPV in 66%, whereas cytology demonstrated positive infection in only 14%. It is estimated that in the past 20 years the number of infected individuals has increased approximately 700%. The increasing incidence and the awareness of the relationship between HPV infection and early cervical intraepithelial neoplasia have been the stimuli for expanding research efforts into this complex group of viruses.

Recent advances in molecular biology have identified more than 50 subtypes of HPV,

which differ from one another in their amino acid sequences. At least 12 different subtypes of HPV have been involved in genital infection. HPV 6, 11, 16, 18, 31, 33, 35, and 39 are the most frequently identified. HPV types 16 and 18 may be associated with aneuploid, premalignant, or malignant lesions of the female genital tract. Types 6 and 11 are more commonly associated with benign, euploid lesions. Clinically, HPV typing is a research tool, and the test sensitivity is amplified by use of the polymerase chain reaction before identifying the specific type with the DNA probe. Condyloma acuminatum is definitely a sexually transmitted disease spread by skin-to-skin contact. Autoinoculation also occurs. The virus can be shed from both macroscopic and microscopic lesions. It is highly contagious, with 25% to 65% of sexual partners developing the infection. Oriel discovered that 60% of adults develop the disease following intercourse with a partner who was actively shedding the virus. The average incubation period is 3 months, with a wide range of 1 to 8 months. As with other sexually transmitted diseases, peak incidence occurs between the ages of 15 and 25 years.

In the majority of women, the diagnosis of

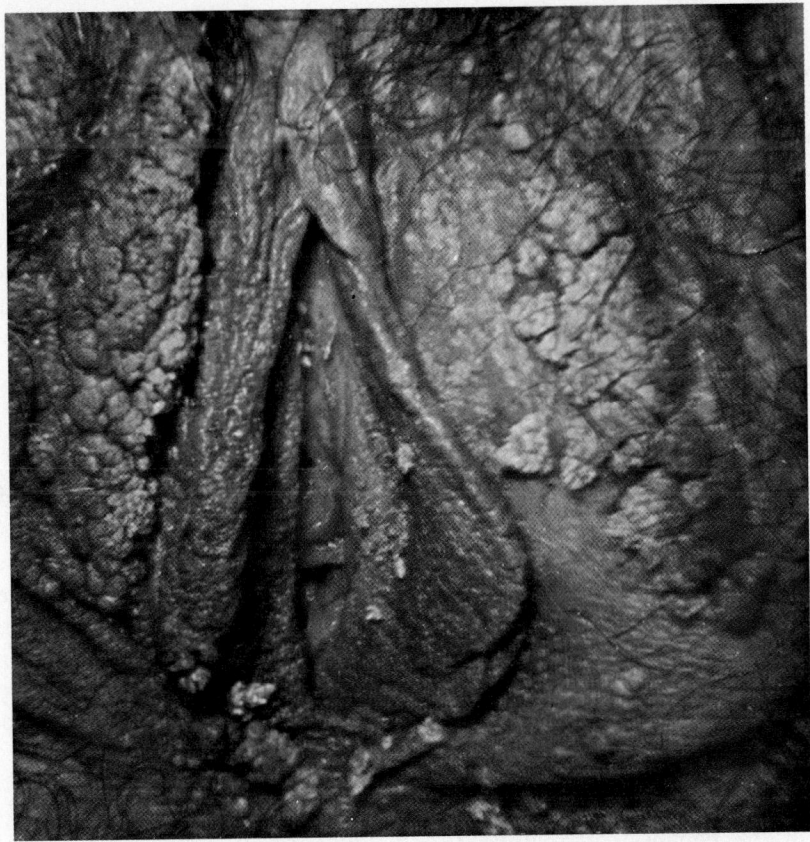

FIGURE 21-8
Condyloma acuminatum. Often small, younger lesions are present with larger older lesions. (From Friedrich EG: Vulva disease, ed 2, Philadelphia, 1983, WB Saunders Co.)

overt condyloma acuminatum can be made by direct inspection. The warts tend to occur on moist skin. Pedunculated warts are friable and tend to bleed following minor trauma. Initial infections usually begin in the vestibule and adjacent areas of the labia. However, all adjacent, moist epithelium may be involved with condyloma, including the vagina, cervix, urethra, bladder, and rectum. Initial lesions are pedunculated, soft papules approximately 2 to 3 mm in diameter and 10 to 20 mm long. They may occur as a single papule or in clusters. As the infection progresses by means of autoinoculation, many different presentations may evolve (Figure 21-8). Lesions vary from pinhead-sized papules to large cauliflower-like masses that may grow to several centimeters in diameter. Uncomplicated condylomata acuminata are usually asymptomatic. Occasionally they become secondarily infected, producing pain, odor, and a tendency to bleed easily. Condylomata in the cervix tend to be flat and bleed on

contact. The presence of condylomata of the cervix is best discovered by colposcopic examination. Perianal warts occur in approximately 20% of women with condyloma acuminatum. Subclinical HPV infection of the cervix, vagina, or vulva may be discovered by applying 3% to 5% acetic acid to the epithelium. Often, HPV-infected cells appear shiny white in color, with the area of infection having irregular borders and sometimes satellite lesions. Subclinical infection is often discovered by routine cytology, with koilocytosis (cells with perinuclear halos) being the classic finding. In sophisticated DNA studies, 10% of women with normal smears have HPV identified, while greater than 90% are associated with HPV DNA.

Several conditions are known to predispose women to infection with HPV. They include immunosuppression, diabetes, pregnancy, and local trauma. Often, preexisting vulvovaginitis has provided the moist, excoriated skin on which the HPV colonizes.

The management of the individual case depends on the location, size, and extent of the condyloma and whether the woman is pregnant. Most clinicians attempt to treat the patient until the macroscopic lesions disappear. No present therapy of HPV eliminates subclinical infection from the surrounding epithelium. There is a wide range of therapeutic choices, including chemical, cautery, and immunologic therapy. For many years, the standard treatment of condyloma acuminatum has been topical podophyllin resin as a 25% solution with benzoin in alcohol. Podophyllin is painted directly on the lesion at weekly intervals for 4 to 6 weeks. Generally lesions slough within 5 to 7 days without associated scarring. Although some physicians advise that the podophyllin be washed off after 4 hours of contact, this is difficult because of the benzoin base. Podophyllin has produced neuropathy, bone marrow depression, and fetal death when absorbed systemically; therefore, it should not be used by pregnant women, intravaginally, or in large amounts over excoriated vulvar skin. Podofilox, 0.5 solution (Condylox), may be self-administered and has the advantage of being less caustic. Another of the chemical alternatives to podophyllin is trichloroacetic acid, which is preferable for small vaginal lesions. Small papules turn white within 60 seconds of being painted with trichloroacetic acid. The patient may experience a sharp burning pain for up to 15 minutes following application. Another chemical alternative is topical 5-fluorouracil (5-FU). The major drawback of 5-FU treatment is local irritation of the skin and vaginal mucosa. When 5-FU is used to treat cervical or vaginal lesions, it is important to avoid contact with vulvar skin so that it does not become ulcerated.

Lesions larger than 2 to 3 cm are best treated by cryotherapy, electrocautery, or laser therapy. It is sometimes best to surgically shave the condyloma and then apply thermal injury to the virus in the base of the lesion. Bellina reported that 65% of women treated with laser therapy for cervical condyloma did not have condyloma recurrence for 24 months following therapy. Ferenczy has been an advocate for laser treatment of the condyloma acuminatum of the penis in sexual partners of women with the disease.

To date, effective treatment of condyloma acuminatum with immunotherapy has been disappointing. Interferon, because of its antiviral and antiproliferative properties, was postulated to be an ideal drug to treat HPV infection. Regretfully, interferons, when given parenterally, result in severe systemic symptoms similar to a viral illness in most women. Interferon treatment of HPV has been tried by topical creams and direct injection into the condylomata. However, this type of therapy is expensive and involves a prolonged course of treatment. In two studies using topical cream, the results of therapy were not significantly different from controls.

Genital Ulcers

Herpes, granuloma inguinale (donovanosis), lymphogranuloma venereum, chancroid, and syphilis all may present as ulcerations in the genital area. However, their etiologies, disease courses, and treatments are vastly different. Table 21-4 lists some of their major characteristics. Table 21-5 contrasts the major laboratory tests used in the differential diagnosis of genital ulcers.

Genital Herpes

Genital herpes is a recurrent, sexually transmitted disease that has reached epidemic proportions. Judging by either incidence or prevalence, it is among the most frequent sexually transmitted diseases, with somewhere between 500,000 and 2 million new cases of herpes estimated to occur per year and the prevalence of genital herpes is estimated to be between 10 and 30 million cases per year in the United States. Herpes is highly contagious, with 75% of sexual partners of infected individuals contracting the disease. It is estimated that 1 out of 200 asymptomatic American women are shedding herpesvirus from their reproductive tracts. Depending on the population studied, the incidence of serum antibodies against herpes in adult women varies from 50% to 100%. A seroepidemiologic survey of the prevalence of herpes simplex virus type II infection found a prevalence of 18% in women ages 35 to 50. Recently, it has been hypothesized that the ulceration associated with herpes genital infection may facilitate infection with the human immunodeficiency virus.

The herpes epidemic has fostered major changes in the sexual mores of our society. Recurrent genital herpes is not a debilitating physical disease, yet to the individual woman it

TABLE 21-4
Clinical Features of Genital Ulcers

	Syphilis	Herpes	Chancroid	Lymphogranuloma Venereum	Donovanosis
Incubation period	2-4 weeks (1-12 weeks)	2-7 days	1-14 days	3 days-6 weeks	1-4 weeks (up to 6 months)
Primary lesion	Papule	Vesicle	Papule or pustule	Papule, pustule, or vesicle	Papule
Number of lesions	Usually one	Multiple, may coalesce	Usually multiple, may coalesce	Usually one	Variable
Diameter (mm)	5-15	1-2	2-20	2-10	Variable
Edges	Sharply demarcated, elevated, round or oval	Erythematous	Undermined, ragged, irregular	Elevated, round or oval	Elevated, irregular
Depth	Superficial or deep	Superficial	Excavated	Superficial or deep	Elevated
Base	Smooth, nonpurulent	Serous, erythmatous	Purulent	Variable	Red and rough ("beefy")
Induration	Firm	None	Soft	Occasionally firm	Firm
Pain	Unusual	Common	Usually very tender	Variable	Uncommon
Lymphadenopathy	Firm, nontender, bilateral	Firm, tender, often bilateral	Tender, may suppurate, usually unilateral	Tender, may suppurate, loculated, usually unilateral	Pseudoadenopathy

From Holmes KK, Mårdh PA, Sparling PF, et al, editors: Sexually transmitted diseases, ed 2, New York, 1990, McGraw-Hill Book Co.

TABLE 21-5
Laboratory Tests for the Diagnosis of Genital Ulcer Adenopathy Syndrome

	Syphilis	Herpes	Chancroid	Lymphogranuloma Venereum	Donovanosis
Microscopy	Dark-field examination	Antigen detection	Gram stain has low sensitivity and specificity	Not available	Giemsa- or Wright-stained tissue smears and sections
Culture	Not available	Cell culture	Sensitive, selective media available	Cell culture	Not available
Serology	RPR/VDRL, FTA-ABS, MHA-TP	Rarely useful (primary herpes)	Experimental	Complement fixation, immunofluorescent antibody tests	Not available

From Holmes KK, Mårdh PA, Sparling PF, et al, editors: Sexually transmitted diseases, ed 2, New York, 1990, McGraw-Hill Book Co.

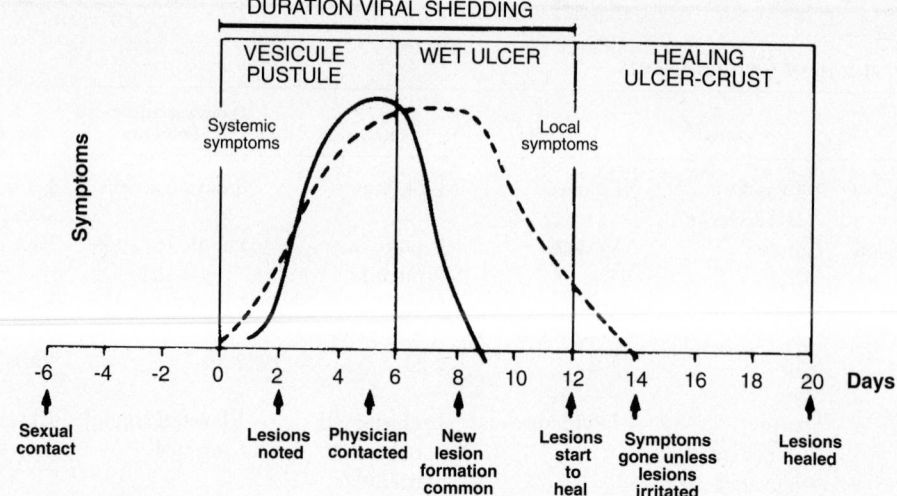

FIGURE 21-9
Schematic graph of clinical course of primary genital herpes. (From Corey L: Genital herpes. In Holmes KK, Mårdh PA, Sparling PF, et al, editors: Sexually transmitted diseases, New York, 1984, McGraw-Hill Book Co.)

may present an overwhelming psychologic burden. Not only are there minor concerns over the association of herpesvirus and malignant transformation of squamous epithelium, but there is anxiety over the rare yet disastrous consequence of fetal and neonatal transmission of the disease. The major consequence of recurrent herpes is the psychologic burden. To the individual patient there is an immense sense of social isolation and a reluctance to initiate a sexual relationship. This results in a decrease in self-esteem, depression, and, most important, a feeling of loss of control due to the inability to predict the time of the next recurrence. Luby and Klinge and Bierman have excellent reviews of the psychologic fears and anxieties created by herpes and the perception of its being "an incurable disease."

There are two distinct types of herpes simplex virus—type I (HSV-I) and type II (HSV-II). As a broad generalization, HSV-I tends to infect epithelium above the waist, and HSV-II tends to cause ulceration below the waist. However, depending on the series, HSV-I may cause pelvic infections between 13% and 40% of the time. From a molecular biologic standpoint the classification of HSV-I and HSV-II is an oversimplification. Multiple strains of each virus have been discovered. From a clinical standpoint the only important difference is that the frequency of recurrence is 4 times greater

following a primary infection with HSV-II in comparison to HSV-I.

The primary infection by herpes is both a local and a systemic disease (Figure 21-9). The majority of initial genital infections occur in women between the ages of 15 and 35. The incubation period is between 3 and 7 days, with an average of 6 days. Often the patient experiences paresthesias of the vulvar skin before vesicle formation. Usually there are multiple vesicles that become shallow, superficial ulcers over a large area of the vulva. There is often simultaneous involvement of the vagina and cervix (Figure 21-10). Patients experience multiple crops of ulcers for 2 to 6 weeks. Often the ulcers coalesce; however, the ulcers heal spontaneously without scarring. Viral shedding may occur for 2 to 3 weeks after vulvar lesions appear. Positive cultures for herpesvirus may be obtained from the cervix in 75% of women and from the urine in 50% of women with primary infections. The vast majority of women have severe vulvar pain, tenderness, and inguinal adenopathy.

Systemic symptoms, including general malaise and fever, are experienced by 70% of women during the primary infection. Rarely there is central nervous system infection, with the reported mortality from herpes encephalitis being approximately 50%. Primary infections of the urethra and bladder may result in acute

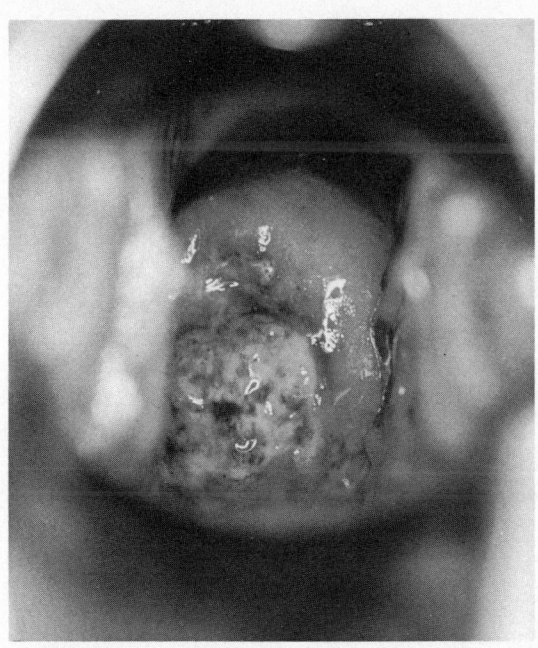

FIGURE 21-10
Primary herpes involving cervix. Necrotic exophytic mass is seen on posterior lip. This was clinically thought to be invasive carcinoma. Herpes simplex virus culture was positive. Lesion spontaneously disappeared. (From Kaufman RH and Faro S: Clin Obstet Gynecol 28:154, 1985.)

urinary retention, necessitating catheterization. The symptoms of vulvar pain, pruritus, and discharge peak between days 7 and 11 of the primary infection. The average woman experiences severe symptoms for approximately 14 days. The severity of symptoms necessitates hospitalization for approximately 10% of women. Occasionally a primary pelvic infection is subclinical.

Recurrent genital herpes is a local disease, and the symptoms are much less severe. In 50% of women the first recurrence occurs within 6 months of the initial infection. Corey et al. estimates that if a women's initial genital infection was HSV-II that she has an approximately 80% chance of having a recurrence within 12 months. On the average a woman will have four recurrences during the first year. In contrast, if the initial pelvic infection was HSV-I, there is a 55% chance of a recurrence within 1 year, with the average rate of recurrence slightly less than one episode. There is a general clinical opinion that recurrences are frequently related to the onset of a menstrual period or emotional stress. To generalize, most clinical manifestations of recurrent infection are half as severe as those of primary infections. That is, vulvar involvement is usually unilateral, recurrent attacks last an average of 7 days, and viral shedding occurs for approximately 5 days. The ability to successfully culture herpesvirus from the cervix during that period varies from 20% to 60%, depending on the study cited. Recurrent herpetic ulcers are small—1 to 5 mm in diameter (Figure 21-11). A common feature of recurrence is a prodromal phase of sacroneuralgia, vulvar burning, tenderness, and pruritus for a few hours to 5 days before vesicle formation. The probability and frequency of recurrence of herpes is related to the HSV serotype.

The herpesvirus resides in a latent phase in the dorsal root ganglia of S-2, S-3, and S-4. Corey et al. reviewed the two current hypotheses regarding the etiology of recurrent attacks. The "ganglion trigger theory" proposes a constant viral replication in the privileged immune site of the dorsal root ganglia. Unknown stimuli, possibly hormonal, trigger the release of virus, which travels in a retrograde fashion via the peripheral nerves to the female genital organs. The alternate "skin trigger theory" proposes a regular production and retrograde flow of virus from the nerve ganglion down the sensory axon. Normally, local immunity inactivates the virus and recurrence results from a local immunologic defect.

The clinical diagnosis of genital herpes usually can be made by simple clinical inspection. Women come to the physician when they develop symptoms from vulvar ulcers. Herpetic ulcers are painful when touched with a cotton-tipped applicator, whereas the ulcers of syphilis are painless. Of the laboratory tests, viral cultures of the lesions are the most accurate in confirming the diagnosis. The estimated failure rate for a culture of the herpesvirus from a recognized lesion is between 10% and 20%. Most herpesvirus cultures will become positive within 2 to 4 days of inoculation. Rapid immunologic tests (10% to 30% false negatives) or cytologic studies (30% false negatives) are significantly less reliable than viral cultures. The sensitivity and specificity of the ELISA test is competitive with any other detection technique in populations with a high prevalence of herpetic infection. Serologic tests are only helpful in determining whether a patient has been infected in the past with herpesvirus. Obviously,

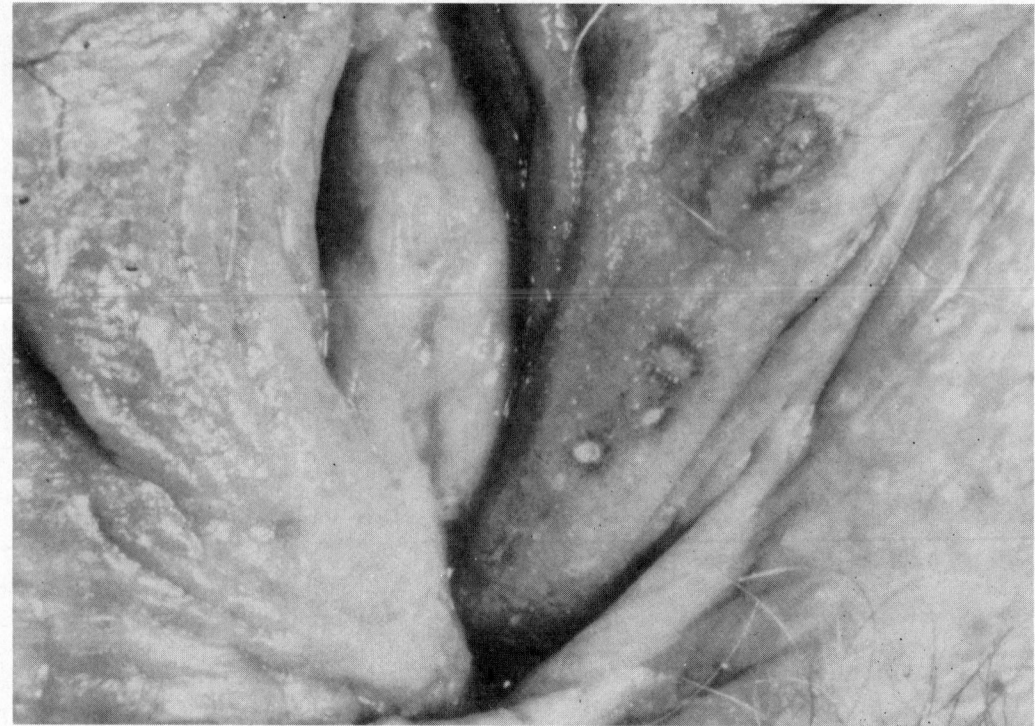

FIGURE 21-11
Recurrent herpes genitalis. Superficial ulcers are noted following rupture of vesicles. (From Kaufman RH and Faro S: Clin Obstet Gynecol 28:156, 1985.)

cultures for other sexually transmitted diseases should be obtained, as they may coexist with herpes.

Approximately 10% of women with primary infection have symptoms severe enough to require hospitalization. Common indications for hospitalization include severe headache, central nervous system involvement, extreme pain, difficulty in walking, and severe pain on urination or acute urinary retention.

The treatment of choice for either severe primary genital herpes or herpes genitalis in an immunosuppressed woman is intravenous acyclovir (5 mg/kg every 8 hours for approximately 5 days). The drug is given as an infusion over approximately 1 hour. Acyclovir (Zovirax) is an antiviral agent that is a purine nucleoside analogue. The drug is concentrated in cells infected with virus and produces its desired action by the inhibition of viral DNA synthesis. The drug is available in oral, topical, and intravenous preparations. The pharmacology of intravenous acyclovir is similar to that of aminoglycosides, although they do not share similar structures. Care must be taken that the patient has normal renal function. Side effects of intravenous acyclovir include local phlebitis and a transient increase in serum creatinine levels in 15% of cases.

If the patient does not require hospitalization, first episodes of genital herpes infections may be treated with oral acyclovir. Large, collaborative, double-blind studies published by Nilsen, Mertz, and Bryson and their co-workers documented that oral acyclovir 200 mg 5 times daily for 5 days was extremely efficacious in primary episodes of genital herpes. Acyclovir significantly reduced the median duration of viral shedding, time to crusting and healing of lesions, and the duration of both constitutional symptoms and local pain as compared with times for control subjects. The clinical course of the disease was shortened approximately 1 week. Treating the patient with oral acyclovir for 5 to 10 days during the primary infection did not influence viral latency—that is, either the frequency of or time to first recurrence. The Centers for Disease Control (CDC) recommends acyclovir 400 mg orally 5 times a day for 10 days for the first clinical episode of herpes proctitis. Many experts are using higher doses of acyclovir to treat herpetic infections in women with immunodeficiencies, especially HIV.

Topical acyclovir in a 5% ointment is sometimes prescribed for primary episodes. The ointment is applied to blisters every 3 to 4 hours for 7 days. Topical acyclovir does decrease the duration of viral shedding by 60% and the duration of pain and healing by approximately 2 days. Because of the possibility of spreading the infection with topical medication, the oral drug is preferred. Topical acyclovir therapy is believed to be less effective than therapy with the oral preparation.

The major fears of women with recurrent genital herpes are the rate of recurrence and possible transmission of the disease to their sexual partners. Women should be instructed to abstain from sexual intercourse from the time of prodromal symptoms or the time that lesions appear until the time that all lesions have completely reepithelialized. Active viral shedding may occur from the time of the prodromal period and does occur in women with ulcers even though the ulcers have crusted over. Oral acyclovir has been shown to be beneficial in reducing the duration of ulcerative lesions and in reducing the time that the virus can be isolated from these lesions. The recommended dose of acyclovir is 200 mg orally 5 times per day. It is interesting that patient-initiated therapy has been found to be superior to therapy ordered by a physician because patients initiate therapy earlier in the course of their disease.

Patients with frequent episodes of recurrent genital herpes may be successfully treated with prophylactic oral acyclovir. Douglas et al. studied 91 women given 200 mg acyclovir tablets (two to five tablets daily) for 4 months and 47 placebo recipients. The median time to first clinical recurrence was 120 days in the acyclovir group versus 18 days in women receiving the placebo. Alternative studies have used a dosage of 400 mg twice a day with improved patient compliance. After acyclovir had been discontinued, the recurrence rate returned to the same frequency as the pretreatment rate. Mertz et al. have published studies of a chronic daily oral acyclovir regimen for as long as 24 months. The average number of recurrences was 1.8 per year in those subjects taking acyclovir, while the placebo group averaged 11.4 recurrences per year.

There are areas of concern in the use of oral acyclovir to suppress recurrent disease. Resistant strains of herpesvirus have been identified from women treated with suppressive acyclovir. To date the prevalence of infection with these resistant strains has not increased, even in immunocompromised patients. Acyclovir is a drug with minimal toxicity, and recent reports have documented use for as long as 48 months, helping to establish the long-term safety of the drug. Also, acyclovir does not alter the rate of asymptomatic shedding of the virus. Therefore, the drug probably does not influence the transmission of the disease to sexual partners.

A vaccine would be the logical approach for optimum prevention of herpes. There have been extensive attempts to develop a safe vaccine. To date researchers have not been successful. It is important that the vaccine be free of viral DNA because of the potential oncogenicity of the viral genetic material. However, there is promise that a successful vaccine against surface glycoproteins will be developed in the future.

Granuloma Inguinale (Donovanosis)

Granuloma inguinale, also known as donovanosis, is a chronic, ulcerative, bacterial infection of the skin and subcutaneous tissue of the vulva. Rarely the vagina and cervix are involved in advanced, untreated cases. Granuloma inguinale is common in tropical climates such as New Guinea and the Caribbean islands, but fewer than 100 cases are reported each year in the United States.

This chronic disease is caused by a gram-negative, nonmotile, encapsulated rod—*Calymmatobacterium granulomatis*. This bacterium shares common antigens with *Klebsiella*. It cannot be cultured on standard media, and serologic tests are nonspecific. This disease can be spread both as a sexually transmitted disease and through close nonsexual contact. However, it is not highly contagious, and chronic exposure is usually necessary to contract the disease. The incubation period is extremely variable—from 1 to 12 weeks. The disease is found in 10% to 50% of sexual partners with the disease. However, it is also found in young children and elderly women who historically are not sexually active. Thus, some experts hypothesize that the disease may be secondary to autoinoculation following trauma to the infected area.

The initial growth of granuloma inguinale is an asymptomatic nodule. The skin over the

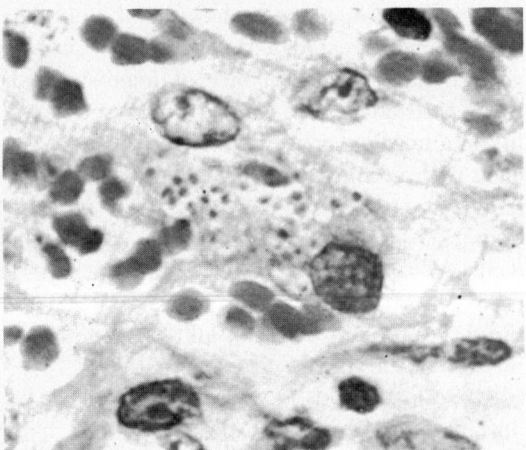

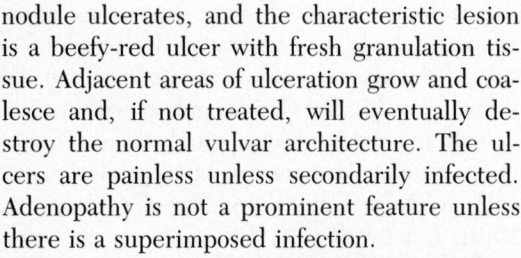

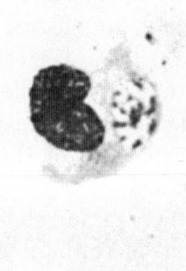

FIGURE 21-12
Donovanosis. Biopsy specimen shows intracytoplasmic Donovan bodies. (H&E stain.) (From Hart G: Donovanosis. In Holmes KK, Mårdh PA, Sparling PF, et al, editors: Sexually transmitted diseases, New York, 1984, McGraw-Hill Book Co.)

FIGURE 21-13
Donovanosis. Crust preparation from biopsy specimen shows single cell with many intracytoplasmic Donovan bodies. (Giemsa stain.) (From Hart G: Donovanosis. In Holmes KK, Mårdh PA, Sparling PF, et al, editors: Sexually transmitted diseases, New York, 1984, McGraw-Hill Book Co.)

nodule ulcerates, and the characteristic lesion is a beefy-red ulcer with fresh granulation tissue. Adjacent areas of ulceration grow and coalesce and, if not treated, will eventually destroy the normal vulvar architecture. The ulcers are painless unless secondarily infected. Adenopathy is not a prominent feature unless there is a superimposed infection.

In endemic areas the disease is usually diagnosed by its clinical manifestations. The diagnosis is established by identifying Donovan bodies in smears and specimens taken from the ulcers (Figure 21-12). Both the deep aspects of the ulcer crater and the fresh edge of an expanding lesion should be sampled. The pathognomonic Donovan bodies are clusters of dark-staining bacteria with a bipolar (safety pin) appearance found in the cytoplasm of large mononuclear cells (Figure 21-13). Special silver stains highlight the Donovan bodies. However, even a brief period of previous antibiotic therapy may result in an absence of Donovan bodies in women who have granuloma inguinale. The differential diagnosis includes lymphogranuloma venereum, vulvar carcinoma, syphilis, chancroid, genital herpes, and other granulomatous diseases.

Granuloma inguinale may be managed by a wide range of oral broad-spectrum antibiotics. Tetracycline is the most popular choice and should be prescribed for a minimum of 2 to 3 weeks (500 mg orally every 6 hours). The initial response to antibiotic therapy should be apparent within the first 7 days. However, optimal clinical response usually takes 3 to 5 weeks to ensure that the lesions have healed completely. It is best to continue antibiotics until a complete clinical response is noted with healing of the ulcerative lesions. Alternate antibiotic therapy such as an aminoglycoside has been used in refractory cases. Rarely, medical therapy fails and surgical excision is required.

Lymphogranuloma Venereum

Lymphogranuloma venereum (LGV) is a chronic infection of lymphatic tissue produced by *Chlamydia trachomatis*. It is found most commonly in the tropics. Cases occur infrequently in the United States, with fewer than 500 new cases being reported each year. The majority of cases are reported to occur in men. In most series the ratio of males to females with the disease is approximately 5:1. The vulva is the most frequent site of infection in women, but the urethra, rectum, and cervix may also be involved. Subclinical infection is common. Studies have demonstrated positive complement fixation tests in more than 50% of prostitutes without demonstrable disease. This sexually transmitted disease is produced by serotypes L_1, L_2, and L_3 of *C. trachomatis*. These serotypes are similar to the serotypes that produce trachoma. The incubation period is between 4 and 21 days.

There are three distinct phases of vulvar and perirectal LGV. The primary infection is a shallow, painless ulcer of the vestibule or labia. Occasionally this ulcer is near the urethra or rectum. The ulcer heals rapidly without therapy. The patient usually consults a physician during the secondary phase of the disease, which begins 1 to 4 weeks after the primary infection. The secondary phase is marked by painful adenopathy in the inguinal and perirectal areas. Two thirds of women have unilateral adenopathy, and half have systemic symptoms, including general malaise and fever. When the disease is not treated, the infected nodes become increasingly tender, enlarged, matted together, and adherent to overlying skin, forming bubos. A classic clinical sign of LGV is the double genitocrural fold or "groove sign" (Figure 21-14), a depression between groups of inflamed nodes. Within 7 to 15 days the bubo will rupture spontaneously and form multiple draining sinuses and fistulas. These are classic signs of the tertiary phase of the infection. Extensive tissue destruction of the external genitalia and anorectal region may occur during the tertiary phase. This tissue destruction and secondary extensive scarring and fibrosis may result in elephantiasis, multiple fistulas, and stricture formation of the anal canal and rectum.

Diagnosis is established by culture of pus or aspirate from a tender lymph node. With the recent development of monoclonal antibodies for *Chlamydia*, the diagnosis may be confirmed with this technique using fluid aspirated from an infected node. The complement fixation antibody titer is the most frequently used serum method for diagnosis. Antibody titers greater than 1:64 are indicative of active infection. The Frei skin test has been abandoned because of its low sensitivity. The differential diagnosis of LGV includes syphilis, chancroid, granuloma inguinale, vulvar carcinoma, genital herpes, and Hodgkin's disease.

Oral tetracycline or erythromycin (500 mg every 6 hours) for 3 to 6 weeks is commonly prescribed for the disease. The CDC recommends doxycycline 100 mg bid for at least 21 days as the preferred treatment. Fluctuant

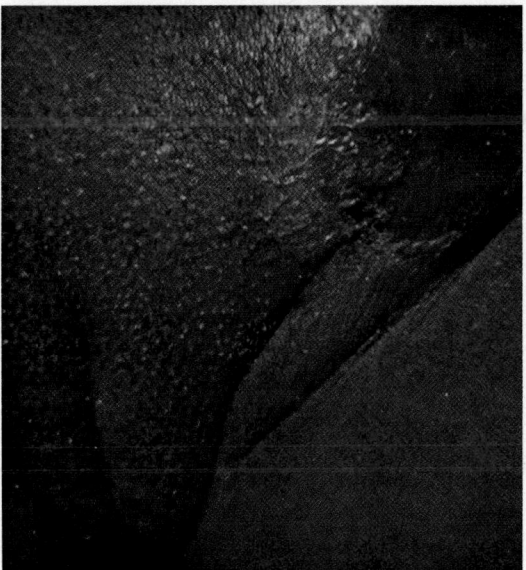

FIGURE 21-14
Lymphogranuloma venereum bubo with "groove" sign. (From Friedrich EG: Vulvae disease, ed 2, Philadelphia, 1983, WB Saunders Co.)

nodes should be aspirated to prevent sinus formation. However, incision and drainage are contraindicated. The late sequelae of the destructive tertiary phase of LGV often require extensive surgical reconstruction. It is important to administer antibiotics during the perioperative period.

Chancroid

Chancroid is a sexually transmitted, acute, ulcerative disease of the vulva. The soft chancre of chancroid is always painful and tender. In comparison, the hard chancre of syphilis is usually asymptomatic. The clinical importance of chancroid is enhanced by recent reports that the genital ulcers of chancroid facilitate the transmission of HIV infection. Chancroid is a common disease in the third world, but until the early 1980s it was rarely discovered in the United States. Recently there has been a substantial increase in reported cases in the United States, with 5047 reported in 1987. The disease is more common in males than females, with the male-to-female ratio varying from 5:1 to 10:1 in most series.

Chancroid is caused by *Haemophilus ducreyi*, a highly contagious, small, gram-negative rod. *H. ducreyi* is a nonmotile, facultative anaerobe. This bacterium on Gram stain exhibits a classic appearance of streptobacillary chains, or what has been described as an extracellular "school of fish." The incubation period is short—usually 3 to 6 days. Tissue trauma and excoriation of the skin must precede initial infection because *H. ducreyi* is unable to penetrate and invade normal skin.

Women with chancroid who consult a physician have solitary or multiple ulcers, most commonly of the vulvar vestibule and rarely of the vagina or cervix. The initial lesion is a small papule. Within 48 to 72 hours the papule evolves into a pustule and subsequently ulcerates. Multiple papules and ulcers may be in different phases of maturation secondary to autoinoculation. The painful ulcers are shallow with a characteristic ragged edge. The ulcers have a dirty, gray, necrotic exudate, and there is an absence of induration at the base (the soft chancre). Approximately 50% of women develop acutely tender inguinal adenopathy, usually within the first 2 weeks of an untreated infection. In most cases the inguinal adenopathy is unilateral, on the same side of the vulva as the preponderance of infection. Nodes that are fluctuant should undergo needle aspiration to prevent rupture of the abscess.

The diagnosis is made by Gram stain and culture of purulent material or by aspiration of tender lymph nodes. *H. ducreyi* may be difficult to grow in culture, depending on the experience of the bacteriology laboratory. Tissue biopsy helps to differentiate chancroid from the other common sexually transmitted diseases that produce vulvar ulcers, including genital herpes, syphilis, lymphogranuloma venereum, and donovanosis.

For years tetracycline was the standard treatment for chancroid. Recently Hammond et al. reported bacterial resistance to tetracycline. Therefore, the CDC recommends erythromycin base 500 mg orally every 6 hours for 7 days or ceftriaxone 250 mg intramuscularly in a single dose. Alternative regimens include trimethoprim-sulfamethoxazole 160 to 800 mg, one double-strength tablet, orally 2 times a day for 7 days; or amoxicillin 500 mg plus clavulanic acid 125 mg (Augmentin) orally every 8 hours for 7 days. Sexual partners should be treated in a similar fashion. Many other antibiotics, including second- and third-generation cephalosporins, are active against *H. ducreyi*. Recent studies have shown that the quinolones such as ciprofloxacin in a dosage of 500 mg orally every 12 hours for 3 days are excellent drugs. *H. ducreyi* is very sensitive to quinolones.

Successful antibiotic therapy results in both symptomatic and objective improvement within 5 to 7 days of initiating therapy. Approximately 10% of women whose ulcers initially heal have a recurrence at the same site. Women with HIV infection have an increased rate of failure to the standard treatments for chancroid and therefore often require more prolonged therapy. Approximately 18% of patients with chancroid in large urban areas in the United States are concurrently infected with HIV. *H. ducreyi* is resistant to multiple antibiotics. Therefore, susceptibility testing of bacterial isolates should be performed on patients who do not respond to therapy.

Syphilis

Syphilis is a chronic disease produced by the spirochete *Treponema pallidum*. The initial infection primarily involves mucous membranes. Syphilis remains one of the important sexually transmitted diseases in the United States. Epidemiologists speculate that only one out of four new cases of syphilis is reported. During the past 10 years the incidence of primary and secondary syphilis has increased 34% in the United States. The CDC estimated that in 1990 there were 130,000 cases of primary and secondary syphilis in the United States. Even with mandatory screening, congenital syphilis also continues to be a public health problem. Careful follow-up has documented that mothers experiencing the tragedy of stillbirth or neonatal death from syphilis usually have not received prenatal care. Syphilis should be included in the differential diagnosis of all genital ulcers and cutaneous rashes of unknown etiology.

Sir William Osler emphasized that syphilis was the great imitator of clinical medicine. He taught that if a physician had mastered all the systemic manifestations of syphilis, he would understand clinical medicine. The present discussion will deal with the gynecologic manifestations of the disease.

T. pallidum is an anaerobic, elongated, tightly wound spirochete. Because of its extreme thinness, it is difficult to detect by light microscopy. Therefore, spirochetes are diagnosed by use of a specially adapted technique—dark-field microscopy (Figure 21-15). These organisms have the ability to penetrate

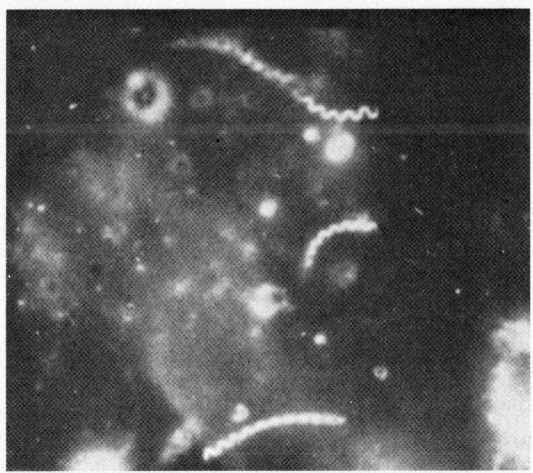

FIGURE 21-15
Dark-field microscopic appearance of *T. pallidum*. (From Larsen SA, McGrew BE, Hunter EF, et al: Syphilis serology and dark field microscopy. In Holmes KK, Mårdh PA, Sparling PF, et al, editors: Sexually transmitted diseases, New York, 1984, McGraw-Hill Book Co.)

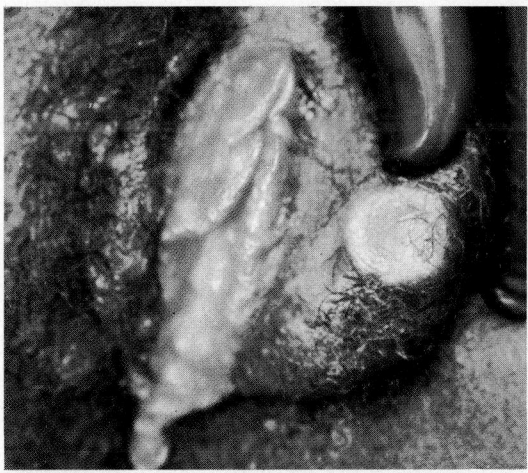

FIGURE 21-16
Hard chancre of primary syphilis. (From Kissane JM: Bacterial diseases. In Kissane JM, editor: Anderson's pathology, vol 1, St Louis, 1985, Mosby–Year Book, Inc.)

either skin or mucous membranes. The incubation period is between 10 and 90 days, with the average being 3 weeks. They replicate every 30 to 36 hours, which accounts for the comparatively long incubation period.

Syphilis is a moderately contagious disease. Approximately 10% of patients contract the disease from a single sexual encounter with an infected partner. Similar studies have documented that 30% of individuals become infected following a 1-month exposure to a sexual partner with primary or secondary syphilis. Patients are contagious during primary, secondary, and probably the first year of latent syphilis.

Serologic tests have been the foundation of screening programs to detect early syphilis, and there are two types of serologic tests—the nonspecific, nontreponemal and the specific, antitreponemal antibody tests. The nonspecific tests such as the VDRL (Venereal Disease Research Laboratories) slide test and the RPR (rapid plasma reagin) card test are inexpensive and easy to perform. These tests evaluate the patient's serum for the presence of reagin antibodies as they react with an antigen from beef heart. Approximately 1% of patients have technical or biologic false positive results with the nonspecific tests. Many conditions produce biologic false positive results, including a recent

febrile illness, pregnancy, immunization, chronic active hepatitis, malaria, sarcoidosis, intravenous drug use, and autoimmune diseases such as lupus erythematosus or rheumatoid arthritis. Biologic false positive serum tests usually are of extremely low titers (< 1:8).

If a nonspecific test result is positive, the significance of this result must be confirmed by a specific antitreponemal test. Specific tests are more sensitive; however, occasionally they may also produce false positive results. Most false positive results occur among women with lupus erythematosus. The standard for specific tests had been the TPI (*Treponema* immobilization test). It has largely been replaced by the FTA-ABS (fluorescent-labeled *Treponema* antibody absorption), the MHA-TP (microhemagglutination assay for antibodies to *T. pallidum*), and the HATTS (hemagglutination treponemal test for syphilis).

Clinically, syphilis is divided into primary, secondary, and tertiary stages. The classic finding of primary syphilis is a hard chancre (Figure 21-16). The chancre is a painless ulcer, with an indurated base that develops at the site of entry of the spirochete. The spirochetes of *T. pallidum* are capable of entering the body only through ulcerations or defects in the mucous membranes or skin. The chancre is often solitary and painless and is usually found on the vulva, vagina, or cervix. However, a recent increase in extragenital primary lesions has been reported, including lesions of the mouth, anal canal, and nipple of the breast. A primary chancre develops approximately 3 weeks after sexual contact with an infected partner. The incubation period for primary syphilis may vary widely, from 10 to 100 days. The ulcer heals spontaneously within 2 to 6 weeks even without antibiotic treatment. Confirmation that the ulcer is primary or secondary syphilis depends on identification of *T. pallidum* by dark-field microscopy from wet smears of the ulcer. Special preparations must be made to obtain suitable smears. It is important to clean and abrade the ulcer with gauze before obtaining the serum for the slides. Nontender regional adenopathy develops during the first week of clinical disease. Primary chancres of the cervix or the vagina will often fail to produce symptoms and, thus, will go undiscovered.

Serologic tests for syphilis generally become positive 4 to 6 weeks after exposure—thus 1 to 2 weeks after development of the chancre. At the time of positive dark-field identification of *T. pallidum* from a primary chancre, approximately 70% of women will have a positive serologic test. If the serologic test result remains negative for 3 months, it is unlikely that the ulcer was syphilis.

Secondary syphilis is the result of hematogenous dissemination of the spirochetes and thus is a systemic disease. Secondary syphilis develops between 6 weeks and 6 months (with an average of 9 weeks) after the primary chancre. During an attack of secondary syphilis, which if untreated will last 2 to 6 weeks, there is a multitude of systemic symptoms depending on the major organs involved. The classic rash of secondary syphilis is red macules and papules over the palms of the hands and the soles of the feet (Figure 21-17). Vulvar lesions include mucous patches and condyloma latum associated with painless lymphadenopathy. The vulvar lesions of condyloma latum are large, raised, flattened, grayish-white areas (Figure 21-18). On wet surfaces of the vulva, soft papules that often coalesce form ulcers. These ulcers are larger than herpetic ulcers and are not tender unless secondarily infected.

The latent stage of syphilis follows the secondary stage and varies in duration from 2 to 20 years. The majority of women who are diagnosed as having syphilis are discovered by positive blood tests during the latent stage of the disease. During the first 3 to 4 years of the latent phase an individual may experience relapses of secondary syphilis. Women with

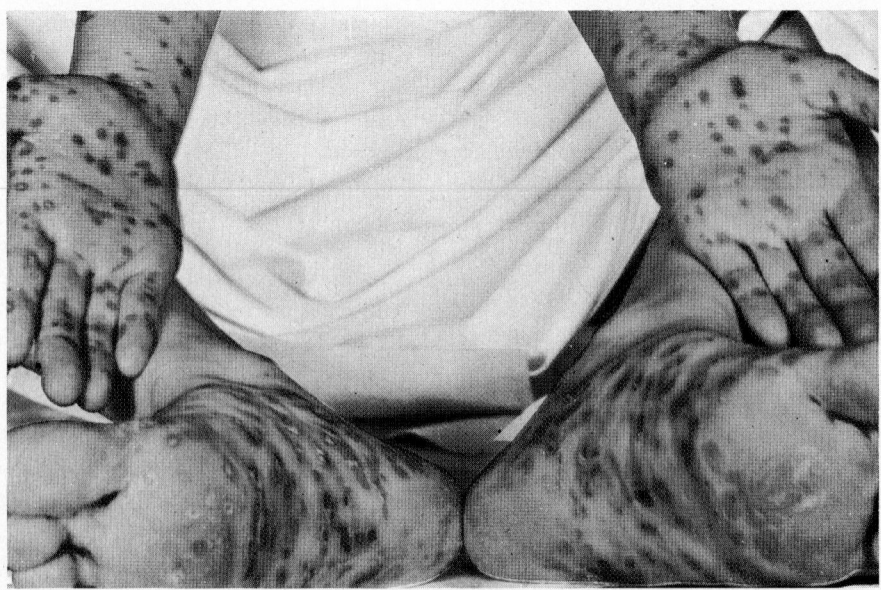

FIGURE 21-17
Rash of secondary syphilis. Red maculopapular lesions involve palms and soles. (From Kissane JM: Bacterial diseases. In Kissane JM, editor: Anderson's pathology, St Louis, 1985, Mosby–Year Book, Inc.)

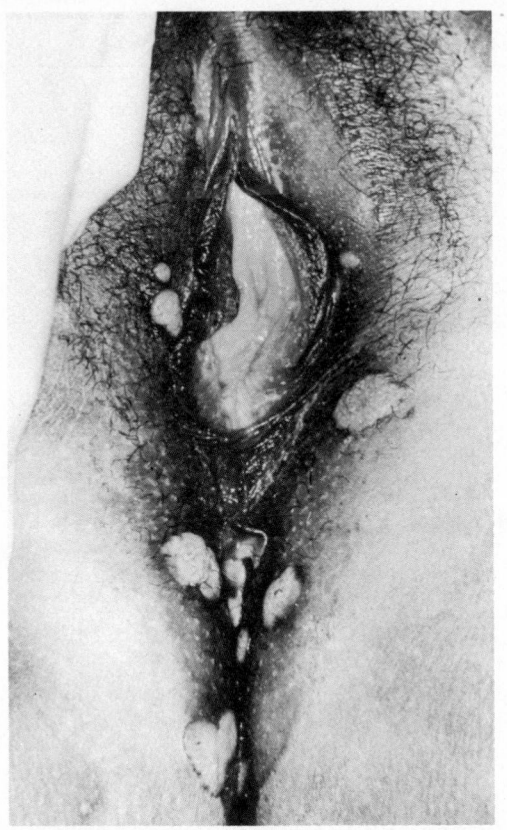

FIGURE 21-18
Multiple lesions of condylomata lata on vulva
and perineum. Dark-field microscopic findings
were positive. (From Gardner HL: Venereal
diseases. In Gardner HL and Kaufman RH, editors: Benign diseases of the vulva and vagina,
ed 2, Chicago, 1981, Mosby–Year Book, Inc.)

syphilis in the primary or secondary stages and
during the first year of latent syphilis are believed to be infectious.

The tertiary phase of syphilis is devastating
in its potentially destructive effects on the central nervous, cardiovascular, and musculoskeletal systems. Tertiary syphilis develops in approximately 33% of patients who are not appropriately treated during the primary, secondary,
or latent phases of the disease. The manifestations of late syphilis include optic atrophy,
tabes dorsalis, generalized paresis, aortic aneu-
rysm, and gummas of the skin and bones. A
gumma is similar to a cold abscess with a necrotic center and the obliteration of small vessels by endarteritis.

Penicillin is the drug of choice for syphilis.
T. pallidum is exquisitely sensitive to penicillin. However, because of the slow replication
time of the spirochete, blood levels must be
maintained for 7 to 14 days. The CDC recommends 2.4 million units of benzathine penicillin G in a single session for early syphilis (primary and secondary syphilis and the first year
of latent syphilis). Patients who are allergic to
penicillin should receive oral tetracycline 500
mg every 6 hours for 15 days. Standard treatment protocols for syphilis are detailed in the
box on p. 656.

All women with early syphilis should have
repeat, quantitative, nontreponemal serum antibody tests every 3 months for the first year
following therapy. These women should have a
spinal tap to detect asymptomatic neurosyphilis
and should receive further therapy. For long-
term follow-up the same serologic tests should
be ordered. The test should also be obtained
from the same laboratory. The VDRL and RPR
are equally valid, but RPR titers tend to be
slightly higher than VDRL titers. With successful treatment the VDRL titer will become
nonreactive or at most be reactive with a lower
titer within 1 year. There is a 1% to 2% chance
that the patient will not exhibit a fourfold titer
decline, and these cases are considered therapeutic failures. These women should be treated
once again. Patients with syphilis lasting longer
than 1 year should have quantitative VDRL titers for 2 years following therapy because their
titers will decline more slowly. A specific test
for syphilis, such as the FTA-ABS, remains reactive indefinitely.

Syphilis often involves the central nervous
system. The diagnosis is complicated and there
is no established diagnostic test that is a gold
standard for neurosyphilis. Women with syphilis of greater than 12 months' duration should
have an examination of their cerebrospinal fluid
(CSF) to rule out asymptomatic neurosyphilis.
Concurrent HIV infection should be considered in all patients with syphilis. Simultaneous
syphilis and HIV infection alters the natural
history of syphilis, with earlier involvement of
the central nervous system. Serologic tests may
be negative or confusing and, following penicillin treatment for syphilis, patients should be
followed with quantitative titers at more frequent intervals.

Vulvar Irritation Caused by Vaginitis

Anatomic distribution of symptoms occasionally creates a semantic misinterpretation of the

CENTERS FOR DISEASE CONTROL RECOMMENDED TREATMENT OF SYPHILIS (1989)

Early syphilis (primary, secondary, and early latent syphilis of less than 1 year's duration)

Recommended regimen

Benzathine penicillin G, 2.4 million units intramuscularly, one dose

Alternative regimen (penicillin-allergic nonpregnant patients)

Doxycycline, 100 mg orally twice a day for 2 weeks

or

Tetracycline, 500 mg orally four times a day for 2 weeks

If follow-up or compliance unsure, patient should have skin testing for penicillin allergy and be desensitized if necessary

If follow-up and compliance ensured, erythromycin, 500 mg orally four times a day for 2 weeks, can be used.

Late latent syphilis of more than 1 year's duration, gummas, and cardiovascular syphilis.

Recommended regimen

Benzathin penicillin G, 7.2 million units total, administered as three doses of 2.4 million units intramuscularly, given 1 week apart for 3 consecutive weeks

Alternative regimen (penicillin-allergic nonpregnant patients)

Doxycycline, 100 mg orally twice a day for 4 weeks

or

Tetracycline, 500 mg orally four times a day for 4 weeks

If patient is allergic to penicillin, alternate drugs should be used only after cerebrospinal fluid examination has excluded neurosyphilis.

Neurosyphilis

Recommended regimen

Aqueous crystalline penicillin G, 12-24 million units administered 2-4 million units every 4 hours intravenously for 10-14 days

Alternative regimen (if outpatient compliance ensured)

Procaine penicillin 2-4 million units intramuscularly daily

and

Probenecid, 500 mg orally four times a day; both drugs for 10-14 days

Many authorities suggest addition of benzathine penicillin, 2.4 million units intramuscularly and weekly for three doses, after completion of these neurosyphilis treatment regimens.

Syphilis in pregnancy

Penicillin regimen appropriate for stage of syphilis

Pregnant women with history of penicillin allergy should be skin tested and desensitized if necessary.

---

clinical reality. This is true for vulvar disease. The first symptom of vaginal infection is often vulvar pruritus, and the first sign of vaginal infection may be secondary erythema and edema of the vulvar skin. Often, self-medication for a vaginal infection may produce irritation of the vulva. Women whose chief complaint is vaginal itching or burning have symptoms because of irritation of the vestibule and adjacent vulvar epithelium. The sensory nerve endings are more numerous in the vulvar skin than in the vagina. The presence of excessive vaginal fluid is not appreciated until the fluid flows from the vagina onto the vulva.

A semantic compromise is to term most vaginal infections as vulvovaginitis. This is especially true with candidiasis and the profuse internal discharge that becomes external and accompanies *Trichomonas* vaginal infections. There is a separate clinical entity of primary cutaneous candidiasis, but it is rare and is most often found in diabetics. In this condition, the vulva appears beefy red, the labia are edematous, and the skin of the vulva has fissures and often small vesicles and pustules. The skin involvement of primary candidiasis is most prominent on the labia and the genitocrural folds.

The differential diagnosis for women with

symptoms of vulvovaginitis is complex. Discharge, burning, and pruritus are the common symptoms, and signs of vulvar irritation include erythema and excoriation of the vulvar skin. Discharge may be caused by either a cervical or vaginal infection. Vulvar irritation may be produced by primary or secondary infections, a primary skin irritant, or contact dermatitis. Physiologic fluids such as urine and normal cervical and vaginal secretions may cause maceration of the vulvar skin if the epithelium remains constantly moist, such as in the situation produced by tight-fitting synthetic fabric undergarments, especially panty hose.

The clinical symptoms of vulvovaginitis are usually not helpful in establishing the etiology. A careful history for contact allergens must be obtained. Often vaginal spermicides, soaps, perfumes, and feminine hygiene sprays will cause skin irritation. The cervical and vaginal secretions should be examined under the microscope for infection. The diagnosis of primary vulvar skin infections should be entertained.

First and foremost in alleviating the symptoms of vulvovaginitis is emphasis on keeping the vulvar skin dry. The patient should be encouraged to wear loose-fitting cotton undergarments. Treatment of vaginal infection is important and will be discussed in the next section.

VAGINITIS

Vaginal discharge resulting from primary infections of the vagina is the most common gynecologic symptom. Other symptoms associated with vaginal infection include superficial dyspareunia, dysuria, odor, and vulvar burning and pruritus. A gynecologist in private practice will see on the average two to four patients per day with vaginal infections. There are three common infections of the vagina—one produced by a fungus (candidiasis), another by a protozoon *(Trichomonas)*, and the third a synergistic bacterial infection (bacterial vaginosis). Relative prevalence differs depending on the population being studied. However, in a group of middle-class women in the reproductive range, bacterial vaginosis represents approximately 50% of cases, whereas candidiasis and *Trichomonas* infection each constitute approximately 25% of cases. Vaginal discharge resulting from viral infections such as herpes was discussed earlier in the chapter. Vaginitis in prepubertal and postmenopausal women is discussed in chapters dedicated to gynecologic

problems in those age groups (Chapters 10 and 40). Atrophic vaginitis is secondary to low levels of circulating estrogens. However, this condition predisposes women to secondary infection due to the thin atrophic lining of the vaginal canal.

The vaginal environment has been described as both a dynamic and a delicate ecosystem. The normal vaginal pH is 3.8 to 4.2. The maintenance of an optimum pH balance involves a complex interplay of hormonal, microbiologic, and other unknown factors. In reproductive-age women, estrogen stimulates the glycogen content of vaginal epithelial cells. The glycogen is metabolized to lactic acid and other short-chain organic acids, principally by the lactobacilli but also by other vaginal bacteria and enzymes. This interplay maintains the acidic environment of the vagina at a pH of approximately 4.0, which in turn limits the growth of potentially pathogenic bacteria and protozoa. One of the most helpful diagnostic aids in the differential diagnosis of vaginitis is to measure vaginal acidity with pH indicator paper. A vaginal pH of greater than 5.0 indicates bacterial vaginosis or *Trichomonas* infection or possibly an atrophic vaginal discharge. A vaginal pH of less than 4.5 represents either a physiologic discharge or a fungal infection. Cervical mucus, vaginal fluids produced during sexual excitement, and semen are all of a neutral or basic pH and may temporarily change the normal acidity. Semen has been found to buffer vaginal acidity for 6 to 8 hours following intercourse. Douching has little effect on vaginal pH. To maintain the vaginal ecosystem, the individual must attempt to maintain an appropriate concentration of *Lactobacillus acidophilus*. Hughes recently discovered that only 4 out of 16 commercially available over-the-counter products contained the appropriate *Lactobacillus acidophilus* that produced hydrogen peroxide.

Normal physiologic vaginal discharge consists of cervical and vaginal epithelium, normal bacterial flora, water, electrolytes, and other chemicals. The quantitative concentration of bacterial organisms is 10^8 to 10^9 colonies per milliliter of vaginal fluid. Döderlein in 1894 was the first to study the bacterial flora. Recently Larsen and Galask as well as Bartlett and Polk have published extensive reviews of both qualitative and quantitative studies of normal bacterial flora of the vagina. Bartlett and Polk serially sampled several women throughout the same cycle. They discovered that the concentration of anaerobic and aerobic bacteria varied considerably during the menstrual cycle. Qualitatively the number of bacterial species varied from 17 to 29. Anaerobic bacteria were quantitatively the most prevalent—5 times more common than aerobic bacteria.

Lactobacillus, an aerobic gram-positive rod,

is found in 62% to 88% of asymptomatic women. Other common aerobic bacteria are diphtheroids, streptococci, *Staphylococcus epidermidis*, and *Gardnerella vaginalis*. The most common gram-negative bacillus is *E. coli*. Anaerobic bacteria have been detected in approximately 80% of women, the most prevalent being *Peptococcus*, *Peptostreptococcus*, and *Bacteroides* species (Table 21-6). *Candida* species and mycoplasmas are also common inhabitants of asymptomatic women.

The ultimate diagnosis of the etiology of vaginitis depends on examination of the vaginal secretions under the microscope and measurement of vaginal pH. Nevertheless it is helpful to generalize about the classic characteristics of normal secretions and the three common vaginal infections (Table 21-7).

Normal vaginal secretions are white, floccular or curdy, and odorless. In a woman with a normal or physiologic discharge it is important to note that the vaginal discharge is present only in the dependent portions of the vagina. Pathologic discharges usually involve the anterior and lateral walls of the vagina. Godley has recently quantified normal vaginal secretions. Although the amount varies with the day of the menstrual cycle, asymptomatic women averaged 1.6 g every 8 hours. If the vaginal discharge is white and curdy, fungal infections are more likely. Gray-white discharges that are thin and usually profuse indicate a differential diagnosis of *Trichomonas* or bacterial vaginosis. Vaginal discharges that have a foul odor are usually caused by either *Trichomonas* or bacterial vaginosis.

There has been recent interest in studying the pathophysiology of vaginal infections with the increased emphasis and funding for the

TABLE 21-6
Bacterial Vaginal Flora among Asymptomatic Women without Vaginitis

Organism	Range of Recovery (%)
Facultative organisms	
Gram-positive rods	
Lactobacilli	50-75
Diphtheroids	40
Gram-positive cocci	
Staphylococcus epidermidis	40-55
Staphylococcus aureus	0-5
Beta-hemolytic streptococci	20
Group D streptococci	35-55
Gram-negative organisms	
Escherichia coli	10-30
Klebsiella sp.	10
Other organisms	2-10
Anaerobic organisms	
Peptococcus sp.	5-65
Peptostreptococcus spp.	25-35
Bacteroides spp.	20-40
Bacteroides fragilis	5-15
Fusobacterium sp.	5-25
Clostridium sp.	5-20
Eubacterium sp.	5-35
Veillonella sp.	10-30

From Eschenbach DA: Clin Obstet Gynecol 26:187, 1983.

TABLE 21-7
Appearance of Vaginal Discharge

	Normal	Bacterial Vaginosis	Trichomoniasis	Candidiasis
Discharge present at introitus	No	Yes	Yes	No
Color	White	Gray	Yellow-gray	White
Viscosity	High	Low	Low	High
Consistency	Floccular	Homogenous	Homogenous	Floccular
Presence in vagina	Dependent portion	Adherent to vaginal walls	Adherent to vaginal walls	Adherent to vaginal walls

From Eschenbach DA: Clin Obstet Gynecol 26:186, 1983.

study of sexually transmitted diseases. During the next 5 years research will emphasize local changes in substances that afford nonspecific protection from vaginal infection, such as lysozymes, lactoferrin, zinc, fibronectin, and complement.

Bacterial Vaginosis (Nonspecific Vaginitis)

Bacterial vaginosis, referred to as nonspecific vaginitis by many, is the most frequent infectious vaginitis. The majority of experts consider it to be a sexually transmitted disease. The incubation period is 5 to 10 days following exposure.

Concepts of the etiology of this disease have changed over the past few years. An associated semantic debate concerning the best descriptive name for the type of vaginitis caused by one or more bacteria has accompanied the changing concepts. Twenty-five years ago the offending organism was called *Haemophilus* or *Corynebacterium vaginale*. Subsequently a specific species was named after Herman Gardner and called *Gardnerella vaginalis*. The latter is classified as a gram-negative, small bacillus. In practice the organism is a coccobacillus that is gram variable (sometimes gram positive, sometimes gram negative), depending on the age of the cultures. As more sophisticated culture techniques have been developed, it is apparent that *G. vaginalis* may be recovered from the vaginas of 30% to 40% of asymptomatic women. Similarly, *G. vaginalis* may be cultured from 40% of women who have been successfully treated for bacterial vaginosis.

Holmes and Eschenbach and their colleagues from Seattle proposed that nonspecific vaginitis was a symbiotic infection of anaerobic bacteria and *Gardnerella*, both organisms contributing to produce the clinical symptoms. They discovered that the prevalence and concentration of *Gardnerella* organisms were increased from 10^4 bacteria per milliliter in asymptomatic women to 10^7 bacteria per milliliter in symptomatic women. Concentrations of anaerobic bacteria increased tenfold in symptomatic women. The name of the infection was therefore changed from nonspecific vaginitis to bacterial vaginosis. Associated with the increase in anaerobic bacteria was a decrease in the concentration of lactobacilli and also the presence of lactobacilli species that produce hydrogen peroxide. To further complicate the picture, several groups have recently reported the association of vaginal *vibrios* in approximately 50% of symptomatic women. These small, curved anaerobic rods are from the *Mobiluncus* group, and their exact role in the production of vaginal infection is unclear.

Women with bacterial vaginosis have the most uniform spectrum of symptoms of all the types of infectious vaginitis (Table 21-8). The most frequent symptom is an unpleasant vaginal odor, which patients describe as "musty" or "fishy." The odor is often sensed following intercourse, when the alkaline semen results in a release of aromatic amines.

The vaginal discharge associated with bacterial vaginosis is thin and gray-white. Some observers have characterized the discharge as similar to a small cup of milk that has been poured into the vagina. Speculum examination reveals that the discharge is mildly adherent to the vaginal walls, in contrast to a physiologic discharge, which is discovered in the most dependent areas of the vagina. The vaginal dis-

TABLE 21-8
Major Categories of Vaginitis

	C. albicans	*C. glabrata*	*Gardnerella*	*Trichomonas*
Symptom	Itch	Burn	Odor	Discharge
Mucosal erythema*	+++	+	None	Variable
pH	4-5	4-5	5-6	6-7
Wet smear	Budding filaments	Spores only	Clue cells	Many white blood cell protozoa

From Friedrich EG: Am J Obstet Gynecol 152:248, 1985.
*Degree of severity: +, mild; +++, severe.

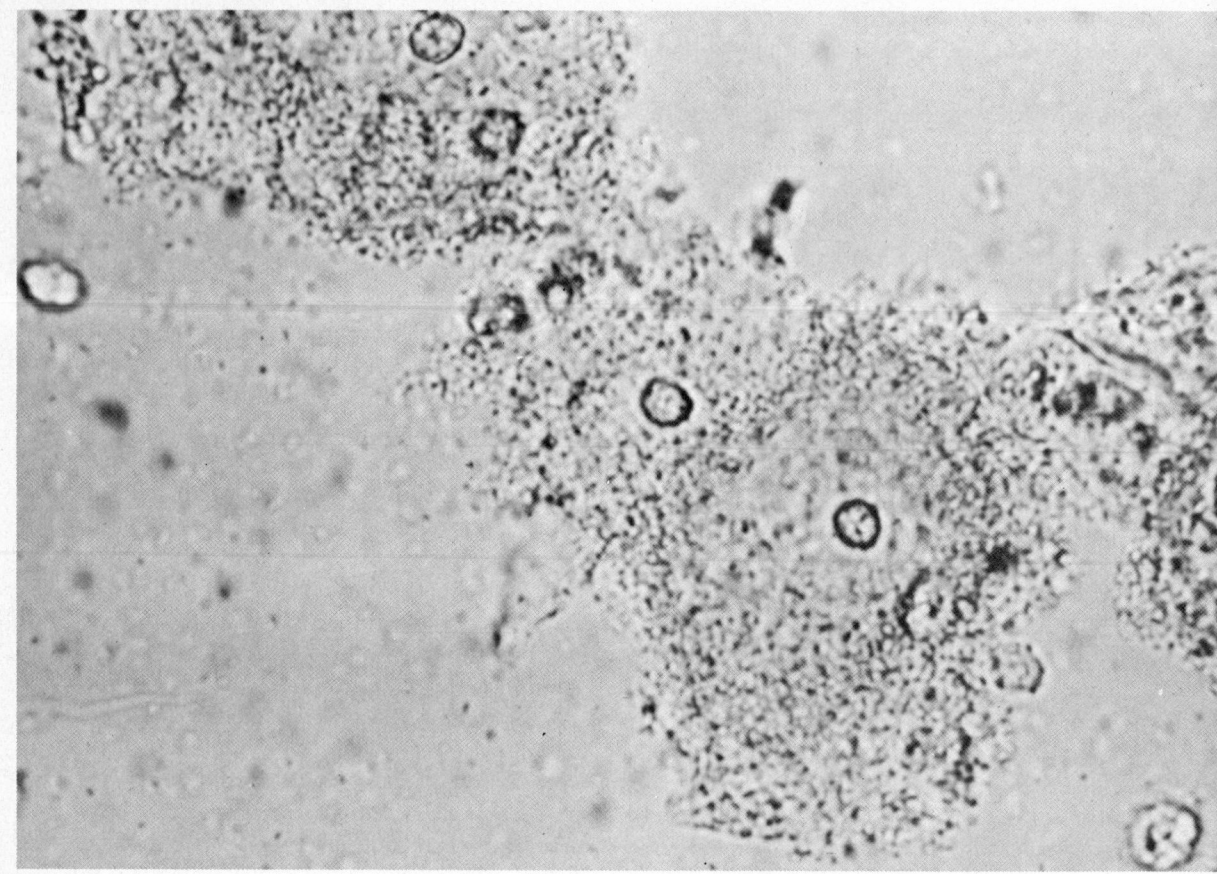

FIGURE 21-19
Vaginal epithelial cells from woman with bacterial vaginosis. These are typical clue cells, being heavily covered by coccobacilli, with loss of distinct cell margins. (×400.) (From Holmes KK: Lower genital tract infections in women: cystitis/urethritis, vulvovaginitis, and cervicitis. In Holmes KK, Mårdh PA, Sparling PF, et al, editors: Sexually transmitted diseases, New York, 1984, McGraw-Hill Book Co.)

charge is frothy in approximately 10% of women, and it is rare to have associated vulvar irritation.

The diagnosis of bacterial vaginosis is confirmed by a saline wet smear. The classic findings on wet smear are clumps of bacteria and "clue cells," which are vaginal epithelial cells with clusters of bacteria adherent to their external surfaces (Figure 21-19). The bacteria give the clue cells a granular or stippled appearance by obscuring their cellular borders. The percentage of clue cells may vary widely, ranging from 2% to 50% of infected women. The wet smear also demonstrates a comparative lack of inflammatory cells and lactobacilli. Leukocytes are not nearly as frequent as epithelial cells underneath the microscope. If inflammatory cells are visualized on wet smear,

there is usually associated cervical infection or *Trichomonas vaginalis* infection. In experimental studies where vaginal biopsies have been performed in women with bacterial vaginosis, there is no histologic evidence of vaginal inflammation. In summary, for scientific studies, the Seattle group has established four criteria for the diagnosis of bacterial vaginosis: (1) a homogeneous vaginal discharge is present; (2) the vaginal discharge has a pH equal to or greater than 4.7; (3) the vaginal discharge has an aminelike odor when mixed with potassium hydroxide; and (4) a wet smear of the vaginal discharge demonstrates clue cells greater in number than 20% of the number of the vaginal epithelial cells.

The vaginal pH associated with bacterial vaginosis is 5.0 to 6.0. When 10% potassium hydroxide is placed on the vaginal speculum or a glass slide containing vaginal secretions, an aromatic amine will be vaporized. A positive "whiff test" may be obtained with either bacterial vaginosis or *Trichomonas* infection. It is usually more prominent with bacterial infections because of the amount of anaerobic metabolism. The common aromatic amines are cadaverine and putrescine, both of which result from anaerobic metabolism. In all likelihood, bacterial vaginosis is a sexually transmitted disease. The *Gardnerella* organism may be recovered from approximately 90% of male partners. Women with multiple sexual partners are in a high-risk group for the disease. It has been postulated that the associated increased prevalence and concentration of anaerobic bacteria in the vagina may also predispose certain women to upper tract pelvic infection.

The treatment of choice for bacterial vaginosis is metronidazole (Protostat, Flagyl), 500 mg twice daily for 7 days. Metronidazole has excellent activity against anaerobic bacteria, and its hydroxy metabolite is active against *G. vaginalis*. Pfeifer et al. found clinical cures in 80 of 81 women treated with metronidazole but mediocre response to ampicillin, tetracycline, or sulfa cream. More important, facultative *Lactobacillus* organisms return after treatment with metronidazole but not with ampicillin. Most investigators report a cure rate of approximately two out of three women with a 1-week course of ampicillin 500 mg every 6 hours. Blackwell et al. have recently contrasted treatment of 7 days of metronidazole with a regimen of 2 g of metronidazole divided over 12 hours. They described a 95% cure rate with 7 days versus a 75% cure rate with single-day therapy. Purdon et al. found similar results with 67% of women treated with single-day therapy and 86% of patients cured receiving the 7-day course. Women who are allergic to flagyl, or resistant cases, should be treated with clindamycin, either 450 mg every 6 hours for 7 days or as a topical 2% vaginal cream. Alternate treatment regimens to metronidazole or clindamycin include amoxicillin 500 mg plus clavulanic acid (Augmentin) every 8 hours for 7 days or cephradine 500 mg every 6 hours for 7 days.

Bump et al. have added to the therapeutic dilemma by a study of prevalence and persistence of *G. vaginalis* in asymptomatic women over a 6-month period. They believe that the *Gardnerella* bacterium is indigenous flora and is often transient. They advise not treating a patient unless she exhibits classic symptoms.

Concurrent treatment of the male partner is most controversial. The literature is divided on this subject. We favor treating the male partner if there is recurrent vaginitis or any suspicion of associated upper genital tract infection.

Trichomonas Vaginal Infection

Trichomonas vaginalis is a protozoon that inhabits the vagina and lower urinary tract, especially Skene's ducts in the female. The relative importance of *Trichomonas* as a cause of vaginitis has decreased since the introduction of metronidazole 30 years ago. It is estimated that there are between 2.5 and 3 million cases of vaginitis secondary to *Trichomonas* infection in the United States each year. *Trichomonas* vaginal infection is the most prevalent nonviral sexually transmitted disease of women. *Trichomonas* is the etiologic factor for approximately one in four episodes of infectious vaginitis.

Many women who harbor *Trichomonas* in their vaginal secretions are free of symptoms. McLellan et al. discovered that only one out of two women with positive vaginal cultures had symptoms of a vaginal discharge. In the same study only one out of six women complained of vulvar pruritus. Positive wet smears or cultures for *Trichomonas* are reported in 5% to 15% of asymptomatic gynecology patients, with a much higher percentage being found in women attending a sexually transmitted disease clinic. Trichomoniasis is definitely a sexually transmitted disease, with the protozoa being isolated from 30% to 40% of male partners of women with a positive culture and approximately 85% of female partners of a male with a positive culture. The incubation period for *Trichomonas* infection is 4 to 28 days. *Trichomonas* is a hardy organism and will survive for up to 24 hours on a wet towel and up to 6 hours on a surface. However, experimental studies have established that successful vaginal infection depends on the deposition of an inoculum of several thousand organisms. Thus it is unlikely that infection may be related to exposure from infected towels or swimming pools.

Trichomonas vaginitis is caused by the anaerobic, flagellated protozoon, *T. vaginalis* (Figure 21-20). There are other species of *Trichomonas* that reside in the oral pharynx and

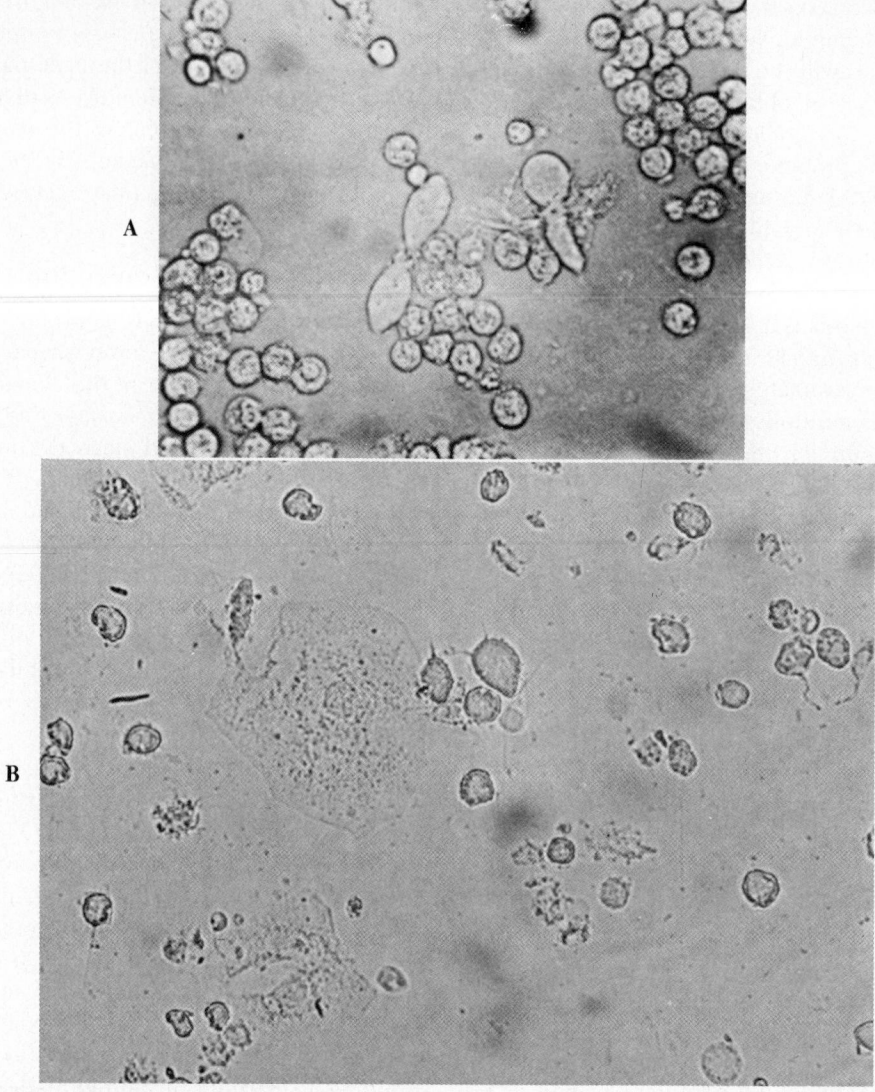

FIGURE 21-20
A and **B,** Trichomonads in wet mount prepared with physiologic saline. (**A** from Gardner HL: Trichomoniasis. In Gardner HL, Kaufman RH, editors: Benign diseases of the vulva and vagina, ed 2, Chicago, 1981, Mosby–Year Book, Inc. **B** from Friedrich EG: Vulvar disease, ed 2, Philadelphia, 1983, WB Saunders Co.)

rectum. These species are site specific and do not produce disease in the vagina. *T. vaginalis* resides in the paraurethral glands of both the male and female. Before systemic medication, reinfection occurred not only from an infected partner but from the patient's own urethra and Skene's ducts.

T. vaginalis is a unicellular protozoon that is normally fusiform in shape. This organism exists only in the trophozoite form or vegetative cell. It is slightly larger than a white blood cell.

Three to five flagella extend from one end of the organism. The flagella provide the active movement of the protozoon, with the direction of motion usually toward the end with the flagella. The *Trichomonas* organism assumes a spherical shape in an acidic environment (Figure 21-21). Motion is then restricted to waves of the undulating membrane of the protozoon.

Vaginitis from *Trichomonas* is a disease primarily of women in the reproductive years. The normal highly acidic vaginal environment

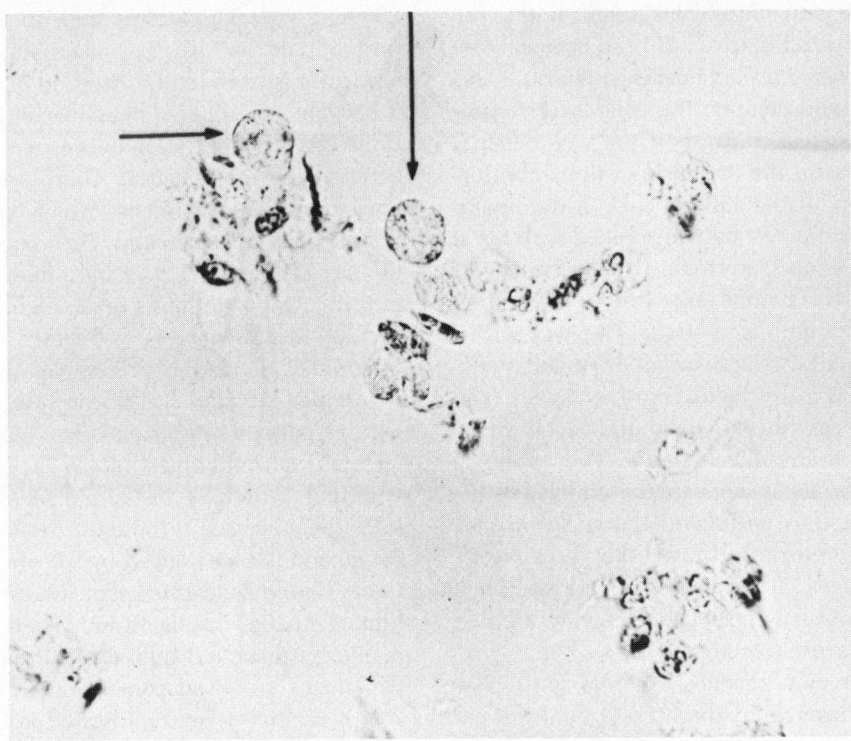

FIGURE 21-21
"Balled-up" trichomonads *(arrows)* in urinary sediment. (From Gardner HL: Trichomoniasis. In Gardner HL and Kaufman RH, editors: Benign diseases of the vulva and vagina, ed 2, Chicago, 1981, Mosby–Year Book, Inc.)

is resistant to *Trichomonas* infection. When lactobacilli predominate in the vaginal fluid, a woman will not develop symptoms. However, menstrual blood, semen, or other vaginal pathogens that transform the vaginal pH to a more basic level favor the growth of *Trichomonas* organisms.

Trichomonas produces a wide variety of patterns of vaginal infection. Women may or may not have symptoms and signs of acute or chronic infection. The primary symptom of *Trichomonas* vaginal infection is profuse vaginal discharge. Patients often complain that the copious discharge makes them feel "wet." The discharge may be white, gray, yellow, or green. The classic discharge of *Trichomonas* infection has been termed "frothy" (with bubbles) and often has an unpleasant odor. However, a frothy discharge is only noted in 10% to 25% of women with proven *Trichomonas* infection.

This discharge is not diagnostic, because it may be seen also with nonspecific bacterial vaginal infections.

Associated with the acute vaginal discharge are erythema and edema of the vulva and vagina. The classic sign of a strawberry appearance of the upper vagina and cervix is rare and is noted in less than 10% of women. Approximately 25% of women experience vulvar pruritus. Vulvar skin involvement is limited to the vestibule and labia minora, which helps to distinguish it from the more extensive vulvar involvement of monilial vulvovaginitis. Women with chronic infection often have a malodorous discharge as their only complaint. Dysuria is a symptom in approximately one out of five women with symptomatic *Trichomonas* infection.

The diagnosis of *Trichomonas* vaginal infection is confirmed by examination of vaginal fluid mixed with physiologic saline under the microscope (see Figure 21-20). To optimally visualize *Trichomonas* organisms, it is best to use high power and dampen the condenser to produce the greatest contrast. If the wet smear is fresh and warm, the organisms will exhibit forward motion. If the slide is cold, if the organisms are surrounded by white blood cells, or if the saline is too hypertonic, the *Trichomonas* organisms will assume an ovoid configuration and exhibit minimal motion. The wet smear usually contains a large number of inflammatory cells and many vaginal epithelial cells. The only other vaginitis with an abundance of white blood cells is atrophic vaginitis. The epithelial cells are normal in appearance and have distinct edges. It is postulated that *Trichomonas* excretes a cytotoxic substance that lyses intracellular bridges. This may explain the large number of normal epithelial cells on wet smear seen with severe infection.

The accuracy of diagnosis by wet smear varies widely throughout the literature. If the patient is symptomatic, the sensitivity of a saline wet preparation is 80% to 90%. Therefore a culture for *Trichomonas* is rarely indicated. Attempts to diagnose *T. vaginalis* infection by Papanicolaou (Pap) smear results in an error rate of at least 50%. There is a large number of both false positive and false negative reports. A complementary laboratory test to the wet smear is the measurement of pH of the vaginal fluid with colorimetric paper. The vaginal pH associated with *T. vaginalis* is between 5.0 and 7.0. Krieger has recently reported a comparison study of direct wet-mount Pap smear slides, fluorescein-conjugated monoclonal antibodies, and two culture media. In this study he used the culture results as the gold standard and found that the wet mount discovered 60%, Pap smears 56%, and the monoclonal antibodies 86% of infections. Importantly, the Pap smear also identified seven women who were false positives and 18 who were suspicious for *Trichomonas* in which the cultures were negative. The fluorescein-conjugated monoclonal antibody test (which takes approximately 1 hour) and another new test, the direct enzyme immunoassay (which requires only an ordinary light microscope), are both promising for improving office diagnosis of *Trichomonas* infection.

Metronidazole (Flagyl, Protostat) is the treatment of choice for *T. vaginalis* infection. Metronidazole is marketed in the United States as 250 and 500 mg tablets and an intravenous preparation for severe anaerobic infections. The drug is completely absorbed orally and has a half-life of 8 hours. Phenobarbital decreases the serum concentration approximately 50% by activating liver enzymes. There are two standard treatment regimens, which yield similar results of an approximately 90% cure rate. Single-day therapy is 1 g of metronidazole in the morning and another 1 g at night. Alternate therapy is 250 mg every 8 hours for 7 days. Single-day therapy is preferable, because it is less expensive and has fewer side effects and greater patient compliance. The major side effects of metronidazole therapy include nausea, vomiting, a metallic taste, and secondary yeast infections. Nausea is the most frequent complication and is experienced by 5% of women. Patients should be warned that metronidazole inhibits ethanol metabolism. Therefore, they may experience a disulfiram-like reaction if the two drugs are used concurrently. Metronidazole is relatively contraindicated in the first trimester of pregnancy because of possible mutagenesis. Several reports have noted an association between chronic high-dose metronidazole treatment and pulmonary cancers in mice. However, studies of humans have not confirmed any relationship between metronidazole therapy and oncogenesis. The asymptomatic female who has *Trichomonas* identified in the lower female genital urinary tract definitely should be treated. Extended follow-up studies have shown that one out of three asymptomatic females will become symptomatic within 3 months. Furthermore, there is speculation that *Trichomonas* may be a vector for viral or bacterial pelvic infections. Obviously, all sexually transmitted diseases have common epidemiologic backgrounds, and finding one dictates appropriate studies to rule out colonization or infection with another sexually transmitted disease. Frequently, vaginal infections are a mixed infection, with *Trichomonas* and bacterial vaginosis occurring simultaneously in the same individual.

One of the continuing debates regarding therapy is treatment of the asymptomatic male partner. Gardner and Dukes documented a 2.5-fold greater reinfection rate when the sexual partner was not treated. Some physicians elect to treat the male partner only when the vaginitis is recurrent. We believe that *Trichomonas* infection should be treated in a similar fashion to any sexually transmitted disease.

Thus it is our practice to treat male sexual partners with 2 g of metronidazole (single-day therapy).

Women who have recurrence have in most cases either been reinfected or complied poorly with therapy. Recently a few resistant strains of *Trichomonas* have been documented. These resistant cases usually respond to daily doses of 1 to 2 g of metronidazole for 7 days. If this is not successful, either a combination of oral and topical therapy or high-dose intravenous therapy is indicated. High-dose intravenous metronidazole may produce ataxia and neuropathy. A clue to a woman with resistant strains of *Trichomonas* is that when a wet smear is obtained 3 to 5 days after therapy, the *Trichomonas* organisms are larger and plumper than normal.

If a woman is allergic to metronidazole, topical clotrimazole, an imidazole derivative, is the appropriate drug. Friedrich has advocated douching with hypertonic (20%) saline solution to reduce the vaginal inoculum.

Candida Vaginitis

Candida vaginitis is produced by a ubiquitous, airborne, gram-positive fungus. The vast majority of cases are caused by *Candida albicans*, with 5% to 20% of vaginal fungal infections produced by *C. glabrata* or *C. tropicalis*. However, the percentage of infections related to the latter two species has increased in recent years. *Candida* species are part of the normal flora of approximately 25% of women, being a commensal saprophytic organism on the mucosal surface of the vagina. Its prevalence in the rectum is three to four times greater and in the mouth two times greater than in the vagina. When the ecosystem of the vagina is disturbed, *C. albicans* becomes an opportunistic pathogen. Lactobacilli inhibit the growth of fungi in the vagina. However, when the relative concentration of lactobacilli declines, rapid overgrowth of *Candida* species occurs. Following the traditional 10 to 14 days of oral broad-spectrum antibiotics, the percentage of women who have vaginal colonization with *Candida* increases threefold.

Vulvovaginal candidiasis has a variety of names, such as "moniliasis." This term is semantically incorrect, because the name is reserved for plant pathogens. Candidiasis is also often referred to as a yeast infection because of its similarity to true yeast cells.

Candida vaginitis has several features unlike those of protozoal or bacterial vaginitis. *Candida* is rarely found in a mixed infection with *Trichomonas* or bacterial vaginosis. *Candida* vulvovaginitis is not associated with other sexually transmitted diseases and is not seen more frequently in STD clinics. Unlike other vaginal infections, there is no direct relationship between the number of organisms and the patient's signs and symptoms. Some women with a small amount of yeast may have extensive symptoms. It has been postulated that such patients may be hypersensitive to the fungus. Also, candidiasis is not considered a sexually transmitted disease. However, 10% of male partners have concomitant symptomatic penile infection. Treatment of the male partners does not reduce the recurrence rate.

Vaginitis caused by fungal infection is primarily a disease of the childbearing years. The greatest enigma of this condition is the recurrence rate after an apparent cure, varying from 20% to 80% of women.

C. albicans is responsible for 80% to 95% of vaginal fungal infections. The organisms develop filamentous (hyphae and pseudohyphae) and ovoid forms, termed conidia, buds, or spores. In contrast, *C. glabrata* does not produce filamentous forms. Merkus et al. and Montes and Wilborn have reported studies of the pathophysiology of *Candida* infections as viewed with the electron microscope. The filamentous forms of *C. albicans* have the ability to penetrate the mucosal surface and become intertwined with the host cells (Figure 21-22). This results in secondary hyperemia and limited lysis of tissue near the site of infection.

C. albicans, although normally not pathogenic, may overgrow the vagina because of a number of well-established host factors that enhance growth of the fungus. Hormonal factors, depressed immunity, and antibiotic use are the three most important. The hormonal changes associated with both pregnancy and menstruation favor growth of the fungus. The prevalence of *Candida* vaginitis increases throughout pregnancy, probably as a result of the high estrogen levels. The literature was originally mixed with respect to the relationship between oral contraceptives and candidiasis. Oriel et al. discovered more positive cultures, but fewer symptoms, in women taking oral contraceptives. Presently with low-dose estrogen oral contraceptives there is no increase in the incidence of fungal vaginitis. Women tend to report recurrent episodes of vaginitis immediately preceding and

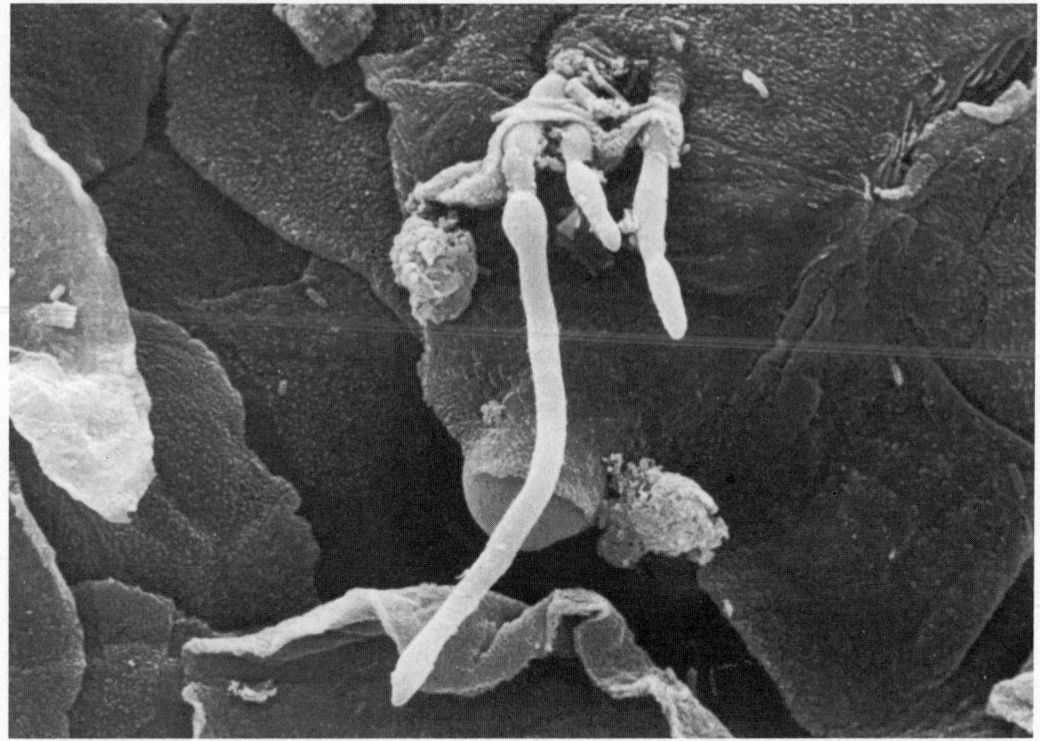

FIGURE 21-22
Scanning electron microscopy of intraluminal debris of specimen of vagina wall taken from patient with vaginal candidiasis. (×3,500) Hyphae of *C. albicans* penetrate epithelial layers of vaginal surface. (From Merkus JMWM, Bisschop MPJM, and Stolte LAM: Obstet Gynecol Surv 40:499, 1985. © by Williams & Wilkins, 1985.)

immediately following their menstrual periods. Broad-spectrum antibiotics, especially those that destroy lactobacilli (penicillin, tetracycline, cephalosporins), are notorious for precipitating acute episodes of *C. albicans* vaginitis. Women with diabetes mellitus, or even a low renal threshold for sugar, have a higher incidence of this disease. Obesity and debilitating disease are other predisposing factors. Women who use the contraceptive sponge with nonoxynol-9 have an increased incidence of vaginal infections secondary to *C. albicans.*

Probably the most important host factor is depressed cell-mediated immunity. Women who take high levels of corticosteroids and women with AIDS often experience recurrent *Candida* vulvovaginitis. For years authors have written of an X-factor that predisposed certain women to recurrent vaginitis. This X-factor is most likely a subtle defect in cell-mediated immunity.

Since fungal vaginitis is usually vulvovagini-tis, the predominant symptom is pruritus. This may be accompanied by vulvar burning, external dysuria, and dyspareunia, depending on the degree of vulvar skin involvement. The vaginal discharge is white or whitish-gray, highly viscous, and described as granular or floccular. It does not have an odor. The amount of discharge is highly variable. The vulvar signs include erythema, edema, and excoriation. With extensive skin involvement, pustules may extend beyond the line of erythema. During speculum examination a cottage cheese–type discharge is often visualized with adherent clumps and plaques (thrush patches) attached to the walls of the vagina. These clumps or raised plaques are usually white or yellow. The pH of the vagina associated with this infection is below 4.5.

The diagnosis is established by obtaining a wet smear of vaginal secretion and mixing this with 10% to 20% potassium hydroxide (Figure 21-23). The alkali rapidly lyse both red blood

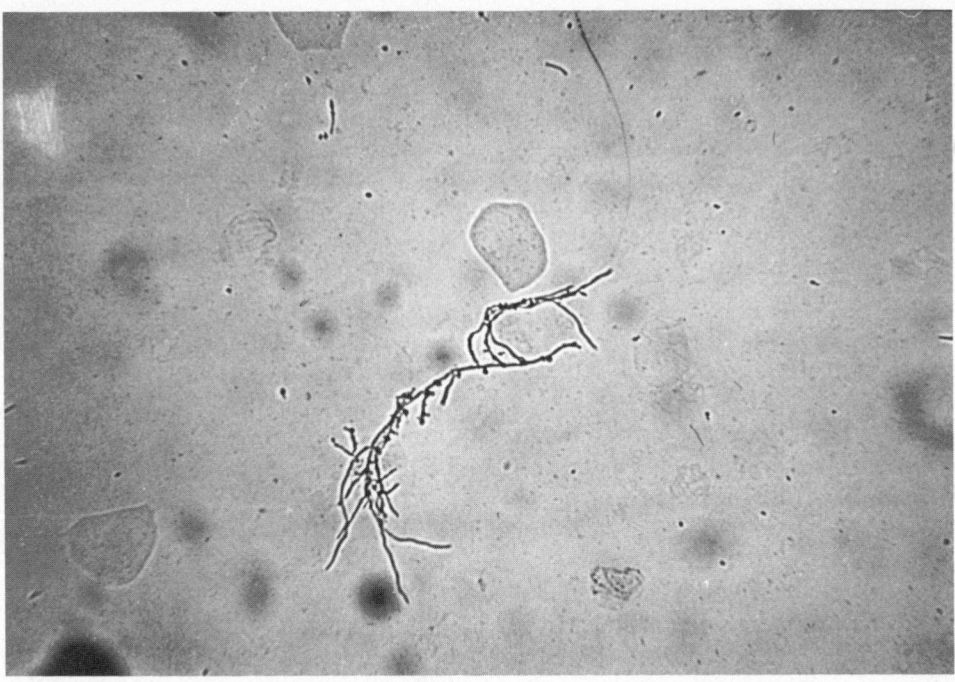

FIGURE 21-23
Microscopic appearance of vaginal smear in a case of vaginal candidiasis. Potassium hydroxide preparation; yeast cells and pseudomycelia. (×320). (From Merkus JMWM, Bisschop MPJM, and Stolte LAM: Obstet Gynecol Surv 40:495, 1985. © by Williams & Wilkins, 1985.)

cells and inflammatory cells. It is important always to use a coverslip, because potassium hydroxide will destroy the glass lens of the microscope. Active disease is associated with filamentous forms, mycelia and/or pseudohyphae, rather than spores. However, it may be necessary to search the slide and scan many different microscopic fields to identify hyphae or pseudohyphae. The average concentration of organisms is 10^3 to 10^4 per milliliter, but as stated previously, there is no direct relationship between the concentration of organism and the severity of the signs and symptoms. The microscopic diagnosis of fungal infection has a sensitivity of approximately 65%. A negative smear does not exclude *Candida* vulvovaginitis. The diagnosis can be established by culture with either Nickerson or Sabouraud medium. These cultures will become positive in 24 to 72 hours and are a simple office procedure, because they can be grown at room temperature. A new 2-minute test, which is a slide latex agglutination method, has recently been developed. The sensitivity of this test is approximately 70% to 75%.

The treatment of choice for *Candida* vaginitis is the topical application of one of the synthetic imidazoles—miconazole (Monistat), clotrimazole (Lotrimin, Mycelex), butoconazole (Femstat), or one of the triazoles, such as the topical terconazole (Terazol) or the oral medication fluconazole (Diflucan). These compounds are marketed in an array of carrier vehicles, primarily as suppositories or creams. They exert their action by changing the permeability of the surface membrane of the fungus. The most recent therapeutic advance has been found in several comparative studies that have documented equal effectiveness between the traditional 7-day therapy and the newer 3-day therapy. The newer 3-day or 1-day therapy is less expensive and provides improved patient compliance. Symptom cure rates are greater than 90%; however, approximately 20% of women will have positive cultures when followed for 4 to 6 weeks after therapy. Marketing studies demonstrate that most practitioners prefer the traditional 7 days of therapy and are reluctant to change their prescribing habits to a shorter course of therapy.

668   GENERAL GYNECOLOGY

Before the introduction of synthetic imida-zoles, polyenes, primarily nystatin (Mycosta-tin), were the standard therapy. Nystatin was prescribed for 10 to 14 days and resulted in clinical cure rates of approximately 80%. Povi-done-iodine douche has been used for years, but when used alone it is only 60% effective.

One of the most perplexing problems in clin-ical gynecology is recurrent vaginal infection caused by *C. albicans*. Often it is difficult to distinguish a relapse from a reinfection. It is important first to confirm that the woman's symptoms are not the result of drug sensitivity. Some investigators hypothesize that an allergic response of the vagina may be a predisposing factor to recurrent infections. There have been small series which report beneficial effects from hyposensitization by following immunotherapy with subcutaneous injections of *C. albicans* al-lergen. A screening test for diabetes should be performed. The vaginal discharge should be cultured and the identity of the fungus species determined. Horowitz et al. have demon-strated a twofold rate of recurrence with *C. tropicalis*, because this organism is not as sus-ceptible to the imidazoles as *C. albicans*. Simi-larly, *C. glabrata* infections are often resistant to imidazoles. The latter fungus produces a clinical syndrome of vulvar burning with little to no vaginal discharge. Both *C. tropicalis* and *C. glabrata* should be treated with topical gen-tian violet.

Sobel and Eschenbach have each reported clinical trials for recurrent or persistent vul-vovaginal candidiasis using ketoconazole (400 mg daily), an oral preparation. Both studies re-ported greater than 50% recurrence rates after the drug was discontinued. Liver toxicity is a worrisome side effect of ketoconazole; thus it is unlikely that it will be prescribed for long peri-ods for vaginal infection. Treatment of the male partner and elimination of *Candida* species from the gastrointestinal tract have not been beneficial in alleviating the problem.

Potential therapy for recurrent disease in-cludes gentian violet, boric acid, povidone-io-dine douching, and dietary changes. Painting the vagina with 1% gentian violet is messy, and patients must be warned to wear a minipad so that their clothes will not be stained. The va-gina should not be treated with gentian violet at intervals of less than 3 to 4 days, for the pa-tient may develop a chemical "burn." Van Slyke et al. recommended that 600 mg boric acid in gelatin capsules be placed high in the vagina twice a day. Boric acid is toxic when taken orally. However, studies have demon-strated minimal absorption following placement in the vagina. Douching with povidone-iodine is sometimes helpful as adjunctive therapy to other methods. There are anecdotal reports of successful therapy with instructions to restrict sugar in the diet. Optimal treatment of recur-rent vaginal infections related to *C. albicans* of-ten involves therapy similar to treating recur-rent urinary tract infections. The patient must be provided with enough medication so that she is able to self-treat at the first suggestion of recurrent symptoms or signs. Also, prophylac-tic treatment either immediately before or fol-lowing menses or at the first sign of recurrence is often beneficial.

TOXIC SHOCK SYNDROME

Toxic shock syndrome (TSS) is an acute, fe-brile illness leading to dysfunction of multiple organ systems, produced by a bacterial exo-toxin. The cardinal feature of the disease is the abrupt onset and the rapidity with which the clinical signs and symptoms may present and progress. A woman with TSS may develop rapid onset of hypotension associated with mul-tiorgan system failure. TSS was first described in 1978 by Todd as a sometimes fatal sequela of *Staphylococcus aureus* infection in children. In the early 1980s more than 95% of the reported cases of TSS were diagnosed in previously healthy, young (< 30 years), menstruating fe-males. *S. aureus* has been isolated from the va-gina in more than 90% of these cases.

Recently, approximately 50% of cases of TSS are related to menses. In cases of menses-re-lated TSS there is a history of the presence of a foreign body in the vagina, such as a tampon, diaphragm, or contraceptive sponge. Nonmen-strual TSS may be a sequela of focal staphylo-coccal infection of the skin and subcutaneous tissue, usually following a surgical procedure. TSS related to a surgical wound occurs early in the postoperative course, usually within the first 48 hours.

In summary, there are three requirements for the development of TSS: (1) the woman must be colonized or infected with *S. aureus*, (2) the bacteria must produce TSS toxin 1 (TSST-1) and/or related toxins, and (3) the tox-ins must have a route of entry into the systemic circulation.

The mortality of reported cases is high—2%

to 8%. If women continue to use tampons when the vagina is colonized with *S. aureus,* the recurrence rate may be 33%. It has been reported that one woman experienced five episodes of the disease. There appears to be no pattern to these recurrent episodes. Interestingly, women with menstrual-related TSS do not respond immunologically to TSST-1 as do women with nonmenstrual-related TSS. It is very rare for a women with nonmenstrual TSS to have a recurrence.

The signs and symptoms of TSS are produced by a specific exotoxin named toxin 1. Toxin 1 is a simple protein with a molecular weight of 22,000. It is accepted as the underlying cause of the disease. Whether this toxin acts alone, in association with other toxins or endotoxins, or acts only as the initiator of in vivo release of other substances such as interleukin-1 or tumor necrosis factor is presently being investigated. The primary effects of this toxin are to produce increased vascular permeability and thus profuse leaking of fluid (capillary leak) from the intravascular compartment into the interstitial space and associated profound loss of vasomotor tone resulting in decreased peripheral resistance.

Studies of the bacteriology of the vagina of normal menstruating females have documented that 5% to 17% of women are colonized with *S. aureus.* Approximately 5% test positive when the culture is obtained at midcycle, and the percentage increases to 10% to 17% during the menses. Rarely are blood cultures positive for *S. aureus* in a woman with TSS. Thus the exotoxin is believed to be absorbed directly from the vagina. It is possible that microulcerations produced by use of tampons facilitate the toxin's entry into the systemic circulation. The risk of nonmenstrual TSS is definitely increased in women who use barrier contraceptives such as the diaphragm, cervical cap, or sponge containing nonoxynol 9. The matched odds ratio for these three types of barrier contraceptives was 14.9 (95% confidence intervals 4.3 to 52.2).

Because of the severity of the disease, gynecologists should have a high index of suspicion for TSS in a woman who has an unexplained fever and a rash during or immediately following her menstrual period. The syndrome has a wide range of symptoms. The varying degree of severity of both symptoms and signs depends on the magnitude of involvement of individual organs. Most women experience a prodromal flulike illness for the first 24 hours. Between days 2 and 4 of the menstrual period, the patient experiences an abrupt onset of a high temperature associated with headache, myalgia, sore throat, vomiting, diarrhea, a generalized skin rash, and often hypotension. It is important to consider that not all women with TSS experience the full-blown manifestations of the disease. The rigid criteria developed by the CDC are used for epidemiologic studies. Clinically, many women present with a "forme fruste" of TSS, with low-grade fever and dizziness rather than hypotension.

The most characteristic manifestations of TSS are the skin changes. During the first 48 hours the skin rash appears similar to an intense sunburn. During the next few days the erythema will become more macular and look like a drug-related rash. From days 12 to 15 of the illness, there is a fine, flaky, desquamation of skin over the face and trunk with sloughing of the entire skin thickness of the palms and soles. The vaginal mucosa is hyperemic during the initial phase of the syndrome. During pelvic examination, patients complain of tenderness of the external genitalia and vagina. Myalgia, vomiting, and diarrhea are experienced by more than 90% of women with TSS. Many abnormal laboratory findings are associated with the disease, and again they reflect the severity of involvement of individual organ systems (see the box on p. 670).

The management of a classic case of severe TSS demands an intensive care unit and the skills of an expert in critical care medicine. The first priority is to eliminate the hypotension produced by the exotoxin. Copious amounts of intravenous fluids are given while pressure and volume dynamics are monitored with a pulmonary artery catheter. Mechanical ventilation is required for women who develop adult respiratory distress syndrome.

When the patient is initially admitted to the hospital, it is important to obtain cervical, vaginal, and blood cultures for *S. aureus.* Although there is no controlled series documenting its efficacy, it is prudent to wash out the vagina with saline or dilute iodine solution to diminish the amount of exotoxin that may be absorbed into the systemic circulation.

Women with TSS should be treated with a beta-lactamase-resistant antistaphylococcal antibiotic for 10 to 14 days. Possible antibiotic choices include beta-lactamase-resistant penicillins (oxacillin or nafcillin), cephalosporins, and aminoglycosides. If the diagnosis is ques-

LABORATORY ABNORMALITIES IN EARLY TOXIC SHOCK SYNDROME*

Present in >85% of Patients

Coagulase-positive staphylococci in cervix or vagina

Immature and mature polymorphonuclear cells >90% of WBCs

Total lymphocyte count <650/mm^3

Total serum protein level <5.6 mg/dl

Serum albumin level <3.1 g/dl

Serum calcium level <7.8 mg/dl

Serum creatinine clearance >1.0 mg/dl

Serum bilirubin value >1.5 mg/dl

Serum cholesterol level ≤120 mg/dl

Prothrombin time >12 seconds

Present in >70% of Patients

Platelet count <150,000/mm^3

Pyuria >5 WBCs per high-power field

Proteinuria ≥2

  (BUN) >20 mg/dl

Aspartate aminotransferase (formerly SGOT) > 41 U/L

From Chesney PJ, Davis JP, Purdy WK, et al: Clinical manifestations of toxic shock syndrome, JAMA 246:746, 1981. Copyright 1981, American Medical Association.
*Results were available for at least 18 patients per category with the following exceptions: cervicovaginal cultures (12 patients), cholesterol level (15 patients), and prothrombin time (14 patients).

tionable, it is best to include the use of an aminoglycoside to obtain coverage for possible gram-negative sepsis. Antibiotic therapy probably has little effect on the course of an individual episode of TSS. However, Helgerson et al. have found that antibiotics definitely decrease the risk of recurrence of TSS. In their series only one recurrent case of TSS was documented among 53 different women. The reported risk of recurrence without antibiotic therapy is approximately 33%.

For severe cases of TSS, Todd et al. have recommended early administration of pharmacologic doses of parenteral corticosteroids. However, most centers no longer give corticosteroids. Dopamine or dobutamine infusions are titrated to obtain optimal perfusion pressures. Others have advocated naloxone (Narcan) for treatment of severe hypotension. In summary, the treatment of TSS depends on the severity of involvement of individual organ systems. Not all patients develop a temperature of greater than 38.9° C and hypotension. Thus clinicians and patients should be aware of the "forme fruste" manifestations of the syndrome. The foundation of treatment of the disease is prompt and aggressive management because of the rapidity with which the disease may progress.

It is possible to significantly decrease the incidence of TSS by a change in use of catamenial products. Women should be encouraged to change tampons every 4 to 6 hours. The intermittent use of external pads is also good preventive medicine. Women will usually accept the recommendation to wear external pads during sleep. The incidence of TSS has decreased dramatically with the removal of superabsorbing tampons from the market.

ACQUIRED IMMUNE DEFICIENCY SYNDROME

Acquired immune deficiency syndrome (AIDS) is the advanced disease state manifestation of a viral infection by the human immunodeficiency virus (HIV). This virus has a predilection for cells of the immune system, specifically "helper" lymphocytes (lymphocytes with CD_4 marker) and monocytes. Infection of these cells leads to a breakdown of the body's immune system, particularly cell-mediated immunity. Clinically, the AIDS patient is affected by a series of opportunistic infections and neoplasms that are eventually lethal. The virus may also infect cells of other organ systems, such as the central nervous system, producing AIDS-dementia complex; and cells of the gastrointestinal tract, producing malabsorption, weight loss, and diarrhea. HIV infection has been called the most important epidemic of the twentieth century. The disease was first recognized in 1981 in a small cluster of patients with an unexplained defect of cellular immunity and *Pneumocystis carinii* pneumonia. The etiologic agent, human immunodeficiency virus, was identified in 1983. By the end of 1991, 10 years after the disease's first description, the CDC has estimated that approximately 1.5 million people in the United States will have been infected by HIV and 270,000 cases of AIDS will have been reported.

AIDS is ubiquitous and has been reported from every state in the United States and from every continent. Although it is most likely underreported in African countries, it has been estimated that there will be 1 million cases of AIDS reported worldwide by the year 2000. The World Health Organization (WHO) has estimated that by the year 2000 there will be between 18 and 20 million people infected with HIV.

In the United States approximately 11% of AIDS victims are women. However, in other countries up to one half of all victims of AIDS are female. AIDS is one of the five leading causes of death in reproductive-age women. Black and Hispanic women have comprised a disproportionate percentage (72%) of the women suffering from AIDS in the late 1980s. The CDC has estimated that 72% of the women who have died from AIDS in the late 1980s have been black or Hispanic. Studies have found that the prevalence of HIV in the American population ranges from as little as 0.02% in blood donors and university students to as much as 6.3% of individuals in urban sexually transmitted disease clinics, and 6.7% of women admitted for acute pelvic inflammatory disease at San Francisco General Hospital.

In the United States high-risk populations for AIDS include homosexual men, intravenous drug users and their sexual partners, and hemophiliacs. Transmission of the virus occurs by both horizontal and vertical routes. There are three primary methods of contracting the virus: intimate sexual contact, use of contaminated needles or blood products, and perinatal transmission from mother to child. When there is transmission of the virus through contamination of bodily fluids, it is more commonly virus within the cellular portion of the inoculum, rather than free virus that leads to infection. The further advanced a person's disease state, the more viral particles present and the more infectious the inoculum becomes.

HIV is a newly described lentivirus. Lentiviruses are a family of retroviruses, which are RNA viruses that contain reverse transcriptase. The reverse transcriptase enzyme translates viral RNA into DNA, which is then incorporated into the DNA of the host cell. Pseudonyms for HIV include human T cell leukemia virus (HTLV-3), lymphadenopathy virus (LAV), and AIDS-related virus (ARV). HIV primarily infects and affects T_4, or helper, lymphocytes with a CD_4 marker on the cell surface. This protein marker is the primary receptor for the virus. However, the virus can also attach and infect other cells that may lack the CD_4 marker, including monocytes, fibroblasts, neurons, and renal, hepatic, intestinal, and other cells. Once the virus is incorporated into the cell, the RNA of the viral core is translated into DNA and incorporated into the host's genome. The virus then may lie dormant in a latency period or may induce the production of new viral proteins and new virus. For most human cells the production of new virus is a cytotoxic process.

There are two subtypes of HIV: HIV-1 and HIV-2. HIV-2 is found primarily in humans in west Africa. Both HIV viruses have a similar lipid outer coat and similar RNA that codes for three genes. The viruses differ slightly in the products of these genes. In addition, there are multiple strains of HIV-1 virus. The strains differ in the various regulatory proteins that they code. Since vaccines are usually directed against specific proteins, the multiple strains of HIV make the development and production of a vaccine very difficult. HIV mutates and develops into new strains within an individual after he or she is infected. As HIV mutates, it may become more infectious or more pathologic to specific tissues, such as the CNS. The mutation to more pathogenic strains of HIV is one mechanism by which a patient may advance from being an asymptomatic carrier of the virus to an individual with the advanced disease state of AIDS.

Among the proteins made by HIV virus is a core protein, P_{24}, which is measured clinically as a serum marker. Another set of proteins made by the virus have been called the "nef" proteins. These are responsible for down-regulation of the virus and inhibition of viral replication. Escape from nef control by mutating strains of HIV is another factor responsible for the progression of the disease.

The CDC has classified HIV infection according to a patient's symptomatology. Four groups of patients have been described. *Group I* patients are individuals who are in the initial viremic period. The initial viremia may last for up to 6 weeks, during which time high levels of free virus may be found in the blood as well as the CNS. Antibodies to HIV are at a low level. The infected individual may be asymptomatic or may suffer an acute, mononucleosis-like illness. After 4 to 6 weeks, HIV antibody levels begin to rise and viral antigen levels decline. *Group II* patients are individuals in the dormant or latent period, which follows the initial viremic phase. The period of latency may last for 10 years or more with rare, intermittent viremic spikes. Ninety-nine percent of HIV-infected individuals fall into group II. During this asymptomatic period, 2% to 10% of individuals per year will undergo progression of disease. *Group III* disease is a generalized lymphadenopathy. *Group IV* disease is clinical AIDS. Clinical AIDS may be manifest by opportunistic infection, malignancy, weight loss and diarrhea, or central nervous system symptoms. The progression from group II to group III and group IV disease is characterized by a gradual rise in viral proteins and free virus in blood and secretions, as well as a decline in the CD_4 lymphocyte count. A normal count is greater than 800 cells per microliter. A CD_4 count of less than 200 per microliter is usually associated with opportunistic infections.

There are two very rare patterns of HIV infection. One is an initial high level of antibody with a low-level viremia. There is subsequent loss of detectable viral antigen in the blood and later loss of circulating antibody. In these rare cases there are still low levels of viral DNA within lymphocytes. The small levels are only detected by the extremely sensitive and specific polymerase chain reaction (PCR) technique. This technique utilizes enzymes to detect small amounts of DNA. The second rare pattern of HIV infection is a low-level viral antigenemia with a prolonged (1 to 4 years) period of minimal HIV antibody production. The subject is thus infectious but may test negative for HIV antibody.

The duration of the latency period, or the length of time individuals are in group II, is affected not only by the nef regulatory gene and the degree of the viral mutation, but also by host immunity. Host immunity is primarily via production of antibody against the HIV virus and via CD_8 cell, or killer lymphocyte, activity against infected CD_4 cells. When the host mechanisms are overwhelmed and the virus has mutated to pathogenic strains, the last stage of the disease, clinical AIDS, begins.

The symptoms of clinical AIDS are caused by a decline in the number and quality of the CD_4 lymphocytes. The CD_4 lymphocyte modulates almost all immune functions in the human immune system. The wide spectrum of immunologic dysfunction has been categorized by Seligmann et al. (see the box, above right). Monocytes are also infected by HIV. These

---

IMMUNOLOGIC ABNORMALITIES IN AIDS

A. Abnormalities that characterize the syndrome
   1. Lymphopenia
   2. Selective T cell deficiency based on a quantitative reduction, with the antigenic subset designated by T_4 or Leu_3 monoclonal antibodies
   3. Decreased or absent delayed cutaneous hypersensitivity to both recall and new antigens
   4. Elevated serum immunoglobulins, predominantly IgG and IgA in adults and including IgM in children
   5. Increased spontaneous immunoglobulin secretion by individual B lymphocytes
B. Consistently observed abnormalities
   1. Decreased in vitro lymphocyte proliferative responses
      a. Mitogens
      b. Antigens
      c. Alloantigens, autoantigens
   2. Decreased cytotoxic responses
      a. Natural killer cells
      b. Cell-mediated cytotoxicity (T cell)
   3. Decreased ability to mount a de novo antibody response to a new antigen
   4. Altered monocyte function
   5. Elevated serum levels of immune complexes
C. Other reported abnormalities
   1. Increased levels of acid-labile alpha-interferon
   2. Antilymphocyte antibodies
   3. Suppressor factors
   4. Increased levels of beta$_2$-microglobulin and alpha$_1$-thymosin; decreased serum thymulin levels

From Seligmann M, Chess L, Fahey HL, et al: AIDS—an immunologic reevaluation, N Engl J Med 311:1287, 1984. Reprinted by permission of The New England Journal of Medicine.

---

cells circulate throughout the body and then migrate after 1 to 4 days into peripheral tissues, including the CNS, carrying the virus with them.

As patients enter into an active disease state and the CD_4 count drops, general systemic symptoms often develop. The patient may experience leukoplakia, thrush, weight loss, diarrhea, fever, fatigue, and thrombocytopenia. Patients with CD_4 counts between 500 and 800 cells per microliter are more susceptible to community-acquired pneumonia, gastroenteritis, and general viral infections. As the CD_4 count drops below 500, patients may develop malignancies, most commonly Kaposi's sarcoma and lymphoma. Before the AIDS epidemic, Kaposi's sarcoma was an extremely rare neoplasm of connective tissue and blood cells. It is usually a slow-growing cancer involving purple or reddish nodules or plaques on the skin and epithelium of the gastrointestinal tract. Kaposi's sarcoma associated with AIDS may involve lymph nodes and occasionally has a rapid downhill course. However, most individuals with Kaposi's sarcoma usually die of opportunistic infections. Interestingly, Kaposi's sarcoma is found much more commonly in men than in women. Twenty-three percent of male homosexual patients with AIDS develop Kaposi's sarcoma, compared to 3% of male heterosexual AIDS victims and 1% of women with the disease. As the CD_4 count drops below 200 cells per microliter, opportunistic infections are found with increasing frequency. *P. carinii* pneumonia has been a common infection in AIDS patients. Pentamidine has been found to be an effective prophylactic agent in decreasing the incidence of this pneumonia. The clinical course in patients who develop *P. carinii* pneumonia varies from intermittent, slowly progressive disease to a fulminating infection with respiratory collapse and death in a few days.

Other common opportunistic infections in AIDS patients are listed in the box, above right, including disseminated viral, fungal, parasitic infections as well as disseminated bacterial infections. Symptomatic infections with the following organisms are less common—*Listeria monocytogenes, Nocardia asteroides;* viruses—Epstein-Barr virus, adenovirus.

Patients with AIDS often develop symptoms involving the CNS. One third of patients with HIV infection will initially present with CNS symptoms, and 80% to 90% of all AIDS patients eventually develop some aspect of the AIDS dementia complex (ADC) during their disease course. This syndrome is characterized by acute and subacute meningoencephalitis, peripheral neuropathy, cortical atrophy, dementia, memory loss, and a variety of psychiatric dysfunctions. Patients who present with CNS symptoms must be evaluated for infection, since many of the opportunistic infections of AIDS involve the CNS.

COMMON OPPORTUNISTIC INFECTIONS IN AIDS PATIENTS

Bacteria

Mycobacterium tuberculosis
Mycobacterium avium-intracellulare
Mycobacterium fortuitum
Salmonella sp.
Legionella pneumophila

Fungi

Cryptococcus carinii
Candida sp.
Aspergillus sp.
Histoplasma capsulatum
Coccidioides immitis

Parasites

Pneumocystis carinii
Toxoplasma gondii
Cryptosporidium sp.
Isospora belli
Strongyloides stercoralis

Viruses

Cytomegalovirus
Herpes simplex virus
Varicella-zoster virus
JC virus (progressive multifocal leukoencephalopathy)

From Curran JW, Gold J, and Jaffe HW: The acquired immunodeficiency syndrome (AIDS). In Holmes KK, Mårdh PA, Sparling PF, et al, editors: Sexually transmitted diseases, ed 2, New York, 1990, McGraw-Hill Book Co.

The screening test for AIDS is an enzyme-linked immunosorbent assay (ELISA) that tests for antibodies against the HIV virus. There are biologic false positive and false negative results related to nonspecific test factors and infections by viruses with similar antigens. The sensitivity of the ELISA test is approximately 95%, and the specificity is 99.7%. Thus, in a population group with a low disease prevalence for AIDS, of 100 positive ELISA tests, 99% may be false positive with 1 true positive result. False positive results are more common in multiparous women and women taking oral contraceptives. A more specific assay, the Western blot technique, is used to investigate individuals with persistently positive ELISA tests. The Western blot technique identifies antibodies to proteins of a specific molecular weight; it is, therefore, more specific than the ELISA test. The most specific test is the polymerase chain reaction (PCR) which tests specifically for HIV viral DNA.

Treatment of AIDS has evolved around two themes, prevention and chemotherapy. From the clinician's perspective the major aspect of prevention involves education and contraceptive counseling. Education should be of how the disease is sexually transmitted. "Safe sex," a term used frequently in the lay press, is a misnomer. "Safer sex" to avoid HIV infection includes the use of condoms and spermicides. Condom use will prevent HIV infection in the great majority of cases. It is not 100% effective, however. Latex condoms rather than "natural membrane" condoms should be used. Condoms made from animal intestines will not prevent viral transmission. The additional use of nonoxynol 9 will afford more protection against the HIV virus, as well as being more effective than condoms alone as a contraceptive agent. Nonoxynol 9 can be found in spermicides, foam, vaginal sponges, and spermicidal gels. This agent destroys HIV. Education should also include information about risk factors that increase the likelihood of acquiring the infection, including sex when the individual has ulcers or abrasions or sexual promiscuity.

The acceptance of the use of condoms by the general population is yet to be determined. Preliminary studies of the effectiveness of the massive education campaigns about "safe sex" have shown disappointing results. In one study of 759 women attending a contraception clinic, 77% thought that condoms would be a "good idea" to prevent sexually transmitted diseases. However, only 21% of couples used them and only 14% of couples used both condoms and foam to prevent HIV infection. Vaginal condoms, condoms that fit within the woman's vagina, have also been developed. The acceptance of these condoms has yet to be determined.

The treatment of AIDS currently focuses on chemotherapeutic agents that attack the virus' life cycle. The most effective agents currently are the nucleoside analogues, which inhibit the reverse transcriptase enzyme necessary for the virus to affect the host's DNA. Zidovudine (ZDV), 3'-asido-3'-deoxythymidine, is the most widely used drug of this group. Zidovudine is currently given when an individual's CD_4 count drops below 500 cells per microliter. Given prophylactically at this time, it prolongs the disease-free interval, helps maintain the CD_4 count, and inhibits viral antigen levels within the blood. Zidovudine has also been found to decrease the incidence and severity of AIDS dementia complex, as well as decrease the severity of opportunistic infections. When zidovudine is given to patients with AIDS, life span is prolonged and the severity of the illness is decreased. The most important side effect of this drug is a dose-related bone marrow suppression in 1% to 10% of patients. Zidovudine is expensive, and once started, patients need to take it for the rest of their lives. Resistance to zidovudine therapy also exists.

Other areas of chemotherapeutic research against the HIV include the development of agents that may inhibit viral attachment, disrupt translation of viral proteins, and affect regulation of the "nef" genes. Vaccine development for HIV is a difficult goal. The lack of an animal model for HIV as well as the multiple strains of HIV-1 virus have been two important impediments to the development of the vaccine.

For the gynecologist there are special concerns for the patient who has HIV infection. Because of the susceptibility to generalized systemic infections, patients with HIV frequently present with vaginal symptoms. Genital herpes is a common problem for patients with HIV infection. Acyclovir can be used safely with this disease and does not interfere with zidovudine. Acyclovir dosages may need to be increased when treating acute herpetic infection in HIV patients, from 200 mg to 400 mg 5 times a day. Dosages greater than 200 mg 3 times a day are often necessary for suppressive therapy. Vaginal candidal infections are a frequent problem in patients with HIV infection. Chronic antifungal suppression is often necessary. The development of mucocutaneous candidiasis is a marker for advancing disease.

There is currently an increase in the incidence of syphilis in the United States, and the ulcer of primary syphilis increases the susceptibility to HIV infection. In addition, the effect of HIV on syphilis, because of the generalized immunosuppression, may be a more rapid progression of disease and a relative refractory response to standard antibiotic treatment. In 1988 the CDC made recommendations for treating syphilis in the presence of HIV. For early syphilis the treatment is the same as for individuals without HIV. However, serum markers should be retested at monthly intervals until a twofold dilution is seen. If there is not a twofold dilution, or if there is an increase in antisyphilis titer, then the patient should be considered refractory to treatment and the patient's CSF should be examined. Any patient with syphilis of unknown duration or latent syphilis should have a CSF examination. The CDC has recommended that neurosyphilis be considered in the differential diagnosis of neurologic disease in HIV-positive patients.

Several studies have noted an increase in human papillomavirus (HPV) infection among HIV-positive patients. Widespread HPV infections throughout the lower genital tract have been noted by several authors. An increased incidence of abnormal Pap smears with HPV-related atypia has also been noted among HIV-infected women. More recently, several investigators have remarked on an increase in cervical intraepithelial neoplasia (CIN) among HIV patients. Patients with HIV infection and concomitant HPV infection should be screened carefully for CIN.

Clinicians are legitimately concerned when treating patients with HIV infection about becoming infected themselves. Medical ethics dictate that patients be treated without prejudice for their disease. The American College of Obstetricians and Gynecologists has restated that it is unethical to refuse to "accept or continue to care" for persons solely on the basis of their HIV status. However, it is also in a physician's interest to take adequate precautions from becoming infected. Since over 90% of HIV-infected individuals are asymptomatic, and many patients do not know that they are HIV positive, we advise precautions be taken at all times. The CDC has recommended "universal blood and body fluid precautions" to minimize the risk of HIV infections. These are summarized in the box, above right. Infection may occur after exposure to contaminated substances, body fluids, or secretions through any break in the skin. Abrasions or cuts on the hands, arms, or face as well as ulcers on the mucous membrane are susceptible sites for infection. Thus, gowns and face and eye protection are advisable in all cases.

During operative procedures, studies have suggested that approximately 10% of gloves will be punctured. Double gloving decreases that rate by 60% to 80%. Thus, double gloving will allow an individual only a 2% to 4% risk of hand contamination during any surgical case. The greatest risk of glove perforation occurs in surgeries longer than 3 hours with greater than

UNIVERSAL BLOOD AND BODY FLUID PRECAUTIONS

1. All blood and body fluids from all patients should be considered potentially infectious for HIV.
2. Barrier precautions such as masks and gowns should be used whenever contact with body fluids is anticipated.
3. Gloves should be worn when touching mucous membranes or nonintact skin, handling blood or body fluids, or touching surfaces contaminated with fluids.
4. Gloves and/or gowns should be changed after each contact.
5. Eyes, mouth, and nose should be protected by face shields, masks, and/or goggles during any procedure that may involve splashing of body fluids.
6. All blood and body fluids should be washed from hands and other skin surfaces immediately and completely even after gloves have been worn.
7. Never recap, bend, or break needles by hand or attempt to remove needles from disposable syringes.
8. Puncture-resistant disposable containers should be available and nearby at all times and, if possible, at every work site.
9. Resuscitation bags or mouthpieces should be available for emergency resuscitation in all appropriate places.

300 ml blood loss. If a needle puncture occurs through the skin, HIV infection may also occur. It is estimated that seroconversion will occur in 0.03% to 0.9% of needle punctures. Thus, HIV infection is extremely rare from a needle puncture. It is estimated that by the end of 1991, there were less than 50 health care workers who have developed HIV infection from exposures related to medical care. This is to be contrasted with a study from San Francisco General Hospital that indicated that cutaneous and parenteral exposures during surgeries occurred in 6.4% of cases despite precautions. The low number of reported HIV conversions compared to the high number of exposures is indicative of the difficulty of becoming infected from slight exposure.

Clinicians are often asked about the risk of developing AIDS from transfusion. In 1985 routine screening of all blood products for HIV was instituted in the United States. The current risk of developing HIV infection from blood transfusion is estimated to be 1:150,000 units transfused.

CERVICITIS

With the current epidemic of sexually transmitted diseases, cervical infections have drawn increasing interest from both clinicians and epidemiologists. The cervix may be a reservoir for *Neisseria gonorrhoeae, Chlamydia trachomatis,* and *Mycoplasma* species. Often the patient is asymptomatic, even though the cervix is colonized with either gonorrheal or chlamydial organisms. The cervix acts as a barrier between the bacterial flora of the vagina and the bacteriologically sterile endometrial cavity and oviducts. Viral infections of the cervix such as herpes simplex and human papillomavirus are frequently associated with the development of cervical intraepithelial neoplasia. Whether this relationship is induction or promotion of neoplasia remains a matter of debate.

The semantics of cervical infections have recently been dramatically revised. Colposcopy has demonstrated that the redness that was believed to be inflammation is often the capillary bed below an area of ectopic columnar epithelia (ectopy). Cervicitis used to be diagnosed erroneously when the clinician was viewing an area of metaplasia or erosion. Therefore descriptive clinical terms such as acute cervicitis, chronic cervicitis, and follicular and hypertrophic cervicitis have been abandoned. In a similar fashion the histologic diagnosis of chronic cervicitis is so prevalent that it should be considered the norm for parous women of reproductive age. Current terminology emphasizes the site of cervical infection. Endocervicitis is usually secondary to bacterial infection with either *C. trachomatis* or *N. gonorrhoeae* or with viral agents such as herpes simplex or human papillomavirus. The most common site of *Chlamydia* infection in the female reproductive tract is the columnar cells of the endocervix. Ectocervical infections are generally either a virus or *Trichomonas vaginalis.* The histopathology of endocervicitis is characterized by a severe inflammatory reaction in the mucosa and submucosa. The tissues are infiltrated with a large number of polymorphonuclear cells and monocytes, and occasionally there is associated epithelial necrosis. Recently, Mecsei et al. have reported that mild cellular atypia on Papanicolaou smears may be related to chlamy-

dial infection. Approximately 20% of their patients with positive *C. trachomatis* cultures had associated mild cellular atypia. The Pap smears reverted to normal in 18 of the 23 patients following tetracycline therapy.

The pathophysiologic relationship between cervical mucus and both lower and upper genital tract infections is beginning to be elucidated. Mucus is much more than a simple physical barrier; it exerts a definite bacteriostatic effect. Mucus may also act as a competitive inhibitor with bacteria for receptors on the endocervical epithelial cells. Cervical mucus also contains antibodies and inflammatory cells that are active against various sexually transmitted organisms. The present debate concerning the effect of oral contraceptives on the prevalence of serious upper tract pelvic infection may yield insight into the pathophysiology of cervical infection. Women taking oral contraceptives have a twofold to threefold increase in incidence of positive endocervical cultures for *C. trachomatis.* There are several hypotheses to explain this association. It may relate to differences in sexual activity. Alternatively, the cervical ectopy produced by oral contraceptives may preferentially facilitate adherence of *Chlamydia* organisms (Figure 21-24). Cultures of *Chlamydia* may be more productive from smears of columnar cells. The higher prevalence may simply reflect a higher isolation rate.

The cervix may become infected by a wide variety of viral, protozoal, and fungal organisms. All of the sexually transmitted diseases may produce ulcerative lesions of the cervix. However, the principal infections of the cervix are caused by *N. gonorrhoeae, C. trachomatis,* genital herpes, and human papillomavirus. This section will focus on mucopurulent cervicitis and techniques to diagnose common cervical infections. The clinical diagnosis of mucopurulent cervicitis may be easily established. It is hoped that by diagnosing and treating mucopurulent cervicitis the prevalence of upper genital tract pelvic infection will be curtailed. The cervix remains the major reservoir for chronic colonization with *Chlamydia.*

Mucopurulent Cervicitis

Brunham et al. have recently described objective criteria to diagnose endocervical infections. They have suggested the term *mucopurulent cervicitis* for the clinical diagnosis of ac-

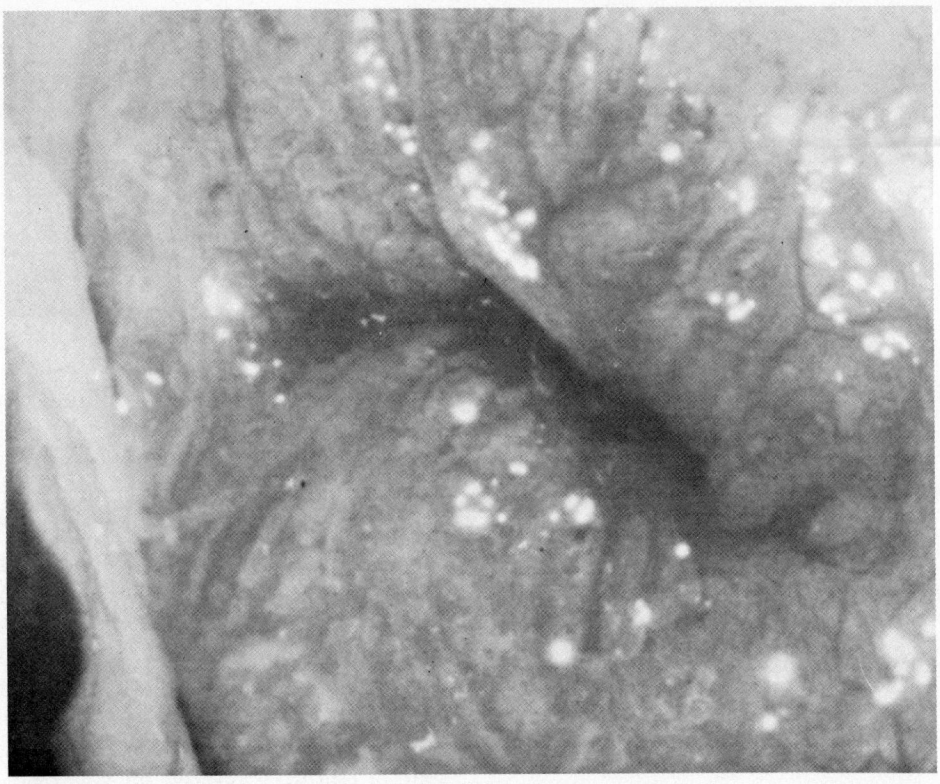

FIGURE 21-24
Colpophotograph of cervix infected with *Chlamydia trachomatis*, showing proliferation and dilation of subepithelial capillaries in zone of ectopy. (From Holmes KK: Lower genital tract infections in women: cystitis/urethritis, vulvovaginitis, and cervicitis. In Holmes KK, Måardh PA, Sparling PF, et al, editors: Sexually transmitted diseases, New York, 1984, McGraw-Hill Book Co.

tive cervical infection. Mucopurulent cervicitis is directly analogous to, and the female counterpart of, urethritis in men. Two simple, definitive, objective criteria have been developed to establish this diagnosis—gross visualization of yellow mucopurulent material on a white cotton swab and the presence of 10 or more polymorphonuclear leukocytes per microscopic field (magnification ×1000) on Gram-stained smears obtained from the endocervix. The third criterion used was erythema and edema in an area of cervical ectopy, bleeding secondary to endocervical ulceration, or friability when the smear was obtained. In their original study, the Seattle group discovered that 40% of patients with sexually transmitted diseases had mucopurulent cervicitis (24% diagnosed by grossly visualized purulent material and 16% without mucopus but positive Gram stains of cervical mucus). However, the sensitivity, specificity, and positive predictive value of objective criteria have varied markedly in follow-up studies.

The prevalence of mucopurulent cervicitis depends on the population being studied. Approximately 30% to 40% of women attending clinics for sexually transmitted diseases and 8% to 10% of women in university student health clinics have the condition. Greater than 60% of women with this disease are asymptomatic. Symptoms that suggest cervical infection include vaginal discharge, deep dyspareunia, and postcoital bleeding.

C. trachomatis is the cause of cervical infection in most women with mucopurulent cervicitis (Figure 21-25). In the initial study in Seattle, *Chlamydia* organisms were isolated from specimens of 20 of 40 women with mucopurulent cervicitis but only 2 of 60 without mucopurulent cervicitis. Subsequent studies have documented that up to two thirds of women with mucopurulent cervicitis have a positive endocervical chlamydial culture. Mucopurulent cervicitis is present in approximately 12% of women in whom no cervical pathogen can be

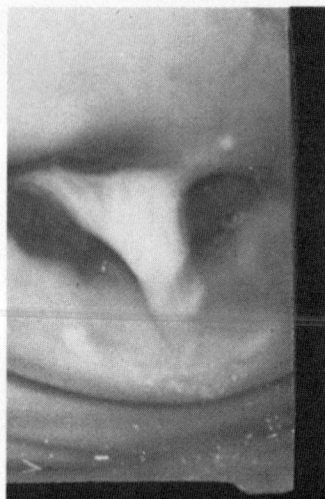

FIGURE 21-25
Mucopurulent cervicitis caused by *C. trachomatis*. (From Holmes KK, Mårdh PA, Sparling PF, et al, editors: Sexually transmitted diseases, ed 2, New York, 1990, McGraw-Hill Book Co.)

identified. The presence of active herpes infection was correlated with ulceration of the exocervix but not mucopus. *N. gonorrhoeae* was frequently isolated in this study, but its presence was not statistically significantly associated with either mucopus or 10 or more inflammatory cells per high-powered field. The mean number of inflammatory cells with positive gonorrheal cultures was 1.9 per high-powered field.

Special care must be taken in obtaining the cervical smears to establish a diagnosis of mucopurulent cervicitis. Initially a large cotton swab is used to absorb the vaginal secretions from the upper vagina and wipe away the mucus from the exocervix. Next a small white cotton swab is inserted into the endocervical canal. It is inspected grossly for the presence of yellow purulent material, gross pus from the endocervix being similar to the purulent urethral discharge in a male. Subsequently, the swab is rolled on a glass slide, and the slide is dried and Gram stained. The slide is scanned to identify strands of cervical mucus containing areas of inflammatory cells. If 10 or more polymorphonuclear leukocytes are seen at a magnification of 1000, a positive diagnosis has been made. A culture for gonorrheal organisms should also be obtained, as the two organisms

will be found simultaneously in approximately one third of cervical infections. Menstruation or the presence of vaginal squamous cells destroys the validity of the slide. Pandya and Cohen have discovered that endocervical leukocytes are a normal physiologic response to the deposition of sperm in the cervical canal. Therefore, if sperm are present, leukocyte presence indicates only a physiologic response of the cervix and not a pathologic reaction.

The treatment of choice for mucopurulent cervicitis if *N. gonorrhoeae* is not found on Gram stain or endocervical culture is oral tetracycline 500 mg every 6 hours for at least 7 days. Doxycycline, 100 mg twice a day for 1 week, is an alternate oral therapy with better patient compliance. If a patient is allergic to tetracycline, erythromycin base, 500 mg every 6 hours for 7 days, or erythomycin ethylsuccinate, 800 mg every 6 hours for 7 days, is acceptable. Another alternative is trimethoprim 160 mg plus sulfamethoxazole 800 mg twice a day for 10 days. The male partner should receive identical therapy. Obviously, if the Gram stain or culture is positive for gonorrhea, tetracycline treatment alone is not sufficient because of the possibility of tetracycline-resistant *N. gonorrhoeae*. Thus, the patient should be treated with either ceftriaxone, 250 mg intramuscularly, or spectinomycin, 2 g intramuscularly, in a single dose.

The genital mycoplasmas, *Mycoplasma hominis* and *Ureaplasma urealyticum*, are frequently isolated from both the vagina and endocervix. Colonization rates as high as 75% have been reported. The exact role of genital mycoplasmas in producing either bacterial vaginosis or active cervical infection is unclear. Paavonen et al. reported that genital mycoplasmas do not produce mucopurulent cervicitis.

Detection of Pathogenic Cervical Bacteria

Neisseria Gonorrhoeae

The diagnosis of cervical infection from *N. gonorrhoeae* is made by culture of the endocervical mucus. The majority of women who are colonized with gonorrhea are asymptomatic. Therefore, it is important to routinely screen women at high risk for gonorrheal infection by culture. Gram staining of the endocervical mucus is diagnostic for only 50% of women with positive cultures for *N. gonorrhoeae* because other bacteria may appear similar on Gram stain. Thus culture of endocervical mucus directly on modified Thayer-Martin or similar medium is the diagnostic standard. A cotton swab should be rotated deep in the endocervical canal for 15 to 20 seconds. A single endocervical culture will detect approximately 85% of cervical infections. A culture from a second consecutive endocervical cotton swab will increase detection approximately 7% to 10%. If a separate rectal swab specimen is cultured, the accuracy of diagnosing gonorrhea increases to 93%. Additional cultures of the pharynx, urethra, and ducts of accessory sex glands may be obtained depending on the patient's symptoms and sexual habits. Although transport media are available, it is important for the culture to reach the laboratory within 24 hours or there will be a loss of sensitivity. Growth of *N. gonorrhoeae* in culture is best at 37° C and in an environment between 2% and 10% carbon dioxide. Cultures should be obtained as a test of effective therapy approximately 5 to 7 days after completion of antibiotic therapy.

It is important to test positive cultures for sensitivity to penicillin. Penicillinase-producing strains of *N. gonorrhoeae* cause approximately 4% to 6% of gonorrheal infections in the United States. However, these strains are common in Africa and Asia, and the prevalence is much higher in selected inner-city urban areas in the United States. Solid-phase enzyme immunoassay procedures such as the Gonozyme test for antigens do not depend on the viability of the organisms. Metaanalysis has demonstrated that the sensitivity of the Gonozyme test ranges from 73% to 100% with a specificity of 94% to 99%. The sensitivity rate is lower in females than in males. Disadvantages of this test are that multiple steps are involved, which take over 1 hour, and that results must be interpreted by a spectrophotometer. The one major advantage of antigen detection is that the test is valuable for clinics that are a considerable distance from the bacteriologic laboratory in which a culture cannot be done within 24 hours. The enzyme immunoassay test is not affected by transport or storage in the refrigerator for up to 14 days.

The treatment for gonococcal urethritis and cervicitis recommended by the CDC was changed in September 1989. These changes were based on the increasing trends of the development of antibiotic-resistant *N. gonorrhoeae*, including penicillinase-producing *N. gonorrhoeae*, tetracycline-resistant *N. gonorrhoeae*, and strains with chromosomally mediated resistance to multiple antibiotics, including penicillin and spectinomycin. Two other considerations are given high priority when choosing an antibiotic: single-dose efficacy and simultaneously treating coexisting chlamydial infection, which has been found to simultaneously colonize women with gonorrhea in up to almost 50% of cases. The present recommended regimen is ceftriaxone, 250 mg intramuscularly one time. The 250 mg dose is preferred because, optimistically, it may delay the emergence of antibiotic-resistant strains and is effective for mucosal gonorrhea regardless of the anatomic location. For patients who are allergic to ceftriaxone, the number-one alternative is spectinomycin, 2 g intramuscularly in a single dose, combined with tetracycline therapy (see the box on p. 680). In addition to this regimen, the CDC recommends also treating with oral tetracycline hydrochloride, 500 mg four times daily for 7 days, or oral doxycycline, 100 mg twice daily for 7 days, because almost 50% of patients with gonorrhea have coexisting chlamydial infection. Follow-up cultures should be obtained 4 to 7 days after completion of treatment. Culture specimens should be obtained from the rectum of all women who have been treated for gonorrhea, regardless of whether rectal gonorrhea was documented before therapy. Women with positive cultures for gonorrhea should have a serologic test for syphilis in 4 to 6 weeks, even though patients with incubating syphilis are usually cured by antibiotic combinations of ceftriaxone and tetracycline. Similarly, patients should be offered informed consent and testing for HIV infection.

Chlamydia trachomatis

The standard technique used to identify *C. trachomatis* infection is isolation of this intracellular organism in tissue culture. Because *C. trachomatis* is an obligatory intracellular organism, it is mandatory to obtain epithelial cells to maximize the percentage of positive cultures. A dacron, rayon, or calcium alginate swab is placed in the endocervical canal. It is rotated for 15 to 20 seconds to gently abrade the columnar epithelium. Recently the cytobrush, which was developed primarily to enhance

CENTERS FOR DISEASE CONTROL RECOMMENDED TREATMENT OF UNCOMPLICATED ANOGENITAL GONORRHEA IN ADULTS (1989)

Recommended regimen

Ceftriaxone, 250 mg intramuscularly once
plus
Doxycycline, 100 mg orally twice a day for 7 days

Alternative regimens

1. Spectinomycin, 2 g intramuscularly as single dose (preferred alternative)
2. Ciprofloxacin,* 500 mg orally once
3. Norfloxacin,* 800 mg orally once
4. Cerfuroxime axetil, 1 g orally once with probenecid, 1 g
5. Cefotaxime, 1 g intramuscularly once
6. Cefitzoxime, 500 mg intramuscularly once

All alternative regimens followed by doxycycline, 100 mg orally twice a day for 7 days.

Comments

If infection is known not to be caused by penicillin-resistant gonorrhea, a penicillin such as amoxicillin (3 g orally) with 1 g probenecid followed by doxycycline may be used.

For patients who cannot take tetracycline (e.g., pregnant women), erythromycin may be substituted (erythromycin base or stearate, 500 mg orally four times a day for 7 days, or erythromycin ethylsuccinate, 800 mg orally four times a day for 7 days).

*Quinolones are contraindicated during pregnancy.

sampling of endocervical cells for cytology, has been discovered to be the optimal instrument for appropriate sampling of *Chlamydia* as well. The swab is placed in an antibiotic containing transport medium and stored at 4° C. It is important to perform the definitive culture within 24 hours. Freezing and thawing of the transport medium decrease the eventual yield of positive cultures. Cultures are incubated on McCoy cell monolayers. Subsequently, in approximately 48 to 72 hours, the monolayers are stained and examined microscopically for inclusions. The exact sensitivity of culture techniques is not known. Most experts estimate the sensitivity to be approximately 75%, depending primarily on the adequacy of sampling infected epithelial cells. Laboratories that routinely add a blind second passage following negative cultures may identify approximately 15% of additional infections.

Rapid, simple, and sensitive methods to detect chlamydial antigens have been introduced. These tests are less expensive than culture and are most appropriate for screening when the prevalence of infection exceeds 10%. One test uses fluorescein-conjugated monocolonal antibodies to detect elementary bodies of *C. trachomatis*. This slide test may be performed on endocervical smears and takes less than 30 minutes to complete. Tam et al. and Stamm et al. have published large series comparing this monocolonal antibody test with traditional tissue culture methods. For women the rapid slide test (MicroTrak, Syva) has a sensitivity of 86% to 93% and a specificity of 93% to 99%. False positive and false negative results were discovered in slide specimens containing a limited number of organisms. This slide test is approximately one-third as expensive as cell culture techniques. There is only one major drawback to the direct test. There is a subjective assessment in reading the immunofluorescence, which necessitates several hours of training by laboratory personnel. The ELISA takes about 3 to 4 hours, requires a spectrophotometer, and has a sensitivity of 70% to 96% and a specificity of 90% to 98%. It is approximately half the cost of the direct fluorescent antibody test. Attempts have been made to diagnose chlamydial cervical infection from routine Pap smears. However, at best this is an insensitive, nonspecific method to judge acute cervical inflammation and will be positive in only approximately one out of four infected females. Nucleic acid probes using DNA hybridization methods are under development. However, comparative clinical studies are not yet available.

_____ **KEY POINTS** _____

- The three most prevalent primary viral infections of the skin of the vulva are genital herpes, condyloma acuminatum, and molluscum contagiosum.

- From 10% to 20% of adult women experience the symptoms of dysuria, frequency, and urgency each year. About 50% of women with these symptoms do not have significant bacteriuria.

- The most frequent pathogens causing acute urethral syndrome are *Escherichia coli, Staphylococcus saprophyticus, Chlamydia trachomatis,* and *Neisseria gonorrhoeae.*

- Women with pyuria and a "sterile" urine culture often have infection with chlamydial or gonorrheal organisms.

- Approximately 2% of adult women develop enlargement of both Bartholin's glands. More than 85% of these women will develop symptoms during their reproductive years.

- The treatment of choice for a symptomatic cyst or abscess is the development of a fistulous tract from the dilated Bartholin's duct to the vestibule.

- Excision of Bartholin's duct and gland is indicated for persistent deep infection, multiple recurrences of abscesses, or enlargement of the gland in a woman over the age of 40.

- Pediculosis pubis, an infestation by the crab louse *Phthirus pubis,* is characterized by constant itching, predominantly vulvar involvement, and the finding of eggs and lice by visual inspection. It may be treated by topical application of lindane (Kwell) or 5% permethrin dermal cream (Nix).

- Scabies, an infection by the itch mite *Sarcoptes scabiei,* is characterized by intermittent pruritus, most commonly in the hands, wrists, breasts, vulva, and buttocks. It is diagnosed by a scraping of the papules, vesicles, or burrows in which the mites live and inspection under the microscope. It may be treated by topical application of lindane (Kwell) or 5% permethrin dermal cream (Nix).

- Condyloma acuminatum is a sexually transmitted disease spread by skin-to-skin contact. It is caused by the human papillomavirus (HPV). Autoinoculation also occurs. It is a highly contagious disease, with 25% to 65% of sexual partners developing the infection.

- The probability and frequency of recurrence of herpes is related to the HSV serotype.

- Oral acyclovir has been shown to be beneficial in reducing the duration of herpetic ulcerative lesions and in reducing the time that the virus can be isolated from these lesions.

- Herpes is highly contagious, with 75% of sexual partners contracting the disease. The prevalence of genital herpes is estimated to be between 10 and 30 million cases.

- Herpes genital infections are caused by both type I and type II virus. HSV-I is found in 13% to 40% of cases.

- The incubation period of primary herpes is 3 to 7 days, with an average of 6 days, and ulcers last for 2 to 6 weeks in multiple crops. Systemic symptoms for primary herpes are experienced by 70% of women. Secondary or recurrent genital herpes will occur in 50% of women by 6 months after the initial infection and last for approximately 7 days. A woman with HSV-II has an 80% chance of recurrence within 12 months.

- Granuloma inguinale (donovanosis) may be managed by a wide range of oral broad-spectrum antibiotics. Tetracycline is the most popular choice and should be prescribed for a minimum of 2 to 3 weeks.

- The treatment for lymphogranuloma venereum is oral tetracycline or erythromycin, 500 mg every 6 hours for 3 to 6 weeks.

- The treatment of chancroid is oral trimethoprim 160 mg and sulfamethaxole 800 mg every 12 hours for 10 days or oral erythromycin 500 mg every 6 hours for 10 days.

- Dark-field microscopy rather than normal light microscopy is used for detection of syphilis because of the extreme thinness of the spirochete *Treponema pallidum*.

- Nonspecific tests for syphilis, the VDRL and RPR, have a 1% false positive rate. Therefore, specific tests such as the FTA-ABS, HATTS, and MHA-TP must be employed when a positive nonspecific test result is encountered.

- Tertiary syphilis develops in approximately 33% of patients who are not appropriately treated during the primary, secondary, or latent phases of the disease.

- After successful treatment of syphilis the VDRL titer will become nonreactive or, at most, reactive with at least a fourfold titer decline within 1 year. The FTA-ABS may remain reactive indefinitely.

- Women with syphilis of greater than 12 months' duration should have an examination of their cerebrospinal fluid to rule out asymptomatic neurosyphilis.

- In middle-class women in the reproductive age range, bacterial vaginosis represents approximately 50% of vaginitis, while candidiasis and *Trichomonas* infection represent approximately 25% each.

- The normal vaginal environment is a dynamic and delicate ecosystem, with a pH of 3.8 to 4.2.

- A vaginal pH of greater than 5.0 indicates atrophic vaginitis, bacterial vaginosis, or *Trichomonas* infection, whereas a vaginal pH of less than 4.5 is either a physiologic discharge or fungal in etiology.

- *Trichomonas* is a hardy organism and will survive for up to 24 hours on a wet towel and up to 6 hours on a wet surface. However, since a large inoculum is needed for infection, it is unlikely that infection is related to exposure from infected towels or swimming pools. *Trichomonas* vaginitis is treated with oral metronidazole (Flagyl).

- The criteria for the diagnosis of bacterial vaginosis are (1) the a homogeneous vaginal discharge is present; (2) the vaginal discharge has a pH equal to or greater than 4.7; (3) the vaginal discharge has an aminelike odor when mixed with potassium hydroxide; and (4) a wet smear of the vaginal discharge demonstrates clue cells greater in number than 20% of the number of the vaginal epithelial cells.

- Dysuria is a symptom in approximately one of five women with symptomatic *Trichomonas* infection.

- Bacterial vaginosis is treated by oral metronidazole (Flagyl), 500 mg twice daily for 7 days.

- *Candida albicans* causes the majority of fungal vaginitis. It is found on most mucosal and skin surfaces and is the normal flora of approximately 25% of women, but it becomes an opportunistic pathogen when the normal ecosystem of the vagina is disturbed. *Candida* vaginitis is treated by means of topical application of one of the synthetic imidazoles or triazoles.

- A negative wet smear of the vagina does not exclude *Candida* vulvovaginitis. The diagnosis can be established by culture with either Nickerson or Sabouraud medium.

- The risk of recurrence of toxic shock syndrome (TSS) without antibiotic therapy is approximately 33%.

- Studies of the vagina of normal menstruating females have documented 5% to 17% colonization with *Staphylococcus aureus* with 5% at midcycle and 10% to 17% during the menses.

- The initial rash of TSS over the first 48 hours is similar in appearance to an intense sunburn. Over the next several days it evolves into a macular rash with fine, flaky desquamation over the face and trunk and sloughing of the entire skin thickness over the palms and soles.

- Women with TSS should be treated with beta-lactamase-resistant antistaphylococcal antibiotics for 10 to 14 days.

- Individuals with HIV infection may shed the virus throughout the asymptomatic phase of their disease, which may last for several years. Every year 2% to 10% of these patients will develop AIDS.

- There are three primary methods of contracting HIV: intimate sexual contact; use of contaminated needles or blood products, especially in hemophiliacs; and perinatal transmission from mother to child.

- The immune defects of AIDS are caused by infection of CD_4 lymphocytes (helper T cells) by the HIV virus.

- Sperm-induced leukocyte presence in the endocervical mucus is a physiologic response.

- Culture is the standard technique for diagnosis of *Neisseria gonorrhoeae* because Gram stain smears are positive for only 50% of women with positive cultures. Sensitivity should also be evaluated, because approximately 2% of gonorrheal infections in the United States are resistant to penicillin.

- Culture of a second consecutive endocervical cotton swab will increase detection of *Neisseria gonorrhoeae* approximately 7% to 10%.

- Cultures should be obtained as a test of effective therapy for gonorrhea approximately 5 to 7 days after completion of antibiotic therapy.

- Symptoms that suggest cervical infection include vaginal discharge, deep dyspareunia, and postcoital bleeding. *Chlamydia trachomatis* is the major etiologic agent in women with mucopurulent cervicitis.

- The standard technique used to identify *Chlamydia trachomatis* infection is isolation of this intracellular organism in tissue culture. The cultures are incubated on McCoy cell monolayers.

- Because *Chlamydia trachomatis* is an obligatory intracellular organism, it is mandatory to obtain epithelial cells to maximize the percentage of positive cultures.

BIBLIOGRAPHY

Abramowicz M, editor: Treatment of sexually transmitted diseases, Med Lett 28:23, 1986.

Abrams AJ: Lymphogranuloma venereum, JAMA 205:199, 1968.

Anderson JR: Gynecologic manifestations of AIDS and HIV disease, Female Patient 14:57, 1989.

Baker DA, Douglas JM, Buntin DM, et al: Topical podofilox for the treatment of condylomata acuminata in women, Obstet Gynecol 76:656, 1990.

Baker DA, Gonik B, Milch PO, et al: Clinical evaluation of a new herpes simplex virus ELISA: a rapid diagnostic test for herpes simplex virus, Obstet Gynecol 73:322, 1989.

Barrasso R, De Brux J, Croissant O, and Orth G: High prevalence of papillomavirus-associated penile intraepithelial neoplasia in sexual partners of women with cervical intraepithelial neoplasia, N Engl J Med 317:916, 1987.

Bartlett JG and Polk R: Bacterial flora of the vagina: quantitative study, Rev Infect Dis 6:S67, 1984.

Beard CM, Noller KL, O'Fallon M, et al: Lack of evidence for cancer due to use of metronidazole, N Engl J Med 301:519, 1979.

Bellina JH: The use of the carbon dioxide laser in the management of condylomata acuminatum with eight-year follow-up, Am J Obstet Gynecol 147:375, 1983.

Bergeron C, Ferenczy A, and Richart R: Underwear: contamination by human papillomaviruses, Am J Obstet Gynecol 162:25, 1990.

Berkley SF, Hightower AW, Broome CV, and Reingold AL: The relationship of tampon characteristics to menstrual toxic shock syndrome, JAMA 258:917, 1987.

Bierman SM: Recurrent genital herpes simplex infection: a trivial disorder, Arch Dermatol 121:513, 1985.

Blackwell AL, Phillips I, Fox AR, et al: Anaerobic vaginosis (non-specific vaginitis): clinical, microbiological, and therapeutic findings, Lancet 2:1379, 1983.

Bolan RK, Sands M, Schachter J, et al: Lymphogranuloma venereum and acute ulcerative proctitis, Am J Med 72:703, 1982.

Bongard F, Landers DV, and Lewis F: Differential diagnosis of appendicitis and pelvic inflammatory disease, Am J Surg 150:90, 1985.

Boothby RA, Carlson JA, Rubin M, et al: Single application treatment of human papillomavirus infection of the cervix and vagina with trichloroacetic acid: a randomized trial, Obstet Gynecol 76:278, 1990.

Britigan BE, Cohen MS, and Sparling PF: Gonococcal infection: a model of molecular pathogenesis, N Engl J Med 312:1683, 1985.

Brock BV, Selke S, Benedetti J, et al: Frequency of asymptomatic shedding of herpes simplex virus in women with genital herpes, JAMA 263:418, 1990.

Brook I: Aerobic and anaerobic microbiology of Bartholin's abscess, Surg Gynecol Obstet 169:32, 1989.

Brown D, Kaufman RH, and Gardner HL: *Gardnerella vaginalis* vaginitis, J Reprod Med 29:300, 1984.

Brown ST, Nalley JF, and Kraus SJ: Molluscum contagiosum, Sex Transm Dis 8:227, 1981.

Brumfitt W, Gargan RA, and Hamilton-Miller MJT: Periurethral enterobacterial carriage preceding urinary infection, Lancet 824, 1987.

Brunham RC, Paavonen J, Stevens CE, et al: Mucopurulent cervicitis—the ignored counterpart in women of urethritis in men, N Engl J Med 311:1, 1984.

Bryson YJ, Dillon M, Lovett M, et al: Treatment of first episodes of genital herpes simplex virus infection with oral acyclovir: a randomized double-blind controlled trial in normal subjects, N Engl J Med 308:916, 1983.

Bump RC and Buesching WJ III: Bacterial vaginosis in virginal and sexually active adolescent females: evidence against exclusive sexual transmission, Am J Obstet Gynecol 158:935, 1988.

Bump RC and Copeland WE: Urethral isolation of the genital mycoplasmas and *Chlamydia trachomatis* in women with chronic urologic complaints, Am J Obstet Gynecol 152:38, 1985.

Bump RC, Zuspan FP, Buesching WJ, et al: The prevalence, six-month persistence and predictive values of laboratory indicators of bacterial vaginosis (nonspecific vaginitis) in asymptomatic women, Am J Obstet Gynecol 150:917, 1984.

Carpenter JL, Back A, Gehle D, et al: Treatment of chancroid with erythromycin, Sex Transm Dis 8:192, 1981.

Caussy D and Goedert JJ: The epidemiology of human immunodeficiency virus and acquired immunodeficiency syndrome, Semin Oncol 17:244, 1990.

Centers for Disease Control: Sexually transmitted disease treatment guidelines 1985, MMWR 35(suppl 4):1, 1985.

Centers for Disease Control: Recommendations and reports: sexually transmitted diseases: treatment guidelines, MMWR 38:28, 1989.

Centers for Disease Control: AIDS in women—United States, MMWR 39:845, 1990.

Centers for Disease Control: Risk for cervical disease in HIV-infected women—New York City, MMWR 39:846, 1990.

Chapel TA: The signs and symptoms of secondary syphilis, Sex Transm Dis 7:161, 1980.

Charles D: Syphilis, Clin Obstet Gynecol 26:125, 1983.

Chesney PJ: Clinical aspects and spectrum of illness of toxic shock syndrome: overview, Rev Infect Dis 11:S1, 1989.

Chesney PJ, Davis JP, Purdy WK, et al: Clinical manifestations of toxic shock syndrome, JAMA 246:741, 1981.

Chin J, Sato PA, and Mann JM: Projections of HIV infections and AIDS cases to the year 2000, Bull WHO 68:1, 1990.

Cho JY, Ahn MO, and Cha KS: Window operation: an alternative treatment method for Bartholin gland cysts and abscesses, Obstet Gynecol 76:886, 1990.

Chu SY, Buehler JW, and Berkelman RL: Impact of the human immunodeficiency virus epidemic of mortality in women of reproductive age, United States, JAMA 264:255, 1990.

Committee on Ethics: Human immunodeficiency virus infection: physician's responsibilities, ACOG Comm Opin 85, 1990.

Corey L, Adams HG, Brown ZA, et al: Genital herpes simplex virus infections: clinical manifestations, course, and complications, Ann Intern Med 98:958, 1983.

Dan BB: Prevention and treatment of toxic shock syndrome: a retrospective look, JAMA 252:3411, 1984.

Davis GD: Management of Bartholin duct cysts with the carbon dioxide laser, Obstet Gynecol 65:279, 1985.

Davis JP, Vergeront JM, Amsterdam LE, et al: Long-term effects of toxic shock syndrome in women: sequelae, subsequent pregnancy, menstrual history, and long-term trends in catamenial product use, Rev Infect Dis 11:S50, 1989.

Dismukes WE, Wade JS, Lee JY, et al: A randomized, double-blind trial of nystatin therapy for the candidiasis hypersensitivity syndrome, N Engl J Med 323:1717, 1990.

Dodson RF, Fritz GS, Hubler WR, et al: Donovanosis: a morphologic study, J Invest Dermatol 62:611, 1974.

Douglas CP: Lymphogranuloma venereum and granuloma inguinale of the vulva, J Obstet Gynaecol Br Cmmwlth 69:871, 1962.

Douglas JM, Critchlow C, Benedetti J, et al: A double-blind study of oral acyclovir for suppression of recurrences of genital herpes simplex virus infection, N Engl J Med 310:1551, 1984.

Drew WL, Blair M, Miner RC, et al: Evaluation of the virus permeability of a new condom for women, Sex Transm Dis 17:110, 1990.

Droegemueller W, Adamson DG, Brown D, et al: Three-day treatment with butoconazole nitrate for vulvovaginal candidiasis, Obstet Gynecol 64:530, 1984.

Elion GB: Mechanism of action and selectivity of acyclovir, Am J Med 73:7, 1982.

Ellerbrock TV, Bush TJ, Chamberland ME, and Oxtoby MJ: Epidemiology of women with AIDS in United States, 1981 through 1990: a comparison with heterosexual men with AIDS, JAMA 265: 2971, 1991.

Eschenbach DA: Vaginal infection, Clin Obstet Gynecol 26:186, 1983.

Eschenbach DA, Hillier S, Critchlow C, et al: Diagnosis and clinical manifestations of bacterial vaginosis, Am J Obstet Gynecol 158:819, 1988.

Eschenbach DA, Hummel D, and Gravett MG: Recurrent and persistent vulvovaginal candidiasis: treatment with ketoconazole, Obstet Gynecol 66:248, 1985.

Ferenczy A: Laser therapy of genital condylomata acuminata, Obstet Gynecol 63:703, 1984.

Fineberg HV: Education to prevent AIDS: prospects and obstacles, Science 239:592, 1988.

Fitzpatrick JE, Tyler H, and Gramstad ND: Treatment of chancroid: comparison of sulfamethoxazole trimethoprim with recommended therapies, JAMA 246:1804, 1981.

Fiumara NJ: Treatment of primary and secondary syphilis, JAMA 243:2500, 1980.

Friedland GH: Early treatment for HIV: the time has come, N Engl J Med 322:1000, 1990.

Friedrich EG: Vulvar disease, ed 2, Philadelphia, 1983, WB Saunders Co.

Friedrich EG: Vaginitis, Am J Obstet Gynecol 152:247, 1985.

Gaisin A and Heaton CL: Chancroid: alias the soft chancre, Int J Dermatol 14:188, 1975.

Galgiani JN: Fluconazole, a new antifungal agent, Ann Intern Med 113:177, 1990.

Gardner HL: *Haemophilus vaginalis* vaginitis after twenty-five years, Am J Obstet Gynecol 137:385, 1980.

Gardner HL and Dukes CD: Clinical and laboratory effects of metronidazole, Am J Obstet Gynecol 89:990, 1964.

Gardner HL and Kaufman RH, editors: Benign diseases of the vulva and vagina, ed 2, Chicago, 1981, Mosby–Year Book, Inc.

Gayle HD, Kelling RP, Garcia-Tunon M, et al: Prevalence of the human immunodeficiency virus among university students, N Engl J Med 323:1538, 1990.

Gerberding JL, Littell C, Tarkington A, et al: Risk of exposure of surgical personnel to patients' blood during surgery at San Francisco General Hospital, N Engl J Med 322:1788, 1990.

Godley MJ: Quantitation of vaginal discharge in healthy volunteers, Br J Obstet Gynaecol 92:739, 1985.

Goedert JJ, Biggar RJ, Weiss SH, et al: Three-year incidence of AIDS in five cohorts of HTLV-III-infected risk group members, Science 231:992, 1986.

Goldberg LH, Kaufman R, Conant MA, et al: Episodic twice-daily treatment for recurrent genital herpes, Am J Med 85(suppl 2A):10, 1988.

Goldman P: Metronidazole, N Engl J Med 303:1212, 1980.

Greenberg MD, Rutledge LH, Reid R, et al: A double-blind, randomized trial of 0.5% podofilox

Greene WC: The molecular biology of human immunodeficiency virus type 1 infection, N Engl J Med 324:308, 1991.

Gwinn M, Pappaioanou M, George JR, et al: Prevalence of HIV Infection in childbearing women in the United States: surveillance using newborn blood samples, JAMA 265: 1704, 1991.

Hammond GW, Lian CJ, Wilt JC, et al: Antimicrobial susceptibility of *Haemophilus ducreyi,* Antimicrob Agents Chemother 13:608, 1978.

Hammond GW, Slutchuk M, Scatliff J, et al: Epidemiological, clinical, laboratory and therapeutic features of an urban outbreak of chancroid in North America, Rev Infect Dis 2:867, 1980.

Haseltine WA: Silent HIV infections, N Engl J Med 320:1487, 1989.

Helgerson SD, Mallery BL, and Foster LR: Toxic shock syndrome in Oregon, JAMA 252:3402, 1984.

Hillier S, Krohn MA, Watts DH, et al: Microbiologic efficacy of intravaginal clindamycin cream for the treatment of bacterial vaginosis, Obstet Gynecol 76:407, 1990.

Holmes KK: Lower genital tract infections in women: cystitis, urethritis, vulvovaginitis, and cervicitis. In Holmes KK, Mårdh PA, Sparling PF, et al, editors: Sexually transmitted diseases, ed 2, New York, 1990, McGraw-Hill Book Co.

Holmes KK, Mårdh PA, Sparling PF, et al, editors: Sexually transmitted diseases, ed 2, New York, 1990, McGraw-Hill Book Co.

Horowitz BJ, Edelstein SW, and Lippman L: *Candida tropicalis* vulvovaginitis, Obstet Gynecol 66:229, 1985.

Hoth DF Jr and Myers MW: Current status of HIV therapy. I. Antiretroviral agents, Hosp Pract, 26:174, 1991.

Howard RJ: Human immunodeficiency virus testing and the risk to the surgeon of acquiring HIV, Surgery 171:22, 1990.

Hughes VL and Hillier SL: Microbiologic characteristics of Lactobacillus products used for colonization of the vagina, Obstet Gyncol 75:244, 1990.

Jaffe HW: The laboratory diagnosis of syphilis, Ann Intern Med 83:846, 1975.

Johannisson G, Lowhagen GB, and Lycke E: Genital *Chlamydia trachomatis* infection in women, Obstet Gynecol 56:671, 1980.

Johnson JR and Stamm WE: Urinary tract infections in women: diagnosis and treatment, Ann Intern Med 111:906, 1989.

Johnson MA and Webster A: Human immunodeficiency virus infection in women, Br J Med 96:129, 1989.

Johnson RE, Nahmias AJ, Magder LS, et al: A seroepidemiologic survey of the prevalence of herpes simples virus type 2 infection in the United States, N Engl J Med 321:7, 1989.

Kaplowitz LG, Baker D, Gelb L, et al: Prolonged continuous acyclovir treatment of normal adults with frequently recurring genital herpes simplex virus infection, JAMA 265:747, 1991.

Kaufman RH and Faro S: Herpes genitalis: clinical features and treatment, Clin Obstet Gynecol 28:152, 1985.

Keay S, Teng N, Eisenberg M, et al: Topical interferon for treating condyloma acuminata in women, J Infect Dis 158:934, 1988.

Kessler HA and Harris AA: Therapy for human immunodeficiency virus infection—1989, Clin Neuropharmacol 13:1, 1990.

Kissane JM, editor: Anderson's pathology, St Louis, 1985, Mosby–Year Book, Inc.

Kit S, Trkula D, Qavi H, et al: Sequential genital infections by herpes simplex viruses types 1 and 2: restriction nuclease analyses of viruses from recurrent infections, Sex Transm Dis 10:67, 1983.

Kiviat NB, Paavonen JA, Brockway J, et al: Cytologic manifestations of cervical and vaginal infections, JAMA 253:989, 1985.

Klein RS and Friedland GH: Transmission of human immunodeficiency virus Type 1 (HIV-1) by exposure to blood: defining the risk, Ann Intern Med 113:729, 1990.

Kraus SJ and Stone KM: Management of genital infection caused by human papillomavirus, Rev Infect Dis 12:S620, 1990.

Krebs HB: Treatment of vaginal condylomata acuminata by weekly topical application of 5-fluorouracil, Obstet Gynecol 70:68, 1987.

Krieger JN, Tam MR, Stevens CE, et al: Diagnosis of trichomoniasis: comparison of conventional wet-mount examination with cytologic studies, cultures, and monoclonal antibody staining of direct specimens, JAMA 259:1223, 1988.

Lal S and Nicholas C: Epidemiological and clinical features in 165 cases of granuloma inguinale, Br J Vener Dis 46:461, 1970.

Langenberg A, Benedetti J, Jenkins J, et al: Development of clinically recognizable genital lesions among women previously identified as having "asymptomatic" herpes simplex virus type 2 infection, Ann Intern Med 110:882, 1989.

Larsen B and Galask RP: Vaginal microbial flora: composition and influences of host physiology, Ann Intern Med 96:926, 1982.

Lee YH, Rankin JS, Alpert S, et al: Microbiological investigation of Bartholin's gland abscesses and cysts, Am J Obstet Gynecol 129:150, 1977.

Levy JA: Human immunodeficiency viruses and the pathogenesis of AIDS, JAMA 261:2997, 1989.

Levy JA: Changing concepts in HIV infection: challenges for the 1990s, AIDS 4:1051, 1990.

Livengood CH III, Thomason JL, and Hill GB: Bacterial vaginosis: treatment with topical intravaginal clindamycin phosphate, Obstet Gynecol 76:118, 1990.

Louv WC, Austin H, Alexander WJ, et al: A clinical trial on nonoxynol-9 for preventing gonococcal and chlamydial infections, J Infect Dis 158:518, 1988.

Louv WC, Austin H, Perlman J, and Alexander WJ: Oral contraceptive use and the risk of chlamydial and gonococcal infections, Am J Obstet Gynecol 160:396, 1989.

Luby ED and Klinge V: Genital herpes: a pervasive psychosocial disorder, Arch Dermatol 121:494, 1895.

Lukehart SA, Hook EW III, Baker-Zander SA, et al: Invasion of the central nervous system by *Treponema pallidum:* implications for diagnosis and treatment, Ann Intern Med 109:855, 1988.

Lutzner MA: The human papillomaviruses: a review, Arch Dermatol 119:631, 1983.

Lytle CD, Carney PG, Vohra S, et al: Virus leakage through natural membrane condoms, Sex Transm Dis 17:58, 1990.

Malviya VK, Deppe G, Pluszczynski R, and Boike G: Trichloroacetic acid in the treatment of human papillomavirus infection of the cervix without associated dysplasia, Obstet Gynecol 70:72, 1987.

Martin R, Wentworth BB, Coopes S, et al: Comparison of Transgrow and Gonozyme for the detection of *Neisseria gonorrhoeae* in mailed specimens, J Clin Microbiol 19:893, 1984.

Matta H, Thompson AM, and Rainey JB: Does wearing two pairs of gloves protect operating theatre staff from skin contamination? Br Med J 297:597, 1988.

McLellan R, Spence MR, Brockman M, et al: The clinical diagnosis of trichomoniasis, Obstet Gynecol 60:30, 1982.

Mecsei R, Haugen OA, Halvorsen LE, and Dalen ARE: Genital *Chlamydia trachomatis* infections in patients with abnormal cervical smears: effect of tetracycline treatment on cell changes, Obstet Gynecol 73:317, 1989.

Merkus JMWM, Bisschop MPJM, and Stolte LAM: The proper nature of vaginal candidosis and the problem of recurrence, Obstet Gynecol Surv 40:493, 1985.

Mertz GJ, Critchlow CW, Benedetti J, et al: Double-blind placebo-controlled trial of oral acyclovir in first-episode genital herpes simplex virus infection, JAMA 252:1147, 1984.

Mertz GJ, Eron L, Kaufman R, et al: Prolonged continuous versus intermittent oral acyclovir treatment in normal adults with frequently recurring genital herpes simplex virus infection, Am J Med 85(suppl 2A):14, 1988.

Mertz GJ, Jones CC, Mills J, et al: Long-term acyclovir suppression of frequently recurring genital herpes simplex virus infection: a multicenter double-blind trial, JAMA 260:201, 1988.

Mindel A, Carney O, Freris M, et al: Dosage and safety of long-term suppressive acyclovir therapy for recurrent genital herpes, Lancet I:926, 1988.

Mindel A, Faherty A, Hindel D, et al: Prophylactic oral acyclovir in recurrent genital herpes, Lancet 2:57, 1984.

Moller BR, Jorgensen AS, From E, et al: *Chlamydia*, mycoplasmas, ureaplasmas, and yeasts in the lower genital tract of females, Acta Obstet Gynecol Scand 64:145, 1985.

Montes LF and Wilborn WH: Fungus-host relationship in candidiasis, Arch Dermatol 121:119, 1985.

Moran JS and Zenilman JM: Therapy for gonococcal infections: options in 1989, Rev Infect Dis 12:S633, 1990.

Morton RS: Metronidazole in the single-dose treatment of trichomoniasis in men and women, Br J Vener Dis 48:525, 1972.

Navia BA, Jordan BD, and Price RW: The AIDS dementia complex. I. Clinical features, Ann Neurol 19:517, 1986.

Nilsen AE, Aasen T, Halsos AM, et al: Efficacy of oral acyclovir in the treatment of initial and recurrent genital herpes, Lancet 2:571, 1982.

Norris SJ: In vitro cultivation of *Treponema pallidum*: independent confirmation, Infect Immun 36:437, 1982.

Nuovo GJ and Pedemonte BM: Human papillomavirus types and recurrent cervical warts, JAMA 263:1223, 1990.

Oriel JD: Natural history of genital warts, Br J Vener Dis 47:1, 1971.

Oriel JD: The increase in molluscum contagiosum, Br Med J 294:74, 1987.

Oriel JD, Partridge BM, Denny MJ, et al: Genital yeast infections, Br Med J 4:761, 1972.

Orkin M, Epstein E, and Maibach HI: Treatment of today's scabies and pediculosis, JAMA 236:1136, 1976.

Paavonen J, Miettinen A, Stevens CE, et al: *Mycoplasma hominis* in cervicitis and endometritis, Sex Transm Dis 10:276, 1983.

Paavonen J and Wolner-Hanssen P: *Chlamydia trachomatis:* a major threat to reproduction, Hum Reprod 4:111, 1989.

Pandya IJ and Cohen J: The leukocytic reaction of the human cervix to spermatozoa, Fertil Steril 43:417, 1985.

Peterman TA and Curran JW: Sexual transmission of human immunodeficiency virus, JAMA 256:2222, 1986.

Pfeifer TA, Forsyth PS, Durfee MA, et al: Nonspecific vaginitis: role of *Haemophilus vaginalis* and treatment with metronidazole, N Engl J Med 298:1429, 1978.

Phillips RS, Hanff PA, Holmes MD, et al: *Chlamydia trachomatis* cervical infection in women seeking routine gynecologic care: criteria for selective testing, Am J Med 86:515, 1989.

Purdon A, Hanna JH, Morse PL, et al: An evaluation of single-dose metronidazole treatment of *Gardnerella vaginalis*, Obstet Gynecol 64:271, 1984.

Quinn TC, Goodell SE, Mkrtichian E, et al: *Chlamydia trachomatis* proctitis, N Engl J Med 305:195, 1981.

Ranki A, Krohn M, Allain JP, et al: Long latency precedes overt seroconversion in sexually transmitted human-immunodeficiency-virus infection, Lancet II:589, 1987.

Redondo-Lopez V, Lynch M, Schmitt C, et al: *Torulopsis glabrata* vaginitis: clinical aspects and susceptibility to antifungal agents, Obstet Gynecol 76:651, 1990.

Reeves WC, Corey L, Adams HG, et al: Risk of recurrence after first episodes of genital herpes, N Engl J Med 305:315, 1981.

Reichman RC, Badger GJ, Mertz GJ, et al: Treatment of recurrent genital herpes simplex infections with oral acyclovir: a controlled trial, JAMA 251:2103, 1984.

Reichman RC, Oakes D, Bonnez W, et al: Treatment of condyloma acuminatum with three different interferons administered intralesionally, Ann Intern Med 108:675, 1988.

Reingold AL, Broome CV, Gaventa S, et al: Risk factors for menstrual toxic shock syndrome: results of a multistate case-control study, Rev Infect Dis 11:S35, 1989.

Resnick L, Veren K, Salahuddin SZ, et al: Stability and inactivation of HTLV-III/LAV under clinical and laboratory environments, JAMA 255:1887, 1986.

Reudy J, Schechter M, and Montaner JSG: Ziovudine for early human immunodeficiency virus (HIV) infection: who, when, how? Ann Intern Med 112:721, 1990.

Richart RM and Nuovo GJ: Human papillomavirus DNA in situ hybridization may be used for the quality control of genital tract biopsies, Obstet Gynecol 75:223, 1990.

Ridgway GL and Taylor-Robinson D: Current problems in microbiology. I. Chlamydial infections: which laboratory test? J Clin Pathol 44:1, 1991.

Rigg D, Miller MM, and Metzger WJ: Recurrent allergic vulvovaginitis: treatment with *Candida albicans* allergen immunotherapy, Am J Obstet Gynecol 162:332, 1990.

Rogers MF, Ou CY, Rayfield M, et al: Use of the polymerase chain reaction for early detection of the proviral sequences of human immunodeficiency virus in infants born to seropositive mothers, N Engl J Med 320:1649, 1989.

Rolfs RT and Nakashima AK: Epidemiology of primary and secondary syphilis in the United States, 1981 through 1989, JAMA 264:1432, 1990.

Schlievert PM, Blomster DA, and Kelly JA: Toxic shock syndrome *Staphylococcus aureus:* effect of tampons on toxic shock syndrome toxin 1 production, Obstet Gynecol 64:666, 1984.

Schmid GP: Treatment of chancroid, 1989, Rev Infect Dis 12:S580, 1990.

Schmid GP, Sanders LL, Blount JH, et al: Chancroid in the United States: reestablishment of an old disease, JAMA 258:3265, 1987.

Schmitt C, Sobel J, and Meriwether C: Comparison of 0.8% and 1.6% terconazole cream in severe vulvovaginal candidiasis, Obstet Gynecol 76:414, 1990.

Schneider A, Sterzik K, Buck G, and DeVilliers EM: Colposcopy is superior to cytology for the detection of early genital human papillomavirus infection, Obstet Gynecol 71:236, 1988.

Schwarcz SK, Zenilman JM, Schnell D, et al: National surveillance of antimicrobial resistance in *Neisseria gonorrhoeae*, JAMA 264:1413, 1990.

Schwartz B, Gaventa S, Broome CV, et al: Nonmenstrual toxic shock syndrome associated with barrier contraceptives: report of a case-controlled study, Rev Infect Dis 11:S43, 1989.

Scotti RJ and Ostergard DR: The urethral syndrome, Clin Obstet Gynecol 27:515, 1984.

Seligmann M, Chess L, Fahey HL, et al: AIDS—an immunologic reevaluation, N Engl J Med 311:1286, 1984.

Shacter B: Treatment of scabies and pediculosis with lindane preparations: an evaluation, J Am Acad Dermatol 5:517, 1981.

Shafer MA, Chew KL, Kromhout LK, et al: Chlamydial endocervical infections and cytologic findings in sexually active female adolescents, Am J Obstet Gynecol 151:765, 1985.

Sjöberg I and Hakansson S: Endotoxin in vaginal fluid of women with bacterial vaginosis, Obstet Gynecol 77:265, 1991.

Sobel JD: Management of recurrent vulvovaginal candidiasis with intermittent ketoconazole prophylaxis, Obstet Gynecol 65:435, 1985.

Sobel JD, Schmitt C, and Meriwether C: Clotrimazole treatment of recurrent and chronic candida vulvovaginitis, Obstet Gynecol 73:330, 1989.

Spitzer M, Krumholz BA, and Seltzer VL: The multicentric nature of disease related to human papillomavirus infection of the female lower genital tract, Obstet Gynecol 73:303, 1989.

Sprott MS, Ingham HS, Pattman RS, et al: Characteristics of motile curved rods in vaginal secretions, J Med Microbiol 16:175, 1983.

Spruance SL, Stewart JCB, Rowe NH, et al: Treatment of recurrent herpes simplex labialis with oral acyclovir, J Infect Dis 161:185, 1990.

Stamm WE, Guinan ME, Johnson C, et al: Effect of treatment regimens for Neisseria gonorrhoeae on simultaneous infection with Chlamydia trachomatis, N Engl J Med 310:545, 1984.

Stamm WE, Harrison HR, Alexander ER, et al: Diagnosis of Chlamydia trachomatis infections by direct immunofluorescence staining of genital secretions, Ann Intern Med 101:638, 1984.

Stapleton A, Latham RH, Johnson C, and Stamm WE: Postcoital antimicrobial prophylaxis for recurrent urinary tract infection: a randomized, double-blind, placebo-controlled trial, JAMA 264:703, 1990.

Stone KM and Whittington WL: Treatment of genital herpes, Rev Infect Dis 12:S610, 1990.

Straus SE, Croen KD, Sawyer MH, et al: Acyclovir suppression of frequently recurring genital herpes: efficacy and diminishing need during successive years of treatment, JAMA 260:2227, 1988.

Straus SE, Takiff HE, Seidlin M, et al: Suppression of frequently recurring genital herpes: a placebo-controlled double-blind trial of oral acyclovir, N Engl J Med 310:1545, 1984.

Sweet RL and Gibbs RS: Infectious diseases of the female genital tract, ed 2, Baltimore, 1990, Williams & Wilkins.

Tam MR, Stamm WE, Handsfield H, et al: Culture-independent diagnosis of Chlamydia trachomatis using monoclonal antibodies, N Engl J Med 310:1146, 1984.

Taplin D, Meinking TL, Porcelain SL, et al: Permethrin 5% dermal cream: a new treatment for scabies, J Am Acad Dermatol 15:995, 1986.

Taylor E, Barlow D, Blackwell AL, et al: Gardnerella vaginalis, anaerobes, and vaginal discharge, Lancet 1:1376, 1982.

Tidy JA, Mason WP, and Farrell PJ: A new and sensitive method of screening for human papillomavirus infection, Obstet Gynecol 74:410, 1989.

Todd JK, Ressman M, Caston SA, et al: Corticosteroid therapy for patients with toxic shock syndrome, JAMA 252:3399, 1984.

Tofte RW and Williams DN: Toxic shock syndrome: evidence of a broad clinical spectrum, JAMA 246:2163, 1981.

Toomey KE and Barnes RC: Treatment of Chlamydia trachomatis genital infection, Rev Infect Dis 12:S645, 1990.

Valdiserri RO, Arena VC, Proctor D, et al: The relationship between women's attitudes about condoms and their use: implications for condom promotion programs, Am J Public Health 79:499, 1989.

Van Slyke KK, Michel VP, and Rein MF: Treatment of vulvovaginal candidiasis with boric acid powder, Am J Obstet Gynecol 141:145, 1981.

Vejtorp M, Bollerup AC, Vejtorp L, et al: Bacterial vaginosis: a double-blind randomized trial of the effect of treatment of the sexual partner, Br J Obstet Gynaecol 95:920, 1988.

Vesterinen E, Meyer B, Cantell K, et al: Topical treatment of flat vaginal condyloma with human leukocyte interferon, Obstet Gynecol 63:535, 1984.

Wager GP: Toxic shock syndrome: a review, Am J Obstet Gynecol 146:93, 1983.

Washington AE, Gove S, Schachter J, et al: Oral contraceptives, Chlamydia trachomatis infection, and pelvic inflammatory disease, JAMA 253:2246, 1985.

Wilkin JK: Molluscum contagiosum venereum in a women's outpatient clinic: a venereally transmitted disease, Am J Obstet Gynecol 128:531, 1977.

Word B: Office treatment of cyst and abscess of Bartholin's gland duct, South Med J 61:514, 1968.

Zenker PN and Rolfs RT: Treatment of syphilis, 1989, Rev Infect Dis 12:S590, 1990.

Upper Genital Tract Infections

Canaliculus. A small, canal-like opening forming a channel for ascension of bacteria from the lower to the upper genital tract.

Commensal Bacteria. An organism that may exist in the genital tract without actually causing disease.

Fitz-Hugh–Curtis Syndrome. A syndrome of perihepatic inflammation that develops in 5% to 10% of women with acute pelvic inflammatory disease, originating from transperitoneal or vascular dissemination of either *Neisseria gonorrhoeae* or *Chlamydia trachomatis*.

"Iatrogenic" Pelvic Inflammatory Disease. An upper genital tract infection secondary to a penetration of the cervical mucus barrier caused by an operative procedure.

Nonoxynol-9. A chemical detergent used in spermicidal preparations that is also bactericidal and viricidal.

Penicillinase-Producing Gonorrhea. Strains of *N. gonorrhoeae* that become resistant to penicillin by acquiring a resistance factor plasmid that enables the gonococcus to produce an enzyme that destroys penicillin.

Hydrosalpinx. A collection of watery, sterile fluid in the fallopian tube, an end stage of a pyosalpinx.

Pelvic Inflammatory Disease. A nonspecific term, used in gynecology, that most commonly refers to inflammation caused by infection in the upper genital tract; often used synonymously with the term *acute salpingitis*.

Silent Pelvic Inflammatory Disease. Asymptomatic inflammation of the upper genital tract usually related to chlamydial infection.

Tuboovarian Complex. A collection of pus within an anatomic space created by adherence of adjacent organs, involving the oviducts, ovaries, and occasionally the intestines.

This chapter considers upper genital tract infections. The primary focus is on acute pelvic inflammatory disease, which is one of the ultimate devastations of sexually transmitted diseases. Although this discussion considers the epidemiology, diagnosis, and treatment of acute pelvic inflammatory disease, the hope of the future is the prevention of the sexually transmitted diseases. The direct and indirect monetary costs of pelvic inflammatory disease are estimated to be in the billions of dollars in the United States each year. The financial sequelae of ectopic pregnancies, chronic pain, and infertility cannot be measured. This chapter will also consider uncommon causes of upper genital tract infection, such as tuberculosis and actinomycosis. For more detail of the infections with *Neisseria gonorrhoeae* and *Chlamydia trachomatis*, the reader is referred to Chapter 21.

ENDOMETRITIS

Nonpuerperal endometritis is an obscure chronic infection of the lining of the uterus. The obstetric counterpart of an acute endometritis that develops following a delivery or an abortion is well known. Since acute pelvic inflammatory disease is an ascending infection along the mucosa of the reproductive tract, endometritis must be an intermediate state of ascending infection from the endocervical canal. Regretfully, the temporal development of endometritis has not been studied extensively in women with either mucopurulent cervicitis or acute pelvic inflammatory disease. Many of the pertinent clinical questions, such as the time it takes for an ascending infection to colonize various areas of the upper genital tract, remain unanswered.

Chronic endometritis is often undiagnosed unless there is a high degree of suspicion by both the clinician and the pathologist. Paavonen et al. have found that 72% of women with laparoscopically proven acute pelvic inflammatory disease had associated histologic evidence of endometritis. Similar studies have found that 40% of women with mucopurulent cervicitis and 58% of women with positive endocervical cultures for either *C. trachomatis* or *N. gonorrhoeae* have concomitant endometritis.

The pathophysiology of endometritis is straightforward. A cervical infection leads to canalicular spread of organisms from the endocervix to the endometrium and subsequently to the endosalpinx. Microorganisms that have been commonly associated with chronic endometritis include *C. trachomatis, N. gonorrhoeae, Streptococcus agalactiae*, cytomegalovirus, and herpes simplex virus. Paavonen et al. have found a correlation between serum antibody levels of *Mycoplasma hominis* and *C. trachomatis* and the prevalence of endometritis.

Many women with chronic endometritis are asymptomatic. Conversely, when endometritis coexists with acute pelvic inflammatory disease, it is difficult to differentiate whether inflammation of the oviducts or of the endometrium is producing the pelvic symptoms. The classic symptom of chronic endometritis is intermenstrual vaginal bleeding. Some women experience postcoital bleeding or menorrhagia. Other women complain of a dull, constant lower abdominal pain. Chronic endometritis is a rare cause of infertility.

The diagnosis of chronic endometritis is established by endometrial biopsy and culture. It is possible to have a positive endometrial culture and at the same time a negative endocervical culture. The histologic findings of chronic endometritis are an inflammatory reaction of monocytes and plasma cells in the endometrial stroma (five plasma cells per high-power field). In severe cases, diffuse inflammatory infiltrates of lymphocytes and plasma cells are seen throughout the endometrial stroma. This may be associated with lymphoid follicles and stromal necrosis. No correlation has been found between the presence of polymorphonuclear leukocytes and chronic endometritis.

The treatment of chronic endometritis is oral tetracycline 2 g per day or Vibramycin 100 mg twice daily for 10 days. Many women have clinically persistent endometritis following treatment of acute pelvic inflammatory disease if they are not given either a tetracycline or erythromycin as part of their primary therapy.

PELVIC INFLAMMATORY DISEASE

Pelvic inflammatory disease is a gynecologic condition that lacks a precise definition. The term is used most commonly to refer to inflammation caused by an infection in the upper genital tract. Thus it may include infection of any or all of the following anatomic locations: the endometrium (endometritis), the oviducts (salpingitis), the ovary (oophoritis), the uterine wall (myometritis), the uterine serosa and broad ligaments (parametritis), and the pelvic peritoneum. Many authors prefer the term *salpingitis* because infection of the oviducts is the most characteristic and common component of pelvic inflammatory disease. Importantly, most long-term sequelae of pelvic inflammatory disease result from destruction of the tubal architecture by the infection. In most clinical situations the terms acute *salpingitis* and *pelvic inflammatory disease* are used synonymously to describe an acute infection. *Chronic pelvic inflammatory disease* is a term that has largely been abandoned because the long-term sequelae of acute infection, such as adhesions and hydrosalpinx, are bacteriologically sterile. With the exception of infection with extremely rare organisms, such as tuberculosis or actinomycosis, pelvic infections are not chronic.

The present and growing epidemic of sexually transmitted diseases and corresponding pelvic inflammatory disease is a major public health concern. In the United States estimates of the direct and indirect costs of pelvic inflammatory disease and its sequelae total $3.5 billion a year. Presently it is estimated that there are approximately 1 million cases of acute pelvic inflammatory disease a year in this country. The disease annually generates approximately 2.5 million visits to physicians, 250,000 to 300,000 inpatient hospital admissions, and

150,000 operative procedures in the United States for conditions directly related to acute pelvic infection. To reduce both the medical and economic impacts of acute pelvic inflammatory disease, emphasis must be placed on aggressive therapy for lower genital tract infection, and early diagnosis and treatment of upper genital tract infection as well as treatment of sexual partners and education to prevent recurrent infection.

In more than 99% of cases, acute pelvic inflammatory disease results from ascending infection from the bacterial flora of the vagina and cervix. This ascending infection occurs along the mucosal surface, where the bacteria colonize and infect the endometrium and fallopian tubes. Acute pelvic inflammatory disease is rare in the woman without menstrual periods, such as the pregnant, premenopausal, or postmenopausal woman. The process sometimes extends to the surface of the ovaries and nearby peritoneum and rarely into the adjacent soft tissues, such as the broad ligament and pelvic blood vessels. In less than 1% of cases, acute pelvic inflammatory disease results from transperitoneal spread of infectious material from a perforated appendix or intraabdominal abscess. Hematogenous and lymphatic spread to the tubes or ovaries is another remote possibility. Acute pelvic inflammatory disease is usually a polymicrobial infection that is a mixture of aerobic and anaerobic bacteria clinically appearing as a single complex infection. Therapeutic strategies and regimens are broadspectrum, seeking to suppress aerobic and anaerobic organisms. More than 20 species of microorganisms have been cultured from direct aspiration of purulent material from infected tubes. This is unlike an infection in many other areas of the body, which usually is caused predominantly by one species of microorganism.

Approximately 85% of cases are spontaneous infections in sexually active females of reproductive age. The other 15% of infections follow procedures that break the cervical mucus barrier, allowing the vaginal flora the opportunity to colonize the upper genital tract. These procedures include endometrial biopsy, curettage, intrauterine device insertion, and hysteroscopy. Spontaneous pelvic inflammatory disease is extremely rare in women who are not sexually active or amenorrheic. When pelvic inflammatory disease is found in the postmenopausal women, genital malignancies, diabetes, and/or concurrent intestinal disease are usually found. Acute pelvic inflammatory disease occurs annually in 1% to 2% of young, sexually active women. Pelvic inflammatory disease is the most common serious infection of women aged 16 to 25, and the morbidity produced by it exceeds that produced by all other infections for this age group.

One in four women with acute pelvic inflammatory disease experiences medical sequelae. Following acute pelvic inflammatory disease, the rate of ectopic pregnancy increases sixfold to tenfold, and the chance of developing chronic pelvic pain increases fourfold. In the United States each year 26,100 ectopic pregnancies and 90,000 new cases of chronic abdominal pain are directly related to pelvic inflammatory disease (Table 22-1). The incidence of infertility following acute pelvic inflammatory disease varies widely (6% to 60%) depending on the severity of the infection, the number of episodes of infection, and the age of the

TABLE 22-1
Incidence of PID and Associated Sequelae for Women Aged 15 to 44 Years

Age (years)	Pelvic Inflammatory Disease			Number of Ectopic Pregnancies	Number of Infertile Women
	Number of Hospitalized Cases	Number of Outpatient Cases	Number of Surgical Procedures		
15-19	42,000	158,000	—	4100	—
20-24	72,100	271,300	—	7050	—
25-29	62,700	236,000	—	6150	—
30-34	43,200	162,600	—	4200	—
35-39	26,700	100,400	—	2600	—
40-44	20,500	77,100	—	2000	—
TOTAL	267,200	1,005,400	118,900	26,100	200,000

From Washington AE, Arno PS, and Brooks MA: JAMA 255:1736, 1986. Copyright 1986, American Medical Association.

patient. Weström reported that hospitalized patients have an incidence of infertility due to tubal obstruction of 11.4% after one episode of pelvic inflammatory disease, 23.1% after two episodes, and 54.3% after three or more episodes. Women with one episode of acute pelvic inflammatory disease are also more susceptible to developing repeat infection. It is difficult to distinguish whether this tendency is related primarily to mucosal damage or to reinfection by a potentially infected mate. Grimes has estimated that 0.29 deaths per 100,000 women aged 15 to 44 are directly related to pelvic inflammatory disease.

The clinical symptoms and signs of acute pelvic inflammatory disease vary considerably and are usually nonspecific. Thus the clinical diagnosis made from symptoms, signs, and even laboratory data is often incorrect. Ideally, laparoscopy with direct visualization of the internal female organs would not only improve the diagnostic accuracy but also afford the opportunity for direct cultures of purulent material, which might help to establish optimum therapy. Although laparoscopy is being used more extensively in the early diagnosis of acute pelvic inflammatory disease, in practice most women do not undergo this procedure because of the expense.

Etiology

Acute pelvic inflammatory disease is usually a polymicrobial infection caused by organisms ascending from the vagina and cervix along the mucosa of the endometrium to infect the mucosa of the oviduct. Bacterial organisms cultured directly from tubal fluid commonly include N. gonorrhoeae, C. trachomatis, endogenous aerobic and anaerobic bacteria, and, rarely, genital Mycoplasma species. Direct cultures have proven that tubal infections are polymicrobial from inception and throughout the active infectious process. Sweet discovered an average of seven different species in his series of intraabdominal cultures performed via the laparoscope. However, the type and number of species vary depending on the stage of the disease when the culture is obtained. For example, gonorrheal organisms are frequently cultured during the first 24 to 48 hours of the disease but are often absent later. Similarly, fewer organisms are cultured late in the disease, and anaerobic bacteria tend to predominate.

It used to be common practice to divide pelvic inflammatory disease into gonococcal and nongonococcal disease depending on the recovery of N. gonorrhoeae from the endocervix. Laparoscopic studies have demonstrated a correlation of no better than 50% between endocervical and tubal cultures. Thus endocervical cultures are a crude index at best of the type of upper genital tract infection, and this practice has been abandoned.

Multiple studies have demonstrated a wide range of positive cultures from women with acute pelvic inflammatory disease. The organisms differ depending on the geographic location of the study, the prevalence of lower genital tract disease, the population studied, the duration of symptoms, the severity of the disease, and the number of previous episodes of acute pelvic inflammatory disease. Sweet has summarized the literature by stating that in approximately one third of women with acute pelvic inflammatory disease, N. gonorrhoeae is the only organism recovered by direct tubal or cul-de-sac culture. One third have a culture positive for N. gonorrhoeae plus a mixture of endogenous aerobic and anaerobic flora, and the remaining one third have only aerobic and anaerobic organisms cultured directly from the intraperitoneal surfaces of the upper genital tract (Table 22-2). One must add to this generalization that approximately 20% of all women with salpingitis have tubal cultures positive for Chlamydia. The two organisms N. gonorrhoeae and C. trachomatis coexist in the same individual 25% to 40% of the time.

Because of the virulence of N. gonorrhoeae in both in vitro and in vivo studies, its major role in pelvic inflammatory disease is well established. Approximately 15% of women with cervical infection by N. gonorrhoeae subsequently develop acute pelvic inflammatory disease. Approximately 50% of women with endocervical cultures positive for N. gonorrhoeae at the time of acute pelvic inflammatory disease will have the same organism cultured from the fallopian tubes. If N. gonorrhoeae is the only organism cultured from the tubes, a patient will usually respond rapidly to treatment.

The virulence of the strain or colony type of N. gonorrhoeae helps to predict the incidence of upper genital tract infection. Transparent colonies of N. gonorrhoeae on culture medium attach more readily to epithelial cells and thus produce tubal infection more frequently than opaque-appearing colonies. Immunologic studies have demonstrated that an antibody against

TABLE 22-2

Studies of Patients with Isolation of *N. gonorrhoeae*, Anaerobes, and Aerobes from Culdocentesis Aspirates of Women with Acute PID*

		Culdocentesis		
No. of Patients	Endocervical *N. gonorrhoeae* (%)	*N. gonorrhoeae* only (%)	*N. gonorrhoeae* plus Anaerobes and Aerobes (%)	Anaerobes and Aerobes Only (%)
104	56 (54)	12 (22)	18 (32)	26 (46)
30	24 (80)	5 (21)	5 (21)	14 (58)
54	21 (39)	6 (28)	1 (5)	5 (24)
17	16 (94)	5 (31)	5 (31)	6 (38)
26	13 (50)	4 (31)	4 (31)	4 (31)
20	13 (65)	—	1 (5)	18 (95)

From Sweet RL: Sex Transm Dis 13:193, 1986.
*Results expressed as number (percentage) with indicated isolate.

TABLE 22-3

Comparison of *C. trachomatis* and *N. gonorrhoeae* Cervical Isolation and *N. gonorrhoeae* Tubal Isolation among Women with Acute PID

		Cervical Infection		Tubal/Peritoneal Infection*
First Author of Study	No. of Patients	*C. trachomatis*	*N. gonorrhoeae*	*N. gonorrhoeae*
Henry-Suchet	17	(38%)	0/4	1/4 (25%)
Møller	166	(22%)	9 (5%)	
Mårdh	60	(38%)	4 (5%)	
Gjønnaess	65	(46%)	5 (8%)	0/65
Mårdh	63	(36%)	11 (17%)	1/14 (7%)
Adler	78	(5%)	14 (18%)	
Ripa	206	(33%)	39 (19%)	
Osser	209	(47%)	41 (20%)	
Paavonen	106	(25%)	27 (25%)	
Paavonen	101	(32%)	25 (25%)	
Paavonen	228	(30%)	60 (26%)	
Eilard	22	(27%)	7 (32%)	1/22 (5%)
Bowie	43	(51%)	15 (35%)	
Eschenbach	204	(20%)	90 (44%)	7/54 (13%)
Sweet	39	(5%)	18 (46%)	8/35 (23%)
Cunningham	104		56 (54%)	30/104 (29%)
Thompson	30	(10%)	24 (80%)	10/30 (33%)
TOTAL	1741	400/1365 (29%)	445/1728 (26%)	58/328 (18%)

From Eschenbach DA: Acute pelvic inflammatory disease, vol 1. In Gynecology and obstetrics, Philadelphia, 1985, Harper & Row, Publishers, p. 8.
*Isolation of *N. gonorrhoeae* from the peritoneum of the total number of women studied.

the outer membrane protein of the gonococcus develops in approximately 70% of women following severe pelvic infection. The lack of significant antibody titers may help explain why teenagers are more likely to develop upper genital tract disease than women in their late 20s.

There is an extremely wide variation in the recovery rates of *N. gonorrhoeae* depending on the geographic location of the study (Table 22-3). The highest recovery rates occur in young, urban, black females in the United States.

The gonococcus produces an intense inflammatory reaction in the tubes, which causes narrowing or occlusion of the tubal lumen because of the presence of necrotic debris and purulent material. This cellular destruction is much more extensive than the reaction associated with a chlamydial infection.

Penicillinase-producing *N. gonorrhoeae* organisms were first identified 15 years ago. These strains of gonorrhea become resistant to penicillin by acquiring a resistance factor plasmid that enables the gonococcus to produce an enzyme that destroys penicillin. In 1983 another form of resistance to penicillin, chromosomally mediated, was first reported. By 1989, 6% of gonorrhea strains were resistant to penicillin.

C. trachomatis is an intracellular, sexually transmitted bacterial pathogen. This organism is the leading cause of acute pelvic inflammatory disease in Sweden. A recent report from Edinburgh found a ratio of chlamydial to gonococcal PID diagnosed by laparoscopy of 4:1. However, there is a widespread difference in isolation rates depending on the series and the geographic location (Table 22-4). One of the primary reasons that chlamydial organisms were not recovered in early studies in the United States was the reluctance to perform a biopsy of the fallopian tubes to obtain culture material. *Chlamydia* has recently become more prevalent than gonorrhea. From 20% to 40% of sexually active women have antibodies against *C. trachomatis*. From 10% to 30% of women with acute pelvic inflammatory disease who do not have cultures positive for *Chlamydia* have evidence of acute chlamydial infection by serial antibody titer testing. Overall, *Chlamydia* is involved in at least 40% of the hospitalized patients with PID. Recent studies have shown upper tract chlamydial infection increases the risk of an ectopic pregnancy from 3 to 6 times compared with women without chlamydial infection.

C. trachomatis infection of either the lower or upper genital tract is seen most frequently in young women who are sexually active. Clinically, *Chlamydia* produces a mild form of salpingitis with an insidious onset. Whereas gonorrhea remains in the fallopian tubes for at most a few days in untreated patients, *Chlamydia* may remain in the fallopian tubes for months after initial colonization of the upper

TABLE 22-4
C. trachomatis Infection among Women with PID

First Author of Study	No. of Patients	C. trachomatis		
		Present in Cervix	Present in Tubes/Peritoneum	Antibody Titer IgM or Fourfold IgGΔ
Adler	78	4 (5%)		24/78 (31%)*
Sweet	39	2 (5%)	0/35	5/22 (23%)
Thompson	30	3 (10%)	3/30 (10%)	
Eschenbach	100	20 (20%)	1/54 (2%)	15/74 (20%)
Møller	166	37 (22%)		34 (20%)
Paavonen	106	27 (25%)		19/72 (26%)
Eilard	22	6 (27%)	2 (9%)	
Paavonen	228	69 (30%)		32/167 (19%)
Paavonen	101	32 (32%)		18 (18%)
Mårdh	63	19/53 (36%)	6/20 (30%)	
Ripa	156	52 (33%)		37/80 (46%)
Henry-Suchet	16	6 (38%)	4/17 (24%)	
Mårdh	60	23 (38%)		22/60 (37%)
Gjønnaess	65	26/56 (46%)	5/31 (16%)†	24/60 (40%)
Osser	111	52 (47%)		37/72 (51%)
Bowie	43	22 (51%)		
Skaug	34	19 (56%)		16 (47%)
TOTAL	1418	419/1399 (30%)	21/209 (10%)	281/986 (28%)

From Eschenbach DA: Acute pelvic inflammatory disease, vol 1. In Gynecology and obstetrics, Philadelphia, 1985, Harper & Row, Publishers, p. 9.
Δ, Antibody change.
*Criteria of antibody response not given.
†Additional women had *C. trachomatis* organisms in the peritoneum but not in the cervix.

TABLE 22-5

Evidence of Genital *Mycoplasma* Infection among Women with Acute Salpingitis

Isolate/First Author of Study	Cervical Isolation (%)	Tubal Isolation (%)	Antibody Change (%)
M. hominis			
Sweet	73	4	
Eschenbach	72	4	20
Mårdh and Weström	62	8	
Thompson	60	17	
Møller	55		30
Mårdh			12
U. urealyticum			
Eschenbach	81	2	18
Mårdh and Eström	56	4	
Sweet	54	15	
Thompson	33	20	
Henry-Suchet	24	17	
Sweet		9	

From Eschenbach DA: Acute pelvic inflammatory disease, vol 1. In Gynecology and obstetrics, Philadelphia, 1985, Harper & Row, Publishers, p. 11.

genital tract. In experimental studies the salpingitis produced by *Chlamydia* is confined to the tubal mucosa. Chlamydiae probably produce a disruption of the tubal mucosa by an immunopathologic mechanism rather than by a direct cytotoxicity, as is the case with *N. gonorrhoeae*.

The past 5 years have produced a clinical awareness of a syndrome often called *silent PID*. This is an asymptomatic inflammation of the upper genital tract associated with chlamydial infection. The sequelae of repeated asymptomatic chlamydial infections is tubal infertility and ectopic pregnancy.

The role of genital mycoplasmas in the etiology of acute pelvic inflammatory disease is unclear. Cervical cultures positive for both *Mycoplasma hominis* and *Ureaplasma urealyticum* may be obtained from the majority of young, sexually active women. The rate of isolation of genital mycoplasmas from the cervix is approximately 75% and similar in populations of women who are sexually active both with and without pelvic inflammatory disease.

Direct tubal cultures demonstrated *M. hominis* in 4% to 17% and *U. urealyticum* in 2% to 20% of women with acute pelvic inflammatory disease (Table 22-5). However, serologic studies in women with acute pelvic inflammatory disease have demonstrated that approximately

one woman in four develops a significant rise in antibody titers to these organisms. Experimental inoculation of the cervix of the Grivet monkey demonstrated that the route of spread of mycoplasmas is via the parametria rather than the mucosa. Thus the primary upper genital tract infection is in the parametria and the tissue surrounding the tubes, not in the tubal lumen. This fact may help to explain the low success rate of direct tubal cultures. Histologically, *Mycoplasma* does not appear to produce damage to the tubal mucosa. In summary, in vitro and in vivo studies suggest that *Mycoplasma* may be a commensal bacterium rather than a pathogen in the oviducts.

The endogenous aerobic and anaerobic flora of the vagina frequently ascend to colonize and infect the upper reproductive tract. Direct cultures of purulent material from the tubal lumen or posterior cul-de-sac have demonstrated a wide range of organisms (Table 22-6). The most common aerobic organisms are nonhemolytic *Streptococcus*, *Escherichia coli*, group B *Streptococcus*, and coagulase-negative *Staphylococcus*. Anaerobic organisms tend to predominate over aerobes, and the most common anaerobic organisms are *Bacteroides* species, *Peptostreptococcus*, and *Peptococcus*. Anaerobic organisms are almost ubiquitous in pelvic abscesses associated with acute pelvic inflammatory disease.

TABLE 22-6
Nongonococcal, Nonchlamydial Bacteria Recovered from the Upper Genital Tract of 74 Patients with Acute Salpingitis at San Francisco General Hospital

Species	No. of Isolates
Bacteroides species	48
Bacteroides bivius	35
Peptococcus asaccharolyticus	38
Peptococcus prevotii	16
Peptostreptococcus anaerobius	24
Veillonella parvula	19
Gardnerella vaginalis	30
Escherichia coli	18
Nonhemolytic streptococci	16
Group B streptococci	16
Coagulase-negative staphylococci	22

From Sweet RL: Sex Transm Dis 13:194, 1986.

Presently there is a controversy as to which species of *Bacteroides* is the predominant agent in acute disease. Some investigators have discovered primarily *Bacteroides fragilis*, whereas others believe *Bacteroides bivius* is the most important anaerobe. With recent emphasis on the predominant anaerobic flora associated with bacterial vaginosis, there has been speculation that this condition predisposes women to acute pelvic inflammatory disease. This hypothesis is plausible and epidemiologically interesting but is difficult to prove. In slightly fewer than 20% of cases of salpingitis, no organism will be cultured from the fallopian tubes.

Risk Factors

Risk factors are important considerations in both the clinical management and prevention of upper genital tract infections. The woman who is classically at highest risk is the menstruating teenager who has multiple sexual partners, does not use contraception, and lives in an area with a high prevalence of sexually transmitted disease. There is a strong correlation between the incidence of sexually transmitted disease and acute pelvic inflammatory disease in any given population. The age distribution of uncomplicated sexually transmitted disease is usually the same as that for acute pelvic inflammatory disease.

In epidemiologic studies, age at first intercourse, marital status, and number of sexual partners are all gross indicators of the frequency of exposure to sexually transmitted diseases. Having multiple sexual partners increases the chance of acquiring acute pelvic inflammatory disease approximately fivefold, and women who are not sexually active rarely acquire upper genital tract infection. The frequency of intercourse with a monogamous partner is not a risk factor. Women with a monogamous partner who has had a vasectomy appear to have a lower incidence of the disease. A recent study by Lidegaard and Helms from Denmark found age at first intercourse and coital frequency to correlate strongest with the incidence of pelvic inflammatory disease.

The incidence of acute pelvic inflammatory disease decreases with advancing age. Acute pelvic inflammatory disease is a condition of young females, with 75% of cases occurring in women less than 25 years of age. The risk that a sexually active adolescent female will develop acute pelvic inflammatory disease is 1 in 8. This risk factor decreases to 1 in 80 for women over the age of 25. Obviously the sexual habits of teenagers, including contact with multiple partners and lack of contraception, predispose them to sexually transmitted diseases and, correspondingly, acute pelvic inflammatory disease. However, relative youth in itself also increases the incidence of acute pelvic inflammatory disease. For unknown reasons young women with colonization of the cervix by *Chlamydia* have a higher incidence of upper genital tract infection than older women do. An unproven hypothesis to explain the increased infection rate in teenagers includes the comparative lack of antibody protection and the wider area of cervical columnar epithelium, which allows colonization by *C. trachomatis* and *N. gonorrhoeae*.

Stone et al. have tabulated (Table 22-7) both proven and hypothetical methods of preventing sexually transmitted disease and acute pelvic inflammatory disease. Both clinical and laboratory studies have documented that the use of contraceptives changes the relative risk of developing acute pelvic inflammatory disease. Weström has developed an arbitrary risk rating scale in which the risk of developing acute pelvic inflammatory disease in sexually active women not using contraception is assigned a score of 1. The corresponding risk among

TABLE 22-7
Methods of Preventing STDs, Mechanisms of Action, and Efficacy

Method	Mechanism	Efficacy in Prevention of STDs
Behavioral		
Monogamy	Decreases likelihood of exposure to infected persons	Not well studied; theoretical efficacy
Reducing number of partners	Decreases likelihood of contact with infectious agents	
Avoiding certain sexual practices		
Inspecting and questioning partners		
Barriers		
Condom	Protects partner from direct contact with semen, urethral discharge, or penile lesion	Effective in vitro barrier to chlamydiae, CMV, HSV, and HIV
	Protects wearer from direct contact with partner's mucosal secretions	Appears to decrease risk of acquiring urethral/cervical GC, PID, cervical cancer, and male urethral *Ureaplasma* colonization
		Effect on risk of acquiring NGU not established
Spermicide	Chemically inactivates infectious agents	Nonvaginal use has not been studied
		Inactivates gonococci, syphilis spirochetes, trichomonads, HSV, ureaplasmas, and HIV in vitro
		Appears to decrease risk of acquiring cervical GC, PID, and cervical cancer; chlamydiae studies in progress
Diaphragm/spermicide	Mechanical barrier covers cervix	Diaphragm alone has not been studied
	Used with spermicides	Appears to decrease risk of acquiring cervical GC and PID
Vaccines	Induce antibody response that renders host immune to disease	Commercially available hepatitis B vaccine is safe and effective
		Results of clinical trials of gonococcal and herpes simplex vaccines not encouraging
		Gonococcal, HIV, and HSV vaccines research in progress
Oral antibiotics	Kill infectious agent on or shortly after exposure before infection is established	No studies among women or civilian men
Penicillin		
Sulfathiazole		Appears to decrease risk of acquiring GC and hard and soft chancre, but use not recommended
Tetracycline analogues		
Local	Flushes infectious agents out of urethra and washes infectious agents of genital skin and mucous membranes	Poorly studied
Postcoital urination		
Postcoital washing		
Postcoital antiseptic douching	Inactivates and washes infectious agents out of vagina	Poorly studied

From Stone KM, Grimes DA, and Magder LS: JAMA 255:1764, 1986. Copyright 1986, American Medical Association.
CMV, Cytomegalovirus: *HSV,* herpes simplex virus; *HIV,* human immunodeficiency virus; *GC,* gonorrhea; *PID,* pelvic inflammatory disease; *NGU,* nongonococcal urethritis.

women wearing an IUD is 2 to 4; among women using oral contraceptives, 0.3; and among women using a barrier method of contraception, 0.4.

Barrier methods—condoms, diaphragms, and spermicidal preparations—are effective both as mechanical obstructive devices and as chemical barriers. Nonoxynol 9, the material ubiquitous in spermicidal preparations, is both bactericidal and viricidal. Laboratory tests have demonstrated that Nonoxynol 9 kills *N. gonorrhoeae*, genital *Mycoplasma* species, *Trichomonas vaginalis*, *Treponema pallidum*, herpes simplex virus, and human immunodeficiency virus (HIV). The porosity of latex in condoms is more than 1000 times smaller than viral particles. Thus routine condom use prevents deposition and transmission of infected organisms from the semen to the endocervix. In contrast, frequent vaginal douching increases the relative risk of PID 3.6-fold over women who douche less frequently than once a month.

Oral contraceptive use has two preventive effects: a lower incidence of acute pelvic inflammatory disease and a milder form of upper genital tract infection when it does occur. The decrease in incidence of upper genital tract infection is believed to be secondary to thicker cervical mucus produced by the progestin component of oral contraceptives, which inhibits sperm and bacterial penetration. The decrease in duration of menstrual flow accompanying oral contraceptive use theoretically creates a shorter interval for bacterial colonization of the upper tract. Wolner-Hanssen et al. correlated laparoscopic findings of women with acute pelvic inflammatory disease and contraceptive use in a case-controlled study. Not only was there less pelvic inflammatory disease in the oral contraceptive group, but also the spread of inflammation to the fallopian tubes seemed to be inhibited in oral contraceptive users (Table 22-8). Washington et al. have urged caution in the conclusion that oral contraceptives protect against all forms of acute pelvic inflammatory disease. A twofold to threefold increase in the prevalence of endocervical infection by *C. trachomatis* has been demonstrated in multiple epidemiologic studies of women using oral contraceptives. Whether the colonization of the endocervix results in more upper genital tract disease is presently being studied.

Multiple case-controlled studies have shown an increased risk of acute pelvic inflammatory

TABLE 22-8

Comparison of Laparoscopic Findings with Type of Contraceptive Use in 738 Women with Signs and Symptoms Suggestive of Acute Salpingitis

Laparoscopic Findings	Contraceptive Method*		
	Oral Contraceptive (%)	Intrauterine Device (%)	Reference† (%)
Salpingitis	171 (59.8)	183 (80.6)	190 (84.4)
Nonsalpingitis	115 (40.2)	44 (19.4)	35 (15.6)

From Wohner-Hanssen P, Svensson L. Mårdh P-A, et al: Obstet Gynecol 66:234, 1985. Reprinted with permission from the American College of Obstetricians and Gynecologists.

*Relative risk of oral contraceptive use versus reference = 0.27 χ_1^2 = 36.9, $P < .0001$); relative risk of IUD use versus reference = 0.77 (95% confidence interval .47 to 1.26, χ_1^2 = 1.1, $P = .28$); and relative risk of oral contraceptive versus IUD use = 0.36 (95% confidence interval .24 to .54, χ_1^2 = 25.7, $P < .0001$).

†Reference = barrier methods or no contraception.

disease in women who wear an IUD. There has been just criticism of some of the early epidemiologic studies for their selection of control groups and the bias of including women with Dalkon Shields in their statistics. Nevertheless, the risk of acute pelvic inflammatory disease in women who wear an IUD is approximately 2 to 3 times greater for the first 4 months after an IUD is inserted than in women who do not use contraceptives.

Acute salpingitis occurring in a woman with a previous tubal ligation is rare. Phillips and D'Ablaing reported the incidence of acute pelvic inflammatory disease developing in the proximal stump of previously ligated fallopian tubes as 1 in 450 women hospitalized for acute salpingitis (Figure 22-1).

Epidemiologic studies have documented that previous acute pelvic inflammatory disease is a definite risk factor for future attacks of the disease. Approximately 25% of women with acute pelvic inflammatory disease subsequently develop acute tubal infection. Ten years ago this reinfection was believed to be "chronic infection" or exacerbations of a "latent" tubal process. Direct cultures have proven that the disease is another primary infection. This increased risk may be related to the sexual habits of the woman involved or to an untreated male partner. Studies have documented that greater

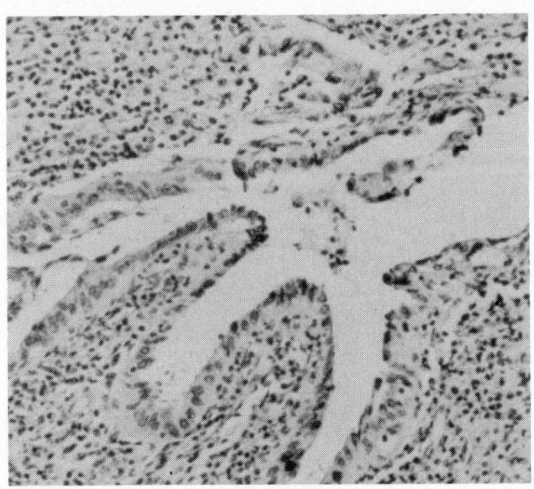

FIGURE 22-1
Tubal mucous membrane of proximal stump with lamina propria extensively infiltrated by numerous acute and chronic inflammatory cells in woman with a previous tubal ligation. (From Phillips AJ and D'Ablaing G: Obstet Gynecol 67:56S, 1986. Reprinted with permission from The American College of Obstetricians and Gynecologists.)

than 80% of male contacts are not treated. Approximately 50% of men with sexually transmitted diseases are free of symptoms, and thus they do not seek treatment. Also, the microscopic tubal damage produced by the initial upper genital tract infection may facilitate repeat infection.

Transcervical penetration of the cervical mucus barrier with instrumentation of the uterus is a risk factor, for it may initiate "iatrogenic" acute pelvic inflammatory disease. Approximately 1 million first trimester abortions are performed each year in the United States. The incidence of upper genital tract infection associated with this procedure is approximately 1 in 200 cases. Thus 5000 cases of acute upper tract infection will result each year from pregnancy terminations. Recent practice has emphasized the use of prophylactic antibiotics in high-risk cases to attempt to decrease the incidence of iatrogenic acute pelvic inflammatory disease.

Symptoms and Signs

Patients with acute pelvic inflammatory disease present with a wide range of nonspecific clinical symptoms. This great variation in clini-

cal presentation is exemplified by the extremes of asymptomatic women versus women with diffuse peritonitis and a life-threatening illness. Since the diagnosis is usually based on clinical criteria, there is both a high false positive rate and a high false negative rate. The differential diagnosis of acute pelvic inflammatory disease includes lower genital tract pelvic infection, ectopic pregnancy, torsion or rupture of an adnexal mass, acute appendicitis, and endometriosis.

Laparoscopic studies of women with a clinical diagnosis of acute pelvic inflammatory disease have established the inadequacy of diagnosis by the usual criteria of history and physical and laboratory examination. In these studies approximately 20% to 25% of women had no identifiable intraabdominal or pelvic disease. Another 10% to 15% of patients were found to have other pathologic conditions, such as ectopic pregnancy, acute appendicitis, or torsion of the adnexa. In one of these studies Jacobson reported a series of 814 women in whom laparoscopy was done because of clinically suspected acute pelvic inflammatory disease. The clinical diagnosis was confirmed at laparoscopy in 532 women (65%). This study also documented the laparoscopic findings in 98 women with a false positive clinical diagnosis of acute pelvic inflammatory disease and 91 cases of false negative clinical diagnosis of acute pelvic inflammatory disease (Tables 22-9 and 22-10). Another interesting finding of laparoscopic studies is the lack of correlation between the number and intensity of symptoms and the severity of tubal inflammation. Women with *C. trachomatis* infections may exhibit minor symptoms but have a severe inflammatory process visualized by laparoscopic examination. Criteria for establishing the severity of acute pelvic inflammatory disease by laparoscopic examination are listed in Table 22-11.

Historically, the diagnosis of acute pelvic inflammatory disease was not established unless the patient had the triad of fever, elevated erythrocyte sedimentation rate, and adnexal tenderness or a mass. Only 17% of laparoscopically identified cases have this classic triad. Jacobson described the reverse logic that has been applied to the syndrome of acute pelvic inflammatory disease. He points out that the disorder had been made to fit the criteria established for it and not vice versa, as is usually the clinical practice. Thus reliance on stringent

TABLE 22-9
Laparoscopic Findings in Patients with False Positive Clinical Diagnosis of Acute PID but with Pelvic Disorders Other than PID

Laparoscopic Finding	No.
Acute appendicitis	24
Endometriosis	16
Corpus luteum bleeding	12
Ectopic pregnancy	11
Pelvic adhesions only	7
Benign ovarian tumor	7
Chronic salpingitis	6
Miscellaneous	15
TOTAL	98

From Jacobson LJ: Am J Obstet Gynecol 138:1007, 1980.

TABLE 22-10
Laparoscopy/Laparotomy Diagnoses in Patients with False Negative Clinical Diagnosis of Acute PID by Laparoscopy

Clinical Diagnosis	Visual Diagnosis: Acute PID (No.)
Ovarian tumor	20
Acute appendicitis	18
Ectopic pregnancy	16
Chronic salpingitis	10
Acute peritonitis	6
Endometriosis	5
Uterine myoma	5
Uncharacteristic pelvic pain	5
Miscellaneous	6
TOTAL	91

From Jacobson LJ: Am J Obstet Gynecol 138:1007, 1980.

clinical criteria for establishing the diagnosis of the disease would result in the majority of cases being overlooked and not treated. Obviously, more frequent and liberal use of diagnostic laparoscopy is an important advance in the management of the disease. Laparoscopy allows precise diagnosis and also the opportunity to collect culture material from the site of the infection. However, in practice the majority of women with acute pelvic inflammatory disease do not undergo laparoscopy because of the expense of this invasive technique.

Hager and Eschenbach have established clinical criteria for acute pelvic inflammatory

TABLE 22-11
Severity of Disease by Laparoscopic Examination

Severity	Findings
Mild	Erythema, edema, no spontaneous purulent exudate*; tubes freely movable
Moderate	Gross purulent material evident; erythema and edema more marked; tubes may not be freely movable, and fimbria stoma may not be patent
Severe	Pyosalpinx or inflammatory complex Abscess†

From Hager WD, Eschenbach DA, Spence MR, et al: Obstet Gynecol 61:114, 1983. Reprinted with permission from The American College of Obstetricians and Gynecologists.
*The tubes may require manipulation to produce purulent exudate.
†The size of any pelvic abscess should be measured.

TABLE 22-12
Salpingitis: Clinical Criteria for Diagnosis

Criteria	
Abdominal direct tenderness, with or without rebound tenderness	
Tenderness with motion of cervix and uterus	All 3 necessary for diagnosis
Adnexal tenderness	
	plus
Gram stain of endocervix— positive for gram-negative, intracellular diplococci	
Temperature (>38° C)	
Leukocytosis (>10,000)	
Purulent material (white blood cells present) from peritoneal cavity by culdocentesis or laparoscopy	1 or more necessary for diagnosis
Pelvic abscess or inflammatory complex on bimanual examination or on sonography	

From Hager WD, Eschenbach DA, Spence MR, et al: Obstet Gynecol 61:114, 1983. Reprinted with permission from the American College of Obstetricians and Gynecologists.

disease. (Table 22-12). These uniform criteria were adopted by the Obstetrical and Gynecologic Infectious Disease Society. Hadgu and Weström published a multivariate logistic re-

TABLE 22-13
Frequency of Various Symptoms as Reported by Patients in Acute PID and Visually Normal Groups (first-time PID patients)

| | Laparoscopic Diagnosis | | | | |
| | Acute PID (No. = 414) | | Normal (No. = 138) | | |
Symptom	Number	Percent	Number	Percent	P Value
Lower abdominal pain	411	99.3	135	97.8	NS
Vaginal discharge	287	69.3	85	61.6	NS
Temperature ≥38° C	142	34.4	34	24.6	0.05
Irregular bleeding	165	40.0	54	39.1	NS
Urinary symptoms	82	19.8	29	21.0	NS
Vomiting	43	10.4	13	9.4	NS
Protitis symptoms	30	7.3	4	2.9	NS
Other	33	8.0	8	5.8	NS

From Hadgu A, Weström L, Brooks CA, et al: Am J Obstet Gynecol 155:956, 1986.

TABLE 22-14
Frequency of Various Objective Findings at Admission in Acute PID and Visually Normal Groups

| | Laparoscopic Diagnosis | | | | |
| | Acute PID (No. = 414) | | Normal (No. = 138) | | |
Clinical Findings at Admission	Number	Percent	Number	Percent	P Value
Bimanual examination					
Marked tenderness	395	95.4	128	92.8	NS
Palpable mass or swelling	198	47.8	36	26.1	0.001
Erythrocyte sedimentation rate >15 mm/h	336	81.2	78	56.5	0.001
Abnormal vaginal discharge	337	81.4	80	58.0	0.001
Fever (38° C)	146	35.3	21	15.2	0.001

From Hadgu A, Weström L, Brooks CA, et al: Am J Obstet Gynecol 155:956, 1986.

gression analysis of symptoms, signs, and laboratory findings of women laparoscopically diagnosed as having their first episode of acute pelvic inflammatory disease. This mathematic model correctly predicted 87% of cases and had an overall correct classification rate of 76%. The frequencies of various symptoms, signs, and laboratory data from this series of 414 women are depicted in Tables 22-13 and 22-14.

Pain in the lower abdomen and pelvis is by far the most frequent symptom of acute pelvic inflammatory disease. In all large series, more than 90% of women present with diffuse bilateral lower abdominal pain. This pain is usually described as constant and dull. On occasion the pain may become cramping, and it is accentuated by motion or sexual activity. Generally the pain is of short duration, usually less than 7 days. If the pain has been present for longer than 3 weeks, it is unlikely that the patient has acute pelvic inflammatory disease. Approximately 75% of patients with acute pelvic inflammatory disease have an associated endocervical infection and coexistent purulent vaginal discharge. Abnormal vaginal bleeding, especially spotting or menorrhagia, is noted in about 40% of patients. The latter symptom often leads to a suspected diagnosis of ectopic pregnancy. Nausea and vomiting are relatively late symptoms in the course of the disease.

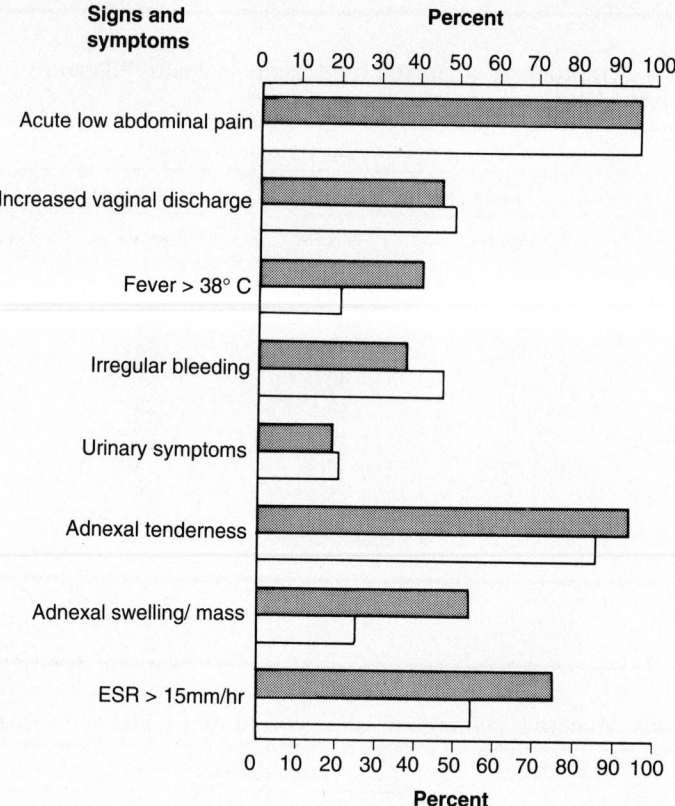

FIGURE 22-2

Comparison of frequency of symptoms, signs, and laboratory findings between patients with acute pelvic inflammatory disease (PID) *(dotted bars)* and suspected PID without pelvic pathology *(open bars)* by laparoscopic examination. (From Jacobson LJ: Am J Obstet Gynecol 138:1008, 1980.)

When one compares the frequency of individual symptoms and signs between women with laparoscopically proven acute pelvic inflammatory disease and those without the disease, there is no significant difference with the exception of fever (Figure 22-2). Acute pelvic inflammatory disease often occurs with minimum symptoms. Approximately 50% of women who are infertile as a result of tubal obstruction do not remember ever having symptoms of acute pelvic infection.

The symptoms of acute pelvic infection secondary to *N. gonorrhoeae* are of rapid onset, and the pelvic pain usually begins a few days after the onset of a menstrual period. Acute pelvic infection caused by *C. trachomatis* alone often has an indolent course with slow onset, less pain, and less fever.

Five to ten percent of women with acute pelvic inflammatory disease develop symptoms of perihepatic inflammation—the Fitz-Hugh–Curtis syndrome. The condition is often mistakenly diagnosed as either pneumonia or acute cholecystitis. Persistent symptoms and signs include right upper quadrant pain, pleuritic pain, and tenderness in the right upper quadrant when the liver is palpated. Liver transaminases may be elevated. Fitz-Hugh–Curtis syndrome develops from transperitoneal or vascular dissemination of either the gonococcus or *Chlamydia* organism to produce the perihepatic inflammation. Currently, *Chlamydia* produces the majority of cases. Other organisms, including anaerobic streptococci and coxsackievirus, have also been associated with this syndrome. Laparoscopy may be useful in the diagnosis of this syndrome. The liver capsule will appear inflamed with classic "violin" string adhesions to the parietal peritoneum beneath the diaphragm. Treatment is the same as the treatment for salpingitis.

Women with laparoscopically confirmed acute pelvic inflammatory disease are often afebrile. Only one out of three women with acute pelvic inflammatory disease presents with a temperature greater than 38° C. Lower abdominal and pelvic tenderness during examination is the hallmark of acute pelvic inflammatory disease. Most women with acute pelvic inflammatory disease have tenderness to direct palpation in the lower abdomen and sometimes may have rebound tenderness. Bilateral tenderness of the parametria and adnexa is usually discovered during pelvic examination. This tenderness is especially noted with movement of the uterus or cervix during the pelvic examination. An ill-defined adnexal fullness is frequently noted. This may represent edema, inflammatory adhesions to either the small or large intestine, or an adnexal complex or abscess. The incidence of true adnexal abscess is approximately 10% in women with acute pelvic inflammatory disease.

Diagnosis

Direct visualization via the laparoscope is the most accurate method of diagnosis of acute pelvic inflammatory disease. Laparoscopy is also indispensable in the clinical research of the disease. Nevertheless the diagnosis of the majority of episodes of acute pelvic inflammatory disease is made on the basis of clinical history and physical examination. Laboratory tests may be obtained, but their results lack sufficient sensitivity and specificity to make them an important factor in establishing the diagnosis. For example, the criteria of the infectious disease society (see Table 22-12) assign a minor role to positive laboratory data. Since clinical symptoms and signs are nonspecific for the disease, when the diagnosis is based on clinical criteria, there is a high percentage of both false positive and false negative rates. Because of the long-term sequelae of the disease, clinicians readily accept that they are treating many women who actually do not have pelvic infection, in order not to omit treating women with early or mild disease.

Leukocytosis is not a reliable indicator of acute pelvic inflammatory disease, nor does it correlate with the need for hospitalization or the severity of tubal inflammation. Less than 50% of women with acute pelvic inflammatory disease have a white blood cell count of greater than 10,000 cells per milliliter. For years, erythrocyte sedimentation rate was a standard laboratory test for women with acute pelvic inflammatory disease. This laboratory test is nonspecific. The sedimentation rate is elevated, greater than 15 mm per hour, in approximately 75% of women with laparoscopically confirmed acute pelvic infection. However, 53% of women with pelvic pain and visually normal pelvic organs have an elevated erythrocyte sedimentation rate. Similarly, the sedimentation rate is a crude indicator of severity of disease and is no longer used to guide therapy.

Women with acute pelvic inflammatory disease should have a sensitive test for human chorionic gonadotrophin to help in the differential diagnosis of ectopic pregnancy. About 3 to 4 of every 100 women who are admitted to a hospital with a diagnosis of acute pelvic infection have an ectopic pregnancy. The diagnosis is often made by aspirating nonclotting bloody fluid by culdocentesis or by diagnostic laparoscopy.

Because most cases of upper genital tract infection are associated with and preceded by lower genital tract infection, it is important to examine the endocervical mucus for inflammatory cells, perform a Gram stain, and culture for both *N. gonorrhoeae* and *C. trachomatis*. A positive gram-stained smear of the endocervical mucus is nonspecific, and a negative smear does not rule out upper tract infection. However, Scandinavian studies have found that acute pelvic inflammatory disease is rare without a concomitant increase in inflammatory cells in the vagina and the cervix. Because acute pelvic inflammatory disease is usually secondary to a sexually transmitted disease, it is ideal to examine, culture, and smear urethral secretions from the male partner. Often this step is not performed for a variety of nonmedical reasons. The Centers for Disease Control has emphasized the importance of treating partners of women with sexually transmitted disease.

European investigators have measured plasma protein levels, "acute phase reactants" including C-reactive protein, and antichymotrypsin to help in the diagnosis of acute pelvic inflammatory disease. These tests are only slightly more sensitive than the sedimentation rate. Other investigators have found that measuring specific genital isoamylases in peritoneal fluid is the best nonculture laboratory test for the disease. These isoamylases may be electrophoretically separated from pancreatic and salivary isoamylases. These enzymes are decreased or absent in peritoneal fluid in cases of acute pelvic inflammatory disease. The major disadvantage of this diagnostic technique is that the test requires several hours to complete.

Ultrasonography is of limited value for patients with mild or moderate pelvic inflammatory disease. Thus ultrasonography should not be routinely ordered for women with acute disease. However, ultrasonography is helpful in distinguishing an adnexal abscess. Ultrasonography is also a noninvasive diagnostic aid for patients who are so tender during pelvic examination that the physician cannot determine the presence or absence of a pelvic mass. Ultrasonography is neither specific nor sensitive in distinguishing the etiology of a pelvic mass.

Culdocentesis sometimes helps in the diagnosis of acute pelvic inflammatory disease when purulent peritoneal fluid is aspirated. With acute pelvic inflammatory disease, the white blood count of peritoneal fluid is greater than 30,000 cells per milliliter. The white blood cell count of women without peritoneal inflammation is less than 1000 cells per milliliter. In some cases endometrial biopsy may be helpful in confirming the diagnosis of coexisting endometritis.

Laparoscopy, as already noted, is the gold standard in the diagnosis of acute pelvic inflammatory disease. Direct visualization of the pelvic organs is the most accurate method of diagnosis. The appearance of the pelvic organs may vary from red, indurated, edematous oviducts, to pockets of purulent material, to a large pyosalpinx or tuboovarian abscess. In recent years there has been increasing use of the laparoscope in women with acute pelvic pain. Laparoscopy is definitely indicated for patients who are not responding to therapy, both to confirm the diagnosis and to obtain cultures of purulent material.

Management

The two most important goals of the medical therapy of acute pelvic inflammatory disease are the resolution of symptoms and the preservation of tubal function. Antibiotic therapy should be started as soon as cervical cultures have been obtained and the diagnosis is suspected; only early diagnosis and early treatment will help reduce the number of women who suffer from the long-term sequelae of the disease. Some studies have suggested that early treatment improves long term fertility. In the management of acute pelvic inflammatory disease, one should not forget the treatment of the male partner and education for the prevention of the disease, including the use of proper contraceptives, which help to reduce the rate of upper genital tract infection.

The choice of antibiotic therapy for an infectious disease is usually based on culture and sensitivity of bacteria obtained directly from the site of the infection. This approach may be accomplished via laparoscopy. However, in most cases this is not financially feasible. Thus selection of antibiotic protocols is largely empirical. In addition to financial factors, laparoscopy is not without its risks. If every woman with acute salpingitis were to undergo laparoscopy, there would be 14 deaths directly associated with this diagnostic technique in the United States each year.

Empirical antibiotic protocols should cover a wide range of bacteria including *N. gonorrhoeae*, *C. trachomatis*, anaerobic rods and cocci, gram-negative aerobic rods, gram-positive aerobes, and *Mycoplasma* species (Table 22-15). Selection of one antibiotic protocol over another will often depend on the clinical history (Table 22-16). For example, acute pelvic inflammatory disease following an operative procedure is usually caused by endogenous flora of the vagina.

Grimes analyzed more than 25 million prescriptions written between 1966 and 1983 in the United States for treatment of acute pelvic infections. He discovered that most women were treated as outpatients and received only a single antibiotic. Less than one third of women received tetracycline to treat possible chlamydial infection. It is hoped that these statistics change as the polymicrobial etiology of acute pelvic inflammatory disease receives greater appreciation.

In the United States, for economic reasons, most women with acute pelvic inflammatory disease are not hospitalized. In Scandinavia, with a different health care system, the vast majority of women are treated as inpatients. Studies have documented a 10% to 20% treatment failure rate (persistence of symptoms and signs) for women receiving oral antibiotics as outpatients. Inpatient failure rates with intravenous antibiotics are approximately 5% to 10%.

TABLE 22-15
Microorganisms Isolated from the Fallopian Tubes of Patients with Pelvic Inflammatory Disease

Type of Agent	Organism
Sexually transmitted disease	*Chlamydia trachomatis*
	Neisseria gonorrhoeae
	Mycoplasma hominis
Endogenous agent	*Streptococcus* species
Aerobic or facultative	*Staphylococcus* species
	Haemophilus species
	Escherichia coli
Anaerobic	*Bacteroides* species
	Peptococcus species
	Peptostreptococcus species
	Clostridium species
	Actinomyces species

From Weström L: Sex Transm Dis 11:439, 1984.

TABLE 22-16
Probability of PID Being Associated or Not Associated with STD

	Risk of Indicated Type of PID	
Factor	Probably STD Associated	Probably Not STD Associated
Age <25 years	+++	+
Age >30 years	+	+++
Mild disease	+++	—
Severe disease	+	+++
Abscess formation	+	+++
Numerous sexual partners	+++	+
Symptoms in partners	+++	—
Use of IUD	+	+++
Earlier PID episode	++	+++
Good general condition	+++	+
Poor general condition	+	+++

From Weström L: Sex Transm Dis 11:439, 1984.
+++, most likely; ++, likely; +, less likely.

Presently in the United States approximately three out of every four women with acute pelvic infection are being treated as outpatients for their disease. The Centers for Disease Control (CDC) has recommended patients receive cefoxitin, 2 g IM, plus probenecid, 1 g orally, concurrently, or ceftriaxone 250 mg IM plus a 10-14 day course of doxycycline or tetracycline

CENTERS FOR DISEASE CONTROL— AMBULATORY MANAGEMENT OF PID

Recommended Regimen

Cefoxitin 2 g intramuscularly plus probenecid, 1 g orally concurrently or ceftriaxone 250 mg intramuscularly, or equivalent cephalosporin plus doxycycline 100 mg orally 2 times a day for 10 to 14 days, or tetracycline 500 mg orally 4 times a day for 10 to 14 days.

Alternative for Patients Who Do Not Tolerate Doxycycline

Erythromycin, 500 mg orally 4 times a day for 10 to 14 days may be substituted for doxycycline/tetracycline. This regimen, however, is based on limited clinical data.

From Centers for Disease Control: MMWR 38(8S):29, 1989.

(see box above). The CDC recommends that all patients receive tetracycline because of the high prevalence of *chlamydia*. Treatment by one drug alone without tetracycline does not cover the possibility that *C. trachomatis* is present. The failure rate of outpatient oral therapy may be related to noncompliance, reinfection, or inadequate antibiotic coverage for penicillinase-producing or chromosomally mediated resistant *N. gonorrhoeae* or facultative or anaerobic organisms involved in upper genital tract infection that are resistant to the drug prescribed. Thus culture with sensitivity testing is imperative.

It is important to reexamine women within 48 to 72 hours of initiating outpatient therapy to evaluate the response of the disease to oral antibiotics. The patient should be hospitalized when the therapeutic response is not optimal. If the disease is responding well, approximately 2 weeks after therapy another specimen should be cultured to test for clinical cure.

Both rectal and pharyngeal gonorrheal infections are more difficult to cure than endocervical infections. Handsfield reports that pharyngeal gonorrhea is the most difficult to cure, with a cure rate of 50% to 70%. The CDC advises using ceftriaxone in a single dose of 250 mg for infections of either gastrointestinal anatomic site plus doxycycline 100 mg orally 2 times a day for 7 days. However for consistancy, we treat with doxycycline for 10-14 days.

Ideally, every woman with acute pelvic in-

INDICATIONS FOR HOSPITALIZING PATIENTS WITH PELVIC INFLAMMATORY DISEASE

- Nulliparity
- Presence of tuboovarian complex or abscess
- Pregnancy
- Uncertain diagnosis
- Gastrointestinal symptoms
- Peritonitis in upper quadrants
- Presence of an intrauterine device
- History of operative or diagnostic procedures
- Inadequate response to outpatient therapy

flammatory disease would be hospitalized for the first few days of antibiotic treatment. Because this therapy is not practical financially, it is important to develop a list of criteria or indications for hospitalization (see box above). If possible, young nulliparous women should be hospitalized with their first episode of acute pelvic inflammatory disease. This would ensure maximum levels of antibiotics in the hope of preventing microscopic tubal damage. An almost absolute indication for hospitalization is an adnexal mass. Outpatient therapy does not provide high enough levels of appropriate antibiotics to successfully penetrate an abscess cavity. The association of a viable pregnancy and pelvic inflammatory disease, without a foreign body being inserted into the uterus, is a rare event. However, the second trimester uterus is a fertile ground for severe pelvic infection since infection does not become localized. A patient may develop widespread signs and symptoms of sepsis before the subtle inflammatory changes in the pelvis are recognized.

Women for whom the definitive diagnosis of acute pelvic inflammatory disease is questionable are best admitted to the hospital. Any large series of 100 consecutive suspected cases of pelvic inflammatory disease will include three or four patients with ectopic pregnancy and three or four patients with acute appendicitis. Both the wide clinical spectrum of pelvic inflammatory disease and the difficulty of establishing a correct diagnosis without direct visualization of the pelvic organs are uncertainties that are best clarified in the hospital. The foundation of outpatient therapy of acute pelvic

inflammatory disease is broad-spectrum oral antibiotics. If the patient presents with gastrointestinal symptoms, such as nausea and vomiting, there is a good chance that she will not be able to tolerate her medications. Acute peritonitis in the right upper quadrant, especially liver tenderness without hepatomegaly, is another indication for hospital admission.

Acute pelvic inflammatory disease associated with the presence of an IUD is usually more advanced at the time of diagnosis than infection without a foreign body. Both patient and physician delays in diagnosis are not unusual. Often women misinterpret the early signs and symptoms of an infection as being related to the IUD. Pelvic infections with an IUD in place and pelvic infections following operative or diagnostic procedures often are due to anaerobic bacteria. Thus it is best to hospitalize these patients and use intravenous antibiotics. The IUD should be removed and cultured as soon as appropriate levels of intravenous antibiotics have been obtained. Finally, if a therapeutic response or compliance with oral medications has not been optimal, the patient should be admitted for intravenous antibiotic therapy.

In September 1989 the CDC published their most recent guidelines for inpatient treatment of acute pelvic inflammatory disease. Their recommendations have been widely accepted with only minor modifications. Their protocols stress the polymicrobial etiology of acute pelvic infection, the increasing importance of C. trachomatis, and the emergence of penicillin-resistant N. gonorrhea. Thus each protocol includes at least two antibiotics (see box on the facing page). With both intravenous protocols the CDC recommends a minimum of 4 days of therapy and continuation of the intravenous antibiotics at least 48 hours after the patient's fever abates. When the patient has a mass, we add ampicillin to clindamycin and gentamycin. However, for patients without a mass, we switch to oral antibiotics when the symptoms have diminished and the patient has been afebrile for 24 hours.

Regimen A (see box) is a combination of intravenous doxycycline and intravenous cefoxitin. It is excellent for community-acquired infection because it treats both gonorrhea and chlamydial infection. Doxycycline and cefoxitin provide excellent coverage for N. gonorrhoeae, C. trachomatis, and also penicillinase-producing N. gonorrhoeae. Cefoxitin is an excellent

CENTERS FOR DISEASE CONTROL— RECOMMENDED REGIMENS FOR INPATIENT THERAPY FOR ACUTE PID

Recommended Regimen A

Cefoxitin 2 g intravenously every 6 hours, or cefotetan intravenously 2 g every 12 hours plus doxycycline 100 mg every 12 hours orally or intravenously. This regimen is given for at least 48 hours after the patient clinically improves. After discharge from hospital, doxycycline is continued at 100 mg orally 2 times a day for a total of 10 to 14 days.

Recommended Regimen B

Clindamycin intravenously 900 mg every 8 hours, plus gentamicin loading dose intravenously or intramuscularly (2 mg/kg) followed by a maintenance dose (1.5 mg/kg) every 8 hours. This regimen is given for at least 48 hours after the patient improves. After discharge from hospital, doxycycline is continued at 100 mg orally 2 times a day for 10 to 14 days total. Continuation of clindamycin, 450 mg orally, 4 times daily, for 10 to 14 days, may be considered as an alternative. Continuation of medication after hospital discharge is important for the treatment of possible *C. trachomatis* infection. Clindamycin has more complete anaerobic coverage. Although limited data suggest that clindamycin is effective against *C. trachomatis* infection, doxycycline remains the treatment of choice for patients with chlamydial disease. When *C. trachomatis* is strongly suspected or confirmed as an etiologic agent, doxycycline is the preferable alternative. In such instances, doxycycline therapy may be started during hospitalization if initiation of therapy before hospital discharge is thought likely to improve the patient's compliance.

From Centers for Disease Control: MMWR 38(8S):1, 1989.

antibiotic against *Peptococcus, Peptostreptococcus,* and *E. coli.* The disadvantage of this combination is that the two drugs are less than ideal for a pelvic abscess or for anaerobic infections. In a comparative trial of the two regimens, Walters and Gibbs found no difference in clinical cure.

Doxycycline should be included in the regimen of follow-up oral therapy. Sweet observed 17 women with pelvic inflammatory disease who initially had endometrial cultures positive for *Chlamydia.* Clinically, 16 of 17 women responded to treatment with cephalosporins alone. However, posttreatment endometrial cultures remained positive for *Chlamydia* in 12 of 13 women. Therefore without tetracycline or erythromycin a patient may appear free of symptoms but may still be harboring *Chlamydia.*

Regimen B is a combination of clindamycin and an aminoglycoside (gentamicin). Regimen B has the advantage of providing excellent coverage for anaerobic infections and facultative gram-negative rods. Therefore it is preferred for patients with an abscess, IUD-related infections, and pelvic infections after a diagnostic or operative procedure. We prefer triple coverage with the addition of a penicillin. Studies have demonstrated that high intravenous levels of clindamycin, such as 900 mg every 8 hours, provide activity against 90% of bacterial strains of *Chlamydia.* It is important with aminoglycoside therapy to obtain peak and trough serum levels. Peak levels should be approximately 8 μg/ml and trough levels less than 2 μg/ml. Peak and trough levels should be obtained after 24 hours of intravenous therapy and approximately every 4 days thereafter. The incidence of aminoglycoside toxicity is 2% to 3%, and approximately 25% of women require an adjustment in their intravenous dosage. Aztreonam, a new monobactam, has antibiotic spectrum similar to the aminoglycosides but without renal toxicity. It is, however, much more expensive. It may be given in a dose of 2g IV q 8h. A third generation cephalosporin may also be used instead of an aminoglycoside in a patient with renal disease.

In summary, neither regimen A nor regimen B is uniformly effective for all patients. To date there are not sufficient clinical data to suggest superiority of one regimen over another, either with respect to initial response or subsequent fertility. One must individualize using the clinical history, which will generally indicate the types of microorganisms causing the disease.

Operative treatment of acute pelvic inflammatory disease has decreased markedly in the past 10 years. Operations are restricted to life-threatening infections, ruptured tuboovarian abscesses, drainage of a pelvic abscess that is pointing into the cul-de-sac, persistent masses

TABLE 22-17

Epidemiologic Correlates of Tuboovarian Abscesses (TOAs) Diagnosed Clinically and those of TOAs Confirmed Surgically

Patient Category (No. of Patients)	No. of Patients (%) with Indicated Epidemiologic Correlate			
	Nulliparous	Prior History of Gonorrhea	Prior History of Salpingitis	IUD Usage
TOA clinically diagnosed only (160)	90 (56)	48 (30)	52 (32.5)	53 (33)
TOA surgically confirmed (72)	30 (42)	23 (32)	24 (33)	23 (32)
TOA not excised (20)	9 (45)	6 (30)	6 (30)	4 (20)
TOA excised (52)	21 (40)	17 (33)	18 (35)	19 (36)
TOTAL (232)	120 (52)	71 (31)	76 (33)	76 (33)

From Landers DV and Sweet RL: Rev Infect Dis 5:878, 1983.

in some older women for whom future child-bearing is not a consideration, and removal of a persistent symptomatic mass. Because of the techniques of in vitro fertilization, every effort is made to perform conservative surgery and preserve ovarian and uterine function in women who have not completed their families. Unilateral removal of a tuboovarian complex or an abscess is a frequent conservative operation for acute pelvic inflammatory disease. Similarly, drainage of a cul-de-sac abscess via a culpotomy incision results in preservation of the reproductive organs.

Recently there have been reports of small series of percutaneous aspiration or drainage of pelvic abscesses under ultrasonic guidance. Percutaneous aspiration under ultrasonic guidance may be transvaginal or transabdominal. This technique has initially shown positive results. However, fertility and ectopic pregnancy rates after percutaneous transvaginal drainage are unknown at this time. Long-term recurrence and sequelae need to be evaluated before this technique is accepted as a therapeutic standard. Laparoscopic aspiration of tuboovarian complexes is investigational at this time. It has shown good results, but does not have greater benefit than percutaneous ultrasound-guided aspiration of abscess cavities. Laparoscopic aspiration obviously carries more operative risks than ultrasound-guided aspiration.

Rigorously defined, an abscess is a collection of pus within a newly created space. In contrast, a tuboovarian complex is a collection of pus within an anatomic space created by adherence of adjacent organs. Clinically, they are treated in similar fashions. Landers and Sweet

TABLE 22-18

Presenting Symptoms and Findings among 232 Patients with Tuboovarian Abscess

Symptom/Finding	No. of Patients in Indicated Group (%) with Presenting Symptom or Finding	
	Medically Treated (No. = 175)	Surgically Treated (No. = 57)
Acute pain	158 (90)	48 (84)
Chronic pain	29 (17)	14 (25)
Fever/chills	86 (49)	31 (53)
Vaginal discharge	53 (30)	11 (19)
Abnormal uterine bleeding	37 (21)	11 (19)
Nausea	44 (25)	17 (30)
Vomiting	23 (13)	13 (23)
Temperature >100° F	102 (58)	37 (65)
White blood cell count >10,000/mm^3	114 (72)	44 (77)

From Landers DV and Sweet RL: Rev Infect Dis 5:879, 1983.

published a large series of 232 women with tuboovarian abscesses or complexes initially treated conservatively with antibiotics (Tables 22-17 and 22-18).

Unilateral tuboovarian abscesses were discovered in 164 (71%) of the women. Seven women (3%) suffered acute rupture of their tuboovarian abscesses. There was no statistical difference between the incidence of unilateral tuboovarian abscess in women with IUDs and those without IUDs. Landers and Sweet described a 20% rate of early treatment

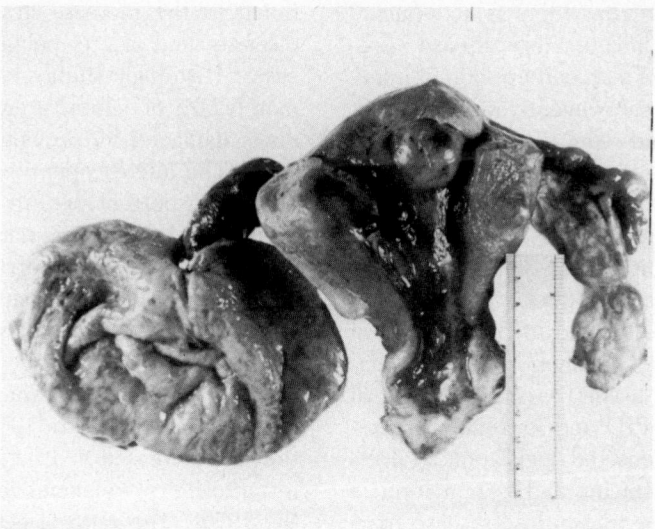

FIGURE 22-3
Pyosalpinx. Right tube is markedly enlarged and contains 50 ml of creamy pus. Tubal wall is thickened. (From Janovski NA, editor: Color atlas of gross gynecologic and obstetric pathology New York, 1969, McGraw-Hill, Inc, p 131.)

failure after 48 to 72 hours of antibiotic therapy as a result of persistent pain or enlargement of the tuboovarian abscess or complex. In addition, 31% required an operation several weeks to months following their acute infections. A fact that was brought to light from this study was that even though women had prior tuboovarian abscesses, 14% subsequently experienced an intrauterine pregnancy.

Abscesses caused by acute pelvic inflammatory disease contain a mixture of anaerobes and facultative or aerobic organisms (Figure 22-3). The environment of an abscess cavity results in a low level of oxygen tension. Therefore anaerobic organisms predominate and have been cultured from 60% to 100% of reported cases. Landers and Sweet noted that in 68% of their cases the abscess decreased in size if the antibiotic protocol contained clindamycin, versus a decrease in mass size in only 37% of cases when clindamycin was not included in the antibiotic therapy. Basic investigations have discovered that clindamycin penetrates the human neutrophil, and it is possible that this property facilitates the level of clindamycin within the abscess. Clindamycin is also stable in the abscess environment, which is not true of many other antibiotics. Thus a combination of clindamycin and an aminoglycoside is considered the gold standard for treatment of tuboovarian abscess. This combination does not treat the enterococcus, and ampicillin should be added if there is suspicion that this organism is involved. Metronidazole is an effective alternative to clindamycin for anaerobic infections. If abscesses do not promptly respond to parenteral broad-spectrum antibiotics, drainage is imperative.

Sequelae

Before antibiotic therapy, the mortality associated with acute pelvic inflammatory disease was 1%. Grimes has estimated that there is presently one death every other day in the United States directly related to pelvic inflammatory disease. Most of these deaths result from rupture of tuboovarian abscesses. The mortality today is 5% to 10% for ruptured tuboovarian abscesses even with modern medical and operative therapy. Each year approximately 40 women die of ectopic pregnancy in the United States, and at least 50% of these ectopic implantations are secondary to the tubal damage produced by acute salpingitis.

Recurrent acute pelvic inflammatory disease is experienced by approximately 25% of women. Younger women become reinfected twice as often as older women. A great challenge to health care providers is to educate women with pelvic inflammatory disease to reduce their chances of a second episode of infection. It is essential that preventive medicine include treatment and education of the male partner. Selection of contraceptives that will reduce the chance of upper genital tract infections and liberal prescriptions for treatment of lower genital tract disease for these women are also important. Because sequelae to PID, both overt and silent, are related to the number of infections, prevention cannot be overemphasized. In response to the escalating financial and human cost of PID and its relation to recurrence, Sweden enacted legislation in 1988 mandating partner tracing and examination of women with sexually transmitted disease, particularly those with cultures positive for *chlamydia*. Because the majority of PID in the United States is related to sexually transmitted diseases, increased attention to partner treatment and education is appropriate.

The number of ectopic pregnancies has more than doubled over the past 20 years. This increased rate is directly parallel and proportional to the increase in sexually transmitted diseases and acute pelvic inflammatory diseases. Histologic studies estimate that approximately 50% of ectopic pregnancies occur in oviducts damaged by previous salpingitis (Figure 22-4). The microscopic tubal damage either retards transport of or entraps fertilized ovum, thereby producing implantation in the tube rather than the endometrial cavity. Weström, in a prospective long-term follow-up of women with acute salpingitis in Sweden, discovered a rate of 1 ectopic pregnancy to every 24 intrauterine pregnancies for women treated for acute pelvic infection in the 1960s. In a later study the rate increased to 1 ectopic pregnancy to 16 intrauterine pregnancies for women treated in the 1970s. The ratio of ectopic pregnancies to intrauterine pregnancies was 1 to 147 in a controlled group of women who had not experienced tubal infection.

The chance that a women will develop chronic pelvic pain following acute salpingitis is 4 times greater than the risk for control subjects. Approximately 20% of women with acute pelvic infections subsequently develop chronic

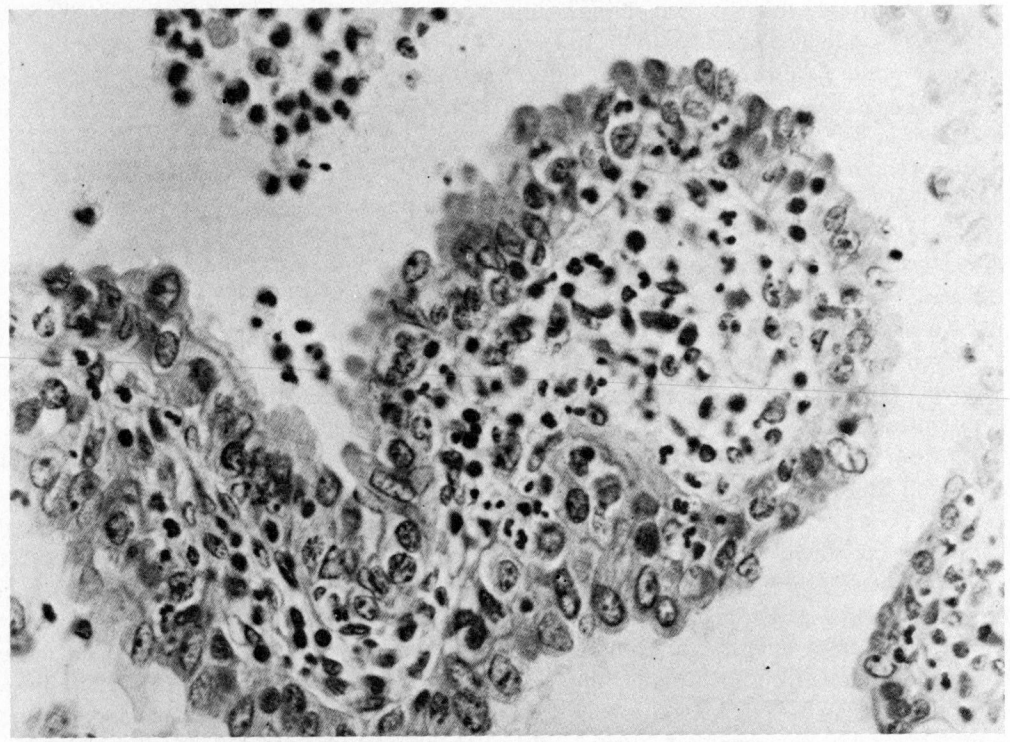

FIGURE 22-4
Microscopic appearance of salpingitis. (From Gompel C and Silverberg SG, editors: Pathology in gynecology and obstetrics, ed 2, Philadelphia, 1977, JB Lippincott Co, p 253.)

pelvic pain, versus approximately 5% in a control group without pelvic infection. Among women with chronic pelvic pain, approximately two out of three are involuntarily infertile, and a similar percentage have deep dyspareunia. Chronic pelvic pain may be caused by a hydrosalpinx, a collection of sterile, watery fluid in the fallopian tube. A hydrosalpinx is the end-stage development of a pyosalpinx. Chronic pain often develops in a woman even though she may have had a normal pelvic examination when examined 4 to 8 weeks following her acute infection. The pain may be related to adhesions surrounding the ovary. The hypothesis has been advanced that the chronic dull pain is secondary to menstrual cycle–related changes in the volume of the ovary, which produce tension in the surrounding adhesions. Some women with chronic pelvic pain benefit from long-term progestin or danazol therapy. All women with chronic pelvic pain believed to be caused by acute pelvic inflammatory disease should undergo laparoscopy to establish the diagnosis and rule out other diseases, such as endometriosis. Conservative surgery for this sequela via either laparoscopy or celiotomy is often successful.

Acute pelvic infection is one of the major causes of female infertility. Epidemiologic studies estimate that between 4% and 13% of women either are infertile or have an operative procedure secondary to acute pelvic inflammatory disease. In one survey of women not using contraception, 15% of the women considered themselves sterile as a result of salpingitis. Before antibiotic therapy, 50% to 75% of women who had experienced upper genital tract infections were sterile.

The sequelae of infections vary from a patent oviduct, to peritubular and periovarian adhesions that may hinder ovum pickup, to complete tubal obstruction. Tubal obstructions that are secondary to infection are commonly found at the fimbrial end or the cornual region of the oviduct. An alarming factor that has been documented with chlamydial infection is the tubal damage from subacute pelvic inflammatory disease. Patton et al. found essentially equally severe tubal damage, adhesion, degeneration of endosalpingeal structures, and cilia dysfunction in women with acute chlamydial PID and women with silent chlamydial infection.

Weström has presented long-term follow-up statistics for women with pelvic inflammatory

TABLE 22-19

Reproductive Events After One or More Tubal Infections in 1000 Women 15 to 34 Years of Age (Lund, 1960-1974) Followed to First Pregnancy or, if Not Pregnant, for 8 Years

	No./1000 Women
Pregnant	
Intrauterine	624
Ectopic	41
Not pregnant	
Voluntarily	171
Involuntarily	
Tubal occlusion	126
Other causes	38

From Weström L: Am J Obstet Gynecol 138:888, 1980.

TABLE 22-20

Percent Infertility Because of Tubal Occlusion after Mild, Moderately Severe, and Severe Infections in Women with One Episode of Salpingitis and Exposure to Chance of Pregnancy

Inflammatory Changes	% Infertility Postsalpingitis in Age Group		
	15-24 Years	25-34 Years	Total
Mild	5.8	7.8	6.1
Moderately severe	10.8	22.0	13.4
Severe	27.3	40.0	30.0

From Weström L: Am J Obstet Gynecol 138:888, 1980.

disease in Sweden (Table 22-19). He discovered that the infertility rate was significantly lower in the younger group than in the older group following a single episode of infection (Table 22-20). Women with mild episodes of acute pelvic inflammatory disease were 7 times less likely to suffer tubal obstruction than women with severe disease. The infertility rate increased directly with the number of episodes of acute pelvic infection (Table 22-21). The latter is not surprising, because the prevalence of most long-term sequelae is directly proportional to the number of episodes of acute pelvic inflammatory disease.

TABLE 22-21
Percent of Infertility Because of Tubal Occlusion after One, Two, and Three or More Episodes of Salpingitis in Women Exposed to a Chance of Pregnancy

No. of Infections	% Infertility Postalpingitis in Age Group		
	15-24 yr	25-34 yr	Total
1	9.4	19.2	11.4
2	20.9	31.0	23.1
3+	51.6	60.0	54.3

From Weström L: Am J Obstet Gynecol 138:880, 1980.

ACTINOMYCES INFECTION

Actinomyces is a rare cause of upper genital tract infection. *Actinomyces israelii* is the most common species found and is a gram-positive anaerobe, which is difficult to culture. To successfully culture this organism, an anaerobic environment must be maintained for 2 to 3 weeks.

A. israelii is discovered either by histologic examination or culture from women with tuboovarian abscesses. There are many large series of tuboovarian abscesses without a single case of *A. israelii* described. Most cases described have been in women wearing an IUD. Usually *A. israelii* is part of a polymicrobial infection, and whether its role is primary or secondary in the infectious process is unknown.

Recently there has been a controversy as to the significance of discovering actinomycetes on a Papanicolaou smear of women wearing an IUD. Burkman et al. reported that women with a positive smear had a 3.5-fold risk of hospitalization for acute pelvic inflammatory disease. Also, these investigators found that when women developed acute infections, there was a higher tendency to develop tuboovarian abscesses. Other investigations have disagreed with this hypothesis. It is controversial whether women without IUDs have actinomycetes on a Papanicolaou smear less often than women with an IUDs. Many clinicians who find a woman with an IUD and actinomycetes on Pap smear will remove the IUD and treat with penicillin.

Although some investigators suggest that actinomycetes produce a chronic endometritis

with an associated foul-smelling discharge, the diagnosis of *Actinomyces* infection is usually not made until a tuboovarian abscess is examined by the pathologist. Then the classic "sulfur granules" are observed histologically.

Although much has been written about chronic draining sinuses with *Actinomyces* infection, this complication is unusual in gynecology. However, when this organism is present, the patient should receive oral penicillin for 12 weeks following an operative procedure.

TUBERCULOSIS

Tuberculosis of the upper genital tract, primarily chronic salpingitis and chronic endometritis, is a rare disease in the United States. Most gynecologists will practice a lifetime and not encounter a single case. However, it is a frequent cause of chronic pelvic inflammatory disease and infertility in other parts of the world. Thus it should be suspected in immigrants, especially those from Asia, the Middle East, and Latin America.

Pelvic tuberculosis may be produced by either *Mycobacterium tuberculosis* or *Mycobacterium bovis*. The primary site of infection for tuberculosis is usually the lung. Early in the course of pulmonary infection the bacteria spread hematogenously, and the infection becomes located in the oviduct. Subsequently the bacilli usually spread to the endometrium and occasionally to the ovaries. However, the oviducts are the primary and predominant site of pelvic tuberculosis. In Third World countries without pasteurization of milk, bovine tuberculosis produces primary infections in the human gastrointestinal tract. Subsequent lymphatic or hematogenous dissemination results in pelvic tuberculosis.

The predominant presentations of this chronic infection are infertility and abnormal uterine bleeding. Mild to moderate chronic abdominal and pelvic pain occur in 35% of women with the disease. Advanced cases are often accompanied by ascites. Some women may be asymptomatic. The findings at pelvic examination are normal in approximately 50% of cases. The remaining patients have mild adnexal tenderness and bilateral adnexal masses, with an inability to manipulate the adnexa because of scarring and fixation.

Tuberculous salpingitis should be suspected

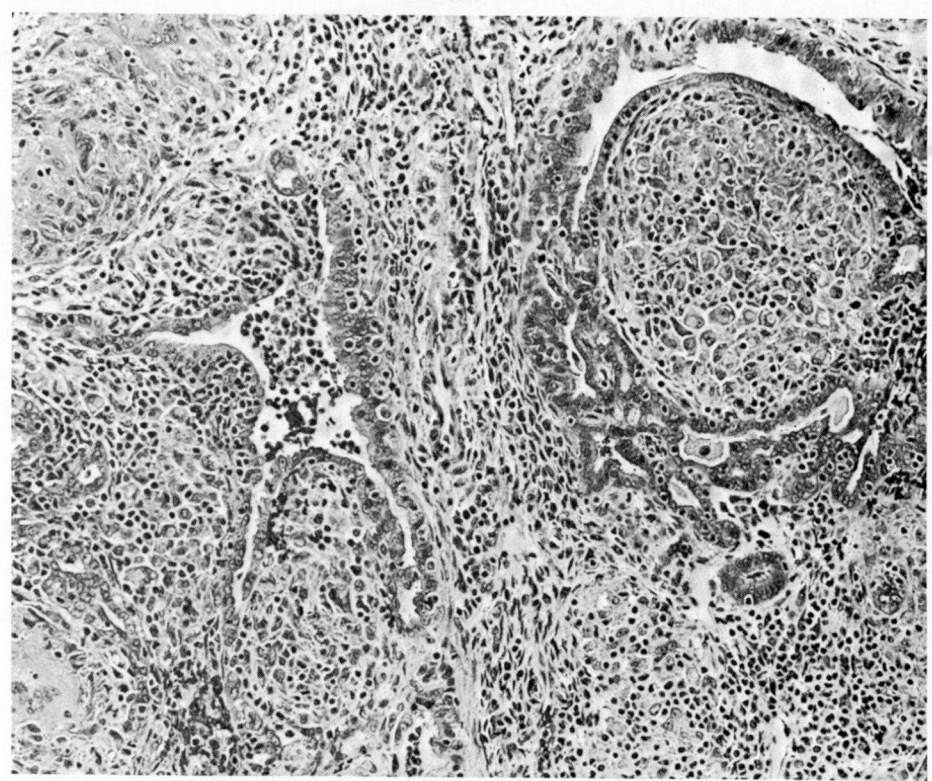

FIGURE 22-5
Tuberculous salpingitis: Langhans' giant cell granuloma. (From Gompel C and Silverberg SG, editors: Pathology in gynecology and obstetrics, ed 2, Philadelphia, 1977 JB Lippincott Co, p 258.)

when a patient is not responding to conventional antibiotic therapy for acute bacterial pelvic inflammatory disease. Results of a tuberculin skin test will be positive. However, approximately one in three women does not have evidence of pulmonary tuberculosis on chest x-ray films. The diagnosis may be established by performing an endometrial biopsy late in the secretory phase of the cycle. A portion of the endometrial biopsy should be sent for culture and animal inoculation, while the remaining portion should be examined histologically. The findings of classic giant cells, granulomas, and caseous necrosis confirm the diagnosis (Figure 22-5). Approximately two out of three women with tuberculous salpingitis will have concomitant tuberculous endometritis. Pelvic tuberculosis may not be diagnosed until laparotomy or celiotomy, when the characteristic changes may be visualized. The distal ends of the oviduct remain everted, producing a "tobacco pouch" appearance. When the diagnosis has been established, the patient should have a chest x-ray examination, intravenous pyleogram, serial gastric washings, and urine cultures for tuberculosis. Approximately 10% of women with pelvic tuberculosis have concomitant urinary tract tuberculosis.

Treatment of pelvic tuberculosis is medical, with a combination of two antibiotics for 24 months. Occasionally a woman becomes pregnant following medical therapy. However, infertility is the more common sequela. Combination therapy is used to decrease the rate of drug-resistant organisms. Present antibiotic therapy includes isoniazid (INH) (300 mg per day) and ethambutol (Myambutol) (1200 mg per day). Operative therapy is reserved for women with persistent pelvic masses, women with resistant organisms, women over 40 years of age, and women whose endometrial cultures remain positive.

_____ **KEY POINTS** _____

- The diagnosis of chronic endometritis is established by the finding of plasma cells on endometrial biopsy.

- Acute pelvic inflammatory disease is usually caused by a polymicrobial infection of organisms ascending from the vagina and cervix, traveling along the mucosa of the endometrium to infect the mucosa of the oviduct. The primary bacterial organisms cultured from tubal fluid and mucosa include *Neisseria gonorrhoeae*, *Chlamydia trachomatis*, endogenous aerobic and anaerobic bacteria.

- Approximately one in four women with acute pelvic inflammatory disease experiences further medical sequelae.

- Approximately 15% of women with cervical infection by gonorrhea subsequently develop pelvic inflammatory disease. The virulence of the strain of *N. gonorrhoeae* helps to predict the incidence of upper genital tract infection.

- *C. trachomatis* is rapidly becoming the most prevalent organism causing pelvic inflammatory disease. The salpingitis it produces is insidious in onset.

- Upper tract chlamydial infection increases the risk of an ectopic pregnancy from 3 to 6 times compared with women without chlamydial infection.

- There is a strong correlation between the incidence of sexually transmitted disease within a population and the incidence of acute pelvic inflammatory disease.

- Acute pelvic inflammatory disease is a condition of young menstruating women, with 75% of cases occurring in women younger than 25 years of age. The risk for a sexually active adolescent female is 1 in 8. This decreases to 1 in 80 for women over the age of 25.

- When pelvic inflammatory disease is found in the postmenopausal woman, genital malignancies, diabetes, and/or concurrent intestinal disease is usually found.

- Oral contraceptive use provides a twofold preventive effect in inhibiting the development of pelvic inflammatory disease. One mechanism may be the thickening of cervical mucus caused by the progestin component of the oral contraceptives. The other may be the decrease in the duration of menstrual flow, which creates a shorter interval for bacterial colonization of the upper genital tract.

- Because acute pelvic inflammatory disease has a wide range of nonspecific clinical symptoms, there is both a high false positive rate and a high false negative rate when the diagnosis is based on clinical findings and laboratory results.

- Approximately 20% to 25% of women have no identifiable intraabdominal or pelvic disease by laparoscopy when diagnosed as having acute pelvic inflammatory disease on the basis of history or physical or laboratory examination.

- Pain in the lower abdomen and pelvis is the most frequent symptom of acute pelvic inflammatory disease, and in all large series more than 90% of women with the diagnosis have some type of abdominal pain.

- Seventy-five percent of patients with acute pelvic inflammatory disease have an associated endocervical infection and coexistent purulent vaginal discharge.

- Nausea and vomiting are comparatively late symptoms in the course of acute pelvic inflammatory disease.

- From 5% to 10% of women with acute pelvic inflammatory disease develop perihepatic inflammation, Fitz-Hugh–Curtis syndrome.

- The treatment of Fitz-Hugh–Curtis syndrome is the same treatment as that of pelvic inflammatory disease.

- Approximately one third of women with acute pelvic inflammatory disease present with a temperature greater than 38° C.

- The incidence of true adnexal abscess is approximately 10% in women with acute pelvic inflammatory disease.

- Less than 50% of women with acute pelvic inflammatory disease have a white blood cell count of greater than 10,000 cells per milliliter.

- Laparoscopy is the optimum method to accurately establish the diagnosis of acute pelvic inflammatory disease.

- Women who are being treated as outpatients for acute pelvic inflammatory disease should be reexamined within 48 to 72 hours of initiation of therapy to evaluate the response of the disease to oral antibiotics.

- Surgical treatment for acute pelvic inflammatory disease is restricted to life-threatening infections, ruptured tuboovarian abscesses, drainage of a pelvic abscess that is pointing into the cul-de-sac, persistent masses in some older women for whom future childbearing is not a consideration, and removal of a persistent symptomatic mass. Unilateral removal of a tuboovarian complex or abscess is a frequent conservative operation for acute pelvic inflammatory disease for women desiring future childbearing.

- If a pelvic abscess does not respond to parenteral broad-spectrum antibiotics, drainage is imperative.

- Recurrent acute pelvic inflammatory disease is experienced by approximately 25% of women. The chance that a woman will develop chronic pelvic pain following acute pelvic inflammatory disease is 4 times greater than the risk for control subjects.

- Because sequelae to PID both overt and silent are related to the number of infections, prevention cannot be overemphasized.

- The chance that a women will develop chronic pelvic pain after acute salpingitis is 4 times greater than the risk for control subjects.

- Chronic pelvic pain may be caused by a hydrosalpinx, a collection of sterile, watery fluid in the fallopian tube.

- *Actinomyces* is a rare cause of upper genital tract infection. *Actinomyces israelii* is the most common species found and is a gram-positive anaerobe, which is difficult to culture.

- Pelvic tuberculosis may be produced by either *Mycobacterium tuberculosis* or *Mycobacterium bovis.* The primary sites of infection are the lung and the gastrointestinal tract.

- The predominant presentations of tuberculous salpingitis are infertility and abnormal uterine bleeding.

BIBLIOGRAPHY

Ahmad MM: IUDs and actinomyces, IPPF Med Bul 21:3, 1987.

Bell TA and Holmes KK: Age-specific risks of syphilis, gonorrhea, and hospitalized pelvic inflammatory disease in sexually experienced U.S. women, Sex Transm Dis 11:291, 1984.

Bulger EA and Parenti DM: The quinolines, Drug Ther Apr:131, 1989

Burkman R, Schlesselman S, McCaffrey L, et al. The relationship of genital tract actinomycetes and the development of pelvic inflammatory disease, Am J Obstet Gynecol 143:585, 1982.

Burnakis TG and Hildebrandt NB: Pelvic inflammatory disease: review with emphasis on antimicrobial therapy, Rev Infect Dis 8:86, 1986.

Centers for Disease Control: STD treatment guidelines 1989, MMWR 38(8S)1, 1989.

Chow JM, Yonekuram L, Richwald GA, et al: The association between *Chlamydia trachomatisa* and ectopic pregnancy, JAMA 263:3164, 1990.

Conway D, Caul EO, Hull MGR, et al: Chlamydial serology in fertile and infertile women, Lancet 1:191, 1984.

Dan BB: Sex, lives, and *Chlamydia* rates, JAMA 263:3191, 1990.

Darling MRN, Golan A, and Rubin A: Colpotomy drainage of pelvic abscesses, Acta Obstet Gynecol Scand 62:257, 1983.

Dodson MG: Acute PID: diagnosis and management, Med Aspect Human Sexual Aug:26, 1990.

Dodson MG and Faro S: The polymicrobial etiology of acute pelvic inflammatory disease and treatment regimens, Rev Infect Dis 7:S696, 1985.

Eschenbach DA: Epidemiology and diagnosis of acute pelvic inflammatory disease, Obstet Gynecol 55:142S, 1980.

Eschenbach DA: New concepts of obstetric and gynecologic infection, Arch Intern Med 142:2039, 1982.

Eschenbach DA: Acute pelvic inflammatory disease, vol 1. In Gynecology and obstetrics, Philadelphia, 1985, Harper & Row, Publishers.

Gompel C and Silverberg SG, editors: Pathology in gynecology and obstetrics, ed 2, Philadelphia, 1977, JB Lippincott Co.

Grifo JA, Jeremias J, Ledger WJ, and Witkin, SS: Interferon-gamma in the diagnosis and pathogenesis of pelvic inflammatory disease, Am J Obstet Gynecol 160:26, 1989.

Grimes DA: Deaths due to sexually transmitted diseases, JAMA 255:1727, 1986.

Grimes DA, Blount JH, Patrick J, et al: Antibiotic treatment of pelvic inflammatory disease, JAMA 256:3233, 1986.

Hadgu A, Weström L, Brooks CA, et al: Predicting acute pelvic inflammatory disease: a multivariate analysis, Am J Obstet Gynecol 155:954, 1986.

Hager WD: Follow-up of patients with tubo-ovarian abscess(es) in association with salpingitis, Obstet Gynecol 61:680, 1983.

Hager WD, Eschenbach DA, Spence MR, et al: Criteria for diagnosis and grading of salpingitis, Obstet Gynecol 61:113, 1983.

Handsfield HH: Problems in the treatment of bacterial sexually transmitted diseases, Sex Transm Dis 13:179, 1986.

Holmes KK, Mårdh P-A, Sparling PF, and Wiesner PJ editors: Sexually transmitted diseases, ed 2, New York, 1990, McGraw Hill, Inc.

Jacobson LJ: Differential diagnosis of acute pelvic inflammatory disease, Am J Obstet Gynecol 138:1006, 1980.

Janovski NA, editor: Color atlas of gross gynecologic and obstetric pathology, New York, 1969, McGraw-Hill, Inc.

Landers DV, Wolner-Hanssen P, Paavonen J, et al: Combination antimicrobial therapy in the treatment of acute pelvic inflammatory disease, Am J Obstet Gynecol 164:849, 1991.

Landers DV and Sweet RL: Tubo-ovarian abscess: contemporary approach to management, Rev Infect Dis 5:876, 1983.

Lidegaard O and Helm P: Pelvic inflammatory disease: the influence of contraceptive, sexual, and social life events, Contraception 41:475, 1990.

Lurie DK, Plzak L, and Deveney CW: Management of intraabdominal abscesses, Infec Surg Aug:477, 1988.

Paavonen J, Aine R, Teisala K, et al: Chlamydial endometritis, J Clin Pathol 38:726, 1985.

Paavonen J, Kiviat N, Brunham RC, et al: Prevalence and manifestations of endometritis among women with cervicitis, Am J Obstet Gynecol 152:280, 1985.

Paavonen J, Miettinen A, Stevens CE, et al: *Mycoplasma hominis* in cervicitis and endometritis, Sex Transm Dis 10:276, 1983.

Pastorek JG Jr.: Antimicrobial therapy for PID, Contemp Obstet Gynecol 30:31, 1989.

Patton DL, Moore DE, Spandoni LR, et al: A comparison of the fallopian tube's response to overt and silent salpingitis, Obstet Gynecol 73:622, 1989.

Peterson HB, Galaqid EI, and Zenilman JM: Pelvic inflammatory disease: review of treatment options, Rev Infect Dis 12(S6):S656, 1990.

Phillips AJ and D'Ablaing G: Acute salpingitis subsequent to tubal ligation, Obstet Gynecol 67:55S, 1986.

Pine L, Curtis EM, and Brown JM: *Actinomyces* and the intrauterine contraceptive device: aspects of the fluorescent antibody stain, Am J Obstet Gynecol 152:287, 1985.

Rice RJ, Biddle JW, JeanLouis YA, et al: Chromosomally mediated resistance in *Neisseria gonorrhoeae* in the United States: results of surveillance and reporting, 1983-1984, J Infect Dis 153:340, 1986.

Ristuccia AM and Cunha BA, editors: Antimicrobial therapy, New York, 1984, Raven Press.

Schaefer G: Female genital tuberculosis, Clin Obstet Gynecol 19:223, 1976.

Scott GR, Thompson G, Smith IW, et al: Infection with *Chlamydia trachomatis* and *Neisseria gonorrhoeae* in women with lower abdominal pain admitted to a gynaecology unit, Br J Obstet Gynaecol 96:473, 1989.

Sellers J, Mahony J, Goldsmith C, et al: The accuracy of clinical findings and laparoscopy in pelvic inflammatory disease, Am J Obstet Gyneol 164:113, 1991.

Siegenthaler WE, Bonetti A, and Luthy R: Aminoglycoside antibiotics in infectious diseases, Am J Med 80(suppl. 6B):2, 1986.

Soper DE, Brockwell NJ, and Dalton HP: False-positive cultures of the cul-de-sac associated with culdocentesis in patients undergoing elective laparoscopy, Obstet Gynecol 77:134, 1991.

Stacey C, Munday P, Thomas B, et al: *Chlamydia trachomatis* in the fallopian tubes of women without laparoscopic evidence of salpingitis, Lancet 336:960, 1990.

Stone KM, Grimes DA, and Magder LS: Primary prevention of sexually transmitted diseases, JAMA 255:1763, 1986.

Sweet RL: Pelvic inflammatory disease, Sex Transm Dis 13:192, 1986.

Sweet RL, Blankfort-Doyle M, Robbie MO, et al: The occurrence of chlamydial and gonococcal salpingitis during the menstrual cycle, JAMA 255:2062, 1986.

Sweet RL and Gibbs RS: Infectious diseases of the female genital tract, ed 2, Baltimore, 1990, Williams & Wilkins.

Sweet RL, Schachter J, and Robbie MO: Failure of β-lactam antibiotics to eradicate *Chlamydia trachomatis* in the endometrium despite apparent clinical cure of acute salpingitis, JAMA 250:2641, 1983.

Sweet RL, Yonekura ML, Hill G, et al: Appropriate use of antibiotics in serious obstetric and gynecologic infections, Am J Obstet Gynecol 146:719, 1983.

Teisala K, Heinonen PK, and Punnonen R: Laparoscopic diagnosis and treatment of acute pyosalpinx, J Reprod Med 35:19, 1990.

Teisala K, Heinonen PK, and Punnonen R: Transvaginal ultrasound in the diagnosis and treatment of tubo-ovarian abscess, Br J Obstet Gynaecol 97:178, 1990.

Toth A, O'Leary WM, and Ledger W: Evidence for microbial transfer by spermatozoa, Obstet Gynecol 59:556, 1982.

Vasilev SA, Roy S, and Essin DJ: Pelvic abscesses in postmenopausal women, Surg Gynecol Obstet 169:243, 1989.

Walters MD, Eddy CA, Gibbs RS et al: Antibodies to *Chlamydia trachomatis* and risk for tubal pregnancy, Am J Obstet Gynecol 159:942, 1988.

Walters MD and Gibbs RS: A randomized comparison of gentamicin-clindamycin and cefoxitin-doxycycline in the treatment of acute pelvic inflammatory disease, Obstet Gynecol 75:867, 1990.

Washington AE, Arno PS, and Brooks MA: The economic cost of pelvic inflammatory disease, JAMA 255:1735, 1986.

Washington AE, Gove S, Schachter J, et al: Oral contraceptives, *Chlamydia trachomatis* infection, and pelvic inflammatory disease, JAMA 253:2246, 1985.

Weström L: Incidence, prevalence, and trends of acute pelvic inflammatory disease and its consequences in industrialized countries, Am J Obstet Gynecol 138:880, 1980.

Weström L: Introductory address: treatment of pelvic inflammatory disease in view of etiology and risk factors, Sex Transm Dis 11:437, 1984.

Weström L: Pelvic inflammatory disease and other sexually transmitted diseases, Cur Opin Obstet Gynecol 1:5, 1989.

Winkler B, Reumann W, Mitao M, et al: Chlamydial endometritis, Am J Surg Pathol 8:771, 1984.

Wolner-Hanssen P, Eschenbach DA, Paavonenj J, et al: Association between vaginal douching and acute pelvic inflammatory disease, JAMA 263:1936, 1990.

Wolner-Hanssen P, Svensson L, Mårdh P-A, et al: Laparoscopic findings and contraceptive use in women with signs and symptoms suggestive of acute salpingitis, Obstet Gynecol 66:233, 1985.

23 Preoperative Management

_____ KEY TERMS AND DEFINITIONS _____

Antisialagogue. An agent that decreases the production and amount of saliva.

Effective Period. The first 3 hours of decreased tissue resistance following a surgical insult. Prophylactic antibiotics must be at the site of damaged tissue during this interval.

Informed Consent. An agreement by the patient that she understands the following: the nature and extent of the disease process, the nature and extent of the contemplated operation, the anticipated benefits and results of the surgery including a conservative estimate of successful outcome, the risks and potential complications of the operative procedure, and alternative methods of therapy.

Minidose Heparin. A low dose (5000 units) of heparin given 2 hours preoperatively and usually every 8 to 12 hours postoperatively, subcutaneously, as a prophylactic agent to decrease the incidence of venous thrombosis.

Nosocomial Infection. An infection acquired in a hospital.

Prophylactic Antibiotics. The administration of antibiotics to patients without evidence of infection to prevent postoperative morbidity related to infection.

Preoperative evaluation is a challenge to the gynecologist, for it involves both the art and the science of clinical medicine. Optimum preparation involves two personality traits: compulsive attention to detailed planning and a deep empathy for the patient. Preoperative planning can be divided into three basic aspects: obtaining preoperative information, reducing the patient's anxieties and fears, and obtaining informed consent. Francis D. Moore states that the first aphorism of preoperative preparation is to avoid "surprises." This dictum should be applied to protect both the patient and the physician.

The gynecologist, as leader of the surgical team, has an obligation to prepare the patient, her family, and the hospital personnel, including nurses, anesthesiologists, and the operating room team, concerning the anticipated details surrounding the surgical procedure. The majority of gynecologic operations are elective and thus allow sufficient time to prepare. However, even in emergency situations, preoperative

preparation should be as detailed as possible because shortcuts during an emergency can result in further compromise to the patient.

For the patient, there are no small, insignificant, or minor operations. Almost any operation is a major event in her life. Associated with an elective operation are the anxiety and apprehension of hospitalization coupled with the ambivalence of deciding whether to have the operation. To help her decide, it is important for the physician to outline the natural history of the gynecologic disease so that the patient is able to understand the benefits of surgery. Most women have questions concerning the return of normal body functions and the cosmetic changes produced by the operation; these questions must be discussed. As always, the physician is an educator. His or her goal should be to outline for the patient the reason and approximate time frame for each preoperative step and procedure. If the patient is ambivalent concerning the need for a surgical procedure, this often may be resolved by suggesting that she seek a second opinion. Many third-party payer programs insist that patients obtain a second opinion before elective gynecologic operations.

There are not many events that assault human dignity as much as admission to a hospital for an elective operation. The woman is usually stripped of her clothing, bombarded with questions, given multiple enemas, and shaved of pubic hair. It is important for the physician to protect the patient's privacy and human dignity during the preoperative period. The gynecologist must appreciate that the preoperative period is one of great psychologic stress for the patient. The time of the anticipated surgical procedure is a catalyst for emotional responses ranging from vulnerability and helplessness to the grief produced by anticipated loss of a reproductive organ. The physician-patient relationship is far more than the legally described contractual one. An important aspect of the relationship that builds confidence is the physician's encouragement of the patient to be a partner in the mutual goal of a return to normal function. The understanding and trust built between the patient and physician during the preoperative period will help the patient cope with the stress of the postoperative period.

One of the most important aspects of the preoperative preparation is a discussion with the physician before the procedure. Ideally the physician, the patient, and her family meet without other members of the hospital staff. During this time, it is important for the physician to answer all the patient's questions as well as those of her family and not skip details. It is acceptable to answer a question with the statement, "I don't know." Patients admire the honesty this expresses. The gynecologist must remember that just as he or she studies the patient for both verbal and nonverbal information, so does the patient watch the gynecologist. Gentleness and patience are essential for the gynecologist to display at this time. Sincere interest may be reinforced by eye-to-eye contact and a gentle touch of the hands.

A thorough and detailed history and physical examination, considering the entire patient, not just the pelvis, detect approximately 90% of the facts pertinent to the surgical procedure. Preoperative laboratory screening tests discover fewer than 10% of significant surgical risk factors. It is an established surgical axiom that operative morbidity and mortality are directly proportional to preexisting conditions. Known or unsuspected medical illnesses may affect the operation, anesthesia, and postoperative course and in rare instances may preclude the procedure altogether. Also, it is important to evaluate the influence of gynecologic disease on other organ systems. For example, is a pelvic mass producing obstruction of the ureters?

This chapter outlines the preoperative preparations for gynecologic operations for benign disease. Emphasis is placed on obtaining a standard history, performing a physical examination, and educating the patient and family (including obtaining informed consent). Special considerations of women with concurrent common medical disease are also included. Two recurrent themes are stressed in the chapter: avoiding surprises during each step in the preoperative period and alleviating the patient's fears and anxiety. This chapter is not intended to be an exhaustive discussion of all medical and surgical conditions that may have some impact on preoperative planning. Rather, the focus is on common preoperative problems faced in benign gynecologic surgery. Cost containment strategies have placed increasing emphasis on same-day admission for most major gynecologic operations. This practice has abruptly changed the timing of many preoperative events. Laboratory tests, electrocardiograms, and x-ray examinations are performed on an outpatient basis the week before surgery. Even preparation of the large intestine must be performed at home.

PREOPERATIVE HISTORY

A detailed history not only obtains information but also helps to relieve the patient's fears and anxieties. If the history is obtained in an unhurried manner, the process is reassuring to the patient. The patient should perceive the gynecologist as a gentle and reassuring clinician rather than a detective trying to rapidly solve a crime. The extent and depth of the general history are modified to a minor degree by the age and general health of the woman and the operation contemplated. However, even minor operations may have major complications. Therefore it is best to be overprepared. The possibility of degenerative multiple organ disease necessitates a detailed review before any surgical procedure in geriatric patients. Even for an emergency operation a detailed history is important.

For elective operations the preoperative history is taken on two separate occasions. The interview occurs initially in the physician's office several days or weeks before the operation and is repeated 1 to 3 days before the procedure is done. The interval is valuable, for it gives the patient an opportunity to reconsider her decision. Similarly, the physician uses the time to collect necessary information, such as records of previous surgical procedures. In reviewing the history the second time, often the patient recalls important information that she omitted during the initial history. For example, she may have recently talked to a sister who has a history of excessive bleeding during an operation.

There are two purposes in obtaining an optimum history from the patient. The first is to put the patient at ease; the second is to cover a formalized and extremely thorough set of questions. The two processes demand time and gentle consideration of the patient's anxiety. It is best to let the patient ramble at first. Subsequently the physician may direct the questions to a standard format. Obviously the format must be covered in a systematic manner so that essential areas are not omitted.

Although this chapter does not review all the components of a complete history (see Chapter 5), it is advantageous to group questions under the specific organ systems: pulmonary, cardiovascular, renal, hepatic, metabolic, endocrine, hematologic, and immunologic. Several specific questions should be included to fill any holes and to cross-check on the review of symptoms. These questions cover problems with surgery, anesthesia, or bleeding in the patient or her family. An example is, "Are there personal or family histories of bleeding problems?"

The next general category is drug allergy and current medications. Questions must be constructed so as to include both prescribed and over-the-counter medications. Many women do not consider aspirin or oral contraceptives as medication; therefore specific questions regarding these substances are needed. General questions regarding smoking, exercise tolerance, and recent upper respiratory infections are often grouped together.

The woman's contraceptive history, including any recent change, must be known. Over the years there has been no greater embarrassment in the operating room than the realization that a recent contraceptive practice has been abandoned and the patient is pregnant. Included with the contraceptive history are key questions concerning possible exposure to the human immodeficiency virus (HIV). Also, the physician should estimate the probability of blood transfusion and together with the patient decide whether autologous blood should be donated for possible transfusion.

PHYSICAL EXAMINATION

The preoperative physical examination should answer three basic questions: Has the primary gynecologic disease process changed since the initial diagnosis? What is the impact of the primary gynecologic disease on other organ systems? What deficiencies in other organ systems may affect the proposed surgery and hospitalization? A pelvic examination performed the day before surgery may demonstrate that a myoma has undergone acute degeneration or an ovarian cyst may have ruptured and "disappeared." Pelvic masses adherent to the large intestine suggest the necessity of mechanical cleansing of the bowel before surgery. A patient with cardiac murmurs from rheumatic heart disease needs antibiotic prophylaxis against subacute bacterial endocarditis.

The most important feature of the pre-operative physical is that it should be performed in a thorough and compulsive manner. The gynecologist should use the same sequence each time to help focus attention on the evaluation of each organ system.

The physical examination is best performed in the physician's office or in the hospital setting in the privacy of a room with a single bed or examining table. Then the patient need not worry about being embarrassed by hospital personnel or visitors entering the hospital room during the physical examination. To diminish the patient's anxiety, the physical examination should not be performed in silence. Conversation with the patient may involve further history taking or questions and answers about the proposed operation. Gentle palpation is important. A gentle touch helps to build the trust and confidence that are the foundation of the physician-patient relationship.

Two important axioms should be stressed. First, in emergency situations it is imperative to perform a complete physical examination. This examination should include an evaluation of the patient's blood pressure and pulse in both the recumbent and sitting positions; orthostatic hypotension and tachycardia are crude indexes of a decrease in circulating intravascular volume. Second, it is important to perform a pelvic examination the day before the operation and again in the operating room immediately before the surgical incision. Pelvic masses sometimes "disappear" when the bladder and gastrointestinal tracts are empty. These measures help avoid surprises.

STANDARD LABORATORY PROCEDURES

The general purpose of preoperative laboratory procedures is to identify conditions that will alter or aid in perioperative management. Specifically, screening tests are used to find unsuspected, asymptomatic diseases that may affect, alter, or postpone the anticipated surgical procedure. Preoperative laboratory tests also help to establish the extent of known disease that may influence the scheduling of elective surgery. Gynecologists should individualize their preoperative approach to patients and select specific tests for each patient. The downside of multiple routine preoperative testing is that it increases the likelihood of false positive results, especially if the disease has a low prevalence in the population being tested. A false positive test has many negative features, including anxiety for the patient, additional testing, financial cost, and often delays in the operation. Some special laboratory procedures are used to determine the effects of pelvic disease on other organ systems. Special laboratory tests, such as intravenous pyelograms or barium enemas, are discussed later.

Presently there is an extensive debate over which preoperative laboratory procedures should be standard. Attention has been drawn to the cost-benefit ratio of preoperative screening. Although the cost of each individual test is usually low, the aggregate costs are substantial. Often the cost argument is overcome by the individual gynecologist's concern to practice defensive medicine in the present medicolegal climate. Many preoperative laboratory tests are ordered simply by convention, for years being standard orders in an individual's or hospital's practice.

Kaplan et al. have retrospectively studied the usefulness of preoperative laboratory procedures. They estimate that 60% of the routinely ordered tests, such as differential cell count, platelet count, and 12-factor automated multiple analyses, would not have been performed if tests had been ordered only for an indication discovered by history or physical examination. Most important, only 0.22% of these tests demonstrated an abnormality that might influence perioperative management (Figure 23-1). These authors predict that rigid cost-benefit analysis will soon affect physicians' habits of routine preoperative testing. The final conclusion in their assessment of 2000 patients undergoing elective operations was that in the absence of specific indications, routine preoperative laboratory tests do not significantly contribute to patient care and could be eliminated.

Two of the most important considerations in the choice of preoperative tests are the age of the patient and the extent of the surgical procedure. Ideally, preoperative laboratory procedures should be determined in each patient based on the findings of both a complete history and a physical examination. Most important, abnormal results from any laboratory test should result in some change in perioperative management. Regretfully, unexpected abnormalities in many standard preoperative laboratory tests are frequently overlooked or ignored.

Preoperative complete blood count and urinalysis are required by nearly all hospitals. By far the most important of these for gynecologists is the test for anemia. A woman should not be admitted for elective gynecologic surgery with a low hematocrit level that will necessitate transfusion during the perioperative period, unless a delay in surgery is contraindicated or medical therapy to improve the hematocrit level has been unsuccessful. The results of the urinalysis, white blood cell count, and differential count rarely alter management. A blood sample should be sent to the blood bank for typing and screening for unusual antibodies before major gynecologic surgery, to replace the expensive routine typing and cross-match. However, it is important that the blood bank have the capability of providing cross-matched blood within a reasonable period of time if serious intraoperative bleeding does occur. Routine clotting studies are not cost effective unless indicated by history and physical examination.

It is beneficial to order the following three blood screening tests in women over age 40 or in women who have positive family histories or questionable past histories of hepatic or renal

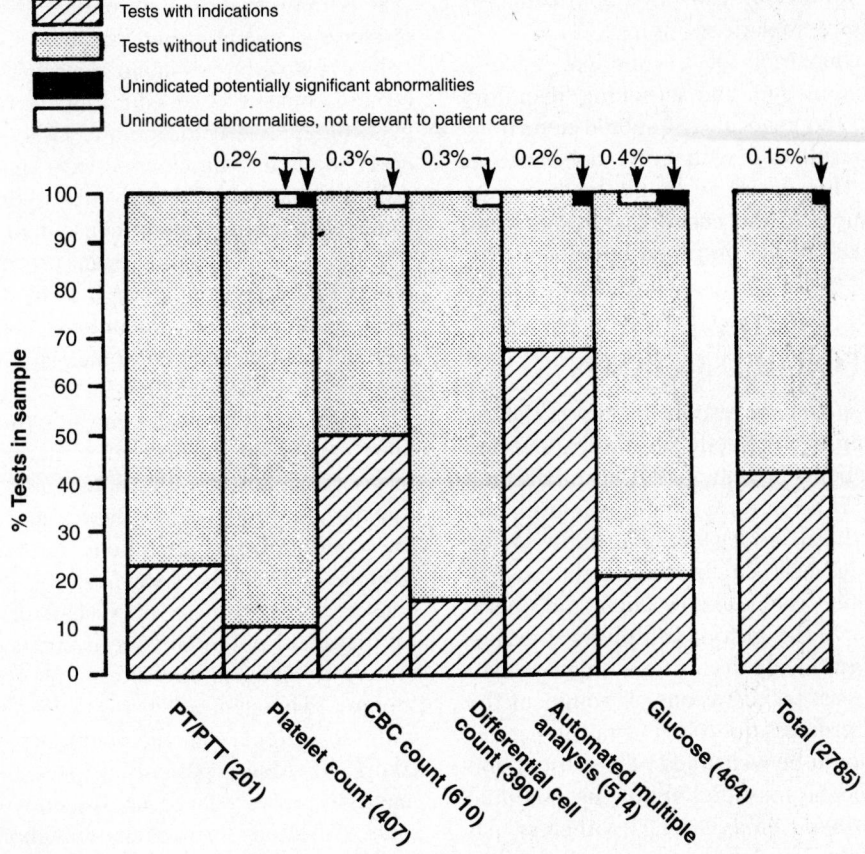

FIGURE 23-1
Proportions of indicated and unindicated preoperative tests, drawn to scale. Numbers in parentheses represent sample sizes used. *PT/PTT*, Prothrombin time/partial thromboplastin time; *CBC*, complete blood cell. Automated multiple analysis is six factor. (From Kaplan EB, Scheiner LB, Boeckmann AJ, et al: JAMA 253:3578, 1985.)

disease: blood urea nitrogen (BUN) or creatinine, blood sugar, and serum transaminase. A preoperative creatinine or BUN is especially important if the patient is going to be treated with antibiotics excreted by the kidneys. A test for human chorionic gonadotrophin may be appropriate, depending on contraceptive and sexual history. Menstrual history is at best an imperfect indication of early pregnancy. Serum electrolytes are ordered in women taking diuretics or for those with a history of renal disease or heart disease. Serum electrolytes should be evaluated for patients with vomiting, diarrhea, ileus, bowel obstruction, or any condition that affects water or electrolyte balance.

The tradition of ordering chest x-ray films on all patients has been seriously questioned. Roizen performed a detailed cost analysis of routine chest x-ray films and determined the practice was not cost effective unless the patient was over age 60 or had known pulmonary or cardiac disease. Rucker et al., in a similar study, concluded that a history and physical examination are sufficient to screen patients and chest x-ray films need be ordered only for patients with positive findings. In the latter study of 368 patients without risk factors, only one had a positive chest x-ray finding, and that finding did not alter the surgical procedure.

A baseline preoperative electrocardiogram has been found to be cost effective in asymptomatic women only after age 50. It sometimes detects a recent asymptomatic myocardial infarction or serious cardiac arrhythmias. The results of several screening tests should be reviewed during the office visit just before hospitalization. These include a Pap smear on all patients and mammography, depending on the patient's age and risk factors. Testing the stool for occult blood in women over age 40 detects bleeding from a colon cancer in approximately 2 of 1000 asymptomatic women.

At the conclusion of a complete history, physical examination, and screening laboratory procedures, the gynecologist should determine whether consultation with other specialists is necessary. This decision should be based on the seriousness of the concurrent disease and the complexity of the proposed operation.

PATIENT-FAMILY EDUCATION AND INFORMED CONSENT

One of the primary responsibilities of the gynecologic surgeon is to educate the patient and her family about the anticipated hospitalization and surgical procedure. Giving this information is both an ethical and legal responsibility. More important, in most circumstances the patient and her family want to know about the operation. Similar to the history and physical examination, educational discussions should take place on at least two occasions. Throughout the educational process, questions from the patient or family should be welcomed. The patient and family should be informed about the potential use of intravenous fluids, urinary catheters, nasogastric tubes, and monitoring equipment. Physicians often take these devices for granted, not realizing such equipment may cause anxiety and fears in lay persons not familiar with modern postoperative care.

Educating the patient is a great step in relieving anxiety. If the patient is aware of the sequence of events following admission, the stress of this time becomes more tolerable. It is difficult to overeducate the patient on details of the hospitalization, the operating room, and recovery room routines. Psychologic preparation of the family is equally important, and arrangements should be made for a meeting with family members immediately following the operation. An informed family is one of the surgeon's greatest assistants. An uninformed family will often harass the entire health care delivery team.

Few concepts bring more anxiety, concern, and fear to the physician than the doctrine of informed consent. In the present medicolegal climate, the absence of informed consent is cited as a major problem in many lawsuits. Some critics have pointed out that true informed consent would involve sending the patient to medical school and then through several hours of intensive discussion.

It is important to differentiate the concepts of consent and informed consent. Consent involves a simple yes-or-no decision, while informed consent is an educational process. If a gynecologist were to operate without consent, he or she would be vulnerable to charges of assault and battery. The right of an adult woman to have final authority to consent to an operation has over 200 years of legal precedent. The preoperative consent form that is standard in most hospitals simply documents that consent, hopefully informed consent, has been obtained.

To obtain informed consent, the surgeon must explain to the patient in understandable terms the following: the nature and extent of the disease process; the nature and extent of the contemplated operation; the anticipated benefits and results of the surgery, including a conservative estimate of successful outcome; the risks and potential complications of the operative procedure; and alternative methods of therapy. The gynecologist should also discuss with the patient what the operation will not accomplish. Many patients expect surgery to magically cure a large constellation of symptoms. Questions from the patient should be encouraged and welcomed. After being educated and considering the information, the patient acquires an understanding of the risks and benefits of the proposed surgery and may make a "fully informed" decision and give informed consent for the operation to be performed.

The possibility of unanticipated pathologic conditions should be discussed with the patient and permission obtained on the written consent form for the most extensive operative procedure that may be necessary. Patients readily accept the necessity of freedom of judgment by the gynecologist during the operation as to the extent of the surgical procedure needed, depending on what is discovered during surgery. For example, written permission to remove both fallopian tubes and ovaries along with the uterus should be obtained in the event that extensive adnexal disease is an unanticipated finding.

One of the greatest dilemmas in the doctrine of informed consent is the extent and depth of discussions concerning potential complications of an operation. Attorneys who specialize in defending gynecologists in medical malpractice litigation strongly advise discussing all major complications, including death from surgery and rare, serious complications, such as urinary tract fistulas following hysterectomy. Wingo et al., from the Centers for Disease Control, reviewed the overall mortality associated with hysterectomy in the United States. This study, which gathered data from approximately 40% of the gynecologic operations performed each year, documented an overall mortality of 12 per 10,000 hysterectomy procedures. The death rate per 10,000 operations was higher in women who were pregnant (29 per 10,000) and women with cancer (38 per 10,000), whereas if the surgery were performed for benign gynecologic disease, there were 6 deaths per 10,000 operations. To protect the gynecologist, the final discussion of the informed consent process should be witnessed by a family member and another member of the health delivery team. Highlights of this discussion should be documented by a paragraph written by the gynecologist in the progress notes of the chart.

ADMISSION AND PREOPERATIVE ORDERS

The admission and preoperative orders should communicate the gynecologist's preoperative preparation for his or her patient. To avoid omissions, it is important to develop a systematic method of writing preoperative orders. A simple outline is depicted in the box above. The orders should be individualized depending on the previous history and physical examination obtained as an outpatient, the patient's age, and the extent of the proposed surgical procedure. Unusual or infrequent orders should be written in specific detail to avoid confusion by nursing and other hospital personnel. Because of the increasing emphasis on same-day admission to the hospital, many procedures and orders are accomplished on an outpatient basis. Therefore it is important to give the patient a specific list of instructions for the 24 hours before surgery.

The first two or three lines of the order sheet should include the reasons for admission, the proposed operation, and a list of the patient's diseases. Further orders are subdivided into four broad categories: general measures, medication, laboratory tests, and preventive therapies.

General measures include orders for activity, diet, and vital signs. The patient should have nothing by mouth (NPO) for at least 6 hours before elective surgery. If the patient's operation is not scheduled until the middle of the af-

---

SAMPLE ADMISSION AND PREOPERATIVE ORDERS

A. General measures
   1. Activity
   2. Diet
   3. Vital signs
   4. NPO after midnight
B. Medications
   1. Pain
   2. Sleep
   3. Prophylactic antibiotics
   4. Special (for medical illness)
C. Laboratory tests
   1. Routine
   2. Special
   3. Blood for typing and screening
   4. Pregnancy test
D. Preventive therapies
   1. Elastic stockings
   2. Enemas until clear
   3. Adequate hydration

---

ternoon, it is acceptable for the patient to have an early liquid breakfast.

The second category of orders is for medications. The three common subgroups of medications are for pain, sleep, and antibiotics. When prophylactic antibiotics are ordered, the time of injection should ensure that significant blood and tissue levels will be present at the time of bacterial contamination during the surgical procedure. An additional subgroup is special medications for specific medical illness. It is presumed that the anesthesiologist will write orders for preoperative medication to alleviate anxiety and reduce tracheobronchial secretions.

The third major group of orders involves preoperative laboratory tests. This group includes standard laboratory tests, specifically indicated laboratory tests or procedures, such as an intravenous pyelogram, or blood samples for typing and screening for unusual antibodies.

The fourth and last group of orders involves preventive therapies. Thrombophlebitis remains a major complication of gynecologic surgery. Patients often are advised to wear elastic stockings up to the knee to help overcome venous stasis. Prophylactic subcutaneous heparin is indicated in women at high risk for thromboembolic disease. Because the lower intestinal tract should be empty before an operation, it is appropriate to order enemas to cleanse the lower intestine. Patients who have been NPO for a prolonged period or have lost fluid from cleansing of the gastrointestinal tract should be given intravenous fluids before induction of anesthesia to ensure proper hydration. One of the time-honored traditions in gynecologic surgery has been douching the evening before the operation. The medical value of this habit is unproved. Amstey and Jones found no advantage to washing the vagina with an iodine solution. The vagina recolonizes with similar quantitative bacterial counts within 30 to 60 minutes. Another unnecessary order involves having the patient empty her bladder before going to the operating room, because catheterization should be performed before the pelvic examination on the operating room table. If removal of hair is necessary for the operation, it should be clipped immediately before the operation.

CONSULTATION WITH THE ANESTHESIOLOGIST

The preoperative interaction between the patient and the anesthesiologist is most important. For the patient, both the reassurance of meeting the anesthesiologist and their exchange of information greatly alleviate anxiety. For the anesthesiologist, it is an opportunity to obtain necessary medical information, evaluate the patient, determine the risk of the perioperative period, and write preoperative medication orders. This meeting has traditionally occurred the afternoon or evening before surgery. However, with emphasis on cost containment and greater use of outpatient facilities, and with admission to the hospital the morning of the operation, this meeting frequently occurs on an outpatient basis several days before surgery. Recently, anesthesiologists have assumed more responsibility for postoperative pain management, primarily using epidural narcotics. This subject should be discussed with the patient.

Anesthesiologists classify surgical procedures according to the patient's risk of mortality. Dripps, in 1961, first published guidelines to determine the risk of death related to major operative procedures. This Physical Status Scale (Table 23-1) has been adopted by the American Society of Anesthesiologists. An emergency operation doubles the mortality risks for classes 1, 2, and 3, produces a slightly

TABLE 23-1
Dripps–American Society of Anesthesiologists Classification

Class	Description
1	A normal healthy patient
2	A patient with mild-to-moderate systemic disease
3	A patient with severe systemic disease with limited activity but not incapacitated
4	A patient with incapacitating, constantly life-threatening systemic disease
5	A moribund patient not expected to survive 24 hours with or without operation

Adapted from Anesthesiology 24:111, 1963. From Jewell ER, Persson AV: Surg Clin North Am 65:4, 1985.

increased risk in class 4, and does not change the risk in class 5. Hirsch is of the opinion that 5% to 10% of the total perioperative mortality rate is directly related to anesthetic problems. The majority of deaths due to anesthesia are ascribable to human error.

A problem frequently encountered by both gynecologists and anesthesiologists is whether to continue or interrupt medications that the patient is taking. If the drug is prescribed for a medical illness, it is best to continue the drug through the perioperative period. The physician must determine whether the drug will adversely affect the course of either the anesthesia or the surgery and whether it will interact with other drugs to be given during the procedure. It is acceptable to have the patient take oral medications the morning of surgery. The 30 to 60 ml of water needed to swallow the oral medication is negligible compared to gastric fluid volumes. Roizen has listed several drugs as special exceptions to routine administration before the operation, for they interfere or interact with either anesthesia or surgery. This list includes monoamine oxidase inhibitors, nicotinic acid, insulin, corticosteroids, and anticoagulants.

Three special gynecologic situations should be considered by the anesthesiologist in his or her choice of general or conduction anesthesia. Spinal anesthesia should be avoided during rectovaginal fistula repairs so that the surgeon may judge the "tightness" of the external sphincter in consideration of performing a relaxing sphincterectomy incision. It has also been our clinical impression that the incidence of spinal head-

TABLE 23-2

Drugs and Doses Used for Preoperative Premedication

Classification	Drug	Typical Adult Dose (mg)	Route of Administration*
Barbiturates	Secobarbital	50-150	Oral, IM
	Pentobarbital	50-150	Oral, IM
Narcotics	Morphine	5-15	IM
	Meperidine	50-100	IM
Benzodiazepines	Diazepam	5-10	Oral
	Lorazepam	2-4	Oral, IM
Butyrophenones†	Droperidol	1.25	IV
Antihistamines	Diphenhydramine	25-75	Oral, IM
	Promethazine	25-50	IM
	Hydroxyzine	50-100	IM
Anticholinergics	Atropine	0.3-0.6	IM
	Scopolamine	0.3-0.6	IM
	Glycopyrrolate	0.1-0.3	IM
H$_2$-antagonists	Cimetidine	300	Oral, IM, IV
	Ranitidine	150	Oral
Antacids	Particulate	15-30 ml	Oral
	Norparticulate	15-30 ml	Oral
Stimulants of gastric motility	Metoclopramide	5-10	Oral, IM, IV

*IM, Intramuscular; IV, intravenous.
†Recommended for use as an antiemetic to be administered near the conclusion of surgery.
Modified from Miller RD: Anesthesia, ed 2, New York, 1986, Churchill Livingstone, Inc, p 394.

ache may be increased in operations performed in the extreme lithotomy position. Finally, the choice of conduction anesthesia for surgery on an adnexal mass must take into account the possibility of upper abdominal exploration and biopsy if the adnexal mass is malignant.

The primary goals of preoperative medication are to relieve anxiety, protect against allergic reactions, and produce sedation, analgesia, and, it is hoped, amnesia. The general types of drugs used for premedication include barbiturates, narcotics, tranquilizers, sedatives, hypnotics, anticholinergics, antihistamines, and H$_2$-receptor antagonists (Table 23-2). Sedation is easy to accomplish; however, relief of anxiety does not invariably accompany sedation. Narcotics and sedatives are contraindicated in patients with chronic respiratory or liver disease.

Stoelting has outlined ideal preoperative medications for the majority of patients (see box on p. 23-10). He recommends flurazepam orally the evening before surgery followed by diazepam and cimetidine orally 1 to 2 hours before induction of anesthesia. For an antisiala-

gogue effect, atropine or scopolamine is given intramuscularly immediately before the patient is transported to the operating room. This alleviates the dry-mouth feeling produced by anticholinergics given 1 or 2 hours before surgery. If the central nervous system effects of atropine and scopolamine are worrisome, glycopyrrolate is the drug of choice. The latter drug has the advantage of producing minimal cardiovascular and visual side effects.

PROPHYLACTIC ANTIBIOTICS

When a significant risk of postoperative infection exists, the use of prophylactic antibiotics in gynecologic surgical procedures has become standard practice. Wound infections and pelvic cellulitis continue to be frequent and important causes of postoperative morbidity. Gynecologic operations produce both hypoxic tissue and collections of bloody and serous fluids, both of which are excellent culture media. Rigidly defined, prophylactic antibiotic use involves the administration of antibiotics to women without evidence of pelvic infection to

RECOMMENDED PREOPERATIVE MEDICATION FOR ADULT PATIENTS PRIOR TO ELECTIVE SURGERY

1. Patient interview by anesthesiologist the day before surgery
2. Flurazepam (oral) to treat insomnia the night before surgery
3. Diazepam or lorazepam orally 1 to 2 hours before induction of anesthesia
4. Substitute morphine intramuscularly for number 3 if analgesia is desired
5. Scopolamine intramuscularly 1 to 2 hours before induction of anesthesia if reliable sedation and amnesia are desired—otherwise otherwise do not administer an anticholinergic, or follow recommendation number 8
6. Cimetidine orally 1 to 2 hours before induction of anesthesia
7. Metoclopramide orally 1 to 2 hours before induction of anesthesia—not routine at present
8. Glycopyrrolate (intramuscular) when patient is ready to be transported to the operating room if an antisialagogue effect is desired

From Stoelting RK: Psychological preparation and preoperative medication. In Miller RD, editor: Anesthesia, ed 2, New York, 1986, Churchill Livingstone, Inc. Reprinted by permission.

prevent postoperative morbidity related to infection. The major use of prophylactic antibiotics is in operations such as vaginal hysterectomy, following which there is potential for a high incidence of postoperative pelvic cellulitis. The goal of antibiotic therapy is to prevent infection by the endogenous flora of the lower female reproductive tract. Prophylactic antibiotics are given occasionally when the incidence of postoperative infection is low but the results of the surgical procedure would be severely compromised if an infection did occur, such as with reconstructive operations on the fallopian tubes. Presently, approximately 40% of all antibiotics used in hospitals are ordered as prophylaxis.

The use of prophylactic antibiotics in gynecologic surgery has been the subject of much debate. As in any discussion of preventive medicine, one has to evaluate the benefits, risks, and costs. In general, the use of prophylactic antibiotics results in fewer operative site infections (abdominal wound and pelvic cellulitis), reduced febrile morbidity, and shorter hospital stays. The major risk of allergic or toxic reactions is small, especially with a short course of prophylactic antibiotics. The increased cost of the antibiotics is justified by a lower total cost from a shorter hospitalization. Certainly the economic costs of prolonged hospitalization for even a minor postoperative infection are substantial.

The foundation of our understanding of prophylactic antibiotics is the classic study of John Burke published in 1961. He stressed the fact that maximum antibacterial activity in subcutaneous wounds results from a combination of host resistance and antibiotics. His experimental studies proved that the antibiotic must be present in damaged tissue at the time of contamination with bacteria or shortly thereafter. Burke termed the first 3 hours of decreased tissue resistance following a surgical insult as the *effective period*. He found that there was no protective effect in preventing the development of subcutaneous wound infections if the antibiotics were given later than 3 hours following bacterial contamination.

Subsequent studies have documented two other important facts concerning prophylactic antibiotics in gynecology. First, the goal of prophylactic antibiotics is to reduce the total number of bacteria present in the operative incision. It is not necessary to kill all of the bacteria. Second, for prophylaxis to be successful, adequate tissue levels of antibiotics need to be maintained only for the duration of the operation. The normal endogenous vaginal flora has 1×10^8 bacteria per milliliter of vaginal secretions, consisting of a wide spectrum of both aerobic and anaerobic organisms. Thus, theoretically, the choice of a single·antibiotic for prophylaxis in gynecology is a most difficult one. Ideally the drug chosen as a prophylactic antibiotic should be nontoxic, inexpensive, and effective against most organisms encountered in the endogenous flora.

There is abundant literature supporting the use of prophylactic antibiotics in gynecology. At least 48 studies summarize the data from more than 3000 women who received prophylactic antibiotics for vaginal hysterectomy. The results of these studies show that the incidence of febrile morbidity was reduced from 40% to 15% and the incidence of pelvic infection from 25% to 5%. The results of 30 studies of 2165 women having abdominal hysterectomies are not as decisive. Some studies demonstrated no significant improvement, whereas positive studies demonstrated less dramatic declines in febrile morbidity, pelvic infection, and wound infection. The average reduction in febrile morbidity was 12%, and the average reduction in operation site infection, 5%. In many studies it is difficult to determine whether the investigators equated postoperative fever with postoperative infection.

No center or expert has demonstrated the antibiotic of choice for prophylaxis in gynecology. It is most difficult to compare one prophylactic antibiotic with another. Not only are there differences in methodology between studies, but also differences in terminology between definitions of febrile morbidity and documented pelvic infections. There do not seem to be significant differences no matter which modern, single broad-spectrum antibiotic (ampicillin, tetracyclines, cephalosporins) is used. Presently, first- or second-generation cephalosporins are the most popular choice for prophylactic antibiotics in gynecology (e.g., a single dose of first-generation cefazolin [Kefzol], 1 to 2 g intramuscularly or intravenously 30 minutes before the operation, or second-generation cefoxitin [Mefoxin], 1 to 2 g intramuscularly or intravenously immediately before the operation). Often nursing personnel give prophylactic antibiotics prematurely by optimistically anticipating when the patient will go to the operating room. This practice may result in lower than desirable antibiotic levels during the time of bacterial contamination.

There is universal agreement that the third-generation cephalosporins should be reserved as alternatives to aminoglycosides for life-threatening infections. With the wide spectrum of bacteria involved in the constantly changing ecologic system of the vagina, a single antibiotic does not have the spectrum to be bactericidal or bacteriostatic against all the bacteria present. The important feature sought in a prophylactic antibiotic is an ability to reduce the total number of bacteria present in the bacterial innoculum; it does not have to affect all organisms. A reduction in overall number allows the woman's natural defense mechanisms to eradicate the remaining bacteria.

Shapiro et al. performed a cost-benefit analysis of prophylactic antibiotics for both abdominal and vaginal hysterectomy. At the time of their study, 1983, they estimated the excessive cost per patient with infection or febrile morbidity was $1777 for vaginal hysterectomies and $716 for abdominal hysterectomies. They performed a randomized, placebo-controlled clinical trial of 515 patients, giving three injections of a cephalosporin for prophylaxis. The computer program estimated the cost savings of prophylactic antibiotics as $492 per patient with vaginal hysterectomy and $102 per patient for abdominal hysterectomy. These calculations included the cost of the prophylactic antibiotics (Table 23-3).

Recent emphasis has focused on an extremely short duration of therapy for prophylactic antibiotics. Comparative studies have documented that single-dose therapy is as effective as 24 hours of antibiotics. No advantage

TABLE 23-3

Derivation of Excess Costs for In-Hospital Infectious Morbidity After Vaginal or Abdominal Hysterectomy

Cost Variable	With Morbidity	Without Morbidity	Difference	Excess Cost ($)
Vaginal hysterectomy				
Hospital stay (days)*	9.16	7.35	1.81	507
Bacterial cultures (no.)	3.04	2.04	1.00	30
Antimicrobials ($)	1276	36	1240	1240
TOTAL ($)				1777
Abdominal hysterectomy				
Hospital stay (days)*	8.78	7.99	0.79	221
Bacterial cultures (no.)	2.47	1.26	1.21	36
Antimicrobials ($)	580	121	459	459
TOTAL ($)				716

From Shapiro M, Schoenbaum SC, Tager IB, et al: JAMA 249:1291, 1983. Copyright 1983, American Medical Association.
*Geometric mean.

exists to continuing prophylactic antibiotics beyond the immediate operative period. This short duration of administration also reduces cost and complications. The incidence of serious complications, such as drug allergy and resistant bacteria, is directly related to the length of administration of the antibiotic. With prophylactic antibiotics the major concern is the potential threat of increasing bacterial resistance. This results in two problems: more nosocomial infections with resistant organisms and alterations of the normal vaginal flora. If infection does develop following prophylactic antibiotics, one must obtain cultures and select antibiotic coverage different from the antibiotic used for prophylaxis. Another potential complication from prophylactic antibiotics is pseudomembranous enterocolitis secondary to *Clostridium difficile* infection. This complication usually follows chronic use of antibiotics, but rarely it may occur after a short exposure to antibiotics.

Many factors affect the risk of postoperative infection. The most important include the length of the operation, whether the woman is premenopausal or postmenopausal, obesity, indigency, malnutrition, immunosuppression, the use of prophylactic antibiotics, and the operative approach. Most studies have not documented that prophylactic antibiotics decrease the incidence of serious pelvic infections such as pelvic abscess. Since this is a rare complication, however, the studies performed to date are not large enough to eliminate a beta error. Some studies have questioned the benefits of prophylactic antibiotics in operative procedures that last more than 3½ hours.

In summary, prophylactic antibiotics are the standard of care for vaginal or abdominal hysterectomies and gynecologic operations that carry a substantial risk of postoperative infection. The most popular choice is a first- or second-generation cephalosporin, such as cefazolin or cefoxitin. Whatever broad-spectrum antibiotic is selected, the gynecologist must know the pharmacokinetics of the drug. The half-life of the antibiotic is important in selecting the proper timing and route of preoperative administration and the possible necessity of an intraoperative dose for longer operations. The amount of antibiotic bound to plasma proteins is important, for it determines the concentration of free antibiotic in the tissues (Table 23-4). The antibiotic selected should be active against the majority of endogenous flora of the vagina. The drug should be present at the time of surgical insult, and it should be used only during the time of the operative procedure.

THROMBOEMBOLIC DISEASE

Thrombophlebitis of either the pelvic or the leg veins is a frequent complication of gynecologic surgery (Table 23-5). Classically the three major pathophysiologic changes that facilitate the development of thrombophlebitis and pulmonary embolus are venous injury, circulatory stasis, and hypercoagulable conditions. Many aspects of pelvic surgery predispose to thrombophlebitis, including venous stasis, surgical injury to the walls of large veins, and often associated anaerobic infection. Because of the significant morbidity and mortality associated with a postoperative pulmonary embolus, every effort should be made to reduce the incidence of thrombophlebitis. Although the initial venous injury most often occurs at the time of the operation, approximately 15% of symptomatic emboli do not occur until the first week following discharge from the hospital.

During the perioperative period the patient should be evaluated for factors that place her at increased risk for thromboembolic disease. Such factors include a history of previous thrombophlebitis or embolus, family history of hypercoagulability, malignant disease, previous radiation therapy, morbid obesity, venous disease, edema of the legs, active pelvic infection, use of oral contraceptives up to the time of the operation, and length of preoperative hospitalization (Table 23-6). Lengthy surgical procedures, especially associated with profuse bleeding, are also significant risk factors.

Various means are used to prevent thromboembolic disease. The first prophylactic measure to reduce the incidence of embolic disease is to discontinue oral contraceptives 4 weeks before *major* elective operations. Oral contraceptives decrease the concentration of the body's major coagulation inhibitor, antithrombin III. Oral contraceptives also modify the effect of plasminogen activator, which activates the fibrinolytic defense system. Several clotting factors are elevated by oral contraceptive use, but the importance of this elevation in thrombogenesis has not been established. There is no evidence of increased venous thrombosis with estrogen doses used for menopausal replacement therapy. Thus replacement estrogen does

TABLE 23-4
Pharmacologic Properties of Cephalosporins

	Peak Serum Concentration (μg/ml)		Half-Life (minutes)	Protein Binding (%)
	Intravenous*	Intramuscular†		
Parenteral (1g dose)				
Cephalothin	15	20	40	70
Cephapirin	15	20	40	45
Cephradine	15	15	20	10
Cefazolin	80	60	100	80
Cefamandole	55	25	40	80
Cefoxitin	30	20	40	70
Cefotaxime	50	20	60	40
Moxalactam	90	25	120	50

From Thompson RL and Wright AJ: Mayo Clin Proc 58:82, 1983.
*At 30 minutes after rapid infusion.
†At 30 minutes after intramuscular injection.

TABLE 23-5
Incidence of Venous Thrombosis After Gynecologic Operations with I-Fibrinogen Scanning

Reference	No. of Patients	Type of Operation	Incidence of Leg Vein Thrombosis
Adolf et al.	75	Major	29
Ballard et al.	55	Major benign disease	29
Clayton et al.	231	Major	16
Endl and Auinger	43	Major	37
Walsh et al.	100	Vaginal hysterectomy	7
	117	Abdominal hysterectomy	13
	23	Wertheim's operation	25
	22	Other malignant disease	45

From Bonnar J: Clin Obstet Gynecol 28:433, 1985.

TABLE 23-6
Assessment of Risk of Venous Thromboembolism in Gynecologic Patients

Thromboembolic Complications	Low Risk (Under 40 years; operative procedures less than 30 minutes; no immobilization)	Moderate Risk (Over 40 years; estrogen therapy; operative procedures more than 30 minutes; varicose veins; obesity; postoperative infection)	High Risk (Previous thromboembolism; abdominal or pelvic operation for malignant disease; immobilization)
Calf vein thrombosis	<3%	10%-30%	30%-60%
Proximal vein thrombosis	<1%	2%-8%	6%-12%
Pulmonary embolism	<0.01%	0.1%-0.7%	1%-2%

From Bonnar J: Clin Obstet Gynecol 28:435, 1985.

not have to be discontinued. Other empiric prophylactic measures include elastic stockings, early ambulation, leg exercises in bed, and elevating the foot of the bed. Support hose should be thigh high so as to avoid venous stasis at the knee. The appearance of the support hose probably serves more of a teaching function to remind patients and nursing personnel of the importance of ambulation and exercise to prevent venous stasis.

The key decision for the prophylaxis of thromboembolic diseases is whether to order prophylactic mini-heparin, intraoperative dextran, or pneumatic inflated sleeve devices (Chapter 24). It is our practice to order mini-heparin for the patient at substantially high risk. Subcutaneous heparin (dose of 5000 units) with 0.5 mg of dihydroergotamine mesylate (Embolex) is given 2 hours before the operation and every 8 to 12 hours thereafter throughout the hospital stay. Critics of prophylactic heparin argue that it may reduce the incidence of venous thrombosis in the calf but has little or no effect in preventing embolic phenomena from pelvic veins. Another problem is that some women are fully anticoagulated by the mini-heparin dose of 5000 units every 8 to 12 hours and thus may experience excessive bleeding during or following the operative procedure. Some women, especially the obese or extremely thin patient, should have their dosage of subcutaneous heparin adjusted according to activated partial thromboplastin time.

Collins et al. performed a metaanalysis, reviewing more than 70 randomized trials of perioperative subcutaneous heparin in over 16,000 general surgery, orthopedic, and urologic patients. This study demonstrated that subcutaneous heparin prevents approximately two thirds of deep venous thrombosis and 50% of all deaths from pulmonary emboli. The most striking data in this study related the reduction in death directly to pulmonary emboli, with 19 deaths in the patients given perioperative heparin and 55 deaths in the control group.

Poller et al. have advocated an alternative anticoagulation prophylaxis using a small, fixed oral dose of warfarin, 1 mg daily. This regimen is used in England and the warfarin is begun approximately 14 days before surgery. This small dose does not result in appreciable changes in coagulation tests, especially prothrombin time, and the authors have not experienced trouble with bleeding during surgery. Extensive experience with this regimen will

determine if it is safer and as efficacious as subcutaneous heparin.

The other major alternative to anticoagulation is pneumatic compression modalities, including stockings and air pumps. These devices not only prevent stasis and the endothelial injury that may occur with extreme venous distention, but also stimulate the fibrinolytic system.

GASTROINTESTINAL TRACT

Gastrointestinal symptoms are rare in women being evaluated for elective operations for benign gynecologic conditions. However, if the patient has such symptoms, the gynecologist should consider preoperative endoscopy and radiologic studies of the gastrointestinal tract. The impact of nausea, vomiting, or diarrhea on serum electrolytes and on the nutritional status of the patient also needs to be evaluated.

In this era of cost containment, a barium enema and flexible colonoscopy need not be routinely performed on all patients with adnexal masses. These tests do help to establish the differential diagnosis among diverticulitis, carcinoma of the colon, and endometriosis. Therefore a barium enema and endoscopy are indicated if there is a left-sided adnexal mass in a woman over age 40, a positive stool guaiac test, or bowel symptoms. Again, the evaluation of each patient must be individualized in an attempt to determine if a primary gynecologic process is pressing on the bowel or directly invading the large intestine.

The preoperative nutritional state of the patient must be assessed. Many women with pelvic cancer need hyperalimentation before an elective operation. The two most common complications of parenteral nutrition are sepsis and metabolic abnormalities.

Proper mechanical cleansing of the gastrointestinal tract is important before every elective gynecologic operation. The patient should not have eaten for 6 hours before surgery. Clear liquids are emptied from the stomach within minutes; however, fatty foods greatly delay gastric emptying. Obviously, incomplete preparation of the upper gastrointestinal tract increases the risk of aspiration, which is a serious complication of anesthesia and operations.

Preoperative enemas to mechanically cleanse the large bowel are one of the simplest of preoperative orders. When properly performed, the cleansing enemas hasten the return of normal bowel function postoperatively and help to reduce the incidence of fecal impaction during the immediate postoperative period. An empty large bowel also facilitates the accuracy of the pelvic examination with the patient under anesthesia. It is important that enemas are given early on the evening before the operation so that most gas and all fluid and stool are properly expelled from the distal colon. If an enema is given the morning of the operation and the colon subsequently is not totally evacuated, the patient is likely to expel the contents during the operation. As stated, the physician and patient must be adaptive, since preoperative preparation often occurs in the outpatient setting.

If there is a suspicion that the operation will necessitate entry into the lumen of the large intestine, both mechanical cleansing and antibiotics to reduce the bacterial count of the colon should be ordered. Colon and rectal surgeons have debated for years about the best methods to accomplish this. Traditionally, mechanical preparation has been accomplished by 3 days of liquid diet, cathartics, and enemas. Recently, almost all gynecologists have modified their mechanical preparation to a single day of an oral gut lavage solution (GOLYTELY and bisacodyl) (Table 23-7). GOLYTELY is ingested at a rate of 1.5 L per hour until diarrheal effluent is clear, usually within 3 to 6 hours. Patients' compliance with GOLYTELY is facilitated if is chilled. Beck et al. have contrasted the standard 3-day bowel preparation with GOLYTELY the day before surgery. Quantitative stool cul-

TABLE 23-7
GOLYTELY Formulation

Components	Concentration
Polyethylene glycol 4000 (PEG)	59.1 g/L
Sodium sulfate (Na_2SO_4)	40 mmol/L
Potassium chloride (KCl)	10 mmol/L
Sodium chloride (NaCl)	25 mmol/L
Sodium bicarbonate ($NaHCO_3$)	20 mmol/L
Distilled water*	
Parabens†	
Final osmolarity	280-300 mosm/L

From Beck DE, Harford FJ, and DiPalma JA: Dis Colon Rectum 28:492, 1985.
*Distilled to a final volume of 1000 ml.
†Methylparabens 0.2 g; prophylparabens 0.1 g.

TABLE 23-8
Mechanical and Antibiotic Preparation of Intestine

Day Before the Operation	Day of the Operation
GoLYTELY orally 1.5 L/hour until effluent is clear	Cefoxitin 2 g IV or IM 30 minutes before the operation
Neomycin 1 g and erythromycin base 1 g orally at 2, 4, and 10 PM	

tures obtained before and after preparation of the bowel and intraoperatively were similar. The GOLYTELY preparation was preferred by patients primarily because it produced less abdominal distress. The patients experienced less weight loss, and superior mechanical cleansing of the colon was discovered at their operations.

In summary, the advantages of oral gut lavage are that it is rapid and safe with negligible water and sodium absorption or intestinal secretion. The alternative choices concerning antibiotic coverage have focused on whether to reduce the high bacterial count inside the bowel lumen (neomycin 1 g and erythromycin base 1 g, each given three or four times the day before the operation) or to use parenteral prophylactic antibiotics as to obtain high tissue levels before possible contamination by colon bacteria. We believe both types of antibiotic prophylaxis are important and both should be utilized (Table 23-8).

URINARY TRACT

The lower urinary tract is in close anatomic proximity to the pelvic organs. Both benign and malignant gynecologic diseases frequently produce anatomic distortion, partial obstruction, hydroureter, or hydronephrosis. Preoperative evaluation may include both radiologic and blood chemistry studies. A decade ago many gynecologists ordered a routine preoperative intravenous pyelogram (IVP) before all major gynecologic operations in an attempt to identify anatomic or functional abnormalities of the lower urinary tract. Recently, indications for a preoperative IVP have become more restricted in women without pelvic malignancy or large pelvic masses, such as leiomyomata.

An IVP helps to diagnose congenital abnormalities of the urinary tract. Congenital urinary anomalies are rare but are more common in women with congenital anomalies of the reproductive tract. If only a single kidney is visualized by an IVP, it is important to determine if the other kidney is congenitally absent or nonfunctioning. The presence of a pelvic kidney is important information in the differential diagnosis of a large, fixed adnexal mass. The presence of a double ureter is another anomaly discovered by preoperative radiologic studies. Preoperative knowledge of a double ureter is advantageous in anatomic identification of structures in the retroperitoneal space.

A preoperative IVP also helps to confirm the patency of the lower urinary tract. It is important to establish whether the enlargement, inflammation, or displacement of the gynecologic organs has produced distortion, obstruction, and possibly associated chronic infection in the corresponding area of the urinary tract. For example, when a uterus is enlarged to the pelvic brim with myomas, hydronephrosis is noted in approximately one third of patients. Common indications for the preoperative IVP with benign gynecologic disease include cervical myomas, lateral projection of uterine myomas, adnexal masses that are fixed and adherent, complete uterine prolapse, and large pelvic masses that produce urinary symptoms. However, a preoperative IVP will not give the gynecologist information that will necessarily reduce the incidence of operative injury to the ureters. During the operation the ureters must be identified along their entire course. The exact incidence of ureteral injury associated with benign surgery is unknown, for many injuries do not produce symptoms. However, Symmonds and others have estimated that ureteral injury occurs in 0.5% to 2.5% of all gynecologic operations.

One serious problem with IVPs is an allergic reaction to the radiologic contrast medium. Approximately 5% to 8% of women have an allergic reaction during an IVP, with 1% to 2% of these reactions being life-threatening. The fatality rate with IVPs is estimated to be approximately 1 in 100,000 procedures. Lasser et al. have reported that in pretreating patients with oral corticosteroids, giving methylprednisolone, 32 mg, 12 hours and 2 hours before the injection of intravenous contrast material significantly reduces the incidence of allergic reaction. This treatment is an alternative to using monomeric non-ionic iodinated compounds as the contrast media, with a lower incidence of allergic reactions. These compounds are new and expensive and have an osmolarity approximately 50% less than standard medications.

Another serious concern in ordering an IVP is the possibility of clinically significant nephrotoxicity being caused by the contrast material. Parfrey et al. found that this risk did not occur in nondiabetic patients with preexisting renal insufficiency or in diabetic patients with normal renal function. However, when the patient has both these high risk factors, diabetes and renal disease, the risk is 9% of developing acute renal insufficiency after an IVP, compared with a risk of 1.6% for control subjects.

Insufficient renal function is a major risk factor in elective operations because of the patient's decreased ability to excrete drugs. Women with insufficient renal function do poorly if they develop perioperative infections. Patients with azotemia have a threefold greater risk of adverse drug reactions than women with normal renal function. However, renal insufficiency is very infrequent in an asymptomatic woman under age 40, especially compared to the incidence of unsuspected respiratory disease. The frequency of abnormal serum BUN or creatinine levels is directly dependent on the patient's age. If all patients are screened regardless of whether the history is positive or negative for renal disease, the incidence of abnormal values is 2.5% in women under age 40, 5% in women ages 40 to 59, and 7.5% in women over age 60. Baseline and interval tests of renal function in women who are going to be treated with aminoglycosides are necessary and valuable studies.

More than 32,000 Americans have received renal transplant operations. Thus the gynecologist may encounter such a woman in his or her practice. These women need sufficient supplemental amounts of parenteral corticosteroids (hydrocortisone, 300 mg total over 24 hours) during the perioperative period to protect against acute adrenal insufficiency.

RESPIRATORY SYSTEM

The goals of the preoperative assessment of the respiratory system are to identify women at risk for developing postoperative pulmonary complications and to prescribe appropriate preoperative therapy to reduce these risks. Only rarely a patient cannot be anesthetized and well oxygenated intraoperatively. The surgeon's goal should be to avoid postoperative pulmonary complications. Similar to the evaluation of other organ systems, the history and physical examination are the most important parts of the pulmonary evaluation. Pulmonary function tests of lung volumes and flow rates are indicated to evaluate women with history or physical findings suggestive of restrictive or obstructive pulmonary disease.

Preoperative assessment must determine if the patient has the pulmonary reserve to overcome the normal postoperative decrease in pulmonary function. Women who have mildly compromised preoperative pulmonary function are especially susceptible to develop significant postoperative atelectasis, which occurs following approximately 10% of gynecologic operations. Women with severely diminished pulmonary reserve sometimes develop fulminating postoperative respiratory failure. Predisposing factors that increase the incidence of atelectasis include obesity, smoking, pulmonary disease, and advanced age. Increased pain, the supine position, abdominal distention, and sedation also contribute to decreased lung volumes and reduced dynamic measurements of pulmonary function for the postoperative patient.

Important questions in the history relate to smoking, recent upper respiratory infection, cough, amount of sputum production, degree of dyspnea, wheezing, and most important, exercise tolerance. In women with known respiratory disease, a complete medication history should be obtained, including antibiotics, bronchodilators, mucolytic agents, and corticosteroids. If either oral or inhalation corticosteroids have been taken during the past 6 to 9 months, the patient needs parenteral hydrocortisone to cover adrenal insufficiency during the perioperative period. The history should also include questions about exposure to industrial air pollution.

Obesity is a significant independent risk factor for postoperative complications. A weight of greater than 30% over ideal body weight increases pulmonary complications twofold by reducing the functional residual capacity by approximately 15%.

If the woman is currently a smoker, the risk of postoperative pulmonary complications increases approximately sixfold. The basic defense mechanisms of the lungs, such as the ciliary action of the epithelial cells that line the respiratory tract, are significantly impaired by smoking. Even young women with "normal lungs" who smoke one-half pack of cigarettes a day are at an increased risk. Ideally, patients should abstain from smoking for 2 to 4 weeks preoperatively. However, even a few days of abstinence from nicotine decreases excessive sputum production. Smoking is most detrimental in women with chronic bronchitis or chronic obstructive pulmonary disease.

Traditionally, anesthesiologists have insisted on at least a 10-day interval between an upper respiratory infection and the date of an elective operation. If the patient has productive sputum, the amount of sputum is estimated, purulent sputum cultured, and appropriate antibiotics given. However, a dramatic change in this practice may be forthcoming in women without underlying pulmonary disease. In a recent editorial, Fennelly and Hall state that little evidence shows that anesthesia in adult patients with an upper respiratory tract infection results in respiratory complications. This editorial challenges the medical community to perform a randomized study to resolve this controversy.

During the physical examination, special attention should be given to findings of tachypnea, wheezing, rales, and prolonged expiration. Direct observation of exercise tolerance, such as climbing a flight of stairs, is helpful in evaluating the extent of pulmonary reserve. This is a crude index of pulmonary function. Patients with any positive findings on history or physical examination should have a chest x-ray examination and in selected cases arterial blood gases and pulmonary function tests. Preoperative pulmonary function tests should be performed on patients with a productive sputum (more than 2 ounces per day), age greater than 65 years, 20 pack-years or greater smoking history, obesity, asthma, and chronic obstructive pulmonary disease. Lockwood has estimated the extent of respiratory disease and the probability of pulmonary complications from the results of pulmonary function tests. If arterial blood gases are measured, the oxygen tension should exceed 65 mm Hg, and the carbon dioxide tension should be less than 45 mm Hg.

Pulmonary function tests help both to assess the pulmonary reserve and to identify the extent to which the dysfunction is reversible. Pulmonary function tests that measure lung volumes and flow rates help to distinguish restrictive defects or a decrease in the amount of lung tissue from obstructive defects in which there is a reduction and prolongation of airflow during expiration. The two most common pulmonary function tests used for screening are vital capacity and forced expiratory volume in 1 second. A woman with a vital capacity volume of less than 50% of the predicted normal for her age and body size should have more extensive testing for significant lung disease. Similarly, the forced expiratory volume in 1 second should be greater than 75% of the predicted normal volume.

Twenty-five million Americans have asthma. Thus this condition is frequently encountered during the preoperative evaluation. Asthma increases the incidence of perioperative respiratory problems approximately fourfold. Ideally, an asthmatic patient should have elective surgery when she is free of wheezing and has optimal pulmonary status, as measured by pulmonary function tests. Preoperative preparation of patients with asthma or other chronic obstructive pulmonary disease includes cessation of smoking; instruction in incentive spirometry, bronchodilators, chest physiotherapy, and postural drainage; adequate hydration; and antibiotics for purulent sputum for several days before the anticipated surgery. Ideally, patients should discontinue smoking at least 8 weeks before surgery. Realistically, only one of four patients will adhere to this recommendation. Improvements in pulmonary function by intensive treatment several days before an operation should be documented by serial pulmonary function tests. Prophylactic lung expansion programs are effective in decreasing the risk of postoperative atelectasis in high-risk individuals. Gilmour has emphasized that the major factors in postoperative respiratory morbidity are underlying pulmonary disease and the associated decrease in functional respiratory capacity normally produced by the events surrounding an operation.

DIABETES MELLITUS

Diabetes mellitus is encountered more frequently in women undergoing gynecologic surgery than any other disease of the endocrine system. Elective operations should be scheduled for the diabetic patient only if she is in nutritional balance and under good diabetic control. The stress of an operation and of anesthesia often produces changes in glucose tolerance and insulin resistance. There is a threefold increase in morbidity and a doubling of mortality if an operation is performed in diabetic patients in poor control. The basic goal of the operative team is to control the blood glucose level perioperatively.

During the perioperative period the additional release of catecholamines, cortisol, growth hormone, and glucagon may produce hyperglycemia. The combined effects of these three hormones tend to elevate the blood sugar levels by 20 to 40 mg/100 ml. The principal postoperative complications in diabetic patients are increased operative site infections and wound disruptions. The increase in infection rate is believed to be secondary to a decrease in both cellular and humoral responses to bacteria. The increased incidence of wound disruptions is due to a decreased tensile strength during healing.

Preoperative evaluation requires meticulous attention to the details of the patient's disease during the history and physical examination. Important questions center around the severity of the diabetes, types of medications, and recent diabetic control, including blood and urine glucose levels. Specific inquiries should be made about the complications of chronic diabetes, especially those affecting the cardiovascular and renal systems. During the physical examination, attention should be directed toward the diagnosis of peripheral neuropathy. Diabetic neuropathy may be the explanation of persistent pain during the perioperative period. Autonomic neuropathy may cause postoperative gastrointestinal or genitourinary dysfunction. Autonomic dysfunction also predisposes the diabetic patient to cardiac arrest. Preoperative blood studies should include some measurement of recent diabetic control, such as hemoglobin A_{1C} or glycosylated proteins (e.g., fructosamine), and complete electrolyte, renal, and liver profiles. An electrocardiogram (ECG) and chest x-ray film should be obtained regardless of the woman's age. The major morbidity in diabetic patients related to surgery usually results from chronic vascular and end-organ damage, not acute changes in glucose control. Thus the cardiovascular, renal, and central nervous systems should be the focus of concern. In a recent shift in clinical opinion, rigid perioperative control of blood glucose levels is not as beneficial as previously believed.

The medical sequelae of diabetes mellitus, such as renal and cardiac insufficiency, peripheral neuropathy, and peripheral vascular disease, are related to both the severity and the chronicity of the disease. The patient's history will help to differentiate mild insulin-dependent diabetes from severe insulin-dependent diabetes. When diabetes is treated with oral agents, consideration should be directed to preoperative dosage. Long-acting sulfonylureas have long half-lives and should be discontinued 3 days before surgery. Short-acting sulfonylureas should be discontinued 24 hours before operation. During major elective surgery, mildly diabetic patients are usually treated with small doses of regular insulin.

There are three current rationales of perioperative management of insulin-dependent diabetes. The general goals of all regimens are to avoid ketosis, hypoglycemia, and hyperosmolar conditions. Women with type I diabetes are much more prone to develop ketoacidosis and hypoglycemia than women with type II diabetes. The first regimen uses no insulin and no glucose. This method is appropriate only for diabetic women under excellent control whose proposed surgery will have a short operative time, with limited disruption of gastrointestinal function. The second regimen is the administration of one third to one half of a woman's usual insulin dosage given subcutaneously the morning of surgery. An intravenous infusion of 5% dextrose at 125 ml per hour is begun 1 hour before surgery. The availability of rapid bedside measurements of blood sugar allows the adjustment of blood sugar levels by supplemental intravenous regular insulin. The third regimen is one of rigid glucose control. The goal of the rigid protocol is to maintain the blood glucose level between 100 and 200 mg/100 ml throughout the perioperative period. Patients are admitted 48 to 72 hours before surgery and placed on a continuous intravenous infusion of regular insulin. Levels of blood glucose are obtained at frequent intervals and insulin adjusted until a steady state is obtained. Thereafter the blood glucose level is measured at least every 4 hours.

CARDIOVASCULAR DISEASE

The vast majority of women with heart disease who have compensated cardiac function tolerate surgery well. The presence of congestive failure is the single most predictive factor of cardiovascular complications during the perioperative period. If a patient with cardiac disease is not in failure and does not have severe coronary artery disease, she will do as well as a woman without heart disease. Elective surgery should be scheduled only when a patient is not in cardiac failure and her blood pressure is under proper control. Physiologically, surgery and anesthesia decrease cardiac output by reducing cardiac function and decreasing effective intravascular volume. The stress of surgery results in increased production of catecholamines, cortisol, and antidiuretic hormone. Anesthetic agents depress myocardial function and have varying effects on the autonomic nervous system and peripheral vascular tone. Surgery and anesthesia are an additional burden to a cardiovascular system without adequate reserve.

The severity of cardiac disease may be assessed in the history by questions regarding exercise tolerance, dyspnea, chest pain, and orthopnea. On physical examination an abnormal heart rate or rhythm, cardiac size, murmurs, and signs of cardiac failure should be noted. A large, appropriately sized blood pressure cuff should be obtained for obese women. Routine ECGs obtained on postmenopausal women may diagnose asymptomatic myocardial infarctions or serious arrhythmias, which will necessitate postponing elective surgery. When women with severe heart disease have major surgery, optimum control of fluid balance and filling pressures are determined by arterial lines and Swan-Ganz catheters. For example, a preoperative history of pulmonary edema is associated with an approximately 40% chance of developing postoperative congestive heart failure.

In 1977 Goldman et al. published a classic study predicting perioperative cardiac risk. Their study involved 1001 patients over age 40. By multivariate analysis, they identified factors related to life-threatening cardiac complications (Table 23-9). Using Goldman's criteria, patients can be rated via a numerical score (Table 23-10) as to the risk of cardiac death or significant cardiac morbidity. With the length of life increasing, more elderly women are candidates for gynecologic surgery. Age is an important risk factor. The risk of postoperative cardiac death is tenfold greater in women over age 70.

HYPERTENSIVE DISEASE. Women with controlled essential hypertension in the absence of cardiac or renal complications are not at an increased risk for major problems with elective surgery. However, women with poorly controlled hypertension and a diastolic pressure greater than 110 mm Hg should have

TABLE 23-9

Cardiac Risk Factors for Patients Going to Surgery

Criteria	Finding	Points
History	Age over 70	5
	Myocardial infarction in previous 6 months	10*
Physical examination	Third heart sound or jugular venous distention	11*
	Significant aortic stenosis	3
Electrocardiogram (ECG)	*Any* rhythm other than normal sinus	7
	Premature atrial contractions on last preoperative ECG	7*
	More than five premature contractions per minute on *any* previous ECG	7
General status	Oxygen tension less than 60 mm Hg, carbon dioxide tension (P_{CO_2}) greater than 50 mm Hg	3*
	Potassium (K^+) less than 3.0 mEq/L, bicarbonate (HCO_3) less than 20 mEq/L	
	Blood urea nitrogen (BUN) greater than 50 mg/dl, creatinine greater than 3.0 mg/dl	
	Abnormal serum glutamic-oxaloacetic transaminase (SGOT) or signs of chronic liver disease	
Operation	Emergency surgery	4*
	Intraperitoneal, thoracic, or major vascular procedure	3
TOTAL POSSIBLE		60

Adapted from Goldman L, Caldera DL, Nussbaum SR, et al: N Engl J Med 297:845, 1977. From Salem DN, Homans D, McNally JW, et al: Cardiology. In Molitch ME, editors: Management of medical problems in surgical patients, Philadelphia, 1982, FA Davis Co, p 75.
*Risk factors that may be altered by preoperative intervention or delay in surgery.

TABLE 23-10

Cardiac Risk Classes for Patients Going to Surgery

Risk Class	Point Score	No or Minor Complications (%)	Life-Threatening Complications* (%)	Cardiac Death (%)
I	0-5	99	0.7	0.2
II	6-12	93	5	2
III	13-25	86	11	2
IV	>26	22	22	56

Adapted from Goldman L, Caldera DL, Southwick FS, et al: Medicine 57:357, 1978. From Salem DN, Homans D, McNally JW, et al: Cardiology. In Molitch ME, editor: Management of medical problems in surgical patients, Philadelphia, 1982, FA Davis Co, p 76.
*Myocardial infarction, ventricular tachycardia, pulmonary edema.

more intense medical management of their hypertension before elective surgery. No increased risk of cardiovascular complications from surgery occurs in women with mild to moderate hypertension when the diastolic blood pressure is less than 110 mm Hg. During the induction of anesthesia, there is a potential abrupt rise of blood pressure of 20 to 50 mm Hg. This transient hypertension is experienced during intubation in 6% of normotensive patients and 17% of women with hypertension. Rapid hemodynamic fluctuations are directly related to morbidity in hypertensive women. Major differences between preoperative and intraoperative blood pressures correlate directly with episodes of myocardial ischemia.

Antihypertensive medication should be continued throughout the perioperative period. The only exception is monoamine oxidase inhibitors, which should be discontinued for at least 2 weeks before surgery. Discontinuing some antihypertensive agents is potentially harmful. For example, if beta-blockers are withdrawn, patients may develop a hypersensitivity to adrenergic stimulation and an exacerbation of ischemic heart disease. Similarly, patients taking clonidine develop abrupt hypertensive rebound if the drug is withdrawn. Diuretic therapy need not be discontinued before surgery. Potential hazards of diuretics include a relative hypovolemia and hypokalemia. Although diuretics often produce hypokalemia, and associated arrhythmias are a major concern in women with organic heart disease, they are rarely seen in women without significant heart disease.

CORONARY ARTERY DISEASE. Medically significant coronary artery disease is a problem of older women. It is most unusual for a premenopausal woman to have ischemic heart disease unless she has diabetes, hyperlipidemia, severe hypertension, or a strong family history of coronary disease. Nevertheless, women over age 50 often have elective gynecologic surgery. Thus considerations of angina and previous myocardial infarctions are essential in planning elective surgery.

Unstable angina of less than 3 months' duration is a strong contraindication to an elective operation. Conversely, women with stable angina without a previous history of myocardial infarction do not have an increased risk of infarction during operations. When a woman has had a myocardial infarction, it is important to delay an elective operation for at least 6 months. The excessive mortality associated with a noncardiac operative procedure within 3 months of an acute myocardial infarct is 27% to 37%. Following a 6-month interval the chance of a reinfarction is 4% to 6% with elective operations. No advantage exists in delaying surgery longer than 6 months, because the woman's risk remains constant for the rest of her life.

The induction of anesthesia is an especially vulnerable period of time for myocardial ischemia. Myocardial ischemia occurs when the heart has to increase its rate and respond to an increase in systemic blood pressure. Recurrent myocardial infarctions are infrequently accompanied by chest pains, and one third occur on the third or fourth postoperative day. Thus

women with coronary artery disease should be closely monitored both hemodynamically and electro-cardiographically for at least 4 days postoperatively.

The potential dangers of operations in a woman with multiple premature ventricular contractions (PVCs) are only significant if the PVCs are associated with a decrease in left ventricular function.

VALVULAR HEART DISEASE. The major perioperative consideration in women with valvular heart disease is the use of prophylactic antibiotics to reduce the incidence of subacute bacterial endocarditis developing from a bacteremia associated with the surgical procedure. Even without antibiotic coverage, this is a rare complication. However, because of the substantial morbidity and mortality associated with bacterial endocarditis, antibiotic prophylaxis is the standard of care. Patients with valvular heart disease who are at significant risk during surgery are women with aortic and mitral stenosis. Physiologically, these lesions are similar in that the fixed cardiac output may lead to decompensation secondary to the need for changes in cardiac performance during surgical procedures.

Women with heart disease who should receive antibiotic coverage include women with congenital or acquired valvular heart disease, high-pressure congenital cardiac shunts, operatively repaired congenital defects or heart valves, and previous episodes of endocarditis. The incidence of rheumatic fever has declined recently, and mitral valve prolapse is presently the leading indication for endocarditis prophylaxis. Mitral valve prolapse is a common finding, being diagnosed in 6% to 8% of women having gynecologic surgery. The incidence of bacterial endocarditis is three-fold to eightfold higher in women with mitral valve prolapse than in the general population. We believe that it is mandatory to give antibiotic prophylaxis only to those women with the classic form of mitral valve prolapse, leaflet thickening and redundancy. In a study on mitral insufficiency, Marks et al. identified them as the group at highest risk. The risk of bacterial endocarditis is low if the extent of mitral valve prolapse is an isolated systolic click. An appropriate antibiotic coverage for gynecologic surgery is ampicillin (2 g intramuscularly or intravenously) and gentamicin (1.5 mg/kg of body weight intramuscularly) approximately 1 hour before the operation. Depending on the time of expected bacteremia, often the same dosage of both drugs is repeated 8 hours later. If the woman is allergic to ampicillin, vancomycin (1 g given slowly intravenously) may be substituted.

Special consideration should be given to women with valvular heart disease who are receiving chronic oral anticoagulation. It is preferable to discontinue the oral medication 48 to 72 hours before surgery. Anticoagulation is accomplished during the perioperative period with heparin. Oral medication is usually resumed approximately 72 hours postoperatively.

THE MORNING OF THE OPERATION

Preoperative Note

A brief preoperative note helps to serve as a final summary of preoperative preparation. This abbreviated checklist should summarize important findings in the preoperative history, physical examination, and laboratory screening tests. This note is designed to assure that no step has been forgotten and to summarize in a few words pertinent details for other individuals who subsequently attend the patient. The surgeon should make a brief notation that all the patient's questions have been answered and that both patient and physician are in agreement over the proposed operative procedure.

Shaving

Many centers have abandoned the ancient ritual of shaving the abdomen and vulvar areas the day before surgery. Shaving is not necessary unless dense hair presents a mechanical problem in preoperative washing of the skin. Multiple studies have documented a twofold to threefold increase in infection rate directly related to perioperative shaving. Cruse and Foord studied approximately 63,000 operations over a 10-year period and found a 0.9% incidence of infection when patients were not shaved as opposed to 2.5% when they were shaved. Razors produce macroscopic and microscopic nicks and cuts that allow a protective environment for colonization by skin bacteria. Depilatory agents often produce intense burning if used on the perineum. In general, gyne-

cologists should abandon the humiliating and crude procedure of preoperative shaving. If the hair is mechanically in the way, it should be clipped just before the operation.

Reassurance

Many women are extremely anxious on the morning of their operation and admission to the hospital the morning of surgery usually intensifies their anxiety. In many hospitals this process offers little emotional support to the individual patient, but rather gives her the opinion that she is being "herded" by low-level hospital employees. The physical presence of "her" gynecologist when she enters the operating room provides great reassurance. The kindness of touching the patient's hand or standing by her side as the induction of anesthesia begins is never forgotten.

Pelvic Examination

After the patient is asleep or the conduction anesthesia has taken effect, the gynecologic surgeon has two important responsibilities: performing the preoperative pelvic examination and supervising the positioning of the patient. A pelvic examination following catheterization and just before surgical incision should be standard practice, regardless of the type or extent of the proposed gynecologic operation. The relaxation of the abdominal wall produced by anesthesia and the advantage of an empty bladder and lower intestinal tract affords the surgeon the optimum environment for performing a pelvic examination. The findings may change the choice of incision or operative approach. Following the pelvic examination, it is sometimes beneficial to measure the depth and direction of the uterine cavity with a metal sound. This procedure helps to distinguish the uterus from adnexal pathology. Before draping the patient, the gynecologist should make sure that the patient is properly positioned on the operating room table. This is especially true to obtain good exposure in the lithotomy position. Pressure points should be avoided to protect against neuromuscular and skin injury, especially over bony prominences.

_____ **KEY POINTS** _____

- The goals of preoperative planning are to obtain appropriate information, reduce the patient's anxieties and fears, and obtain informed consent.

- Eye-to-eye contact and gentle touching of the hands are appropriate and effective ways to express the physician's sincere interest in caring for the patient.

- A detailed history and physical examination will detect approximately 90% of the information pertinent to the surgical procedure.

- Cost containment strategies have placed increasing emphasis on same-day admission for most patients having major gynecologic operations.

- Surgical morbidity and mortality are directly proportional to the amount of a patient's preexisting medical disease.

- It is important in taking the history to ask specifically about oral contraceptives, as well as nonprescription medicine, such as aspirin, for they are often not considered "medicines" by the patient.

- Included with the contaceptive history are key questions concerning possible exposure to the human immunodeficiency (AIDS) virus.

- The most important feature of the preoperative physical examination is that it be performed in a thorough and compulsive manner.

- The choice of which preoperative tests to perform should be based on the age of the patient and the extent of the surgical procedure, as well as details from the history and physical examination.

- Routine clotting studies are not cost effective unless indicated by history or physical examination.

- Blood urea nitrogen and creatinine measurements should be ordered preoperatively if there is a history suggestive of renal disease or the woman is over age 40.

- Routine chest x-ray films are not cost effective unless the patient is over age 60 or has findings in the history or physical examination suggestive of cardiac or respiratory disease.

- A baseline preoperative electrocardiogram is appropriate and cost effective in women over age 50.

- Serum electrolyte levels should be evaluated for patients with vomiting, diarrhea, ileus, bowel obstruction, or any condition that affects water or electrolyte balance.

- An operation without consent makes the gynecologist vulnerable to charges of assault and battery, except in an emergency.

- Highlights of the discussion regarding informed consent should be documented by a paragraph written by the gynecologist in the progress notes of the chart.

- Perioperative shaving of the patient is inappropriate because studies have documented a twofold to threefold increase in infection rate related to shaving. If the hair will interfere with the operation, it should be clipped immediately before the operation.

- Douching the evening before surgery is not an effective way of cleaning the vagina and is not necessary. Emptying the bladder before going to the operating room is also unnecessary because catheterization should be performed before surgery.

- Oral contraceptives should be discontinued 4 weeks before major elective surgery. Postmenopausal replacement estrogens need not be discontinued.

- The factors that make a woman at high risk for thromboembolic disease include a previous history of thromboembolic disease, a family history of hypercoagulability, malignant disease, previous radiation therapy, obesity, venous disease, active pelvic infection, and lengthy preoperative hospitalization.

- Patients at high risk for thromboembolic disease should be considered as candidates for prophylactic heparin in a dose of 5000 units of subcutaneous heparin combined with 0.5 mg of dihydroergotamine mesylate 2 hours before operation and every 8 to 12 hours afterward for 5 to 7 days or until the patient is fully ambulatory.

- The primary goals of preoperative medication are to relieve anxiety, protect against allergic reactions, and produce sedation, analgesia, and, it is hoped, amnesia.

- Antibiotic prophylaxis works by reducing the number of bacteria present, not by killing all bacteria. To be effective, the antibiotic must be present at the time of tissue injury or shortly thereafter.

- Oral medications that a patient may be taking for a specific condition or illness may be taken the morning before surgery with 30 to 60 ml of water.

- Barium enema and endoscopy need not be performed routinely on all patients with adnexal masses. These tests are indicated in women over age 40 with left-sided masses, women with positive stool guaiac tests, or women with bowel symptoms.

- If there is a possibility that the pelvic pathology may necessitate entry in the lumen of the large intestine, both mechanical cleansing of the bowel and antibiotics to reduce the bacterial count should be ordered before surgery.

- Allergic reactions to the radiologic contrast medium occur during intravenous pyelograms in approximately 5% to 8% of women.

- Factors that increase the incidence of atelectasis include obesity, smoking, pulmonary disease, and advanced age.

- A weight of greater than 30% over ideal body weight increases pulmonary complications twofold, primarily by reducing the functional residual capacity by up to 15%.

- If a woman is currently a smoker, her risk of postoperative pulmonary complications increases approximately sixfold.

- Ideally an asthmatic patient should undergo an elective surgical procedure when she is free of wheezing and in optimal pulmonary status, as measured by pulmonary function tests.

- If preoperative arterial blood gases are measured, the oxygen tension should exceed 65 mm Hg, and the carbon dioxide tension should be less than 45 mm Hg.

- Asthma increases the incidence of perioperative respiratory problems approximately fourfold.

- There is a threefold increase in morbidity and a doubling of mortality if surgery is performed on diabetic patients who are in poor glucose control.

- The preoperative workup of a diabetic patient should include electrolyte levels, renal panel, liver profiles, an electrocardiogram, and a chest x-ray film, regardless of the woman's age.

- In a recent shift in clinical opinion, rigid perioperative control of blood glucose levels are not as beneficial as previously believed.

- The presence of congestive failure is the single most predictive factor of cardiovascular complications during the perioperative period.

- No increased risk of cardiovascular complications from surgery occurs in women with mild to moderate hypertension when the diastolic blood pressure is less than 110 mm Hg.

- The excessive mortality associated with noncardiac surgery within 3 months of an acute myocardial infarction is 27% to 37%.

- The recommended protocol for bacterial endocarditis prophylaxis is ampicillin, (2 g intramuscularly or intravenously) and gentamicin (1.5 mg/kg intramuscularly or intravenously) 1 hour before the operation.

BIBLIOGRAPHY

Aitkenhead AR: Awareness during anaesthesia: what should the patient be told? Anaesthesia 45:351, 1990.

Amstey MS and Jones AP: Preparation of the vagina for surgery, JAMA 245:839, 1981.

Applebaum PS and Grisso T: Assessing patients' capacities to consent to treatment, N Engl J Med 319:1635, 1988.

Astedt B: Does estrogen replacement therapy predispose to thrombosis? Acta Obstet Gynecol Scand Suppl 130:71, 1985.

Beck DE, Harford FJ, and DiPalma JA: Comparison of cleansing methods in preparation for colonic surgery, Dis Colon Rectum 28:491, 1985.

Bettmann MA: Radiographic contrast agents—a perspective. N Engl J Med 317:891, 1987.

Bird BJ, Chrisp DB, and Scrimgeour G: Extensive preoperative shaving: a costly exercise, NZ Med J 97:727, 1984.

Bone RC: Ventilation/perfusion scan in pulmonary embolism: "the emperor is incompletely attired," JAMA 263:2794, 1990.

Bonnar J: Venous thromboembolism and gynecologic surgery, Clin Obstet Gynecol 28:432, 1985.

Breslow MJ, Miller CF, and Rogers M, editors: Perioperative management, St Louis, 1990, Mosby–Year Book, Inc.

Burke JF: The effective period of preventive antibiotic action in experimental incisions and dermal lesions, Surgery 50:161, 1961.

Burns ER and Lawrence C: Bleeding time: a guide to its diagnostic and clinical utility, Arch Pathol Lab Med 113:1219, 1989.

Caprini JA, Scurr JH, and Hasty JH: Role of compression modalities in a prophylactic program for deep vein thrombosis, Sem Thromb Hemost 14(S1):77, 1988.

Cartwright PS, Pittaway DE, Jones HW, et al: The use of prophylactic antibiotics in obstetrics and gynecology: a review, Obstet Gynecol Surv 39:537, 1984.

Collins R, Scrimgeour A, Yusuf S, et al: Reduction in fatal pulmonary embolism and venous thrombosis by perioperative administration of subcutaneous heparin, N Engl J Med 318:1162, 1988.

Cruse PJ and Foord R: A 10-year prospective study of 62,939 wounds, Surg Clin North Am 60:27, 1980.

Dajan AS, Bisno AL, Chung KJ, et al: Prevention of bacterial endocarditis: recommendations by the American Heart Association, JAMA 264:2919, 1990.

Daly MP: The medical evaluation of the elderly preoperative patient, Prim Care 16:361, 1989.

Devereux RB, Kramer-Fox R, and Kligfield P: Mitral valve prolapse: causes, clinical manifestations, and management, Ann Intern Med 111:305, 1989.

Erban SB, Kinman JL, and Schwartz JS: Routine use of the prothrombin and partial thromboplastin times, JAMA 262:2428, 1989.

Fennelly ME and Hall GM: Anaesthesia and upper respiratory tract infections—a non-existent hazard? Br J Anaesth 64:535, 1990.

Galandiuk S, Polk HC, Jagelman DG, and Fazio VW: Reemphasis of priorities in surgical antibiotic prophylaxis, Surg Gynecol Obstet 169:219, 1989.

Gerding DN: Disease associated with Clostridium difficile infection, Ann Intern Med 110:255, 1989.

Gilmour IJ: Perioperative respiratory care, Urol Clin North Am 10:65, 1983.

Goldman DR, Brown FH, Levy WK, et al, editors: Medical care of the surgical patient, Philadelphia, 1982, JB Lippincott Co.

Goldman L, Caldera DL, Nussbaum SR, et al: Multifactorial index of cardiac risk in noncardiac surgical procedures, N Engl J Med 297:845, 1977.

Goldman L, Caldera DL, Southwick FS, et al: Cardiac risk factors and complications in non-cardiac surgery, Medicine 57:357, 1978.

Guillebaud J: Surgery and the pill, Br Med J 291:498, 1985.

Hirsch HA: Prophylactic antibiotics in obstetrics and gynecology, Am J Med 78(suppl 6B):170, 1985.

Hirsh RA: An approach to assessing perioperative risk. In Goldman DR, Brown FH, Levy WK, et al, editors: Medical care of the surgical patient, Philadelphia, 1982, JB Lippincott Co.

Hubbell FA, Greenfield S, Tyler JL, et al: The impact of routine admission chest x-ray films on patient care, N Engl J Med 312:209, 1985.

Jackson CV: Preoperative pulmonary evaluation, Arch Intern Med 148:2120, 1988.

Jewell ER and Persson AV: Preoperative evaluation of the high-risk patient, Surg Clin North Am 65:3, 1985.

Kaplan EB, Sheiner LB, Boeckmann AJ, et al: The usefulness of preoperative laboratory screening, JAMA 253:3576, 1985.

Kelley MA, Carson JL, Palevsky HI, and Schwartz JS: Diagnosing pulmonary embolism: new facts and strategies, Ann Intern Med 114:300, 1991.

Lasser EC, Berry CC, Talner LB, et al: Pretreatment with corticosteroids to alleviate reactions to intravenous contrast material, N Engl J Med 317:845, 1987.

Lavie CJ, Khandheria BK, Seward JB, et al: Factors associated with the recommendation for endocarditis prophylaxis in mitral valve prolapse, JAMA 262:3308, 1989.

Lockwood P: Lung function test results and the risk of post-thoracotomy complications, Respiration 30:529, 1973.

Lockwood P: The principles of predicting the risk of post-thoracotomy function-related complications in bronchial carcinoma, Respiration 30:329, 1973.

Lutomski DM, Djuric PE, and Draeger RW: Warfarin therapy: the effect of heparin on prothrombin times, Arch Intern Med 147:432, 1987.

Marks AR, Choong CY, Chir MBB, et al: Identification of high-risk and low-risk subgroups of patients with mitral-valve prolapse, N Engl J Med 320:1031, 1989.

National Blood Resource Education Program Expert Panel: The use of autologous blood, JAMA 263:414, 1990.

Norman J: Preoperative patient assessment: general assessment, Br Med Bull 42:247, 1988.

Panton ONM, Atkinson KG, Crichton EP, et al: Mechanical preparation of the large bowel for elective surgery, Am J Surg 149:615, 1985.

Parfrey PS, Griffiths SM, Barrett BJ, et al: Contrast material–induced renal failure in patients with diabetes mellitus, renal insufficiency, or both: a prospective controlled study, N Engl J Med 320:143, 1989.

Pennock JL: Perioperative management of drug therapy, Surg Clin North Am 63:1049, 1983.

Piscitelli JT, Simel DL, and Addison A: Who should have intravenous pyelograms before hysterectomy for benign disease? Obstet Gynecol 69:541, 1987.

Polak JF, Cutter SS, and O'Leary DH: Deep veins of the calf: assessment with Doppler flow imaging, Radiol 171:481, 1989.

Poller A, McKernan A, Thomson JM, et al: Fixed minidose warfarin: a new approach to prophylaxis against venous thrombosis after major surgery, Br Med J 295:1309, 1987.

Roizen MF: Preoperative evaluation of patients with diseases that require special preoperative evaluation and intraoperative management. In Miller RD, editor: Anesthesia, vol 1, ed 2, New York, 1986, Churchill Livingstone, Inc.

Roizen MF: Routine preoperative evaluation. In Miller RD, editor: Anesthesia, vol 1, ed 2, New York, 1986, Churchill Livingstone, Inc.

Rucker L, Frey EB, and Staten MA: Usefulness of screening chest roentgenograms in preoperative patients, JAMA 250:3209, 1983.

Salem DN, Homans D, McNally JW, et al: Cardiology. In Molitch ME, editor: Management of medical problems in surgical patients, Philadelphia, 1982, FA Davis Co.

Shapiro M, Munoz A, Tager IB, et al: Risk factors for infection at the operative site after abdominal or vaginal hysterectomy, N Engl J Med 307:1661, 1982.

Shapiro M, Schoenbaum SC, Tager IB, et al: Benefit-cost analysis of antimicrobial prophylaxis in abdominal and vaginal hysterectomy, JAMA 249:1290, 1983.

Simel DL, Matchar DB, and Piscitelli JT: Routine intravenous pyelograms before hysterectomy in cases of benign disease: possibly effective, definitely expensive, Am J Obstet Gynecol 159:1049, 1988.

Stoelting RK: Psychological preparation and preoperative medication. In Miller RD, ed: Anesthesia, vol 1, ed 2, New York, 1986, Churchill Livingstone, Inc.

Sundram CJ: Informed consent for major medical treatment of mentally disabled people, N Engl J Med 318:1368, 1988.

Symmonds RE: Ureteral injuries associated with gynecologic surgery: prevention and management, Clin Obstet Gynecol 19:632, 1976.

Taberner DA, Poller L, Thomson JM, et al: Randomized study of adjusted versus fixed low dose heparin prophylaxis of deep vein thrombosis in hip surgery, Br J Surg 76:933, 1989.

Toy PTCY, Strauss RG, Stehling LC, et al: Predeposited autologous blood for elective surgery: a national multicenter study, N Engl J Med 316:517, 1987.

White RH, McGahan JP, Daschbach MM, and Harling RP: Diagnosis of deep vein thrombosis using duplex ultrasound, Ann Intern Med 111:297, 1989.

Wingo PA, Huezo CM, Rubin GL, et al: The mortality risk associated with hysterectomy, Am J Obstet Gynecol 152:803, 1985.

KEY TERMS AND DEFINITIONS

Adynamic (Paralytic) Ileus. A temporary loss of intestinal peristalsis that may lead to a functional intestinal obstruction.

Antipyretic. A drug or device to lower body temperature.

Atelectasis. Imperfect expansion of the lung.

Cuff Cellulitis. One of many terms used for the cellulitis caused by an infection from endogenous bacteria in the serosanguineous fluid that collects in the retroperitoneal space at the vaginal apex.

Dihydroergotamine. A venotonic drug exerting a selective constrictive effect on capacitance blood vessels with only minimum constrictive effects on resistance vessels.

Duplex Ultrasound. A high-resolution ultrasound technique using real time and Doppler, rapidly becoming the preferred method for the diagnosis of proximal venous thrombosis.

Homan's Sign. Discomfort behind the knee on forced dorsiflexion of the foot; a sign of thrombophebitis in the calf.

Impedance Plethysmography. A noninvasive screening method using changes in blood volume, as measured by changes in electrical resistance, for the detection of deep vein thrombophlebitis.

Latzko's Operation. A technique for repair of a fistula at the vaginal apex that includes partial colpocleisis with denudation of the vaginal mucosa surrounding the fistula and subsequent multilayer closure without entering the bladder.

Lymphocyst. A local collection of lymphatic fluid.

Necrotizing Fasciitis. A virulent, rapidly progressing soft tissue infection that is sometimes fatal.

Phlebography (Venography). Radiography of the venous system, the most accurate current method of detecting deep vein thrombophlebitis.

Shock. A condition in which circulatory insufficiency prevents adequate vascular perfusion of vital organs.

Therapeutic Window. The range of effective blood concentration of a medication before undesired side effects occur.

Thrombophlebitis. The process of venous thrombosis formation, secondary coagulation of blood, and fibrin formation in the presence of venous stasis.

Ventilation/Perfusion Scan (V/Q Scan). A noninvasive imaging technique that is the first step in establishing or excluding the diagnosis of pulmonary embolus.

Ventilation Scintigraphy. A technique of injection of small radioactive pharmaceuticals of technetium or xenon gas used to detect pulmonary emboli.

Wound Dehiscence. Disruption of any layers of the surgical incision caused by a failure of normal healing. The peritoneum remains intact.

Wound Evisceration. Complete breakdown of the healing process through all levels of the incision, with omentum or bowel presenting through the incision.

Postoperative complications may occur even after minor operations. The period of hospitalization following an operation often is as important in ensuring a successful outcome as the preoperative preparation and the operation itself. The goal of postoperative care is to restore the woman to normal physiologic and psychologic health. Some problems are inherently nonpreventable, and therefore early recognition and treatment are necessary. If minor complications are overlooked, they may evolve into major problems for both the patient and her physician.

During the first 24 hours following an operation, the cardiovascular, renal, and respiratory systems should be closely monitored. If the patient is in good health and has had a gynecologic operation for a benign disease, she may be moved to an inpatient room after being monitored for 1 to 3 hours in the recovery room. The expert monitoring and skilled assistance of an intensive care unit are preferable for patients with coexisting illness or extensive operations for malignancy.

An outline of general guidelines for postoperative orders for a woman following an abdominal or vaginal hysterectomy is included in the box below. Flexibility and individual considerations should take precedence over standard orders, but the guidelines can help the physician develop his or her own preferences.

Two major considerations in the postoperative course are pyrexia and blood loss. The causes of fever encompass the majority of postoperative complications. All gynecologic organs are endowed with a rich blood supply. Thus hemorrhage and hematoma formation are also frequent postoperative complications.

POSTOPERATIVE FEVER

The exact definition of postoperative febrile morbidity varies greatly among authors. Although a normal temperature is usually below 37° C, most definitions use a temperature greater than 38° C as the febrile indicator of morbidity. It is not unusual for gynecologic patients to have a mild temperature elevation during the first 72 hours of the postoperative period, especially during the late afternoon or evening. Approximately 75% of patients develop a temperature greater than 37°, which is usually not associated with an infectious process. Approximately 25% of women after abdominal hysterectomy and 35% following vaginal hysterectomy exhibit febrile morbidity. Agents that produce fever are either endogenous or exogenous pyrogens.

The physician's primary goal in examining the postoperatively febrile patient is to determine whether the fever is caused by an infection. Some conditions necessitate active intervention, whereas others are self-limiting. Approximately 20% of postoperative fevers are directly related to infection, and 80% are related to noninfectious causes. Thus it is imperative not to empirically treat a postoperatively febrile patient with broad-spectrum antibiotics; in addition, it is usually unnecessary to give antipyretics to lower the temperature of an adult. As Duff has emphasized, fever is a phylogenic host response to infection in fish, lizards, and in higher mammals, including humans. Fever may be a beneficial response to the host.

Fever is a common postoperative finding, especially a mild temperature elevation during the first 48 to 72 hours following an operation. The cause of a postoperative fever may be simple and common, such as atelectasis or dehydration, or unusual, such as malignant hyperthermia or thyroid storm. The temporal relationship of the *onset* of a patient's febrile response to common postoperative complications

---

SAMPLE POSTOPERATIVE ORDERS

1. Admit to recovery area; to postoperative room when awake and vital signs are stable
2. Diagnosis: abdominal hysterectomy for myomas
3. Condition: stable
4. Vital signs: q15min ×4, q30min ×2, q1h ×4, q4h
5. No known allergies
6. I & O (intake and output)
7. Turn, cough, and deep breathe in bed q2h
8. Dangle feet this evening
9. Ambulate in halls ×4 on postop. day 1
10. IV solutions: 5% dextrose and lactated Ringer's solution 125 ml/h
11. NPO (nothing by mouth)
12. Medications: PCA (patient-controlled analgesic) pump for narcotics (see Table 24-19 for specific dosage)
    50 mg promethazine (Phenergan) IM q4-6h, prn, nausea, pain
13. Foley catheter to gravity drainage
14. Hematocrit on postop. days 1 and 3

TABLE 24-1
Time of Usual Onset of Fever for Various Postoperative Complications

Causes	Day 1	2	3	4	5	6	1 Week or More
Atelectasis	→→→→		→				
Pneumonia		→→→	→				→
Wound infection							
Streptococcal							
or	→→→		→				
Clostridial							
Other bacterial					→→→		→
Ovarian abscess							→
Cuff cellulitis			→→→			→	
Phlebitis							
Superficial			→→→			→	
Deep			→→→				→
Urinary tract							
infection			→→→				→
Ureteral or							
bladder injury					→→→		→

is depicted in Table 24-1. Fever is the most common diagnostic problem in the postoperative patient. Common causes of a fever include atelectasis, pneumonia, urinary tract infection, nonseptic phlebitis, wound infection, and operative site infection. Two intraoperative factors that dramatically increase the risk of postoperative fever are an operative time longer than 2 hours and the necessity for intraoperative transfusion.

Workup for Fever

The initial workup for a postoperatively febrile patient should emphasize the most common problems. Medical students memorize the five Ws in the differential diagnosis: wind (atelectasis), water (urinary tract infection), wound (infection or hematoma), walk (superficial or deep vein phlebitis), and wonder drugs (drug-induced fever).

The proper workup of a postoperative fever, similar to that of any problem in gynecology, involves the three classic steps of history, physical examination, and laboratory evaluations. A chart review and history from the patient may highlight preoperative problems that might cause fever: intraoperative complications, such as aspiration of gastric or oral contents; placement of foreign bodies, such as drains; recent infusion of blood products or drugs; and known allergies. The physical examination emphasizes examination of the lungs for atelectasis or pneumonia; the wound and operative site for infection or hematoma formation; the costovertebral angles for tenderness, which might suggest pyelonephritis; and veins in the arms for superficial phlebitis and deep veins in the legs for deep vein phlebitis.

The findings of the history and physical examination and considerations of cost containment all influence the extent of laboratory tests ordered. The three most commonly ordered laboratory tests are complete blood count (CBC), chest roentgenogram, and urinalysis. Other common tests include a sputum and urine Gram smear and culture and serial blood cultures. Refractory patients may need tests of liver function or special imaging studies, such as an intravenous pyelogram, computed tomography (CT), or magnetic resonance imaging (MRI), to detect problems such as compromised ureters, abscesses, or foreign bodies.

Each major complication will be discussed in detail later in the chapter. However, several specific generalizations concerning the type and characteristics of fever patterns should be emphasized. Atelectasis is the cause of more than 90% of fevers occurring in the first 48 hours after operation. Patients who develop fever as a result of foreign bodies, such as plastic intravenous lines or Foley catheters, are afebrile for several days, then experience an abrupt temperature spike. In contrast, wound or pelvic infections, which are usually clinically diagnosed from the fourth to seventh postoperative days, in retrospect are associated with a low-grade fever that begins early in the postoperative period. An empiric trial of intravenous heparin for 72 hours is often a diagnostic and therapeutic trial for pelvic thrombophlebitis in refractory cases of postoperative fever of unknown origin.

A patient with a drug-induced fever both feels better and does not look as ill as her temperature course indicates. The tachycardia associated with the elevated temperature is usually much less than usually anticipated with a similar temperature secondary to inflammation or infection. The presence of eosinophilia suggests a drug-induced fever. However, it is often a diagnosis of exclusion. Presumptive evidence of a drug-induced fever is established when the fever disappears after discontinuation of the drug. The diagnosis can only be confirmed by challenging the patient with the medication again after the fever has subsided. Clinically, this latter technique is not pragmatic.

Superficial thrombophlebitis often produces an enigmatic fever. Thus it is important to empirically change any intravenous lines that have been in place for longer than 48 hours. Febrile transfusion reactions generally are caused by leukocyte or platelet antibodies. As long as a major blood type incompatibility is not found, treatment may be conservative.

The basic fever workup should be repeated at intervals until the diagnosis is established. The patient should be reexamined and selective laboratory tests reordered. Rare causes of postoperative fever include malignant neoplasms, pelvic thrombophlebitis, halothane hepatitis, thyroid storm, and malignant hyperthermia.

It is important to consider that fever is a potential beneficial physiologic response to the patient. Therefore, unless the adult is markedly symptomatic secondary to the elevated temperature, it is not necessary to order an antipyretic medication.

MANAGEMENT OF A FALLING HEMATOCRIT

Postoperative bleeding is one of the most feared postoperative complications because it not only prolongs the hospital stay, but also in rare cases may lead to the patient's death. Significant bleeding in the first 24 hours often necessitates reoperation. This complication is discussed along with the management of shock and pelvic hematomas later in the chapter.

Vital signs should be ordered at frequent intervals during the first 24 hours to detect hypovolemia secondary to postoperative bleeding. However, following an operation, sizable amounts of unrecognized intraperitoneal or retroperitoneal bleeding sometimes are present without the patient having subjective symptoms or appreciable changes in her vital signs or urine output. Thus a hematocrit is necessary at two times during the postoperative course. We prefer a hematocrit at 24 and 72 hours following the operative procedure. A hematocrit drawn 24 hours following an operation may not give a true reflection of postoperative blood loss. The normal physiologic response to the stress of the operation and tissue destruction is a release of increased levels of aldosterone and antidiuretic hormone. The higher levels of aldosterone produce an increase in both sodium and water retention, while increased levels of antidiuretic hormone promote free water retention. Depending on the type and amount of intraoperative and postoperative intravenous fluids, the hematocrit on the first postoperative day may be misleading and reflect fluid changes rather than postoperative hemorrhage. The hematocrit from the third postoperative day is a more valid measurement of postoperative change. Hematocrits should be obtained in a standard fashion so as to eliminate sampling errors. For example, hematocrit samples drawn from central lines or during blood gas determinations often give false values because of the heparin or saline flush solutions.

After the effects of the operative blood loss are subtracted from the preoperative hematocrit, each further reduction in hematocrit of 3 to 5 points reflects a postoperative hemorrhage of approximately 500 ml. The safe level of postoperative anemia is a controversial issue. Certainly it is not identical to the level needed before an operation. Most young, healthy women without complicating medical illness will tolerate hematocrits of 20% to 22% without needing transfusion. These patients should be observed for orthostatic changes in their vital signs. Obviously the site of the hematoma should be discovered by abdominal and bimanual examination (see discussions on the diagnosis and management of wound and pelvic hematomas).

In summary, the morbidity and mortality of a surgical procedure is directly related to the amount of intraoperative and postoperative blood loss and not the corresponding level of preoperative anemia.

RESPIRATORY COMPLICATIONS

Alterations of pulmonary function are an expected physiologic change in women having general anesthesia and operations that open the peritoneal cavity. Of importance, respiratory complications directly cause 25% of deaths in women who die during the first 7 postoperative days.

Atelectasis

The term *atelectasis* is derived from two Greek words that mean "imperfect expansion." The severity of atelectasis ranges from lack of expansion of a small group of terminal bronchioles and alveoli to complete collapse of a lung. In most patients, atelectasis is the failure to maintain patency of the small pulmonary airways and alveoli. Atelectasis is a common complication, developing after a pelvic operation in approximately 10% to 20% of women without any risk factors. Atlectasis is the most common cause of postoperative fever. The incidence of atelectasis depends on the number of predis-

posing risk factors in the population studied and the vigor with which the clinical diagnosis is established.

Ninety percent of all postoperative respiratory complications are related to atelectasis. The immediate postoperative period is characterized by a decrease in functional residual capacity and lung compliance (Figure 24-1). Thus the work of breathing is increased. Microatelectasis is most common where small airways (less than 1 mm in diameter) become blocked by secretions. When small airways remain closed, the gas distal to the obstruction is absorbed, resulting in atelectasis. These changes occur during the first 72 hours following an operation. When atelectasis becomes progressive and involves a large area of lung tissue, there is an associated decrease in oxygen saturation and a decrease in arterial oxygen pressure (Po_2). This is associated with a normal to low arterial carbon dioxide pressure (Pco_2).

Wellman has listed both nonpulmonary and pulmonary factors that favor premature airway closure and development of atelectasis (see box on p. 754). The supine position decreases the functional residual capacity approximately 20% as compared with the erect position. Obesity, smoking, age greater than 60 years, prolonged operative time, and coexisting medical conditions, such as cardiac or lung disease and pulmonary infection, all predispose patients to atelectasis. In one study, 40% of obese women demonstrated radiologic evidence of atelectasis

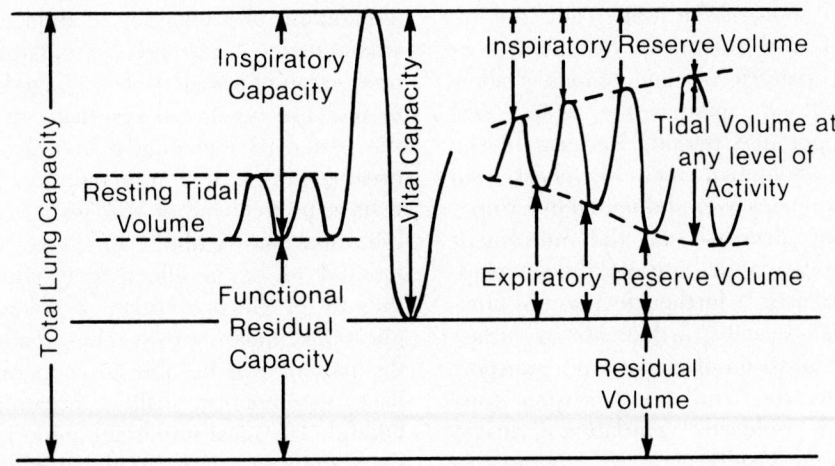

FIGURE 24-1
Graphic illustration of lung volumes and capacities. (From Wellman JJ: Respiratory care in the surgical patient. In Lubin MF, Walker HD, and Smith RB, editors; Medical management of the surgical patient, Stoneham, Mass, 1982, Butterworth Publishers, p 285. Used with permission.)

NONPULMONARY AND PULMONARY FACTORS THAT FAVOR PREMATURE AIRWAY CLOSURE AND ATELECTASIS

Nonpulmonary Factors

Supine position
Obesity
Increased abdominal girth (ileus, pneumoperitoneum)
Breathing at low lung volumes
    Bindings around the chest and abdomen
    Incisional pain
    Sedative narcotic drugs
    Prolonged effect of paralyzing drugs
    Immobility
    Excessively high concentrations of oxygen
      for prolonged periods

Pulmonary Factors

Interstitial edema
Loss of surfactant with air space instability
Airway obstruction
    Inflammation with swelling of bronchial
      and interbronchial tissue
    Constriction of bronchial smooth muscle
    Retained secretions

From Wellman JJ: Respirator care in the surgical patient. In Lubin MF, Walker HK, and Smith RB, editors: Medical management of the surgical patient, Stoneham, MA, 1982, Butterworth Publishers, p 288. Used with permission.

in their postoperative chest roentgenograms.

In normal breathing there are periodic, involuntary, deep inspirations that help to expand all areas of the lung. Pain, the supine position, and abdominal distention contribute to a pattern of monotonous shallow breathing without spontaneous deep sighs in the postoperative period. Because of the pain of an abdominal incision, chest wall breathing dominates over abdominal breathing. The resultant decrease in the movement of the diaphragm contributes to the development of atelectasis. A further decrease in functional residual capacity, a decrease in surfactant, and a depression of mucociliary transport all contribute to ventilation/perfusion mismatches and reduced ventilation/perfusion ratios. The end results are gas trapping, atelectasis, and vascular shunting. In the majority of individuals, microatelectasis is patchy and localized to small areas. However, the severity of atelectasis varies and may involve a complete lung.

Pulmonary blood flow depends greatly on gravity. A greater proportion of pulmonary blood flows to dependent areas of the lungs in the supine patient. This increased blood flow, combined with the atelectasis in dependent areas, results in an increased impairment of oxygenation, as well as a decrease in the elimination of carbon dioxide.

The endotracheal tube may contribute to the development of atelectasis. Even correctly placed endotracheal tubes have been associated with destruction of cilia in the respiratory tract epithelium. Women with nasogastric tubes have a higher incidence of atelectasis, more commonly related to a decrease in deep breathing than to aspiration of stomach contents.

Atelectasis may present as the classic triad of fever, tachypnea, and tachycardia developing within the first 72 hours following an operation. On physical examination, tubular breathing, decreased breath sounds, and moist inspiratory rales may be heard. These findings are most prominent over the bases of the lung. If the condition progresses, an increase in productive cough and leukocytosis result. Chest x-ray films may demonstrate a patchy infiltrate with elevations of the diaphragm. There may be a corresponding shift of the trachea and mediastinum in atelectasis, involving a large segment of the lung.

Atelectasis usually resolves spontaneously by the third to fifth postoperative day. Nevertheless, major efforts are made to prevent atelectasis, especially in high-risk individuals. The foundations of prevention of atelectasis are the encouragement of uneven ventilation and the production of episodes of prolonged inspiration to increase functional residual capacity. Thus the patient is encouraged to walk, take deep breaths, cough, turn from side to side, and remain semierect rather than supine. Early mobilization and ambulation have been documented to be as effective as chest physical therapy in the prevention of pulmonary complications. Keeping pain relief to a level where the patient will be able to cooperate and not have monotonous shallow breathing is also helpful. The most important aid to prevent and treat atelectasis is a simple bedside incentive spirometry device. Many patients need encouragement by the hospital staff to use these devices effectively.

If atelectasis does not clear, the patient should be treated with chest physical therapy, intermittent positive pressure breathing, aerosol therapy, or intermittent continuous positive airway pressure by mask. Bronchoscopy may be indicated to remove large mucus plugs.

Pneumonia

Postoperative pneumonia is commonly associated with atelectasis, because bacterial infections often begin in collapsed areas of the lungs. The infections lead to increased water in the lungs, increased elastic resistance, and decreased lung compliance. In animals the inhalation of infected material does not produce pneumonia without associated atelectasis. In a similar animal experiment the injection of an intravenous bolus of bacteria was found to cause pneumonia in selectively localized areas of the lung that were obstructed. Predisposing factors to the development of pneumonia include chronic pulmonary disease, heavy cigarette smoking, obesity, advanced age, nasogastric tube, long operative procedures, and debilitating illnesses.

The symptoms and signs of pneumonia are fever, tachypnea, and productive purulent sputum. The classic physical finding of pneumonia is coarse rales over the infected area. The patient usually has a higher temperature and more systemic toxicity than does a woman with atelectasis. Chest roentgenograms often demonstrate a diffuse, patchy infiltrate of the lung. Gram stain of the sputum helps to differentiate between bacterial colonization and infection. In cases of pneumonia the smear contains a large number of inflammatory cells with both intracellular and extracellular bacteria.

The management of pneumonia is similar to the management of atelectasis, with the addition of parenteral antibiotics. The initial choice of parenteral antibiotics is usually based on the Gram stain and subsequently on sputum cultures. Two other special conditions should be considered in any case of postoperative pneumonia. Aspiration pneumonia results when contents of the mouth (mucus and bacteria) that have a physiologic pH are inhaled and subsequently produce bacterial pneumonia. The other problem is pneumonitis produced by aspiration of gastric fluid (sterile and highly acidic), which produces a severe chemical pneumonitis. The latter condition does not usually involve bacterial infection.

CARDIOVASCULAR PROBLEMS

Hemorrhagic Shock

Shock is defined as a condition in which circulatory insufficiency prevents adequate vascular perfusion of vital organs. Systemic hypotension results in poor tissue perfusion and reduced capillary filling. If this pathophysiologic state is neglected, prolonged hypotension results in oliguria, progressive metabolic acidosis, and multiple organ failure. Shock may be produced by hemorrhage, cardiac failure, sepsis, and anaphylactic reactions. Shock from postoperative hemorrhage is usually seen in the first few hours following the operation. Hypovolemia may be secondary to several factors in the perioperative period, including the patient being volume deficient preoperatively, unreplaced blood loss during surgery, extracellular fluid loss during surgery, inadequate fluid replacement, or continued blood loss following the surgical procedure.

The vast majority of perioperative cases of shock are related to hemorrhage secondary to inadequate hemostasis. The development of shock from acute blood loss depends on the rate of bleeding; for example, a slow venous ooze may produce a large amount of blood loss but not produce shock. In general, it takes a reduction of 20% of the blood volume to produce shock in a reproductive age female. Rapid loss of 20% of the blood volume produces mild shock, whereas a loss of greater than 40% of blood volume results in severe shock. Actual measurement of intraoperative blood loss is imprecise even with extensive use of suction equipment. Studies have demonstrated that 15% to 45% of surgical blood loss is absorbed on the drapes, laparotomy pads, and other areas. The level of blood in the suction bottle does not always accurately represent the patient's loss from the procedure.

Hypotension in the immediate postoperative period may be secondary to the residual effects of anesthesia or oversedation. For example, elderly patients often experience prolonged vasodilation secondary to the sympathetic blockade produced by epidural or spinal anesthesia.

The most common cause of postoperative bleeding is either a ligature that has slipped or hemorrhage from a vessel that retracted during the operation. Such bleeding may come from an artery or vein or may be related to a bleeding diathesis. The differential diagnosis of postoperative hemorrhagic shock includes condi-

CLASSIFICATION OF SHOCK

I. Hypovolemic
   A. External loss (e.g., blood, plasma, water)
   B. Sequestration—distributive abnormality
      1. Intravascular
         a. Arteriolar resistance loss (e.g., spinal shock)
         b. Capacitance pooling, venous system (e.g., endotoxin)
      2. Extravascular
         a. Exudative (e.g., peritonitis)
         b. Traumatic (e.g., hematoma)
II. Cardiogenic
   A. Intrinsic power
      1. Focal (e.g., infarct or aneurysm)
      2. Generalized (e.g., drug effect or ischemia)
   B. Extrinsic factors
      1. Obstructive (e.g., pulmonary embolus)
      2. Compressive (e.g., cardiac tamponade)
III. Peripheral vascular
   A. Neural factors (e.g., neurogenic shock—fainting)
   B. Humoral factors (e.g., anaphylactic shock, histamine shock)

From Greenfield LJ: Shock. In Hardy JD, editor: Complications in surgery and their management, ed 4, Philadelphia, 1981, WB Saunders Co, p 34.

tions such as pneumothorax, pulmonary embolus, massive pulmonary aspiration, myocardial infarction, and acute gastric dilation. The box above lists the differential diagnoses of shock. The differential diagnosis of ineffective coagulation includes sepsis, fibrinolysis, diffuse intravascular coagulation, and a previously unrecognized coagulation defect, such as von Willebrand's disease. Inadequate hemostasis sometimes develops from excessive transfusion. Thrombocytopenia, impaired platelet function, and a decrease in factors V, VIII, and XI occur with massive transfusions (greater than 5 units of blood).

Tachycardia and decreased urine output are two early signs of hypovolemia caused by hidden internal bleeding. The body's adrenergic response to hemorrhage includes perspiration, tachycardia, and peripheral vasoconstriction. Urine output decreases to less than 25 ml per hour as a result of poor perfusion of the kidneys. Urine osmolality is an excellent test to help determine the etiology of the oliguria. With further loss of blood the patient becomes agitated, appears weak, and develops skin pallor and cold and clammy extremities, and the systolic blood pressure drops below 80 mm Hg. Again, because of adaptive cardiovascular changes, it takes a rapid loss of approximately one third of the blood volume to produce significant hypotension.

After an operation both intraperitoneal and retroperitoneal bleeding often occur without significant local symptoms. Extraperitoneal bleeding may present as bleeding from the vaginal vault if the vaginal cuff was left open. There may be mild flank or back tenderness with rebound on abdominal palpation. However, abdominal distention, muscle rigidity, and shoulder pain are late signs of intraperitoneal hemorrhage. The diagnosis of significant postoperative bleeding may be confirmed by serial changes in hematocrits or by paracentesis. However, it is important to caution that marked changes in hematocrit and hemoglobin require time to develop. Bimanual examination with the patient under anesthesia will help in the diagnosis of silent retroperitoneal bleeding immediately before reoperation. An intravenous pyelogram will sometimes demonstrate obliteration of the psoas shadow and deviation of the ureter by a large retroperitoneal hematoma.

The goals of management of a woman who has developed postoperative shock are to replace and restore the effective circulating blood volume and establish normal cellular perfusion and oxygenation. The first priority is to provide adequate ventilation; poor respiratory gas exchange is the most frequent cause of death in these patients. The second, almost simultaneous, priority is rapid fluid replacement with adequate amounts of blood and crystalloid solution (normal saline or lactated Ringer's solution). The three-to-one rule suggests a ratio of 3 ml of crystalloid solution for every 1 ml of blood loss. Moss and Gould, in a review of plasma expanders, strongly expressed that no good evidence has documented any benefits of colloid solutions over crystalloid solutions in the treatment of shock. The optimal fluid replacement is a fluid evenly distributed throughout multiple body compartments. They concluded that optimal replacement included packed red blood cells and a balanced electrolyte solution, such as lactated Ringer's solution or normal saline.

TABLE 24-2
Available Blood Components

Component	Content	Vol. (ml)	Indications	Risk	Comments
Whole blood	All components	500	Massive acute blood loss	Hepatitis, volume overload	Consider component therapy
Packed cells	Red cells	200	Blood replacement	Hepatitis, allosensitization	Increases hematocrit 3%-5%
Frozen plasma	Clotting factors	200	DIC,* factor and immunoglobulin deficiency	Hepatitis	Increase fibrinogen 10 mg/dl per unit infused
Platelet concentrate	Platelets	50	Hereditary and acquired thrombocytopenia	Rh isoimmunization	Increase platelet count 7500 μl per unit infused
Cryoprecipitate	I, V, VIII, XIII	40	DIC, von Willebrand's hemophilia A	Hepatitis	Increase fibrinogen 10 mg/dl per unit infused
Factor concentrates	VIII, IX	20	Hemophilia A, IX deficiency	Hepatitis	1 unit equals factor activity in 1 ml pooled plasma

From American College of Obstetricians and Gynecologists: Blood component therapy, ACOG Tech Bull 78:1, Washington DC, 1984, ACOG.
*DIC, Disseminated intravascular coagulation.

The goals of fluid replacement are to obtain a systolic blood pressure that is similar to preoperative readings, maintain urine output greater than 30 ml per hour, and maintain a pulmonary wedge pressure between 10 and 15 mm Hg. Table 24-2 lists types of blood components used for replacement therapy. To monitor the rapid replacement of large volumes of intravenous fluid, a Swan-Ganz catheter is usually inserted to determine pulmonary artery pressure, pulmonary wedge pressure, central venous pressure, and cardiac output. These values allow adjustments in the rate of vascular volume replacement. A Foley catheter facilitates measurement of hourly urine outputs. We prefer a Swan-Ganz catheter over a traditional central venous pressure line. However, if one is using a central venous pressure line, it is important to measure the pressure with the patient at a 45- degree angle. Studies have demonstrated that in the supine position, the volume of intravascular depletion will be severely underestimated by a central venous pressure measurement.

Returning a patient to the operating room to control hemorrhage is often a difficult decision. However, this decision should not be postponed, and the patient should have an explor-atory operation as soon as possible after volume replacement. During this operation excellent anesthesia, a full selection of surgical instruments, and the value of good assistance cannot be overemphasized. Proper exposure is paramount for the success of this operation. Initially the old clots are removed, and further bleeding is reduced by direct pressure over the pelvic vessels. A systematic search is conducted in an effort to identify the individual vessels that are bleeding. Often the offending artery or vein cannot be identified, or friability of the tissues results in further bleeding.

Bilateral ligation of the hypogastric arteries is an effective operation to control persistent postoperative pelvic hemorrhage. This procedure results in a reduction of pulse pressure, which allows a stable clot to form at the site where the pelvic vessels are injured. Classically, two ligatures are placed and tied around each hypogastric artery (Figure 24-2). The major potential complication of this procedure is injury to the hypogastric vein. If there is generalized oozing, thrombocytopenia, disseminated intravascular coagulation, or factor VIII deficiency should be suspected. If these conditions are excluded, venous oozing from small vessels in the pelvis may be controlled by local

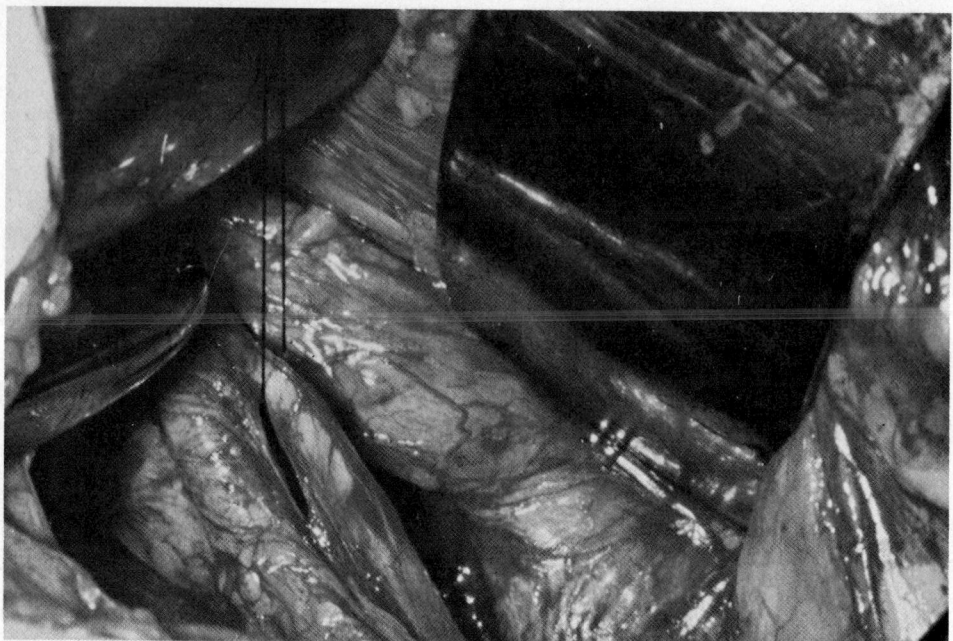

FIGURE 24-2
Ligation of internal iliac artery. Double loop is being directed toward bifurcation of common iliac artery. (From Breen JL, Gregori CA, and Kindzierski JA: Hemorrhage in gynecologic surgery. In Shaefer G and Graber EA, editors: Complications in obstetric and gynecologic surgery, Hagerstown, Md, 1981, Harper & Row, Publishers, Inc, p 439.)

application of microfibrillar collagen (Avitene).

Intraoperative rapid autologous blood transfusion is a commonly available technique that is used extensively in cardiovascular and trauma surgery. Regretfully, it is underused or rarely performed by gynecologists. Recently, Grimes has described a simple device that can adapt this technique for use in any operating room. The major complication of rapid autologous transfusion is a 10% hemolysis rate. The risks of air embolism or infusion of particulate matter have virtually been eliminated. Rapid autologous transfusion is contraindicated in advanced pelvic infection or malignancy.

Many centers prefer using angiographic embolization instead of hypogastric artery ligation. To permit visualization of a bleeding vessel, a flow of 1 ml per minute is required. Rosenthal and Colapinto have described treatment of recurrent postoperative hemorrhage or hemorrhage late in the postoperative course (7 to 14 days), performed with angiographic arterial embolization. Either absorbable gelatin sponge, which produces vascular occlusion for 10 to 30 days, or metal coils with Dacron fibers, which produce permanent occlusion, may be used.

Hematomas

This section will describe the management of wounds or pelvic hematomas that develop slowly and are diagnosed after the first postoperative day. The incidence of hematomas is directly related to the extent to which meticulous hemostasis is obtained intraoperatively. Hematomas result from intermittent or slow, continuous venous bleeding and are self-limited. Eventually the pressure of the expanding hematoma will exceed the venous pressure, and a stable clot will form. The extent of the hematoma is determined partially by the potential size of the compartment into which the bleeding occurs. Retroperitoneal or broad ligament hematomas may contain several units of blood. The diagnosis of a wound or pelvic hematoma is usually suspected on the morning of the third postoperative day when the laboratory reports an unexpectedly low hematocrit. The patient may have mild to moderate tenderness over the affected area. By the fifth postoperative day the hematoma liquefies and is easier to outline during bimanual examination. The differential diagnosis between an uninfected hematoma and a hematoma that has become secondarily infected is difficult before its incision and drainage. Both clinical situations produce tenderness and fever secondary to the inflammation surrounding the hematoma. The diagnosis of most retroperitoneal hematomas may be made by physical examination. Most important is a careful rectovaginal examination. Rarely, radiologic imaging studies are indicated when the hematoma cannot be palpated.

Hematomas less than 5 cm in diameter may be treated conservatively. Larger hematomas should be drained via an extraperitoneal approach as soon as they liquefy. If not treated by incision and drainage, most hematomas will become secondarily infected even when the patient is treated with parenteral antibiotics. Effective drainage of most pelvic and broad ligament hematomas usually can be accomplished vaginally. Whenever a surgeon punctures a hematoma with a syringe and needle to confirm the diagnosis, incision and drainage should be performed soon afterward, since introduction of the needle from the vagina to the hematoma results in inoculation of the hematoma with vaginal flora.

Any operation is accompanied by the potential risk of an unrecognized retained sponge or laparotomy pad. The exact incidence of this worrisome complication is difficult to establish but is estimated to be between 1 in 1200 and 1 in 1500 laparotomies. Most often the sponge counts at surgery have been correct. When this complication is discovered during the first postoperative week, the patient usually has a tender pelvic mass that is infected. When this mass is discovered after the immediate postoperative course, patients are often asymptomatic or exhibit minimal tenderness. The possibility of a retained foreign body should be considered in the differential diagnosis of pelvic hematomas and abscesses.

Thrombophlebitis and Pulmonary Embolus

Superficial Thrombophlebitis

Superficial thrombophlebitis is one of the most frequently occurring postoperative complications and is most commonly associated with intravenous catheters. Superficial thrombophlebitis is frequently overlooked or disregarded as a cause of postoperative fever. However, this diagnosis should be suspected when-

ever an intravenous line with antibiotics or hypertonic solutions has been used. Women with established superficial varicosities in the lower extremities are especially susceptible because of localized stasis or pressure during the operative procedure and inactivity during the first 24 hours after operation. Patients with superficial thrombophlebitis of the legs may also have concomitant deep venous disease. Thus the finding of superficial thrombophlebitis does not eliminate the necessity to consider deep venous thrombosis as well.

Detailed basic investigations have identified fibrin sheaths surrounding intravenous catheters in 60% to 100% of patients studied. The exact fate of the several inches of clot and fibrin sheath after the removal of the intravenous catheter is uncertain. Venography studies have found that these clots and fibrin sheaths do not break up on catheter removal but initially remain in situ. Intravenous catheters are an important source of nosocomial infections. Approximately 30% of all hospital-acquired bacteremias are secondary to intravenous lines. The most serious complication of intravenous catheter use is infection of the thrombus, producing suppurative phlebitis or catheter sepsis. The initial infection may occur via the bloodstream or via bacteria from the skin reaching the thrombus along the catheter line. When frank pus is expressed, the treatment of suppurative phlebitis includes excising the infected vein.

The natural history of intravenous catheter–associated phlebitis has been documented by Hershey et al. The classic symptoms of phlebitis are those of inflammation of the subcutaneous tissue along the course of a vein or over the area of merging varicosities. The patient develops a painful, tender, erythematous induration (nodule or core). In the majority of severe cases there is associated fever. However, milder forms may not involve fever. In studying 202 episodes of superficial phlebitis, Hershey et al. discovered that the disease develops relatively rapidly, giving few symptoms or signs that allow removal of the catheter to prevent the disease (Figures 24-3 and 24-4). After the process has begun, the inflammation does not consistently terminate with removal of the catheter. In their study, more than 40% of cases occurred 24 hours or more after withdrawal of the intravenous line. Nevertheless, the duration of phlebitis is prolonged if the

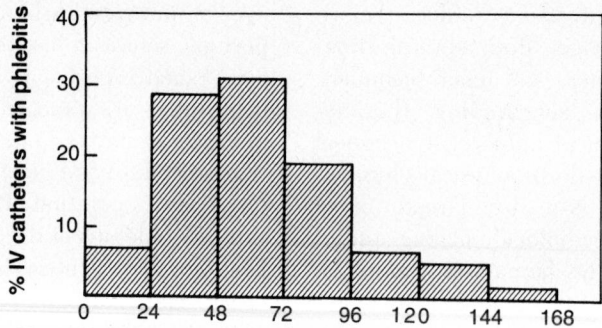

Hours after insertion that phlebitis was diagnosed

FIGURE 24-3
Hours after insertion that phlebitis was diagnosed. Time of diagnosis of phlebitis from time of intravenous catheter insertion. (From Hershey CO, Tomford JW, McLaren CE, et al: Arch Intern Med 144:1374, 1984, Copyright 1984, American Medical Association.)

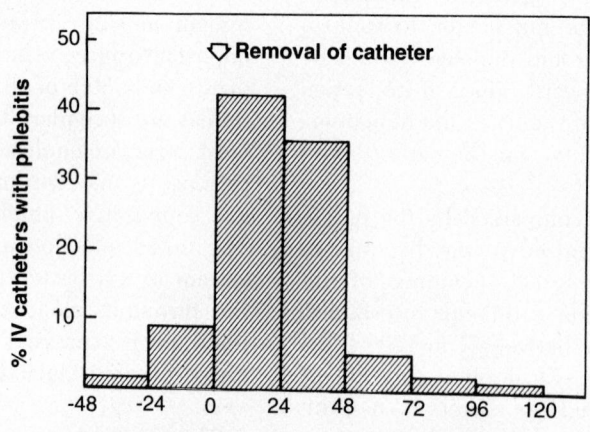

Hours before or after removal of IV catheter

FIGURE 24-4
Distribution of intravenous catheter–induced phlebitis relative to interval between diagnosis of phlebitis and removal of catheter. (From Hershey CO, Tomford JW, McLaren CE, et al: Arch Intern Med 144:1374, 1984, Copyright 1984, American Medical Association.)

catheter is not immediately removed when the diagnosis of superficial phlebitis is made. The authors recommended that all intravenous catheters be removed and replaced at 48-hour intervals regardless of whether signs or symptoms of superficial phlebitis are present. In addition, the use of an intravenous team decreased the incidence of catheter-associated phlebitis from 32% to 15% in their series. Strict aseptic techniques should be used during catheter insertion. Catheters inserted into the hand or forearm, through which antibiotics are infused, should be changed at least every 36 hours. In summary, venous catheters should be removed at the first sign of induration, erythema, or edema.

The clinical management of mild superficial thrombophlebitis includes rest, elevation, and local heat. Moderate to severe superficial thrombophlebitis may be treated with a nonsteroidal antiinflammatory agent such as ibuprofen (Motrin, 800 mg every 8 hours). The rare case of proximal progression of the inflammatory process should be treated with therapeutic doses of intravenous heparin and antibiotics.

Deep Vein Thrombophlebitis

Thrombophlebitis is a common postoperative complication in which the initial pathophysiology usually begins during the operation. It is the process of venous thrombosis formation occurring in any deep vein, secondary to coagulation of blood, and fibrin formation in the presence of venous stasis. Generally, thromboembolic complications occur early in the postoperative course—50% within the first 24 hours and 75% within 72 hours. Approximately 15% occur after the seventh postoperative day. Thus the potential threat is present even after the woman is discharged from the hospital.

Venous thrombosis and pulmonary embolus are the direct causes of approximately 40% of deaths in gynecologic cases. The incidence of fatal pulmonary emboli following gynecologic operations is between 0.1% and 0.8%. Because patients often die within a few hours of the appearance of initial symptoms, emphasis must be placed on prevention rather than treatment of this complication. Pulmonary embolus is not the only major consequence of deep venous thrombophlebitis. Many women develop chronic venous insufficiency or "postphlebitic syn-

drome" of the legs as a major sequela following thrombophlebitis. The resulting damage to valves of the deep veins produces shunting of blood to superficial veins, chronic edema, pain on exercise, and skin ulceration.

The reported incidence of deep vein thrombosis with gynecologic operations varies from 7% to 45%, with an average of approximately 15%. Fatal pulmonary emboli occur in approximately 1% of these cases. Walsh et al. found the incidence of deep venous thrombosis to be 7% following vaginal hysterectomy, 13% after abdominal hysterectomy for benign disease, 25% following Wertheim hysterectomy, and 45% following extensive gynecologic cancer operations. The incidence of thrombophlebitis is directly dependent on risk factors such as the type and duration of operation, the age of patient, history of deep vein thrombophlebitis, peripheral edema, amount of blood lost at operation, restrictions in preoperative ambulation, obesity, immobility, malignancy, sepsis, severe diabetes, and conditions that produce venous stasis, such as ascites and heart failure (Table 24-3). Older and obese women have an increased incidence of thrombophlebitis be-

TABLE 24-3
Risk Categories of Thromboembolism in Gynecologic Operations

Risk Category	Low Risk	Medium Risk	High Risk
Age	40 years	40 years	50 years
Contributing factors			
Operation	Uncomplicated or minor	Major abdominal or pelvic	Major, extensive malignant disease
Weight		Moderately obese—75 to 90 kg or >20% above ideal weight	Morbidly obese— >115 kg or >30% above ideal weight
			Previous venous thrombosis
			Varicose veins
			Cardiac disease
			Diabetes (insulin dependent)
Calf vein thrombosis	2%	10%-35%	30%-60%
Iliofemoral vein thrombosis	0.4%	2%-8%	5%-10%
Fatal pulmonary emboli	0.2%	0.1%-0.5%	1%
Recommended prophylaxis	Early ambulation	Low-dose heparin or intermittent pneumatic compression	Low-dose heparin or intermittent pneumatic compression

From Mattingly RF and Thompson JD, editors: Te Linde's operative gynecology, ed 6, Philadelphia, 1985, LB Lippincott Co, p 106.

cause of dilation of their deep venous system. The length of the surgical procedure also has an important influence on the development of thrombophlebitis. If the operation is 1 to 2 hours, approximately 15% of women develop the disease; if the surgery is longer than 3 hours, the risk is greater than 45%.

The process of thrombosis most often begins in the deep veins of the calf. It is estimated that 75% of pulmonary emboli originate from a thrombus that began in the leg veins. If one leg is involved, the other leg has thrombophlebitis in approximately 33% of women. Usually the thrombophlebitis remains localized and the clot lyses spontaneously, and the patient is free of symptoms. In approximately 1 in 20 cases the process extends centrally to the veins of the upper leg and pelvis. Involvement of the femoral vein often results in swelling caused by obstruction of this large vein. Pulmonary emboli from calf veins alone are rare, with only 4% to 10% of pulmonary emboli originating from this area. In contrast there is a 50% risk of a pulmonary embolus if thrombophlebitis of the femoral vein is not treated.

In 1854 Virchow described the three key predisposing or precipitating factors in the production of thrombi: an increase in coagulation factors, damage to the vessel wall, and venous stasis. Subsequent studies have documented that all three events occur with gynecologic operations. Blood flow in the iliac vein decreases by approximately 55% during an operation. After an operation a patient normally undergoes several changes that produce hypercoagulability, including increases in the following: factors VIII, IX, and X, number of platelets, platelet aggregation and adherence, fibrinogen, and thromboplastin-like substance from tissue necrosis.

Kakkar has described the cascade of events leading to the development of thrombophlebitis. The initial event in the cascade was stasis. Stasis leads to localized anoxia with subsequent generation of thrombi at the anoxic site. This produces changes in the lining of the vessel with exposure of the basement membrane and platelet adhesion and local coagulation. Kakkar further postulated that the interaction of this process with activators of fibrinolysis and inhibitors of coagulation determines and regulates whether fibrin is deposited and a venous thrombus develops. Thus the most important event in thrombophlebitis is the generation of

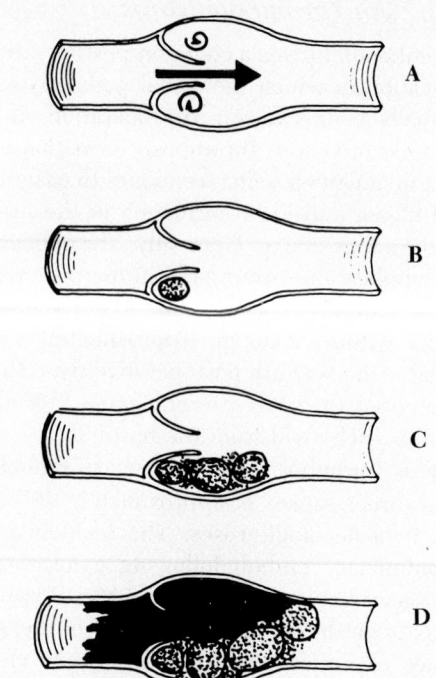

FIGURE 24-5
Stages in development of thrombus in valve pocket of deep veins of leg. **A,** Stasis in valve pocket results in thrombin generation. **B,** Platelet aggregation and fibrin formation. **C,** Propagation of platelet-fibrin nidus. **D,** Blockage of venous flow with resultant retrograde extension. (From Bloom AL, and Thomas DP, editors: Haemostases and thrombosis, Edinburgh, 1981, Churchill Livingstone, Inc., p 684.)

thrombi in the presence of venous stasis. A thrombus may generate in an area of stasis, or it may generate wherever a vessel wall is damaged during the operative procedure with resultant exposure of the subendothelial collagen, to which platelets will adhere.

The site of initial formation of the thrombus is most often near the base of a valve cusp in the calf of the leg (Figure 24-5). The thrombus propagates and grows by repetitive layers of platelet aggregation and deposition of fibrin from fibrinogen. The most recently formed portion of the propagating thrombi are free floating (not attached to the vein) and are most likely to become pulmonary emboli. The body attempts to repair the area of thrombosis through an invasion of fibroblasts from the vein wall to encompass the base of the thrombus. Eventually the thrombus is attached to the vein wall, the area is reepithelialized, organization occurs, and symptoms resolve.

The signs and symptoms of deep vein thrombophlebitis depend directly on the severity and extent of the process. Many localized cases of deep vein thrombophlebitis in the calf are asymptomatic and are only recognized by screening procedures such as scanning for thrombus formation using fibrinogen labeled with iodine 125 (^{125}I) or duplex ultrasonography. However, even extensive areas of deep vein thrombophlebitis may be asymptomatic, and the first sign may be the development of a pulmonary embolus.

Studies using ^{125}I-labeled fibrinogen to screen the legs have documented that approximately one out of two patients who develop deep vein thrombophlebitis following gynecologic operation is totally free of symptoms. Among women who develop signs and symptoms, approximately 68% have induration of the calf muscles, 52% have minimum edema, 25% have calf tenderness, and 11% develop a difference of more than 1 cm in diameter of the leg. Homans' sign is present in 10%, and differential pain over the calf with a blood pressure cuff is present in approximately 40%. The clinical diagnosis of iliofemoral thrombosis is much easier, and the patient usually develops severe symptoms due to obstruction of venous return. Usually there is an acute onset of severe pain, swelling, and a sensation that the leg will "burst."

The clinician must have a high degree of suspicion to begin the diagnostic workup for deep vein thrombophlebitis. One disturbing fact is that the more symptomatic the disease, the more adherent the thrombus. Thus patients with symptoms are less likely to develop pulmonary emboli. A clinical clue is the persistence of a low-grade fever with unexplained tachycardia. The tachycardia is often more rapid than one would expect with a low-grade fever. Physical examination of the legs produces false positive findings in approximately 50% of cases. Thus, if the signs and symptoms are suspicious, the diagnosis should be confirmed by one of the imaging techniques currently available to detect deep vein thrombophlebitis.

Presently, ascending venography (phlebography) is the gold standard—the most accurate method—for detecting deep vein thrombophlebitis (Figure 24-6). However, duplex ultrasonography, the combination of Doppler and real-time B-mode ultrasound, is rapidly replacing venography as the preferred method for diagnosis of deep vein thrombophlebitis. The diagnostic accuracy of venography is estimated to be 95% for peripheral disease and 90% for iliofemoral thrombophlebitis. The major drawback is that this imaging procedure is quite painful when there is extravasation of the contrast material into the tissue.

Scanning the leg with ^{125}I-labeled fibrinogen is an excellent method to screen women for occult thrombi. The test has been used extensively in research protocols; however, as with venography, it is also being replaced by duplex ultrasonography. Initially, the patient is given an oral dose of potassium iodide to block the thyroid gland. The test is performed by repetitive scanning of the leg for radioactivity for several days after the single intravenous injection of 100 μCi of ^{125}I-labeled fibrinogen. The test result is positive when the area of thrombophlebitis incorporates the radioactive fibrinogen into the propagating thrombus. This test correlates 85% to 95% with venography. The test is not diagnostic above the midthigh because of the amount of radiation emanating from the femoral artery and urinary bladder.

Duplex ultrasonography is a noninvasive screening test for deep vein thrombosis. Real-time ultrasound imaging provides visualization of the larger veins while sensitive Doppler ultrasound is focused simultaneously on the suspicious vessel. The technology depends on changes in venous flow for a positive diagnosis. In a recent metaanalysis of published studies, White et al. documented that the sensitivity of duplex ultrasonography to detect proximal thrombi is 95% (confidence intervals, 92% to 98%) and the specificity is 99% (confidence intervals, 98% to 100%). The authors predict that duplex ultrasonography will supplant venography as the gold standard for diagnosis. The advantages of this method are that it is noninvasive, easy to use, highly accurate, objective, simple, and reproducible. The main disadvantage of duplex ultrasonography is its limited accuracy when investigating small vessels in the calf.

Lensing et al., in a prospective study of 220 patients, used compressibility of the vein as the sole criterion for diagnosis of deep vein throm-

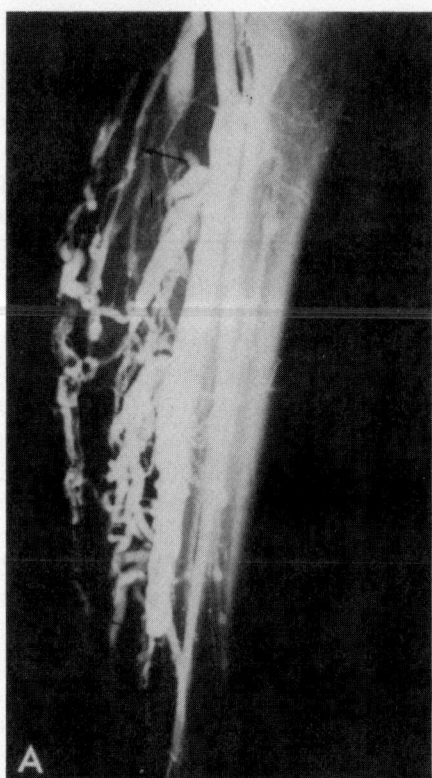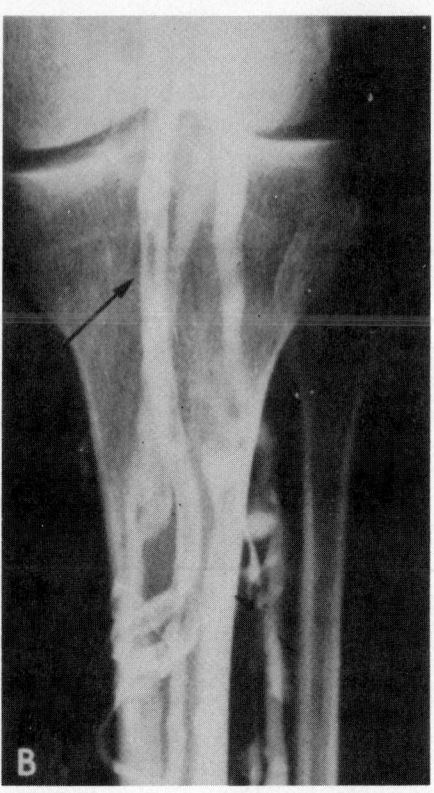

FIGURE 24-6
A, Phlebogram showing small thrombi in veins of calf, which are usually of no clinical significance. **B,** Thrombi in deep vein of calf showing extension into popliteal vein. (From Bonnar J: Clin Obstet Gynecol 28:439, 1985.)

TABLE 24-4
Comparison of Ultrasonographic and Venographic Results in 66 Patients with Proximal Vein Thrombosis and 143 Patients without Venous Thrombosis*

| | Venogram | |
Ultrasonographic Result	Proximal Vein Thrombosis	Normal
Noncompressible†	66	1
Compressible	0	142

From Lensing AWA, Prandoni P, Brandjes D, et al: N Engl J Med 320:342, 1989.
*The sensitivity of noncompressibility for the detection of proximal vein thrmbosis was 100% (95% confidence interval, 95% to 100%); the specificity was 99% (95% confidence interval, 97% to 100%).
†Noncompressible denotes an inability to compress the common femoral vein, popliteal vein, or both with the transducer probe.

bosis (Table 24-4). For all patients in their study, for both proximal vein and calf vein thrombosis, the sensitivity was 91% and the specificity was 99%.

Impedance plethysmography is another non-invasive screening method to detect deep vein thrombosis. A pneumatic cuff is applied around the thigh, and changes in blood volume are measured by changes in electrical resistance (impedance). Impedance is reduced with venous thrombi. This method has at least a 15% false negative rate and a 20% false positive rate. As with duplex ultrasonography, the accuracy of this method to detect thrombi of small vessels is limited.

The objectives of clinical management of deep vein thrombophlebitis associated with gynecologic operations are preventive medicine, early detection, and early therapy. In reality all antithrombotic therapy, whether with heparin or warfarin sodium (Coumadin), is prophylactic, since the therapeutic agent interrupts progression of the disease (thrombus formation) but does not actively resolve the disease process.

The National Institutes of Health (NIH) Consensus Conference has published recommended guidelines for prevention of venous thrombosis and pulmonary embolism in gynecology. For the low-risk patient under 40 years of age with an operative procedure of less than 30 minutes' duration, early ambulation and graduated compression stockings are "sufficient prophylaxis." Women at moderate to high risk undergoing gynecologic operations for benign conditions can be managed with low-dose heparin, dextran, external pneumatic compression, or a combination of these with comparable results (Table 24-5). The NIH Consensus Conference stated that data are not conclusive to determine the optimal management of high-risk patients with malignant disease.

Low-dose heparin (5000 IU given prophylactically 2 hours before operation and every 8 to 12 hours subcutaneously thereafter) reduces substantially the frequency and morbidity of deep vein thrombophlebitis (Chapter 23). Two studies of patients with benign gynecologic conditions have documented a reduction in the incidence of deep vein thrombosis: one from 23% to 6% and the other from 29% to 4%. Wound hematomas were reported in 7% of cases in one series; however, they occur much less frequently if low-dose heparin is given every 12 hours. Low-dose heparin prolongs the activated partial thromboplastin time more than 1.5 times control values in 10% to 15% of women. Furthermore, 6% experience an associated thrombocytopenia with low-dose heparin.

A multicentered investigation of prophylaxis of postoperative thrombosis in 880 patients has suggested that a combination of 0.5 mg of dihydroergotamine mesylate plus 5000 IU of heparin (Embolex) every 12 hours is more effective than either drug given alone (Table 24-6). Dihydroergotamine is a venotonic drug that exerts a selective constrictive effect on capacitance blood vessels (veins and venules) with only minimum effects on resistance vessels (arteries and arterioles). Thus its prophylactic effect is via correction of venous stasis and increase of venous return from the lower extremities. In this large series the placebo group had an incidence of deep vein thrombophlebitis of 24.4%, whereas the group given dihydroergot-

amine alone had an incidence of 19.4%, the group given heparin alone 16.8%, and the group given a combination of heparin and dihydroergotamine 9.4%. Dihydroergotamine is contraindicated for patients with sepsis, hypertension, or atherosclerotic vascular disease. The medical community has been reluctant to adopt the combination of ergot and heparin, and most gynecologists choose to use heparin alone.

An alternative to low-dose heparin for prevention of deep vein thrombosis is the intravenous infusion of dextran, either 40,000 or 70,000 molecular weight. Protocols for the use of dextran differ. However, usually 500 ml is infused during the operation, with 500 ml given during the first 6 hours after the operation and another 500 ml on the first postoperative day. Dextran is expensive, and anaphylaxis occurs in approximately 1 in 3500 patients. Dextran's method of action is not understood. It may decrease platelet adhesion, or it may decrease blood viscosity.

Several studies have documented that external pneumatic intraoperative and postoperative compression of the legs by pneumatic inflated sleeve devices decreases the incidence of deep vein thrombosis to approximately one third of that in control patients. These mechanical devices not only increase venous return from the legs but also are believed to increase endogenous fibrinolysis. Pneumatic compression devices develop waves of pressure between 30 and 50 mm Hg that progress along the legs' length every 10 to 12 seconds. Women at high risk for deep vein thrombophlebitis should be treated with both low-dose heparin and pneumatic compression devices. The cost for external pneumatic compression is approximately the same as the cost for low-dose heparin, and either is approximately 50% of the cost for prophylactic dextran.

In a double-blind randomized trial, Hull et al. (1990) demonstrated that 5 days of heparin therapy was as effective as 10 days. Repeat venous thromboembolic events were similar in women receiving the shorter course of therapy. The authors believe that oral Coumadin may be started on the first day of heparin therapy; thus patients may have a shorter hospital stay. Approximately 1% of patients on full-dose heparin develop thrombocytopenia, platelet counts less than 100,000. If thrombocytopenia develops, heparin should be discontinued because of

TABLE 24-5

Antithrombotic Agents and Procedures in Venous Thromboembolism

Agent	Mechanism of Action	Onset of Action
Heparin, 25,000-35,000 units per day	Prevents extension of active, established venous thromboembolism by inhibiting thrombin activity via the cofactor (ATIII)*	Immediate
Heparin, 10,000-15,000 units per day	Prevents formation of venous thrombi by inhibiting factor Xa activity via the cofactor (ATIII)	Immediate
Warfarin	Inhibits proper synthesis of vitamin K–dependent coagulation factors (II, VII, IX, X)	4-5 days
Dextran	Inhibits platelet function and fibrin polymerization	Immediate
Aspirin	Inhibits platelet function by suppressing prostaglandin synthesis	Hours
External pneumatic leg compression	Prevents venous stasis, activates fibrinolytic system	Immediate

From Hyers TM, Hull RD, and Web JG: Chest 89:26S, 1986.
*ATIII, Antithrombin III.

TABLE 24-6

Comparison of Deep Vein Thrombosis (DVT) Incidence Rates for All Patients

Treatment Group	No. of Patients	Frequency (%) With DVT	Frequency (%) Without DVT	Pairwise Comparisons, Exact *P* Level by Group* 2	3	4	5
Dihydroergotamine mesylate, 0.5 mg, and heparin sodium, 5000 IU	181	17 (9.4)	164 (90.6)	0.0241	0.0241	0.0174	0.0011
Dihydroergotamine mesylate, 0.5 mg. and heparin sodium 2500 IU	190	32 (16.8)	158 (83.2)	—	1.0000	0.3575	0.0908
Heparin sodium, 5000 IU	190	32 (16.8)	158 (83.2)	—	—	0.6209	0.0908
Dihydroergotamine mesylate, 0.5 mg	93	18 (19.4)	75 (80.6)	—	—	—	0.2566
Placebo	90	22 (24.4)	68 (75.6)	—	—	—	—

From Multicenter Trial Committee: JAMA 251:2963, 1984. Copyright 1984, American Medical Association.
*One-tailed tests used when comparing a combination with a component or with a lower dose or when making comparisons with a placebo. All other tests are two tailed.

Application	Route of Administration	Contraindication
Treatment of established pulmonary embolism and deep vein thrombosis	IV or subcutaneous	Severe active bleeding documented; hypersensitivity; heparin-induced thrombocytopenia and thrombosis
Prevention of venous thromboembolic disease in selected postoperative patients	Subcutaneous	Established venous thromboembolic disease documented; hypersensitivity; heparin-induced thrombocytopenia and thrombosis
Long-term treatment of established disease; prevention of disease	Oral	Severe active bleeding; pregnancy
Prevention of venous thromboembolic disease in selected high-risk patients	IV	Established venous thromboembolism; congestive heart failure; dextran hypersensitivity
Possible prevention in selected high-risk orthopedic patients	Oral	Established venous thromboembolism; sensitivity to aspirin (e.g., triad asthma)
Prevention in high-risk patients	Local application	Established venous thromboembolism; severe peripheral arterial disease with compromised tissue viability, skin ulcers.

the potential risk of paradoxical thrombosis.

For the future there is the promise that new, low-molecular-weight heparins or heparinoids will be available with similar antithrombin effects but fewer hemorrhagic complications.

Heparin is the drug of choice for the initial treatment of deep vein thrombosis or pulmonary embolism once the diagnosis is confirmed. An initial loading dose of 5000 IU is given intravenously, followed by continuous infusion of 1000 to 1500 IU per hour. The dosage of continuous intravenous heparin should be adjusted to prolong the Lee-White clotting time to 2 to 3 times control values or, alternatively, to prolong an activated partial thromboplastin time to 1.5 to 2 times control values. Continuous heparin infusion is preferred over periodic bolus injections because there are fewer hemorrhagic complications. The half-life of heparin on the average is 1 to 2 hours after intravenous injection. Heparin should be continued for 7 to 10 days. Oral warfarin (Coumadin), 15 mg daily, should be begun after approximately 1 week of heparin therapy. Following 2 to 3 days of 10 to 15 mg of Coumadin daily, the prothrombin time will usually be prolonged to 1.5 to 2 times the control value. This therapeutic level of 1.5 to 2 times normal control should be maintained by appropriate downward adjustment of the Coumadin dosage. The biologic half-life of Coumadin is 2 to 3 days. Anticoagulation with Coumadin should be continued for approximately 3 to 6 months.

Pulmonary Embolus

The accurate diagnosis of pulmonary embolus is essential for the prevention of death from lack of treatment or from unnecessary anticoagulation therapy. Autopsy studies have documented that pulmonary emboli are undiagnosed clinically in approximately 50% of patients who experience this complication. Approximately 10% of patients with a pulmonary embolus die within the first hour. The mortality of patients with correctly diagnosed and treated pulmonary emboli is 8%, in contrast to approximately 30% if the disease is not treated. Anticoagulation therapy is also dangerous, so there is the associated risk of heparin treatment if a false positive diagnosis is made. Heparin is the leading cause of drug-related deaths in hos-

TABLE 24-7

Symptoms and Signs of Pulmonary Embolus

	Patients with Finding (%)
Symptoms	
Predisposing factors*	94
Dyspnea	84
Pleuritic chest pain	74
Apprehension	59
Cough	53
Hemoptysis	30
Syncope	14
Signs	
Tachypnea	92
Rales	58
Accentuation of pulmonic valve closure	53
Tachycardia	44
Cyanosis	20

From Blinder RA and Coleman RE: Radiol Clin North Am 23:392, 1985. Data from the Urokinase Pulmonary Embolism Trial—a national cooperative study, Circulation 47 (suppl II):1, 1973.
*Prolonged immobilization, postoperative state, congestive heart failure, carcinomatosis, and so on.

pitalized patients. Most pulmonary emboli in gynecologic patients originate from thrombi in the pelvic and femoral veins.

The signs and symptoms of pulmonary embolus are nonspecific, and similar symptoms are caused by many other forms of cardiorespiratory disease. No combination of symptoms or signs is pathognomonic for pulmonary embolus, and many patients are asymptomatic. Nevertheless, they do alert the physician to the possibility of a pulmonary embolus, thus allowing a proper diagnostic workup to establish or rule out the disease. A national study of 327 patients with an angiographically proven pulmonary embolus found that chest pain, dyspnea, and apprehension are the most common symptoms. The dyspnea is often of abrupt onset. The triad of shortness of breath, chest pain, and hemoptysis is seen in less than 20% of patients with proven pulmonary embolus. Tachypnea, rales, and an increase in the second heart sound over the pulmonic area are the most frequently found signs of pulmonary emboli (Table 24-7). Shock and syncope are associated with massive pulmonary emboli.

Routine laboratory data, such as electrocardiograms (ECGs), chest x-ray films, and blood gas analyses, are important because they may contribute to the overall clinical impression, but individually or collectively they are not diagnostic. Less than 15% of ECGs demonstrate significant changes with a pulmonary embolus. Diminished pulmonary vascular markings may be a suspicious finding on a chest film. In the final analysis, only imaging studies are of central importance in confirming the diagnosis of pulmonary embolus. However, the chest x-ray film may be helpful in the differential diagnosis by demonstrating other pulmonary complications, and the ECG helps to differentiate the symptom complex from myocardial infarction. The three most common findings on chest x-ray examination with a pulmonary embolus are infiltrate, pleural effusion, and atelectasis, although these findings are nonspecific. The majority of women with pulmonary emboli demonstrate hypoxemia on blood gas determinations, but as with other routine tests, these findings do not occur invariably. The clinical manifestations of pulmonary embolus are produced primarily by occlusion of the large branches of the pulmonary arteries by embolic material. Pathophysiologically, associated reflex bronchial constriction and vasoconstriction intensify the symptomatology.

The first step in imaging techniques to establish or exclude the diagnosis of pulmonary embolus is a ventilation/perfusion lung scan. This test is safe and relatively easy to perform. The scan involves the injection of small radiocolloid particles into the circulation. They are trapped in small vessels, and their distribution depends on regional pulmonary blood flow. Ventilation scintigraphy uses radioactive pharmaceuticals of technetium aerosol or xenon gas. The combination of lack of symmetry and a mismatch in the ventilation scan is the abnormality that leads to the diagnosis. The results of the ventilation/perfusion scan constitute the critical point in the differential diagnosis. In patients with a suspected pulmonary embolus, 40% will have a normal scan. A normal result effectively rules out the diagnosis of pulmonary embolus.

The results of 933 patients involved in the multicenter Prospective Investigation of Pulmonary Embolism Diagnosis (PIOPED) have recently been published. This report found that 4% of patients with normal or near-normal perfusion lung scans subsequently were discov-

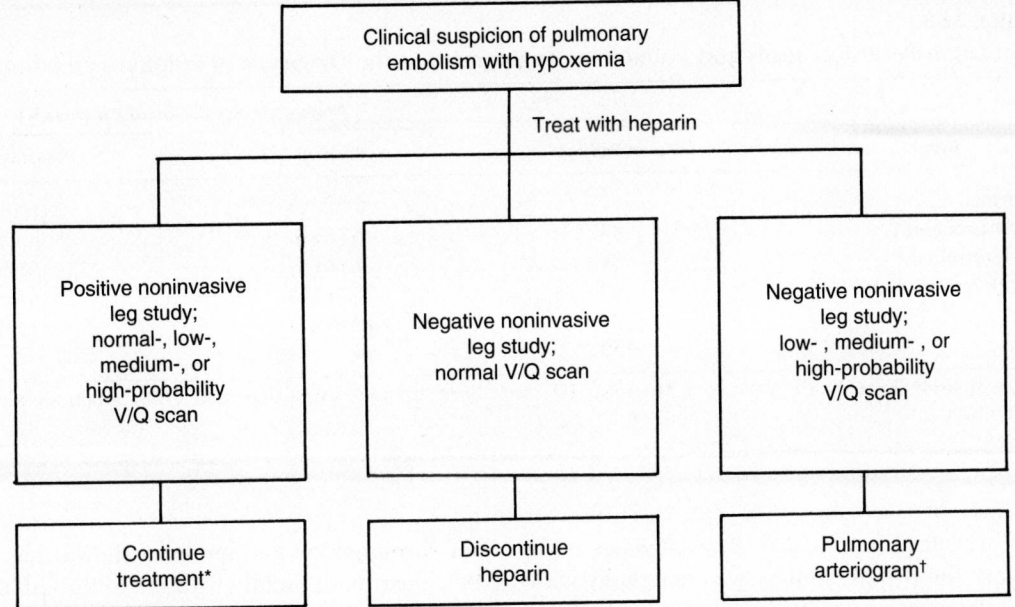

FIGURE 24-7

Algorithm for diagnostic evaluation of pulmonary embolus. Asterisk (*) indicates that treatment should be continued only if high-quality, noninvasive leg study can be performed. If one doubts quality of noninvasive study, venogram should be done. Dagger (†) indicates that, in selected patients with highly suspected pulmonary embolus (e.g., those with previously documented embolus), high-probability ventilation/perfusion (V/Q) scan might be accepted as proof of pulmonary embolus without angiogram. (Redrawn from Bone RC: JAMA 263:2794, 1990.)

ered to have pulmonary emboli. This study emphasized a high sensitivity of 98% but a low specificity of 10% for ventilation/perfusion scans in the diagnosis of pulmonary embolus. The authors pointed out that almost all patients with acute pulmonary embolus had abnormal scans, but so did most patients without emboli. Therefore Bone has suggested the algorithm shown in Figure 24-7 for the diagnostic evaluation and management of a patient with pulmonary embolus.

Ventilation/perfusion scans have a high sensitivity but a variable specificity for the diagnosis of pulmonary embolus. For example, other cardiorespiratory diseases such as asthma may result in regional areas of decreased perfusion. If the scan documents multiple segments or lobar perfusion defects with a ventilation mismatch, the probability of pulmonary emboli is greater than 85%. At this point, treatment is indicated without further imaging studies. However, ventilation/perfusion scans with less extensive

perfusion abnormalities or matching ventilation defects do not reliably exclude the diagnosis of pulmonary embolus. McBride et al. studied 150 patients with clinically suspected pulmonary emboli, 56 of whom had pulmonary embolus documented by angiography. The presence or absence of pulmonary emboli could not be confidently predicted by ventilation/perfusion scans in the majority of patients (Table 24-8). Thus most patients subsequently had pulmonary angiography in the diagnostic workup of suspected pulmonary emboli.

Pulmonary angiography is the gold standard—the most definitive test presently available to detect pulmonary emboli. This test is not ordered routinely because of the potential morbidity (hypotension and cardiac dysrhythmias) and risk of death associated with its use. Most deaths are directly related to pulmonary hypertension and right ventricular dysfunction. Approximately 5% of patients experience complications from this test, and the mortality is

TABLE 24-8

Ventilation/Perfusion Scans and Pulmonary Angiograms in the Diagnosis of Pulmonary Embolus

Ventilation/Perfusion Scan Result	No. of Patients	Angiogram Result, No. of Patients (%)	
		Positive	Negative
Normal	7	0 (0)	7 (100)
Low probability	44	6 (13.6)	38 (86.4)
Indeterminate	38	7 (18.4)	31 (81.6)
Moderate probability	40	25 (62.5)	15 (37.5)
High probability	21	18 (85.7)	3 (14.3)
TOTAL	150	56	94

From McBride K, LaMorte WW, and Menzoian JO: Arch Surg 121:755, 1986. Copyright 1986, American Medical Association.

approximately 2 per 1000. The clinician must balance the risk of pulmonary angiography with the risk of anticoagulation in the individual patient. The significance of this imaging technique is unquestioned if one accepts intraluminal filling defects for the definitive diagnosis of pulmonary embolus. A series of 960 patients yielded only two false positive tests. Digital subtraction pulmonary angiography and radiolabeled platelet scanning are promising but still experimental imaging techniques. Echocardiography, Doppler ultrasonography, and MRI are complementary diagnostic techniques that may identify differences in regional pulmonary blood flow.

The management of the vast majority of patients with pulmonary emboli is by full-dose intravenous heparin therapy, similar to the management of deep vein thrombophlebitis. Recently, some women have been treated with thrombolytic therapy (streptokinase-urokinase) or recombinant human tissue–type plasminogen activator. However, this therapy is more expensive and more dangerous than heparin. Thrombolytic therapy works by transforming plasminogen to plasmin. Goldharber et al. completed a randomized controlled study comparing urokinase and the new recombinant human tissue–type plasminogen activator. The latter was found to act more rapidly and to be safer than urokinase. Thrombolytic therapy is indicated in patients with massive pulmonary emboli (angiographically, greater than 50% obstruction of the pulmonary arterial bed) with associated moderate to severe hemodynamic embarrassment. Random trials of heparin versus thrombolytic therapy have shown that emboli clear more rapidly with initial thrombolytic therapy. A thrombolytic agent is infused intravenously for the first 12 to 24 hours, and heparin therapy is continued for 7 to 10 days. The clinical assumption is that approximately 7 days are needed for the intravascular venous thrombus to become firmly attached to the vein's side wall. All patients with pulmonary emboli should have warfarin therapy after heparin treatment for 3 to 6 months. Treatment of a massive pulmonary embolus in an unstable patient involves a choice of thrombolytic therapy, pulmonary artery embolectomy, transvenous catheter embolectomy, and/or filter placement in the inferior vena cava.

URINARY TRACT PROBLEMS

Inability to Void

Many women experience an inability to void or an incomplete emptying of the bladder during the postoperative period. Inability to void is more frequent and lasts longer after an operation that involves the urethra or bladder neck. The etiology of postoperative voiding problems is complex. The major pathophysiologic change is the direct trauma and edema produced by the surgical procedure in the perivesical tissues. The differential diagnosis includes anxiety, mechanical interference, obstruction by swelling and edema, neurologic imbalance, and tranquilizer-associated detrusor hypotonia.

The patient's initial attempts at voiding should be made *in privacy* to minimize performance anxiety and should be made in a sitting position. It is best not to remove the Foley catheter until the patient is ambulatory. Most women have difficulty in completely emptying their bladder either on a bedpan or in a semirecumbent position during the first 24 hours following abdominal hysterectomy. Catheter drainage keeps the bladder at rest and avoids acute bladder distention with resulting detrusor dysfunction and possibly retrograde reflux of urine. The age-old tradition of intermittent clamping and releasing of the Foley catheter to regain bladder tone is often counterproductive. We do not believe in this technique, since it is not based on sound physiologic principles and, most important, overdistention is possible, which would compound voiding difficulties.

Most problems with voiding resolve without medication and with time. If mechanical obstruction is not suspected to be a major factor, intermittent straight catheterization is indicated. This will result in a lower incidence of urinary tract infection and a more rapid return to normal function than periodic replacement and removal of a Foley catheter for the evaluation of residual urine volume. Although bacteriuria occurs secondary to intermittent catheterization, development of pyelonephritis is rare unless the patient has concomitant vesicourethral reflux. Patients especially appreciate intermittent self-catheterization because it gives them control over a part of their postoperative care.

Rarely, medications may be given to patients who experience prolonged periods of inability to void. Reflex urethral spasm is common after plastic surgery to repair an enterocele or rectocele. Urethral spasm may be diminished by an alpha-adrenergic receptor blocking agent, phenoxybenzamine (Dibenzyline), in a dosage of 10 mg every 8 hours. However, hypotension is commonly associated with this drug. Bladder hypotonia may occur as a result of overdistention, prolonged inactivity, or use of medications such as beta-blockers. Bladder hypotonia may be treated with bethanechol (Urecholine) in a dosage of 25 to 50 mg every 8 hours. Urecholine effectively produces detrusor contractions. This medication is prescribed rarely and only to those patients who have had operations on the bladder neck. It is used late in their postoperative course when postoperative edema has begun to regress, usually 5 to 7 days.

Infection

The most commonly acquired infection in the hospital and the most frequent cause of gram-negative bacteremia in hospitalized patients is catheter-associated urinary tract infection. Approximately 40% of nosocomial infections are urinary tract infections, and 60% of these are directly related to an indwelling urethral catheter. One percent of patients with infections from bladder catheters will develop bacteremia. However, patients without catheters may develop overdistention and bladder atony as a result of pain. Overdistention produces a temporary paralysis of the detrusor activity that may take several days to resolve. The atonic bladder is also prone to urinary tract infection. Thus, after a gynecologic operation, the patient is susceptible to urinary tract infection either with or without a Foley catheter in place.

The normal uroepithelium inhibits adherence of surface bacteria to the walls of the urethra and bladder. A Foley catheter disrupts this property, and surface bacteria are able to colonize the lower urinary tract. The incidence of a positive culture increases dramatically with time. After a Foley catheter has been in place for 36 hours, approximately 20% of women have bacterial colonization, and after 72 hours, more than 75% have positive cultures. Women with an indwelling catheter in place develop urinary tract infections at the rate of approximately 5% per 24 hours; this increases to 50% of women after 7 days of continuous catheterization.

Catheter-related urinary tract infections are related to the patient's age. In one study, 30% of women over age 50 developed an infection, compared with 16% of those postoperative women younger than age 50. Diabetes increased the incidence of catheter-related urinary tract infections threefold. The incidence of infection is directly related to the length of time the catheter is in place. Daifuku and Stamm performed a series of cultures and documented that rectal or urethral colonization precedes lower urinary tract infection by 24 to 48 hours (Table 24-9). The incidence of a positive urine culture after a single in-and-out catheterization is approximately 4%.

Sterile technique used during insertion, strict aseptic catheter care, and maintenance of a closed drainage system are all important steps to reduce the incidence of infection through re-

TABLE 24-9

Occurrence of Antecedent Urethral or Rectal Bacterial Colonization in Patients with Catheter-Associated Urinary Tract Infections

	Women		Men	
	Urethral Colonization	Rectal Colonization	Urethral Colonization	Rectal Colonization
Gram-positive cocci	4/5	5/5	3/12	2/12
Gram-negative rods	6/9	7/9	1/4	3/4
Candida	2/4	2/4	1/1	0/1
All microorganisms	12/18	14/18	5/17	5/17

From Daifuku R and Stamm WE: JAMA 252:2029, 1984. Copyright 1984, American Medical Association.

duced colonization. Bacteria ascend from the exterior to the bladder either via the lumen of the catheter or around the outside of the catheter. A sterile, closed drainage system is the best single prophylactic measure to reduce the incidence of urinary tract infections. In one study, strict closed drainage reduced the rate of infection from 80% to 23%. Studies have documented a lower risk of infection with a suprapubic, transabdominal urinary catheter. The latter technique also decreases patient discomfort and permits earlier spontaneous voiding. Systemic prophylactic antibiotics exert a short-term effect, decreasing the initial incidence of infection. However, the negative effect of prophylactic antibiotics is an increased emergence of antibiotic-resistant bacteria. Therefore prophylactic antibiotics are not used to "cover a catheter" except in immunocompromised patients. With catheterization for longer than 3 weeks, all patients have bacterial colonization regardless of the use of prophylactic antibiotics.

The symptoms of urinary tract infection usually develop 24 to 48 hours after the Foley catheter is removed. Of interest, the signs and symptoms associated with a catheter acquired lower urinary tract infection are not nearly as pronounced or as specific as those associated with cystitis unrelated to catheter use. Patients with lower urinary tract infections usually do not have fever but experience urinary frequency and mild dysuria, which are difficult to distinguish from normal postoperative discomfort. Women with upper urinary tract infections usually have a high fever, chills, and flank pain. If urinary tract symptoms persist after appropriate antibiotic therapy, one should obtain an intravenous pyelogram to evaluate the possibility of obstruction in the urinary tract. Ob-

struction of the ureter without associated infection may be asymptomatic or produce only mild flank tenderness. No appreciable change will be noted in urinary output with an isolated unilateral ureteral obstruction.

The diagnosis of urinary tract infection is established by urinalysis and urine culture. It is important to identify white blood cells and bacteria with the microscope. However, women with high-volume urine outputs may demonstrate minimal findings on urinalysis but have a positive urine culture. Stark and Maki have emphasized that a bacterial concentration of 10^2 organisms per milliliter in a catheterized specimen is significant. In their studies more than 95% of patients with 10^2 colony-forming units per milliliter subsequently developed the standard criterion of infection, which is 100,000 colonies per milliliter for a midstream culture.

We recommend 3 days of antibiotic therapy for a woman who has developed cystitis after catheter use. Single-dose antibiotic treatment is reserved for nonpregnant women with an uncomplicated urinary tract infection unrelated to catheter use.

To reduce the incidence of urinary tract infection, the Foley catheter should be used judiciously. When possible, use of a suprapubic catheter or intermittent in-and-out catheterization is preferable to continuous drainage with a Foley catheter. If a Foley catheter is used, retrograde flow of urine from the bag to the bladder during ambulation should be avoided. Preventive measures, such as aseptic care of the catheter and a closed, sterile drainage system, are also important. Modern practice is not to treat catheter-associated urinary tract infections unless the patient is febrile. Prophylactic antibiotics are not used unless the patient is immunosuppressed, for they often result in a urinary tract infection with a *Proteus* or *Pseudomonas* species rather than the more common *Escherichia coli*.

Urinary Fistula

Vesicovaginal and ureterovaginal fistulas are infrequent yet troublesome complications of operations for benign gynecologic conditions. In recent series, gynecologic operations have been found to be the cause of approximately 75% of urinary tract fistulas. Surprisingly, it is not the difficult cancer operation but rather the simple total abdominal hysterectomy for benign disease, such as myomas or abnormal bleeding, that is the most frequent cause of this complication. Fistulas following gynecologic operations are secondary to abdominal hysterectomy in 75% of cases and to vaginal operations in the remaining 25%. The exact incidence of injury to the ureter associated with gynecologic operations is unknown because many patients do not exhibit symptoms. However, it has been estimated that ureteral injury occurs as frequently as 1 per 200 abdominal hysterectomies.

The classic clinical symptom of a urinary tract fistula is the painless and almost continuous loss of urine, usually from the vagina. On occasion the uncontrolled loss of urine is not continuous but may be related to change in position or posture. When urine loss is intermittent and related to position, one should suspect a ureterovaginal rather than vesicovaginal fistula. Urinary incontinence may be present within a few hours of the operative procedure. This symptom is secondary to a direct surgical injury to the bladder or ureter that was not appreciated during the operative procedure. The majority of fistulas become symptomatic 8 to 12 days and occasionally as late as 25 to 30 days after an operation. Occlusion of the blood supply from clamping or figure-of-8 sutures produces avascular necrosis and subsequent sloughing of the urogenital tissue. Pelvic examination often reveals a small reddened area of granulation tissue at the site of the fistula.

The differential diagnosis of a ureterovaginal fistula includes spontaneous loss of peritoneal fluid or serosanguineous fluid from the retroperitoneal space. A small fistula may be localized by placing a tampon in the vagina and instilling a dilute solution of methylene blue dye into the urinary bladder. This will also help differentiate between a vesicovaginal fistula and a ureterovaginal fistula. If the blue coloring is discovered on the tampon, then a defect in the bladder should be suspected. If the tampon is not colored, 1 to 2 ml of indigo carmine should be injected intravenously. The subsequent finding of blue coloring on the tampon is presumptive evidence of a ureterovaginal fistula. An intravenous pyelogram should be obtained in either case to detect obstruction of the ureter and diagnose compound (ureter and bladder) fistulas.

As with most other postoperative complications, preventive medicine is paramount. Optimum operative technique should emphasize the standard axioms in the prevention of urinary tract injury: the patient should have an empty bladder, and the physician should obtain adequate exposure of the site. Sharp dissection should be made along tissue planes with proper traction and countertraction. When operating near the bladder or ureter, bleeding vessels should be ligated individually rather than with random clamping of tissue. With extensive dissection of the periureteral tissue, care should be taken to avoid interference with the longitudinal vascular supply of the ureter. Opening of the dome of the bladder and palpation with the index finger and thumb may help to identify the proper surgical plane in the most difficult cases where anatomic landmarks are obscure. The urinary system, especially the bladder, is very "forgiving" if given a short period of rest to recover. If trauma to the bladder is suspected, continuous catheter drainage for 3 to 5 days often results in spontaneous healing of multiple defects.

When leakage from the urinary tract is first discovered, the bladder should be drained with a large-bore Foley catheter. Ureteral injuries should be treated with retrograde ureteral catheters. Approximately 20% of bladder injuries and 30% of ureteral injuries heal spontaneously without further operations. In these cases, splinting of the urinary tract facilitates healing of the defect before epithelization of the aberrant tract occurs, which would result in a true fistula. Spontaneous healing usually occurs within the first 4 weeks. With a ureteral fistula, follow-up intravenous pyelograms should be ordered at 3, 6, and 12 months to detect delayed ureteral strictures.

Operative repair should usually be delayed 2 to 4 months after the initial injury to obtain optimum results. The workup of a patient before operative repair of a vesicovaginal fistula includes intravenous pyelography, cystoscopy, and biopsy of the fistula's margins if carcinoma is suspected. Cystoscopy is mandatory and should be performed for two reasons: to establish that edema and inflammation have subsided around the fistulous tract and to establish the relationship of the fistulous tract to the trigone of the bladder, especially the ureteral orifices. Occasionally, repair of a fistula within 1 cm of the ureteral orifice compromises the ureter, and the ureter must be reimplanted into the bladder.

Operative repair of a vesicovaginal fistula is usually accomplished via a multilayered closure performed by the vaginal route. The principles for a successful operation include adequate exposure, dissection and mobilization of each tissue layer; excision of the fistulous tract; closure of each layer without tension on the suture line; and excellent hemostasis with closure of the dead space. Reliable bladder drainage is provided to avoid tension on the suture line for approximately 10 days. Latzko's operation is the simplest means of repairing a fistula at the vaginal apex. This technique of partial colpocleisis involves denudation of the vaginal mucosa surrounding the fistula and subsequent multilayer closure without entering the bladder. The primary disadvantage of the procedure is postoperative shortening of the vagina.

Many ureteral injuries discovered during the immediate postoperative period will heal when treated by percutaneous nephrostomy and ureteral catheters. Ureterovaginal fistulas that do not heal spontaneously are usually repaired 2 to 3 months after the original operation. The surgeon has several choices as to the operative technique. However, most persistent ureterovaginal fistulas involving the lower third of the ureter are repaired by reimplanting the ureter into the bladder.

GASTROINTESTINAL COMPLICATIONS

Ileus

Minor disturbances in gastrointestinal function are a normal consequence of anesthesia. The patient usually experiences nausea for approximately 12 hours, passes flatus some time during the first 3 postoperative days, and has a spontaneous bowel movement by the third or fourth postoperative day.

Ileus is an inhibition of the normal propulsive reflexes of the bowel that are regulated by the autonomic nervous system. Ileus causes a functional intestinal obstruction. Adynamic (paralytic) ileus is a normal event defined as an ileus of minor to moderate degree. It may be expected to follow any intraperitoneal or pelvic operation. An uncomplicated ileus may last 24 to 48 hours in the stomach, only a few hours in the small intestines, and 48 to 72 hours in the colon. The incidence and duration of adynamic ileus are less following vaginal hysterectomy than with abdominal hysterectomy. If adynamic ileus persists longer than 5 days, a diagnosis of mechanical bowel obstruction should be strongly considered.

Adynamic ileus is believed to result from a lack of coordinated motor activity of the intestine, which results in disorganized, propulsive activity. Electrical activity is present, but the basic defect is continuous activity of the intrinsic inhibitor neurons in the wall of the small intestine. Usually the process is generalized, but occasionally it may be localized, involving only an isolated loop of small intestine.

Major factors that result in intensification of adynamic ileus are peritoneal contamination by purulent material or blood, extensive handling of the small intestine, retroperitoneal surgery, metabolic diseases such as uremia, ganglionic blocking agents, and inadequate replacement of fluids or electrolytes, specifically potassium. Early feeding of the postoperative patient may intensify adynamic ileus and certainly will not improve the condition. Air swallowing that accompanies chewing gum, ice cubes in the mouth, or drinking carbonated beverages via a straw may contribute to the problem. Other factors predisposing to the development of ileus include obesity, advanced age of the patient, preoperative immobility, prolonged use of narcotics, and the removal of large pelvic-abdominal masses. The duration of the surgical procedure does not directly influence the severity of the ileus.

The classic symptoms of ileus include absence of flatus, abdominal distention, and obstipation. These symptoms are often associated with nausea and effortless vomiting. Bowel sounds may be hypoactive or absent. This condition may be associated with abdominal tenderness, and the abdomen is usually tympanic to percussion. Nausea and vomiting persisting longer than 24 hours after operation constitute cause for concern. The difference between small bowel obstruction and adynamic ileus is a

TABLE 24-10
Differential Radiographic Findings in Ileus and Mechanical Obstruction

Adynamic Ileus	Mechanical Obstruction
Small and large bowel are distended in proportion to each other	In small-bowel obstruction there is dilated small bowel proximal to site of obstruction: in colonic obstruction the colon is distended and small-bowel distention is present with incompetent ileocecal valve
Air-fluid levels in small bowel are infrequent; when present, they are at the same levels	Air-fluid levels are common and at different levels in the bowel
Quantitative difference in small-bowel distention	Greater small-bowel distention than with ileus
Small-bowel distention in central part of abdomen with colon in periphery	Small-bowel distention present in central part of abdomen; no peripheral large-bowel distention

From Buchsbaum HJ and Mazer J: The gastrointestinal tract. In Buchsbaum HJ and Walton LA, editors: Strategies in gynecologic surgery, New York, 1986 Springer-Verlag New York, Inc, p 100.

subtle one, for adynamic ileus is normally associated with partial obstruction of the small intestine.

Diagnostic films of the abdomen (supine, erect, and lateral) help to establish the correct diagnosis (Table 24-10). In a woman with adynamic ileus, the intestinal gas is scattered throughout the gastrointestinal tract, including the small intestine and colon. Air-fluid levels, if present, tend to be at the same level.

Watkins and Robertson have suggested that the oral administration of radiocontrast material may be both a therapeutic and diagnostic test. After preliminary abdominal films were obtained, 120 ml of 66% diatrizoate meglumine, 10% diatrizoate sodium (Gastrografin) was administered orally or via nasogastric tube. The osmolality of the radiocontrast material is approximately 6 times greater than that of normal saline. Thus a large amount of fluid enters the small bowel and acts as a direct stimulant of peristalsis. They noted that passage of

liquid stool occurred within a few hours in patients with adynamic ileus (Table 24-11). This material, unlike barium, is nontoxic if it accidentally contaminates the peritoneal cavity during an operation for bowel obstruction.

Adynamic ileus is a self-limiting condition that responds to gastrointestinal rest and time. During the period of watchful expectancy, adequate fluid and electrolyte replacement is necessary. Patients experience mild cramping and passage of flatus and regain their appetite with the return of normal peristalsis. If adequate bowel sounds are present, a rectal tube, Fleet's enema, or rectal suppository may facilitate the initial passage of flatus. Some advocate the routine postoperative administration of a wetting agent, such as simethicone (Mylicon) to reduce surface tension of intestinal mucus and liberate entrapped gas. Opinions are mixed as to whether such an agent reduces the incidence or intensity of adynamic ileus.

Severe cases of ileus should be treated with intravenous fluids and gastrointestinal and nasogastric suctioning. Nasogastric suction prevents progression of the intestinal distention. During periods when nasogastric suctioning is used, special attention should be given to correct replacement of fluid and electrolytes (Tables 24-12 and 24-13). The use of drugs that stimulate peristalsis is usually ineffective. A rare but worrisome complication of prolonged ileus is massive dilation of the cecum. This condition may be treated medically by evacuating the air with colonoscopy.

Intestinal Obstruction

Adhesions are the most common cause of intestinal obstruction postoperatively. Less common causes are hernias, mesenteric defects, intussusception, volvulus, and neoplasm. Large raw areas of the pelvis with hypoxic tissue facilitate the attachment of small intestine following pelvic operations. Fortunately the fibrous adhesions that form during the first 2 to 3 weeks after an operation are soft and filmy. Thus intestinal strangulation during the postoperative period is extremely rare. Dense adhesions may develop several months after an operation. In their review of bowel obstruction, Ratcliff et al. point out that gynecologic operations are the most common cause of small-bowel obstruction in women. The incidence of intestinal obstruction depends on the type of gynecologic operation performed. Approximately two women in

TABLE 24-11

Study of 47 Cases of Adynamic Ileus Treated with Ingestion of Contrast Material

	Average	Range
Interim from operation to time of study	4.2 days	2-14 days
Approximate duration of ileus	35 hours	12-96 hours
Transit time from ingestion to large bowel	3 hours 20 minutes	25 minutes 6 hours
Transit time from ingestion to first stool	6 hours 20 minutes	1-18 hours
Duration of hospitalization after study	3.8 days	1-8 days
Obstetric-gynecologic patients	2.8 days	1-7 days

From Watkins DT and Robertson CL: Am J Obstet Gynecol 152:451, 1985.

TABLE 24-12

Average Daily Volume and Electrolyte Concentrations of Gastrointestinal Secretions

	Volume (ml/day)	Electrolyte Concentrations (mEq/L)		
		Na^+	K^+	Cl^-
Saliva	1000-1500	10-40	10-20	6-30
Gastric juice	2000-2500	60-120	10-20	10-30
Hepatic bile	600-800	130-155	2-12	80-100
Pancreatic juice	700-1000	150-155	5-10	30-50
Duodenal secretions	300-800	90-140	2-10	70-120
Jejunal and ileal secretions	2000-3000	125-140	5-10	100-130
Colonic mucosal secretions	200-500	140-148	5-10	60-90
TOTAL	8000-10,000			

From Buchsbaum HJ and Mazer J: The gastrointestinal tract. In Buchsbaum HJ and Walton LA, editors: Strategies in gynecologic surgery, New York, 1986, Springer-Verlag New York, Inc, p 103.

TABLE 24-13

Composition of Intravenous Solutions

Solutions	Glucose (g/L)	Na	Cl	HCO₃	K	Ca	Mg	HPO₄	NH₄
					(mEq/L)				
Extracellular fluid	1000	140	102	27	4.2	5	3	0.3	
5% Dextrose and water	50								
10% Dextrose and water	100								
0.9% Sodium chloride (normal saline)		154	154						
0.45% Sodium chloride (half-normal saline)		77	77						
0.21% Sodium chloride (¼ normal saline)		34	34						
3% Sodium chloride (hypertonic saline)		513	513						
Lactated Ringer's solution		130	109	28*	4	2.7			
0.9% Ammonium chloride		168							168

From Miller TA and Duke JH: Fluid and electrolyte management. In Dudrick SJ, Baue AE, Eiseman B, et al, editors: Manual of preoperative and postoperative care, ed 3, Philadelphia, 1983, WB Saunders Co, p 47.
*Present in solution as lactate but is metabolized to bicarbonate.

TABLE 24-14

Differential Diagnosis Between Postoperative Ileus and Postoperative Obstruction

Clinical Features	Postoperative Ileus	Postoperative Obstruction
Abdominal pain	Discomfort from distention but not cramping pains	Cramping, progressively severe
Relationship to previous operation	Usually within 48-72 hours of operation	Usually delayed; may be 5-7 days for remote onset
Nausea and vomiting	Present	Present
Distention	Present	Present
Bowel sounds	Absent or hypoactive	Borborygmi with peristaltic rushes and high-pitched tinkles
Fever	Only if related to associated peritonitis	Rarely present unless bowel becomes gangrenous
Abdominal x-ray film	Distended loops of small and large bowels; gas usually present in colon	Single or multiple loops of distended bowel, usually small bowel with air-fluid levels
Treatment	Conservative with nasogastric suction, enemas, cholinergic stimulation	Partial: conservative with nasogastric decompression; or Complete: surgical

From Mattingly RF and Thompson JD, editors: Te Linde's operative gynecology, ed 6, Philadelphia, 1985, JB Lippincott Co, p 102.

1000 develop an obstruction after a benign gynecologic operation, whereas approximately 8% develop intestinal obstruction after radical cancer operations. Intestinal obstruction occurs in the small intestine in approximately 80% of cases and in the colon in the remaining 20%. As mentioned previously, the differential diagnosis between bowel obstruction and ileus is a difficult one (Table 24-14).

The acute symptoms of intestinal obstruction present most commonly between the fifth and seventh postoperative day. The majority of patients have a short period of normal intestinal function before the onset of symptoms. Women with bowel obstruction appear to have more toxicity and more acute distress than women with ileus. The abdominal pain is intermittent, colicky, and sharp in nature. The colicky pain usually lasts from 1 to 3 minutes. Associated symptoms include vomiting, abdominal distention, and constipation. Bowel sounds are loud, high pitched, and metallic. Occasionally they may be heard without a stethoscope. Nasogastric drainage is more profuse than in patients with severe adynamic ileus. A patient with a small-bowel obstruction may have a bowel movement, eliminating fecal material that already existed in the colon.

Abdominal x-ray films demonstrate a stepladder appearance—multiple air-fluid levels throughout the small intestine with an absence of gas in the colon and rectum. Pneumoperitoneum from an exploratory celiotomy usually persists for 7 to 10 days. Thus free air under the diaphragm is not diagnostic of perforation of a hollow viscus in a postoperative patient. Obstruction of the colon may be diagnosed by retrograde infusion of contrast material or by flexible endoscopy.

The foundation of early treatment of postoperative intestinal obstruction is decompression of the small intestine and adequate replacement of fluids and electrolytes. On some occasions, such as with a ruptured tuboovarian abscess, a nasogastric tube should be used in the immediate postoperative period for its prophylactic value. Decompression may be accomplished by means of a nasogastric tube or, preferably, a long tube (Miller-Abbott or Cantor tube). Serial monitoring of white blood cell counts with differentials should be performed. Repeat abdominal x-ray examinations at regular intervals are used to assess the degree of intestinal distention. Expectant management is successful in many patients. In the series by Wolfson et al., less than 40% of 112 patients with small-bowel obstruction due to adhesions required operation. Conservative therapy was most successful in those patients in whom the long intestinal drainage tube was successfully advanced from the stomach into the small intestine.

The major cause of morbidity and death with bowel obstruction is delay in diagnosis with resultant strangulation and secondary sepsis. Women who develop strangulation experience a dramatic increase in the intensity of abdominal pain, and it becomes continuous. Generally, strangulation of the small bowel is associated with localized peritoneal irritation, increase in temperature, and marked leukocytosis.

Fecal impaction is most often seen in elderly patients. It results from loss of peristalsis in the colon, with an impaired perception of rectal fullness. Fecal impaction is a humiliating experience to the patient. She may have either diarrhea around the impaction or obstipation. Treatment involves obtaining partial analgesia with lidocaine jelly and, subsequently, manually fragmenting and extracting the fecal mass.

Rectovaginal Fistula

Rectovaginal fistulas and fecal incontinence secondary to complete perineal tears are most commonly obstetric complications and are only rarely associated with gynecologic operations. In general, rectovaginal fistulas following hysterectomy or repair of an enterocele are usually located in the upper third of the vagina, while those secondary to a posterior colporrhaphy are in the lower third of the vagina. Other causes of rectovaginal fistula are carcinoma, radiation therapy, perirectal abscess, inflammatory bowel disease, lymphogranuloma venereum, and trauma.

Fistulous tracts between the rectum and vagina usually present 7 to 14 days after an operation. The first warning may be the rectal passage of several blood clots, indicating that a hematoma has ruptured into the rectum. Distressing symptoms include involuntary passage of gas and, depending on the size of the opening, the passage of fecal material from the vagina. Associated with these two classic symptoms are chronic, foul-smelling vaginal discharge and subsequent dyspareunia. Aside from the physical symptoms of the anatomic defect, these fistulas cause severe emotional distress because they affect almost every aspect of the patient's daily life.

The diagnosis is not difficult to establish, and only very small openings present a diagnostic problem. What appears to be granulation tissue in the posterior aspect of the vagina is the dark-red rectal mucosa, which stands out in contrast to the lighter vaginal mucosa. Usually the defect may be successfully defined with a small, malleable metal probe. If this is not successful, a Foley catheter should be placed in the rectum. Methylene blue dye or milk may then be instilled into the rectum with a tampon in the vagina, as is done for the diagnosis of a vesicovaginal fistula.

For initial treatment the patient should be obstipated with a low-residue diet and diphenoxylate hydrochloride (Lomotil). Approximately one in four anatomic defects heals spontaneously before epithelialization of the tract. Hyperalimentation may be helpful in the closure of some fistulas by allowing the patient to abstain from oral intake.

Timing of the operative repair is important. Repairs should not be undertaken before 8 to 12 weeks after the injury. The gynecologist should inspect the area surrounding the fistula to make sure that the tissues are free of edema, induration, and infection. Preoperative evaluation includes visualization of the entire vagina and sigmoidoscopy of the rectal mucosa for attempts to discover more than one opening. A barium enema or flexible endoscopy is important if there is any suspicion of coexistence of Crohn's disease.

The operative technique employed depends on the size and location of the fistula. Standard operative principles include removal of the entire fistulous tract and closure of tissue layers without tension on the suture line. In the repair of large rectovaginal fistulas in the lower part of the vagina, it is usually easier to convert the rectovaginal fistula into a fourth-degree laceration. Diverting colostomy should be used for all radiation-induced fistulas, the majority of fistulas associated with inflammatory bowel disease, and some large postoperative fistulas at the apex of the vagina. Postoperative care is minimal in that the patient may be discharged from the hospital after the first bowel movement. The stool should be kept soft with low-residue diets and stool softeners for the first 2 weeks after the operation.

WOUND COMPLICATIONS

Infection

Most major wound infections prolong a hospital stay approximately 6 to 8 days. In their extensive review of 23,649 operations, Cruse and Foord determined that the incidence of abdominal wound infection varied depending on risk factors; however, for abdominal hysterectomy the incidence was approximately 5%. In a population of women not at high risk, the incidence of infection should be approximately 1% to 2%.

The pathophysiology of wound infection depends on an interaction of two factors: the number and virulence of bacterial contamination and the resistance of the patient. Inoculation of bacteria into the wound occurs in the operating room during the operative procedure. There is a wide spectrum of common, endogenous bacteria that produces wound infections, including most gram-positive cocci and both aerobic and anaerobic rods. Small numbers of bacteria are present in all surgical wounds; however, bacterial growth is facilitated by decreased tissue oxygen and excessive amounts of necrotic tissue. The primary source of bacterial contamination of an abdominal wound may be exogenous to the patient, such as a break in sterile technique, or endogenous, such as purulent material from a pelvic abscess.

Both local and systemic factors contribute to the level of host resistance and thus to the incidence of wound infections. Local factors are more significant and include the presence of hematomas, necrotic tissue, foreign bodies, dead space, use of cautery, and decreased local tissue perfusion. Systemic factors include obesity, diabetes, liver disease, malnutrition, immunosuppression, defects in the reticuloendothelial system, age, and the duration of preoperative hospitalization. Pitkin discovered that the incidence of postoperative wound infection is increased eightfold when the woman's preoperative weight exceeds 200 pounds. Corticosteroid therapy may deplete systemic protein and suppress the inflammatory phase of the healing process. However, after the first 5 days of wound healing, corticosteroid therapy has no effect on an uninfected wound.

The first symptom of most wound infections appears between the fifth and the tenth postoperative day. Wound infection may occur as late as several months following surgery, but more than 90% of cases present within the first 2 weeks of the postoperative period. The first sign is usually fever, followed by tachycardia and varying degrees of increased tenderness and pain. As the infection progresses, many wounds develop areas that are either fluctuant or firm, and some develop crepitus. The incision is swollen, erythematous, edematous, and tender. Occasionally, subcutaneous gas may be seen on radiographic examination. Later in the course of the infection there may be associated spontaneous purulent drainage from the wound

Fever during the first 24 to 48 hours is usually secondary to atelectasis. However, two rare types of wound infections are so virulent that they produce toxicity within the first 48 hours: those produced by *Clostridium* species and acute beta-hemolytic streptococcal infection. Clinically, wound infections secondary to beta-hemolytic streptococci appear swollen and red and have an odorless discharge. In contrast, infections secondary to *Clostridium* are boggy and edematous, and the discharge has a sweet odor.

Initial management of any wound infection consists of opening and drainage of the wound. On removal of the skin sutures or skin clips the wound opens easily. Gram stain and both aerobic and anaerobic cultures of the wound should be obtained at this point. These initial cultures are most valuable if the patient does not respond to initial management. In such cases the differential diagnosis would be between infections involving deeper tissue planes and infection for which host resistance has failed even after drainage of the wound.

Once a wound infection has been opened and drained, care is directed toward initial packing of the wound with gauze to effect debridement and periodic irrigation. Rarely are antibiotics needed, unless there is a surrounding cellulitis. If there is a distinct zone of diffuse erythema surrounding a wound infection, the most likely organism is a streptococcal infection, and IV antibiotics are indicated. Systemic antibiotics are always indicated in women with immunosuppression or concomitant diseases with impaired defense mechanisms. Most women with a wound infection will become afebrile within 72 hours after the wound has been opened and debrided.

Prevention is the foundation of any approach to the management of wound infections. Prevention involves consideration of both local and systemic factors, which if unattended, predispose to infection. Prophylactic antibiotics, especially in high-risk cases, definitely decrease the incidence of wound infection. If the wound is grossly contaminated, then delayed primary closure on the third or fourth postoperative day is appropriate. Women who should be considered as candidates for delayed primary closure include those who are immunosupressed or malnourished or who have far-advanced malignancies. Women having operative procedures that involve a simultaneous abdominal and vaginal approach and those with a surgical opening of unprepared large intestine are also candidates for delayed primary closure. In a small series, Brown et al. reported that the latter technique reduced the incidence of wound infection from 23% in a control group to 2% in the group having delayed closure. Delayed secondary closure may be accomplished in previously infected wounds after several days of drainage and debridement. Delayed secondary closure markedly reduces the time necessary for eventual closure of the skin defect.

A virulent, rapidly progressing form of soft tissue wound infection is necrotizing fasciitis. The early symptoms are local pain with systemic symptoms of tachycardia and fever, which are higher than would be expected with an uncomplicated wound infection. As the disease progresses, the wound edges usually darken, with bullae formation adjacent to the wound. Necrotizing fasciitis involves the subcutaneous tissue and superficial fascia. It rapidly expands in the subcutaneous spaces. This condition is a surgical emergency, and patients should have an operation as soon as possible. This extremely rare but potentially fatal condition necessitates wide debridement of all necrotic tissue, high levels of systemic antibiotics, and sometimes hyperbaric oxygen. Stamenkovic and Lew have suggested the use of frozen-section biopsy to help establish the early diagnosis of this condition. Debridement to freely bleeding tissue helps determine the surgical margin.

Dehiscence and Evisceration

Dehiscence is a failure of normal healing and literally means disruption of any of the layers of a surgical incision. The physiologic, biochemical, and structural changes that characterize normal wound healing are complex and, at best, imperfectly understood. However, the most important fact to the clinician is that the strength of the wound increases over time. The strength of a skin incision increases at a rapid and almost constant rate for the first 4 months and at a much slower rate for the first year. Clinically, dehiscence usually means that the incision of the skin, subcutaneous tissue, and fascia has separated, but not the peritoneum.

This complication usually occurs during the first 2 postoperative weeks. Evisceration is a complete breakdown of the healing process through all levels of the abdominal incision, with omentum or bowel presenting through the incision.

The incidence of wound dehiscence is approximately 1 in 200 gynecologic operations. The major short-term result of wound dehiscence is the prolongation of hospital stay. Over the long term, dehiscence predisposes to incisional hernias. Wound dehiscence is a rare cause of surgical mortality, especially in debilitated patients. Wound infection is present in approximately 50% of women with wound disruption. As with wound infections, preventive management is the most important therapeutic consideration. The incidence of dehiscence has decreased with the introduction of synthetic absorbable sutures, such as Dexon and Vicryl (Table 24-15). They are superior to catgut in their more predictable absorption, reduction of tissue reaction, and greater tensile strength (Table 24-16).

Poole has reviewed the literature concerning prevention of disruption of fascial closure. The consensus of authorities is that local factors are much more important in the pathophysiology of wound disruption than systemic factors, although both should be considered in preventive management. Important mechanical factors predisposing to disruption are conditions that increase the tension on the incision line, such as abdominal distention and chronic lung disease, or a technically inadequate closure of the wound. Other factors include obesity, advanced age, malignancy, uremia, liver failure, diabetes, hypoproteinemia, hematoma formation, sepsis, corticosteroids or chemotherapy, prior radiation therapy, and whether the incision is made through an area of a previous incision. Malt has shown that whether an incision is horizontal or vertical has little effect on the incidence of wound disruption. The pathophysiology of fascial dehiscence involves exaggerated collagen lysis in the wound. Clinically the sutures "tear through the fascia" rather than dissolving or becoming "untied." For example, approximating and tying sutures too vigorously, especially a figure-of-8 suture, may lead to strangulation and necrosis of the tissue and subsequent wound dehiscence. Some gynecologists are performing primary mass closure with a continuous monofilament, delayed absorbable suture to avoid this problem.

TABLE 24-15
Classification of Suture Material

Type	Generic Name	Raw Material	Trade Names
Absorbable			
Natural collagen	Plain catgut	Submucosa of sheep intestine	—
	Chromic catgut	+ Buffered chromicizing	—
Synthetics	Polyglycolic acid	Homopolymer of glycolide + Poloxamer 188 coating	Dexon, Dexon-S, Dexon-Plus
	Polyglactin	Copolymer lactic and glycolic acid	Vicryl
		+ Calcium stearate coating	Coated Vicryl
	Polydioxanone	Monofilament	PDS
	Polyglyconate	Monofilament	Maxon
Nonabsorbable			
Natural fiber	Surgical cotton	Twisted natural cotton	—
	Surgical silk	Braided protein, naturally spun by silk worm	—
Synthetics	Nylon	Polyamide polymer	—
		Monofilament	Dermalon, Ethilon
		Multifilament	Neurolon
		Multifilament-silicone treated	Surgilon
	Polypropylene	Polymer of polypropylene	—
		Monofilament	Surgilene, Prolene, NovaFil
	Polybutester	Monofilament	NovaFil
	Polyethylene	Thermoplastic synthetic resin	Dermalene
	Polyester	Polyethylene terephthalate-multifilament	
		Braided-plain	Dacron, Mersilene
		Braided-silcone treated	Ti-Cron
		Braided-polybutilate coated	Ethibond
		Braided-PFTE* (Teflon) coated	Polydek, Ethiflex
		Braided-heavy PFTE (Teflon) impregnated	Tevdek
Metal	Stainless steel wire	Ferrous alloy	—
		Twisted multistrand	Flexon
		Monofilament strand	—
	Silver wire	Silver wire	—

From Sanz L and Smith S: Mechanisms of wound healing, suture material, and wound closure, in Buchsbaum HJ and Walton LA, editors: Strategies in gynecologic surgery, New York, 1986, Springer-Verlag New York, Inc, p 62.
*Polytetrafluoroethylene.

TABLE 24-16
Qualities of Absorbable Sutures

Type	Knot Security	Tensile Strength	Wound Security
Gut	+	++	5-7 days (50%)
Chromic	++	++	10-14 days (50%)
Dexon*	++++	++++	25 days (50%)
Vicryl†	+++	++++	30 days (50%)

From Sanz L and Smith S: Mechanisms of wound healing, suture material, and wound closure. In Buchsbaum HJ and Walton LA, editors: Strategies in gynecologic surgery, New York, 1986,
Springer-Verlag, New York, Inc, p 63.
*Polyglycolic acid.
†Polyglactin.

The classic symptom and sign of an impending wound disruption is the spontaneous passage of serosanguineous fluid from the abdominal incision. Most often this occurs between the fifth and eighth postoperative days. Patients with uninfected wounds generally have been asymptomatic. Patients who develop wound defects often lack the normal "healing ridge" of tissue that can be palpated in normal healing wounds.

Imperative for prevention of wound dehiscence is proper closure of the incision in a woman at high risk for anything less than optimum healing. Although there are many regional preferences for the choice of suture and method of closure, the most popular technique is the Smead-Jones closure with permanent suture (Figure 24-8). Closure with the Smead-Jones technique results in a dehiscence rate of approximately 1 in 1000 operations. With this technique it is important to place individual sutures at least 1 to 1.5 cm away from the adjacent sutures and include at least 2 cm of fascia on either side of the incision. The alternate technique is a mass closure using a monofilament permanent suture material such as nylon or polypropylene (Proline). Delayed primary wound closure 3 to 5 days after the operation should be considered if the wound was contaminated during the procedure, such as with rupture of a tuboovarian abscess. Delayed closure should also be considered for any patient already at high risk for wound complications, such as the malnourished patient, diabetic patient, or the woman who is immunosuppressed.

The treatment of wound disruption depends on the size and the depth of the defect. Simi-

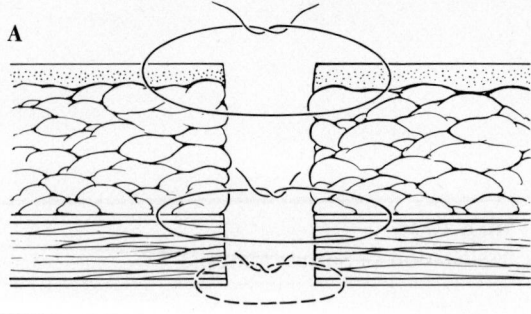

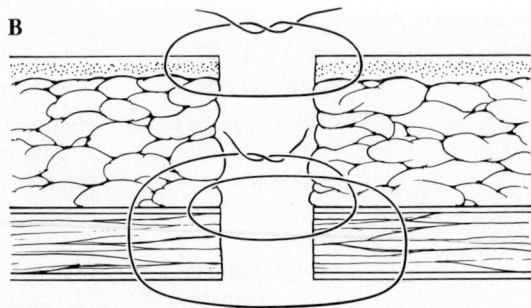

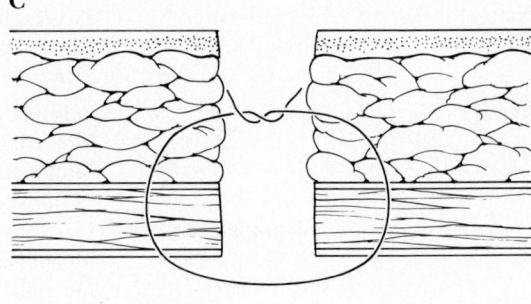

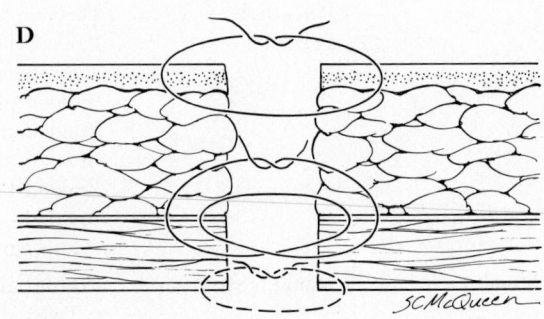

FIGURE 24-8
Types of abdominal incision closures. **A**, Layered. **B**, Smead-Jones. **C**, Through-and-through. **D**, Far-near. (From Braun TE: Wound dehiscence. In Schaefer G and Graber EA, editors: Complications in obstetric and gynecological surgery, Hagerstown, Md, 1981 Harper & Row, Publishers, Inc, p 159.)

lar to the management of wound infections, digital examination of the defect is important so that the full extent of the problem will be recognized. With larger defects the wound edges must be debrided and the wound closed with the Smead-Jones or mass closure technique.

OPERATIVE SITE COMPLICATIONS

Pelvic Cellulitis and Abscess

Infections of the contiguous retroperitoneal space immediately above the vaginal apex are common complications following abdominal or vaginal hysterectomy. However, the frequency of this postoperative complication has dramatically decreased in direct relation to the use of prophylactic antibiotics. These soft tissue infections range in severity from localized, minor cellulitis to large pelvic abscesses and have many names, from "cuff cellulitis" to "infected hematoma." Nevertheless, they are similar to soft tissue infections in other parts of the body and are either a cellulitis or an abscess. These infections prolong hospital stay and increase the cost of patient care. The bacterial spectrum that produces these infections includes aerobic and anaerobic bacteria from both exogenous and endogenous sources. Most postoperative pelvic infections are polymicrobial, usually from endogenous vaginal flora, and approximately 60% to 80% involve anaerobic organisms.

The pathophysiology of development of retroperitoneal infection is straightforward. The classic clamp-crush-cut-and-tie technique used in pelvic surgery produces an abundance of hypoxic and anoxic tissue that helps to establish an optimal environment for infection. This environment is further enhanced by the normal hysterectomy site producing an average of 40 ml of serosanguineous fluid each day during the first 72 postoperative hours. The endogenous flora of the upper vagina colonize and multiply in this retroperitoneal serosanguineous fluid or in pelvic hematomas after the operation.

The major symptoms of an operative site infection are fever and lower quadrant abdominal and pelvic pain. The fever usually becomes prominent between the third and fifth postoperative days. As the infection becomes more severe, the fever becomes spiking in character, the pain intensifies, and the patient develops moderate leukocytosis.

The diagnosis of cuff cellulitis is confirmed by pelvic examination. Pelvic tenderness and induration are prominent during the bimanual examination. A subtle difference exists between normal postoperative pelvic tenderness and induration and the tenderness and induration produced by infection. Postoperative infection is accompanied by an increase in suprapubic pain and perimetrial tenderness. Cuff cellulitis sometimes responds to drainage by opening the vaginal cuff. Appropriate cultures of the site are difficult with cellulitis because of surface contamination. Both persistent cellulitis, or one encompassing a large area, and abscess necessitate parenteral antibiotic therapy. Often a retroperitoneal abscess is diagnosed when the patient has ongoing fever and pelvic tenderness after 2 to 3 days of parenteral antibiotics for a suspected cuff cellulitis.

Because of their polymicrobial etiology, the infections are usually treated with an aminoglycoside (gentamicin, 2 mg/kg intravenously followed by 1.5 mg/kg intravenously every 8 hours in patients with normal renal function) and an antibiotic specific for anaerobic infection (clindamycin, 900 mg intravenously every 8 hours). Metronidazole (Flagyl) may be substituted for clindamycin. An alternative therapy is substitution of a third-generation cephalosporin or the monobactam agent aztreonam (Azactam) for the aminoglycoside. Aztreonam has a similar spectrum of antibiotic coverage with much less renal toxicity; however, it is much more expensive. It is important with an aminoglycoside to obtain peak and trough levels. They should be obtained 30 minutes after intravenous injection or 1 hour after intramuscular injection and 30 minutes before the next dose of the drug. Peak levels should be approximately 8 μg/ml of gentamicin and trough levels less than 2 μg/ml. The prevalence of aminoglycoside toxicity is 2% to 3%, and approximately 25% of women will require an adjustment in intravenous dosage. It is important to obtain peak and trough levels after 24 hours of antibiotic therapy and approximately every 3 to 4 days thereafter. Intravenous antibiotics should be continued until the patient is afebrile for 24 to 48 hours.

Although many pelvic abscesses drain spontaneously, patients should have serial pelvic examinations to determine the most appropriate time to effect operative drainage. Appropriate cultures should be obtained from the center of an abscess cavity when the abscess is operatively incised. If a patient does not become afebrile within 48 hours of proper drainage of a retroperitoneal abscess, a concomitant complication of pelvic thrombophlebitis should be suspected. If pelvic thrombophlebitis is suspected, a 72-hour trial of intravenous heparin therapy may be instituted.

Granulation Tissue

Granulation tissue at the apex of the vaginal vault is a frequent complication following abdominal hysterectomy. Small areas of friable, red granulation tissue are seen at the 6-week postoperative pelvic examination in more than 50% of women. Granulation tissue is more common following abdominal than vaginal hysterectomy and is more frequently found when the vaginal cuff is left open rather than closed.

Recently, Manyonda et al. conducted a prospective randomized trial of women with total abdominal hysterectomies and compared polygalactide (Vicryl) and chromic catgut. In this study 32% of the women developed vault granulation tissue, observed at their 6-week postoperative checkup. Of women who developed granulation tissue at the vault, chromic catgut was implicated twice as frequently as polygalactide suture, 68% versus 32%, respectively.

Excessive granulation tissue is the result of an exaggerated healing response of the vascular-rich pelvic tissues. One of the causes is believed to be inversion of the vaginal epithelium between the margins of the edges of the incision at the apex of the vaginal vault.

Some patients are asymptomatic, but many women experience spotting or a bloody discharge after intercourse. The rare patient may have mild pelvic discomfort. On speculum examination the granulation tissue appears as a polypoid projection hanging from the vaginal suture line. The differential diagnosis includes a prolapsed fallopian tube and recurrent carcinoma in a patient with a pelvic malignancy. The polypoid mass is easily avulsed from the vaginal apex. The remaining areas of granulation tissue should be treated with a chemical cautery (silver nitrate or Monsel's solution) or by cryocautery or electrocautery.

Prolapsed Fallopian Tube

Prolapse of the distal end of the fallopian tube is a rare complication of abdominal or vaginal hysterectomy. It is usually discovered during a routine visit during the first few months following the operation.

Many women with this complication are free of symptoms, but others experience a watery discharge, postcoital spotting, or moderate lower abdominal and pelvic pain. Differing from granulation tissue, the fallopian tube is not friable and is firmly attached. Grasping the fallopian tube with an instrument and applying traction produces much more pain than traction on granulation tissue. Treatment is the destruction of the segment of the fallopian tube protruding through the vaginal vault with cryocautery or the laser. The fallopian tube may be removed during an outpatient procedure using conduction anesthesia. Most clinicians opt for a vaginal approach with ligation of the fallopian tube as high as possible. The stump of the tube is buried retroperitoneally and the vaginal epithelium closed. An alternate treatment is coagulation of the segment of fallopian tube protruding through the vaginal apex with cryocautery. Often the vaginal wall reepithelializes over the area, thereby excluding the tube from any connection with the vaginal cavity.

MISCELLANEOUS COMPLICATIONS

Lymphocyst

A lymphocyst is a local collection of lymphatic fluid within the pelvis resulting from retrograde drainage of lymph. It is a rare complication, found most frequently after pelvic node dissections. In the past this complication occurred in approximately 20% of patients having undergone radical operations. However, with meticulous attention to ligation of distal lymphatic channels and routine postoperative suction drainage of the retroperitoneal space, this complication is now reported in only 1% to 3% of such cases. Conditions that predispose the patient to formation of a lymphocyst are previous radiation and anticoagulation.

Lymphocysts usually present during the first 6 postoperative weeks. They vary greatly in size and seldom become infected. The cyst usually begins anterior and medial to the iliac vessels. As it expands, it may produce obstruction or angulation of the ureter, pressure symptoms on the bladder, or partial venous obstruction. Small lymphocysts, less than 4 cm in diameter, are usually asymptomatic and regress spontaneously within 8 weeks. Larger cysts necessitate treatment either by intermittent aspiration followed by pressure dressings or insertion of an indwelling catheter under ultrasound guidance. Simple incision and drainage are usually unsuccessful because the condition often recurs. Traditional surgical management involves removing a large segment of the wall of the lymphocyst and placing a tongue of omentum in the cavity. Choo et al. have advised peritoneal marsupialization for lymphocysts that do not respond to traditional operative management. Some gynecologic oncologists have postulated that leaving the pelvic peritoneum open after radical hysterectomy and lymph node dissection helps to decrease the incidence of this complication.

Ovarian Abscess

Ovarian abscess is a rare but serious postoperative complication. If the diagnosis is not established, this condition is potentially fatal because of intraperitoneal rupture of the abscess. Ovarian abscesses arise from bacterial colonization of the ovarian cortex. This may occur either via disruption of the ovarian capsule by the presence of a corpus luteum or via an operative disruption, such as cystectomy performed during vaginal hysterectomy.

The disease may follow either a slow, indolent course or a rapidly progressive one. Some patients with this complication present during the first postoperative week with a high fever and severe pain, which are continuous until rupture occurs. Others become afebrile following the operation but return sometime during the first few months with a persistent low-grade fever and mild pain. Chronologically, most ovarian abscesses appear later in the postoperative course than other retroperitoneal abscesses. Ovarian abscesses usually appear 2 to 3 weeks postoperatively, but cases have been reported as late as 3 to 4 months later. Willson and Black, in a classic work describing 28 patients with ovarian abscess, noted that the predominant symptom was abdominal pain associated with persistent tachycardia and high fever. This abscess is found higher in the pelvis than a retroperitoneal abscess at the apex of the vagina.

Initial treatment is medical therapy with intravenous antibiotics; however, most patients do not respond to medical therapy, and operative removal of the adnexa becomes a necessity. Surgical drainage often may not be accomplished transvaginally, and the abdominal approach is preferable. This rare problem should be considered in any woman having a gynecologic operation in which the integrity of the ovarian capsule is disrupted either physiologically or operatively.

Femoral Neuropathy

The femoral nerve is the largest branch of the lumbar plexus and arises from the primary rami of L2, L3, and L4. It provides motor function to several leg muscles, including the quadriceps, and sensory fibers that innervate the anterior and medial surfaces of the thigh and leg. The vascular supply to the femoral nerve may be compromised during an abdominal or vaginal hysterectomy. Rosenblum et al. have described the pathophysiology of this complication as being secondary to continuous pressure, usually by a self-retaining retractor producing ischemic necrosis of the nerve. The vascular circulation of the nerve itself is compromised by diminished blood flow in the vasa nervorum. The most common site of nerve compression is 4 to 6 cm above the inguinal ligament where the nerve pierces the psoas muscle.

Factors that contribute to the development of this complication are thinness, long retractor blades, prolonged operative times and systemic diseases, such as diabetes mellitus, gout, alcoholism, and malnutrition. However, the classic patient who develops this complication is a short, thin, athletic woman who has a transverse incision in which a self-retaining retractor is used. A similar problem may develop after vaginal operations in thin women with exaggerated hip flexion or abduction in the lithotomy position.

Patients with this complication may experience numbness, paresthesias, and difficulty with their gait. Usually these neurologic symptoms develop within the first 24 to 72 hours following an operation. These symptoms are causes of great anxiety to the patient. Because of the inability to lift the leg, climbing stairs is a particular problem. The muscle and sensory function recovers spontaneously over several weeks to several months. The patient should be seen by a physical therapist to facilitate ambulation and prevent muscle atrophy. To prevent this complication, it is important to palpate the lateral pelvic wall and femoral artery after placement of a self-retaining retractor. With the woman in the lithotomy position, one should check for pulsations in the popliteal or posterior tibial vessels. In a thin patient, placing folded towels between the skin surface and the self-retaining retractor helps to prevent this complication by decreasing the depth of penetration of the lateral retractor blades.

ESTROGEN REPLACEMENT

Bilateral salpingo-oophorectomy is often performed on young women for conditions such as pelvic inflammatory disease. National surveys have documented that bilateral castration concomitant with hysterectomy is performed in approximately 25% of premenopausal women undergoing this operation. The possible consequences of estrogen deprivation include vasomotor symptoms, urogenital tissue atrophy (atrophic vaginitis, dyspareunia, and urethral syndrome), and osteoporosis. For premenopausal women an additional risk of castration is the development of atherosclerotic heart disease at an earlier age than for a woman with normal ovarian function. The pathophysiology of premature coronary vascular disease is complex and multifactorial, but the change in the ratio of high-density lipoproteins (HDLs) to low-density lipoproteins (LDLs) is a critical factor.

Estrogen replacement is indicated in the vast majority of premenopausal women having bilateral oophorectomy. The increase in hypercoagulability produced by the doses of estrogen used for postmenopausal symptoms is negligible. Nevertheless, because of the hypercoagulability and injury to the intima of vessels associated with the operative procedure, oral estrogen therapy should not be started immediately after the procedure. Theoretically, estradiol given via a cutaneous patch is acceptable in the immediate postoperative period because of a decrease in the liver's production of clotting factors. A dosage of 0.625 mg of conjugated estrogens daily is sufficient to protect from bone demineralization and osteoporosis. A higher dose may be required to alleviate hot flushes (Chapter 40).

PSYCHOLOGIC COMPLICATIONS

Pain Relief

The proper management of pain during the postoperative period is a primary goal of all surgeons. Most women experience moderate to severe pain during the first 36 to 48 hours following a gynecologic operation. However, pain and suffering are personal, internal events, the

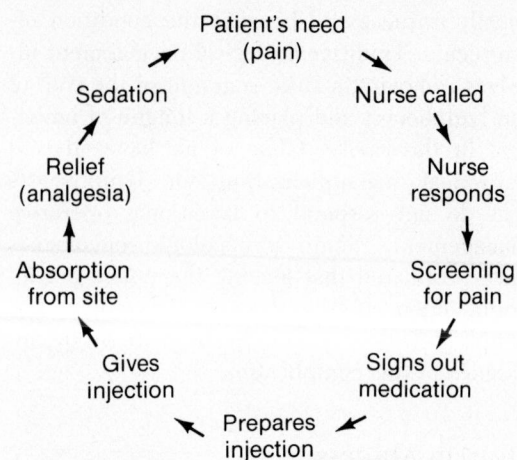

FIGURE 24-9
Pain cycle. (From White PF: Postgrad Med 80:8, 1986.)

extent and presence of which may only be measured by direct communication with the patient.

The current literature documents that pain relief is often treated inadequately in postoperative patients. For many patients who undergo gynecologic operations, dosages of analgesics are prescribed that are less than adequate to relieve pain, and many nurses further reduce the amount of medication. The many misconceptions concerning postoperative pain include the dangers of addiction and the fear of respiratory depression. Recently, Kuhn et al. have emphasized that it is not only physicians and nurses who contribute to ineffective treatment. Patients, such as those having hysterectomy, also contribute by having a lower level of pain relief expectation. These authors believe that pain relief is poor because of inadequate education of patients in what to expect from pain relief. Inadequate pain relief prolongs hospital stay and has adverse psychologic consequences.

White (1986) has presented a schematic diagram of the pain cycle and the potential delays in pain relief with traditional "prn" analgesic regimens (Figure 24-9). Many studies have confirmed that regular-interval preventive pain relief is superior to conventional "on demand" analgesic medication during the first 36 to 48 hours following the operation. Relative potencies of common analgesic medications are listed in Table 24-17. However, there is great variability in absorption. In addition, the therapeutic window (the range of effective blood concentration before undesired side effects occur) is narrow. When 100 mg of meperidine hydrochloride (Demerol) is given every 4 hours intramuscularly, the concentration of the drug in the blood exceeds the minimum level necessary to produce adequate pain relief only 35% of the 4-hour period (Table 24-18).

In White's study, peak concentrations varied as much as fivefold among the 10 different individuals, and the time to reach peak blood level varied as much as sevenfold. Thus patient-controlled analgesic (PCA) systems have become the preferred method of pain relief during the immediate postoperative period (Figure 24-10). PCA systems dramatically decrease patients' anxiety because they are in control rather than the hospital staff. These systems are both safe and effective as long as there is a lockout period, and they help to minimize individual differences in pharmacokinetics. Modern PCA systems minimize the risk of drug overdose and allow the patient to titrate and therefore maximize analgesic effectiveness. In general, patients use the PCA system for approximately 36 to 72 hours until they are tolerating oral liquids. The suggested initial doses for PCA systems using meperidine and morphine are listed in Table 24-19.

During the past 5 years anesthesiologists have been increasingly using intrathecal or epidural opioid injection. Both routes effectively relieve postoperative pelvic pain.

After the first 48 hours, pain relief may be successfully controlled with prostaglandin synthetase inhibitors. Morrison et al. reported in a study of 161 women that 50 mg of flurbiprofen (Ansaid) was as effective as 10 mg of intramuscular morphine for postoperative gynecologic pain. This oral medication was as effective in pain intensity scores, duration of pain relief, and clinical appreciation of pain by the patients.

TABLE 24-17
Relative* Potencies of Analgesics (mg/mg)

	Intramuscular	Oral
Alphaprodine	45	—
Buprenorphine	2.5-5	0.4 (sublingual)
Butorphanol	2-3	—
Codeine	130	200
Fentanyl	0.125	—
Heroin	4	—
Hydromorphone	1.5	7.5
Levorphanol	2	4
Meperidine	75	300
Methadone	10	20
Morphine	10	30-60
Nalbuphine	10	—
Oxycodone	10	30
Pentazocine	60	180
Propoxyphene	240	300
Sufentanil	0.0125	—

From Gorman ES and Warfield CA: Hosp Pract 21:48B, 1986.
*To 10 mg morphine, intramuscular.

TABLE 24-18
Blood Meperidine Concentrations After Intramuscular Administration of 100 mg Every 4 Hours in 10 Patients

	Peak Level (μg/ml)	Time to Peak Level (min)	Minimum Analgesic Concentration* (μg/ml)	Time Level Exceeded Minimum Analgesic Concentration* (min)
Initial postoperative injections				
Mean	0.51	57	0.43	43
Range	0.24-0.82	18-108	0.26-0.85	0-240
SD	0.14	27	0.14	57
Second postoperative day				
Mean	0.77	39	0.49	150
Range	0.51-1.21	18-108	0.28-0.66	54-240
SD	0.23	24	0.10	72

From White PF: Postgrad Med 80:9, 1986.
*Minimum analgesic concentration refers to the minimum level required to provide adequate pain relief.

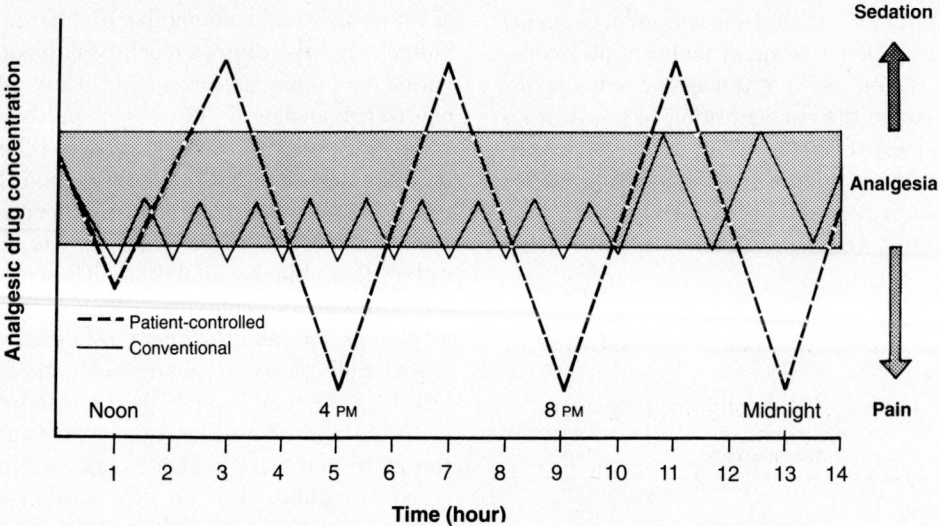

FIGURE 24-10
Theoretic relationships among dosing interval, analgesic drug concentration, and clinical effects when comparing patient-controlled analgesic (PCA) system *(solid lines)* with conventional intramuscular therapy *(dashed lines)*. (Redrawn from White PF: Semin Anesthesiol 4:255, 1985.)

TABLE 24-19
Usual PCA Doses for Meperidine and Morphine*

Drug	Bolus Dose (mg)		Lockout Interval (min)		Basal Infusion (mg/hr)	
	Average	Range	Average	Range	Average	Range
Meperidine	10	5-30	6	5-15	5	5-20
Morphine	1	0.5-3	6	5-15	0.5	0.5-2

From Breslow MJ, Miller CF, and Rogers MC: Perioperative management, St Louis, 1990, Mosby–Year Book, Inc.
*These are suggested as starting doses only. After initiating therapy, titrate dose to analgesia versus sedation.

Psychosexual Problems and Depression

The time both immediately before and after a surgical procedure is a stressful period for all patients. Anxiety and fear are normal responses and should be anticipated by health care providers. Any operation on the female reproductive organs stimulates questions and conflicts concerning body image, feminine identity, sexuality, and possibly future childbearing. The period following a gynecologic operation is one of transition and is a unique psychologic challenge to the patient. The reader should review Chapter 7 to emphasize the problems of loss and grief and the four stages of depression: impact, retreat, acknowledgment, and reconstitu-

tion. After gynecologic operations, every patient needs support to overcome this challenge, and it is important to emphasize that it may take many months to complete the process.

DISCHARGE INSTRUCTIONS

Simple but complete discharge instructions are an important component of postoperative care. The physician should anticipate the most common questions and give the patient explicit instructions. Particular attention should be given to limitations in physical activity, such as heavy lifting, driving a car, climbing stairs, and getting the incision wet. Information should be given about vaginal spotting as sutures dissolve. Appropriate phone numbers should be provided in case of unanticipated complications and to schedule return appointments. One of the most accomplished clinicians of our generation is the internist Eugene A. Stead Jr. He teaches that discharge instructions should not be given on the morning of discharge. Rather, patients should receive these instructions the day before discharge; then a "posttest" is given on the morning of discharge to ensure that the patient understands. Instructions should be given in both verbal and written form.

KEY POINTS

- Postoperative febrile morbidity is related to infection in approximately 20% of cases and noninfectious causes in 80% of cases.

- Atelectasis is the cause of more than 90% of cases of postoperative fever presenting in the first 48 hours.

- Intraoperative factors that dramatically increase the risk of postoperative fever are an operative time longer than 2 hours and intraoperative transfusion.

- The normal physiologic response to the stress of an operation and tissue destruction is release of increased levels of antidiuretic hormone and aldosterone, producing both sodium and water retention.

- Because of the shifts in water balance, the postoperative hematocrit at 72 hours is a more accurate measurement of operative and postoperative blood loss than a hematocrit at 24 hours.

- After subtracting the effects of the operative blood loss from the preoperative hematocrit, a further reduction in hematocrit of 3 to 5 points reflects a postoperative hemorrhage of approximately 500 ml.

- Factors that predispose patients to atelectasis include supine position, obesity, smoking, age greater than 60 years, prolonged operative time, and coexisting medical conditions, such as cardiac disease or pulmonary infection.

- The clinical presentation of fever, tachypnea, and tachycardia within 72 hours of an operation is pathognomonic for atelectasis.

- Early mobilization and ambulation have been documented to be as effective as chest physical therapy in the prevention of pulmonary complications.

- Postoperative pneumonia is commonly associated with atelectasis with predisposing factors including chronic pulmonary disease, heavy cigarette smoking, obesity, older age, nasogastric tubes, long procedures, and debilitating illnesses.

- Postoperative hypovolemia may be secondary to several factors in the perioperative period, including the patient being volume deficient preoperatively, unreplaced blood loss during surgery, extracellular fluid loss during surgery, inadequate fluid replacement, or continued blood loss after the surgical procedure.

- From 15% to 45% of surgical blood loss is absorbed onto drapes, pads, and other areas. Thus blood levels in the suction bottle are inaccurate markers of total operative blood loss.

- The differential diagnosis of hemorrhagic shock in the postoperative patient includes pneumothorax, pulmonary embolus, massive pulmonary aspiration, myocardial infarction, and acute gastric dilation.

- In the healthy reproductive age female, because of normal adaptive changes, it takes a rapid loss of approximately one third of the blood volume to produce significant hypotension.

- The goals of management of shock are to replace and restore effective circulating blood volume and to establish normal cellular perfusion and oxygenation.

- The extent of wound or pelvic hematomas is determined by the potential size of the compartment into which the bleeding occurs.

- Retroperitoneal or broad ligament hematomas may contain several units of blood.

- The incidence of retained sponges or pads is between 1 in 1200 and 1 in 1500 laparotomies. Clinically, they usually present as a tender pelvic mass.

- Approximately 30% of all hospital-acquired bacteremias are secondary to intravenous lines.

- The length of the surgical procedure has an important influence on the development of thrombophlebitis. If the operation is 1 to 2 hours, approximately 15% of women develop the disease; if longer than 3 hours, the risk is greater than 45%.

- Generally, thromboembolic complications occur early in the postoperative course, with 75% occurring within the first 72 hours. Approximately 15% occur after the seventh postoperative day.

- The incidence of fatal pulmonary emboli following gynecologic operations is between 0.1% and 0.8%.

- Superficial thrombophlebitis is a common problem both in the lower extremities and along intravenous catheter sites. The finding of superficial thrombophlebitis does not rule out concomitant inflammation in the deep veins.

- The clinical management of mild superficial thrombophlebitis includes rest, elevation, and local heat. Moderate to severe superficial thrombophlebitis may be treated with nonsteroidal antiinflammatory agents.

- The incidence of thrombophlebitis is directly dependent on the risk factors of type and duration of operation, age of the patient, obesity, immobility, malignancy, sepsis, diabetes, and conditions producing venous stasis.

- Thrombophlebitis most often begins in the deep veins of the calf. Approximately 75% of pulmonary emboli originate from a thrombus that begins in the leg veins and extends to the femoral veins.

- If thrombophlebitis affects one leg, the other leg is involved in approximately 33% of women.

- The three precipitating factors that produce thrombi, as described by Virchow, are an increase in coagulability, damage to the vessel wall, and venous stasis.

- Duplex ultrasonography is rapidly replacing venography as the diagnostic procedure of choice for deep vein thrombophlebitis.

- Recently published guidelines from the NIH Consensus Conference suggest that low-risk patients under 40 years of age who undergo an operation of less than 30 minutes' duration need early ambulation and compression stockings for prophylaxis for deep vein thrombophlebitis. Women at moderate to high risk should be treated with low-dose heparin, dextran, or external pneumatic compression for prophylaxis.

- Low-dose heparin (5000 IU given 2 hours before and every 8 to 12 hours after operation) reduces the incidence of deep vein thrombophlebitis.

- External pneumatic compression of the legs by pneumatic-inflated sleeve devices is as effective as low-dose heparin in the prevention of deep vein thrombophlebitis. It is approximately equal in cost.

- Heparin is the drug of choice for the initial treatment of thrombosis or pulmonary embolus once the diagnosis is confirmed. An intravenous bolus of 5000 IU is given initially, after which an infusion of 1000 to 1500 IU per hour is appropriate.

- Patients with pulmonary emboli have a mortality rate of 30% in untreated cases versus 8% in treated cases.

- Signs and symptoms of pulmonary emboli are nonspecific; however, a national study found the most common to include chest pain, dyspnea, apprehension, tachypnea, rales, and an increase in the second heart sound over the pulmonic area.

- Ventilation/perfusion scans are the first line in imaging techniques to rule out the diagnosis of pulmonary embolus. However, pulmonary angiography is the most definitive test in establishing the diagnosis. Five percent of patients experience complications from pulmonary angiography.

- The etiology of postoperative voiding problems includes anxiety, mechanical interference, obstruction by swelling and edema, neurologic imbalance, and tranquilizer-associated detrusor hypotonia.

- The most commonlyly acquired infection in the hospital and most frequent cause of gram-negative bacteremia in hospitalized patients is catheter-associated urinary tract infection.

- The incidence of positive urine culture after a single in-and-out catheterization is 4%. When a Foley catheter has been in place for 36 hours, approximately 20% of women have bacterial colonization. After 72 hours of catheterization, 75% of patients will have positive cultures.

- Prophylactic antibiotics should not be used with a Foley catheter to cover for the possibility of urinary tract infection unless the patient is immunocompromised.

- We recommend 3 days of antibiotic therapy for a woman who has developed cystitis after catheter use. Single-dose antibiotic treatment is reserved for nonpregnant women with an uncomplicated urinary tract infection unrelated to catheter use.

- It has been estimated that ureteral injury occurs in as many as 1 per 200 women during abdominal hysterectomies.

- Urinary fistulas following gynecologic operations are secondary to abdominal hysterectomy in 75% and to vaginal procedures in the remaining 25%.

- Although symptoms of urinary incontinence may present within a few hours of the operative procedure, the majority of fistulas usually present 8 to 12 days after operation, occasionally as late as 25 to 30 days after operation.

- If there is a suspicion that trauma to the bladder has occurred during an operative procedure, continuous catheter drainage for 3 to 5 days will often result in spontaneous healing of multiple defects.

- Approximately 20% of bladder injuries and 30% of ureteral injuries heal spontaneously without further operation if adequate drainage is obtained.

- Operative repair of a urinary tract fistula should be delayed 2 to 6 months after the initial injury to obtain optimal results. Preoperative workup of such an injury includes intravenous pyelography, cystoscopy, and biopsy of the margins if carcinoma is suspected.

- An uncomplicated ileus may last 24 to 48 hours in the stomach, only a few hours in the small intestines, and 48 to 72 hours in the colon.

- Major factors that result in intensification of adynamic ileus include peritoneal contamination by purulent material or blood, extensive handling of the small intestine, and inadequate replacement of fluids and electrolytes.

- If adynamic ileus persists for longer than 5 days, a diagnosis of mechanical bowel obstruction should be strongly considered.

- Predisposing factors to the development of ileus include obesity, age of the patient, preoperative immobility, and removal of large pelvic and abdominal masses.

- Previous gynecologic operations are the most common cause of bowel obstruction in women.

- Pneumoperitoneum from an exploratory celiotomy usually persists for 7 to 10 days; thus, after operation, free air under the diaphragm is not diagnostic of perforation of a viscus.

- The foundation of early treatment of postoperative intestinal obstruction is decompression of the small intestine, accomplished by nasogastric tube or, preferably, a long tube.

- The etiology of rectovaginal fistula includes gynecologic operations, carcinoma, radiation therapy, perirectal abscess, inflammatory bowel disease, lymphogranuloma venereum, and trauma.

- Postoperative fistulas between the rectum and vagina usually present 7 to 14 days after the procedure.

- After the diagnosis of a rectovaginal fistula has been made, the patient should be obstipated with a low-residue diet and diphenoxylate hydrochloride (Lomotil). Approximately one in four anatomic defects heals spontaneously before epithelialization of the tract.

- Most repairs of rectovaginal fistulas should not be undertaken until 8 to 12 weeks after the operation. The area surrounding the fistula should be free of edema, induration, and infection.

- Symptoms of wound infections occur most commonly between the fifth and tenth postoperative day, with the patient usually exhibiting tachycardia and fever.

- The incidence of wound dehiscence is approximately 1 in 200 gynecologic operations. Wound infection is found in approximately 50% of women with wound disruption.

- The classic symptom and sign of an impending wound disruption is the spontaneous passage of serosanguineous fluid from the abdominal incision.

- If a distinct zone of diffuse erythema surrounds a wound infection, the most likely organism is a beta-hemolytic streptococcus, and intravenous antibiotics are indicated.

- Systemic antibiotics are always indicated in women who have immunosuppression or concomitant diseases with impaired defense mechanisms.

- Delayed secondary closure may be accomplished in previously infected wounds after several days of drainage and debridement. Delayed secondary closure markedly reduces the time necessary for eventual closure of the skin defect.

- Necrotizing fasciitis involves the subcutaneous tissue and superficial fascia. It rapidly expands in the subcutaneous spaces. This condition is a surgical emergency, and patients should have an operation as soon as possible.

- Granulation tissue at the vaginal vault apex often appears as friable, red, polypoid tissue at the 6-week postoperative check. This tissue may be treated with chemical cautery, cryocautery, or electrocautery.

- Ovarian abscesses arise from bacterial colonization of a disrupted ovarian capsule, usually by the presence of a corpus luteum or by surgical disruption during a procedure.

- Ovarian abscesses usually present 2 to 3 weeks postoperatively, but cases have been reported as late as 3 to 4 months.

- Common causes of femoral neuropathy are continuous pressure from self-retaining retractors or exaggerated hip flexion or abduction from the lithotomy position in thin women.

- Patient-controlled analgesic (PCA) systems dramatically decrease patients' anxiety because they are in control rather than the hospital staff. These systems are both safe and effective as long as there is a lockout period, and they help to minimize individual differences in pharmacokinetics.

- After the first 36 to 48 hours, postoperative pain may be successfully controlled with prostaglandin synthetase inhibitors.

- Discharge instructions should be given in both verbal and written forms, and physicians should anticipate patients' most common questions.

BIBLIOGRAPHY

Alvarez RD: Gastrointestinal complications in gynecologic surgery: a review for the general gynecologist, Obstet Gynecol 72:533, 1988.

American College of Obstetricians and Gynecologists: Blood component therapy, ACOG Tech Bull 78:1,1984.

Amoroso P and Greenwood RN: Posture and central venous pressure measurement in circulatory volume depletion, Lancet 11:258, 1989.

Arieff AI: Hyponatremia, convulsions, respiratory arrest, and permanent brain damage after elective surgery in healthy women, N Engl J Med 314:1529, 1986.

Bachmann GA: Psychosexual aspects of hysterectomy, Women's Health Instit 1:41, 1990.

Bandy LC, Addison A, and Parker RT: Surgical management of rectovaginal fistulas in Crohn's disease, Am J Obstet Gynecol 147:359, 1983.

Batres F and Barclay DL: Sciatic nerve injury during gynecologic procedures using the lithotomy position, Obstet Gynecol 62:92S, 1983.

Biello DR: Radiological (scintigraphic) evaluation of patients with suspected pulmonary thromboembolism, JAMA 257:3257, 1987.

Blinder RA and Coleman RE: Evaluation of pulmonary embolism, Radiol Clin North Am 23:391, 1985.

Bone RC: Ventilation/perfusion scan in pulmonary embolism: "The emperor is incompletely attired," JAMA 263:2794, 1990.

Bonnar J: Venous thromboembolism and gynecologic surgery, Clin Obstet Gynecol 28:432, 1985.

Breitenbucher RB: Bacterial changes in the urine samples of patients with long-term indwelling catheters, Arch Intern Med 144:1585, 1984.

Brenner DW, Fogle MA, and Schellhammer PF: Venous thromboembolism, J Urol 142:1403, 1989.

Breslow MJ, Miller CF, and Rogers MC, editors: Perioperative management, St Louis, 1990, Mosby–Year Book, Inc.

Brown SE, Allen HH, and Robbins RN: The use of delayed primary wound closure in preventing wound infections, Am J Obstet Gynecol 127:713, 1977.

Buchsbaum HJ and Walton LA, editors: Strategies in gynecologic surgery, New York, 1986, Springer-Verlag New York, Inc.

Cercenado E, Ena J, Rodriguez-Creixems M, et al: A conservative procedure for the diagnosis of catheter-related infections, Arch Intern Med 150:1417, 1990.

Choo YC, Wong LC, Wong KP, et al: The management of intractable lymphocyst following radical hysterectomy, Gynecol Oncol 24:309, 1986.

Clarke DB and Abrams LD: Pulmonary embolectomy: a 25 year experience, J Thorac Cardiovasc Surg 92:442, 1986.

Clarke-Pearson DL, DeLong ER, Synan IS, et al: Complications of low-dose heparin prophylaxis in gynecologic oncology surgery, Obstet Gynecol 64:689, 1984.

Clarke-Pearson DL, Synan IS, Colemen RE, et al: The natural history of postoperative venous thromboemboli in gynecologic oncology: a prospective study of 382 patients, Am J Obstet Gynecol 148:1051, 1984.

Clarke-Pearson DL, Synan IS, Hinshaw WM, et al: Prevention of postoperative venous thromboembolism by external pneumatic calf compression in patients with gynecologic malignancy, Obstet Gynecol 63:92, 1984.

Condon RE and DeCosse J, editors: Surgical care II, Philadelphia, 1985, Lea & Febiger.

Consensus Conference: Prevention of venous thrombosis and pulmonary embolism, JAMA 256:744, 1986.

Creasman WT, Henderson D, Hinshaw W, et al: Estrogen replacement therapy in the patient treated for endometrial cancer, Obstet Gynecol 67:326, 1986.

Cruikshank MK, Levine MN, Hirsch J, et al: A standard heparin homogram for the management of heparin therapy, Arch Intern Med 151:333, 1991.

Cruse PJE and Foord R: A 5-year prospective study of 23,649 surgical wounds, Arch Surg 107:206, 1973.

Cruse PJE and Foord R: The epidemiology of wound infection, Surg Clin North Am 60:27, 1980.

Cumming PD, Wallace EL, Schorr JB, et al: Exposure of patients to human immunodeficiency virus through the transfusion of blood components that test antibody-negative, N Engl J Med 321:941, 1989.

Daifuku R and Stamm WE: Association of rectal and urethral colonization with urinary tract infection in patients with indwelling catheters, JAMA 252:2028, 1984.

Dalen JE, Paraskos JA, Ockene IS, et al: Venous thromboembolism, Chest 89:370S, 1986.

Deming RH: Current concepts on the adult respiratory distress syndrome, Circ Shock 30:297, 1990.

Dudrick SJ, Baue AE, Eiseman B, et al, editors: Manual of preoperative and postoperative care, ed 3, Philadelphia, 1983, WB Saunders Co.

Duff GW: Is fever beneficial to the host? A clinical perspective, Yale J Biol Med 59:125, 1986.

Dunn LJ and Van Voorhis LW: Enigmatic fever and pelvic thrombophlebitis, N Engl J Med 276:265, 1967.

Fry DE, Milholen L and Harbrecht PJ: Iatrogenic ureteral injury, Arch Surg 118:454, 1983.

Fulkerson WJ, Coleman E, Ravin CF, et al: Diagnosis of pulmonary embolism, Arch Intern Med 146:961, 1986.

Gallup DG: Modifications of celiotomy techniques to decrease morbidity in obese gynecologic patients, Am J Obstet Gynecol 150:171, 1984.

Gallup DG, Nolan TE, and Smith RP: Primary mass closure of midline incisions with a continuous polyglyconate monofilament absorbable suture, Obstet Gynecol 76:872, 1990.

Garcia CR and Cutler WB: Preservation of the ovary: a reevaluation, Fertil Steril 42:510, 1984.

Georgy FM: Femoral neuropathy following abdominal hysterectomy, Am J Obstet Gynecol 123:819, 1975.

Goldharber SZ, Kessler CM, Heit J, et al: Randomized controlled trial of recombinant tissue plasminogen activator versus urokinase in the treatment of acute pulmonary embolism, Lancet 8606:293, 1988.

Gorman ES and Warfield CA: The use of opioids in the management of pain, Hosp Pract 20:48A, 1986.

Grimes DA: A simplified device for intraoperative autotransfusion, Obstet Gynecol 72:947, 1988.

Hall R: Difficulties in the treatment of acute pulmonary embolism, Thorax 40:729, 1985.

Harding GKM, Nicolle LE, Ronald AR, et al: How long should catheter-acquired urinary tract infection in women be treated? A randomized controlled study, Ann Intern Med 114:713, 1991.

Hardy JD, editor: Complications in surgery and their management, ed 4, Philadelphia, 1981, WB Saunders Co.

Hassan AA, Reiff RH, and Fayez JA: Femoral neuropathy following microsurgical tuboplasty, Fertil Steril 45:889, 1986.

Helmkamp BF: Abdominal wound dehiscence, Am J Obstet Gynecol 128:803, 1977.

Hemsel DL: Post-hysterectomy cuff and pelvic cellulitis, Contemp Obstet Gynecol, 32:39, 1990.

Henriksson C, Kihl B, and Pettersson S: Urethrovaginal and vesicovaginal fistula, Acta Obstet Gynecol Scand 61:143, 1982.

Hershey CO, Tomford JW, McLaren CE, et al: The natural history of intravenous catheter–associated phlebitis, Arch Intern Med 144:1373, 1984.

Howkins J and Williams DK: Vault granulations after total abdominal hysterectomy, J Obstet Gynaecol Br Comm 75:84, 1968.

Huisman MV, Buller HR, TenCate JW, et al: Serial impedance plethysmography for suspected deep venous thrombosis in outpatients, N Engl J Med 314:823, 1986.

Hull RD, Raskob GE, and Hirsch J: The diagnosis of clinically suspected pulmonary embolism, Chest 89:417S, 1986.

Hull RD, Raskob GE, Rosenbloom D, et al: Heparin for 5 days as compared with 10 days in the initial treatment of proximal venous thrombosis, N Engl J Med 322:1260, 1990.

Hunt TK, ed: Wound healing and wound infection, New York, 1980, Appleton-Century-Crofts.

Hyers TM, Hull RD, and Web JG: Antithrombotic therapy for venous thromboembolic disease, Chest 89:26S, 1986.

Jorgensen BC, Schmidt JF, Risbo A, et al: Regular interval preventive pain relief compared with on demand treatment after hysterectomy, Pain 21:137, 1985.

Kakkar VV: Pathophysiologic characteristics of venous thrombosis, Am J Surg 150:1, 1985.

Krebs HB: Intestinal injury in gynecologic surgery: a ten-year experience, Am J Obstet Gynecol 155:509, 1986.

Kuhn S, Cooke K, Collins M, et al: Perceptions of pain relief after surgery, Br Med J 300:1687, 1990.

Lensing AWA, Prandoni P, Brandjes D, et al: Detection of deep-vein thrombosis by real-time B-mode ultrasonography, N Engl J Med 320:342, 1989.

Livingston EH and Passaro EP Jr: Postoperative ileus, Dig Dis Sci 35:121, 1990.

Lubin MF, Walker HK, and Smith RB, editors: Medical management of the surgical patient, ed 2, Stoneham, MA, 1988, Butterworth Publishers.

Malt RA: Abdominal incisions, sutures and sacrilege, N Engl J Med 297:722, 1977.

Mann WJ, Arato M, Patsner B, et al: Ureteral injuries in an obstetrics and gynecology training program: etiology and management, Obstet Gynecol 72:82, 1988.

Manyonda IT, Welch CR, McWhinney NA, et al: The influence of suture material on vaginal vault granulations following abdominal hysterectomy, Br J Obstet Gynaecol 97:608, 1990.

McBride K, LaMorte WW, and Menzoian JO: Can ventilation-perfusion scans accurately diagnose acute pulmonary embolism? Arch Surg 121:754, 1986.

McLintock TTC, Aitken H, Downie CFA, et al: Postoperative analgesic requirements in patients exposed to positive intraoperative suggestions, Br Med J 301:788, 1990.

McNeil PM and Sugerman HJ: Continuous absorbable vs. interrupted nonabsorbable fascial closure, Arch Surg 121:821, 1986.

Morrison JC, Harris J, Sherrill J, et al: Comparative study of flurbiprofen and morphine for postsurgical gynecologic pain, Am J Med 80:55, 1986.

Moss GS and Gould SA: Plasma expanders: an update, Am J Surg 155:425, 1988.

Multicenter Trial Committee: Dihydroergotamine-heparin prophylaxis of postoperative deep vein thrombosis, JAMA 251:2960, 1984.

Nichols DH, editor: Clinical problems, injuries, and complications of gynecologic surgery, Baltimore, 1983, Williams & Wilkins.

Notelovitz M, Kitchens C, Ware M, et al: Combination estrogen and progestogen replacement therapy does not adversely affect coagulation, Obstet Gynecol 62:596, 1983.

O'Conor VJ: Review of experience with vesicovaginal fistula repair, J Urol 123:367, 1980.

Orr JW, Orr PF, Barrett JM, et al: Continuous or interrupted fascial closure: a prospective evaluation of no. 1 Maxon suture in 402 gynecologic procedures, Am J Obstet Gynecol 163:1485, 1990.

Parker MM and Parrillo JE: Septic shock, JAMA 250:3324, 1983.

Pasulka PS, Bistrian BR, Benotti PN, et al: The risks of surgery in obese patients, Ann Intern Med 104:540, 1986.

Peterson CE and Kwaan HC: Current concepts of warfarin therapy, Arch Intern Med 146:581, 1986.

PIOPED investigators: Value of the ventilation/perfusion scan in acute pulmonary embolism: results of the Prospective Investigation of Pulmonary Embolism Diagnosis, JAMA 263:2753, 1990.

Pitkin RM: Abdominal hysterectomy in obese women, Surg Gynecol Obstet 142:532, 1976.

Piver MS, Malfetano JH, Lele SB, et al: Prophylactic anticoagulation as a possible cause of inguinal lymphocyst after radical vulvectomy and inguinal lymphadenectomy, Obstet Gynecol 62:17, 1983.

Polak JF, Culter SS, and O'Leary DH: Deep veins of the calf: assessment with doppler flow imaging, Radiology 171:481, 1989.

Poole GV: Mechanical factors in abdominal wound closure: the prevention of fascial dehiscence, Surgery 97:631, 1985.

Ratcliff JB, Kapernick P, Brooks GG, et al: Small bowel obstruction and previous gynecologic surgery, South Med J 76:1349, 1983.

Rayburn WF, Geranis BJ, Ramadei CA, et al: Patient-controlled analgesia for postcesarean section pain, Obstet Gynecol 72:136, 1988.

Rimailho A, Riou B, Richard C, et al: Fulminant necrotizing fasciitis and nonsteroidal anti-inflammatory drugs, J Infect Dis 155:143, 1987.

Roberts JA, Fussell EN, and Kaack MB: Bacterial adherence to urethral catheters, J Urol 144:264, 1990.

Rosenblum J, Schwarz GA, and Bendler E: Femoral neuropathy—a neurological complication of hysterectomy, JAMA 195:115, 1966.

Rosenthal DM and Colapinto R: Angiographic arterial embolization in the management of postoperative vaginal hemorrhage, Am J Obstet Gynecol 151:227, 1985.

Rosenthal DM, Harkins JL, Garzo G, et al: Management of postoperative vaginal hemorrhage, Obstet Gynecol 61:42S, 1983.

Ryan M and Dennerstein L: Hysterectomy and tubal ligation, Adv Psychosom Med 15:180, 1986.

Sabiston DC Jr, editor: Textbook of surgery, Philadelphia, 1986, WB Saunders Co.

Samra SK, Friedman BA, and Beitler PJ: A study of blood utilization in association with hysterectomy, Transfusion 23:490, 1983.

Serradimigni A, Philip F, Elias A, et al: Pulmonary embolism: what happens to the source of the embolus? Haemostatis 16(S3):65, 1986.

Shapiro M, Munoz A, Tager IB, et al: Risk factors for infection at the operative site after abdominal or vaginal hysterectomy, N Engl J Med 307:1661, 1982.

Silva PD and Beguin EA Jr: Intraoperative rapid autologous blood transfusion, Am J Obstet Gynecol 160:1226, 1989.

Sinclair RH and Pratt JH: Femoral neuropathy after pelvic operation, Am J Obstet Gynecol 112:404, 1972.

Sprung CL, Caralis PV, Marcial EH, et al: The effects of high-dose corticosteroids in patients with septic shock, N Engl J Med 311:1137, 1984.

Stamenkovic I and Lew PD: Early recognition of potentially fatal necrotizing fasciitis, N Engl J Med 310:1689, 1984.

Stamm WE: Prevention of urinary tract infections, Am J Med 74:148, 1984.

Stark RP and Maki DG: Bacteriuria in the catheterized patient, N Engl J Med 311:560, 1984.

Stevens CD, Aach RD, Hollinger FB, et al: Hepatitis B virus antibody in blood donors and the occurrence of non-A, non-B hepatitis in transfusion recipients, Ann Intern Med 101:733, 1984.

Symmonds RE: Ureteral injuries associated with gynecologic surgery: prevention and management, Clin Obstet Gynecol 19:623, 1976.

Symmonds RE: Prevention and management of genitourinary fistula, JCE Obstet Gynecol 21:13, 1979.

Tancer ML: The post-total hysterectomy (vault) vesicovaginal fistula, J Urol 123:839, 1980.

Tewes PA, Taylor DR, and Bourke DL: Postoperative pain management. In Breslow MJ, Miller CF, and Rogers MC, editors: Perioperative management, St Louis, 1990, Mosby–Year Book.

Thomas JH: Pathogenesis, diagnosis, and treatment of thrombosis, Am J Surg 160:547, 1990.

Thompson JD: Fallopian tube prolapse after abdominal hysterectomy, Aust NZ J Obstet Gynaecol 20:187, 1980.

Tobin MJ: Respiratory monitoring, JAMA 264:244, 1990.

Turner GM, Cole SE, and Brooks JH: The efficacy of graduated compression stockings in the prevention of deep vein thrombosis after major gynaecological surgery, Br J Obstet Gynaecol 91:588, 1984.

van Ooijen B: Subcutaneous heparin and postoperative wound hematomas, Arch Surg 121:937, 1986.

Wallace D, Hernandez W, Schlaerth JB, et al: Prevention of abdominal wound disruption utilizing the Smead-Jones closure technique, Obstet Gynecol 56:226, 1980.

Walsh JJ, Bomar J, and Wright FW: A study of pulmonary embolism and deep leg vein thrombosis after major gynaecological surgery using labelled fibrinogen-phlebography and lung scanning, J Obstet Gynaecol Br Comm 81:311, 1974.

Walters MD, Dombroski RA, Davidson SA, et al: Reclosure of disrupted abdominal incisions, Obstet Gynecol 76:597, 1990.

Watkins DT and Robertson CL: Water-soluble radiocontrast material in the treatment of postoperative ileus, Am J Obstet 152:450, 1985.

Weaver M, Burdon DW, Youngs DJ, et al: Oral neomycin and erythromycin compared with single-dose systemic metronidazole and ceftriaxone prophylaxis in elective colorectal surgery, Am J Surg 151:437, 1986.

Wetchler SJ and Dunn LJ: Ovarian abscess, Obstet Gynecol Surv 40:476, 1985.

White PF: Patient controlled analgesia: infuser for management of postoperative pain, Semin Anesthesiol 4:255, 1985.

White PF: Pain management (special report), Postgrad Med 80:7, 1986.

White PF: Use of patient-controlled analgesia for management of acute pain, JAMA 259:243, 1988.

White RH, McGahan JP, Daschbach MM, et al: Diagnosis of deep-vein thrombosis using duplex ultrasound, Ann Intern Med 111:297, 1989.

Willson JR and Black JR: Ovarian abscess, Am J Obstet Gynecol 90:34, 1964.

Witters S, Cornelissen M, and Vereecken R: Iatrogenic ureteral injury: aggressive or conservative treatment, Am J Obstet Gynecol 155:582, 1986.

Wolfson PH, Bauer JJ, Gelernt IM, et al: Use of the long tube in the management of patients with small-intestine obstruction due to adhesions, Arch Surg 120:1001, 1985.

Wrenn K: Fecal impaction, N Engl J Med 321:658, 1989.

GYNECOLOGIC ONCOLOGY

Principles of Radiation Therapy and Chemotherapy in Gynecologic Cancer

KEY TERMS AND DEFINITIONS

Adoptive Immunotherapy. The use of extracts derived from sensitized lymphocytes to transfer "immunologic memory" and induce an antitumor response.

Alkylating Agent. A class of antineoplastic agents that covalently link (alkylation) with DNA, which inhibits the growth of dividing cells.

Alpha Particle. A type of particulate radiation that is the same as a helium nucleus.

Antimetabolites. Antineoplastic agents that resemble naturally occurring purines or pyrimidines and interfere with normal cell metabolism.

Antitumor Antibiotic. Antineoplastic agents derived from bacterial or fungal cultures.

B Lymphocyte. A lymphocyte that synthesizes antibodies and is responsible for humoral immunity.

Beta Rays. Low-energy electron radiation produced by radionuclide decay.

Betatron. A circular accelerator for electrons for production of high energy.

Brachytherapy. A form of radiation therapy in which the source is placed close to the tumor. The application may be in the form of needles implanted into the tumor (interstitial) or placed in the vagina or cervical canal (internal).

Cellular Immunity. Cell-mediated immunity in which lymphoid cells directly react with foreign cells or antigens.

Complete Remission. Total disappearance of the tumor for at least 1 month.

Curie (Ci). A measure of the rate of disintegration of radioisotopes. One curie is equivalent to 3.7×10^{10} disintegrations per second.

Cytokine. Soluble mediators produced by cells of the lymphoreticular system that mediate the immune response (also known as lymphokines). Examples include interleukins, interferons, tumor necrosis factor, and colony-stimulating growth factors.

Depth Dose. The specific dose of irradiation absorbed at a given distance beneath the surface.

Electron Volt (eV). A unit of measurement of electromagnetic energy equivalent to 1.6×10^{-12} ergs. MeV = 1 million eV; keV = 1000 eV.

Erythropoietin (epo). A stimulator of bone marrow red cell production.

Fractionation. The practice of dividing radiation therapy treatments into numerous small doses to reduce damage to normal tissues.

Gamma Rays. A form of photon energy produced by the decay of radioactive isotopes.

Granulocyte-Macrophage Colony-Stimulating Factor (GM-CSF). A cytokine capable of stimulating granulocyte and monocyte production.

Gray. A measurement of the dosage of radiation absorbed by tissue. 1 gray = 1 joule per kilogram (100 rads).

Growth Fraction. The proportion of tumor cells in a replicating phase.

Humoral Immunity. Antibody-mediated immunity resulting from antibodies produced in response to a variety of foreign antigens.

Interferon (IFN). A cytokine produced by lymphocytes or fibroblasts in response to viral infection. There are three types: alpha, beta, and gamma, and they may have an antiproliferative effect on tumor cells.

Interleukin (IL). A class of cytokines secreted by monocytes, lymphocytes, and macrophages. They are numerically designated, with six types having been described.

Isodose Curve. A curve connecting points that receive equivalent doses of irradiation.

Linear Accelerator. A machine that accelerates electrons in a straight line to produce high energy.

Linear Energy Transfer (LET). The measurement of the amount of energy transferred by ionizing radiation per unit of distance traveled.

Log Cell Kill. The proportion of cells killed by a particular treatment: 90% equals a 1-log cell kill; 99% equals a 2-log cell kill.

Lymphokine. See cytokine.

Natural Killer (NK) Cells. A type of mononuclear cell that mediates the killing of tumor cells by the immune system.

Neutron. A subatomic particle with mass but no charge, making it a highly penetrating form of radiation.

Partial Objective Response. A more than 50% reduction in the greatest perpendicular dimension of the tumor for at least 1 month.

Passive Immunity. The transfer of specific antibodies to try to increase the immune response.

Photons. Quanta of radiation whose energy is proportional to their frequency and inversely proportional to their wavelength (gamma rays and x-rays).

Progression. Increase in size or spread of tumor in a patient receiving therapy.

Rad. A measurement of the dose of radiation absorbed in tissue equivalent to 100 ergs per gram or 1 centiGray (cGy).

Radiocurability. The ability to cure a malignant tumor with radiation.

Radiosensitivity. The relative response of tumor cells to radiation.

Source-to-Skin Distance (SSD). The distance from the external radiation source to the skin of the patient receiving external therapy.

Stabilization. A term occasionally used to indicate that a tumor has not changed in size while a patient has been receiving therapy.

Systemic-Active Nonspecific Immunotherapy. Use of adjuvant agents, usually of microbiologic origin, to increase cellular and humoral immunity. Examples are bacillus Calmette-Guerin (BCG) and *Corynebacterium parvum* (C-Parvum).

Teletherapy. A form of radiation therapy with the placement of the radioactive source at a distance from the patient (external therapy).

T Lymphocyte. Lymphocytes that exhibit cell surface antigenicity and mediate cellular immunity.

Tumor Necrosis Factor (TNF). A cytokine that mediates endotoxic shock and is capable of inhibiting tumor cell growth.

Vinca Alkaloids. Antineoplastic agents derived from periwinkle plant *(Vinca rosea)* extracts.

X-ray. Electromagnetic radiation formed by accelerated electrons in a vacuum striking a target.

This chapter presents the general principles of radiation therapy and chemotherapy, with particular attention to those concepts, procedures, and drugs used to treat gynecologic cancers. The details of treatment of individual cancers are described separately in the various chapters dealing with specific gynecologic malignancies.

Included with the basic concepts of radiation physics are the types and measurements of radiation energy, the biologic effects of radiation on cells, and the factors that alter these effects. Common radiation sources and their properties are illustrated as they relate specifically to the treatment of gynecologic cancers. Risks and complications are also presented.

Cell growth and division are affected by cancerous processes and by chemotherapeutic treatments. The physician must know the various classes of chemotherapeutic agents, their actions in gynecologic malignancies, and their toxicities. There are also general approaches to be followed in administering chemotherapy, specifically including the monitoring of patients receiving these agents. Finally, some newer techniques involving immunology offer promise in treating gynecologic cancers.

RADIATION THERAPY

Basic Radiation Physics

Radiation physics deals with the measurement of energy that is transferred from the source of the radiation to the tissues or cells being irradiated. One form of ionizing radiation is electromagnetic, which refers to x-rays or gamma rays. These sources of energy have no mass and no electrical charge. They are produced in discrete quanta or photons, and their energy is proportional to their frequency; that is, higher energies are transmitted at a higher frequency of electromagnetic radiation. Since the frequency of a photon is inversely proportional to the wavelength, electromagnetic radiation with shorter wavelengths has a higher frequency and thus a higher energy. The energy that is produced is measured in electron volts (eV); $1 \text{ eV} = 1.6 \times 10^{-12}$ ergs. Various x-ray radiotherapy units can range from 50,000 eV (50 kV) to over 30 million eV (30 meV).

A second source of photon radiation comes from the production of gamma rays (similar to x-rays), which result from the decay of radioactive isotopes. Such decay or disintegration is measured in curies (Ci). One curie is defined as 3.7×10^{10} disintegrations per second, which is equivalent to the disintegration of 1 g of radium.

Regardless of the source of electromagnetic or photon radiation, the transmitted energy from the source diverges as the distance it travels from the source increases. This divergence causes a decrease in energy, and the relationship is described by the inverse square law, which indicates that the energy dose of radiation per unit area decreases proportionately to the square of the distance from the site to the source $(1/d^2)$. For example, the dose of radiation 2 cm from a point source is only one fourth of the value of the dose at 1 cm (Figure 25-1).

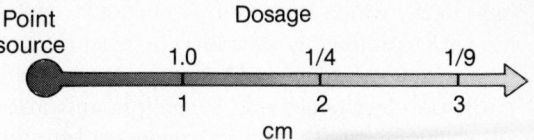

FIGURE 25-1
Radiation effects at various distances from point source of irradiation demonstrating the inverse square law.

In general, x-rays or photons can be generated as a result of rapidly accelerated electrons in a vacuum striking a target. Modern generators that accelerate these electrons at high speed may do so in a circular fashion (betatron) or linearly (linear accelerator). Another type of radiation energy is known as particulate radiation and is produced by subatomic particles with a discrete mass. These particles are usually released by the disintegration of radionuclides. Four common types are alpha particles (the same as a helium nucleus), neutrons, protons, and electrons. Alpha particles produce a large number of ions over a short distance. They currently have little practical use in radiation therapy because of their short range in tissue but are being investigated for intraperitoneal radiation application. Neutrons are highly penetrating and have no charge but have a large mass, and for the purposes of cancer treatment they are usually produced by machines. They cause high-energy collisions with atomic nuclei, principally of hydrogen, in the tissues. The resultant recoil proton loses energy to the surrounding tissue by ionization, which leads to cell death. Protons are positively charged particles, and generators are available for the direct production of protons to yield very high energy beams, which have specialized uses such as in the treatment of pituitary tumors.

Electrons may also be referred to as beta rays, produced by radionuclide disintegration. Electrons can be produced at different energies by machines for various therapeutic applications.

Radiation Biology

Photons (gamma rays or x-rays) act by dislodging orbital electrons from the atoms of the medium or tissue through which they pass. This collision produces a fast electron (Compton effect), which then ionizes molecules along its path, producing secondary electrons and free hydroxyl radicals. The process continues until the electromagnetic beam (photon) loses all of its energy. The cells are damaged by the free hydroxyl radicals and the negatively charged electrons that affect the DNA of the cell. This effect may be lethal and kill the cell, or it can be sublethal, in which case the cell will subsequently undergo repair of the DNA. In addition, free hydroxyl radicals may react with molecular oxygen to form peroxide in the tissues. This adds to the lethal effects of radiation on the cells. As shown by Gray et al., oxygen is important for the tissue effects of photon irradiation. This has practical implications in tumor therapy insofar as cancers tend to have poor blood supplies, which decreases the oxygenation, particularly at the center of large tumors. The effect of photon radiation in these hypoxic areas is therefore diminished.

The rate of loss of energy of an ionizing particle as it traverses a unit length of medium is known as linear energy transfer (LET). In the case of photon irradiation, the loss of energy per hit is small. This is described as low LET irradiation, which often causes a sublethal effect on a single cell and thus necessitates multiple hits to kill the cell, as well as to produce toxic hydroxyl radicals. In the case of particulate radiation with heavy particles, the ionization is known as high LET. Thus neutrons, with their large mass, produce high-energy recoil protons that kill the cell directly on impact, independent of oxygenation. For this reason research has been directed toward the development of neutron generators to try to improve tumor therapy by overcoming the limitation of poor oxygenation of cancer cells.

An important principle is that a given dose of radiation kills a constant fraction of the number of cells irradiated. For example, if 90% of the cells of a tumor are killed with each fraction of radiation delivered, then 10% of the cells would survive. Thus if one were to begin to irradiate a tumor with 10 million cells, there would be 1 million cells surviving after the first fraction, 100,000 cells after the second fraction, 10,000 cells after the third fraction, etc. By the seventh fraction all of the cells would be killed.

As shown in Figure 25-2 there are four phases of the cell cycle. Sinclair and Morton showed that during mitosis the cell is most sensitive to radiation. Thus rapidly dividing cells are the most radiosensitive. It has been dem-

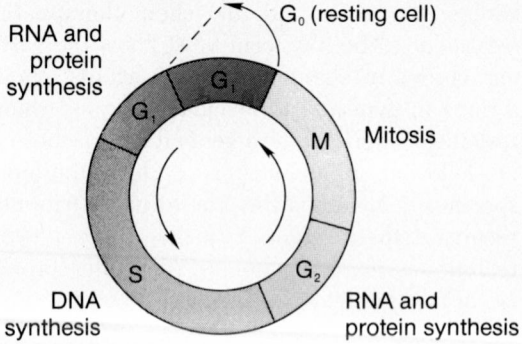

FIGURE 25-2
Phases of the cell. After mitosis (M) there is an interval of variable duration during which there is RNA and protein synthesis and a diploid DNA content $(G_1 \text{ [gap}_1])$. The cell may also enter a prolonged or resting phase (G_0) and then reenter the cycle during DNA synthesis, the (S) phase, in which DNA is duplicated. During $G_2 (\text{gap}_2)$ there again is protein and RNA synthesis. During the M phase the cell divides into two cells, each of which receives a diploid DNA content.

onstrated that dividing radiation treatment into a number of small doses (fractionation) allows for effective treatment of the tumor without increasing the complications of radiation to the normal tissues (bone marrow, intestine, and other rapidly dividing tissues) that would occur with single large doses. The more efficient repair of normal tissue occurring between treatment fractions affords a therapeutic advantage. The measurement of the amount of energy absorbed by tissue is the rad, which is defined as 100 ergs of energy absorbed per gram of tissue. Recently the term *gray* (1 joule per kilogram) has been introduced; 1 gray is equivalent to 100 rads.

Radiation Sources—External and Internal Therapy

In general two techniques are utilized in radiation treatment: brachytherapy (internal) and teletherapy (external). For brachytherapy the radiation source is placed within or adjacent to the target tissue. In the treatment of gynecologic malignant tumors, radioactive needles may be implanted directly into the tissue to be irradiated (interstitial implant), or a tandem containing radioactive sources may be placed within the cervix and uterus accompanied by two vaginal ovoids —one on each side of the

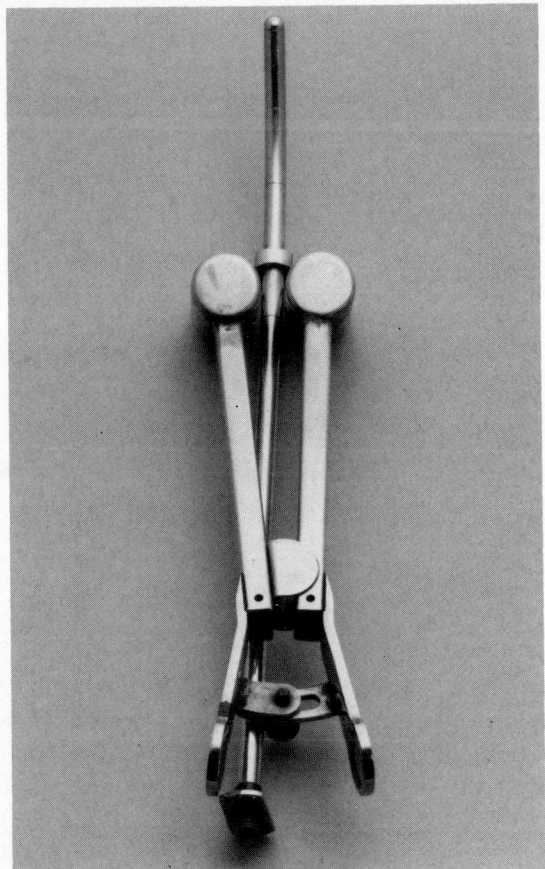

FIGURE 25-3
Fletcher-Suite applicator (tandem and ovoids) used for afterloading internal therapy.

TABLE 25-1
Half-Lives of Commonly Used Isotopes

Radionuclide	Half-Life
Gold 198	2.7 Days
Phosphorus 32	14.3 Days
Iodine 125	60 Days
Iridium 192	74.4 Days
Cobalt 60	5.3 Years
Cesium 137	30 Years
Radium 226	1620 Years

tandem— that also contain radioactive sources (intracavitary therapy). Such an arrangement would be useful for treatment of a cervical tumor or a tumor located near the cervix (Figure 25-3). In such an arrangement the dose delivered to the tissues is determined by the inverse square law. In practice the radioactive sources are placed in the devices after the apparatus has been properly placed within the endocervix and vagina. This "afterloading" technique reduces radiation exposure to the personnel treating the patient.

In brachytherapy various radioisotopes are used for treatment; which ones are chosen depends on the half-life of the radionuclide. In general those with a short half-life (such as gold 198) may be placed within the patient and left permanently, whereas those with a long half-life (cesium 137) are placed temporarily within the patient and then removed after a prescribed dose of irradiation has been administered. Table 25-1 indicates the half-lives of

some of the isotopes commonly used in treating gynecologic cancers. It is also important that a uniform distribution of radiation be achieved in the adjacent tissues to avoid "hot spots," which can lead to excess damage to normal tissue, as well as "cold spots," which can lead to undertreatment of the tumor.

Teletherapy refers to the placement of the radioactive source at a distance from the patient, in which case the machine delivers external radiation to the tumor. With external therapy the source of radiation is located at a distance 5 to 10 times greater than the depth of the tumor being irradiated in order to deliver a uniform dose to the tumor and thus avoid the large dose changes that result because of the inverse square law. This distance is referred to as the source-to-skin distance (SSD).

More recently, with the utilization of different angles and ports of treatment, the concept of source axis distance (SAD) has been introduced; it denotes the distance from the radiation source to the central axis of machine rotation. The patient is positioned so that this axis passes through the center of the tumor, and treatment ports are arranged around this axis to optimize tumor dose and minimize the dose to vital structures.

To focus the beam from the external source, a collimator is used. The collimator prevents scatter and allows for a directed beam of for a given field size (10 × 10 cm, for example) to be applied to the tissue being irradiated (Figure 25-4). In general the higher the energy source of the radiation, the deeper the beam penetrates the tissue. Thus high-energy (shortwavelength) radiation has its predominant effect in deeper tissues and spares the surface or the skin of radiation effect. The term *orthovoltage* refers to machines in the 125,000 to 400,000 eV (125 to 400 keV) range, whereas su-

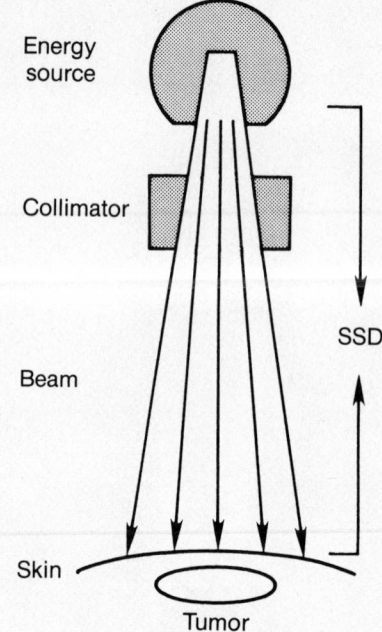

FIGURE 25-4
External therapy unit. Divergence of beam increases with distance from source. (Redrawn from Kase NG and Weingold AB: Principles and practice of clinical gynecology, New York, 1983, John Wiley & Sons.)

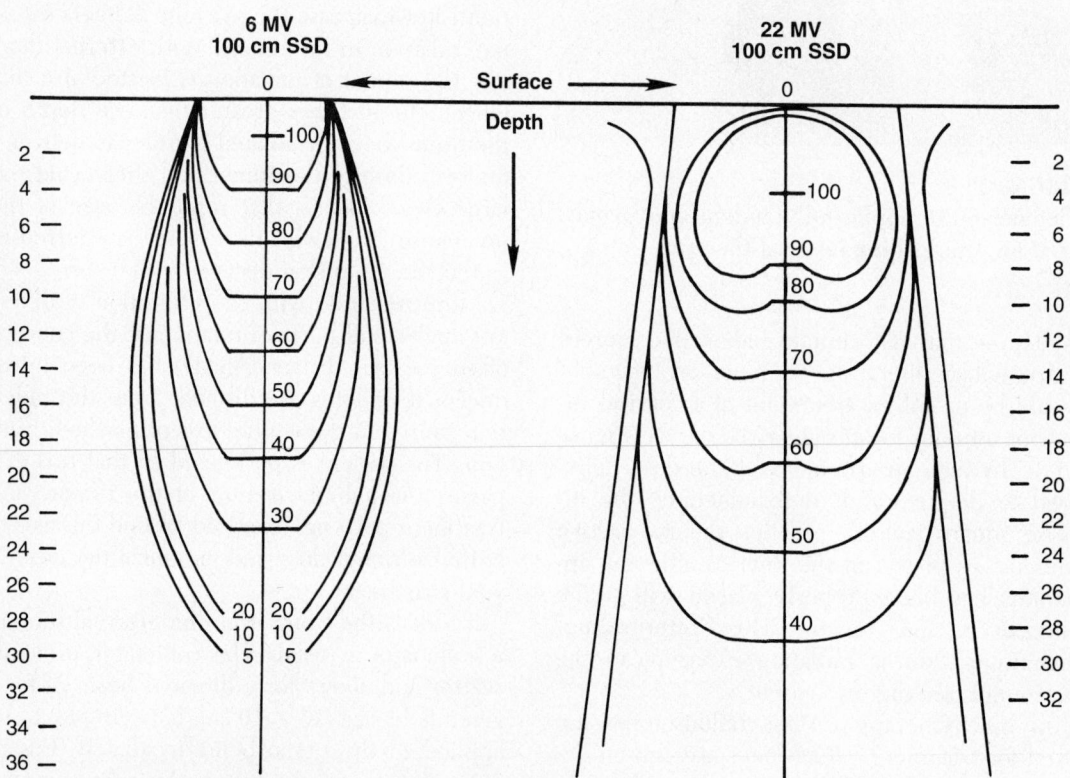

FIGURE 25-5
Comparison of isodose curves and depth-dose distribution for 6 MV and 22 MV betatrons. Note that the higher energy machine delivers radiation to greater depth for same surface dose, and there is considerable skin sparing. (Redrawn from DiSaia PJ and Creasman WT: Clinical gynecologic oncology, ed 2, St Louis, 1984, Mosby–Year Book, Inc.)

pervoltage or megavoltage refers to machines with 2 to 35 million eV (megavolt) range. Cobalt machines (equivalent to 1.25 meV) and 4 to 6 meV machines have similar properties and achieve their maximum dosage at about 0.5 cm beneath the skin; higher energy machines such as the 22 meV have their maximum effect at a depth of about 5 cm beneath the skin.

An isodose curve is a line that connects points in the tissue that receive equivalent dosages of irradiation. Figure 25-5 contrasts the isodose curves for 6 and 22 meV machines. For the 6 meV machine the maximum dose is near the surface, with a more rapid falloff in the deeper tissues, in comparison to the 22 meV machine, which has its maximum dose well beneath the surface. Thus at a given depth the higher dose of radiation can be achieved with 22 meV, sparing the effects of radiation on the skin. These high-energy machines are particularly useful for treating deep tumors and for obese patients. Achieving comparable large doses of irradiation in deep tissue with cobalt or 4 to 6 meV machines produces higher radiation levels on the surface, which can lead to increased skin reaction and eventually subcutaneous fibrosis.

In addition to the energy of the beam, that is determined by the machine producing the radiation, the energy of radiation absorbed at various depths is affected by the size of the field being treated. Larger fields contain more scattered radiation, which leads to a greater dose at a given depth. Figure 25-6 demonstrates the effect of increasing the size of the field with increasing dosage at a given depth for three different types of energy sources.

Thus the radiation dose delivered to the tumor is affected by the energy of the source, the depth of the tumor beneath the surface, and the size of the field undergoing irradiation. With external therapy, usually 160 to 200 rads per day is given five times per week. Recently there has been experimental work evaluating hyperfractionation, which involves smaller multiple doses given more frequently (for example, 120 rads t.i.d. or 160 rads b.i.d.).

As previously noted, the effect of electromagnetic radiation also depends on the oxygenation of the tissue. Recently a number of pharmacologic agents, such as hydroxyurea and metronidazole, have been investigated for their abilities to potentiate the sensitivity to radiation. These radiation sensitizers are not yet used routinely in the treatment of gynecologic malignancies, although certain chemotherapeu-

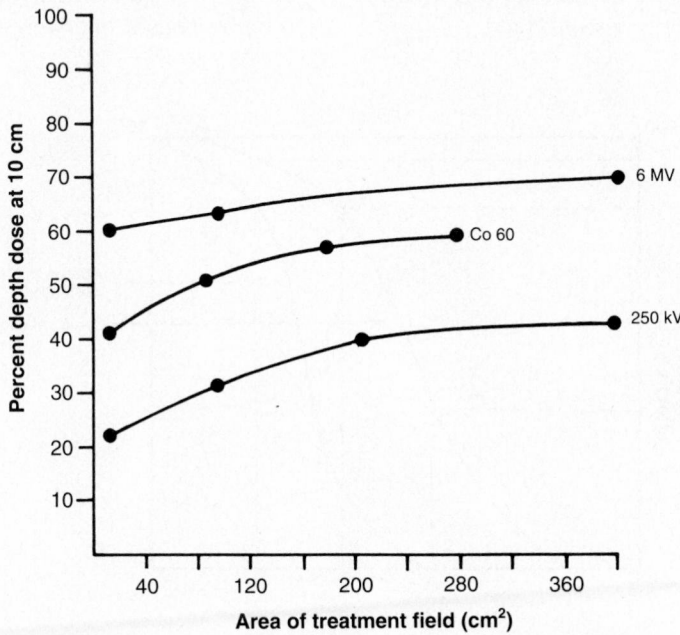

FIGURE 25-6
Variation of depth dose at 10 cm with energy and size of treatment field. (Redrawn from Joslin CAF: Basic parameters of radiotherapy. In Coppleson M, editors: Gynecologic oncology, Edinburgh, 1981, Churchill Livingstone.)

tic agents, particularly cisplatin and 5-fluorouracil, are being tested with radiation treatment to improve response rates (see Chapter 27). Hyperthermia is also being explored to potentiate the therapeutic effectiveness of radiation. It appears to offer the most promise for tumors localized in an area that can effectively and safely tolerate increased temperatures (42° to 43° C). In some studies higher temperatures have been used locally.

Tissue Tolerance and Radiation Complications

Radiation acutely affects tissues undergoing continuous cell replacement, such as the skin, the intestinal mucosa, and the mucosa of the vagina and bladder. These tissues are undergoing rapid division, and radiation given in the fractions noted previously reduces the untoward effects of cell damage on normal tissue and allows for normal healing to occur between treatment fractions. Side effects of radiation include depression of the quantity of circulating white cells, as well as gastrointestinal effects, such as nausea, anorexia, or diarrhea, which usually can be controlled with medication. The skin may be irritated with a "wet reaction," particularly if lower-energy external sources are used; occasionally a treatment program may have to be temporarily discontinued.

Although the acute effects of radiation limit the rate at which the dosage is administered, late effects may occur many years later and can cause permanent damage. Late adverse effects include tissue necrosis and fibrosis, as well as fistula formation, ulceration, and bleeding. These late-stage complications depend on the total dose of the radiation administered, the volume of tissue treated, and also somewhat on the size of the radiation fraction administered with each dose. It is thought that these late effects are due to radiation damage to the vascular tissue and connective tissue. An alternate explanation is that the radiation destroys the cells that are capable of regeneration, which eventually leads to tissue destruction. Second cancers induced after radiation are rare. Arai et al. noted an excess of rectal cancer, bladder cancer, and leukemia among patients with carcinoma of the cervix treated by radiation in comparison with those treated by operation.

It has been observed clinically that the response of the tumor to radiation treatment follows a sigmoid curve, with increasingly effective tumor control associated with increasing dosage (Figure 25-7). A similar dosage effect exists for normal tissues, and the ability of radiation therapy to control tumors depends on the greater tolerance of normal tissues to radiation exposure. Thus if one were to use the level of

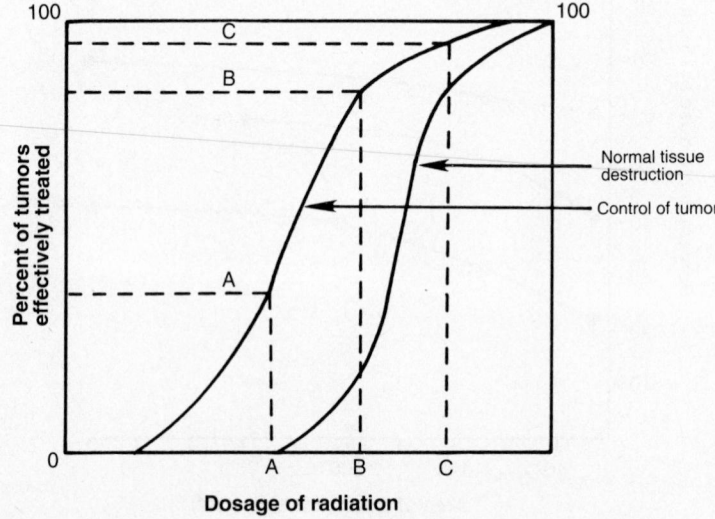

FIGURE 25-7
Concept of tumor control versus complications. At point *A* there are no complications but insufficient control. Point *C* has good control but excess complications. There is reasonable tumor control at *B* with a slight risk of complications.

radiation that causes no normal tissue damage, only a small proportion of tumors would be controlled. Conversely, if one were to use a dosage that could control almost all tumors, massive damage to normal tissue would occur and an unacceptable series of complications and even patient death could follow. The optimum goal is to achieve maximum tumor control with as little risk of damage to normal tissues as possible.

In the treatment of gynecologic malignancies the main sites of radiation damage are the bladder, rectum, and large and small bowel. As a rule, complications of the bladder can occur in the form of radiation cystitis, which can lead to complaints of dysuria and frequency. Hematuria may also occur, and therapy with sclerosing solutions or fulguration through a cystoscope may be necessary. In rare instances urinary diversion may be required. Fistulas between the vagina and bladder or between the vagina and rectum may develop when there has been extensive radiation damage to the intervening tissues. This usually takes place during therapy for large carcinomas of the cervix (see Chapter 27). As a general rule such complications will occur 6 months to 2 years after treatment, although they may occur many years after primary therapy. In addition, the bone marrow of the sacrum and lower vertebrae is compromised by pelvic irradiation, an important consideration if the patient is to receive subsequent chemotherapy.

Damage to the large bowel usually occurs in the form of inflammation (sigmoiditis), which may be associated with severe bleeding and pain. Less severe cases can often be controlled with a low-roughage diet and antispasmodic medication, while more severe cases may require bowel resection or permanent bowel diversion through a colostomy.

Recently Montana and Fowler showed that the risks of proctitis and cystitis are dose related. For example, severe proctitis and cystitis were noted at dosages of 6750 cGy and 6900 cGy respectively, while such complications were not observed in patients whose median dose was 6500 and 6300 cGy. The small bowel also receives irradiation during external therapy for pelvic tumors. In the acute phases of treatment this often leads to bowel irritability, and the patient complains of diarrhea. Long-term complications include fibrosis of the wall of the intestine, which can lead to permanent

TABLE 25-2
Approximate Tolerance of Tissues to Radiation Therapy

Tissue	Approximate Tolerance Dose (rads)
Bladder	6000-7000
Rectum	6000-7000
Vaginal mucosa	7000
Bowel	6000
Cervix	>12,000
Kidney	2000-2300
Liver	2500-3500

narrowing and even obstruction. Occasionally enteric fistulas also develop and bowel perforation may occur. In the latter cases surgical therapy is required, usually to bypass the affected area of the intestine. As a general rule, extensive dissection of irradiated tissue is avoided. Smallbowel injuries are more frequent in patients who have had a previous operation, particularly pelvic surgery.

Spontaneous mobility of the bowel resulting from peristalsis may be decreased by adhesion formation. With reduction of bowel mobility, injury risks from radiation increase, since the loops of small bowel become fixed and are unable to have normal peristalsis, resulting in a higher radiation dose to the affected bowel segment. Table 25-2 presents the *approximate* tolerance of tissues to radiation therapy.

Generalizations regarding tissue tolerance in relation to total dosage must be regarded as only approximations. Multiple factors, as already discussed, influence late effects of radiation on normal tissue, such as dose fractionation, field size, port arrangement, extent of tumor damage to normal tissues, previous operations, concurrent chemotherapy, and other less well-defined elements, including anemia, small vessel pathology, and the patient's nutritional status.

CHEMOTHERAPY

The use of drugs to treat disseminated cancer has developed into an extensive clinical discipline, particularly since the 1950s. Numerous compounds have been tested to treat human tumors, and the first successful effort in gynecologic cancer was the demonstration by Li et al. that the antimetabolite, methotrexate, could cause permanent remission in cases of metastatic trophoblastic disease (Chapter 33). A number of general principles have been developed that provide guidelines for the use of chemotherapeutic agents to treat malignant disease. Many of these principles were developed by Skipper, Bruce, and others and involve an understanding of the cell replication cycle, as well as knowledge of factors that appear to affect the growth and development of tumors.

Cell Kinetics

The cell replication cycle is demonstrated in Figure 25-2. After completion of mitosis, the cell usually enters the gap$_1$ (G$_1$) phase, during which there is a diploid content of DNA and RNA and protein synthesis occurs. This phase is usually of variable length. The G$_1$ phase then leads into a phase of DNA synthesis (S), during which the DNA is duplicated. Then a second mitotic gap develops (G$_2$), during which DNA synthesis ceases and RNA and protein synthesis can again occur. During G$_2$ there is twice the DNA content of a normal cell. G$_2$ then leads into the mitosis (M) phase, during which the cell divides into two daughter cells, each of which contains a normal amount of DNA. Occasionally the cell enters a prolonged resting phase, termed the G$_0$ phase. During this phase the cell is not part of the active replication cycle and the cells are not generally sensitive at this time to chemotherapy or irradiation.

As has been noted previously, irradiation acts principally on the cell by attacking DNA and affecting the mitotic phase. Many chemotherapeutic drugs, such as alkylating agents, have actions similar to those of radiation, but others affect different parts of the cell cycle. In many cases the specific site of action of a cytotoxic agent is unknown. However, in all cases these agents affect not only the tumor cells but also the normal tissues of the body, particularly those undergoing rapid cell replication, such as those of the hematopoietic system, mucosa of the gastrointestinal tract, the vagina, the bladder, germ cells, and skin. All these tissues have particular relevance in patients with gynecologic malignancies, since they have frequently been exposed to radiation, and the resultant toxicity increases their vulnerability to the subsequent effects of chemotherapy.

As is the case in radiation, the proliferating cells are the most susceptible to chemotherapeutic agents. While normal tissues at steady state have cell growth occurring at a rate comparable to cell loss, malignant tumors have a rate of cell growth that greatly exceeds cell loss. The proportion of cells actively involved in proliferation of the tumor is known as the growth fraction (GF). The nondividing tumor cells may have reached a mature stage, may lack essential nutrition, may be anoxic, or may be inhibited by the host or other unknown influences. Different tumors require varying intervals for them to double in size (doubling time). In general, smaller tumors grow more rapidly than larger tumors, and it appears that metastases often grow more rapidly than the primary tumor, in part because they are smaller and in part because of the likelihood that more rapidly dividing cells will be the ones that tend to metastasize. This effect appears to be operative following the administration of cytotoxic agents. These reduce the mass of the tumor, but cell replication then appears to proceed at a faster rate. This has led to the assumption that chemotherapy not only reduces the number of cells but also leads to a smaller tumor mass, which then allows the remaining cells to replicate faster. It is generally estimated that 1 g of tumor tissue is equal to 10^9 cells.

Principles of Therapy

Some of the concepts used in antibiotic therapy of infections have been initially applied to cancer treatment. However, major differences exist. Infections are frequently caused by a single agent or even multiple types of bacteria with specific growth patterns and sensitivities to antibiotics. Although it is believed that a cancer can originate in a single (stem) cell, clinically evident disease is composed of a heterogeneous population of cells with different cell cycle durations and varying growth fractions. Larger tumors are more likely to contain cells resistant to a single cytotoxic agent.

An additional problem with larger tumors is their lower growth fraction, which is associated with a larger proportion of cells in the resting or G$_0$ phase of the cell cycle. These cells are resistant to cytotoxic drugs and may become a source of future growth when they leave the G$_0$ phase to enter the cell replication cycle. Thus smaller tumors, those with a higher growth fraction, and those with a short doubling time are the most sensitive to cytotoxic agents.

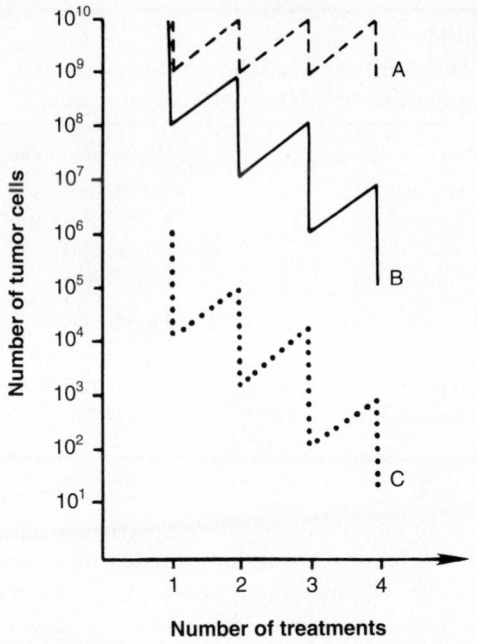

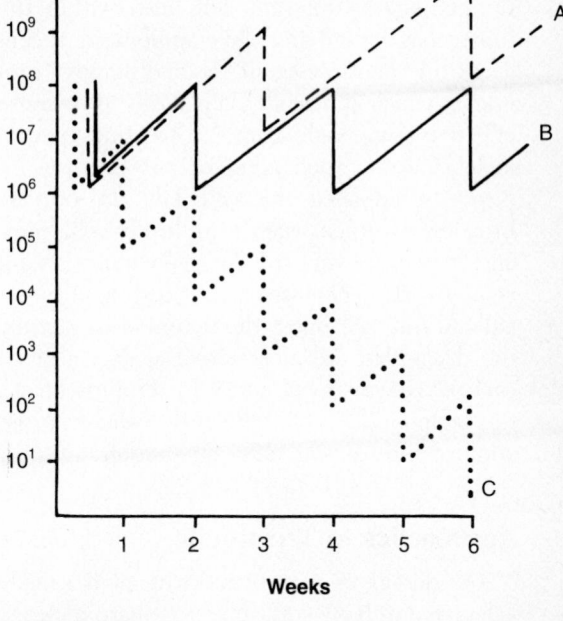

FIGURE 25-8

If treatment is initiated with lower tumor burden, fewer treatment courses are needed. *A*, One log cell kill (90% of cells) with smaller dose of drug. *B*, Two log cell kill (99% of cells) with larger dose of drug, leading to tumor regression. *C*, Two log cell kill (99% of cells) with larger dose of drug applied to smaller tumor burden, leading to more rapid tumor disappearance.

FIGURE 25-9

Importance of treatment frequency is illustrated in this example in which same drug is given at different intervals. *A*, Two log cell kill with recovery with therapy every 3 weeks (tumor progression). *B*, Two log cell kill with recovery with therapy every 2 weeks (no net change in tumor size). *C*, Two log cell kill with recovery with therapy weekly (tumor regression).

Cytotoxic agents kill cancer cells according to first-order kinetics; that is, a given dose kills a constant fraction of malignant cells, similar in concept to that noted previously for radiation therapy. One of the reasons chemotherapy appears selectively to affect cancer tissue more than normal tissue is that malignant tumor cells have a higher growth fraction in comparison to normal cells and are thus more susceptible to the effects of the chemotherapeutic agent. The net effect of the agent depends on the proportion of the cells killed, as well as on the rapidity with which the surviving cells duplicate. The ability of a chemotherapeutic agent to destroy a greater proportion of cancer cells more effectively is enhanced if the agent can be given more frequently. The antitumor effect is also enhanced if a larger dose can be given, which will increase the proportion of the cells killed. However, the dose and frequency are both limited by the tolerance of normal tissues.

Figures 25-8 and 25-9 demonstrate these principles. Starting with a smaller tumor burden (Figure 25-8), and therefore fewer tumor cells, leads to a more rapid elimination of the entire tumor within fewer treatment cycles. This effect of shorter duration of treatment also provides for less time for the development of resistant cell strains. In addition, the selection of an agent that yields a greater cell kill leads to an increased net reduction in tumor mass between treatment cycles, which results in more effective control despite the tumor regeneration that occurs between cycles of chemotherapy. Figure 25-9 demonstrates the effects of frequency of therapy, illustrating that prolonging the interval between the cycles of treatment increases the risk of loss of tumor control and disease progression.

Since the risk of having multiple resistant cell lines increases as the tumor becomes larger, it is important to choose initially a therapeutic program that has the best chance of inducing tumor regression. The potential to treat simultaneously different cell lines within the tumor has led to the development in recent years of multiple-agent chemotherapy programs, which appear in many cases to be more effective than single agents in treating gynecologic cancers. Such combination therapy appears to enhance the cell kill, to provide broader coverage against multiple cell lines, and to help prevent the emergence of resistant cells. In vitro chemosensitivity testing of tumor cells in soft agar offers the potential to identify the drugs that are most active against a given cancer. However, as noted by Phillips et al., the technique is not sufficiently reliable to be applicable to routine clinical situations.

Approaches to Treatment

The dosage of an anticancer agent is usually calculated in body surface area (square meters), which provides a better measure of potential toxicity than body weight, in part because surface area more closely reflects cardiac output and blood flow. Chemotherapeutic agents have varying toxicities, which will be considered in the next section. A major problem with most agents is bone marrow toxicity, along with the resultant necessity to monitor carefully the hemopoietic system. Most gynecologic chemotherapy protocols are administered in cycles that frequently vary from 3- to 4-week intervals. If the blood elements (white cells and platelets) have not recovered adequately by the time the next cycle of chemotherapy is due to be administered, the dosage of the agent or agents must be reduced or the time interval between treatments extended. Table 25-3 shows a schedule of approximate dosage reductions for myelosuppressive agents.

An additional consideration in toxicity of chemotherapeutic agents relates to hepatic metabolism and/or renal excretion. It may be necessary to modify the dosage of the drug administered when either renal or hepatic function is compromised. For example, doxorubicin (Adriamycin) and vincristine are metabolized in the liver, and dosage reductions must be made if the drug is administered to a patient with hepatic dysfunction; methotrexate and cisplatin effects are increased in patients with renal damage, necessitating dosage reduction in such patients; cisplatin not only has its effects intensified in patients with renal damage but also is

TABLE 25-3
A Schedule of Approximate Dosage Reductions for Myelosuppressive Agents

Dose	White blood count
Total dose	$>4000/mm^3$
½ dose	$\geq 3000\text{-}4000 \ mm^3$
¼ dose	$\geq 1500\text{-}3000 \ mm^3$
Withhold dose	$<1000/mm^3$

Dose	Platelet count
Total dose	$>100,000/mm^3$
½ dose	$50,000\text{-}100,000/mm^3$
Withhold dose	$<50,000/mm^3$

toxic to the kidney, requiring particular caution if it is administered to individuals with compromised renal function or patients receiving therapy with aminoglycosides, which are also toxic to the kidney. Methotrexate and cisplatin are also bound to albumin, and this binding is decreased in patients taking sulfonamides or salicylates, both of which increase the toxicity and effects of the chemotherapy.

Various chemotherapeutic agents can be differentially toxic to other organ systems of the body, including the intestine, nervous system, and lungs. The therapist must be aware of the individual adverse affects when administering these agents. The goal of treatment is to provide as high a dosage of the chemotherapeutic agent as possible to produce maximum therapeutic effectiveness without causing unacceptable toxicity and side effects.

In assessment of the effect of chemotherapeutic agents, a number of definitions are used to describe the response of the tumor being treated. A *complete remission* or *response* is total disappearance of the tumor for at least 1 month. A partial *objective response* is the reduction in the size of the tumor greater than 50% in its greatest perpendicular diameter for at least 1 month. *Progression* indicates an increase in tumor size or the appearance of new lesions. Occasionally the term *stabilization* is used to indicate that the disease has not changed in size and no new lesions have appeared. However, clinically the possibility of confusion exists, insofar as stabilization of the disease may be assumed to be due to chemotherapy when the lack of observed increase in size may be related in part to a prolonged doubling time of the tumor.

TABLE 25-4
Karnofsky Performance Status

100 =	Normal, no complaints; no evidence of disease
90 =	Able to carry on normal activity; minor signs or symptoms of disease
80 =	Normal activity with effort; some signs or symptoms of disease
70 =	Cares for self but unable to carry on normal activity or do active work
60 =	Requires occasional assistance but is able to care for most personal needs
50 =	Requires considerable assistance and frequent medical care
40 =	Disabled; requires special care and assistance
30 =	Severely disabled; hospitalization indicated, although death not imminent
20 =	Very sick; hospitalization necessary; active support treatment necessary
10 =	Moribund; fatal process progressing rapidly
0 =	Death

Evaluation of New Agents

In the development of new drugs, serial evaluations are necessary to assess the effectiveness of the drug as well as to ascertain its toxicity. A number of trials are necessary to move a new agent from the point of evaluation to allow it to be used in regular medical practice. Such "phase trials" are defined as follows:

Phase I trial An initial trial to test new drugs at various doses to evaluate toxicity and determine tolerance to the drug. At the various doses tested some therapeutic effects may be observed.

Phase II trials Tests to determine the therapeutic effectiveness and extent of the toxicity of the drug at doses expected to be effective against a specific tumor type.

Phase III trials Trials to compare the drug therapy to treatment currently in use to ascertain if the new therapy is superior.

A standard method frequently used to measure the patient's status in chemotherapy trials is the Karnofsky Performance Status (Table 25-4). In general, patients are not accepted to trials of new agents if their Karnofsky status is 50 or less.

Chemotherapeutic Agents Commonly Used in Gynecologic Cancer

A large number of drugs have been used in the therapy of cancer. In general the agents used in gynecologic oncology can be classified into six groups: alkylating agents, antitumor antibiotics, antimetabolites, vinca (plant) alkaloids, synthetic and miscellaneous compounds, and hormones.

Alkylating Agents

The primary action of these chemicals appears to be via direct interaction with DNA. The process of alkylation leads to the development of positively charged alkyl groups, which react with the negatively charged portion of DNA, leading to interference with DNA function. Cross-linking of DNA also occurs. The alkylating agents affect rapidly dividing cells and are particularly toxic to the bone marrow, leading to severe myelosuppression. They may be administered intravenously or orally and have been used extensively in gynecologic malignancies, particularly in ovarian cancers. The most commonly used agents are cyclophosphamide (Cytoxan), chlorambucil (Leukeran), and phenylalanine mustard (melphalan or Alkeran). In general the effectiveness of these agents appears similar, but there are some variations in toxicity. Phenylalanine mustard not only is acutely toxic to the bone marrow, but also appears to have a cumulative effect on the marrow that may compromise marrow function after its use has been discontinued.

Cyclophosphamide is associated with hemorrhagic cystitis. A urinary metabolite, acrolein, causes urothelial damage. A new structural analog of cyclophosphamide, Ifosfamide, has been evaluated for its marked antitumor effects, which are similar to those of other alkylating agents. However, it is highly toxic to the bladder and urothelium, and severe hemorrhagic cystitis can be prevented by the prophylactic administration of 2-mercaptoethane sulfonate (MESNA), which binds to acrolein and prevents urotoxicity. In addition, it has been noted that therapy with alkylating agents, particularly phenylalanine mustard, is associated with the subsequent risk of the patient's developing acute leukemia. This risk may range from 2% to 10% and appears to be related to the dose, the drug, and the duration of treatment.

Antitumor Antibiotics

Antitumor antibiotics are derived from products of bacterial or fungal cultures. Their mechanism of action is not clearly delineated, but it is thought that they directly attack DNA and appear to be able to produce DNA breaks and also interfere with DNA synthesis and transcription. The ones most commonly used in gynecologic cancer are actinomycin D (Cosmegen), doxorubicin (Adriamycin), and bleomycin (Blenoxane).

Actinomycin D is usually given intravenously often in 5-day courses every 4 weeks. The drug causes severe myelosuppression and can affect the gastrointestinal mucosa, leading to diarrhea and ulcers in the mouth. Alopecia and skin toxicity may also occur. The drug has a potentiating effect with radiation therapy, and this increased activity may be observed even when the drug is given after radiation treatment is completed. The drug is active in ovarian tumors and also widely used to treat trophoblastic disease. It is also sclerosing and has been used to treat malignant pleural effusions.

Doxorubicin must be carefully administered intravenously, since extravasation leads to soft tissue and skin necrosis and ulceration. It is metabolized in the liver, and dosages must be reduced in patients with compromised hepatic function. Myelosuppression occurs regularly with therapeutic doses. Complete alopecia is a common and almost constant side effect. The alopecia is reversible after cessation of the use of the drug, but it tends to be one of the greatest causes of patient distress. The drug also causes cardiomyopathy, which leads to congestive heart failure and can be life threatening. In general, doses are kept below 550 mg/m^2, and cardiac function is often monitored by ultrasound evaluation or radionuclide scans. The drug has widespread use in gynecologic cancers, particularly in sarcomas, ovarian tumors, and endometrial and cervical carcinomas.

Bleomycin may be administered intravenously, intramuscularly, or subcutaneously. It is excreted via the kidney, and some dosage reduction is made if renal function is markedly compromised. The drug does *not* have significant myelosuppressant properties, in contrast to most of the other cytotoxic agents. It is, however, highly toxic to the lungs, and pneumonitis and pulmonary fibrosis may occur. Thus particular care must be used in persons with compromised lung function. The drug is

also toxic to skin and can produce erythema, peeling, and pigmentation. It has been used recently as part of combination therapy with particular effectiveness against ovarian germ cell tumors, and it has been tried for a variety of other gynecologic malignancies, particularly carcinoma of the cervix, but with limited success.

Antimetabolites

Antimetabolites interfere with cell metabolism by competing with naturally occurring purines or pyrimidines, whose chemical structure they resemble. In this way they interfere or prevent vital biochemical reactions.

5-Fluorouracil (5-FU) is a substitute pyrimidine that interferes with DNA synthesis and can also be incorporated into RNA. It is usually given intravenously and is also active orally. It is myelosuppressive, although less so than many other cytotoxic agents used in gynecologic cancer treatment. It causes gastrointestinal side effects (diarrhea) and ulceration of the oral mucosa. It is effectively metabolized in the liver, which has led to its use in hepatic artery infusions for liver metastasis. The clearing of 5-FU from the blood by the liver markedly reduces systemic toxicity in patients receiving these infusions. The drug is extensively used in gynecologic cancer, including ovarian carcinomas, endometrial adenocarcinomas, and some cases of cervical squamous cell carcinomas. It has also been used topically to treat intraepithelial neoplasia of the lower genital tract.

Methotrexate inhibits the enzyme dihydrofolate reductase, preventing the conversion of dihydrofolate to tetrahydrofolate. This prevents metabolic transfer of one carbon unit and inhibits the synthesis of thymidylic acid as well as different purine nucleotides. RNA and DNA syntheses are inhibited, and the drug works primarily in the S phase. Nondividing or resting cells are resistant. The effects of methotrexate can be overcome by the administration of folinic acid (citrovorum factor) 24 hours after methotrexate, which replenishes the tetrahydrofolate. Some chemotherapy protocols have used very high doses of methotrexate to treat the tumor, followed by citrovorum rescue to avoid severe toxic side effects. Figure 25-10 illustrates schematically the action of the drug. Methotrexate is administered intravenously, intramuscularly, or orally. It is excreted in the urine, and dosage adjustments must be made if

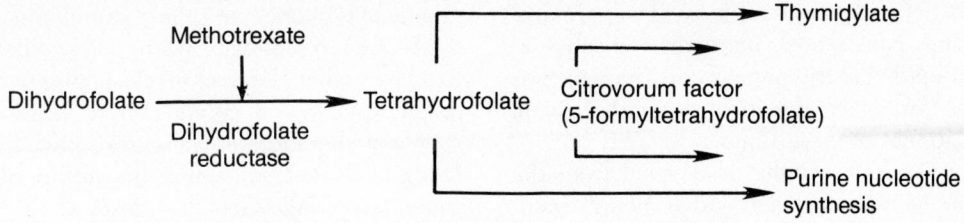

FIGURE 25-10
Schematic of action of methotrexate and reversal by citrovorum factor.

there is decreased renal function. Methotrexate is severely myelosuppressive and causes toxicity to the oral mucosa and intestines, as well as the liver, and an increase in liver enzymes is seen after treatment. The serum levels are also prolonged in patients with ascites or pleural effusion, since these act as a reservoir for the drug. Blood levels of methotrexate can be monitored with radioimmunoassay. The predominant use of the drug in gynecologic cancer has been the effective treatment of trophoblastic disease; it has also been used in cervical and ovarian carcinomas.

Vinca (Plant) Alkaloids

A number of cytotoxic drugs have been isolated from plant extracts. Those in current use in gynecologic oncology include vinblastine and vincristine. These drugs attack the cell during the M phase and cause toxic destruction of the mitotic spindle and thus arrest mitosis. This can result in synchronization of the cell cycle for those cells surviving therapy. The drugs are given intravenously and have different side effects. Vincristine is severely neurotoxic and can produce numbness, motor weakness, and constipation as a result of its autonomic effects. There is little myelosuppression. Vinblastine is myelotoxic, and this tends to be a dose-limiting factor. However, it has less neurotoxicity than vincristine. VP-16 (etoposide) is a recently introduced plant-derived drug that is topoisomerase-II (enzyme) inhibitor, which is involved in DNA synthesis. It appears to have fewer toxic side effects but is myelotoxic. These drugs have been used in ovarian germ cell tumors, as well as in trophoblastic disease.

Synthetic and Miscellaneous Compounds

Recently synthetically produced drugs have been introduced that have antitumor activity. They do not have any single mode of action, and in some instances their mechanism of antitumor activity is unknown. Currently the two synthetic agents most commonly used in gynecologic cancers are cisplatin and hexamethylmelamine.

Cisplatin (cis-diamminedichloroplatinum, cis-DDP) has been found to have wide antitumor activity. It appears to bind to DNA and interfere with DNA synthesis, but its cell cycle specificity has not been clearly defined. It is administered intravenously and is very toxic to the kidney. A high urine output must be maintained during administration to try to reduce kidney toxicity, since the drug is excreted in the urine in its active form. It induces myelosuppression and also causes high-frequency ototoxicity, so that renal and auditory function must be monitored during treatment in addition to peripheral blood counts. Cisplatin induces severe peripheral neuropathy, which may improve somewhat after cessation of therapy but tends to be permanent. Metabolic changes including hypomagnesemia and hypokalemia occur, and seizures have been reported in severe cases. One of the side effects most annoying to the patient is the production of severe nausea with vomiting, which may be controlled in part by antiemetic medication. The drug is widely used in the treatment of ovarian epithelial and germ cell tumors and is currently being tested for the treatment of all types of gynecologic cancers.

New analogs have been introduced, such as carboplatinum, which according to recent studies of Mangioni et al. appear to have comparable activity in ovarian epithelial carcinoma as cisplatin. Carboplatinum is not toxic to the kidneys but appears more suppressive to the bone marrow, especially to platelets.

Hexamethylmelamine is orally active, but its mechanism of antitumor activity is unclear. It is thought to act somewhat similarly to alkylating agents, but it is structurally different from that class of compounds. It is myelosuppressive and causes nausea and vomiting. It is active in ovarian epithelial carcinomas and frequently is used as part of combination chemotherapy in the treatment of these tumors.

Taxol (Taxus brevifolia) is derived from the bark of the Western yew and is being evaluated in the treatment of ovarian carcinoma. It is a potent agent whose administration can be accompanied by severe hypersensitivity reaction and hypotension.

Hormones

Hormone therapy has been effectively developed in the treatment of breast cancer. Estrogen and progesterone receptors have been clearly identified in endometrial carcinomas and have been recently found in other types of gynecologic cancers, particularly ovarian epithelial carcinomas. Progestins such as megestrol (Megace), depo-medroxyprogesterone (Depo-Provera), and 17-OH progesterone caproate (Delalutin), as well as antiestrogens such as tamoxifen, have been used in the treatment of endometrial carcinomas and seem to have their best effects against well-differentiated tumors. Hormonal therapy is also being evaluated in the treatment of some ovarian epithelial carcinomas.

Alternative Modes of Therapy

Many new modes of therapy are being tried, particularly those that are being adapted from trials of nongynecologic tumors; this includes high-dose chemotherapy with autologous bone marrow reinfusion, such as that described by Dauplat et al. Bone marrow is harvested, and then high myelosuppressive chemotherapy doses are administered in the hopes of achieving increased antitumor effect. Subsequently, the patient's bone marrow is reinfused to permit replenishment of the hematopoietic system. This technique has had success in the therapy for breast cancer, but only limited trials have been conducted in cases of gynecologic cancers.

Stimulators of the hematopoietic system are also being used to diminish the toxicity of chemotherapeutic agents; this includes the use of erythropoietin (epo) to overcome the chronic anemia that oftens occurs with chemotherapy. In addition, trials have been initiated with granulocyte-monocyte colony stimulating factor (GM-CSF) to stimulate white cell proliferation to allow higher doses of myelosuppressive chemotherapy to be administered. Alternative routes of chemotherapy administration are also being evaluated, including the intraperitoneal route, which allows higher doses of the agent to be delivered to intraperitoneal tumors, as discussed in Chapter 29.

IMMUNOTHERAPY

It has been shown that many experimental animal tumors are able to elicit an immune response, and the concept of tumor-specific antigens has gained wide acceptance. However, antigens specific for a given gynecologic tumor have not been identified. Nonetheless, it is recognized that an immune response to human tumors does occur. It appears that tumor growth stimulates the major cells of the immune system: the T lymphocyte, B lymphocyte, and macrophage. T lymphocytes are cells that confer cell-mediated immunity, while B lymphocytes are cells associated with antibody production and humoral immunity. Macrophages also act directly on tumor cells, and when activated they can enter into the immune response and become cytotoxic to tumor cells. It has also been observed that immunosuppressed patients, such as kidney transplant recipients, are at greater risk for the development of malignant disease. All of these considerations have led to efforts to utilize the immune system to treat human cancer. In the case of gynecologic malignancies, a number of trials of immunotherapy have been conducted, but currently this modality of treatment is primarily investigational.

Mature T cells circulate to various lymphoid sites where they become activated by antigens. The recognition of the antigens results in T cell activation. Monocytes and macrophages also participate in the cellular immune response, and the activation process produces a number of soluble immune mediators known as *cytokines* or *lymphokines*. With the development of recombinant DNA technology, these substances can be synthesized and a number of them are being evaluated for their potential in tumor therapy. Some of the cytokines produced by the lymphoreticular system have been used, mostly experimentally, in tumor therapy and are discussed in the next section.

Interleukins

Interleukins (IL) are cytokines that are designated numerically. IL-1 is released in response to cell damage. Macrophages and monocytes release it in response to antigens leading to a number of immune messages, including stimulation of IL-2 production, hematopoietic factors, and glucocorticoid release.

IL-2 is produced by T cells and has a primary role of cell-mediated immunity. It is being evaluated as an antitumor agent in gynecologic and other malignancies, particularly ovarian carcinomas. IL-2 stimulates T lymphocytes, natural killer (NK) cells, and lymphokine-activated killer cells (LAK cells) and leads to the secretion of other lymphokines including tumor necrosis factor (see below).

IL-3 stimulates differentiation of myeloid stem cells. IL-4, formerly called B cell stimulating factor-I, stimulates the proliferation of B cells. IL-5 also stimulates B cells and has been termed B cell stimulating factor II. IL-6 is a B cell stimulant as well.

Interferon

Interferons (IFNs) are produced in response to viral infection and act to inhibit viral replication. Three major types of these lymphokines have been described: alpha, beta, and gamma. IFN-alpha is secreted by trophoblasts and may enhance the antiviral response by stimulating cell surface antigens (major histocompatability complex [MHC]). IFN-beta is produced by fibroblasts and also acts to stimulate MHC antigens. IFN-gamma is produced by activated T cells. It appears to have a wide-ranging set of actions, including enhancing MHC expression and inducing cytotoxic T cell maturation. The interferons have also been observed in vitro to inhibit tumor cell proliferation. Interferons bind to cell surface receptors and become biologically active, which can result in antiviral and antiproliferative effects. Their precise mechanism of action is not known, but they appear to interact with T and B cells to augment cellular and humoral immunity.

Tumor Necrosis Factor

Tumor necrosis factor (TNF), a cytokine, induces necrosis of tumor cells in vitro and also appears to act synergistically with interferons. It is a mediator of endotoxic shock and can stimulate hematopoietic cells. Furthermore, it can introduce production of other cytokines, including GM-CSF. TNF appears to be selective for tumor cells, which provides a theoretical advantage over classical chemotherapeutic agents inasmuch as approximately 100 to 10,000 X concentration of TNF is needed to affect normal cells in comparison with malignant cells in vitro. Moreover, TNF can act synergistically with IFN-gamma as well as chemotherapeutic agents such as 5-FU, alkylating agents, and etoposide. However, its administration has also been accompanied by severe toxicity, including shocklike symptoms, fever, and hypotension.

Granulocyte Colony-Stimulating Factor

Granulocyte colony-stimulating factor (G-CSF), a cytokine, promotes growth of granulocytes and is secreted by lymphocytes, as well as macrophages. It is being evaluated for use in patients receiving cytotoxic chemotherapy to stimulate their bone marrow and thus decrease the myelosuppressive response.

Lymphokine-Activated Killer Cells

There are peripheral monocytes that are stimulated in vitro by IL-2 or other agents to produce cells that are cytotoxic to tumor cells but not to normal cells. LAK cells are being tested for application to human tumor therapy.

Various approaches have been taken to augment the immune response to human tumors. One of the most common is active nonspecific immunotherapy, which involves the administration of adjuvant agents, usually of microbiologic origin, to stimulate cell-mediated and humoral immunity, as well as to activate macrophages. Two examples are bacillus Calmette-Guerin (BCG) and *Corynebacterium parvum* (C-Parvum). Both of these produce marked proliferation of lymphocytes and have been tested in gynecologic malignancies, but no therapeutic role has been identified for their routine use. It is thought that the benefits of BCG may be enhanced if it is administered in conjunction with other treatment modalities such as cytotoxic chemotherapy.

A second type of immunotherapy is active specific immunotherapy, which involves the use of tumor cells and their antigens to produce specific tumor immunities. The tumor cells may be modified with chemicals or irradiation and then placed into a growth medium to produce a vaccine to allow active immunization. Immunotherapy may also be given locally, such as BCG treatment of malignant melanoma or the use of dinitrochlorobenzene (DCNB) to treat skin cancers. Widespread granulomas (BCGosis [bacillus calmette-guerinosis]) and death have been described as results of BCG therapy. Efforts are also under way to confer passive immunity. Transfer of specific immunity through extracts of lymphocytes sensitized to tumor antigens is being investigated. Extracts of such "transfer factor" may lead to a type of adoptive immunotherapy by transfer of "immunologic memory" to the patient's lymphocytes. IFN is another substance being evaluated. It has been noted to prevent cancer cell division, perhaps through augmenting the action of natural killer (NK) cells. By preventing the replication of cancer cells, the treatment would gradually lead to tumor regression. Passive transfer of antibodies involves another method of potential immunotherapy involving the transfer of active antibodies against a given tumor. All of these approaches remain investigational at present.

A new investigational form of therapy involves radiolabeled antibodies. For example, Epenetos et al. have given tumor-associated antigens labeled with ^{131}I intraperitoneally to patients with refractory ovarian carcinoma. They have obtained complete remissions in some patients with small-volume disease.

KEY POINTS

- Electromagnetic radiation is a form of energy that has no mass or charge and travels at the speed of light.

- Particulate energy is a form of ionizing radiation consisting of subatomic particles (electrons, neutrons, and protons) whose energy is in part related to their mass and velocity.

- Inverse square law states that the energy measured from a radiation source is inversely proportional to the distance from the source.

- A given dose of radiation kills a constant fraction of tumor cells radiated. The tissue effects of electromagnetic radiation (x-rays and gamma rays) are dependent on oxygenation.

- The effect of photon radiation (low LET) on tissues is altered by tissue oxygenation, while neutron (high LET) radiation is independent of oxygenation.

- The cell replication cycle consists of M (mitosis), G_1 (Gap_1 = RNA and protein synthesis), S (DNA synthesis), and G_2 (Gap_2 = RNA and protein synthesis). When the cell is not in the replication cycle, it is in the G_0 phase.

- The dose of radiation delivered to a tumor depends on the energy of the source, the size of the treatment field, and the depth of the tumor beneath the surface.

- Radiation acts on cells primarily in the M phase, making rapidly proliferating cells the most radiosensitive. Normal tissues recover from the effects of radiation therapy more efficiently than tumor tissue does.

- Cytotoxic chemotherapeutic agents act on various phases of the cell cycle, primarily affecting rapidly proliferating cells, and at a given dose destroy a constant fraction of tumor cells.

- Most chemotherapeutic drugs are severely myelosuppressive, with the exception of bleomycin and vincristine.

- Methotrexate and cisplatin are excreted by the kidney, and their effects are increased in patients with diminished renal function. Because of displacement from serum albumin, both salicylates and sulfa drugs increase toxicity of these agents.

- Vincristine and cisplatin cause severe peripheral neurotoxicity.

- Bleomycin is associated with severe pulmonary toxicity.

- Doxorubicin is associated with severe cardiomyopathy.

- Cisplatin is nephrotoxic and myelosuppressive. Its analog, carboplatin, is also excreted by the kidney but is not nephrotoxic.

- Alopecia can occur with any chemotherapy, but it is total and severe with doxorubicin and actinomycin. Hair growth resumes after cessation of treatment.

- Large tumors tend to have smaller growth fractions and a higher proportion of cells in the resting phase (G_0) of the cycle than small tumors. Tumors consist of a heterogeneous population of cells and have variable growth fractions.

- The major classes of cytotoxic chemotherapeutic agents used in gynecologic oncology are alkylating agents, antitumor antibiotics, antimetabolites, vinca (plant) alkaloids, and specially synthesized compounds.

- Systemic-active nonspecific immunotherapy results from the injection of agents derived from bacteriologic sources mixed with an adjuvant that cause a proliferation of lymphocytes leading to cellular and humoral immunity.

- Active specific immunotherapy is the use of tumor cells and their surface antigens to produce specific tumor immunity.

BIBLIOGRAPHY

Arai A, Nakano T, Fukuhisa K, et al: Second cancer after radiation therapy for cancer of the uterine cervix, Cancer 67:398, 1991.

Beller U, Chachoua A, Speyer JL, et al: Phase IB study of low-dose intraperitoneal recombinant interleukin-2 in patients with refractory advanced ovarian cancer: rationale and preliminary report, Gynecol Oncol 34:407, 1989.

Bellin SL and Selin M: Cisplatin-induced hypomagnesemia with seizures: a case report and review of the literature, Gynecol Oncol 30:104, 1988.

Bruce WR, Meeker RE, and Valeriote FA: Comparison of the sensitivity of normal hematopoietic and transplanted lymphoma colony-forming cells to chemotherapeutic agents administered in vivo, J Natl Cancer Inst 37:233, 1966.

Bunn HF: Recombinant erythropoietin therapy in cancer patients, J Clin Oncol 6:949, 1990.

Byrne A, Mulvihill JJ, Myers MH, et al: Effects of treatment on fertility in long-term survivals of childhood or adolescent cancer, N Engl J Med 317:1315, 1987.

Chabner BA and Myers CE: Clinical pharmacology of cancer chemotherapy. In DeVita VT Jr and Hellman S, editors: Cancer: principles and practice of oncology, Philadelphia, 1982, JB Lippincott Co.

Chambers SK, Chopyk RL, Chambers JT, et al: Development of leukemia after doxorubicin and cisplatin treatment for ovarian cancer, Cancer 64:2459, 1989.

Dauplat J, Legros M, Condat P, et al: High-dose melphalan and autologous bone marrow support for treatment of ovarian carcinoma with positive second-look operation, Gynecol Oncol 34:294, 1989.

DeVita VT: Cell kinetics and the chemotherapy of cancer, Cancer Treat Rep 2:23, 1971.

DeVita VT, Hellman S, and Rosenberg SA: Cancer principles and practice of oncology, ed 3, Philadelphia, 1989, JB Lippincott Co.

Dickson JA: Hyperthermia in the treatment of cancer, Lancet 1:202, 1979.

Erslev AJ: Erythropoietin, N Engl J Med 324:1339, 1991.

Frei E III and Spriggs D: Tumor necrosis factor: still a promising agent, J Clin Oncol 7:291, 1987.

Gray LH, Coger AD, Ebert M, et al: The concentration of oxygen dissolved in tissues at the time of radiation as a factor in radiotherapy, Br J Radiol 26:638, 1953.

Hall EJ: Radiation dose rate: a factor of importance in radiobiology and radiotherapy, Br J Radiol 45:81, 1972.

Hall EJ: Radiobiology for the radiologist, ed 2, Philadelphia, 1978, Harper & Row, Publishers, Inc.

Hamilton TC, Ozols RF, and Longo DL: Biologic therapy for the treatment of malignant common epithelial tumors of the ovary, Cancer 60:2054, 1987.

Herberman RB: Interleukin-2 therapy of human cancer: potential benefits versus toxicity, J Clin Oncol 7:1, 1989.

Joslin CAF: Basic parameters of radiotherapy. In Coppleson M, editor: Gynecologic oncology, Edinburgh, 1981, Churchill Livingstone.

Kelleher MB, Christopherson WA, and Macpherson TA: Desseminated granulomatous disease (BCGosis) following chemoimmunotherapy for ovarian carcinoma, Gynecol Oncol 31:321, 1988.

Lederer CM, Hollander J, and Perlman I: Table of isotopes, New York, 1967, John Wiley & Sons.

Li MC, Hertz R, and Spencer DB: Effect of methotrexate therapy upon choriocarcinoma and chorioadenoma, Proc Soc Exp Biol Med 93:361, 1956.

Mangioni C, Bolis G, Pecorelli K, et al: Randomized trial in advanced ovarian cancer comparing cisplatin and carboplatin, J Natl Cancer Inst 81:1464, 1989.

McGuire WP III, Arseneau J, Blessing JA, et al: A randomized comparative trial of carboplatin and iproplatin in advanced squamous carcinoma of the uterine cervix: a gynecologic oncology group study, J Clin Oncol 7:1462, 1989.

Montana GS and Fowler WC: Carcinoma of the cervix: analysis of bladder and rectal radiation dose and complications, Int J Radiat Oncol Biol Phys 16:95, 1989.

Phillips RM, Bibby MC, and Double JA: Review: a critical appraisal of the predictive value of in vitro chemosensitivity assays, J Natl Cancer Inst 82:1457, 1990.

Plaxe SC, Dottino PR, and Cohen CJ: Therapeutic and metabolic effects of high $(>1 g/m^2)$ systemic cumulative doses of cisplatinum in patients with ovarian carcinoma, Gynecol Oncol 37:250, 1990.

Sinclair WK: Cyclic x-ray responses in mammalian cells in vitro, Radiat Res 33:620, 1968.

Sinclair WK and Morton RA: X-ray sensitivity during cell generation cycle of cultured Chinese hamster cells, Radiat Res 29:450, 1966.

Skipper HE: Biochemical, pharmacologic, toxicological, kinetic, and chemical (subhuman and human) relationships, Cancer 21:600, 1968.

Skipper H, Schabel F, and Wilcox WS: Experimental evaluation of potential anticancer agent XIII on the criterion and kinetics associated with "curability" of experimental leukemia, Cancer Chemother Rep 35:1, 1964.

Stillwell TJ and Benson RC: Cyclophosphamide-induced hemorrhagic cystitis: a review of 100 patients, Cancer 61:451, 1988.

Tucker MA and Fraumeni JF Jr: Treatment-related cancers after gynecologic malignancy, Cancer 60:2117, 1987.

Weiss RB, Donehower RC, Wiernik PH, et al: Hypersensitivity reactions from Taxol, J Clin Oncol 8:1263, 1990.

Wilcox WS: The last surviving cancer cell—the chances of killing it, Cancer Chemother Rep 50:541, 1966.

Young RC: Chemotherapy. In Berek JS and Hacker NF, editors: Practical gynecologic oncology, Baltimore, 1989, Williams & Wilkins.

Intraepithelial Neoplasia of the Cervix

KEY TERMS AND DEFINITIONS

Abnormal Transformation Zone. Area on the cervix or vagina that may contain columnar epithelium and squamous metaplasia and that often contains intraepithelial neoplasia with an abnormal colposcopic pattern.

Acetowhite Epithelium. A colposcopic term to describe epithelium that initially looks normal but appears white after acetic acid application. The area is frequently found to have histologic evidence of human papillomavirus (HPV) infection, in which case the term *subclinical papilloma infection (SPI)* is used.

Carcinoma in Situ. A morphologic alteration of the epithelium that usually precedes, occasionally gives rise to, and is usually present in the vicinity of invasive carcinoma. The full thickness of the epithelium is replaced with dysplastic cells (CIN III).

Cervical Intraepithelial Neoplasia (CIN). A premalignant change in the cervical epithelium that can progress to the development of cervical carcinoma. The degree of change from mild to severe is described as CIN I, CIN II, or CIN III.

Colposcope. An instrument used to magnify and examine the epithelium of the transformation zone to identify abnormal areas in the lower genital tract that warrant biopsy.

Conization. A surgical technique to remove a cone-shaped central core of the cervix for diagnosis or treatment of intraepithelial neoplasia.

Cryotherapy. Freezing of the cervix to destroy abnormal epithelium.

Dysplasia. A term used to describe varying degrees of cervical intraepithelial neoplasia. It may be mild, involving approximately one third of the epithelium (CIN I); moderate, approximately two thirds of the epithelium (CIN II); or severe, full thickness of the epithelium (CIN III).

Endocervical Curettage (ECC). A biopsy procedure used to obtain endocervical tissue for histologic diagnosis.

Flat Wart. An alternate term to describe subclinical human papillomavirus (HPV) infection.

Human Papillomavirus (HPV) Types. A numeric designation given to varying types of HPVs, as determined by their DNA characteristics. New types are being continuously described.

Koilocytosis. A cellular change associated with papillomavirus infection, which includes perinuclear cavitation and nuclear atypicality.

Laser. *L*ight *a*mplification by *s*timulated *e*mission of *r*adiation. A technique that uses energized light to vaporize tissue.

Leukoplakia. A colposcopic term to describe an area that appears white to the naked eye even before application of 3% acetic acid.

Mosaic Pattern. A colposcopic term to describe the rosette appearance of capillary vessels in an abnormal transformation zone.

Native Squamous Epithelium. The normal original squamous epithelium found in the vagina and on the portio of the cervix.

Normal Transformation Zone. Area of columnar epithelium and squamous metaplasia that has a normal colposcopic pattern.

Punctation. A colposcopic term to describe the stippled appearance of capillary vessels in the abnormal transformation zone.

Radiation Dysplasia. A term to describe abnormal cells in the cytologic smear of patients treated by ionizing irradiation for cervical cancer. These patients are at increased risk for recurrent disease.

Satisfactory Colposcopy. A colposcopic examination in which the entire transformation zone, including the squamocolumnar junction, is adequately visualized.

Squamocolumnar Junction. The junction of the squamous epithelium and columnar (glandular) epithelium, usually located near the external cervical os.

Squamous Intraepithelial Lesion (SIL). A cytologic term used to describe abnormal cells according to the Bethesda Classification proposed in 1989.

Squamous Metaplasia. A physiologic process whereby squamous tissue replaces columnar tissue.

Subclinical Papilloma Infection (SPI). An area that looks normal to the naked eye but colposcopically appears white after acetic acid application. It often contains papillomavirus infection.

Because of the accessible location of the cervix and the upper vagina, intraepithelial neoplasia of the cervix has been investigated more than any other premalignant lesion of the female genital tract, and this process has resulted in improved detection and treatment. The development of cytology as a discipline to aid in the detection of neoplasia of the cervix and the colposcope as an instrument to localize the site of the most severe change and allow directed biopsy has contributed to improvement of the management of these disorders. This chapter reviews the morphologic changes that characterize the intraepithelial neoplastic lesions of the cervix. The current concepts of the factors thought to lead to the development of cervical neoplasia, including a detailed consideration of human papillomavirus infection (HPV), are reviewed and the methods of diagnosis and treatment described.

DEFINITIONS AND MORPHOLOGY

The squamocolumnar junction is an important landmark where neoplastic change develops in the cervix. In young adults this intersection between the cervical glandular (columnar) epithelium and the native squamous epithelium is usually located on the exocervix just distal to the external os. During pregnancy and after childbirth this area may enlarge and become more distally located on the portio of the cervix away from the os. After menopause the junction usually recedes and is frequently located in the endocervical canal. Thus in the

normal adult female of reproductive age, there are usually areas of columnar epithelium surrounding the exocervix. During puberty and throughout reproductive life, especially during pregnancy, this exposed columnar epithelium undergoes gradual replacement by squamous epithelium (squamous metaplasia). This process can be readily identified with the colposcope, and the areas of columnar epithelium and squamous metaplasia constitute the normal transformation zone. In contrast, abnormal or neoplastic squamous epithelium can also be found in the transformation zone, which leads to abnormal colposcopic patterns and characterizes the abnormal transformation zone (see colposcopy section).

Numerous terms have been used to describe the premalignant lesions of the cervix. It is important to emphasize that these changes are part of a continuum of slight to severe atypicality which can progress to invasive carcinoma (Figure 26-1). Two terminologies are most commonly used to describe intraepithelial neoplasia. One relies on the term *dysplasia* (mild, moderate, or severe) to describe the early premalignant changes in the epithelium and the term *carcinoma in situ* to describe the most advanced premalignant change. An alternate nomenclature that describes the same histologic features utilizes the terminology of *cervical intraepithelial neoplasia (CIN)* of various grades of severity: CIN I (mild dysplasia), CIN II (moderate dysplasia), and CIN III (severe dysplasia to carcinoma in situ). The term *CIN* was introduced by Richart, who emphasized the concept of a single entity of intraepithelial neo-

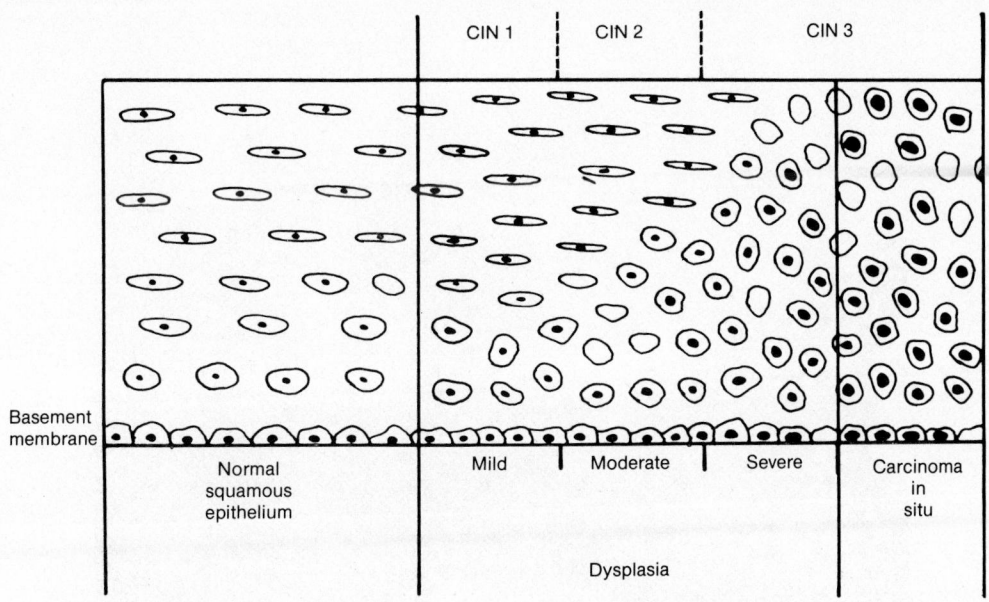

FIGURE 26-1
Diagram of cervical epithelium showing various terminology used to characterize progressive degrees of cervical neoplasia. (Modified from Richart RM: Can J Med Tech 38:177, 1976.)

plasia that has the potential to develop into invasive carcinoma. Many diagnosticians consider severe dysplasia and carcinoma in situ to be comparable lesions. Recently a new terminology has been recommended, "The Bethesda System," which is discussed subsequently (see section on cytology).

The cytologic and histologic features of mild, moderate, and severe dysplasia and carcinoma in situ are illustrated in Figures 26-2 to 26-5. The least disturbance of the squamous epithelium and the lowest proportion of abnormal cells occur in the lesion of mild dysplasia (CIN I). In the case of carcinoma in situ the entire thickness of the epithelium is replaced with abnormal cells, but there is no invasion of the underlying stroma (CIN III). With progression, invasive carcinoma is diagnosed (Figures 26-6 and 26-7). Unfortunately, there is a lack of agreement regarding the precise definition of each category of intraepithelial neoplasia, and there is no sharp morphologic boundary between them, a problem that often leads to disagreements in the diagnosis of the degree of severity of intraepithelial neoplasia. In general, if up to one third of the basal epithelium is abnormal, the term "mild" is applied; up to two thirds, "moderate"; more than two thirds, "se-

vere"; and full thickness, "carcinoma in situ." In addition, carcinoma in situ may develop in the crypts of the glands of the cervix as well as in the surface epithelium. Involvement of the glands leads to a diagnosis of "carcinoma in situ with gland involvement." For purposes of patient management, this entity is the same as carcinoma in situ without gland involvement.

EPIDEMIOLOGY

Potential Factors in Carcinogenesis

Intraepithelial neoplasia of the cervix occurs mainly in young women. The incidence is approximately twice as high in black women as in white. The peak in the age incidence of the disease appeared to be the early 30s, but recently it has been noted to be occurring more frequently in those in their 20s and occasionally younger. Furthermore, it appears that the frequency of the diagnosis of carcinoma in situ has increased in the past 25 years, in part because of the effectiveness of cytologic screening (Pap smear). This has been accompanied by a concomitant decrease in the frequency of invasive carcinoma, as was documented by the studies of Devesa, who demonstrated a drop of approximately 50% in the frequency of cervical carci-

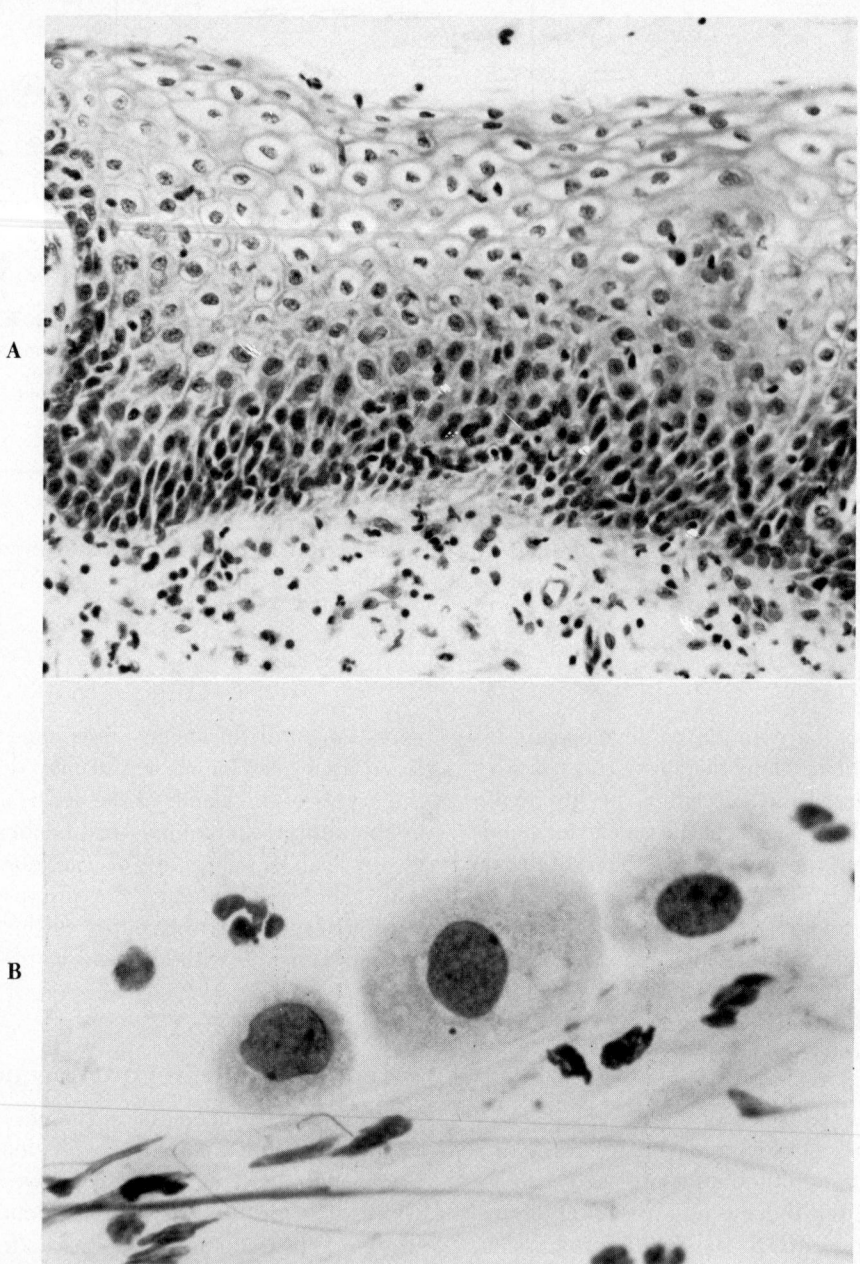

FIGURE 26-2
A, Mild dysplasia (histology) (CIN-I). Undifferentiated cells are confined to lower two to four layers of epithelium. Cells of middle and upper third show nuclear enlargement and irregular nuclei. (H&E stain; ×250.) **B,** Mild dysplasia (cytology). Dysplastic cells have altered nuclear-cytoplasmic ratio, exhibit nuclear enlargement, and have finely granular chromatin structure. (Papanicolaou stain; ×800.)

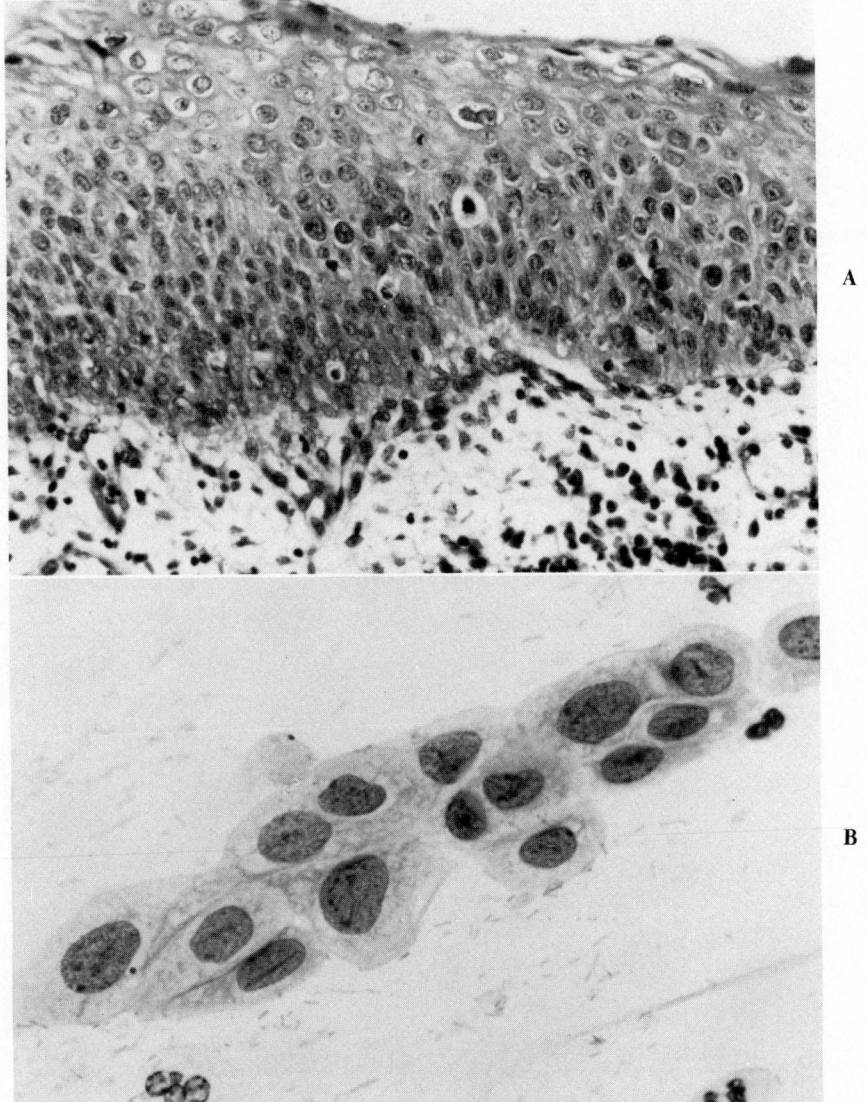

FIGURE 26-3
A, Moderate dysplasia (histology) (CIN-II). Immature cells are confined to lower half of epithelium. Cells of upper half show well-defined cell borders and enlarged, pleomorphic nuclei. (H&E stain; ×300.) **B,** Moderate dysplasia (cytology). Cells derived from moderate dysplasia exhibit altered nuclear-cytoplasmic ratio with less cytoplasm than in cells of mild dysplasia. There may be a uniformly finely granular chromatin pattern, with occasional chromocenter and (as cell at right) irregular nuclear envelope. (Papanicolaou stain; ×800.)

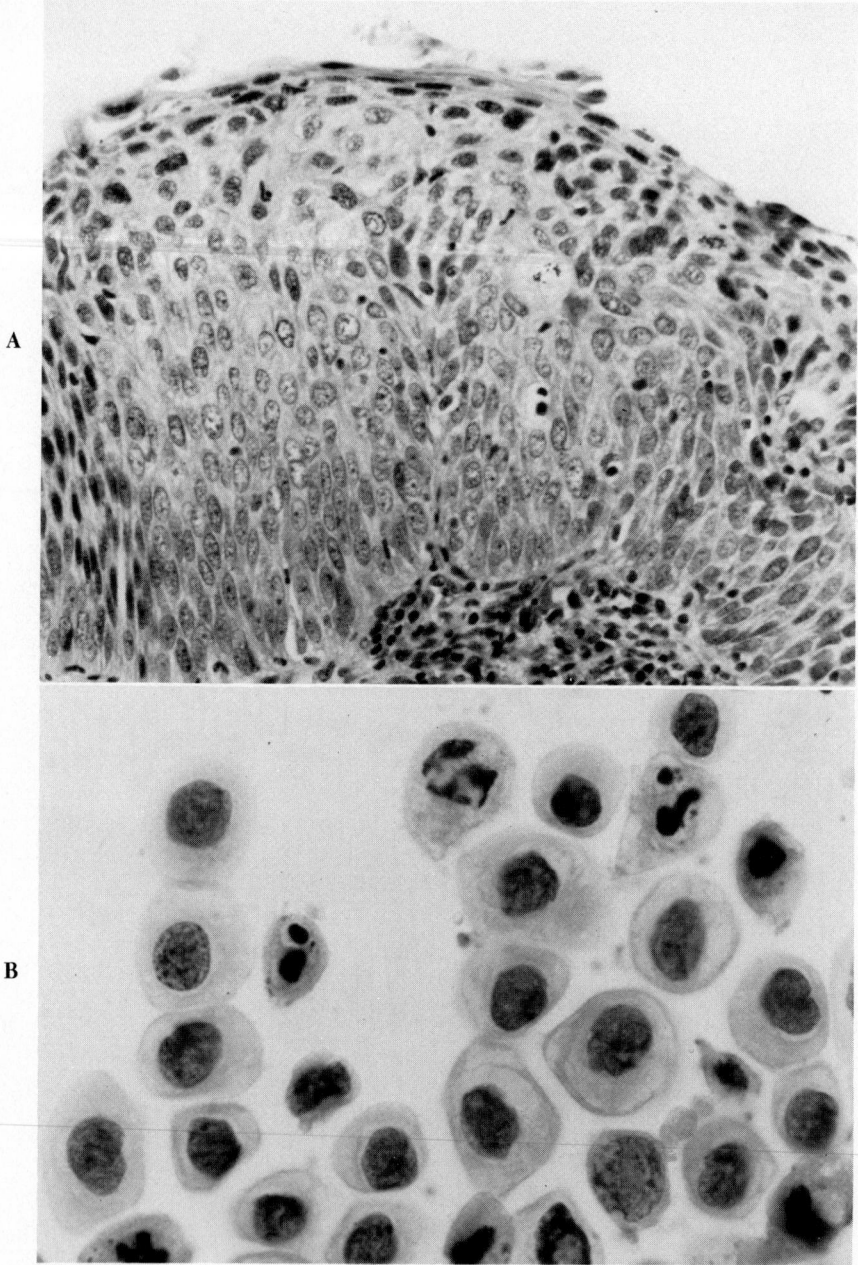

FIGURE 26-4

A, Severe dysplasia (histology) (CIN-III). In this lesion, immature cells with spindle-shaped nuclei replace more than two thirds of the mucosal thickness. Upper layers show evidence of squamous cell differentiation (H&E stain; ×300.) **B,** Severe dysplasia (cytology). Cells derived from a severe dysplasia may exhibit enlarged hyperchromatic nuclei, an irregular nuclear envelope, a course chromatin structure, and less cytoplasm than less severe dysplastic reactions. (Papanicolaou stain, ×1000.)

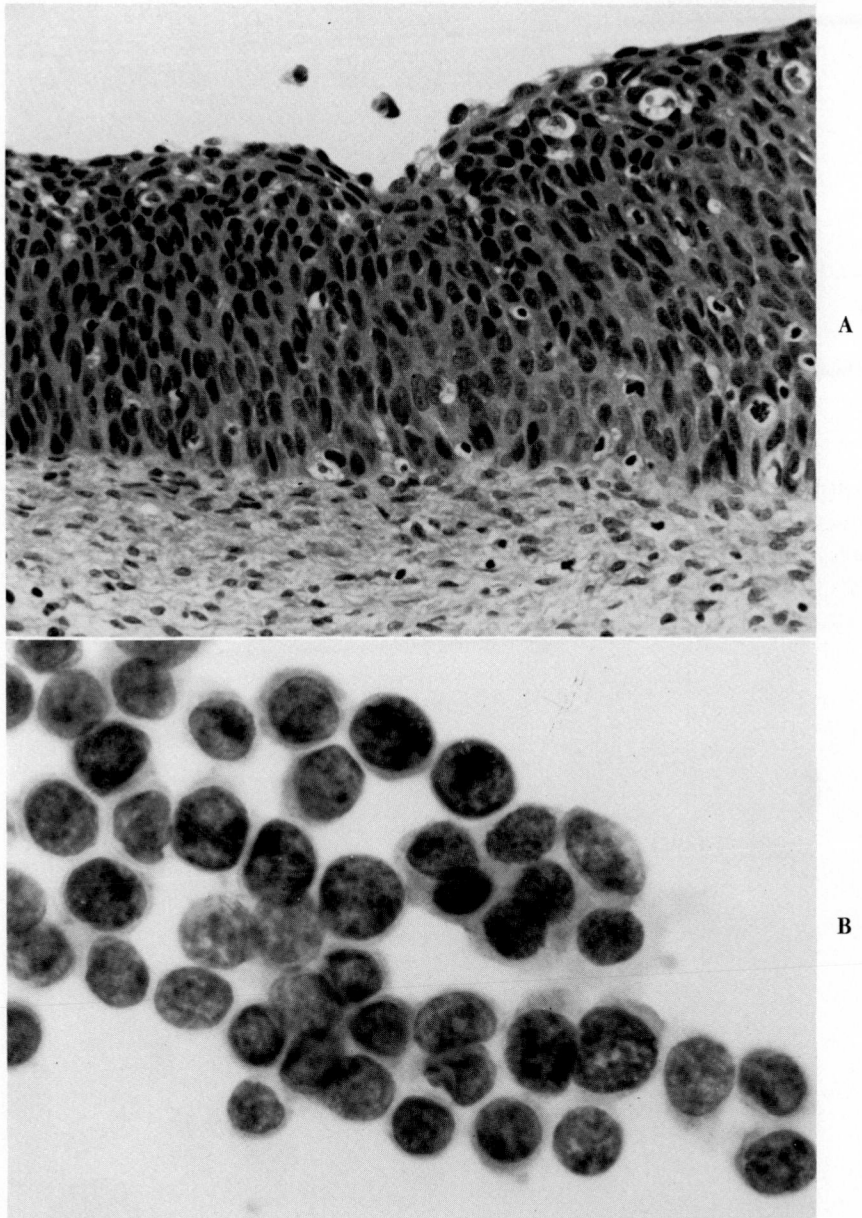

FIGURE 26-5
A, Carcinoma in situ (CIS) (histology). Basal-type cells with elongated nuclei and indistinct cytoplasmic boundaries occupy full thickness of mucosa. No maturation is present. (H&E stain; ×300.) **B,** CIS (cytology). CIS in cytologic sample may reveal groups of primitive cells with scant, ill-defined cytoplasm, nuclei that are round or oval, and a coarsely granular chromatin pattern with distinct chromocenters. Nucleoli are usually absent. (Papanicolaou stain; ×800.)

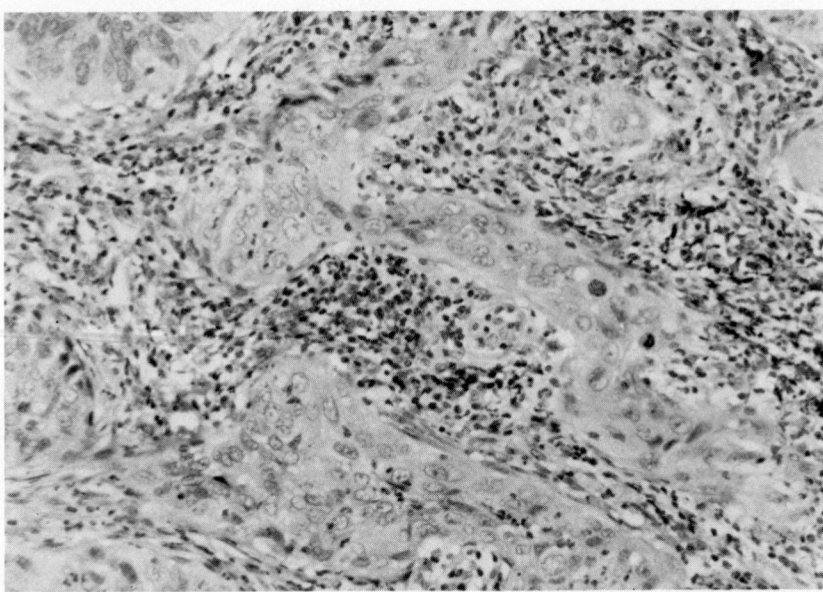

FIGURE 26-6
Invasive squamous carcinoma (histology). Irregular tumor nests infiltrate a stroma rich in inflammatory cells. Tumor cells are pleomorphic. A mitotic figure is seen at left. (H&E stain; ×200.)

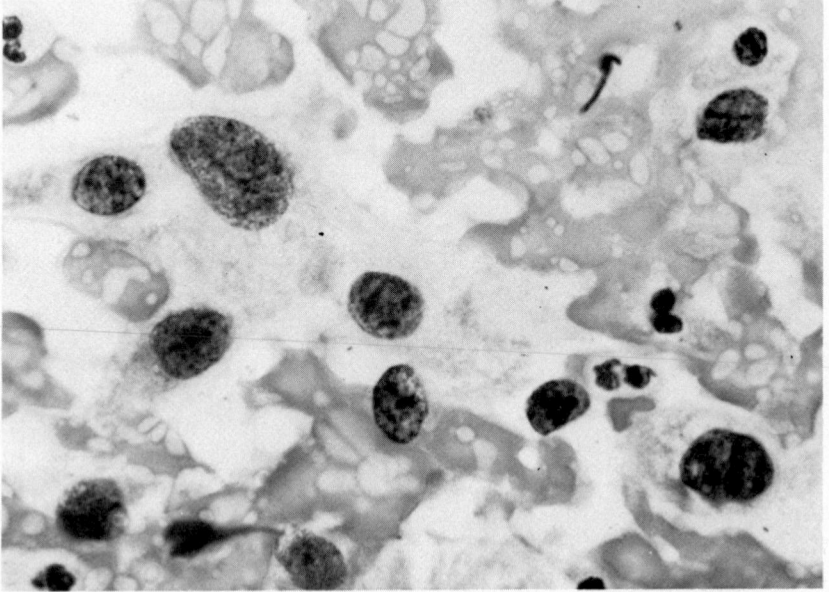

FIGURE 26-7
Invasive squamous cell carcinoma (cytology). Poorly differentiated squamous cell carcinoma may exhibit in the cytologic sample isolated malignant tumor cells with marked variation in nuclear size and shape. Because of the coarse and irregular chromatin pattern, nucleoli are not easily discerned here but are usually evident on direct microscopic examination. Background shows degenerated red blood cells and a few polymorphonuclear leukocytes. (Papanicolaou stain; ×1000.)

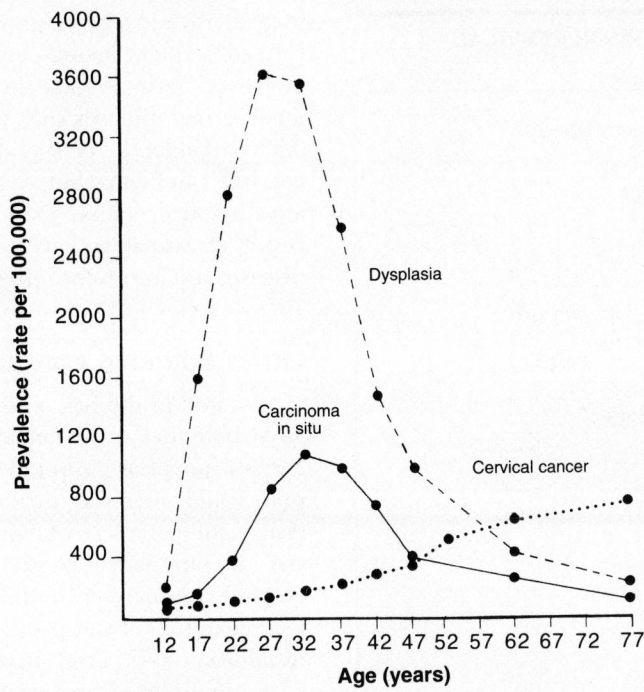

FIGURE 26-8

Graph of prevalence of minor precursors, major precursors, and invasive cancer. Precursors are much more common than invasive cancer. (From Reid R and Fu YS: In Peto R, editor: Banbury Report 21: viral etiology of cervical cancer, Cold Spring Harbor, NY, 1986. Copyright © Cold Spring Harbor Laboratory, 1986.)

noma from 1947 to 1977 in the United States. Figure 26-8 shows the approximate age incidence curves for dysplasia, carcinoma in situ, and invasive cancer. Dysplasia is the most common lesion, with a peak in the age incidence curve in the mid-20s. Carcinoma in situ is much less frequent and peaks at a slightly later age. In contrast, the frequency of invasive cancer is a curve of different shape that appears to plateau in the late 40s and then rises slowly with increasing age. As the individuals move into their 60s, invasive carcinoma becomes more common than carcinoma in situ. These age incidence curves suggest that a large number of atypias (dysplasias) of the cervical epithelium develop during reproductive life yet do not progress to malignancy. On the other hand, some dysplasias progress to cancer, and the risk of such progression increases with the more atypical lesions, such as carcinoma in situ.

The cause of CIN is not known, but a number of factors have been studied regarding their potential role in carcinogenesis. The box on p.

830 outlines the major factors postulated to be related to the development of CIN. Many of these have a venereal association. It is generally agreed that the atypical epithelium develops in the transformation zone of the cervix during the process of squamous metaplasia. Viruses, particularly HPV, are thought to have a major role in the genesis of premalignant lesions. In addition to this pathway of cervical carcinogenesis, it is recognized that some squamous cell cancers can arise de novo in areas outside the transformation zone, as discussed by Burghardt and Ostor. Some of these cancers may contribute to the continuing increased incidence of squamous cell carcinoma of the cervix that occurs in older women (see Figure 26-8).

For many years it has been observed that carcinoma of the cervix occurs more frequently in persons who have sexual intercourse early in their lives, as well as those who begin to have children at an early age. Women who have multiple sex partners are also at increased risk, and the disease is more frequent in young prostitutes. The age at first intercourse appears

POTENTIAL FACTORS IN CERVICAL NEOPLASIA

Epidemiologic Characteristics

Early intercourse
Multiple sex partners
Early marriage
Early childbearing
Prostitution
Male factors—"high-risk" consort
Socioeconomic status, race
Venereal infection

Other Potential Factors

Immune status
Oral contraceptives
Cigarette smoking
Prior radiation
Intrauterine DES exposure
Vitamins A and C

Viral Relations

Papillomavirus
Herpesvirus
Cytomegalovirus

---

particularly important. Herrero et al. recently noted a greater than twofold risk of cervical cancer for those starting intercourse at ages 14 to 15 years compared with those over 20 years, suggesting that the younger patients may be more susceptible to carcinogenic influences. In contrast, squamous cell carcinoma of the cervix is almost unknown in nuns. The disease is also rare among Jewish women, and this has led to speculation that circumcision might reduce the risk of development of the disease, but studies have failed to confirm that circumcision is a factor. Moreover, cervical carcinoma has been noted among Israeli Jews, especially if the usually associated venereal risk factors exist.

The male consort can also be important in the development of the disease. For example, Kessler studied women married to men whose previous wives had developed cervical cancer. This cohort was compared with women married to men whose previous wives had not had cervical cancer. A threefold increased frequency of cervical cancer occurred among the former group.

The occurrence of diseases such as gonorrhea have also been shown to be associated with the frequency of cervical carcinoma. Beral and colleagues noted that an increase in the frequency of gonorrhea in a given group was accompanied by a subsequent increase in cervical carcinoma. However, current data do not indicate a role for venereal diseases such as gonorrhea, *Trichomonas vaginalis,* or syphilis in the genesis of cervical carcinoma but suggest that the causative agent or agents may be transmitted as a result of sexual activity, during which these diseases are also transmitted.

Other Potential Factors

As noted in the box on the left, other factors have potential involvement in the genesis of cervical neoplasia. Alteration in immune function could increase the risk. For example, transplant patients receiving immunosuppressive therapy have been noted to be at increased risk for recurrent genital tract viral infection and recurrent papilloma wart infections. In addition Seski et al. have noted altered cellular immunity as measured by T cell function in lymphocyte toxicity tests in individuals with recurrent papilloma infection. An increase in gynecologic malignancies and cervical carcinoma in immunosuppressed patients has been reported.

Other potential effects in the genesis of CIN have been evaluated with extensive studies of women ingesting oral contraceptives. Vessey et al. suggest that oral contraceptives may increase the risk of CIN in comparison to controls with comparable sexual histories who used an IUD. Beral et al. studied 47,000 women and showed that oral contraceptive users were at increased risk for CIN. The increase in cervical neoplasia was most prominent in those who used oral contraceptives for more than 5 to 10 years. Although these results may be affected by other confounding factors, the patients taking oral contraceptives should have at least annual cytologic screening (see cytology discussion), since they have 2 to 4 times the risk of developing CIN.

Cigarette smoking has also been implicated as a factor. Brinton et al. found a relative risk of 1.5 for the development of cervical neoplasia among women who smoke. Slattery et al. noted a significant increased risk of cervical neoplasia for those who smoke, as well as those who are exposed to "passive smoke." A mechanism was suggested by the studies of Hellberg et al. who found nicotine and its metabolite contine in the cervical mucus of smokers.

Radiation has also been considered as a potential factor in CIN. Cervical dysplasia has been reported in cytologic (Pap) smears in patients after irradiation therapy for carcinoma of the cervix. If these patients with so-called radiation dysplasia are carefully followed, they are found to be at increased risk for the development of recurrent disease compared with those who do not show radiation dysplasia changes. However, it is not clear if this radiation dysplasia is a result of the radiation or is an early morphologic cellular change that precedes the development of recurrent cancer. A definitive role for radiation in the development of CIN has not been established.

Intrauterine diethylstilbestrol (DES) exposure is discussed in detail in Chapter 14. Because of the enlarged transformation zone that occurs in the cervix and occasionally the vagina of these females with concomitant larger areas of squamous metaplasia, there is concern that such patients may be at increased risk for squamous neoplasia. Although such patients require regular medical surveillance for the development of squamous neoplasia, current evidence has not established that DES exposure is a risk factor for cervical squamous neoplasia.

Vitamins have also been evaluated as potential risk factors. Animal studies have suggested that deficiencies in vitamin A can promote neoplasia. Vitamin A deficiencies in humans have been associated with dysplastic-type changes in cytologic smears of the cervix, and these changes have been reversed by vitamin A administration. Some studies have been undertaken to evaluate vitamin A analogues (retinoids) in regard to their ability to prevent or reverse CIN. Surwit et al. studied transretinoic acid in 18 patients with CIN II or III: one third improved, but half experienced severe vaginal burning, which in some cases required discontinuation of the drug. Romney et al. noted a deficiency of vitamin C in patients who had an abnormal Pap smear in comparison to those who had normal smears, and they suggested that vitamin C deficiency might be a factor.

Viral Hypothesis

Human Papillomavirus

Papillomaviruses belong to the Papovaviridae family. They are double-stranded deoxyribonucleic acid (DNA) viruses that replicate within epithelial cells. They are commonly associated with genital warts and have been ex-

tensively studied in the past few years for their potential role in the genesis of CIN. Human papillomavirus (HPV) does not cause systemic infection. For many years there has been indirect evidence for a role of the papillomavirus in CIN. Malignant transformation of papillomas in animals exposed to the papillomavirus has been observed, and human papilloma warts have also been noted to undergo malignant transformation. Like HSV II (see following section), papillomaviruses are sexually transmitted, and infections have been identified in the male partners of infected females; these females appear to be at increased risk for CIN. In addition, papillomaviral infections have been noted by Meisels and Morin to precede invasive carcinoma of the cervix by 27.5 years.

In recent years extensive evidence has accumulated linking HPV to CIN. HPV causes distinct cellular changes, the most common of which is koilocytosis (perinuclear cavitation) (Figure 26-9). These cells are found in genital warts and are frequently identified in areas of intraepithelial neoplasia. Papillomaviral particles have been identified by electron microscopy in the nuclei of koilocytes (Figure 26-10). Some of the morphologic changes of HPV infection mimic the changes of mild dysplasia (CIN I). The rapid increase in knowledge regarding HPV has affected both the diagnosis and the current management of atypias of the cervix. The cytologic and histologic features of HPV infection of the lower female genital tract are illustrated in Figure 26-11.

HPVs are classified by DNA-hybridization techniques, which differentiate the major DNA composition of the viruses. Each type is designated by a number, depending upon the order in which the type is discovered. More than 60 human types have been described, and new ones can be anticipated to be discovered. The subject has been extensively reviewed by Wright and Richart and Crum et al.

Several DNA-hybridization techniques have been used to study and characterize HPVs. One must have a general understanding of these techniques to interpret the varying results of the many studies published. The *Southern blot technique* has been frequently used and was the basis of the characterization of HPV-DNA in vulvar warts and vulvar neoplasia by zur Hausen and other researchers. Regardless of the technique, the identification depends on the hybridization between a spe-

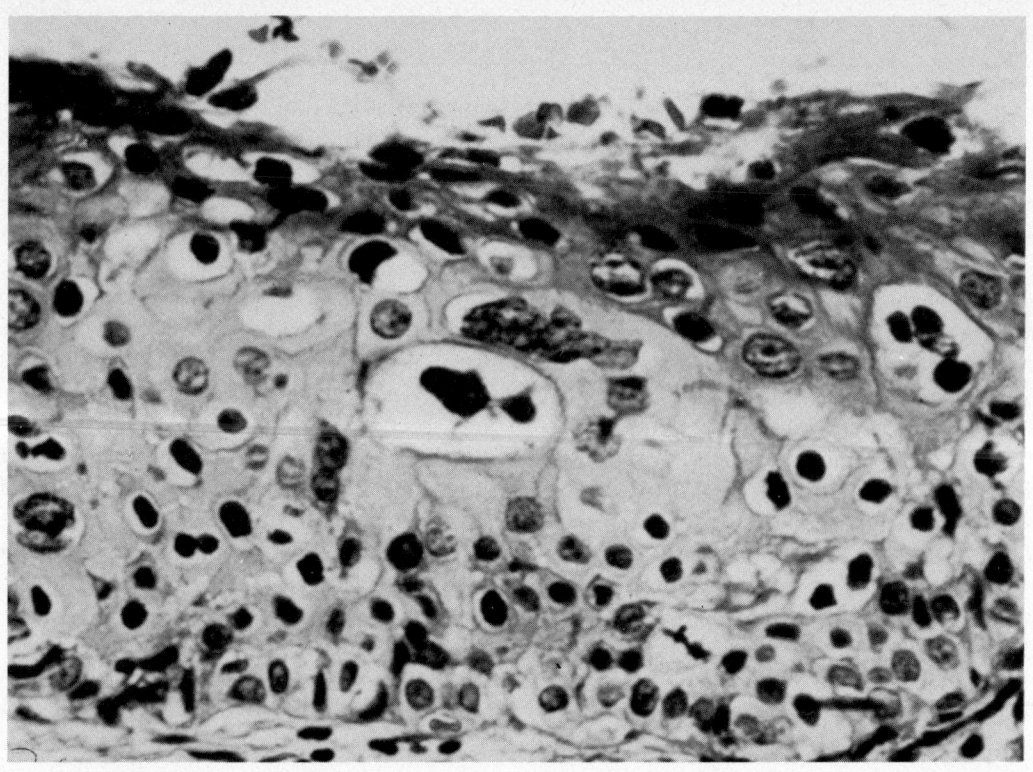

FIGURE 26-9
Human papillomavirus changes: koilocytosis, multinucleation, parakeratosis, and dyskeratosis. (Light microscopy: H&E stain.) (From Grunebaum AN, Sedlis A, Sillman F, et al: Obstet Gynecol 62:448, 1983. Reprinted with permission from The American College of Obstetricians and Gynecologists.)

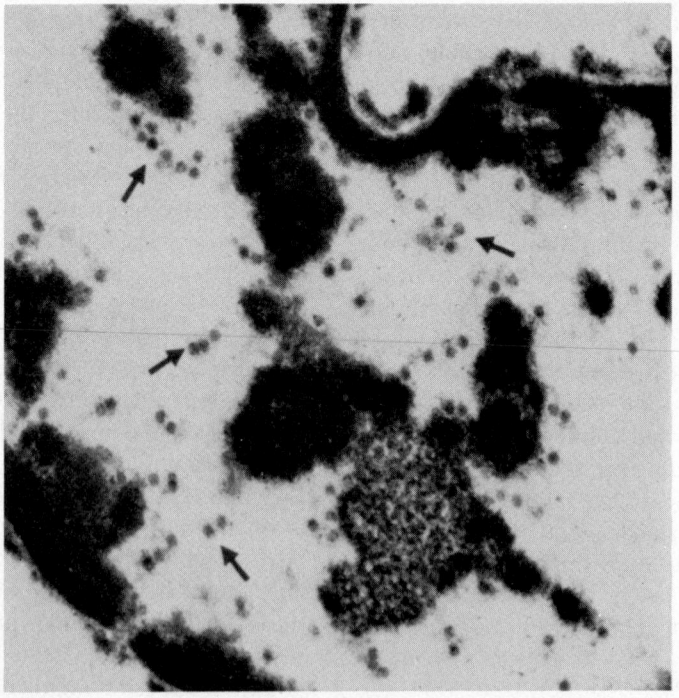

FIGURE 26-10
Higher magnification of Figure 26-9. Human papillomavirus particles *(arrows)* measure 45 to 50 nm within nucleus. (TEM; ×39,900.) (From Grunebaum AN, Sedlis A, Sillman F, et al: Obstet Gynecol 62:448, 1983. Reprinted with permission from The American College of Obstetricians and Gynecologists.)

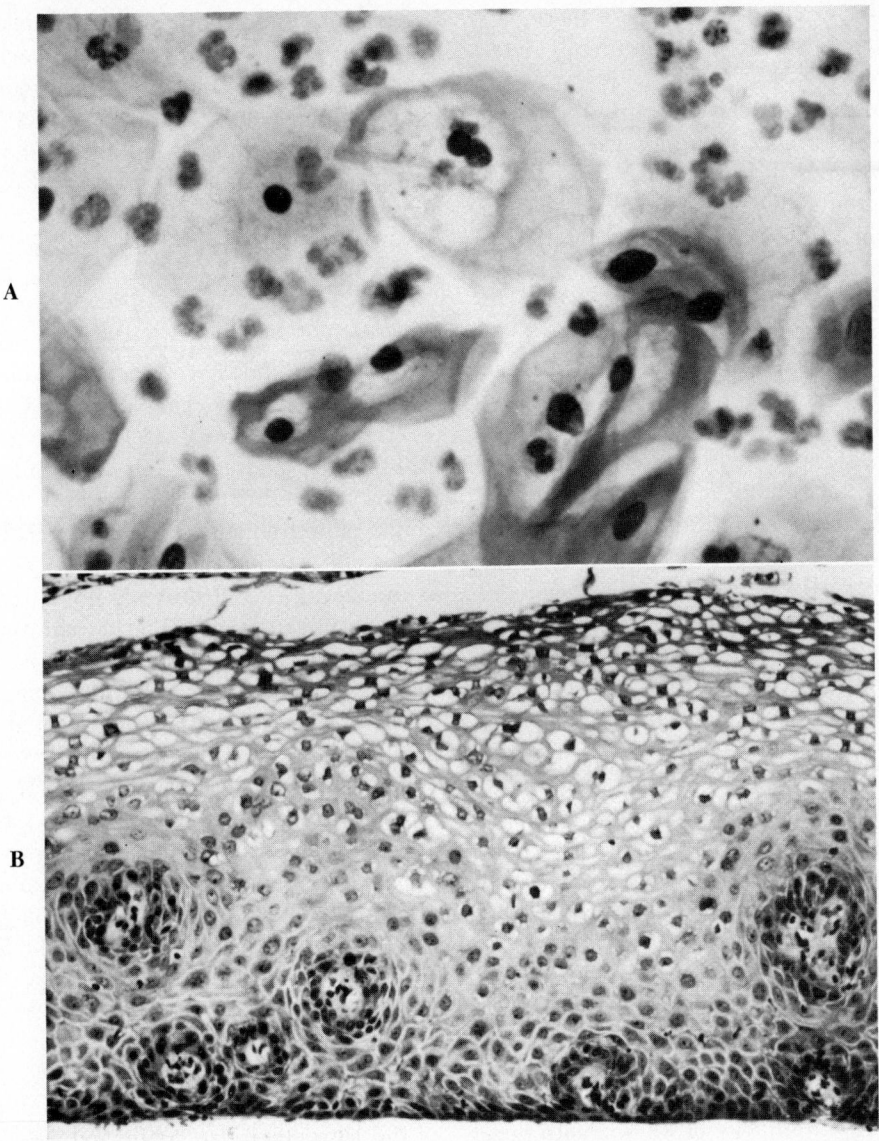

FIGURE 26-11
A, Typical koilocytic cells in HPV infection of uterine cervix. Note cavitation of cytoplasm, binucleation, and pyknotic nuclei. (Papanicolaou stain; ×400.) **B,** Condyloma of uterine cervix. Note koilocytes in superficial layers of epithelium and many binucleated cells. (H&E stain; ×240.) (Courtesy Marluce Bibbo, M.D.)

cific DNA or ribonucleic acid (RNA) probe and the target HPV in the cell. Some studies have used a *dot-blot procedure,* which depends on HPV-DNA hybridization but eliminates the electrophoretic step needed with the Southern blot technique. Both are sensitive but time consuming. Techniques are also available to study formalin-processed tissue sections already fixed in paraffin, called *in situ hybridization.* These can be performed without radioac-

tive probes. However, the technique is much less sensitive than the Southern or the dot-blot procedure. A much more sensitive technique recently introduced is known as the *polymerase chain reaction* (PCR). It involves the enzymatic amplification of DNA sequences and is reported to be capable of detecting a single HPV molecule in a million cells, compared with the Southern blot technique, which is reported to require about one copy per hundred cells. The precise sensitivity and specificity of these various techniques have not been accurately determined.

Numerous studies have reported different HPV types associated with various genital lesions. HPV types 6 and 11 have been associated most frequently with benign condyloma, whereas types 16, 18, and occasionally 31 have often been associated with neoplasia. Some have called the latter "high-risk viruses." HPV 18 has particularly been associated with high-grade CIN lesions, and Kurman et al. suggest this type of virus may be associated with more rapid transition to carcinoma. Many other types have been described less frequently, including HPV 33, 35, 39, 40, 43, 45, 51 to 56, and 58, which appear to be of intermediate risk.

Unfortunately, numerous exceptions exist. For example, HPV 6 and 11 have been described in cervical carcinomas. Willett et al. noted that multiple HPV types were associated with varying degrees of CIN. Moreover, as noted by Kurman et al., diagnostic and therapeutic decisions cannot currently be made on the basis of HPV typing but should be based on morphologic criteria. Nonetheless, commercial kits approved by the Food and Drug Administration (FDA) have become available in the United States. They are based on in situ DNA hybridization, but current evidence indicates they should not be used in patient management because their results are not clinically relevant. The difficulty of basing conclusions on HPV typing was recently emphasized by Tidy et al., who used the sensitive PCR technique and noted HPV 16 in 84% of women with negative cervical cytology, suggesting a more widespread prevalence of this viral type than previously reported. A 1991 Study by Nieminen et al. using commercially available probes for HPV typing concluded no HPV specific types were detected in the various cytologic atypias. Current Centers for Disease Control (CDC) recommendations are that HPV-DNA typing not be used for clinical management.

Nonetheless, the strong associations between HPV and CIN suggest a causative role for the virus. As noted by Koss, HPV is a prime candidate for transforming the cervical epithelial cell. Repeated infections or perhaps other viral infections are needed to promote the change, and environmental or hormonal factors previously discussed may also play a role. These various factors could then combine to lead to genetic changes, producing neoplasia. Such events are supported by the studies of protoon-cogenes by Riou et al., who noted deletion and mutation in the C-ha-*ras* gene in cervical cancers and amplification of C-*myc* gene. Oncogene amplification (Ha- RAS and C-MYC) have been recently reported in CIN III and invasive carcinoma in comparison to normal cervix and CIN I by Pinion et al. Most of these changes were associated with HPV infection.

Herpesvirus

Various studies have related genital tract infections with herpes simplex virus II (HSV II) to cervical carcinoma. The herpesvirus elicits antibody responses in humans, and elevated serum antibody titers to HSV II have been found more frequently among women with premalignant and malignant cervical lesions. Moreover, elevated antibody titers to this virus have also been observed in Jewish women with cervical carcinoma. The virus has been detected in tissues from cervical carcinoma, and viral antigens have also been detected in carcinoma tissues. Cervical carcinoma has also been found to contain antibodies to HSV II antigens. The virus has been found to be capable of transforming mammalian cells in vitro and of producing tumors in experimental animals. Although HSV II is suspect in the etiology of cervical cancer, a definitive cause-and-effect relationship has not been established.

Cytomegalovirus

The cytomegalovirus is the largest member of the Herpetoviridae family and also has been studied for its potential role in cervical carcinogenesis. It is transmitted by sexual contact, and a limited number of seroepidemiologic studies have shown elevated antibody titers in women with cervical cancer. The viral particles have been uncovered in cervical carcinoma biopsies, and in vitro malignant cellular transformation has been observed. Although a potential agent in the etiology of cervical carcinoma, cytomegalovirus has not been as extensively studied as HSV II and is not currently thought to have a major role in cervical carcinogenesis.

DIAGNOSIS AND MANAGEMENT

In considering the changes of intraepithelial neoplasia it must be recognized that the morphology of the cervical epithelium is also altered by HPV infection and that koilocytosis

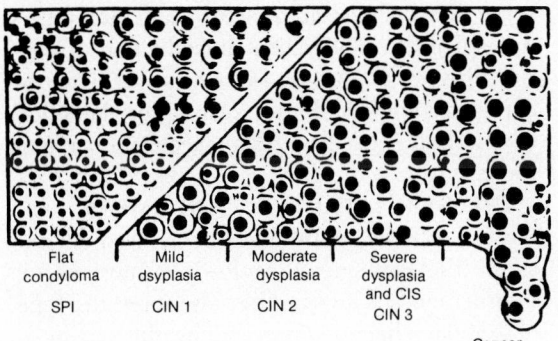

FIGURE 26-12

Schematic model explaining interrelationships between different grades of disorders and showing nomenclature division, according to the proportion of cells exhibiting morphologic features of either late viral expression *(left half)* or premalignant change *(right half)*. (From Reid R and Fu YS: In Peto R, editor: Banbury Report 21: viral etiology of cervical cancer, Cold Spring Harbor, NY, 1986. Copyright © Cold Spring Harbor Laboratory, 1986.)

(see Figure 26-9) can be accompanied by nuclear changes that on cytologic smear and biopsy resemble the alterations normally identified with CIN. Reid et al. have extensively studied HPV infections and their role in neoplasia. They and others have used the term *subclinical papillomavirus infection* (SPI) to describe an entity that is not clinically visible to the naked eye but that can be recognized utilizing the colposcope and staining the vagina and cervix with acetic acid (see colposcopy section). Subclinical HPV infection and clinically evident condyloma constitute important manifestations of HPV infection of the lower genital tract; some of these infections may eventually lead to malignant transformation, as previously discussed. The spectrum of such changes, including SPI, is shown in Figure 26-12, which is a modification of the concept initially introduced by Richart (see Figure 26-1).

The morphologic manifestations of HPV infection, such as koilocytosis and papillomatosis, are most prominent in the early premalignant lesions, such as mild dysplasia (CIN I), and decrease as the more severe alterations of the cervical epithelium occur. Moreover, it appears that some diagnoses reported as dysplasia in the past may in fact have been HPV infection. Furthermore, it is important to emphasize that the detection of HPV does not imply clinical disease. Therapy is limited to women who have clinically evident or symptomatic condyloma or morphologic evidence of neoplasia.

Risks of Progression and Natural History

What are the rates of progression of premalignant lesions of the cervix? Precise data are not available. However, Richart and Barron estimated transit times from mild, moderate, or severe dysplasia to carcinoma in situ to have a median duration of 44 months for all of the dysplasias. The shortest duration of progression was 12 months for severe dysplasia, while the longest was 86 months for mild dysplasia. Koss et al. studied 93 women with untreated CIS and observed that it did progress to invasive carcinoma. However, they also noted that cervical biopsy could occasionally eradicate the lesion, and in addition spontaneous disappearance of carcinoma in situ rarely occurred. In more recent studies of mild and moderate cervical dysplasia, Nasiell et al. used cervical cytology or biopsy to follow women in the Stockholm area from 1962 to 1983. Regression to normal from mild dysplasia occurred in 62% of the cases, while progression to more severe lesions of carcinoma in situ or severe dysplasia occurred in 16%, and two cases of invasive cancer were noted. The remaining 22% had persistence of mild dysplasia. In a similar study of moderate dysplasia, the same authors noted that regression occurred in 54% over 6 years, progression to severe dysplasia or carcinoma in situ in 30%, and persistence of severe dysplasia in 16%. The complexity of the problem was noted by Carmichael and Maskens, who studied 235 women with mild to moderate dysplasia accompanied by HPV infection. In up to 24 months of follow-up, only 9 (5.5%) progressed while 134 (57%) regressed and the remainder were unchanged, suggesting that the progression rate in these HPV lesions may be quite low.

While some have concern in regard to these studies, particularly with diagnoses based only on cytology findings, biopsies were done on many of the patients and the results are consistent with the concept that the risk of progression of CIN is higher for those with high-grade lesions but that spontaneous regression of these lesions can also occur. Current evidence suggests a slow progression to invasive cancer from CIN, but the risk of such progression is small and usually takes many months or years to occur. The studies of McIndoe et al. from the early 1980s indicate the risk is greatly elevated in patients with persistent abnormal cytology after treatment. In their series, 29 of 131 patients (22%) subsequently developed invasive carcinoma. Current techniques do not allow accurate prediction concerning how fast any particular lesion will progress.

Methods of Detection and Diagnosis

The Papanicolaou (Pap) smear has been used widely for about 50 years to screen large populations of women for malignant and premalignant cervical disease. Its usage has been effective to reduce the frequency of invasive carcinoma of the cervix. It is essential to realize that cervical cytology is useful only for screening, and its results do not establish definitive diagnosis. False negative and false positive results can also occur. For example, in the detection of cervical carcinoma it is estimated that approximately 5% to 10% of the cases will be missed by routine cytologic screening because of sampling variation or other technical difficulties that may contribute to a false negative result. Similarly, certain conditions can cause the cells on the smear to appear atypical and mimic neoplastic changes. Examples are severe cervical infection, *Trichomonas vaginalis* infection, herpesvirus infection (which can cause cellular nuclear change), and HPV infections leading to koilocytosis (see Figure 26-9). All these may cause confusion of interpretation of the Pap smear, especially for the less experienced cytologist. Once a Pap smear suggestive of CIN is reported, the patient should be reexamined and the smear repeated to verify the findings. Colposcopic evaluation is performed and a biopsy obtained to establish the diagnosis.

Cytology

TECHNIQUE. The Pap smear is best obtained by taking a direct scrape (sample) from the tissue being studied. This is usually accomplished by exposing the cervix after introducing a speculum into the vagina and using a wood or plastic spatula to scrape the exocervix and endocervix separately so as to include the entire transformation zone (Figure 26-13). Many centers obtain a separate smear initially from the vagina and from the cervix and endocervix (V, vaginal; C, cervical; E, endocervical), and these are placed on a glass slide. The cellular specimen is immediately fixed, either in 90% alcohol or sprayed with fixative. It is important to hold the fixative spray more than 12 inches (30 cm) from the smear and not to allow the smear to air dry before fixing in order to preserve the cellular architecture and not introduce artifacts. The recent introduction of narrow brushes (Figure 26-14) to sample the endocervix has yielded better results for detection of neoplastic cells from this inaccessible area of the cervix.

INTERPRETATION OF THE SMEAR. Numerous classifications have been used to describe the Pap smear results. The most useful information is conveyed by describing the type of cellular changes observed by the cytology. One classification used for many years is demonstrated in the box below. It is very important that the smear be interpreted by laboratories with adequate volumes to maintain diagnostic skills. It is recommended that a cytopathologist annually supervise at least 25,000 cervical smears to achieve this. Cytologists also frequently indicate the type of inflammation or infection that may exist if morphologic changes that allow infectious agents, such as herpesvirus, HPV, *Chlamydia,* or *Trichomonas vaginalis,* to be identified. Figures 26-2 to 26-7 illustrate the various cytologic changes that correspond to the various types of cervical neoplasia that are also demonstrated histologically.

In the past, cervical smears were classified in five categories: class I, benign; class II, inflammation; class III, mild to moderate atypia consistent with dysplasia; class IV, severe atypia consistent with severe dysplasia or carcinoma in situ; and class V, suggestive of invasion of cancer. This classification for Pap smear results has been discarded. Recently in the United States a new terminology has been introduced, the Bethesda System, based on a conference sponsored by the National Institutes of Health (NIH) in 1988 and summarized by Solomon. The Bethesda classification is summarized in the box on p. 838. Currently, some controversy

---

TRADITIONAL CLASSIFICATION OF PAPANICOLAOU SMEAR

Normal
Metaplasia
Inflammation
Minimal atypia—koilocytosis
Mild dysplasia (CIN I)
Moderate dysplasia (CIN II)
Severe dysplasia—carcinoma in situ (CIN III)
Invasive carcinoma

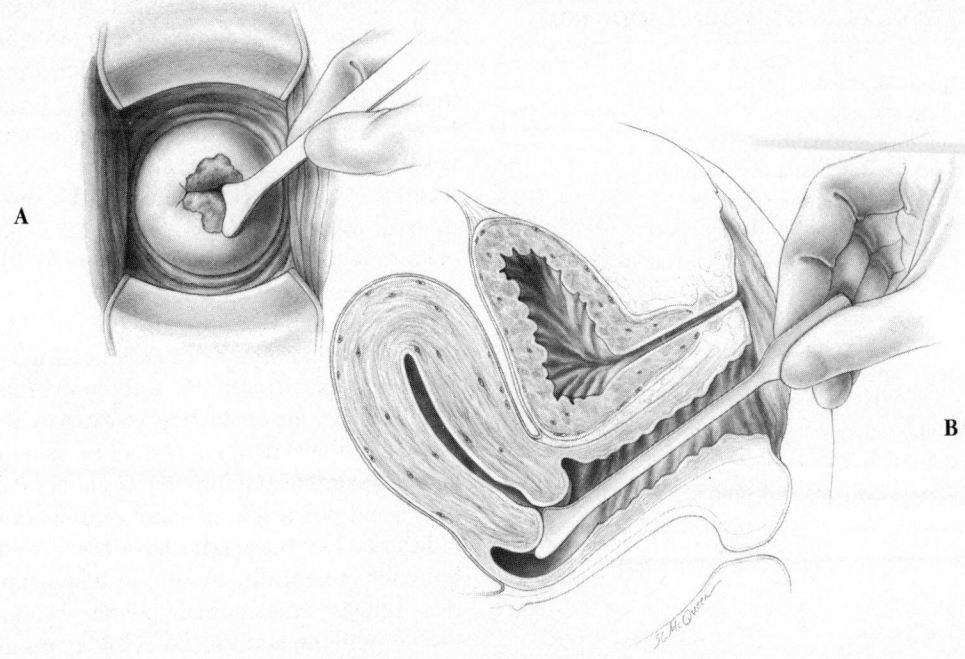

FIGURE 26-13
A, Scrape of endocervix. **B,** Scrape of exocervix.

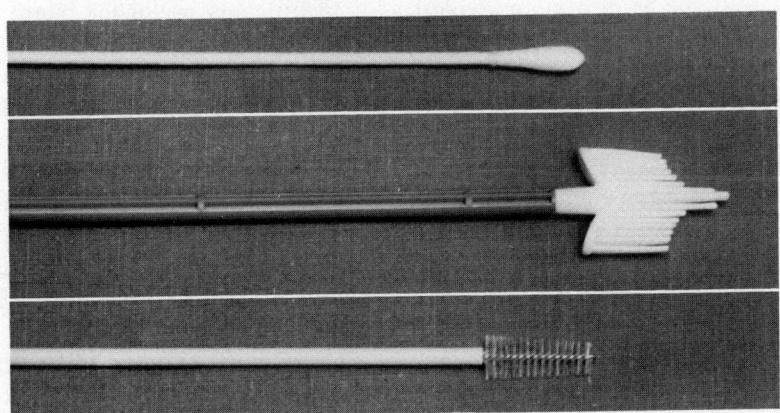

FIGURE 26-14
Narrow brushes for endocervical sampling. *Top,* Q-Tip; *middle,* Cervix Brush (Unimar); *bottom,* Cytobrush (Medscand).

exists among gynecologists and cytologists regarding this terminology, which lumps koilocytosis with intraepithelial neoplasia and provides a two-tier system by combining CIN II and III into the category of high-grade squamous intraepithelial lesion. In this system koilocytosis and mild dysplasia are considered low-grade squamous intraepithelial lesions. Although the system is widely supported, especially among cytologists in the United States, it has not been accepted worldwide and, as recently noted by Koss, may require modification. However,

based on the descriptions in the box on p. 836, the clinician can proceed with diagnosis and management, as well as if the report uses the Bethesda System, since the latter also allows the use of these descriptive terms.

If severe inflammation or infection is present, it should be treated as outlined in Chapter 21. In the case of nonspecific or so-called mild atypia, it is often necessary only to repeat the smear in 4 to 6 months. Similar follow-up is appropriate for women who have only koilocytosis (koilocytic atypia) without neoplas-

BETHESDA CLASSIFICATION (MODIFIED)

Adequacy of smear
Infection type
Squamous abnormalities
    Reactive (inflammatory change)
    Epithelial cell abnormalities
        Atypical type, undetermined
        Squamous intraepithelial lesions (SILs)
            Low grade: HPV or mild dysplasia
                (CIN I)
            High grade: moderate to severe dys-
                plasia–carcinoma in situ (CIN II-
                III)
Glandular cells
    Atypical and source
    Adenocarcinoma and source

tic change. If more severe changes are found, the cytologist may recommend additional diagnostic procedures, such as colposcopy or further biopsy. If the cytologic smear indicates mild or moderate dysplasia or a more atypical lesion, colposcopy is done and usually a biopsy is performed, with therapy dependent on biopsy results.

CYTOLOGIC SCREENING GUIDELINES. The ideal frequency for Pap smear screening is not established, and disagreement exists in regard to the interval between examinations for cytologic screening of the cervix. Much of the disagreement is in regard to the cost-effectiveness of such screening and is based on studies of large populations. For example, the so-called Walton Report from Canada recommended annual smears when the individual becomes sexually active, to be repeated up to age 35. From age 36 on, screening is done only once every 5 years after two negative tests, and beyond age 60 it is discontinued after two negative tests. In contrast, the American College of Obstetricians and Gynecologists (ACOG) and the International Academy of Cytology recommend that cytologic screening start at age 18 or when the individual becomes sexually active and continue annually indefinitely. Development of cervical cancer has been reported to occur within 3 to 4 years after a negative Pap smear. In addition, even after hysterectomy the risk for neoplasia remains. Stuart et al., in a study of 29 cases of vaginal cancer, noted a 5.7-year interval for diagnosis of cancer after hysterectomy when the operation was performed for CIN. When hysterectomy was performed for benign disease, the interval was 13.1 years. A recent retrospective study of women with cervical cancer by Shy et al. suggested an increased risk of cervical cancer if the screening interval exceeds 2 years. Table 26-1 shows a composite of recommended intervals for Pap smear screening.

An additional factor for the physician to consider is the importance of an annual pelvic examination, particularly for women over age 40, which allows for evaluation of ovarian size. In general, for women interested in an effective health maintenance program, an annual Pap smear and pelvic and physical examinations are indicated. For those who have had a hysterectomy for benign disease and in whom the ovaries remain, an annual pelvic examination should be done and vaginal cytology performed every 3 to 5 years.

Biopsy

Instruments useful for biopsy of the cervix are shown in Figure 26-15. The punch biopsy is capable of removing a small tissue sample 2 to 3 mm in size from the cervix. The colposcopically directed biopsy can easily be obtained in the office without anesthesia. Once the biopsy specimen is taken, it is usually fixed immediately in either Bouin's solution or formalin. It is important that each specimen be placed in a separate container and appropriately labeled.

Current convention is to identify the location of the exocervix using the position of the 12 hours of the clock (Figure 26-16). An endocervical curette is used to obtain an endocervical curettage (ECC) specimen. To obtain an ade-

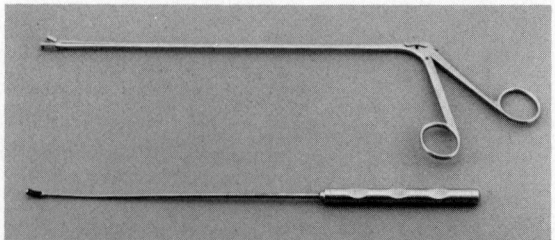

FIGURE 26-15
Cervical biopsy instruments. *Above,* Punch biopsy; *below,* endocervical curette.

TABLE 26-1
Recommendations on the Frequency of Pap Testing

	ACOG (1980)	American Cancer Society (1980)	Canadian Task Force (1982)	International Academy of Cytology (1980)	National Cancer Institute (1980)
Start	Age 18 or when sexually active	Age 20 or when sexually active	When sexually active	Age 18 or when sexually active	When sexually active
Age 18-35	Annually	Annually until two negative tests; then continue every 3 years	Annually if sexually active	—	After two negative tests, continue every 1-3 years
Age 36-60	Annually	At least every 3 years; more frequently if high risk; pelvic examination should be done annually after age 40	After two negative tests, continue every 5 years	Annually	Every 1-3 years
Over age 60	Annually	At least every 3 years; more frequently if high risk; pelvic examination should be done annually	After two negative tests, testing may be stopped	Annually	After two negative tests, testing may be stopped

Modified from American College of Obstetricians and Gynecologists (ACOG) Newsletter, June 1984.

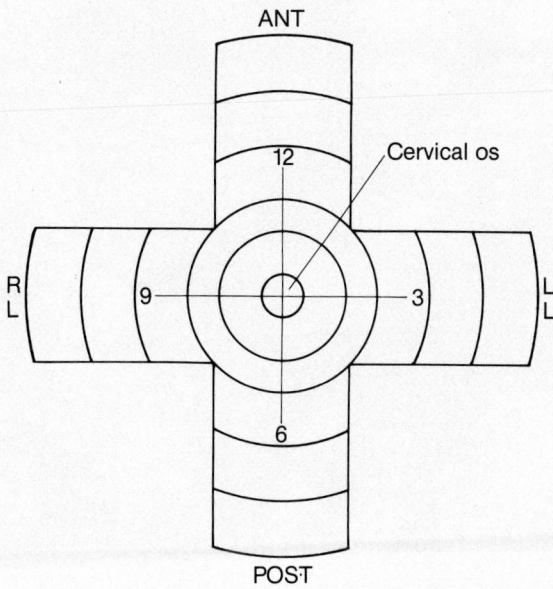

FIGURE 26-16
Diagram using the positions of the 12 hours of the clock; utilized during examination of cervix to record position of any abnormality.

quate sample, the curette is introduced into the endocervix approximately 1 to 2 cm, and firm pressure is applied to obtain a sample from the four quadrants of the endocervix. This part of the procedure often causes discomfort to the patient, and the administration of an oral analgesic is occasionally helpful. Usually the examination can be completed without analgesia. The ECC specimens are grouped together in one container and submitted to pathology, since it is important to only ascertain whether neoplasia exists in the cervical canal. It is not feasible to identify which portion of the canal contains abnormal epithelium.

Colposcopy

The colposcope is a magnifying instrument used to identify those abnormal cervical areas that require biopsy. The pertinent area is the transformation zone, which may be either nor-

mal or abnormal. A normal transformation zone, as previously noted, is the junction of normal columnar epithelium and squamous metaplasia, while the abnormal transformation zone contains patterns that may indicate the presence of neoplastic tissue or a premalignant process.

Colposcopic examination is usually performed at 10 to 16 magnification. After excess mucus is gently wiped away from the cervix and the Pap smear has been taken, 3% acetic acid is applied. The colposcopic examination is usually performed using a green filter. Normal columnar epithelium will often produce a grapelike pattern, while squamous metaplasia appears as a smooth, gray-white epithelium after the application of acetic acid (Figure 26-17). The native squamous epithelium outside the transformation zone has a smooth, red-tan appearance.

An abnormal transformation zone may be marked by white areas with red stippling

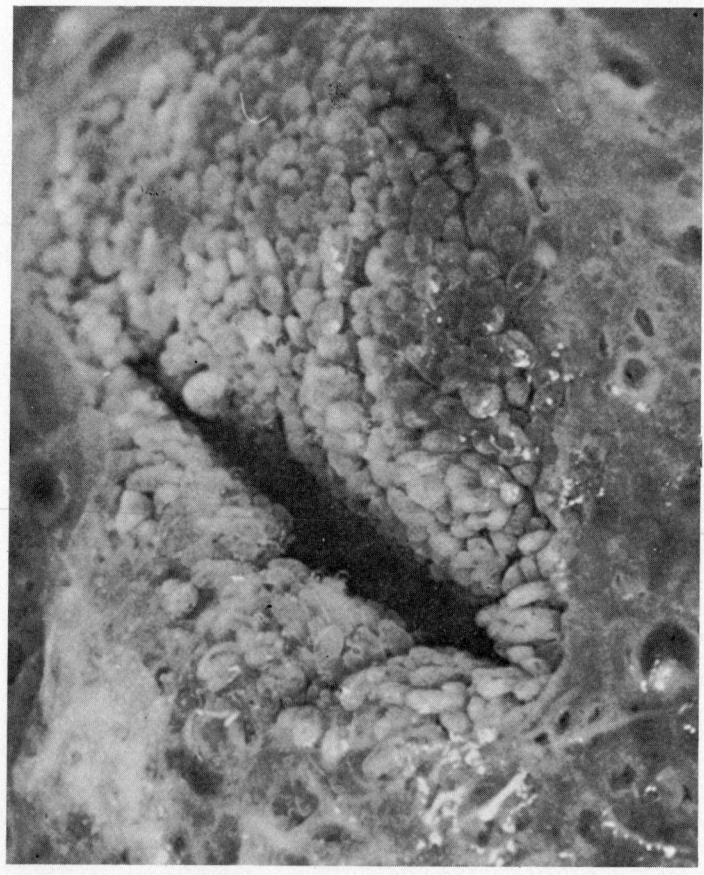

FIGURE 26-17
Typical transformation zone. The distal portion of columnar (grapelike) epithelium is replaced by a crescentic sheet of white metaplastic epithelium. At its inner edge it adjoins columnar epithelium. (From Coppleson M, Pixley E, and Reid B: Colposcopy—a scientific and practical approach to the cervix in health and disease, Springfield, IL, 1971, Charles C Thomas, Publisher.)

(punctation), sharp-bordered lesions with vessels in a mosaic pattern (mosaic), white tissue with sharp borders (white epithelium), or atypical vessels. The white epithelium is seen best after acetic acid application and results from the piling up of cells with an increased nuclear-cytoplasmic ratio. A mosaic pattern results from neovascularization with capillaries running just beneath the surface epithelium, whereas punctation results from capillaries growing perpendicular to the surface. In addition, some areas may appear white before the application of acetic acid (leukoplakia).

The main criteria used by the colposcopist to establish the degree of atypicality and identify the sites for subsequent biopsies are (1) the vascular pattern (arrangement of the capillaries), (2) the distance between the capillaries, (3) the intensity of color tone after the addition of acetic acid, (4) the surface pattern (regular or irregular), and (5) the sharpness of the border of the suspected site in comparison to adjacent tissues. In general, the more severe lesions have a deeper whitish tone and greater width and irregularity in the intracapillary distance. Abnormal vessels may be present in advanced lesions. In addition, the surface appears irregular and the vessels are coarser.

As shown by Rome et al., the high-grade intraepithelial lesions are usually found in large abnormal transformation zones (63 mm^2), whereas small abnormal transformation zones (46 mm^2) are associated with low-grade lesions. A large abnormal transformation zone should heighten the examiner's suspicion of a high-grade lesion and possibly an invasive carcinoma. Similarly, atypical vessels usually indicate a high-grade intraepithelial lesion or invasive cancer.

An additional diagnostic criterion is the presence of *aceto-white epithelium*. This is tissue that initially looks normal but takes a white color after acetic acid is applied. The areas are found outside the transformation zone and, as previously noted, frequently contain HPV infection (SPI, "flat warts," or "flat condyloma"). A clinically evident condyloma is illustrated in Figure 26-18, and an example of intraepithelial neoplasia is shown in Figure 26-19, which demonstrates punctation and variably sized mosaic structures. For a detailed description of the important colposcopic changes of the abnormal transformation zone and their interpretation, the reader should consult an atlas of colposcopy.

Only if the entire transformation zone can be seen colposcopically and if biopsies are obtained from the most abnormal areas is the examination considered technically satisfactory. If the transformation zone extends into the endocervical canal above the examiner's vision, the colposcopic examination is termed unsatisfactory, and diagnostic conization (see later discussion) is usually performed. If the colposcopic examination is technically satisfactory, multiple biopsy specimens are taken of the most abnormal areas. Before initiating outpatient therapy, an ECC is usually performed, even though the entire transformation zone can be seen. A scheme for the colposcopic evaluation of the abnormal Pap smear is shown in the box below. The biopsy results of the abnormal areas are compared with the results of the cytologic examination to verify that the tissue samples appear to be representative of the abnormal cells identified cytologically. Precise agreement between the cytologic and histologic diagnoses is not necessary and often does not occur. However, it is vital that an invasive carcinoma not be missed, and the degree of atypicality found cytologically must be adequately explained by the tissue obtained on biopsy.

MANAGEMENT

General Principles

The general principle to be followed in the therapy of CIN is the eradication of the abnor-

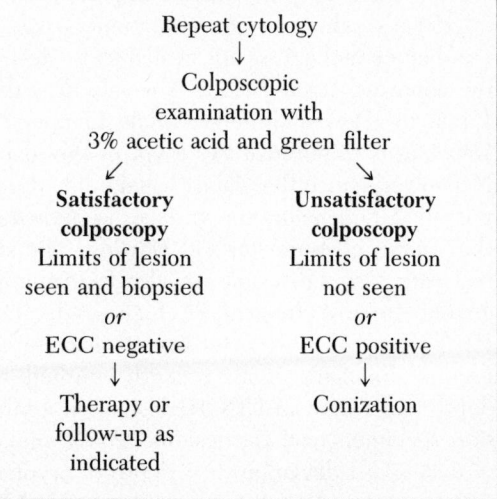

EVALUATION OF ABNORMAL PAP SMEAR

Repeat cytology
↓
Colposcopic
examination with
3% acetic acid and green filter
↙ ↘
Satisfactory   **Unsatisfactory**
colposcopy   **colposcopy**
Limits of lesion   Limits of lesion
seen and biopsied   not seen
or   *or*
ECC negative   ECC positive
↓   ↓
Therapy or   Conization
follow-up as
indicated

ECC, Endocervical curettage.

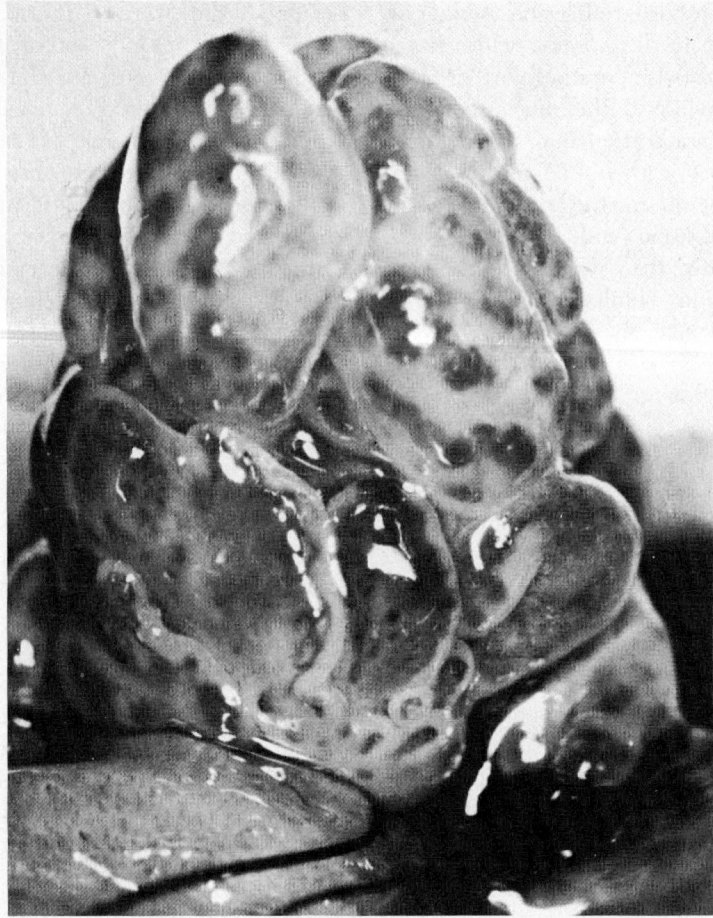

FIGURE 26-18
Condylomata acuminata of the vagina. These wartlike papillomata may be found on the vulva, in the vagina, and on the ectocervix. The vessels appear as dark areas surrounded by whitish epithelium. (×16.) (From Kolstad P and Stafl A: Atlas of colposcopy, Baltimore, 1972, University Park Press.)

mal epithelium. In many instances, this can be accomplished by procedures completed in the physician's office on an outpatient basis. A number of modalities are available to destroy the abnormal tissue, which is usually less than 1 mm to a few millimeters thick. Deeper destruction is required if the crypt of the glands is involved, since the glands usually lie approximately 5 mm below the surface, as shown by the studies of Anderson and Hartley. The size and extent of the lesion are also factors influencing therapy. In general, high grade (CIN III) lesions are more extensive than low-grade lesions. Boonstra et al. recently studied the depth and extent of CIN III lesions in conization specimens. Of the lesions, 97.7% (mean, + 2 standard deviation) had depth of crypt involvement less than 3.6 mm and extended lin-

early to the proximal border less than 19.3 mm from the cervical os. Moreover, similar to previous reports, younger patients had smaller transformation zones with a more ectocervical location. Also, in women over age 50, the depth of the crypt involvement increased significantly, indicating more extensive tissue destruction (if needed) for therapy of older patients.

For outpatient therapy to be effective, a colposcopic examination must be satisfactory and the entire transformation zone visualized. The biopsy results should provide appropriate consistency with the abnormal cells seen cytologically, as well as with the colposcopic appearance of the transformation zone. As shown by Stafl and Mattingly, there is usually no more than one degree of severity in the differ-

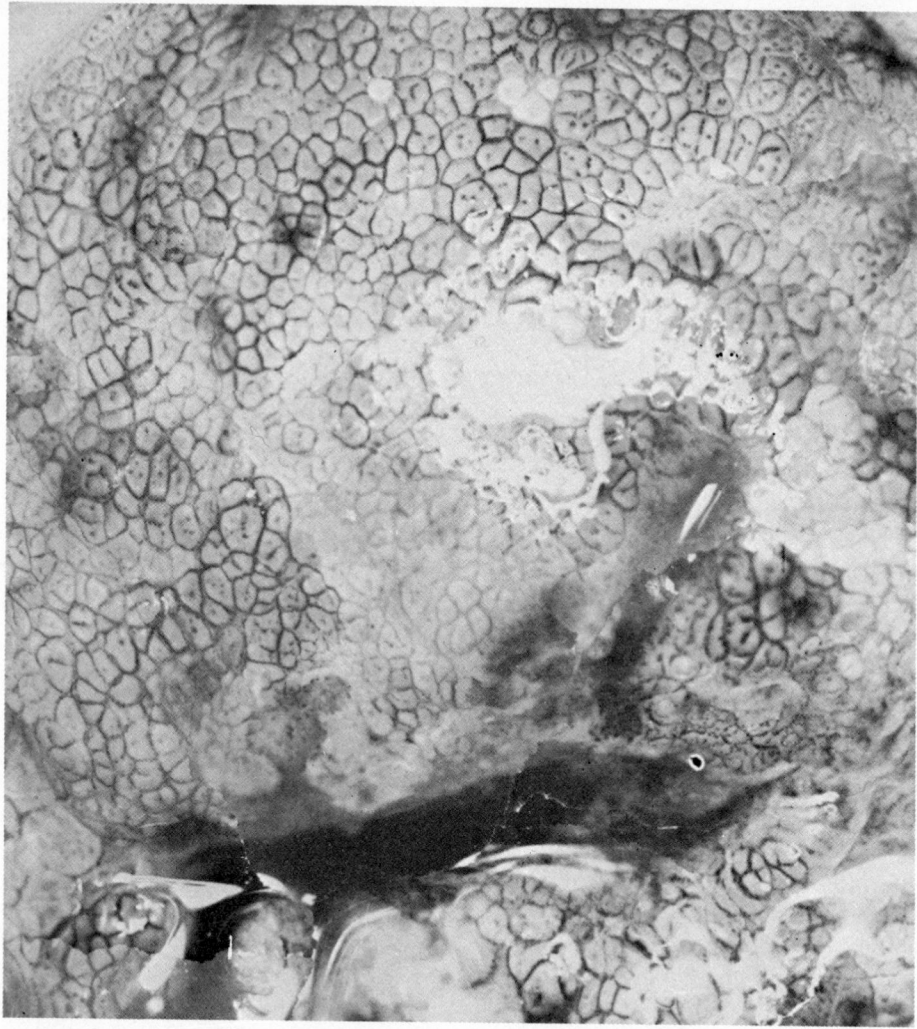

FIGURE 26-19
Extensive in situ carcinoma almost completely covers the visible part of ectocervix. The picture is dominated by coarse but regular mosaic vascular figures with greatly increased intercapillary distance. Atypical vessels are not to be seen. (×8). (From Kolstad P and Stafl A: Atlas of colposcopy, Baltimore, 1972, University Park Press.)

ences of diagnoses (mild dysplasia versus moderate dysplasia) between the colposcopic impression and the biopsy. If the colposcopic examination is technically unsatisfactory, that is, the entire transformation zone cannot be seen, or if there is marked disparity between the cytology and biopsy results, a conization is indicated. The recent studies of McCord et al. reconfirm the necessity of conization if two degrees of discrepancy exist between the cytologic and histologic findings. Hysterectomy is considered only after it is ascertained that the patient does not have invasive cancer and no longer wishes to maintain childbearing function. ECC is performed before outpatient therapy, and it is mandatory that the curettage

results be negative before office therapy is undertaken.

In recommending various treatment modalities, the physician is often faced with the problem of whether or not the cellular atypicalities noted cytologically or on biopsy are potentially premalignant. Furthermore the differentiation of active squamous metaplasia, which is found at puberty and during pregnancy, as well as in instances of tissue repair, can also produce a histomorphologic pattern that may be confused with neoplasia, as can papillomaviral infection (see later discussion). It may be difficult to make an accurate diagnosis using conventional histologic techniques, and marked differences of opinion regarding the correct diagnosis com-

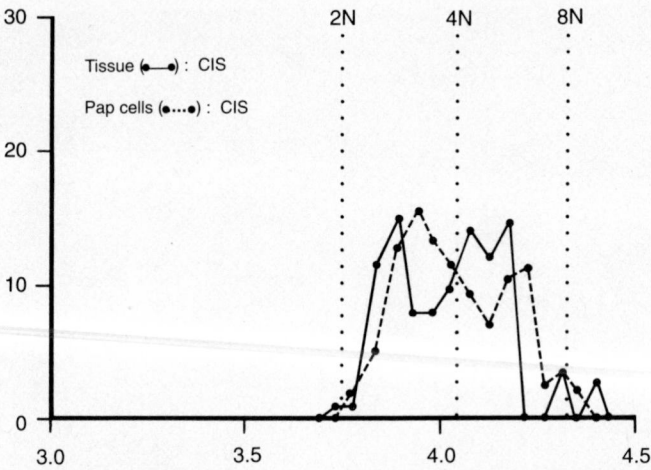

FIGURE 26-20

Histogram showing aneuploid distribution indicating neoplasia. In this case the tissue biopsy and cytology (Pap) results agree; 2N corresponds to a normal diploid pattern.

monly occur. Therefore it is reemphasized that it is important for the therapist to be certain that the histologic biopsy findings appear to explain the morphologic abnormalities found on the cytologic smear and the colposcopic examination.

To help with the problems of morphologic interpretation, efforts have been made to identify authentic premalignant lesions. One laboratory aid is to estimate the ploidy of the lesion by microspectrophotometric measurement of nuclear DNA. A Feulgen stain is used, and the tissue is analyzed by measuring the ploidy of the lesion and comparing the cells under study to normal lymphocytes. The normal lymphocyte has a diploid (2N) distribution, while metaplastic lesions usually are tetraploid (4N); premalignant and malignant lesions have an aneuploid distribution. Figure 26-20 demonstrates the analysis of a Pap smear and biopsy specimen. It should be noted that tetraploid lesions are occasionally also associated with low-grade neoplastic lesions as well. While this technique is primarily a laboratory investigative tool, recent refinements by Bibbo et al. suggest that it can be used for routine diagnostic utilization.

Papillomavirus Infection

If a clinically evident condyloma is identified (see Fig. 26-18), therapy of the affected area is usually undertaken. It is clear that not all HPV infections have premalignant potential. Moreover, some of the infections regress spontane-

ously. A reliable method to identify which lesions have neoplastic potential would be desirable but does not exist at the present time. The finding of koilocytosis on a cytologic preparation or biopsy does not indicate the need for therapy, and such patients sometimes are described as having koilocytic atypia. They should be periodically reevaluated, usually in one-half year. Reid and Fu have noted that SPI with a diploid pattern is seen with koilocytic atypia and metaplastic epithelium, while an aneuploid pattern is shown primarily with CIN that demonstrates little histologic evidence of HPV changes. Viral typing to distinguish HPV is a research tool and, as noted previously, cannot currently be applied for clinical management.

The current inability to differentiate possibly inconsequential from high-risk HPV infections emphasizes the difficulty in choosing therapy of these lesions. If all women with HPV infection were treated to prevent neoplasia, most patients would be treated unnecessarily. Insofar as malignant progression is uncommon and it appears to develop slowly, refinements in identifying the lesions which are premalignant will be needed in the future to provide a guide for therapy. If the female is treated, as has been emphasized by Levine et al., the male sexual partner should be evaluated and treated if condylomas are found. Krebs has noted that two thirds of male partners of females with dysplasia or condyloma have HPV genital warts, which he treated with cryotherapy, laser, or 5-FU. However, in a follow-up study he noted that therapy of the male did not seem to affect the rate of subsequent development of dysplasia in the female partner. However, the futility of trying to eradicate SPI in the female was emphasized by the studies of Riva et al., who performed extensive CO_2 laser vaporization of the lower female genital tract in 25 women with confirmed SPI. Significant febrile and pain morbidity resulted, and 88% of the patients still had evidence of SPI at follow-up examination.

For condylomata involving the cervix and vagina, the laser is often employed. For those only on the cervix, either the laser or cryotherapy is used. Cautery with anesthesia can also be used for cervicovaginal HPV infection and for isolated vaginal or cervical condylomata, local application of podophyllin in benzoin or a resin or application of trichloroacetic acid has been tried (Chapter 21) but occasionally can cause excess tissue slough. It is important that the patient douche 1 to 2 hours after the application to reduce normal tissue destruction. For cervical condyloma, electrocautery is also effective but requires anesthesia for use in the vagina.

Therapy of Intraepithelial Neoplasia—Ablative Treatment

Cryotherapy

Cryotherapy is often used to treat CIN. The freezing process results from rapid expansion of fluid, usually carbon dioxide or nitrous oxide, into the probe (Figure 26-21), which is placed against the cervix. The probe chosen depends on the size of the lesion to be treated, but the flat probes are commonly used, particularly since probes with long endocervical nipples can cause extensive destruction of the endocervix with resulting cervical stenosis. The contact is enhanced by putting water-soluble lubricating jelly on the tip of the probe, which is then applied closely against the cervix. While cryotherapy can be used in other areas, such as the vulva, local anesthesia is usually required, but no anesthesia is required for cervical treatment. Once the gas is released into the probe, an ice ball begins to form and is usually complete in a few minutes. It is important that the ice ball extend 4 to 5 mm beyond the edge of the lesion to ensure adequate freezing and destruction of abnormal epithelium. Usually the ball reaches its maximum size in about 3 to 5

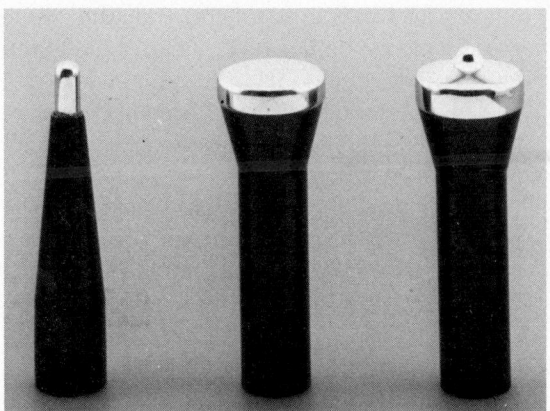

FIGURE 26-21
Three varieties of cryotherapy probes.

minutes, and after the ball thaws, a second freeze is usually carried out, particularly with large lesions and when more extensive tissue necrosis is desired (double-freeze technique). It is sometimes necessary to reapply the probe to a different area to treat larger areas of CIN adequately. For CIN III lesions, Boonstra et al. noted failures at the 3 and 9 o'clock positions (see Figure 26-16), presumably because of increased vascularity from cervical vessels, if the freeze lasted less than 5 minutes. They advocate the double-freeze technique.

Initial cure rates approximate 90% and averaged 89% for 4549 patients summarized from the literature in a review by Charles and Savage. Some have reported higher failure rates for carcinoma in situ (CIN III) using cryotherapy. This in part appears to be due to the extensive transformation zone usually seen with these lesions. There is also concern about the use of cryotherapy in lesions that involve the cervical crypts (gland involvement) on the grounds that such deep tissue might escape the effects of freezing. Anderson et al. noted that cure rates were lower after a single cryotreatment with high-grade lesions, particularly with endocervical involvement. Rates of cure with cryotherapy increase with the experience of the therapist as well as with the use of the double-freeze technique. In addition, results can be improved if careful follow-up is carried out and the patient is treated a second time, if needed.

After initial cryotherapy a follow-up examination is carried out in 4 months. Further evaluation is in accordance with the guidelines discussed for all CINs, that is, a smear every 6 months for 1 year to 18 months and, after three or four successive negative smears, annual follow-up indefinitely. It is recommended that ECC be performed at least once after freezing to be certain there is no disease in the canal after freezing.

A number of reports on the development of invasive carcinoma after cryotherapy have appeared and emphasize the importance of extreme care in being sure not only that CIN alone is being treated but also that all abnormal tissue is adequately destroyed and that appropriate postcryosurgery follow-up occurs. Townsend et al. reviewed 66 cases of invasive cancer following outpatient cryotherapy and found errors in workup and diagnosis in most. Nonetheless it may be more hazardous to treat very large lesions with cryotherapy since many series report higher cryotherapy failure rates with large CIN III lesions.

Possible complications in addition to recurrence of neoplasia following cryotherapy include infertility and cervical stenosis. Although both have been reported, there is no clear evidence of an increased risk of these adverse outcomes in patients treated with cryotherapy. Recurrent treatments or extensive therapy of the endocervical canal does increase the risk because of the more extensive destruction of the normal endocervix.

Laser Therapy

In recent years the laser has become widely used for the treatment of subclinical papillomavirus infection and intraepithelial neoplasia. The instrument is used in conjunction with the colposcope. The energy from the laser beam is absorbed by water with resultant vaporization of the target tissue. The laser beam is controlled by a small "joystick," and the spot size of the laser can be varied but is usually less than 1 mm. Different degrees of power are available, and for therapy of intraepithelial neoplasia approximately 25 to 35 watts are utilized. Most reports express the treatment mode as a power density, that is, watts per square centimeter. Because therapy results in tissue vaporization, the resultant smoke must be evacuated with vacuum suction; thus a speculum with a special smoke evacuator is used to clear the operative field. This may be of particular importance to the therapist who is treating papillomaviral infections because of the risk of spread of these viruses to individuals who are exposed to the vaporized tissues. Graduated millimeter probes can be used to gauge the depth of the laser crater.

Reports have varied on the effectiveness of the laser to treat CIN. Current practice is to carry therapy to a depth of 5 to 7 mm and to use a power density of over 600 W/cm^2. The treatment is more effective at higher power densities. However, the complications of pain and bleeding are also related to the power density and depth of treatment. If bleeding occurs during therapy, it can easily be controlled by coagulating the site by defocusing the laser beam and using a lower power density. Healing in the laser crater is usually complete in 4 to 6 weeks, and the site is covered with metaplastic squamous tissue within 2 months. A particular advantage of the laser is that the transformation zone is more likely to remain visible colposcopically after treatment than is true with cryosurgery, following which the squamocolumnar junction is usually located in the endocervical canal.

Stanhope et al. treated lesions with the laser to a depth of 5 to 7 mm, as recommended earlier, and extended the treatment approximately 3 to 5 mm beyond the abnormal (non-iodine-staining) epithelium. These authors noted only a 9% failure rate of CIN III after such therapy. Baggish et al. summarized the results from 3070 women treated by laser vaporization over 10 years: 94% were free of disease at 1 year. Bleeding during the procedure was controlled by defocusing the laser beam, but delayed bleeding in 4 to 10 days required additional treatment in 170 (5.5%) of the patients. Cervical stenosis was rare (6 cases).

The laser is also frequently used to perform conization (see later section).

Cautery

Electrocautery was the mainstay of outpatient therapy of CIN before the advent of cryosurgery and laser therapy. Cryotherapy became popular because it usually causes less discomfort and also with less posttherapy vaginal discharge than cautery. Cervical stenosis can result from electrocautery or repeated cryotherapy if there is extensive treatment into the endocervical canal.

The treatment can be accomplished with a hot wire unit generating heat to the cervix or an electrodiathermy unit, which requires current to be passed through the tissues and electrical grounding of the patient. The treatment is carried out with sufficient depth to destroy cervical glands.

Chanen and Rome reported the results of cautery in 864 patients, 63% of whom had CIN III, with an overall success rate of 97.5%. In their treatment they used general anesthesia (day surgery) and colposcopically determined the areas to be treated. They also dilated the cervix during anesthesia to prevent subsequent stenosis. Only patients in whom the entire transformation zone can be visualized are treated. However, after therapy the squamocolumnar junction is usually located in the cervical canal, similar to the results after cryotherapy. According to Chanen and Rome, increased adverse effects of treatment on fertility or parturition are not observed. A disadvantage of this approach is the requirement for general anesthesia. However, effective outpatient therapy can be achieved without anesthesia, as noted by Deigan et al. from Canada, who treated 776 patients with electrocautery (hot wire pistol cautery) using colposcopic guidance. They achieved an overall initial eradication of CIN in approximately 90% of cases (92% for carcinoma in situ). Subsequent recurrences were usually treated with hot cautery. They required that the transformation zone be totally visualized, as is true for cryotherapy and laser therapy.

Electrocautery is much less expensive than the laser and appears able to yield comparable therapy results to cryosurgery. Kauraniemi et al. in Finland have utilized routine outpatient electrocautery to destroy the entire transformation zone in the cervices of a large population of women and reported that these individuals have lower rates of invasive carcinoma and CIN than those who did not have routine electrocautery.

Summary of Ablative Management

Ablative therapy of intraepithelial neoplasia depends on adequate destruction of all abnormal tissues. Prerequisites are that the transformation zone should be completely visualized colposcopically with no neoplasia on ECC, that treatment should be carried out to a depth to reach the cervical crypts, and that it should also extend a few millimeters

beyond the transformation zone to include normal-appearing tissue. Many authors have reported increased failure rates with high-grade lesions and carcinoma in situ (CIN III) with cryotherapy, but this is partly because these high-grade lesions cover larger areas of the cervix and extend more deeply into the cervical crypts. Success rates overall approximate 90%, and proven success has been obtained with the laser by treating to a depth of 5 to 7 mm at power densities greater than 600 W/cm^2 and extending the treatment 3 to 4 mm beyond the abnormal epithelium. Similar area and depth requirements exist for electrocautery.

Results for cryotherapy are optimized providing the ice ball extends 3 to 5 mm beyond the transformation zone, and using the double-freeze technique. Ferenczy noted that lesions smaller than 3 cm could be equivalently treated by cryosurgery or laser but that larger lesions or those that extended up to 5 mm into the cervical canal faired better with laser treatment. Less vaginal discharge is usually noted after laser, but it also is accompanied by higher rates of bleeding and risks of pelvic infection. Providing the entire transformation zone can be seen, the ECC results are negative, and a careful colposcopic protocol is followed, cryosurgery and electrocautery can be used as inexpensive and successful modalities for CIN therapy. Larger lesions, particularly those that begin to extend onto the vagina, can be treated with the laser.

Operative Excisional Therapy

Conization

Conization of the cervix is performed for diagnostic purposes if the colposcopic examination is unsatisfactory, if there is uncertainty regarding the presence of invasive disease, if the ECC results are positive, or if the cells seen on cytologic examination are not adequately explained by the biopsy specimens. If the biopsy suggests the possibility of microinvasion or if invasion cannot be confirmed, conization is performed for definitive diagnosis. A conization for treatment is carried out when childbearing function is to be maintained or when a patient prefers operative therapy less extensive than hysterectomy and is willing to adhere to a strict protocol for follow-up.

TECHNIQUE. The extent of the transforma-

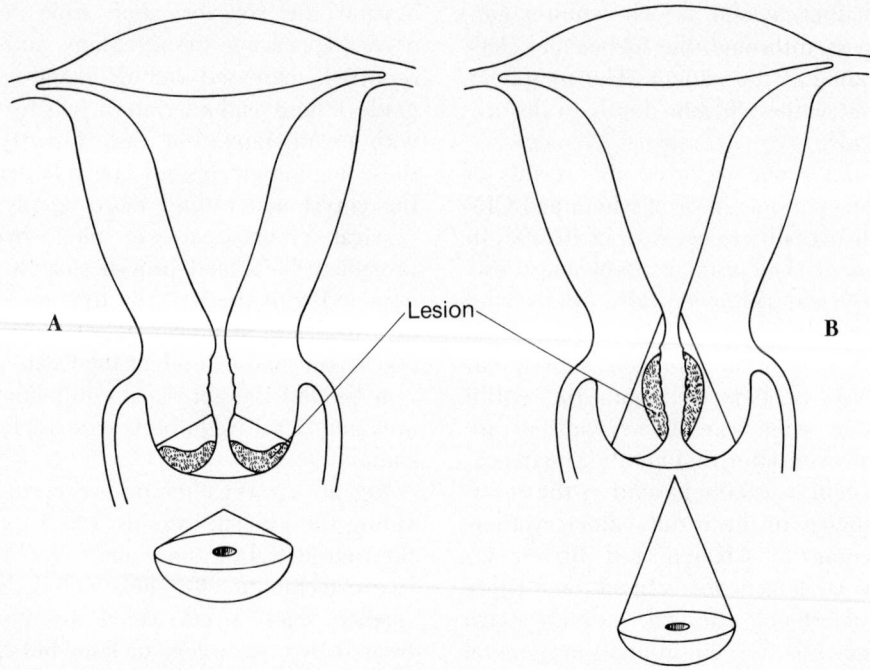

FIGURE 26-22
A, Cone biopsy for CIN of exocervix. Limits of lesion were identified colposcopically. **B,** Cone biopsy for endocervical disease. Limits of lesions were not seen colposcopically. (Redrawn from DiSaia PJ and Creasman WT: Clinical gynecologic oncology, St Louis, 1984, Mosby–Year Book, Inc.)

tion zone on the exocervix is outlined by use of the colposcope. In addition, it is advisable to stain the cervix with iodine (Lugol's or Schiller's solution) to outline the limits of the resection margin of the cone. Since normal squamous epithelium contains glycogen and stains dark brown with iodine, whereas neoplastic tissue fails to stain, care must be taken not to denude the normal epithelium with the blade of the speculum or an abrasive, since this will also lead to nonstaining. The degree to which the cone extends into the endocervical canal depends on the extent of the transformation zone. If the upper limits of the transformation zone cannot be seen, then the colposcopy is "unsatisfactory" and conization is performed in an attempt to have the upper margins of the cone include the transformation zone. If the upper limits cannot be seen in the endocervical canal or the ECC results are positive, the operation is adjusted so as to place the apex of the cone higher in the canal than in instances where the upper part of the transformation zone can be visualized, as illustrated in Figure 26-22.

The procedure can be done with a scalpel

(cold knife cone) or the laser, or more recently with an electrocautery loop. The laser has become more popular, since some believe it reduces blood loss in comparison to the cold knife conization, as reported by Larsson et al.

After the resection limits of the operative conization specimen have been determined, absorbable sutures (Vicryl, Dexon catgut) are usually placed at the 3 and 9 o'clock positions on the cervix to reduce blood loss by ligating the descending cervical branches of the uterine artery. Some therapists use dilute vasopressin (1 ml in 100 ml sterile saline) and inject it into the stroma of the cervix to reduce bleeding from the bed of the cone. The endocervical canal is sounded and the cone cut so as to keep the apex below the internal os. It is sometimes helpful to leave the sound or cervical dilator in the canal during the procedure to serve as a guide for the cold knife cone. The posterior part of the cone (3 to 9 o'clock) is cut first so the resultant blood loss does not obscure the operative field. The upper margin of the cone is usually dissected free with scissors, and the 12 o'clock position of the cone identified for the pathologists with a margin suture.

An ECC is performed after the completion of the conization, and, if indicated, uterine curettage is done. Husseinzadeh et al. noted if the postconization ECC was positive, residual disease was present in 24 of 30 (80%) of the hysterectomy specimens. It is advisable for one of the members of the operative team to examine the cone with the pathologist to ensure proper orientation. Individual arterial bleeding vessels are ligated, and the edge of the cone margin is repaired with interrupted figure-of-eight sutures. In the past the so-called Sturmdorf hemostatic suture, which turns the edge of the cervix into the canal, was widely used. This suture should not be used as it may bury abnormal cervical epithelium and also interferes with future colposcopic follow-up examination. It is advisable to sound the cervix at about 3 and 6 weeks after the procedure to help avoid stenosis.

COMPLICATIONS. As previously noted, bleeding is the major short-term complication of conization. Long-term complications that have been of concern include cervical stenosis, infertility, loss of cervical mucus, and an increase in adverse pregnancy outcome (incompetent cervix). Definitive data are not available concerning the degree of risk of these adverse outcomes, but they are thought to be related in part to the height of the cone, that is, the degree to which the endocervical glands are removed. Buller and Jones evaluated infertility and pregnancy outcome in 166 patients and found no evidence of an increased rate of infertility or alteration of pregnancy outcome as a complication of the operation. In contrast, a case-control study from England of 66 matched patients found a statistically significant association between conization and preterm delivery (17% versus 3%) and the risk of pregnancy loss was even more frequent among their patients with second pregnancies. Currently, no specific conclusions can be drawn regarding these risks. Patients desiring future childbearing function who need to undergo conization should be made aware of the potential risks of infertility, preterm labor, and cervical stenosis, but they can also be advised that the data are ambiguous concerning these risks.

LASER CONIZATION. The laser has also been used frequently to perform conization. The procedure is done with the patient under light general anesthesia or sometimes with a paracervical block. The cervix is usually infiltrated with dilute vasopressin, and lateral sutures are placed as described previously. The cone's limits are marked on the exocervix with shots from the laser, which is then used at 20 to 50 watts to cut through the cervix and remove a conical-shaped specimen by manipulating the cervix with a hook and forceps. The cone's apex can be removed with a scissors. The surgeon must be careful, especially with a sharply retroverted uterus, not to penetrate too deeply into the cervix with the laser because of possible perforation through the cervical wall. McIndoe et al. treated 196 patients by laser conization at approximately 5000 W/cm^2 (most therapists use lower power densities). All their patients satisfied colposcopic and morphologic criteria for laser vaporization, but histologic evaluation of the cone specimens showed two microinvasive carcinomas and one adenocarcinoma in situ. Baggish et al. summarized the results of 954 patients after laser conization: 97% had no disease at follow-up. Complications included bleeding up to 2 weeks after the procedure, which occurred approximately twice as often compared with vaporization. Cervical stenosis occurred in about 1% of the patients. Cervical incompetence has also been reported but was not observed in the summary series reported by Baggish et al. Howell et al. report in their series that laser cone introduces coagulation artifact making it less reliable than a cold knife conization.

LOOP DIATHERMY CONIZATION. This technique involves the use of an electrosurgical unit with both cutting and coagulation currents. It has been termed LEEP (loop electrosurgical excision procedure) or LLETZ (large loop excision transformation zone). Various-sized loops and cautery tips (Figure 26-23) can be used to cut the cone after colposcopy is completed. The cervix is often infiltrated with dilute vasopressin and local anesthetic. Lateral sutures can be used but are not necessary. The loop is passed across the cervix beneath the transformation zone, as described by Whiteley and Olah. The entire procedure can be accomplished in a few minutes, and any bleeding from the cervical base is coagulated. Most experience has been published from the United Kingdom. Mor-Yosef et al., in a study of 50 patients, found the cone size comparable with that obtained with the laser, and complications of bleeding and infection were also comparable. Whiteley and Olah treated 80 patients and noted secondary hemorrhage in three (3.7%). At 6 months the squamocolumnar junction was

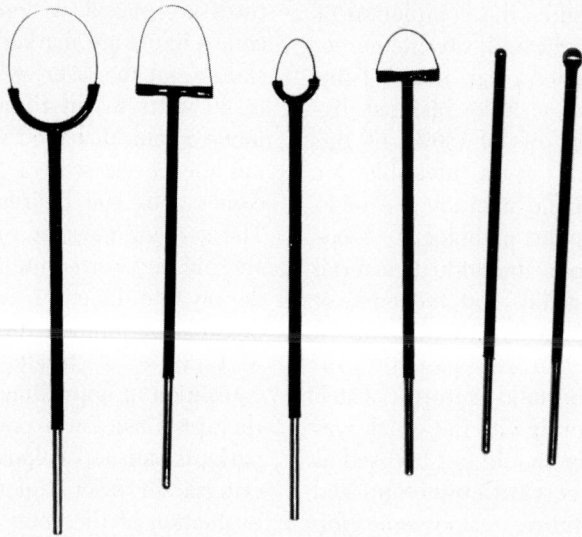

FIGURE 26-23
Different types of diathermy loops and cautery balls. (From Mor-Yosef S, Lopes A, Pearson S, and Monaghan JM: Obstet Gynecol 75:884, 1990.)

visible in 91% of the patients. This technique began to be popularized in 1990, and its effectiveness and risks (coagulation artifact of the specimen) have not been studied in detail.

FOLLOW-UP. If the margin of the conization specimen is free of neoplastic epithelium, the patient still requires long-term follow-up since new lesions can develop. If the margins of the cone specimen are involved with neoplasia, the patient is considered for further treatment with hysterectomy, since there is an increased risk of failure in these cases. However, some patients with "positive" cone margins are found to have residual disease at subsequent hysterectomy. To select which patients with positive margins might need further operation, Buxton et al. used endocervical cytologic sampling. They noted that none of 35 patients with negative cytology but with positive cone margins after conization had residual disease at hysterectomy. In contrast, 16 of 28 women with positive conization margins and subsequent positive cervical cytology had histologic evidence of disease in their hysterectomy specimens. The authors advocate follow-up rather than immediate hysterectomy for those with positive cone margins. This recommendation is particularly appropriate for women who want to preserve childbearing function.

At the time of 5-year follow-up examination, Ahlgren et al. noted 98% cure rates if the margin of the cervical conization was free, while the rate fell to 70% for those with positive margins. Kolstad and Klem followed 1128 patients for 15 to 25 years. Twenty-five of their patients had conization margins involved with neoplastic disease, and four of them eventually developed recurrence, some as long as 6 years after therapy. However, the remaining 21 were free of disease up to 15 years. These data emphasize that it is not always mandatory to perform hysterectomy if the margins of the cone are involved with CIN. This is particularly true if the ectocervical margins are involved, since subsequent outpatient therapy can usually eradicate any residual CIN at this site.

In the past it has been customary to perform the hysterectomy within 48 hours of conization or to wait more than 6 weeks to reduce the risk of postoperative infection at the time of the hysterectomy. Recent evidence from Webb and Symmonds as well as others suggests that it is not necessary to operate within these intervals. It is thought to be advisable to prescribe prophylactic antibiotics, such as cephalosporin, during the hysterectomy to reduce infections. Kolstad and Klem also noted that conization and hysterectomy were approximately equivalent in their effectiveness in treating carcinoma in situ. Conization was done in 795 patients, and with 5 to 25 years of follow-up, recurrences of carcinoma in situ occurred in 2.3%, whereas invasive cancer occurred in 0.9% (seven patients). For the 238 patients treated by hysterectomy, recurrence of carcinoma in situ occurred in 1.2% and invasive cancer in 2.1%. The recurrent carcinoma in situ or invasive cancer developed up to 10 years after primary treatment. These data indicate that conization is approximately as effective as hysterectomy for treatment of carcinoma in situ, particularly if the surgical margins are free. However, long-term follow-up is mandatory because of the risk of subsequent development of neoplasia. It should be emphasized that good results presented for conization are partly due to adequate pretherapy colposcopic evaluation.

Because of the apparent increased risk of invasive disease in older patients, Killackey et al. recommend that all patients over age 50 with a biopsy diagnosis of carcinoma in situ undergo conization to rule out invasive disease. In their series, 3 of 16 patients (19%) so treated were found to have unsuspected invasive carcinoma despite adequate colposcopic evaluation with cytology and negative ECC results.

Hysterectomy

Hysterectomy is performed for treatment of CIN if childbearing function is not to be preserved and if there is no evidence of invasive disease (Chapter 27 discusses invasive carcinoma). If neoplastic epithelium is found in the resection margin of the cervical cone, hysterectomy is sometimes performed. The need to perform hysterectomy following conization must be individualized depending on the clinicopathologic circumstances, including the patient's willingness to be followed and desire to preserve childbearing function. A vaginal hysterectomy is usually performed, or if the abdominal route is chosen, a class I hysterectomy (as described in Chapter 27) is done. The limits of the abnormal epithelium are defined before operation using the colposcope and iodine solution (Lugol's or Schiller's solution). If the vagina is involved with neoplasia, it is important to extend the surgical margins to include the abnormal vaginal tissue. It is important to remove the entire cervix, but resecting normal upper vagina does not improve therapeutic outcome. Follow-up is required after hysterectomy as after conization, since the patient is at risk for the development of lower genital tract intraepithelial neoplasia years later.

Other Modalities

In some instances, none of the previously described modalities is utilized and alternate forms of treatment may be tried. For example, this could arise in an elderly patient who has extensive CIN involving the vagina and cervix and in whom prolonged follow-up is difficult. Local radiation (tandem and ovoids, Chapter 25) has been used in some circumstances as definitive treatment but is very rarely used today, particularly with the availability of the laser. Local chemotherapy with 5-fluorouracil (5-FU) is described in Chapter 25 and is also occasionally tried for patients with recurrent cervicovaginal lesions or with recurrent condyloma. On an experimental basis, interferon gel has been used and has not been demonstrated to be efficacious.

ABNORMAL PAP SMEAR IN PREGNANCY

When an abnormal Pap smear is discovered initially in a pregnant patient, evaluation is more complicated than in the nonpregnant patient because of the increased vascularity of the cervix, the presence of the fetus, and morphologic changes (edema, decidual reaction, etc.) in the cervix that develop as pregnancy progresses. Colposcopic evaluation in the pregnant patient is best performed by physicians with extensive experience. CIN is not treated during pregnancy; therapy is postponed until the postpartum period. The prime objective in the pregnant patient with an abnormal Pap smear is to perform an adequate evaluation to rule out the invasive carcinoma.

Many years ago DePetrillo et al. introduced a scheme (Figure 26-24) for the evaluation of the abnormal Pap smear during pregnancy utilizing colposcopy. Insofar as the cervix everts during pregnancy, the squamocolumnar junction is more easily visible for evaluation. This circumstance also lessens the need for an ECC, which increases the risk of interrupting the pregnancy. When a patient has abnormal cytologic findings during pregnancy and the colposcopic examination is within normal limits, these examinations are periodically repeated, usually every 6 to 10 weeks depending upon the severity of the lesion. If there is neither evidence of neoplasia nor indication of a lesion requiring biopsy, the patient is followed and evaluated postpartum. If the colposcopic exam-

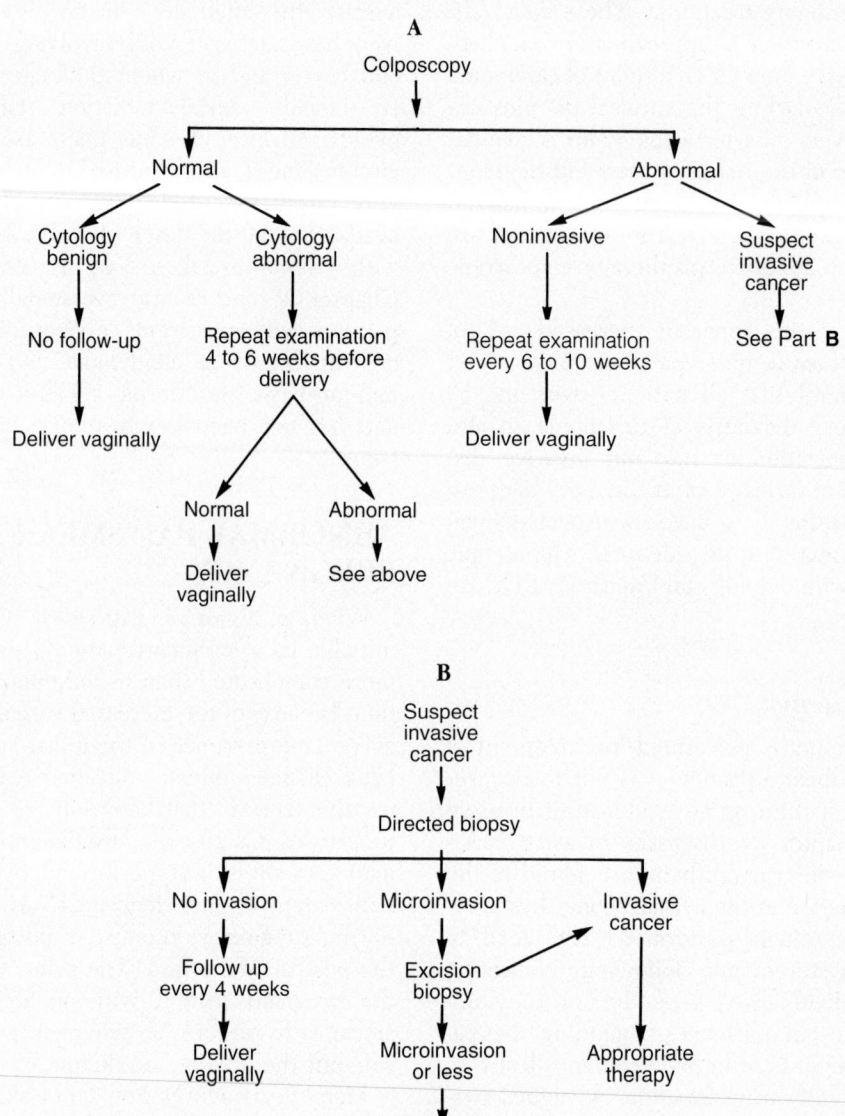

FIGURE 26-24
Scheme for evaluation of abnormal Pap smear during pregnancy utilizing colposcopy. **A,** Screening evaluation of abnormal Pap smear in pregnancy. **B,** Schematic of evaluation when an invasive lesion is suspected. (Modified from DePetrillo AD, Townsend DE, Morrow CP, et al: Am J Obstet Gynecol 121:441, 1975.)

ination is abnormal, a biopsy is usually taken of the most abnormal area to confirm the cytologic and colposcopic findings, and the examination (including Pap smear) and colposcopy are repeated periodically until the patient delivers. Then definitive evaluation is performed

in the postpartum period. A major problem arises if the patient has an undetected invasive lesion. In all circumstances a directed biopsy is needed, and then the management is carried out as outlined in Figure 26-24, *B.*

In a study of 401 pregnant patients, Benedet

et al. noted that the antepartum colposcopic impression was within one degree of the postpartum diagnosis in 87% of the women. Of the nine invasive cancers, five were found in 83 patients over age 30 (6%), in contrast to 3 of 318 patients (1%) under age 30. These authors advocate biopsies for all patients over age 30 or if there is an indication of carcinoma in situ or a more severe lesion. They omit biopsy for the patients under age 30 if the colposcopy and cytology suggest a lesion less severe than carcinoma in situ. Such management, however, requires extensive experience with colposcopy by the examiner.

If microinvasion is suspected, either conization or excision of the abnormal area is carried out. If following this procedure there is no evidence of invasive carcinoma, the patient may deliver vaginally and the necessary treatment is performed in the postpartum period. If invasive cancer is discovered, management is carried out in accordance with the guidelines in Chapter 27. Wedge resection or conization is needed if there is cytologic suspicion of invasion not explained by colposcopically directed biopsy or if the colposcopic pattern suggests invasion but the biopsy did not confirm its presence. The conization (or wedge resection of the poorly visualized or colposcopically abnormal area) in the pregnant patient is usually less extensive than that in the nonpregnant patient. Conization should be avoided because of the risk of blood loss and the potential of disturbing the pregnancy. If conization must be performed, most therapists prefer to carry it out in the second trimester.

DePetrillo et al. evaluated 300 pregnant patients with abnormal cytologic smears and found it necessary to perform conization only on three. Hannigan et al. summarized the literature on the treatment of 448 patients by conization during pregnancy and noted that approximately 9% had serious blood loss (more than 500 ml) and required blood transfusion. In their summary pregnancy losses did not appear to be increased for women who underwent conization. The authors noted that their data did not substantiate the need to perform conization in the second trimester, as generally practiced. Currently the precise risk of coniza-

tion to the fetus is not known.

There are studies, as reported by Kiguchi et al., to suggest that CIN has higher regression rates when detected in pregnant women than in nonpregnant individuals. The precise reason for this is not known, but two explanations are generally offered: (1) the low-grade intraepithelial changes, particularly those with mild dysplasia recorded during pregnancy, may represent cytologic changes that occur as a consequence of pregnancy itself, and (2) intraepithelial lesions may be removed during the trauma of vaginal delivery.

FOLLOW-UP

After treatment for CIN a patient requires long-term follow-up. As has been previously discussed, the recurrence of intraepithelial neoplasia in the cervix, vagina, or vulva can take place many years after treatment. The risk of development of neoplasia is also small (about 3%) but is ever present. Generally the initial screening examination is performed 3 to 4 months after therapy. For low-grade lesions, generally three negative examinations are sufficient and a patient is placed on a schedule of annual follow-up thereafter. Berget and Lenstrup recommend a fourth 6-month examination, since their review of the literature suggested that 75% of recurrences are detected within the first 21 months; therefore this more extensive follow-up is indicated, particularly for high-grade lesions such as carcinoma in situ (CIN III). In contrast, Hatch et al., in a follow-up study of intraepithelial neoplasia with cryotherapy, noted that 90% of their failures were detected in the first two examinations. In their study the failure rate was highest in the CIN III group, again emphasizing the importance of more intensive and prolonged follow-up for high-grade lesions.

The posttherapy evaluation includes both cytology and colposcopy. If the initial lesion occupied the endocervical canal, many therapists advise a routine ECC as part of the initial posttherapy evaluation. The use of an endocervical brush improves the detection of abnormal endocervical cells. However, biopsies are usually performed only when indicated as a result of the cytologic and colposcopic examinations.

_____ **KEY POINTS** _____

- Intraepithelial neoplasia is a spectrum of premalignant changes in the epithelium of the cervix that histologically show varying degrees of cellular atypia. Numerous terms are used to describe the severity of the atypias, but there is no clearly defined boundary between them.

- During reproductive life the squamocolumnar junction is usually on the portio of the cervix near the external os. It may be found farther away from the os during and after pregnancy and usually recedes into the endocervical canal after menopause.

- Pap smear (cytology) screening appears to have decreased the frequency of invasive carcinoma of the cervix by 50% in the past 25 years.

- Many cases of cervical intraepithelial neoplasia (CIN) do not progress. Some spontaneously regress, but all have the potential for progression to malignancy.

- The risk of progression for CIN I (mild dysplasia) to a higher grade lesion is approximately 16%.

- High-grade lesions (carcinoma in situ [CIN III]) are at greater risk for malignant progression and usually are found in larger abnormal transformation zones.

- Carcinoma in situ with gland involvement does not require hysterectomy for treatment.

- The cause of CIN is not known but appears to be associated with sexual activity.

- Females with multiple sex partners are at increased risk for CIN, and males with multiple sex partners increase the risk of neoplasia for a female sex partner.

- Females starting intercourse at a younger age (14 to 15 years) are at increased risk for CIN compared with those starting after age 20.

- Cigarette smoking appears to increase the risk of CIN.

- Prolonged oral contraceptive use (more than 5 years) is associated with an increased risk of cervical neoplasia.

- Herpes simplex virus II (HSV II) has been suspected to increase the risk of CIN, but a definitive causative role has not been identified.

- Human papillomavirus (HPV) infection is associated with an increased risk of CIN. Types 6 and 11 are often associated with benign condyloma, while types 16, 18, and occasionally 31 are found in specimens with neoplastic changes.

- Immunosuppressed patients are at an increased risk for genital HPV infection and CIN.

- HPV infection can progress to CIN. However, HPV infections also spontaneously regress.

- Currently, HPV typing is not useful to make treatment choices for CIN or to decide which patients with HPV infection should be treated.

- The false negative rate for properly performed cytology smears is 5% to 10%.

- The colposcope is used to evaluate the cervix if an abnormal Pap smear is present. Usually multiple biopsy specimens of an abnormal transformation zone are needed for an adequate evaluation.

- Colposcopic and cytologic findings do not establish a diagnosis; biopsy is necessary.

- Endocervical curettage (ECC) should be performed before outpatient therapy is undertaken for CIN.

- Before outpatient therapy for CIN, the entire transformation zone must be seen, the ECC results must be negative, and the evaluation must be adequate to rule out the presence of invasive carcinoma.

- The crypts of the endocervical glands are located as deep as 5 mm beneath the surface.

- Atypical cells seen on the biopsy specimen should be of similar magnitude (within one degree) of abnormality as those seen on cytologic smears before therapy is begun. If the discrepancy is 2 or more degrees, a conization should be performed.

- In the determination of the ploidy of a cell, those cells with an aneuploid content are neoplastic, cells with a tetraploid content may be metaplastic, and diploid cells are normal.

- Therapy of all HPV infections would result in treatment of many women to try to prevent a few cases of invasive carcinoma of the cervix.

- Conization of the cervix should be performed if colposcopy is unsatisfactory, if the biopsy results do not explain the cytologic findings, if the ECC sample has neoplastic cells, or if there is suspicion of invasive or microinvasive disease.

- The diagnosis of microinvasion requires a conization specimen.

- Conization is usually performed for therapy of carcinoma in situ if childbearing function is to be preserved.

- Young patients with CIN tend to have smaller transformation zones with an ectocervical location when compared with older patients, who have larger areas of neoplasia and more cervical crypt involvement.

- The goal of treatment in CIN is eradication of all abnormal tissue.

- Laser therapy, cryotherapy, and electrocautery have been reported to have equivalent results and lead to eradication of the lesions in about 90% of the patients with carcinoma in situ after initial therapy.

- Cryosurgery has been less effective than other modalities in treating large lesions as well as high-grade (carcinoma in situ [CIN III]) lesions. The effectiveness of cryotherapy is enhanced by treating for 3 to 4 mm beyond the abnormal epithelium and using a double-freeze technique.

- Cervical stenosis and infertility may result from outpatient therapy of CIN if large areas of the endocervix are destroyed.

- Laser therapy of CIN is usually done to a depth of 5 to 7 mm and extends 3 to 4 mm beyond the boundary of the abnormal epithelium. Higher power densities and greater depths of treatment increase the complications of bleeding and pain.

- Conization for the therapy of CIN is as effective as hysterectomy, especially if the margins are free of disease.

- Hysterectomy is not always necessary if the margins of the conization specimen contain neoplastic tissue, especially low-grade lesions.

- Hysterectomy may be performed for therapy of CIN if childbearing function is not to be preserved and there is no evidence of invasive disease.

- Evaluation of the abnormal Pap smear in pregnancy is conducted primarily to rule out the presence of invasive carcinoma. CIN is treated in the postpartum period.

- Follow-up of patients treated for CIN consists of colposcopy and cytology.

- Follow-up is done initially 3 to 4 months after initial therapy for CIN and then every 6 months.

- When three consecutive examinations on patients with low-grade lesions or four consecutive examinations on patients with high-grade lesions are negative, annual follow-up is instituted and continued indefinitely.

- The risk of long-term development (up to 10 years) of neoplasia following initial therapy is about 3%.

- Most short-term recurrences of neoplasia occur within 1 to 2 years after initial treatment.

BIBLIOGRAPHY

Ahlgren M, Ingemarsson I, Lindgerg LG, et al: Conization as treatment of carcinoma in situ of the uterine cervix, Obstet Gynecol 46:135, 1975.

American College of Obstetricians and Gynecologists Newsletter, June 1984.

Andersen ES, Thorup K, and Larsen G: The results of cryosurgery for cervical intraepithelial neoplasia, Gynecol Oncol 30:21, 1988.

Anderson MC and Hartley RB: Cervical crypt involvement by intraepithelial neoplasia. Obstet Gynecol 55:546, 1980.

Baggish MS, Dorsey JH, and Adelson M: A ten-year experience treating cervical intraepithelial neoplasia with the CO_2 laser, Am J Obstet Gynecol 161:60, 1989.

Benedet JL, Selke PA, and Nickerson KG: Colposcopic evaluation of abnormal Papanicolaou smears in pregnancy, Am J Obstet Gynecol 157:932, 1987.

Beral V: Cancer of the cervix: a sexually transmitted infection? Lancet 1:1037, 1974.

Beral V, Hannaford P, and Kay C: Oral contraceptive use and malignancies of the genital tract, Lancet 2(8624): 1331, 1988.

Berget A and Lenstrup C: Cervical intraepithelial neoplasia. Examination, treatment and follow-up, Obstet Gynecol Surv 40:545, 1985.

Bibbo M, Alenghat E, Bahr GF, et al: A quality-control procedure on cervical lesions for the comparison of cytology and histology, J Reprod Med 28:811, 1983.

Boonstra H, Aalders JG, Koudstaal J, et al: Minimum extension and appropriate topographic position of tissue destruction for treatment of cervical intraepithelial neoplasia, Obstet Gynecol 75:227, 1990.

Boonstra H, Koudstaal J, Oosterhuis JW, et al: Analysis of cryolesions in the uterine cervix: application techniques, extension, and failures, Obstet Gynecol 75:232, 1990.

Brinton LA, Schairer C, Haenszel WB, et al: Cigarette smoking and invasive cervical cancer, JAMA 255:3265, 1986.

Bryson SCP, Lenehan P, and Lickrish GM: The treatment of grade 3 cervical intraepithelial neoplasia with cryotherapy: an 11-year experience, Am J Obstet Gynecol 151:201, 1985.

Buller RE and Jones HW: Pregnancy following cervical conization, Am J Obstet Gynecol 142:506, 1982.

Burghardt E and Ostor AG: Site and origin of squamous cervical cancer: a histomorphologic study, Obstet Gynecol 62:117, 1983.

Buxton EJ, Luesley DM, Wade-Evans T, and Jordan JA: Residual disease after cone biopsy: completeness of excision and follow-up cytology as predictive factors, Obstet Gynecol 70:529, 1987.

Caglar H, Ayhan A, and Hreshchyshyn MM: CO_2 laser therapy for cervical intraephithelial neoplasia, Gynecol Oncol 22:46, 1985.

Campion MS, Singer A, and Clarkson PK: Increased risk of cervical neoplasia in consorts of men with penile condyloma acuminata, Lancet 1:943, 1985.

Carmichael JA and Maskens PD: Cervical dysplasia and human papillomavirus, Am J Obstet Gynecol 160:916, 1989.

Chanen W and Rome RM: Electrocoagulation diathermy for cervical dysplasia and carcinoma in situ: a 15-year survey, Obstet Gynecol 61:673, 1983.

Charles EW and Savage EW: Cryosurgical treatment of cervical intraepithelial neoplasia, Obstet Gynecol Surv 35:539, 1980.

Coppleson M, Pixley E, and Reid B: Colposcopy—a scientific and practical approach to the cervix in health and disease, Springfield, Ill, 1971, Charles C Thomas, Publisher.

Cramer DW: The role of cervical cytology in declining morbidity and mortality of cervical cancer, Cancer 34:2018, 1974.

Cramer DW and Cutler SJ: Incidence and histopathology of malignancies of the female genital organs in the United States, Am J Obstet Gynecol 118:443, 1974.

Crum C, Fu YS, Kurman RJ, et al: Editorial Board Symposium: Practical approach to cervical human papillomavirus-related intraepithelial lesions, Int J Gynecol Pathol 8:388, 1989.

Crum CP and Levine RU: Review: human papillomavirus infection and cervical neoplasia: new perspectives, Int J Gynecol Pathol 3:376, 1984.

Day NE: Effect of cervical cancer screening in Scandinavia, Obstet Gynecol 63:714, 1984.

Deigan EA, Carmichael JA, Ohlke ID, et al: Treatment of cervical intraepithelial neoplasia with electrocautery: a report of 776 cases, Am J Obstet Gynecol 154:255, 1986.

DePetrillo AD, Townsend DE, Morrow CP, et al: Colposcopic evaluation of the abnormal Papanicolaou test in pregnancy, Am J Obstet Gynecol 121:441, 1975.

Devesa SS: Descriptive epidemiology of cancer of the uterine cervix, Obstet Gynecol 63:605, 1984.

DiSaia PJ and Creasman WT: Clinical gynecologic oncology, ed 3, St Louis, 1989, Mosby–Year Book, Inc.

Fenoglio CM and Ferenczy A: Etiologic factors in cervical neoplasia, Semin Oncol 9:349, 1982.

Ferenczy A: Comparison of cryo- and carbon dioxide laser therapy for cervical intraepithelial neoplasia, Obstet Gynecol 66:793, 1985.

Ferenczy A, Mitao M, Nagai N, et al: Latent papillomavirus and recurring genital warts, N Engl J Med 313:784, 1985.

Grunebaum AN, Sedlis A, Sillman F, et al: Association of human papillomavirus infection with cervical intraepithelial neoplasia, Obstet Gynecol 62:448, 1983.

Hannigan EV, Whitehouse HH III, Atkinson WD, et al: Cone biopsy during pregnancy, Obstet Gynecol 60:450, 1982.

Hatch KD, Shingleton HM, Austin JM Jr, et al: Cryosurgery of cervical intraepithelial neoplasia, Obstet Gynecol 57:692, 1981.

Hatch KD, Shingleton HM, Orr JW, et al: Role of endocervical curettage in colposcopy, Obstet Gynecol 65:403, 1985.

Hellberg D, Valentin J, and Nilsson S: Smoking and cervical intraepithelial neoplasia—an association independent of sexual and other risk factors? Acta Obstet Gynecol Scand 65:625, 1986.

Herbst AL: The Bethesda System for cervical/vaginal cytologic diagnoses: a note of caution, Obstet Gynecol 76:449, 1990.

Herrero R, Brinton LA, Reeves WC, et al: Sexual behavior, venereal diseases, hygiene practices, and invasive cervical cancer in a high-risk population, Cancer 65:380, 1990.

Hollyhock VE, Chanen W, and Wein R: Cervical function following treatment of intraepithelial neoplasia by electrocoagulation diathermy, Obstet Gynecol 61:79, 1983.

Howell R, Hammond R, and Pryse-Davies J: The histologic reliability of laser cone biopsy of the cervix, Obstet Gynecol 77:905, 1991.

Husseinzadeh N, Shbaro I, and Wesseler T: Predictive value of cone margins and post-cone endocervical curettage with residual disease in subsequent hysterectomy, Gynecol Oncol 33:198, 1989.

Jones JM, Sweetnam P, and Hibbard BM: The outcome of pregnancy after cone biopsy of the cervix: a case-control study, Br J Obstet Gynaecol 86:913, 1979.

Kauraniemi T, Rasanen-Virtanen U, and Hakama M: Risk of cervical cancer among an electrocoagulated population, Am J Obstet Gynecol 131:533, 1978.

Kessler F: Etiologic concepts in cervical carcinogenesis, Gynecol Oncol 12:S7, 1981.

Kiguchi K, Bibbo M, Hasegawa T, et al: Dysplasia during pregnancy. a cytologic follow-up study, J Reprod Med 26:66, 1981.

Killackey MA, Jones WB, and Lewis JL Jr: Diagnostic conization of the cervix: review of 460 consecutive cases, Obstet Gynecol 67:766, 1986.

Kolstad P and Klem V: Long-term follow-up of 1121 cases of carcinoma in situ, Obstet Gynecol 48:125, 1976.

Kolstad P and Stafl A: Atlas of colposcopy, Baltimore, 1972, University Park Press, p 91.

Koss LG: Dysplasia: a real concept or misnomer? Obstet Gynecol 51:374, 1978.

Koss LG: The new Bethesda System for reporting results of smears of the uterine cervix, JNCI 82:988, 1990.

Koss LG, Stewart FW, Foote FW, et al: Some histological aspects of behavior of epidermoid carcinoma in situ and related lesions of the uterine cervix: a long-term prospective study, Cancer 16:1160, 1963.

Krebs HB: Management of human papillomavirus associated genital lesions in men, Obstet Gynecol 73:312, 1989.

Krebs HB and Helmkamp BF: Does the treatment of genital condyloma in men decrease the treatment failure rate of cervical dysplasia in the female sexual partner? Obstet Gynecol 76:660, 1990.

Kurman RJ, Schiffman MH, Lancaster WD, et al: Analysis of individual human papillomavirus types in cervical neoplasia: a possible role for type 18 in rapid progression, Am J Obstet Gynecol 159:293, 1988.

Kwikkel HJ, Bezemer PD, Helmerhorst ThJM, et al: Predictive value of a positive endocervical curettage in diagnosis and treatment of CIN, Gynecol Oncol 24:162, 1986.

Kwikkel HJ, Helmerhorst ThJM, Bezemer PD, et al: Laser or cryotherapy for cervical intraepithelial neoplasia: a randomized study to compare efficacy and side effects, Gynecol Oncol 22:23, 1985.

Larsson G, Gullberg B, and Grundsell H: A comparison of complications of laser and cold knife conizations, Obstet Gynecol 62:213, 1983.

Levine RU, Crum CP, Herman E, et al: Cervical papillomavirus infection and intraepithelial neoplasia: a study of male sexual partners, Obstet Gynecol 64:16, 1984.

McChance DJ, Campion MJ, Clarkson PK, et al: Prevalence of human papillomavirus type 16 DNA sequences in cervical intraepithelial neoplasia and invasive carcinoma of the cervix, Br J Obstet Gynaecol 92:1101, 1985.

McCord ML, Stovall TG, Summitt RL, et al: Discrepancy of cervical cytology and colposcopic biopsy: Is cervical conization necessary? Obstet Gynecol 77:715, 1991.

McIndoe WA, McLean MR, Jones RW, and Mullins PR: The invasive potential of carcinoma in situ of the cervix, Obstet Gynecol 64:451, 1984.

McIndoe GA, Robson MS, Tidy JA, et al: Laser excision rather than vaporization: the treatment of choice for cervical intraepithelial neoplasia, Obstet Gynecol 74:165, 1989.

Meisels A and Morin C: Human papillomavirus and cancer of the uterine cervix, Gynecol Oncol 12:S111, 1981.

Mitchell H, Drake N, and Medley G: Prospective evaluation of risk of cervical cancer after cytological evidence of human papillomavirus infection, Lancet 1:573, 1986.

Moller BR, Johannesen P, Osther K, et al: Treatment of dysplasia of the cervical epithelium with an interferon gel, Obstet Gynecol 62:625, 1983.

Mor-Yosef S, Lopes A, Pearson S, and Monaghan JM: Loop diathermy cone biopsy, Obstet Gynecol 75:884, 1990.

Nasiell K, Nasiell M, and Vaclavinkova V: Behavior of moderate cervical dysplasia during long-term follow-up, Obstet Gynecol 61:609, 1983.

Nasiell K, Roger V, and Nasiell M: Behavior of mild cervical dysplasia during long-term follow-up, Obstet Gynecol 67:665, 1986.

Nieminen P, Soares VRX, Aho M, et al: Cervical human papillomavirus deoxyribonucleic acid and cytologic evaluations in gynecologic outpatients, AM J Obstet Gynecol 164:1265, 1991.

Pinion SB, Kennedy JH, Miller RW, et al: Oncogene expression in cervical intraepithelial neoplasia and invasive cancer of the cervix, Lancet 337:819, 1991.

Porreco R, Penn I, Droegemueller W, et al: Gynecologic malignancies in immunosuppressed organ transplant recipients, Obstet Gynecol 45:359, 1975.

Rapp F and Jenkins FJ: Genital cancer and viruses, Gynecol Oncol 12:S25, 1981.

Reid R and Fu YS: Is there a morphologic spectrum linking condyloma to cervical cancer? In Banbury Report 21: Viral etiology of cervical cancer, Cold Spring Harbor, NY, 1986, Cold Spring Harbor Laboratory.

Reid R, Stanhope R, Herschman BR, et al: Genital warts and cervical cancer. I. Evidence of an association between subclinical papillomavirus infection and cervical malignancy, Cancer 50:377, 1982.

Richart RM: Cervical intraepithelial neoplasia and the cervicologist, Can J Med Tech 38:177, 1976.

Richart RM and Barron BA: A follow-up study of patients with cervical dysplasia, Am J Obstet Gynecol 105:386, 1969.

Richart RM and Townsend DE: Outpatient therapy of cervical intraepithelial neoplasia with cryotherapy or CO_2 laser. In Advances in clinical obstetrics and gynecology, Baltimore, 1982, Williams & Wilkins.

Riou G, Barrois M, Sheng ZM, et al: Somatic deletions and mutations of c-Ha-*ras* gene in human cervical cancers, Oncogene 2:329, 1988.

Riva JM, Sedlacek TV, Cunnane MF, and Mangan CE: Extended carbon dioxide laser vaporization in the treatment of subclinical papillomavirus infection of the lower genital tract, Obstet Gynecol 73:25, 1989.

Rome RM, Urcuyo R, and Nelson JH: Observations on the surface area of the abnormal transformation zone associated with intraepithelial and early invasive squamous cell lesions of the cervix, Am J Obstet Gynecol 129:565, 1977.

Romney SL, Dattagupta C, Basu J, et al: Plasma vitamin C and uterine cervical dysplasia, Am J Obstet Gynecol 151:976, 1985.

Sasson IM, Haley NJ, Hoffman D, et al: Cigarette smoking and neoplasia of the uterine cervix: smoke constituents in cervical mucus (letter), N Engl J Med 312(5):315, 1985.

Savage EW, Matlock DL, Salem FA, et al: The effects of endocervical gland involvement on the cure rates of patients with cervical intraepithelial neoplasia undergoing cryosurgery, Gynecol Oncol 14:194, 1982.

Seski JC, Reinhalter ER, and Silva JH: Abnormalities of lymphocyte transformations in women with condyloma acuminata, Obstet Gynecol 51:188, 1978.

Shy K, Chu J, Mandelson M, et al: Papanicolaou smear screening interval and risk of cervical cancer, Obstet Gynecol 74:838, 1989.

Slattery ML, Robison LM, Schuman KL, et al: Cigarette smoking and exposure to passive smoke are risk factors for cervical cancer, JAMA 261:1593, 1989.

Solomon D: The 1988 Bethesda System for reporting cervical/vaginal diagnoses: a National Cancer Institute Workshop, JAMA 262:931, 1989.

Stafl A and Mattingly RF: Colposcopic diagnosis of cervical neoplasia, Obstet Gynecol 41:168, 1973.

Stanhope CR, Phibbs GD, Stuart GCE, et al: Carbon dioxide laser surgery, Obstet Gynecol 61:624, 1983.

Stuart GCE, Allen HH, and Anderson RJ: Squamous cell carcinoma of the vagina following hysterectomy, Am J Obstet Gynecol 139:311, 1981.

Surwit EA, Graham V, Droegemueller W, et al: Evaluation of topically applied transretinoic acid in the treatment of cervical intraepithelial neoplasia, Am J Obstet Gynecol 143:821, 1982.

Syrajanen K: Cervical papillomavirus infection progressing to invasive cancer in less than three years, Lancet 1:510, 1985.

Tidy JA, Mason WP, and Farrell PJ: A new and sensitive method of screening for human papillomavirus infection, Obstet Gynecol 74:410, 1989.

Tidy JA, Parry GCN, Ward P, et al: High rate of human papillomavirus type 16 infection in cytologically normal cervices, Lancet 1:434, 1989.

Townsend DE, Richart RM, Marks E, et al: Invasive cancer following outpatient evaluation and therapy for cervical disease, Obstet Gynecol 57:145, 1981.

Vessey MP, McPherson K, Lawless M, et al: Neoplasia of the cervix uteri and contraception: a possible adverse effect of the pill, Lancet 2:930, 1983.

Walton RJ: The Task Force on Cervical Cancer Screening Program, Can Med Assoc J, Oct 1, 1982.

Webb MJ, and Symmonds RE: Radical hysterectomy: influence of recent conization on morbidity and complications, Obstet Gynecol 53:290, 1979.

Weitzman GA, Korhonen MO, Reeves KO, et al: Endocervical brush cytology: an alternative to endocervical curettage? J Reprod Med 33:677, 1988.

Wentz WB and Reagan JW: Clinical significance of post irradiation dysplasia of the uterine cervix, Am J Obstet Gynecol 106:812, 1970.

Whiteley PF and Olah KS: Treatment of cervical intraepithelial neoplasia: experience with the low-voltage diathermy loop, Am J Obstet Gynecol 162:127, 1990.

Willett GD, Kurman RJ, Reid R, et al: Correlation of the histologic appearance of intraepithelial neoplasia of the cervix with human papillomavirus types, Int J Gynecol Pathol 8:18, 1989.

Wright TC and Richart RM: Review: role of human papillomavirus in the pathogenesis of genital tract warts and cancer, Gynecol Oncol 37:151, 1990.

zur Hausen H: Human papillomavirus and their possible role in squamous cell carcinoma, Can Top Microbiol Immunol 78:1, 1977.

Malignant Diseases of the Cervix

KEY TERMS AND DEFINITIONS

Adenoma Malignum. A virulent adenocarcinoma of the cervix that histologically consists of glands that appear well differentiated.

Barrel-Shaped Cervix. A cervix containing a large carcinoma, *generally* of endocervical origin, that has replaced much of the cervix, causing it to widen (usually more than 6 cm).

Brachytherapy. A form of radiation therapy in which the source is placed close to the tumor. The application may be in the form of needles implanted into the tumor (interstitial therapy) or into the vagina or cervical canal (internal therapy). For cervical tumors an intracervical tandem and vaginal ovoids (colpostats) are usually used.

Cordotomy. A neurosurgical operation for relief of pain of the lower extremity in cases of recurrent cervical carcinoma. It interrupts the lateral spinothalamic tract.

Endophytic. A term used to describe a tumor that begins in the cervical canal and penetrates internally into the cervix.

Exophytic. A term used to describe a cervical tumor that grows on the outside surface of the cervix (exocervical part).

Extrafascial Hysterectomy. An operation that develops the pubocervical fascia to allow total removal of the cervix and uterus (class I hysterectomy).

Fletcher-Suit Applicator. A system that delivers brachytherapy to cervical carcinomas by use of a tandem in the cervical canal and ovoids (colpostats) in the vagina.

Glassy Cell Carcinoma. A virulent adenosquamous carcinoma that occurs in the cervix and metastasizes early in the course of the disease.

Microinvasive Carcinoma. A small (stage IA) carcinoma detected by microscopic examination with little or no risk of spread to regional lymph nodes.

Modified Radical Hysterectomy. An operation that removes the uterus and cervix and some paracervical tissues but does not dissect the ureters distal to the uterine artery (class II hysterectomy).

Pelvic Exenteration. An extensive pelvic operation usually employed to treat a central pelvic recurrence of cervical carcinoma after radiation. A total exenteration involves removal of the bladder, uterus, cervix, and rectum. An anterior exenteration spares the rectum, while a posterior exenteration spares the bladder.

Persistent Tumor. The identification of invasive disease at the site of primary therapy less than 6 months after therapy.

Point A. A term used in radiation therapy of carcinoma of the cervix to identify a point 2 cm above the external os of the cervix and 2 cm lateral to the cervical canal.

Point B. A term used in the radiation treatment of carcinoma of the cervix to identify a point 3 cm lateral to point A or 5 cm from the cervical canal.

Radical Hysterectomy. An operation that removes the uterus, upper third of the vagina, cervix, and paracervical-parametrial tissues. The pelvic ureters are dissected to the uterovesical junction. It is usually combined with a pelvic lymph node dissection (class III hysterectomy).

Recurrent Tumor. The identification of invasive disease 6 months or more after therapy.

Summary of Stages of Carcinoma:

I: Tumor confined to the cervix

IA: Microinvasion (preclinical)

IB: All other cases confined to cervix

IIA: Tumor spread to the vagina—upper two thirds

IIB: Tumor spread to paracervical tissue but not to pelvic walls

IIIA: Tumor spread to lower third of vagina

IIIB: Tumor spread to pelvic wall or obstruction of either ureter by tumor

IV: Tumor spread to mucosa of bladder or rectum or outside the pelvis

Teletherapy. A form of radiation therapy with placement of the radioactive source at a distance from the patient (external therapy). It is usually used to treat the pelvis and occasionally the paraaortic nodes in patients with cervical carcinoma.

Verrucous Carcinoma. A warty appearing, well-differentiated squamous malignancy that rarely metastasizes.

Malignancies of the cervix are almost always carcinomas, and a summary of the more common histologic types are shown in the box below. Approximately 85% to 90% of these tumors are squamous cell carcinomas, and from 10% to 15% are adenocarcinomas. The proportion of adenocarcinomas has increased in recent decades, partly because of a decrease in the frequency of occurrence of squamous cell carcinomas. The cause of squamous cell carcinomas of the cervix is unknown, but there is a close association with early and frequent sexual contact and cervical viral infection, as detailed in Chapter 26. According to the American Cancer Society, the frequency of cervical cancer has been steadily decreasing, in part because of the effect of widespread screening for premalignant cervical changes by cervical cytology (Pap smear). Approximately 13,500 cases of cervical cancer occur in the United States annually, making it the third most frequent malignancy of the lower female genital tract after endometrial and ovarian carcinomas. Approximately 6000 deaths annually result from cervical cancer, which is less than the 12,400 for ovarian cancer but higher than the 4000 observed for endometrial cancer.

This chapter will detail the various types of cervical carcinomas and consider their natural history, methods of diagnosis and evaluation, and the details of therapy. Primary sarcomas and melanomas of the cervix are extremely rare and are not considered separately.

MAJOR CATEGORIES OF CERVICAL CARCINOMA

Squamous Cell Carcinomas

Large cell (keratinizing or nonkeratinizing)
Small cell
Verrucous

Adenocarcinomas

Typical (endocervical)
Endometrioid
Clear cell
Adenoid cystic (basaloid cylindroma)
Adenoma malignum

Mixed Carcinomas

Adenosquamous
Glassy cell

HISTOLOGIC TYPES

Varieties of squamous cell carcinoma of the cervix are illustrated in Figure 27-1. An early form, microinvasive carcinoma, is considered separately in the next discussion. Most squamous cell carcinomas of the cervix are reported to be of the large cell, nonkeratinizing type, but many are keratinized, and squamous pearls may be seen. About 5% are small cell carcinomas, and these tend to be more virulent than the other types. Van Nagell et al. noted that small cell carcinomas tend to have higher recurrence rates and more distant spread than squamous cell carcinomas, with poorer patient survival rates. The degree of differentiation of

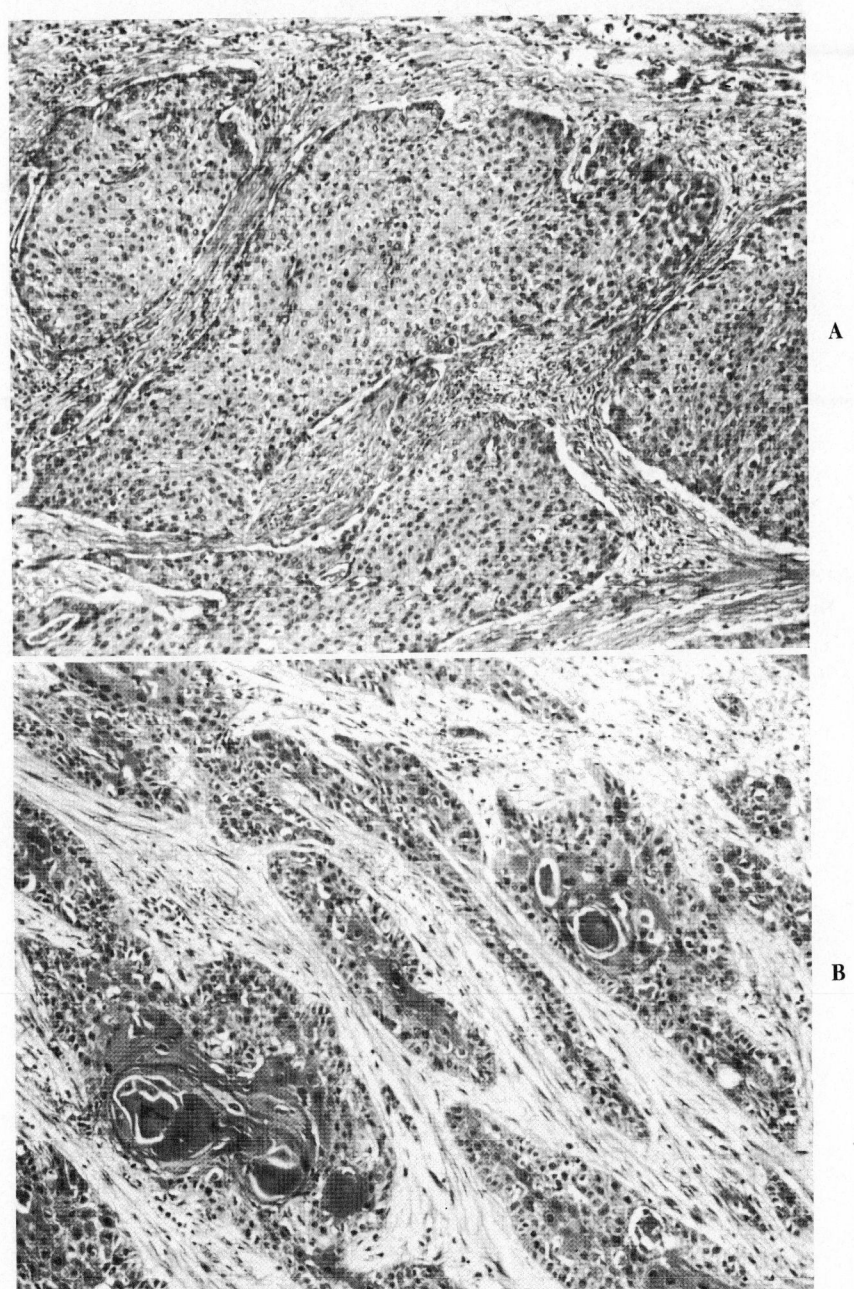

FIGURE 27-1

A, Large cell, nonkeratinizing squamous cell carcinoma. Discrete islands of uniform, large cells with abundant cytoplasm are separated by fibrous stroma. (×160.)
B, Keratinizing squamous cell carcinoma. Irregular nests of squamous cells forming several pearls are separated by fibrous stroma. The nests have pointed projections. (×160.) (From Clement PB and Scully RE: Semin Oncol 9:251, 1982.)

Continued.

C

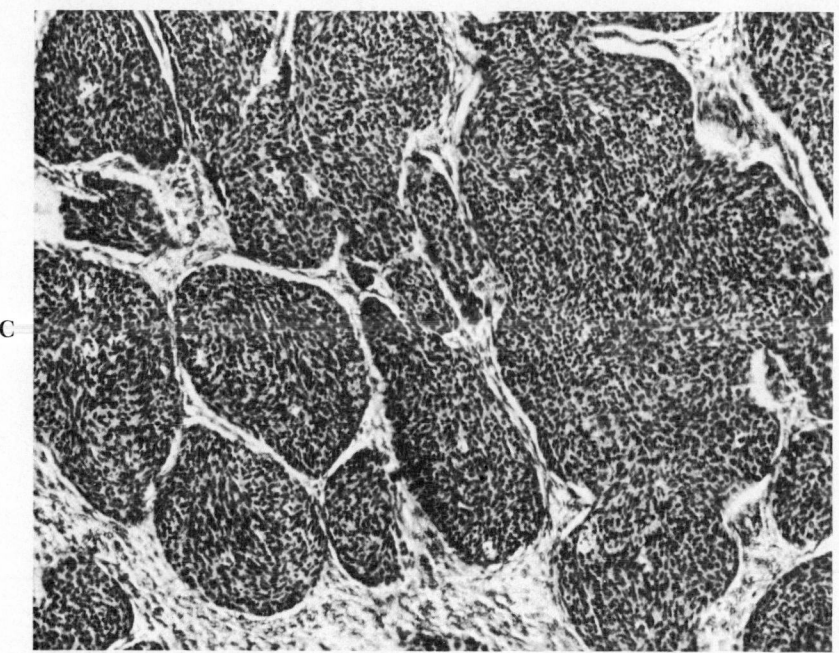

FIGURE 27-1, cont'd.
C, Small cell, nonkeratinizing squamous cell carcinoma. Nests are composed of cells with scant cytoplasm and small, round to spindle-shaped nuclei. (×160.) (From Clement PB and Scully RE: Semin Oncol 9:251, 1982).

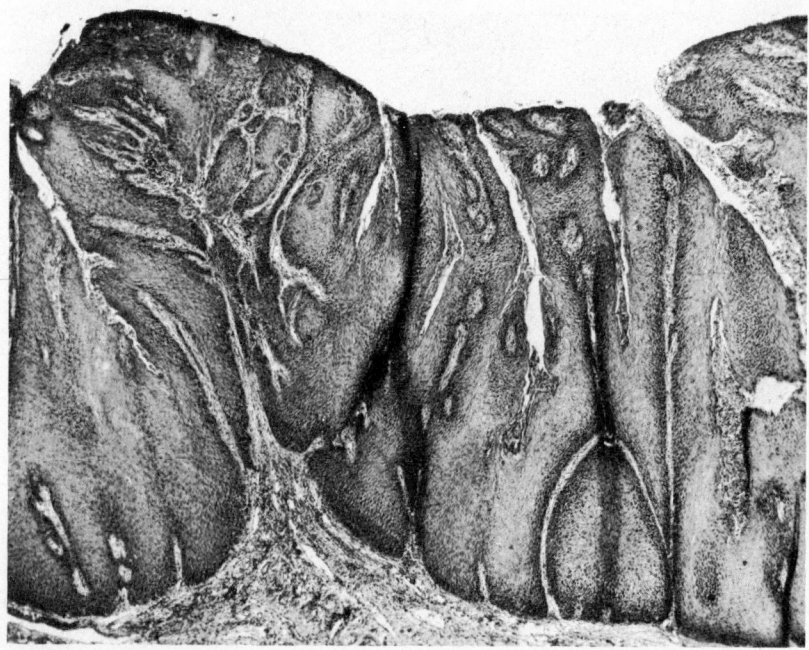

FIGURE 27-2
Verrucous carcinoma. Downgrowns of papillae have broad bases. Tumor cells are well differentiated. (×34.) (From Clement PB and Scully RE: Semin Oncol 9:251, 1982.)

tumors is usually designated by three grades: G1, well differentiated; G2, intermediate; and G3, undifferentiated. Occasionally a four-grade classification is used. However, there is no consensus on the value of tumor grade as a major prognostic factor for squamous cell carcinoma of the cervix.

A rare variety of squamous cell carcinoma is the so-called verrucous carcinoma, which is morphologically similar to those found in the vulva (Chapter 30). These warty tumors appear as large, bulbous masses (Figure 27-2). They rarely metastasize but unfortunately may be accompanied by the more virulent, typical squamous cell carcinomas, in which case metastatic spread is more likely.

Adenocarcinomas may have a number of histologic varieties. The typical variant often contains intracytoplasmic mucin and is related to the mucinous cells of the endocervix (endocervical pattern) (Figure 27-3). However, on occasion the cells contain little or no mucin, and then the tumor may resemble an endometrial carcinoma (endometrioid pattern). It may be difficult histologically to ascertain if these carcinomas arise in the cervix or endometrium. Endocervical tumors more frequently stain positive for carcino-

embryonic antigen (CEA) than do endometrial tumors, and this histochemical observation has been used to try to distinguish the tumors microscopically by an immunoperoxidase reaction.

A rare but important variety of adenocarcinoma is the adenoma malignum. These innocuous-appearing tumors consist of well-differentiated glands (Figure 27-4) that vary in size and shape and infiltrate the stroma. Despite their bland histologic appearance, these tumors tend to be deeply invasive and metastasize early. They are extremely virulent. According to McGowan et al., patients with Peutz-Jeghers syndrome are at increased risk for development of these tumors.

Clear cell adenocarcinomas of the cervix are histologically identical to those of the ovary (Chapter 29) and vagina (Chapter 31). They are uncommon in the cervix and can also be associated with intrauterine diethylstilbestrol (DES) exposure (Chapter 14), although they also often develop spontaneously in the absence of DES exposure.

Adenoid cystic carcinomas are rare. Berchuk and Mullin summarized 88 cases reported in the literature. These tumors are aggressive and

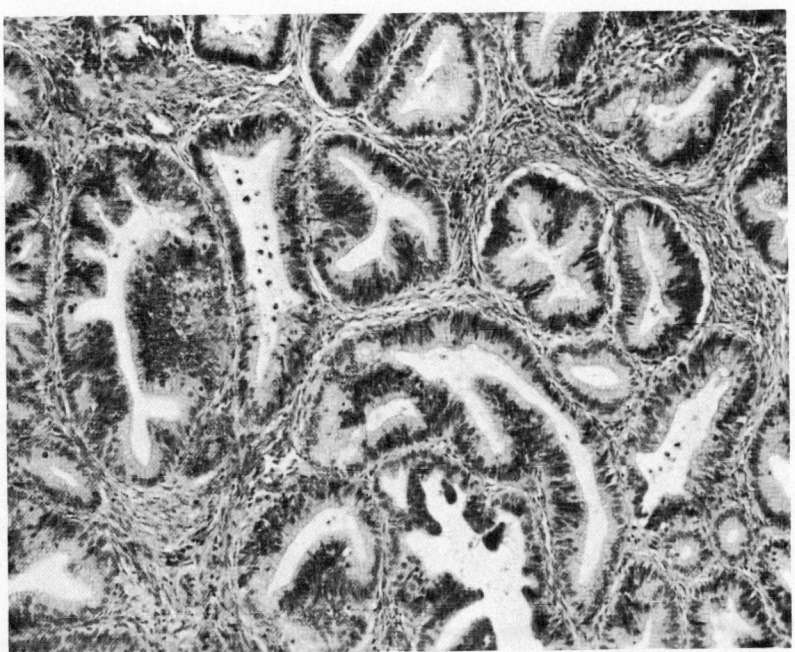

FIGURE 27-3
Typical adenocarcinoma. Irregular glands are lined by stratified mucin-containing epithelium. Mitotic figures are numerous. (×160.) (From Clement PB and Scully RE: Semin Oncol 9:251, 1982.)

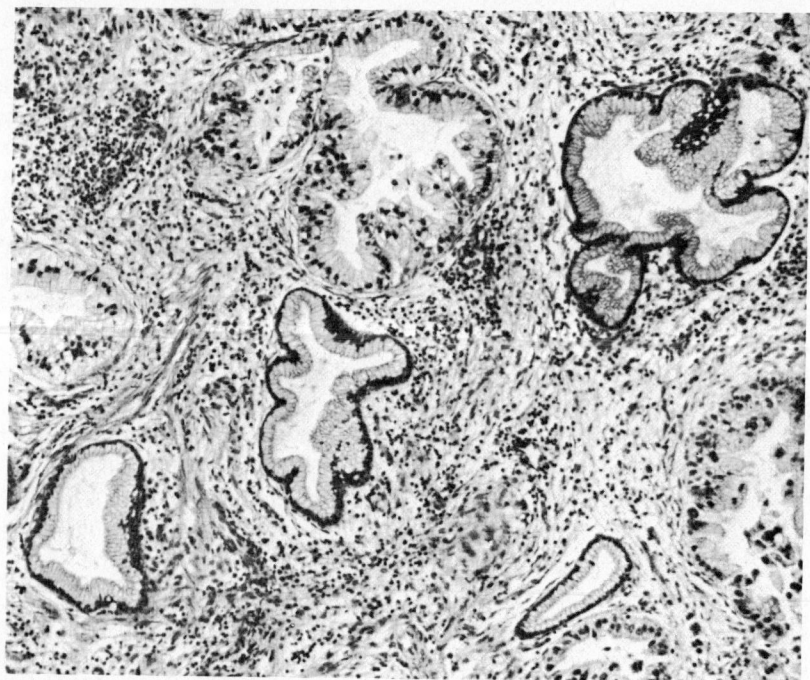

FIGURE 27-4
Adenoma malignum. Glands are mostly well differentiated, appearing normal except for their irregular shapes. A few obviously malignant glands are also present. (×160.) (From Clement PB and Scully RE: Semin Oncol 9:251, 1982.)

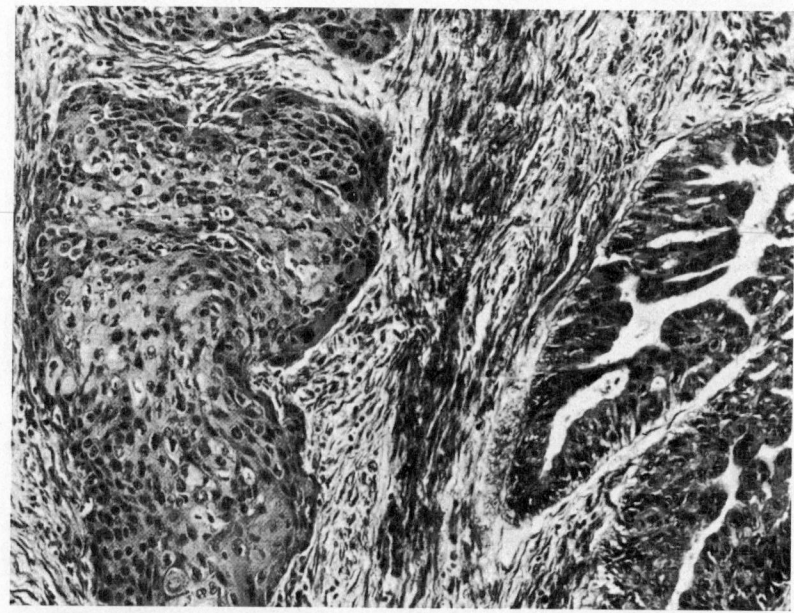

FIGURE 27-5
Well-differentiated adenosquamous carcinoma. Glandular structure lies adjacent to nest of nonkeratinizing, large squamous cells. (×400.) (From Clement PB and Scully RE: Semin Oncol 9:251, 1982.)

may resemble cylindromas of salivary gland or breast origin and histologically may resemble basal cell carcinomas of the skin (adenoid basal, or basaloid, carcinomas). Most patients with these tumors are over age 60 years. The basaloid variety appears to be less aggressive. King et al. reported four unusual cases in women under age 40. One patient was noted to survive more than 5 years.

Adenosquamous carcinomas, as the name implies, consist of both squamous carcinoma and adenocarcinoma elements in varying proportions (Figure 27-5). They occur frequently in pregnant women. A particularly virulent variety is termed *glassy cell carcinoma* (Figure 27-6). This is an undifferentiated tumor consisting of large cells containing cytoplasm with a ground-glass appearance. Glassy cell carcinomas tend to metastasize early to lymph nodes as well as to distant sites, and usually have a fatal outcome.

MICROINVASIVE CARCINOMA OF THE CERVIX

Microinvasive carcinoma of the cervix requires special consideration, since it is part of the spectrum of cervical neoplasia between intraepithelial carcinoma (Chapter 26) and frankly invasive carcinoma. As the name implies, these are tiny lesions that have begun to invade the cervical stroma (Figure 27-7), but they can often be treated by less extensive measures than those required for invasive cancers. In the International Federation of Gynecology and Obstetrics (FIGO) staging classification, these preclinical carcinomas are designated as stage IA.

A major problem in gynecologic oncology is that there is no uniform agreement on the appropriate definition of microinvasive carcinoma. The ideal definition is one that would have widespread clinicopathologic applicability and describe an early invasive lesion that has little or no risk of spread beyond the cervix, such as to regional pelvic lymph nodes. It is important to consider some of the definitions that have been used to describe this entity and also to consider the results of therapy that have been obtained. The important factors that have provided points of disagreement concerning the definition of microinvasive carcinomas of the cervix are the depth of stromal invasion, the presence or absence of vascular or lymphatic space involvement (capillary-like spaces), the presence or absence of tumor confluence, and the lateral extent (width) of the lesion.

FIGO (1985) defines a stage IA lesion as a

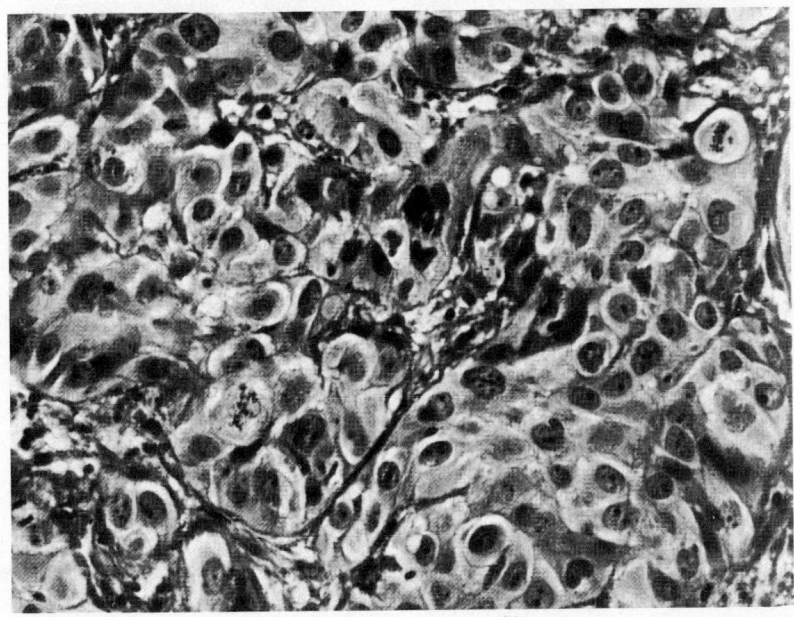

FIGURE 27-6
Glassy cell carcinoma. Cells have sharp borders, ground-glass-type cytoplasm, and nuclei containing prominent nucleoli. (×1000.) (From Clement PB and Scully RE: Semin Oncol 9:251, 1982.)

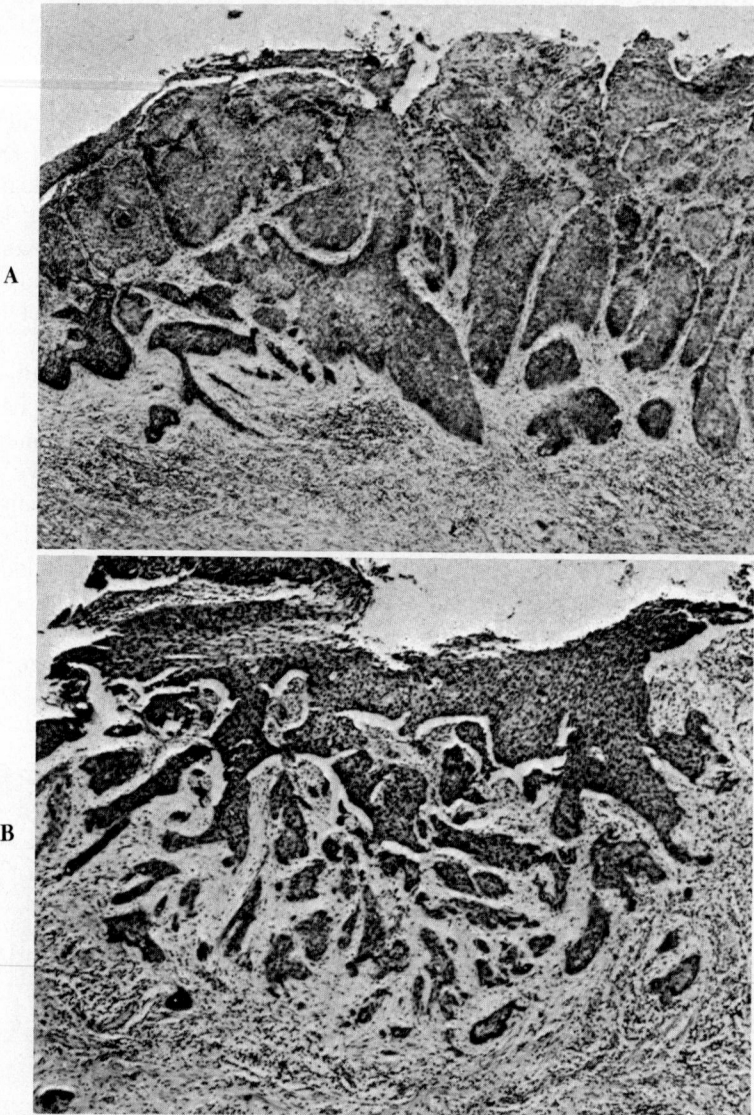

FIGURE 27-7
A, Tumor with only 0.5 mm of invasion. (×40.) **B,** Example of so-called spray pattern with multiple invasive nodules in stroma. Invasion is only 1 mm. (×50.) (From Creasman WT, Fetter BF, Clarke-Pearson DL, et al: Am J Obstet Gynecol 153:164, 1985.)

preclinical cervical carcinoma and divides microinvasion into two categories: stages IA1 and IA2. Stage IA1 is minimal stromal invasion that most authorities believe can be treated as a carcinoma in situ. Stage IA2 is a microinvasive tumor whose dimensions are less than 5 mm depth of invasion and 7 mm width. It is not clear whether this definition provides reliable criteria for lack of risk of tumor spread to regional nodes. Recently, Greer et al. evaluated this definition in 17 patients who satisfied the FIGO definition of stage IA2 but had residual tumor at subsequent radical hysterectomy. In contrast, Kolstad summarized 411 patients with stage IA2, 245 of whom were treated by hysterectomy and 166 by more radical therapy. Two patients had node metastases, and four died. The poor outcome occurred primarily in those with vascular space involvement. Kolstad recommends conservative therapy if the margins of the cone are clearly negative and there is no lymphatic or vascular space involvement. However, the difficulty of using the stage IA2 category as a guide to therapy was emphasized in a report by Burghardt et al., who studied microinvasive carcinomas in 445 patients. Of 101 Stage IA2, 41 on reexamination were reclassified as stage IB. Five with stage IA2 developed recurrence while none of the 38 classified as stage IB recurred.

The Society of Gynecologic Oncologists in 1974 described microinvasive carcinoma of the cervix as "a lesion in which the neoplastic epithelium invades the stroma in one or more places to a depth of 3 mm or less below the basement membrane of the epithelium and in which lymphatic or vascular involvement is not demonstrated." Currently available studies indicate that almost all lesions meeting the latter definition will not have spread beyond the cervix, but the definition, while widely used, definition does not provide sufficient precision for many clinical situations.

In regard to lesion depth, Creasman et al., Hasumi et al., and van Nagell et al., in separate studies, reported only one pelvic metastasis in 232 patients with cervical carcinomas that invaded to less than 3 mm from the basement membrane. In a different study, Leman et al. found no lymph node spread in 51 cases with up to 5 mm of invasion, but their measurements were made from the *surface* of the epithelium rather than from the basement membrane. With depth of invasion greater than 3 mm from the basement membrane, a higher proportion of patients have tumor involvement of lymphatic and vascular spaces and an increased risk of spread of tumor to regional pelvic nodes, but this risk remains quite small. Furthermore, the impact of tumor confluence or lymphatic or vascular space involvement may not be as important as previously reported by many authorities. Creasman et al. summarized 267 cases from the literature with less than 3 mm of invasion from the basement membrane, of which 40 (17%) had capillary-like space involvement and none had tumor in pelvic nodes. Furthermore confluence was noted in 10 of 74 cases (14%), and in none was there spread to regional nodes. For tumors with 3 to 5 mm invasion the risk of spread increases.

A further refinement has been reported by investigators from Western Europe, who used a meticulous three-dimensional microscopic study to calculate the *volume* of neoplastic tissue. This is obtained by step-sectioning the conization or hysterectomy specimens and measuring 50 to 60 slides per case. The technique is too laborious and expensive for routine use. Burghardt and Holzer defined microinvasion as a tumor volume of less than 500 mm^3. In some cases vascular space involvement did occur. This three-dimensional technique has been modified by many to a two-dimensional model that limits the extent of neoplastic tissue to 50 mm^2, or 5 × 10 mm. Using the 50 mm^2 criterion, Lohe et al. reported no positive nodes in 134 cases studied in numerous centers in Western Europe. This two-dimensional definition has the advantage of considering both the depth of invasion and the width of tumor and provides a general guide that is used by many pathologists for determination of microinvasive disease.

These area measurements provide the general guidelines but there are other factors to consider when undertaking conservative treatment for suspected microinvasive tumors. First, the diagnosis of microinvasive tumor cannot be made on the basis of a biopsy specimen alone and a cervical conization must be performed. Second, if the margin of the cervical cone specimen contains neoplastic epithelium, the risk of invasive tumor in the remaining uterus is increased. Third, endocervical tumors have an increased risk of being associated with invasion, and this frequently occurs when the exocervix is covered with normal squamous epithelium. If the second or third situation exists,

Larsson et al. recommend that the patient be treated as having a frankly invasive tumor. On the other hand, these Scandinavian workers and others have reported that authentic microinvasive carcinoma can be effectively treated by conization as well as simple hysterectomy. For example, no tumor recurrences were noted among 25 cases of microinvasive disease that penetrated from the basement membrane up to 4 mm and extended laterally up to 8 mm; all were treated only by conization. One recurrence was observed in 30 similar patients treated by simple hysterectomy. This recurrence was located centrally and successfully treated when diagnosed. None of the patients treated conservatively died of the disease, with follow-up in some instances as long as 19 years.

In considering the therapy of microinvasive carcinoma of the cervix, the clinician must weigh the risk that an invasive lesion may be mistakenly treated by conservative means. If invasive carcinoma is present, it can usually be successfully treated by means of a radical or modified radical hysterectomy (see later discussion). The risk of death or serious morbidity from such operation is probably on the order of 1%, and the risk of error or misdiagnosis of a lesion should be comparably small.

At present a patient suspected of having microinvasive carcinoma of the cervix should first have conization of the cervix. If the lesion is less than 35 mm^2, the patient should be treated by conservative means, which is usually a simple hysterectomy, particularly if invasion from the basement membrane is less than 3 mm. If the lesion is less than 50 mm^2 and there is only infrequent capillary-like space involvement, such conservative treatment is usually adequate, but the risk of failure increases for lesions that invade more than 3 mm from the basement membrane. The presence of capillary-like space involvement does not preclude conservative therapy, but the risk of invasive disease or future recurrence increases with capillary-like space involvement and larger lesions. Conservative therapy, including simple hysterectomy, should not be attempted if the conization margins are not adequately free of neoplastic tissue. In addition, an exclusive endocervical location of the microinvasive tumor increases the risk of the tumor's behaving like an invasive carcinoma. All patients must be followed indefinitely with periodic physical and cytologic (Pap smear) examinations, since recurrences may develop late and have been noted more than 15 years after primary therapy. The 5-year survival rate following appropriately chosen therapy of microinvasive carcinoma of the cervix should approach 100%.

CARCINOMA OF THE CERVIX

Clinical Considerations

Patients with carcinoma of the cervix characteristically present with abnormal bleeding or brownish discharge, frequently noted following douching or intercourse and also occurring spontaneously between menstrual periods. The patients often have a history of not having had a cervicovaginal cytologic smear for many years. Other symptoms, such as back pain, loss of appetite, and weight loss, are late manifestations of the disease and occur only when there is extensive spread of cervical carcinoma. These patients tend to be in their 40s to 60s, with a median age of 54 years noted worldwide by Pettersson et al. It is more frequent in blacks than whites in the United States (Figure 27-8). Beyond age 45 there is a slight increase in the frequency of the disease in whites, but the condition continues to be more common in blacks. Preinvasive intraepithelial carcinoma of the cervix (Chapter 26) occurs primarily in women in their 20s and 30s and recently has become much more common among those in

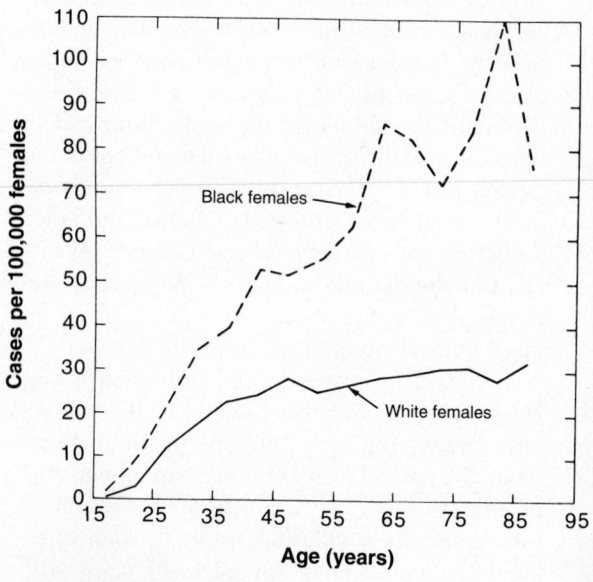

FIGURE 27-8
Age-specific incidence rates for invasive carcinoma of uterine cervix in black and white women. (From Henson D and Tarone R: Am J Obstet Gynecol 129:525, 1977.)

TABLE 27-1
Clinical Stages of Carcinoma of the Cervix Uteri (FIGO, Revised 1985)

Stage	Characteristics
I	Carcinoma is strictly confined to cervix (extension to corpus should be disregarded)
IA	Preclinical carcinoma
IA1	Minimal microscopically evident stromal invasion
IA2	Microscopic lesions no more than 5 mm depth measured from base of epithelium surface or glandular from which it originates, and horizontal spread not to exceed 7 mm
IB	All other cases of stage I; occult cancer should be marked "occ"
II	Carcinoma extends beyond cervix but has not extended to pelvic wall; it involves vagina, but not as far as lower third
IIA	No obvious parametrial involvement
IIB	Obvious parametrial involvement
III	Carcinoma has extended to pelvic wall; on rectal examination there is no cancer-free space between tumor and pelvic wall; tumor involves lower third of vagina; all cases with hydronephrosis or nonfunctioning kidney should be included, unless they are known to be due to another cause
IIIA	No extension to pelvic wall, but involvement of lower third of vagina
IIIB	Extension to pelvic wall, or hydronephrosis or nonfunctioning kidney due to tumor
IV	Carcinoma has extended beyond true pelvis or has clinically involved mucosa of bladder or rectum
IVA	Spread of growth to adjacent pelvic organs
IVB	Spread to distant organs

their 20s, leading to a gradual increase in the incidence of invasive carcinoma in younger patients.

The diagnosis of cervical carcinoma is established by biopsy of the tumor; a specimen can be easily obtained at office examination. A Kevorkian, Eppendorf, Tishler, or similar punch biopsy instrument (see Chapters 26 and 31) is convenient to use. Occasionally it is necessary to biopsy nodularity or induration in the vagina near the cervix to ascertain the limit of tumor spread and to define a correct tumor stage, as described later. If the patient's cytologic smear is suggestive of invasive carcinoma with no gross lesion visible and endocervical curettage does not demonstrate carcinoma, or if an adequate biopsy specimen to establish carcinoma cannot be obtained, then cervical conization should be performed.

Staging

The staging of carcinoma of the cervix depends primarily on the pelvic examination, and the designation may be modified by general physical examination, by chest x-ray examination, by intravenous pyelogram, or CT scan and is not changed based on operative findings, as occurs with ovarian carcinoma. Table 27-1 shows the definition of the four stages of cervical carcinoma according to FIGO (revised in 1985), and the various types of tumor distribution that may be observed in the various stages are illustrated in Figure 27-9.

To summarize, stage I tumors are confined to the cervix; stage II have spread to the vagina (upper two thirds) or paracervical areas or both but not to the pelvic wall; stage III involves spread to the lower third of the vagina or to the pelvic wall or evidence of ureteral obstruction or nonfunctioning of the kidney caused by tumor; and stage IV tumors have spread to the mucosa of the bladder or rectum or outside the pelvis.

Natural History and Spread

Carcinoma of the cervix is initially a locally infiltrating cancer that spreads from the cervix to the vagina and paracervical and parametrial areas. Grossly the tumors may be ulcerated (Figure 27-10), similar to carcinomas occurring elsewhere in the female genital tract, and may have an exophytic growth pattern or cauliflower-like appearance extruding from the cervix. The tumors usually produce abnormal bleeding and staining early in the course of the disease. Alternatively, they may be endo-

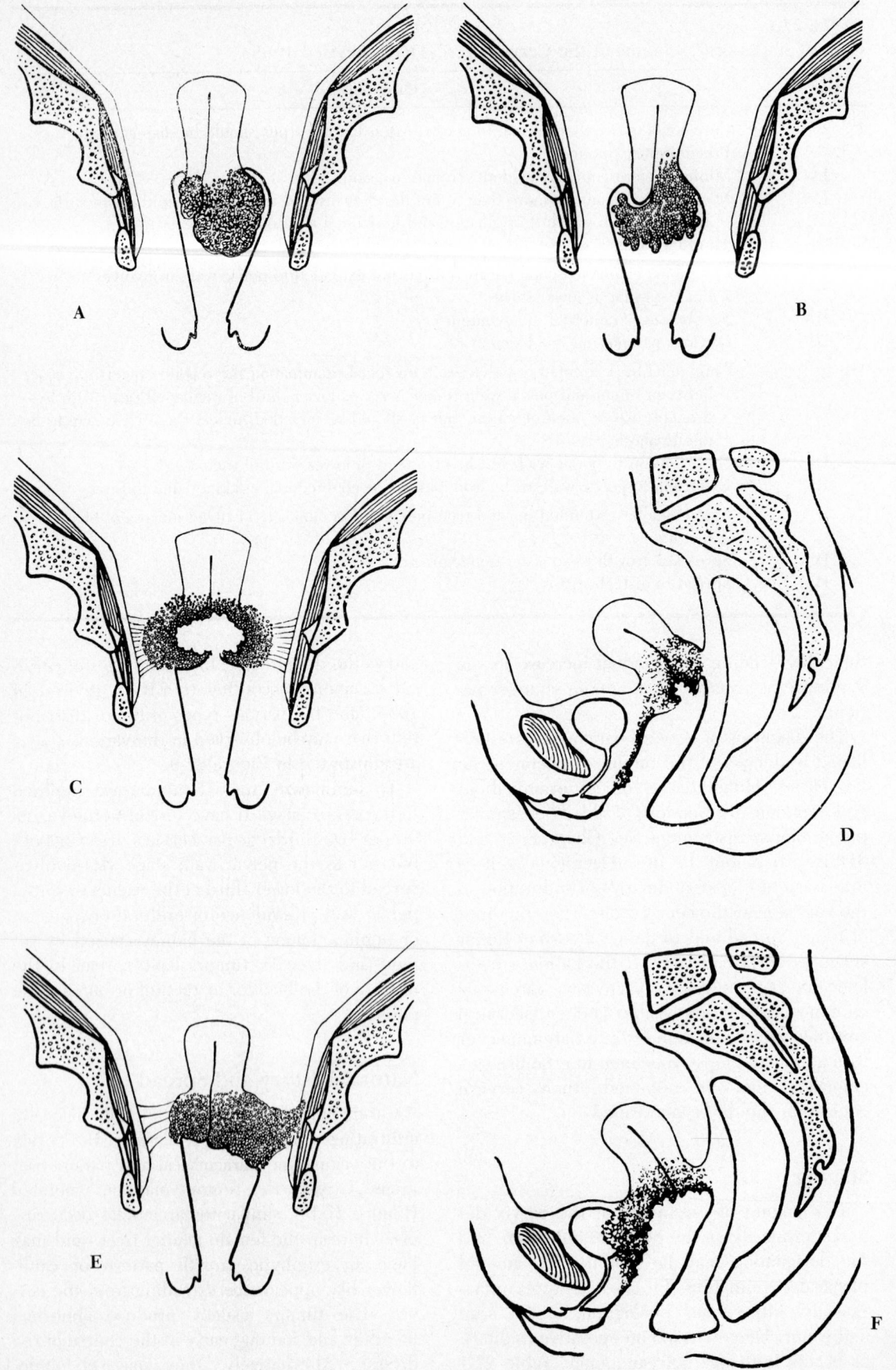

FIGURE 27-9

Staging of cervical carcinoma. **A,** Stage IB; nodular cervix. **B,** Stage IIA: carcinoma extending into left vault. **C,** Stage IIB: parametrium involved on both sides, but carcinoma has not invaded pelvic wall; endocervical crater. **D,** Stage IIIA: submucosal involvement of anterior vaginal wall and small, papillomatous nodule in its lower third. **E,** Stage IIIB: parametrium involved on both sides; at left, carcinoma has invaded pelvic wall. **F,** Stage IVA: involvement of bladder. (From Pettersson F and Bjorkholm E: Semin Oncol 9:289, 1982.)

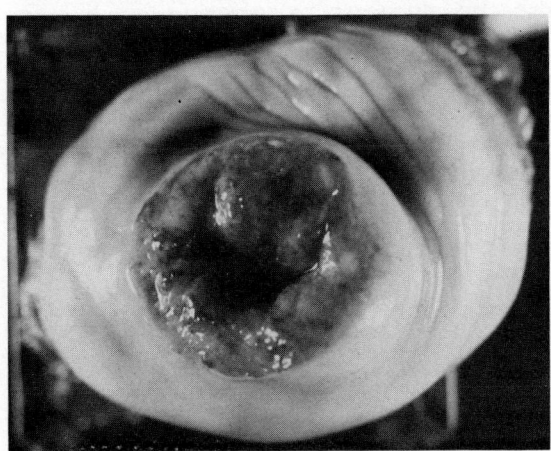

FIGURE 27-10

Carcinoma of cervix (gross specimen)

phytic, in which case they remain asymptomatic, particularly in the early stage of development, and tend to be deeply invasive into the cervix when diagnosed. They usually start initially from an endocervical location and often fill the cervix and lower uterine segment, resulting in a barrel-shaped cervix. The latter tumors tend to metastasize to regional pelvic nodes, and because of the tendency of late diagnosis, they are often more advanced than the exophytic variety. The primary path for distant spread is through lymphatics to the regional pelvic nodes. Blood-borne metastases from cervical carcinomas do occur, but they are less frequent and usually are seen late in the course of the disease.

Initially, cervical carcinoma spreads to the primary pelvic nodes, which include the pericervical (ureteral) node, which lies near the intersection of the uterine artery and ureter; the hypogastric (internal iliac) and external iliac nodes, which lie along their respective vessels; and the nodes in the obturator fossa near the vessels and nerve. From this primary group, tumor spread proceeds secondarily to the common iliac and paraaortic nodes. Rarely the inguinal nodes or the presacral nodes may be involved; the latter are particularly at risk for tumors that grow into the area of the rectum. The distribution of lymph node involvement was studied in detail in 26 cases of untreated carcinoma of the cervix by Henriksen (Figure 27-11) (five stage I, six stage II, eight stage III, and seven stage IV). All were examined at autopsy, and the primary pelvic group had the highest frequency of metastases with distal sites also involved, but less frequently. An important distal node that becomes involved after the paraaortic group is the left scalene node, that is the left supraclavicular node. A clinical correlation is that biopsy of this node is frequently performed in the assessment of advanced cervical carcinoma to clarify whether the tumor has spread outside the abdomen. In addition to nodal spread, hematogenous spread of cervical carcinoma occurs primarily to the lung, liver, and, less frequently, bone (see recurrence section).

Prognostic Factors

Clinical stage is the most important determinant of prognosis for carcinoma of the cervix. Table 27-2 demonstrates the collated results for 31,543 cases treated worldwide between 1979 and 1981. Almost 70% of the tumors are in stage I or II, about 25% in stage III, and fewer than 5% in stage IV. Age appears to be a factor, insofar as those under age 40 have a lower rate of survival than those between ages 40 and 69. This was recently emphasized by the studies of Dattoli et al., who noted a 5-year survival of 54% for those with stage IB who were younger than age 40, compared with 91% for older patients.

Numerous other factors have been evaluated to ascertain their importance in predicting the behavior of cervical carcinoma. These include

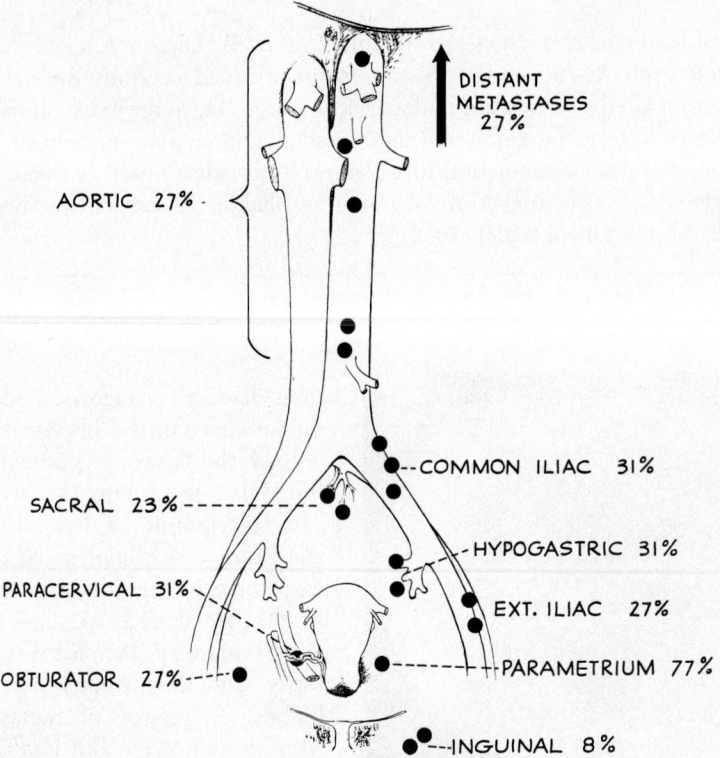

FIGURE 27-11

Frequency of lymph node metastases in cervical carcinoma. Incidence of node group involvement in 26 nontreated cases of cervical carcinoma. (From Henriksen E: Am J Obstet Gynecol 58:924, 1949.)

TABLE 27-2

Carcinoma of the Uterine Cervix: Distribution by Stage and 5-Year Survival Rates for Patients Treated in 1979 to 1981

| | Patients Treated | | 5-year Survival | |
Stage	No.	%	No.	%
I	10,912	34.6	8265	75.7
II	10,765	34.1	5877	54.6
III	8255	26.2	2527	30.6
IV	1386	4.4	101	7.3
No stage	225	0.7	106	47.1
TOTAL	31,543	100.0	16876	53.5

Modified from Pettersson F, Coppleson M, Creasman W, et al: Twentieth Annual Report on the Results of Treatment in Gynecologic Cancer, Stockholm, 1988, International Federation of Gynecology and Obstetrics.

tumor grade, depth of invasion, histologic type, presence of lymph-vascular (capillary-like) space involvement, and status of regional pelvic nodes. Many of these factors, however, are interrelated; that is, the stage of the tumor closely correlates with the status of the regional pelvic nodes. For example, in a summary of 6560 cases,

Plentl and Friedman noted a frequency of 15% positive pelvic nodes in 3391 cases of stage I, 29% in 2952 cases of stage II, and 47% in 217 cases of stage III. Percentages based on a single series of patients are not available for paraaortic node involvement, but in a multiinstitutional review of 290 patients by Lagasse et al., the proportion was 6% in stage I, 19% in stage IIA, and 33% in stages IIB and III; overall, 29% of the patients in stage II and higher had positive paraaortic nodes.

Within stage IB, lesion size has proved to be a very effective predictor of tumor behavior, as has the depth of tumor invasion into the stroma. The importance of lymph-vascular (capillary-like) space involvement in the prognosis of cervical carcinoma is not clear. Most studies indicate that capillary-like space involvement by tumor worsens the prognosis. Using a multivariate analysis of stage I tumors, Boyce et al. and Crissman et al. found that vasculocapillary space involvement was the only major histologic parameter of importance that correlated with survival in two studies totalling 218 patients. Delgado et al., in a cooperative Gynecologic Oncology Group study, analyzed 645 patients with stage I disease who had radical hysterectomy and node dissections at 33 institutions. The presence of pelvic node metastases independently correlated with lymph-vascular space involvement, depth of invasion, parametrial involvement, and patient age. In a follow-up GOG study the authors noted disease-free interval following therapy also correlated with lesion size, capillary-lymphatic space involvement, and depth of tumor invasion. Similar correlations for lesion size, capillary-like space involvement, and depth of invasion were noted by Gauthier et al. Recent molecular studies indicate that overexpression of the C-*myc* protooncogene is also associated with a poor prognosis.

ADENOCARCINOMAS OF THE CERVIX

Cervical adenocarcinomas occur in women of all ages, but the typical mucinous variety occurs primarily in women in their 50s. These tumors appear to have a different etiology than squamous cell carcinomas of the cervix insofar as there does not appear to be relationship to sexual transmission or a viral infection. Milsom and Friberg noted that patients with adenocarcinoma tend to be nulliparous or of low parity, are more often diabetic, and are older than patients with squamous cell carcinoma. In contrast, patients with clear cell adenocarcinoma of the cervix are often younger, particularly individuals who are exposed to DES in utero (Chapter 14). The prognosis of adenocarcinoma may be worse within comparable stages than for squamous cell carcinoma (Table 27-3), but this is debatable. Kleine et al., in a study of 145 patients with adenocarcinoma, noted poorer survival rates, particularly in patients with stage I or II disease. However, Davidson et al., in a study of 120 patients, and Leminen et al., in a study of 106, observed no difference. A 1991 study of 203 patients by Hopkins and Morley suggests poor survival in all stages for patients with adenocarcinoma in comparison to squamous cell carcinoma. Prognosis is related not only to the stage of the tumor but also to tumor grade and size and depth of stromal invasion. Berek et al. reported that the size of the adenocarcinoma, its degree of differentiation, and the depth of stromal invasion all

TABLE 27-3
Five-Year Survival Rates for Carcinoma of the Cervix by Treatment Modalities

	Radiation		Radiation Plus Operation	
Stage	Adeno. (n = 974)	Squamous (n = 13,106)	Adeno. (n = 241)	Squamous (n = 1660)
I	51.6%	66.7%	71.2%	78.9%
II	36.5%	51.5%	55.4%	63.3%
III	20.5%	29.8%	27%*	41.8%
IV	7.0%	7.0%	—	—
TOTAL AVERAGE	32.0%	43.0%	64.1%	70.0%

Modified from Pettersson F, Coppleson M, Creasman W, et al: Twentieth Annual Report on the Results of Treatment in Gynecologic Cancer, Stockholm, 1988, International Federation of Gynecology and Obstetrics.
*Only 11 cases treated.

correlated with the frequency of metastases to lymph nodes and thus patient survival. For adenocarcinomas with less than 2 mm of invasion, there was no lymph node metastases, while the frequency was greater than 50% for tumors that invaded more than 10 mm. Similarly, among stage I tumors less than 2 cm in diameter, all pelvic lymph node studies were negative for tumor, while larger tumors had an increasing proportion of positive nodes as tumor size or dedifferentiation increased. Therapy is considered in subsequent discussions. However, data from the Twentieth Annual Report from FIGO (Table 27-3) suggest that adenocarcinomas of the cervix may not be as curable by radiation alone as are squamous cell carcinomas.

MANAGEMENT

Pretherapy Evaluation

Once the patient has been diagnosed as having an invasive carcinoma of the cervix, pretreatment evaluation is conducted to determine the extent of disease, to arrive at an accurate clinical staging, and to plan the program of therapy. The usual evaluation consists of a thorough history and physical examination, routine blood studies (including a complete blood count and blood chemistries—chem-17), and an electrocardiogram for those age 40 or older. An intravenous pyelogram (IVP) or computed tomography (CT) scan and chest x-ray examination are part of this pretherapy evaluation. Demonstration of an obstructed ureter or nonfunctioning kidney caused by tumor automatically assigns the case at least to stage III (see Table 27-1). A barium enema test is sometimes performed, particularly in the case of large tumors, to have a baseline study for those who will be receiving radiation treatment.

The CT scan is a much more expensive examination than IVP but has the advantage of being able to provide the therapist with greater information concerning possible tumor spread to lymph nodes, particularly in cases of higher-stage disease. Goldman et al. found that the CT scan and IVP provide approximately equivalent information for cases of stages I and IIA carcinoma of the cervix but that CT was superior in stage IIB and above, not only in diagnosing a greater proportion of obstructed ureters, but also in helping to detect enlarged pelvic and paraaortic nodes that were suspicious for involvement of tumor. However, the CT scan is not particularly useful to detect the parametrial extent of cervical carcinoma, which is evaluated more reliably by pelvic examination. Magnetic resonance imaging (MRI) (Chapter 8) has also been used to evaluate local spread, but experience is limited and the test is not in widespread use currently to evaluate patients with cervical carcinoma. Only the status of the ureters and kidneys affects the assignment of tumor stage. The suggestion of tumor in retroperitoneal nodes by CT scan does not affect tumor stage, since the convention of staging relies only on clinical examination and the results of generally available radiologic tests (i.e., IVP and chest x-ray examination). Many therapists substitute the results of the evaluation of the kidney and ureters as determined by CT scan for the IVP findings in the assignment of clinical stage so that both a CT scan and IVP need not be performed. For low-stage tumors of small diameter (less than 2 cm), particularly those that are not endocervical, the less expensive IVP is sufficient.

A pelvic examination for determining tumor stage is usually performed with anesthesia to assess accurately the extent of disease. Cystoscopy is also performed at this time to rule out extension of tumor to the bladder. The results are usually normal for tumors that initially appear to be of low stage (i.e., I or IIA). Sigmoidoscopy is also often performed, particularly in patients with larger tumors, in patents with tumors posterior and near the rectum, or in patients who have symptoms referable to the lower bowel. Additional diagnostic tests, such as radionuclide scans of liver or bone and CT scan of the chest, are performed only as specifically indicated. In the past many patients, particularly those with large tumors, were also studied with lymphangiography. This test consists of injection of radiopaque dye into the lymphatics of the dorsum of the foot, which results in opacification of the pelvic and paraaortic nodes with defects in the nodes suggestive of tumor spread. The technique has been hampered by a high false negative rate that in some series has been reported to be 50%; it has now been replaced at most centers by CT analysis.

If a pelvic or paraaortic node appears to be involved with tumor by CT scan, further evaluation is indicated. If possible, fine-needle aspiration of the suspicious node should be performed under CT guidance. Bandy et al. used CT guidance to evaluate the pelvic and paraaortic nodes in 41 patients with primary or metastatic carcinoma of the cervix, and a fine-needle aspirate was obtained with a 20- to 22-gauge needle. The results were submitted for cytologic examination. These authors reported that the technique was successful in correctly diagnosing 67% of metastatic nodes that were 1.5 cm in diameter or greater. Nash et al. obtained similar results in 177 aspirations, with a reported sensitivity of 68%; since there were no false positive results, their specificity and positive predictive value were 100%. If the fine-needle aspiration does not yield a positive diagnosis of a suspicious node, particularly those in the paraaortic area, many therapists will proceed with open biopsy removal of the node through a retroperitoneal approach (see the discussions of therapy of high-stage tumors). The advantage of the retroperitoneal approach is that subsequent radiation therapy results in less bowel injury than a transperitoneal approach.

A scalene node biopsy of the left supraclavicular area is sometimes performed for evaluation of tumor spread. In a study of 40 patients, Brandt and Lifshitz performed this procedure on individuals who had metastatic paraaortic nodes or palpable scalene nodes. Of 25 patients with metastatic paraaortic nodes, 7 (28%) had metastasis to the scalene node. In reviewing the literature of 225 cases, it was noted that 11.6% had positive scalene nodes. Vasilev and Schlaerth used the procedure before paraaortic irradiation for positive nodes and found 4 of 17 patients had a positive scalene evaluation indicative of systemic disease. The diagnostic step is particularly useful in high-stage disease or in cases of patients with pelvic tumor recurrence who are being considered for exenterative therapy.

Low-Stage (IB - IIA) Disease

After pretherapy evaluation has been completed, treatment is usually planned jointly by a gynecologic oncologist and a radiation therapist. Radical hysterectomy and radiation therapy are equally effective as treatments for low-stage disease, and comparable survival statistics have been reported for stage IB and early stage IIA (i.e., minimal spread to the vagina). Numerous studies have been conducted to try to ascertain which tumors will respond preferentially either to radiation or to operation, but no reliable method of predicting which modality is optimum for a given tumor has been devel-

oped. Five-year survival rates from some centers of approximately 80% to 90% have been reported for stage IB and 70% to 80% for stage IIA with either radiation or radical hysterectomy; these statistics are somewhat better than most recently published, collated worldwide percentages (Table 27-2).

Both modalities have advantages and disadvantages. Operation allows preservation of ovarian function and completion of therapy in one hospitalization and may cause less vaginal radiation fibrosis and compromise of sexual function. It also permits a thorough exploration of the abdomen. The best results are obtained when operation is performed on small tumors, particularly those that are exophytic. Short-term complications such as infection, thromboembolic disease, and rarely fistula formation may occur, but there are few long-term complications (see later discussion). Short-term serious complications will occur in 1% to 2% of cases. Patients selected for hysterectomy are usually younger and in general in better health and thus are better able to tolerate a major surgical procedure. Patients who have had salpingitis or inflammatory bowel disease or who have unexplained pelvic masses are also treated by operation because of the increased risk of complications with extensive radiation. Radiation therapy is also widely used to treat low-stage carcinomas of the cervix and is the usual therapy for high-stage disease (stage IIB and above). Attempts have been made to combine full radiation treatment with radical hysterectomy, but this leads to frequent severe complications, including lack of healing and fistula formation. Einhorn et al. have reported promising effective combined results by using preliminary brachytherapy alone followed by radical hysterectomy, primarily for stage IB disease.

Operative Therapy: Radical Hysterectomy, Pelvic Node Dissection

Radical hysterectomy and bilateral pelvic lymphadenectomy are effective for treatment of many stage IB and some early stage IIA cancers. It is important that the operation remove the same volume of tissues that receive cancerocidal doses of radiation in cases for which radiation is the sole therapy. The amount of tissue removed, particularly in the paracervical and parametrial areas near the ureter, depends on the extent and location of the tumor. Piver et al. defined five classes to describe the extent

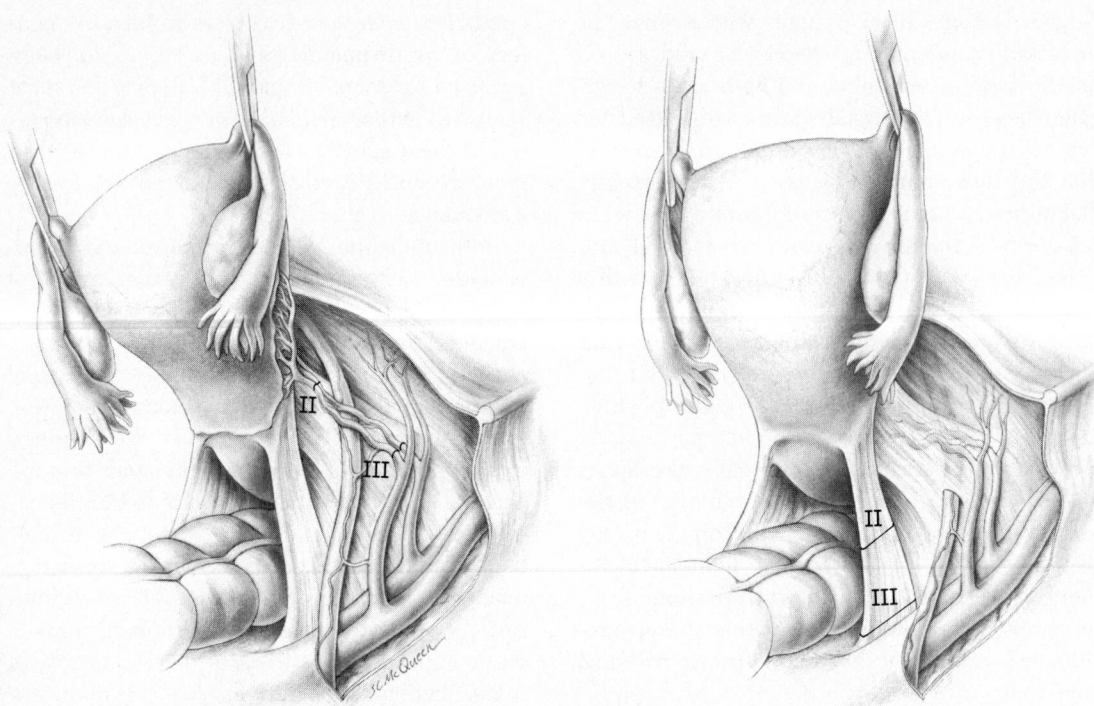

FIGURE 27-12
Classes II and III radical hysterectomy with points of dissection shown (see text).

of the operation. Class I is a hysterectomy that guarantees the removal of the entire cervix and uterus by lateral retraction of the ureters. The ureter is not disturbed from its bed, but the specimen is removed without dissection into the cervix. In many instances this is described as an *extrafascial hysterectomy*, the type used after preoperative radiation for treatment of a barrel-shaped cervix (see later discussion). A class II operation (Figure 27-12) removes more paracervical tissue than class I, but the ureters are retracted laterally yet are not dissected from their attachments distal to the uterine artery, and the uterosacral ligaments are ligated approximately halfway between the uterus and rectum. The operation is usually performed with pelvic lymphadenectomy and is often termed a *modified radical hysterectomy*. The operation is useful to treat small invasive carcinomas of the cervix that exceed the criteria for microinvasive carcinomas. This procedure may also be used to treat small, central cervical recurrences of carcinoma that are diagnosed following radiation therapy of the primary tumor. A class III operation is also performed with pelvic lymphadenectomy, and in this case the uterine artery is ligated at its origin from the anterior division of the

hypogastric artery, and the uterosacrals are ligated deep in the pelvis near the rectum (Figure 27-12). This operation is usually termed a *radical hysterectomy* (Meigs-Wertheim hysterectomy) and is performed for stage IB and occasionally stage IIA carcinomas of the cervix.

Class IV and V operations are infrequently performed. The former involves a complete dissection of the ureter from its bed and sacrifice of the superior vesical artery, with resulting partial loss of blood supply to the ureter and bladder. A class V operation involves resection of the distal ureter or bladder or both with reimplantation of the ureter into the bladder (ureteroneocystotomy). Both class IV and V operations are designed to remove small, central recurrent disease and would be attempted to avoid an anterior exenteration (see following discussion) to preserve the bladder. Although extensive data are not available, results of the latter two procedures are accompanied by high complication rates.

Preoperative preparation for a patient who is to undergo radical hysterectomy includes the same basic considerations for anyone undergoing a major procedure. Mechanical cleansing of the bowel is usually performed; mini-heparin

(5000 IU every 12 hours) is frequently prescribed or graduated-compression leg stockings (Kendall) to reduce the risk of thromboembolism. Prophylactic antibiotics are also frequently prescribed (see Chapter 23). During the course of the operation care is taken not to grasp the ureters with instruments such as forceps to avoid damaging the periureteral capillary blood supply. In addition, following removal of the pelvic nodes, suction catheters are left in the retroperitoneal space, and the upper and lower margins of the excised lymphatic tissue (near the femoral vessels inferiorly and the common iliac vessels superiorly) are ligated to reduce the risk of lymphocyst formation. Ovarian function may be preserved in younger patients if there is little likelihood of postoperative radiation. Many surgeons prefer a suprapubic cystotomy, which is more convenient for the patient and less likely to be accompanied by postoperative infection than a transurethral catheter. If a pelvic node dissection is not performed, particularly in an obese patient, a radical hysterectomy can also be accomplished vaginally (Shauta-Aumreich procedure). This operation has been more widely practiced in Europe than in the United States.

In stage I cases treated by radical hysterectomy and node dissection, the results obtained are related primarily to the status of the pelvic nodes, as well as the surgical resection margins around the primary tumor (ideally more than 1 cm). If the pelvic nodes are free of tumor, the 5-year survival rate can be expected to exceed 90%, whereas if the nodes are found to contain tumor, the 5-year survival rate drops to 45% to 50%. Lerner et al. reported a 5-year survival rate (life table technique) of 93.4% for 108 patients using class III hysterectomy for stage IB carcinomas of the cervix. All but five of these tumors were less than 5 cm in diameter. Six patients experienced prolonged bladder dysfunction after operation. Only one postoperative ureterovaginal fistula developed, and there were no postoperative deaths, indicating that excellent results can be obtained with operation, particularly if the patients are carefully selected. If the patient is found to have obvious spread of gross disease to pelvic nodes, the studies of Potter et al. suggest it is preferable to cease the operation and complete radiation therapy to improve pelvic control of tumor.

Numerous studies have been published evaluating low-dose preoperative radiation followed by radical hysterectomy and pelvic node dissection. The technique has been particularly widely used in Western Europe, and Einhorn et al. evaluated the Swedish experience comparing complete treatment with full radiation therapy alone, or preoperative partial radiation (two intracavitary radiums) and radical hysterectomy for patients under age 41 with stage IB or IIA carcinoma of the cervix. A significant ($P < 0.004$) improvement was noted in stage IB for the combined-therapy group as compared with radiation alone (5-year survival rate: 96% versus 81%). No significant difference was noted in stage IIA. Current data have not clearly established the superiority of this combined therapy to single-modality therapy with either radiation or radical hysterectomy, but the combination technique is used in many treatment centers. Calais et al. used combined therapy for tumors less than 4 cm in diameter in 70 patients and reported a 10-year survival of 96%, an excellent result.

Postoperative Therapy and Care

If the pelvic nodes are found to contain metastatic tumor following radical hysterectomy, it is current practice at most centers to add external pelvic radiation (teletherapy). Usually, approximately 50 Gy (5000 rads) are delivered by megavoltage radiation. Unfortunately, current data do not establish that this practice improves patient survival. A collaborative study by Zander et al. from Europe demonstrated no advantage of radiation following radical hysterectomy for those found to have metastatic tumor in the pelvic nodes. Similarly, Martimbeau et al. noted a 5-year survival rate of 53% among the patients treated at the Norwegian Radium Hospital with radiation therapy who had tumor involvement in nodes following radical hysterectomy, which is similar to that for patients with positive nodes who do not undergo irradiation. Although those receiving radiation therapy do not appear to have improved survival, they do appear to have a decreased rate of local tumor recurrence. Kinney et al. performed a matched retrospective analysis of adjuvant radiotherapy in 185 patients and noted no differences in survival. Soisson et al. also noted no improved survival with fewer pelvic recurrences in their series of 72 patients who tended to fail with distant metastases, indicating the need for effective systemic therapy. Similar results were reported by Remy et al. on 32 patients with stage IB carcinoma post radical hysterectomy with tumor found in their pelvic nodes, suggesting that pelvic irradiation reduces the risk of pelvic recurrence without extending survival. The number of positive nodes appears to have prognostic importance. Inoue and Morita noted decreasing 5-year survival in patients with stage IB cervical carcinoma as follows: no nodes, 92%; one node, 91%; two to three nodes, 71%; and four or more nodes, 50%. Survival appeared to improve in patients with one node who had postoperative radiotherapy, but a control group was not available for comparison.

Following radical hysterectomy many patients experience long-term complications that may be expected to accompany such extensive surgery. In previous years fistulas from the urinary tract, particularly ureterovaginal fistulas, were reported in 5% to 8% of patients, but in recent years this has been reported to be less than 1%. The improvement has been the result of administration of antibiotics, the postoperative use of retroperitoneal suction catheters to prevent serosanguineous collections, and avoidance of direct manipulation of the ureter to avoid injury to the periureteral blood supply.

Many patients suffer postoperative bladder dysfunction. In part this appears to be due to disruption of the sympathetic nerve supply to the bladder. However, the dysfunction is often temporary, and current evidence indicates that fibrosis and edema of the bladder, as well as surgical trauma, play a role in long-term bladder dysfunction. Low et al. noted an increase in bladder pressure with a decrease in urethral pressure (see Chapter 20) following radical hysterectomy. There was reduced bladder compliance with detrusor instability. The bladder can develop hypotonicity, and overdistention can then become a problem. If overdistention of the bladder and infection are avoided, progressive improvement of bladder function usually occurs. Forney correlated the degree of bladder dysfunction after radical hysterectomy with the extent of resection of the cardinal ligament. Those who had a complete resection of cardinal ligaments could void satisfactorily in an average of 51 days, in comparison to 20 days for those with only partial resection of the ligaments. All the patients experienced a decrease in bladder sensation. In a few patients the decrease in bladder sensation can be permanent. For patients in whom it is temporary, recovery occurs

after continuous drainage of the bladder with an indwelling catheter. Westby and Asmussen observed that by 1 year after operation, a slight decrease in urethral pressure persists but that the decrease is not as great as that noted immediately after operation. After 1 year the postoperative changes and bladder function usually recover.

Radiation Treatment

The majority of patients with carcinoma of the cervix are treated by radiation. The principles of external megavoltage treatment (teletherapy) and local implants (brachytherapy) are reviewed in Chapter 25. External beam radiation is administered in fractions so as to destroy the tumor without causing permanent damage to normal tissues. This delivers uniform dosages to the entire pelvis, including the regional pelvic nodes. The local implant delivers its highest energy in the region of the cervix and surface of the vagina, and paravaginal and paracervical tissues. The radiation from the implant diminishes according to the inverse square law, and the uterus and cervix serve as a receptacle for arranging and holding the intracavitary applicator stem (tandem) and accompanying vaginal applicators (ovoids) in a fixed and optimum position for delivering the desired radiation dosimetry (Fletcher-Suit applicator, see Figure 25-3).

Current technique usually involves delivering about 40 rads per hour to point A with shielding on the posterior ovoids to protect the rectum. The tandem and ovoids are inserted with the patient anesthetized, and a pack is placed in the vagina to stabilize the apparatus and increase the distance from the mucosa of the bladder and rectum. After the position of the applicator has been confirmed to be satisfactory by x-ray films, the radioactive sources, such as cesium 137, are inserted (afterloading technique). Other types of applicators are available, but the principle of delivering intense radiation to the cervix and paracervical areas is the same. The goal is to increase the total dosage of radiation to the maximum allowable to achieve tumor control without introducing a major risk of complications and injury to adjacent normal tissue. The specific protocols followed in various treatment centers differ, and individualization for specific patients is often needed depending on the stage and size of the cervical tumor as well as the patient's local

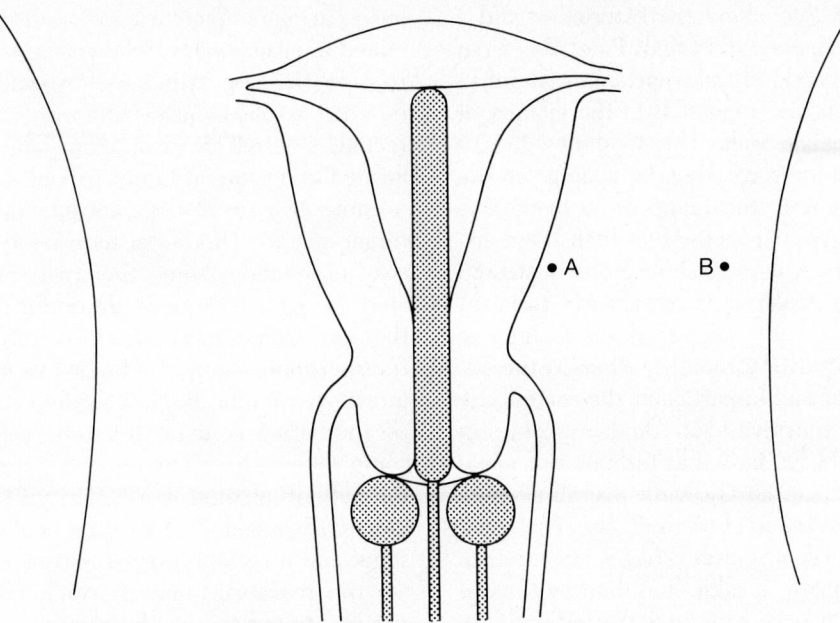

FIGURE 27-13
Points A and B with central stem (tandem) and two ovoids in place.

TABLE 27-4
Approximate Radiation Therapy Dosages for Carcinoma of the Cervix*

Stage	External Therapy	Local Implant† (mg hr)
IB (small, 1 cm)	Optional 40 Gy with central shield and decrease in implant dosage	8000-10,000 alone
IB (bulky, 3 cm)	20 Gy external first plus up to 20 Gy parametrial	6000-7500
	or	
	40-45 Gy	4500-5500
IB (barrel, 6 cm)	Radiation and surgery (see text)	
IIA	Similar to bulky stage IB	
IIB	Up to 50 Gy; may have additional boost to parametrial disease up to 6 Gy	4500-5500
III	50 Gy; may have additional boost to parametrial disease up to 10 Gy	4500
IVA	Individualized or similar to stage III	

*Average dosages will vary among patients and treatment centers.
†Usually done in two applications.

anatomy. In general, for tumors extending beyond the cervix, external therapy is given first both to treat the regional pelvic nodes and to shrink the central tumor mass, which then is more amenable for a local implant (Table 27-4). External therapy is also often prescribed initially in many cases of stage IB carcinoma to shrink the tumor before brachytherapy. In some patients external therapy leads to excessive shrinkage of the vaginal apex, making safe, effective implantation of local radiation sources difficult. This can be a problem particularly in older or postmenopausal patients. In some instances the central pelvis is shielded during external radiation therapy to allow for subsequent higher dosages from the implant. Occasionally, interstitial therapy in the form of needles implanted into the area of the tumor is needed to achieve effective local tumor control.

In calculating the dosages of radiation, two arbitrary reference points, A and B, are frequently used (Figure 27-13). Point A is defined to be located 2 cm above the external os and 2 cm lateral to the cervical canal. Point B is 5 cm lateral to the cervical canal and 3 cm lateral to point A which places point B in the vicinity of the lateral pelvic wall. The total dosage depends on tumor stage, but in general at the pelvic wall it is in the range of 50 to 65 Gy, with the higher dosages used for high-stage disease. At point A it varies but approximates 85 Gy. The normal cervix is particularly resistant to radiation and can tolerate doses as high as 200 to 250 Gy over 2 months, whereas the adjacent bladder and in particular the rectum are much more sensitive, and their exposure in general should be limited at the point of maximum radiation to 80 Gy, with overall average dosages in the range of 65 to 70 Gy. The small bowel can be damaged at dosages above 45 to 50 Gy, especially if adhesions limit intestinal mobility and a large volume is treated.

A general scheme for treating the various stages of carcinoma of the cervix by radiation is summarized in Table 27-4. The sum of external radiation therapy (Gy/10) plus the implant dose (mg hr/1000) equals approximately 10. At many treatment centers this sum varies from 9.0 to 10.0, and in general as the sum increases, the risk of complications from radiation therapy increases (see following discussion). In addition, as the volume of tissue that receives high doses of radiation increases, the risk of complications also increases. Therapeutic results with radiation therapy are generally similar to those with surgery for low-stage disease, and representative values are shown in Table 27-2. However, recently reported results from some centers are superior to those in Table 27-2. For example, Perez et al. studied results for 975 patients and reported 5-year survival rates of 85% for stage IB, 70% for stage IIA, 68% for stage IIB, and 45% for stage III. In a follow-up of that study, Sommers et al. noted failures in 376 of 1054 patients, and the failure pattern, as expected, correlated with stage. The median survival for those who failed more than 3 years after therapy was 22.5 months, compared with less than 12 months for those who failed earlier.

PARAAORTIC RADIATION. The field of external radiation is often extended from the pelvis to include the paraaortic nodes, particularly for high-stage disease (IIB or greater). The risk of paraaortic metastases in these cases is approximately 30%. Most therapists prefer to treat individuals in whom there is evidence of spread to paraaortic nodes. As noted previously, at many centers a CT scan is often obtained to evaluate advanced cervical carcinoma. In cases that appear to have suspected paraaortic node involvement by tumor, a CT scan–directed, fine-needle aspiration biopsy is performed to document tumor spread. However, a negative test result does not guarantee lack of tumor spread. Therefore, to provide more precise information, some therapists have evaluated the paraaortic node by performing a pretherapy laparotomy. Unfortunately, such a transperitoneal approach lends to a high rate of intestinal complications if subsequent paraaortic irradiation is given. In some series severe complications have been noted in a majority of the patients treated, particularly if the dose of radiation exceeded 5000 rads. Lagasse et al. suggested a retroperitoneal approach to evaluate the paraaortic nodes, which reduced the risk of intraperitoneal adhesions and provided a basis for selection of patients for paraaortic irradiation.

Current evidence suggests that a few patients with microscopic metastases in paraaortic nodes or a single large metastasis that can be resected will benefit from radiation treatment. Potish et al. noted only two severe complications in 81 patients who received 4350 to 5075 rads of paraaortic radiation. However, the patients in their series had not undergone prior surgical exploration. Using a combined retroperitoneal operation and radiation approach, Berman et al. estimated a 3-year survival rate of 25% for patients with tumor involvement in paraaortic common iliac nodes. Most centers treat with 4500 to 5000 rads (45 to 50 Gy). Major reasons for failure in these cases are systemic dissemination of tumor outside the radiation field and failure to control the primary tumor, especially in cases in which the cervical carcinoma is a large, bulky lesion. Podczaski et al. reported a 5-year survival of 31% in 33 patients with positive paraaortic or high common iliac nodes treated with dosages of 4250 to 5100 cGy.

Some have suggested an approach that would include paraaortic radiation for all patients with high-stage lesions (stage IIB or greater). In theory such a procedure would benefit approximately 7% of the patients, that is, 30% of those with tumor in the nodes and 25% of those who survive 3 years. The problem of resistant, bulky, primary pelvic carcinoma (see later discussion) remains, and a large number of patients who do not have tumor in the paraaortic nodes would receive unnecessary radiation. The optimum mode of management of these patients has not yet been defined.

ALTERNATE APPROACHES AND CHEMO-RADIATION. To improve the results of radiation treatment, new and other approaches are constantly being evaluated. Techniques include the use of hyperthermia and also radiation sensitizers (discussed in Chapter 25) to improve the tumoricidal effects of radiation without a comparable increase in effects on normal tissues. In the therapy of cervical carcinoma, hydroxyurea has been studied as a radiation potentiator by Piver et al., who treated 40 patients with stage IIB carcinoma of the cervix with hydroxyurea or a placebo. All were without paraaortic node metastases, proven at exploratory laparotomy. An improved actuarial survival rate of 94% was noted for the hydroxyurea group, in comparison to 53% for the placebo group. Unfortunately, severe complications, such as thrombocytopenia and severe sepsis, are recurrent problems. Leibel et al. reported a recent randomized trial of another radiation sensitizer, misonidazole. It did not improve survival in high-stage disease.

Induction chemotherapy with cisplatin 50 mg/m^2, Mitomycin C 10 mg/m^2, vincristine 1 mg/m^2, and bleomycin 10 units given over 21 days was administered by Dottino et al. to 28 patients with stages IB to IVA disease prior to operation. There were 35% complete and 65% partial responses with 4 patients free of disease at operation.

Newer techniques also include concomitant chemotherapy with drugs such as *cis*-platinum (cisplatin) during irradiation. Runowicz et al. reported very encouraging preliminary results on 32 evaluable patients with tumors greater than 4 cm in diameter. They administered cisplatin (20mg/m^2) continuously for 5 days every 3 weeks during radiation treatment. Twenty had high-stage tumors (IIB, III, or IV). There were 29 complete responses with a 28-month survival rate of over 80%. Most patients received four courses of cisplatin with future courses prevented by bone marrow depression. In addition, chemotherapy-radiation treatments have also been tried to improve results in patients with paraaortic node involvement, but long-term results are not available. Podczaski et al. noted two late bowel injuries in patients receiving extended-field irradiation with 5-fluorouracil (5-FU) and cisplatin.

The use of radiation sources that are not impeded by tumor hypoxia, such as fast neutrons (see Chapter 25), is also under study. Maruyama et al. showed an improved 5-year survival rate (54%) for patients with stage IIIB carcinomas of the cervix using neutrons for brachytherapy (californium 252), which were given before conventional teletherapy (photons). The results of a large series of patients treated in various centers by neutron therapy are not currently available.

RADIATION COMPLICATIONS. Complications experienced by the patient following radiation therapy are related to dosage, volume treated, and sensitivity of the various tissues receiving radiation. The patient's habitus and presence of diseases that affect circulation, such as diabetes and high blood pressure, increase the risk, as does prior intraabdominal operation. Acute minor complications, such as diarrhea and nausea, subside after radiation therapy is completed. Complications usually arise in 1 to 2 years but can occur as early as 6 months or as late as many years after radiation therapy is completed. Scarring of normal tissues can lead to severe radiation fibrosis.

The treatment of radiation complications depends on the symptoms and site of the complication. Vaginal or cervical ulcerations occasionally occur, and local treatment with topical antibiotics and estrogen creams is usually satisfactory. Postradiation cystitis may manifest itself as urinary frequency or dysuria. After infection has been ruled out, symptomatic treatment is undertaken with drugs such as antispasmodics or urinary analgesics (e.g., phenazopyridine [Pyridium], 100 mg three times daily), and these are prescribed until the symptoms clear. Occasionally hemorrhagic cystitis occasionally develops and this may require hospitalization for continuous bladder irrigation or instillation of agents to control bleeding, such as silver nitrate or sometimes fulguration of the bleeding points. In cases of hematuria, recurrent tumor should first be ruled out. Periureteral fibrosis can lead to ureteral obstruction and loss of kidney function. In this case recurrent tumor is often also responsible, and it is important for the clinician to rule out recurrent carcinoma before ascribing the cause of urinary obstruction to radiation fibrosis.

Bowel complications tend to be more frequent than urinary complications. Proctosigmoiditis can lead to diarrhea, severe pain on defecation, or gastrointestinal bleeding. Conservative therapy with stool softeners and a low-roughage diet may suffice; occasionally local corticosteroids (Cort enema) are of assistance. Fistulas or rectal ulcerations are occasionally seen in the area adjacent to the tip of the cervix, which is also the area maximally radiated during the local vaginocervical implant. If a fistula develops, or in cases of ulceration or severe bleeding and pain, a diverting colostomy is required. Serious small bowel complications may occur, leading to obstruction, fistula formation, or necrosis. The use of parenteral nutrition and intravenous hyperalimentation has provided an excellent mechanism to help deal with these problems.

The rate of complications also is related to the frequency of cure, especially for high-stage disease. Montana et al. noted a 19.5% complication rate in the therapy of 251 patients with stage II disease, and the risk of complications increased with dose. For example, patients with complications had a mean dose of 7877 rads to point A, in comparison to 7593 rads for those without complications. In a follow-up study, the risk of proctitis was also related to increasing doses of external beam treatment. The balancing of the risk of complication with increasing radiation dosage to improve cure rates was further demonstrated by Orton and Wolf-Rosenblum, who studied patients with stages IIB and III carcinoma of the cervix. Higher dosages had been used in persons who survived 5 years, and their complication rate was 21%, in comparison to only 6% for those who did not survive 5 years.

Adenocarcinomas

The appropriate therapy of adenocarcinoma of the cervix has been debated, and many therapists use the same approaches as have been described for squamous cell carcinoma. Some reports have suggested that these tumors may be more resistant to radiation than comparable squamous cell carcinomas of the cervix. There are no data from randomized studies, but recent collated data from the Twentieth Annual Report on Results of Treatment of Gynecologic Cancer (see Table 27-3) support the impression of a worse prognosis, stage for stage, for adenocarcinoma of the cervix as does the 1991 report of Hopkins and Morley. Furthermore, these results suggest that, particularly for low-stage tumor, the combination of operation and radiation is preferable to radiation alone. Patients who are able to receive only radiation do worse, in part because the larger and more extensive tumors are chosen to be radiated. As shown by Weiss and Lucas, larger tumors tend to be poorly differentiated and have a higher frequency of node metastases. Duk et al. reported the tumor marker CA-125, usually used for ovarian carcinoma (Chapter 29), may predict prognosis in cervical adenocarcinoma, since patients with elevated levels had a worse prognosis.

Although many authors have reported comparable survival statistics for adenocarcinoma of the cervix following operation alone or radiation alone, the desirability of utilizing a combined modality has recently been supported in a study of 211 cases of pure or typical adenocarcinoma of the cervix by Moberg et al. in which stage IB or IIA cases were treated by either full radiation alone or partial radiation (two local implants into the cervix and vagina) followed by radical hysterectomy within 3 months. The overall 5-year survival rates for patients with stage IB were 79% and 92%, respectively, and stage IIA, 46% and 67%, respectively, suggesting that a combined radiation and surgical approach gives superior results but definitive conclusions cannot be drawn regarding the optimal treatment of low-stage adenocarcinoma. Radiation alone is used for higher-stage tumors.

Bulky Stage IB Carcinomas

Bulky tumors of the cervix over 4 to 6 cm in diameter, particularly those of an endocervical location, give rise to a barrel-shaped cervix. Because of the large volume of hypoxic tumor, such lesions are believed to be more resistant to conventional ionizing radiation, which requires oxygen (Chapter 25). This leads to an increased risk of radiation failure and local tumor recurrence. To avoid those risks a combined radiation and surgical approach has been used. Usually 4000 rads at approximately 180 rads per day external therapy is given, followed by one or two intracavitary implants and in 4 to 6 weeks an extrafascial (class I) hysterectomy is performed. Gallion et al. compared such combined therapy with radiation treatment alone for stage IB barrel-shaped cervical lesions and noted improved results with the combined approach (16% recurrence rate versus 47% for radiation alone). Maruyama et al. combined external and brachytherapy for 80 patients with bulky or barrel-shaped stage IB tumors followed in 6 weeks by extrafascial hysterectomy.

This yielded a 5-year survival of 84%. Pelvic control was excellent, and most failures resulted from distant metastases. This approach is also used for low-stage adenocarcinomas of the cervix.

Cervical Stump Tumors

Some patients undergo supracervical hysterectomy for nonmalignant disease. The operation was more frequently practiced years ago, but it is occasionally done even today in some cases, such as severe sepsis, to avoid a more extensive operative procedure. Carcinomas that subsequently develop in the cervical stump pose special problems because of the shortness of the cervical canal and absence of the uterus, both of which curtail the effective use of brachytherapy, especially insertion of an intracervical tandem. There is also the risk that bowel adhesions to the apex of the vagina and cervix will increase the chances of radiation complications, and a pretherapy barium study of the small and large bowel may be helpful to identify loops that adhere to the cervical apex. For patients with small stage IB tumors, an operative approach similar to radical hysterectomy can be considered. However, most patients are treated with radiation therapy. External treatment is emphasized because of the difficulty of an optimum intracavitary implant. A transvaginal cone may also be used to supplement external pelvic therapy. Effective treatment of cervical stump carcinoma can be achieved, and an overall 5-year survival rate of 45% in 173 patients was reported by Wolff et al. Stage for stage, the survival rates are comparable to those achieved for invasive carcinoma of the cervix, but because of the prior supracervical hysterectomy, there is an increased risk of complications.

Carcinoma of the Cervix Inadvertently Removed at Simple Hysterectomy

Unfortunately the situation occasionally arises in which a patient undergoes simple total hysterectomy and an invasive carcinoma of the cervix is found after operation. Optimum radiation treatment of the cancer is not possible, since the uterus and cervix are no longer present and the receptacle for a tandem has been removed. The therapist can subsequently perform a radical operation, removing the tissues that would normally be removed at radical

hysterectomy, including the regional pelvic nodes. Such an approach has been utilized particularly in younger patients. More commonly, however, the patient is treated with radiation therapy. Usually external therapy is initiated and supplemented with local brachytherapy with vaginal colpostats. Heller et al. reported a 5-year survival rate of 70% for 25 patients. Similar results were reported in an older series by Davy et al., but the survival rate decreased to 38% if tumor was transected at the initial operation.

Carcinoma of the Cervix in Pregnancy

Rarely an invasive carcinoma of the cervix is discovered in a pregnant patient. In the past it has been thought that pregnancy may have an adverse effect on cervical carcinoma, but this has not proven to be the case. Within each stage, survival statistics are similar in pregnant and nonpregnant women. An additional concern has been that the delivery of a fetus through a cervix that is replaced by carcinoma might worsen the prognosis. Although there has been concern in the past about tumor dissemination in such cases, there is no clear evidence to indicate that tumor dissemination is caused by the birth process. The major risk to the patient of delivery through a cervix containing invasive carcinoma is the risk of hemorrhage as a result of tearing of the tumor during cervical dilation and delivery.

A problem arising in pregnancy is whether a patient with an abnormal cytologic smear has intraepithelial neoplasia or invasive cancer. In general, if the cytologic and histologic findings of colposcopically directed biopsies are comparable and suggest intraepithelial neoplasia or carcinoma in situ, the patient is observed and delivered, with final evaluation and therapy completed approximately 6 weeks after delivery, as outlined in Chapter 26. Even if there is a question of microinvasion, a patient so diagnosed in the last trimester of pregnancy is usually followed and evaluated further after delivery. Cervical conization during pregnancy can lead to severe complications, particularly hemorrhage and also loss of the fetus. If it is necessary to perform a conization or a wedge resection of the cervix during pregnancy, it is probably best to perform this during the second trimester, when the risks of fetal loss and hemorrhage are minimal. For patients in whom invasive cancer is diagnosed, a therapeutic plan must be developed to deliver appropriate care, with regard also for the outcome of the pregnancy.

The therapy of invasive carcinoma of the cervix during pregnancy is influenced by the stage of the disease, the time in pregnancy the cancer is diagnosed, and the beliefs and desires of the patient in terms of initiating therapy that can interrupt the pregnancy as opposed to postponing the therapy until fetal viability is achieved. If the carcinoma is diagnosed in the first trimester or early in the second trimester (before 20 weeks), treatment is preferably undertaken immediately because of the concern that a delay of over 4 months would lead to tumor progression or spread. If the patient has resectable tumor (stage IB or early IIA), then effective treatment consists of radical hysterectomy and node dissection (class III). This procedure can usually be carried out without difficulty on a pregnant woman, especially before the twentieth week. Although an enlarged uterus can interfere with the operative field, increased uterine motility and edema of the pelvic tissue planes help to simplify the procedure for the experienced surgeon. Pregnancy does increase the risk of blood loss. For higher-stage tumors therapy is begun with external beam radiation (teletherapy), and usually in 4 to 6 weeks this leads to spontaneous abortion. The dosage of external therapy prescribed varies depending on the stage of the tumor, but approximately 40 to 50 Gy is given. Following abortion the uterus involutes, and an implant (brachytherapy) is performed. If the pregnancy does not spontaneously abort, dilation and curettage, prostaglandin-assisted delivery, or rarely hysterotomy may be necessary to empty the uterus before brachytherapy. Alternatively, if the initial tumor was small and has completely regressed, an extrafascial hysterectomy or modified radical hysterectomy (class I or II) may be performed.

For patients beyond the twentieth week of gestation a decision regarding initiating therapy immediately or delaying therapy until fetal viability must be made. If it is desired to continue the therapy, assessment must be made of the health of the fetus and its maturity. These are determined by appropriate ultrasound studies and amniotic fluid analysis to ensure fetal lung maturity. Delivery is usually accomplished by cesarean section, and after this, therapy is completed by operation or radiation with the same

considerations of tumor stage and size for patients who are treated before the twentieth week of pregnancy. If immediate treatment is to be undertaken, hysterotomy is first performed and then operation or radiation therapy completed. Overall, treatment results in pregnant patients are similar to those in nonpregnant patients, stage for stage. The reader should be aware that some published studies on dealing with carcinoma of the cervix in pregnancy include cases treated as long as 1 year postpartum, which assumes the carcinoma was present during pregnancy. Hacker et al. summarized the results of 1249 cases reported in various series in the literature. Overall, a 5-year survival rate of 49.2% was recorded for pregnant patients, in comparison to 51% for nonpregnant patients treated during the same period of time. Their statistics included not only patients treated during pregnancy but also those treated up to 6 months after delivery, and the postpartum group had the poorest survival statistics. Survival was most closely related to stage, as expected, and persons diagnosed during the first trimester had a better prognosis than those diagnosed during the third trimester.

RECURRENCES

Approximately one third of patients treated for cancer of the cervix will experience tumor recurrence, which is defined as the reappearance of tumor 6 months or more after therapy. Earlier identification of tumor indicates persistent rather than recurrent disease. Metastases can occur anywhere, but most are in the pelvis (centrally in the vagina or cervix or laterally near the pelvic walls) or less frequently distally in the periaortic nodes, lung, liver, or bone. It should be noted that liver, lung, and distal bone metastases outside the pelvis likely result from hematogenous tumor spread.

The symptoms caused by recurrence depend on the site and extent of metastatic disease. Vaginal discharge and abnormal bleeding are often symptoms of an early central pelvic recurrence. Malaise, loss of appetite, and general symptoms associated with widespread metastatic disease are usually late manifestations of recurrence. Lateral pelvic recurrences often have a retroperitoneal component, which can lead to sciatic nerve irritation and cause severe pain around the distribution of the sciatic nerve in back of the leg as well as loss of muscle strength causing the patient to walk with a limp. Unilateral leg edema frequently accompanies such metastases, or leg swelling may occur from fibrosis of lymphatics following operation or radiation. In addition, tumor recurrence can also cause ureteral obstruction, leading to unilateral or bilateral compromise of kidney function. Low back pain frequently occurs. Symptoms of pulmonary or hepatic disease will develop, with progressive metastases in these areas. In addition, it should be remembered that the pattern of recurrence depends not only on the natural history of the tumor, but also on the initial treatment utilized. For example, some tumors appear to be cured in the pelvis after radiation, only to recur later at a distant site as a result of blood-borne metastases.

Patients treated for carcinoma of the cervix are examined according to the same schedule as patients with other malignancies: every 3 months the first year, every 4 months the second year, every 6 months from years 3 to 5, and yearly thereafter. More frequent examinations are done if abnormal symptoms or signs develop. Examination consists of vaginal and cervical cytology (Pap smear), as well as complete physical and pelvic examinations. Generally, chest x-ray films are obtained annually, and an IVP is also performed annually, particularly during the first 3 years after treatment, when the majority of recurrences will develop. Special studies, such as CT scans, are ordered as indicated. A recently introduced blood test for squamous cell carcinoma (SCC) antigen has promise as an added modality to follow patients with squamous cell carcinoma who have detectable levels of the antigen in their blood. Holloway et al. noted elevated levels in 72 of 153 patients (53%) and found the test useful for following patients who initially had elevated levels. Once recurrent disease is suspected, verification is usually obtained by biopsy of an accessible mass or CT–directed thin-needle aspiration, depending on the location of the tumor recurrence.

Pelvic Recurrences

Approximately 50% of the recurrences of squamous cell carcinoma will develop in the pelvis. Other major sites are the abdomen and paraaortic nodes, liver, lung, and bone. Recurrences of adenocarcinoma are less frequent in the pelvis and are more likely to be at distant sites, such as the lung or supraclavicular areas.

For patients who were initially treated by operation, radiation is usually prescribed for pelvic recurrences, and approximately 50 Gy whole pelvic irradiation is given. Supplemental interstitial or intracavitary radiation is also prescribed, depending on the size and location of recurrence in the pelvis. For patients who were initially treated with radiation who have developed a pelvic recurrence, surgical eradication of the tumor should be considered, since further effective radiation is not possible and limited surgical resection of the pelvic recurrence will not lead to a cure but will often cause severe complications of wound healing and intestinal and urinary fistulas.

Pelvic Exenteration

Exenterative therapy for central pelvic tumor recurrence is an extensive operative procedure used only if preoperative evaluation suggests that the patient's condition can be cured by this procedure. Exenteration is not performed for palliation. Three types of operation may be used. *Anterior pelvic exenteration* is the removal of the bladder, uterus, cervix, and part or all of the vagina. *Posterior pelvic exenteration* is the removal of the anus and rectum and resection of the uterus, cervix, and all or part of the vagina. *Total exenteration* is combined anteroposterior exenteration to remove all the pelvic contents.

Before an exenterative operation is undertaken, the patient is thoroughly evaluated for any evidence of disease spread outside the pelvis. A CT scan is usually performed, and radiologic studies, such as barium enema and IVP, are done, particularly if a CT scan is not performed. Liver function tests are done, and, if indicated, radionuclide scans (including liver and bone scans) are performed. If there is suspicion of spread outside of the pelvis, a supraclavicular (scalene) node biopsy is undertaken. Assuming that the disease appears to be confined to the pelvis, operation is performed. Initially, a thorough abdominal exploration is carried out to be sure the tumor is resectable. Biopsy specimens of any enlarged lymph nodes or suspicious areas outside the pelvis are taken, and frozen-section studies are performed, including evaluation of the operative margins. Usually total exenteration is performed, and a colostomy is created for feces and an intestinal pouch (ileal bladder) for urine. The recent introduction of a continent urinary pouch has contributed to patient comfort; the operation is well described by Penalver et al. Generally the urinary stoma is located in the abdomen on the right side and the intestinal stoma on the left side. The use of intestinal stapling devices sometimes allows preservation of the rectal sphincter and anal function.

Severe postoperative and intraoperative complications can occur with this extensive procedure, and perioperative mortalities as high as 10% to 20% have been reported in the past. Infection and bowel obstruction are the major risks. However, current surgical techniques of preoperative bowel preparation, use of antibiotics, careful intraoperative fluid and volume monitoring, and the use of parenteral nutrition have reduced the immediate postoperative mortality to less than 5%. The use of a peritoneal graft or an omental flap, created from the right or left side of the omentum and placed in the pelvis to protect the denuded pelvic floor, can promote healing, help to avoid bowel obstruction, and reduce postoperative morbidity. Occasionally, gracilis myocutaneous grafts are used both to create a new vagina and to bring a new blood supply to the previously irradiated pelvis, which aids in wound healing. Morley et al. reported a 5-year survival of 61% in 100 patients ages 21 to 74 years. No patients with positive nodes in the specimen survived.

Nonpelvic Recurrences

Recurrences outside of the pelvis can be treated with radiation, operation, or chemotherapy. Localized recurrences in areas not previously irradiated are occasionally treated by means of radiation. Resection of the metastasis is rarely done, and it is usually restricted to a localized lesion that occurs 3 to 4 years after primary therapy on the assumption that such a solitary metastasis can be effectively treated with local resection. However, in general, distant metastases are usually manifestations of systemic disease and are not cured with local therapy.

Chemotherapy

Chemotherapy is usually prescribed for patients with unresectable pelvic recurrences following radiation therapy or for patients with disseminated metastatic disease. A variety of chemotherapeutic agents, either singly or in combination, have been used to treat recurrent squamous cell carcinoma of the vagina with generally poor results. Part of the problem is that in many of the cases there is often compromise of renal function due to ureteral obstruction or loss of bone marrow due to prior pelvic irradiation that reduces the dosage of chemotherapeutic agent that can be administered. In addition, squamous cell carcinomas in general have proven to be resistant to many chemotherapy programs.

Short-term responses of recurrent squamous cell carcinoma of the cervix have been reported with various multiple-agent protocols and the best results appear to be obtained with protocols that contain cisplatin. Bloch et al. reported on the use of bleomycin and cisplatin in 17 patients and obtained an overall 53% response rate, only one case of which represented a complete response. The median survival time was 8 months. A more active program appears to be the use of cisplatin with continuous infusion of 5-fluorouracil, which has been successfully employed in squamous cell carcinomas of the head and neck. Recently Rotmensch et al. utilized intravenous cisplatin, 100 mg/m^2, followed by 5-fluorouracil, 1000 mg/m^2 per day for 3 to 5 days of continuous infusion, and the regimen was given every 3 to 4 weeks. Among the 25 patients so treated, the overall response rate was 52%, and complete response comprised 20% (five patients). The median survival time was 40 weeks. The successful treatment of recurrent squamous cell carcinoma of the cervix will depend on the introduction of new agents and different therapeutic approaches than are currently available. However, as noted, chemotherapy may provide a useful adjuvant to radiation therapy. A different adjuvant use was suggested by Lai et al., who gave adjuvant chemotherapy with cisplatin, vinblastine, and bleomycin. In 40 patients with extensive tumors or positive nodes after radical hysterectomy and node dissection, the 3-year survival was 75% for those who received chemotherapy, compared with 47% for those who did not.

Advanced Disease

As noted previously, pelvic pain can be a severe problem in patients with recurrent carcinoma of the cervix, especially when there is irritation or invasion of nerve trunks by tumor.

This often becomes a particularly serious problem in patients with pelvic recurrence, where back pain and lower limb pain are often severe. Analgesics, including narcotics, are used as needed to control pain. Continuous intravenous infusion of narcotics, such as morphine, is occasionally very helpful. Local nerve blocks are also used, and in selected cases neurosurgical procedures, such as cordotomy (interruption of the lateral spinothalamic tract), provide the patient with excellent pain relief. Unfortunately, the operation also has potential severe side effects, such as bladder atony.

In addition to pain, urinary or intestinal fistulas or obstruction may develop. In certain selected cases this is relieved with an operation to divert the feces or urine, although if possible an operation is avoided in patients with advanced disease. Urinary diversion is generally avoided, since persons who undergo such a diversion frequently have prolonged periods of severe pain from metastatic disease in comparison to patients who do not have diversion and who succumb to uremia. The decision to use an operative approach to provide palliation to these patients depends on their activity status and near-term prognosis. The appropriate management of these difficult therapeutic problems requires sensitive and close interaction among the physician, allied health workers, and the patient and her family.

Sarcomas

Very rare sarcomas of the cervix have been reported. Brand et al. summarized 21 cases of sarcoma botryoides with encouraging results using multiagent chemotherapy followed by operation. A report by Daya and Scully suggests that patients with these tumors may have a better prognosis than those with tumors of similar histology arising in the vagina (Chapter 31).

―――――――――― **KEY POINTS** ――――――――――

- Carcinomas of the cervix are predominantly squamous cell carcinomas (85% to 90%), and about 10% to 15% are adenocarcinomas.

- Squamous cell carcinomas appear to have a viral and venereal association, whereas adenocarcinomas do not. In the United States squamous cell carcinoma is more frequent in blacks than in whites.

- Cervical carcinoma is the third most frequent malignancy of the lower female genital tract, after endometrial and ovarian cancer, and the second most frequent cause of death, after ovarian cancer.

- The definitive diagnosis of microinvasive carcinoma is established by means of cervical conization, not biopsy. The margins of the cone should be free of neoplastic epithelium before conservative therapy is undertaken.

- Microinvasive carcinoma of the cervix should be effectively treated by total hysterectomy, with a 5-year survival rate of almost 100%, but recurrent neoplasia can develop after 5 years. However, a precise and reliable definition of microinvasion is controversial.

- The prognosis of squamous cell carcinoma of the cervix is related to tumor stage and size and depth of invasion. The prognosis of adenocarcinoma of the cervix is related to tumor stage, size, grade, and depth of invasion. Large adenocarcinomas tend to be poorly differentiated. Younger patients, less than age 40 years, have a worse prognosis than older patients.

- Metastases to regional pelvic nodes in stage I squamous carcinomas correlate with lesion size, depth of invasion, presence of capillary lymphatic space involvement, and correlate inversely with patient age.

- Cervical carcinomas are locally invasive tumors that spread primarily to the pelvic tissues and then to the pelvic and paraaortic lymph nodes. Less frequently, hematogenous spread to the liver, lung, and bone occurs.

- The risk of the spread of cervical carcinoma to pelvic nodes is 15% for stage I, 29% for stage II, and 47% for stage III. For the paraaortic nodes, percentages are 6% for stage I, 19% for stage II, and 33% for stage III.

- Stage IB carcinomas of the cervix may be treated equally effectively by radical hysterectomy and pelvic node dissection or radiation. The 5-year survival rate is approximately 80%. If lymph nodes are free of tumor, the 5-year survival rate is approximately 90%, and if the nodes contain metastatic tumor, 50%. Improved overall survival rates have been reported for patients with tumors less than 4 cm in diameter treated by preliminary brachytherapy followed by radical hysterectomy.

- During radical hysterectomy the ureter should never be grasped with surgical instruments so as to avoid damaging the periureteral blood supply.

- Operation is often used for treating stage IB to stage IIA carcinomas of the cervix, particularly for smaller tumors and for younger patients to preserve their ovarian function. Operation produces less scarring and vaginal fibrosis than does irradiation. Operation is preferred for women with pelvic mass, pelvic infection, or history of conditions such as inflammatory bowel disease, which increase the risk for radiation complications.

- High-stage tumors are treated by irradiation. Improved regression appears feasible with combined irradiation and chemotherapy.

- Urinary fistulas follow radical hysterectomy in approximately 1% of cases.

- Most cancers of the cervix are treated by irradiation (teletherapy and brachytherapy). Radiation dosages vary with tumor size and stage but approximate 50 to 65 Gy at point B and 85 Gy at point A.

- Improved cure rates of cervical cancers are obtained with increased dosages, which also lead to an increased frequency of complications. Large increments in dosage increase complications without increasing cure rates.

- Complications following radiation are related to dosage and volume of tissue treated and include radiation inflammation of the bladder or bowel, which may lead to pain, bleeding, or, infrequently, fistula formation. The normal cervix is resistant to radiation, and the dose can be as high as 200 to 250 Gy over 2 months. The bladder and rectum can be injured at average dosages in the range of 65 to 70 Gy. Overall moderate to severe radiation complications for treatment of all stages approximate 10%.

- Radiation complications of the intestine are more frequent than bladder complications. Both tend to occur more than 1 year after therapy.

- Worldwide 5-year survival rates reported for patients with carcinomas of the cervix are as follows: stage I, 78%; stage II, 57%; stage III, 31%; and stage IV, 8%.

- Survival rates of patients with adenocarcinoma appear to be slightly lower than rates for those with squamous cell carcinomas. Patients with low-stage disease are usually treated by means of combined radiation and operation.

- Pregnancy does not adversely affect the survival rate for women with carcinoma of the cervix, stage for stage.

- Approximately one third of patients treated for cervical carcinoma develop tumor recurrence, and most of these recurrences are located in the pelvis.

- Patients whose recurrences occur more than 3 years after primary therapy have a better prognosis than those with earlier recurrence.

- Pelvic exenteration in carefully selected patients with central pelvic recurrence can lead to a 5-year survival of 50% or better.

- Chemotherapy of squamous cell carcinoma of the cervix does not produce long-term cures, but response rates of approximately 50% (partial and complete) have been obtained with multiple-agent regimens that contain cisplatin.

- Leg pain following the distribution of the sciatic nerve or unilateral leg swelling is often an indication of pelvic recurrence of carcinoma of the cervix.

BIBLIOGRAPHY

Abell MR and Ramirez JA: Sarcomas and carcinosarcomas of the uterine cervix, Cancer 31:1176, 1973.

Alvarez RD, Soong S-J, Kinney WK, et al: Identification of prognostic factors and risk groups in patients found to have nodal metastasis at the time of radical hysterectomy for early-stage squamous cell carcinoma of the cervix, Gynecol Oncol 35:130, 1989.

Bandy LC, Clarke-Pearson DL, Silverman PM, et al: Computed tomography in evaluation of extrapelvic lymphadenopathy in carcinoma of the cervix, Obstet Gynecol 65:73, 1985.

Benson WL and Norris HJ: A critical review of the frequency of lymph node metastasis and death from microinvasive carcinoma of the cervix, Obstet Gynecol 49:632, 1977.

Berchuk A and Mullin TJ: Cervical adenoid cystic carcinoma associated with ascites, Gynecol Oncol 22:201, 1985.

Berek JS, Hacker NF, Fu YS, et al: Adenocarcinoma of the uterine cervix: histologic variables associated with lymph node metastasis and spread, Obstet Gynecol 65:46, 1985.

Berman ML, Keys H, and Creasman W: Survival and patterns of recurrence in cervical cancer metastatic to periaortic lymph nodes, Gynecol Oncol 19:8, 1984.

Bloch B, Nel CP, Kriel A, et al: Combination chemotherapy with cisplatin and bleomycin in advanced cervical cancer, Cancer Treat Rep 68:891, 1984.

Boyce JG, Fruchter RG, Nicrasti AD, et al: Vascular invasion in stage I carcinoma of the cervix, Cancer 53:1175, 1984.

Brand E, Berek JS, and Hacker N: Controversies in the management of cervical adenocarcinoma, Obstet Gynecol 71:261, 1988.

Brand E, Berek JS, Nieberg RK, and Hacker NF: Rhabdomyosarcoma of the uterine cervix, Cancer 60:1552, 1987.

Brandt B III and Lifshitz S: Scalene node biopsy in advanced carcinoma of the cervix uteri, Cancer 47:1920, 1981.

Burghardt E and Holzer E: Diagnosis and treatment of microinvasive carcinoma of the cervix uteri, Obstet Gynecol 153:641, 1977.

Calais G, Le Floch O, Chauvet B, et al: Carcinoma of the uterine cervix stage Ib and early stage II: prognostic value of the histological tumor regression after initial brachytherapy, Int J Radiat Oncol Biol Phys 17:1231, 1989.

Choo YC, Choy TK, Wong LC, et al: Potentiation of radiotherapy by cis-dichlorodiamine platinum (II) in advanced cervical carcinoma, Gynecol Oncol 23:94, 1986.

Clement PB and Scully RE: Carcinoma of the cervix: histologic types, Semin Oncol 9:251, 1982.

Creasman WT, Fetter BF, Clarke-Pearson DL, et al: Management of stage Ia carcinoma of the cervix, Am J Obstet Gynecol 153:164, 1985.

Crissman JD, Makuch R, and Budhraja M: Histopathologic grading of squamous carcinoma of the uterine cervix: an evaluation of 70 stage Ib patients, Cancer 55:1590, 1985.

Dattoli MJ, Gretz HF III, Beller U, et al: Analysis of multiple prognostic factors in patients with stage Ib cervical cancer: age as a major determinant, Int J Radiat Oncol Biol Phys 17:41, 1989.

Davidson SE, Symonds RP, Lamont D, and Watson ER: Does adenocarcinoma of uterine cervix have a worse prognosis than squamous carcinoma when treated by radiotherapy? Gynecol Oncol 33:23, 1989.

Davy M, Bentzen H, and Jahren R: Simple hysterectomy in the presence of invasive cervical cancer, Acta Obstet Gynecol Scand 56:105, 1977.

Daya DA and Scully RE: Sarcoma botryoides of the uterine cervix in young women: a clinicopathological study of 13 cases, Gynecol Oncol 29:290, 1988.

Delgado G, Bundy BN, Fowler WC, et al: A prospective surgical pathological study of stage I squamous carcinoma of the cervix: a gynecologic oncology group study, Gynecol Oncol 35:314, 1989.

Delgado G, Bundy B, Zaino R, et al: Prospective surgical-pathologic study of disease-free interval in patients with stage IB squamous cell carcinoma of the cervix: a Gynecologic Oncology Group study, Gynecol Oncol 38:352, 1990.

Dottino PR, Plaxe SC, Beddoe AM, et al: Induction chemotherapy followed by radical surgery in cervical cancer, Gynecol Oncol 40:7, 1991.

Duk JM, De Bruijn HWA, Groenier KH, et al: Adenocarcinoma of the uterine cervix: prognostic significance of pretreatment serum CA-125, squamous cell carcinoma antigen, and carcinoembryonic antigen levels in relation to clinical and histopathologic tumor characteristics, Cancer 65:1830, 1990.

Einhorn N, Patek E, and Sjoberg B: Outcome of different treatment modalities in cervix carcinoma stages Ib and IIa: observations in a well-defined Swedish population, Cancer 55:949, 1985.

Forney JP: The effect of radical hysterectomy on bladder physiology, Am J Obstet Gynecol 138:374, 1980.

Gallion HH, van Nagell JR, Donaldson ES, et al: Combined radiation therapy and extrafascial hysterectomy in the treatment of stage Ib barrel-shaped cervical cancer, Cancer 56:262, 1985.

Gallup DG, Harper RH, and Stock RJ: Poor prognosis in patients with adenosquamous cell carcinoma of the cervix, Obstet Gynecol 65:416, 1985.

Gauthier P, Gore I, Shingleton HM, et al: Identification of histopathologic risk groups in stage Ib squamous cell carcinoma of the cervix, Obstet Gynecol 66:569, 1985.

Goldman SM, Fishman EK, Rosenshein NB, et al: Excretory urography and computed tomography in initial evaluation of patients with cervical cancer: are both evaluations necessary? AJR 143:991, 1984.

Greer BE, Figge DC, Tamimi HK, et al: Stage IA_2 squamous carcinoma of the cervix: difficult diagnosis and therapeutic dilemma, Am J Obstet Gynecol 162:1406, 1990.

Hacker NF, Berek JS, and Lagasse LD: Carcinoma of the cervix associated with pregnancy, Obstet Gynecol 59:735, 1982.

Hasumi K, Sakamoto A, and Sugano H: Microinvasive carcinoma of the uterine cervix, Cancer 45:928, 1980.

Heller PB, Barnhill DR, Mayer AR, et al: Cervical carcinoma found incidentally in a uterus removed for benign indications, Obstet Gynecol 67:187, 1986.

Henriksen E: The lymphatic spread of carcinoma of the cervix and of the body of the uterus, Am J Obstet Gynecol 58:924, 1949.

Henson D and Tarone R: An epidemiologic study of cancer of the cervix, vagina, and vulva based on the Third National Cancer Survey in the United States, Am J Obstet Gynecol 129:525, 1977.

Holloway RW, To A, Moradi M, et al: Monitoring the course of cervical carcinoma with the squamous cell carcinoma serum radioimmunoassay, Obstet Gynecol 74:944, 1989.

Hopkins MP and Morley GW: A comparison of adenocarcinoma and squamous cell carcinoma of the cervix, Obstet Gynecol 77:912, 1991.

Inoue T and Morita K: The prognostic significance of number of positive nodes in cervical carcinoma stages Ib, IIa, and IIb, Cancer 65:1923, 1990.

King LA, Talledo OE, Gallup DG, et al: Adenoid cystic carcinoma of the cervix in women under age 40, Gynecol Oncol 32:26, 1989.

Kinney WK, Alvarez RD, Reid GC, et al: Value of adjuvant whole-pelvis irradiation after Wertheim hysterectomy for early-stage squamous carcinoma of the cervix with pelvic nodal metastasis: a matched-control study, Gynecol Oncol 34:258, 1989.

Kjorstad K, Martinbeau PW, and Iversen T: Stage Ib carcinoma of the cervix, The Norwegian Radium Hospital: results and complications. III. Urinary and gastrointestinal complications, Gynecol Oncol 15:42, 1983.

Kleine W, Rau K, Schwoeorer D, et al: Prognosis of the adenocarcinoma of the cervix uteri: a comparative study, Gynecol Oncol 35:145, 1989.

Kolstad P: Follow-up study of 232 patients with stage Ia1 and 411 patients with stage Ia2 squamous cell carcinoma of the cervix (microinvasive carcinoma), Gynecol Oncol 33:265, 1989.

Lagasse LD, Creasman WT, and Shingleton HM: Results and complications of operative staging in cervical cancer: experience of the Gynecologic Oncology Group, Gynecol Oncol 9:90, 1980.

Lai C-H, Lin T-S, Soong Y-K, et al: Adjuvant chemotherapy after radical hysterectomy for cervical carcinoma, Gynecol Oncol 35:193, 1989.

LaPolla JP, Schlaerth JB, Gaddis O, et al: The influence of surgical staging on the evaluation and treatment of patients with cervical carcinoma, Gynecol Oncol 24:194, 1986.

Larsson G, Alm P, Gullberg B, et al: Prognostic factors in early invasive carcinoma of the uterine cervix, Am J Obstet Gynecol 146:145, 1983.

Leibel S, Bauer M, Wasserman T, et al: Radiotherapy with or without misonidazole for patients with stage IIIb or stage IVa squamous cell carcinoma of the uterine cervix: preliminary report of a radiation therapy oncology group randomized trial, Int J Radiat Oncol Biol Phys 13:541, 1987.

Leman MH, Benson WL, Kurman RJ, et al: Microinvasive carcinoma of the cervix, Obstet Gynecol 48:571, 1976.

Leminen A, Paavonen J, Forss M, et al: Adenocarcinoma of the uterine cervix, Cancer 65:53, 1990.

Lerner HM, Jones HW, and Hill EC: Radical surgery for the treatment of early invasive carcinoma (stage Ib): review of 15 years' experience, Obstet Gynecol 56:413, 1980.

Lohe KJ, Burghardt E, Hillemanns HG, et al: Early squamous cell carcinoma of the uterine cervix. II. Clinical results of a cooperative study in the management of 419 patients with early stromal invasion and microcarcinoma, Gynecol Oncol 6:31, 1978.

Low JA, Mauger GM, and Carmichael JA: The effect of Wertheim hysterectomy on bladder and urethral function, Am J Obstet Gynecol 139:826, 1981.

Martimbeau PW, Kjorstad KE, and Iversen T: Stage Ib carcinoma of the cervix, The Norwegian Radium Hospital. II. Results when pelvic nodes are involved, Obstet Gynecol 60:215, 1982.

Maruyama Y, van Nagell JR, Donaldson E, et al: Neutron brachytherapy is better than conventional radiotherapy in advanced cervical cancer, Lancet 1:1120, 1985.

Maruyama Y, van Nagell JR, Yoneda J, et al: Dose-response and failure pattern for bulky or barrel-shaped stage Ib cervical cancer treated by combined photon irradiation and extrafascial hysterectomy, Cancer 63:70, 1989.

McGowan L, Young RH, and Scully RE: Peutz-Jeghers syndrome with "adenoma malignum" of the cervix, Gynecol Oncol 10:125, 1980.

McKelvey JL and Goodlin RR: Adenoma malignum of the cervix: a cancer of deceptively innocent histological pattern, Cancer 16:549, 1963.

Milsom I and Friberg LG: Primary adenocarcinoma of the uterine cervix: a clinical study, Cancer 52:942, 1983.

Moberg PJ, Einhorn N, Silfversward C, et al: Adenocarcinoma of the uterine cervix, Cancer 57:407, 1986.

Montana GS and Fowler WC: Carcinoma of the cervix: analysis of bladder and rectal radiation dose and complications, Int J Radiat Oncol Biol Phys 16:95, 1989.

Montana GS, Fowler WC, Varia MA, et al: Analysis of results of radiation therapy for stage II carcinoma of the cervix, Cancer 55:956, 1985.

Montana GS, Fowler WC, Varia MA, et al: Carcinoma of the cervix, stage III: results of radiation therapy, Cancer 57:148, 1986.

Morley GW, Hopkins MP, Lindenauer SM, and Roberts JA: Pelvic exenteration, University of Michigan: 100 patients at 5 years, Obstet Gynecol 74:934, 1989.

Nash JD, Burke TW, Woodward JE, et al: Diagnosis of recurrent gynecologic malignancy with fine-needle aspiration cytology, Obstet Gynecol 71:333, 1988.

Orton CG and Wolf-Rosenblum S: Dose dependence of complication rates in cervix cancer radiotherapy, Int J Radiat Oncol Biol Phys 12:37, 1986.

Penalver MA, Bejany DE, Averette HE, et al: Continent urinary diversion in gynecologic oncology, Gynecol Oncol 34:274, 1989.

Perez CA, Camel HM, Kuske RR, et al: Radiation therapy alone in the treatment of carcinoma of the uterine cervix: a 20-year experience, Gynecol Oncol 23:127, 1986.

Pettersson F and Bjorkholm E: Staging and reporting of cervical carcinoma, Semin Oncol 9:287, 1982.

Pettersson F, Coppleson M, Creasman W, et al, editors: Twentieth Annual Report on the Results of Treatment in Gynecologic Cancer, Stockholm, 1988, International Federation of Gynecology and Obstetrics.

Piver MS, Barlow JJ, Vongtama V, et al: Hydroxyurea: a radiation potentiator in carcinoma of the uterine cervix: a randomized double-blind study, Am J Obstet Gynecol 147:803, 1983.

Piver MS, Rutledge F, and Smith JR: Five classes of extended hysterectomy for women with cervical cancer, Obstet Gynecol 44:265, 1974.

Plentl AA and Friedman EA: Lymphatic system of the female genitalia, Philadelphia, 1971, WB Saunders Co.

Podczaski E, Stryker JA, Kaminiski P, et al: Extended-field radiation therapy for carcinoma of the cervix, Cancer 66:251, 1990.

Potish R, Adcock L, Jones T, et al: The morbidity and utility of periaortic radiotherapy in cervical carcinoma, Gynecol Oncol 15:1, 1983.

Potish R, Twiggs LB, Adcock LL, et al: Effect of cis-platinum on tolerance to radiation therapy in advanced cervical cancer, Am J Clin Oncol 9:387, 1986.

Potter ME, Alvarez RD, Shingleton HM, et al: Early invasive cervical cancer with pelvic lymph node involvement: to complete or not to complete radical hysterectomy? Gynecol Oncol 37:78, 1990.

Riou G, Barrois M, Le MG, et al: C-myc proto-oncogene expression and prognosis in early carcinoma of the uterine cervix, Lancet April 1987, p 761.

Rotmensch J, Rosenshein NB, and Woodruff JD: Cervical sarcoma: a review, Obstet Gynecol Surv 38:456, 1983.

Rotmensch J, Senekjian EK, Javaheri G, et al: Evaluation of bolus high dose cis-platinum and continuous 5-fluorouracil intravenous infusion for metastatic and recurrent squamous cell carcinoma of the female genital tract, Gynecol Oncol 29:76, 1988.

Runowicz CD, Wadler S, Rodriguez-Rodriguez L, et al: Concomitant cisplatin and radiotherapy in locally advanced cervical carcinoma, Gynecol Oncol 34:395, 1989.

Senekjian EK, Young JM, Weiser P, et al: Utility of squamous cell carcinoma antigen (SCC) in patients with cervical squamous cell carcinoma (abstract), Gynecol Oncol 23:248, 1986.

Silverberg E, Boring CC, and Squires TS: Cancer statistics, 1990, CA 40:1, 1990.

Soisson AP, Soper JT, Clarke-Pearson DL, et al: Adjuvant radiotherapy following radical hysterectomy for patients with stage Ib and IIa cervical cancer, Gynecol Oncol 37:390, 1990.

Sommers GM, Grigsby PW, Perez CA, et al: Outcome of recurrent cervical carcinoma following definitive irradiation, Gynecol Oncol 35:150, 1989.

Thar TL, Million RR, and Daly JW: Radiation treatment of carcinoma of the cervix, Semin Oncol 9:299, 1982.

Timmer PR, Aalders JG, and Bouma J: Radical surgery after preoperative intracavitary radiotherapy for stages Ib and IIa carcinoma of the uterine cervix, Gynecol Oncol 18:206, 1984.

van Nagell JR, Maruyama Y, Donaldson ES, et al: Phase II clinical trial using californium 252 fast neutron brachytherapy, external pelvic radiation and extrafascial hysterectomy in the treatment of bulky, barrel-shaped stage Ib cervical cancer, Cancer 57:1918, 1986.

van Nagell JR, Powell DE, Gallion HH, et al: Small cell carcinoma of the uterine cervix, Cancer 62:1586, 1988.

Vasilev SA and Schlaerth JB: Scalene lymph node sampling in cervical carcinoma: a reappraisal, Gynecol Oncol 37:120, 1990.

Weiss RS and Lucas WE: Adenocarcinoma of the cervix, Cancer 57:1996, 1986.

Westby M and Asmussen M: Anatomical and functional changes in the lower urinary tract after radical hysterectomy with lymph node dissection as studied by dynamic urethrocystography in simultaneous urethrocystometrics, Gynecol Oncol 21:261, 1985.

Wolff JP, Lacour J, Chassagne D, et al: Cancer of the cervical stump: a study of 173 patients, Obstet Gynecol 39:10, 1972.

Zander J, Baltzer RJ, Lohe KJ, et al: Carcinoma of the cervix: an attempt to individualize therapy—results of a 20-year cooperative study, Am J Obstet Gynecol 139:752, 1981.

Neoplastic Diseases of the Uterus

--- KEY TERMS AND DEFINITIONS ---

Adenoacanthoma. A variant of endometrial carcinoma that contains epithelium resembling squamous metaplasia in addition to adenocarcinoma.

Adenosquamous Carcinoma. A virulent form of endometrial carcinoma that contains tissue resembling squamous cell carcinoma in addition to adenocarcinoma.

Clear Cell Endometrial Carcinoma. A virulent form of endometrial carcinoma that histologically is similar to clear cell adenocarcinomas that arise in the ovary, cervix, and vagina.

Endolymphatic Stromal Myosis (ESM). A term that describes a low-grade (<10 mitoses/10 hpf) endometrial stromal sarcoma.

Endometrial Carcinoma Grade. A pathologic classification that describes the degree of differentiation of endometrial carcinoma. G1, well differentiated; G2, intermediate; G3, poorly differentiated.

Endometrial Carcinoma Stage. A clinical classification that describes the extent of spread of endometrial carcinoma:
Stage I: Tumor confined to the uterine corpus.
Stage II: Tumor involving the corpus and cervix.
Stage III: Tumor spreading outside the uterus but confined in the pelvis.
Stage IV: Tumor spreading outside the pelvis or into the mucosa of the bladder or rectum.

Endometrial Hyperplasia. A general term that encompasses a variety of proliferative endometrial patterns. Hyperplasia often occurs with abnormal bleeding during times of anovulation. Unless there is cytologic atypia, the hyperplasias are not generally considered to be premalignant.

• **Adenomatous Endometrial Hyperplasia.** A variant of hyperplasia that involves proliferation of the glands of the endometrium, resulting in crowding of the glands and irregularities in their shape.

• **Atypical Hyperplasia.** A variant of endometrial hyperplasia that is premalignant. The glands are often severely crowded and have abnormal outpouchings (architectural atypia), or there may be an abnormal appearance to the epithelial cells of the glands (cytologic atypia). The degree of atypia is occasionally further described as mild, moderate, or severe.

• **Complex Hyperplasia.** A term recently adopted by The International Society of Gynecologic Pathologists to define glandular proliferation similar to adenomatous hyperplasia without atypia. Its premalignant potential is low.

• **Cystic Endometrial Hyperplasia.** A variant of hyperplasia in which the glands are markedly dilated and lined by relatively uniform epithelial cells without cytologic atypia. It frequently occurs in the perimenopausal period. When many glands are greatly dilated, the term *Swiss-cheese hyperplasia* is sometimes used.

• **Simple Hyperplasia.** A term recently adopted by ISGYP used to describe a variant of endometrial cystic hyperplasia consisting of dilated glands and abundant stroma.

Heterologous Uterine Sarcoma. A sarcoma consisting of mesenchymal elements foreign to the uterus, that is, chondrosarcoma, osteosarcoma, liposarcoma, and rhabdomyosarcoma.

Homologous Uterine Sarcoma. A sarcoma consisting of mesenchymal elements normally found in the uterus, that is, leiomyosarcoma and endometrial stromal sarcoma.

Leiomyosarcoma. A smooth muscle malignancy with >5 mitoses/10 hpf and bizzare cells with nuclear atypia.

Malignant Mixed Müllerian Tumor (MMMT). A uterine malignancy consisting of both adenocarcinoma and sarcomatous elements. De-

pending on the appearance of the sarcomatous element, it is designated as a homologous MMMT or a heterologous MMMT.

Serous Endometrial Carcinoma. A virulent form of endometrial carcinoma that histologically resembles papillary serous adenocarcinoma of the ovary.

Endometrial carcinoma is the most common malignancy of the lower female genital tract in the United States. Approximately 33,000 new cases develop in the United States each year, according to recent figures from the National Cancer Institute SEER Program. This is about 1.5 times the frequency of ovarian cancer and almost 3 times the number of new cases of cervical cancer. However, the fewest deaths (4000) occur annually from uterine cancer, in comparison with cervical or ovarian cancer. Overall, about 1 woman in 100 will develop this disease during her life.

This chapter reviews the clinical and pathologic features of endometrial neoplasia (hyperplasias and carcinomas). The factors that contribute to the development of these diseases and the appropriate methods of management are discussed separately for the endometrial hyperplasias and the invasive carcinomas. Sarcomas of the uterus and their clinical behavior and therapy are also presented.

EPIDEMIOLOGY

Adenocarcinoma of the endometrium affects women primarily in the perimenopausal and postmenopausal years and is most frequently diagnosed in those between the ages of 50 and 65. However, these cancers can also develop in young women during their reproductive years, and about 5% of the cases are diagnosed in women under 40. Figure 28-1 plots the incidence curve for cancers of the endometrium according to age. The curve rises sharply after age 45 and peaks between 55 and 69; then there is a gradual decrease. Atypical endometrial hyperplasia may develop into endometrial carcinoma after unopposed estrogen stimulation of the endometrium. Recent data suggest a second pathway insofar as some endometrial cancers appear to develop without prior hyperplasia and these non–estrogen-related carcinomas tend to be poorly differentiated and ag-

gressive tumors (see later discussion).

Hyperplasia develops primarily in women 40 to 60 years old. Gusberg and Kaplan studied 191 patients with endometrial hyperplasia; approximately 40% were 40 to 50 years old, 25% were 50 to 60, and 15% were under age 40.

Factors that increase the risk of developing endometrial carcinoma (and endometrial hyperplasia) are many. Unopposed estrogen stimulation appears to be a primary factor, increasing the risk 4 to 8 times for a woman using estrogens alone for menopausal replacement therapy. The risk increases with higher doses of estrogen (greater than 0.625 mg conjugated estrogens) and more prolonged use but can be markedly reduced with the use of progestin (see Chapter 40). Similarly, combination (progestin-containing) oral contraceptives decrease the risk. Other conditions leading to long-term estrogen stimulation, including the polycystic ovary syndrome (Stein-Leventhal syndrome) and feminizing ovarian tumors, are also associated with increased risk of endometrial carcinoma. Recent data suggest that patients with breast cancer who receive the anti-estrogen tamoxifen are at increased risk of developing endometrial carcinoma.

MacMahon defines three of the most important factors as obesity, nulliparity, and late menopause (over the age of 52 years). The risk for endometrial carcinoma increased 3 times for those 21 to 50 pounds overweight and 10 times for those more than 50 pounds overweight. Nulliparous women have twice the risk in comparison with those with one child and 3 times in comparison with those with five or more children. Elwood et al. noted that the risk for women whose menopause occurred after age 52 was 2.4 times that for women whose menopause occurred before age 49.

Various other factors have been found or postulated. Diabetes increases the risk by 2.8. Hypertension has frequently been reported to be a risk factor, and many obese patients do

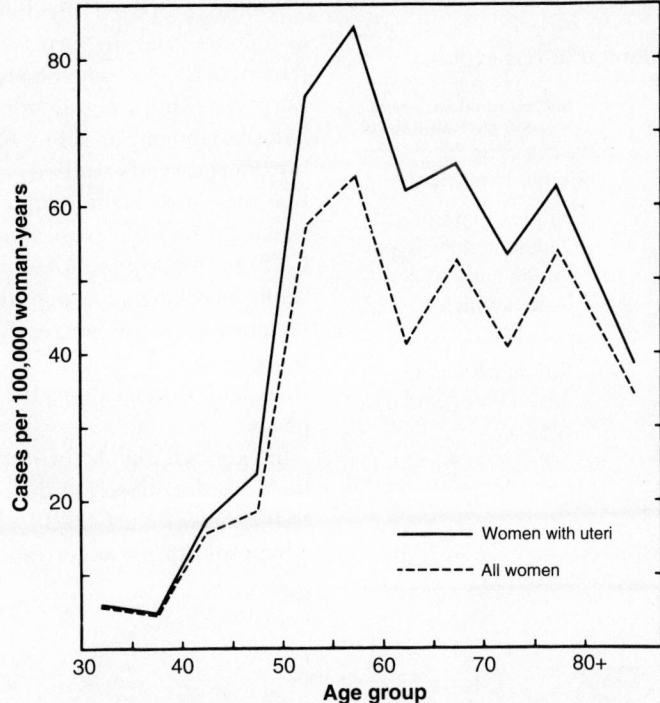

FIGURE 28-1
Incidence curve for carcinoma of the endometrium by age. (From Elwood JM, Cole P, Rothman KJ, and Kaplan SD: J Natl Cancer Inst 59:1055, 1977.)

have hypertension. Currently hypertension has not been established as a significant risk factor, and prior pelvic irradiation also has not been established as a risk factor. Regarding racial factors, the incidence of endometrial cancer among white women is approximately twice the rate in black women. Recent oncogene studies by Berchuck et al. indicate that HER-2/*neu* overexpression is associated with advanced metastatic disease. The box on the right summarizes the risk factors for endometrial carcinoma with estimates of the increased relative risk. The risk factors have recently been extensively reviewed by Parazzini et al.

ENDOMETRIAL HYPERPLASIA

The normal morphologic changes that occur in the endometrium during the menstrual cycle are reviewed in Chapter 4. Endometrial hyperplasia occurs during periods of long-term unopposed estrogen stimulation, such as anovulation, particularly around the time of menopause. Normally, perimenopausal bleeding is characterized by "skips and delays." Marked increases in the quantity of menstrual flow or more frequent bleeding can have multiple causes (Chapter 6), including endometrial hy-

ENDOMETRIAL CARCINOMA RISK FACTORS

Increases the Risk	Diminishes the Risk
Unopposed estrogen stimulation	Ovulation
Unopposed menopausal estrogen (4-8×) replacement therapy	Progestin therapy
	Combination oral contraceptives
Menopause after 52 years (2.4×)	Menopause prior to 49 years
Obesity (3×, 21-50 lb; 10×, over 50 lb)	Normal weight
Nulliparity (2-3×)	Multiparity
Diabetes (2.8×)	
Feminizing ovarian tumors	
Polycystic ovarian syndrome	
Tamoxifen therapy for breast cancer	

perplasia and occasionally endometrial carcinoma. There is no universally accepted terminology for hyperplasias of the endometrium.

TABLE 28-1

Classifications of Endometrial Hyperplasias

Traditional	International Society of Gynecologic Pathologists
Cystic hyperplasia	Simple hyperplasia
Adenomatous hyperplasia	Complex hyperplasia (adenomatous hyperplasia without cytologic atypia)

Atypical adenomatous hyperplasia
  Architectural atypia (mild, moderate, severe)
  Cytologic atypia (mild, moderate, severe)
	Atypical hyperplasia (adenomatous hyperplasia with cytologic atypia)

Vellios proposed the following classification of endometrial hyperplasias: cystic endometrial hyperplasia, adenomatous endometrial hyperplasia, atypical adenomatous hyperplasia, and carcinoma in situ. Kurman and Norris introduced and studied a new terminology that has just been adopted by the International Society of Gynecologic Pathologists (IS-GYP) to describe endometrial hyperplasias and their premalignant potential. Because both terminologies are currently in use, they will be considered in detail. Table 28-1 summarizes both classifications for endometrial hyperplasia.

In general the term *cystic hyperplasia* has been used to describe dilation of the endometrial glands (Figure 28-2), which often occurs in a hyperplastic endometrium in a menopausal or

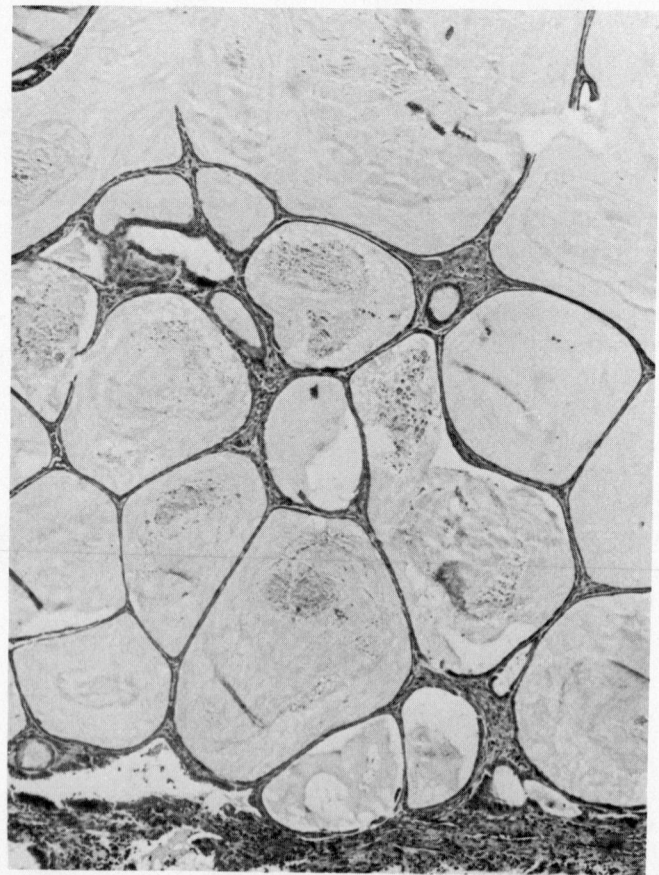

FIGURE 28-2

Cystic hyperplasia. (×79.) (From Christopherson WM and Gray LA: Premalignant lesions of the endometrium: endometrial hyperplasia and adenocarcinoma in situ. In Coppleson M, editor: Gynecologic oncology. Edinburgh, 1981, Churchill-Livingstone. Reprinted by permission.)

postmenopausal woman (cystic atrophy). It is also referred to as *Swiss-cheese hyperplasia* and is considered to be weakly premalignant.

The term *adenomatous hyperplasia* describes alterations in the appearance of the glands of the endometrium and has provided great confusion in gynecologic pathology, particularly regarding premalignant potential.

The degree to which hyperplasia is premalignant is related primarily to its cellular atypicality. Welch and Scully described two types of atypia, architectural and cytologic, and further described them as mild, moderate, or severe. Architectural atypia refers to crowding and alterations in the shape of the glands. Cytologic atypia refers to nuclear atypia, piling up of the epithelium, development of epithelial bridges. Recent evidence indicates that the degree of cytologic atypia is the predominant determinant of premalignant potential (see Natural History).

Figure 28-3 demonstrates glandular crowding and outpouching in adenomatous hyperplasia. This architectural atypia is marked by epithelial stratification and by crowding, budding, and branching of the glands. Cytologic atypia is the major determinant of premalignant potential of endometrial hyperplasia. Progressive cytologic atypia is marked by irregular cell size, high nuclear/cytoplasmic ratio, prominent nucleoli, occasional nuclear pleomorphism, mitoses, and abnormal chromatin configuration. Figure 28-4 shows an endometrium with severe cytologic atypia and marked irregularity of the nuclei.

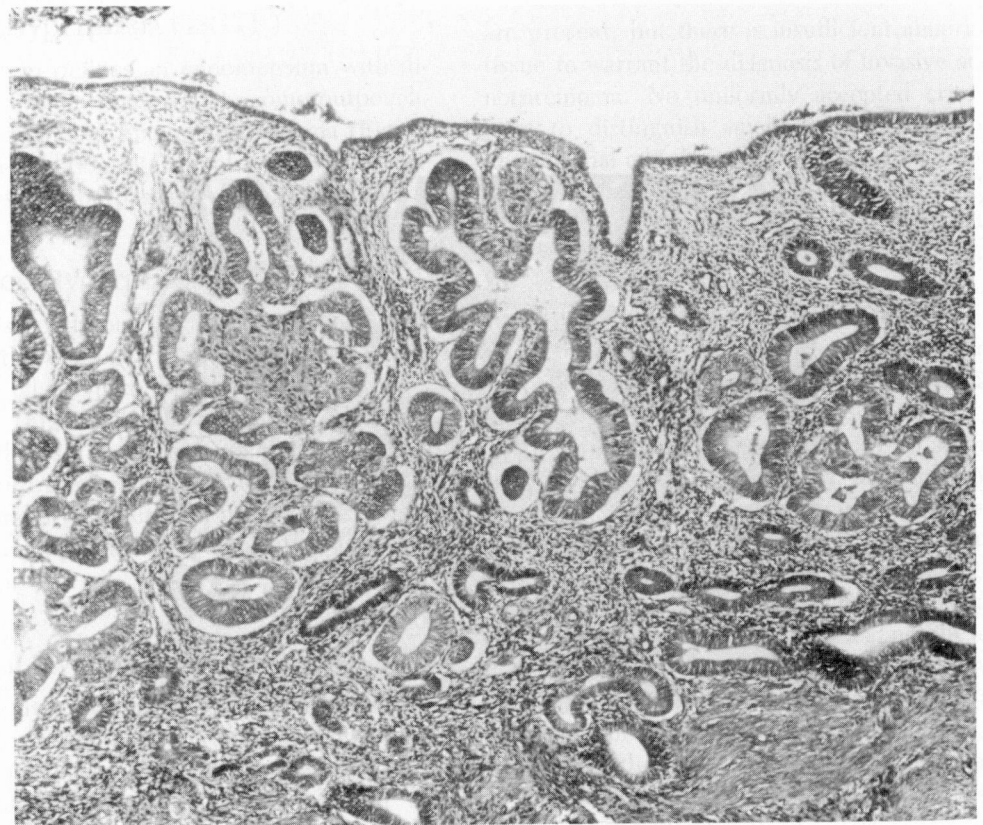

FIGURE 28-3
Glandular crowding and outpouching in adenomatous hyperplasia. (×79.) (From Christopherson WM and Gray LA: Premalignant lesions of the endometrium: endometrial hyperplasia and adenocarcinoma in situ. In Coppleson M, editor: Gynecologic oncology, Edinburgh, 1981, Churchill-Livingstone. Reprinted by permission.)

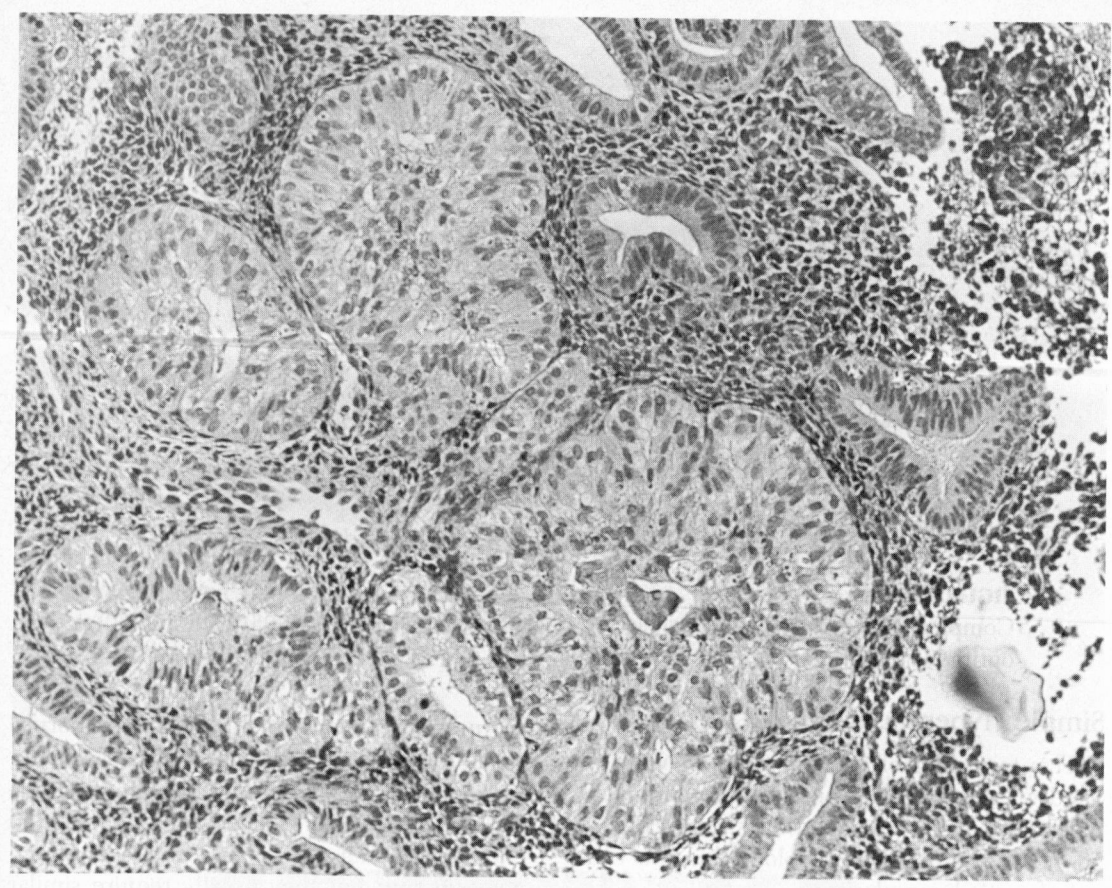

FIGURE 28-7
Carcinoma in situ of the endometrium. There is a small focus and no stromal invasion. (×192.) (From Christopherson WM and Gray LA: Premalignant lesions of the endometrium: endometrial hyperplasia and adenocarcinoma in situ. In Coppleson M, editor: Gynecologic oncology, Edinburgh, 1981, Churchill-Livingstone. Reprinted by permission.)

polyp is often histologically more severe than that found in nonpolypoid areas of the endometrium.

The clinician must consult directly with the pathologist interpreting the endometrial histologic picture to be certain of the terminology used. The lack of uniform terminology, the fact that the demarcations between various diagnostic categories are not sharply defined, and the presence of multiple patterns in the same endometrial tissue make this communication essential.

Natural History

The rate at which endometrial hyperplasia progresses to endometrial carcinoma has not been accurately determined. Studies address-

ing this area have been retrospective, based on samples obtained from dilation-and-curettage (D&C) specimens at a single institution, and are therefore not necessarily generalizable. Kurman et al. studied 170 patients with endometrial hyperplasia diagnosed by D&C at least 1 year before hysterectomy. Table 28-2 shows the results of their study. Overall, most of the hyperplasias regressed, whereas the atypical hyperplasias (those with cytologic abnormalities) had the highest risk for progression to carcinoma. A few patients in each category became pregnant after medical therapy. The endometrial carcinomas that developed from the atypical endometrial hyperplasias were grade 1 (well differentiated), and the atypical endometrial hyperplasia regressed in 15 patients after withdrawal of estrogen ther-

TABLE 28-2
Endometrial Hyperplasia Follow-up

Type	Number	Age	(Mean)	Regressed*	Progressed No. of Cases	Progressed Mean (Years)	Follow-up (Years)
Simple hyperplasia†	93	17-71	(42)	74 (80%)	1	11	1-26.7 10 pregnancies
Complex hyperplasia‡	29	20-67	(39)	23 (79%)	1	8.3	2-26 3 pregnancies
Atypical hyperplasia	48	20-70	(40)	28 (58%)	11	4.1	1-25 3 pregnancies

From Kurman RJ, Kaminski PF, and Norris HJ: Cancer 56:403, 1985.
*A total of 34 patients with simple hyperplasia, 7 with complex hyperplasia, and 15 with atypical hyperplasia had no further therapy.
†Benign proliferation of the glands.
‡Greater crowding of glands—no cytologic atypia present.

apy. This study provides additional evidence that many endometrial hyperplasias spontaneously regress and that progression to cancer from atypical lesions usually takes years.

Diagnosis and Endometrial Sampling

Abnormal vaginal bleeding is the most frequent symptom of endometrial hyperplasia. In younger patients, hyperplasia may develop during anovulatory bleeding and may even be detected after prolonged periods of oligomenorrhea or amenorrhea. It can occur at any time during the reproductive years but is most common with abnormal bleeding in the perimenopausal period, although it also occurs in women taking menopausal estrogen replacement therapy without an accompanying progestin.

Diagnosis may be made from tissue samples obtained during office endometrial sampling or at D&C. The sampling instruments (see Chapter 8) are introduced through the cervical os into the endometrial cavity. Many patients tolerate office endometrial sampling without an analgesic agent, but paracervical block can be an effective anesthetic aid, particularly in nulliparous women or at the time of D&C. Some patients benefit from an oral antiprostaglandin taken about 30 minutes before biopsy.

Bibbo et al. summarized the effectiveness of various instruments in diagnosing endometrial hyperplasias and carcinoma. Over 90% of en-

TABLE 28-3
Diagnostic Accuracy of Sampling Technique for Endometrial Hyperplasias

Sampling Technique	No. of Cases	Diagnostic Accuracy (%)
Endocervical aspiration	148	71
Isaacs cell sampler	50	62
Vabra curettage	84	91
Endocervical aspiration and VCE*	140	20
Vakutage	140	88

Adapted from Bibbo M, Kluskens L, Azizi F, et al: J Reprod Med 27:622, 1982.
*Vaginal, cervical, and endocervical cytology.

dometrial carcinomas can be successfully detected with procedures that sample the endometrial cavity directly. Endometrial hyperplasias are less successfully detected (Table 28-3), but up to 90% can be diagnosed if endometrial tissue is obtained from the uterine cavity. Screening procedures that obtain tissue are more reliable than those which rely on endometrial cytologic features since endometrial hyperplasia is particularly difficult to diagnose from the morphology of the epithelial cells, alone.

Recent studies with transvaginal ultrasound suggest that this modality may be of use to detect endometrial abnormalities. Granberg et al., in a study of 205 women with postmenopausal bleeding, noted that those women whose endometrium measured less than 9 mm in thickness did not have carcinoma at curettage, while those with cancer measured 18.2 ±6.2 mm and those with atrophic endometriun 3.4 ±1.2 mm. They preliminarily suggest curettage could be avoided in those whose endometrium measures <5 mm. Osmers et al., in a study of 103 women with postmenopausal bleeding and 283 women without postmenopausal bleeding, noted carcinomas were present in those whose endometrium was 4 mm or more. They recommend those whose endometrium is >4 mm should have an endometrial sampling, including asymptomatic women. Further studies are needed to define the optimal thickness to warrant endometrial sampling, but the technique of vaginal ultrasound appears to be very promising in patient evaluation.

Koss et al. studied the endometria of 2586 asymptomatic women, 98% of whom were older than 45 years. Only 16 carcinomas and 17 cases of hyperplasia were detected. These authors concluded that the endometrial sampling procedure was probably not cost-effective in asymptomatic women. In addition, endometrial hyperplasia did *not* always precede endometrial carcinoma, suggesting two different pathways for carcinoma development. These are, first, endometrial hyperplasia occurring after long-term estrogen stimulation leading to carcinoma, and second, endometrial adenocarcinoma developing without prior endometrial hyperplasia. These non−estrogen-stimulated cancers tend to be less well differentiated and to have a poorer prognosis.

Management

The therapy employed for endometrial hyperplasia depends on the degree of atypicality of the hyperplasia and the patient's age. In addition, the risk of carcinoma development without cytologic atypia from the studies of Kurman is about 2%. Therapy for young women in their 20s and 30s is usually conservative and directed toward preservation of childbearing function. After a D&C, providing no further symptoms develop, a patient with hyperplasia without atypia can simply be managed by long-term follow-up. Kurman's studies showed that most endometrial hyperplasias without cytologic aty-

pia regress. Such lesions include simple and complex hyperplasias, as well as adenomatous hyperplasias, and these are frequently removed by D&C alone. Endometrial sampling should be repeated if abnormal bleeding occurs; otherwise, endometrial sampling should be performed in 6 months. Usually progestin (Provera), 10 mg daily for 10 days, or an estrogen-progestin combination (oral contraceptives) will induce monthly withdrawal bleeding in young women who are having anovulatory and irregular menstrual bleeding, and these patients are also followed with endometrial sampling in 6 months (Figure 28-8, *A*).

Patients with atypical hyperplasia (cytologic atypia) require therapy even though about half of hyperplasias with cytologic atypia can regress spontaneously. However, given the risk of transition to carcinoma, atypical hyperplasia (cytologic) requires treatment. Mild atypia can be treated with a progestin (Provera), 10 mg bid continuously or for 10 to 14 days monthly, or an estrogen-progestin oral contraceptive if contraception is desired. Women with moderate to severe atypia and who desire preservation of childbearing function are treated with higher dose progestin therapy. Gal et al. used megestrol acetate (Megace), 40 mg orally per day, to treat 52 postmenopausal women with adenomatous hyperplasia, atypical hyperplasia, or adenocarcinoma in situ. Their data demonstrate the efficacy of progestin treatment for severe atypia. The patient should remain amenorrheic and should have long-term follow-up and periodic sampling, at least every 6 months (Figure 28-8, *A*).

Younger patients with chronic anovulation and hyperplasia who desire children may be treated effectively by induction of ovulation with clomiphene citrate (Clomid) (see Chapter 39), especially if the hyperplasia is mildly atypical. Weight reduction for very obese patients is also advised.

For older patients the risk of carcinoma increases. For example, Kurman et al. studied the uterus of patients after curettage had been performed, and atypical (cytologic) hyperplasia was found in the curettings. In their study, 11% of those under age 35, 12% of those 36 to 54, and 28% of those over age 55 with atypical hyperplasia were found to have carcinoma in their uterus. Thus older patients with moderate or severe cytologic atypical hyperplasia generally require hysterectomy. In addition, those who fail progestin therapy and especially those with severe cytologic atypia should also be considered for hysterectomy. (Figure 28-8, *B*) Ferenczy and Gelford followed 85 patients with endometrial hyperplasia, 65 without and 20 with cytologic atypia, treated with medroxyprogesterone. Eighty percent of the former group regressed, and none developed carcinoma. Of those with severe atypia, only 25% regressed while 25% developed carcinoma, and 50% persisted. This emphasizes the importance of cytologic atypia in the response to medical therapy. If hysterectomy is medically unadvisable, long-term high-dose progestin therapy can be used (megestrol acetate 40 to 160 mg/day or its equivalent depending on the endometrial response). Periodic sampling (every 6 months) of the endometrium is also performed. High-dose progestin therapy does carry the risk of thrombophlebitis. An alternative approach is depo Provera (depo medroxyprogesterone acetate) 200 mg IM initially followed by 100 mg IM every 2 weeks two times, and 100 mg IM monthly for 6 months. The patient will remain amenorrheic after therapy, but sampling of the endometrium should be performed at 6-month intervals.

Figure 28-8, *A* and *B* displays a flow chart as a guide to the management of endometrial hyperplasia. It is important to emphasize that the diagnoses are not precisely defined, and these proliferative disorders are a continuum from mild abnormalities to malignant change.

ENDOMETRIAL CARCINOMA

Symptoms, Signs, and Diagnosis

Postmenopausal bleeding and abnormal perimenopausal bleeding are the primary symptoms of endometrial carcinoma. A routine cytologic examination (Papanicolaou smear) from the exocervix, which screens for cervical neoplasia, detects endometrial carcinoma in only about 50% of the cases. In Procope's study of postmenopausal bleeding, endometrial carcinoma was responsible for at least 14% of the cases.

The diagnosis of endometrial carcinoma is established by histologic examination of the endometrium. Initial diagnosis can frequently be made on an outpatient basis, with an endometrial biopsy. If endometrial carcinoma is found,

endocervical curettage is performed to rule out invasion of the endocervix.

If adequate outpatient evaluation cannot be obtained or if the diagnosis or cause of the abnormal bleeding is not clear from the tissue obtained, a fractional D&C should be performed. The endocervix is first sampled with a curette to rule out cervical involvement by endometrial cancer (invasion of the cervical stroma by tumor should be demonstrated), and then a sound is used to determine uterine depth. A complete uterine curettage is then performed.

Histologic Types

Almost all endometrial carcinomas are adenocarcinomas. The various types are listed in the box below.

Figure 28-9 illustrates typical adenocarcinomas of the endometrium and demonstrates varying degrees of differentiation (G1, well differentiated; G2, intermediate differentiation; G3, poorly differentiated). Occasionally the tumor takes a papillary form, in which case the term *papillary endometrial carcinoma* is applied.

Squamous epithelium commonly coexists with the glandular elements of endometrial carcinoma. If the squamous element comprises at least 10% of the tumor and appears benign as in squamous metaplasia, the term *adenoacanthoma* is used; the prognosis is similar to that for an adenocarcinoma of comparable differentiation (Figure 28-10). If the squamous component appears malignant, the term *adenosquamous carcinoma* is used (Figure 28-11). Usually adenosquamous tumors tend to be less well differentiated and have a poorer prognosis

---

ENDOMETRIAL PRIMARY ADENOCARCINOMAS

Typical endometrioid adenocarcinoma
    Adenoacanthoma (squamous metaplasia)
    Adenosquamous carcinoma
    Papillary endometrial carcinoma
Clear cell carcinoma
Serous carcinoma
Secretory carcinoma
Mucinous carcinoma
Squamous carcinoma

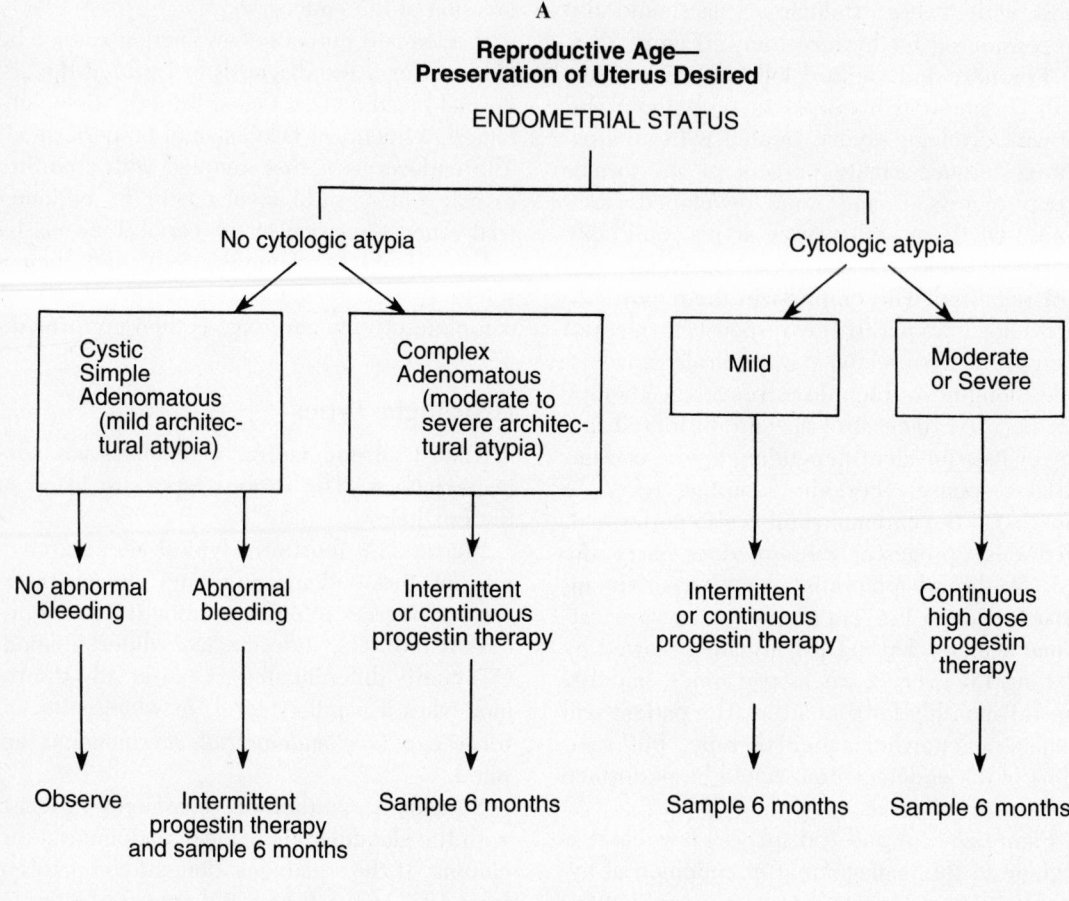

A

**Reproductive Age—
Preservation of Uterus Desired**

ENDOMETRIAL STATUS

No cytologic atypia

Cytologic atypia

Cystic
Simple
Adenomatous
(mild architec-
tural atypia)

Complex
Adenomatous
(moderate to
severe architec-
tural atypia)

Mild

Moderate
or Severe

No abnormal
bleeding

Abnormal
bleeding

Intermittent
or continuous
progestin therapy

Intermittent
or continuous
progestin therapy

Continuous
high dose
progestin
therapy

Observe

Intermittent
progestin therapy
and sample 6 months

Sample 6 months

Sample 6 months

Sample 6 months

B

**Post Reproductive Years
or Uterine Preservation Not Desired**

ENDOMETRIAL STATUS

No cytologic atypia

Same as chart A for
medical therapy, or hysterectomy
for recurrent hyperplasia
or abnormal bleeding

Mild

Moderate
or Severe

Same as chart A,
or hysterectomy

Hysterectomy

FIGURE 28-8, A and B
Schematic diagram for endometrial hyperplasia management for **A**, reproductive
and **B**, post reproductive patients.

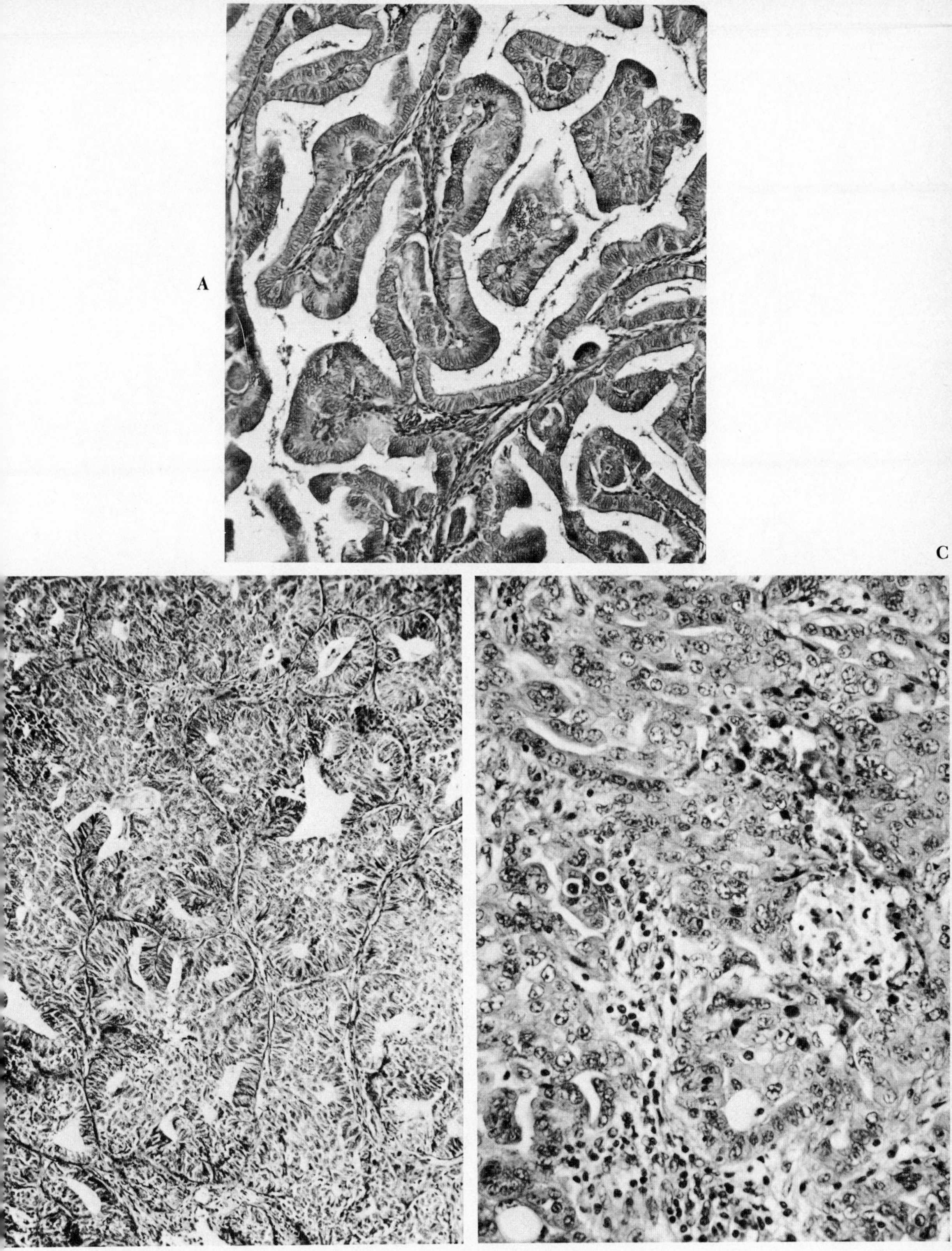

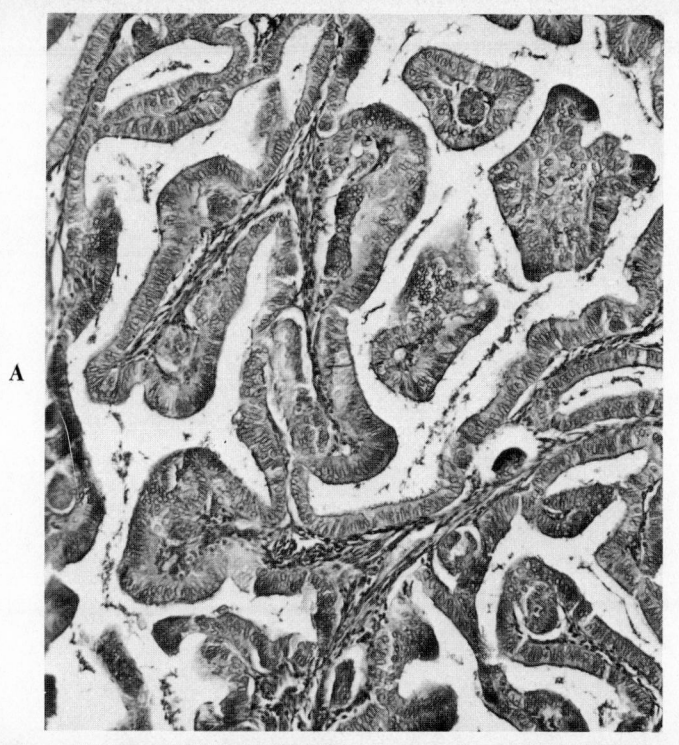

FIGURE 28-9

A, Well-differentiated adenocarcinoma of endometrium. The glands are confluent. (×130.) **B,** Moderately differentiated adenocarcinoma of endometrium. The glands are more solid, but some lumens remain. (×100.) **C,** Poorly differentiated adenocarcinoma of endometrium. The epithelium shows solid proliferation with only a rare lumen. (×100.) (From Kurman RJ and Norris HJ: Endometrial neoplasia: hyperplasia and carcinoma. In Blaustein A, editor: Pathology of the female genital tract, ed 2, New York, 1982, Springer-Verlag.)

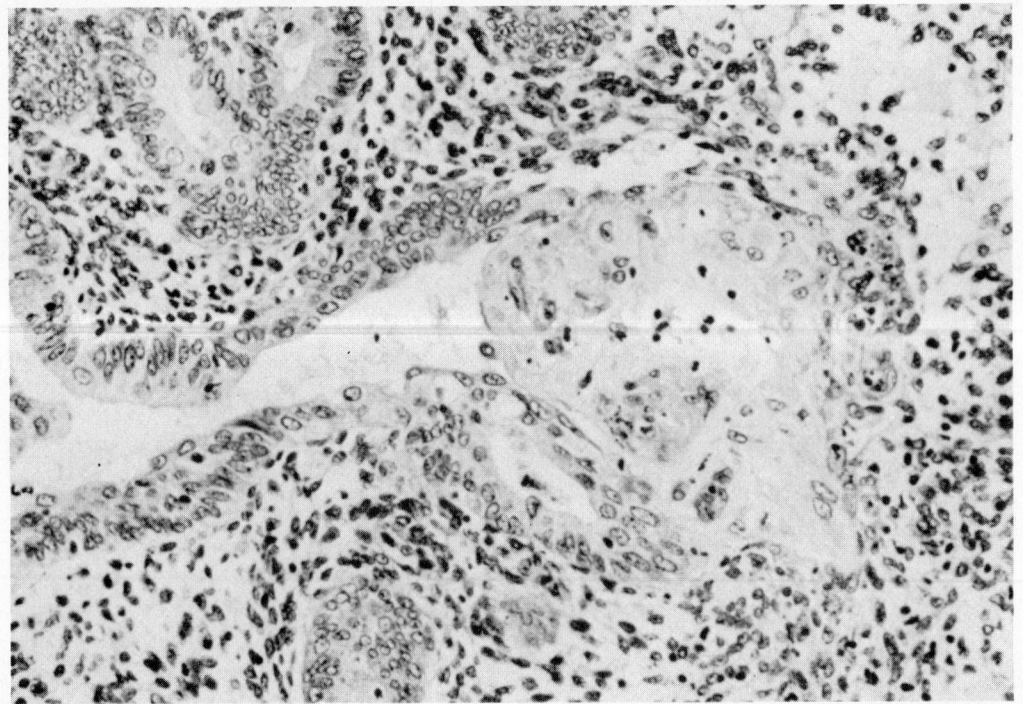

FIGURE 28-10
Adenoacanthoma of endometrium. Adenocarcinoma with squamous metaplasia. (From Gompel C and Silverberg SG: Pathology in gynecology and obstetrics, ed 3, Philadelphia, 1985, JB Lippincott Co.)

FIGURE 28-11
Adenosquamous carcinoma of endometrium. Malignant appearing glandular and squamous elements are present. (×150.) (From Reagan JW and Fu YS: Pathology of endometrial carcinoma. In Coppleson M, editor: Gynecologic oncology, Edinburgh, 1981, Churchill-Livingstone. Reprinted by permission.)

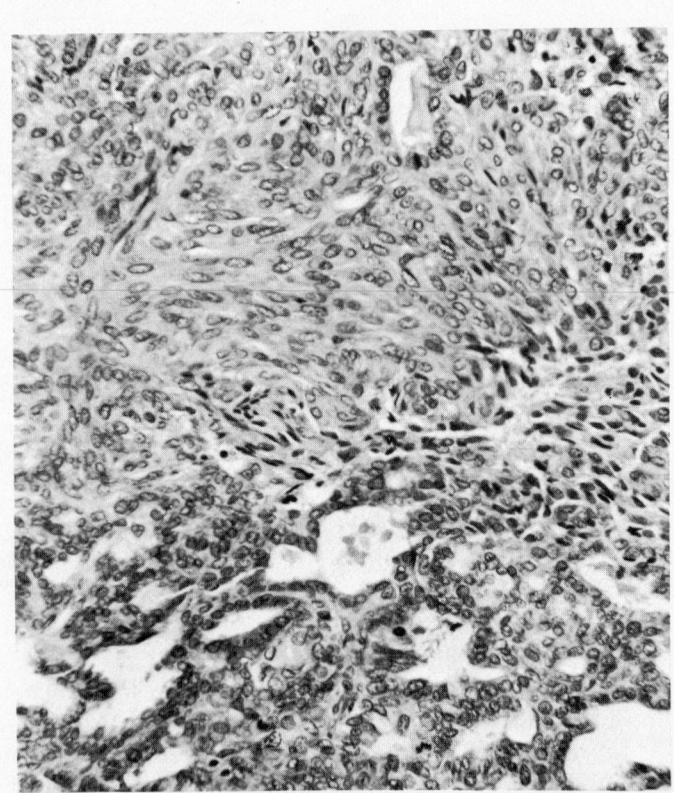

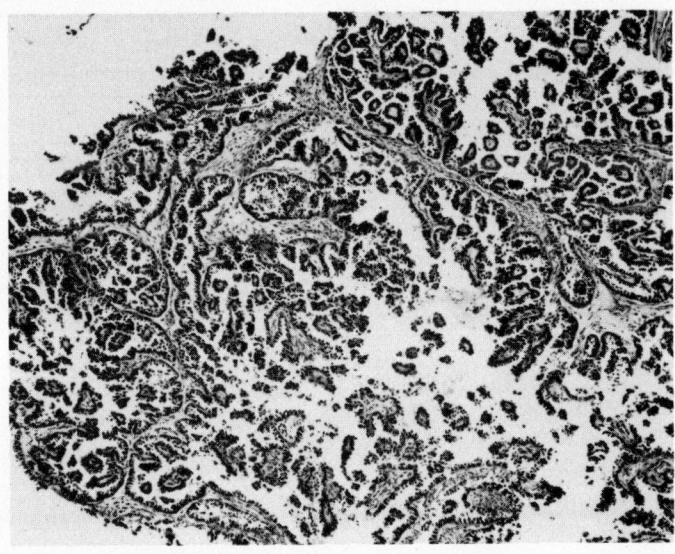

FIGURE 28-12
Serous carcinoma characterized by a complex papillary architecture resembling serous carcinoma of the ovary. (From Kurman RJ: Blaustein's pathology of the female genital tract, ed 3, New York, 1987, Springer-Verlag.)

than typical adenocarcinomas or adenoacanthomas. Reagan reported a 5-year survival of only 19% for adenosquamous carcinoma, much less than the results reported for endometrial carcinoma in general. Some authors prefer the term *adenocarcinoma with squamous elements* and describe the degree of differentiation of both the glandular and the squamous components. However, currently available data do not allow conclusions regarding which system of nomenclature provides the most precise clinical information.

Clear cell adenocarcinomas of the endometrium are rare. Histologically they resemble clear cell adenocarcinomas of the ovary, cervix, and vagina. Endometrial clear cell tumors tend to develop in postmenopausal women and carry a prognosis much worse than typical endometrial adenocarcinomas. Survival rates of 39% to 55% have been reported, much less than the 65% or better usually recorded for endometrial carcinoma. Abeler and Kjorstad reviewed 97 cases and noted the best prognosis (90%) for those without myometrial invasion. Patients whose tumors had blood vessel invasion experienced a 15% 5-year survival.

Serous carcinomas are also highly virulent and uncommon endometrial carcinomas. Histologically they demonstrate epithelial anaplasia and papillary growth (Figure 28-12). These tumors closely resemble papillary serous carcinomas of the ovary. Christopherson et al. reported that 21% of women with stage I papillary serous endometrial carcinomas died within 5 years, in comparison with only 6% of those with typical endometrial adenocarcinomas.

Secretory carcinomas are extremely rare, occurring primarily in premenopausal patients. They are diagnosed in the presence of progestational stimulation, and corpus luteum is frequently detected in the ovary of patients with this tumor. These tumors have been reported in postmenopausal patients and thus can develop in the absence of a demonstrable progestational effect. The prognosis is good; Christopherson et al. reported an overall 5-year survival of 87%.

Mucinous carcinomas are also extremely rare; only a few cases have been reported as primary endometrial tumors. They can be confused with primary mucinous carcinomas of the ovary, cervix, or bowel. They usually occur in postmenopausal women and may be associated with estrogen replacement therapy. They appear to have a good prognosis.

Primary squamous cell carcinoma of the endometrium is also very rare and usually occurs in postmenopausal women. Approximately 20 cases have been reported, and they have usually been associated with pyometra. The prognosis is poor, and White et al. documented no 5-year survivors.

TABLE 28-4

FIGO Staging Classification of Endometrial Carcinoma (1971-1988)

Stage	Characteristic
I	Confined to corpus
IA	Uterine cavity ≤8 cm G1: Well-differentiated tumor G2: Moderately differentiated tumor G3: Poorly differentiated tumor
IB	Uterine cavity >8 cm G1, G2, or G3
II	Involvement of corpus and cervix
III	Extension outside uterus but not outside true pelvis; may involve bladder or parametrium but not mucosa of bladder or rectum
IV	Extends outside true pelvis or involves mucosa of bladder or rectum

TABLE 28-5

Corpus Cancer Staging (Adopted 1988)

Stages	Characteristic
IA G123	Tumor limited to endometrium
IB G123	Invasion to <½ myometrium
IC G123	Invasion to >½ myometrium
IIA G123	Endocervical glandular involvement only
IIB G123	Cervical stromal invasion
IIIA G123	Tumor invades serosa and/or adnexae, and/or positive peritoneal cytology
IIIB G123	Vaginal metastases
IIIC G123	Metastases to pelvic and/or paraaortic lymph nodes
IVA G123	Tumor invasion of bladder and/or bowel mucosa
IVB	Distant metastases including intraabdominal and/or inguinal lymph node

Staging

Tables 28-4 and 28-5 demonstrate the staging classifications of the International Federation of Gynecology and Obstetrics (FIGO) for endometrial carcinoma. Table 28-4 shows the classification in use from 1971 to 1988. In 1988 a new classification was introduced (Table 28-5) that relies on an operative evaluation with particular emphasis in stage I on myometrial invasion. Figure 28-13 displays the various stages of endometrial carcinoma based on the varying degrees of uterine involvement according to the new FIGO system. For patients who are treated primarily with radiation, the older staging system is applied. There is limited experience with the new system, so that all survivals quoted in the remainder of this chapter will be based on currently available data using the 1971 to 1988 system.

Prognostic Factors

Many variables affect the behavior of endometrial adenocarcinomas. These variables can be conveniently divided into clinical and pathologic factors. The clinical determinants are patient age at diagnosis, race, and clinical tumor stage. The pathologic determinants are tumor grade, histologic type, uterine size, depth of myometrial invasion, microscopic involvement of vascular spaces in the uterus by tumor, and

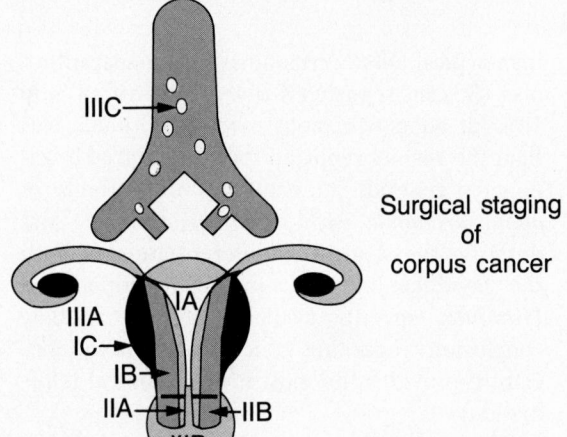

Surgical staging of corpus cancer

FIGURE 28-13

Schematic for surgical staging for endometrial carcinoma according to 1988 FIGO definitions (Table 28-5). Courtesy of Dr. James Orr, Watson Clinic, Lakeland, Florida.

spread of tumor outside the uterus to the retroperitoneal lymph nodes, peritoneal cavity, or uterine adnexa. In addition, steroid receptor hormone content affects prognosis.

Clinical Factors

A number of studies have shown that younger women with endometrial carcinoma have an improved prognosis. Christopherson et al. reported a 95% 10-year survival among 115 women under age 50 treated for stage I endometrial carcinomas, a rate that is much higher than the 74.5% for all the patients in their series. In a different study of patients with all stages of endometrial carcinoma, the same authors noted that older patients had tumors of a higher stage and grade than younger patients. The finding of malignant endometrial cells in routine cervical-vaginal cytology (Pap smear) is a poor prognostic factor. DuBeshter et al. recently noted that among 66 women with suspicious or malignant endometrial cells in their cervical smears, only 2 were stage IA while 24 had a stage III-IV disease (1988 revised FIGO staging).

White patients have a higher survival rate than black patients, a finding partially explained by higher-stage and higher-grade tumors among black women. The 10-year survival of black patients in the series of Christopherson et al. was 27%, in comparison with 64% for white patients. Forty-two percent of the black women, in comparison with only 12% of the white women, died of disease within 10 years.

Tumor stage is a well-recognized prognostic factor for endometrial carcinoma (Table 28-6). Fortunately, most cases are diagnosed in stage I, which provides a favorable prognosis.

Pathologic Factors

The histologic grade of the tumor is a major determinant of prognosis. Endometrial carcinomas are divided into three grades: grade 1, well differentiated; grade 2, intermediate differentiation; and grade 3, poorly differentiated. Table 28-7 shows the survival of 811 patients with endometrial carcinoma related to tumor grade and demonstrates the worsening of prognosis with advancing tumor grade.

The histologic type of the endometrial carcinoma is also related to prognosis, with the best prognosis associated with typical adenocarcinomas, as well as adenoacanthomas and secretory carcinomas. Approximately 80% of all endometrial carcinomas fall into the favorable category. Poor prognostic histologic types are papillary carcinomas, clear cell carcinomas, and adenosquamous carcinomas, as previously noted. Table 28-8 summarizes the 5-year survivals for stage I cases of various cell types.

Uterine size and myometrial invasion have been correlated with the prognosis of endometrial carcinomas. As shown in Table 28-4, uterine size changes the pre-1988 staging of uterine

TABLE 28-6

Carcinoma of the Corpus Uteri, 1979-1981: 5-year Survival in Collected Series of Patients, Distribution by Stage ($n = 14,906$)

Stage	5-year Survival (%)	Proportion of Cases (%)*
I	72	74
II	56	14
III	32	6
IV	11	3
OVERALL	65	

Modified from Pettersson F, Coppleson M, Creasman WT, et al: Annual report on the results of treatment in gynecologic cancer Vol 20, Stockholm, 1988, The International Federation of Gynecology and Obstetrics.
*3.5% not staged.

TABLE 28-7

Five-year Survival in Carcinoma of the Endometrium Related to Histologic Grade

Grade	Number	% Alive
1	455	84.1
2	264	73.9
3	92	51.1
TOTAL	811	77.1

Modified from Connelly PJ, Alberhasky RC, Christopherson WM, et al: Obstet Gynecol 59:569, 1982. Reprinted with permission from The American College of Obstetricians and Gynecologists.

cancer within the category of stage I. However, uterine size is not as major a determinant of prognosis as is tumor grade. The degree of myometrial invasion does correlate with the risk of tumor spread outside the uterus, but the higher grade and higher stage tumors in general have the deepest myometrial penetration. The importance of tumor grade and myometrial invasion is also illustrated by a study of their relationship to the spread of adenocarcinoma of the endometrium to the retroperitoneal pelvic and paraaortic lymph nodes. Recent studies of 142 patients by Schink et al. indicate that tumor size is prognostic. Only 4% of those with tumors ≤ 2 cm in size had lymph node metastases. The rate increased to 15% for those with tumors > 2 cm to 35% when the entire endometrial cavity was involved.

Peritoneal cytology has been studied as a prognostic factor, and the results are conflicting. For example, in a study of 567 surgical

TABLE 28-8

Survival at 5 Years for Stage I Endometrial Cancer According to Subtype

Subtype	Alive (%)	DOD* (%)
Adenocarcinoma with squamous metaplasia†	88	6
Adenocarcinoma, NSF‡	80	6
Serous papillary	70	21
Adenosquamous	53	33
Clear cell	44	51

From Christopherson WM, Connelly PJ, and Alberhasky RC: Cancer 51:1705, 1983.
*Dead of disease
†Adenoacanthoma
‡No specific features; including secretory carcinoma

stage I cases, Turner et al. found that positive peritoneal cytology was an independent prognostic factor. In contrast, Grimshaw et al. evaluated 322 clinical stage I cases and found that positive peritoneal cytology was an adverse prognostic factor, but they did not find it to be an independent risk factor when other variables were considered.

PATTERNS OF SPREAD OF ENDOMETRIAL CARCINOMA. Plentl and Friedman noted four major channels of lymphatic drainage from the uterus that serve as sites for extrauterine spread of tumor: (1) a small lymphatic branch along the round ligament that runs to the inguinal femoral nodes, (2) branches from the tubal and (3) ovarian pedicles (infundibulopelvic ligaments), which are large lymphatics that drain into the paraaortic nodes, and (4) the broad ligament lymphatics that drain directly to the pelvic nodes. The pelvic and paraaortic node drainage sites (2, 3, and 4) are the most important clinically. In addition, direct peritoneal spread of tumor can occur through the uterine wall or via the lumen of the fallopian tube. Clinically, therefore, the clinician must assess the retroperitoneal nodes, the peritoneal cavity, and the uterine adnexa for the spread of endometrial carcinoma (Figure 28-14).

Recently extensive studies by the Gynecologic Oncology Group have elucidated both the frequency of lymph node metastases in endometrial carcinoma and the pathologic factors that modify this risk in stage I disease. Tumor grade, size of the uterus, and degree of myometrial invasion were studied. Table 28-9 illustrates the frequency of lymph node metastases according to uterine size and tumor grade. There are differences in the proportion of positive nodes between stage IB and IA

TABLE 28-9

FIGO Staging and Nodal Metastasis

	Metastasis	
Staging	Pelvic	Aortic
IA G1 (n = 101)	2 (2%)	0 (0%)
G2 (n = 169)	13 (8%)	6 (4%)
G3 (n = 76)	8 (11%)	5 (7%)
IB G1 (n = 79)	3 (4%)	3 (4%)
G2 (n = 119)	12 (10%)	8 (7%)
G3 (n = 77)	20 (26%)	12 (16%)

From Creasman WT, Morrow CP, Bundy BN, et al: Cancer 60:2035, 1987. Reprinted with permission.

(pre-1988 staging) cases, as well as tumor grade. Table 28-10 shows the effects of tumor grade and depth of myometrial invasion. The frequency of nodal involvement becomes much greater with higher-grade tumors and with greater depth of myometrial invasion. The risk of lymph node involvement appears to be negligible for endometrial carcinoma involving only the endometrium. With invasion of the inner third of the myometrium there is negligible risk of node involvement for grade 1 and grade 2 cases. If the outer third of the myometrium is involved, the risk of nodal metastases is greatly increased. These data emphasize the importance of myometrial invasion and tumor spread providing the basis for the new (1988) FIGO Operative Staging System. Table 28-11 summarizes the risk of nodal metastases based on the most recent GOG studies published by Creasman et al. In a more recent GOG study, Morrow et al. noted that for patients without metastases at operation, the greatest risk of future recurrence was grade 3 histology. Further-

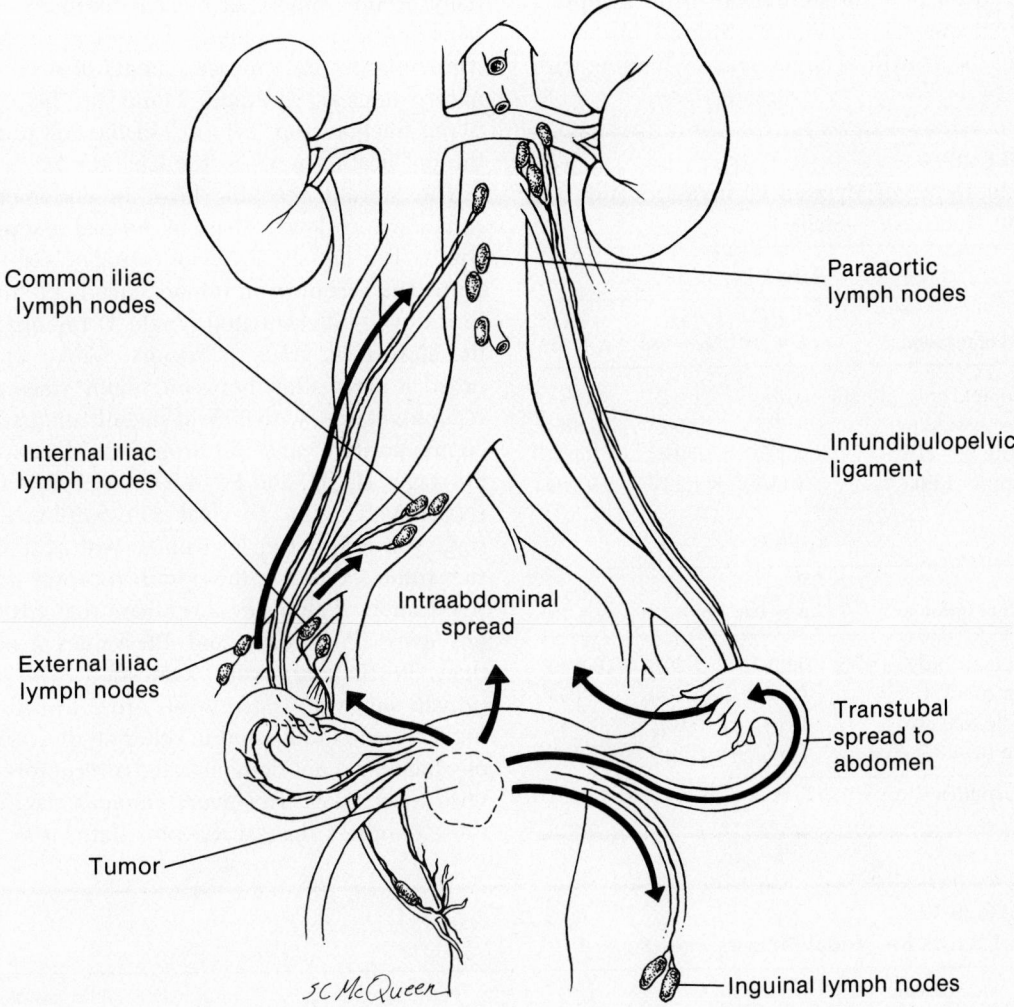

FIGURE 28-14
Spread of endometrial carcinoma. The major pathways of tumor spread are illustrated (see text).

more, among 48 patients with histologically documented aortic node metastases, 47 were found to have positive pelvic nodes, adnexal metastases, or tumor invasion to the outer one third of the myometrium, emphasizing the poor prognostic aspects of these three findings.

STEROID HORMONE RECEPTORS. Because the endometrium is sensitive to estrogen and progesterone stimulation, extensive studies have been done of steroid hormone receptors in endometrial carcinoma. Steroid hormones affect the growth of target cells by binding with

steroid receptors in the cell. The receptor steroid complex then interacts with DNA in the cell nucleus, stimulating the synthesis of messenger RNA (mRNA), which acts in the cytoplasm to stimulate protein synthesis.

Traditionally it has been thought that the steroid receptor is initially located primarily in the cytoplasm. Recent histochemical studies, however, indicate that steroid receptors initially occupy almost all nuclear locations. The biochemical measurement of estrogen receptor content represents measurements of predominantly nuclear receptors found in the cytoplasm fraction (the "cytosol") of the cell during the purification process (see Chapter 4).

The steroid receptor level in endometrial carcinoma is lower than in normal endometrium. The highest levels of estrogen and progesterone receptors in tumors have been found in the well-differentiated (grade 1) tumors and the lowest in grade 3 tumors. Vihko et al. noted a correlation between tumor stage and receptor status, with 65% of stage I tumors "receptor positive" and the proportion decreasing for stages II, III, and IV to 50%, 17%, and 0%, respectively. The survival rate within each stage was also better for women with receptor-rich tumors than for those with receptor-negative tumors. Palmer et al. noticed that ER values over 70 fmol/mg and PR values greater than 30 fmol/mg were associated with improved survival. These levels are 2 to 3 times higher than cutoffs used in other studies, some of which have not demonstrated a receptor-survival association. However, Palmer's data and those of others suggest receptor status is an im-

TABLE 28-10
Grade, Depth of Myometrial Invasion, and Node Metastasis—Stage I

Pelvic

Depth of Invasion	G1 n = 180	G2 n = 288	G3 n = 153
Endomet. only (n=86)	0(0%)	1(3%)	0(0%)
Inner (n=281)	3(3%)	7(5%)	5(9%)
Middle (n=115)	0(0%)	6(9%)	1(4%)
Deep (n=139)	2(11%)	11(19%)	23(34%)

Aortic

Depth of Invasion	G1 n = 180	G2 n = 288	G3 n = 153
Endomet. only (n=86)	0(0%)	1(3%)	0(0%)
Inner (n=281)	1(1%)	5(4%)	2(4%)
Middle (n=115)	1(5%)	0(0%)	0(0%)
Deep (n=139)	1(6%)	8(14%)	15(23%)

Adapted from Creasman WT, et al: Cancer 60:2035, 1987.

TABLE 28-11
Risk Factors for Nodal Metastases—Stage I

Factor	Pelvic	Aortic
Low Risk Grade 1 Endometrium only No intraperitoneal spread	0/44 (0%)	0/44 (0%)
Moderate Risk Grade 2 or 3 Invasion to middle ⅓	15/268 (6%)	6/268 (2%)
High Risk Invasion to outer ⅓	21/116 (18%)	17/118 (15%)

Adapted from Creasman WT, Morrow CP, Bundy BN, et al: Cancer 60:2035, 1987.

portant parameter for endometrial carcinoma prognosis. In a study of 309 tumors, Kleine et al. performed a multivariate analysis of survival and found progesterone receptor status, not estrogen receptor status, the most significant prognostic factor after clinical stage. Receptor status also appears to influence tumor response to progestational therapy. It is therefore advisable to obtain a steroid receptor measurement on the tissues of primary endometrial adenocarcinoma.

Evaluation

When the patient's disease is diagnosed as adenocarcinoma of the endometrium, fractional D&C or endometrial biopsy and endocervical curettage are usually performed to ascertain tumor grade, uterine size, and cervical involvement. A uterine sound is then introduced to determine the depth of the uterus. In some cases conization may be necessary to define accurately cervical involvement when planning treatment, since microscopic tumor found on endocervical curettage without invasion of the cervical stroma is not conclusive evidence of cervical involvement. It should be noted that the post-1988 tumor stage (see Table 28-5) requires ascertainment of cervical stromal invasion to define stage IIB.

In addition to the usual routine preoperative evaluation, the patient should have a chest x-ray examination, intravenous pyelogram, barium enema, and liver function studies and/or an abdominal pelvic CT scan. A formal staging procedure with the patient under anesthesia (as performed for cervical carcinoma, Chapter 27) is not necessary, but if the uterus is enlarged or adnexal spread or bladder or rectosigmoid involvement seems possible, a clinical staging examination with anesthesia, including cystoscopy and proctoscopy, is performed. The estrogen and progesterone receptor content of the tumor should be evaluated, usually with the hysterectomy specimen for patients who undergo surgery or with tissue obtained from D&C if radiation is to be used. Recent reports indicate that the measurement of antigen CA-125, usually used in cases of ovarian carcinoma, may be useful. If elevated preoperatively, it usually indicates extrauterine disease. It is also a useful marker for those with serous carcinoma of the endometrium.

Management

Stage I

Both operation and irradiation have been used effectively to treat carcinoma of the endometrium. For patients in satisfactory physical condition, a surgical procedure is the primary treatment modality, with irradiation used as an adjunct. For patients who cannot medically tolerate an operation, irradiation alone can be used. However, irradiation as the sole method of therapy yields inferior results, as Bickenbach et al. noted, with an 87% 5-year survival rate for patients with stage I carcinoma treated by an operation alone, in comparison with a 69% survival rate for those treated with irradiation alone.

Most patients with stage I carcinoma of the endometrium undergo hysterectomy. Sometimes preoperative irradiation is used before operation to increase the likelihood of sterilization of small tumor deposits outside the uterus and reduce the risk of tumor dissemination resulting from surgical manipulation. However, initial operation followed by irradiation, when needed, allows accurate surgical and histologic assessment of (1) tumor spread in the uterus, (2) degree of penetration into the myometrium, and (3) extrauterine spread to retroperitoneal nodes, adnexa, and/or the peritoneal cavity. This is the approach that will be used for cases that will be staged according to the 1988 FIGO system (see Table 28-5).

The operation performed for stage I carcinoma depends on tumor grade determined preoperatively, intraoperative findings, and results of pathologic examination of the removed hysterectomy specimen. The extent of the operative approach is based on the relative risk of spreading disease outside the uterus.

STAGE I, GRADE 1. The risk of spread of grade 1 tumor to pelvic nodes is extremely small (see Table 28-10). Operatively the abdomen is explored through a lower abdominal vertical incision, peritoneal cytology is sampled, and an extrafascial total abdominal hysterectomy with bilateral salpingo-oophorectomy is performed. Before the hysterectomy, clamps are placed across both fallopian tubes to obtain traction on the uterus and allow its manipulation during surgery. In theory this reduces the risk of dissemination of endometrial tumor cells. Routine sampling of retroperitoneal nodes is not performed in these cases, but any clinically enlarged pelvic or paraaortic lymph nodes are removed for histologic evaluation. The surgical specimen should be opened in the operating room and a frozen section performed if there is evidence of deep myometrial penetration. Doering et al. have shown that visual inspection of the opened uterus in the operating room accurately determines the depth of invasion confirmed microscopically in 91% of 148 cases. The technique of opening and sampling the uterus with demonstration of the depth of tumor invasion is shown in Figure 28-15, *A* and *B*. If deep penetration is present or

if there is a well-differentiated tumor penetrating into the outer one third of the uterus, the tumor could have microscopic areas advanced beyond grade 1, in which case lymph node dissection would be indicated. Goff and Rice noted that gross examination alone is less reliable for estimating depth of myometrial invasion for grade 2 or 3 tumors, and they suggest a frozen section be performed, particularly for high grade tumors. If the patient has only grade 1 tumor and the pathologic evaluation shows no deep penetration of the myometrium, the operation is concluded for grade I cases.

If peritoneal cytologic sampling shows tumor

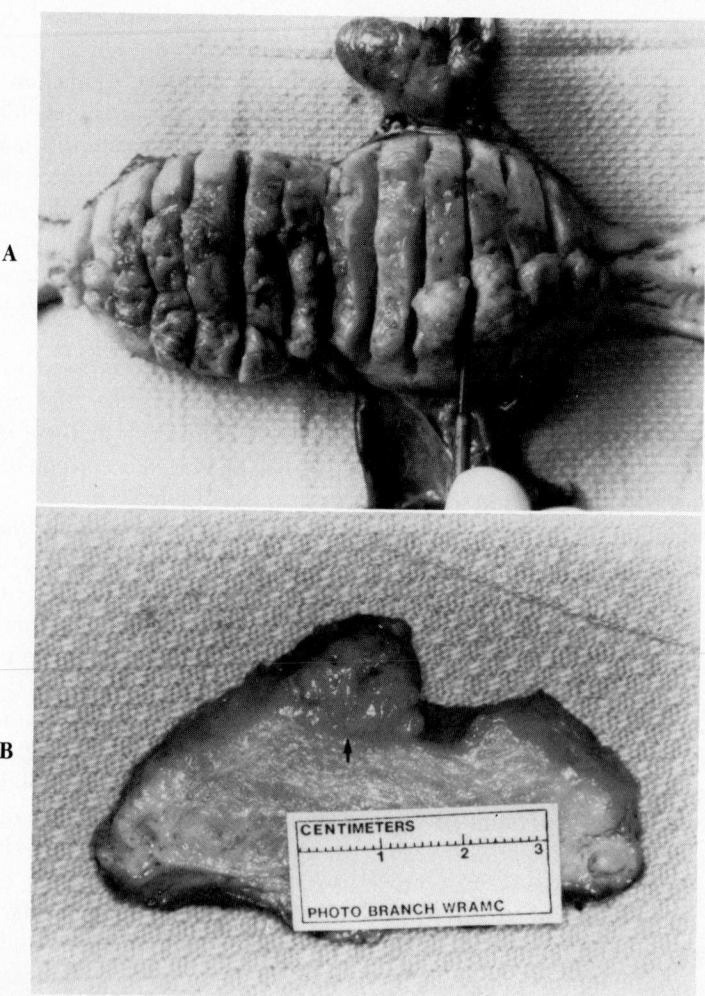

FIGURE 28-15
A, Technique for intraoperative assessment of the depth of myometrial invasion. **B,** Cross section of uterine wall demonstrating superficial myometrial invasion. Arrow shows tumor-myometrial junction. (From Doering DL, Barnhill DR, Weiser EB, et al: Obstet Gynecol, 74:930, 1989.)

cells and there is no indication for external irradiation or brachytherapy, 15 mCi of ^{32}P may be given intraperitoneally 2 to 3 weeks postoperatively (Chapter 29). However, the efficacy of ^{32}P in endometrial carcinoma has not been established. If there is deep myometrial invasion, postoperative irradiation delivered via vaginal implant provides a surface dose to the vagina of approximately 5000 to 6000 rads (50 to 60 Gy). External pelvic irradiation should be considered if there is tumor penetration close to the peritoneal surface (see later discussion). However, such situations are rare in stage I, grade I adenocarcinoma of the endometrium.

STAGE I, GRADES 2 AND 3. Insofar as there is a definite risk of nodal tumor spread for grade 2 and particularly grade 3, the operative approach often includes sampling of the paraaortic and pelvic nodes. This is usually done for grade 2 cases with invasion to the inner one half or for grade 3 cases with invasion to the inner one third of the myometrium. These are only rough guidelines, and the decision to do a pelvic and paraaortic node sampling is also affected by the degree of operative risk, including the patient's obesity and medical risk factors. Node sampling is usually performed in patients with poor prognostic cell types (clear cell, serous, adenosquamous). For node sampling, the aorta and iliac vessels are identified and palpated, and any enlarged nodes up to the level of the third portion of the duodenum as it crosses the aorta are identified and removed. If no enlarged nodes are encountered, the retroperitoneal space along the pelvic wall is opened, and the ureters are retracted medially. The lymph node tissue over the external iliac vessels and obturator spaces is removed, with particular emphasis on any enlarged nodes identified in this area or along the common iliac artery. The peritoneum over the aorta is incised. The ureter is retracted laterally, as is the inferior mesenteric artery; the lymph node tissue over the anterior part of the aorta and vena cava is removed up to the level of the duodenum (Figure 28-16).

Use of postoperative irradiation depends on the pathologic findings. If the peritoneal results of cytologic testing are positive,^{32}P may be given. For grade 2 tumors that invade the myometrium to the middle third or beyond or for grade 3 tumors that invade the myometrium

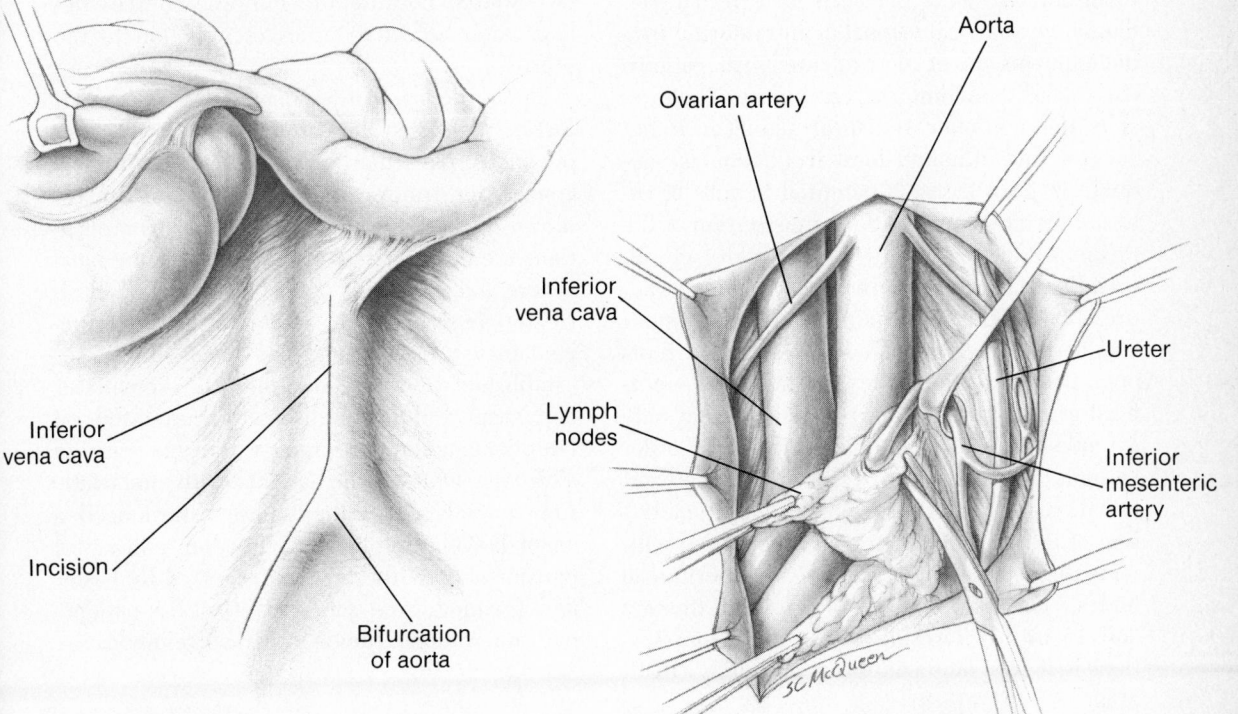

FIGURE 28-16
Removal of lymph node tissue. The technique of removal of retroperitoneal paraaortic nodes is demonstrated with the important anatomic landmarks.

even superficially, full pelvic irradiation is usually given to treat the pelvic nodes, in view of the high risk of spread. However, if the pelvic nodes are free of tumor, local vaginal irradiation alone may be sufficient. For grade 2 tumors confined to the inner third of the myometrium or grade 3 tumors only in the endometrium, vaginal irradiation is usually prescribed. If the nodes are found to contain tumor, external irradiation encompasses the area from which the tumor-bearing node was removed. Current data do not prove that administration of paraaortic irradiation increases the length of patient survival when metastatic tumor is identified in the paraaortic nodes, but such irradiation of 45-50 Gy is usually given.

Adnexal spread of tumor is usually managed by external pelvic irradiation, usually extended to include the entire abdomen, since transperitoneal seeding is likely.

RADIATION THERAPY CONSIDERATIONS.

As just discussed, radiation therapy is prescribed for stage I endometrial carcinomas preoperatively, postoperatively, or as the sole therapy for patients unable to undergo surgery. However, current data conflict as to the efficacy of preoperative versus postoperative treatment and also as to the need for external irradiation versus local vaginal or intrauterine irradiation. Onsrud et al. evaluated 386 patients with stage I endometrial carcinoma. Their results did not offer statistical significance but suggest that although local irradiation is adequate in most cases, a potential benefit of external therapy exists in deep penetration of the myometrium. Similarly, Meerwaldt et al. found only a small number of locoregional failures (23 of 326) in patients who had a tumor confined to the uterus and who received postoperative irradiation. They did not treat superficial grade I tumors and pointed out that only a randomized trial could identify those other patients who might do well without adjuvant radiation. As shown previously, deep penetration of the myometrium is also associated with increased spread of tumor to retroperitoneal nodes. The combination of external therapy and 15 mCi ^{32}P resulted in bowel complications in four of nine patients reported by Heath et al.

A recent study of 605 patients by Kucera et al. demonstrated the efficacy of postoperative irradiation in improving survival in stage I patients and also provided useful guidelines for therapy. They administered vaginal irradiation only (3200 cGy) to the vaginal surface to 376 patients with inner one-third myometrial involvement regardless of grade or for middle one-third involvement for grade I cases. No pelvic irradiation was given to these patients with a good prognosis, and the 5-year survival was 91.8%. External pelvic irradiation to give a total dose of 5400 to 5600 cGy was prescribed for patients with grade 2 or 3 tumors that penetrated to the middle one third of the myometrium or for all grades that penetrated to the outer one third. The 5-year survival for these 229 high-risk patients was 87.8%, almost as good as the 91.8% for those with good prognostic factors. A recent study of 86 patients by Stryker et al. suggests 4250 cGy whole-pelvis radiotherapy may be adequate following total abdominal hysterectomy and bilateral salpingo-oophorectomy for patients with disease confined to the uterus or occultly extending to the cervix.

For intrauterine radiation treatment of endometrial carcinoma, small radium capsules (Heyman) are often used. The uterus is packed with multiple small sources of radiation, and the myometrial wall is distended, as shown in Figure 28-17. A system of multiple sources is used in preference to a single linear intracavitary source because the multiple sources deliver more effective doses of radiation to the uterus.

Paraaortic irradiation may also be used. It carries with it an increased risk of bowel complications, particularly if the patient has undergone prior transperitoneal exploration or removal of the paraaortic nodes. Such complications are dose related and usually become most severe above dosages of 5000 cGy. Potish et al. treated 48 women with 4500 to 5075 cGy to the paraaortic areas; 22 had had nodal metastases established at operation, and the remainder had suspected nodal disease documented on lymphangiogram. Overall, a salvage rate of 47% was achieved in patients with metastatic tumor. Only one patient (2%) experienced a small bowel complication. Further efficacy of paraaortic node therapy was reported by Feuer and Calanog, who salvaged 10 of 15 patients with microscopic tumor in paraaortic nodes.

Stage II

Three therapeutic options have been employed for the treatment of stage II carcinoma of the endometrium that also involves the endocervix: (1) primary operation (radical hyster-

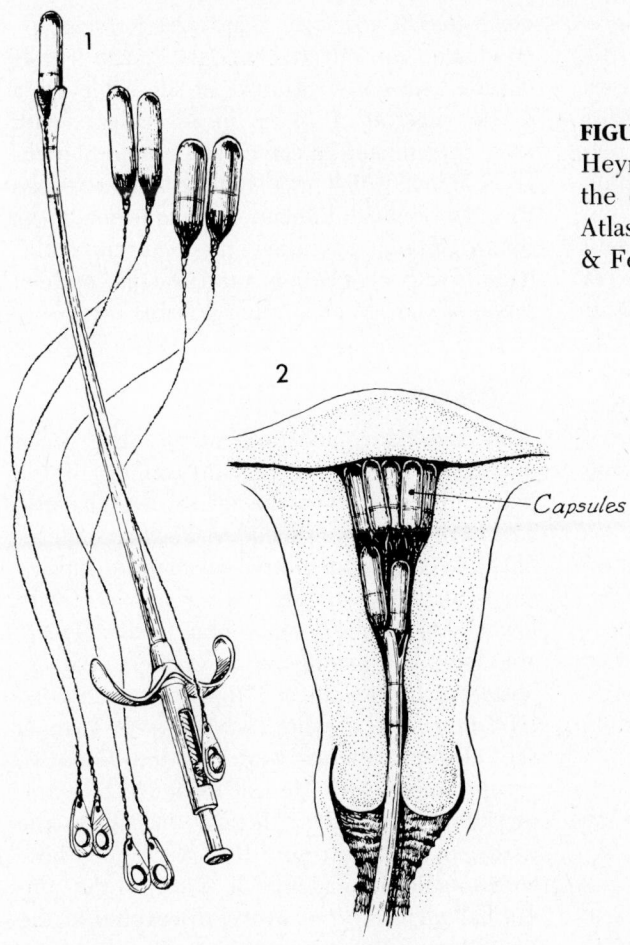

FIGURE 28-17
Heyman's capsules used to pack and distend the endometrial cavity. (From Wheeless CR: Atlas of pelvic surgery, Philadelphia, 1981, Lea & Febiger.)

ectomy and pelvic node dissection), (2) primary irradiation (intrauterine and vaginal implant and external irradiation) followed by an operation (extrafascial hysterectomy), and (3) irradiation as the sole method of management. Because tumor involves the cervix, as well as the endometrium, in stage II carcinoma, dissemination of malignancy from both sites must be considered.

Radical hysterectomy and pelvic node dissection have been used as effective therapy and have resulted in a 75% 5-year survival for the 26 patients treated by Homesley et al. and 65% for the 20 patients reported by Wallin et al. External irradiation is usually added if the pelvic nodes are involved with tumor. For grade 1 tumors, particularly those with less than one-third myometrial invasion, no postoperative irradiation is used.

Most patients with stage II carcinoma of the endometrium are treated with a combination of radiation and extrafascial hysterectomy. A widely used protocol includes external radiation (45 Gy) and a single brachytherapy implant usually followed in 4 to 6 weeks by extrafascial total abdominal hysterectomy, bilateral salpingo-oophorectomy, and paraaortic node sampling. Podczaski et al. noted that those with gross cervical tumor had a poor prognosis and were likely to have extrauterine disease at operation. For patients with cervical involvement on biopsy but no gross tumor, Trimble and Jones found radiation treatment by a single implant alone followed by a hysterectomy to be effective, and they added external therapy depending on the nodal findings and myometrial invasion. Anderson reported on 54 patients with stage II tumors and found a 70.6% survival in patients treated by abdominal hysterectomy followed by radiation.

If the patient is able to tolerate an operation, removal of the uterus improves prognosis and survival. If the patient is unable to tolerate an operation, irradiation alone (combined uterine and vaginal local irradiation and external therapy) is utilized (see later discussion). Most patients with stage II adenocarcinoma of the endometrium are elderly and obese and thus are not good candidates for radical hysterectomy. However, for good operative candidates, especially younger, thin patients and those with "occult" cervical involvement rather than gross clinical disease, radical hysterectomy and pelvic node dissection are appropriate. Radiation therapy is added for higher grade lesions, patients with deep myometrial invasion (beyond the inner third), or those with evidence of spread of tumor to regional pelvic nodes. Most frequently the initial irradiation for patients with stage II adenocarcinoma of the endometrium consists of uterine packing and radiation therapy to the cervix and the upper portion of the vagina (see Figure 28-17). For higher grade lesions and those grossly involving the cervix, external irradiation is added, followed by extrafascial hysterectomy. For well-differentiated tumors or only microscopic involvement of the cervix, an extrafascial hysterectomy with selective lymph node sampling is performed after intrauterine irradiation. External irradiation is added postoperatively, depending on the pathologic findings.

Radiation Therapy as the Sole Treatment of Stage I or II

Occasionally irradiation is used alone to treat stage I or II adenocarcinoma of the endometrium. Landgren et al. used Heyman packing with vaginal ovoids and two or three applications to treat stage I carcinomas. Either a dosage of 6000 mg-hours of radium was given to the uterus, or this dosage was reduced to 2500 mg-hours and supplemented later with 4000 rads of external radiation therapy. The best results were obtained with radium packing alone. This series was not randomized, but an improved result with the added external therapy was not demonstrated. The 5-year survival for stage I patients was approximately 75% in comparison with 55% for stage II patients. Later the same authors noted that treatment by uterine packing (6000 mg-hours) provided greater pelvic control of stage I disease than did 4000 rads of external irradiation in combination with only 2500 mg-hours of uterine packing.

Patanaphan et al. reported a 56% 5-year survival for 32 patients treated by irradiation in stage I and 40% for those in stage II. Tumor grade was not a significant factor in survival rate. Andersen et al. reported an overall 5-year survival rate of 49.6% for all stages, broken down to 65% for stage I and 42% for stage II. Irradiation can effectively control stage I or II disease. Recently, Ahmad et al. achieved a 5-year survival of 74.5% in 16 patients with stage II endometrial carcinoma treated by radiation alone, which was similar to their results with operation and radiation. Eradication of the tumor through operation, however, in combination with irradiation remains the optimal mode of management when possible.

Stage III

In stage III carcinoma the disease has spread outside the uterus but remains confined to the pelvis. These tumors do not involve the mucosa of the rectum or bladder. They account for only 7% of all endometrial carcinomas and occur in patients who are older than those with lower stage tumors and often medically less able to undergo an operation. Aalders et al. reported on the results of 175 patients with stage III tumor, 52% of whom were over 60 years of age. These patients were divided into two groups: those with clinical evidence of extra-uterine spread before therapy (usually to the vagina or parametrium, 108 cases) and those with subclinical evidence of spread to the adnexa (fallopian tube or ovary) discovered at the time of operation in a patient believed to have stage I or II carcinoma initially (but IIIA by the new operative classification, 67 cases.) Operative eradication of microscopic tumor was of major prognostic importance in these cases; eradication was usually possible if the tumor involved only the uterine adnexa. The optimal therapy, when possible, was a total abdominal hysterectomy and bilateral salpingo-oophorectomy followed by external irradiation (40 to 50 Gy). If there was vaginal extension of cervical disease, the cervical field was shielded at 20 Gy and subsequent brachytherapy was administered to the vagina, bringing the vaginal surface dose to 60 Gy. For patients who could not undergo surgery, packing of the uterus was done as described (Figure 28-17), followed by external irradiation therapy. Those with subclinical spread of tumor had a much better 5-year survival (40%) than those with overt clinical stage III disease (16%). Pliskow et al. noted a 5-year survival of 27% for 22 patients with stage III disease with the best results for those treated by operation and irradiation.

For intraperitoneal metastatic disease, Greer

and Hamburger used whole abdominal irradiation in 31 patients. In 27 of the patients with residual tumor less than 2 cm, a 5-year survival of 63% was noted. These authors recommend that such salvage therapy could be effective for individuals with endometrial carcinoma, particularly stage III disease, providing tumor reduction surgery results in residual tumor under 2 cm in diameter, as shown in the data for ovarian epithelial carcinoma.

The patients with stage III endometrial carcinoma with the best prognosis have tumor spread only to the fallopian tubes or ovaries or both (Stage IIIA). This has been emphasized in a recent report by Greven et al., who noted a 60% 5-year survival for those with adnexal involvement and only 45% for those with parametrial or pelvic peritoneal involvement. If possible, therapy should include operative eradication of macroscopic tumor. This is combined with radiotherapy, the dosage and delivery system of which depend on the extent of tumor. If there is no extensive involvement of the cervix and paracervical areas, initial Heyman packing can be done before hysterectomy and external beam therapy. For tumor that extends into the vagina and paravaginal tissues, intracavitary irradiation is combined with external therapy, followed by hysterectomy if technically feasible. For tumor extending to the pelvic wall or patients in poor medical condition, usually only irradiation therapy is possible.

Stage IV

Approximately 3% of endometrial carcinomas are at stage IV, and many of these patients have tumor metastases outside the pelvis. In a series of 83 patients from the Norwegian Radium Hospital, Aalders et al. reported that the lung was the main site of extrauterine spread (36% of the cases), which is consistent with the generalized pattern of recurrent adenocarcinoma of the endometrium. They utilized hysterectomy to achieve local control of stage IV disease, usually followed by postoperative external irradiation therapy. Progestational therapy (17α-hydroxyprogesterone caproate, 1000 mg intramuscularly daily for 1 week, weekly for 3 months, and every other week for at least 1 year) was also prescribed for 17 patients, two of whom survived 3 and 13 years, respectively. Progestins were also used in 30 patients with

pulmonary metastases, and 8 had a complete remission (disappearance) of metastatic tumor. Complete remission occurred in 7 patients with grade 2 tumors and in 1 patient with grade 3, but progression occurred in 11 of 13 patients with grade 3 carcinoma, a finding that is consistent with the observation that poorly differentiated adenocarcinomas are least responsive to progestational therapy. The 5-year survival was 10% for all 83 cases, similar to the general experience (see Table 28-6).

Individualization of therapy is necessary for the patient with stage IV endometrial carcinoma. If feasible, the uterus, tubes, and ovaries are removed to achieve local control. Irradiation therapy is administered as an adjunct or, if necessary, as the sole therapy for palliation to achieve pelvic control of disease. Progestational agents are particularly useful in the case of well-differentiated tumors.

Recurrent Adenocarcinoma of the Endometrium

Most recurrences of adenocarcinoma of the endometrium occur within 3 years of diagnosis, and 90% occur within 5 years of diagnosis. Since 10% of recurrences will occur more than 5 years after initial diagnosis, patients with adenocarcinoma of the endometrium need prolonged follow-up. In the series of Aalders et al. involving 379 patients, half of the recurrences were in the pelvis and vagina; the most frequent sites of nonpelvic metastases were lung (17%), upper portion of the abdomen (10%), and bone (6%). Irradiation was the primary treatment of localized recurrent disease in patients who had an operation alone as the initial treatment, but operative excision of resectable nodules was also done when feasible. Progestational agents are added as initial treatment, particularly for disseminated disease. The 5-year survival rate for those patients who received progestins with other forms of treatment for grade 1 and grade 2 recurrences was 26%, in comparison with 14% for those who did not. For undifferentiated tumors the comparable survival was 9%.

CHEMOTHERAPY. Chemotherapy for endometrial carcinoma has primarily involved the use of progestins, as well as cytotoxic agents. Unfortunately, no clearly effective program of cytotoxic chemotherapy has emerged. Progestins have been used frequently, and responses of 10% to 30% have been reported. Responses are more likely in well-differentiated tumors, as well as those recurring at distant sites not previously treated, such as the lung.

Steroid hormone receptor content of tumor has been studied in relation to chemotherapeutic response. It has been shown that the well-differentiated tumors also have the highest content of estrogen and progestin steroid hormone receptors. Ehrlich et al. reported that progesterone and estrogen receptor levels correlate with grade of tumor—84% of grade 1 tumors were progesterone receptor positive, 55% of grade 2, and 22% of grade 3. The content of receptor correlated with response to progestin treatment; none of the 15 patients with receptor-negative tumors responded to progestational therapy, yet seven of eight with receptor-positive tumors responded. Numerous and various dosage schedules have been employed, including 17α-hydroxyprogesterone (Delalutin), discussed earlier; medroxyprogesterone (Depo-Provera), 400 mg intramuscularly weekly for 3 months, and then every 2 weeks; and oral megestrol acetate (Megace), 160 to 320 mg daily. Kohorn summarized many case reports from the literature and noted that responses were approximately 15% for poorly differentiated tumors and 32% for well-differentiated tumors. The results do not appear to depend on the type of progestin administered.

Recently antiestrogens, such as tamoxifen, have been added to treat recurrent endometrial carcinoma. A regimen of 5 days of therapy (10 mg orally twice daily) was associated with increased receptor content of endometrial carcinoma in the patients studied. Carlson et al. noted that only 13 of 25 tumors were progesterone receptor positive before tamoxifen therapy, whereas 21 of 25 tumors became positive after tamoxifen. These observations raise the possibility of combining tamoxifen and progestin therapy to improve the results of treatment.

Cytotoxic chemotherapy. A number of cytotoxic agents have been used to treat endometrial carcinoma. No effective salvage therapy has emerged, however, and combinations of cisplatin, doxorubicin (Adriamycin), and cyclophosphamide (Cytoxan) or 5-fluorouracil (5-FU) are usually employed.

There is some evidence that combined chemohormonal therapy provides better results. Ayoub et al. showed that 3 weeks of ta-

moxifen 20 mg PO daily alternating with 3 weeks of Provera 200 mg daily plus Cytoxan 400 mg/m^2 IV on days 1 and 8, Adriamycin 30 mg/m^2 IV day 1 and 5-fluorouracil 400/m^2 IV days 1 and 8 (CAF) gave significantly better results in a randomized trial than CAF alone. The combined chemohormonal therapy was also effective in reducing the frequency of relapses when used adjuvantly in high-risk cases (ER-negative, grade 3 tumors). Effective chemohormonal results were also reported by Hoffman et al. using Cytoxan (250 to 500 mg/m^2), Adriamycin (30 mg/m^2), and platinum (50 mg/m^2) (CAP) with megestrol acetate (40 to 160 mg PO daily). Of 15 patients, 4 had complete responses in their studies.

Some have tried progestin therapy as an adjuvant to improve therapeutic results in endometrial carcinoma, but a recent randomized trial reported by Vergote et al. confirmed previous reports that adjuvant progestin therapy has no demonstrated value for the treatment of endometrial carcinoma.

Newer approaches and agents are needed to deal with metastatic and recurrent adenocarcinoma of the endometrium. Multiple-agent regimens utilizing cyclophosphamide, doxorubicin, and platinum and/or 5-FU combined with hormonal therapy appear to offer occasional effective results.

Post Treatment Estrogen Replacement Therapy

Since estrogens have been implicated in the genesis of many endometrial carcinomas, it has usually been advised to avoid estrogen replacement therapy (ERT) (see Chapter 40) in these patients. However, recent studies by Creasman et al. suggest that those receiving ERT do not have a demonstrably increased risk of tumor recurrence and are protected against the complications of estrogen lack, i.e., osteoporosis, coronary artery disease, etc. In a nonrandomized study of 221 patients with stage I disease, 47 received ERT and 174 did not. Recurrence occurred in 26 (14.7%) of the non-ERT group and in 1 (2.1%) of the ERT group. Moreover, in a 5-year followup, 26 of the non-ERT group had died in comparison with only 1 of the ERT group, suggesting the ERT group was protected. Further studies are needed, but these data do suggest that ERT may be administered to those treated for Stage I endometrial carcinoma without increased risk of tumor recurrence and with likely health benefits. The patient needs to be informed of the various risks and benefits.

SARCOMAS

Uterine sarcomas are much less frequent than endometrial carcinomas, particularly in Western countries where carcinoma of the endometrium has become so common. Sarcomas comprise less than 5% of uterine malignancies. Numerous terms have been used to describe the many histologic types. One useful classification is based on determination of the resemblance of the sarcomatous elements to mesenchymal tissue normally found in the uterus (homologous sarcomas) in contrast to tissues foreign to the uterus (heterologous sarcomas). Homologous types include leiomyosarcomas, endometrial stromal sarcomas, and rarely angiosarcomas. Heterologous types include rhabdomyosarcomas, chondrosarcomas, osteosarcomas, and liposarcomas. These sarcomas may exist exclusively or may be admixed with epithelial adenocarcinoma, in which case the term *malignant mixed müllerian tumor* (MMMT) is applied. The box on the right shows a morphologic classification for uterine sarcomas. No uniformly defined staging criteria exist for these tumors, and the most widely used definitions are similar to those for endometrial carcinoma, that is, stage I, confined to the corpus; stage II, corpus and cervix involved; stage III, spread outside the uterus but confined to the pelvis; and stage IV, spread outside the true pelvis or into the mucosa of the bladder or rectum. Therapy for the more commonly occurring types will be discussed, including leiomyosarcomas, endometrial stromal sarcomas, and malignant müllerian mixed tumors.

Homologous Sarcoma

Leiomyosarcoma

Among the uterine sarcomas, leiomyosarcomas are the most common, occurring somewhat more frequently than mixed malignant müllerian tumors. In summarizing 1089 uterine sarcomas from the literature, Piver and Lurain noted that leiomyosarcomas comprised 45% of the group. The determination of malignancy is made in part by ascertaining the number of mitoses in 10 high-power fields (hpf), as well as the presence of cytologic atypia, abnormal mi-

---

MODIFIED CLASSIFICATION OF UTERINE SARCOMAS

I. Pure sarcoma
  A. Homologous
    1. Smooth muscle tumors
      a. Leiomyosarcoma
      b. Leiomyoblastoma
      c. Metastasizing tumors with benign histologic appearance
        (1) Intravenous leiomyomatosis
        (2) Metastasizing uterine leiomyoma
        (3) Leiomyomatosis peritonealis disseminata
    2. Endometrial stromal sarcomas
      a. Low grade: endolymphatic stromal myosis (ESM)
      b. High grade: endometrial stromal sarcoma (ESS)
  B. Heterologous
    1. Rhabdomyosarcoma
    2. Chondrosarcoma
    3. Osteosarcoma
    4. Liposarcoma
  C. Other sarcomas
II. Malignant mixed müllerian tumors (MMMT)
  A. Homologous (carcinosarcoma): Carcinoma + Homologous sarcoma
  B. Heterologous: Carcinoma + Heterologous sarcoma
III. Müllerian adenosarcoma
IV. Lymphoma

Modified from Clement P and Scully RE: Pathology of uterine sarcomas. In Coppleson M, editor: Gynecologic oncology, New York, 1981, Churchill Livingstone, p 591. Reprinted by permission.

---

totic figures, as well as nuclear pleomorphism (Figure 28-18). Vascular invasion and extrauterine spread of tumor are associated with worse prognoses. A finding of more than 5 mitoses/10 hpf with cytologic atypia leads to a diagnosis of leiomyosarcoma; when there are 4 mitoses/10 hpf or less, the tumors usually have a more benign clinical course. The prognosis worsens for tumors with over 10 mitoses/10 hpf. The presence of bizarre cells may not necessarily establish the diagnosis (Figure 28-19) because they

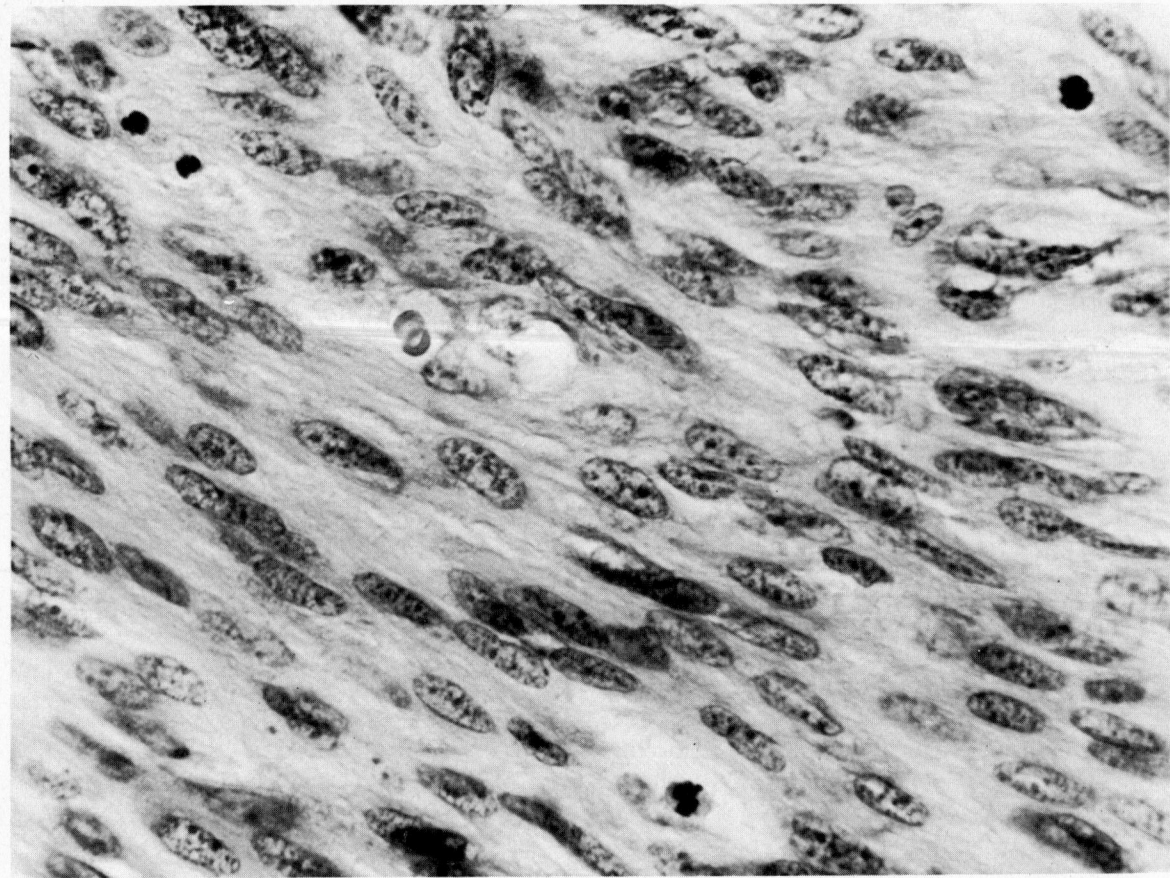

FIGURE 28-18
Leiomyosarcoma. Nuclear hyperchromatism and mitotic figures are present. (×660.) (From Clement PB and Scully RE: Pathology of uterine sarcomas. In Coppleson M, editor: Gynecologic oncology, Edinburgh, 1981, Churchill-Livingstone. Reprinted by permission.)

can occasionally be seen in benign leiomyomas and in patients receiving progestational agents. Furthermore, it is important to note that an increase in mitotic count in leiomyomas occurs in pregnancy as well as during oral contraceptive use. This can occasionally cause confusion in the histologic diagnosis. Leiomyosarcomas tend to occur in patients in their 50s and occasionally in conjunction with leiomyomas, although leiomyosarcomas usually infiltrate diffusely into the myometrium.

The development of leiomyosarcoma from leiomyoma is rare. Leibsohn and co-workers noted that among 1423 patients who had hysterectomies for presumed leiomyomas with a uterine size comparable with a 12-week pregnancy or larger, the risk of sarcoma increased with age, being 0.4% for those in their 30s to 1.4% for those in their 50s.

Premenopausal patients have been reported to have a better prognosis than postmenopausal patients. Usually the patient has an enlarged pelvic mass, occasionally accompanied by pain or vaginal bleeding. Leiomyosarcomas are suspected if the uterus undergoes rapid enlargement, particularly in patients in the perimenopausal or postmenopausal age group. It is also occasionally possible to detect uterine sarcomas with ultrasound using a vaginal probe, because of the enhancement of the sarcoma image as a consequence of increased vascularity as illustrated in Figure 28-20, *A*. In addition, with a fibroid, there is acoustic shadowing as shown in Figure 28-20, *B*.

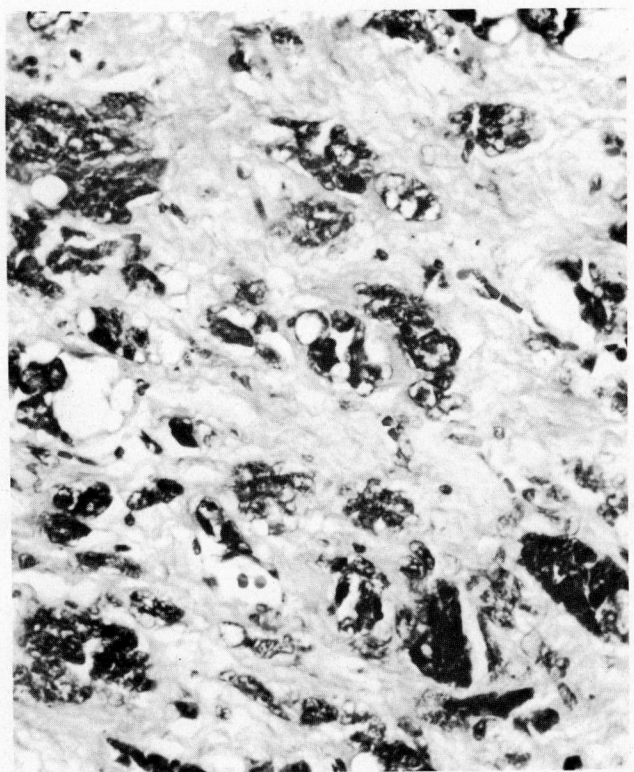

FIGURE 28-19
Leiomyoma with bizarre nuclei. No mitoses are present. (×256.) (From Clement
PB and Scully RE: Pathology of uterine sarcomas. In Coppleson M, editor: Gynecologic oncology, Edinburgh, 1981, Churchill-Livingstone. Reprinted by permission.)

Treatment consists of surgical removal of all
disease if possible. Mitotic rate is important in
determining prognosis. With increasing mitotic
rate the prognosis becomes worse. For patients
with well-documented leiomyosarcoma the
overall 5-year survival rate is about 20%; for
those with stage I and II tumors it is approximately 40%.

The most important aspect of treatment is
removal of the tumor, usually by total abdominal hysterectomy with bilateral salpingo-
oophorectomy (TAH-BSO). Irradiation therapy
has been used to treat residual pelvic disease
but is of unproved value. Salazar et al. noted
that irradiation therapy appeared to decrease
the risk of pelvic recurrence of tumor but did
not significantly improve survival rates. Radiation is usually not prescribed for these tumors.
Chemotherapy usually consists of Adriamycin-
containing combinations. Berchuck et al. reported responses of only 16% to chemotherapy
for these tumors.

In addition to local pelvic recurrences, distant metastases are frequent and most often occur in the lungs or intraabdominally. These are
preferably treated by multiple-agent chemotherapy. Occasionally a patient of reproductive
age has an unsuspected leiomyosarcoma diagnosed in a leiomyoma removed at myomectomy. Usually in such cases, hysterectomy is
subsequently performed, but a few cures have
been reported in individuals who have had no
further treatment beyond myomectomy; a complete, accurate histologic assessment is vital to
ascertain the risk. Pregnancy can increase the
mitotic rate in smooth muscle tumors, which
should be remembered when myomas are removed from pregnant or recently pregnant patients.

The clinician should be aware of variations of
smooth muscle tumors that are not leiomyosarcomas or benign leiomyomas. These tumors include leiomyoblastoma, intravenous leiomyomatosis, metastasizing uterine leiomyoma, and

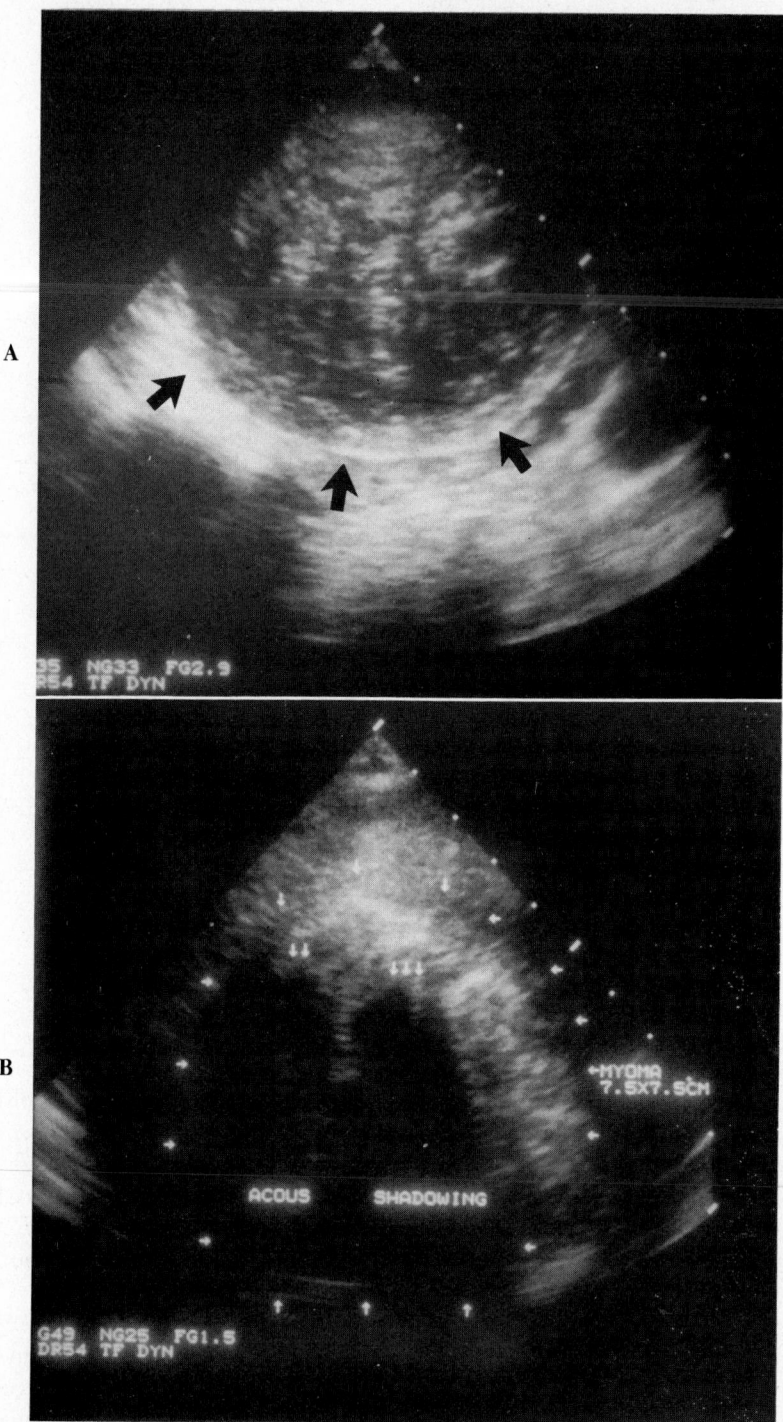

FIGURE 28-20

A, Transvaginal ultrasound image of uterine sarcoma; posterior wall enhancement *(arrows);* no acoustic shadowing. **B,** Transvaginal ultrasound depicting a myoma (fibroid) between the arrows. The arrows at the top point to acoustic shadowing, which is a typical characteristic of a fibroid. (Courtesy Dr. Zubie Sheikh, Department of Obstetrics & Gynecology, The University of Chicago.)

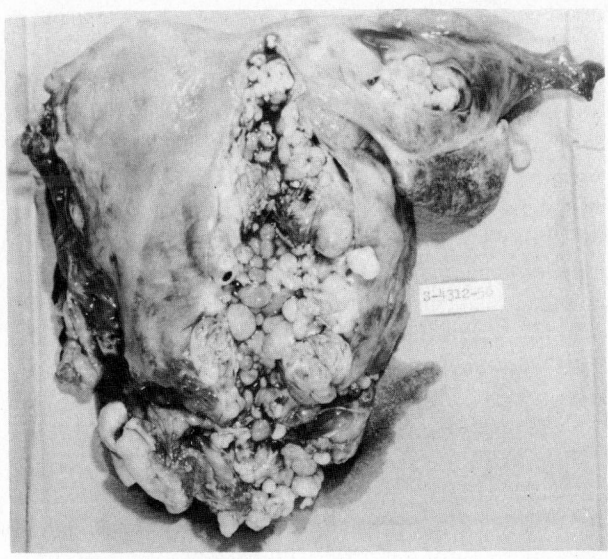

FIGURE 28-21
Intravenous leiomyomatosis replacing most of the uterus and extending into the broad ligaments and adjacent veins. (From Norris HJ and Zaloudek CJ: Mesenchymal tumors of the uterus. In Blaustein A, editor: Pathology of the female genital tract, ed 2, New York, 1982, Springer-Verlag.)

leiomyomatosis peritonealis disseminata. Leiomyoblastomas are rare smooth muscle tumors that grossly resemble leiomyomas. They contain epithelial-like cells with spindle-shaped cells characteristic of smooth muscle tumors. Usually the mitotic rate is less than 5/10 hpf, and these tumors should be regarded as low-grade sarcomas for which operative removal is the preferred therapy. Intravenous leiomyomatosis is also rare and is usually a condition characterized by intravenous extension of smooth muscle tissue outside the uterus (Figure 28-21). Wormlike projections of the tumor may be found in vascular spaces in the broad ligament or extending even into the vena cava. Occasionally smooth muscle nodules are found outside the pelvis either in lymph nodes or in the lungs, in which case the term *metastasizing leiomyoma* is used. Removal of the uterus and the extrauterine lesion, if possible, is the treatment of choice, although leaving some tissue in cases of intravenous leiomyomatosis does not appear to lead to spread of the disease. Very rarely, small nodes of leiomyoma are found in the peritoneal cavity (leiomyomatosis peritonealis disseminata). The condition is usually found during pregnancy and regresses after delivery. However, it can exist in the absence of pregnancy, in which case it may require operative removal.

Endometrial Stromal Sarcoma

Overall, stromal tumors comprise about 10% of uterine sarcomas. Their behavior correlates primarily with mitotic rate, and they usually are divided into low-grade and high-grade tumors.

LOW GRADE—ENDOLYMPHATIC STROMAL MYOSIS. Endolymphatic stromal myosis is the least frequent among the uterine sarcomas, leiomyosarcomas, and malignant mixed müllerian tumors. The tumor consists of cells that resemble those of the uterine stroma, with a spindlelike appearance somewhat resembling fibrous sarcoma. Endolymphatic stromal myosis is diagnosed if the mitotic rate in the tumor is less than 5/10 hpf. Occasionally these tumors have 10 mitoses/10 hpf. Despite the comparatively innocuous appearance and prolonged clinical course, these tumors can be fatal.

Piver et al. summarized a comparative study of 152 cases of endolymphatic stromal myosis. The patients with this tumor were 20 to 70 years of age, but almost three fourths were under age 50. Most had abnormal vaginal bleeding, and pelvic examination frequently revealed a large, irregularly shaped uterus. Occasionally the diagnosis is made on tissue obtained at diagnostic D&C. Press and Scully reported six cases associated with chronic estrogen stimulation and suggested that unopposed estrogen stimulation might increase the risk of these tumors.

The predominant mode of treatment is surgical and usually consists of total abdominal hysterectomy and bilateral salpingo-oophorectomy. Occasionally for tumors that spread to the cervix or paracervical areas a more radical procedure is performed, and a major effort is made to remove all gross disease. Long-term survivors are common, and 5-year survival of 100% was reported for the 15 patients originally described by Norris and Taylor; it was 88% in the collaborative series collected by Piver et al. for patients with tumors confined to the uterus.

Recurrence. Endolymphatic stromal myosis tends to recur locally in the pelvis or peritoneal cavity and frequently spreads to the lungs. In treating metastatic disease it should be remembered that these tumors contain estrogen and progestin steroid hormone receptors and are sensitive to progestational therapy. Megestrol acetate (Megace), medroxyprogesterone (Provera), and 17α-hydroxyprogesterone caproate (Delalutin) have been used. Complete resolution of the pulmonary lesions has been reported, and dosages of progestational drugs used are comparable to those for endometrial carcinoma. Nine patients reported by Thatcher and Woodruff were all living without evidence of disease 2 to 8 years after treatment, even though five had disease beyond the uterus at the time of initial operation. In view of the potential reappearance of disease, it is advisable to continue progestational therapy indefinitely after successful initial treatment of metastatic disease.

Irradiation has also been used to treat recurrences of these tumors, especially in the pelvis, with resolution of all residual tumor, but extensive experience with irradiation treatment is not available. Systemic chemotherapy with cytotoxic agents has not been reported generally to be effective, although complete response to doxorubicin (Adriamycin) has been reported.

HIGH GRADE—ENDOMETRIAL STROMAL SARCOMA. Endometrial stromal sarcomas are high-grade stromal tumors that behave aggressively and have a poor prognosis; microscopically more than 10 mitoses/10 hpf are present, and frequently 20 or more mitoses/10 hpf are present. Most series have reported 100% fatalities, although Vongtama et al. reported survival of over 60% for 24 patients with stage I and 1 patient with stage II disease. All cases of endolymphatic stromal myosis were eliminated, and treatment consisted of either operation alone or operation plus irradiation.

Patients with endometrial stromal sarcoma have abnormal bleeding or a pelvic mass. The tumor can occur at any age during reproductive life but tends to be primarily diagnosed in women under age 50 years. Operative removal of the tumor is the treatment of choice, but in view of the frequently poor survival rate, adjuvant therapy is occasionally considered. Unfortunately current data do not show a beneficial effect of adjuvant therapy in uterine sarcomas. A randomized trial using Adriamycin for stage I or II uterine sarcomas was reported for the Gynecologic Oncology Group (GOG) by Omura et al. and showed no benefit to the treated group.

Recurrence. Recurrences are common in the pelvis, lung, and abdomen. If there has not been prior irradiation and the recurrence is confined to the pelvis, usually pelvic irradiation is prescribed. If there is disseminated disease, multiple-agent chemotherapy is then used.

Malignant Mixed Müllerian Tumors

Malignant mixed müllerian tumors (MMMTs) are aggressive malignancies that comprised about 40% of uterine sarcomas. As shown in the box on p. 889, these tumors consist of carcinomatous and sarcomatous elements native to the uterus that may resemble the endometrial stroma of smooth muscle (homologous tumor or carcinosarcoma) or of sarcomatous tissues foreign to the uterus (heterologous). Spanos et al. reviewed 188 patients with mixed mesodermal tumor and found both the prognosis and the pattern of survival similar for both homologous and heterologous tumors. Unlike patients with endometrial stromal sarcoma or leiomyosarcoma, those with MMMT tend to be older and primarily postmenopausal, usually beyond the age of 62 years. Prior pelvic irradiation has been identified as a predisposing factor and was experienced by 17 of the 136 patients reviewed by Norris and Taylor. The heterologous and homologous tumors occur with approximately equivalent frequency. These tumors spread into the myometrium and then to the pelvis, to the abdomen including the peritoneum, and frequently to the lungs and pleura, a pattern similar to the spread of endometrial carcinoma.

A common symptom is postmenopausal bleeding, often accompanied by a large uterus.

Occasionally the diagnosis is made in tissue removed with D&C, and the tumor may appear to be a polypoid excrescence from the cervix; diagnosis may be made also by vaginal ultrasound examination.

As is true for other sarcomas, the primary treatment for MMMT is operative removal of the uterus. An additional problem is the older age of these patients. The extent of the tumor and the depth of myometrial invasion are important prognostic factors. Those with deep myometrial invasion are more likely to have spread of MMMT to pelvic or paraaortic nodes, as in endometrial carcinomas. Patients with tumors confined to the uterus and little or no myometrial spread have the best prognosis. TAH and BSO are completed with stage I tumors; more extensive procedures are occasionally attempted for stage II tumors, as well as for those with early extrauterine spread. Nielson et al. reported a 5-year survival of 58% for these tumors when the disease was confined to the uterus.

Because of the poor results with operation alone, supplemental treatment with irradiation or chemotherapy has been advocated. Perez et al. used preoperative intracavitary irradiation (5000 mg-hours) followed by TAH and BSO and then supplemented with full pelvic irradiation for stage I and stage II MMMT. The pelvic disease was eradicated, but distant metastases were common. Although irradiation may augment the beneficial effects of operation, particularly for the carcinomatous elements of MMMT, systemic dissemination of disease is common. Current evidence fails to support a survival advantage for those receiving pelvic irradiation, although the frequency of pelvic recurrence is thought to be reduced. Full control depends on the identification of an effective program of chemotherapy to control systemic disease, particularly because lung metastases are so common in uterine sarcomas.

Müllerian Adenosarcoma

Müllerian adenosarcoma is a rare low-grade malignancy composed of both a sarcomatous stroma (homologous) and a proliferation of benign glandular elements that are intimately associated. It occurs predominantly in women older than 60 years. Ten cases were described initially by Clement and Scully. TAH with BSO is the treatment of choice.

Lymphoma

On rare occasions the uterus can be the original site for lymphoma, or, more commonly, involvement of the uterus may be the initial presentation of disseminated lymphoma. About 40 cases of primary lymphoma of the uterus have been reported. They are usually treated by irradiation.

Chemotherapy

It is evident from available data that treatment beyond operative resection and irradiation therapy is needed to achieve control of uterine sarcomas. Once resection has been accomplished, cytotoxic chemotherapy is considered as an adjuvant to improve survival, particularly with high-grade tumors. Unfortunately, few data are available, and conflicting results have been reported. Marchese et al. studied 38 patients with sarcomas. Six with complete resection received adjuvant chemotherapy, primarily with vincristine, actinomycin D, and cyclophosphamide, and had a 5-year survival of 61%; survival was 15% for 23 patients with complete resections who did not receive chemotherapy. Confounding factors, such as tumor histologic findings and stage, were not controlled.

No single program has proved superior for the treatment of endometrial stromal sarcoma, leiomyosarcoma, or mixed müllerian malignant tumor, with the exception of progestin therapy to treat low-grade endometrial stromal sarcoma (endolymphatic stromal myosis). Thus chemotherapy programs for these sarcomas can be considered together.

Azizi et al. treated six cases of metastatic leiomyosarcoma with vincristine, 1.2 mg/m^2 weekly for 7 to 8 weeks; doxorubicin, 20 to 25 mg/m^2 intravenously for 3 days; and dacarbazine (DTIC), 250 mg/m^2 for 5 days every 3 weeks. Three complete responses lasting up to 2 years and one partial response were observed. Hannigan et al. used vincristine, actinomycin D, and cyclophosphamide (Cytoxan) (VAC protocol, Chapter 29) and noted a 13% complete response rate and 16% partial response rate in 74 patients with advanced metastatic uterine sarcomas. A large collaborative trial was recently conducted by the Gynecologic Oncology Group and reported by Omura et al. The best responses were obtained for patients with lung metastases who received doxorubicin and DTIC. Current evidence suggests that a multidrug program that includes doxorubicin (Adriamycin) offers the greatest potential for inducing remission of uterine sarcomas. Cisplatin also appears to have some effectiveness. Peters et al. reported response in 8 of 11 patients treated with cisplatin (100 mg/m^2) and Adriamycin (40 to 60 mg/m^2) every 3 weeks.

_____ KEY POINTS _____

- Endometrial carcinoma is the most common malignancy of the lower female genital tract. In the United States about 1 woman in 100 will develop the disease.

- More deaths occur from ovarian and cervical cancer than from endometrial cancer.

- Most women who develop endometrial cancer are between 50 and 65 years of age.

- The primary symptom of endometrial carcinoma is postmenopausal bleeding.

- Chronic unopposed estrogen stimulation of the endometrium leads to endometrial hyperplasia and in some cases adenocarcinoma. Other important predisposing factors include obesity, nulliparity, late menopause, and diabetes.

- The risk of a woman developing endometrial carcinoma is increased 3 times if she is 21 to 50 pounds overweight and 10 times if she is more than 50 pounds overweight. Nulliparous women have twice the risk of those with one child and 3 times the risk of those with five or more children. Menopause after 52 years of age increases the risk by 2.4 times in comparison with menopause before age 49 years. Diabetes raises the risk by a factor of 2.8. Tamoxifen therapy for patients with breast cancer also appears to increase the risk.

- Prognosis in endometrial carcinoma is related to tumor grade, tumor stage, and histologic type.

- Endometrial carcinoma can develop without preexisting endometrial hyperplasia, particularly in older patients and those with less well-differentiated tumors.

- Younger women with endometrial cancer have a better prognosis than older women.

- Most endometrial hyperplasias regress without treatment.

- Cytologic atypia in endometrial hyperplasia is the most important factor in determining premalignant potential.

- Older patients with atypical hyperplasia are at increased risk for malignant progression in comparison with younger patients.

- Adenocarcinoma of the endometrium is detected only in about 50% of the cases by routine cervical-vaginal cytologic study (Papanicolaou smear).

- Initially, endometrial carcinoma spreads outside the uterus, to the retroperitoneal, pelvic, and paraaortic lymph nodes, to the adnexa, and then to the peritoneal cavity.

- A key determinant of risk of nodal spread of endometrial carcinoma is depth of myometrial invasion.

- Well-differentiated (grade I) endometrial carcinomas usually contain measurable levels of steroid hormone receptors, whereas poorly differentiated (grade 3) tumors usually do not contain measurable levels of receptors.

- Receptor-positive endometrial carcinomas have a better prognosis than do those that are receptor negative.

- Ninety percent of recurrences of adenocarcinoma of the endometrium occur within 5 years.

- Overall survival rates for patients with adenocarcinoma of the endometrium by stage are as follows: stage I, 72%; stage II, 56%; stage III, 32%; stage IV, 11%.

- Histologic variants of endometrial carcinoma with a poor prognosis include adenosquamous carcinoma, serous carcinoma, and clear cell carcinoma.

- The most frequent sites of distant metastasis of adenocarcinoma of the endometrium are the lung, retroperitoneal nodes, and abdomen.

- Progestin therapy results in responses of 10% to 30% in recurrent endometrial carcinoma. The highest response rates are in tumors with elevated sex steroid receptor levels, well-differentiated tumors, and recurrences at sites not previously irradiated.

- Hormonal therapy (progestin-antiestrogen) combined with cytoxic chemotherapy appears to give better response rates for recurrent or metastatic endometrial carcinoma than chemotherapy alone.

- Uterine sarcomas comprise less than 5% of uterine malignancies.

- The optimal treatment of resectable endometrial carcinoma or uterine sarcoma is by operation that includes total abdominal hysterectomy and bilateral salpingo-oophorectomy. Supplemental irradiation or chemotherapy is prescribed depending on the extent of the disease and the histologic features of the tumor.

- Uterine sarcomas are treated primarily by removal of the uterus, tubes, and ovaries.

- Mitotic rate is an important prognostic factor in uterine leiomyosarcomas and is worse for those with more than 10 mitoses/10 hpf. Tumors with 5 to 9 mitoses/10 hpf have a low malignant potential.

- Endometrial stromal sarcomas are virulent sarcomas with 10 or more mitoses/10 hpf. For tumors with less than 10 mitoses/10 hpf, the prognosis is improved, and a diagnosis of endolymphatic stromal myosis or low-grade stromal sarcoma is made if there are less than 5 mitoses/10 hpf.

- Recurrences of uterine sarcomas are most frequent locally in the pelvis, the abdomen, and the lungs.

- Metastatic endolymphatic stromal myosis (low-grade stromal sarcoma) is treated with progestin therapy initially. More than half will resolve.

- Chemotherapeutic regimens that include doxorubicin (Adriamycin) and cisplatin are prescribed for metastatic sarcomas; complete responses are rare and usually temporary.

BIBLIOGRAPHY

Aalders JG, Abeler V, and Kolstad P: Clinical (stage III) as compared to subclinical intrapelvic extrauterine tumor spread in endometrial carcinoma: a clinical and histopathological study of 175 patients, Gynecol Oncol 17:64, 1984.

Aalders JG, Abeler V, and Kolstad P: Stage IV endometrial carcinoma: a clinical and histopathological study of 83 patients, Gynecol Oncol 17:75, 1984.

Aalders JG, Abelar V, and Kolstad P: Recurrent adenocarcinoma of the endometrium: a clinical and histopathological study of 379 patients, Gynecol Oncol 17:85, 1984.

Abeler VM and Kjorstad KE: Clear cell carcinoma of the endometrium: a histopathological and clinical study of 97 cases, Gynecol Oncol 40:207, 1991.

Ahmad K, Kim YH, Deppe G, et al: Radiation therapy in stage II carcinoma of the endometrium, Cancer 63:854, 1989.

Andersen ES: Stage II endometrial carcinoma: prognostic factors and the results of treatment, Gynecol Oncol 38: 220, 1990.

Andersen WA, Peters WA, Fechner RE, et al: Radioactive alternatives to standard management of adenocarcinoma of the endometrium, Gynecol Oncol 16:383, 1983.

Ayoub J, Audet-Lapointe P, Methot Y, et al: Efficacy of sequential cyclical hormone therapy in endometrial cancer and its correlation with steroid hormone receptor status, Gynecol Oncol 31:327, 1988.

Azizi F, Bitran J, Javehari G, et al: Remission of uterine leiomyosarcomas treated with vincristine, adriamycin and dimethyl-triazeno-imidazole-carboxamide, Am J Obstet Gynecol 133:379, 1979.

Barter JF, Smith EB, Szpak CA, et al: Leiomyosarcoma of the uterus: clinicopathologic study of 21 cases, Gynecol Oncol 21:220, 1985.

Berchuck A, Rodriguez G, Kinney RB, etal.: Overexpression of HER-2/*neu* in endometrial cancer is associated with advanced stage disease, AM J Obstet Gynecol 164: 15, 1991.

Berchuck A, Rubin SC, Hoskins WJ, et al: Treatment of uterine leiomyosarcoma, Obstet Gynecol 71:845, 1988.

Bibbo M, Kluskens L, Azizi F, et al: Accuracy of three sampling technics for the diagnosis of endometrial cancer and hyperplasias, J Reprod Med 27:622, 1982.

Bokhman JV: Two pathogenic types of endometrial carcinoma, Gynecol Oncol 15:10, 1983.

Bruckman JE, Bloomer WD, Marck A, et al: Stage III adenocarcinoma of the endometrium: two prognostic groups, Gynecol Oncol 9:12, 1980.

Carlson JA, Allegra JC, Day TG, et al: Tamoxifen and endometrial carcinoma: alterations in estrogen and progesterone receptors in untreated patients and combination hormonal therapy in advanced neoplasia, Am J Obstet Gynecol 149:149, 1984.

Chambers JT, MacLusky N, Eisenfield A, et al: Estrogen and progestin receptor levels as prognosticators for survival in endometrial cancer, Gynecol Oncol 31:65, 1988.

Chen SS and Lee L: Retroperitoneal lymph node metastases in stage I carcinoma of the endometrium: correlation with risk factors, Gynecol Oncol 16:319, 1983.

Christopherson WM, Alberhasky RC, and Connelly PJ: Carcinoma of the endometrium. I. A clinicopathologic study of clear cell adenocarcinoma and secretory carcinoma, Cancer 49:1511, 1982.

Christopherson WM, Connelly PJ, and Alberhasky RC: Carcinoma of the endometrium. V. An analysis of prognosticators in patients with favorable subtypes and stage I disease, Cancer 51:1705, 1983.

Christopherson WM and Gray LA: Premalignant lesions of the endometrium: endometrial hyperplasia and adenocarcinoma in situ. In Coppleson M, editor: Gynecologic oncology, Edinburgh, 1981, Churchill Livingstone.

Clement PB and Scully RE: Müllerian adenosarcoma of the uterus, Cancer 34:1138, 1974.

Clement PB and Scully RE: Pathology of uterine sarcomas. In Coppleson M, editor: Gynecologic oncology, Edinburgh, 1981, Churchill Livingstone.

Cohen CJ, Bruckner HW, Deppe G, et al: Multidrug treatment of advanced and recurrent endometrial carcinoma: a Gynecologic Oncology Group study, Obstet Gynecol 63:719, 1984.

Connelly PJ, Alberhasky RC, and Christopherson WM: Carcinoma of the endometrium. III. Analysis of 865 cases of adenocarcinoma and adenoacanthoma, Obstet Gynecol 59:569, 1982.

Cramer DW, Cutler SJ, and Christine B: Trends in the incidence of endometrial cancer in the United States, Gynecol Oncol 2:130, 1974.

Creasman WT: New gynecologic cancer staging, Obstet Gynecol 75:287, 1990.

Creasman WT: Estrogen replacement therapy: Is previously treated cancer a contraindication? Obstet Gynecol 77:308, 1991.

Creasman WT, Morrow CP, Bundy BN, et al: Surgical pathologic spread patterns of endometrial cancer, Cancer 60:2035, 1987.

Creasman WT, Henderson D, Hinshaw W, et al: Estrogen replacement therapy in the patient treated for endometrial cancer, Obstet Gynecol 67: 326, 1986.

Doering DL, Barnhill DR, Weiser EB, et al: Intraoperative evaluation of depth of superficial invasion in stage I endometrial carcinoma, Obstet Gynecol 74:930, 1989.

DuBeshter B, Warshal DP, Angel C, et al: Endometrial carcinoma: the relevance of cervical cytology, Obstet Gynecol 77: 458, 1991.

Eifel PJ, Ross J, Hendrickson M, et al: Adenocarcinoma of the endometrium: analysis of 256 cases with disease limited to the uterine corpus: treatment comparison, Cancer 52:1026, 1983.

Ferenczy A and Gelfand M: The biologic significance of cytologic atypia in progestin-treated endometrial hyperplasia, Am J Obstet Gynecol 160:126, 1989.

Feuer GA and Calanog A: Endometrial carcinoma: treatment of positive paraaortic nodes, Gynecol Oncol 27:104, 1987.

Fornander T, Cedermark B, Mattsson A, et al: Adjuvant tamoxifen in early breast cancer: occurrence of new primary cancers, Lancet 1(8630): 117, 1989.

Gal D, Edman CD, Vellios F, et al: Long-term effect of megestrol acetate in the treatment of endometrial hyperplasia, Am J Obstet Gynecol 146:316, 1983.

Gallion HH, van Nagell JR, Powell DF, et al: Stage I serous papillary carcinoma of the endometrium, Cancer 63:2224, 1989.

Goff BA and Rice LW: Assessment of depth of myometrial invasion in endometrial adenocarcinoma, Gynecol Oncol 38: 46, 1990.

Granberg S, Wikland M, Karlsson B, et al: Endometrial thickness as measured by endovaginal ultrasonography for identifying endometrial abnormality, Am J Obstet Gynecol 164: 47, 1991.

Greer BE and Hamburger AD: Treatment of intraperitoneal metastatic adenocarcinoma of the endometrium by the whole-abdomen moving-strip technique and pelvic boost irradiation, Gynecol Oncol 16:365, 1983.

Greven KM, Curran WJ, Whittington R, et al: Analysis of failure patterns in stage III endometrial carcinoma and therapeutic implications, Int J Radiat Oncol Biol Phys 17:35, 1989.

Grimshaw RN, Tupper WC, Fraser RC, et al: Prognostic value of peritoneal cytology in endometrial carcinoma, Gynecol Oncol 36:97, 1990.

Gusberg SB and Kaplan AL: Precursors of corpus cancer. IV. Adenomatous hyperplasia as stage 0 carcinoma of the endometrium, Am J Obstet Gynecol 87:662, 1963.

Hannigan EV, Freedman RS, Elder KW, et al: Treatment of advanced uterine sarcoma with vincristine, actinomycin D, and cyclophosphamide, Gynecol Oncol 15:224, 1983.

Heath R, Rosenman J, Varia M, et al: Peritoneal fluid cytology in endometrial cancer: its significance and the role of chromic phosphate (P^{32}) therapy, Int J Radiat Oncol Biol Phys 15:815, 1988.

Hendrickson M, Ross J, Eifel P, et al: Uterine papillary serous carcinoma: a highly malignant form of endometrial adenocarcinoma, Am J Surg Pathol 6:93, 1982.

Hoffman MS, Roberts WS, Cavanagh D, et al: Treatment of recurrent and metastatic endometrial cancer and cisplatin, doxorubicin, cyclophosphamide, and megestrol acetate, Gynecol Oncol 35:75, 1989.

Homesley HD, Boronow RC, and Lewis JL: Stage II endometrial adenocarcinoma, Obstet Gynecol 49:604, 1977.

Kauppila A, Jänne O, Kujansuu E, and Vihko R: Treatment of advanced endometrial adenocarcinoma with a combined cytotoxic therapy: predictive value of cytosol estrogen and progestin receptor levels, Cancer 46:2162, 1980.

Kleine W, Maier T, Geyer H, et al: Estrogen and progesterone receptors in endometrial cancer and their prognostic relevance, Gynecol Oncol 38: 59, 1990.

Kohorn EI: Gestagens and endometrial carcinoma, Gynecol Oncol 4:398, 1976.

Koss LG, Schreiber K, Oberlander SG, et al: Detection of endometrial carcinoma and hyperplasia in asymptomatic women, Obstet Gynecol 64:1, 1984.

Kucera H, Vavra N, and Weghaupt K: Benefit of external irradiation in pathologic stage I endometrial carcinoma: a prospective clinical trial of 605 patients who received postoperative vaginal irradiation and additional pelvic irradiation in the presence of unfavorable prognostic factors, Gynecol Oncol 38: 99, 1990.

Kurman RJ, Kaminski PF, and Norris HJ: Behavior of endometrial hyperplasia: a long-term study of "untreated" hyperplasias in 170 patients, Cancer 56:403, 1985.

Kurman RJ and Norris HJ: Endometrial neoplasia: hyperplasia and carcinoma. In Blaustein A, editor: Pathology of the female genital tract, ed 3, New York, 1987, Springer-Verlag.

Kurman RJ and Norris HJ: Evaluation of criteria for distinguishing atypical endometrial hyperplasia from well-differentiated carcinoma, Cancer 49:2547, 1982.

Kurman RJ and Scully RE: Clear cell carcinoma of the endometrium, Cancer 37:872, 1976.

Lee RB, Burke TW, and Park RC: Estrogen replacement therapy following treatment for stage I endometrial carcinoma, Gynecol Oncol 36:189, 1990.

Leibsohn S, Mishell DR, d'Ablaing G, and Schlaerth JB: Leiomyosarcomas in a series of hysterectomies performed for presumed uterine leiomyomata, Am J Obstet Gynecol 162: 968, 1990.

MacMahon B: Risk factors for endometrial cancer, Gynecol Oncol 2:122, 1974.

Malfetano JH: Tamoxifen-associated endometrial carcinoma in postmenopausal breast cancer patients, Gynecol Oncol 39: 82, 1990.

Marchese MJ, Liskow AS, Crum CP, et al: Uterine sarcomas: a clinicopathologic study, 1965-1981, Gynecol Oncol 18:299, 1984.

Meerwaldt JH, Hoekstra CJM, van Putten WLJ, et al: Endometrial adenocarcinoma, adjuvant radiotherapy tailored to prognostic factors, Int J Radiat Oncol Biol Phys 18:299, 1990.

Melhem MF and Tobon H: Mucinous adenocarcinoma of the endometrium: a clinico-pathological review of 18 cases, Int J Gynecol Pathol 6:347, 1987.

Melin JR, Wanner L, Schulz DM, et al: Primary squamous cell carcinoma of the endometrium, Obstet Gynecol 53:115, 1979.

Mishell DR: Contraception, N Engl J Med 320:777, 1989.

Moore DH, Fowler WC, Walton LA, and Droegemueller W: Morbidity of lymph node sampling in cancers of the uterine corpus and cervix, Obstet Gynecol 74:180, 1989.

Morrow CP, Bundy BN, Kurman RJ, et al: Relationship between surgical-pathological risk factors and outcome in clinical stage I and II carcinoma of the endometrium: a Gynecologic Oncology Group study, Gynecol Oncol 40: 55, 1991.

Neven P, De Muylder X, van Belle Y, et al: Tamoxifen and the uterus and endometrium (Letters to the Editor) Lancet, Feb 19, 1989.

Nielsen SN, Podratz KC, Scheithauer BW, and O'Brien PC: Clinicopathologic analysis of uterine malignant mixed müllerian tumors, Gynecol Oncol 34:372, 1989.

Norris HJ and Parmley T: Mesenchymal tumors of the uterus. V. Intravenous leiomyomatosis: a clinical and pathologic study of 14 cases, Cancer 36:2164, 1975.

Norris HJ and Taylor HB: Postirradiation sarcomas of the uterus, Obstet Gynecol 26:689, 1965.

Norris HJ and Taylor HB: Mesenchymal tumors of the uterus. I. A clinical and pathologic study of 53 endometrial stromal tumors, Cancer 19:755, 1966.

Omura GA, Major FJ, Blessing JA, et al: A randomized study of Adriamycin with and without dimethyl-triazeno-imidazole-carboxamide in advanced uterine sarcomas, Cancer 52:626, 1983.

Omura GA, Blessing JA, Major FJ, et al: A randomized clinical trial of adjuvant Adriamycin in uterine sarcomas: a gynecologic oncology group study, J Clin Oncol 3:1240, 1985.

Onsrud M, Aalders J, Abeler V, et al: Endometrial carcinoma with cervical involvement (stage II): prognostic factors and value of combined radiological-surgical treatment, Gynecol Oncol 13:76, 1982.

Onsrud M, Kolstad P, and Normann T: Postoperative external pelvic irradiation in carcinoma of the corpus, stage I: a controlled clinical trial, Gynecol Oncol 4:222, 1976.

Osmers R, Völksen M, and Schauer A: Vaginosonography for early detection of endometrial carcinoma? Lancet 335: 1569, 1990.

Palmer DC, Muir IM, Alexander AI, et al: The prognostic importance of steroid receptors in endometrial carcinoma, Obstet Gynecol 72:388, 1988.

Parazzini F, LaVecchia C, Bocciolone L, et al: Review. The epidemiology of endometrial cancer, Gynecol Oncol 41:1, 1991.

Patanaphan V, Salazar OM, and Chougule P: What can be expected when radiation therapy becomes the curative alternative for endometrial cancer? Cancer 55:1462, 1985.

Patsner B, Mann WJ, Cohen H, and Loesch M: Predictive value of preoperative serum CA-125 levels in clinically localized and advanced endometrial carcinoma, Am J Obstet Gynecol 158:399, 1988.

Peters WA, Rivkin SE, Smith MR, and Tesh DE: Cisplatin and Adriamycin combination chemotherapy for uterine stromal sarcomas and mixed mesodermal tumors, Gynecol Oncol 34:323, 1989.

Pettersson F, Coppleson M, Creasman WT, et al: Annual report on the results of treatment in gynecologic cancer, vol 20, Stockholm, 1988, International Federation of Gynecology and Obstetrics.

Piver MS and Lurain JR: Uterine sarcomas: clinical features and management. In Coppelson M, editor: Gynecologic oncology, Edinburgh, 1981, Churchill Livingstone, p. 608.

Piver MS, Rutledge FN, Copeland L, et al: Uterine endolymphatic stromal myosis: a collaborative study, Obstet Gynecol 64:173, 1984.

Plentl AA and Friedman EA: Lymphatic system of the female genitalia, Philadelphia, 1971, WB Saunders Co.

Pliskow S, Penalver M, and Averette H: Stage III and stage IV endometrial carcinoma: a review of 41 cases, Gynecol Oncol 38: 210, 1990.

Podczaski ES, Kaminski P, Manetta A, et al: Stage II endometrial carcinoma treated with external-beam radiotherapy, intracavitary application of cesium, and surgery, Gynecol Oncol 35:251, 1989.

Potish RA, Twiggs LB, Adcock LL, et al: Paraaortic lymph node radiotherapy in cancer of the uterine corpus, Obstet Gynecol 65:251, 1985.

Press MF and Scully RE: Endometrial "sarcomas" complicating ovarian thecoma, polycystic ovarian disease and estrogen therapy, Gynecol Oncol 21:135, 1985.

Procope BJ: Aetiology of postmenopausal bleeding, Obstet Gynaecol Scand 50:311, 1971.

Schink JC, Rademaker AW, Miller DS, et al: Tumor size in endometrial cancer, Cancer 67:2791, 1991.

Silverberg E et al: Cancer statistics, 1990 in Ca-A Cancer Journal for Clinicians, Vol 40, No 1, January/February 1990.

Sorbe G and Smeds A-C: Postoperative vaginal irradiation with high dose rate afterloading technique in endometrial carcinoma stage I, Int J Radiat Oncol Biol Phys 18:305, 1990.

Spanos WJ, Wharton JT, Gomez L, et al: Malignant mixed müllerian tumors of the uterus, Cancer 53:311, 1984.

Stryker JA, Podczaski E, Kaminski P, et al: Adjuvant external beam therapy for pathologic stage I and occult stage II endometrial carcinoma, Cancer 67:2872, 1991.

Surwit EA, Fowler WC, and Rogoff EE: Stage II carcinoma of the endometrium, Obstet Gynecol 52:97, 1978.

Surwit EA, Joelsson I, and Einhorn N: Adjunctive radiation therapy in the management of stage I cancer of the endometrium, Obstet Gynecol 58:590, 1981.

Swenerton KD, Chrumka K, Patterson AHG, et al: Efficacy of tamoxifen in endometrial cancer, Progr Cancer Res Ther 31:417, 1984.

Thatcher SS and Woodruff JD: Uterine stromatosis: a report of 33 cases, Obstet Gynecol 59:428, 1982.

Tiltman AJ: Mucinous carcinoma of the endometrium, Obstet Gynecol 55:244, 1980.

Tosi P, Sforza V, and Santopietro R: Estrogen receptor content, immunohistochemically determined by monoclonal antibodies, in endometrial stromal sarcoma, Obstet Gynecol 73:75, 1989.

Trimble EL and Jones HW: Management of stage II endometrial adenocarcinoma, Obstet Gynecol 71:323, 1988.

Tseng PC, Sprance HE, Carcangiu ML, et al: CA-125, NB/70K, and lipid-associated sialic acid in monitoring uterine papillary serous carcinoma, Obstet Gynecol 74:384, 1989.

Tsukamoto N, Kamura T, Matsukuma K, et al: Endolymphatic stromal myosis: a case with positive estrogen and progesterone receptors and good response to progestins, Gynecol Oncol 20:120, 1985.

Turbow MM, Ballon SC, Sikic BI, et al: Cisplatin, doxorubicin and cyclophosphamide chemotherapy for advanced endometrial carcinoma, Cancer Treat Rep 69:465, 1985.

Turner DA, Gershenson DM, Atkinson N, et al: The prognostic significance of peritoneal cytology for stage I endometrial cancer, Obstet Gynecol 74:775, 1989.

Vellios F: Endometrial hyperplasia, precursors of endometrial cancer. In Sommers SC, editor: Pathology annual, East Norwalk, Conn, 1972, Appleton-Century-Crofts, p 201.

Vergote I, Kjorstad K, Abeler V, et al: A randomized trial of adjuvant progestagen in early endometrial cancer, Cancer 64:1011, 1989.

Vihko R, Isotalo H, Kauppila A, et al: Endocrine indicators of endometrial and ovarian tumor aggressiveness. In Bresciani F, et al, editor: Progr Cancer Res Ther 31:377, 1984.

Vongtama V, Karlen JR, Piver MS, et al: Treatment results and prognostic factors in stage I and II sarcomas of the corpus uteri, Am J Roentgenol Rad Ther Nucl Med 126:139, 1976.

Wallin TE, Malkasian GD, Gaffey TA, et al: Stage II cancer of the endometrium: a pathologic and clinical study, Gynecol Oncol 18:1, 1984.

Welch WR and Scully RE: Precancerous lesions of the endometrium, Hum Pathol 8:503, 1977.

Wilson TO, Podratz KC, Gaffey TA, et al: Evaluation of unfavorable histologic subtypes in endometrial adenocarcinoma, Am J Obstet Gynecol 162:418, 1990.

Wheeless CR: Atlas of pelvic surgery. Philadelphia, 1981, Lea & Febiger.

Wheelock JB, Krebs HB, Schneider V, et al: Uterine sarcoma: an analysis of prognostic variables in 71 cases, Am J Obstet Gynecol 151:1016, 1985.

White AJ, Buchsbaum HJ, and Macasaet MA: Primary squamous cell carcinoma of the endometrium, Obstet Gynecol 41:912, 1973.

Yoonessi M and Hart WR: Endometrial stromal sarcomas, Cancer 40:898, 1977.

Neoplastic Diseases of the Ovary

KEY TERMS AND DEFINITIONS

Adenoma. A benign ovarian epithelial tumor consisting of glandular (adenomatous) elements.

Adenofibroma. An epithelial tumor that consists of glandular elements and large amounts of ovarian stromal (fibroblast) elements.

Alpha-fetoprotein. A secretory product from endodermal sinus tumors that can be measured in serum and serves as a specific tumor marker.

Borderline Tumors. A term used to describe an epithelial carcinoma of low malignant potential (grade 0). The malignant cells do not invade the stroma.

Brenner Tumor. An epithelial neoplasm that consists of cells resembling urothelium and so-called Walthard nests of the ovary. These are mixed with ovarian stroma.

Carcinoid. A rare type of teratoma that histologically resembles the carcinoid tumors that arise in the gastrointestinal tract.

Clear Cell Tumor (Mesonephroma). An ovarian neoplasm that consists of clear cells (containing glycogen) or "hobnail" cells. Histologically they resemble clear cell tumors that arise in the endocervix, endometrium, and vagina.

Cyst. A descriptive term added as a prefix to the designation of epithelial tumors to indicate the presence of cystlike spaces, for example, cystadenoma.

Cytoreductive Surgery. The practice of reducing the bulk of carcinomatous tissue and removing, if possible, all gross disease.

Dermoid. A benign cystic germ cell tumor (cystic teratoma) that may contain elements of all three germ cell layers. It is the most common ovarian neoplasm in those under 30 years of age.

Dysgerminoma. The most common of ovarian malignant germ cell tumors. It consists of primitive germ cells.

Endodermal Sinus Tumor. A malignant germ cell tumor. It is derived from germ cells and recapitulates extraembryonic tissue and may resemble the yolk sac of the rodent placenta.

Endometrioid Tumor. An ovarian epithelial tumor whose cells resemble those of the uterine endometrium.

Epithelial Stromal Tumors. The most common type of ovarian neoplasms. It is derived from the surface (coelomic) epithelium and ovarian stroma. Have previously been termed *common epithelial tumors.*

Fibroma. The most common benign ovarian solid tumor composed of stromal cells (fibroblasts). In some cases it is associated with benign ascites and hydrothorax (Meigs' syndrome).

Germ Cell Tumor. The second most common type of ovarian neoplasm after epithelial tumors. Germ cell tumors contain cells that recapitulate embryonic tissues (ectoderm, mesoderm, or endoderm) or extraembryonic elements.

Gonadoblastoma. A rare tumor that arises in abnormal (dysgenetic) gonads and consists of sex-cord stromal elements and germ cells.

Granulosa-Thecal Cell Tumor. A sex-cord stromal tumor that often secretes estrogens and consists of granulosa cells (sex cord) and ovarian stromal cells (thecal cells or fibroblasts).

Immature Teratoma. A teratoma with malignant (immature) embryonic elements (ectoderm, mesoderm, or endoderm).

Krukenberg Tumor. A tumor metastatic to the ovary consisting of signet-ring cells that usually originate from the gastrointestinal tract, most frequently the stomach, and then from the large intestine.

Mucinous Tumor. An ovarian epithelial tumor whose cells contain mucin and resemble those of the endocervix.

Ovarian Neoplasm. An ovarian tumor that is not physiologic and will not regress with time. It may be benign or malignant.

Papillary. A descriptive term added to the designation of epithelial tumors if papillary-like projections are present, for example, papillary cystadenocarcinoma.

Papillary Serous Carcinoma of the Peritoneum. A variant of widespread peritoneal carcinomatosis with a papillary serous appearance and small (<4 cm) ovaries, also termed *serous surface papillary carcinoma of the ovary.*

Pseudomyxoma Peritonei. Intraperitoneal spread of mucin-secreting cells that originate from ovarian mucinous cystadenoma or cystadenocarcinoma or mucoceles of the appendix that lead to recurrent abdominal masses and bowel obstruction.

Second-Look Operation. A laparotomy with extensive biopsy sampling and cytologic sampling of the peritoneal cavity, as well as evaluation of the retroperitoneal nodes. It is usually performed after chemotherapy in a patient who is clinically in remission.

Serous Tumor. An ovarian epithelial tumor whose cells resemble those of the fallopian tube.

Sertoli-Leydig Cell Tumor. A rare sex-cord stromal tumor with male elements. It often causes virilization.

Sex-Cord Stromal Tumors. A class of ovarian tumors in which the constituents of the ovary or testes are recapitulated.

Small Cell Carcinoma. A highly virulent, usually fatal ovarian malignancy occurring in young women, frequently accompanied by hypercalcemia.

Stages of Ovarian Cancer:
   Stage I: Confined to one or both ovaries.
   Stage II: Extension to pelvic structures.
   Stage III: Extension outside of pelvis or to retroperitoneal or inguinal nodes.
   Stage IV: Extension outside of peritoneal cavity or to liver parenchyma—pleural effusion with malignant cells.

Struma Ovarii. A specialized ovarian teratoma that consists of thyroid tissue as a major or exclusive component. It may rarely produce sufficient thyroid hormone to induce hyperthyroidism.

Teratoma. An ovarian germ cell tumor that recapitulates any one or all of tissues of the ectoderm, mesoderm, or endoderm. The tissues can be benign (mature) or malignant (immature).

Thecoma. A benign ovarian stromal tumor consisting of thecal cells.

Ovarian cancer is the second most common malignancy of the lower part of the female genital tract, occurring less frequently than cancers of the endometrium but more frequently than cancers of the cervix. However, it is the most frequent cause of death from gynecologic neoplasms. The 1990 data of the National Cancer Institute SEER Program suggest that approximately 20,500 new cases of ovarian cancer will be diagnosed yearly in the United States, and there will be 12,500 deaths. A major contributing factor to the high death rate from relatively few cases is the late detection of the disease because of the intraabdominal location of the ovary and the fact that these cancers often do not cause symptoms until the malignancy is widespread. The incidence of ovarian cancer (Figure 29-1) rises with age, becoming most

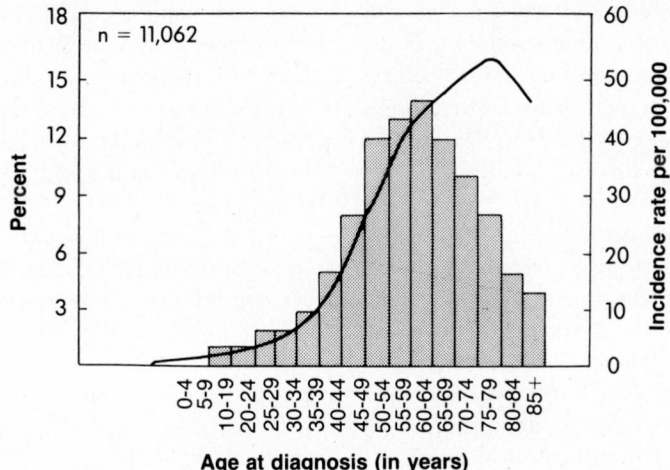

FIGURE 29-1
Ovarian cancer incidence rates by age, 1973 to 1982. (From Yancik R, Ries LG, and
Yates JW: Am J Obstet Gynecol 154:639, 1986.)

marked beyond 50 years, with a gradual increase continuing to age 70 years followed by a
decrease for those over age 80. Moreover, Yancik et al. noted that those over 65 were more
likely to have their cancers diagnosed at an advanced stage, leading to a worse prognosis and
poorer survival compared to those under age
65 years.

Despite numerous epidemiologic investigations, a clear-cut cause of ovarian cancer has
not been defined. A number of theories have
been advanced. It is thought that these malignancies are related to frequent ovulation, and
therefore women who ovulate regularly appear
to be at higher risk. Included are those with a
late menopause, a history of nulliparity, or late
childbearing. Conversely, women who have
had several pregnancies or who have used oral
contraceptives appear to have some protection
against ovarian cancer. Casagrande et al. related the development of ovarian cancer to
"ovulatory age," that is, the number of years
during which the patient has ovulated. This
number would be reduced by pregnancy,
breast-feeding, or oral contraceptive use. In
addition, talcum powder used on the perineum
has been postulated to increase the risk, presumably by migration of the irritant powder
through the vagina, cervix, and fallopian tubes
to the peritoneal surface of the ovary. Subclinical mumps infection before menarche has
been suggested as potentially increasing the
risk of ovarian cancer. Cramer et al. found

women with ovarian cancer to have a diet high
in animal fat in comparison with control subjects.

In a recent case control study Hartge et al.
showed a familial history of breast cancer and a
personal history of breast cancer were risk factors. Data from Piver et al. indicate familial
ovarian cancers are lethal, with 92% of the patients dead. Half of the 148 families had 3 or
more affected members, while in some cases it
was a sister/sister or mother/daughter. Bian-
nual screening with vaginal ultrasound and the
tumor marker CA-125 (see later discussion)
have been advocated for screening these high-
risk patients. Unfortunately, carcinomatosis
throughout the abdomen has developed in
some of these individuals despite prophylactic
removal of the ovaries, and present evidence
does not warrant routine prophylactic
oophorectomy in those whose mothers developed ovarian cancer although vaginal ultrasound
does appear to be a promising diagnostic tool for
screening patients who are at increased risk or
are difficult to examine. Although women with
one or even two first degree relatives with ovarian carcinoma are probably at some increased
risk for ovarian cancer development, there are
no adequate population-based studies to provide data on the specific magnitude of the risk.
Current data suggest daughters whose mothers
had ovarian cancer have a small increased risk,
and they should be monitored, if possible, with
vaginal ultrasound after age 35.

There are geographic and racial differences in the distribution of ovarian cancers. These cancers occur most frequently in industrialized and affluent countries such as the United States and Western Europe, and less frequently in Asia and Africa. The disease is more frequent among white than black women. Finally, patients with ovarian carcinoma have an increased risk of developing breast and endometrial cancer. The major factors, however, appear to be related to the frequency of ovulation and residence in an industrialized country.

The following describes the classification and histology of the major ovarian neoplasms. Pertinent microscopic findings, clinical behavior, and appropriate therapy are presented.

CLASSIFICATION OF OVARIAN NEOPLASMS

The most widely used classification of ovarian neoplasms is that of the World Health Organization. This classification, along with frequency of occurrence of the primary ovarian neoplasms, is shown in Table 29-1.

The epithelial stromal (common epithelial) tumors are the most frequent ovarian neoplasms. They are believed to arise from the surface (coelomic) epithelium. Germ cell tumors are the second most frequent of the ovarian neoplasms and are the most common among young women. There are a large variety of histologic types. They may be composed of

extraembryonic elements or may have features that resemble any or all of the three embryonic layers (ectoderm, mesoderm, or endoderm). These tumors are the main cause of ovarian malignancy in young women, particularly those in their teens and early 20s. Sex-cord stromal tumors are the third most frequent and contain elements that recapitulate the constituents of the ovary or testis. These tumors may secrete sex steroid hormones or may be hormonally inactive. Lipid (lipoid) cell tumors are extremely rare and histologically resemble the adrenal gland. Gonadoblastomas consist of germ cells and sex-cord stromal elements. They occur in individuals with dysgenetic gonads, particularly when a Y chromosome is present. All these ovarian neoplasms are discussed in this chapter.

Soft tissue tumors not specific to the ovary, such as hemangioma or lipoma, are rare and are categorized according to the criteria for soft tissue tumors arising elsewhere in the body. Unclassified tumors, as the name implies, cannot be placed in any of the preceding categories. One example is small cell carcinoma, which is a highly virulent cancer affecting primarily young women. Metastatic tumors to the ovary arise elsewhere in the reproductive tract, as well as in distant sites. Tumorlike conditions refer to enlargements of the ovary, such as extensive edema, pregnancy luteoma, endometriomas, and follicular or luteal cysts, none of which are true neoplasms. With the exceptions of metastatic tumors and small cell carcinoma of the ovary, none of these latter conditions are considered further in this chapter.

EPITHELIAL STROMAL OVARIAN NEOPLASMS

According to Scully, two thirds of ovarian neoplasms are epithelial tumors; malignant epithelial tumors account for about 85% of ovarian cancers. As stated earlier, it is believed that these tumors arise from the surface (coelomic) epithelium and adjacent ovarian stroma. Table 29-2 summarizes the five cell types that most commonly comprise epithelial ovarian tumors, indicating their relative frequency.

Epithelial tumors can be categorized as benign (adenoma), malignant (adenocarcinoma), or of an intermediate form, known as *borderline malignant adenocarcinoma* or *tumor of low malignant potential.* The term *papillary* or the

TABLE 29-1
Frequency of Ovarian Neoplasms (WHO Classification)

Class	Approximate Frequency (%)
Epithelial stromal (common epithelial) tumors	65
Germ cell tumors	20-25
Sex-cord stromal tumors	6
Lipid (lipoid) cell tumors	<0.1
Gonadoblastoma	<0.1
Soft tissue tumors (not specific to ovary)	
Unclassified tumors	
Secondary (metastatic) tumors	
Tumorlike conditions (not true neoplasm)	

TABLE 29-2
Epithelial Ovarian Tumor Cell Types

	Approximate Frequency (%)	
	All Ovarian Neoplasms	Ovarian Cancers
Serous	20-50	35-40
Mucinous	15-25	6-10
Endometrioid	5	15-25
Clear cell (mesonephroid)	<5	5
Brenner	2-3	Rare

Modified from Scully RE: Tumors of the ovary and maldeveloped gonads. In Atlas of tumor pathology, fascicle 16, series 2, Washington, DC, 1979, Armed Forces Institute of Pathology.

prefix *cyst* (as in cystadenoma) is used when the tumor has, respectively, papillae or cystic structures. The suffix *fibroma* (as in adenofibroma) is added when the ovarian stroma predominates, with the exception of a Brenner tumor, which normally contains a large amount of ovarian stroma.

Well-differentiated serous tumors (Figure 29-2, *A* and *B*) consist of ciliated epithelial cells that resemble those of the fallopian tube. Serous tumors (Figure 29-2, *C*) are the most frequent ovarian epithelial tumors. The malignant forms account for up to 40% of ovarian cancers; the benign forms (serous cystadenomas) occur primarily during the reproductive years; the borderline tumors occur in women 30 to 50 years of age; the carcinomas occur in women over 40 years of age.

Mucinous tumors (Figure 29-3, *A* and *B*) consist of epithelial cells filled with mucin; most are benign. These cells resemble cells of the endocervix or may mimic intestinal cells, which can pose a problem in the differential diagnosis of tumors that appear to originate from the ovary or intestine. Benign mucinous tumors are found primarily during the reproductive years, and mucinous carcinomas (Figure 29-3, *C*) usually occur among those in the 30- to 60-year age range. Overall they can account for about one fourth of ovarian tumors and up to 10% of ovarian cancers.

Endometrioid tumors (Figure 29-4), as the name implies, consist of epithelial cells resembling those of the endometrium. In the ovary these neoplasms are less frequent (approximately 5%) than either the serous or mucinous tumors, but the malignant variety can account for about 20% of ovarian carcinomas. Endometrioid carcinomas usually occur in women in their 40s and 50s. They may be seen in conjunction with endometriosis and ovarian endometriomas, although an origin from endometriosis is rarely demonstrated. Most endometrioid carcinomas arise directly from the surface epithelium of the ovary, as do the other epithelial tumors.

Clear cell (mesonephroid) tumors contain cells with abundant glycogen (Figure 29-5, *A*) and so-called *hobnail* cells (Figure 29-5, *B*), in which the nuclei of the cells protrude into the glandular lumen. Tumors with identical histologic features are found in the endometrium, cervix, and vagina, the latter two often associated with intrauterine diethylstilbestrol (DES) exposure. Clear cell ovarian tumors are not related to DES exposure and comprise about 5% of ovarian cancers. They occur primarily in women 40 to 70 years of age.

The major cell types of ovarian epithelial tumors recapitulate the müllerian-derived epithelium of the female reproductive system (serous—endosalpinx; mucinous—endocervix; endometrioid—endometrium). This differentiation occurs even though the ovary is not derived directly from the müllerian ducts (Chapter 2). The clear cell tumors also mimic this müllerian tendency, frequently being admixed with endometrioid carcinomas, as well as with ovarian endometriomas.

Brenner tumors (Figure 29-6) consist of cells that resemble the transitional epithelium of the bladder and Walthard nests of the ovary. There is abundant stroma. These tumors constitute only 2% to 3% of all ovarian tumors.

In addition to the cell types shown in Table 29-2, epithelial tumors may be classified as undifferentiated if the tumor consists of poorly differentiated epithelial cells not characteristic of any particular cell type. They may be considered unclassifiable if they cannot be placed in any of the categories shown in Table 29-2.

Many epithelial ovarian tumors can be bilateral, and the risk of bilaterality is an important consideration in therapy, particularly when an ovarian tumor is discovered in a young woman of reproductive age. Widely varying

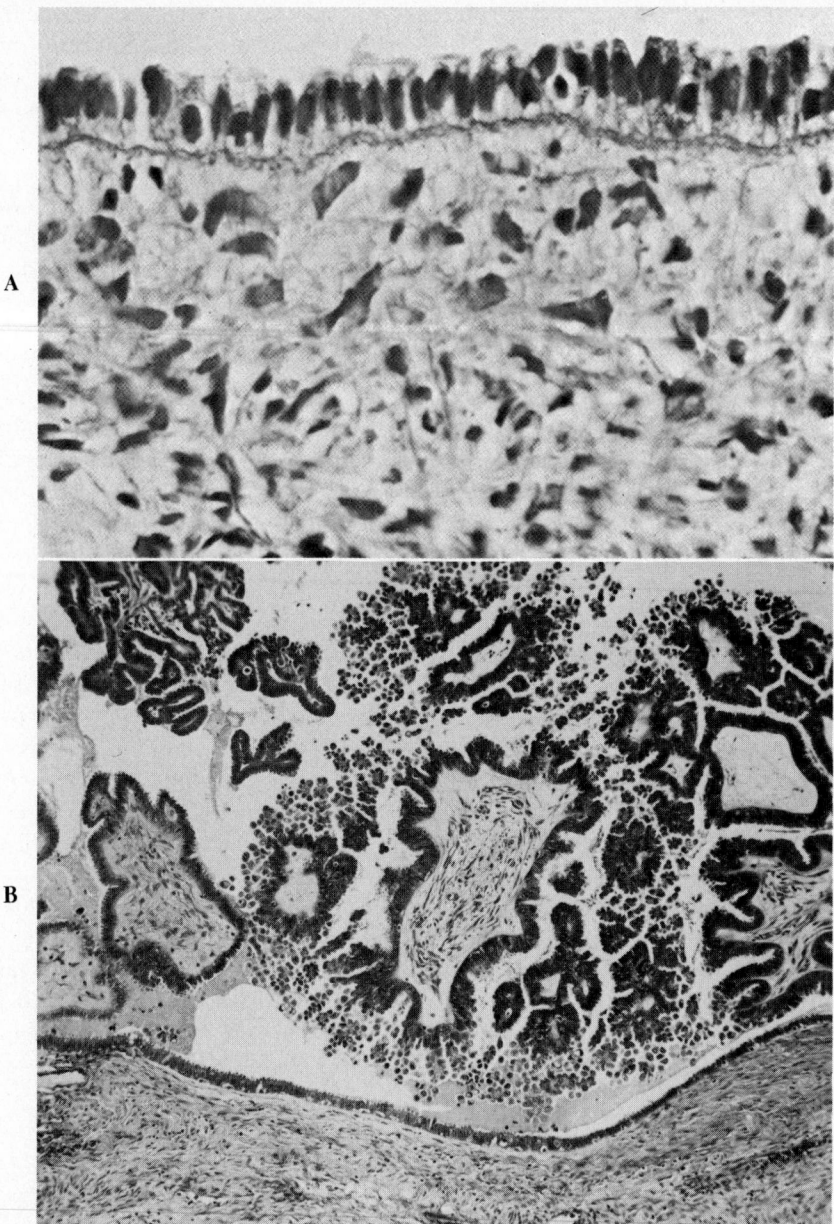

FIGURE 29-2
A, Ciliated epithelium of a well-differentiated serous tumor. (×800.) **B,** Serous papillary cystadenoma of borderline malignancy. The epithelium resembles that of the fallopian tube, and a well-developed papillary pattern is present. (×80.)

percentages have been reported for bilaterality in ovarian tumors, and the most widely quoted are summarized in Table 29-3. Malignant epithelial tumors tend to involve both ovaries more frequently than do benign epithelial tumors. Serous tumors also tend to be bilateral more frequently than do mucinous tumors.

Benign Epithelial Ovarian Tumors— The Adnexal Mass

As noted in Chapter 6, enlargement of the ovary beyond 5 cm is considered abnormal. However, age and menstrual status must also be considered before the appropriate course of action is chosen. A 5- to 8-cm ovarian mass in a woman with regular menses, even if she is in

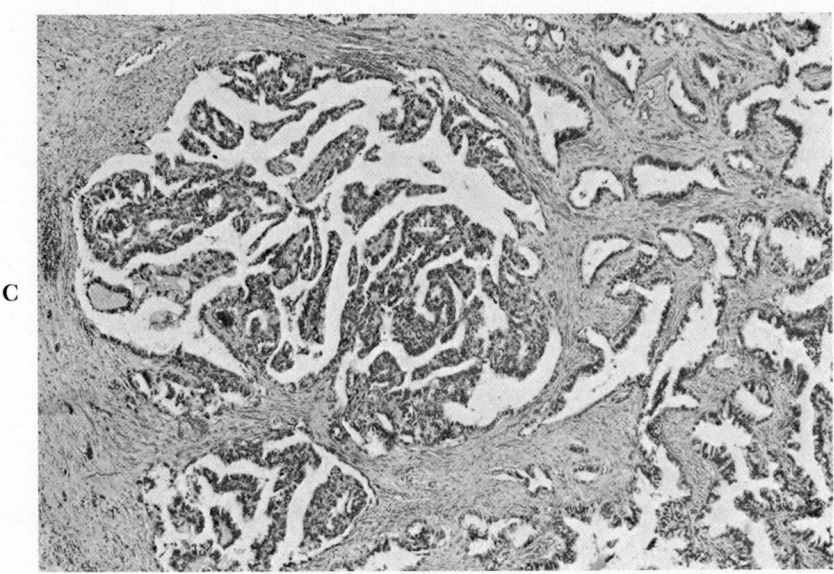

FIGURE 29-2, cont'd.

C, Serous papillary adenocarcinoma. (×50.) The neoplastic epithelium invades the stroma. (**A** and **C** From Serov SF, Scully RE, and Sobin LH: Histologic typing of ovarian tumors. Geneva, 1973, World Health Organization. **B,** Courtesy Dr. R. E. Scully.)

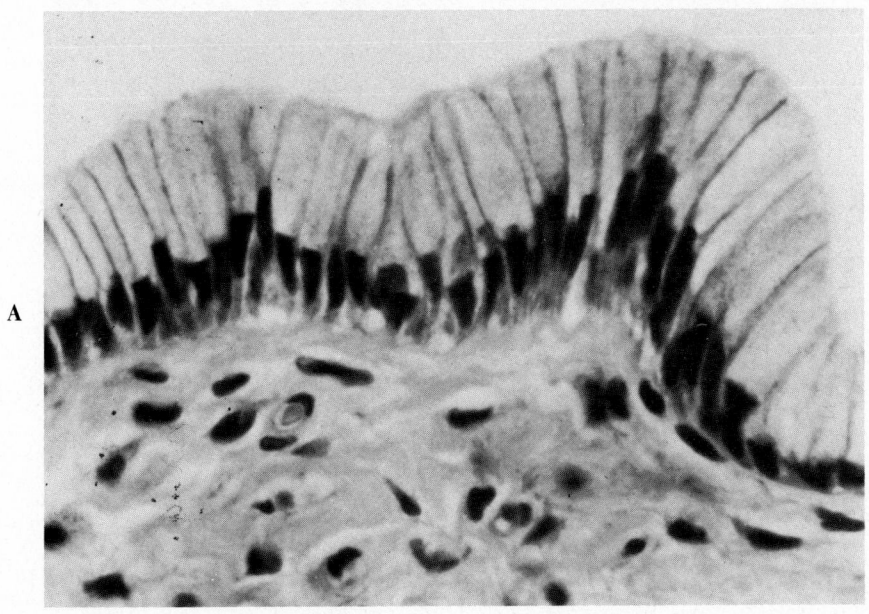

FIGURE 29-3

A, Mucinous cystadenoma. (×800.)   *Continued.*

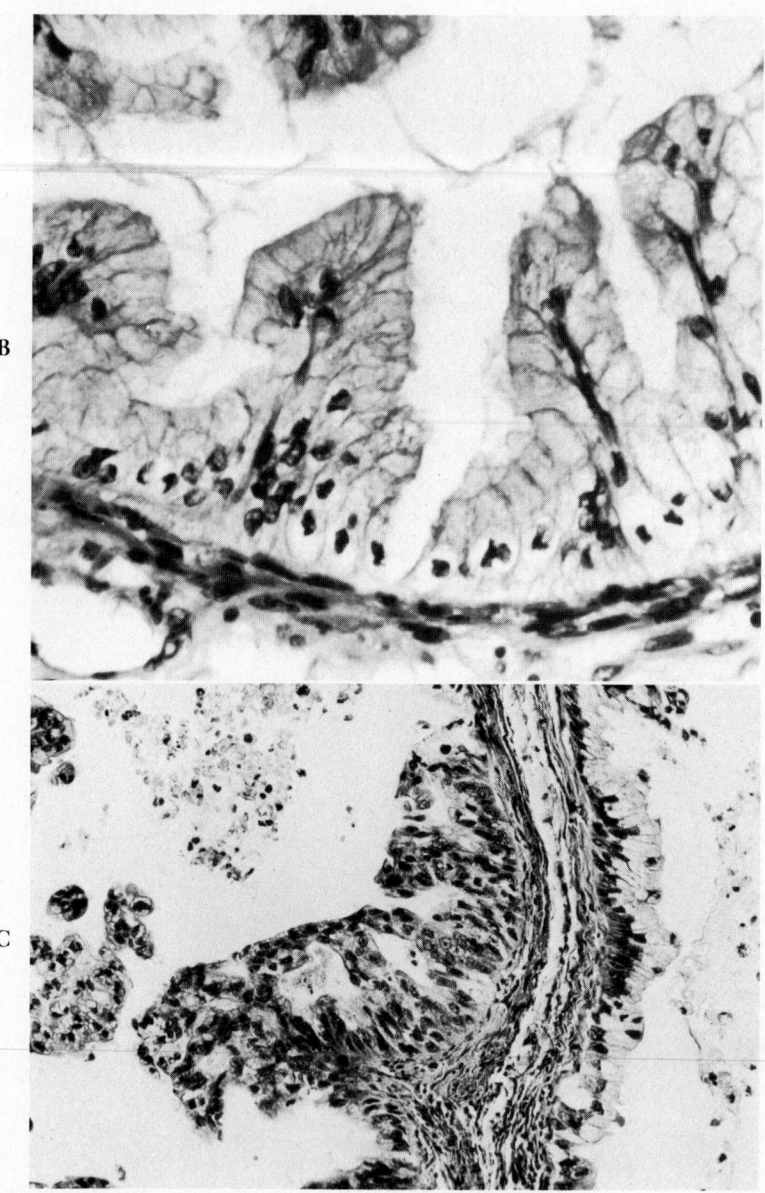

FIGURE 29-3, cont'd.
B, Mucinous borderline tumor. Epithelium resembles that of the endocervix. **C,** Mucinous carcinoma. (×120.) Incomplete stratification of cells and atypicality is present. (**A** and **C** From Serov SF, Scully RE, and Sobin LH: Histologic typing of ovarian tumors. Geneva, 1973, World Health Organization. **B,** Courtesy Dr. R.E. Scully.)

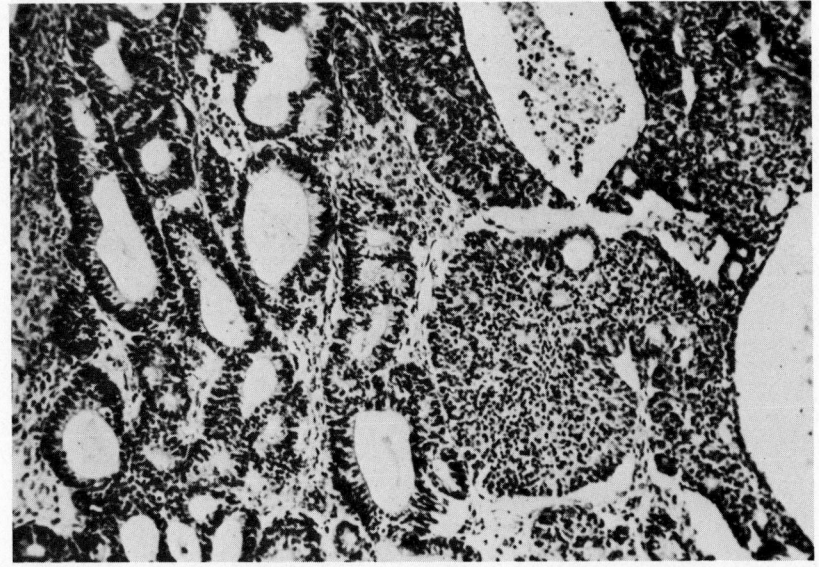

FIGURE 29-4
Endometrioid carcinoma. Tubular glands are lined by stratified endometrium. (×80.) (From Meadowbrook Staff Journal 1:148, 1968. Courtesy Dr. R.E. Scully.)

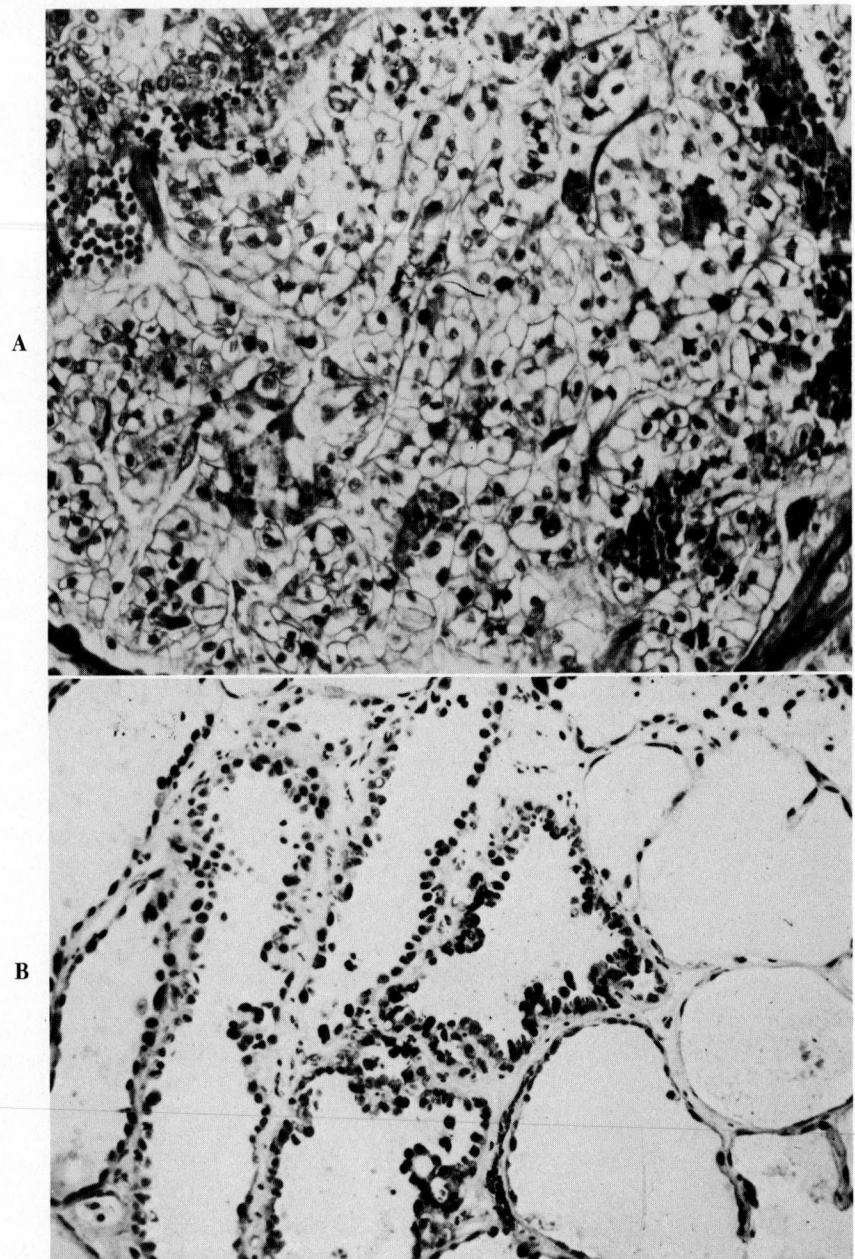

FIGURE 29-5
A, Clear cell adenocarcinoma. (×200.) Solid pattern of abundant polyhedral tumor cells containing abundant clear cytoplasm is present. **B,** Clear cell adenocarcinoma. (×200.) *Left:* Hobnail cells with scant cytoplasm; protruding nuclei line shows tubules. *Right:* Cysts lined by flattened tumor cells. (**A** from Barlow JF and Scully RE: Cancer 20:1405, 1967. **B** from Meadowbrook Staff Journal 1:148, 1968. Courtesy Dr. R.E. Scully.)

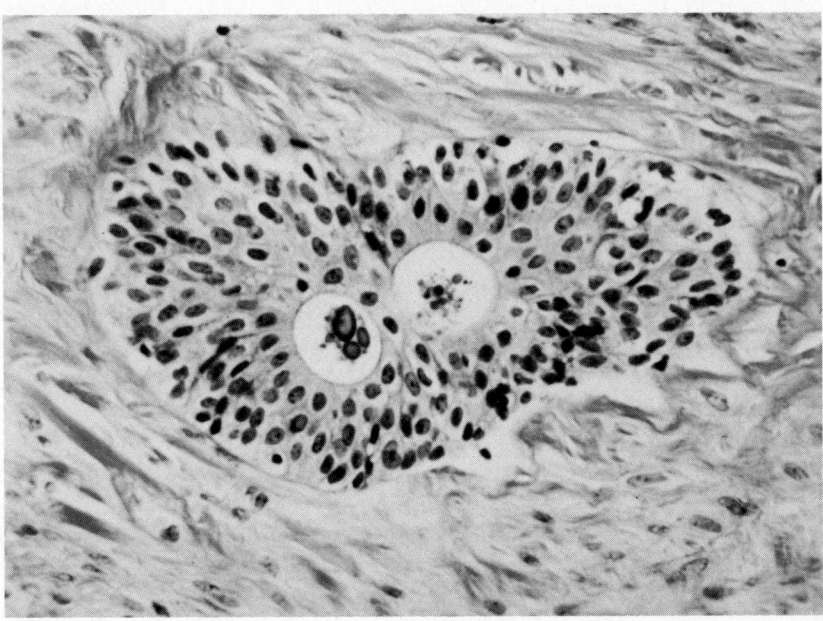

FIGURE 29-6
Brenner tumor. (×350.) Note nest of transition-like epithelium containing spaces with eosinophilic material. (From Atlas of tumor pathology, fascicle 16, series 2, Washington DC, 1979, Armed Forces Institute of Pathology.)

her 40s, is frequently a functioning ovarian cyst, such as a follicular or corpus luteum cyst. It will usually regress spontaneously during a subsequent menstrual cycle. Enlargements of this type in young patients in their 20s or early 30s do not automatically require immediate operative intervention and can be observed for two menstrual cycles. An exception would be a mass in a patient who is taking oral contraceptives, in which case a neoplastic mass is most likely. Unilocular 5- to 8-cm cysts are likely to be functional (Chapter 16), whereas multilocular or partially solid tumors are more likely to be neoplastic. An ultrasound examination, preferably with a vaginal probe, helps to differentiate these lesions.

Occasionally it is discovered that the adnexal mass is paraovarian. In a study of 168 paraovarian tumors, Stein et al. noted that 3 (2%) were malignant. The 3 cysts all had solid components, and the cysts were 8 to 12 cm size in patients 19 to 48 years of age.

Beyond the age of 40 years the risk of malignancy rises. Further evaluation by ultrasound is needed if follow-up without operation is contemplated. The ovary shrinks during the menopause and normally is about 1.5 to 2.0 cm in size. According to Rodriguez, transvaginal ul-

TABLE 29-3
Bilaterality of Ovarian Tumors

Type of Tumor	Occurrence (%)
Epithelial tumors	
Serous cystadenoma	10
Serous cystadenocarcinoma	33-66
Mucinous cystadenoma	5
Mucinous cystadenocarcinoma	10-20
Endometrioid carcinoma	13-30
Benign Brenner tumor	6
Germ cell tumors	
Benign cystic teratoma (dermoid)	12
Immature teratoma (malignant)	2-5
Dysgerminoma	5-10
Other malignant germ cell tumors	Rare
Sex-cord stromal tumors	
Thecoma	Rare
Sertoli-Leydig cell tumor	Rare
Granulosa-theca cell tumor	Rare

trasound can reliably detect an ovary greater than 1.5 cm. Higgins et al. estimated the upper limit of the volume of a postmenopausal ovary was about 8 cm^3 in comparison with 18 cm^3 for the premenopausal ovary. Ten of their patients who exceeded these criteria and had solid or complex echo patterns all had neoplastic tumors, and one carcinoma was discovered.

Ultrasound has helped to define criteria to allow conservative follow-up of some adnexal masses. Goldstein et al. studied 42 postmenopausal patients whose ultrasound scans showed unilocular cysts less than 5 cm in diameter. Twenty-eight were explored, and none had malignancy. Fourteen were followed for up to 6 years with no change in ultrasound appearance. Finkler et al. noted that the addition of CA-125 serum assay (see later discussion) to their ultrasound criteria in postmenopausal women increased the accuracy of preoperative evaluation. In a study of 182 patients Vasilev et al. noted that 22% of benign pelvic masses were associated with elevated CA-125 values (>35 U/ml) and that conditions such as endometriosis give false positive results. However, for patients over the age of 50, a value of greater than 35 U/ml usually indicates malignancy. In a clinical pathologic study to define ultrasound criteria of malignancy, Granberg et al. studied the ovarian tumors in 1017 women. Of 296 with unilocular cysts, only 1 was malignant, this had visible papillary formations on the cyst wall, and 60% of these women were over age 40. In contrast, malignancy rates were 8% (20 of 229) for multilocular cysts, 65% (147 of 201) for multilocular-solid tumors, and 39% (31 of 80) for solid ovarian masses. In a follow-up study of 180 women, the authors noted that 45 of 45 unilocular cysts were benign. Larger numbers and additional studies are needed, but these data indicate the value of vaginal ultrasound in the evaluation of adnexal masses.

In summary, in postmenopausal women, unilocular cysts less than 5 cm in diameter are usually benign. Those with solid elements; or multiloculated; over 5 cm; or with elevated CA-125 in the postmenopausal patient usually should be explored. Certainly the concept that a "palpable" postmenopausal ovary requires operative intervention is no longer valid. The decision for follow-up will require a balanced consideration of the patient's age, operative risk, and ultrasound characteristics of the mass, as recently noted by Sparks and Varner.

Most nonmalignant epithelial ovarian tumors are observed initially as asymptomatic unilateral adnexal masses that can be treated by oophorectomy or occasionally cystectomy (see section on benign cystic teratomas later in this chapter). Some have recommended bisecting the opposite ovary to rule out bilaterality in the case of benign epithelial ovarian tumors (see Table 29-3), but in view of the risk of adhesions and infertility in these young patients, wedge resection of the contralateral ovary in the case of any benign epithelial ovarian neoplasm is not recommended if the contralateral ovary appears normal. In a woman beyond her reproductive years, especially in the presence of a serous cystadenoma, which tends to be bilateral, abdominal hysterectomy and bilateral salpingo-oophorectomy are usually performed.

Mucinous tumors can become particularly large and reach sizes up to 30 cm. Possible complications of mucinous cystadenoma are perforation and rupture, which can lead to the deposit and growth of mucin-secreting epithelium in the peritoneal cavity (pseudomyxoma peritonei, discussed later under borderline mucinous tumors).

Adenofibromas consist of fibrous and epithelial elements. The epithelial component may be serous, mucinous, clear cell, or endometrioid—the architectural subtypes of these benign ovarian tumors. Their appearance will depend on the predominant histologic features— epithelial or fibrous. These tumors are also managed by simple excision. Endometriomas are considered in Chapter 18.

Brenner tumors (see Figure 29-6) are rare and often incidental findings when oophorectomy is performed for an indication other than ovarian enlargement. Most often, these tumors occur in women in their 40s and 50s, but both younger and older patients have been found to have them. Brenner tumors are almost always benign and can usually be managed by oophorectomy. When the ovary is palpably enlarged, approximately 5% of Brenner tumors will prove to be malignant. These tumors often occur in perimenopausal and postmenopausal women, in which case hysterectomy and bilateral salpingo-oophorectomy are indicated. Unfortunately, malignant Brenner tumors appear to have a poor prognosis despite this operative therapy, and an effective program of chemotherapy has not been developed.

The differential diagnosis for and approach to an adnexal mass in female patients of various ages are discussed in Chapter 6. Ovarian enlargement in the premenarchal female is usually the result of a germ cell tumor, which may be malignant but is usually benign (see later discussion of germ cell tumors). During the reproductive years ovarian neoplasms are usually benign. For the patient in her 20s or 30s most ovarian enlargements can be approached operatively through a lower abdominal transverse (Pfannenstiel) incision, unless there is a possibility of malignancy, such as a solid tumor or one with papillae viewed on ultrasound examination. The risk of trying to do this by laparoscopic excision was emphasized in a recent report by Maiman et al. They conducted a national survey and discovered 42 cases of ovarian malignancy in patients who had laparoscopic aspiration and/or excision of an adnexal mass that subsequently proved to be malignant. In these cases, as well as in women over age 40 or those with a large mass extending out of the pelvis and into the abdomen, a vertical incision is indicated. The tumor must be removed intact, and if malignancy is present, as is more likely in older patients, a thorough surgical evaluation is indicated (outlined in the section on epithelial carcinoma).

A frozen section should be obtained if gross examination of the ovarian tumor is at all suspicious for malignancy. For women of reproductive age, if the diagnosis of malignancy is suspected but uncertain even after a frozen section is obtained, the operation should be terminated after removal of the ovarian tumor. A second procedure can be performed if malignancy is confirmed after detailed histologic study of the permanent sections. This is preferable to risking an unnecessary hysterectomy or bilateral salpingo-oophorectomy in a patient who desires to preserve childbearing function.

Epithelial Carcinomas

Diagnosis, Staging, Spread, and Preoperative Evaluation

Ovarian carcinomas are usually diagnosed by detection of an adnexal mass on pelvic examination. Unfortunately the diagnosis is frequently made only after the disease has spread beyond the confines of the ovary. Scully estimates that the risk of malignancy in a primary ovarian tumor rises to about 33% in a woman over the age of 45, whereas it is less than 1 in 15 for women who are 20 to 45 years of age. In general, over half of ovarian carcinomas occur in women beyond the age of 50. In a hospital-based study of ovarian neoplasms in 861 women, Koonings et al. noted the risk of malignancy was 13% in premenopausal women but rose to 45% in postmenopausal women. In their study, benign ovarian neoplasms were most common among those 20 to 29 years of age.

Patients with ovarian carcinoma frequently develop ascites, and a swollen abdomen may be their first symptom, either due to ascites or tumor spread. Vague lower abdominal discomfort is a frequent complaint, but severe pain is not a prominent symptom. Vaginal cytologic testing can detect ovarian carcinoma cells because of their transmigration through the tubes, uterus, and cervix into the vagina. However, an ovarian carcinoma is rarely initially detected from vaginal cytologic smears. The diagnosis is established by histologic examination of the tumor tissue removed at operation. Occasionally the initial diagnosis is suggested by examination of ascitic fluid obtained at paracentesis, which may reveal cells characteristic of ovarian epithelial malignancy.

The clinical staging of ovarian cancer (Table 29-4) is designed according to the criteria of the International Federation of Gynecology and Obstetrics (FIGO) and is based on the results of operative exploration. The system was modified in 1985.

Before operative exploration, the patient with suspected ovarian carcinoma has the preoperative workup usual for a major abdominal operation (Chapter 23). Additional diagnostic studies include a CT scan of the abdomen to search for retroperitoneal node enlargement and a barium enema or colonoscopy. The latter is of particular importance for evaluation of the possibility of a primary colon carcinoma, which may be found initially as an adnexal mass in the older patient. An endoscopic examination is performed if there is evidence of gastrointestinal bleeding or the suggestion of rectosigmoid disease. An upper gastrointestinal tract series is also obtained if there are upper gastrointestinal symptoms or evidence of gastrointestinal bleeding. Preoperative blood tests are not sufficiently specific to be a screening tool, but they can be useful. Bast et al. studied the ovarian antigen designated CA-125 in serum and found it to be elevated in approximately 80% of carcinoma cases. If the CA-125 level is elevated at the time of operation, the test is useful for following the progress of the patient with ovarian carcinoma after treatment and demonstrating the response to therapy or detecting tumor progression. Occasionally the level of the isoenzyme lactic acid dehydrogenase (LDH) is elevated, but this test is not specific. Newer tumor markers, such as CA 19-9 and urinary gonadotrophin fragment, are being investigated.

TABLE 29-4
Staging of Ovarian Carcinomas (FIGO)
Modified 1985

Stage	Characteristics
I	Growth limited to the ovaries. Growth limited to one ovary; no ascites present containing malignant cells. No tumor on the external surface; capsule intact.
IB	Growth limited to both ovaries; no ascites present containing malignant cells. No tumor on the external surfaces; capsules intact.
IC	Tumor either stage IA or IB but with tumor on surface of one or both ovaries; or with capsule ruptured; or with ascites present containing malignant cells; or with positive peritoneal washings.
II	Growth involving one or both ovaries with pelvic extension.
IIA	Extension and/or metastases to the uterus and/or tubes.
IIB	Extension to other pelvic tissues.
IIC	Tumor either stage IIA or IIB, but with tumor on surface of one or both ovaries; or with capsules(s) ruptured; or with ascites present containing malignant cells; or with positive peritoneal washings.
III	Tumor involving one or both ovaries with peritoneal implants outside the pelvis and/or positive retroperitoneal or inguinal nodes. Superficial liver metastasis equals stage III. Tumor is limited to the true pelvis but with histologically proven malignant extension to small bowel or omentum.
IIIA	Tumor grossly limited to the true pelvis with negative nodes but with histologically confirmed microscopic seeding of abdominal peritoneal surfaces.
IIIB	Tumor of one or both ovaries with histologically confirmed implants of abdominal peritoneal surfaces, none exceeding 2 cm in diameter. Nodes are negative.
IIIC	Abdominal implants greater than 2 cm in diameter and/or positive retroperitoneal or inguinal nodes.
IV	Growth involving one or both ovaries with distant metastases. If pleural effusion is present, there must be positive cytology to allot a case to stage IV. Parenchymal liver metastasis equals stage IV.

Preoperatively a program to cleanse the bowel is instituted in case intestinal resection is required. In one program the patient is given a liquid diet 48 hours preoperatively. One widely used program utilizes GoLYTELY. Neomycin sulfate 1 g, with 1 g erythromycin base, is given 3 times (3 PM, 7 PM, and 11 PM) on the day before surgery. However, the important principle is mechanical cleansing of the bowel (see Chapter 23). Treatment with prophylactic low-dose heparin (mini-heparin) is advisable to reduce the risk of thromboembolism. The patient usually receives heparin, 5000 IU intramuscularly, 2 hours before surgery and every 12 hours thereafter.

In a consideration of therapy for ovarian epithelial carcinoma, knowledge of its natural path of spread is important. The tumors spread along the peritoneal surface to involve ovarian, parietal, and intestinal peritoneal surfaces, as well as the undersurface of the diaphragm, particularly on the right side (Figure 29-7). This knowledge is particularly important because tumors that appear at operation to be confined to the ovary may have small areas of diaphragmatic involvement as the sole site of extraovarian spread. Such a tumor should be classified as a stage III ovarian carcinoma (see Table 29-4). Lymphatic dissemination is also a prominent part of disease spread (Figure 29-8), and it is particularly important to note that the paraaortic nodes are at risk through lymphatics that run parallel to the ovarian vessels. Knapp and Friedman noted that, of 26 patients with ovarian cancer apparently limited to the ovary, 19% had paraaortic involvement and all had poorly differentiated tumors. Piver et al. noted that approximately 10% of apparent stage I ovarian tumors had paraaortic node metastases; the risk was greatest for women with poorly differentiated tumors. In a recent study of 180 patients, Burghardt et al. observed that the proportion of positive nodes rose with higher stage tumors: 24% in stage I, 50% in stage II, and 73.5% in stages III and IV. Five-year survivals were 58% for those with one node and dropped to 28% for those with more than one node.

The prognosis for patients with ovarian carcinoma is related to tumor stage, tumor grade, cell type, and the amount of residual tumor after resection. In addition, recent studies of flow cytometry indicate that the ploidy of the tumor is prognostic with aneuploidy being a

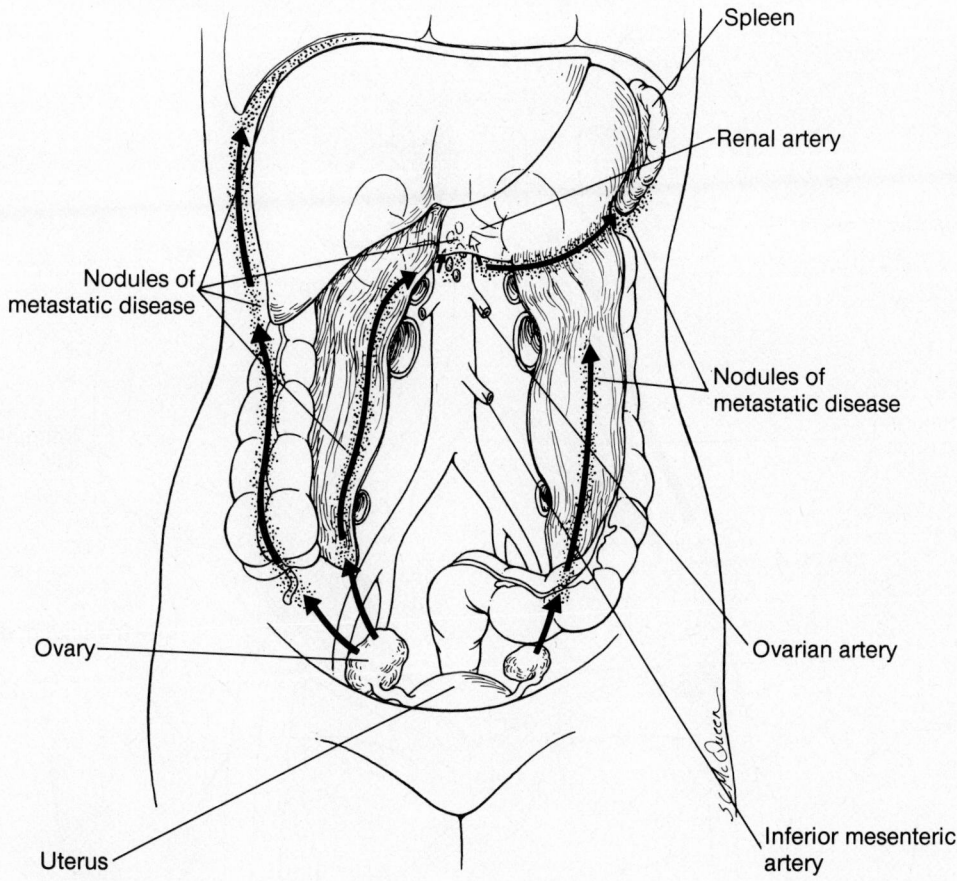

FIGURE 29-7
Peritoneal spread of ovarian cancer. Portions of omentum, small intestine, and transverse colon have been resected. (From Knapp RC, Berkowitz RS, and Leavitt T Jr: Natural history and detection of ovarian cancer. In Gynecology and obstetrics, vol 4, Philadelphia, 1986, JB Lippincott Co.)

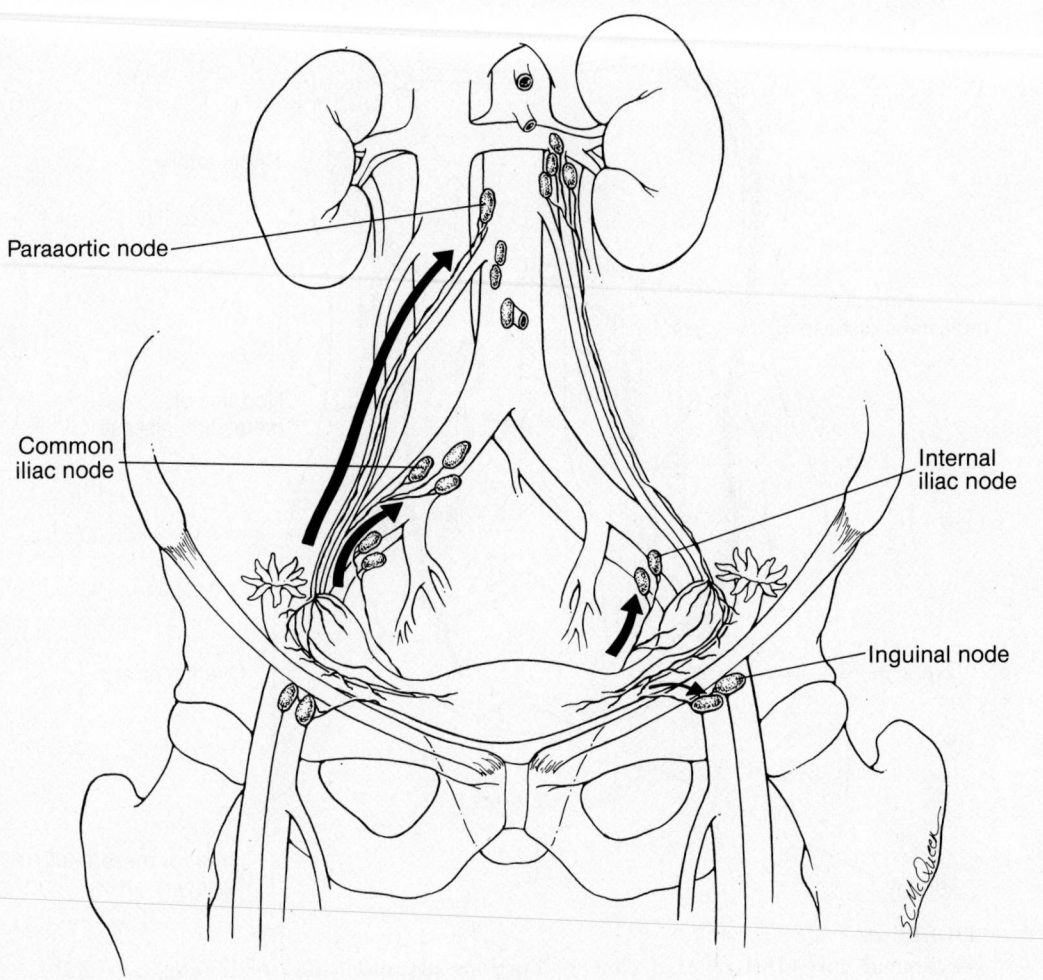

FIGURE 29-8
Lymph nodes draining ovaries. Primary routes of spread to the pelvic and paraaortic nodes are illustrated. (Redrawn from Musumeci R: Cancer 40:1444, 1977).

negative prognostic factor. Klemi et al. noted an independent prognostic association with the DNA index and S phase fraction. A better prognosis was observed if the proportion of S phase cells was less than 11% or if the DNA index (the relative DNA content of aneuploid cells compared with diploid) was less than 1.3. Genetic studies by Slamon et al. have shown that the proto-oncogene HER-2/*neu* is found to be amplified in ovarian and breast cancers. In 87 cases of ovarian cancers, gene amplification was found to correlate with survival, that is, for 1 copy, 1879 days; 2 to 5 copies, 959 days; and more than 5 copies, 243 days. Richardson (Table 29-5) summarized the historical results of therapy for ovarian cancer from a number of institutions according to stage.

Cell type has been reported to be an important factor in prognosis, as shown in Figure 29-9, which summarizes the 20-year survival rate of a group of patients. The most common

invasive epithelial cancers, serous carcinomas, have the worst prognosis; prognosis is better for mucinous, endometrioid, and clear cell tumors, although clear cell carcinomas do have a

TABLE 29-5

Five-Year Survival in 5254 Cases of Ovarian Cancer (1973-1975)*

Stage	Proportion of Cases (%)	5-Year Survival (%)
I	25.2	66.4
II	17.6	45.0
III	39.5	13.3
IV	17.8	4.1

Modified from Richardson GS, Scully RE, Nikrui N, et al: N Engl J Med 312:415, 1985. Reprinted with permission of The New England Journal of Medicine.
*Overall 5-year survival is 30.6%.

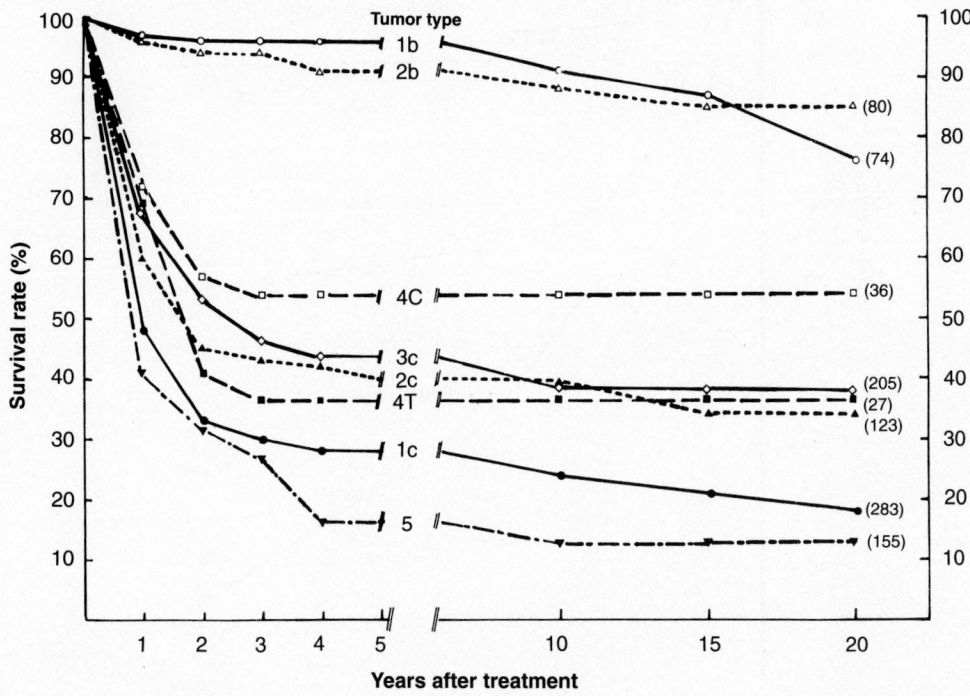

FIGURE 29-9
Survival rates for 983 patients with all stages of ovarian cancer by histologic type. *1b*, (74 cases) Serous, low malignant potential (74 cases); *2b*, Mucinous, low malignant potential (80 cases); *1c*, Serous carcinoma (283 cases); 2c, Mucinous carcinoma (123 cases); *3c*, Endometrioid carcinoma (205 cases); *4c*, Clear cell (36 cases); *4T*, Tubulocystic pattern of clear cell (27 cases); *5*, (155 cases) Undifferentiated (155 cases). (Redrawn from Aure JC, Hoeg K, and Kolstad P: Obstet Gynecol 37:1, 1971. Reprinted with permission from The American College of Obstetricians and Gynecologists.)

poor prognosis as well. However, it should be noted that both stage and grade affect these observations, insofar as serous tumors tend to be more poorly differentiated and discovered at a higher stage than are mucinous tumors, which tend to be of lower grade and/or stage.

In addition to stage, the grade of the tumor is a major determinant of patient prognosis. Figure 29-10 demonstrates the survival of 442 patients with ovarian carcinoma by grade, with a markedly worse prognosis for poorly differentiated tumors (grade 3). The relationship between grade and survival also exists when the results are examined separately for each stage of disease. Grade 0 (borderline) tumors have the best prognosis (see Figure 29-9).

The size of residual nodules and the presence or absence of tumor after operation have been shown to be related to the survival of patients treated for ovarian carcinoma. Aure et al., in their classic studies, (Figure 29-11) noted a 5-year survival of over 30% for stage III tumors that were completely resected, in comparison with 10% when resection was incomplete. The 5-year survival of incompletely resected stage II tumors was approximately 18%. Patients with small postoperative residual tumors have a better prognosis than those with larger diameter residual tumors. Frequently used categories are microscopic (present on biopsy, but not grossly), less than 0.5 cm, 0.5 to 2.0 cm, and greater than 2.0 cm.

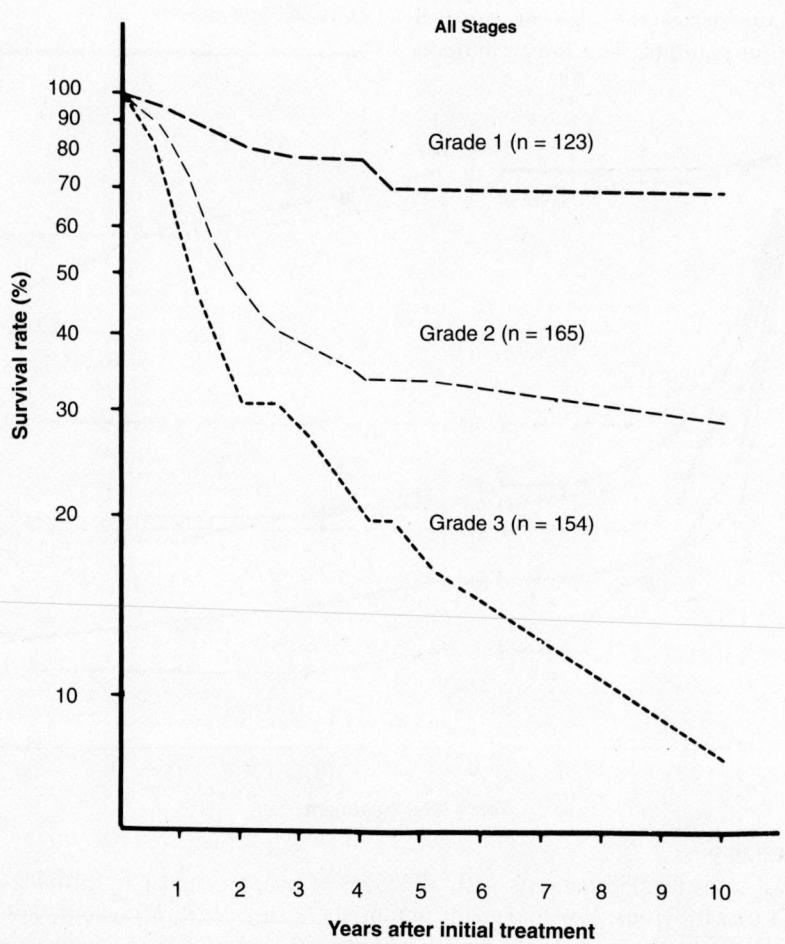

FIGURE 29-10
Survival rates for patients with ovarian cancer by tumor grade. Survival curves for the complete series according to the histologic degree of differentiation. All differences between curves are highly significant. (From Sorbe B, Frankendal B, and Veress B: Obstet Gynecol 59:576, 1982. Reprinted with permission from the American College of Obstetricians and Gynecologists.)

Management

BORDERLINE OVARIAN TUMORS (OVARI-AN CARCINOMAS OF LOW MALIGNANT PO-TENTIAL). Approximately 20% of ovarian epithelial cancers fit into the category of tumors of low malignant potential (grade 0) and are associated with excellent prognosis regardless of stage. Most studies have been confined to borderline tumors of the serous (see Figure 29-2, *B*) and mucinous (see Figure 29-3, *B*) varieties, which are the most common of borderline tumors, but other epithelial types (see Table 29-2) can occur. The cells of these epithelial tumors do not invade the stroma of the ovary. It is extremely important that the ovarian tumor be thoroughly sampled by the pathologist to be certain that a borderline tumor is not mixed with invasive elements. Numerous studies have confirmed that borderline tumors have a slower growth rate than do invasive ovarian carcinomas, and the patients have a prolonged survival time (see Figure 29-9).

Since these tumors tend to occur in young women during the reproductive years, it is desirable to ascertain the safety of conservative therapy for patients with borderline stage 1A tumors (confined to one ovary). Julian and Woodruff reported a 100% 5-year survival rate in 34 patients treated for stage I borderline serous tumors; the 5-year survival rates were 80% to 86% for 30 patients with stage II to IV borderline ovarian serous tumors (survival rates corrected for individuals dying of unrelated illnesses). Twenty-five patients had their tumors confined to one ovary (Table 29-6). All were younger than 30 years, and as can be seen from the table, unilateral adnexectomy was as effective as more radical surgery. Lim-Tan et al. recently reported on 33 cases of stage I serous borderline tumors initially treated by cystectomy. Only 3 of 33 patients undergoing cystectomy had recurrence or persistence, and these 3 patients had positive resection margins and/or multiple cysts present in the ovary, emphasizing the effectiveness of conservative operation. However, for most stage IA cases, unilateral adnexectomy is performed, and if the opposite ovary looks normal, no biopsy or wedge resection is done. In some cases patients are found to have small ovaries

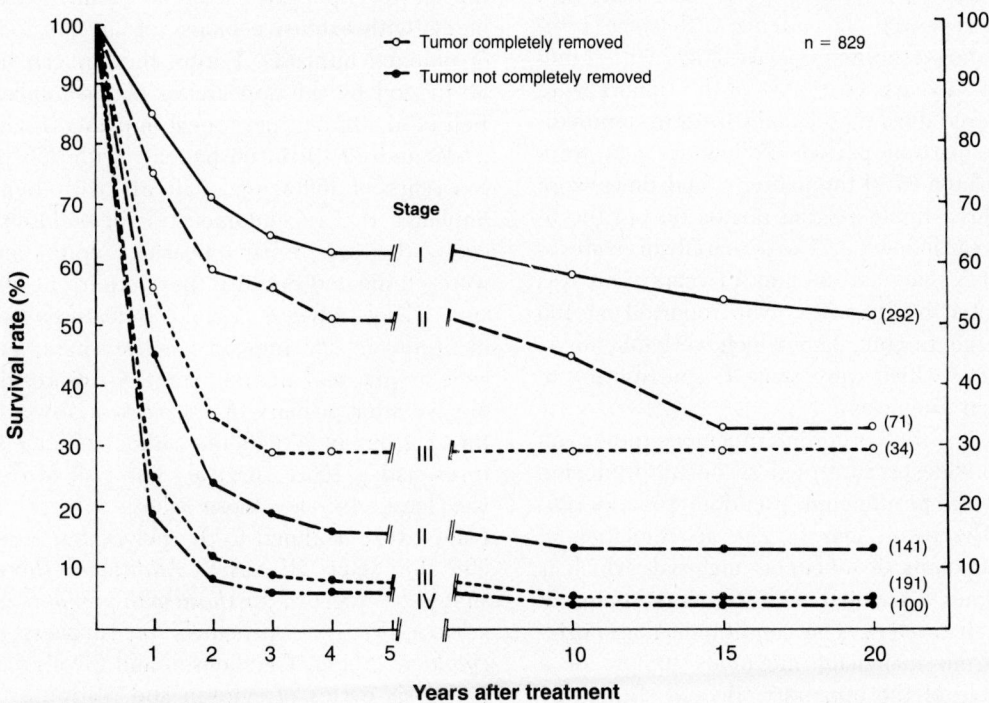

FIGURE 29-11
Survival rate for 829 patients with ovarian cancer in relation to stage and operability (number of patients in parentheses). (From Aure JC, Hoeg K, and Kolstad P: Obstet Gynecol 37:1, 1971. Reprinted with permission from The American College of Obstetricians and Gynecologists.)

TABLE 29-6
Conservative Versus Total Ablative Operation for 25 Patients with Stage IA, Grade 0 Ovarian Papillary Serous Cystadenocarcinoma

Surgery	Number	5-Year Salvage
Unilateral adnexectomy	15	15
Hysterectomy and bilateral adnexectomy	10	9*

Modified from Julian CG and Woodruff JD: Obstet Gynecol 40:860, 1972. Reprinted with permission from The American College of Obstetrics and Gynecology.
*One patient died of other disease.

(less than 4 cm in diameter) and widespread papillary serous carcinoma in the abdomen. In such cases the term *serous surface papillary carcinoma of the ovary* or *papillary serous carcinoma of the peritoneum* is applied. Fromm et al. reported on 74 patients and found survival improved if the patients were treated postoperatively with combination chemotherapy (see later discussion for therapy of high stage carcinoma of the ovary).

Mucinous borderline tumors also are associated with an excellent prognosis. Hart and Norris reviewed 97 patients with stage I tumors who were 9 to 70 years of age with a median of 35 years. Over 10% of the tumors were discovered during pregnancy or in the immediate postpartum period. Follow-up data were available on 87 of the patients, and there were only three tumor-related deaths during the 5- to 10-year follow-up. The actuarial survival was 98% at 5 years and 96% at 10 years. This was also noted by Bostwick, who reported on 109 borderline tumors, 33 of which were mucinous, and all of which were stage I, contributing to the good prognosis.

Rupture of a borderline mucinous tumor can lead to widespread growth of mucin-producing cells in the peritoneum (pseudomyxoma peritonei). The result may be the accumulation of large amounts of mucinous material, which is sometimes associated with recurrent bouts of bowel obstruction. This condition can also originate from malignant mucinous tumors or a mucocele of the appendix. Recent studies by Young et al. suggest pseudomyxoma peritonei usually arise in the appendix. It tends to recur and to require repeated laparotomy. Chemotherapy and mucolytic agents have been tried but are not well tested. Long-term therapy is currently unavailable. Greene et al. reported that mucinous material was easier to remove after irrigation of the abdomen with 5% dextrose and water. Jones and Homesley reported a complete remission following eight courses of cyclophosphamide (Cytoxan), 500 mg/m^2; doxorubicin (Adriamycin), 50 mg/m^2; and cisplatin, 50 mg/m^2.

Conservative therapy for borderline tumors with preservation of childbearing function may be carried out by unilateral oophorectomy if the following criteria are met: the tumor is confirmed to be at stage IA; extensive histologic sampling of the tumor confirms it to be grade 0 (borderline); the contralateral ovary appears normal; biopsy specimens of areas of omental or peritoneal nodularity are negative; and results of peritoneal cytologic tests are negative for tumor cells.

For borderline tumors beyond stage I, both irradiation therapy and chemotherapy, primarily with alkylating agents, have been prescribed to attempt to improve survival. However, as noted in Figure 29-9, the 5-year survival of patients with all stages of borderline tumors is high (over 90%) after resection alone. Effective removal of all gross disease remains the most important factor in primary treatment, with extensive biopsy of any peritoneal or omental implants. Future therapy can then be judged by the appearance of the implants. Bell et al. studied peritoneal implants (Figures 29-12 and 29-13) in 56 patients with 368 person-years of follow-up. Patients with benign implants, that is, endometriosis or endosalpingosis (benign tubal-appearing epithelium), were eliminated because they require no therapy. Three adverse histologic features were identified in the implants: invasiveness, cytologic atypia, and mitotic count. Gross residual disease after primary operation was also a factor. A group of 27 patients without adverse features had a 100% survival. The risk of death was least (4%) for those whose invasive implants were confined to the pelvis, but rose to 20% for stage III cases. *Additional therapy should be reserved for those with implants with adverse features, primarily invasiveness and cytologic atypia.* Gershenson and Silva recommend six cycles of cytoxan and platinum (see later discussion) for patients with invasive implants. As noted in many studies, including those of Chambers et al., adjuvant therapy has not been demonstrated to be generally beneficial in those with borderline tumors. Histologic

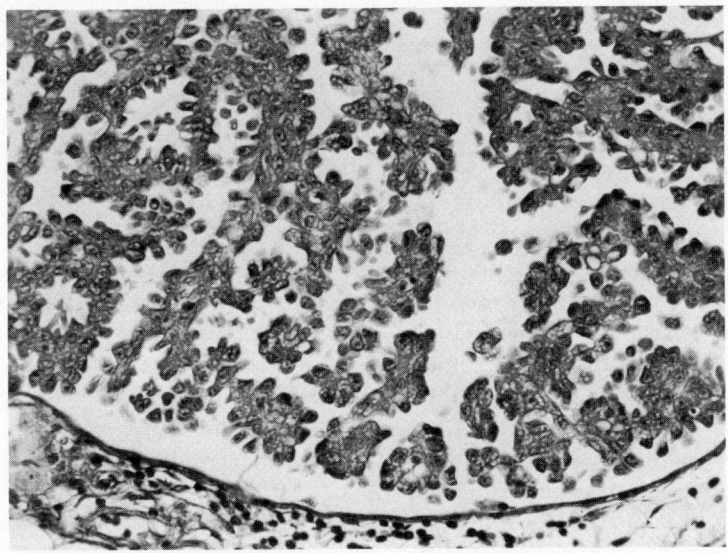

FIGURE 29-12
Noninvasive implant of epithelial type. Branching papillae and detached clusters of polygonal cells showing moderate cytologic atypicality are present (H&E; ×313). (From Bell DA, Weinstock MA, Scully RE: Cancer 62:2212, 1988.)

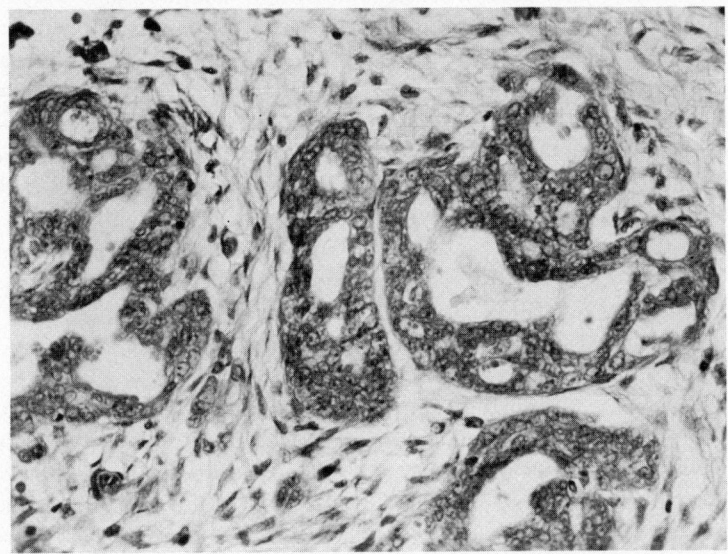

FIGURE 29-13
Invasive implant. Glands with an irregular contour lined by severely atypical epithelial cells with extensive intraglandular bridging are present (H&E, ×313). (From Bell DA, Weinstock MA, and Scully RE: Cancer 62:2212, 1988.)

examination of the implants appears to provide a basis to choose patients who might benefit from therapy.

INVASIVE EPITHELIAL CARCINOMAS. The primary principle for treatment of ovarian epithelial carcinoma is removal of all resectable gross disease. The patient's abdomen is explored through a vertical incision, which is extended well into the upper part of the abdomen, if needed. If ascitic fluid is present, it is sent for cytologic evaluation; if ascites is not present, 200 to 400 ml of normal saline solution with 1 ml (1000 IU) of heparin is used to obtain cytologic samples from the peritoneum by separately irrigating at least the pelvis, upper abdomen, and right and left paracolic gutters before any resection is done. The extent of the disease is established by evaluating the entire peritoneal cavity, with biopsy specimens taken of any suspicious nodules and with excision, rather than lysis, of all adhesions, since adhesions between bowel and other peritoneal surfaces may contain tumor deposits. A total abdominal hysterectomy, bilateral salpingo-oophorectomy, and appendectomy as well as infracolic omentectomy, are performed if technically possible. When there is no gross disease outside the pelvis, paraaortic and pelvic lymph node sampling is *usually* performed, with care taken to remove enlarged nodes. Current evidence indicates that if the bulk of the disease can be reduced to residual masses less than 2 cm in diameter (preferably smaller), the patient's response to postoperative therapy will be improved.

It may occasionally be necessary to resect bowel to relieve impending obstruction or to remove a tumor nodule and thereby eliminate all gross disease from the peritoneal cavity. Studies from the Gynecologic Oncology Group (GOG) summarized by Buchsbaum et al. emphasized that many ovarian carcinomas that clinically appeared to be of low stage initially were actually determined to be high-stage tumors after adequate operative exploration. Partial cystectomy may be necessary, but total cystectomy and urinary diversion are not indicated. Heintz et al. noted prognosis was improved for younger patients (age ≤50 years), those with good initial performance status (Karnofsky >80, Table 25-4), as well as those whose disease could be cytoreduced to less than 1.5 cm. Adverse factors were large metastases before initial operation, ascites, and peritoneal carcinomatosis.

One exception to the required removal of the uterus and opposite ovary occurs in the case of well-differentiated (grade 1) ovarian tumors confined to one ovary (stage IA). DiSaia et al. outlined criteria for preserving childbearing function in a young woman with stage IA, grade 1 ovarian epithelial carcinoma, as follows:

1. Tumor confined to one ovary
2. Tumor well differentiated (grade 1) with no invasion of capsule, lymphatics, or mesovarium
3. Peritoneal washings negative
4. Omental biopsy specimen negative
5. Young woman of childbearing years with strong desire to preserve reproductive function
6. Agreement to close follow-up with consideration of excision of contralateral ovary after childbearing function is completed

These criteria can be applied to all types of epithelial ovarian tumors but are more likely to be satisfied in the case of mucinous tumors, which are more frequently well differentiated and unilateral than serous carcinomas. Some advocate wedge resection of a normal-appearing contralateral ovary. However, this is unlikely to uncover an occult tumor. It appears more prudent to follow the patient closely for any evidence of future ovarian enlargement. Vaginal ultrasound can be a very useful diagnostic aid. Such an approach reduces the risks of postoperative adhesions leading to infertility and also prevents cutting into microscopic tumor at the time of wedge resection. If such a tiny tumor were present, it would presumably be discovered at an early stage during close follow-up and could then be removed intact.

LOW-STAGE OVARIAN CARCINOMAS

Stage I. Most patients with stage I tumors are treated according to the surgical principles already outlined. It is important to emphasize that careful assessment of the subdiaphragmatic areas (by direct visualization if possible) and inspection of the entire peritoneum and the retroperitoneal paraaortic and pelvic nodes are important, particularly in view of the risk of diaphragmatic and nodal spread in tumors that initially appear to be at stage I. Since unsuspected metastases to the paraaortic nodes appear to occur most frequently in poorly differentiated tumors, the paraaortic and pelvic nodes should be sampled and any enlarged nodes removed in all apparent stage I cases that appear on frozen section to be less well differentiated than grade 1. In addition, the omentum, uterus, tubes, and contralateral ovary are removed.

Rupture of ovary. Occasionally during removal a stage I ovarian carcinoma is inadvertently ruptured (stage IC, Table 29-4). There are conflicting opinions as to the potential adverse effects on patient prognosis. It is possible, for example, that the higher-grade and larger tumors, which are more difficult to remove, also tend to rupture, suggesting that most tumors that rupture also initially had the worst prognosis. In general the spilled fluid and all residual tumor should be removed promptly from the operative field following rupture (see later discussion).

Stage II. Stage II ovarian cancer is initially treated by removal of the uterus, tubes, and ovaries, which usually leads to resection of all gross disease in stage IIA carcinoma (tumor involving uterus or tubes or both). With extension to other pelvic tissues (stage IIB), subtotal removal of tumor may be the only feasible operative outcome. An omentectomy (infracolic) is performed, and the pelvic and paraaortic nodes are sampled in view of the risk of retroperitoneal spread, which is highest for grade 3 tumors.

Postoperative management. After operative therapy is completed, a decision must be made as to whether the patient will receive additional treatment with irradiation or chemotherapy. Guthrie et al. evaluated 656 patients treated for epithelial ovarian carcinomas that had been totally excised. Most carcinomas were at stage I or II, and patients were randomly assigned to receive postoperative treatment of radiation therapy alone, chemotherapy alone, radiation therapy and chemotherapy, or no postoperative therapy. Follow-up was for at least 2 years. Approximately 20% of the tumors were borderline malignancies, and the rest were invasive carcinomas. Perhaps surprisingly, the lowest frequency of death or recurrence was noted in the group receiving no postoperative therapy (2%), whereas in the other groups the death or recurrence incidence was 14% to 17%. Thus this study showed no benefit for adjuvant therapy in completely excised stage I and II carcinomas, emphasizing the importance of a control-nontreatment group in adjuvant therapy trials.

Radioactive colloids have been used postop-

eratively in an attempt to improve survival rates in patients with stage I disease or with no gross residual tumor after operation. Currently ^{32}P, a primary beta emitter, is used. The material is introduced through a catheter inserted into the peritoneal cavity 3 to 4 weeks postoperatively, and usually 15 mCi of ^{32}P in 500 ml of saline solution is injected and distributed widely throughout the peritoneal cavity. The distribution of the material is usually checked by the instillation of a small amount of radiopaque dye such as Hypaque or radioactive technetium (^{99}Tc) to ensure uniform distribution throughout the peritoneal cavity. Radioactive gold (^{198}Au) has also been used in the past as a radioactive colloid. However ^{198}Au produces greater tissue penetration because of gamma ray emission (see Chapter 25) with associated damage to normal tissue. Its use is associated with more posttherapy complications; as a result, ^{32}P is primarily used today.

For patients with completely resected stage II disease or poorly differentiated stage I tumors, adjuvant chemotherapy is often prescribed. In the past an alkylating agent such as melphalan, in a dosage of 1 to 2 mg/kg given in divided doses for 5 days orally every 5 weeks, has been used for 1 year. Hreshchyshyn et al. reported a collaborative study of 86 patients with stage I ovarian carcinomas and noted the fewest recurrences (6%) in those who received melphalan compared with 17% for those who received pelvic irradiation and 30% for the no-therapy group. No benefit was demonstrated for patients with stage IA grade 1 tumors.

Unfortunately, alkylating agent administration is also associated with an increased risk of subsequently developing leukemia, which is related to the dose and duration of alkylating agent treatment. This risk increases from about 2% within 4 years of therapy to as great as 10% 8 years after treatment. Recent data by Kaldor et al. indicate that alkylating agents, as well as cisplatin and doxorubicin, used for ovarian cancer were associated with an increased risk of leukemia that was not seen after radiotherapy. This risk must be balanced against the potential benefits of improved survival when adjuvant therapy with alkylating agents is prescribed for patients with completely resected disease. For this reason, if adjuvant chemotherapy is to be used, some prefer a multiple-agent regimen containing cisplatin (see later discussion of postoperative chemotherapy). Such treatment is used also for stage II cases, particularly if there is residual disease after operation.

Two case-control randomized studies by Young et al. provide some guidelines for therapy of patients with low-stage disease. For patients with stage IA (confined to one ovary) and well-differentiated to moderately differentiated tumors (grades 1 or 2) the results of (1) observation and (2) melphalan 0.2 mg/kg/day for 5 days every 4 to 6 weeks for up to 12 cycles were compared. The 5-year survival results were similar, 91% and 95%, so that for these patients no further therapy is indicated.

In the second trial 141 patients with stage I poorly differentiated (grade 3) or IC tumors, as well as stage II resectable tumors (residual <2 cm), were treated with melphalan or ^{32}P. The 5-year survivals were comparable—80% in both groups. Because of the risk of leukemia with melphalan, ^{32}P appears to be a better choice. However, there was no control group of observation in the second trial, and as noted by the work of Guthrie et al., such a comparison group would be needed to demonstrate unequivocally that patients with no gross disease after operation do in fact benefit from such adjuvant therapy.

A recent study by Dembo et al. of 519 stage I patients found that adverse factors were grade of tumor, dense pelvic adherence (no invasion but adhesion), or over 250 ml of ascites. Patients without these features had a 98% 5-year survival. It appears that patients with stage I grade 3 tumors should have postoperative therapy, but data are unclear for stage I grade 2 patients.

External irradiation has been used extensively as treatment for ovarian carcinoma, particularly stage II disease. Dembo and Bush used pelvic irradiation (4500 rads to the midpoint of the pelvis) plus upper abdominal radiation, including the liver and diaphragm (2250 rads), to treat stage IB, stage II, and asymptomatic stage III ovarian cancer. They found abdominopelvic irradiation to be superior to pelvic irradiation alone or pelvic irradiation plus adjuvant chemotherapy with an alkylating agent. Over 78% of the patients treated with abdominopelvic irradiation survived at least 5 years, in comparison with 50% of those in the other treatment group. The therapy was most effective for those without gross residual disease at the completion of resection. Comparable survival results were achieved by Leers and

Kock in 127 patients with stages I, II, and III whom they treated with postoperative irradiation. However, 5 patients required operation for bowel complications, and 2 died.

The results with postoperative irradiation have not been confirmed by other treatment centers, and a randomized trial of radiation therapy versus chemotherapy for low-stage ovarian cancer has not been conducted. Data comparing the use of postoperative chemotherapy versus postoperative pelvic irradiation for patients with meticulously documented stage II disease are also not available. An additional concern regarding the use of external therapy is that the therapy compromises bone marrow function because wide areas of pelvic bone marrow are irradiated. There is also an increased risk of bowel complications if subsequent surgery is required. In general, chemotherapeutic doses must be reduced by half for patients who have had prior pelvic irradiation. In contrast, a second or third regimen of chemotherapy can be given, frequently at full doses, after primary treatment with cytotoxic agents.

ADVANCED EPITHELIAL CARCINOMAS (STAGES III AND IV). A maximal surgical resection, as previously outlined, is completed to minimize the amount of residual disease in the case of advanced ovarian cancer. Griffiths et al. subsequently showed that survival was improved for those women with residual tumor nodules of 1.5 cm or less after cytoreduction, and Aure et al. noted an improved 5-year survival of 30% for patients with stage III ovarian cancers with no residual disease after resection (see Figure 29-11). The desirability of reducing the size of the residual tumor is clear from many studies, but some of the reported results may be affected by the fact that tumors that are less advanced or less invasive are also the ones most amenable to successful cytoreductive procedures. Heintz also reported that diffuse peritoneal carcinomatosis and the presence of ascites worsen the prognosis. As previously noted, bowel resection may be needed to complete effective removal of tumor, but this procedure is not advisable if large residual tumors would be left after intestinal resection is completed. Partial cystectomies may be necessary in some cases, but urinary diversions are not recommended.

For patients who are cachectic or those who are undergoing extensive operative procedures leading to prolonged periods of compromised bowel function, total parenteral nutrition (hyperalimentation) via a centrally placed intravenous catheter that will allow delivery of 2000 to 3000 calories daily (20% dextrose, amino acids, and lipid for essential nutrients) is advised. For short-term therapy, a peripheral vein may be used and hyperalimentation accomplished with 10% dextrose and lipids, but phlebitis will eventually develop, and only about half as many calories can be administered in this manner. Patients treated with hyperalimentation are better able to tolerate intestinal resection and also appear to be more resistant to the adverse effects of subsequent chemotherapy.

As noted previously (p. 956), the term *serous surface papillary carcinoma of the ovary* is applied to cases of small (<4 cm) ovaries and widespread peritoneal tumor. These tumors, as noted by Altaras et al., often elaborate CA-125 and appear to respond best to platinum-based chemotherapy following maximal surgical debulking.

It has recently been noticed that some high grade ovarian carcinomas have predominant (>50%) histologic patterns that resemble transitional cell carcinoma (TCC) of the urinary bladder. Robey et al. compared the results of 18 stage III TCCs with 35 high-grade stage III epithelial tumors. All 53 cases had residual disease after initial operation. Those with the TCC pattern had a greatly improved prognosis with 17 of 18 (94%) responding to chemotherapy and 15 of 18 (83%) alive 4 to 10 years after treatment. In comparison, 27 of 35 (77%) of the patients with non-TCC high-grade tumors were dead of disease in an average of 2.5 years.

Postoperative chemotherapy. Until the late 1970s, chemotherapy for ovarian carcinoma was usually in the form of a single alkylating agent (melphalan, cyclophosphamide [Cytoxan], or chlorambucil (see Chapter 25). The choice of the particular agent did not appear to affect results, and complete response rates of 10% to 20% were reported, with overall responses (complete plus partial) on the order of 50%. In 1978 Young et al. reported a randomized clinical trial comparing melphalan with a four-drug combination of hexamethylmelamine, cyclophosphamide, methotrexate, and 5-fluorouracil. They noted a 75% response rate in patients treated with four drugs in comparison with 54% in those treated with melphalan alone. Subsequently it was shown that multiple-agent regimens with cisplatin produce better results than a single alkylating agent. The results of a few studies reported in the early 1980s are summarized in Table 29-7. As can be seen from this table, initial response rates are on the order of 90%, but by 4 to 5 years after treatment the survival has decreased to about 30% or less. A 5-year follow-up of 103 stage III and stage IV cases by Belinson et al. show survival in stage III of 27% and in stage IV of only 7%. Decker et al., in their 2-year study of 21 patients, used only two agents, intravenous cyclophosphamide (1000 mg/m^2) and intravenous cisplatin (50 mg/m^2) given every 4 weeks and obtained results comparable with the three- and four-drug regimens. This was confirmed in subsequent studies, including an evaluation of 349 patients by Omura et al. The patients all had less than 1 cm of residual disease, and

TABLE 29-7

Examples of Responses to Platinum-containing Regimens in Ovarian Epithelial Carcinoma

Study (First Author)	Drugs	Patients (No.)	% Initial Response (CR + PR)	% Survival	Duration of Study (Years)
Decker 1982	Cytox & Plat	21		62	2
Bruckner 1983	Hexa, Cytox, Plat, Adria	37		43	3
Wharton 1984	Melph, Plat	46		43	4
Cohen 1983	Cytox, Adria, Plat	64		56	2
	Hexa, Cytox, Plat, Adria	37		30	5
Neijt 1984	Hexa, Cytox, Plat, Adria	92	91	30 (approx)	4 (approx)
Vogl 1983	Cytox, Hexa, Plat, Adria	38	92	30 (approx)	4 (approx)
Greco 1981	Hexa, Cytox, Adria, Plat	46	95	NA	NA

CR, Complete response; *PR*, partial response; *NA*, not available; *Cytox*, cyclophosphamide (Cytoxan); *Plat*, cisplatin *Hexa*, hexamethylmelamine, *Adria*, doxorubicin (Adriamycin); *Melph*, melphalan.

there was no therapeutic advantage in the addition of doxorubicin (Adriamycin) to cyclophosphamide (Cytoxan) and cisplatin to avoid increased toxicity with apparently comparable benefit. The combination of Cytoxan (750 to 1000 mg/m^2) and cisplatin (50 to 100 mg/m^2) is frequently used for primary treatment. A recent randomized study by Conte et al. suggests that combination therapies with cisplatin or its analogue carboplatin at comparable doses have similar therapeutic effects.

All the studies indicate that the response rate is related to the amount of residual disease postoperatively, with the best results achieved for patients with minimal or no observable disease after resection. However, some patients with large residual tumors and stage III or IV disease have also achieved complete remission with multiple-agent programs containing platinum. Chemotherapy is usually begun 2 to 4 weeks postoperatively. Current evidence also indicates that younger patients achieve results superior to those of older patients. It is not clear at present to what degree platinum-containing regimens including newer agents such as carboplatin (see Chapter 25) will produce a long-term cure of ovarian carcinomas. Other modalities, such as intraperitoneal administration, may offer a therapeutic advantage (see later discussion).

Evaluation of Chemotherapy Results: Second-look Procedures

Chemotherapy is usually administered every 3 to 4 weeks. The patient is monitored with careful physical examination; blood tests to measure hematologic, liver, and kidney functions; and radiologic studies, such as chest x-ray examinations, ultrasound tests, or (usually) computed tomography (CT) scans of the abdomen and the pelvis. If tumor is suspected on CT scan, needle biopsy can frequently document the presence of persistent or recurrent disease. A negative CT scan, however, does not indicate complete clinical response. Goldhirsch et al. noted in 1983 that 5 of 26 patients with tumor nodules larger than 1 cm had negative CT scans, and the examination was most effective (80%) for detecting metastasis in retroperitoneal nodes. In 1989 Reuter et al. reported improved results of 8% false negatives using newer equipment with CT slices at 10- to 15-mm intervals. CA-125 levels are used to monitor the course of the patient with carci-

noma. A value greater than 35 U/ml is positive and is found in approximately 80% of patients with ovarian cancer. It may be predictive of recurrent disease, but high false negative rates preclude its use exclusively for monitoring patients. Hunter et al. noted that patients on multiagent-cisplatinum therapy whose CA-125 returned to normal levels (<35 u/ml) within 65 days of primary operation had an improved survival over those who did not. Buller et al. calculated that CA-125 followed an exponential regression curve in successfully treated patients. This provides the possibility of mathematically estimating early in treatment the patient's response to chemotherapy. Usually a second-look laparotomy is employed to evaluate the patient who appears to have had a complete response to chemotherapy, although the use of this procedure is controversial.

Occasionally the problem arises of a patient who was incompletely resected at initial operation, usually because an ovarian cancer was not suspected preoperatively. Some therapists advocate reexploration to achieve maximum debulking. An alternative approach was suggested by Lawton et al., who administered 3 cycles of platinum-based multiagent chemotherapy to 36 incompletely resected ovarian cancer patients. They concluded such neoadjuvant therapy improved the likelihood of successful resection and subsequent effectiveness of chemotherapy.

Some therapists perform a laparoscopy before second-look laparotomy. If gross tumor is not visualized and biopsy specimens and cytologic sampling through the laparoscope are negative, an exploration is then performed. Many prefer to use only the second-look laparotomy not only to confirm the presence or absence of tumor but also to remove residual tumor. The steps of an adequate second-look laparotomy are as follows:

1. Exploratory laparotomy is done with sampling of any free peritoneal fluid for cytologic study.
2. Saline washings for cytologic evaluation are taken from the pelvis and abdomen, usually separately from each hemidiaphragm, and from the gutters lateral to the ascending and descending colon. The hemidiaphragms can be effectively sampled by scraping with a tongue depressor and spreading the scrapings on a slide, fixing them in the operating room, and sending them for analysis.

3. Multiple-biopsy specimens are taken of any adhesions and nodules suggestive of tumor, as well as areas that previously contained tumors, with particular attention to the areas of residual disease noted at initial laparotomy.

4. Biopsy specimens are taken from the cul-de-sac and bladder peritoneum, the areas of the infundibulopelvic ligament, and the upper part of the abdomen, including the omentum along the transverse colon.

5. Any residual omentum is removed.

6. The retroperitoneal paraaortic and pelvic nodes from which biopsy specimens had not previously been taken or that have become enlarged are sampled for histologic evaluation.

There are conflicting opinions regarding the value and indications of second-look laparotomy in the therapy of ovarian cancer. Initially it was thought that those who were found to be free of disease could then have treatment safely discontinued. However, subsequent studies have shown that many patients with negative second-look operation eventually develop recurrent disease. Early studies of second-look laparotomy showed about half (25% to 75%) of the patients thought clinically and radiologically to be free of disease actually had persistent disease at second-look operation. In a study by Berek et al. of 56 stage III or stage IV patients, almost half had visible disease, and in a series of 135 patients reported by Podratz et al., including those with lower-stage disease, only 58% had a negative second-look procedure. More recent data from Walton et al. show that few patients who initially have stage I or II disease have positive second-look procedures, and they recommend the operation not be done for those with low-stage tumors, a result confirmed by Sonnendecker. However, in Walton's study of stage I and stage II cases, 13% did have positive findings at second-look operation. Carmichael et al. noted a positive second-look operation was more likely in patients with high-stage tumors (IV > III), those who had microscopic disease at the end of the initial operation, older patients (>60 years of age), or those with poor performance status. In a GOG Cooperative Study of 186 stage III patients who initially had less than 3 cm of residual disease after primary operation, Creasman et al. noted 49% had a negative second look. Favorable factors were low tumor grade, no residual disease af-

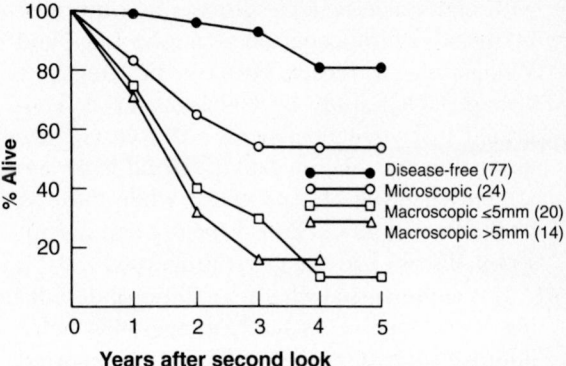

FIGURE 29-14
Survival rates for patients with ovarian carcinomas, second-look procedures. (From Podratz KC, Malkasian GD, Hilton JF, et al: Am J Obstet Gynecol 152:230, 1985.)

ter primary operation, and young age (<55 years).

Timing of the operation has varied in recent times. Hainsworth reported that 96% of chemotherapy responses occur within 6 months, an observation confirmed by Lund et al., who thought that if a response to chemotherapy is to occur, it will be evident after 6 cycles of platinum-based treatment. Currently most therapists have shortened the time of chemotherapy so that second-look operation usually takes place after 6 cycles rather than 12 cycles.

SURVIVAL RESULTS AFTER SECOND-LOOK OPERATION. The survival of patients after second-look operation varies with the findings, as noted by Friedman and Weiss. Recurrence rates have varied from 5% to 57% after negative second-look procedures. Podratz et al. (Figure 29-14) in a series of 135 patients noted a 5-year survival rate of over 80%, although some of his patients had lower-stage disease. Podczaski noted that half of 28 stage III patients with negative second look had recurrence. In a recent study Rubin et al. noted a high (45%) rate of recurrence in patients with negative second-look laparotomy. Those initially with higher-stage and higher-grade tumors are more likely to recur after second-look operation.

In general, survival results decrease if microscopic disease is found and progressively deteriorate if gross disease is found. Survival is also related to the grade of the tumor. Those with low-grade microscopic disease at second-look operation have survival rates superior to those with high-grade residual disease, as confirmed by the studies of Copeland et al. and Lund and Williamson. A recent Gynecologic Oncology Group (GOG) study by Creasman et al. confirmed that younger patients (<55 years), low grade tumors, and negative second-look laparotomy had the best prognosis while those ≥ 55 years, with grade 2 or 3 tumors and macroscopic disease had the worst prognosis.

It is controversial whether additional debulking at the time of second-look operation helps improve survival rates. Hoskins et al. reported on 67 patients who underwent second-look operation. Of these, 16 were found to have minimal disease and had a 5-year survival rate of 62% in comparison with a 51% 5-year survival rate for 17 patients who were successfully cytoreduced to microscopic disease. The authors concluded that additional operative debulking was indicated if the patients could be successfully reduced to microscopic disease. Some patients are discovered to have recurrent ovarian carcinoma years after primary therapy. Recent studies by Markman et al. and others indicate that secondary platinum-based regimens are more likely to produce a response if the patient initially responded to a platinum regimen and was at least 2 years from the completion of initial therapy. The likelihood of response increases the longer the interval since primary treatment.

A randomized clinical trial is needed to demonstrate the optimal management of patients after second-look operation and also to determine the potential value of the procedure. In view of known failure rates even after negative second-look procedure, some have continued systemic treatment for 3 cycles after a negative second look and 6 cycles if microscopic disease is present. Neijt et al. noted 36-month survival rates of 75% and 65% respectively after this protocol. Recently great attention has been given to the potential advantages of intraperitoneal chemotherapy. In addition, efforts have been made with intraperitoneal radiation and whole abdominal radiation (WAR), which are considered later in this section.

INTRAPERITONEAL THERAPY. Intraperitoneal instillation of chemotherapeutic agents has been tried recently to increase the effect of cytotoxic drugs on the tumor within the abdominal cavity. High intraperitoneal concentrations are achieved with instillation of the drug into the peritoneal cavity. Eventually serum levels comparable to those seen after intravenous therapy are obtained. The drug can be instilled with a catheter similar to that used for peritoneal dialysis. One modification is shown in Figure 29-15, A, in which a needle is allowed subcutaneous access through the skin into the port to administer the chemotherapy intraperitoneally through the catheter. The advantages of the pharmacokinetics of intraperitoneal therapy have been recently reviewed by McClay and Howell.

In brief, the drug is administered into the peritoneal cavity (Figure 29-15, B), and the total intraperitoneal drug exposure is a function of its concentration in the cavity and the length of time it takes the drug to escape the peritoneal cavity. Thus the effectiveness of the drug is increased by higher intraperitoneal concentrations and longer residence within the peritoneal cavity before escaping into the systemic circulation. The ideal agent would be one that slowly leaves the peritoneal cavity but then is rapidly metabolized once it reaches the systemic circulation, thus reducing side effects of the agent. In general, peritoneal absorption is decreased as molecular weight increases and lipid solubility decreases. In addition, drugs that are highly ionized at physiologic pH absorb more slowly from the peritoneal cavity than un-ionized agents. With these considerations, various drugs are being studied to develop the most effective intraperitoneal regimens. In general, 2 liters of fluid containing the therapeutic drugs are administered through the system as shown in Figure 29-15, B, in about 30 minutes to obtain a widespread distribution. Most trials of intraperitoneal chemotherapy for ovarian cancer have been used with combinations containing cisplatin. Sodium thiosulfate is given systemically to reduce the nephrotoxic effect of the absorbed cisplatin. Howell et al. treated 25 patients with cisplatin, cytoarabine, and doxorubicin. Patients with residual disease less than 2 cm had immediate survival of more than 49 months compared with only 8 months for those with residual tumors greater than 2 cm. In a recent study Markman et al. obtained complete responses in patients whose disease was <1 cm in diameter. Piver et al. used cisplatin, cytoarabine, and bleomycin in 31 patients with residual disease at second-look operation. Of 15 patients with disease less than 1 cm in diameter, 5 had complete responses, proven at a third-look operation. However, agents such as Adriamycin and bleomycin cause acute peritoneal reactions, making them difficult to use by this route. More recently Reichman et al. used cisplatin

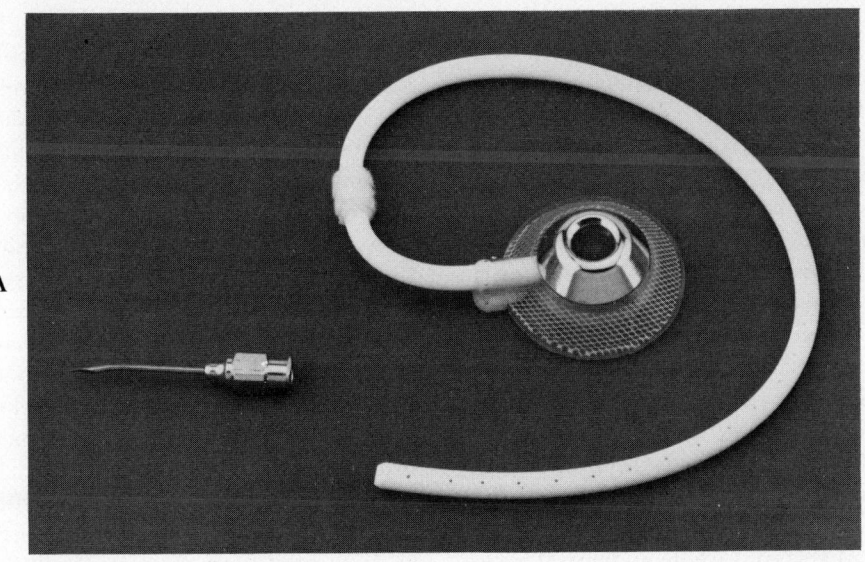

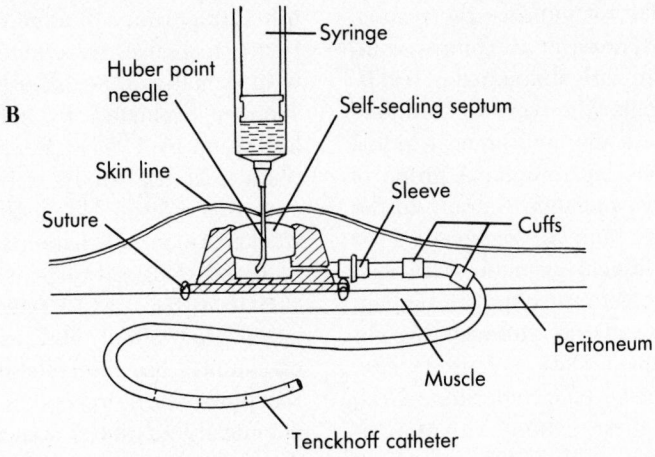

FIGURE 29-15
A, Peritoneal catheter with access port for infusion of drugs. **B,** Totally impaired peritoneal access system (Port-A-Cath, Pharmacia Deltec, Inc.) (**B,** From McClay EF and Howell SB: Gynecol Oncol 36:1, 1990.)

(100 mg/m^2) and etoposide (VP-16) (200 mg/m^2) intraperitoneally monthly for 6 months on 57 patients. A documented complete response occurred in 12 (21%), but the ultimate effect of this treatment on survival is not known. In a phase II trial, Kirmani et al. treated 37 patients with IP cisplatin (200 mg/m^2) and IP VP-16 (350 $\text{mg/m}^2)$ with Thiosulfate intravenous protection for a median of 6 cycles every 4 weeks. Twenty-four of the patients were clinically free of disease at the end of therapy, and 9 of 11 who were reexplored were free of disease. These studies suggest a potential role of second-look operation, if residual disease can be reduced to small volumes, which would then theoretically be more susceptible to intraperi-

toneal chemotherapy treatment. Antibody-guided intraperitoneal irradiation therapy is briefly considered in the section on immunotherapy. Nonspecific intraperitoneal ^{32}P is discussed in the irradiation treatment section.

IRRADIATION THERAPY. Intraperitoneal installation of radioactive ^{32}P has also been used to improve survival. Soper et al. treated 23 patients who had minimal disease at second- or third-look operation. Of these, 10 were free of disease 13 to 94 months after treatment, but there were three bowel complications requiring operation. In a study of 31 patients with negative second-look operation, Spencer et al. treated 14 patients with ^{32}P and noted no recurrences with 2 to 4 years follow-up compared with 4 of 17 recurrences among those who received no therapy. The differences between these groups, however, did not attain statistical significance.

Whole abdominal radiation (WAR) has also been studied to improve salvage, with varying results and a high frequency of bowel complications, often serious and requiring operative intervention. Morgan et al. suggested an alternative to traditional whole abdominal radiation, which is usually given at the rate of 160 to 200 cGy per day. They treated patients with a program of hyperfractionation, that is, 80 cGy twice a day, and noted no bowel complications. On the other hand, Goldhirsch et al. studied whole abdominal radiation in 45 patients who had pathologic complete responses. A group of 24 received whole abdominal radiation and the remainder no therapy. The addition of irradiation did not improve the results. In a recent study, Menczer et al. compared intraperitoneal cisplatin with abdominal pelvic irradiation in individuals who were in complete clinical remission with minimal or no residual disease at second-look laparotomy. A group of 18 patients received irradiation therapy to the abdomen and pelvis, and 19 received three courses of intraperitoneal cisplatin with systemic thiosulfate protection. A statistically significant difference in overall survival was observed at 36 months (76.6% versus 44.4%), suggesting an advantage to intraperitoneal cisplatin treatment in these patients in comparison with irradiation. Similar effectiveness of chemotherapy over radiotherapy in these patients was recently reported by Bruzzone et al. Because of the risk of complications and the lack of extensive data regarding its effectiveness, whole abdominal radiation is generally not used in these cases.

Complications and Alternative Considerations

MALIGNANT EFFUSIONS. Patients with ovarian cancer frequently develop ascites or hydrothorax or both, requiring repeated drainage by paracentesis or thoracentesis. Occasionally sclerosing solutions are used in the thoracic cavity to prevent reaccumulation of fluid, with resultant adherence of the pleural surfaces. Nitrogen mustard, tetracycline, and quinacrine have all been used successfully for this purpose.

IMMUNOTHERAPY. Immunotherapy agents, such as *Corynebacterium parvum* (C-Parvum),

and bacille Calmette-Guérin (BCG) have been administered to try to augment the immunologic response and promote tumor resistance in the host. These agents have also been used in combination with cytotoxic chemotherapy, and preliminary improved results have been reported; long-term studies are not available. New approaches with intraperitoneal immunotherapy are being evaluated with such agents as interferon, lymphokine-activated killer (LAK) cells, interleukin-2 tumor necrosis factor (TNF), and other immunomodulators. Further studies are needed to define the effectiveness of these and other immunologic modifiers on ovarian cancer (see Chapter 25). The use of monoclonal antibodies as a form of site-directed therapy is also being investigated. Epenetos et al. have used tumor-associated antigens linked to ^{131}I to treat recurrent ovarian carcinoma. After intraperitoneal administration to 24 patients, responses were noted primarily in those with small-volume disease, with some responses evaluated by follow-up laparoscopy lasting up to 3 years. Berek et al. conducted a phase I-II trial of IP cisplatinum (60 mg/m^2) and α-Interferon (25 × 10^6 IV) given every 4 weeks. Among 18 patients there were 3 complete and 4 partial responses.

HORMONE RECEPTORS. Holt et al. have noted that about 50% of ovarian epithelial carcinomas have detectable levels of estrogen receptors. These receptors are similar physicochemically to those noted in breast and endometrial carcinomas. However, their presence in ovarian carcinomas does not, in general, appear to correlate with tumor differentiation or clinical behavior. Hormone therapy with progestins and antiestrogens such as tamoxifen has been tried, and a few isolated reports of responses or stabilization of disease have been reported.

HUMAN TUMOR STEM CELL ASSAY. The in vitro method of human tumor stem cell assay was developed by Salmon et al. in 1978. The test is based on the growth of cultured cells in vitro, which are then tested against a variety of chemotherapeutic agents. Such clonogenic assays may someday provide useful clinical information regarding drug selection for chemotherapy in gynecologic malignancies, but at present they are not reliable for regular clinical use.

SUMMARY

Therapy for epithelial ovarian carcinoma is based on removal of all gross disease and sampling of areas at high risk for spread in the peritoneal cavity and retroperitoneal nodes. Postoperative therapy is employed depending on the stage and grade of the primary tumor. For accurately staged cases, postoperative ^{32}P is used in low-stage tumors, such as stage IC carcinomas where there is a risk of intraperitoneal tumor seeding but no residual disease.

External irradiation has been effective in tumor treatment, especially in accurately documented stage II cases, but its use usually compromises bone marrow function and interferes with the future use of chemotherapy. Single-agent alkylating therapy has been employed as adjunctive treatment for poorly differentiated tumors, such as stage I, grade 3, or for stage II cases without residual tumor, but such treatment carries with it a high risk of subsequent development of leukemia, which may reach 10% by 8 years after therapy.

Multiple-agent chemotherapy, usually Cytoxan and cisplatin, is used for treatment of high-stage tumors and for patients with residual disease after initial tumor resection. It is accompanied by multiple short- and long-term toxic side effects but results in initial response rates in advanced cases that may exceed 90%. Five-year survival rates drop to 30% or less. Intraperitoneal therapy, especially for small residual disease, may improve these results. Long-term randomized trials will be needed to improve rates of salvage and to optimize therapy for epithelial ovarian carcinomas.

SMALL CELL CARCINOMA

Dickerson et al. described a new and virulent type of ovarian malignancy that occurs in young women, usually between the ages of 15 and 30 years. Because of its histologic appearance, it has been designated a small cell carcinoma. The tumor is often but not always accompanied by hypercalcemia. Most patients have died, although a few stage I survivors have been reported, some of whom have been treated with adjuvant multiagent chemotherapy. However, for advanced-stage disease, even in most stage I cases, the course of the tumor has been fatal. Senekjian et al. suggested multiagent chemotherapy may be of benefit.

GERM CELL TUMORS

These tumors are derived from the germ cells of the ovary. As a group they are the sec-

WHO CLASSIFICATION OF GERM CELL TUMORS

Dysgerminoma
Endodermal sinus tumor
Embryonal carcinoma
Polyembryoma
Choriocarcinoma
Teratomas
  Immature
  Mature
    Solid
    Cystic
      Dermoid cyst (mature cystic teratoma)
      Dermoid cyst with malignant transformation
  Monodermal and highly specialized
    Struma ovarii
    Carcinoid
    Struma ovarii and carcinoid
    Others
Mixed forms

ond most frequent of ovarian neoplasms, and they account for about 20% to 25% of all ovarian tumors. The classification of germ cell tumors according to the World Health Organization (WHO) designation is shown in the box above.

The most frequent germ cell tumor is the benign cystic teratoma (dermoid); overall, only 2% to 3% of germ cell tumors are malignant. Among the malignant germ cell tumors, the most frequent is the dysgerminoma, which accounts for about 45% of malignant germ cell tumors. Next in frequency are the immature teratomas and then endodermal sinus tumors. In female patients under age 30, germ cell tumors are the most frequent ovarian neoplasm, and about one third of the germ cell tumors encountered in those under age 21 are malignant.

The histogenesis of germ cell tumors has been extensively studied and summarized by Talerman. Figure 29-16 shows the theory of the histogenesis of these tumors—that they originate from the primitive germ cell and then gradually differentiate to mimic the developmental tissues of embryonic origin (ectoderm, mesoderm, or endoderm) and the extraembryonic tissues (yolk sac and trophoblast). Germ cell tumors that originate in the ovary have homologous counterparts in the testes, that is, dysgerminoma and seminoma. Germ cell tumors are usually unilateral, with the exception of teratomas and dysgerminomas (see Table 29-3). The morphologic and clinical aspects of each of the various types of germ cell tumors will be separately considered.

Teratomas

Teratomas consist of tissues that recapitulate the three layers of the developing embryo (ectoderm, mesoderm, and endoderm). One or more of the layers may be represented, and the tissues can be mature (benign) or immature (malignant). Chromosomal studies indicate that teratomas appear to arise from a single germ and have an XX karyotype. In the older literature, terms such as *malignant teratoma* and *teratocarcinoma* were used to denote the malignant variety of these tumors, but these terms have been replaced by the nomenclature shown in the box on p. 967.

Benign Cystic Teratomas (Dermoids)

Benign cystic teratomas are the most common germ cell tumors and account for 25% of all ovarian neoplasms. They primarily occur during the reproductive years but may occur in postmenopausal women and in children. The risk of malignant transformation (see later discussion) is markedly increased if these tumors are found in postmenopausal women. One of the interesting facets of teratomas is their ability to produce adult tissue, including skin, bone, teeth, hair, and dermal tissue. The presence of calcified bone or teeth allows the tumor to be diagnosed preoperatively with ultrasound or radiography, the latter having been reported to detect dermoids preoperatively in about one third of the cases (Figures 29-17 and 29-18).

Dermoids are usually unilateral, but 10% to 15% are bilateral. The outside wall of the tumor tends to be smooth with a yellowish appearance caused by the sebaceous fatty material that fills the tumor. Hair is also a prominent feature once the cyst is opened (Figure 29-19). Usually the tumors are asymptomatic, but they can cause severe pain if there is torsion or if the sebaceous material perforates the cyst wall, leading to a reactive peritonitis. This rare complication is severe and can occur during pregnancy. Microscopically a number of adult tissues are seen (Figure 29-20).

Treatment of the reproductive-age female patient or of the child consists of either cystectomy or unilateral oophorectomy. In most cases it should be possible to remove only the cyst

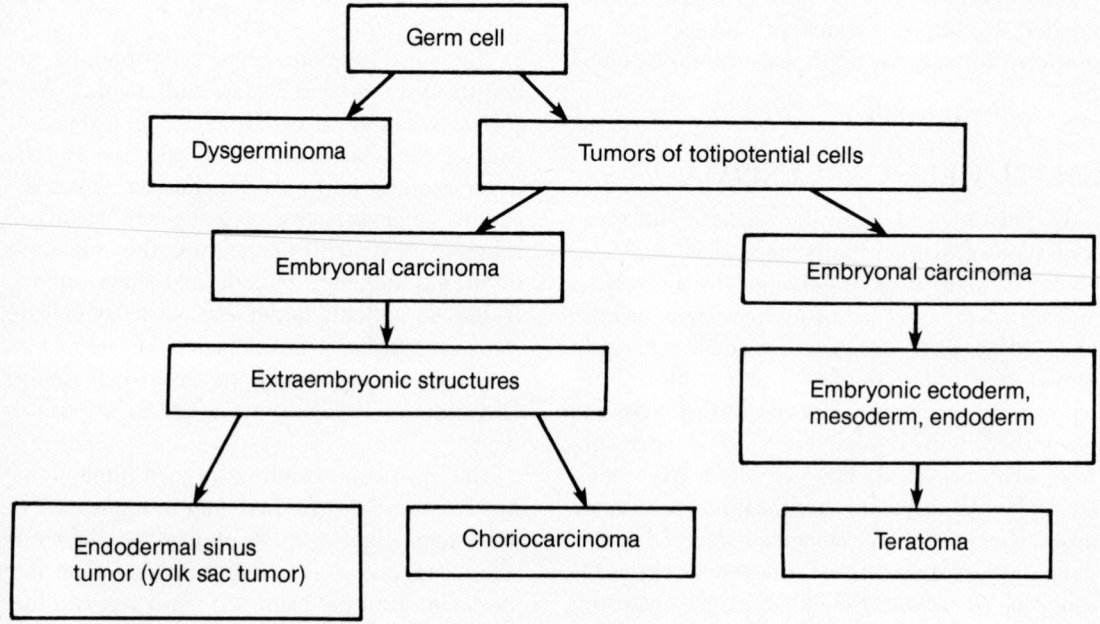

FIGURE 29-16
Histogenesis of germ cell tumors. (Modified from Talerman A: Germ cell tumors of the ovary. In Blaustein A, editor: Pathology of the female genital tract, New York, 1982, Springer-Verlag)

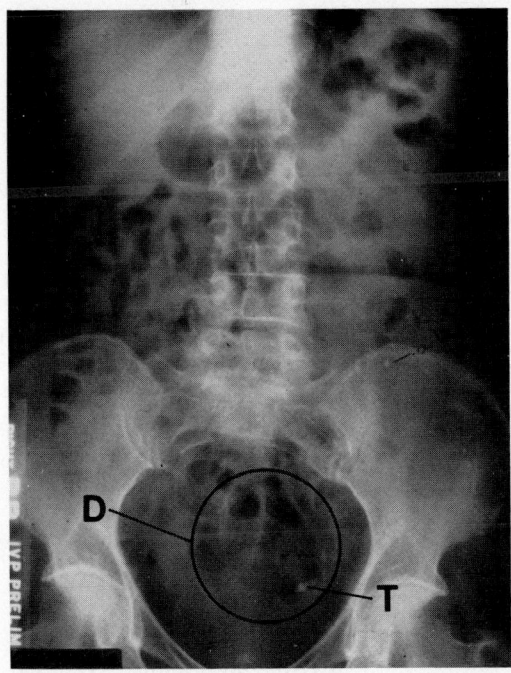

FIGURE 29-17
X-ray film of a dermoid. *D*, Dermoid; *T*, tooth. (Courtesy Dr. E.K. Senekjian.)

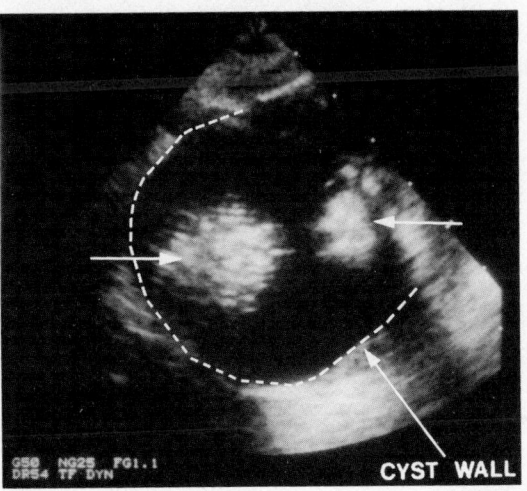

FIGURE 29-18
Transvaginal ultrasound image of an ovarian dermoid cyst. The arrows indicate balls of hair. (Courtesy Dr. Zubie Sheikh, The University of Chicago, Department of Obstetrics & Gynecology.)

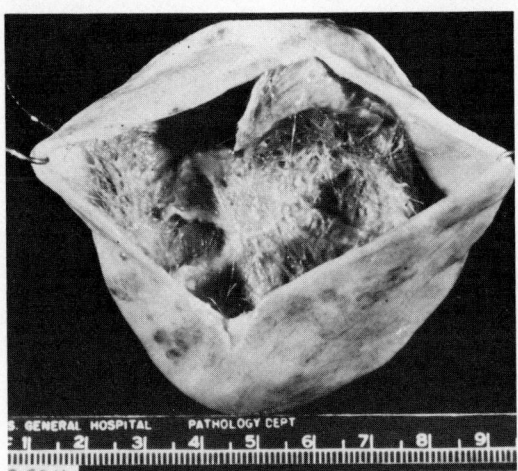

FIGURE 29-19
Gross specimen of a dermoid cyst that was filled with sebaceous material and hair. (Courtesy Dr. R.E. Scully.)

and preserve normal ovarian tissue. The technique is demonstrated in Figure 29-21. The opposite ovary should be inspected. If it is grossly normal, nothing further need be done. In the past, bivalving of a normal-appearing ovary was suggested to rule out a contralateral dermoid, but this procedure results in a high risk of adhesions and subsequent infertility. Doss et al. studied 148 women with ovarian teratomas who

had a grossly normal-appearing contralateral ovary. Ninety of them had a biopsy or tissue removed from the opposite normal-appearing contralateral ovary, and no dermoid was detected. The 58 other patients did not have a surgical procedure on the contralateral ovary, and subsequently only one of these patients (0.6% of the total) required laparotomy for a dermoid. These data strongly reinforce the de-

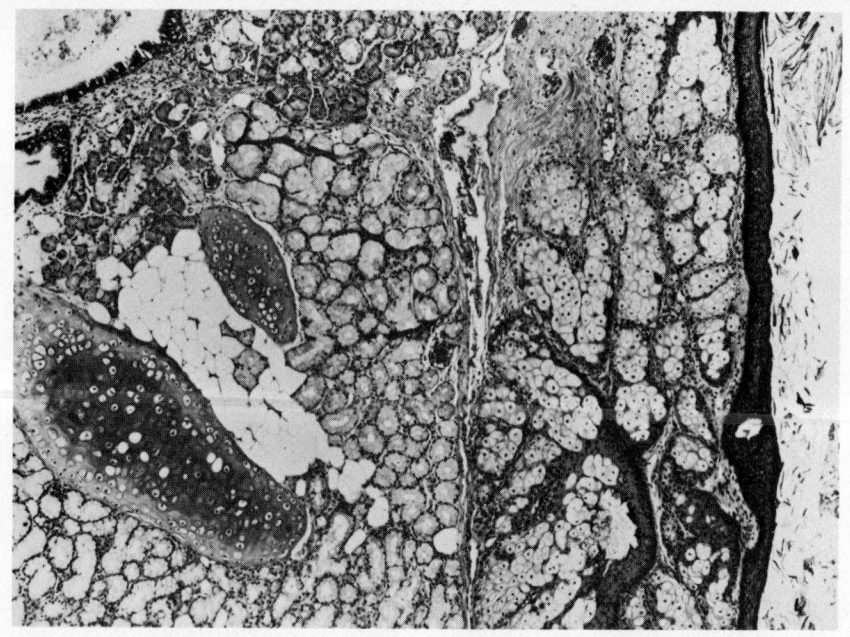

FIGURE 29-20
Photomicrograph of dermoid. Cartilage is shown *(right)* lined by epidermis and accompanying appendages *(left)*. (×50.) (From Serov SF, Scully RE, and Sobin LH: Histologic typing of ovarian tumors. Geneva, 1973, World Health Organization.)

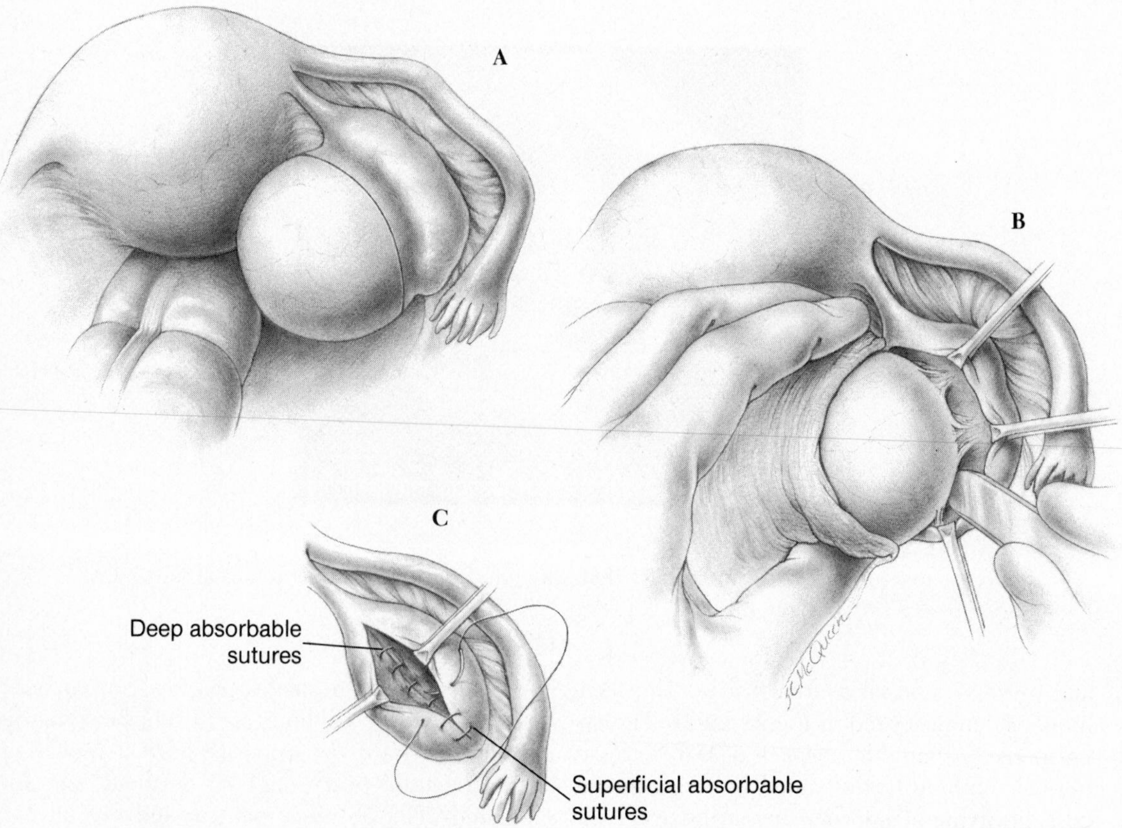

A

B

C

Deep absorbable
sutures

Superficial absorbable
sutures

FIGURE 29-21
Shelling out of teratoma. **A,** Scalpel incision in ovary at intersection of dermoid and normal ovary. **B,** Dermoid being separated. Note how upper part peels away. **C,** Reconstruction of normal ovary.

sirability of inspecting only the contralateral ovary if it appears grossly normal. In women beyond childbearing years, therapy for a dermoid usually consists of removal of the uterus, both tubes, and the ovaries.

Occasionally teratomas may be solid and may consist only of adult tissues, leading to the diagnosis of solid, mature teratoma. These benign germ cell tumors are rare.

A cystic teratoma can undergo malignant degeneration, which usually occurs in the squamous epithelial elements of the dermoid, producing a squamous cell carcinoma. It is a rare complication estimated to occur in fewer than 2% of these tumors, most frequently in postmenopausal women. If the malignant tissue has spread beyond the confines of the ovary, the prognosis is poor. In such cases additional therapy for squamous cell carcinoma with irradiation or chemotherapy or both are indicated.

Immature Teratomas

Immature teratomas are malignant and account for up to 20% of the malignant ovarian tumors found in women under the age of 20 but less than 1% of all ovarian cancers. They have not been documented to occur in women after menopause. They consist of immature embryonic structures that can be admixed with mature elements.

The prognosis for patients with immature teratomas is related to the stage (FIGO) and grade of the tumor. The grade of the tumor is based on the degree of immaturity of the various tissues. Grade 3 tumors consist of the most immature tissues and often have a high proportion of immature neuroepithelium. Figure 29-22 shows the survival of patients with immature teratomas by stage and grade before the advent of modern chemotherapy. Because these tumors occur in young women, preservation of childbearing function is an important consideration. Kurman and Norris reported that patients with stage IA immature teratoma had a 10-year actuarial survival of 70% after unilateral salpingo-oophorectomy; this rate is comparable to that recorded after bilateral salpingo-oophorectomy. The opposite ovary is rarely involved by immature teratoma, although a benign cystic teratoma (dermoid) is present in about 10% of cases. If the opposite ovary appears grossly normal, unilateral salp-

ingo-oophorectomy alone is adequate. If there is extension of tumor outside the ovary, implants and metastases should be extensively sampled and graded histologically to decide on therapy. The retroperitoneal nodes also should be evaluated and sampled, especially for grades 2 and 3 cases.

Multiple-agent chemotherapy has greatly improved the outlook for patients with immature teratoma. A widely used protocol is the so-called VAC regimen (vincristine, 1.5 mg/m^2 given intravenously weekly for 12 weeks and actinomycin D, 0.5 mg, with cyclophosphamide [Cytoxan] 5 to 7 mg/kg/day given intravenously daily for 5 days every 4 weeks). Gershenson et al. noted excellent chemotherapy results with immature teratoma. Of 21 patients stages I to III treated with VAC, 18 survived. The progression-free survival rate was significantly better for those who received postoperative chemotherapy in comparison with those who did not (approximately 90% versus 10%). All 22 patients who underwent second-look laparotomy were free of disease. Conversion of metastatic immature teratoma (grades 2 and 3) after chemotherapy to mature elements (grade 0) has been reported by DiSaia et al. Mature elements require no further therapy. Another effective chemotherapy is vinblastine, bleomycin, and cisplatin (VBP) (see "Endodermal Sinus Tumors").

Chemotherapy is indicated for metastatic immature teratoma (other than grade 0). For stage IA tumors that are composed of grade 2 or 3 elements, adjunctive chemotherapy is indicated because of the associated poor prognosis for tumors of these grades (see Figure 29-22). If metastatic disease is noted at primary operation, a second-look procedure is performed after completion of chemotherapy, usually in 6 months. For patients with grade 1 primary tumors with or without grade 0 implants, no further therapy is needed. (See later discussion on chemotherapy of germ cell tumors.)

Specialized Germ Cell Tumors— Struma Ovarii and Carcinoids

Specialized ovarian germ cell tumors are rare; two types are commonly recognized (see box on p. 967): the struma ovarii and carcinoids. Struma ovarii are dermoids with thyroid tissue exclusively or as a major component.

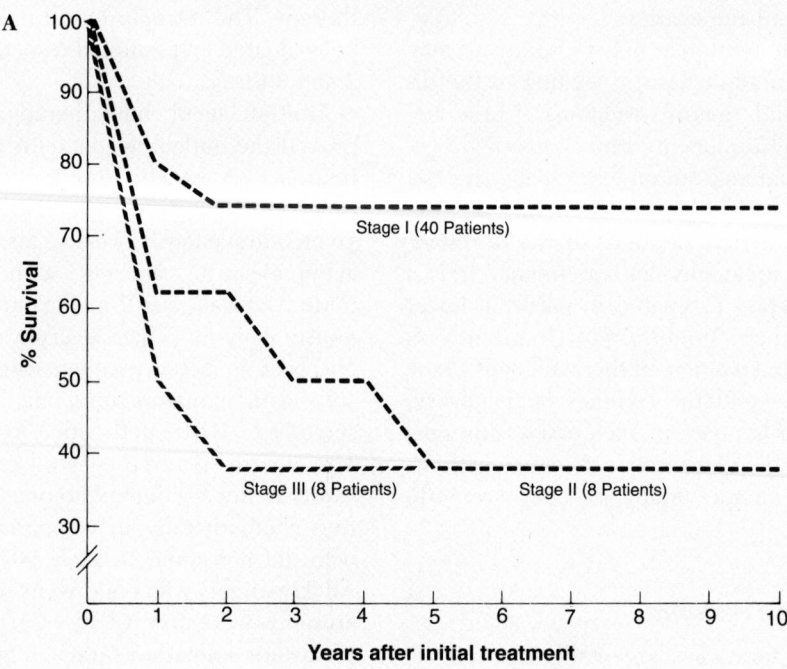

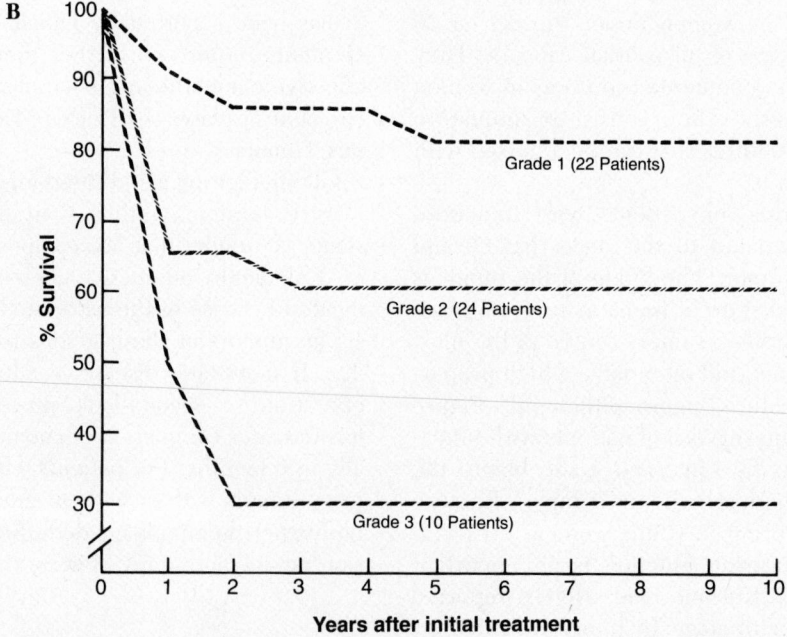

FIGURE 29-22
A, Actuarial survival of 56 patients with malignant teratoma by neoplasm stage. **B,** By neoplasm grade. (From Norris HJ, Zirkin JH, and Benson WL: Cancer 37:2359, 1976.)

The thyroid tissue can be functional, leading to clinical hyperthyroidism. Most of these tumors are benign, but malignant changes are possible. Metastatic disease, if present, has been reported to be effectively treated with ^{131}I, as is thyroid carcinoma.

Carcinoids are ovarian teratomas that histologically resemble similar tumors in the gastrointestinal tract. Carcinoids are rare and are unilateral in the ovary. In about 30% of cases a true carcinoid syndrome will develop, and 5-hydroxyindoleacetic acid (5-HIAA) can be detected and used to monitor the tumor postoperatively. These tumors occur primarily in older women and tend to grow slowly; the prognosis after hysterectomy and bilateral salpingo-oophorectomy is excellent. For a young woman desiring preservation of childbearing function, a stage IA carcinoid can be treated by unilateral salpingo-oophorectomy.

Dysgerminomas

Dysgerminomas are the most common type of malignant germ cell tumors. They consist of primitive germ cells with stroma infiltrated by lymphocytes (Figure 29-23). They are analogous to seminoma in the male testis, and they comprise about 1% of ovarian malignancies. Dysgerminomas occur primarily in women under the age of 30. The tumor is often discovered during pregnancy. Some arise in dysgenetic gonads (see later discussion of gonadoblastomas). Unlike other malignant germ cell tumors, dysgerminomas are bilateral in about 10% of cases (see Table 29-3); therefore sampling of the contralateral ovary is indicated in cases of apparent stage IA dysgerminoma. The prognosis is related to tumor size (improved if less than 15 cm), unilaterality, encapsulation (not ruptured), lack of spread to retroperitoneal nodes, and lack of ascites. If all these criteria are present, the prognosis in stage IA cases is excellent (greater than 90% 5-year survival). Fortunately about two thirds of the cases present as stage IA.

Insofar as patients with dysgerminoma are young, preservation of childbearing function is desirable, if possible. The tumor can spread within the peritoneal cavity and to retroperito-

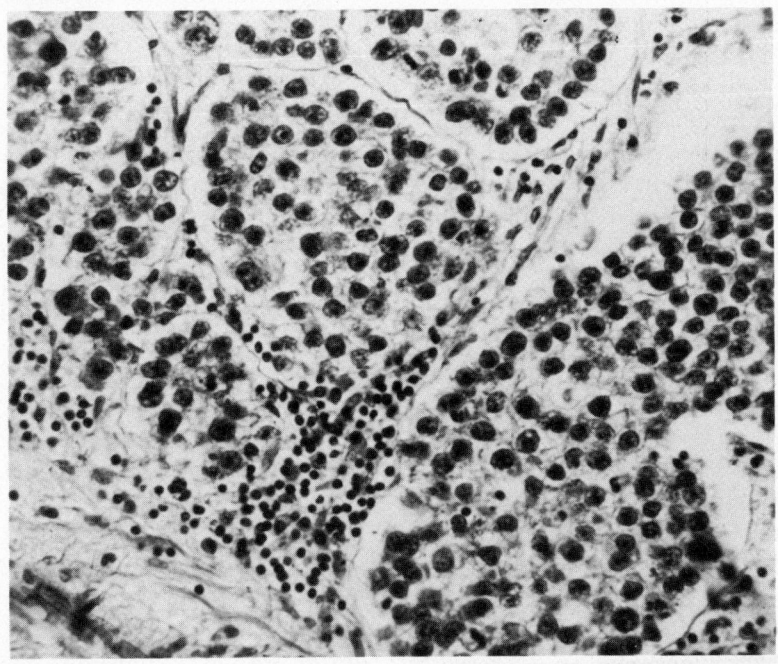

FIGURE 29-23
Dysgerminoma. (×300.) Dysgerminoma cells are demonstrated, as well as infiltration of stroma by lymphocytes. (From Scully RE: Germ cell tumors of the ovary and fallopian tube. In Meigs JV and Sturgis SH, editors: Progress in gynecology, vol 4, New York, 1963, Grune & Stratton.)

neal nodes, a more likely occurrence with larger dysgerminomas. If the tumor is confined to one ovary, a unilateral salpingo-oophorectomy should be performed and the abdomen thoroughly explored to determine the presence of intraperitoneal and retroperitoneal spread. Pelvic and paraaortic nodes should be sampled and any enlarged nodes excised. The contralateral ovary should have a wedge biopsy even if it appears normal. If frozen section indicates pure dysgerminoma and there is no evidence of spread outside the primary tumor, only a unilateral salpingo-oophorectomy is indicated. Patients so treated have a 5-year survival in excess of 90%. Assadourian and Taylor noted that unilateral salpingo-oophorectomy was as effective as more radical treatment for unilateral dysgerminoma. There can be a recurrence in as many as 20% of cases, primarily in tumors over 15 cm, but most of these tumors can be effectively treated by an additional operative procedure or irradiation or chemotherapy. These tumors are extremely radiosensitive and can be cured with less than 3000 cGy, a dosage used to treat extraovarian residual tumor after primary surgery or for recurrence.

Thomas et al. recommend 2500 cGy for radiotherapy of dysgerminoma and 3500 cGy if the mass is over 15 cm. For stage IA cases they advocate unilateral salpingo-oophorectomy. Although recurrences may reach 20%, cure rates with subsequent treatment reach 100%, similar to seminoma of the testes. The authors advocate chemotherapy for advanced disease in patients desiring to preserve fertility. In a recent report from the Radiumhemmet, Bjorkholm et al. achieved a 5-year survival of 83%. For cases treated with megavoltage since 1963, there were no deaths in their series. Among their stage IA cases treated with unilateral adnexectomy and unilateral external radiation with blocking of the contralateral side, 14 women subsequently gave birth to 21 children.

Patients treated conservatively should be closely followed up and periodic CT scans performed to monitor the abdominal cavity and retroperitoneal nodes. Occasionally the serum lactic dehydrogenase (LDH) is elevated as a nonspecific tumor marker as recently summarized by Schwartz and Norris. Lymphangiography has also been frequently employed to check on the status of the retroperitoneal nodes.

The successful therapy of germ cell tumors with VAC (see previous section on immature teratoma), as well as VBP (see later section on endodermal sinus tumor) and other multiple-agent regimens, has improved the prognosis and results of all germ cell tumors. Effective regressions have been accomplished and menstrual and childbearing function have been preserved in many of these patients after successful chemotherapy. Wu et al. reported 6 normal pregnancies among 12 married women previously treated successfully by chemotherapy for malignant germ cell tumors.

It is important to emphasize that these considerations apply to pure dysgerminoma. Other germ cell elements may coexist with these tumors (mixed germ cell tumor), in which case the prognosis is markedly worse. Some of the reports in the earlier literature of poor prognosis with unilateral dysgerminoma were probably unrecognized cases of mixed germ cell tumors, such as would be suggested if alpha-fetoprotein is found elevated in a case thought to be dysgerminoma (see later discussion). However, minor elevations of HCG have been reported in pure dysgerminoma. If the levels exceed 100 mIU/ml, the tumor probably contains choriocarcinoma elements and should be considered a mixed germ cell tumor.

Endodermal Sinus Tumors (Yolk Sac Tumors)

The endodermal sinus tumor, which comprises 10% of malignant germ cell tumors, in part resembles the yolk sac of the rodent placenta, thus recapitulating extraembryonic tissues (see Figure 29-16). One typical histologic pattern is shown in Figure 29-24. Other terms have been applied to this tumor, including mesonephroma and embryonalcarcinoma, but these terms are no longer used. The tumor secretes alpha-fetoprotein, which is a specific marker that is useful in identifying and following these tumors clinically.

These rapidly growing tumors occur in females between 13 months and 45 years of age. A median age of 19 years at diagnosis was noted by Kurman and Norris. Stage IA cases can be treated by unilateral adnexectomy. Before modern chemotherapy, the tumor was usually fatal, even if it was confined to one ovary. Therefore patients with endodermal sinus tumor should undergo chemotherapy postoperatively. The VAC protocol (see previous

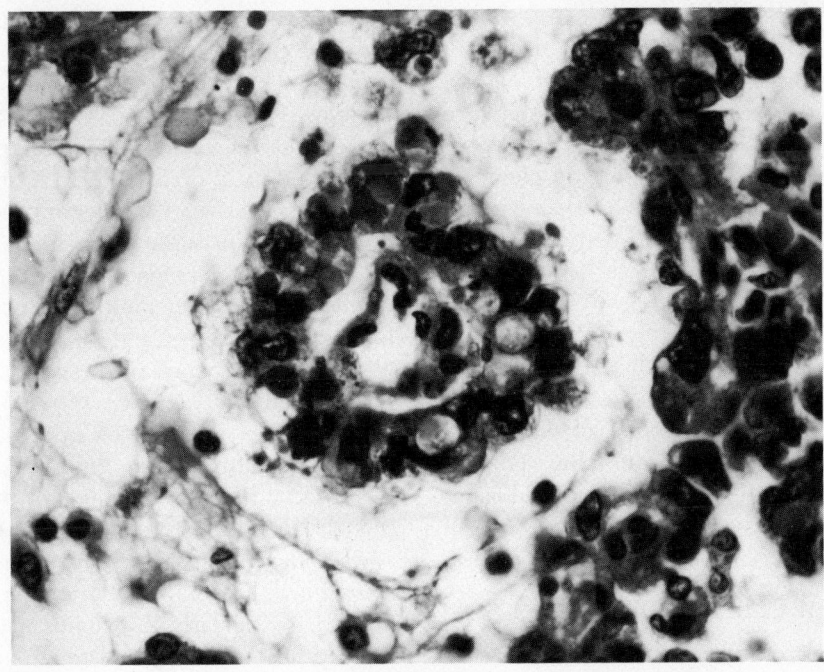

FIGURE 29-24
Schiller-Duvall body associated with numerous hyaline droplets in an endodermal sinus tumor. (×350.) (From Kurman RJ and Norris HJ: Hum Pathol 8:551, 1977. Reprinted with permission from WB Saunders Co, Philadelphia, 1977.)

section on immature teratoma) has been widely used. Another effective regimen has been a 5-day program: actinomycin D, 10g/kg/day; 5-fluorouracil (5-FU), 8 mg/kg/day up to 500 mg; and cyclophosphamide (Cytoxan), 7 mg/kg/day up to 450 mg (Act-FU-Cy). Forney noted regression of endodermal sinus tumor with this program and also reported subsequent pregnancy in a patient so treated. Einhorn and Donahue initially reported a potent combination of vinblastine, 12 mg/m^2 intravenously every 3 weeks for four doses; bleomycin, 20 units/m^2 (maximum dose, 30 units/m^2) intravenously given weekly for seven doses and an eighth course on week 10; and cisplatin (*cis*-platinum), 20 mg/m^2 daily for 5 days given every 3 weeks for up to four courses (VBP). This regimen has been found to be effective in treating patients with metastatic germ cell tumors of the testis and in inducing remissions in endodermal sinus tumors. Multiple-agent chemotherapy is needed, and of the 41 patients reported by Gershenson et al., all of the 21 who survived had received multiple-agent chemotherapy with one of these protocols. VBP or etoposide plus platinum are prob-

ably used most frequently. Good results have been reported also with the older VAC regimen.

Choriocarcinomas

Nongestational choriocarcinoma is a highly malignant rare germ cell tumor resembling extraembryonic tissues. Like gestational choriocarcinoma (see Chapter 33), it consists of malignant cytotrophoblasts and syncytiotrophoblasts; human chorionic gonadotrophin (HCG) is a useful tumor marker. Most patients developing this tumor primarily in the ovary are under the age of 20. The disease was usually fatal in the past and does not appear to respond to single-agent chemotherapy, such as methotrexate or actinomycin D, with the same frequency as gestational trophoblastic disease. This lack of response may be due in part to the occurrence of these tumors in combination with other malignant germ cell tumors (mixed germ cell tumor), and on occasion the other germ cell elements may not be histologically recognized. Multiple-agent chemotherapy is advisable.

Embryonal Carcinomas

An embryonal carcinoma is a rare malignant germ cell tumor composed of primitive embryonal cells. It occurs in young females between the ages of 4 and 28 years. Kurman and Norris summarized 15 cases. Trophoblastic elements may be present, and both HCG and alpha-fetoprotein have been reported to be present.

Polyembryomas

Polyembryomas are exceedingly rare tumors that are usually found in the testes. They can occur in the ovary and consist of embryonal bodies that resemble early embryos. Trophoblastic elements with HCG and placental lactogen secretion have been reported.

Mixed Germ Cell Tumors

Mixed germ cell tumors are combinations of any of the previously described germ cell tumors of the ovary. They can be bilateral if dysgerminoma elements are involved; otherwise they are unilateral. Treatment of apparent stage IA mixed germ cell tumors consists of unilateral adnexectomy. A wedge biopsy of the opposite ovary is performed in women desiring to preserve reproductive function if dysgerminoma is present. Multiple-agent chemotherapy with VAC or with vinblastine, bleomycin, and *cis*-platinum (VBP), as previously described, is recommended. The most frequently found elements in mixed germ cell tumors are dysgerminomas and teratomas. Survival of patients with mixed germ cell tumors is related primarily to the immaturity of the constituent tissues; it can reach 100% for small mixed germ cell tumors. It is diminished for women with large tumors or with a predominance of endodermal sinus elements, choriocarcinoma, or grade 3 immature teratoma.

SUMMARY AND CONSIDERATIONS OF CHEMOTHERAPY FOR MALIGNANT GERM CELL TUMORS

As noted, the advent of modern multiagent chemotherapy has vastly improved the prognosis of these tumors. The most frequently employed regimens have been VAC (see previous section on immature teratoma) or VBP (see previous section on endodermal sinus tumor) or EP (etoposide 100 mg/m^2 per day IV for 5 days and cisplatin 20 mg/m^2 per day for 5 days

every 3 weeks). Although the optimal approach for these tumors is not certain, those cases that require adjuvant treatment usually receive 4 to 6 cycles. For cases in which a tumor marker is present and elevated, chemotherapy is usually prescribed for 2 cycles after the tumor marker becomes negative. Childbearing potential can be preserved in these individuals. In a report of 40 patients Gershenson et al. noted 27 had normal menses after multiagent chemotherapy for germ cell tumors, and 11 of 16 patients who attempted pregnancy were successful in bearing 22 children.

The role of second-look operation in these tumors is controversial. Pippitt et al. recommend second-look operation after the patient is thought to be free of tumor, but Gershenson advised that in the high proportion of negative second-look procedures, the operation was not needed, particularly if a tumor marker is elevated prior to therapy and reverts to a normal value. In addition, a recurrence, if it develops, can usually be effectively treated with chemotherapy. In most cases second-look operation would appear to be most useful to determine further therapy in patients without a tumor marker who have advanced-stage disease at initial operation.

GONADOBLASTOMAS (GERM CELL SEX CORD–STROMAL TUMORS)

The term *gonadoblastoma* was introduced by Scully in 1953 to describe a tumor that consists of germ cell and sex cord–stromal elements. Approximately 100 cases have been reported. The germ cells usually resemble dysgerminoma, whereas the sex cord–stromal elements may consist of immature granulosa and Sertoli cells. Leydig cells and luteinized cells may be present. The tumor usually occurs in patients with abnormal (dysgenetic) gonads. Most patients have a female phenotype but may be virilized. These patients have a Y chromosome detected in their karyotype, and patients with gonadal dysgenesis and a Y chromosome are at risk for the development of gonadoblastoma or malignant germ cell tumors, predominantly dysgerminoma, which may occur in an individual as young as 6 months of age. Removal of these gonads is indicated when they are discovered. Both gonads should be removed, and if the presence of pure gonadoblastoma is confirmed, the prognosis is excellent, since these tumors have not been reported to metastasize.

SEX CORD–STROMAL TUMORS

The sex cord–stromal tumors are derived from the sex cords of the ovary and the specialized stroma of the developing gonad. The elements can have a male or female differentiation, and some of these tumors are hormonally active. The group accounts for about 6% of ovarian neoplasms and the majority of hormonally functioning ovarian tumors. For the female derivatives the sex cord component is the granulosa cell, and the stromal component is the theca cell or fibroblast. For the male counterpart the similar components are the Sertoli cell and the Leydig cell. Granulosa-theca cell tumors and Sertoli-Leydig cell tumors tend to behave as low-grade malignancies. Their clinical and morphologic aspects will be separately considered.

Granulosa-Theca Cell Tumors

Granulosa cell tumors consist primarily of granulosa cells and a varying proportion of theca cells or fibroblasts or both. One characteristic microscopic pattern is shown in Figure 29-25, which demonstrates the so-called *Call Exner bodies*, eosinophilic bodies surrounded by granulosa cells. Functional granulosa cell tumors are primarily estrogenic. About 5% occur before puberty, and they can be one of the causes of precocious puberty, but the tumors have been described in women of all ages. In postmenopausal women these tumors can produce elevated levels of blood estrogens, uterine bleeding, and occasionally endometrial carcinoma. It is estimated that about 5% of the granulosa cell tumors in adults are associated with endometrial carcinoma. In menstruating women the functional granulosa cell tumor can produce abnormal menstrual patterns, menorrhagia, and even amenorrhea.

These tumors can become large and may present as a ruptured mass, leading to laparotomy for an acute abdomen with hemoperitoneum. Because of the low-grade malignant character of these tumors, recurrences are frequently more than 5 years after primary therapy. In general, prognosis does not correlate with the histologic pattern of the tumor. A total of 90% of granulosa cell tumors present as stage I. Advanced clinical stage, the presence

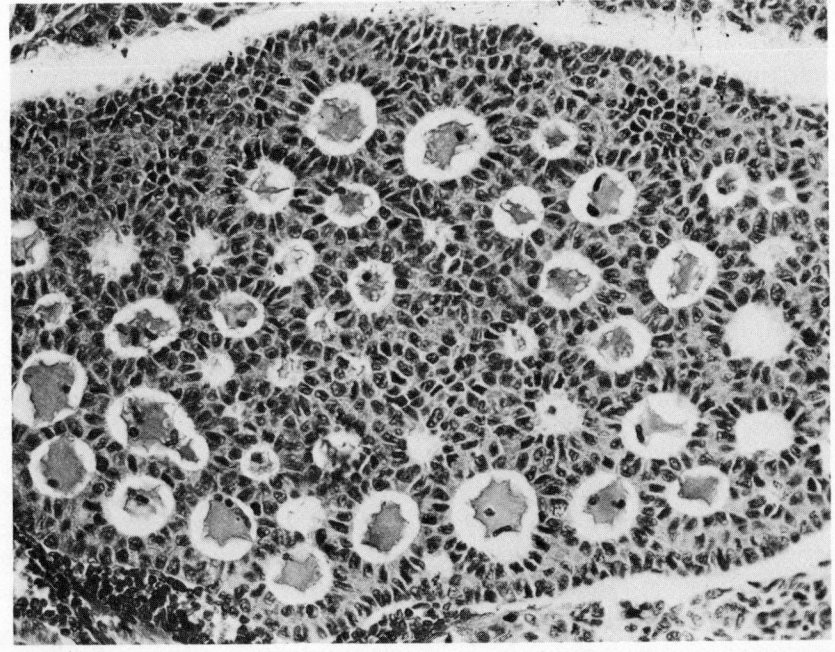

FIGURE 29-25
Granulosa cell tumor. (×460.) (From Scully RE and Morris J: Functioning ovarian tumors. In Meigs JV and Sturgis SH, editors: Progress in gynecology, vol 3, New York, 1957, Grune & Stratton.)

of tumor rupture, a large primary tumor (greater than 15 cm), and a high mitotic rate have been associated with a poorer prognosis. Overall 10-year survival rates of 90% have been reported. Recent studies by Klemi et al. and others suggest that most granulosa cell tumors have a diploid pattern and a low (<60%) S phase fraction when analyzed by flow cytometry. Those with an aneuploid pattern had a worse prognosis in the study of Klemi et al. However, it is important to recognize that granulosa cell tumors can be confused histologically with poorly differentiated adenocarcinomas, and the latter would also have an aneuploid pattern, as well as a poor prognosis.

The primary therapeutic approach is the operative removal of the tumor. Since these tumors are rarely bilateral (less than 5%), stage IA tumors can be treated by unilateral adnexectomy with biopsy of the contralateral ovary to rule out bilaterality. Lack et al. reported 10 cases of granulosa cell tumors in premenarchal female patients, all of whom were treated by unilateral salpingo-oophorectomy. Two tumors were ruptured. All 10 of the patients were surviving with no evidence of disease 2 to 33 years after therapy. Evans et al. did note a higher recurrence rate among women who were treated by unilateral salpingo-oophorectomy for stage IA cases in comparison with those treated with bilateral salpingo-oophorectomy. This finding has led to the recommendation that women of reproductive age treated for granulosa cell tumor by unilateral salpingo-oophorectomy have close follow-up. The removal of the contralateral ovary is considered after reproductive function is completed or if there is evidence of ovarian enlargement. Recent studies by Lappohn et al. suggest that the peptide hormone, inhibin, is secreted by some granulosa cell tumors and serum measurements could serve as a tumor marker.

Although radiation and chemotherapy have been employed for the treatment of recurrent or metastatic granulosa cell tumors, there is insufficient experience to warrant conclusions regarding their effectiveness. Complete responses to chemotherapy have been reported in patients using multiple-agent protocols, including cisplatin, 50 mg/m^2, and doxorubicin (Adriamycin), 50 mg/m^2, as well as in patients receiving Act-FU-Cy or vinblastine, bleomycin, and cisplatin (see previous section on endodermal sinus tumor).

Thecomas and Fibromas

Thecomas are benign tumors that consist entirely of stroma (theca) cells. They occur in women predominantly in the perimenopausal and menopausal years. These tumors can be associated with estrogen production but not as frequently as are granulosa cell tumors. Removal of the tumor alone is adequate treatment in women in the reproductive years. For older women, total abdominal hysterectomy and bilateral salpingo-oophorectomy are performed. Rarely, thecomas have been reported to be malignant, and these are most likely fibrosarcomas. A closely related tumor is the fibroma, which is the most common benign solid ovarian tumor and accounts for 4% of all ovarian tumors. Like the thecoma, it can occur at any age but is more common in older women; it does not secrete hormones. These tumors contain spindle cells, and the tumors can grow to a large size. They are benign, and excision is adequate treatment. These tumors are associated with ascites in about 40% of cases if the tumor exceeds 10 cm, according to Samanth and Black. They can also be responsible for hydrothorax with a benign ascites (Meigs' syndrome), which regresses following tumor removal.

Sertoli-Leydig Cell Tumors (Androblastomas)

Sertoli-Leydig cell tumors are very rare. Sertoli (sex cord) and Leydig (stromal) cells are present in varying amounts, and the tumor may consist almost entirely of either Sertoli or Leydig cells (Figure 29-26). These tumors tend to occur in young women of reproductive age and frequently are the cause of masculinization and hirsutism. The symptoms of virilization usually regress after tumor removal, but temporal hair recession and a deeper voice tend to remain. Rarely they have been reported also to have estrogenic activity, leading to the same symptoms and signs as granulosa cell tumors. The tumors tend to behave as low-grade malignancies, and 5-year survival is reported to vary from 70% to 90%. Poorly differentiated types tend to have a poor prognosis, as do higher stage tumors. Young and Scully reviewed 207 cases. Seventy-five percent were 30 years of age or younger, and fewer than 10% were over 50 years old. One third had evidence of androgen excess. Both ovaries were involved in only three cases. The well-differentiated tu-

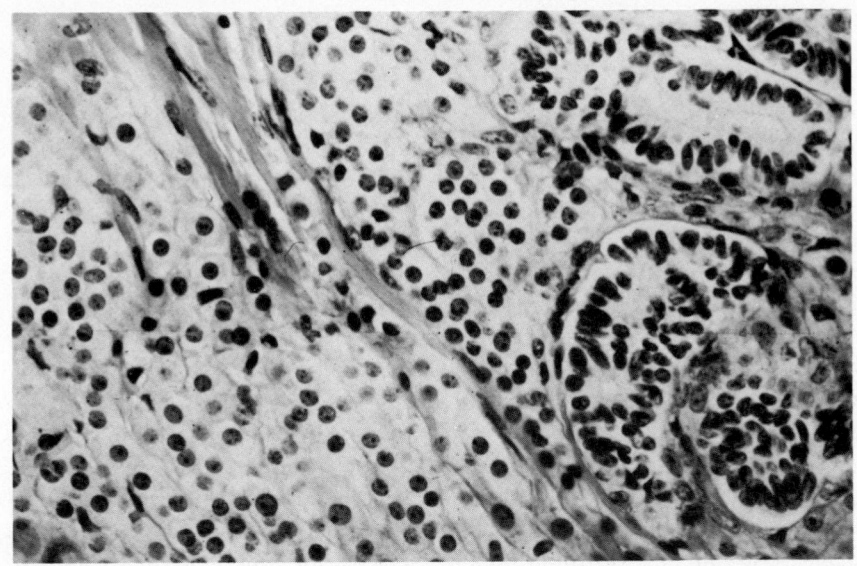

FIGURE 29-26
Sertoli-Leydig cell tumor. Tubules of Sertoli cells *(right)* and Leydig cells *(left)* are shown. (×250.) (Courtesy Dr. R.E. Scully.)

mors behaved clinically as benign tumors, whereas recurrence or extrauterine spread was noted occasionally in women with intermediate differentiation (11%) and frequently in those with poor differentiation (59%). Of 164 patients available for follow-up, 18% had metastasis or recurrence. There is insufficient experience to provide guidelines for therapy. Irradiation for localized pelvic disease has been beneficial, and chemotherapy with agents such as VAC (see previous section on immature teratoma) would be considered for disseminated disease or in the case of undifferentiated tumors.

Gynandroblastomas

Gynandroblastomas are rare sex cord–stromal tumors consisting of both female and male cell types.

Sex Cord Tumors with Annular Tubules

Sex cord tumors with annular tubules (SC-TAT) are unusual. As suggested by the name, there is a prominent tubular pattern. Features of both Sertoli and granulosa cell tumors are present. Recently 74 cases were reviewed by Young et al. Twenty-seven of them were associated with mucocutaneous pigmentation and gastrointestinal tract polyposis (Peutz-Jeghers

syndrome). The tumors may have estrogenic manifestations. Those associated with Peutz-Jeghers syndrome are benign, and those not associated with this syndrome can be malignant. It is of interest that 4 of the 74 cases reported by Young et al. were associated with a virulent form of cervical adenocarcinoma (adenoma malignum).

Leydig Cell and Hilus Cell Tumors

Leydig cell and hilus cell tumors are rare and are composed of Leydig cells or cells of the ovarian hilus. Their cytoplasm contains hyaline bodies known as *crystalloids of Reinke*. They usually cause virilization and are benign. They tend to be small (under 6 cm) and develop primarily in perimenopausal women.

LIPID (LIPOID) TUMORS

Lipid tumors are infrequently occurring ovarian tumors composed of large cells that resemble Leydig cells, luteinized cells, or cells that arise in the adrenal cortex. About 100 tumors have been reported. These tumors usually cause virilization but have also been associated with excess cortisol production. There is not enough experience with them to delineate an effective form of treatment. However, metastases of lipid cell tumors have been reported.

METASTATIC OVARIAN TUMORS

Tumors from distant primary sites can metastasize to the ovary. Frequently metastases are from primary tumors that originate elsewhere in the female reproductive tract, particularly from the endometrium and fallopian tube. Distant sites of origin occur most frequently from the breast and gastrointestinal tract. Metastatic tumors from the gastrointestinal tract to the ovary can be associated with sex hormone production, which usually leads to estrogenic manifestations. One special type of metastatic ovarian tumor is known as *Krukenberg's tumor,* which histologically consists of nests of mucin-filled signet-ring cells in a cellular stroma (Figure 29-27). The most common gastrointestinal tract origin for these tumors is the stomach,

and the next frequent is the large intestine. However, breast metastases to the ovary can on occasion give the same histologic picture. A few cases of Krukenberg's tumors have been described with no apparent distant primary malignancy, suggesting the rare possibility of a primary ovarian tumor with the histologic features of a Krukenberg's tumor. A primary gastrointestinal tract malignancy should be considered in older women with an adnexal mass, particularly if it is bilateral and solid. Pretherapy evaluation to rule out a gastrointestinal tract or breast primary tumor is indicated. The tumor should be removed when discovered, and the primary site should be treated. The prognosis is poor, and it is rare for a patient to survive for 5 or more years after treatment of these tumors.

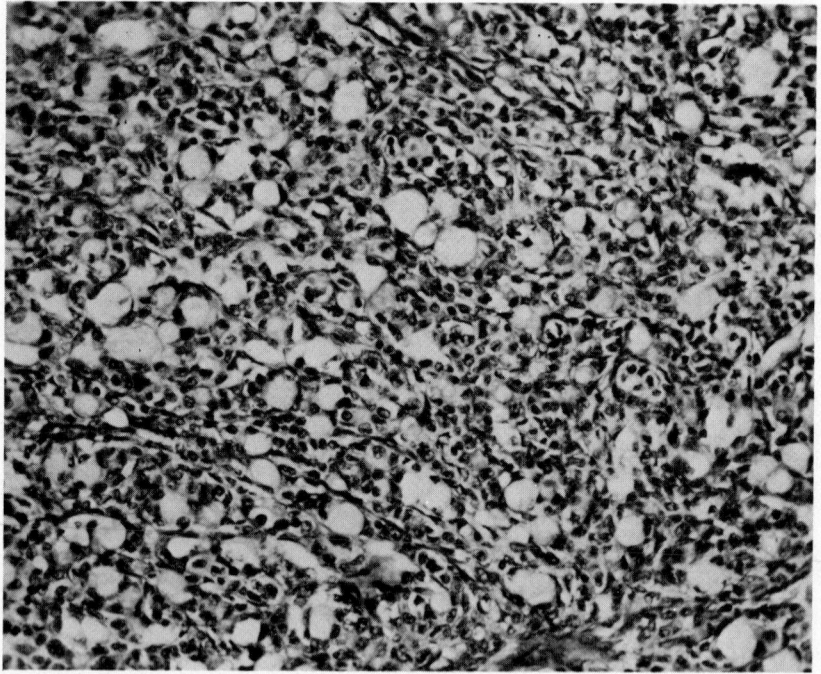

FIGURE 29-27
Krukenberg tumor. (×256.) Mucin-filled signet-ring cells are present. (Courtesy Dr. R.E. Scully.)

_____ KEY POINTS _____

- Ovarian cancer is the leading cause of death from gynecologic cancer, but it occurs less frequently than endometrial cancers.

- Ovarian cancers of women older than age 65 are diagnosed at a more advanced stage, leading to a worse prognosis than for younger women.

- Patients with ovarian cancer are at increased risk of developing breast cancer and endometrial cancer. It is important that the follow-up of ovarian cancer patients include monitoring for breast cancer.

- Epithelial tumors are the most frequent ovarian neoplasm. They account for two thirds of all ovarian neoplasms and 85% of ovarian cancers.

- The major ovarian epithelial tumor cell types recapitulate müllerian-type epithelium (serous-endosalpinx, mucinous-endocervix, and endometrioid-endometrium).

- Serous ovarian neoplasms are the most common type of epithelial tumors. Serous adenocarcinomas tend to be high grade, are the most virulent, and have the worst prognosis of epithelial adenocarcinomas. They are bilateral in 33% to 66% of cases.

- A cystic adnexal mass less than 8 cm in diameter in a menstruating female is most frequently functional.

- The normal postmenopausal ovary is approximately 1.5 to 2 cm in diameter.

- The risk of an ovarian tumor being malignant is about 33% in a woman over age 45, whereas it is less than 1 in 15 for those 20 to 45 years of age. More than half of ovarian cancers occur in women beyond the age of 50.

- A vaginal ultrasound finding of a unilocular cyst of 5 cm or less in a perimenopausal woman can usually be followed without operative intervention.

- The primary mode of spread of epithelial carcinoma is transcoelomic to the visceral and parietal peritoneum and diaphragm and to the retroperitoneal nodes.

- The risk of retroperitoneal node spread of epithelial carcinoma in apparent stage I cases is greatest for poorly differentiated tumors, for which the risk can reach 10% to 20%. The risk of retroperitoneal node spread increases in higher-stage cases.

- The prognosis of a patient with ovarian epithelial carcinoma is related primarily to tumor stage and tumor grade, as well as to the amount of residual tumor remaining after primary resection.

- The 5-year survival rate for patients with borderline epithelial ovarian carcinoma (grade 0) is close to 100% for stage I cases and over 90% for all stages.

- The overall 5-year survival rate for patients with stage I ovarian carcinoma is 65%. For stage I, grade 1, survival is reported to be over 80%.

- Alkylating agent administration is accompanied by an increased risk of subsequent development of leukemia, which can reach almost 10% 8 years after therapy.

- Computed tomographic scan for patients with ovarian cancer can be approximately 80% to 90% effective for detecting tumor in retroperitoneal nodes. The test is much less successful for detecting intraabdominal disease.

- The ovarian antigen CA-125 is useful in helping to monitor patients with ovarian carcinoma. Reaction to the antigen is positive in about 80% of cases.

- The initial response rate of ovarian epithelial carcinomas treated with cisplatin (platinum-containing) multiple-agent chemotherapy is over 90%, but the proportion of patients who survive drops to around 30% in 4 years. Initial treatment is usually with cyclophosphamide and cisplatin.

- Approximately half of patients thought initially to be clinically free of disease are found at second-look laparotomy to have gross or microscopic tumor. The operation, if performed, is usually done after 6 months of chemotherapy.

- The 5-year survival rate after negative second-look operation is about 50% to 80%.

- Survival after second look is related to tumor grade and size of residual disease. Younger patients also have a more favorable prognosis.

- Complete responses to intraperitoneal chemotherapy have been observed in patients with recurrent ovarian tumor. Those with small volume disease (microscopic disease or ≤5 mm) have the best responses.

- Germ cell tumors are the second most common type of ovarian neoplasms and account for about 20% to 25% of all ovarian tumors.

- In young women under age 30 the most frequent ovarian neoplasm is a germ cell tumor, and about one third of these germ cell tumors are malignant under age 21.

- The most common germ cell tumor is the benign cystic teratoma (dermoid). It is bilateral in 10% to 15% of the cases. Approximately 30% are calcified.

- For women under age 30 the most common ovarian neoplasm is the dermoid.

- Malignant germ cell tumors are usually unilateral except dysgerminomas, which are bilateral in about 10% of the cases.

- Dysgerminomas are the most common malignant germ cell tumors and account for 1% to 2% of ovarian cancers.

- The prognosis for a patient with immature teratoma is related to tumor grade and tumor stage. These tumors are the second most common type of malignant germ cell tumor.

- The 5-year survival or stage IA pure dysgerminoma treated by unilateral salpingo-oophorectomy is over 90%.

- Pure dysgerminomas are radiosensitive and curable by irradiation therapy or chemotherapy. Favorable prognostic factors include size under 15 cm, encapsulation without rupture, lack of ascites, and no spread to retroperitoneal nodes. About two thirds of cases present as stage IA.

- Patients with immature teratoma stage IA grade 2 or 3 should receive postoperative adjuvant chemotherapy.

- Patients with endodermal sinus tumors have a median age of 19. These tumors can be followed by measuring serum levels of alpha-fetoprotein. They should be treated with chemotherapy even in stage IA.

- Multiple-agent chemotherapy has improved the survival in patients with malignant germ cell tumors, preserving childbearing function in most cases. Commonly used protocols include VAC (vincristine, actinomycin D, and Cytoxan), VBP (vinblastine, bleomycin, and platinum), and EP (etoposide and platinum).

- Gonadoblastomas are sex cord–stromal germ cell tumors that arise in dysgenetic gonads in patients with a Y chromosome. They are cured by removal.

- Granulosa cell tumors and Sertoli-Leydig tumors usually behave as low-grade malignancies, but there may be late recurrences.

- Fibroma is the most common benign solid ovarian tumor.

- The most frequent sites of origin of tumors metastatic to the ovary are the lower reproductive tract, the gastrointestinal tract, and the breast.

BIBLIOGRAPHY

Abdulhay G, DiSaia PJ, Blessing JA, et al: Human lymphoblastoid interferon in the treatment of advanced ovarian epithelial malignancies: a Gynecologic Oncology Group study, Am J Obstet Gynecol 152:418, 1985.

Abeler V, Kjorstad KE, and Nesland JM: Small cell carcinoma of the ovary: a report of six cases, Int J Gynecol Pathol 7:315, 1988.

Altaras MM, Aviram R, Cohen I, et al: Primary peritoneal papillary serous adenocarcinoma: clinical and management aspects, Gynecol Oncol 40:230, 1991.

Assadourian LA and Taylor HB: Dysgerminoma: an analysis of 105 cases, Obstet Gynecol 33:370, 1969.

Aure JC, Hoeg K, and Kolstad P: The clinical and histologic studies of ovarian carcinoma: long-term follow-up of 990 cases, Obstet Gynecol 37:1, 1971.

Averette HE and Donato DM: Ovarian carcinoma: advances in diagnosis, staging, and treatment, Cancer 65:703, 1990.

Belinson JL, Lee KR, Jarrell MA, and McClure M: Management of epithelial ovarian neoplasms using a platinum-based regimen: a 10-year experience, Gynecol Oncol 37:66, 1990.

Bell DA, Weinstock MA, and Scully RE: Peritoneal implants of ovarian serous borderline tumors: histologic features and prognosis, Cancer 62:2212, 1988.

Berek JS, Hacker NF, Lagasse LD, et al: Second-look laparotomy in stage III epithelial ovarian cancer: clinical variables associated with the disease status, Obstet Gynecol 64:207, 1984.

Berek JS, Knapp RC, Malkasian GD, et al: CA-125 serum levels correlated with second-look operations among ovarian cancer patients, Obstet Gynecol 67:685, 1986.

Berek JS, Welander C, Schink JC, et al: A phase I-II trial of intraperitoneal cisplatin and α-Interferon in patients with persistent epithelial ovarian cancer, Gynecol Oncol 40:237, 1991

Bertelsen K, Jakobsen A, Andersen JE, et al: A randomized study of cyclophosphamide and *cis*-platinum with or without doxorubicin in advanced ovarian carcinoma, Gynecol Oncol 28:161, 1987.

Bezwoda WR, Seymour L, and Dansey R: Intraperitoneal recombinant interferon 2B for recurrent malignant ascites due to ovarian cancer, Cancer 64:1029, 1989.

Bjorkholm E, Lundell M, Gyftodimos A, and Silfversward C: Dysgerminoma: the Radiumhemmet Series 1927-1984, Cancer 65:38, 1990.

Bjorkholm E and Silfversward C: Prognostic factors in granulosa cell tumor, Gynecol Oncol 11:261, 1981.

Bostwick DG, Tazelaar HD, Ballon SC, et al: Ovarian epithelial tumors of borderline malignancy: clinical and pathologic study of 109 cases, Cancer 58:2052, 1986.

Bruckner HW, Cohen CJ, Goldberg JD, et al: Cisplatin regimens and improved prognosis of patients with poorly differentiated ovarian cancer, Am J Obstet Gynecol 145:653, 1983.

Bruzzone M, Repetto L, Chiara S, et al: Chemotherapy versus radiotherapy in the management of ovarian cancer patients with pathological complete response or minimal residual disease at second look, Gynecol Oncol 38:392, 1990.

Buchsbaum HJ, Brady MF, Delgado G, et al: Surgical staging of carcinoma of the ovaries, Surg Gynecol Obstet 169:226, 1989.

Buller RE, Berman ML, Bloss JD, et al: CA-125 regression: a model for epithelial ovarian cancer response, Am J Obstet Gynecol 165:360, 1991.

Burghardt E, Girardi F, Lahousen M, et al: Patterns of pelvic and paraaortic lymph node involvement in ovarian cancer, Gynecol Oncol 40:103, 1991.

Carmichael JA, Shelley WE, Brown LB, et al: A predictive index of cure versus no cure in advanced ovarian carcinoma patients: replacement of second-look laparotomy as a diagnostic test, Gynecol Oncol 27:269, 1987.

Casagrande JT, Louie EW, Pike MC, et al: "Incessant ovulation" and ovarian cancer, Lancet 2:170, 1979.

Chadha S, Cornelisse CJ, and Schaberg A: Flow cytometry DNA ploidy analysis of ovarian granulosa cell tumor, Gynecol Oncol 36:240, 1990.

Chambers JT, Merino MJ, Kohorn EI, and Schwartz PE: Borderline ovarian tumors, Am J Obstet Gynecol 159:1088, 1988.

Chen SS and Lee L: Incidence of para-aortic and pelvic lymph node metastases in epithelial carcinoma of the ovary, Gynecol Oncol 16:95, 1983.

Chen SS and Lee L: Prognostic significance of morphology of tumor and retroperitoneal lymph nodes in epithelial carcinoma of the ovary, Gynecol Oncol 18:87, 1984.

Cohen CJ, Goldberg JD, Holland JF, et al: Improved therapy with *cis*-platinum regimens for patients with ovarian carcinoma (FIGO stages III and IV) as measured by surgical end-staging (second-look operation), Am J Obstet Gynecol 145:955, 1983.

Columbo N, Sessa C, Landoni F, et al: Cisplatin, vinblastine and bleomycin, combination chemotherapy in metastatic granulosa cell tumor of the ovary, Obstet Gynecol 67:265, 1986.

Conte PF, Bruzzone M, Carnino F, et al: Carboplatin, doxorubicin, and Cyclophosphamide versus Cisplatin, Doxorubicin, and Cyclophosphamide: a randomized trial in stage III-IV epithelial ovarian carcinoma, J Clin Oncol 9:658, 1991.

Copeland LJ, Gershenson DM, Wharton JT, et al: Microscopic disease at second-look laparotomy in advanced ovarian carcinoma, Cancer 55:472, 1985.

Cramer DW, Welch WR, Hutchinson GB, et al: Dietary animal fat in relation to ovarian cancer risk, Obstet Gynecol 63:833, 1984.

Cramer DW, Welch WR, Scully RE, et al: Ovarian cancer and talc: a case-control study, Cancer 50:372, 1982.

Creasman WT: New gynecologic cancer staging, Obstet Gynecol 75:287, 1990.

Creasman WT, Gall S, Bundy BN, et al: Second-look laparotomy in the patient with minimal residual stage III ovarian cancer (a Gynecologic Oncology Group study), Gynecol Oncol 35:378, 1989.

Creasman WT and Soper JT: Assessment of the contemporary management of germ cell malignancies of the ovary, Am J Obstet Gynecol 153:828, 1985.

Curry SL, Smith JP, and Gallagher HS: Malignant teratoma of the ovary: prognostic factors and treatment, Am J Obstet Gynecol 131:845, 1978.

Decker DG, Fleming TR, Malkasian GD, et al: Cyclophosphamide plus *cis*-platinum in combination: treatment program for stage III or IV ovarian carcinoma, Obstet Gynecol 60:481, 1982.

Dembo AJ, Bush RS, Beale FA, et al: Ovarian carcinoma: improved survival following abdominopelvic irradiation in patients with a completed pelvic operation, Am J Obstet Gynecol 134:793, 1979.

Dembo AJ, Bush RS, Beale FA, et al: The Princess Margaret Hospital study of ovarian cancer: stages I, II and asymptomatic III presentations, Cancer Treat Rep 63:249, 1979.

Dembo AJ, Bush RS, and DeBoer G: Therapy in stage I ovarian cancer, Am J Obstet Gynecol 141:231, 1981.

Dembo AJ, Davy M, Stenwig AE, et al: Prognostic factors in patients with stage I epithelial ovarian cancer, Obstet Gynecol 75:263, 1990.

Dickerson GR, Kline IW, and Scully RE: Small cell carcinoma of the ovary with hypercalcemia: a report of 11 cases, Cancer 49:188, 1982.

DiSaia PJ, Saltz A, Kagan AR, et al: Chemotherapeutic retroconversion of immature teratoma of the ovary, Obstet Gynecol 49:347, 1977.

DiSaia P, Townsend DE, and Morrow CP: The rationale for less than radical treatment for gynecologic malignancy in early reproductive years, Obstet Gynecol Surv 29:581, 1974.

Doss N, Forney JP, Vellios F, et al: Covert bilaterality of mature ovarian teratomas, Obstet Gynecol 50:651, 1977.

Einhorn LH and Donahue J: *Cis*-diamminedichloroplatinum, vinblastine, and bleomycin combination chemotherapy in disseminated testicular cancer, Ann Intern Med 87:87, 1977.

Epenetos AA, Munro AJ, Stewart S, et al: Antibody guided irradiation of advanced ovarian cancer with intraperitoneally administered radiolabeled monoclonal antibodies, J Clin Oncol 5:1890, 1987.

Evans AT, Gaffey TA, and Malkasian GD: Clinical pathologic review of 118 granulosa and 82 theca cell tumors, Obstet Gynecol 55:231, 1980.

Finkler NJ, Benacerraf B, Lavin PT, et al: Comparison of serum CA-125, clinical impression, and ultrasound in the preoperative evaluation of ovarian masses, Obstet Gynecol 72:659, 1988.

Forney JP: Pregnancy following removal and chemotherapy of ovarian endodermal sinus tumor, Obstet Gynecol 52:360, 1978.

Friedman JB and Weiss NS: Second thoughts about second-look laparotomy in advanced ovarian cancer, N Engl J Med 322:1079, 1990.

Fromm GL, Gershenson DM, and Silva EG: Papillary serous carcinoma of the peritoneum, Obstet Gynecol 75:89, 1990.

Gershenson DM: Menstrual and reproductive function after treatment with combination chemotherapy for malignant ovarian germ cell tumors, J Clin Oncol 6:270, 1988.

Gershenson DM: Second-look laparotomy in endodermal sinus tumor: a report of two patients with normal levels of alpha-fetoprotein and residual tumor at reexploration (a Letter to the Editor), Obstet Gynecol 74:683, 1989.

Gershenson DM, Copeland LJ, De Junco G, et al: Second-look laparotomy in the management of malignant germ cell tumors of the ovary, Obstet Gynecol 67:789, 1986.

Gershenson DM, Copeland LJ, Kavanagh JJ, et al: Treatment of metastatic stromal tumors of the ovary with cisplatin, doxorubicin, and cyclophosphamide, Obstet Gynecol 70:765, 1987.

Gershenson DM, Del Junco G, Herson J, et al: Endodermal sinus tumor of the ovary: the MD Anderson experience, Obstet Gynecol 61:194, 1983.

Gershenson DM, Del Junco G, Silva EG, et al: Immature teratoma of the ovary, Obstet Gynecol 68:624, 1986.

Gershenson DM and Silva EG: Metastatic serous ovarian tumors of low malignant potential, Cancer 65:578, 1990.

Goldhirsch A, Greiner R, Dreher E, et al: Treatment of advanced ovarian cancer with surgery, chemotherapy, and consolidation of response by whole-abdominal radiotherapy, Cancer 62:40, 1988.

Goldhirsch A, Triller JF, Greiner R, et al: Computed tomography prior to second-look operation in advanced ovarian cancer, Obstet Gynecol 62:630, 1983.

Goldstein SR, Subramanyam B, Snyder JR, et al: The postmenopausal cystic adnexal mass: the potential role of ultrasound in conservative management, Obstet Gynecol 73:8, 1988.

Granberg S, Wikland M, and Jansson I: Macroscopic characterization of ovarian tumors and the relation to the histologic diagnosis: criteria to be used for ultrasound evaluation, Gynecol Oncol 35:139, 1989.

Granberg S, Norström A, and Wikland M: Tumors in the lower pelvis as imaged by vaginal sonography, Gynecol Oncol 37:224, 1990.

Greco FA, Julian CG, Richardson RL, et al: Advanced ovarian cancer: brief intensive combination chemotherapy and second-look operation, Obstet Gynecol 58:199, 1981.

Greene MH, Boice JD, Greer BE, et al: Acute nonlymphocytic leukemia after therapy with alkylating agent for ovarian cancer: a study of five randomized clinical trials, N Engl J Med 307:1416, 1982.

Griffiths CT: Surgical resection of tumor bulk in the primary treatment of ovarian carcinoma, Natl Cancer Inst Monogr 42:101, 1975.

Guthrie D, Davy MLJ, and Philips PR: A study of 656 patients with "early" ovarian cancer, Gynecol Oncol 17:363, 1984.

Hacker NF, Berek JS, Burnison CM, et al: Whole abdominal radiation as salvage therapy for epithelial ovarian cancer, Obstet Gynecol 65:60, 1985.

Hainsworth JD, Grosh WM, Burnett LS, et al: Advanced ovarian cancer: long-term results of treatment with intensive cisplatin-based chemotherapy of brief duration, Ann Intern Med, 108:165, 1988.

Hart WR and Norris HJ: Borderline and malignant mucinous tumors of the ovary: histologic criteria and clinical behavior, Cancer 31:1031, 1973.

Hartge P, Schiffman MH, Hoover R, et al: A case-control study of epithelial ovarian cancer, Am J Obstet Gynecol 161:10, 1989.

Heintz APM, Van Oosterom AT, Baptist J, et al: The treatment of advanced ovarian carcinoma: clinical variables associated with prognosis, Gynecol Oncol 30:347, 1988.

Higgins RV, van Nagell JR, Donaldson ES, et al: Transvaginal sonography as a screening method for ovarian cancer, Gynecol Oncol 34:402, 1989.

Holt JA, Caputo TA, Kelly KM, et al: Estrogen and progestin binding in cytosols of ovarian carcinoma, Obstet Gynecol 53:50, 1979.

Hoskins WJ, Rubin SC, Dulaney E, et al: Influence of secondary cytoreduction at the time of second-look laparotomy on the survival of patients with epithelial ovarian carcinoma, Gynecol Oncol 34:365, 1989.

Howell SB, Pfeifle CE, Wung WE, et al: Intraperitoneal cis-diamminedichloroplatinum with systemic thiosulfate protection, Cancer Res 43:1426, 1983.

Hreshchyshyn MM, Park RC, Blessing JA, et al: The role of adjuvant therapy in stage I ovarian cancer, Am J Obstet Gynecol 138:139, 1980.

Hunter VJ, Daly L, Helms M, et al: The prognostic significance of CA-125 half-life in patients with ovarian cancer who have received primary chemotherapy after surgical cytoreduction, Am J Obstet Gynecol 163:1164, 1990.

Iversen O-E and Skaarland E: Ploidy assessment of benign and malignant ovarian tumors by flow cytometry, Cancer 60:82, 1987.

Jacobs A, Deppe G, and Cohen CJ: Combination chemotherapy of ovarian granulosa cell tumor with cis-platinum and doxorubicin, Gynecol Oncol 14:294, 1982.

Jones CM III and Homesley HD: Successful treatment of pseudomyxoma peritonei of ovarian origin with cis-platinum, doxorubicin, and cyclophosphamide, Gynecol Oncol 22:257, 1985.

Julian CG, Barrett JM, Richardson RC, et al: Bleomycin, vinblastine, and cis-platinum in the treatment of advanced endodermal sinus tumors, Obstet Gynecol 56:396, 1980.

Julian CG and Woodruff JD: The biologic behavior of low-grade papillary serous carcinoma of the ovary, Obstet Gynecol 40:860, 1972.

Kaldor JM, Day NE, Pettersson F, et al: Leukemia following chemotherapy for ovarian cancer, N Engl J Med 322:1, 1990.

Kallioniemi O-P, Punnonen R, Mattila J, et al: Prognostic significance of DNA index, multiploidy, and S-phase fraction in ovarian cancer, Cancer 61:334, 1988.

Kamiya N, Mizuno K, Kawai M, et al: Simultaneous measurement of CA 125, CA 19-9, tissue polypeptide antigen, and immunosuppresive acidic protein to predict recurrence of ovarian cancer, Obstet Gynecol 76:417, 1990.

Kim DS and Park MI: Maternal and fetal survival following surgery and chemotherapy of endodermal sinus tumor of the ovary during pregnancy: a case report, Obstet Gynecol 73:503, 1989.

Kirmani S, Lucas WE, Kim S, et al: A phase II trial of intraperitoneal cisplatin and etoposide as salvage treatment for minimal residual ovarian carcinoma, J Clin Oncol 9:649, 1991.

Klemi PJ, Joensuu H, Maenpaa J, and Kilholma P: Influence of cellular DNA content on survival in ovarian carcinoma, Obstet Gynecol 74:200, 1989.

Klemi PJ, Joensuu H, and Salmi T: Prognostic value of flow cytometric DNA content analysis in granulosa cell tumor of the ovary, Cancer 65:1189, 1990.

Knapp RC and Friedman EA: Aortic lymph node metastases in early ovarian cancer, Am J Obstet Gynecol 119:1013, 1974.

Kohorn EI, Schwartz PE, Chambers JT, et al: Adjuvant therapy in mixed müllerian tumors of the uterus, Gynecol Oncol 23:212, 1986.

Koonings PP, Campbell K, Mishell DR, and Grimes DA: Relative frequency of primary ovarian neoplasms: a 10-year review, Obstet Gynecol 74:921, 1989.

Koulos JP, Hoffman JS, and Steinhoff MM: Immature teratoma of the ovary, Gynecol Oncol 34:46, 1989.

Kurman RJ and Norris HJ: Embryonal carcinoma of the ovary: a clinical pathogenic entity distinct from endodermal sinus tumor resembling embryonal carcinoma of the adult testes, Cancer 38:2420, 1976.

Kurman RJ and Norris HJ: Malignant germ cell tumors of the ovary, Hum Pathol 8:551, 1977.

Lack EE, Perez-Atayde AR, Murthy ASK, et al: Granulosa theca cell tumors in premenarcheal girls: a clinical and pathologic study of 10 cases, Cancer 48:1846, 1981.

Lappohn RE, Burger HG, Bouma J, et al: Inhibin as a marker for granulosa-cell tumors, N Engl J Med 321:790, 1989.

Lawton FG, Redman CWE, Luesley DM, et al: Neoadjuvant (cytoreductive) chemotherapy combined with intervention debulking surgery in advanced, unresected epithelial ovarian cancer, Obstet Gynecol 73:61, 1989.

Leers WH and Kock HCLV: The evaluation of postoperative irradiation in patients with early-stage ovarian cancer, Gynecol Oncol 28:41, 1987.

Lim-Tan SK, Cajigas HE, and Scully RE: Ovarian cystectomy for serous borderline tumors: a follow-up of 35 cases, Obstet Gynecol 72:775, 1988.

Linder D et al: Pathogenetic origin of benign ovarian teratomas, N Engl J Med 292:63, 1975.

Lucas WE, Markman M, and Howell SB: Intraperitoneal chemotherapy for advanced ovarian cancer, Am J Obstet Gynecol 152:474, 1985.

Lund B, Hansen M, Hansen OP, and Hansen HH: High-dose platinum consisting of combined carboplatin and cisplatin in previously untreated ovarian cancer patients with residual disease, J Clin Oncol 7:1469, 1989.

Lund B and Williamson P: Prognostic factors for outcome of and survival after second-look laparotomy in patients with advanced ovarian carcinoma, Obstet Gyncol 76:617, 1990.

Maiman M, Seltzer V, and Boyce J: Laparoscopic excision of ovarian neoplasms subsequently found to be malignant, Obstet Gynecol 77:563, 1991.

Malfetano JH: The appendix and its metastatic potential in epithelial ovarian cancer, Obstet Gynecol 69:396, 1987.

Markham M, Cleary S, Howell SB, et al: Complications of extensive adhesion formation after intraperitoneal chemotherapy, Surg Gynecol Obstet 162:445, 1986.

Markman M, Hakes T, Reichman B, et al: Intraperitoneal cisplatin and cytarabine in the treatment of refractoy or recurrent ovarian carcinoma, J Clin Oncol 9:204, 1991.

Markman M, Rothman R, Hakes T, et al: Second-line platinum therapy in patients with ovarian cancer previously treated with cisplatin, J Clin Oncol 9:389, 1991.

Masood S, Heitmann J, Nuss RC, and Benrubi GI: Clinical correlation of hormone receptor status in epithelial ovarian cancer, Gynecol Oncol 34:57, 1989.

McClay EF and Howell SB: A review: intraperitoneal cisplatin in the management of patients with ovarian cancer, Gynecol Oncol 36:1, 1990.

Menczer J, Ben-Baruch G, Modan M, and Brenner H: Intraperitoneal cisplatin chemotherapy versus abdominopelvic irradiation in ovarian carcinoma patients after second-look laparotomy, Cancer 63:1509, 1989.

Menczer M, Modan M, Brenner J, et al: Abdominal pelvic irradiation for stage II-IV ovarian carcinoma patients with limited or no residual disease at second-look laparotomy after completion of cis-platinum-based combination chemotherapy, Gynecol Oncol 24:149, 1986.

Mishell DR: Contraception, N Engl J Med 320:777, 1989.

Morgan L, Chafe W, Mendenhall W, and Marcus R: Hyperfractionation of whole-abdomen radiation therapy: salvage treatment of persistent ovarian carcinoma following chemotherapy, Gynecol Oncol 31:122, 1988.

Nam J, Chambers JT, Schwartz PE, et al: Urinary gonadotropin fragment, a new tumor marker, Gynecol Oncol 39:352, 1990.

Neijt JP, ten Bokkel Huinink WW, van der Burg ME, et al: Randomized trial comparing two combination chemotherapy regimens (CHAP-5 v CP) in advanced ovarian carcinoma, J Clin Oncol 5:1157, 1987.

Nichols CR, Tricot G, Williams SD, et al: Dose-intensive chemotherapy in refractory germ cell cancer: a phase I/II trial of high-dose carboplatin and etoposide with autologous bone marrow transplant, J Clin Oncol 7:932, 1989.

Norris HJ, Zirkin HJ, and Benson WL: Immature (malignant) teratoma of the ovary: a clinical and pathologic study of 58 cases, Cancer 37:2359, 1976.

Omura GA, Bundy BN, Berek JS, et al: Randomized trial of cyclophosphamide plus cisplatin with or without doxorubicin in ovarian carcinoma: a Gynecologic Oncology Group study, J Clin Oncol 7:457, 1989.

Ozols RF: Intraperitoneal therapy in ovarian cancer: time's up, J Clin Oncol 9:197, 1991.

Panici PB, Scambia G, Baiocchi G, et al: Predictive value of multiple tumor marker assays in second-look procedures for ovarian cancer, Gynecol Oncol 35:286, 1989.

Parker LM: Leukemia after treatment of ovarian cancer with alkylating agents, N Engl J Med 308:1422, 1983.

Pippit CH, Cain JM, Hakes TB, et al: Primary chemotherapy and the role of second-look laparotomy in non-dysgerminoma germ cell malignancies of the ovary, Gynecol Oncol 31:268, 1988.

Piver MS, Baker TR, Mettlin C, et al: Familial Ovarian Cancer Registry Newsletter, Roswell Park Memorial Institute, September, 1987.

Piver MS, Barlow JJ, Lele SB, et al: Intraperitoneal chromic phosphate in peritoneally confirmed stage I ovarian adenocarcinoma, Am J Obstet Gynecol 144:836, 1982.

Piver MS, Lele SB, Marchetti DL, et al: Surgically documented response to intraperitoneal cisplatin, cytarabine, and bleomycin after intravenous cisplatin-based chemotherapy in advanced ovarian adenocarcinoma, J Clin Oncol 6:1679, 1988.

Podczaski E, Manetta A, Kaminski P, et al: Survival of patients with ovarian epithelial carcinomas after second-look laparotomy, Gynecol Oncol 36:43, 1990.

Podratz KC, Malkasian GD, Hilton JF, et al: Second-look laparotomy in ovarian cancer: evaluation of pathologic variables, Am J Obstet Gynecol 152:230, 1985.

Podratz KC, Malkasian GD, Wieand HS, et al: Recurrent disease after negative second-look laparotomy in stages III and IV ovarian carcinoma, Gynecol Oncol 29:274, 1988.

Reichman B, Markman M, Hakes T, et al: Intraperitoneal cisplatin and etoposide in the treatment of refractory/recurrent ovarian carcinoma, J Clin Oncol 7:1327, 1989.

Reimer RR, Hoover R, Fraumeini JF, et al: Acute leukemia after alkylating-agent therapy of ovarian cancer, N Engl J Med 297:177, 1977.

Reuter KL, Griffin T, and Hunter RE: Comparison of abdominopelvic computer tomography results and findings at second-look laparotomy in ovarian carcioma patients, Cancer 63:1123, 1989.

Richardson GS, Scully RE, Nikrui N, et al: Common epithelial cancer of the ovary, N Engl J Med 312:415, 1985.

Robey SS, Silva EG, Gershenson DM, et al: Transitional cell carcinoma in high-grade high-stage ovarian carcinoma, Cancer 63:839, 1989.

Rodriquez MH, Platt LD, Medearis AL, et al: The use of transvaginal sonography for evaluation of postmenopausal ovarian size and morphology, Am J Obstet Gynecol 159:810, 1988.

Rubin SC, Hoskins WJ, Saigo PE, et al: Prognosis of surgical complete responders following platinum-based chemotherapy for epithelial ovarian cancer (EOC), Abstract, Gynecol Oncol, 1991 (in press).

Samanth KK and Black WC: Benign ovarian stromal tumors associated with free peritoneal fluid, Am J Obstet Gynecol 197:538, 1970.

Schneider J, Erasun F, Hervas JL, et al: Normal pregnancy and delivery 2 years after adjuvant chemotherapy for grade III immature ovarian teratoma, Gynecol Oncol 29:245, 1988.

Schwartz PE and Morris JM: Serum lactic dehydrogenase: a tumor marker for dysgerminoma, Obstet Gynecol 72:511, 1988.

Schwartz PE and Smith JP: Treatment of ovarian stromal tumors, Am J Obstet Gynecol 125:402, 1976.

Scully RE: Gonadoblastoma: a gonadal tumor related to dysgerminoma (seminoma) and capable of sex hormone production, Cancer 6:455, 1953.

Scully RE: Tumors of the ovary and maldeveloped gonads. In Atlas of tumor pathology, fascicle 16, series 2, Washington, DC, 1979, Armed Forces Institute of Pathology.

Scully RE: Sex cord–stromal tumors. In Blaustein A, editor: Pathology of the female genital tract, New York, 1982, Springer-Verlag.

Selby P, Buick RN, and Tannock I: A critical appraisal of the "human tumor stem-cell assay," N Engl J Med 308:129, 1983.

Senekjian EK, Wesier PA, Talerman A, and Herbst AL: Vinblastine, cisplatin, cyclophosphamide, bleomycin, doxorubicin, and etoposide in the treatment of small cell carcinoma of the ovary, Cancer 64:1183, 1989.

Serov SF, Scully RE, and Sobin LH: Histological typing of ovarian tumors, Geneva, 1973, World Health Organization.

Shakfeh AM and Woodruff JD: Primary ovarian sarcomas: report of 46 cases and review of literature, Obstet Gynecol Surv 42:331, 1987.

Slamon DJ, Godolophin W, Jones LA, et al: Studies of the HER-2/*neu* protooncogene in human breast and ovarian cancer, Science 244:707, 1989.

Soper JT, Hunter VJ, Daly L, et al: Preoperative serum tumor-associated antigen levels in women with pelvic masses, Obstet Gynecol 75:249, 1990.

Soper JT, Wilkinson RH, Bandy LC, et al: Intraperitoneal chromic phosphate ^{32}P as salvage therapy for persistent carcinoma of the ovary after surgical testing, Am J Obstet Gynecol 156:1153, 1987.

Sorbe B, Frankendal B, and Veress B: Importance of histologic grading in the prognosis of epithelial cancer, Obstet Gynecol 59:576, 1982.

Sparks JM and Varner RE: Ovarian cancer screening, Obstet Gynecol 77:787, 1991.

Spencer TR, Marks RD, Fenn JO, et al: Intraperitoneal ^{32}P after negative second-look laparotomy in ovarian carcinoma, Cancer 63:2434, 1989.

Stein AL, Koonings PP, Schlaerth JB, et al: Relative frequency of malignant paraovarian tumors: should paraovarian tumors be aspirated? Obstet Gynecol 75:1029, 1990.

Swanson SA, Norris HJ, Kelsten ML, and Wheeler JE: DNA content of juvenile granulosa tumors determined by flow cytometry, Int J Gynecol Pathol 9:101, 1990.

Talerman A: Germ cell tumors of the ovary. In Blaustein A, editor: Pathology of the female genital tract, New York, 1982, Springer-Verlag.

Thomas GM, Dembo AJ, Hacker NF, and DePetrillo AD: Review: current therapy for dysgerminoma of the ovary, Obstet Gynecol 70:268, 1987.

Troche V and Hernandez E: Neoplasia arising in dysgenetic gonads, Obstet Gynecol Surv 41:74, 1986.

Vasilev SA, Schlaerth JB, Campeau J, and Morrow CP: Serum CA-125 levels in preoperative evaluation of pelvic masses, Obstet Gynecol 71:751, 1988.

Vogl SE, Pagano M, Kaplan BH, et al: Cisplatin-based chemotherapy for advanced ovarian cancer: high overall response rate with curative potential only in women with small tumor burdens, Cancer 51:2024, 1983.

Von Hoff DD, Kronmal R, Salmon SE, et al: A Southwest Oncology Group study for the use of a human tumor cloning assay for predicting response in patients with ovarian cancer, Cancer 67:20, 1991.

Walton L, Ellenberg SS, Major F, et al: Results of second-look laparotomy in patients with early-stage ovarian carcinoma, Obstet Gynecol 70:770, 1987.

Wharton JT, Edwards CL, and Rutledge FN: Long-term survival after chemotherapy for advanced epithelial ovarian carcinoma, Am J Obstet Gynecol 148:997, 1984.

Wick MR, Mills SE, Dehner LP, et al: Serous papillary carcinomas arising from the peritoneum and ovaries, Int J Gynecol Pathol 8:179, 1989.

Willemse PHB, Aalders JG, Bouma J, et al: Long-term survival after vinblastine, bleomycin, and cisplatin treatment in patients with germ cell tumors of the ovary: an update, Gynecol Oncol 28:268, 1987.

Willemse PHB, Oosterhuis JW, Aalders JG, et al: Malignant struma ovarii by ovariectomy, thyroidectomy, and ^{131}I administration, Cancer 60:182, 1987.

Wu PC, Huang RL, Lang JH, et al: Treatment of malignant ovarian germ cell tumors with preservation of fertility: a report of 28 cases, Gynecol Oncol 40:2, 1991.

Yancik R, Ries LG, and Yates JW: An analysis of surveillance, epidemiology, and end results program data, Am J Obstet Gynecol 154:639, 1986.

Young RH, Gilks CB, and Scully RE: Mucinous tumors of the appendix associated with mucinous tumors of the ovary and pseudomyxoma peritonei, Am J Surg Pathol 15(5):415, 1991.

Young RH, Welch WR, Dickerson GR, et al: Ovarian sex cord tumor with annular tubules, Cancer 50:1384, 1982.

Young RH and Scully RE: Ovarian Sertoli-Leydig cell tumors: a clinicopathological analysis of 207 cases, Am J Surg Pathol 9:543, 1985.

Young RC, Walton LA, Ellenberg SS, et al: Adjuvant therapy in stage I and stage II epithelial ovarian cancer: results of two prospective randomized trials, N Engl J Med 332:1021, 1990.

Zambetti M, Escobedo A, Pilotti S, and De Palo G: *Cis*-platinum/vinblastine/bleomycin combination chemotherapy in advanced or recurrent granulosa cell tumors of the ovary, Gynecol Oncol 36:317, 1990.

KEY TERMS AND DEFINITIONS

Carcinoma in Situ. Premalignant epithelial change throughout the full thickness of the vulvar epithelium. It is also comparable to vulvar intraepithelial neoplasia (VIN) III.

Keyes Punch. An instrument used to biopsy the vulva.

Lichen Sclerosus. A vulvar abnormality usually characterized by thinning of the epithelium with a loss of subcutaneous adnexal structures, hyalinization of the superficial dermis, and lymphocytic infiltrates below the zone of dermal homogenization.

Melanoma Level. A system (I to V) used to define the depth or level to which a malignant melanoma invades the epithelium.

Microinvasive Vulvar Carcinoma. A controversial term used to describe a superficially invasive carcinoma of the vulva that is not expected to be associated with lymph node metastasis. Usually the invasion is less than 1 mm into the stroma.

Paget's Disease of the Vulva. A vulvar atypicality containing large cells with pale cytoplasm similar to Paget cells seen in the breast. The squamous epithelium is studded with large cells containing clear cytoplasm and pleomorphic nuclei with prominent nucleoli. It may be associated with malignancy of the vulva and other sites.

Radical Vulvectomy. An operation that removes the entire vulva, including subcutaneous and fatty tissue, the labia minora and majora, perineal skin, and clitoris, to treat cancer.

Simple Vulvectomy. An operation that removes the skin of the vulva, including the labia majora and minora, the clitoris, and perineal skin.

Stages of Vulvar Cancer:

  Stage I: Less than 2 cm in diameter and confined to the vulva and/or perineum.

  Stage II: Over 2 cm in diameter and confined to the vulva and/or perineum.

  Stage III: Extends to the anus and/or lower urethra, and/or unilateral regional node metastasis.

  Stage IV: Spreads to the bladder or rectum or pelvic bone or upper urethra or nonvulvar sites, or bilateral regional node metastases

Verrucous Carcinoma. An infrequent well-differentiated squamous carcinoma with a gross wartlike appearance that is curable with a local operation.

Vulvar Atypia. A mild, moderate, or severe neoplastic or dysplastic change in the vulvar squamous epithelium. It may also be termed *vulvar intraepithelial neoplasia (VIN I, II, or III)*.

Cancer of the vulva accounts for about 4% of malignancies of the lower female genital tract, which ranks it fourth in frequency among these malignancies, after cancers of the endometrium, ovary, and cervix.

Well-defined predisposing factors for the development of vulvar carcinoma have not been identified. In general, premalignant and malignant changes frequently arise at multifocal points on the vulva. Occasionally invasive carcinoma arises from areas of carcinoma in situ, similar to the mechanism in cervical squamous cell carcinoma (Chapter 27). However, many cases of squamous cell carcinoma of the vulva

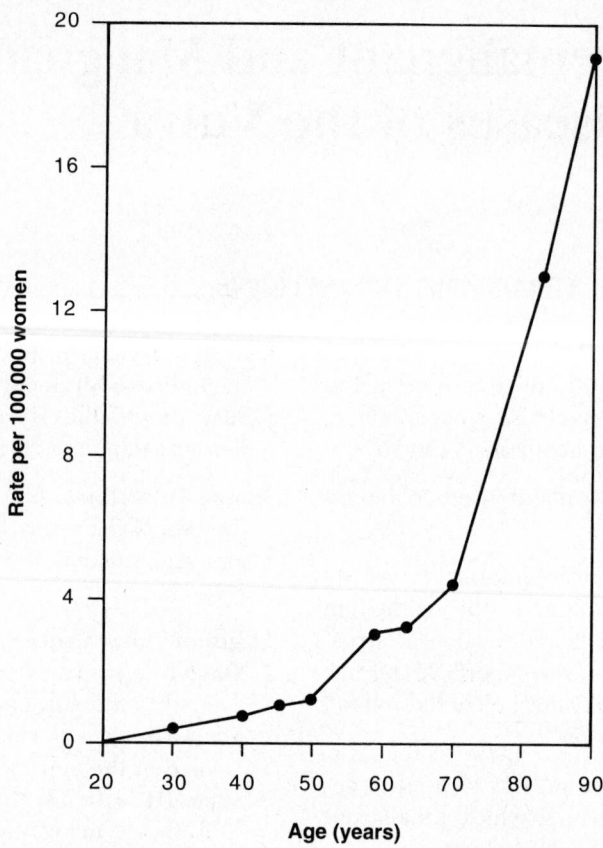

FIGURE 30-1
Age incidence curve for carcinoma of vulva in white women in the United States. (Adapted from Menczer J, Voliovitch Y, Modan B, et al: Am J Obstet Gynecol 143:893, 1982.)

appear to develop in the absence of premalignant changes in the vulvar epithelium. Condyloma acuminatum (human papillomavirus) has been noted in many patients with carcinoma of the vulva. At present, however, a sexually transmitted origin for carcinoma of the vulva has not been demonstrated. Other factors, such as granulomatous disease of the vulva, diabetes, hypertension, and obesity, have all been suggested as etiologic factors, but current data do not support their involvement in the genesis of vulvar carcinoma. One case control study by Mabuchi et al. implicated the environment as a potential contributing cause insofar as those who worked as domestic servants or were employed in laundry or cleaning plants were at an increased risk for vulvar carcinoma. In addition, carcinoma of the vulva does occur with increasing frequency in those who have been treated for squamous cell carcinoma of the cervix or vagina, presumably as a result of the increased risk of carcinogenesis in the squamous

epithelium of the lower genital tract in these patients.

Most vulvar malignancies are squamous cell carcinomas. Although this is a disease of older women, Franklin and Rutledge noted that 15% of cancers of the vulva in their series occurred in women under the age of 40. The incidence of squamous cell carcinoma of the vulva in the United States increases progressively with age (Figure 30-1). More than half of patients with carcinoma of the vulva are 60 to 79 years of age at the time of diagnosis. While most patients with carcinoma of the vulva are older than 60, those with carcinoma in situ of the vulva are usually 10 to 15 years younger, that is, 40 to 55 years of age. In recent years premalignant changes of the vulva are being seen with increasing frequency among younger patients, often in their twenties and thirties, possibly as a result of an increasing rate of multiple sexual contacts and increased venereal-viral infections in the population. An increase in the frequency of invasive carcinoma of the vulva, however, has not yet been detected, but it may well develop in future years.

This chapter reviews the clinical and pathologic aspects of premalignant vulvar lesions and vulvar atypias. This is followed by consideration of the diagnosis, natural history, and management of invasive cancers of the vulva, which includes not only the squamous cell carcinomas but also the rarer melanomas and sarcomas.

VULVAR ATYPIAS

Specific Conditions

The diagnosis and treatment of premalignant conditions of the vulva have been confusing in the past because of the lack of a uniform definition of the various lesions encountered. Recently the International Society for the Study of Vulvar Diseases (ISSVD) has provided a new standard nomenclature that has also been adopted by the International Society for Gynecologic Pathology (ISGYP) (see box below). For comparison, the classification before 1985 is also shown. A number of ambiguous terms have been eliminated. For example, terms such as *leukoplakia* and *leukoplakic vulvitis*

have been discarded, and terms such as *Bowen's disease, erythroplasia of Queyrat*, and *carcinoma simplex* are all grouped under the term *carcinoma in situ* or *vulvar intraepithelial neoplasia (VIN)*.

Vulvar Atypias—Intraepithelial Neoplasia

Although the term vulvar dystrophy is no longer in official use (see box), it is widespread in gynecologic literature and therefore is briefly reviewed in this chapter.

Two types of vulvar dystrophy have been previously described: lichen sclerosus (still in use) and hyperplastic dystrophy (no longer used). Hyperplastic dystrophy has been defined as existing with or without cellular atypia (dysplastic change). In current terminology if premalignant change exists, it is termed *dysplasia* (mild, moderate, or severe) or *carcinoma in situ* (VIN I, II, or III). The nonpremalignant squamous changes that used to be termed *hyperplastic dystrophy* now fall into the classification of *squamous hyperplasia*.

Lichen sclerosus (Figure 30-2) is a change in the vulvar skin that often appears whitish. Microscopically the epithelium becomes markedly thinned with a loss or blunting of the rete ridges. In some cases there is also a thickening or hyperkeratosis of the surface layers (Figure 30-3). This is not a premalignant condition, but it tends to be multifocal and can recur. Inflammation is usually present. Hart et al. studied 107 patients with lichen sclerosus, and only one followed for 12 years eventually developed vulvar carcinoma. Five of the patients in their series had vulvar carcinoma at the time lichen sclerosus was diagnosed. Twelve other patients subsequently developed malignancies at other sites, such as the cervix, colon, breast, ovary, and endometrium. Patients with lichen sclerosus are not at increased risk for the development of vulvar carcinoma, but there appears to be potential for developing malignancies at other sites and also for lichen sclerosus to recur.

Hyperplastic dystrophy changes involve elongation and widening of the rete ridges, which may be confluent (Figure 30-4). There may also be hyperkeratotic surface layers, and the tissue grossly often is whitish or reddish.

Atypical changes may appear in the vulvar epithelium. These changes are usually marked

---

CLASSIFICATION OF VULVAR ATYPIAS

Classification Before 1985

Hyperplastic dystrophy
  Without atypia
  With atypia (mild, moderate, or severe)

Lichen sclerosus

Mixed dystrophy (lichen sclerosus with hyperplastic dystrophy)
  Without atypia
  With atypia (mild, moderate, or severe)

Current (After 1985) Classification of Vulvar Atypias

Intraepithelial atypias
  VIN I   Mild dysplasia
  VIN II   Moderate dysplasia
  VIN III Severe dysplasia—carcinoma in situ

Lichen sclerosus

Squamous hyperplasia—not otherwise specified

Miscellaneous specific diagnoses (benign dermatoses—Paget's disease)

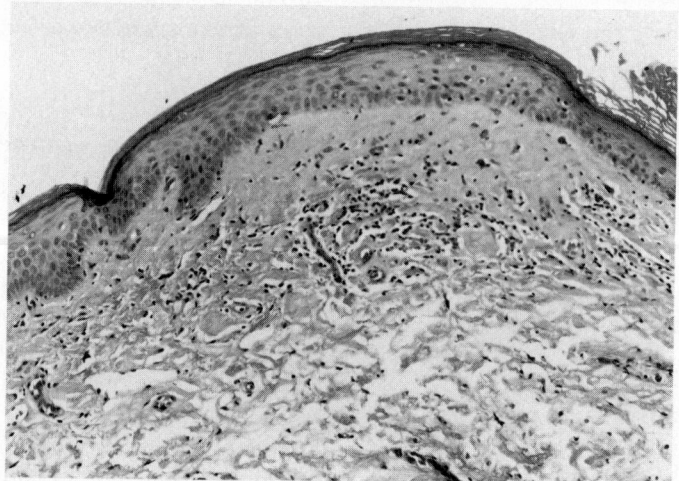

FIGURE 30-2

Lichen sclerosus et atrophicus. Homogenous collagen in the papillary dermis is accompanied by a scattered lymphocytic infiltrate and atrophy of the epithelium. (H&E ×80.) (Courtesy Dr. Anthony Montag, The University of Chicago.)

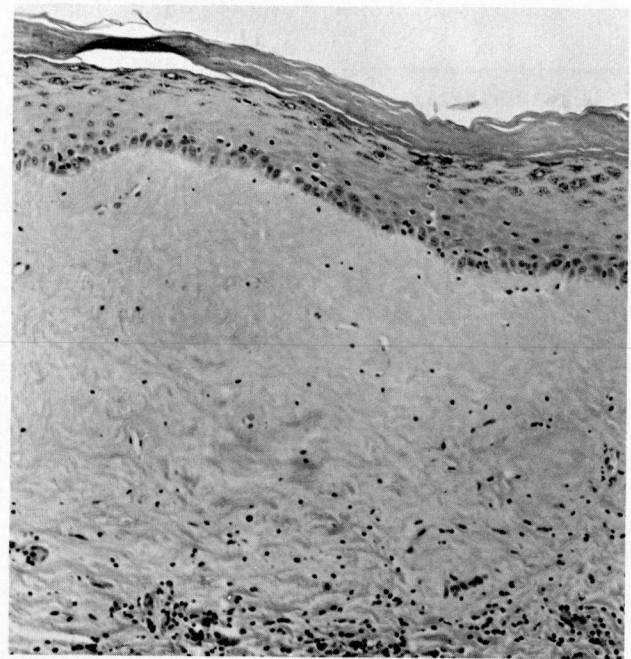

FIGURE 30-3

Lichen sclerosus. Hyperkeratosis is occasionally present. (From Friedrich EG and Wilkinson EJ: The vulva. In Blaustein A, editor: Pathology of the female genital tract, New York, 1982, Springer-Verlag.)

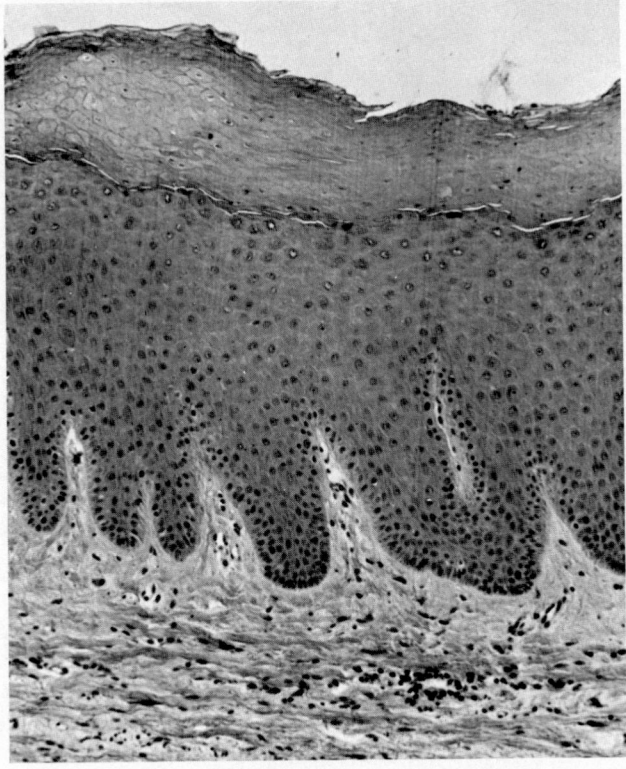

FIGURE 30-4
Hyperplastic dystrophy, benign. Hyperkeratosis, acanthosis, and mild inflammation are present. (From Friedrich EG and Wilkinson EJ: The vulva. In Blaustein A, editor: Pathology of the female genital tract, New York, 1982, Springer-Verlag.)

by a loss of maturation process usually seen in squamous epithelium as well as an increase in mitotic activity and in the nuclear-cytoplasmic ratio (Figure 30-5). Mild dyplasia (atypia) is diagnosed if these changes involve the lower third of the epithelium; moderate dysplasia (atypia) if half to two thirds of the epithelium is involved; and severe dysplasia (atypia) if over two thirds of the epithelium is affected. Carcinoma in situ involves full thickness of the epithelium. The term *VIN I* is used for mild atypia, *VIN II* for moderate atypia, and *VIN III* for severe atypia, as well as carcinoma in situ. It is sometimes difficult to distinguish between squamous hyperplasia and intraepithelial neoplasia. Crum has suggested that intraepithelial neoplasia of the vulva almost always contains nuclei which are fourfold or greater different in size, while differences in the size of nuclei in condyloma or non-neoplastic epithelia are threefold or less. Furthermore, abnormal mitoses are usually observed in vulvar intraepithelial neoplasia.

Carcinoma in Situ (VIN III)

Carcinoma in situ is diagnosed if the full thickness of the epithelium is abnormal (Figure 30-6, A). Occasionally the process may histologically resemble carcinoma in situ of the cervix, and in many lesions there are multinucleated cells, abnormal mitoses, an increased density in cells, and an increase in the nuclear-cytoplasmic ratio. Studies of the chromosome distribution of these lesions have indicated that they are aneuploid as measured by DNA analysis using the microspectrophotometric techniques described in Chapter 26.

Paget's Disease

Paget's disease is a rare intraepithelial disorder that occurs in the vulvar skin and histologically resembles Paget's disease in the breast. Paget cells are large pale cells (Figure 30-7). The cells often occur in nests and infiltrate upward through the epithelium. Frequently, histologic abnormalities of the apocrine glands of

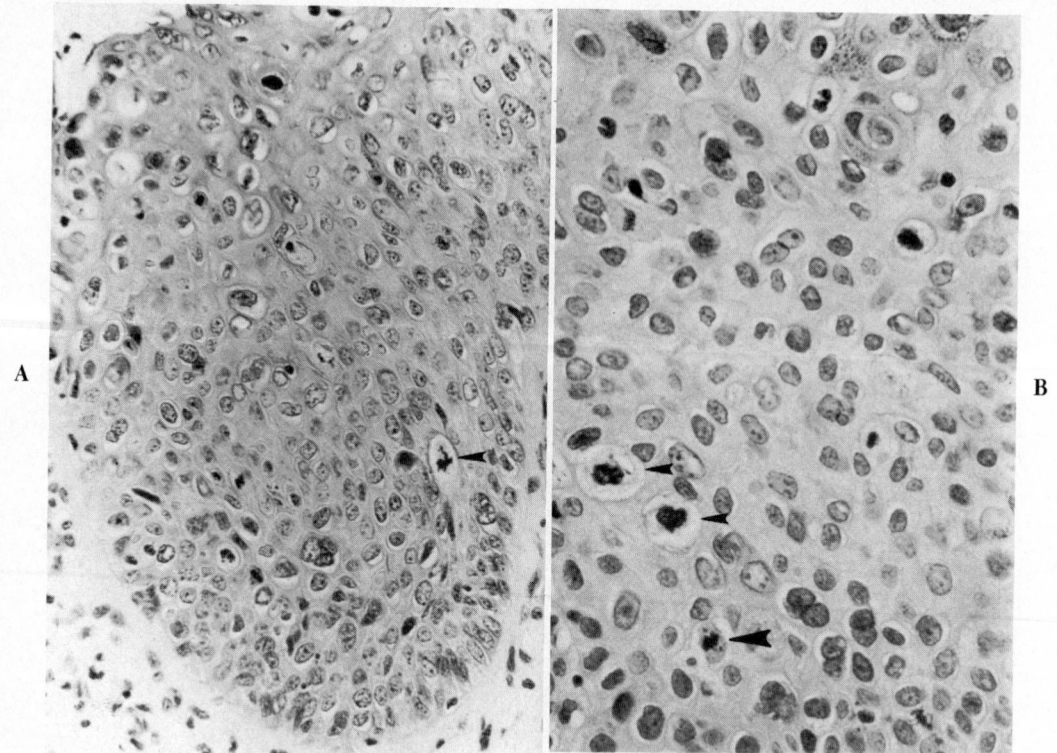

FIGURE 30-5
A, Vulvar intraepithelial neoplasia from which HPV type 16 was isolated. Characteristic features displayed here include abnormal mitoses (a two-group metaphase is denoted by the arrow), a full-thickness population of abnormal cells and abnormal differentiation. Superficial cells contain perinuclear halos, which in contrast to condylomata are small and concentric. **B,** The higher-power photomicrograph of vulvar intraepithelial neoplasia illustrates the marked variability in nuclear size and staining with both enlarged nuclei and multinucleated cells. Coarsely clumped mitoses *(small arrows)* and a three-group metaphase *(large arrow)* are present. (From Crum CP: Pathology of the vulva and vagina, New York, 1987, Churchill-Livingstone.)

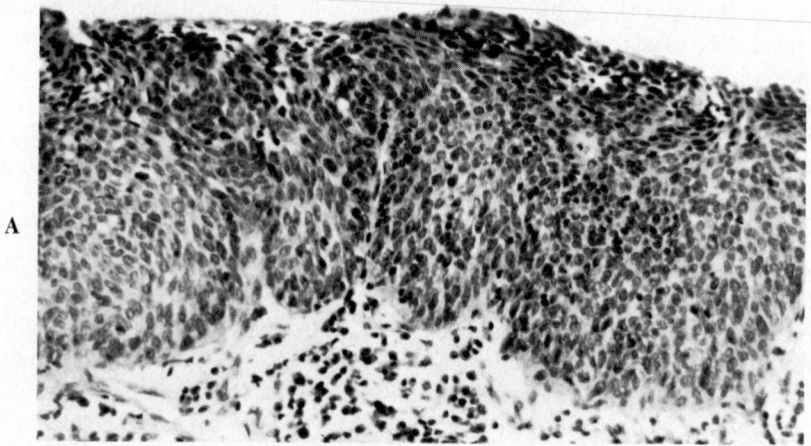

FIGURE 30-6
For legend see opposite page.

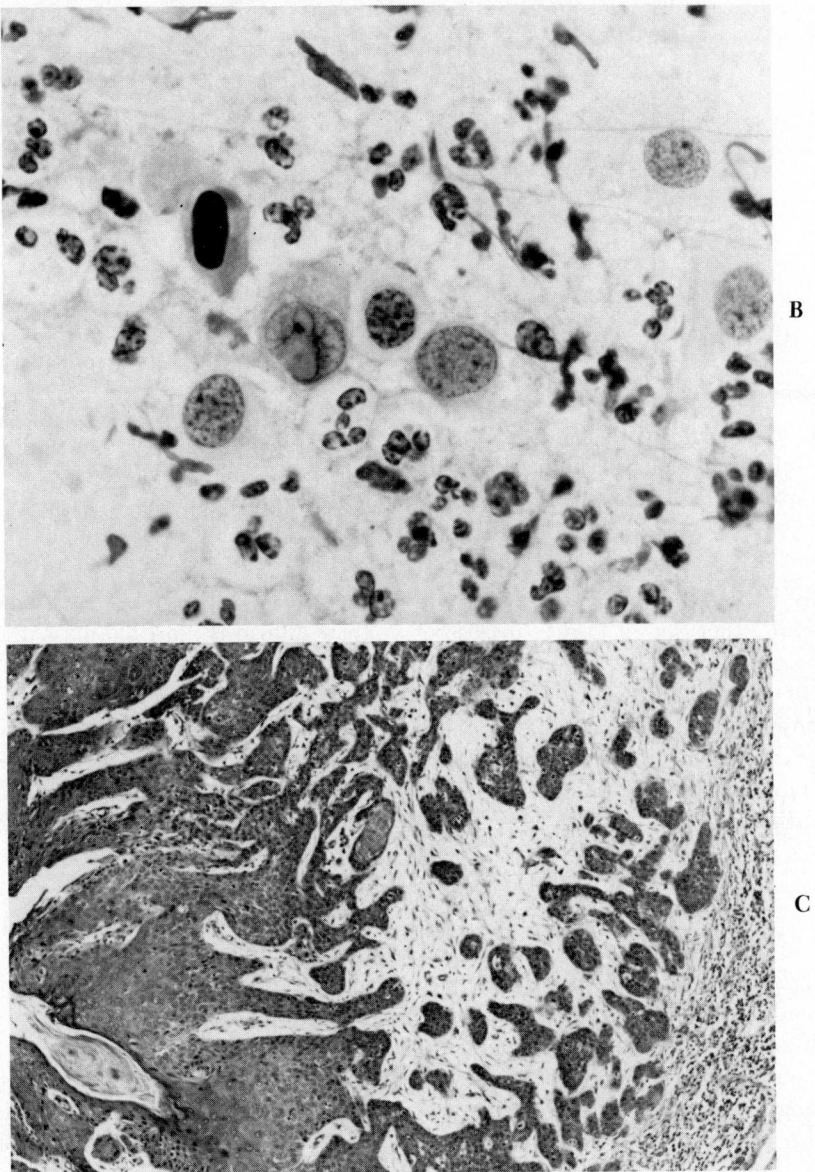

FIGURE 30-6
A, Carcinoma in situ, histology. Full thickness of epithelium is replaced by hyperchromatic cells with poorly defined cellular borders. (×80.) **B,** Carcinoma in situ,
cytology. Cells derived from carcinoma in situ of vulva may exhibit varying sizes
and shapes as depicted in this photomicrograph. Note variation in nuclear pattern
from one nucleus to another. Degenerated polymorphonuclear leukocytes are
present in background. (×800.) **C,** Invasive squamous carcinoma, histology. Tumor
nests and cords infiltrate stroma. The squamous nature of tumor is more apparent
on surface *(left),* where cells have abundant dense cytoplasm. Keratin is also seen.
(×80.)

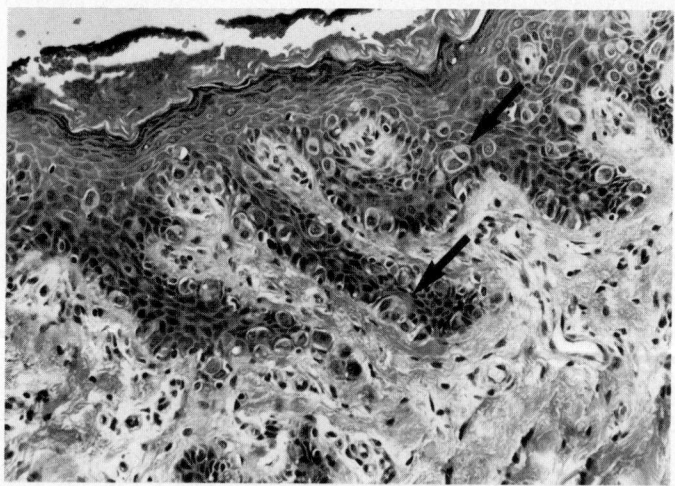

FIGURE 30-7
Vulvar epidermis with Paget's disease. Malignant cells *(arrows)* are seen infiltrating the epidermis and spreading along the dermal-epidermal junction. (H&E ×160.) (Courtesy Dr. Anthony Montag, The University of Chicago.)

the skin may be noted in these lesions. There is an increased association of Paget's disease of the vulva with invasive carcinoma at other sites. Paget's disease of the vulva tends to spread, often in an occult fashion. Extension to apparently normal skin will often occur after surgical therapy, particularly if Paget's cells are identified at the resection margin.

Diagnosis

Clinical Presentation

Atypias of the vulva present with a variety of symptoms and signs. Irritation or itching is common, although some patients may not complain of these symptoms. The vulva often has a whitish change due to a thickened keratin layer. In the past the term *leukoplakia* was used. This term, denoting a premalignant change in the vulvar epithelium, has been discarded in part because most whitish lesions of the vulva are not premalignant. When lichen sclerosus is present, there is usually a diffuse whitish change to the vulvar skin (Figure 30-8). The vulvar skin often appears thin, and there may be scarring and contracture. In addition, fissuring of the skin is often present, accompanied by excoriation secondary to itching. Areas of squamous hyperplasias (formerly called *hyperplastic dystrophy without atypia*) also appear as whitish lesions in general, but the tissues of the vulva usually appear thickened and

the process tends to be more focal or multifocal than diffuse (Figure 30-9). A biopsy is necessary to establish the diagnosis.

Abnormal areas of vulvar atypia or intraepithelial neoplasia may also appear as red nodules or pigmented areas on the vulva. However, the clinical appearance of vulvar intraepithelial neoplasia is variable. Wilkinson and Friedrich estimate that about one third of patients with carcinoma in situ will present with pigmented lesions, emphasizing the importance of a biopsy to establish the diagnosis. The lesions tend to be discrete and multifocal, and they occur more frequently in those who have had squamous cell neoplasia of the cervix. In addition, reddish nodules may also be foci of Paget's disease, as well as carcinoma in situ. Paget's disease often has a reddish, eczematoid appearance. It should be reemphasized that these conditions cannot be accurately diagnosed from their clinical appearance, and biopsies are needed.

Diagnostic Methods

A number of aids are available to help the physician establish the diagnosis of vulvar abnormalities. Along with cytology (Pap smear) and the colposcope, the toluidine blue test can be used before biopsy. In general, the cytologic evaluation of the vulva has often not been helpful, in part because the vulvar skin is thick

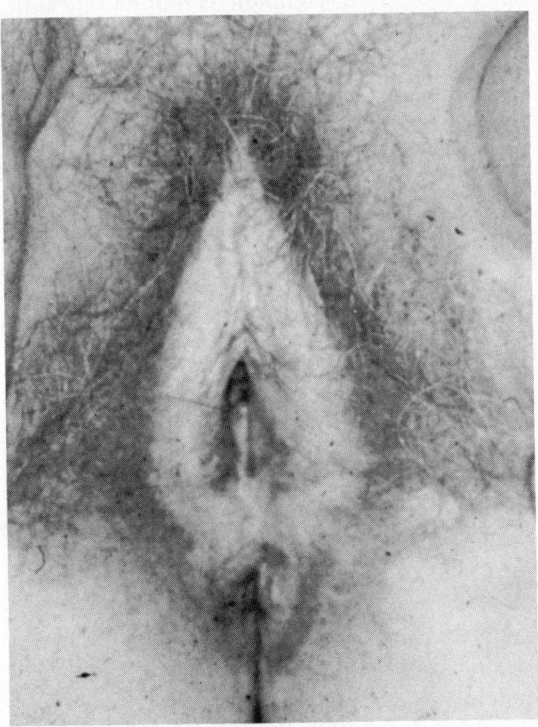

FIGURE 30-8
Vulva, lichen sclerosus. Tissue of labia minora and perineum has white, brittle "cigarette paper" appearance. (From Kaufman RH, Gardner HL, and Merrill JA: Diseases of the vulva and vagina. In Romney SL, et al, editors: Gynecology and obstetrics, New York, 1980, McGraw-Hill Book Co.)

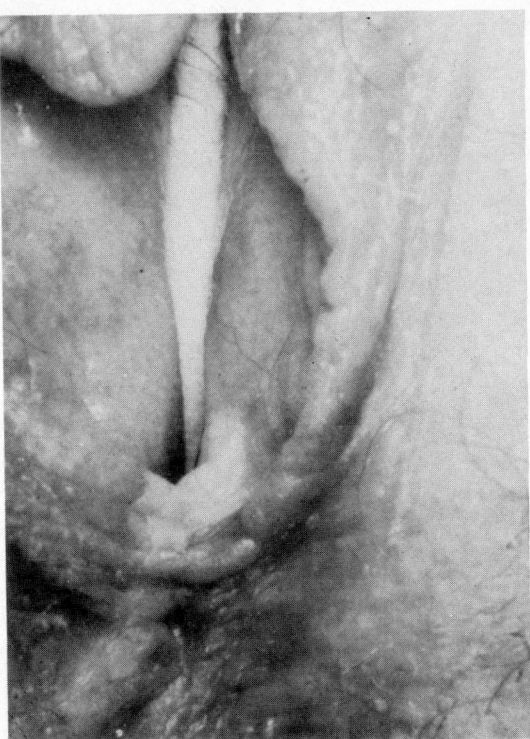

FIGURE 30-9
Vulva, hyperplastic dystrophy. Sharply demarcated, raised, white area is noted at lower tip of white pointer. (From Kaufman RH, Gardner HL, and Merrill JA: Diseases of the vulva and vagina. In Romney SL, et al, editors: Gynecology and obstetrics. New York, 1980, McGraw-Hill Book Co.)

and keratinized and does not shed cells as readily as the epithelium of the vagina and cervix. However, in some cases, particularly if there is ulceration of the vulva, a cytologic smear can be helpful diagnostically (Figure 30-6, *B*). A tongue depressor moistened with normal saline or tap water is scraped over the surface portion of the vulva to be sampled, and the specimen is placed on a glass slide and then fixed.

An additional diagnostic aid is the toluidine blue test, which is nonspecific and stains nuclei in the superficial part of the epithelium. Normally the superficial keratin layers of the vulva do not contain nuclei. The test is performed by applying 1% aqueous solution toluidine blue to the vulva. It is allowed to dry for at least 1 minute, and then 1% acetic acid is applied and the excess gently removed with a cotton swab. The areas that retain a blue stain should be bi-

opsied. (About two thirds of vulvar atypias retain the dye.) However, ulceration and fissures of the skin also stain, and a positive test does not always indicate a premalignant condition.

Colposcopy of the vulva is difficult because the characteristic changes in vascular appearance and tissue patterns that are seen in the cervix are not present (Chapter 26). Nevertheless, the magnification of the colposcope can be used to help follow patients with intraepithelial neoplasia of the vulva, as well as to examine the vulva to identify the discrete whitish or pigmented areas that warrant biopsy. The colposcope is not used for routine vulvar examination but is primarily employed for those who are being evaluated or followed for vulvar atypia or intraepithelial neoplasia.

Biopsy of the vulva can be conveniently accomplished with a Keyes dermal punch (Figure

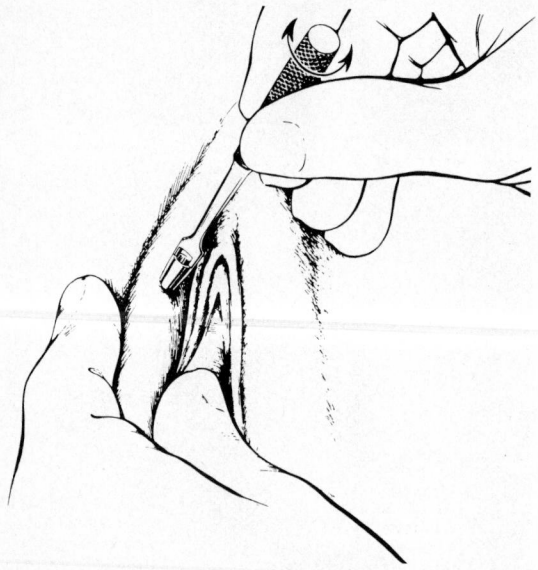

FIGURE 30-10
Diagnostic Keyes punch biopsy. (From Friedrich EG: Vulvar disease, ed 2, Philadelphia, 1983, WB Saunders Co.)

30-10). Usually a 4 to 5 mm diameter punch is used. Each area to be biopsied is to be performed is infiltrated with local anesthesia using a fine 25-gauge needle. The punch is then rotated and a downward pressure applied so that a disc of tissue is circumscribed. When the entire thickness of the skin has been incised, the specimen is elevated with forceps and then removed with a sharp scissors. Occasionally a larger biopsy is needed, in which case a larger field is anesthetized and a small scalpel or cervical punch biopsy (Figure 26-15) is used to obtain the specimen. Usually little bleeding is encountered, and it can generally be controlled by applying silver nitrate or ferrous subsulfate (Monsel's solution). Depending on the size of the atypical area and the variety of atypical appearing areas, one or multiple biopsies may be needed.

Management

Vulvar Atypias

Most vulvar atypias have pruritus as the major symptom, so the relief of itching is often the main concern of the patient. Once the correct diagnosis has been established by biopsy, appropriate therapy can be undertaken. Most whitish lesions will be benign, as lichen sclero-sus is the most common condition encountered.

Topical testosterone is employed for atrophic conditions of the vulva, particularly in cases of lichen sclerosus. An effective preparation is 2% testosterone proprionate in petrolatum, which is used twice daily. Once daily is often sufficient maintenance after the first week. Side effects, such as clitoral hypertrophy and increased hair growth, can occur. If there are undesirable side effects with testosterone, then local progesterone cream is sometimes tried. Those who have a beneficial response to testosterone should be continued on the medication indefinitely. Often testosterone cream twice weekly is a sufficient maintenance dose.

The control of local irritation of the vulva is discussed in Chapter 17. In addition to local measures to diminish irritation (cotton underclothes, avoidance of strong soaps and detergents, and avoidance of synthetic undergarments), topical fluorinated corticosteroids are helpful to control itching. Frequently used preparations are 0.025% or 0.1% triamcinolone acetonide (Aristocort, Kenalog), fluorocinolone acetonide (Synalar), or 0.01% or 0.1% betamethasone valerate (Valisone). These are usually applied twice daily to control the itching, which is often relieved in 1 to 2 weeks. Unfortunately the prolonged use of fluorinated topical steroids can lead to vulvar atrophy and contraction. Thus once the symptoms of itching are controlled, the dosage of topical corticosteroids is tapered off, or if long-term therapy is needed, a nonfluorinated compound such as 1.0% hydrocortisone is used to avoid vulvar contraction. Occasionally 1% hydrocortisone is sufficient for initial therapy. In some cases the corticosteroids are not successful, and numerous types of topical therapy need to be tried to control symptoms. Gentle soaps such as Basis are helpful. Burow's solution (5% solution of aluminum acetate) is frequently used as a wet dressing to help control irritation and itching. Three percent Doak's Tar in petrolatum or in 1% hydrocortisone ointment is also occasionally of use for severe cases.

In some patients with lichen sclerosus, severe contracture of the vulva, particularly in the area of the posterior fourchette, will occur with concomitant scarring and tenderness. Intercourse may then become painful in these patients. Woodruff et al. have described a useful surgical technique to treat these vaginal

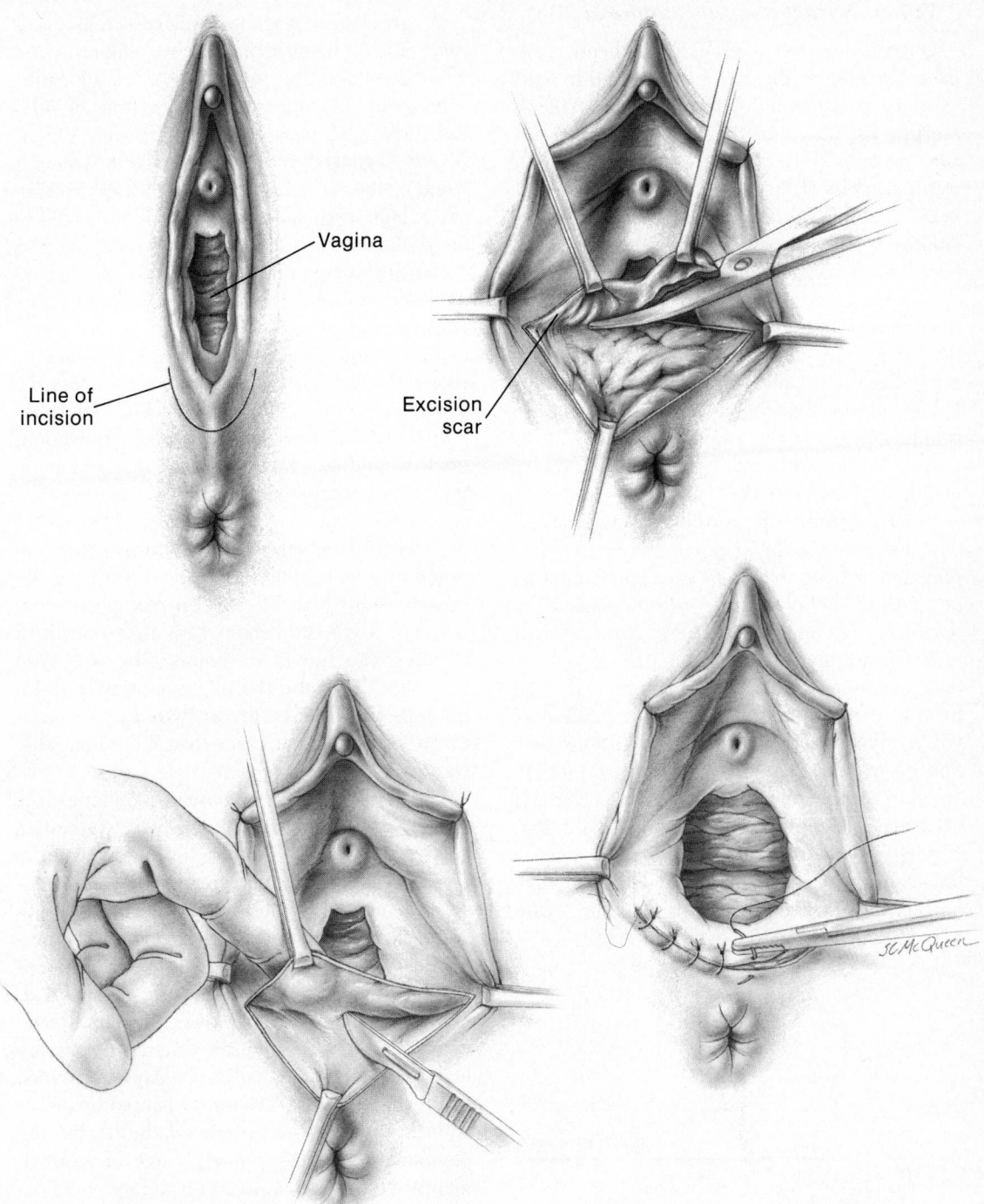

FIGURE 30-11
Surgical correction of perineal scars. (From Woodruff JD and Julian CJ: Surgery of the vulva. In Ridley JH: Gynecologic surgery: errors, safeguards, salvage, Baltimore, 1974, Williams & Wilkins.)

outlet disorders by plastic repair of the perineum. The contractured and fissured area in the posterior fourchette is excised, which results in an elliptical defect. This defect is then closed by undermining the distal 3 to 4 cm of the posterior vaginal mucosa and suturing the freed mucosa to the perineal skin (Figure 30-11).

Vulvar Intraepithelial Neoplasia

Once the diagnosis of VIN has been established by biopsy, therapy is performed to eradicate the area containing the neoplasia. The clinician must be aware that the progress of vulvar atypia (mild dysplasia—VIN I) to moderate dysplasia (VIN II) to severe dysplasia and carcinoma in situ (VIN III) and then to invasive carcinoma is not as well documented for vulvar neoplasia as it is for squamous cell neoplasia of the cervix. Moreover, vulvar neoplasia is frequently multifocal, requiring treatment of several areas. An additional complication is that some cases originally diagnosed as intraepithelial neoplasia have been reported to regress spontaneously. Finally, areas contiguous to the vulva are frequently involved in intraepithelial neoplasia (Figure 30-12).

In 1972 Friedrich reported Bowenoid atypia (histologically similar to carcinoma in situ) in a pregnant patient that regressed spontaneously postpartum. Others also reported spontaneous regression of this lesion. These spontaneously regressing lesions tend to be discrete elevations in young women. Some may be explained by recent studies of nuclear DNA content of vulvar atypias that suggest not all lesions with this designation are premalignant. Fu et al. noted that only four of eight cases of vulvar atypia had an aneuploid (neoplastic) distribution. A polyploid distribution was noted in four of the cases, which is consistent with a benign process, whereas aneuploidy is consistent with intraepithelial neoplasia.

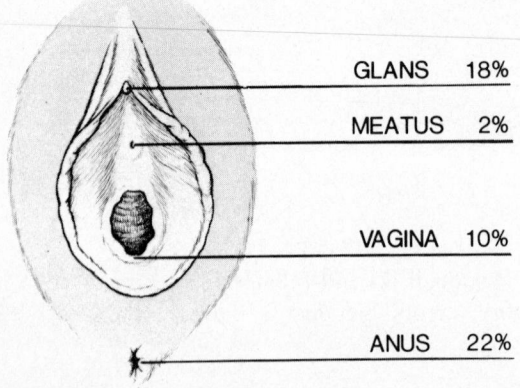

GLANS	18%
MEATUS	2%
VAGINA	10%
ANUS	22%

FIGURE 30-12
Frequency of involvement of contiguous structures by carcinoma in situ. (From Friedrich EG: Vulvar disease, ed 2, Philadelphia, 1983, WB Saunders Co.)

Progression of VIN to invasive carcinoma is rare and has been estimated by Wilkinson and Friedrich to occur in about 6% of all cases. Moreover, a comparable proportion of VIN cases spontaneously regress. Although VIN is being diagnosed more commonly in younger women, the risk of progression to invasive cancer is higher for those who are older as well as for those who are immunosuppressed, such as transplant recipients. Chafe et al. studied 69 patients with a diagnosis of VIN treated by surgical excision. Unsuspected invasion was found in 13 patients. The median age was 36 years for those without invasive carcinoma, whereas the median age was 58 years ($p = .003$) for those with invasion found in the excision specimen, emphasizing the increased risk of invasion in the older patients. Furthermore, the risk of invasion was higher in those who had raised lesions with irregular surface patterns. Thus patients who were older and those with irregular raised lesions had the greatest risk of unrecognized invasive carcinoma. Less than one third of vulvar carcinomas are found to be associated with VIN. Thus the risk of progression from intraepithelial disease to invasive carcinoma is much less for vulvar cases than for comparable cervical disease (Chapter 26).

The potential role of human papillomavirus (HPV) has begun to be extensively studied in cases of VIN and is more fully reviewed in Chapter 26. HPV vulvar infection is widespread and is associated histologically with koilocytosis (nuclear cellular changes and a perinuclear halo) and may also occur with intraepithelial neoplasia (Figure 30-13). Crum et al. found that older patients (over 45 years of age) with VIN did not show the stigmas of papillomavirus infection in vulvar biopsy specimens, whereas those with VIN accompanied by either koilocytosis or condyloma, produced by the papillomavirus, had a median age of approximately 31 years. Invasive vulvar carcinoma occurred in five patients, all of whom were over the age of 45. This suggests that papillomavirus may be involved in the genesis of VIN, but the viral infection may not necessarily lead directly to vulvar carcinoma. The rates of progression from VIN to invasive carcinoma are not established. However, current evidence suggests that the potential of VIN to develop into invasive cancer is low. Buscema et al. followed 102 patients with vulvar carcinoma in situ for 1 to 15 years without treatment, and four patients developed invasive disease, two of whom were

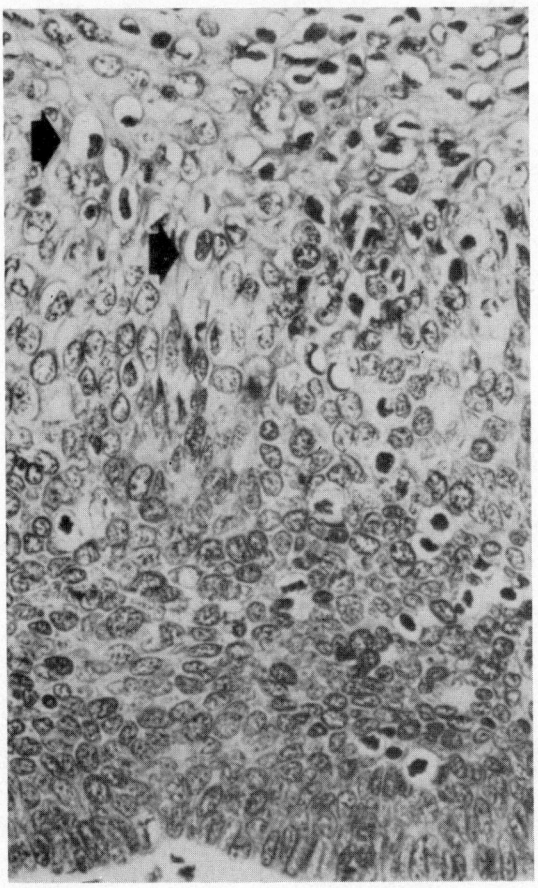

FIGURE 30-13
Vulvar intraepithelial neoplasia with koilocytosis. Lower half of lesion contains pleomorphism and abnormal mitoses. Upper half contains koilocytotic atypia with numerous halo cells *(arrows)*. (From Crum PC, Liskow A, Petras P, et al: Cancer 54:1429, 1984.)

immunosuppressed. Unfortunately, current techniques do not allow prediction of which lesions of VIN are at the greatest risk for progression to invasive disease.

Currently HPV types 6 and 11 are generally recognized as being found most frequently in benign vulvar warts, whereas primarily HPV types 16, 18, 31, 33, and 35 are more frequently associated with intraepithelial neoplasia or invasive carcinoma. Crum has estimated that perineal warts develop in more than 1 million women per year in the United States, and perhaps as many as 10% of all women harbor HPV infection. An additional complication is that HPV type 16 infection is not always accompanied by histologic evidence of VIN. Moreover, HPV types 6, 11, and 16 can be re-

covered from a single site, including those that show only condyloma, as well as those that show carcinoma. Thus a unique role for HPV types in VIN has not been elucidated. At the current state of our knowledge, therapy should be based on histologic findings and not on the presence or absence of HPV infection or specific HPV types. Studies by Buscema et al. suggest that HPV type 16 is frequently found in vulvar neoplasia.

THERAPY. The problem of the management of vulvar HPV infection is particularly complicated, since it is extremely prevalent and the risk of progression from HPV infection to VIN is extremely small. Planner et al. evaluated 148 women with cytologic evidence of vulvar HPV infection and found that two thirds of them had pruritus and dyspareunia. Results of the biopsy revealed that 11 of the 148 women had VIN. Follow-up showed spontaneous regression of HPV infection in 56 patients, whereas VIN III developed in 2 and invasive cancer eventually developed in 1. It appears that the best approach is to restrict therapy to individuals with clinically bothersome symptoms such as warts or to eradicate lesions with VIN, particularly VIN II and III. Cytologic or histologic evidence of an asymptomatic HPV infection, such as koilocytosis, is not an indication for therapy.

Long-term follow-up is needed in view of the risk of recurrence of disease. As noted, the treatment is complicated by the fact that many lesions are multifocal, and wide and separate areas may be affected. Most lesions of intraepithelial neoplasia of the vulva tend to be posterior, predominantly in the perineal area. Surgical removal has been effectively used, but the type of operation has changed in recent years. In the past, simple vulvectomy was widely practiced to treat carcinoma in situ of the vulva, but this disfiguring operation is now infrequently used, particularly since the disease is occurring in younger women. To improve the cosmetic result and sexual function, Rutledge and Sinclair introduced the method of "skinning vulvectomy." This removes the superficial vulvar skin, preserving the clitoris, and replaces the removed skin with a split-thickness vulvar graft. In many cases, however, such extensive surgery is not needed, and the abnormal area of the vulva can often be removed with wide local excision. Sixty-two of the patients in the series reported by Buscema were treated with local excision; 68% showed no recurrence. For comparison, in 28 patients treated by vulvectomy, 70% showed no recurrence. The risk of recurrence is higher if neoplastic epithelium is found at the resection margin. Friedrich noted a 10% risk of recurrence if the surgical margins were free of disease in comparison to a 50% risk if the surgical margins were involved with neoplasia. However, since recurrence may develop even if the resection margins are negative, long-term follow-up is mandatory.

Alternatives to operations have been introduced. The carbon dioxide laser has recently been utilized to treat VIN, usually to a depth of about 3 mm. This results in eradication of the abnormal vulvar tissue and healing without scarring. Most patients require a single treatment, but some patients require two to four, particularly those with large or multiple lesions. A few patients can be treated on an outpatient basis with local anesthesia, but most require either general or regional anesthesia. Current evidence indicates that laser therapy is as effective as surgical excision in most situations, but some patients have needed an excision after laser treatment to control disease. The laser is particularly useful for younger patients. It is essential to be certain that the patient does not have invasive disease before utilizing the laser. Therefore the therapist should be experienced in the diagnosis and treatment of vulvar disease before utilizing laser ablation. Treatment is usually carried out to a depth of 3 to 4 mm, and healing is usually complete within 2 to 3 weeks. Leuchter et al. treated 142 patients with carcinoma in situ of the vulva. Of the 42 treated by laser, 17% had recurrence; 4 (25%) of the 16 treated with vulvectomy and 15 (33%) of 45 treated by local excision also had recurrence. In view of the risk of unsuspected carcinoma in older patients as noted by the studies of Chafe et al., those over the age of 45 and those with raised or irregular lesions should, if possible, have an excision performed and have the entire tissue submitted for histologic evaluation.

5-Fluorouracil (5-FU) cream has been used successfully to treat carcinoma in situ of the vulva. While such therapy has been reported to be successful in approximately 75% of the cases, the treatment causes severe vulvar edema and pain over a 6-week period; for that reason it is not usually prescribed. Reid et al. marginally improved their results of laser ablation for vulvar disease by adding posttherapy 5-FU, but the outcome was not uniformly successful.

Paget's Disease of the Vulva

Paget's disease is generally seen in postmenopausal women and appears grossly as a diffuse erythematous eczematoid lesion that has usually been present for a prolonged time. Itching is a common problem. The disease is primarily seen in whites, and the average age of the patient is approximately 65 years. The major importance of Paget's disease of the vulva is the frequent association with other invasive carcinomas. They may present as squamous carcinoma of the vulva or cervix or an adenocarcinoma of the sweat glands of the vulva or Bartholin's gland carcinoma. Cases of adenocarcinoma of the gastrointestinal tract accompanying Paget's disease have also been reported. Once a diagnosis of Paget's disease of the vulva is made, it is important for the gynecologist to rule out the presence of malignancy at other sites, including the breast. In a review by Lee et al. a total of 75 cases of Paget's disease of the vulva were identified, and an underlying invasive carcinoma of the adnexal structures of the skin was reported in only 16 (22%) and a carcinoma in situ in 7 (9%). Twenty-two of the patients (29%) had cancer at distant sites, including adenocarcinoma of the rectum, carcinoma of the breast, carcinoma of the urethra, basal cell carcinoma of the skin, and carcinoma of the cervix.

If no local or distant primary malignancy is uncovered, a total vulvectomy is usually performed, as noted in the recent series reported by Curtin et al.. It is important to remove the full thickness of the skin to the subcutaneous fat to be certain that all the skin adnexal structures are excised, as they may have a subclinical malignancy. Bergen et al. evaluated 14 patients with Paget's disease of the vulva treated by operation, usually vulvectomy, skinning vulvectomy with graft, or hemivulvectomy. With a median follow-up of 50 months, all patients were free of disease, although two with positive margins and one with negative margins required treatment for recurrence.

As a rule, other forms of local therapy, such as laser and 5-FU cream, have not been used for vulvar Paget's disease. However, insofar as the disease may recur and multiple surgical procedures can lead to extensive scarring, laser treatment or topical 5-FU has occasionally been tried. Even if resection margins are free of Paget's disease at the time of surgical excision, local recurrence remains a major risk. Those women who have been treated for Paget's disease of the vulva should have as part of their routine follow-up annual examination of the breast, cytologic evaluation of the cervix and vulva, and screening for gastrointestinal disease at least by testing for occult blood in the stool. Progression of Paget's disease of the vulva to invasive adenocarcinoma has been reported, but such cases are rare.

PRIMARY VULVAR MALIGNANCIES

Squamous cell carcinoma
Adenocarcinoma (including Bartholin's gland)
Verrucous carcinoma
Basal cell carcinoma
Melanoma
Sarcoma

MALIGNANT CONDITIONS

Squamous Cell Carcinoma

Squamous cell carcinomas comprise approximately 90% of primary vulvar malignancies, but a variety of other vulvar cancers are encountered; the primary ones are listed in the box on the left. Melanomas account for about 4% to 5% and the other types for the remainder.

Morphology and Staging

Grossly, vulvar carcinomas usually appear as polypoid masses on the vulva (Figure 30-14, *A*).

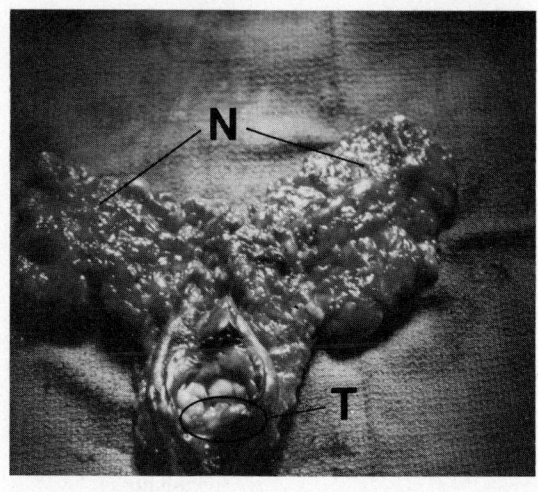

A

FIGURE 30-14
A, Radical vulvectomy specimen. **B,** Vulvectomy with operative incision lines shown. Note groin incisions.

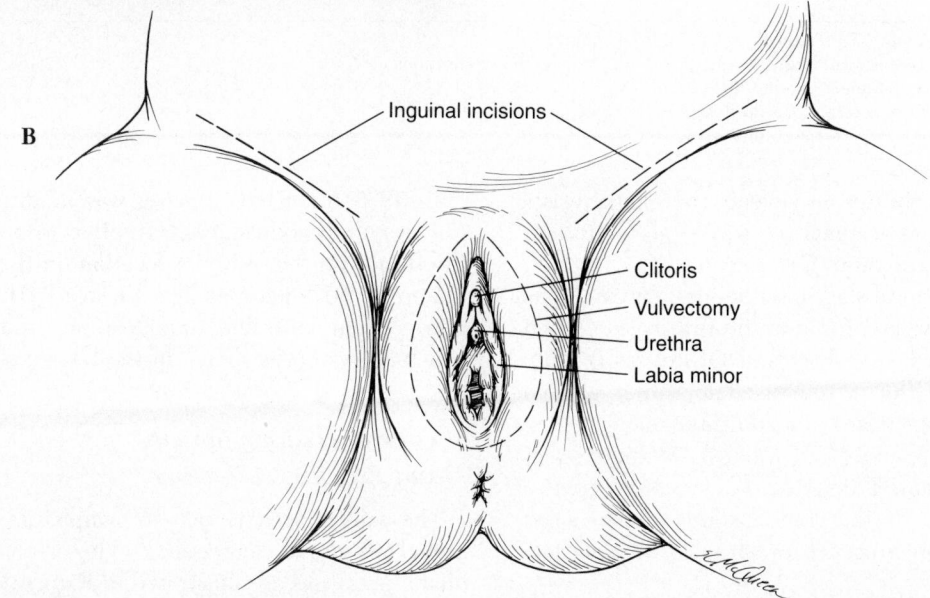

B

Inguinal incisions

Clitoris
Vulvectomy
Urethra
Labia minor

TNM* AND STAGING CLASSIFICATIONS OF CARCINOMA OF THE VULVA

TNM

T Primary Tumor

Tis   Preinvasive carcinoma (carcinoma in situ)

T 1   Tumor confined to the vulva and/or perineum—2 cm or less in diameter

T 2   Tumor confined to the vulva and/or perineum—more than 2 cm in diameter

T 3   Tumor of any size with adjacent spread to the urethra, vagina, anus or all of these

T 4   Tumor of any size infiltrating the bladder mucosa or the rectal mucosa or both, including the upper part of the urethral mucosa or fixed to the anus

N Regional Lymph Nodes

N 0   No nodes palpable

N 1   Unilateral regional lymph node metastases

N 2   Bilateral regional lymph node metastases

M Distant Metastases

M 0   No clinical metastases

M 1   Distant metastases (including pelvic lymph node metastases)

Staging (FIGO)† 1988

Stage 0 Tis   Carcinoma in situ; intraepithelial carcinoma

Stage I   T1 N0 M0   Tumor confined to the vulva and/or perineum— 2 cm or less in greatest dimension. No nodal metastases.

Stage II   T2 N0 M0   Tumor confined to the vulva and/or perineum— more than 2 cm in greatest dimension. No nodal metastases.

Stage III   T3 N0 M0   Tumor of any size with the following:

T3 N1 M0 (1)   Adjacent spread to the lower urethra, the vagina, the anus, and/or the following:

T1 N1 M0 (2)

T2 N1 M0   Unilateral regional lymph node metastases

Stage IVA T1 N2 M0   Tumor invades any of the following:

T2 N2 M0

T3 N2 M0

T4 any N M0   Upper urethra, bladder mucosa, rectal mucosa, pelvic bone, and/or bilateral regional node metastases

Stage IVB any T, any N, M1   Any distant metastases, including pelvic lymph nodes

Creasman WT: Obstet Gynecol 75:287, 1990.
Underlined words indicate changes from the pre-1988 definitions.
*TNM = Tumor–Nodes–Metastases.
†FIGO = International Federation of Gynecology and Obstetrics.

Biopsy of the lesion reveals the characteristic histologic appearance of squamous cell carcinoma (Figure 30-6, *C*).

Four clinical stages are defined for carcinoma of the vulva according to the International Federation of Gynecology and Obstetrics (FIGO), similar to the system used for other gynecologic malignancies. In addition, many centers use the T (tumor), N (nodes), M (metastases) classification; T denotes the size and extent of the tumor, N the clinical status of the nodes, and M the presence or absence of metastatic disease.

In 1988 the FIGO staging was modified to reflect lymph node status, as well as location of the tumor on the vulva. A location on the perineum is no longer alloted to stage III. The new system with the modifications from the pre-1988 system is shown in the box above.

Natural History, Spread, and Prognostic Factors

The vulvar area is rich in lymphatics with numerous cross connections. The main lymphatic pathways are illustrated in Figure 30-15.

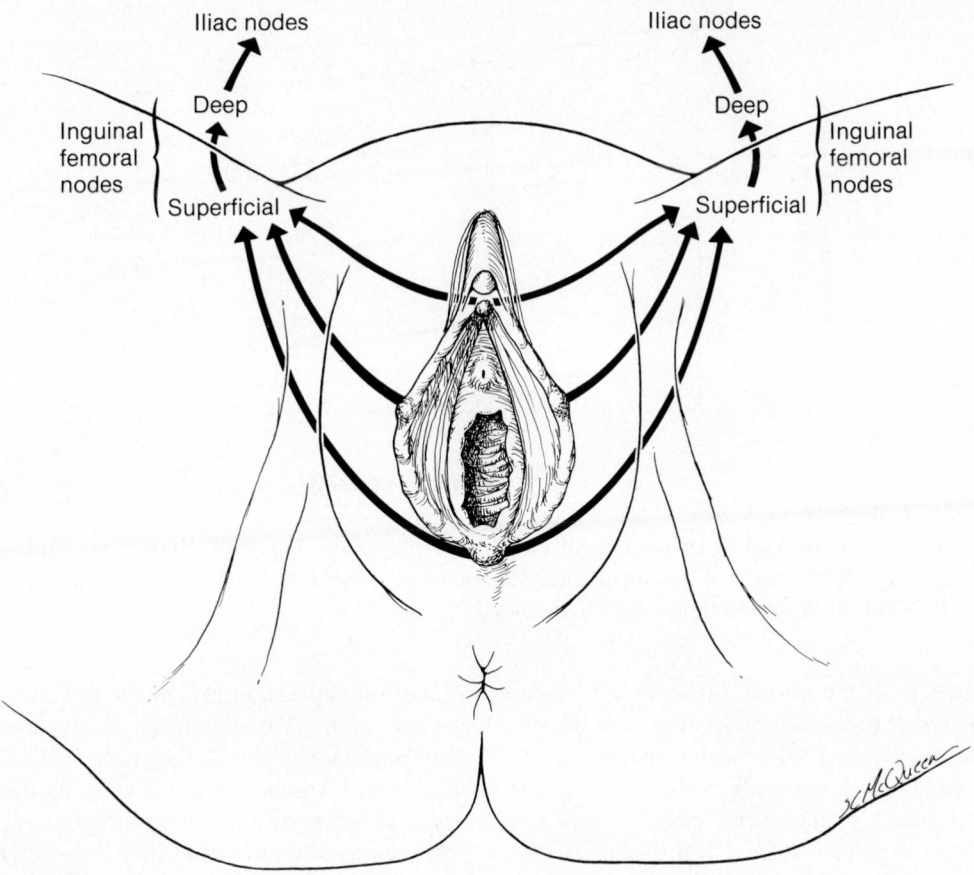

FIGURE 30-15
Vulva lymph drainage. General schematic representation of major drainage channels of vulva.

Tumors located in the middle of either labium tend to drain initially to the ipsilateral femoral-inguinal nodes, whereas perineal tumors can spread to either the left or the right side. Tumors in the clitoral or urethral areas can also spread to either side. From the inguinal-femoral nodes, the lymphatic spread of tumor is cephalad to the deep pelvic iliac and obturator nodes. Although there has been concern in the past that tumors in the clitoral-urethral area would spread directly to the deep pelvic nodes, current evidence indicates that this rarely, if ever, occurs. The characteristics of lymph drainage of the vulva were evaluated by Iverson and Aas, who injected[99m]Tc-colloid subcutaneously into the anterior and posterior labia majora, anterior and posterior labia minora, clitoral area, and perineum. They then measured the radioactivity in the pelvic lymph nodes, which were surgically removed 5 hours later. From the injections in the labia majora and minora, over 98% of the radioactivity was found

in the ipsilateral node and less than 2% on the contralateral side. The anterior labial injections resulted in 92% concentration of radioactivity in the ipsilateral side with 8% on the contralateral side. The clitoral and perineal injections developed a bilateral nodal distribution of radioactivity in all the patients. It is of interest that two thirds of the patients with labial injections had a small amount of detectable radioactivity in the contralateral nodes. Thus anastomoses of the lymphatics do exist, but a direct connection from the clitoris to the deep nodes was not demonstrated.

The prognosis of a patient with vulvar carcinoma is related to the stage of the disease (Figure 30-16), lesion size, as well as the presence or absence of cancer in regional nodes. The worldwide 5-year survival results from the *20th Annual Report on the Results of Treatment of Gynecologic Cancer* are stage I, 69%; stage II, 49%; stage III, 32%; and stage IV, 13%. The presence of carcinoma in regional lymph nodes

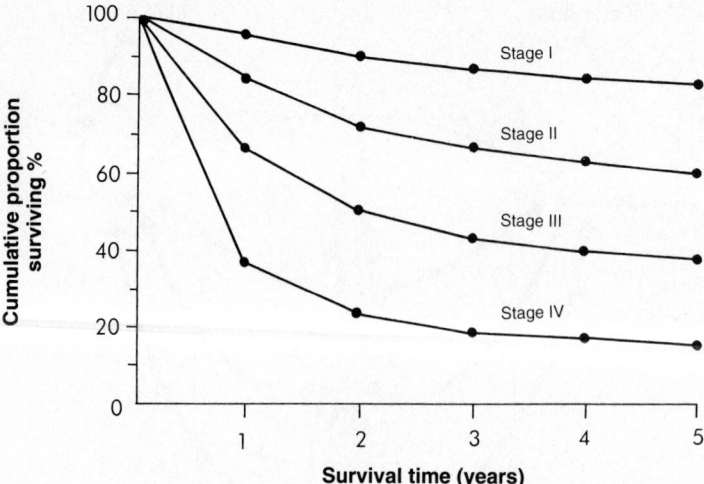

FIGURE 30-16

Stage and survival of carcinoma of vulva. (Adapted from the 20th Report on End Results of Therapy of Gynecologic Malignancies, Stockholm, 1988, International Federation of Gynecology and Obstetrics.)

correlates with the size of the primary lesion, the degree of tumor differentiation, and the extent of involvement of vascular spaces by tumor. Tumor size is usually estimated by the greatest tumor diameter; for example, ≤2 cm or >2 cm separates stage I from stage II disease.

The status of the regional lymph nodes is important prognostically, as well as therapeutically. Numerous studies, including a multicenter collaborative investigation from the Gynecologic Oncology Group (GOG), indicate that tumor stage, location on the vulva, microscopic differentiation, presence or absence of vascular space involvement, and tumor thickness are all important prognostic factors. The GOG study of 272 women was reported by Sedlis et al., and the results shown in Table 30-1 demonstrate the relation of stage to tumor thickness and histologic grade in their study. It should be noted that in this study four grades of differentiation rather than the international system of three grades (well differentiated, moderately differentiated, and poorly differentiated) were used. In addition, these authors noted that labial lesions were associated with 7.4% positive nodes, while clitoral lesions were associated with 27.4% positive nodes. Lesion size is also a factor. Boyce et al. noted in a study of 84 cases that 6 tumors under 1 cm in diameter had no metastases to regional nodes while the proportion rose to 55% for 29 cases over 4 cm in diameter. A 1991 GOG analysis of 588 cases by Homesley et al. emphasized that lesion diameter and groin node status are the primary independent prognostic factors for vulvar carcinoma. Vascular space involvement was also important in the Boyce study, with 72% of 9 cases with vascular invasion showing tumor in regional nodes, compared with 34% of 65 cases without vascular invasion. In a series of 42 patients Hussadeinzadeh et al. noted no metastases to regional nodes in 13 patients with grade I tumors who microscopically had no vascular involvement and whose stromal penetration did not exceed 5 mm. Perineural invasion also appears to be a factor in vulvar tumors as it is in cervical carcinoma (Chapter 26). In a small study of 22 patients Rowley et al. noted no metastases in 20 patients without perineural invasion and in 2 of 2 patients with perineural invasion.

In general, spread to regional nodes has been reported to vary from 0% to 10% in tumors with less than 5 mm invasion, but this statistic is affected by both tumor size and tumor grade. Depth of invasion, tumor diameter and differentiation, and involvement of vascular spaces are important considerations to define appropriate therapy for cancer of the vulva, particularly for "microinvasive" carcinoma (see below).

In assessing the patient, the clinician's evaluation of the regional nodes and whether they are involved with tumor can be a factor in the choice of therapy. In the 1987 GOG study, if the nodes were not palpable and were considered normal by the clinician, 16.5% of cases were found to have positive nodes, whereas the figure rose to 58.6% for those with suspicious

TABLE 30-1
Factors Related to Positive Regional Nodes (272 Cases)

Stage	Percent of Positive Nodes	Grade	Percent of Positive Nodes	Tumor Thickness	Percent of Positive Nodes
I	8.9	1	0	<1mm	3.1
II	25.3	2	8.0	2	8.9
III	31.1	3	24.6	3	18.6
IV	62.5	4	47.7	≥ 4	31

Adapted from Sedlis A, Homesley H, Bundy BN, et al: Am J Obstet Gynecol 156:1159, 1987.

or clinically fixed or ulcerated nodes. Because the new staging system of carcinoma of the vulva (see box on p. 1004) includes the morphologic status of the regional nodes, it is helpful in treatment planning to confirm the status of the nodes with fine-needle aspiration. Using this technique, Crosby et al. found no false positive and only two false negative results among 34 patients evaluated, 19 of whom had positive and 15 negative cytologic fine-needle aspirations. This indicates that the technique can be highly useful, particularly if positive results are obtained.

Stage IA: Carcinoma of the Vulva (Early or Microinvasive Carcinoma)

DEFINITION AND CLINICAL-PATHOLOGIC RELATIONSHIPS. The term *microinvasive carcinoma of the vulva* has no uniformly accepted definition. To identify early tumors unlikely to spread to regional nodes, many authorities have defined microinvasion as a small vulvar tumor less than 2 cm in diameter that invades less than 3 mm. However, varying clinicopathologic results are reported when this definition is used. For example, Hoffman et al. noted no nodal metastases among 43 patients whose tumors invaded less than 2 mm. They noted spread to regional nodes was less likely among tumors with individual tumor tongues spreading into the stroma rather than those that were confluent. In contrast, Hacker et al. reported six of seven tumors with less than 3 mm invasion had spread to regional nodes.

Part of the confusion is due to different reference points from which the depth of invasion is measured, that is, from the surface or basement membrane. Dvoretsky et al. carefully analyzed the microscopic aspects of 36 cases of superficial vulvar carcinoma. They measured the dimension of tumor penetration into the stroma from the surface of the squamous epithelium (neoplastic thickness) (Figure 30-17,A) and also from the tip of the adjacent epithelial ridge (stromal invasion) (Figure 30-17,B). Six of the 36 cases had spread to regional nodes, and all had invaded over 3 mm from the surface. The International Society for the Study of Vulvar Disease has recommended that the term *microinvasion* be dropped and the designation *stage IA* be used for tumors less than 2 cm in diameter with depth of invasion less than 1 mm from the epidermal-stromal junction (basement membrane). Insofar as the vulvar epithelium is often 2 mm thick, this definition would approximate 3 mm of invasion (thickness) measured from the surface. These are important points to remember when reviewing the results of various series reported in the literature. Kneale et al. have pointed out that although there is almost no risk of metastases to regional nodes in stage IA lesions, late recurrence of these tumors can develop years after primary therapy, and in a literature review, eight instances of recurrence were reported in 88 cases of superficial vulvar carcinoma. All tumors were less than 2 cm diameter and invaded less than 1 mm into the stroma measured from the basement membrane.

The presence of carcinoma in situ in the primary lesion decreases the risk of node involvement in these cases. Ross and Ehrman noted only 1 of 35 cases with adjacent CIS had nodal metastases, and this tumor penetrated into the stroma 1.7 mm. In contrast, 5 of 27 cases of superficial stage I cases (2.1 to 5.0 mm penetration) without adjacent CIS had positive nodes. Thus spread to regional nodes is unlikely, particularly if the tumor is well differentiated (grade 1), invades less than 3 mm measured from the surface or has a depth of inva-

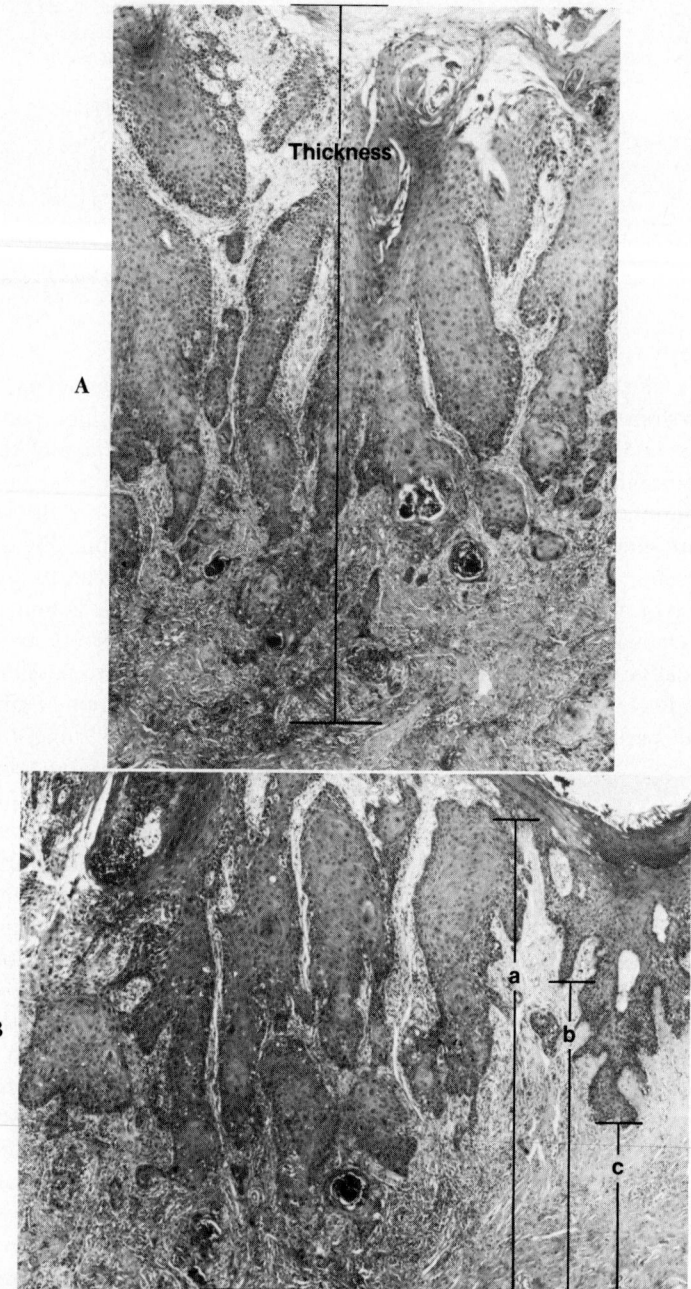

FIGURE 30-17
A, Measurement of neoplastic thickness in squamous cell carcinoma. (×35.) **B,** Superficially invasive squamous cell carcinoma. Reference point used to measure depth of stromal invasion is demonstrated by line *b*. Note striking variation in measurement of stromal invasion, depending on which reference point is chosen (line *a*, *b*, or *c*). (×35.) (From Dvoretsky PM, Bonfiglio TA, Helkamp BF, et al: The pathology of superficially invasive thin vulva squamous cell carcinoma, Int J Gynecol Pathol 3:331, 1984.)

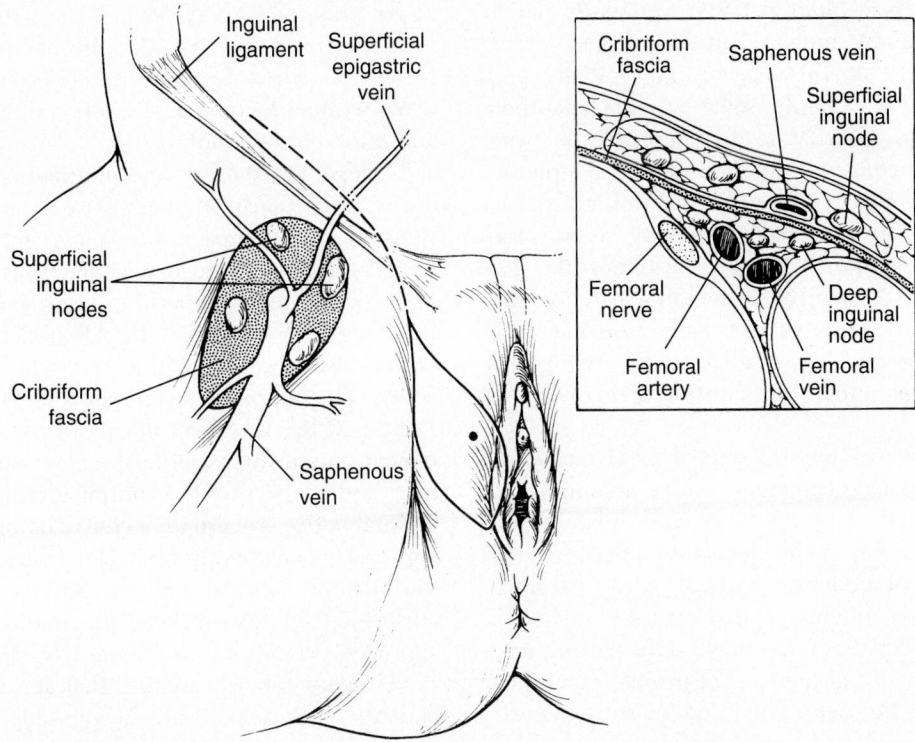

FIGURE 30-18
Early vulvar cancer. Wide local excision with ipsilateral superficial lymph node dissection. Lymph nodes removed are above cribriform fascia. (From Rowley KC, Gallion HH, Donaldson ES, et al: Gynecol Oncol 31:43, 1988.)

sion measured from the adjacent rete pegs of less than 1 mm, and is without vascular space involvement. The presence of carcinoma in situ is a favorable factor. Less well-differentiated tumors or those with vascular involvement or confluence and with greater depths of invasion have an increased risk of lymph node involvement by cancer.

MANAGEMENT. For stage IA lesions satisfying these criteria, therapy may be less extensive than is usually employed for invasive vulvar carcinoma. Wide local excision with or without ipsilateral node dissection, simple vulvectomy without node dissection, and radical vulvectomy without node dissection have all been advocated. Based on available evidence, it would appear prudent that most patients with stage IA carcinoma of the vulva by the criteria previously described should be treated at least with a wide excision to give a margin of 2 to 3 cm. Depending on the location of the tumor, a hemivulvectomy may be needed. The lymph node dissection is omitted or deferred depending on the final pathologic evaluation of the tumor in the surgical specimen. For younger patients, especially with tumors that involve either the labia or the perineum at a distance from the clitoris, an operation that spares the clitoris should be considered. An alternative approach has been suggested by Iverson et al., who recommended a hemivulvectomy with ipsilateral groin dissection for lesions involving the labia. They advocate conventional radical vulvectomy and bilateral groin dissection for medial lesions because of the danger of bilateral spread of the tumor to regional nodes. The latter recommendation is advisable if there is more than 1 mm of invasion (3 mm thickness) and the tumor is more than 2 cm in diameter.

Invasive Carcinoma of the Vulva

Figure 30-14,A shows a typical carcinoma of the vulva, which usually appears as a polyploid mass. The patient frequently complains of a "sore" that has not healed. The patient may also complain of bleeding, but this does not usually occur early in the course of the disease. Unfortunately, the delay in diagnosis is common because older patients frequently fail to seek prompt medical attention, and often, when they do, a biopsy is not initially performed. For example, some patients have their symptoms of irritation or itching treated with various medications to eradicate the symptoms. It is vital that a biopsy be taken of any vulvar lesion before undertaking therapy, as was emphasized earlier. A biopsy of a tumor like that shown in Figure 30-14,A can easily be obtained on an outpatient basis utilizing local anesthesia and biopsy forceps, for example, a Kevorkian punch as illustrated in Chapter 26.

Effective therapy of stage I or II and early stage III vulvar carcinoma can be accomplished with a radical vulvectomy and bilateral inguinal-femoral node dissection. Because the deep pelvic nodes are virtually never involved unless the inguinal nodes are also involved, most therapists now remove only the inguinal femoral nodes at the time of primary operation and treat the deep pelvic nodes subsequently with external radiation if the superficial nodes are involved with tumor.

Until recent times, radical vulvectomy and groin dissection were carried out through a single suprapubic incision that extended between the left and right anterior iliac spines and then an en bloc dissection in continuity with the radical vulvectomy. The operation removes the entire vulva, including the clitoris and subcutaneous tissues. For anteriorly located lesions the distal urethra must be removed occasionally, which can usually be accomplished without loss of urinary continence. However, wound breakdown and infection may affect up to 50% of patients undergoing radical vulvectomy. For that reason, modifications have been introduced to perform the inguinal-femoral node dissection through separate inguinal incisions and then complete the radical vulvectomy. Figure 30-14,A shows the type of specimen that can be obtained through separate groin incisions. The operative incisions are shown in Figure 30-14,B. It appears that an adequate surgical dissection with decreased wound complications can be accomplished by this technique. It is advisable to use suction drainage in the inguinal area until all drainage is complete, which usually takes 7 to 10 days, and drains are frequently also used in the vulvar area. Insofar as vulvar recurrences are the main problem, it is important that an adequate margin, usually 2 to 3 cm, be obtained around the primary tumor

at the time of surgery. Tumor recurrence has occurred rarely in the skin bridge over the symphysis when separate groin incisions are used, without an en bloc dissection of the vulva and intervening lymph tissue.

To lessen extensive and mutilating procedures, particularly in stage I cases, modifications of the approach previously mentioned have been introduced in recent years. Rowley et al. performed wide local excision and superficial inguinal dissection for 20 patients with stage I lesions and a depth of invasion less than 5 mm. The operative technique is illustrated in Figure 30-18. The deep inguinal nodes are removed only if the superficial nodes contain tumor, and in this case the contralateral inguinal-femoral nodes are also dissected. The unilateral approach is most appropriate for labial lesions, but bilateral inguinal node dissections must be performed for lesions near the midline. This approach was initially suggested by DiSaia et al. A recent report updating that series on 50 patients by Berman et al. showed only one patient had succumbed to recurrent carcinoma, and she had a grade 2 lesion with positive regional nodes. Six of the 50 patients had recurrent local CIS or minimally invasive carcinoma, and they were successfully treated subsequently. The approach appears effective and is accompanied by less morbidity than the standard radical vulvectomy.

In treating stage I and stage II tumors of the vulva, the results of histologic evaluation of the inguinal-femoral nodes are important. If these nodes do not contain metastatic tumor, no further therapy is given after the primary operation of radical vulvectomy and bilateral inguinal-femoral node dissection. If the lymph nodes, particularly the upper femoral group, are involved with tumor, the deep pelvic nodes require treatment. A recent national cooperative randomized study of 118 patients suggests radiation is superior. Homesley et al. reported improved survival for those who received radiation (4500 to 5000 rads) to the deep pelvic nodes in comparison with those who had a pelvic node dissection.

The results of therapy in stage I and II disease relate not only to the stage of the disease but also to the status of the regional pelvic nodes. If the nodes do not contain metastatic tumor and the patient can be successfully treated by radical vulvectomy and bilateral node dissection, 5-year survivals of about 95% are reported. Recently Iverson et al. in a series of 424 patients with carcinoma of the vulva noted lymph node metastasis in 10.5% of stage I cases, 30% of stage II, 66% of stage III, and 100% of stage IV. The number of positive nodes in the radical vulvectomy specimen correlates with the size of the primary tumor and also with the patient's survival. In a study of 113 patients, Hacker et al. noted an actuarial 5-year survival of 96% for those with negative nodes, but there was a progressive fall in survival to 94% for those having one positive node; 80% for two positive nodes; and 12% for three or more positive nodes. In various cases that have been studied, the deep pelvic nodes do not contain tumor unless the upper inguinal-femoral nodes contain metastatic disease. The number of nodes involved as well as the size of the metastasis are both important. Hoffman et al. noted that 14 of 15 patients with inguinal lymph node metastasis measuring less than 36 mm^2 survived free of disease 5 years in comparison to 12 of 29 whose lymph node metastases measured more than 100 mm^2. These results should be taken into consideration when planning additional therapy for patients with two positive nodes.

The standard treatment for stage I and II carcinoma of the vulva and resectable stage III tumors that do not involve either the urethra or the anus is radical vulvectomy with bilateral inguinal-femoral lymphadenectomy. Depending on the location of the lesion, modifications can be introduced. For example, a margin of 2 to 3 cm around the primary lesion is required. For lesions located in the posterior perineal area, this can be accomplished without removal of the clitoris. Such "tailoring" of the operative excisions has been introduced, and early results, such as those reported by Burrell et al., appear to indicate effective rates of cure with a "modified radical vulvectomy," providing adequate margins are obtained. For large tumors both groins should be dissected because of the risk, albeit small, of contralateral spread.

If tumor spread to the regional inguinal-femoral nodes is identified, further treatment should be considered. If only one node is microscopically involved with tumor, no further therapy is needed. However, if three or more nodes are involved, pelvic radiation as outlined is usually prescribed. For patients with only two nodes involved, the decision for further therapy will depend on the location of the node and the size of the metastatic deposit of tumor.

However, 5-year survivals of 80% have been recorded for those with two positive nodes and 90% for those with one node, without further therapy beyond primary operation.

Advanced Vulvar Tumors

Large tumors of the vulva, particularly those that encroach on the anal-rectal area or the urethra, require more extensive treatment than radical vulvectomy to achieve effective tumor control. In such instances, removal of the anus or urethra is usually necessary as part of the primary procedure, in which case diversion of the urinary or fecal stream is required (see discussion of exenterative surgery for carcinoma of the cervix, Chapter 27). The best results are achieved by selecting patients with tumors that involve the urethra or anal areas that have not metastasized to regional nodes. Five-year survivals of approximately 50% have been reported. Because of the large defect created in the vulvar area, a gracilis myocutaneous flap from the leg is often applied to the vulvar area to aid in healing.

A newer therapeutic approach has been to treat the large vulvar tumor with external radiation and then after the tumor has been reduced in size, remove it surgically, usually by radical vulvectomy with or without regional lymph node dissection. External radiation is used to deliver approximately 4000 rads to the tumor and 4500 rads to the pelvis and inguinal nodes. Operation is usually performed about 5 weeks after the completion of radiation therapy. Although a large series of patients has not been treated by this technique, a sufficient number have been treated to demonstrate that marked tumor regression does occur. The primary cancer can be eradicated by an operation that does not require diversion of the urine or feces. Boronow summarized the treatment of 26 patients with primary carcinoma of the vaginal vulvar area with this technique and noted a 5-year survival of 80%. Rotmensch et al. recently reported on 16 patients, 13 stage III and 3 stage IV, and achieved an overall 5-year survival of 45% with this technique, somewhat better than might be expected with stage III-IV (see Figure 30-16). Recurrences are more likely if the resection margins were within 1 cm of the tumor. Complications reported include stenosis of the introitus, urethral stenosis, and rectovaginal fistula, but this technique is an effective alternative to primary exenteration for large vulvar vaginal carcinomas and is preferred in most treatment centers.

Radiation Therapy and Recurrences

In a few instances the medical condition of the patient precludes operation, and radiation therapy may be employed as the sole treatment. However, the vulvar skin is prone to radiation dermatitis fibrosis and ulceration, making irradiation, as the sole form of therapy, a less desirable treatment of these tumors. Therefore irradiation is seldom used as the sole treatment of carcinoma of the vulva.

As may be expected, the risk of recurring carcinoma rises as the stage of the disease increases. Podratz et al. in an analysis of 224 patients with vulvar carcinoma noted a recurrence rate of 14% in stage I and 71% in stage IV. Local vulvar recurrences were the most common and occurred in 40 of 74 cases of recurrence (54%). The remaining recurrences were in the groin, pelvis, or distant sites. Radiation therapy or additional operations for local vulvar recurrences usually provide effective control and 5-year survivals of approximately 50%. The risk of recurrence of the disease in the vulva requires careful attention to the surgical resection margins at the time of initial operation.

Combined use of chemotherapy and radiation has been introduced as a new and apparently effective means of treating recurrent and occasionally large primary vulvar carcinomas, particularly in patients who are not good operative candidates. Thomas et al. used 5-FU 1 g/m^2 by continuous IV infusion for 4 to 5 days every 4 weeks during radiation (median therapy 4500 cGy). The combined therapy was the sole treatment in nine patients, six of whom had a complete remission. Of a total of 33 patients, 2 had serious complications: avascular necrosis of the hip and radiation proctitis with stricture. Combined chemotherapy and radiation therapy are being more widely used in the treatment of squamous cell carcinomas of the lower genital tract (Chapter 27). It appears an effective modality either as postoperative adjuvant therapy or for preoperative shrinkage of large tumors before radical vulvectomy.

Treatment of patients with disseminated disease requires chemotherapy but, unfortunately, no chemotherapeutic regimen has been successful in this disease. Squamous cell carcinomas of the female genital tract have generally not been responsive to cytotoxic chemotherapy, and the protocols followed are similar to those described for recurrent squamous cell carcinomas of the cervix (Chapter 27).

Other Vulvar Malignancies

Bartholin's Gland Carcinoma

These are adenocarcinomas which comprise about 1% to 2% of vulvar carcinomas. An enlargement of Bartholin's gland in a postmenopausal patient should raise suspicion for this malignancy. These tumors are treated similarly to primary squamous cell carcinoma of the vulva, and radical vulvectomy with bilateral inguinal-femoral lymphadenectomy is the treatment of choice. If the regional lymph nodes are free of tumor, the prognosis is good. Rosenberg has reported on five cases of adenoid cystic carcinoma of Bartholin's gland treated by operation (usually hemivulvectomy) and postoperative irradiation. Four of the five patients were living and free of disease 28 to 57 months after treatment.

Basal Cell Carcinoma

Basal cell carcinomas can arise in the vulva as they can arise in the skin elsewhere in the body. They are rare and comprise about 2% of vulvar carcinomas. Therapy consists of wide local excision of the lesion, which is generally ulcerated. If the surgical resection margins are free of tumor, the disease is cured.

Verrucous Carcinoma

Verrucous carcinomas of the vulva are also rare. They are a special variant of squamous cell cancer with distinctive histologic features. Clinically they appear as a large condylomatous mass on the vulva. Histologically they consist of mature squamous cells and extensive keratinization with nests that invade the underlying vulvar tissue. It is often necessary to perform multiple biopsies of the condylomatous lesion to establish a diagnosis of malignancy. Radiation therapy is ineffective and can worsen the prognosis by causing anaplastic change in the tumor and is therefore contraindicated. The treatment is operative.

In 24 cases of verrucous carcinoma Japaze et al. noted no lymph node metastases. Some of the primary tumors were as large as 10 cm in diameter. Recurrences developed in nine of the patients, five of whom had prior irradiation. Wide local excision is usually effective therapy. Depending on the size and location of the tumor, simple vulvectomy may be needed, but a radical vulvectomy or inguinal node dissection is not indicated. The 17 cases treated surgically and reported by Japaze et al. had a 5-year survival of 94%. As noted by Crowther et al., it is important to take a large biopsy specimen to establish the diagnosis. This is particularly important when dealing with a malignant-appearing tumor from a biopsy specimen that has been reported as benign. This can lead to incorrect therapy for "condyloma acuminatum." Conversely, too shallow a biopsy may fail to show areas of squamous cell carcinoma that can coexist with verrucous carcinoma. However, in the presence of areas of squamous cell carcinoma, local excision is inadequate therapy. Verrucous tumors with squamous cell carcinoma elements can metastasize to regional nodes, and such tumors should not be treated as true verrucous carcinomas.

Melanoma

Melanoma is the most frequent nonsquamous cell malignancy of the vulva. It comprises about 5% of primary cancers of this area. As is true elsewhere in the body, melanomas arise from junctional or compound nevi. Pigmented lesions of the vulva are usually junctional nevi, and all such lesions should be removed by excision.

Patients with malignant melanoma of the vulva vary widely in age from the late teens to women in their eighties. The average age is approximately 50 years. Clinically, melanomas appear as brown, black, or blue-black masses on the vulva. The lesion can be flat or ulcerated. Occasionally it is nodular, and small, darkly pigmented areas (satellite nodules) may surround the primary lesion. Some melanomas may be without pigment and can grossly resemble squamous cell carcinoma of the vulva. Most melanomas of the vulva occur on the labia minora or the clitoris (Figure 30-19).

Vulvar melanomas if staged, use the same FIGO classification employed for squamous carcinomas (see box, p. 1013). However, recent evidence indicates that staging is not as useful a prognostic indicator as is the depth of invasion. A system for vulvar melanoma analogous to that used by Clark for cutaneous melanomas has been adopted. Five levels (I to V) have

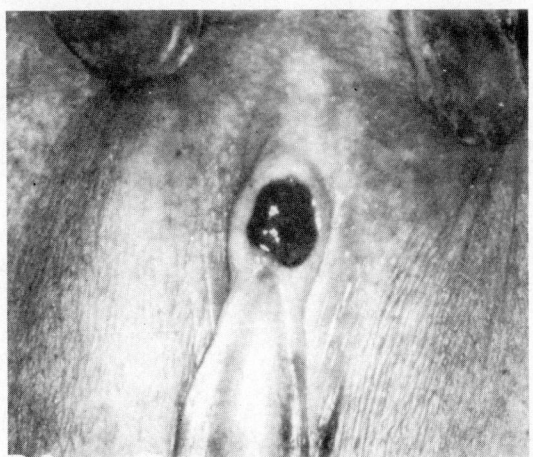

FIGURE 30-19
Nodular melanoma arising directly from glans clitoris. (Courtesy J. McL. Morris, M.D. and John Slade Ely, Professor of Gynecology, Yale University School of Medicine, New Haven, Conn.)

been defined based on the Clark classification. Figure 30-20 shows the depth of invasion for each level of superficial spreading melanoma and nodular melanoma, the two most common varieties of melanomas that occur on the vulva. Superficial spreading melanoma is more common and fortunately has a better prognosis, with a 5-year survival of 71% reported in the series by Podratz et al. The 5-year survival for nodular melanoma, which is more invasive, was only 38%. The level of invasion correlates with survival, which varies from 100% for level II, to 83% for level IV, to 28% for level V.

Tumor thickness is also useful to evaluate the tumor. Breslow et al. reported that overall prognosis is excellent, and spread to regional node is not likely for melanomas whose thickness measured from the surface epithelium to the deepest point of penetration is less than 0.76 mm. Most of these lesions would correspond to level I or level II penetration by the modified Clark system. Stefanon et al., in a study of 28 patients, noted no lymph node metastasis if melanoma thickness was less than 3 mm and the 5-year survival in this group was 50% in comparison with 25% for those whose melanomas were more than 3 mm thick.

The standard therapy for vulvar melanoma has been radical vulvectomy and bilateral inguinal-femoral dissection. Because the tumors are rare, a large clinical experience is not avail-

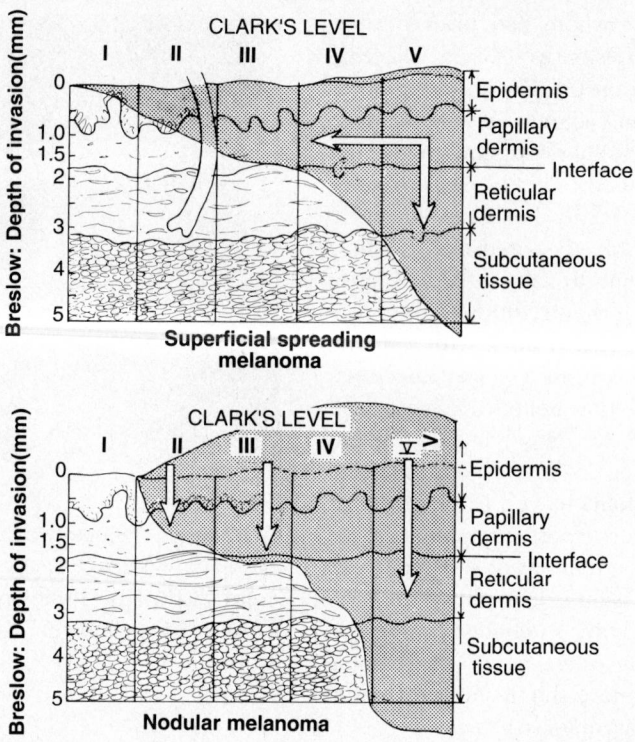

FIGURE 30-20

Level of invasion for superficial spreading melanoma and nodular melanoma. (From Podratz KC, Gaffey TA, Symmonds RE, et al: Gynecol Oncol 16:153, 1983.)

able. It was believed that melanoma of the vulva could metastasize to pelvic nodes, bypassing the inguinal femoral nodes; current evidence indicates that there is no pelvic node involvement without prior inguinal node involvement. A further therapeutic consideration is that patients with melanoma whose pelvic nodes are involved with tumor usually do not survive the disease.

Excision margins have been extensively studied for cutaneous melanomas. Veronesi et al. found that cutaneous melanomas less than 2 mm thick could be adequately treated with a 1 cm margin, which was as effective as a 3 cm margin for these thin lesions. Although comparable data do not exist for vulvar melanomas, the data from cutaneous melanomas suggest that a 1 cm margin could be used for very thin vulvar melanomas. In a report of 36 melanoma cases, Rose et al. noted that wide excision was as effective as radical vulvectomy. They noted that the prognosis was improved in younger patients, presumably because most of them had superficial spreading (good prognosis) rather than nodular (poor prognosis) melanomas. Although firm recommendations from available data are not possible, a reasonable approach

would be to excise a melanoma with a 2 cm margin without node dissection for tumors that are less than 2 mm thick. An excision with a 2 to 3 cm margin combined with node dissection would be carried out for more advanced melanomas.

Long-term results are generally not available for large series of melanoma, but for lesions that correspond to Clark level 1 or 2, that is, less than 0.76 mm thick, a wide local excision results in 5-year survivals in the vicinity of 100%. The prognosis is poor for patients with melanomas more than 3 mm thick. If the regional nodes are negative, survival is greater than 60%, but survival drops to less than 30% if the regional nodes are involved with tumor. Most series of malignant melanoma report overall survivals of approximately 50%.

Distant metastases are frequently noted, and no effective program of chemotherapy has been described. Regressions (but not cures) have been reported with various multiagent cytotoxic programs. Current efforts are devoted to developing an effective program of immunotherapy, particularly in view of the occasional favorable responses reported with agents such as Bacille Calmette-Guérin (BCG).

Sarcoma

Sarcomas of the vulva are extremely rare. Twelve cases were reported by DiSaia et al., and surgical removal of the primary tumor is the treatment of choice. Chemotherapeutic considerations are the same as those for sarcomas of other sites in the female genital tract.

Granular Cell Myoblastomas

Granular cell myoblastoma is also an extremely rare tumor that is almost invariably benign but does morphologically show pleomorphism. Local excision is generally sufficient therapy. The tumor appears as a solitary, firm, nontender, slowly growing nodule in the subcutaneous tissue of the vulva.

KEY POINTS

- Squamous cell carcinoma comprise 90% of primary vulvar malignancies. More than half the patients are over 60 years of age at the time of diagnosis.

- Cancer of the vulva accounts for about 4% of malignancies of the lower female genital tract and is less frequent than uterine, ovarian, and cervical cancers.

- Paget's disease generally occurs in postmenopausal women and is usually treated by simple vulvectomy. Invasive carcinomas at other sites should be ruled out.

- Prolonged use of fluorinated corticosteroids to treat itching accompanying vulvar dystrophy can lead to vulvar contraction.

- Topical testosterone is often beneficial to treat lichen sclerosus but is absorbed systemically and occasionally can produce masculinizing symptoms.

- HPV vulvar infection is common. Intraepithelial neoplasia occurs much less frequently.

- A clear progression of dysplasia-CIS (VIN I, II, and III) to invasive carcinoma in the vulva is not well established. Intraepithelial neoplasia in the vulva may spontaneously regress.

- Intraepithelial neoplasia of the vulva is usually treated by local excision or laser therapy of the atypical area.

- Vulvar carcinomas less than 2 cm in diameter and depth of invasion less than 1 mm (3 mm thickness) rarely metastasize to regional nodes.

- Unilateral vulvar tumors are more likely to metastasize to ipsilateral inguinal-femoral nodes, but contralateral metastases also rarely occur.

- Prognosis in vulvar carcinoma is primarily related to lesion size, stage, and lymph node status.

- The deep pelvic nodes do not become involved with metastatic vulvar cancer unless the inguinal-femoral nodes are affected.

- Most patients with cancer of the vulva are treated by radical vulvectomy and bilateral inguinal-femoral node dissection. The 5-year survival of those with negative nodes is over 95%. With one positive node the 5-year survival is approximately the same, that is, 94%; with two nodes it decreases to 80%; with three or more, to 12%.

- The worldwide 5-year survival for carcinoma of the vulva by stage is I, 69%; II, 49%; III, 32%; and IV, 13%.

- Advanced vulvar tumors encroaching on the urethra and/or anus may be treated by preliminary radiation followed by radical vulvectomy rather than exenteration.

- Verrucous carcinomas are a variant of squamous cancer that does not metastasize to regional nodes. Radiation therapy is contraindicated, and local surgical extirpation is utilized.

- Melanomas comprise 5% of vulvar cancers and are the most frequent non–squamous cell malignancies.

- The overall 5-year survival of patients with vulvar melanoma is about 50%.

- Superficial spreading melanomas tend to occur in younger patients and have a better prognosis than nodular melanomas.

- Prognosis of vulvar melanoma is related to tumor invasion (level) and to tumor thickness.

- Basal cell carcinoma of the vulva is treated by wide local excision.

BIBLIOGRAPHY

Bergen S, DiSaia PJ, Liao SY, et al: Conservative management of extramammary Paget's disease of the vulva, Gynecol Oncol 33:151, 1989.

Berman ML, Soper JT, Creasman WT, et al: Conservative surgical management in superficially invasive stage I vulvar carcinoma, Gynecol Oncol 35:352, 1989.

Boronow RC: Combined therapy as an alternative to exenteration of locally advanced vulvar vaginal cancer, Cancer 49:1085, 1982.

Boronow RC, Hickman BT, Reagan MT, et al: Combined therapy as an alternative to exenteration for locally advanced vulvovaginal cancer, Am J Clin Oncol 10(2):1711, 1987.

Boyce J, Fruchter RG, Kasambilides E, et al: Prognostic factors in carcinoma of the vulva, Gynecol Oncol 20:364, 1985.

Breslow A: Thickness, cross-sectional areas, and depth of invasion in the prognosis of cutaneous melanoma, Ann Surg 172:908, 1970.

Burrell MO, Franklin EW III, Campion MJ, et al: The modified radical vulvectomy: an 8-year experience, Am J Obstet Gynecol 159:715, 1988.

Buscema J, Woodruff JD, Parmley TH, et al: Carcinoma in situ of the vulva, Obstet Gynecol 55:225, 1980.

Buscema I, Naghashfar Z, Sawada E, et al: The predominance of human papillomavirus type 16 in vulvar neoplasia, Obstet Gynecol 71:601, 1988.

Chafe W, Richards A, Morgan L, et al: Unrecognized invasive carcinoma in vulvar epithelial neoplasia (VIN), Gynecol Oncol 31:154, 1988.

Christopherson W, Buchsbaum HJ, Vort R, et al: Radical vulvectomy and bilateral groin lymphadenectomy utilizing separate groin incisions: report of a case with recurrence in the intervening skin bridge, Gynecol Oncol 21:247, 1985.

Chu J, Tamimi HK, Ek M, et al: Stage I vulvar cancer: criteria for microinvasion, Obstet Gynecol 59:716, 1982.

Creasman WT: New gynecologic cancer staging, Obstet Gynecol 75:287, 1990.

Crosby JH, Bryan AB, Gallup D, et al: Fine-needle aspiration of inguinal lymph nodes in gynecologic practice, Obstet Gynecol 73:281, 1989.

Crowther ME, Lowe DG, and Shepherd JH: Verrucous carcinoma of the female genital tract: a review, Obstet Gynecol Survey 43:263, 1988.

Crum CP: Vulvar intraepithelial neoplasia: histology and associated viral changes. In Wilkinson EJ, editor: Pathology of the vulva and vagina, New York, 1987, Churchill Livingstone.

Crum CP and Burkett BJ: Papilloma virus and vulvar vaginal neoplasia, J Reprod Med 34:566, 1989.

Crum PC, Liskow A, Petras P, et al: Vulvar intraepithelial neoplasia (severe atypia and carcinoma in situ), Cancer 54:1429, 1984.

Curtin JP, Rubey SR, Jones WB, et al: Paget's disease of the vulva, Gynecol Oncol 39:374, 1990.

DiSaia PJ, Creasman WT, Rich WM, et al: An alternate approach to early cancer of the vulva, Am J Obstet Gynecol 133:825, 1979.

DiSaia PJ, Rutledge F, and Smith JP: Sarcoma of the vulva—report of 12 patients, Obstet Gynecol 38:180, 1971.

Donaldson ES, Powell DE, Hanson MB, et al: Prognostic parameters in invasive vulvar cancer, Gynecol Oncol 11:184, 1981.

Dvoretsky PM, Bonfiglio TA, Helkamp BF, et al: The pathology of superficially invasive thin vulva squamous cell carcinoma, Int J Gynecol Pathol 3:331, 1984.

Farey RN, McKay PA, and Benedet JL: Radiation treatment of carcinoma of the vulva, 1950-1980, Am J Obstet Gynecol 151:591, 1985.

Figge DC, Tamimi HK, and Greer BE: Lymphatic spread in carcinoma of the vulva, Am J Obstet Gynecol 152:387, 1985.

Franklin EW III and Rutledge F: Epidemiology of epidermoid carcinoma of the vulva, Obstet Gynecol 39:165, 1972.

Friedrich EG: Reversible vulvar atypia: a case report, Obstet Gynecol 39:173, 1972.

Friedrich EG: Vulvar disease, ed 2, Philadelphia, 1983, WB Saunders Co.

Friedrich EG, Wilkinson EJ, Steingraber PH, et al: Paget's disease of the vulva and carcinoma of the breast, Obstet Gynecol 46:130, 1975.

Friedrich EF, Wilkinson EJ, and Fu YS: Carcinoma-in-situ of the vulva: a continuing challenge, Am J Obstet Gynecol 136:830, 1980.

Fu YS, Reagan JW, Townsend DE, et al: Nuclear DNA study of vulvar intraepithelial and invasive squamous neoplasms, Obstet Gynecol 57:643, 1981.

Hacker NF, Berek JS, Lagasse LD, et al: Management of regional lymph nodes and their prognostic influence in vulvar cancer, Obstet Gynecol 61:408, 1983.

Hacker NF, Nieburg RK, Berek JS, et al: Superficially invasive vulvar cancer with nodal metastases, Gynecol Oncol 15:65, 1983.

Hart WR, Norris HJ, and Helwig ED: Relation of lichen sclerosus et atrophicus of the vulva to development of carcinoma, Obstet Gynecol 45:369, 1975.

Helwig EP and Graham JH: Anogenital (extramammary) Paget's disease, Cancer 16:387, 1963.

Hoffman JS, Kumar NB, and Morley GW: Microinvasive squamous cell carcinoma of the vulva: a search for definition, Obstet Gynecol 61:615, 1983.

Hoffman JS, Kumar NB, and Morley GW: Prognostic significance of groin lymph node metastases of squamous carcinoma of the vulva, Obstet Gynecol 66:402, 1985.

Homesley HD, Bundy BN, Sedlis A, and Adcock L: A randomized study of radiation therapy versus pelvic node resection for patients with invasive squamous cell carcinoma of the vulva having positive groin nodes (a Gynecologic Oncology Group Study), Obstet Gynecol 68:733, 1986.

Homesley HD, Bundy BN, Sedlis A, et al: Assessment of current International Federation of Gynecology and Obstetrics staging of vulvar carcinoma relative to prognostic factors for survival (a Gynecologic Oncology Group study), Am J Obstet Gynecol 164:997, 1991.

Husseinzadeh N, Wesseler T, Schneider D, et al: Prognostic factors and the significance of cytologic grading in invasive squamous cell carcinoma of the vulva: a clinicopathologic study, Gynecol Oncol 36:192, 1990.

Husseinzadeh N, Zaino R, Nahhas WA, et al: The significance of histologic findings in predicting nodal metastases in invasive squamous cell carcinoma of the vulva, Gynecol Oncol 16:105, 1983.

Iverson T and Aas M: Lymph drainage from the vulva, Gynecol Oncol 16:179, 1983.

Iverson T, Abler V, and Aalder J: Individual treatment of stage I carcinoma of the vulva, Obstet Gynecol 57:85, 1981.

Iverson T, Elders JG, Christensen A, et al: Squamous cell carcinoma of the vulva: review of 424 patients, 1957-1974, Gynecol Oncol 9:271, 1980.

Japaze H, Dinh TV, and Woodruff JD: Verrucous carcinoma of the vulva: study of 24 cases, Obstet Gynecol 60:462, 1982.

Kneale BL, Cavanagh D, DiPaola GR, et al: Microinvasive cancer of the vulva: report of the ISSVD task force, J Reprod Med 29:454, 1984.

Lee SC, Roth LM, Ehrlich C, et al: Extramammary Paget's disease of the vulva—a clinicopathologic study of 13 cases, Cancer 39:2540, 1977.

Leuchter RS, Hacker NF, Voet RL, et al: Primary carcinoma of the Bartholin gland: a report of 14 cases and review of the literature, Obstet Gynecol 60:361, 1982.

Leuchter RS, Townsend DE, Hacker NF, et al: Treatment of vulvar carcinoma in situ with the CO_2 laser, Gynecol Oncol 19:314, 1984.

Lieb SM, Gallousis S, and Freedman H: Granular cell myoblastoma of the vulva, Gynecol Oncol 8:12, 1979.

Mabuchi K, Bross DS, and Kessler II: Epidemiology of cancer of the vulva: a case-control study. Cancer 55:1843, 1985.

Menczer J, Voliovitch Y, Modan B, et al: Some epidemiologic aspects of carcinoma of the vulva in Israel, Am J Obstet Gynecol 143:893, 1982.

Morrow CP: Melanoma of the female genital tract. In Coppleson M, ed: Gynecologic oncology, Edinburgh, 1981 Churchill Livingstone.

Pettersson F, Coppleson M, Creasman W, et al: Annual report on the results of treatment in gynecologic cancer, vol 20, Stockholm, 1988, International Federation of Gynecology and Obstetrics.

Phillips GL, Twiggs LB, and Okagaki T: Vulvar melanoma: a microstaging study, Gynecol Oncol 14:80, 1982.

Planner RS and Hobbs JB: Intraepithelial and invasive neoplasia of the vulva in association with human papillomavirus infection, J Reprod Med 33:503, 1988.

Plentl AA and Friedman EA: Lymphatic system of the female genitalia, Philadelphia, 1971, WB Saunders Co.

Podratz KC, Gaffey TA, Symmonds RE, et al: Melanoma of the vulva: an update, Gynecol Oncol 16:153, 1983.

Reid R: Superficial laser vulvectomy. III. A new surgical technique for appendage conserving ablation of refractory condylomas and vulvar intraepithelial neoplasia, Am J Obstet Gynecol 152:504, 1985.

Reid R, Greenberg MD, Lörincz AT, et al: Superficial laser vulvectomy. IV. Extended laser vaporization and adjunctive 5-fluorouracil therapy of human papillomavirus-associated vulvar disease, Obstet Gynecol 76:439, 1990.

Rose PG, Piver S, Tsukada Y, et al: Conservative therapy for melanoma of the vulva, Am J Obstet Gynecol 159:57, 1988.

Rosenberg P, Simonsen E, and Risberg B: Adenoid cystic carcinoma of Bartholin's gland: a report of 5 new cases treated with surgery and radiotherapy, Gynecol Oncol 34:145, 1989.

Rotmensch J, Rubin SJ, Sutton HG, et al: Preoperative radiotherapy followed by radical vulvectomy with inguinal lymphadenectomy for advanced vulvar cancer, Gynecol Oncol 36:181, 1990.

Rowley KC, Gallion HH, Donaldson ES, et al: Prognostic factors in early vulvar cancer, Gynecol Oncol 31:43, 1988.

Rutledge F and Sinclair M: Treatment of intraepithelial neoplasia of the vulva by skin excision and graft, Obstet Gynecol 102:806, 1968.

Sedlis A, Homesley H, Bundy BN, et al: Positive groin lymph nodes in superficial squamous vulvar cancer, Am J Obstet Gynecol 156:1159, 1987.

Silverberg E, Boring CC, and Squires TS: Cancer statistics, 1990, CA 40:9, 1990.

Skinner MS, Sternberg WH, Ichinose H, et al: Spontaneous regression of Bowenoid atypia of the vulva, Obstet Gynecol 42:40, 1973.

Stefanon B, Clemente C, Lupi G, et al: Malignant melanoma of the vulva: a clinicopathologic study of 28 cases, Cervix & IFGT 5:223, 1987.

Sutton GP, Stehman FB, Ehrlich CE, et al: Human papillomavirus desoxyribonucleic acid in lesions of the female genital tract: evidence for types 6/11 in squamous carcinoma of the vulva, Obstet Gynecol 70:564, 1987.

Thomas G, Dembo A, and DePetrillo A: Concurrent radiation and chemotherapy in vulvar carcinoma, Gynecol Oncol 34:263, 1989.

Veronesi V, Cascinelli N, Adams J, et al: Thin stage I primary cutaneous malignant melanomas: comparison of excision with margins of 1 or 3 cm, N Engl J Med 318:1159, 1988.

Wilkinson EJ: Pathology of the vulva and vagina, New York, 1987, Churchill Livingstone.

Woodruff JD, Genadry R, and Poliakoff S: Treatment of dyspareunia and vaginal outlet distortions by perineoplasty, Obstet Gynecol 57:750, 1981.

Woodruff JD and Julian CS: Surgery of the vulva. In Ridley JH, editor: Gynecologic surgery: errors, safeguards, salvage, Baltimore, 1974 The Williams & Wilkins Co.

Premalignant and Malignant Diseases of the Vagina

------------------- KEY TERMS AND DEFINITIONS -------------------

Clear Cell Adenocarcinoma. A vaginal or cervical malignancy occurring primarily after 14 years of age. It is often associated with prenatal exposure to diethylstilbestrol (DES), particularly the vaginal cases.

Endodermal Sinus Tumor. A rare adenocarcinoma of the vagina occurring in infants less than 2 years of age.

Field Defect. The propensity of squamous epithelium of the lower genital tract (cervix, vagina, and vulva) to undergo premalignant change.

Laser (*L*ight *A*mplification by *S*timulated *E*mission of *R*adiation). An energized source of light that can be used to vaporize tissue and to treat intraepithelial neoplasia.

Pelvic Exenteration. An extensive pelvic operation usually employed to treat a central pelvic recurrence of cervical carcinoma after radiation. A total exenteration involves removal of the bladder, uterus, cervix, and rectum. An anterior exenteration spares the rectum, while a posterior exenteration spares the bladder.

Pseudosarcoma Botryoides. A benign tumor occurring in the vagina of infants and pregnant women that has a polyploid shape. Microscopically it may be confused with sarcoma botryoides.

Sarcoma Botryoides (Embryonal Rhabdomyosarcoma). A rare, often fatal, malignancy of the vagina that occurs in infants and children.

Vaginal Tumor Stage. A clinical classification that describes the extent of spread of vaginal carcinoma:

Stage I: Limited to vaginal wall

Stage II: Extends to subvaginal tissue

Stage III: Reaches the pelvic wall

Stage IV: Extends beyond the true pelvis or into mucosa of the bladder or rectum

VAIN-1. Vaginal intraepithelial neoplasia of the least severe type (comparable to mild dysplasia), usually occupying the lower one third of the epithelium.

VAIN-2. Vaginal intraepithelial neoplasia of intermediate severity (comparable to moderate dysplasia), usually occupying the lower two thirds of the epithelium.

VAIN-3. Vaginal intraepithelial neoplasia of the most severe type (comparable to severe dysplasia and carcinoma in situ), usually replacing the full thickness of the epithelium.

Premalignant changes in the vagina appear as intraepithelial squamous atypicalities and occur less frequently than comparable lesions in the cervix and vulva. However, the histologic appearance of intraepithelial neoplasia of the vagina is similar to that described for the cervix (Chapter 26). These changes are also similarly designated as dysplasia (mild, moderate, or severe) and carcinoma in situ. The term *VAIN* (vaginal, *VA*; intraepithelial, *I*; neoplasia, *N*) has been used to describe these histologic changes; the comparable categories are VAIN-1 (mild dysplasia), VAIN-2 (moderate dysplasia), and VAIN-3 (severe dysplasia to carcinoma in situ). The cytologic and histologic features of these changes are illustrated in Figure 31-1.

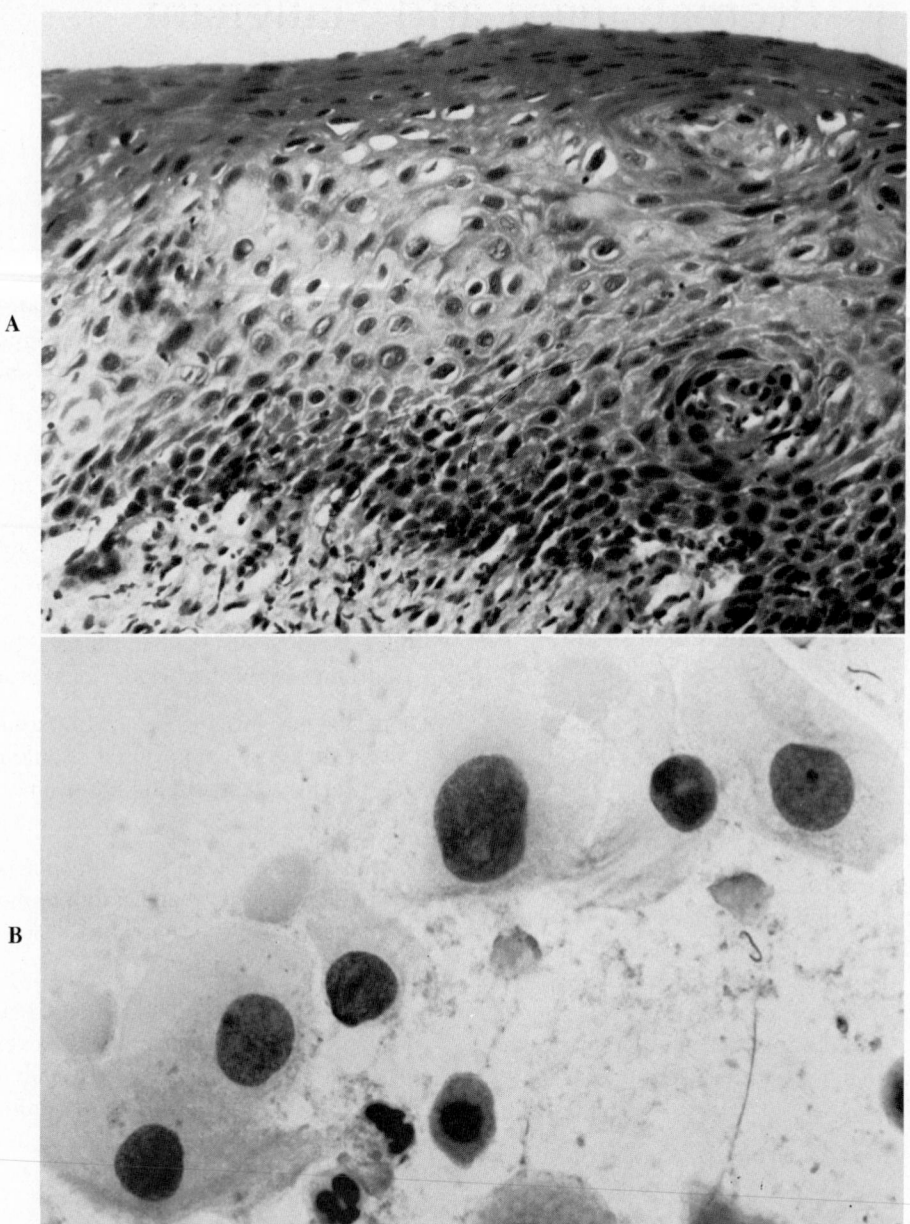

FIGURE 31-1

A, Section of vagina showing dysplasia. Epithelium appears thickened and shows abnormal maturation. Immature, hyperchromatic cells occupy lower two to four layers. Middle and upper third of mucosa show evidence of cytoplasmic differentiation with well-defined cellular borders. Nuclei in these areas are enlarged and pleomorphic. Parakeratosis is apparent on surface. Because immature cells are confined to lower third of mucosa, dysplasia is classified as mild. (H&E stain; ×250.) **B,** Cytologic specimen showing mild dysplasia. Note sheet of dysplastic cells. Cells show well-defined cytoplasmic borders. Nuclei are enlarged, and nuclear contour is smooth. Chromatin is uniformly, finely granular. Focal condensations of chromatin (chromocenters) are present in some nuclei. Nucleoli are not present. (Papanicolaou stain; ×1000.)

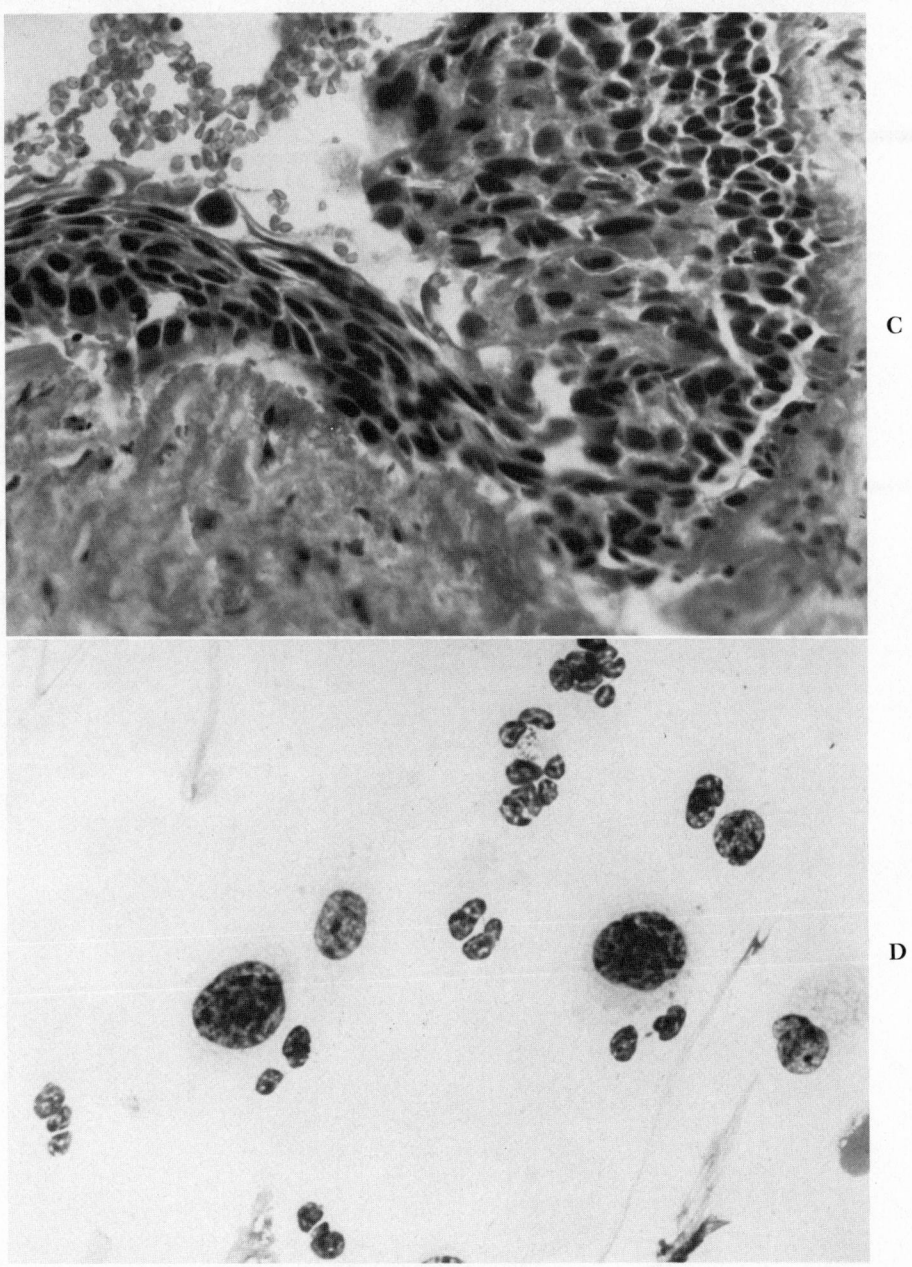

FIGURE 31-1, cont'd
C, Section showing severe dysplasia to carcinoma in situ. Entire epithelial thickness is occupied by hyperchromatic, dysplastic cells. Marked nuclear variation and mitoses are seen. Because of occasional cells with squamous differentiation (spindle-shaped cells, cells with well-defined cytoplasmic borders) in superficial layers, this lesion is sometimes classified as severe dysplasia. In carcinoma in situ immature cells replace the full thickness, and there is no evidence of squamous differentiation on the surface. (H&E stain; ×400.) **D,** Cytologic specimen showing carcinoma in situ. Several isolated immature cells with high nuclear-cytoplasmic ratio and poorly defined cytoplasmic borders can be seen. Chromatin is coarsely granular, and no nucleoli are present. In background are several polymorphonuclear leukocytes and strings of mucus. (Papanicolaou stain; ×1000.)   *Continued.*

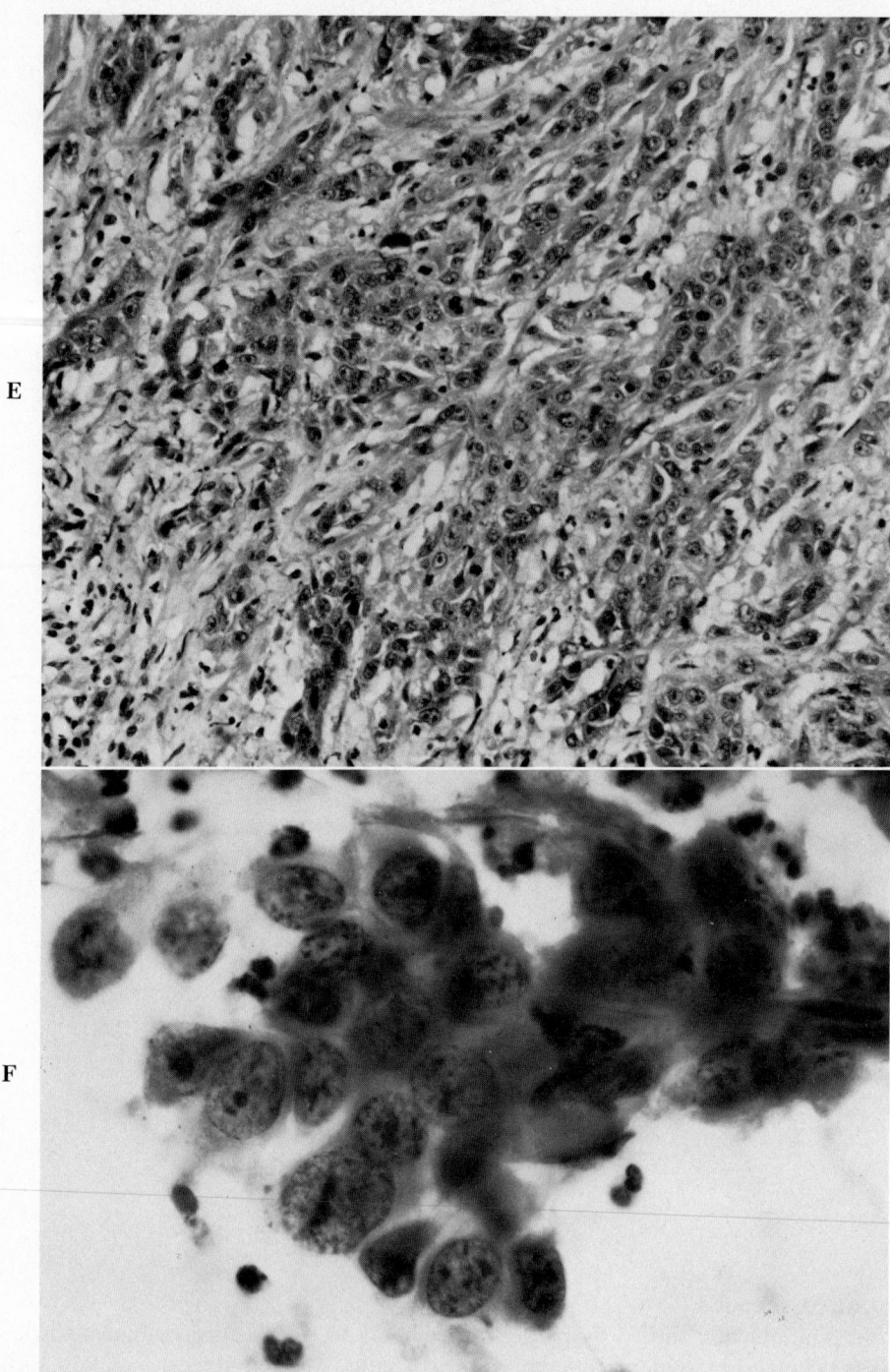

FIGURE 31-1, cont'd
E, Section showing invasive squamous carcinoma. Cords and sheets of poorly differentiated tumor cells infiltrate stroma. Nuclei are pleomorphic, and nucleoli are distinct. Mitotic rate is high. Squamous differentiation (keratin pearl formation, single-cell keratinization) was present in other areas of tumor. (H&E stain; ×200.) **F,** Cytologic specimen showing invasive squamous cell carcinoma. Note aggregate of tumor cells. Cellular boundaries are poorly defined, and nuclear orientation is lacking. Chromatin is irregularly distributed and has areas of clumping and clearing. Note nucleoli in some cells, which were absent in cells of patient with dysplasia and carcinoma in situ. (Papanicolaou stain; ×800.)

TABLE 31-1
Common Primary Vaginal Cancers

Tumor Type	Predominant Age (years)	Clinical Correlations
Endodermal sinus tumor (adenocarcinoma)	<2	Extremely rare, alpha-fetoprotein secretion, often fatal, multimodality therapy
Sarcoma botryoides	<8	Aggressive malignancy, multimodality therapy
Clear cell adenocarcinoma	>14	Associated with intrauterine exposure to DES
Melanoma	>50	Very rare, poor survival
Squamous cell carcinoma	>50	Most common primary vaginal cancer

VAIN occurs more commonly in patients previously treated for cervical intraepithelial neoplasia. The frequency of vaginal premalignancy in these patients is about 1% to 3%. Similarly, there is an increased risk for VAIN in those previously treated for squamous cell neoplasia of the vulva. The tendency to develop premalignant changes in the lower genital tract has been termed a *field defect* and denotes the increased risk of squamous cell neoplasia arising anywhere in the lower genital tract in such individuals. As with the cervix, predisposing factors associated with these changes may include venereal diseases, herpesvirus type II infection, and human papillomavirus infection. Additional risk factors include prior radiation therapy of the genital tract, immunosuppressive therapy in transplant patients, and chemotherapy in patients undergoing treatment for malignant disease.

Primary cancer of the vagina is rare and constitutes less than 2% of gynecologic malignancies. Most vaginal malignancies are metastatic, primarily from the cervix and endometrium. Less commonly, ovarian and rectosigmoid carcinomas, as well as choriocarcinoma, metastasize to the vagina. The most common histologic type of primary vaginal cancer is squamous cell carcinoma, but numerous other types of carcinomas, as well as primary sarcomas, occur. Table 31-1 summarizes the major primary malignancies of the vagina arranged according to the age of occurrence.

PREMALIGNANT DISEASE OF THE VAGINA

Detection and Diagnosis

Since premalignant disease of the vagina is generally asymptomatic, detection depends primarily on cytologic screening (Figure 31-1, *B* and *D*). Most commonly the changes will be observed in patients who have undergone prior therapy for intraepithelial disease of the cervix. Once an abnormal smear from vaginal epithelium is identified, a biopsy is required for histologic identification and verification of the severity of the change (Figure 31-1, *A* and *C*). A colposcopic examination is usually necessary to identify the areas requiring biopsy. As in the case of cervical neoplasia, a repeat Pap smear is taken during the colposcopic examination. Vaginal colposcopic techniques are similar to those described for the cervix. A large speculum is used to aid in visualizing the entire vaginal wall. While the abnormal colposcopic findings resemble those of the cervix (Chapter 26), full visualization of the entire vaginal wall is often difficult and time consuming.

A biopsy is performed with small instruments, such as the Kevorkian or Eppendorf punch biopsy forceps (Figure 31-2), or similar instruments also used for the cervix. Occasionally it is necessary to use a fine instrument, such as a nerve hook, to provide traction on the vaginal epithelium to obtain a biopsy. Most patients experience some discomfort during the biopsy, but usually local anesthesia is not needed, since injection of the anesthetic is often as uncomfortable as the biopsy itself. A less precise method for identifying an area for biopsy is to stain the vaginal epithelium with half-strength Lugol's solution and to take a biopsy specimen from the nonstaining areas. The vaginal epithelium must be adequately estrogenized so that sufficient epithelial glycogen is present for the normal tissue to stain dark brown. Local estrogen cream used for 1 week before examination is frequently helpful in postmenopausal patients and in patients with

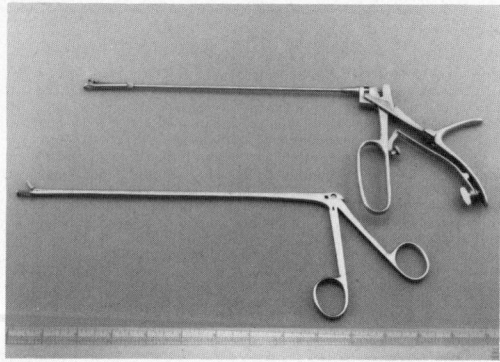

FIGURE 31-2
Eppendorf *(upper)* and Kevorkian *(lower)* punch biopsy instruments.

severe atrophic vaginitis in which atypical cells are first detected on cytologic (Pap) smear.

It is important for the examiner to realize that vaginal neoplasia is often multifocal. While the process is frequently located in the vaginal apex, it can occur anywhere along the vaginal tube, necessitating examination of the vagina in its entirety.

Management

As is true for cervical intraepithelial neoplasia, the abnormal vaginal epithelium must be completely eradicated. Small lesions, particularly those at the vaginal apex in patients who have undergone hysterectomy, usually are excised locally. However, excision of large areas may require skin grafting, and for that reason, other therapeutic modalities are often chosen.

Alternate nonsurgical treatment modalities are also directed toward destruction of all the abnormal epithelium. Radiation therapy, although used in the past, often leads to scarring and fibrosis and is generally not currently recommended for treatment of noninvasive disease. Because of the proximity of the bladder and rectum and the availability of newer modalities, cryotherapy is not used as frequently today as in the past. Widely used nonsurgical approaches include the laser, which is most commonly employed, or 5-fluorouracil (5-FU) cream for widespread multicentric lesions, particularly those with papillomavirus infection.

The carbon dioxide laser allows vaporization of the abnormal tissue. The beam is directed colposcopically. Iodine staining of the vagina can also outline those areas requiring therapy.

Treatment is frequently performed on an outpatient basis with a local anesthetic or analgesic, or both. If the lesions are extensive, general or regional anesthesia may be required. The intensity of therapy is regulated by adjusting the wattage of the laser, most commonly 15 to 20 watts if carried to a depth of 2 to 4 mm. The patient will experience a discharge for a few days after therapy. Healing usually requires a few weeks. Although long-term experience and follow-up with laser treatment of vaginal neoplasia is not available, preliminary results reported by Petrilli et al. show success rates on the order of 90%. Regular follow-up every 4 months, including a Pap smear and colposcopy, is required during the first year and usually 6 to 12 months thereafter.

Five percent 5-FU cream is often used for approximately 7 days. One half of a vaginal applicator (approximately 5 g) is inserted into the vagina nightly. Because the cream is irritating, some protective ointment such as zinc oxide should be applied to the vulva. If excess leakage occurs, less than half of an applicator should be used. In addition, the treatment should be discontinued before 7 days if the patient notes excessive irritation. A cycle of therapy should be repeated in 3 to 4 weeks if the intraepithelial process persists. In some cases the application of 5-FU is continued for 10 to 14 days, in which case the nontherapy interval is increased to 2 or 3 months. Lesions with a thickened white crust (hyperkeratosis) appear to be less sensitive to this treatment. On the other hand, postmenopausal women tolerate only small doses of 5-FU, presumably because of the comparative thinness of the vaginal epithelium. Krebs used one third of an applicator of 5% 5-FU weekly for 10 weeks and noted that 17 of 20 patients with vaginal condyloma were free of disease at 3 months. Three patients received a second cycle, and 16 of 18 were free of disease at 10 to 20 months. Ballon et al. and Petrilli et al. reported success rates of 80% to 90% for patients with vaginal intraepithelial neoplasia after multiple treatment cycles; the method appears particularly useful for patients with multifocal diffuse lesions.

Audet-Lapointe et al. noted that 61 of 66 cases of VAIN occurred in the upper one third of the vagina. For apical lesions, especially after hysterectomy, excision is advisable; for multifocal lesions and condyloma, they used 5-FU. The laser was used to eradicate discreet lesions.

MALIGNANT DISEASE OF THE VAGINA

Symptoms and Diagnosis

Primary vaginal cancers are rare, constituting less than 2% of all gynecologic malignancies, and usually occur as squamous cell carcinomas in women over age 50. To be considered a primary vaginal tumor, the malignancy must arise in the vagina and not involve the external os of the cervix superiorly or the vulva inferiorly. Otherwise the tumor is classified as cervical or vulvar. This is also an important therapeutic consideration, insofar as same management techniques apply to small tumors of the upper one third of the vagina and cervical carcinomas. Tumors of the lower one-third of the vagina are treated similarly to vulvar cancers (Chapter 30). Table 31-2 lists the staging criteria for vaginal cancers according to the International Federation of Gynecology and Obstetrics.

Delay in the diagnosis of these cancers frequently occurs, in part because of their rarity as well as because of a lack of recognition that the abnormal symptoms may be due to a malignancy. The most common symptom of vaginal cancer is abnormal bleeding or discharge. Pain is usually a symptom of an advanced tumor. Urinary frequency is also reported occasionally, particularly in the case of anterior wall tumors, whereas constipation or tenesmus may be reported when the tumors involve the posterior vaginal wall. In general, the longer the delay in diagnosis, the worse the prognosis and the more difficult the therapy. Vaginal cancer is usually diagnosed by direct biopsy of the tumor mass (Figure 31-1, *E*). Abnormal cytologic findings (Figure 31-1, *F*) may prompt a thorough pelvic examination that will lead to diagnosis of vaginal cancer. It is important during the course of the pelvic examination to inspect and palpate the entire vaginal tube and to rotate the speculum carefully to visualize the entire vagina, since often a small tumor may occupy the anterior or posterior vaginal wall.

Tumors of Adult Vagina

Squamous Cell Carcinoma

Squamous cell carcinoma is the most common of the vaginal malignancies and accounts for 90% of primary vaginal cancers. Although reported in women in their 30s, the disease occurs primarily in those over age 50. Most squamous cell carcinomas occur in the upper third of the vagina, but primary tumors in the middle third and lower third are also common. Grossly the tumor appears as a fungating, ulcerating mass, often accompanied by a foul smell and discharge related to a secondary infection. Microscopically (Figure 31-1, *E*) the tumor demonstrates the classic findings of an invasive squamous cell carcinoma infiltrating the vaginal epithelium.

Treatment of these tumors is based on the size, stage, and location. Therapy is limited by the proximity of the bladder anteriorly and the rectum posteriorly. It is also influenced by the location of the tumor in the vagina, which determines the area of lymphatic spread (Figure 31-3).

The lymphatics of the vagina envelop the mucosa and anastomose with lymphatic vessels in the muscularis. Those of the middle to upper vagina communicate superiorly with the lymphatics of the cervix and drain into the pelvic nodes of the obturator and internal and external iliac chains. In contrast, the lymphatics of the distal third of the vagina drain to both the inguinal nodes as well as to the pelvic nodes, similar to the drainage of the vulva. The posterior wall lymphatics anastomose with the rectal lymphatic system and then to the nodes that drain the rectum, such as the inferior gluteal, sacral, and rectal nodes.

MANAGEMENT. Both operation and irradiation therapy have been effective, considering the limits imposed by the proximity to the bladder and rectum and the risk of fistula for-

---

TABLE 31-2

International Federation of Gynecology and Obstetrics (FIGO) Staging Classification for Vaginal Cancer

Stage	Characteristics
0	Carcinoma in situ
I	Carcinoma limited to vaginal wall
II	Carcinoma involves subvaginal tissue but has not extended to pelvic wall
III	Carcinoma extends to pelvic wall
IV	Carcinoma extends beyond true pelvis or involves mucosa of bladder or rectum (bullous edema as such does not assign a patient to stage IV)

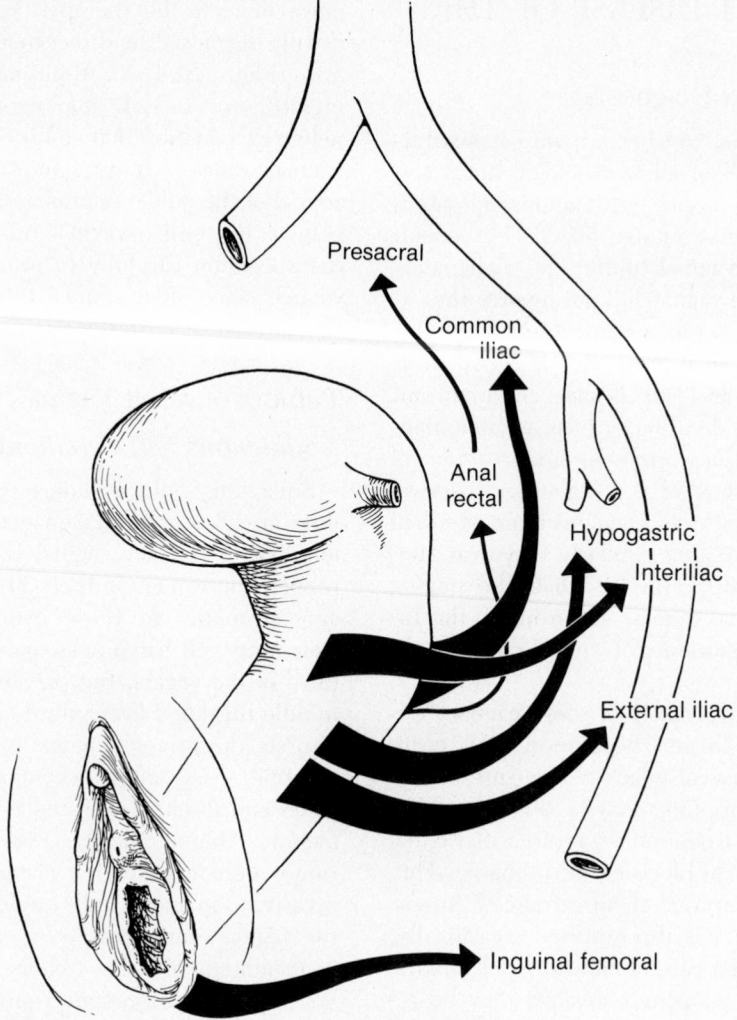

FIGURE 31-3
Lymphatic drainage of vagina. Predominant pathways from various parts of vagina
are shown.

mation from these organs to the vagina. Radiation therapy has been the most frequent mode of treatment. External radiation therapy with megavoltage equipment is initially utilized to shrink the tumor. This is then followed by a local cesium or radium implant placed interstitially with needles or by intracavitary radiation using a tandem or ovoids, similar to the delivery systems used for cervical carcinoma (particularly in the case of a tumor in the upper one third of the vagina if the cervix is present) (Chapter 27). The treatment is individualized depending on tumor size and stage. Some therapists have advocated using only local sources of radiation if the primary carcinoma is small (under 2 cm) and accessible to needle implantation.

For larger lesions the dosage of the external component of radiation therapy is increased, with a concomitant reduction in the local vaginal component of treatment of the primary tumor. Usually a total tumor dose of approximately 7500 cGy is administered. Implants cannot be done in some patients with stage III or IV carcinoma; in such cases only external therapy can be used, and a central "boost" is given after an initial 5000 rads (50 Gy) whole-pelvic treatment (Table 31-3). Spirtos et al., in a study of 23 stage I patients, noted only two local recurrences, and both patients had tumor dosages less than 7500 cGy. However, Perez et al. noted increasingly severe complications if the vaginal dose exceeded 9800 cGy. Kucera and Vavra, in a series

TABLE 31-3
Summary of Average Dosages* for Treatment of Vaginal Carcinoma

	External Therapy	Implant (Interstitial)
Stage I		
Small tumors (<2 cm)	May omit	6000-7000 cGy, 6-7 days
All Others	4000 cGy, whole pelvis	3000-4000 cGy, 3-4 days
Stage II	4000-5000 cGy, whole pelvis	3000-4000 cGy, 3-4 days
Stages III and IV	5000 cGy, whole pelvis; an additional 1000-2000 cGy through reduced field if implant not possible	2000 cGy, by implant if possible

Modified from Nori D, Hilaris BS, Stanimir G, et al: Int J Radiat Oncol Biol Phys 9:1471, 1983.
*1 cGy = 1 rad.

of 434 patients treated with irradiation, noted results were best for low stage tumors, those in the upper one third of the vagina and if the tumor was well-differentiated.

For localized tumors in the upper one third of the vagina, radical hysterectomy and vaginectomy can be effective, especially in younger patients. In most instances, radical pelvic surgery, including removal of the bladder (anterior exenteration) or removal of the rectum (posterior exenteration), or both (total exenteration), is necessary only in patients with localized recurrence after radiation therapy. Initially the tumors usually recur locally, as in squamous cell carcinoma of the cervix and vulva, but distant metastases also occur, as in vulvar and cervical cancers. An effective chemotherapy program for recurrent squamous cell vaginal carcinoma has not been developed. A variety of regimens for squamous cell carcinoma utilizing multiple-agent chemotherapy is usually employed, similar to those for squamous cell carcinoma of the cervix (Chapter 27).

SURVIVAL. Overall 5-year survival rates for patients with primary carcinoma of the vagina have been reported to be approximately 45%. Table 31-4 demonstrates that survival is related to stage.

Clear Cell Adenocarcinoma

Clear cell adenocarcinomas in young women have been seen more frequently since 1970 as a result of the association of many of these cancers with intrauterine exposure to diethylstilbestrol (DES). The nonmalignant manifesta-

TABLE 31-4
Stage and Survival from Collated Series of Squamous Cell Carcinoma of Vagina

	Patient (no.)	5-Year Survival (no.)	Percentage
Stage I	95	67	71
Stage II	174	81	47
Stage III	63	16	25
Stage IV	40	3	8
TOTAL	372	167	45

Adapted from Benedet JL, Murphy KS, Fairey RN, et al: Obstet Gynecol 62:715, 1983. Reprinted with permission from The American College of Obstetricians and Gynecologists.

tions of this exposure are discussed in Chapter 14.

MANAGEMENT. Therapeutic considerations are similar to those for squamous cell carcinoma, taking into account the young age of the patients undergoing therapy. Cervical clear cell adenocarcinomas are treated like primary cervical carcinomas (Chapter 27). The results of therapy for both vaginal and cervical clear cell adenocarcinoma in young women will be discussed together in this section. These tumors are also staged according to the FIGO classification (see Tables 27-3 and 31-2). The majority (80%) have been diagnosed as stage I or II. The overall results of therapy, based on the stage of the tumor at the time of treatment, are shown in Table 31-5. As can be seen, the survival rate is related directly to the stage of the tumor, similar to other gynecologic malignancies at these sites.

TABLE 31-5
5- and 10-Year Survival Rates for 547 Patients
with Clear Cell Adenocarcinoma of the Vagina
and Cervix

Stage	5-Year Survival (%)	10-Year Survival (%)
I	93	87
IIA	80	66
IIB	58	49
II (vagina)	83	67
III	37	12
IV	0	0

**FAVORABLE FACTORS IN SURVIVAL OF
PATIENTS WITH CLEAR CELL
ADENOCARCINOMA**

Low stage
Older age
Tubulocystic histologic pattern
Small tumor diameter
Reduced depth of invasion
Regional lymph nodes free of tumor

In general, operation is the primary treatment modality because of the young age of the patients. For stage I and early stage II tumors, radical hysterectomy with partial or complete vaginectomy, pelvic lymphadenectomy, and replacement of the vagina with split-thickness skin grafts has been the most common approach. In most cases, ovarian function is preserved. In addition, efforts have been made to preserve fertility in patients who have small tumors of the vagina by the use of local irradiation of the primary tumor and immediate adjacent tissues to spare the ovaries. Since metastases to regional pelvic nodes can occur even with small stage I tumors, retroperitoneal lymph node dissections are usually performed before local therapy.

Usually local excision of the tumor has been performed before irradiation to facilitate local application. Senekjian et al. in 1987 have noted that the survival of patients with small vaginal tumors treated by local excision and then local irradiation is comparable to those with conventional extensive therapy. The best candidates are those with tumors less than 2 cm in diameter, a predominant tubulocystic pattern (Figure 31-4, A) and depth of invasion less than 3 cm. After wide local excision, a laparotomy is performed to sample the pelvic nodes to rule out tumor spread. If these are negative, local irradiation can then be given. Eight pregnancies have been reported in five patients locally treated. Larger tumors, however, have been treated with full pelvic irradiation, in addition to an intracavitary implant. In a few instances exenterative surgery has been successfully performed, but as noted in 1989 by Senekjian et al., this procedure is preferably applied to central recurrences after primary irradiation. Local

vaginal excision as the sole therapy is not usually adequate for small tumors since the tumor frequently recurs.

SURVIVAL. Three predominant histologic patterns are found in patients with clear cell adenocarcinoma (Figure 31-4). In addition, a number of prognostic factors have been identified. The older patients (over 19 years of age) have been found to have a more favorable prognosis in comparison to younger subjects (under 15 years of age). This difference is associated with a more favorable outcome for those with the tubulocystic pattern of clear cell adenocarcinoma, which is the most frequent histologic pattern found in older patients. In addition, smaller tumor diameter and superficial depth of invasion correlate with improved patient survival. If the regional pelvic nodes are free of tumor, the prognosis is also more favorable. It is more likely that the regional pelvic lymph nodes will be free of tumor if other factors are favorable (see box above).

Clear cell adenocarcinomas can spread locally as well as by lymphatics and blood vessels. Metastases to regional pelvic nodes are found in about one sixth of stage I cases. The spread to regional pelvic nodes becomes more frequent in higher-stage tumors. Depending on the location of the tumor recurrence, therapy has consisted of additional radical surgery or extensive radiation in localized pelvic disease and systemic chemotherapy in cases of metastatic disease. Multiple-agent cytotoxic chemotherapy is usually prescribed. Cisplatin, 75 to 100 mg/m^2 with 3 to 5 days of continuous infusion, and 5-FU, 1 gm/m^2 every 3 to 4 weeks, are currently recommended. Unfortunately, no single agent or combination of chemotherapeutic agents has emerged as an effective therapy.

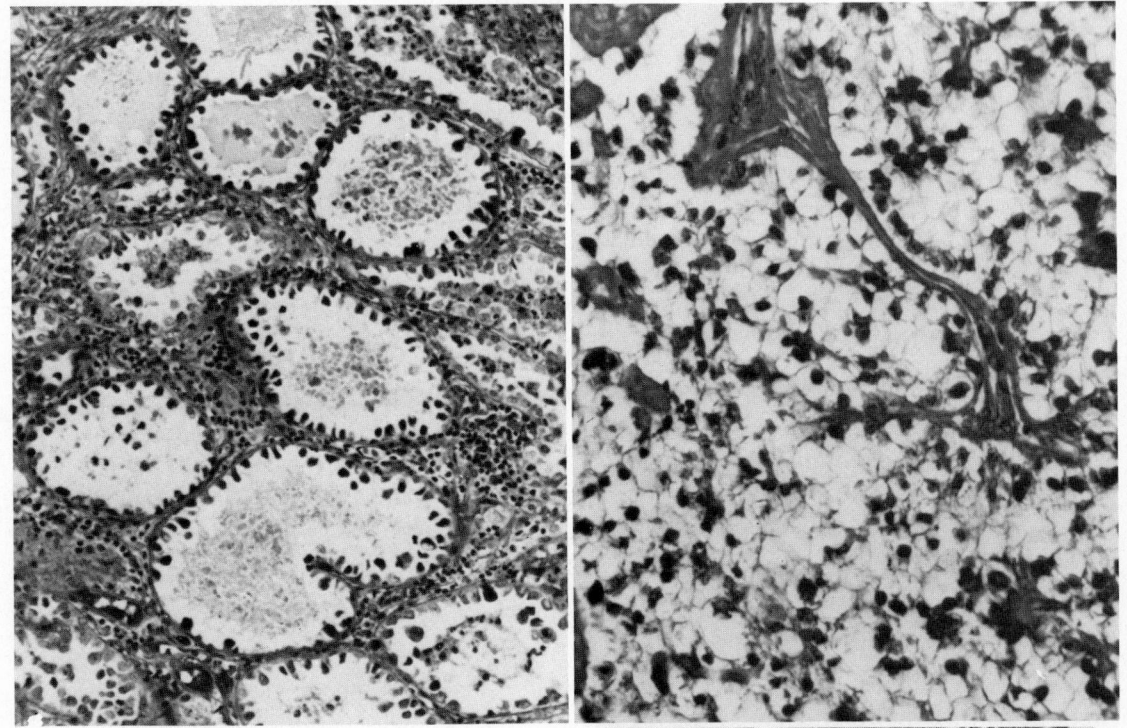

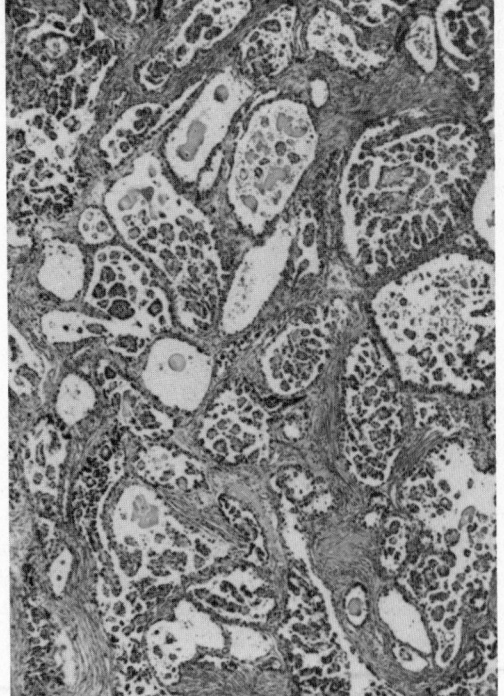

FIGURE 31-4
Clear cell adenocarcinoma. **A,** Tubulocystic cell pattern. Note hobnail cells extruding into lumina of tubular structures. (H&E stain; ×180.) **B,** Solid pattern. (H&E stain; ×300.) **C,** Papillary pattern. (H&E stain; ×50.) (**A** and **B** from Scully RE, Robboy SJ, and Herbst AL: Ann Clin Lab Sci 4:222, 1974, Copyright 1974, Institute for Clinical Science; **C** from Scully RE, Robboy SJ, and Welch WR: Pathology and pathogenesis of diethylstilbestrol-related disorders of the female genital tract. In Herbst AL, editor: Intrauterine exposure to diethylstilbestrol in the human, Washington, DC, 1978, American College of Obstetricians and Gynecologists.)

Prolonged follow-up is necessary for these patients, since recurrences have been reported as long as 19 years after primary therapy, particularly in the lungs and supraclavicular areas.

Malignant Melanoma

Vaginal melanomas are rare. The tumors occur in adult patients predominantly (average age 60 years). They tend to be deeply invasive in the vagina, although histologically they may resemble other melanomas, such as those of the vulva. However, patients with vaginal melanoma have a worse prognosis than those with vulvar melanoma.

MANAGEMENT. Treatment usually consists of radical surgery with wide excision of the vagina and dissection of the regional nodes (pelvic or inguinal-femoral, or both), depending on the location of the lesion. Adjunctive radiotherapy and chemotherapy have also been used.

SURVIVAL. Local recurrence is common, and the disease is usually fatal. Chung et al. reported a 5-year survival of only 21% in a series of 19 patients. Reid et al. noted 17.4% 5-year survival in 15 patients, but the prognosis improved for those with tumors less than 3 cm in diameter. More recently, Borazjani et al. noted improved survival for patients whose tumors had less than six mitoses per 10 hpf.

Vaginal Tumors of Infants and Children

Endodermal Sinus Tumor (Yolk-Sac Tumor)

This type of adenocarcinoma is a rare germ cell tumor that usually occurs in the ovary (Chapter 29). The tumor secretes alpha-fetoprotein (AFP), which provides a useful tumor marker to monitor patients treated for these neoplasms. Approximately 20 cases of this unusual malignancy originating in the vagina of infants, predominantly those under 2 years of age, have been reported. The tumor is aggressive, and most patients have died. Young and Scully reported six patients who were free of disease 2 to 9 years after operation or irradiation, or both, with vincristine, actinomycin D, and cyclophosphamide (VAC; Chapter 29) chemotherapy. Copeland et al. reported similar good results with combination chemotherapy and excision. Recently, Collins et al. noted tu-

mor regression in a 5-month-old patient after VAC therapy alone.

Sarcoma Botryoides (Embryonal Rhabdomyosarcoma)

This rare sarcoma is usually diagnosed in the vagina of a young female. Rarely does it occur in a young child over 8 years of age, although cases in adolescents have been reported. The most common symptom is abnormal vaginal bleeding, with an occasional mass at the introitus (Figure 31-5). The tumor grossly will resemble a cluster of grapes forming multiple polypoid masses.

The tumors are believed to begin in the subepithelial layers of the vagina and expand rapidly to fill the vagina. These sarcomas often are multicentric. Histologically, they have a loose myxomatous stroma with malignant pleomorphic cells and occasional eosinophilic rhab-

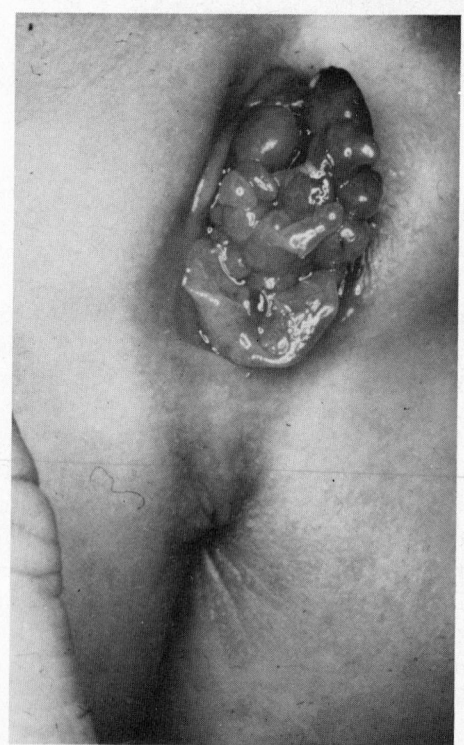

FIGURE 31-5
Sarcoma botryoides protruding through vaginal introitus. (From Herbst AL: Cancer of the vagina. In Gusberg SB and Frick HC, editors: Gynecologic cancer, ed 5, Baltimore, 1978, Williams & Wilkins. © 1978 by The Williams & Wilkins Co, Baltimore.)

domyoblasts that often contain characteristic cross-striations (strap cells) (Figure 31-6).

These virulent tumors have been treated in the past by radical surgery, such as pelvic ex-

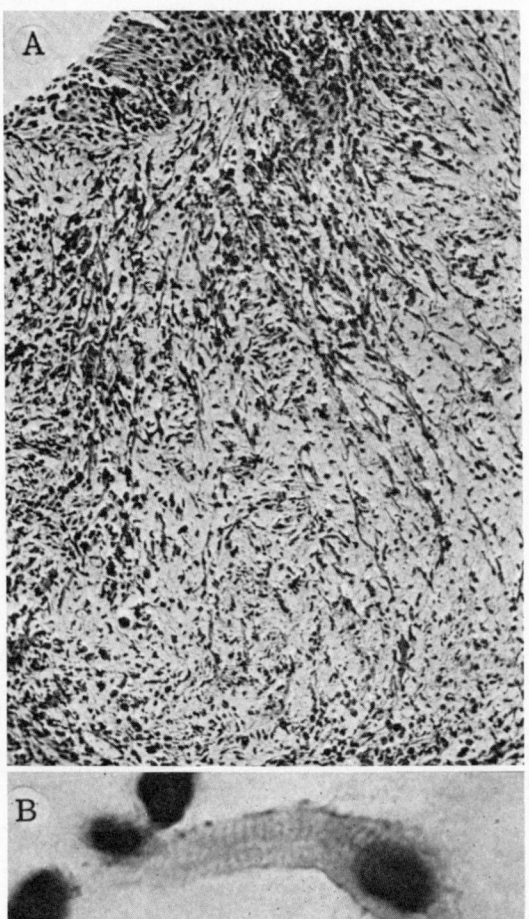

FIGURE 31-6
Section showing sarcoma botryoides. Note rhabdomyoblasts and strap cells. (From Hilgers RD, Malkasian GD, and Soule EH: Am J Obstet Gynecol 107:484, 1970.)

enteration. However, effective control with less radical surgery has been achieved with a multimodality approach consisting of multiagent chemotherapy (VAC), usually combined with operation. Radiation therapy has also been used. Hays et al. reported recently on 21 patients with vaginal rhabdomyosarcomas who received chemotherapy. Seven relapsed, five of whom had residual disease after incomplete resection. One had disseminated disease. In 17 patients who received chemotherapy for 8 to 48 weeks, a delayed excision could be performed. Long-term survival data for a large number of patients are not available, but such a combined approach appears to result in effective treatment with less mutilating surgery. A multimodality approach including chemotherapy was used by Flamant et al. in 17 females with rhabdomyosarcoma of the vagina or vulva. At the time of their 1990 report 15 appeared cured and 11 of 12 pubescent females have had menses, while 2 have successfully conceived and delivered healthy children. This was emphasized in a recent report from the Intergroup Rhabdomyosarcoma Study (IRS) by Maurer et al. They found VAC to be effective for disease confined to the vagina without nodal spread. Therapy was effective without irradiation for disease that was locally resected, suggesting for these patients chemotherapy plus operation can be effective therapy.

Pseudosarcoma Botryoides

A rare, benign vaginal polyp that resembles sarcoma botryoides is found in the vagina of infants or pregnant women. Although large atypical cells may be present microscopically, strap cells are absent. Grossly these polyps do not resemble the grapelike appearance of sarcoma botryoides. They are called *pseudosarcoma* botryoides. Treatment by local excision is effective.

_____ KEY POINTS _____

- Predisposing factors associated with the development of vaginal intraepithelial neoplasia include infection with herpesvirus II and papillomavirus, prior radiation therapy to the vagina, and immunosuppression.

- The tendency of intraepithelial squamous neoplasia to develop anywhere in the lower female genital tract is termed *field defect* and describes the increased risk of premalignant changes occurring in the cervix, vagina, or vulva.

- Most cases of vaginal intraepithelial neoplasia (VAIN) occur in the upper one third of the vagina.

- VAIN can be treated by excision, laser, or 5-fluorouracil (5-FU). Excision is often used if the apex is involved, particularly after hysterectomy; laser is generally used for discreet lesions; and 5-FU cream for diffuse multicentric disease.

- The most common primary vaginal malignancy is squamous cell carcinoma (90%).

- Most cancers occurring in the vagina are metastatic.

- Vaginal cancers constitute less than 2% of gynecologic malignancies.

- Radiation therapy is the most frequently used modality for treatment of squamous cell carcinoma of the vagina.

- Overall 5-year survival of patients treated for squamous cell carcinoma of the vagina is approximately 45%.

- Clear cell adenocarcinoma is associated with prenatal DES exposure and has an improved prognosis if the patient is over age 19 years, has a predominant tubulocystic tumor pattern, and has low-stage disease.

- Local therapy for small stage I clear cell adenocarcinomas of the vagina is best considered if the tumor is less than 2 cm in diameter, invades less than 3 mm, and is predominantly of the tubulocystic histologic type. A staging laparotomy to rule out pelvic node spread should be negative.

- The overall 5-year survival of patients treated for clear cell adenocarcinoma is approximately 80%, in part due to the high proportion of low-stage cases.

- Vaginal melanomas are usually fatal. They occur primarily in patients over age 50 years.

- Endodermal sinus tumors occur in infants under age 2 years. They secrete alpha-fetoprotein and are usually treated by multiagent chemotherapy followed by operative excision.

- Sarcoma botryoides occurs primarily in children under age 8 years. It is treated by a multimodality approach using multiagent chemotherapy with operative removal and occasionally irradiation.

BIBLIOGRAPHY

Allyn DL, Silverberg SG, and Salzberg AM: Endodermal sinus tumor of the vagina: report of a case with 7-year survival and literature review of so-called "mesonephromas," Cancer 27:1231, 1971.

Andersen ES: Primary carcinoma of the vagina: a study of 29 cases, Gynecol Oncol 33:317, 1989.

Andersen WA, Sabio H, Durso N, et al: Endodermal sinus tumor of the vagina, Cancer 56:1025, 1985.

Audet-Lapointe P, Body G, Vauclair R, et al: Vaginal intraepithelial neoplasia, Gynecol Oncol 36:232, 1990.

Ballon SC, Roberts JA, and Lagasse LD: Topical 5-fluorouracil in the treatment of intraepithelial neoplasia of the vagina, Obstet Gynecol 54:163, 1979.

Benedet JL, Murphy KS, Fairey RN, et al: Primary invasive carcinoma of the vagina, Obstet Gynecol 62:715, 1983.

Borazjani G, Prem KA, Okagaki T, et al: Primary malignant melanoma of the vagina: a clinicopathological analysis of 10 cases, Gynecol Oncol 37:264, 1990.

Chung AF, Casey MJ, Flannery JT, et al: Malignant melanoma of the vagina: report of 19 cases, Obstet Gynecol 55:720, 1980.

Collins HS, Burke TW, Heller PB, et al: Endodermal sinus tumor of the infant vagina treated exclusively by chemotherapy, Obstet Gynecol 73:507, 1989.

Copeland LJ, Gershenson DM, Saul PB, et al: Sarcoma botryoides of the female genital tract, Obstet Gynecol 66:262, 1985.

Copeland LJ, Sneige N, Ordonez NG, et al: Endodermal sinus tumor of the vagina and cervix, Cancer 55:2558, 1985.

Dewhurst J: Genital malignancies in the prepubertal child. In Coppleson M, editor: Gynecologic oncology, New York, 1981, Churchill Livingstone, Inc.

Elliott GB, Reynolds HA, and Fidler HK: Pseudosarcoma botryoides of cervix and vagina in pregnancy, J Obstet Gynaecol Br Comm 74:728, 1967.

Flamant F, Gerbaulet A, Nihoul-Fekete C, et al: Long-term sequelae of conservative treatment by surgery, brachytherapy, and chemotherapy for vulval and vaginal rhabdomyosarcoma in children, J Clin Oncol 8:1847, 1990.

Frick HC, Jacox HW, and Taylor HC: Primary carcinoma of the vagina, Am J Obstet Gynecol 101:695, 1968.

Gallup DG and Morley GW: Carcinoma in situ of the vagina: a study and review, Obstet Gynecol 46:334, 1975.

Hays DM, Shimada H, Raney RB, et al: Clinical staging and treatment results in rhabdomyosarcoma of the female genital tract among children and adolescents, Cancer 61:1893, 1988.

Herbst AL and Anderson D: Recent advances in clear cell adenocarcinoma of the vagina and cervix secondary to intrauterine exposure to DES, Semin Surg Oncol 6:343, 1990.

Herbst AL, Green TH, and Ulfelder H: Primary carcinoma of the vagina: an analysis of 68 cases, Am J Obstet Gynecol 106:210, 1970.

Herbst AL and Scully RE: Adenocarcinoma of the vagina in adolescence, Cancer 25:745, 1970.

Herbst AL, Ulfelder H, and Poskanzer DC: Adenocarcinoma of the vagina, N Engl J Med 284:878, 1971.

Hilgers RD: Pelvic exenteration for vaginal embryonal rhabdomyosarcoma: a review, Obstet Gynecol 45:175, 1975.

Krebs H-B: Treatment of vaginal condylomata acuminata by weekly topical application of 5-fluorouracil, Obstet Gynecol 70:68, 1987.

Kucera H and Vavra N: Radiation management of primary carcinoma of the vagina: clinical and histopathological variables associated with survival, Gynecol Oncol 40:12, 1991.

Maurer HM, Beltangady M, Gehan EA, et al: The Intergroup Rhabdomyosarcoma Study: a final report, Cancer 6:209, 1988.

Miettinen M, Wahlstrom T, Vesterinen E, et al: Vaginal polyps with pseudosarcomatous features: a clinicopathologic study of seven cases, Cancer 51:1148, 1983.

Mitchell M, Talerman A, Sholl JS, et al: Pseudosarcoma botryoides in pregnancy: report of a case with ultrastructural observations, Obstet Gynecol 70:522, 1987.

Nori D, Hilaris BS, Stanimir G, et al: Radiation therapy of primary vaginal carcinoma, Int J Radiat Oncol Biol Phys 9:1471, 1983.

Perez CA, Arneson AN, Dehner LP, et al: Radiation therapy in carcinoma of the vagina, Obstet Gynecol 44:862, 1974.

Perez CA, Camel HM, Galakatos AE, et al: Definitive irradiation in carcinoma of the vagina: long-term evaluation of results, Int J Radiat Oncol Biol Phys 15:1283, 1988.

Perticucci S: Diagnostic, prognostic, and therapeutic considerations in invasive carcinoma of the vagina, Obstet Gynecol 40:843, 1972.

Petrilli ES, Townsend DE, Morrow CP, et al: Vaginal intraepithelial neoplasm: biologic aspects and treatment with topical 5-fluorouracil and the carbon dioxide laser, Am J Obstet Gynecol 38:321, 1980.

Piver MS and Rose PG: Long-term follow-up and complications of infants with vulvovaginal embryonal rhabdomyosarcoma treated with surgery, radiation therapy, and chemotherapy, Obstet Gynecol 71:435, 1988.

Plentl AA and Friedman EA: Lymphatic system of the female genitalia, Philadelphia, 1971, WB Saunders Co.

Prempree T, Viravathana T, Slawson RG, et al: Radiation management of primary carcinoma of the vagina, Cancer 40:109, 1977.

Pride GL, Schultz AE, Chuprevich TW, et al: Primary invasive squamous carcinoma of the vagina, Obstet Gynecol 53:218, 1979.

Reid GC, Schmidt RW, Roberts JA, et al: Primary melanoma of the vagina: a clincopathologic analysis, Obstet Gynecol 74:190, 1989.

Scully RE, Robboy SJ, and Herbst AL: Vaginal and cervical abnormalities, including clear cell adenocarcinoma related to prenatal exposure to stilbestrol, Ann Clin Lab Sci 4:222, 1974.

Scully RE and Welch WR: Pathology of the female genital tract after prenatal exposure to diethylstilbestrol. In Herbst AL and Bern HA, editors: Developmental effects of diethylstilbestrol (DES) in pregnancy, New York, 1981, Thieme-Stratton.

Senekjian EK, Frey KW, Anderson D, and Herbst AL: Local therapy in stage I clear cell adenocarcinoma of the vagina, Cancer 60:1319, 1987.

Senekjian EK, Frey KW, and Herbst AL: Pelvic exenteration in clear cell adenocarcinoma of the vagina and cervix, Gynecol Oncol 34:413, 1989.

Senekjian EK, Frey KW, Stone C, and Herbst AL: An evaluation of stage II vaginal clear cell adenocarcinoma according to substages, Gynecol Oncol 31:56, 1988.

Spirtos NM, Doshi BP, Kapp DS, and Teng N: Radiation therapy for primary squamous cell carcinoma of the vagina: Stanford University experience, Gynecol Oncol 35:20, 1989.

Sulak P, Barnhill D, Heller P, et al: Nonsquamous cancer of the vagina, Gynecol Oncol 29:309, 1988.

Townsend DE: Intraepithelial neoplasm of the vagina. In Coppleson M, editor: Gynecologic oncology, New York, 1981, Churchill Livingstone, Inc.

Wharton JT, Fletcher GH, and Delclos L: Invasive tumors of the vagina. In Coppleson M, editor: Gynecologic oncology, New York, 1981, Churchill Livingstone, Inc.

Young RH and Scully RE: Endodermal sinus tumor of the vagina: a report of nine cases and review of the literature, Gynecol Oncol 18:380, 1984.

<table>
<tr><td>CHAPTER
32</td><td></td></tr>
</table>

Malignant Disease of the Fallopian Tube

KEY TERMS AND DEFINITIONS

Hydrops Tubae Profluens. A symptom complex of abnormal vaginal discharge preceded by pain and a mass that may disappear after the discharge is noted. This complex occasionally occurs in patients with tubal carcinoma.

Primary Tubal Carcinoma. An adenocarcinoma usually of papillary or medullary variety arising within the lumen of the oviduct. A transition can often be demonstrated between nonneoplastic and malignant tubal epithelium.

Primary cancers of the fallopian tube are the rarest of female genital tract malignancies, and almost all are adenocarcinomas. This malignancy comprises approximately 0.3% to 1.1% of all gynecologic cancers. Approximately 80% to 90% of fallopian tube malignancies are metastatic from other sites, usually arising in the ovary or uterus and occasionally in the gastrointestinal tract. Metastatic carcinomas are approximately 10 times as frequent as primary tumors. Approximately 1000 cases of primary fallopian tube carcinoma have been reported, mostly from studies comprising individual cases or small series of patients treated at a single center. This heterogeneity of data, combined with lack of a uniform staging system for these very rare cancers, has made it difficult to provide precise information regarding their optimal management. This chapter reviews current information, with particular emphasis on diagnosis, natural history, and management.

ETIOLOGY AND AGE DISTRIBUTION

The etiology of adenocarcinoma of the fallopian tube is unknown. It has been postulated that chronic salpingitis and prior pelvic inflammatory disease are associated factors. However, pelvic inflammatory disease is common, and the carcinomas rare, suggesting that other factors are involved.

The disease primarily affects older women, the average age being in the 50s, with a range from 18 to 80 years. Podzcaski and Herbst summarized the age distribution of 188 cases reported in the literature since 1970 (Figure 32-1) and noted an average age of 54.9 years.

DIAGNOSIS

These tumors are usually asymptomatic, and the diagnosis is most frequently made only after the patient has undergone surgical exploration. The most commonly reported sign is abnormal or excessive vaginal bleeding or discharge, which occurs in about 50% of the patients. Pain is less frequently reported. Occasionally an adnexal mass is noted. Abnormal vaginal discharge and bleeding, combined with lower abdominal pain and an adnexal mass in the postmenopausal woman, are considered pathognomonic for the diagnosis of tubal malignancy. Unfortunately, these three conditions rarely exist together, which is why the diagnosis is frequently made postoperatively. The term *hydrops tubae profluens* has been used to describe the abnormal discharge and pain that presumably result from blockage of the distal part of the fallopian tube. Subsequent peristalsis produces the discharge, occasionally accompanied by the disappearance of the mass secondary to the expulsion of fluid from the dilated tube. The disease should be strongly sus-

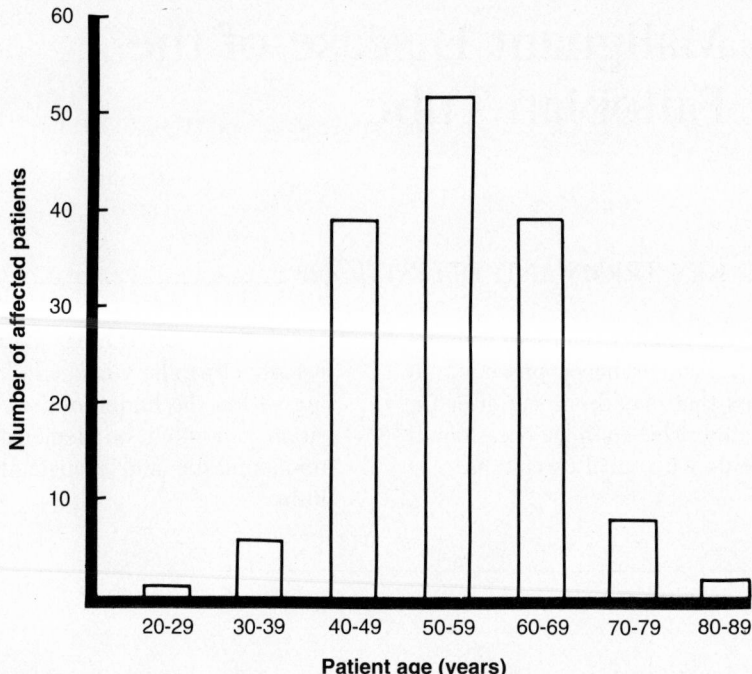

FIGURE 32-1

Histogram illustrating age distribution of patients with tubal carcinomas. (From Podczaski E and Herbst AL: Cancer of the vagina and fallopian tube. In Knapp RC and Berkowitz RS, editors: Gynecologic oncology, New York, 1983, Macmillan Publishing Co.)

pected in anyone with these findings. Vaginal cytology may show malignant adenocarcinoma cells in cases of tubal cancer. However, vaginal cytology is usually negative; Benedet et al. found it to be positive in only 10% of their 40 patients, although Hirai et al. reported preoperative cytology was positive in 6 (40%) of their 15 cases.

The diagnosis of tubal carcinoma should be considered in any patient with vaginal cytology positive for adenocarcinoma in whom the diagnosis of endometrial carcinoma has been excluded, although ovarian and endocervical adenocarcinomas are other possibilities. The diagnosis should also be suspected in patients with postmenopausal uterine bleeding for whom dilation and curettage fail to reveal the cause. Laparoscopy can be of benefit in establishing the diagnosis for such patients. Vaginal ultrasound may also aid in preoperative diagnosis.

PATHOLOGY

On gross examination the fallopian tube containing primary adenocarcinoma often apears dilated and may resemble a hydrosalpinx until the tube is opened, revealing an infiltrating tumor (Figures 32-2 and 32-3). Sometimes it is difficult to be certain that the tumor is of tubal origin, and confusion with metastatic carcinoma, particularly from the ovary, can be a diagnostic problem. In 1950 Hu, Taymor, and Hertig suggested the following criteria to allow the diagnosis of primary tubal carcinoma:

1. The primary tumor is grossly within the lumen of the tube.
2. The mucosa of the tube is involved with the tumor, which displays a papillary (or medullary) pattern.
3. A transition can be demonstrated between the malignant and nonmalignant tubal epithelium (if the tubal wall is involved to a great extent).

Figures 32-4 and 32-5 demonstrate a primary tubal carcinoma showing a papillary-alveolar pattern. These tumors can arise in either tube with approximately equal frequency and occasionally may be bilateral.

CLINICAL STAGING

No widely accepted staging system exists for fallopian tube carcinoma. The tumor spreads in

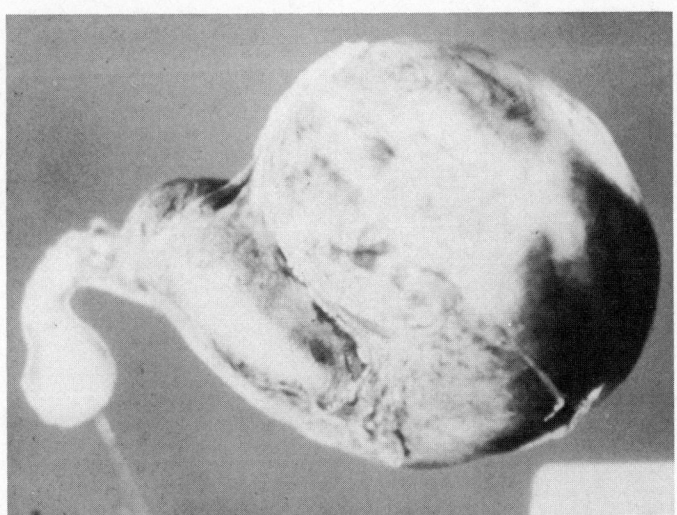

FIGURE 32-2
External appearance of fallopian tube with primary adenocarcinoma. (From Podczaski E and Herbst AL: Cancer of the vagina and fallopian tube. In Knapp RC and
Berkowitz RS, editors: Gynecologic oncology, New York, 1983, Macmillan Publishing Co. [Courtesy Freidoon Azizi, M.D.])

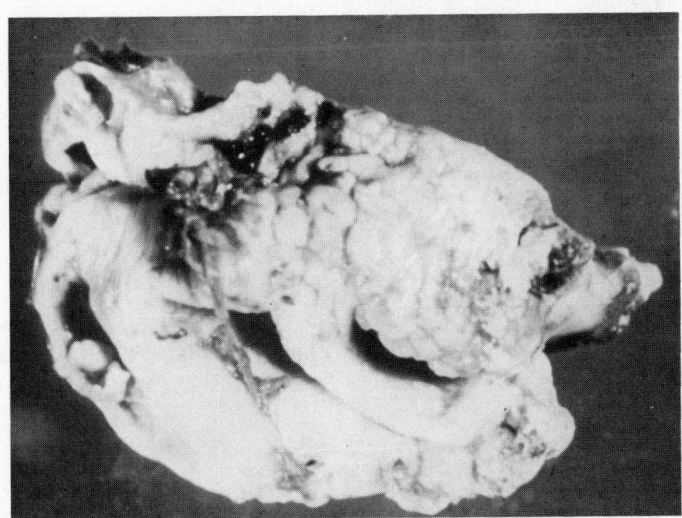

FIGURE 32-3
Cross section through fallopian tube demonstrating primary adenocarcinoma.
(From Podczaski E and Herbst AL: Cancer of the vagina and fallopian tube. In
Knapp RC and Berkowitz RS, editors: Gynecologic oncology, New York, 1983,
Macmillan Publishing Co. [Courtesy Freidoon Azizi, M.D.])

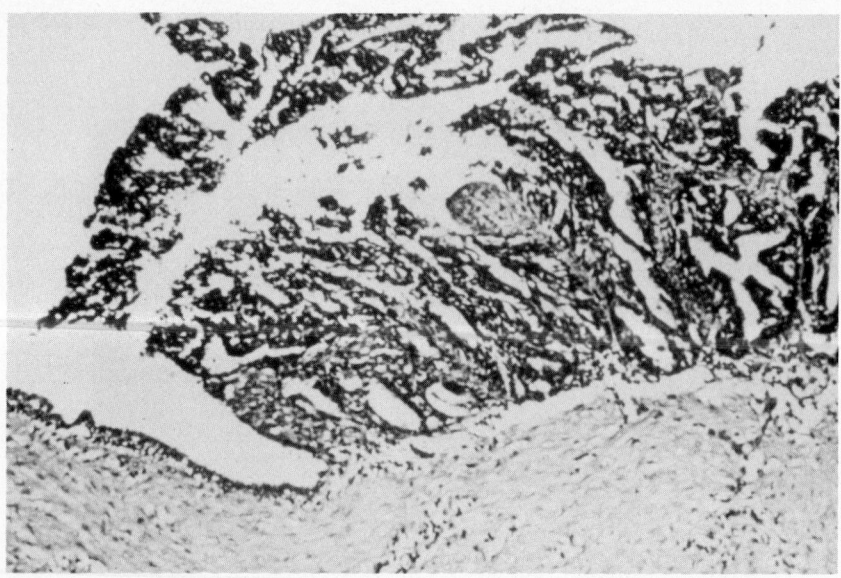

FIGURE 32-4
Microscopic appearance of well-differentiated papillary adenocarcinoma of fallopian tube. (From Podczaski E and Herbst AL: Cancer of the vagina and fallopian tube. In Knapp RC and Berkowitz RS, editors: Gynecologic oncology, New York, 1983, Macmillan Publishing Co. [Courtesy Elizabeth Alenghat, M.D.])

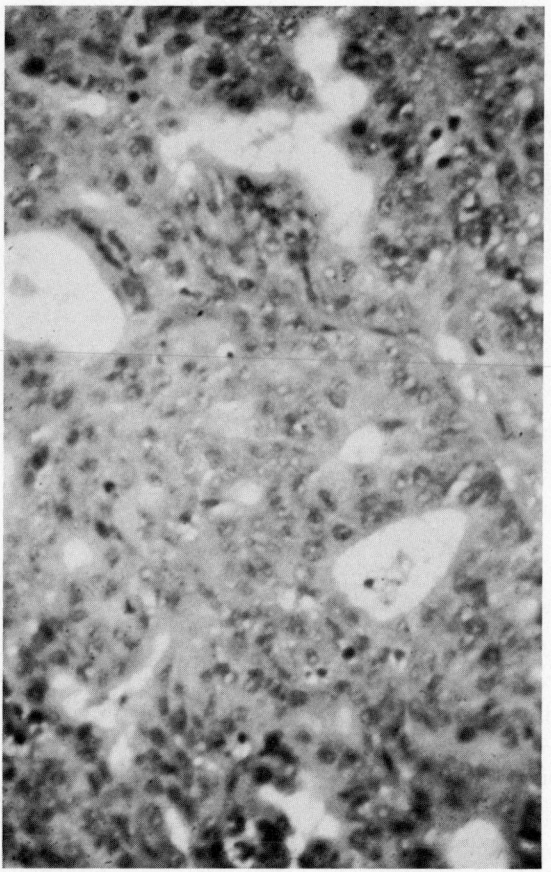

FIGURE 32-5
Poorly differentiated tubal carcinoma with a predominantly solid growth pattern. (From Azizi F and Johnston GA: Female Patient 7:42, 1982.)

a manner similar to epithelial carcinoma of the ovary. Therefore many authors have suggested a staging system for fallopian tube carcinoma based on that used for primary ovarian carcinomas. A suggested system is shown in Table 32-1.

NATURAL HISTORY

The carcinoma is initially confined to the lumen of the tube but can penetrate to the serosa and then spread intraperitoneally to involve the surface of the bowel, the omentum, and the parietal peritoneum, similar to ovarian carcinoma. The peritoneum is the most frequent site of metastatic spread of tubal carcinoma. In addition, lymphatic spread occurs, particularly

TABLE 32-1
Suggested Staging System for Tubal Carcinoma*

Stage	Characteristics
I	Tumor confined to one or both tubes, not involving the serosa
IA	One tube
IB	Both tubes
IC	Positive peritoneal washings or ascitic fluid positive for malignant cells
IIA	Tumor involving one or both tubes and spread to either the ovary or the uterus
IIB	Tumor extends to other pelvic tissues
III	Tumor involves one or both tubes with intraperitoneal spread, including retroperitoneal nodes
IV	Tumor involves one or both tubes with metastases outside the peritoneum or to the parenchyma of the liver (pleural fluid containing malignant cells allows assignment to stage IV)

*Not officially adopted by the International Federation of Gynecology and Obstetrics (FIGO).

to the paraaortic nodes. Tamini and Figge noted metastases to the paraaortic nodes in 5 of 15 patients, and these nodes were the only site of metastatic disease in two patients. Thus the retroperitoneal nodes must also be considered as sites of common spread in the management of these cancers, similar to considerations for ovarian epithelial carcinomas.

Prognosis in tubal carcinoma is related to the extent ("stage") of disease (Table 32-1). In addition, Asmussen et al., noted in a study of 33 cases that vessel invasion was a negative factor. In a study of 115 patients, Peters et al. noted that depth of invasion of the tubal wall was also a factor for those with disease confined to the tube.

MANAGEMENT

As noted previously, the diagnosis of primary tubal carcinoma is most frequently made at the time of surgical exploration. Once the diagnosis is established, frequently by frozen section, a thorough operative staging procedure is carried out, including a total abdominal hysterectomy and bilateral salpingo-oophorectomy. Perito-

neal cytology testing is performed using 200 to 300 ml of normal saline solution mixed with 0.5 ml (5000 IU) of heparin to prevent clotting of any blood present in the fluid. If there is no evidence of intraperitoneal spread, a paraaortic node biopsy should be performed to rule out extrapelvic spread. This is particularly important in cases of large or poorly differentiated tumors, in view of the fact that these carcinomas can metastasize to the paraaortic nodes without evidence of intraperitoneal spread. An omentectomy should also be performed. As emphasized by Podratz et al., meticulous staging is important both for optimal effective treatment and to help decide if additional postoperative therapy is advisable.

Because of the varied experience in the treatment of these malignancies, a number of therapeutic approaches have been suggested. The value of postoperative radiation therapy or chemotherapy is not established at present, although those modalities have been reported to be effective. In the case of a stage I carcinoma, in which the cancer is confined to the tubal lumen and peritoneal cytology is negative, therapy usually consists only of primary operation. If there is positive peritoneal cytology (stage IC), postoperative intraperitoneal ^{32}P is advisable or whole-abdominal radiation is used. If there is spread of tumor outside of the tube to the pelvis, postoperative radiation including the paraaortic nodes has also been considered, depending on the extent of disease discovered at surgery. Brown et al. recommend abdominopelvic radiation postoperatively providing there is no residual disease greater than 2 cm^2 after operation.

For intraperitoneal disease or for recurrent metastatic carcinoma, chemotherapy usually is considered. Traditionally, alkylating agents have been prescribed, since these were active against ovarian epithelial carcinomas and presumed effective in tubal carcinomas. However, combination chemotherapy with cisplatin is now usually prescribed. Deppe et al. reported two patients with widespread disseminated fallopian tube carcinoma who were treated with *cis*-diamminedichloroplatinum (cisplatin, 50 mg/m^2) and doxorubicin (Adriamycin, 37.5 mg/m^2) as well as a progestin, megestrol acetate (Megace, 160 mg daily). One patient also received cyclophosphamide (Cytoxan, 400 mg/m^2). At a second-look procedure 10 to 13 months later, both patients showed no evidence of disease. In a multicenter analysis, Peters et al. noted a significant improvement in patient survival for "stage III" disease with combination chemotherapy, primarily platinum, Cytoxan, and Adriamycin, as recently reported by Morris et al., from M.D. Anderson Cancer Center. Because platinum combinations appear to be superior to single-agent alkylating therapy for ovarian carcinoma (Chapter 29), they should also be utilized in disseminated fallopian tube carcinoma. Rose et al., from Roswell Park Memorial Institute, found second-look laparotomy is an important prognostic factor and recommend its use.

No definitive conclusions can yet be drawn regarding the results of therapy. Sedlis noted a 5-year survival of 38% for all stages of tubal carcinoma. Patients with tubal carcinoma confined to the tube have the best prognosis, expecting a 70% to 80% 5-year survival. High-grade tumors are thought to behave more ag-gressively, but definitive data relating tumor grade to survival are lacking.

OTHER TUMORS

Sarcomas of the fallopian tube are extremely rare. They may be mixed, containing carcinomatous elements (carcinosarcoma), or may have heterologous sarcomatous tissue, in which case the term *mixed mesodermal tumors* is used. These tumors' behavior is similar to that of other sarcomas and mixed müllerian tumors within the uterus (Chapter 28). Treatment consists of surgery, with removal of the uterus and tube, and follow-up chemotherapy, usually with a regimen including doxorubicin (Adriamycin). Choriocarcinoma of the tube has also been reported and is believed to result from trophoblastic disease associated with ectopic pregnancy. The same considerations of therapy apply to these lesions as for trophoblastic disease elsewhere (Chapter 33).

────────── KEY POINTS ──────────

- Ninety percent of tubal cancers are metastatic, mostly from the ovary, uterus, or gastrointestinal tract.

- Only 10% of patients with fallopian tube carcinoma have positive vaginal cytology.

- Primary tubal carcinoma is the rarest gynecologic malignancy (0.3% to 1.1%), with only approximately 1000 cases reported.

- The diagnosis of tubal carcinoma is usually made at operation.

- The average age of patients with tubal carcinoma is 55 years.

- The most common site of spread of tubal carcinoma is to the peritoneum and retroperitoneal lymph nodes.

- Overall 5-year survival for all stages of primary tubal carcinoma is approximately 40%.

- The diagnosis of tubal carcinoma should be considered for anyone with vaginal cytology positive for adenocarcinoma in whom the diagnosis of endometrial carcinoma has been excluded. It should also be considered for anyone with postmenopausal uterine bleeding in whom a D&C fails to reveal the cause.

- The triad of abnormal bleeding, adnexal mass, and watery discharge in a postmenopausal woman is suggestive of tubal carcinoma.

- Prognosis in tubal carcinoma is related to extent ("stage") of disease, vascular invasion histologically, and, for tumors confined to the tube, depth of invasion.

- Combination chemotherapy using cisplatin improves survival in disseminated or recurrent fallopian tube carcinoma.

BIBLIOGRAPHY

Asmussen M, Kaern J, Kjoerstad K, et al: Primary adenocarcinoma localized to the fallopian tubes: report on 33 cases, Gynecol Oncol 30:183, 1988.

Benedet JL, White GW, Fairey RN, and Boyes DA: Adenocarcinoma of the fallopian tube, Obstet Gynecol 50:654, 1977.

Brown MD, Kohorn EI, Kapp DS, et al: Fallopian tube carcinoma, Int J Radiat Oncol Biol Phys 11:583, 1985.

Deppe G, Bruckner HW, and Cohen CJ: Combination chemotherapy for advanced carcinoma of the fallopian tube, Obstet Gynecol 56:530, 1980.

Erez S, Kaplan AL, and Wall JA: Clinical staging of carcinoma of the uterine tube, Obstet Gynecol 30:547, 1967.

Hershey DW, Fennell RH, and Major FJ: Primary carcinoma of the fallopian tube, Obstet Gynecol 57:367, 1981.

Hirai Y, Kaku S, Teshima H, et al: Clinical study of primary carcinoma of the fallopian tube: experience with 15 cases, Gynecol Oncol 34:20, 1989.

Hu CY, Taymor ML, and Hertig AT: Primary carcinoma of the fallopian tube, Am J Obstet Gynecol 59:58, 1950.

Kol S, Gal D, Friedman M, and Paldi E: Case report: preoperative diagnosis of fallopian tube carcinoma by transvaginal sonography and CA-125, Gynecol Oncol 37:129, 1990.

Morris M, Gershenson DM, Burke TW, et al: Treatment of fallopian tube carcinoma with cisplatin, doxorubicin, and cyclophosphamide, Obstet Gynecol 76:1020, 1990.

Peters WA, Andersen WA, Hopkins MP, et al: Prognostic features of carcinoma of the fallopian tube, Obstet Gynecol 71:757, 1988.

Phelps HM and Chapman KE: Role of radiation therapy in treatment of primary carcinoma of the uterine tube, Obstet Gynecol 43:669, 1974.

Podczaski E and Herbst AL: Cancer of the vagina and fallopian tube. In Knapp RC and Berkowitz RS, editors: Gynecologic oncology, ed 2, New York, 1990, Macmillan Publishing Co.

Podratz KC, Podczaski ES, Gaffey TA, et al: Primary carcinoma of the fallopian tube, Am J Obstet Gynecol 154:1319, 1986.

Rose PG, Piver MS, and Tsukada Y: Fallopian tube cancer: the Roswell Park experience, Cancer 66:2661, 1990.

Schiller HM and Silverberg SG: Staging and prognosis in primary carcinoma of the fallopian tube, Cancer 28:389, 1971.

Sedlis A: Primary carcinoma of the fallopian tube, Obstet Gynecol Surv 16:209, 1961.

Sedlis A: Carcinoma of the fallopian tube, Surg Clin North Am 58:121, 1978.

Tamini HK and Figge DC: Adenocarcinoma of the uterine tube: potential for lymph node metastases, Am J Obstet Gynecol 141:132, 1981.

Wu JP, Tanner WS, and Fardal PM: Malignant mixed müllerian tumor of the uterine tube, Obstet Gynecol 41:707, 1981.

Yoonessi M: Carcinoma of the fallopian tube, Obstet Gynecol Surv 34:257, 1979.

Gestational Trophoblastic Disease

KEY TERMS AND DEFINITIONS

Androgenesis. Impregnation of an inactive egg by a paternal haploid sperm that duplicates its chromosomes to provide a diploid complement. This results in a complete mole.

Choriocarcinoma. A morphologic term applied to a highly malignant type of trophoblastic neoplasia in which both the cytotrophoblast and syncytiotrophoblast grow in a malignant fashion.

Complete Mole. A molar pregnancy with swelling of all placental villi. Fetal tissues are absent.

Gestational Trophoblastic Disease (GTD). The spectrum of diseases resulting from the abnormal proliferation of trophoblast associated with pregnancy.

Gestational Trophoblastic Tumor (GTT). A term applied to gestational diseases that have neoplastic potential, including invasive mole, choriocarcinoma, and placental-site trophoblastic tumor. It can be either nonmetastatic or metastatic.

Hydatidiform Mole. A placental abnormality involving swollen placental villi and trophoblastic hyperplasia with loss of fetal blood vessels. There are two types: partial and complete.

Invasive Mole. A variant of hydatidiform mole in which the hydropic villi invade into the myometrium or blood vessels. It may spread to extrauterine sites.

Partial Mole. A molar pregnancy with some normal and some swollen villi plus fetal, cord, and/or amniotic membrane elements.

Placental-Site Trophoblastic Tumor. A rare type of GTT arising in the uterus that secretes human placental lactogen (HPL) and human chorionic gonadotrophin (HCG) and is often resistant to chemotherapy.

Prognostic Scoring System. An international system for calculating the prognosis of GTT and its response to chemotherapy. Results are usually divided into low, middle, and high risk.

Stages of GTT:
I: Confined to corpus uteri
II: Metastases to the pelvis and vagina
III: Metastases to the lungs
IV: Distant metastases (liver, brain, etc.)

Theca Lutein Cysts. Enlargements of the ovary occurring with hydatidiform moles and consisting of theca lutein cells. Usually they regress after treatment of the mole.

Gestational trophoblastic disease (GTD) refers to the spectrum of proliferative abnormalities of the trophoblast associated with pregnancy. These neoplasias have been known for hundreds of years, and they are unique in that they secrete human chorionic gonadotrophin (HCG). The availability of extremely sensitive and specific radioimmunoassays (RIA) or enzymatic immunoassays (EIA) to measure HCG al-lows prediction of the status of the disease, permitting refinement of its classification and thus improving understanding of its pathophysiology and monitoring treatment. The initial use of methotrexate in 1956 by Li, Hertz, and Spencer to successfully treat malignant trophoblastic disease completely altered the prognosis of patients with these tumors and represented a milestone in the cure of human tumors by chemotherapeutic agents.

This chapter presents the current classification of GTDs and the factors that appear to be associated with their development. The methods of diagnosis, appropriate therapy, and necessary follow-up of these patients are reviewed.

CHARACTERISTICS

Trophoblastic tissue normally shares certain characteristics with malignancies, such as the ability to divide rapidly, to invade locally, and occasionally to metastasize to distant sites such as the lung, yet these activities usually cease at the end of pregnancy, and the trophoblast disappears. However, in GTD, abnormal growth and development continue beyond the end of pregnancy.

MORPHOLOGY

Hydatidiform Mole

A hydatidiform mole has three morphologic characteristics: (1) a mass of vesicles (distended villi) that appear as large, grapelike dilations (Figure 33-1); (2) a loss of fetal blood vessels, which are either diminished or absent from the villi; and (3) hyperplasia of the syncytiotrophoblast and cytotrophoblast.

The terms *complete mole* and *partial mole* have been used to describe the variations of molar pregnancies. Vassilakos et al. noted that these two conditions appear to have different morphologic presentations and are developmentally distinct. With a complete mole, all placental villi are swollen and the fetus, cord, and amniotic membrane are absent. In partial molar pregnancy, only some chorionic villi are swollen, whereas others appear normal and fetal tissues are present, such as amniotic membrane, cord, or even occasionally a full-term fetus, although the fetus is usually chromosomally abnormal (see following discussion). With a partial mole the trophoblastic hyperplasia is limited to the syncytiotrophoblast.

The genetics of molar pregnancy has been extensively studied. Chromosomal banding techniques have provided useful information regarding the development of these tumors. In normal pregnancy, half the chromosomes of the conceptus are paternal and the other half maternal, resulting in a diploid content. In complete mole, only paternal chromosomes are believed to be present; there are 46 chromosomes and nearly always 46, XX, although a few moles with 46, XY karyotype have been reported. The development of complete mole appears to result from the fertilization of an "empty egg," one with an absent or inactive nucleus. The haploid paternal set of chromosomes from the sperm impregnate the inactive egg. These paternal chromosomes then duplicate to give the diploid number, a process known as *androgenesis*, the development of an "embryo" due only to chromosomes from an X-bearing sperm (Figure 33-2). In the rare case of complete mole with an XY chromosomal content, the "empty egg" is fertilized by two haploid sperm, one X bearing and one Y bearing.

Incomplete, or partial, moles are usually triploid and have 69 chromosomes of both maternal and paternal origin. The most common mechanism for the origin of partial mole (Figure 33-3) is a haploid egg being fertilized by two sperm, resulting in three sets of chromosomes. Alternatively, triploidy could result when an abnormal diploid sperm fertilizes the haploid egg. It is also possible for an abnormal diploid egg to be fertilized by a haploid sperm, but this latter mechanism usually results in an abnormal conceptus with congenital abnormalities rather than a partial mole. Partial mole is often difficult to diagnose and may be present with a fetus as a missed abortion in the second trimester. Although such fetuses are usually abnormal, Watson et al. noted that some partial moles have occurred with phenotypically normal fetuses. In such cases the uterus is small for dates. As recently noted by Lage et al., a few partial moles are diploid, and these very rare cases may be less sensitive to chemotherapy than triploid moles when subsequent GTT develops (see below).

Partial moles are rarely associated with the subsequent development of GTT, and Berkowitz et al. observed that 9.9% of their 81 patients with partial mole subsequently developed nonmetastatic GTT. Bagshawe et al. recently noted that neoplasia requiring chemotherapy occurs in approximately 1 in 200 cases of partial mole, compared with 1 in 12 after a complete mole. However, Rice et al. noted 16 of 240 partial moles (6.6%) had malignant *sequelae*, all of which responded to chemotherapy. Despite rare subsequent malignancy, patients with partial moles need the same follow-up as those with complete mole.

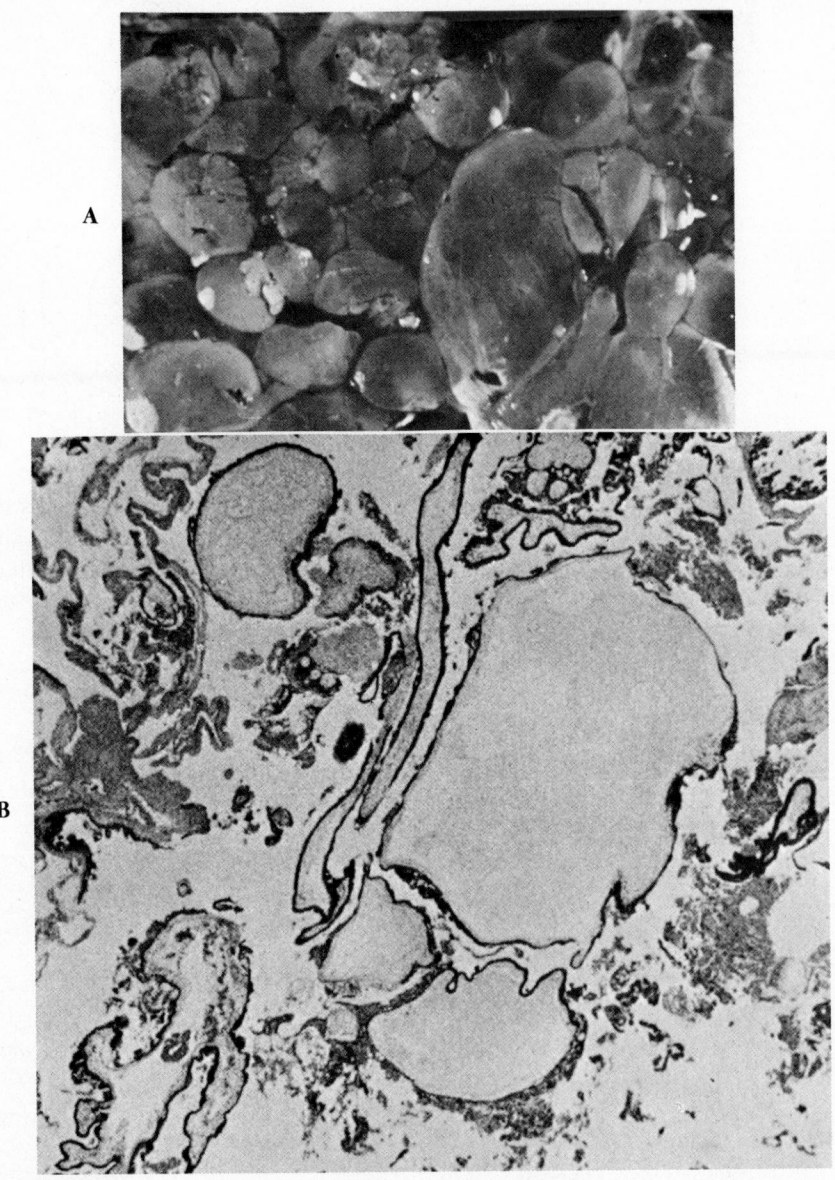

FIGURE 33-1
A, Hydatidiform mole. A few vesicles approach 1 cm in diameter. The background is formed by smaller vesicles. **B,** Hydatidiform mole aborted by suction curettage. A large intact vesicle is near the center. Many vesicles, however, have been ruptured and have collapsed. (From Bigelow B: Gestational trophoblast disease. In Blaustein A, editor: Pathology of the female genital tract, ed 2, New York, 1982, Springer-Verlag New York, Inc.)

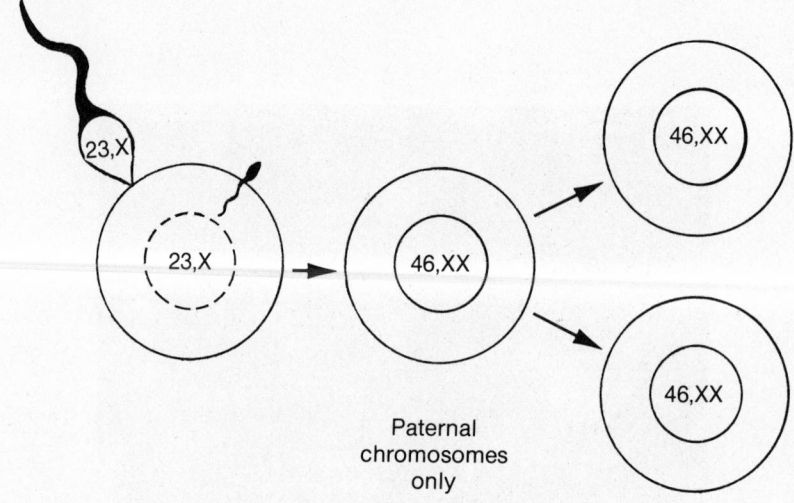

FIGURE 33-2
Paternal chromosomal origin of a complete classic mode (46,XX). Left to right, entry of normal sperm with haploid set of 23,X into egg whose 23,X haploid set is lost; egg is "taken over" by paternal chromosomes, which duplicate (without cell's division) to reach requisite complement of 46. Observe that virtually the same result can be obtained through a fertilization by two sperm gaining entry into an "empty egg" (dispermy). (From Szulman AE and Surti U: Clin Obstet Gynecol 27:172, 1984.)

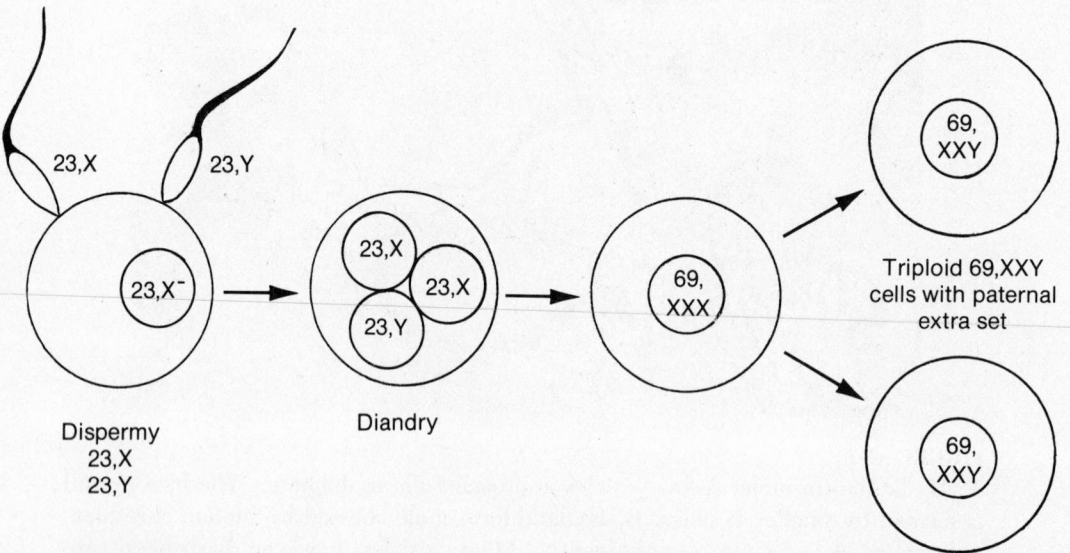

FIGURE 33-3
Triploid chromosomal origin of partial mole (69,XXY—dispermy). Fertilization of an egg equipped with a normal 23,X complement by two independently produced sperm (dispermy) to give total of 69 chromosomes. Observe that triploidy can also result through fertilization by sperm carrying father's total complement of 46,XY. (From Szulman AE and Surti U: Clin Obstet Gynecol 27:172, 1984.)

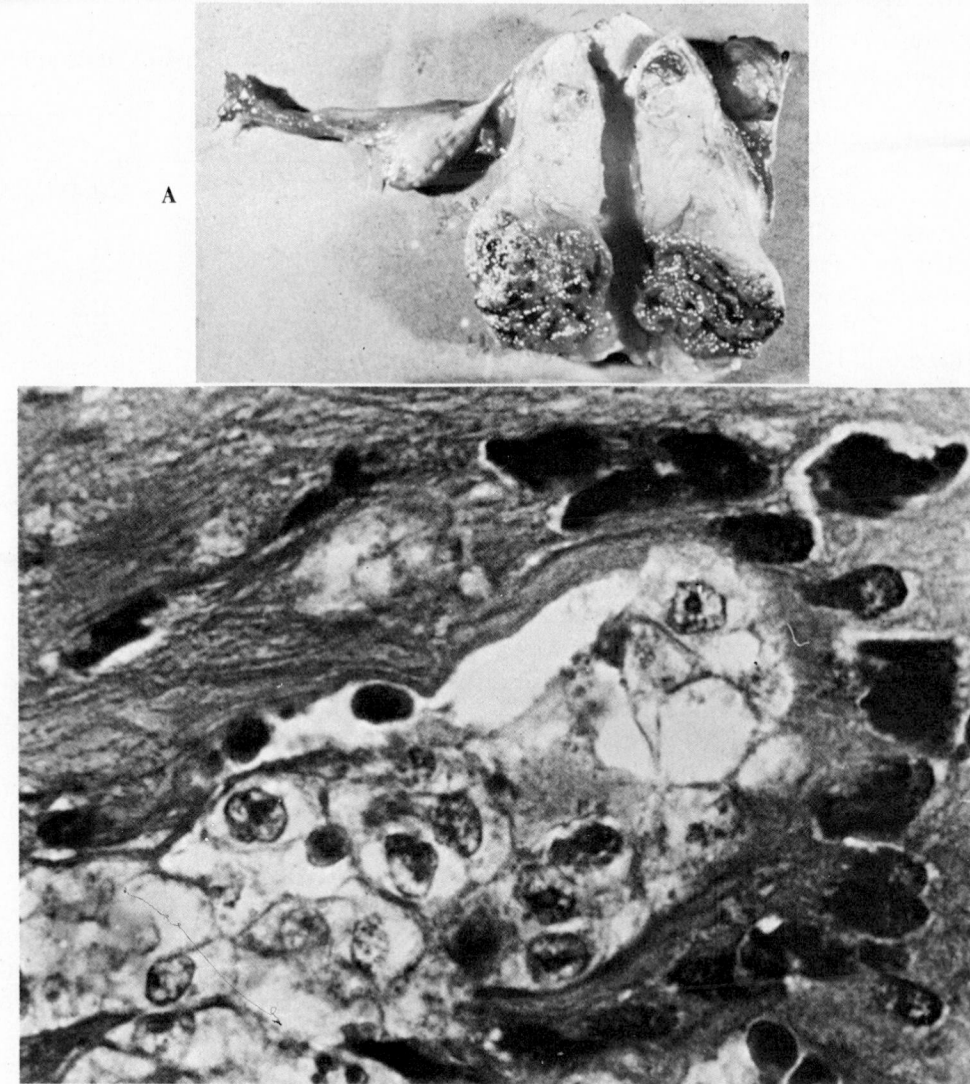

FIGURE 33-4
A, Choriocarcinoma. Hermorrhagic tumor occupies lower uterine segment and cervix. Smaller foci of choriocarcinoma can be seen in left and right fundal walls. **B,** Choriocarcinoma, high-power view. Central pale cytotrophoblast is surrounded by syncytiotrophoblasts. Nuclei are pleomorphic. (From Bigelow B: Gestational trophoblast disease. In Blaustein A, editors: Pathology of the female genital tract, ed 2, New York, 1982, Springer-Verlag New York, Inc.)

Choriocarcinoma

Choriocarcinomas are malignancies that occur after or in association with pregnancy, although the same histologic tumor can develop without pregnancy as a primary neoplasm in the ovaries or in the testes in men. The prognosis for primary gonadal choriocarcinomas is worse than for those associated with gestation.

The diagnosis is made histologically, and the term is applied to the finding of malignant cytotrophoblast and syncytiotrophoblast. Chorionic villi are absent. These tumors (Figure 33-4) tend to be hemorrhagic and necrotic.

Most choriocarcinomas develop after molar pregnancies but can occur in association with other pregnancies. Trophoblastic tissue normally regresses within 2 to 3 weeks after delivery, including cells that have spread to the lung. The normal processes leading to this regression are unknown, but the finding of trophoblastic cells in the uterus more than 3 weeks after delivery should lead one to consider the possibility of choriocarcinoma.

Placental-Site Trophoblastic Tumor

The term *placental-site trophoblastic tumor* (trophoblastic pseudotumor) was introduced by Young and Scully to describe a rare variety of tumor that consists of excessive groups of mononucleate and multinucleate trophoblastic cells at the implantation site accompanied by an inflammatory cell reaction. Histocytochemical studies have shown that the cells of these tumors tend to stain more for human placental lactogen (HPL) than for HCG, and both HCG and HPL should be monitored. The tumor can lead to hemorrhage and uterine perforation, requiring hysterectomy. As noted by Finkler et al., if this neoplasm is diagnosed by endometrial curettage, the patient should have a hysterectomy. Chemotherapy is usually administered for metastatic disease but is less effective with these tumors than with other gestational trophoblastic tumors, which is another reason for prompt operative treatment. The EMA/CO regimen (see below) has been reported by Dessau et al. to produce long-term survival.

EPIDEMIOLOGY AND INCIDENCE

Extensive investigation has been performed to ascertain the factors that enhance the occurrence of trophoblastic disease. The major areas that have been evaluated are geographic distribution and socioeconomic factors, maternal age, race, history of fetal wastage or prior hydatidiform mole, and ABO blood groupings.

Hydatidiform Mole

There is wide variation in the reported incidence of hydatidiform mole, with the most accurate statistics derived from population-based studies rather than from those based on hospital referral center data. The rates are usually expressed in terms of molar gestations per numbers of pregnancies. In the United States the rate is estimated to be approximately 0.75 per 1000. The rates from Southeast Asia are 1.5 to 2.5 times higher with much larger variations, and rates up to 8 per 1000 have been reported. The high rates reported in some studies are derived from hospital-based rather than population-based statistics. As already noted, hydatidiform mole develops because of abnormal fertilization. A few reports note molar pregnancies occurring among female siblings. An additional risk factor is a history of prior hydatidiform mole, which increases the risk of

TABLE 33-1
Relationship of Age to Risk of Hydatidiform Mole

Age	Risk
Less than 20	1.53
20-24	1.17
25-29	1
30-34	1.04
35-39	1.33
40-44	2.66
45-49	24.89
Over 50	80.76

Adapted from Buckley JD: Clin Obstet Gynecol 27:153, 1984.

subsequent mole by 20 to 40 times. Recurrent spontaneous abortion is also a risk factor, as shown by the studies of Acaia et al., and there is a suggestion that they are associated with twins.

The increased frequency among those with lower socioeconomic status, as well as in underdeveloped areas, particularly in Southeast Asia, has led to the suggestion that poor nutrition is a factor in the development of this disease. However, evidence is conflicting, and as noted by Grimes, a dietary etiology for hydatidiform mole is not supported by current data.

The risk appears to vary with race and ethnic origin. In Southeast Asia the rates are double for Eurasians as compared to those of Chinese, Malaysian, or Indian origin. A decreased rate has also been reported among blacks in the United States in comparison to whites, and rates are higher among those of Latin American origin. Mexicans and Filipinos appear to have elevated rates in comparison to Japanese and Chinese.

Maternal age is an extremely important risk factor. The lowest rates are among those in their 20s and 30s, with a great increase in those over 40, after which the risk progressively increases with age. There is also an increase in risk among those under the age of 20 years, but the magnitude is not nearly so great as it is among older women. A summary of age risks for hydatidiform mole is shown in Table 33-1.

Choriocarcinoma

Choriocarcinoma primarily occurs in about 3% to 5% of those who have had a prior complete hydatidiform mole, and the risk factors for molar pregnancy also apply to choriocarcinoma. In Western countries choriocarcinomas are reported at rates between 0.014 and 0.1 per 1000 pregnancies. The rate in the United States is about 1 per 20,000 pregnancies. Although most choriocarcinomas occur after complete molar pregnancies, choriocarcinomas have developed after normal pregnancy (1 per 40,000 term pregnancies). The disease also follows incomplete abortion and ectopic pregnancy. The risk factors for complete mole, particularly maternal age and pregnancy loss, are indirectly associated with choriocarcinoma. An additional factor for choriocarcinoma has been found among ABO blood groups. Some studies, including those of Bagshawe, have shown that women with type A blood married to men with type O, and vice versa, are at higher risk for choriocarcinoma in comparison to matings of other blood groups. No differential in the risk for hydatidiform mole for ABO blood groups has been demonstrated.

CLINICAL CLASSIFICATION OF GTD

The histologic terminology used to describe GTD may be confusing, since the terms were based on the morphologic appearance of the abnormal tissue. With the use of sensitive and specific radioimmunoassays for HCG and modern diagnostic techniques, clinical terminology more useful in describing GTD has been found, as shown in the box below. This terminology allows the physician to describe all forms of GTD and also offers an effective way of analyzing the treatment and the biologic behavior of these abnormal trophoblastic conditions.

CLASSIFICATION OF GESTATIONAL TROPHOBLASTIC DISEASE (GTD)

Hydatidiform mole
  1. Complete
  2. Incomplete

Gestational trophoblastic tumor (GTT)
  1. Nonmetastatic
  2. Metastatic
    a. Low risk
    b. High risk

CLINICAL ASPECTS OF GTD

Hydatidiform Mole

Symptoms and Signs

The most common presenting symptom is abnormal bleeding in a patient who has experienced delayed menses and seems to be pregnant. Abnormal bleeding is present in almost all patients, and associated symptoms often mimic an incomplete or threatened abortion. Occasionally the patient notices a swollen villus that has been passed from the uterus. The uterus is frequently large for dates; Curry et al. noted this change in about half of their patients with molar pregnancy. However, as many as one fourth of the patients may have a uterus small for dates. Sequelae appear to be more common among those with an enlarged uterus. In about 20% of the patients, an additional physical finding is enlargement of the ovaries (theca lutein cysts), which is associated with a higher frequency of future sequelae (approximately 50%) as compared to less than 15% for those without ovarian enlargement. The development of these theca lutein cysts is believed to be secondary to the luteinizing hormone–like effect of excessive HCG stimulation on the ovary. However, in a study of 102 patients with theca lutein cysts, Montz et al. noted that cyst growth did not correlate with changes in HCG concentrations and that some persisted after HCG disappeared from the circulation. Three of the cysts ruptured; the remaining spontaneously regressed.

Nausea and vomiting are common complaints, as is true in normal pregnancy, and hyperemesis gravidarum has been reported. Additionally, preeclamptic toxemia may occur in as many as one fourth of the patients, although its frequency has been reported to be less in many series.

Insofar as molar pregnancies are frequently diagnosed in the latter part of the first trimester of pregnancy, GTD should be considered in any patient with signs of toxemia during this time or during the early part of the second trimester. In addition, laboratory manifestations of hyperthyroidism have been reported, but clinical manifestations of hyperthyroidism are rare. The changes are in part due to the production of thyrotrophin-like hormone by the abnormal trophoblastic tissue, although a weak thyroid-stimulating hormone action for HCG has also been hypothesized. These changes are reversible and usually abate after treatment of trophoblastic disease. The signs and symptoms

SYMPTOMS AND SIGNS OF HYDATIDIFORM MOLE

Abnormal bleeding in early pregnancy
Lower abdominal pain
Toxemia before 24 weeks of gestation
Hyperemesis gravidarum
Hyperthyroidism (rare)
Uterus large for dates (50%)
Enlargement of ovaries (20%)
Absent fetal heart tones and fetal parts
Expulsion of swollen villi

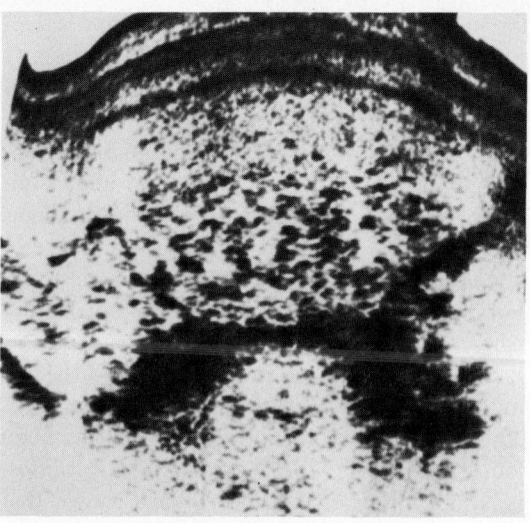

FIGURE 33-5
Ultrasound of uterus demonstrating "snowstorm" appearance of hydatidiform mole.

of hydatidiform moles are summarized in the box above.

Clinically the behaviors of partial and complete moles differ. Complete mole is the more common and also has a more serious prognosis, with increased risk for the subsequent development of a GTT. Partial moles usually present as an incomplete or missed abortion. Szulman and Surti analyzed the characteristics of 200 moles, both complete and partial; their results are summarized in Table 33-2. HCG levels tend to be lower in partial moles.

Diagnosis

In a patient suspected of having a molar pregnancy, the most valuable diagnostic aid is ultrasound (Figure 33-5). The examination usually reveals absence of a fetus (in the case of a complete mole) and characteristic swollen villi that produce a snowstorm-like pattern. The examination may also demonstrate ovarian enlargement secondary to the development of a theca lutein cyst. If a fetal sac is detected, the possibility of a partial mole still exists. However, beyond the seventh week a fetal heart should be detected by ultrasound; its absence may suggest a missed abortion. If hydropic villi are present, it is possible that a blood clot in the uterus has been mistaken for a fetal sac. If there is doubt concerning the presence of fetal tissue and the existence of a partial mole, follow-up sonographic examinations are indicated.

The measurement of HCG is an integral part of the diagnosis and evaluation of the patient suspected of having GTD. Immunoassays (RIA or EIA) allow the measurement of extremely small amounts of HCG in blood and urine, as little as 2 to 5 mIU/ml. The levels in normal pregnancy reach a peak at about 10 to 14 weeks and rarely exceed levels of 100,000 mIU/ml. They can be higher in twin gestation, are frequently elevated in GTD, and may appear elevated in patients whose dates are not accurate. With molar pregnancy it is possible that the level of HCG may not be elevated, so that a single determination is not diagnostic and will not necessarily differentiate normal pregnancy, multiple pregnancy, and GTD. However, a level in excess of 100,000 mIU/ml suggests GTD. The HCG levels tend to be elevated above normal pregnancy values in complete mole, whereas partial mole tends to produce lower levels.

Management

Once the diagnosis of molar pregnancy is made, the uterus should be evacuated. Medical problems, such as anemia due to blood loss, pregnancy-induced hypertension, pulmonary insufficiency, and hyperthyroidism, should be evaluated and, when necessary, corrected. Hyperemesis gravidarum may develop, necessitating antiemetic and intravenous therapy. Occasionally, disseminated intravascular coagulation (DIC) occurs, leading to a consumptive coagulopathy that requries correction, as well as prompt uterine evacuation. Preevacuation

TABLE 33-2
Complete Versus Partial Hydatidiform Moles

	Complete Mole		Partial Mole	
Clinical presentation and average gestational age	Molar pregnancy 16 weeks	48%	Molar pregnancy 19.7 weeks	8%
	Spontaneous abortion		Spontaneous abortion	
	13.7 weeks	40%	14.4 weeks	49%
	Missed abortion 19.5 weeks	6%	Missed abortion 24.8 weeks	43%
Preeclampsia		6%		8%
Uterus large for dates		33%		11%

Adapted from Szulman AE and Surti U: Clin Obstet Gynecol 27:172, 1984.

chest x-ray examination is performed to rule out the spread of GTD to the lungs and also for comparison in future follow-up. Unless a viable fetus is found, the pregnancy should be promptly terminated. If hyperthyroidism is present, it should be treated before operative removal of the molar tissue. Theca-lutein cysts usually regress spontaneously in a few months and do not require therapy unless an acute episode (e.g., rupture) occurs.

Acute pulmonary insufficiency may also occur. Acute dyspnea and cyanosis may develop, usually within 4 hours of evacuation. As noted by Cotton et al., this risk is greatest in patients whose uterus is more than 16 weeks' gestation size. Trophoblastic embolization and fluid overload with blood volume expansion appear to contribute to the picture of cardiac decompensation and pulmonary edema. If there are signs of pulmonary distress, arterial PO_2 should be monitored. In severely compromised patients ventilatory assistance, monitoring of pulmonary arterial pressure, and management in an intensive care unit may be needed. As noted by Kelly et al., respiratory failure can occur, and these authors recommend extracorporeal perfusion be considered for those patients who develop right to left shunting.

Goldstein et al. have advocated the use of prophylactic cytotoxic chemotherapy to prevent the neoplastic sequelae of molar pregnancy. However, this practice has not gained widespread acceptance because giving chemotherapy at the time of evacuation of the mole exposes the patient to toxic drugs, even though most patients with hydatidiform mole do not require further treatment. Approximately 80% of the patients require only uterine evacuation as definitive therapy. If sequelae do develop,

which is a risk for the remaining 20%, chemotherapy can then be used.

The most effective and widely used method of emptying the uterus of a molar pregnancy is suction curettage. In many instances the molar pregnancy will have already begun to abort, and suction can complete the process. Intravenous oxytocic agents are used during the evacuation and immediately postoperatively to aid in uterine contraction and to help reduce blood loss. However, it is not advisable to use oxytocic drugs before evacuation of the molar pregnancy because of the risk of disseminating abnormal trophoblastic cells. If possible, a large suction curette (12 mm) should be used to aid in evacuation. The operator should begin the evacuation in the lower part of the uterus near the cervix and gradually extend it toward the fundus.

Previously for uterine enlargement beyond the size of a 16-week pregnancy, hysterotomy was used to evacuate a hydatidiform mole. However, suction evacuation has proven to be safe and effective even with a larger uterus. After evacuation by suction curettage is complete, a sharp curettage should be gently performed to ensure completion of the procedure.

If the patient has completed childbearing, hysterectomy may be considered as primary therapy for molar pregnancy. This is particularly desirable treatment in patients at greater risk for GTT following the molar pregnancy, especially older patients with ovarian lutein cysts or an enlarged uterus. Since the ovarian lutein cysts regress after termination, it is not necessary to remove them, although older patients or those with risk factors for ovarian carcinoma may wish to consider elective removal. In an analysis of 358 patients with hydatidiform mole, Schlaerth et al. primarily used suction evacuation with an 11 mm curette followed by gentle curettage in 88% of their patients. Major complications included infection, toxemia, anemia, and postevacuation respiratory insufficiency.

Follow-up

After evacuation of the uterus of a molar pregnancy (or in the rare case of therapy by hysterectomy), the patient should be carefully monitored for the potential development of malignant sequelae, specifically gestational trophoblastic tumor (GTT). The key to monitoring is the serial determination of β-HCG in the patient's serum. While pregnancy tests can measure HCG, their lack of sensitivity and specificity requires an assay for β-HCG. In most laboratories this assay has a sensitivity of 2 to 5 mIU/ml. Abnormal regression of the HCG levels following therapy for hydatidiform mole is an early indication in the 20% of patients who will develop GTT.

Evaluation of the patient should include the data summarized in the box below, which also allow identification of those at higher risk for GTT. The risk of GTT is increased in those with a large uterus, high HCG level, lutein cysts, and a history of molar pregnancy and toxemia, as well as in older exposed patients, particularly individuals over 40. The risk of sequelae is less in the absence of these factors and also if fetal tissue is present (partial mole).

BASELINE DATA FOR PATIENT WITH MOLAR PREGNANCY

HCG serum level (preevacuation)
Chest x-ray
Age
Uterine size
Presence or absence of ovarian theca-lutein
 cysts
Presence or absence of fetal tissue
History of prior molar pregnancy
Assessment for medical complications
 Anemia
 Toxemia
 Hyperemesis
 Hyperthyroidism
 Pulmonary compromise

To follow the course of the disease after evacuation of a molar pregnancy, the physician must carefully monitor the HCG levels. A normal regression curve is shown in Figure 33-6. There is a gradual decline after evacuation of hydatidiform mole, reaching a normal range usually by the fourteenth week after evacuation. However, in some instances the level returns to normal after a longer interval. Adequate monitoring consists of weekly HCGs until the level reaches normal values. The patient must not become pregnant, and usually oral contraceptives are prescribed. There has been some suggestion in the literature that birth control pills might increase the risk of GTT, but data from Morrow et al. suggest that birth control pills are safe and effective in this situation. A recent study by Deicas et al. indicates that oral contraceptives actually offer a therapeutic advantage with fewer patients developing GTT who used birth control pills.

After the initial pelvic examination a repeat evaluation is performed, usually every 2 weeks until the uterus and ovaries have returned to normal size. Theca-lutein cysts characteristically resolve within 2 months, but Montz et al. showed they may last as long as 4 months. However, patients with the high-risk factors listed earlier are approximately 10 times more likely to develop the sequelae of neoplasia in comparison to those without these factors. Once the HCG reaches undetectable levels, it is preferable to monitor them every 3 months for 6 to 12 months, after which the patient may be advised that she can safely attempt another pregnancy.

There may be an abnormal regression curve after evacuation (Figure 33-7), and in such instances the patient requires therapy for GTT. A rise in HCG (a doubling over a 2-week period) or a plateau in HCG (failure to decrease over a 3-week interval) indicates the presence of postmolar trophoblastic tumor. The box on p. 1054 outlines the management of hydatidiform mole, including the indications for chemotherapy.

Gestational Trophoblastic Neoplasia

Incidence and Diagnosis

As has been noted, malignancy (gestational trophoblastic tumor, GTT) develops after approximately 20% of complete hydatidiform moles. Conversely, about half the cases of GTT arise after molar pregnancy, while one fourth occur after normal pregnancy and one fourth

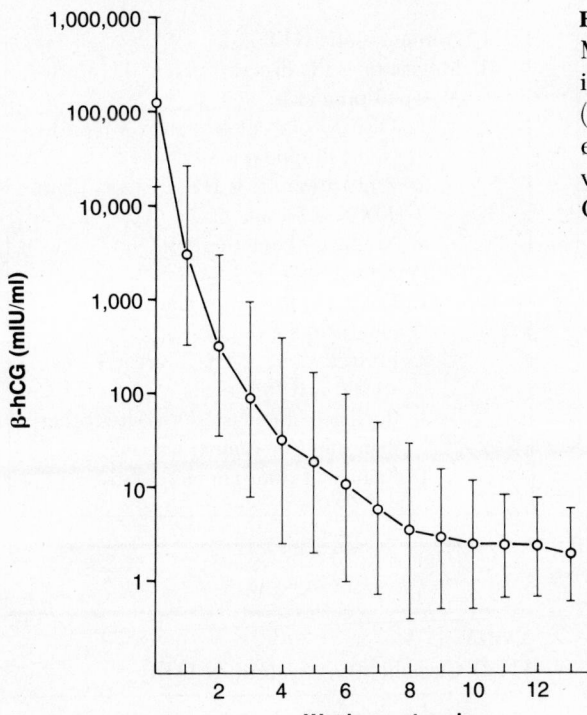

FIGURE 33-6
Mean value and 95% confidence limits describing normal postmolar β-HCG regression curve. (From Schlaerth JB, Morrow CP, Kletzky OA, et al: Obstet Gynecol 58:478, 1981. Reprinted with permission from The American College of Obstetricians and Gynecologists.)

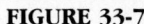

FIGURE 33-7
Mean value and 95% confidence limits for serum β-HCG titers obtained weekly after molar pregnancy in 38 patients whose regression curve deviated early in follow-up from normal regression curve, represented by stippled area. (From Schlaerth JB, Morrow CP, Kletzky OA, et al: Obstet Gynecol 58:478, 1981. Reprinted with permission from The American College of Obstetricians and Gynecologists.)

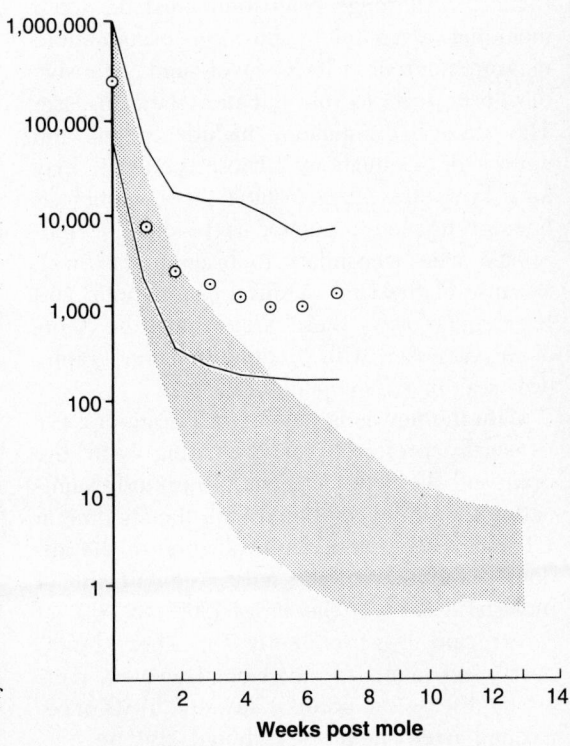

MANAGEMENT OF HYDATIDIFORM MOLE

HCG weekly serum determination until normal for two values, then monthly for 1 year

Chest x-ray examination initially and repeat if abnormal or if HCG plateaus or rises

Contraception for 1 year

Pelvic examination every 2 weeks until normal, then every 3 months

Initiate chemotherapy if:
HCG level increases or plateaus
Metastatic disease is present
Choriocarcinoma is diagnosed on tissue
HCG level still elevated 6 months after molar evacuation
HCG levels greater than 20,000 mIU/ml more than 4 weeks after evacuation
Elevated HCG is detected after normal levels are reached

PROGNOSTIC CLASSIFICATION OF GTT

I. Nonmetastatic GTT
II. Metastatic GTT: disease outside the uterus
  A. Good prognosis
    1. Disease present less than 4 months (short duration)
    2. Pretreatment β-HCG less than 40,000 mIU/ml
    3. No prior chemotherapy
  B. Poor prognosis
    1. Disease present more than 4 months (long duration), or
    2. Pretreatment β-HCG greater than 40,000 mIU/ml, or
    3. Presence of metastases to sites other than lungs or vagina, or
    4. Failure of prior chemotherapy

after abortion or ectopic pregnancy. Therefore patients who continue to have abnormal bleeding after any pregnancy should have a β-HCG assay performed. Once GTT is diagnosed, chemotherapy is initiated unless complications, such as uterine hemorrhage or perforation, arise that require hysterectomy.

First, a thorough evaluation must be done, including a complete physical examination, measurement of β-HCG level, and extensive diagnostic tests to rule out metastatic disease. The physical examination includes pelvic and neurologic evaluations. These patients may have symptoms of metastatic disease, such as hemoptysis (due to pulmonary lesions), or neurologic signs (secondary to brain metastases). Because of the fatal ramifications of brain and liver metastases, these areas must be thoroughly assessed with a computed tomography (CT) scan or radionuclide brain scan.

With the new generation of CT scanners, CT is usually preferred for evaluating both the brain and the liver. A pelvic ultrasound examination should be combined with the abdominal CT scan to complete the evaluation of the abdomen and pelvis. The most frequent site of metastatic GTT is the lungs (80% to 90% of cases), and less frequently the liver, brain, ovary, and vagina are involved. However, metastatic disease can occur at any site. Tests of renal and liver chemistries should also be performed, in addition to a hematologic profile.

TABLE 33-3
FIGO Classification System of GTT

Stage	Anatomic Location
I	Confined to corpus uteri
II	Metastases outside uterus to vagina or pelvic structures
III	Metastases to lungs
IV	Distant metastases

Depending on the location of the disease, the duration of symptoms, the level of HCG, and a history of prior chemotherapy, it is possible to categorize the patient as having low-risk or high-risk GTT, as outlined in the box above. It has been stated that associated term pregnancy results in high-risk GTT, but evidence by Olive et al. from the Brewer Trophoblastic Disease Center indicates that GTT after term pregnancy may be considered as low risk unless one of the poor prognosis factors listed is also present.

Two methods have been adopted to classify GTT: firstly, clinical staging and secondly, the prognostic scoring, suggested by Bagshawe. The International Federation of Gynecology and Obstetrics (FIGO) anatomic staging system is shown in Table 33-3 and allows a comparison of treatment results from various centers. The prognostic scoring system is shown in Table 33-4. It provides another mechanism evaluating clinical and pathologic variables of GTT and

TABLE 33-4
Prognostic Scoring System for GTT

Factor	Score*			
	0	1	2	4
Age (years)	<39	>39		
Antecedent pregnancy	H. Mole	Abortion	Term	
Interval between end of antecedent pregnancy and start of chemotherapy (months)	<4	4-6	7-12	>12
HCG (IU/L)	$<10^3$	10^3-10^4	10^4-10^5	$>10^5$
ABO groups		O or A	B or AB	
Largest tumor, including uterine (cm)	<3	3-5	>5	
Site of metastases		Spleen, kidney	GI tract, liver	Brain
Number of metastases		1-3	4-8	>8
Prior chemotherapy			1 drug	≥2 drugs

Reproduced with permission from Bagshawe KD: J Reprod Med 29:813, 1984.
*Low risk, ≤4; medium risk, 5-7; high risk ≥8.

then summing them to provide a score that predicts chemotherapy resistance.

Although no large published series have used the prognostic scoring system, Gordon et al. recently noted that patients with a score of 8 or higher required multiagent chemotherapy. In another study, Mortakis and Braga noted the response to multiagent chemotherapy correlated with the scoring system. For patients with a score less than 12, 17 of 17 responded to multiagent chemotherapy (see following discussion). For the 11 patients who had scores higher than 12, only 3 responded, 5 responded to secondary therapy, and 3 died. In 1989 Bagshawe et al. summarized results on 487 patients. In this report a score of 5 or less was considered low risk, and 347 of 348 patients survived. The authors advise that those with medium- and high-risk disease should begin with multiagent chemotherapy. In a study of 53 patients with pathology-documented choriocarcinoma who died, Lurain noted that 51 had scores greater than 8 and that the average score of this high-risk group was 13.

Management

NONMETASTATIC AND GOOD-PROGNOSIS METASTATIC GTT. Single-agent chemotherapy is started for nonmetastatic GTT and good-prognosis (low-risk) metastatic GTT. Many pro-

grams of single-agent chemotherapy have been used, including methotrexate, 0.4 mg/kg body weight (maximum, 30 mg) intravenously or intramuscularly daily for 5 days every 2 weeks; actinomycin D, 10 to 12 mg/kg intravenously daily for 5 days every 2 weeks; or methotrexate, 1 to 1.5 mg/kg intramuscularly or intravenously on days 1, 3, 5, and 7, followed by citrovorum factor rescue (leucovorin), 0.1 to 0.15 mg/kg intramuscularly on days 2, 4, 6, and 8. Pulse actinomycin D, 1.25 mg/m^2 intravenously once every 2 weeks, has also been used. The latter regimen was introduced by Morrow et al. to treat low-risk nonmetastatic disease and has the advantage of being able to be given conveniently on an outpatient basis. It is used for low-risk postmolar trophoblastic neoplasia. Preliminary evidence suggests that it is effective, although it may require a longer treatment time to attain regression of HCG to normal values.

Petrilli et al. reported on single-dose actinomycin D for 31 patients in a cooperative Gynecologic Oncology Group (GOG) study. Twenty-nine (94%) achieved remission after a median of four courses of therapy. Another alternative was reported by Homesley et al., who summarized a GOG study of 63 patients with nonmetastatic GTD. Fifty-one responded completely to weekly intramuscular methotrexate, initially 30 mg/m^2 and increased as tolerated 5 mg/m^2/week to 50 mg/m^2. However, 11 patients failed and subsequently required 5-day actinomycin D therapy.

The 5-day actinomycin D and methotrexate courses have been found to be equally effective, but methotrexate appears to have more toxicity, particularly for the oral mucosa, and the severity of its toxicity increases with liver or renal compromise (Chapter 25). High-dose methotrexate with citrovorum rescue has not proven to be more effective than the other single agents given alone. Some investigators have alternated the 5-day actinomycin D and methotrexate courses in the belief that this results in reduced toxicity and more rapid resolution of the disease. VP-16 (etoposide) has also been effectively used as single-agent therapy.

Patients are treated until a normal β-HCG level has been obtained; then one to two additional courses of chemotherapy are usually given. Although recurrence rates of approximately 5% may be expected after therapy, recurrence more than 1 year after treatment is extremely unusual. Weekly serum HCG determinations are made until three negative β-HCG levels are obtained. Then monthly levels are taken for at least 12 months, after which pregnancy may be attempted. Even with recurrence, chemotherapy can be expected to cure 100% of patients with low-risk nonmetastatic trophoblastic disease. Hysterectomy may be performed in good operative candidates with nonmetastatic GTT who desire no further children or who have uterine disease resistant to chemotherapy.

HIGH-RISK METASTATIC GTT. The treatment of poor-prognosis GTT requires multiple-agent chemotherapy. Until recently, the most frequently utilized protocol was designated MAC, consisting of methotrexate (0.3 mg/kg), actinomycin D (8 to 10 mg/kg), and chlorambucil (oral, 0.2 mg/kg) or cyclophosphamide (3 to 5 mg/kg) given intravenously daily for 5 days. The cycle is repeated in 9 to 14 days as toxicity permits. To repeat the cycle, the white blood cell count must be greater than 3000, granulocytes over 1500, the platelet count more than 100,000, and the liver profile within normal limits.

In a cooperative, randomized GOG study, Curry et al. reported good results for MAC therapy with less toxicity than the modified Bagshawe regimen produces. However, vinblastine, bleomycin, and cisplatin (Einhorn regimen) have also been used for high-risk GTT as for ovarian germ cell tumors (Chapter 29). The chemotherapy of poor-prognosis GTT is continued for three courses after levels become negative, a practice that appears to decrease the rate of relapse. In recent years more effective protocols have been introduced using etoposide (VP-16). A widely used protocol uses *e*toposide, high-dose *m*ethotrexate with citrovorin rescue, *a*ctinomycin D, *c*yclophosphamide, and vincristine (Oncovin) (EMA/CO) (Table 33-5). Bolis et al., in a study of 36 high-risk patients, noted EMA/CO to be effective, including a 64% response rate when used as second-line therapy, which was higher than MAC or other multiagent protocols. EMA/CO is the current treatment of choice for poor-

---

TABLE 33-5
EMA/CO Regimen*

Day	Drug/Dosage	Abbreviation
1	Etoposide; 100 mg/m² IV over 30 minutes	E (etoposide)
	Actinomycin D: 0.5 mg IV push	M (methotrexate)
	Methotrexate: 100 mg/m² IV push	A (actinomycin D)
	200 mg/m² IV infusion in 1000 ml D₅W over 12 hours	
2	Etoposide: 100 mg/m² IV infusion in 250 ml NS over 30 minutes	
	Actinomycin D: 0.5 mg IV push	
	Folinic acid: 15 mg IM every 12 hours for 4 doses beginning 24 hours after starting methotrexate	
8	Cyclophosphamide: 600 mg/m² IV	C (cyclophosphamide)
	Vincristine: 1.0 mg/m² IV push	O (Oncovin)

*Repeat cycle on days 15, 16, and 22 (every 2 weeks).

prognosis GTT. Some therapists have used platinum and etoposide (EP) for high-risk disease.

If brain metastases are diagnosed, 2000 to 3000 rads are given immediately along with systemic chemotherapy. Liver metastases are usually treated by systemic chemotherapy, and intraarterial chemotherapy infusion has been tried.

As many as 20% of patients with poor-prognosis GTT who attain a negative HCG level have a recurrence. In comparison, the recurrence rate for those with good-prognosis GTT is 5%, while those with nonmetastatic GTT have recurrence rates of 1% to 2%.

After a negative HCG level is achieved for three cycles in patients with high-risk GTT, HCG measurements are repeated every 2 weeks for 3 months and then monthly for 1 year. Some therapists continue the measurement of HCG levels every 6 months for as long as 5 years because of the slight risk of late recurrence of the disease. Chest x-ray examinations are also usually repeated every 3 months during the first year of follow-up, but the HCG level is the crucial element in following the patient. A few isolated cases of choriocarcinomas have been reported in the absence of elevated levels of HCG. After 1 year of negative follow-up, the patient may again attempt pregnancy.

Fertility After Treatment for GTT

There is concern, particularly among patients who have been treated for GTD, that a subsequent pregnancy will lead to repeat GTD or recrudescence of the disease. While repeat molar pregnancy is an increased risk (1% to 2%) among these patients, current evidence suggests that normal pregnancy usually results. Data from Rustin et al. indicate no increased frequency of congenital anomalies among infants whose mothers received chemotherapy. Goldstein et al. reported that 67.4% of 929 individuals treated at various centers for GTD subsequently had a normal term delivery, while only 1.4% experienced a recurrent molar pregnancy. A recent study by Green et al. suggests those treated with chemotherapy for a variety of tumors are not at increased risk for having offspring with congenital anomalies. However, the patients receiving Actinomycin D 2-16 mg/m^2 had the greatest frequency of congenital anomalies suggesting further study is indicated for this drug. If pregnancy occurs following GTD, it is important to perform an ultrasound examination early to identify a gestational sac in the uterus, as well as a fetal heart, which should be evident by the seventh week of pregnancy. HCG levels should be obtained after delivery to rule out any recurrence of GTD. Products of conception or placentas should be examined histopathologically.

_____ **KEY POINTS** _____

- The monitoring of trophoblastic disease and its follow-up is accomplished by the measurement of the beta-subunit of HCG by radioimmunoassay (RIA) or enzyme immunoassay (EIA).

- The risk of hydatidiform mole is about 0.75 per 1000 pregnancies in the United States.

- Choriocarcinomas follow 1 in 40,000 term pregnancies and 3% to 5% of complete molar pregnancies.

- Risk factors for molar pregnancy include age (over 40 and under 20 years), geographic location (Southeast Asia and Mexico), and a history of prior molar pregnancy. Choriocarcinoma risk factors are similar, with an increased risk for women with blood type O impregnated by men of type A and those with type A impregnated by men of type O.

- The risk of developing a second molar pregnancy after a primary mole is about 20 to 40 times greater than the initial risk.

- About half the cases of gestational trophoblastic tumor (GTT) follow molar pregnancy, one fourth follow normal pregnancy, and one fourth follow abortion or ectopic pregnancy.

- Complete moles are of paternal origin, are diploid, and carry a 20% risk of GTT sequelae.

- Partial moles are of maternal and paternal origin, are triploid, and rarely are followed by GTT.

- Hydatidiform molar pregnancy should be suspected in a woman with persistent bleeding in the first half of pregnancy, toxemia before 24 weeks' gestation, or hyperemesis. The uterus is large for gestational dates in about half the cases, and ovarian enlargement occurs in about 20%.

- An elevated serum level of HCG is not diagnostic of molar pregnancy but may indicate a multiple gestation or a normal pregnancy with incorrect gestational dates.

- The diagnosis of a molar pregnancy (complete mole) can be established with ultrasound, which displays a "snowstorm" pattern.

- Hydatidiform moles are effectively and safely evacuated from the uterus using suction curettage.

- Medical complications of hydatidiform mole include anemia from blood loss, toxemia, hyperthyroidism, hyperemesis gravidarum, and rarely pulmonary insufficiency.

- In low-risk GTT, the initial serum HCG level is less than 40,000 mIU/ml, the disease is present less than 4 months, metastases involve the lung and vagina only, and there has been no prior chemotherapy. It is usually treated by single-agent chemotherapy.

- In high-risk GTT, one or more of the following are present: the initial serum HCG level is greater than 40,000 mIU/ml, the disease has been present more than 4 months; metastases beyond the lung and vagina are present; and there is failure of prior chemotherapy. It is treated with multiple-agent chemotherapy.

- Recurrence rate for patients treated for GTT whose HCG level reached normal is 5% for good-prognosis metastatic GTT and 1% to 2% for good-prognosis nonmetastatic GTT. However, nonmetastatic GTT and low-risk GTT are 100% curable by chemotherapy.

- Patients with high-risk GTT are successfully treated with chemotherapy in more than 70% of the cases.

- Patients treated for GTT should not become pregnant for at least 1 year after treatment to allow accurate assessment of β-HCG levels.

- Infants born to mothers treated for GTD do not appear to have an increased frequency of congenital anomalies.

BIBLIOGRAPHY

Acaia B, Parazzini F, La Vecchia C, et al: Increased frequency of complete hydatidiform mole in women with repeated abortion, Gynecol Oncol 31:310, 1988.

Atrash HK, Hogue CJR, and Grimes DA: Epidemiology of hydatidiform mole during early gestation, Am J Obstet Gynecol 154:906, 1986.

Bagshawe KD: Some facets of trophoblastic neoplasia in man, J Reprod Fertil (Suppl) 31:175, 1982.

Bagshawe KD: Treatment of high-risk choriocarcinoma, J Reprod Med 29:813, 1984.

Bagshawe KD, Dent J, Newlands ES, et al: The role of low-dose methotrexate and folinic acid in gestational trophoblastic tumours (GTT), Br J Obstet Gynecol 96:795, 1989.

Bagshawe KD, Lawler SD, Paradinas FJ, et al: Gestational trophoblastic tumours following initial diagnosis of partial hydatidiform mole, Lancet 335:1074, 1990.

Bagshawe KD, Rawlings G, Pike MC, et al: The ABO blood groups in trophoblastic neoplasia, Lancet 1:553, 1971.

Bandy LC, Clarke-Pearson DL, and Hammond C: Malignant potential of gestational trophoblastic disease at the extreme ages of reproductive life, Obstet Gynecol 64:395, 1984.

Berkowitz RS, Goldstein DP, and Bernstein MR: Natural history of partial molar pregnancy, Obstet Gynecol 66:667, 1983.

Bigelow B: Gestational trophoblast disease. In Blaustein A, ed: Pathology of the female genital tract, ed 2, New York, 1982, Springer-Verlag New York Inc.

Bolis G, Bonazzi C, Landoni F, et al: EMA/CO regimen in high-risk gestational trophoblastic tumor (GTT), Gynecol Oncol 31:439, 1988.

Buckley JD: The epidemiology of molar pregnancy and choriocarcinoma, Clin Obstet Gynecol 27:153, 1984.

Cotton DB, Bernstein SG, Read SA, et al: Hemodynamic observations in evacuation of molar pregnancy, Am J Obstet Gynecol 138:6, 1980.

Curry SL, Blessing J, DiSaia P, et al: A prospective randomized comparison of methotrexate, dactinomycin, and chlorambucil versus methotrexate, dactinomycin, cyclophosphamide, doxorubicin, melphalan, hydroxyurea, and vincristine in "poor prognosis" metastatic gestational trophoblastic disease: a Gynecologic Oncology Group study, Obstet Gynecol 73:357, 1989.

Curry SL, Hammond CB, Tyrey L, et al: Hydatidiform mole—diagnosis, management and long term follow-up of 347 patients, Obstet Gynecol 45:1, 1975.

Davis JR, Surwitt EA, Garay JP, et al: Sex assignment in gestational trophoblastic neoplasia, Am J Obstet Gynecol 148:722, 1984.

Dawook MY, Teoh ES, and Ratnam SS: ABO blood group in trophoblastic disease, J Obstet Gynaecol Br Comm 78:918, 1971.

Deicas RE, Miller DS, Rademaker AW, et al: The role of contraception in the development of postmolar gestational trophoblastic disease, Obstet Gynecol 78:221, 1991.

Dessau R, Rustin GJS, Paradinas FJ, et al: Surgery and chemotherapy in the management of placental site tumor, Gynecol Oncol 39:56, 1990.

Finkler NJ, Berkowitz RS, Driscoll SG, et al: Clinical experience with placental site trophoblastic tumors at the New England Trophoblastic Disease Center, Obstet Gynecol 71:854, 1988.

Goldstein DP, Berkowitz RS, and Bernstein MR: Reproductive performance after molar pregnancy and gestational trophoblastic tumor, Clin Obstet Gynecol 27:221, 1984.

Gordon AN, Gershenson DM, Copeland LJ, et al: High-risk metastatic gestational trophoblastic disease: further stratification into two clinical entities, Gynecol Oncol 34:54, 1989.

Green DM, Zevon MA, Lowrie G, et al: Congenital anomalies in children of patients who received chemotherapy for cancer in childhood and adolescence, N Engl J Med 325:141, 1991.

Grimes DA: Epidemiology of gestational trophoblastic disease, Am J Obstet Gynecol 150:309, 1984.

Hammond CB and Soper JT: Poor-prognostic metastatic gestational trophoblastic neoplasia, Clin Obstet Gynecol 27:228, 1984.

Homesley HD, Blessing JA, Rettenmaier M, et al: Weekly intramuscular methotrexate for nonmetastatic gestational trophoblastic disease, Obstet Gynecol 72:413, 1988.

Kelly MP, Rustin GJS, Ivory C, et al: Respiratory failure due to choriocarcinoma: a study of 103 dyspneic patients, Gynecol Oncol 38:149, 1990.

Lage JM, Berkowitz, RS, Rice LW, et al: Flow cytometric analysis of DNA content in partial hydatidiform moles with persistent gestational trophoblastic tumor, Obstet Gynecol 77:111, 1991.

Lemonnier M-C, Glezerman V, Auclair R, et al: Choriocarcinoma associated with undetectable levels of human chorionic gonadotropin, Gynecol Oncol 25:48, 1986.

Li MC, Hertz R, and Spencer DB: Effect of methotrexate therapy upon choriocarcinoma and chorioadenoma, Proc Soc Exp Biol Med 93:36, 1956.

Lurain JR: Causes of treatment failure in gestational trophoblastic disease, J Reprod Med 32:675, 1987.

Lurain JR: Chemotherapy of gestational trophoblastic disease. In Deppe G, editor: Chemotherapy of gynecologic cancer, ed 2, New York, 1990, Alan R Liss, Inc.

Lurain JR and Brewer JI: Treatment of high-risk gestational trophoblastic disease with methotrexate, actinomycin D, and cyclophosphamide chemotherapy, Obstet Gynecol 65:830, 1985.

Montz FJ, Schlaerth JB, and Morrow CP: The natural history of theca lutein cysts, Obstet Gynecol 72:247, 1988.

Morrow P, Nakamura R, Schlaerth JB, et al: The influence of oral contraceptives on the post molar HCG regression curve, Am J Obstet Gynecol 151:906, 1985.

Mortakis AE and Braga CA: "Poor prognosis" metastatic gestational trophoblastic disease: the prognostic significance of the scoring system in predicting chemotherapy failures, Obstet Gynecol 76:272, 1990.

Olive DL, Lurain JR, and Brewer JI: Choriocarcinoma associated with term gestation, Am J Obstet Gynecol 148:711, 1984.

Petrilli ES, Twiggs LB, Blessing JA, et al: Single-dose actinomycin D treatment for nonmetastatic gestational trophoblastic disease: a prospective phase II trial of the gynecologic oncology group, Cancer 60:2173, 1987.

Rice LW, Berkowitz RS, Lage JM, et al: Persistent gestational trophoblastic tumor after partial hydatidiform mole, Gynecol Oncol 36:358, 1990.

Rustin GJS, Booth M, Dent J, et al: Pregnancy after cytotoxic chemotherapy for gestational trophoblastic tumors, Br Med J 288:103, 1984.

Schlaerth JB, Morrow CR, Kletzky OA, et al: Prognostic characteristics of serum human chorionic gonadotropin titer regression following molar pregnancy, Obstet Gynecol 58:478, 1981.

Schlaerth JB, Morrow CP, Montz FJ, and d'Ablaing G: Initial management of hydatidiform mole, Am J Obstet Gynecol 158:1299, 1988.

Schlaerth JB, Morrow CP, Nalick RH, et al: Single-dose actinomycin D in the treatment of post molar trophoblastic disease, Gynecol Oncol 19:53, 1984.

Smith EB, Szulman AE, Hinshaw W, et al: Human chorionic gonadotropin levels in complete and partial hydatidiform moles and in nonmolar abortuses, Am J Obstet Gynecol 149:129, 1984.

Szulman AE and Surti U: The syndromes of partial and complete molar gestation, Clin Obstet Gynecol 27:172, 1984.

Vaitukaitis JL, Braunstein GD, and Ross GT: A radioimmunoassay which specifically measures human chorionic gonadotropin in the presence of human luteinizing hormone, Am J Obstet Gynecol 113:751, 1972.

Vassilakos P, Riotten G, and Kajii T: Hydatidiform mole: two entities—a morphologic and cytogenic study with some clinical considerations, Am J Obstet Gynecol 127:167, 1977.

Watson EJ, Hernandez E, and Miyazawa K: Partial hydatidiform moles: a review, Obstet Gynecol Surv 42:540, 1987.

WHO Scientific Group: Gestational trophoblastic diseases, Technical Report Series 692, Geneva, 1983, World Health Organization.

Young RH and Scully RE: Placental-site trophoblastic tumor: current status, Clin Obstet Gynecol 27:248, 1984.

ENDOCRINOLOGY
AND INFERTILITY

Dysmenorrhea and Premenstrual Syndrome

CHAPTER 34

KEY TERMS AND DEFINITIONS

Cervical Stenosis. Narrowing of the cervical canal, often at the level of the internal os, in such a way that menstrual flow is impeded and intrauterine pressure is increased at the time of menses.

Dysmenorrhea. Painful cramping sensation in the lower abdomen often accompanied by other symptoms such as sweating, tachycardia, headaches, nausea, vomiting, diarrhea, and tremulousness. These all occur just before or during the menses. Primary dysmenorrhea begins at or shortly after menarche and is usually not accompanied by pelvic pathologic conditions. Secondary dysmenorrhea arises later and usually is associated with other pelvic conditions.

Mittelschmerz. Midcycle pelvic pain usually related to ovulation. The actual mechanism is not clearly understood.

Pelvic Congestion Syndrome. Vascular engorgement of the uterus and the vessels of the broad ligament and lateral pelvic walls, which may lead to chronic pelvic pain.

Premenstrual Syndrome (PMS). A group of symptoms, both physical and behavioral, that occur in the second half of the menstrual cycle and often interfere with work and personal relationships. They are followed by a period entirely free of symptoms.

Prostaglandin-Synthetase Inhibitors (PGSIs). Substances that block the activity of prostaglandin synthetase, thereby preventing the effect of prostaglandins on tissue. These basically consist of two chemical groups: the arylcarboxylic acids and the arylalkanoic acids.

Dysmenorrhea and premenstrual syndrome afflict a large percentage of women in the reproductive years. These conditions have a negative effect on the quality of the patients' lives and on the lives of their families, and they are also responsible for a huge economic loss as a result of the cost of medications, medical care, and decreased productivity. This chapter will discuss current thinking with respect to the etiology, pathophysiology, and management of these two conditions, which are not always related.

DYSMENORRHEA

Dysmenorrhea is defined as a severe, painful cramping sensation in the lower abdomen often accompanied by other biologic symptoms, including sweating, tachycardia, headaches, nausea, vomiting, diarrhea, and tremulousness, all occurring just before or during the menses. In the past the definition has been subdivided into primary and secondary dysmenorrhea. The term *primary dysmenorrhea* was reserved for women who had no obvious pathologic condition. We currently recognize that these patients are suffering from the effects of endogenous prostaglandins. *Secondary dysmenorrhea*, on the other hand, is associated with pelvic conditions or pathology that causes pelvic pain in conjunction with the menses. Primary dysmenorrhea almost always first occurs in women younger than 20. Indeed, the patient will report pain as soon as she establishes ovulatory cycles. Secondary dysmenorrhea may, of course, occur in women under 20, but it is most often seen in women over 20.

Incidence

A number of studies have attempted to determine the prevalence of dysmenorrhea; a wide range (3% to 90%) has been reported. These studies have been performed on students, teenagers and their mothers, and individuals from various specific populations, such as industrial workers or college students. The best estimate of the prevalence of primary dysmenorrhea is about 75%. Andersch and Milsom surveyed all the 19-year-old women in the city of Gothenburg, Sweden. A total of 90.9% of such women responded to a randomly distributed questionnaire, and 72.4% of these stated that they suffered from dysmenorrhea. In addition, 34.3% of the total population reported mild menstrual symptoms, 22.7% cited moderate symptoms that required analgesia, and 15.4% stated that they had severe dysmenorrhea that clearly inhibited their working ability and that could not be adequately assuaged by general analgesia (Table 34-1). This study verified the work of others who found that women who had vaginally delivered a child, who took birth control pills, or who were smokers were less likely to have dysmenorrhea. Pregnancy itself without actual birth did not seem to alleviate dysmenorrhea, as women who had ectopic pregnancies or spontaneous or voluntary terminations of pregnancy were not relieved of their symptoms, whereas women who delivered babies were.

Oral contraceptive use was noted by these investigators to reduce the prevalence and severity of dysmenorrhea significantly ($P \le .01$). IUD use did not affect prevalence or severity in any measurable way.

Relationship to Menstruation and the Menstrual Cycle

Andersch and Milsom demonstrated a significant positive correlation between the severity of dysmenorrhea and the duration of menstrual flow, amount of menstrual flow, and early menarche. They showed no relationship with the actual duration of the menstrual cycle.

In their series, 38.3% of the patients reported that they had experienced dysmenorrhea for the first time during the first year after menarche, and only 20.8% reported that dysmenorrhea had not occurred until 4 years after menarche.

Family History

Dysmenorrhea has been reported to be significantly increased among mothers and sisters of women with dysmenorrhea.

Pathogenesis of Primary Dysmenorrhea

Although the pathogenesis of dysmenorrhea is still unknown, the fact that there is a close association between an elevated prostaglandin $F_{2\alpha}$ level in the secretory endometrium and the symptoms of dysmenorrhea, including uterine hypercontractility, complaints of severe cramping, and other prostaglandin-induced symptoms, has led to the theory that prostaglandin $F_{2\alpha}$ is associated with the pathogenesis of dysmenorrhea. Prostaglandin-synthetase inhibitors (PGSIs) have been demonstrated to alleviate these symptoms. These substances are nonsteroidal and antiinflammatory. They have been used as analgesics for a number of conditions, including arthritis, and generally are divided into two chemical groups—the arylcarboxylic acids, which include acetylsalicylic acid (aspirin) and fenamates, and the arylalkanoic acids, including the arylpropionic acids (ibuprofen, naproxen, and ketoprofen), as well as the indoleacetic acids (indomethacin). The specific effect of these agents on the uterine musculature is reduction of contractility as measured by reduction of intrauterine pressure.

In 1984 Owen reviewed the effectiveness of

TABLE 34-1

Severity of Primary Dysmenorrhea in a Population of 586 Swedish, 19-year-old Women

Severity	Number	Percent
None	162	27.6
Mild*	201	34.3
Moderate†	133	22.7
Severe‡	90	15.4

Data from Andersch B and Milsom I: Am J Obstet Gynecol 144:655, 1982.

*No systemic symptoms, medication rarely required, work rarely affected.

†Few systemic symptoms, medication required, work moderately affected.

‡Multiple symptoms, poor medication response, work inhibited.

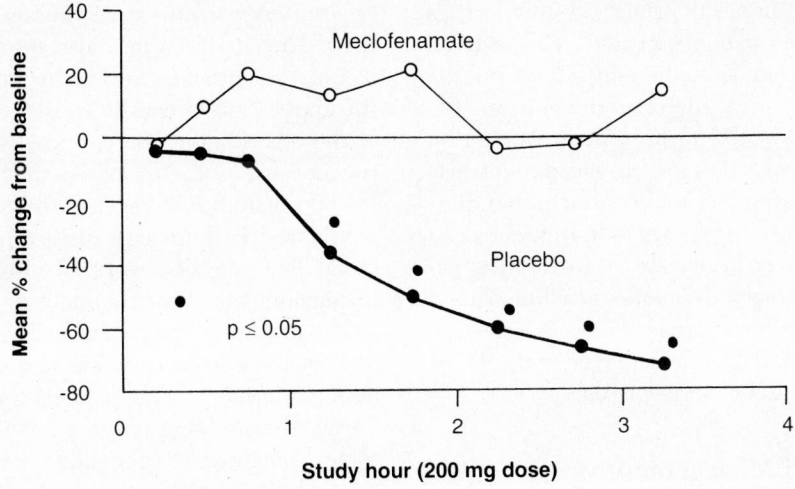

FIGURE 34-1

Average pressure: meclofenamate versus placebo. Redrawn from Smith RP: Obstet Gynecol 70:785, 1987.

PGSIs in the treatment of primary dysmenorrhea. She reviewed 51 trials carried out in 1649 women. More than 72% of the women suffering from dysmenorrhea reported significant pain relief with PGSIs, 18% reported minimal or no pain relief, and 15% showed a placebo response. Owen concluded that PGSI compounds were effective and safe for the majority of women with primary dysmenorrhea. The fenamates seemed to be more effective in providing pain relief than ibuprofen, indomethacin, or naproxen. All the compounds demonstrated minimal PGSI-associated side effects with the exception of indomethacin. In trials with indomethacin the dropout rate was higher primarily because of symptoms involving the central nervous system and gastrointestinal tract.

Smith has demonstrated that the effectiveness of PGSIs is related to tissue concentration. Using meclofenamate in 18 subjects who participated in a double-blind, placebo-controlled, cross-over study, he was able to show a parallel in time response curves between the plasma levels of the drug and decrease in uterine contractility. Figure 34-1 demonstrates the average intrauterine pressure relationships between placebo-treated and drug-treated patients over time. Intrauterine pressure declined 20% to 56% in these patients during meclofenamate therapy.

PGSIs should not be given to patients who have shown previous hypersensitivity to such drugs. It is also contraindicated for individuals

TABLE 34-2
Commonly Used Prostaglandin-Synthetase Inhibitors

Brand Name	Generic Name	Usual Regimen (mg q6h)
Motrin	Ibuprofen	400-800
Naprosyn	Naproxen	250-500
Anaprox	Naproxen sodium	275-550
Ponstel	Mefenamic acid	250-500

who have had nasal polyps, angioedema, and bronchospasm related to aspirin or nonsteroidal antiinflammatory agents. In addition, these agents are contraindicated for individuals with a history of chronic ulceration or inflammatory reaction of the upper or lower gastrointestinal tract and for those with preexisting chronic renal disease. During the use of such agents, autoimmune hemolytic anemia, rash, edema and fluid retention, and central nervous system symptoms, such as dizziness, headache, nervousness, and blurred vision, can occur. In up to 15% of users slight elevation of hepatic enzymes may also be found. Table 34-2 lists some of the PGSIs in common use for the treatment of dysmenorrhea.

Other Therapy

Although PGSIs are the standard therapy available for primary dysmenorrhea, other approaches are possible. Oral contraceptives will relieve the symptoms of primary dysmenorrhea in about 90% of patients treated. This may be because of either a modulating effect on the hypothalamus or a direct reduction in the amount of endometrium present in women on oral contraceptive therapy. If the patient also requires contraception, oral contraceptive therapy may prove to be the treatment of choice.

Analgesics may be necessary in treating patients with primary dysmenorrhea but should be used as back-up drugs when the desired therapeutic effect is not achieved with PGSI medication or oral contraceptives.

Etiology and Management of Secondary Dysmenorrhea

A variety of other conditions cause or are associated with dysmenorrhea. These conditions may occur at any age, and in most cases the pain experienced is either secondary to the pathologic process of the condition or a specific result of the condition. These constitute the so-called secondary dysmenorrhea group of problems and include cervical stenosis, ectopic endometrial tissue, pelvic inflammation, pelvic congestion, conditioned behavior, and stress and tension (see box below).

Cervical Stenosis

Severe narrowing of the cervical canal, particularly at the level of the internal os, may impede menstrual flow, causing an increase in intrauterine pressure at the time of menses. In addition, retrograde menstrual flow through the fallopian tubes into the peritoneal cavity may take place. Thus severe cervical stenosis may eventually be associated with pelvic endometriosis as well. The etiology of cervical stenosis may be congenital or may be secondary to cervical injury, such as with electrocautery,

cryocautery, or operative trauma (i.e., conization). The condition may also result from an inflammatory process caused by infection or by the application of caustic substances. After any of these conditions the cervical canal may narrow because of the formation of scar tissue.

The possibility of cervical stenosis should be considered if there is a history of scant menstrual flow and if severe cramping continues throughout the menstrual period.

The diagnosis is suspected when the external os appears scarred or when it is impossible to pass a uterine sound through the internal os during the proliferative stage of the menstrual cycle. Diagnosis is generally documented by the inability to pass a thin probe of a few millimeters' diameter through the internal os or by hysterosalpingogram, which demonstrates a thin, stringy-appearing canal. If dilation and curettage (D&C) are performed, finding the passage through the internal os with a thin probe is often difficult but can frequently be accomplished with patience. The patient should be anesthetized.

Treatment consists of dilating the cervix; this may be accomplished by D&C with progressive dilators or by the use of progressive *laminaria* tents. In the past the insertion of stem pessaries has been noted to be of some value in such cases. Unfortunately, cervical stenosis often recurs after therapy, necessitating repeat procedures. Pregnancy and vaginal delivery often afford more lasting cure.

Often other problems obstructing the cervix can have a similar presentation. Figure 34-2 shows anteroposterior and lateral views of a hysterogram in an 18-year-old nulliparous woman who had a 2-year history of severe, disabling dysmenorrhea that usually required morphine therapy with each menstrual period. At hysteroscopy she was found to have a tissue band across her internal os, at which site a large endocervical polyp had formed. Transecting the band and removing the polyp completely relieved the dysmenorrhea, and she has had no further symptoms after 3 years.

CAUSES OF SECONDARY DYSMENORRHEA

Cervical stenosis
Endometriosis and adenomyosis
Pelvic infection and adhesions
Pelvic congestion
Conditioned behavior
Stress and tension

Ectopic Endometrial Tissue (Endometriosis)

Ectopic endometrial tissue or endometriosis (including endometriosis and adenomyosis) should be considered when there is a history of pain becoming more severe during menses.

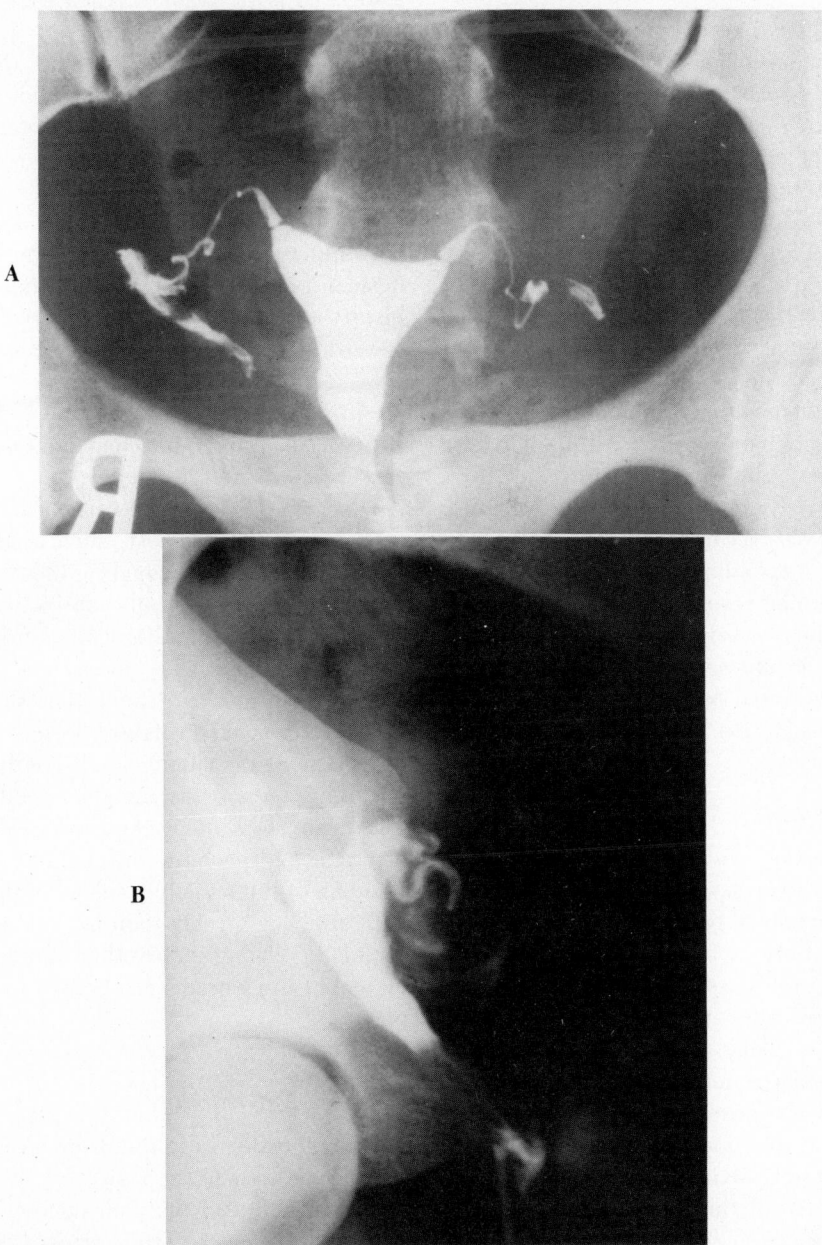

FIGURE 34-2
Hysterogram. **A,** Anteroposterior view and **B,** lateral view, of an 18-year-old patient with severe disabling dysmenorrhea. At hysteroscopy she was found to have a tissue band across the internal os and an endocervical polyp at this site. Removal of the polyp and transection of the band completely relieved the dysmenorrhea.

Frequently dyspareunia and infertility are accompanying symptoms. Pertinent physical findings may include uterosacral ligament nodules or evidence for endometriosis in the vagina or cervix.

Specific diagnosis of endometriosis is made by direct visualization via laparoscopy or laparotomy or by direct biopsy of vaginal or cervical lesions.

Treatment of endometriosis is discussed in Chapter 18. Management should be designed for the patient's specific needs.

Pelvic Inflammation

Pelvic infections secondary to gonorrhea, chlamydia, or other infectious agents may cause pelvic inflammation or pelvic abscess and with healing may be associated with pelvic adhesions that may cause pelvic pain. Often this may be aggravated at menses, causing dysmenorrhea. Infections secondary to other conditions, such as appendicitis or IUD use, may also create a similar response. The pain may be secondary to the congestion and edema that occur normally at menses, which may subsequently be aggravated by the healed inflammatory areas and adhesions.

Pelvic Congestion Syndrome

Pelvic congestion syndrome, which was first described by Taylor several years ago, results from engorgement of pelvic vasculature. The pain is usually burning or throbbing in nature, worse at night, and worse after standing. Physical examination of the vagina and cervix usually reveals vasocongestion with evidence of some uterine enlargement and tenderness. Diagnosis is made by observation of the features noted and by laparoscopy, which not only rules out other causes of pelvic pain but also demonstrates congestion of the uterus and engorgement or varicosities of the broad ligament and pelvic side wall veins. If laparoscopy is used for diagnosis, it is important to observe the broad ligament vasculature as the pressure of the carbon dioxide or nitrous oxide is released. At full pressure during the procedure these vessels may be obliterated but will reappear as pressure is reduced.

The pathophysiology of pelvic congestion syndrome is probably related to tension and psychosomatic problems. Consequently, management relates to careful history of the patient's past and present social situation and, where appropriate, the use of counseling.

Severe cases of pelvic congestion syndrome associated with dysmenorrhea that do not respond to counseling or other medical types of pain management may respond to hysterectomy, although such management should be considered a last resort (see Chapter 6).

Conditioned Behavior

In individuals with strong family histories of dysmenorrhea or in situations where a careful history demonstrates a possibility for societal reward or control because of the symptoms of pain, a conditioned behavior should be considered. It is important to obtain a careful medical and social history and to rule out all other causes of acquired dysmenorrhea.

Diagnosis can often be verified by the use of a personality profile test, such as the Minnesota Multiphasic Personality Index. This test has been used clinically on many different groups of patients and is well standardized. It is frequently necessary to use such a test to demonstrate to the patient that she does indeed fit into such a category.

Treatment of patients with conditioned behavior dysmenorrhea includes reeducation so that the pain is not looked on as a rewarding experience. Teaching the patient an understanding of the pathophysiology of the problem and applying reconditioning techniques are useful. Psychologists or other similarly trained mental health workers can be consulted for this purpose.

Stress and Tension

Dysmenorrhea resulting from stress and tension usually is accompanied by a history of gradual onset, and the pain is generally worse at times, particularly when stress is severe and when there may be a possibility for secondary gain. The pathophysiology is difficult to define; it may be a combination of prostaglandin activity and engorgement.

The treatment is centered on finding the means to relieve stress, which may include education, the teaching of relaxation techniques, counseling, and, on rare occasions, antidepression or tranquilizing medications for short periods of time.

Other Causes

At times dysmenorrhea may be related to unusual pathologic findings. These include small leiomyomas or polyps at the junction of the internal os and lower uterine segment. Such a condition may produce a valvelike effect at the os at the time of menses. Frequently myomas or polyps become engorged or edematous at the time of menses, accentuating the problem. Diagnosis is generally made by history and by hysterosalpingography, hysteroscopy, or D&C. Therapy consists of excising the pathologic tissue. In the case of a myoma a hysterectomy may be necessary.

PREMENSTRUAL SYNDROME

The premenstrual syndrome (PMS) is defined as a group of symptoms, both physical and behavioral, that occur in the second half of the menstrual cycle and that often interfere with work and personal relationships. These are followed by a period entirely free of symptoms. The condition was first described by Frank in 1931. That author attempted to relate symptoms of then so-called *premenstrual tension* with hormonal changes of the menstrual cycle. The term *premenstrual syndrome* was first used by Dalton in 1953. The symptoms do vary from woman to woman, and more than 150 symptoms have been linked with the disorder.

Incidence

Although various reports place the prevalence of PMS at 5% to 95% of menstruating women, it is generally agreed that about 40% of women are significantly affected at one time or another. Severe symptoms occur in only 2% or 3% of women between the ages of 18 and 48.

Symptoms

In a review by O'Brien a number of common somatic and psychological symptoms were enumerated. These are summarized in the box (upper right). In general, somatic symptoms relate to presumed fluid retention, breast tenderness, and various pain constellations, such as headache or pelvic pain. Psychological symptoms vary from irritability and tension to anxiety, aggression, and depression. The personality

---

SYMPTOMS OF PREMENSTRUAL SYNDROME

Somatic Symptoms

Bloated feeling
Feeling of weight increase
Breast pain or tenderness
Skin disorders
Hot flushes
Headache
Pelvic pain
Change in bowel habits

Psychological Symptoms

Irritability
Aggression
Tension
Anxiety
Depression
Lethargy
Insomnia
Change in appetite
Crying
Change in libido
Thirst
Loss of concentration
Poor coordination, clumsiness, accidents

From O'Brien PM: Drugs 24:140, 1982.

---

changes that occur in the second half of the menstrual cycle are so severe in some patients that the term *Dr. Jekyl and Mr. Hyde* is frequently used. In a few instances PMS has been used as a defense in murder trials.

Freeman et al. in a study of 60 women ages 18 to 45 who were newly enrolled in a PMS program at the University of Pennsylvania found that four major history variables explained 34% of the variance of symptom severity using step regression analysis. These were PMS in the patient's mother, low level of exercise, younger age, and more children. These relationships suggested to the authors that familial and stress factors had a role in the syndrome.

Depression is a common complaint in the population in general and also in PMS sufferers during the luteal phase. Mortola et al. have recently shown that 16 PMS patients had marked worsening of scores on the Profile of Mood States and Beck Depression Inventory during the luteal phase compared with 16 controls. However, six patients suffering from endogenous depression had scores threefold higher on both indices than PMS patients who were in the luteal phase. Also, the amplitude of cortisol secretion pulses was higher in the depressed patients than either PMS patients or control patients. The data of this study demonstrate that PMS patients do have more episodes of depression during the luteal phase compared with controls, but these episodes are distinctly different from those suffered by patients with endogenous depression.

In addition, Rapkin et al. have demonstrated that PMS patients show no deficit in cognitive processing and performance, as well as no loss in ability to concentrate and sustain attention and motivation. No such alterations were seen in 10 PMS patients during the luteal phase. Their performance was similar to 9 controls when tested in these areas.

Etiology

When Frank first described the syndrome, he attributed it to estrogen excess. Israel theorized 7 years later that it resulted from an imbalance of estrogen and progesterone. Others have offered theories that the disorder is related to endogenous hormone allergy, hypoglycemia, vitamin B_6 deficiency, prolactin excess, fluid retention, inappropriate prostaglandin activity, elevated monoamine oxidase (MAO), endorphin malfunction, and multiple psychological disturbances. In 1981, Reid and Yen reviewed the subject and concluded that PMS was a multifactorial psychoendocrine disorder. Recently Rossignol and Bonnlander reported on a relationship between caffeine ingestion and the prevalence and severity of PMS. In a study of 841 college women, those with severe symptoms showed a dose dependency relationship. Prevalence odds ratios for demonstrating PMS symptoms varied from 1.3 for consumers of one cup of caffeine-containing beverage to 7.0 for consumers of 8 to 10 cups per day when compared with non-caffeine users.

As yet, however, the specific etiology remains unclear. Nevertheless, it is still worthwhile to review some of the data related to the specific theories that have been considered to offer some insight for therapy.

Steroid Allergy

The first of these theories involved the thought that the condition might be related to an allergy to an endogenous hormone, specifi-

cally progesterone. It had been observed that many women did, indeed, have dermatitis during the luteal phase of the menstrual cycle. In 1962 Rogers reported that 80% of his PMS patients who were desensitized with small amounts of pregnanediol reported some improvement of their symptoms. However, there were no control subjects in his study, and no placebo studies were carried out.

Hypoglycemia and Vitamin Deficiency

One of the older theories of the etiology of PMS related this condition to hypoglycemia. In 1953 Morton et al. reported finding that results of the glucose tolerance test (GTT) revealed flattening, with a delayed hypoglycemia in many patients immediately before or during menses. In such individuals the glucose tolerance level was found to be normal after the menstrual period. Because many patients craved sweets and complained of headaches, he felt there was supportive evidence for a hypoglycemic etiology. He therefore treated 249 volunteers in a New York state prison with high-protein diets. Some individuals received a placebo, while others received medication consisting of a diuretic, caffeine, and vitamin B complex. None of those on the medication regimen required isolation for behavior problems during their premenstrual period even though several had required this before the treatment had begun. In addition, their efficiency at work activities was judged as superior; they performed almost a third more work than they had previously. Although 15% of patients treated with placebo demonstrated an improvement in symptoms, 39% treated with placebo and high-protein diet noted improvement. Patients who were treated with the drug regimen reported a 61% improvement in symptoms, and those treated with drug plus high-protein diet showed a 79% improvement. All individuals reported the greatest improvement in those symptoms that were related to nervousness and other emotional symptoms.

About the same time that the hypoglycemia theory was postulated, it was suggested that there was a vitamin B_6 deficiency in PMS patients as well. Originally it was suggested that a deficiency of vitamins could lead to impaired liver function, thus causing an increase in circulating estrogen. However, groups of women on diets severely lacking in vitamin B during wartime were found to have normal estrogen metabolism. With the discovery that vitamin B_6 is a coenzyme in the biosynthesis of dopamine and serotonin, the possibility that this agent might be involved in the etiology of PMS was raised. Also, in 1973 Adams et al. noted that vitamin B_6 therapy seemed to be associated with improvement of depression in women taking oral contraceptives in a double-blind trial. It was believed that the oral contraceptives caused an abnormal tryptophan metabolism and that vitamin B_6 to some extent reversed this.

One double-blind study by Abraham and Hargrov demonstrated that vitamin B_6 administered in 200 to 800 mg doses daily prevented some of the symptoms of PMS in women with this affliction significantly better than did a placebo. Abraham and Hargrov theorized that deficiencies of vitamin B_6 and magnesium could result in a lower threshold to stress and to a potential hormone imbalance. They also noted that giving vitamin B_6 to a patient raised serum progesterone levels at midluteal cycle. The requirements for pyridoxine may increase with increased estrogen levels partly because estrogen may increase the metabolism of tryptophan via the kynurenine-niacin pathway. In this reaction pyridoxine is required as a cofactor. Estrogen conjugates also competitively inhibit pyridoxine activity. This action may lower brain serotonin levels, which may be involved in causing a depression reaction. However, a previous double-blind study by Stokes and Mendels failed to show any improvement by pyridoxine over placebo in alleviating PMS symptoms. However, only 13 women were studied in this trial.

Doll et al. recently studied 32 women ages 18 to 49 using a double-blind, placebo-controlled, cross-over method. They administered 200 mg of pyridoxine daily and noted a significant beneficial effect on only emotional symptoms (depression, irritability, and tiredness), but on no other PMS symptoms.

Higher doses of pyridoxine should be administered with caution, since neuropathy occurring in several patients treated with as little as 100 to 200 mg daily has been reported. Such symptoms as sensory deficits, paresthesia, numbness, ataxia, and muscle weakness may occur.

Prolactin Effect

Some investigators believe that elevated prolactin may induce PMS symptoms. Kullander and Svanberg and Halbreich et al. actually offered evidence that elevated prolactin levels stimulate PMS symptoms in certain patients. Prolactin is known to affect the breast, and it is suspected to affect the kidneys' ability to excrete water. In 1981 Ylöstalo et al. studied 36 women suffering from PMS, using bromocriptine versus a placebo and norethisterone versus a placebo in a double-blind study. Bromocriptine decreased breast engorgement and irritability, as well as all PMS symptoms in general. These authors noted weight gain during the luteal phase to be smaller in the group treated with either drug than in the placebo group. Norethisterone alleviated breast tenderness and caused a decrease in serum levels of luteinizing hormone (LH), follicle-stimulating hormone (FSH), and progesterone while increasing the serum level of prolactin. Ylöstalo et al. concluded that bromocriptine was more efficient in the treatment of PMS than was norethisterone.

In the same year, Andersch and Hahn studied 34 PMS patients in a double-blind experiment in which patients were given bromocriptine or placebo during the luteal phase of cycles at random, with each patient serving as her own control. Serum prolactin levels were within normal limits without treatment and were significantly reduced by bromocriptine. Serum progesterone levels did not change during any treatment. The administration of any medication (bromocriptine or placebo) considerably improved all the premenstrual symptoms, but results with bromocriptine were not significantly better than with the placebo. These authors concluded that prolactin alone does not seem to cause premenstrual symptoms.

In 1983 Andersch reviewed 14 placebo control studies in which PMS was treated with bromocriptine. Andersch concluded that there was no substantial support that bromocriptine is an effective drug in treating PMS as an entity. He noted that irritability, depression, and anxiety were not significantly improved during treatment with the drug when compared with placebo treatment. The drug, however, was effective in treating premenstrual breast tenderness if the dosage of bromocriptine was above 5 mg per day. He concluded that bromocriptine had a place in the management of PMS only if breast tenderness was a major concern of the patient.

Fluid Retention

For some years fluid retention has been believed to be the single mechanism most likely to be responsible for PMS because fluid retention in the brain could cause mood changes, fluid retention in the breast could cause tenderness, and gastrointestinal symptoms could result from edema of the gastrointestinal tract. It has been difficult, however, to demonstrate relationships between specific symptoms of PMS and luteal phase weight gain. Perceived swelling of the body is difficult to prove unless actual careful weight analysis is utilized. Faratian et al. evaluated 148 menstrual cycles in 52 women, and in each cycle various parameters were measured to determine an objective means of assessing the syndrome. These included daily mood assessment and measurement of body weight, plasma 17β-estradiol levels, and plasma progesterone levels. The abdominal girth was measured carefully in two dimensions: at the level of the umbilicus and at 10 cm below the umbilicus. At the same time these dimensions were subjectively judged by the patient. Mood scores showed a marked shift during the premenstrual phase of each cycle. The symptom of bloatedness was most marked during the premenstrual phase of the cycle. Despite these elevated scores for bloatedness, there was no increase in body weight or measured body dimension changes in any plane during this period. The patient's perception of body size did increase, and a discrepancy between the perceived body size and actual body size was noted. The authors divided their patients into those with predominantly somatic symptoms and those with predominantly psychological symptoms and also studied a control group. No hormonal differences were noted in the three groups.

Sex Steroids

Although sex steroid concentrations in patients with PMS have been quite thoroughly investigated, there is no evidence that these women have impaired corpus luteal function. Estrogen can lead to increased aldosterone levels by stimulating synthesis of angiotensinogen. Progesterone, on the other hand, exerts a natriuretic effect on renal tubules. It is presumed that progesterone blocks aldosterone action at this site. However, if progesterone is given, it causes an increase in aldosterone levels after 48 to 72 hours. This is apparently a compensatory

response to the progesterone-induced sodium loss. Progesterone may be responsible for the observed luteal phase increase in aldosterone, and some authors believe that aldosterone levels are higher in PMS patients who complain of fluid retention. Abraham thinks that this results from vitamin B_6 and magnesium deficiencies and attributes the therapeutic effect of progesterone to its natriuretic effect. If it is accepted that aldosterone levels do increase in PMS, diuretic therapy may have a place.

In a double-blind study, Werch and Kane reported benefit to PMS patients who used a diuretic if the patients had complained of swelling. They suggested that failure of diuretics to relieve symptoms in some PMS patients might relate to patient selection. O'Brien noted that patients treated with the diuretic spironolactone demonstrated decreases in depression, sadness, tension, bloating, loss of libido, aggression, lethargy, and anxiety. Thus, although it is difficult to understand why diuretics alleviate symptoms in certain PMS patients, their success in many cases makes their selective use reasonable.

Prostaglandins

Although prostaglandin substances are definitely related to the symptoms of primary dysmenorrhea, their role in causing symptoms in PMS patients is unclear. In a double-blind, placebo-controlled study, Budoff examined the therapeutic value of one PGSI, zomepirac sodium. The substance reduced by more than half the severity of nine symptoms—cramping, backache, systemic weakness, headache, nausea, leg pain, insomnia, dizziness, and vomiting. In her series there was a strong placebo effect, but the drug proved significantly better than the placebo in relief of all symptoms except insomnia. Of the women in her series, 80% had reportedly missed at least 1 day from their usual activities monthly before therapy. The placebo reduced this loss by 53% and the zomepirac sodium by 77%.

Facchinetti et al. studied naproxen sodium in a double-blind, placebo-controlled, crossover study of 28 women with PMS. They noted that symptoms related to pain that were both premenstrual and menstrual were decreased by the drug but not by the placebo.

It seems likely that some of the symptoms of PMS may be caused by prostaglandin activity or at least are relieved by a PGSI, making it likely that the inclusion of one of these compounds in a treatment regimen of patients with specific symptoms may be useful.

Elevated Monoamine Oxidase (MAO)

One theory of depression is that it may be caused by elevated brain MAO activity and that this may be the result of a deficiency in catecholamines. MAO catalyzes the oxidation of primary amines to aldehydes. Progesterone increases plasma levels of MAO during the luteal phase.

Dalton believes that the cause of PMS lies in a faulty progesterone feedback pathway. Placebo-controlled studies with synthetic progestins have demonstrated little effect in treating PMS symptoms. Dalton favors the use of naturally occurring progesterone for the treatment of PMS and states that the indications for treatment include recurrent symptoms severe enough to interfere with normal activities, risk of suicide, battering or alcoholism, domestic disharmony and stress, and cyclic symptoms after menopause or hysterectomy. She recommends 50 to 100 mg of progesterone daily intramuscularly or 200 to 400 mg daily by progesterone vaginal suppository. Others advocate twice daily vaginal suppositories containing 50 to 100 mg of progesterone each. Dalton begins patients on this regimen 5 days before symptoms are expected and continues until the onset of menses or until the symptoms cease. She notes that in nulliparous women progesterone may cause euphoria, restless energy, insomnia, faintness, and uterine cramps during menstruation. In her patients, symptoms returned 3 months after discontinuation of therapy. She maintains that failure results from improper diagnosis or improper dosage schedule. Such therapy is extremely expensive.

Double-blind studies by Smith and by Sampson failed to show any improvement when progesterone was compared with placebo. Likewise, a randomized, placebo-controlled, double-blind, cross-over study of 168 women suffering from PMS was conducted by Freeman et al. using suppositories containing 400 mg or 800 mg of progesterone or a placebo. No symptoms or cluster of symptoms was relieved significantly by either treatment regimen or the placebo control. There is really no study that supports the use of progesterone for the treatment of PMS.

Endorphins

It has been suggested that increased endorphin levels during the luteal phase inhibit catecholamines and that their abrupt decrease during menses leads to an increase in catecholamine activity. A decrease in catecholamines can be associated with depression, whereas an excess may be associated with irritability, aggression, and even psychotic symptoms. In monkey studies endorphins peak during the luteal phase and fall to imperceptible levels during menses. Cohen et al. administered naloxone, an endorphin antagonist, to volunteers and produced symptoms of irritability, anxiety, tension, and aggressiveness. Progesterone therapy will maintain high levels of endorphin, and this could be a means by which progesterone might be useful in some PMS patients.

Diagnosis

Because the etiology of PMS is still unknown, the diagnosis is made by history. The facts given by the patient may allow the physician to construct a specific treatment regimen for that patient. It is important that the physician have a clear understanding of the patient's symptoms before undertaking therapy. After a complete history and physical examination, the physician should rule out any medical problems that could be influencing the symptomatology. The physician should then ask the patient to keep a diary of her symptoms throughout two menstrual cycles. Although the patient and the physician may focus on the second half of the menstrual cycle, the patient should be encouraged to keep track of all symptoms regardless of the stage of the menstrual cycle. A number of commercial diary sheets and symptom checkoff lists are available, but it is probably better to have the patient write the symptoms she perceives in her own words rather than clue her to specific response patterns. At the end of two cycles the physician should review the symptom diary with the patient and discuss carefully those symptoms that seem to be causing her the most difficulty.

It is important to differentiate PMS from other illnesses with similar symptomatology. Patients with psychiatric disorders, such as different types of depression, anxiety reactions, and psychosis, may present believing that they have PMS. A differentiating aspect is that PMS patients suffer their symptoms *only* during the luteal phase.

No laboratory tests are available to make the diagnosis. Although it has been reported that many patients with PMS suffer thyroid hypofunction, a recent study by Nikolai et al. demonstrated that there was no significant thyroid disease in 44 carefully studied PMS patients compared with 15 normal controls. In addition, treating 22 with L-thyroxine and 22 with placebo led to no differences in relief of symptoms.

The diagnosis of PMS is therefore made by symptom diary and by the elimination of other diagnoses.

Management

Diet and Exercise

The physician should review the patient's diet and initially suggest a high-protein, well-balanced diet. Supplemental vitamins may be used, and the physician may elect to suggest that the patient use a vitamin B_6 (pyridoxine) supplement at the rate of 50 mg per day. It is appropriate to begin with this therapy and add other medications if necessary. The patient should be encouraged to exercise at least 3 to 4 times per week, particularly during the luteal phase.

Diuretics

The physician may elect to add a diuretic to the regimen if the patient's complaints involve bloating and perceived change in body habitus during the luteal phase of the cycle. A potassium-saving diuretic should be selected. The lowest dose possible to achieve symptomatic relief should be used.

Progesterone

Although Dalton advocates the use of naturally occurring progesterone, the fact that progesterone receptors will respond to both synthetic progestins and progesterone implies that any reasonable progestational agent would be appropriate. A regimen of 10 to 30 mg per day of medroxyprogesterone acetate (Provera) or 50 to 100 mg twice a day of progesterone vaginal suppositories can be tried, but to date, no study supports its value.

Some relief of symptoms was noted in a dou-ble-blind, placebo-controlled, cross-over study using estradiol patches (200 micrograms every 3 days) and norethisterone 5 mg (days 19 to 26 of each cycle) when compared with placebo by Watson et al. The authors realized they were suppressing ovulation and that this may have been the mechanism for obtaining symptom relief.

Psychotherapy

Studies in the 1950s showed that 50% of patients improved with psychotherapy alone. However, this is similar to the response rate of many placebo therapies. Certainly if patients have obvious psychiatric problems as detected by history, psychotherapy should be added. It is less effective as a primary therapy.

Psychoactive Drugs

Although continuous use of psychoactive drugs, such as tricyclics and lithium, has not yielded good PMS symptom relief, Smith et al. recently noted in a carefully performed double-blind, placebo-controlled, cross-over study of 19 patients suffering from PMS using alprazolam (Xanax) that the drug significantly relieved the severity of premenstrual nervous tension, mood swings, irritability, anxiety, depression, fatigue, forgetfulness, crying, cravings for sweets, abdominal bloating, cramps, and headaches, compared with the placebo. These investigators prescribed 0.25 mg tid days 20 to 28 of each cycle, tapering to 0.25 mg bid on day 1 and 0.25 mg on day 2. On this regimen in my hands, many patients complain of sleepiness, but 0.25 mg bid and even 0.125 mg bid has proved to be equally effective in many cases. In fact, I usually use 0.25 mg bid days 20 to 28 with one 0.25 mg dose on day 1. Patients with strong tendencies to habituation should not be treated with this regimen.

Other anti-anxiety drugs will probably work as well as alprazolam in the control of PMS symptoms. One such, fluoxetine hydrochloride (Prozac) has been effectively used in several clinics, including mine. Although reports in the literature have not yet appeared, as little as 5 mg of this drug per day, days 20 to 28, seems effective. Fluoxetine hydrochloride should not be given to patients with bipolar depression because it may lead to deepening depression and even suicide.

These newer drugs, however, seem to hold great promise for relieving PMS symptoms when properly used and seem to be required in small doses only.

Danazol

Recently Sarno et al. reported on the apparent effectiveness of danazol in doses of 200 mg qd, days 20 to 28 of each menstrual cycle, in relieving PMS symptoms. Studying 14 patients in a double-blind, placebo-controlled protocol, they found significant relief of symptoms in 11 of the 14 patients, compared with placebo. Because such a small dose given during only the luteal phase will not prevent pregnancy, patients should be cautioned to avoid this agent if pregnancy is contemplated, to avoid the potential of masculinizing a female fetus.

Bromocriptine

Bromocriptine may be used in patients with breast tenderness and may be helpful for some of the other symptoms of PMS, although its use in any individual case will need to be evaluated. A dose of 5 mg per day during the luteal phase is appropriate.

Prostaglandin-Synthetase Inhibitors

For patients who complain of cramping or other systemic symptoms, such as diarrhea or heat intolerance, a trial with a PGSI may be useful. It should be noted, however, that a toxic complication of PGSI use is nonoliguric renal failure. Because it is more likely to occur with PGSI use associated with severe dehydration, the agent should be discontinued if severe diarrhea is present and should not be used with diuretics.

Hysterectomy and Bilateral Oophorectomy

Recently Casper et al. reported complete relief of symptoms in 14 women with severe debilitating symptoms of PMS who had completed their families, had been demonstrated to have relief of symptoms with ovarian-suppressing doses of danazol, and now were treated with total hysterectomy and bilateral oophorectomy followed by continuous low-dose estrogen replacement therapy. Although this approach is not offered as standard therapy for severe PMS, it may be a reasonable alternative for selective cases.

• • •

The physician should be cautious in building a treatment regimen for any individual patient and should attempt to verify the patient's symptoms and to add medications only when relief has not been achieved. Medications that do not seem to be helping should be stopped. Because most agents when scrutinized by double-blind control methods are less than utopian in the treatment of this condition, it is not surprising that individualization of treatment is essential. Some of the newer therapies just mentioned, however, do offer relief of most symptoms and hope for many sufferers.

KEY POINTS

- Primary dysmenorrhea almost always occurs before the age of 20. Secondary dysmenorrhea may occur at any time during the menstrual years.

- Approximately 75% of all women complain of primary dysmenorrhea. Roughly 15% have severe symptoms.

- Pregnancy without vaginal birth does not seem to alleviate primary dysmenorrhea, whereas childbirth does.

- Oral contraceptives reduce the prevalence and severity of dysmenorrhea.

- IUD use does not affect the prevalence or severity of primary dysmenorrhea.

- The severity of primary dysmenorrhea correlates directly with the duration of menstrual flow, amount of menstrual flow, and age at menarche but does not correlate with the duration of the menstrual cycle.

- Among patients who had primary dysmenorrhea, 38% reported onset of symptoms within the first year after menarche.

- Prostaglandin-synthetase inhibitors (PGSIs) are the treatment of choice in primary dysmenorrhea, with 72% of women suffering from dysmenorrhea reporting significant pain relief.

- PGSIs reduced intrauterine pressure 20% to 56% during treatment of patients with dysmenorrhea in one study.

- Approximately 40% of all women suffer considerably from premenstrual syndrome (PMS), with 2% to 3% demonstrating severe symptoms.

- Common historical findings in PMS patients are (1) a history of maternal PMS, (2) low levels of exercise, (3) younger age, and (4) higher parity.

- PMS patients often suffer depression during the luteal phase but not as severe as depression noted by endogenous depression patients when measured by standard depression scales or the amplitude of cortisol secretion pulses.

- PMS patients show no deficit in cognitive function during the luteal phase.

- Bromocriptine is effective primarily in relieving breast tenderness in PMS.

- Although fluid retention–related symptoms are prevalent in patients with PMS, it is difficult to document such retention.

- There is no evidence that women with symptoms of PMS have impaired corpus luteal function.

- The most useful diagnostic tool in caring for PMS patients is a symptom diary.

- There is little objective data to support the concept that vitamin B_6 therapy relieves PMS symptoms.

- There is little objective data to support the concept that progesterone relieves PMS symptoms in most women.

- Recent therapy with psychoactive drugs, such as alprazolam (Xanax) and fluoxetine hydrochloride (Prozac), in relatively small doses given during the luteal phase may be helpful in relieving PMS symptoms. Specific cautions for the use of these agents must be followed.

- In severe cases of PMS involving older women who have completed their families, hysterectomy and bilateral oophorectomy can give symptom relief. Small, constant dosage of estrogen may then be given.

BIBLIOGRAPHY

Abraham GE and Hargrov JT: Effect of vitamin B_6 on premenstrual symptomatology in women with premenstrual tension syndrome: a double blind crossover study, Infertility 3:155, 1980.

Abramson M and Torghele JR: Weight, temperature changes and psychosomatic symptomatology in relation to the menstrual cycle, Am J Obstet Gynecol 81:223, 1961.

Adams PW, Rose DP, Folkard J, et al: Effect of pyridoxine hydrochloride (vitamin B_6) upon depression associated with oral contraception, Lancet 1:897, 1973.

Andersch B: Bromocriptine and premenstrual symptoms. A survey of double blind trials, Obstet Gynecol Surv 38:643, 1983.

Andersch B and Hahn L: Bromocriptine and premenstrual tension: a clinical and hormonal study, Pharmatherapeutica 3:107, 1982.

Andersch B and Milsom I: An epidemiologic study of young women with dysmenorrhea, Am J Obstet Gynecol 144:655, 1982.

Baumann E, Marynick SP, Winters SJ, et al: The effect of osmotic stimuli on prolactin secretion and renal water excretion in normal men and in chronic hyperprolactinemia, J Clin Endocrinol Metab 44:199, 1977.

Bruce J and Russell GFM: Premenstrual tension: a study of weight changes and balances of water, sodium and potassium, Lancet 2:267, 1962.

Budoff PW: Zomepirac sodium in the treatment of primary dysmenorrhea syndrome, N Engl J Med 307:714, 1982.

Casper RF and Hearn MT: The effect of hysterectomy and bilateral oophorectomy in women with severe premenstrual syndrome, Am J Obstet Gynecol 162:105, 1990.

Casson P, Hahn PM, Van Vugt DA, and Reid RL: Lasting response to ovariectomy in severe intractable premenstrual syndrome, Am J Obstet Gynecol 162:99, 1990.

Cohen MR, Cohen RM, Pickar D, et al: Behavioral effect of high dose naloxone administration in normal volunteers, Lancet 1:1110, 1981.

Dalton K: The premenstrual syndrome and progesterone therapy, London, 1977, William Heinemann Medical Books.

Doll H, Brown S, Thurston A, and Vessey M: Pyridoxine (vitamin B_6) and the premenstrual syndrome: a randomized crossover trial, J R Coll Gen Pract 39:364, 1989.

Facchinetti F, Fioroni L, Sances G, et al: Naproxen sodium in the treatment of premenstrual symptoms: a placebo-controlled study, Gynecol Obstet Invest 28:205, 1989.

Faratian B, Gaspar A, O'Brien PM, et al: Premenstrual syndrome, weight, abdominal swelling and perceived body image, Am J Obstet Gynecol 150:200, 1984.

Frank RT: The hormonal causes of premenstrual tension, Arch Neurol Psychol 126:1052, 1931.

Freeman E, Rickels K, Sondheimer SJ, and Polansky M: Ineffectiveness of progesterone suppository treatment for premenstrual syndrome, JAMA 264:349, 1990.

Freeman EW, Sondheimer SJ, and Rickels K: Effects of medical history factors on symptoms severity in women meeting criteria for premenstrual syndrome, Obstet Gynecol 72:236, 1988.

Green R and Dalton K: The premenstrual syndrome, Br Med J 1:1007, 1953.

Halbreich U, Assael M, Ben-David M, et al: Serum prolactin in women with premenstrual syndrome, Lancet 2:654, 1976.

Henzl MR, Ortega-Herrera E, Rodriguez C, and Izu A: Anaprox in dysmenorrhea: reduction of pain in intrauterine pressure, Am J Obstet Gynecol 135:455, 1979.

Herzberg BN: Body composition and premenstrual tension, J Psychosom Res 15:251, 1971.

Israel SL: Premenstrual tension, JAMA 110:172, 1938.

Janowsky DS, Berens SC, and Davis JM: Correlations between mood, weight and electrolyte during the menstrual cycle: renin-angiotensin hypothesis of premenstrual tension, Psychosom Med 35:143, 1973.

Kullander S and Svanberg L: Bromocriptine treatment of the premenstrual syndrome, Acta Obstet Gynecol Scand 58:375, 1979.

Mattes JA and Martin D: Pyridoxine in premenstrual depression, Hum Nutr Appl Nutr 36(2):131, 1982.

Mortola JF, Girton L, and Yen SSC: Depressive episodes in premenstrual syndrome, Am J Obstet Gynecol 161:1682, 1989.

Morton JH, Additon H, Addison RG, et al: A clinical study of premenstrual tension, Am J Obstet Gynecol 65:1182, 1953.

Nikolai TF, Mulligan GM, Gribble RK, et al: Thyroid function and treatment in premenstrual syndrome, J Clin Endocrinol Metab 70:1108, 1990.

O'Brien PM: The premenstrual syndrome: a review of the present status of therapy, Drugs 24:140, 1982.

Owen PR: Prostaglandin synthetase inhibitors in the treatment of primary dysmenorrhea: outcome trials reviewed, Am J Obstet Gynecol 148:96, 1984.

Rapkin AJ, Chang LI, and Reading AE: Mood and cognitive style in premenstrual syndrome, Obstet Gynecol 74:644, 1989.

Reid RL and Yen SSC: Premenstrual syndrome, Am J Obstet Gynecol 139:85, 1981.

Rogers WC: The role of endocrine allergy in the production of premenstrual tension, West J Surg Obstet Gynecol 70:100, 1962.

Rossignol AM and Bonnlander H: Caffeine-containing beverages, total fluid consumption, and premenstrual syndrome, Am J Public Health 80:1106, 1990.

Sampson GA: Premenstrual syndrome: a double blind control trial of progesterone and placebo, Br J Psychiatry 135:209, 1979.

Sarno AP Jr, Miller EJ, and Lundblad EG: Premenstrual syndrome: beneficial effects of periodic, low-dose danazol, Obstet Gynecol 70:33, 1987.

Smith RP: The dynamics of nonsteroidal antiinflammatory therapy for primary dysmenorrhea, Obstet Gynecol 70:785, 1987.

Smith S, Rinehart JS, Ruddock VE, and Schiff I: Treatment of premenstrual syndrome with alprazolam: results of a double-blind, placebo-controlled, randomized crossover clinical trial, Obstet Gynecol 70:37, 1987.

Smith S and Schiff I: The premenstrual syndrome: diagnosis and management, Fertil Steril 52:527, 1989.

Smith SL: Mood and the menstrual cycle. In Sacher EJ, editor: Topics in cycle endocrinology, New York, 1975, Grune & Stratton.

Speroff L and Ramwell P: Prostaglandins in reproductive physiology, Am J Obstet Gynecol 107:1111, 1970.

Stokes J and Mendels J: Pyridoxine and premenstrual tension, Lancet 1:1177, 1972.

Taylor HC: Vascular congestion and hyperemia, their effect on the structure and function in the female reproductive system, Am J Obstet Gynecol 57:211, 1949.

Taylor JW: The timing of menstruation-related symptoms assessed by a daily symptom rating scale, Acta Psychiatr Scand 60:87, 1979.

Watson NR, Studd JWW, Savvas M, et al: Treatment of severe premenstrual syndrome with oestradiol patches and cyclical oral norethisterone, Lancet 2:730, 1989.

Werch A and Kane RE: Treatment of premenstrual tension with metolazone: a double blind evaluation of a new diuretic, Curr Ther Res 19:565, 1976.

Ylikorkala O and Dawood MY: New concepts in dysmenorrhea, Am J Obstet Gynecol 130:833, 1978.

Ylöstalo P, Kauppila A, Puolakka J, et al: Bromocriptine and norethisterone in the treatment of premenstrual syndrome, Obstet Gynecol 58:292, 1982.

Abnormal Uterine Bleeding

————————— KEY TERMS AND DEFINITIONS —————————

Dysfunctional Uterine Bleeding (DUB). Excessive uterine bleeding with no demonstrable organic cause (genital or extragenital). It is most frequently due to abnormalities of endocrine origin, particularly anovulation.

Intermenstrual Bleeding. Bleeding of variable amounts occurring between regular menstrual periods.

Menometrorrhagia. Prolonged uterine bleeding occurring at irregular intervals.

Menorrhagia. Prolonged (more than 7 days) or excessive (greater than 80 ml) uterine bleeding occurring at regular intervals. The term *hypermenorrhea* is synonymous.

Metrorrhagia. Uterine bleeding occurring at irregular but frequent intervals, the amount being variable.

Nonsteroidal Antiinflammatory Drugs (NSAIDs). Drugs that inhibit the synthesis of prostaglandins.

Polymenorrhea. Uterine bleeding occurring at regular intervals of less than 21 days.

Abnormal uterine bleeding can take many forms: infrequent episodes, excessive flow, or prolonged duration of menses and intermenstrual bleeding. Alterations in the pattern or volume of blood flow of menses are among the most common health concerns of women. Infrequent uterine bleeding, defined as *oligomenorrhea* if the intervals between bleeding episodes vary from 35 days to 6 months, and *amenorrhea,* defined as no menses for at least 6 months, are discussed fully in Chapter 36. Excessive or prolonged bleeding will be discussed in this chapter. Recently several new therapeutic modalities have been successfully utilized to treat excessive uterine bleeding, and they will be discussed in this chapter.

To define excessive abnormal uterine bleeding it is necessary to define normal menstrual flow. The mean interval between menses is 28 days (±7 days). Thus if bleeding occurs at intervals of 21 days or less, it is abnormal. The mean duration of menstrual flow is 4 days. Since few women with normal menses bleed more than 7 days, bleeding more than 7 days is considered to be abnormally prolonged (menorrhagia). It is useful to document the duration and frequency of menstrual flow with the use of menstrual diary cards; however, it is difficult to determine the amount of menstrual blood loss (MBL) by subjective means. Several studies have shown that there is poor correlation between subjective judgment and objective measurement of MBL. Hallberg et al. found that 40% of women with blood loss greater than 80 ml considered their menstrual flow to be small or moderate in amount (Figure 35-1), whereas 14% of women with blood loss less than 20 ml thought their menses were heavy. In a study by Chimbira et al, there was also poor correlation between a woman's perception of menstrual blood loss and the actual amount lost. These investigators reported that one third of the menses described as light were more than 80 ml and that about half of those believed to be heavy were less than 80 ml. Determining the number of sanitary pads used is also an unreliable indication of MBL. Grimes found that there is great variability of absorp-

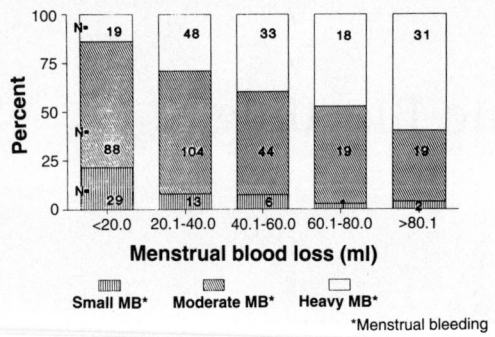

FIGURE 35-1
Subjective judgments of menstrual blood loss.
(From Hallberg L, Högdahl A-M, Nilsson L,
and Rybo G: Acta Obstet Gynecol Scand
45:320, 1966.)

tion among different types of sanitary products
as well as among different devices in the same
package. Fraser et al. reported that the percentage contribution of blood to the total fluid
volume of the menstrual discharge varied extensively among different women, from 1.6%
to 81% with a mean of 36%. Thus the majority
of fluid volume in menstrual discharge is probably derived from endometrial tissue exudate.
These investigators also reported that there
was a very significant correlation between the
total fluid loss and blood loss. Women differ
markedly in their fastidiousness in changing
sanitary products. Thus queries about the passage of blood clots or the degree of inconve-
nience caused by the bleeding are more helpful
than determining the number of pads used in
ascertaining that menorrhagia exists.

Because of the unreliability of subjective assessment, objective methods have been developed to quantify MBL. One method involves
radioisotopic labeling of the patient's red blood
cells. The other, which is the most widely used
technique, involves photometric measurement
to quantify hematin collected onto sanitary
napkins. This alkaline hematin method, originated by Hallberg and Nilsson, has been re-
fined by Newton et al. and van Eijkeren and is
very accurate. Nevertheless the accuracy depends on complete collection of the sanitary
napkins used by the patient. With this technique it has been found in several studies that
the mean amount of MBL in normal women
(women with normal hemoglobin, hematocrit,
and plasma iron) is about 35 ml, with the mean

in various studies ranging from 31 to 44 ml.
About 95% of normal women lose less than an
average of 60 ml of blood during each menses.

In each of these studies of populations of
normal women, there was a wide range of
menstrual blood loss with a marked positive
skewness of the distribution of different volumes (Figure 35-2). In the study by Cole et al.
of 280 women using neither oral contraceptives
nor an IUD, about one third of women lost less
than 20 ml (light) during each menstrual episode, one third lost 20 to 44 ml (medium), and
one third lost more than 45 ml (heavy). These
investigators also reported that there was a significant increase in menstrual blood loss with
increasing parity, but not with age, and that
short women lost less blood than women of
normal or tall height.

Hallberg and Nilsson reported that in normal
women there is little variation in volume of
menstrual blood loss in successive menses of
the same individual (standard deviation [SD],
1.9 ml) during a 1-year period, whereas the
variation between women is great (SD, 15.3
ml) (Figure 35-3). In this study the average loss
of iron in each menses was 13.0 mg. In normal
women about 70% of the total blood loss occurs
during the first 2 days of menses.

Hallberg et al. found that individuals with
blood loss greater than 80 ml have significantly
lower mean hemoglobin, hematocrit, and serum iron levels (Figure 35-4). Therefore an
MBL greater than 80 ml should be regarded as
hypermenorrhea. For practical purposes, if a
patient experiences a change in duration of
flow (e.g., from 3 to 6 days), it must be considered abnormal, even though by definition she
does not have menorrhagia.

Menorrhagia has been reported to occur in
9% to 14 % of healthy women who participated
in the various studies of measurement of
MBL. In women complaining of menorrhagia,
Haynes et al. reported that, as with women
with normal menses, 70% of the blood was
lost within the first 2 days of menses and
92% by the end of the third day. Also, there
was no relation between the number of days
of menstrual bleeding and the total MBL.
The majority of these women with menorrhagia did not have increased duration of
menses but rather had a markedly increased
amount of menstrual flow for the first few days
of menses. Thus the mechanisms responsible
for control of menses are as effective in these

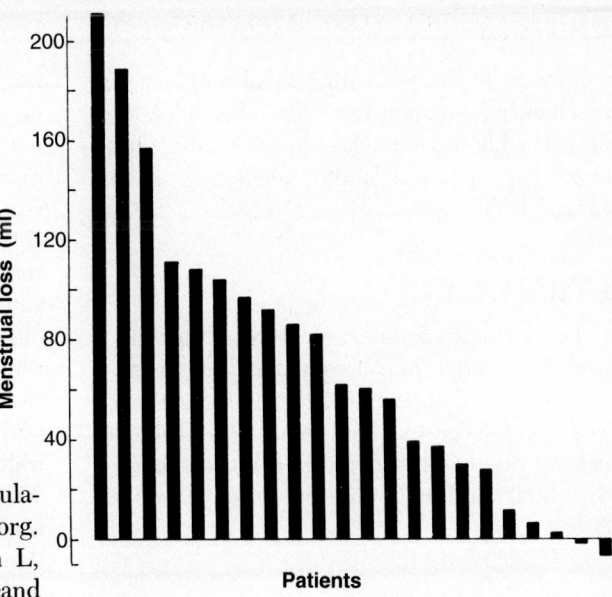

FIGURE 35-2
Distribution of menstrual blood loss in population sample from women living in Göteborg. (From Hallberg L, Högdahl A-M, Nilsson L, and Rybo G: Acta Obstet Gynecol Scand 45:320, 1966.)

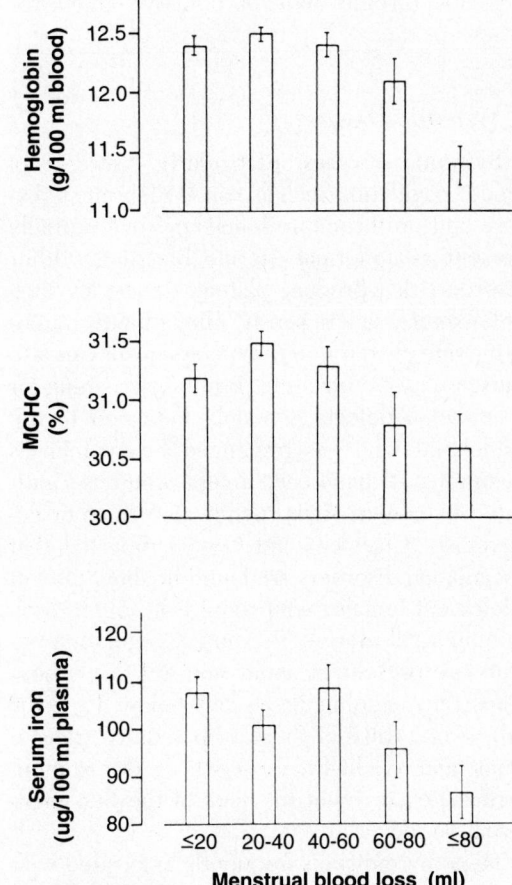

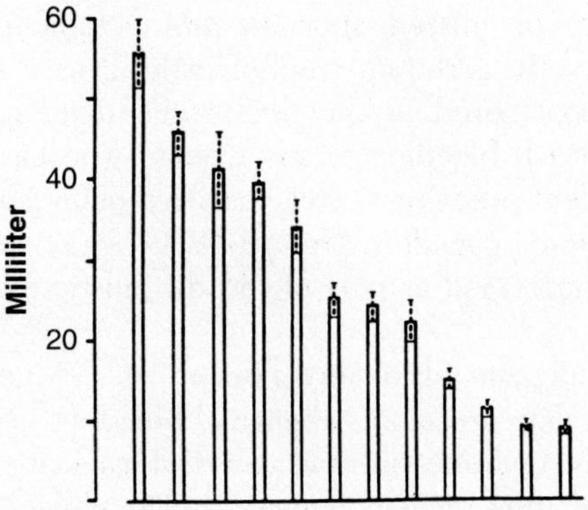

FIGURE 35-3
Menstrual blood loss in 12 subjects. Mean values of 12 periods and standard error of means. (From Hallberg L and Nilsson L: Acta Obstet Gynecol Scand 43:352, 1964.)

FIGURE 35-4
Mean values (±SEM) of hemoglobin concentration, menstrual cycle hematocrit (*MCHC*), and plasma iron concentration in different ranges of menstrual blood loss. (From Hallberg L, Högdahl A-M, Nilsson L, and Rybo G: Acta Obstet Gynecol Scand 45:320, 1966.)

women as in women with normal menses. The mechanisms responsible for the increased menstrual flow are unclear but may result from alterations in prostaglandin metabolism, as discussed later.

ETIOLOGY

The etiology of abnormal uterine bleeding is usually divided into two major categories— organic and dysfunctional (or endocrinologic). The organic causes of abnormal uterine bleeding are discussed in detail in other chapters of this book and will only be briefly outlined here.

Organic Causes

The organic causes can be subdivided into systemic disease and reproductive tract disease.

Systemic Disease

Systemic diseases, particularly disorders of blood coagulation such as von Willebrand's disease and prothrombin deficiency, may initially present as abnormal uterine bleeding. Other disorders that produce platelet deficiency such as leukemia, severe sepsis, idiopathic thrombocytopenic purpura, and hypersplenism can also cause excessive bleeding. Routine screening for coagulation defects is mainly indicated in the adolescent who has prolonged heavy menses beginning at menarche, unless otherwise indicated by clinical signs such as petechiae or ecchymosis. Claessens and Cowell reported that coagulation disorders are found in about 20% of adolescent females who require hospitalization for abnormal uterine bleeding. Coagulation defects are present in about one fourth of those whose hemoglobin levels fall below 10 g/100 ml, in one third of those who require transfusions, and one half of those whose severe menorrhagia occurred at the time of the first menstrual period.

Hypothyroidism is frequently associated with menorrhagia as well as intermenstrual bleeding. Thyroid-stimulating hormone (TSH) should be measured in women with menorrhagia of undetermined etiology. When standard tests of thyroid function are used to diagnose hypothyroidism, the incidence of this disorder among women with menorrhagia has been estimated to

range between 0.3% and 2.5%. Wilansky and Greisman studied 67 clinically euthyroid women with normal serum thyroxine and triiodothyronine levels who had symptoms of severe menorrhagia with a thyrotropin-releasing hormone (TRH) stimulation test. They found that 15 of these women had small but significantly elevated baseline TSH levels as well as significantly elevated TSH responses (>30 mU/L) 30 minutes after TRH infusion. They characterized those women as having early or potential hypothyroidism instead of subclinical hypothyroidism. Treatment of these women with 50 to 200 mg of L-thyroxine daily resulted in normalization of their TSH levels and disappearance of the menorrhagia within 3 to 6 months in all the women treated. If these results are confirmed elsewhere, a sensitive TSH assay and/or a TRH stimulation test should be performed in all women with unexplained menorrhagia. If the test is abnormal, thyroxine therapy is indicated. Although hyperthyroidism is usually not associated with menstrual abnormalities, hypomenorrhea, oligomenorrhea, and amenorrhea have been reported.

Cirrhosis is associated with excessive bleeding secondary to the reduced capacity of the liver to metabolize estrogens. If the patient has hypoprothrombinemia, the tendency toward abnormal bleeding will be increased.

Reproductive Tract Disease

The most common causes of abnormal uterine bleeding during reproductive age are accidents of pregnancy such as threatened, incomplete, or missed abortion and ectopic pregnancy. In addition, trophoblastic disease must be considered in the differential diagnosis of abnormal bleeding in any woman who has had a recent pregnancy, so a sensitive beta–human chorionic gonadotrophin (β-HCG) assay should be performed as part of the diagnostic evaluation.

Malignancies of any portion of the genital tract may present as abnormal bleeding, particularly endometrial and cervical cancer. Less commonly, vaginal, vulvar, and oviductal cancer may produce abnormal bleeding. In addition, rare estrogen-producing ovarian tumors may become manifest by abnormal uterine bleeding. Thus granulosa-theca cell tumors may present with excessive uterine bleeding. Infection of the upper genital tract, particularly endometritis, may present as prolonged menses, although episodic intermenstrual spotting is a more common symptom.

Uterine organic lesions such as submucous myomas, endometrial polyps, and adenomyosis frequently produce symptoms of prolonged and excessive uterine bleeding as well. The mechanisms behind why these lesions cause menorrhagia are unclear. Makarainen and Ylikorkala reported that release of thromboxane and prostacycline from endometrial specimens of normal women and women with menorrhagia associated with leiomyomas was similar. Cervical lesions such as erosions, polyps, and cervicitis may cause irregular bleeding, particularly postcoital spotting. These lesions can usually be diagnosed by visualization of the cervix. In addition, traumatic vaginal lesions, severe vaginal infections, and foreign bodies have been associated with abnormal bleeding.

Foreign bodies in the uterus, such as the IUD, frequently produce abnormal uterine bleeding. Other iatrogenic causes include oral and injectable steroids such as those used for estrogen replacement in the perimenopausal period or for the management of dysmenorrhea, hirsutism, acne, or endometriosis. Tranquilizers may interfere with the neurotransmitters responsible for releasing and inhibiting hypothalamic hormones, thus causing anovulation and abnormal bleeding.

Dysfunctional Causes

After organic, systemic, and iatrogenic causes for the abnormal bleeding are ruled out, the diagnosis of dysfunctional uterine bleeding (DUB) can be made. There are two types of DUB, anovulatory and ovulatory. The predominant cause of DUB in the postmenarcheal and premenopausal years is anovulation secondary to alterations in neuroendocrinologic function. In patients with anovulatory DUB there is continuous estradiol production without corpus luteum formation and progesterone production. The steady state of estrogen stimulation leads to a continuously proliferating endometrium, which may outgrow its blood supply or lose nutrients with varying degrees of necrosis. In contrast to normal menstruation, uniform slough to the basalis layer does not occur, which produces excessive uterine blood flow. Ovulatory DUB occurs most commonly after the adolescent years and before the perimenopausal years.

The incidence of this disorder has been reported to occur in as many as 10% of ovulatory women.

In the past literature, prolonged life of the corpus luteum was reported as a cause for abnormal bleeding (Halban's syndrome). This disorder is associated with a normal-appearing secretory endometrium. It should be differentiated from early pregnancy loss by means of a sensitve serum HCG asssay. Irregular shedding of the endometrium has also been reported to produce menorrhagia. The diagnosis of this disorder is made if a biopsy specimen obtained during the fourth day of the flow reveals both proliferative and secretory endometrium. No recent studies have documented the presence of these two conditions. Thus the prevalence of these disorders, if they actually exist, is uncertain.

In most tissues, following blood vessel damage, the process of hemostasis consists of five actions, some of which occur concomitantly: (1) localized vasoconstriction, (2) platelet adhesion, (3) formation of a platelet plug, (4) reinforcement of the platelet plug with fibrin, and (5) removal of the coagulated material by fibrinolytic mechanisms. The process of hemostasis in the endometrial vessels differs somewhat from the response to vessel damage elsewhere in the body. Morphologic studies by Christiaens et al. have revealed that hemostatic plugs in the endometrium are smaller, have a different morphologly, and persist for a shorter time than those in other tissues.

These investigators found that there are two mechanisms for hemostasis during menstruation. The first, hemostatic plug formation, is the most important mechanism in the functional endometrium. The second, vasoconstriction, is more important in the basalis layer. Since vascular occlusion by both mechanisms is never total, blood leakage continues for several days until endometrial regeneration is completed.

Sheppard et al. performed ultrastructural studies of samples of menstrual fluid obtained from the uterine cavity and vagina of 10 women with normal menses and 10 women with DUB. Fibrin and platelets were found in nearly all samples. No differences were found in the morphology of fibrin and platelets in the samples collected from the two groups of women. Rees et al. reported that there was no significant difference in amounts of coagulation factors or fibrinolytic proteins in the menstrual fluid of women with normal blood loss compared with those with menorrhagia.

Hahn and Rybo reported that there was no difference in the concentrations of fibrinogen-fibrin degradation products in menstrual blood samples obtained form normal women and those with menorrhagia. Rees et al. reported no difference in clotting factors in menstrual fluid between the two groups of women.

Rees et al. performed a histologic study of the endometrium and myometrium in uteri removed by hysterectomy from women with normal and excessive amounts of uterine bleeding. No pathologic findings were found in the specimens. These investigators found no correlation between menstrual blood loss and endometrial and myometrial arterial density and endometrial glandular density. Thus menorrhagia in the absence of pathologic findings does not result from an excessive number of arteries or abnormal distribution of the endometrial glands.

With the discovery that prostaglandins are involved with the regulation of vasodilation and vasoconstriction as well as the clotting process, numerous studies were conducted in the 1980s in which various prostaglandins and their metabolites were measured in endometrial and myometrial samples obtained from normal women and women with menorrhagia. The majority of the studies were performed by two groups in Britain, one in Oxford and the other in Edinburgh, and sometimes the results were contradictory because of differences in methodology. Since PGE_2 produces vasodilation while $PGF_{2\alpha}$ increases vasoconstriction, and thromboxane promotes platelet aggregation while prostacycline inhibits this process, most of the studies measured these prostaglandins or their metabolites. In women with regular ovulatory cycles with normal menstrual blood loss, there was an increase in the amount of both $PGF_{2\alpha}$ and PGE_2 found in the endometrium in the late secretory phase and during menses, with the endometrial $PGF_{2\alpha}/PGE_2$ ratio steadily increasing from midcycle to menses.

Smith et al. found that the levels of $PGF_{2\alpha}$ in persistently proliferative endometria obtained from women with anovulatory DUB were lower than the levels in women with normal secretory endometria. They theorized that progesterone was necessary to increase levels of arachidonic acid, the precursor of $PGF_{2\alpha}$, while estradiol stimulates synthesis of pros-

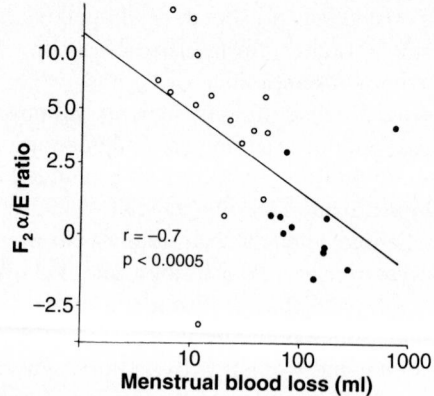

FIGURE 35-5
Correlation between ratio of endogenous concentrations of $PGF_{2\alpha}$ and PGE and menstrual blood loss (MBL). ○, Normal secretory endometrium; ●, persistent proliferative endometrium. (From Smith SK, Abel MH, Kelly RW, and Baird DT: J Clin Endocrinol Metab 55:284, 1982.)

taglandins from arachidonic acid by cyclic endoperoxides. With the absence of progesterone in anovulatory cycles, there are reduced levels of $PGF_{2\alpha}$ with normal levels of PGF_2, resulting in a decreased $PGF_{2\alpha}/PGE_2$ ratio. Since $PGF_{2\alpha}$ binds to receptors in the spiral arteries in the late secretory phase to cause vasoconstriction and control menstrual flow, decreased levels of $PGF_{2\alpha}$ could cause heavier and/or more prolonged bleeding.

These investigators found there was an inverse correlation between the endometrial $PGF_{2\alpha}/PGE$ ratio and the amount of menstrual blood loss (Figure 35-5). $PGF_{2\alpha}$ also stimulates contraction of the smooth muscle cells in the myometrium, and elevated levels of $PGF_{2\alpha}$ are found in the menstrual blood of women with dysmenorrhea. Anovulatory cycles are usually not associated with dysmenorrhea, probably because of the reduced levels of $PGF_{2\alpha}$. Progesterone treatment of women with anovulatory DUB rapidly reduces the amount of menstrual blood loss, probably by stimulating production of arachidonic acid, the precursor of $PGF_{2\alpha}$.

Circulating levels of reproductive hormones are not different in women with ovulatory DUB and those with normal cycles. Various investigators have shown that the increased MBL in women with ovulatory DUB is also associated with reduced uterine synthesis of $PGF_{2\alpha}$

and an increase in synthesis of PGE_2 and prostacycline.

Furthermore, Adelantado et al. reported that PGE receptor concentrations in the myometrium of hysterectomy specimens were significantly greater in women with unexplained ovulatory menorrhagia than in women with normal MBL. Also, there was a direct correlation between the concentration of myometrial PGE receptor concentration and MBL.

Makarainen and Ylikorkala reported that the ratio of release of thromboxane to the metabolite of prostaglandin in endometrial biopsy specimens was inversely related to the amount of MBL in a group of women with menorrhagia. They concluded that the menorrhagia could be due in part to a relative deficiency of thromboxane in the endometrium.

Booney et al. recently reported that there was a significantly greater amount of phospholipase C, but not phospholipase A_2 types 1 and 2, in the endometrium of women with ovulatory menorrhagia. Phospholipases release arachidonic acid from cell membrane phospholipids. Several investigators have reported that there is an increased availability of arachidonic acid in the endometrium of women with ovulatory menorrhagia, in contrast to the decreased amount of this substance in the endometrium of women with anovulatory DUB.

Thus alterations in prostaglandin synthesis and release appear to occur in women with both anovulatory as well as ovulatory DUB. The reasons why these changes occur and their exact causal relation with menorrhagia have not yet been determined.

DIAGNOSIS

When a patient presents with a complaint of abnormal bleeding, it is essential to take a thorough history regarding the frequency, duration, and amount of bleeding, as well as to inquire whether and when the menstrual pattern has changed. This history is extremely important to determine whether the menstrual abnormality is polymenorrhea, menorrhagia (hypermenorrhea), metrorrhagia, menometrorrhagia, or intermenstrual bleeding. Providing the patient with a calender to record her bleeding episodes is a very helpful way to characterize definitively the bleeding episodes. Since there is a poor correlation between a patient's estimate of the amount of blood flow and the measured loss, as well as great variation in the amount of blood and fluid absorbed by different types of sanitary napkins and in the same type of napkin in different individuals, objective criteria should be used to determine if menorrhagia (blood loss more than 80 ml) is present.

Since direct measurement of MBL is not generally available, indirect assessment by measurement of hemoglobin concentration, serum iron levels, and serum ferritin levels is useful. Serum ferritin provides a valid assessment of iron stores in the bone marrow. Additional useful laboratory tests include a sensitive HCG determination, a sensitive TSH assay, and perhaps a TRH stimulation test. For adolescent patients, as well as older women with systemic disease, a coagulation profile should be performed to rule out a coagulation defect. If the woman has regular cycles, it is important to determine whether she is ovulating by obtaining a luteal phase serum progesterone measurement, a daily basal body temperature, or a prementsrual sampling of the endometrium.

In those patients who are ovulating and have menorrhagia, it is important to rule out the presence of a uterine lesion such as a endometrial polyp, submucous leiomyoma, or carcinoma by performing an endocervical curettage, pelvic sonography with a vaginal probe (which also permits measurement of the endometrial thickness), and hysterosalpingography or hysteroscopy. Hysteroscopy, which can be performed in the office or clinic setting with local anesthesia even when the patient is bleeding, is a more accurate diagnostic procedure than a dilation and curettage (D&C). Therefore hysteroscopy should be utilized in all women who have ovulatory menorrhagia to determine if endometrial pathology exists. D&C is a blind technique and does not always detect focal lesions. It has been estimated that D&C misses the diagnosis in 10% to 25% of patients. In a comparison of panoramic hysteroscopy with endometrial biopsy and D&C in a group of 342 women, Gimpelson and Rappold found that hysteroscopy permitted the accurate diagnosis in 60 patients in whom the diagnosis was not made by D&C. Most of these patients had the diagnosis of submucous myomas and endometrial polyps made by hysteroscopy and missed by D&C. March reported that one fourth of patients with a presumptive diagnosis of DUB were found to have uterine lesions at the time of hysteroscopy. Following the diagnosis of a uterine lesion, it is then usually possible to resect the polyp or submucous leiomyoma by operative hysteroscopy.

MANAGEMENT

In the absence of an organic cause for excessive uterine bleeding, it is preferable to use medical instead of surgical treatment, especially if the patient desires to retain her uterus for future childbearing or will be undergoing natural menopause within a short period of time. There are several effective medical methods for treatment of DUB. These include estrogens, progestins (delivered systemically or locally), nonsteroidal antiinflammatory agents, antifibrinolytic agents, danazol, and gonadotrophin-releasing hormone (GnRH) agonists. The type of treatment utilized depends on whether it is used to stop an acute heavy bleeding episode or whether it is given to reduce the amount of MBL in subsequent menstrual cycles. Before instituting long-term treatment, definitive diagnosis is warranted and should be made on the basis of hysteroscopy and directed endometrial biopsies, with definitive treatment determined by the diagnosis.

Estrogens

The rationale for the therapeutic use of estrogen for the treatment of DUB is based on the fact that estrogen in pharmacologic doses causes rapid growth of the endometrium. The bleeding that results from most causes of DUB will respond to such therapy because a rapid growth of endometrial tissue occurs over the denuded and raw epithelial surfaces. To control an acute bleeding episode, the use of oral conjugated estrogen (CE) in a dose of 10 mg a day, administered in four divided doses, is a therapeutic regimen that has been found to be clinically useful. Acute bleeding from most causes is usually controlled by this method. If bleeding is not controlled within the first 24 hours with this dose of estrogen, higher doses of CE (20 mg) may be effective; however, consideration must be given to the fact that an organic cause, such as an accident of pregnancy, may be the cause of the bleeding, and curettage should usually be performed.

Intravenous administration of estrogen is also effective in the acute treatment of menorrhagia. DeVore et al. reported that, compared with women given a placebo, a significantly greater percentage of women had cessation of bleeding 2 hours after the second of two 25 mg doses of conjugated equine estrogens (CEE) were administered intravenously 3 hours apart. There was no significant difference in cessation of bleeding between women administered estrogen and those given a placebo 3 hours after the first infusion. This study indicates that at least several hours are required to induce mitotic activity and growth of the endometrium, whether the estrogen is administered orally or parenterally. Thus intravenous estrogen therapy accompanied by its rapid metabolic clearance does not appear to offer a significant advantage compared with the same dose of estrogen given orally.

Livio et al. reported that 6 hours after infusion of an average dose of 30 mg of CEE to individuals with a prolonged bleeding time due to renal failure, the bleeding time was significantly shortened. In this study, measurements of various clotting factors were unchanged after CEE infusion. Therefore the mechanism whereby intravenous CEE controls bleeding is unknown. No studies indicate that intravenous estrogen acts quicker or is more effective than high doses of oral estrogen. The latter route of administration is less costly, is easier to administer, and therefore is preferred.

Usually estrogen therapy reduces the amount of uterine bleeding within the first 24 hours after treatment is initiated. However, because most patients with an acute heavy bleeding episode bleed because of anovulation, progestin treatment is also required. Therefore, after bleeding has ceased, oral estrogen therapy is continued at the same dosage, and a progestin, usually medroxyprogesterone acetate (MPA) 10 mg once a day, is added. Both hormones are administered for another 7 to 10 days, after which treatment is stopped to allow withdrawal bleeding, which may have an increased amount of flow but is rarely prolonged because estrogen therapy controls only the acute bleeding episode and is not curative. Before instituting long-term treatment following the withdrawal bleeding episode, one of several alternate treatment modalities should be used.

A more convenient regimen to stop acute bleeding than the sequential high-dose estrogen-progestin regimen is the use of a combination oral contraceptive containing both estrogen and progestin. Four tablets of an oral contraceptive containing 50 μg of estrogen taken every 24 hours in divided doses will usually provide sufficient estrogen to stop acute bleeding and simultaneously provide progestin. Treatment is continued for at least 1 week after the bleeding stops. This regimen is successful and convenient and is thus the preferred method of some clinicians. However, in one study it was found not to be as effective as the use of high doses of CE. A theoretical reason for this difference might be the fact that the combined use of estrogen and progestin does not afford as rapid endometrial growth as estrogen alone, because the progestin decreases the synthesis of estrogen receptors and increases estradiol dehydrogenase in the endometrial cell, thus inhibiting the growth-promoting action of estrogen.

Progestins

Progestins, therefore, not only stop endometrial growth but also support and organize the endometrium in such a way that an organized slough occurs after their withdrawal. In the absence of progesterone, erratic unorganized breakdown of the endometrium occurs. With progesterone or progestin treatment, an organized slough to the basalis layer allows a rapid cessation of bleeding. In addition, progestins stimulate arachidonic acid formation in the endometrium, increasing the $PGF_{2\alpha}/PGE$ ratio. Thus progestins usually do not stop the acute bleeding episode but produce a normal bleeding episode following their withdrawal.

Anovulatory patients are difficult to treat, and a prolonged regimen of progestins may be administered for 14 to 21 days each month so that the amount of withdrawal bleeding will be reduced. Fraser reported that administration of two oral progestins, norethindrone and MPA, in high doses of 5 to 10 mg three times a day, significantly reduced MBL by 40% to 50% in women with both ovulatory and anovulatory DUB. In women with ovulatory DUB the progestins were given from cycle days 12 to 25, whereas the anovulatory group received progestins from days 5 to 25. Prolonged use of these high doses of progestins may cause unpleasant adverse effects, including tiredness, mood changes, and weight gain, as well as unfavorably alter the lipid profile. To eliminate these effects, local administration of progestins can be utilized.

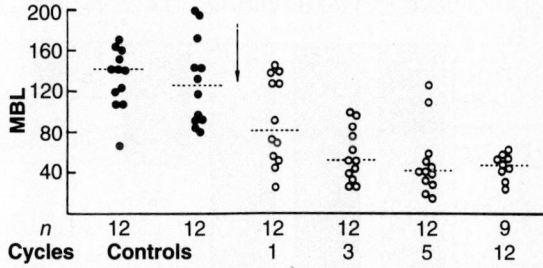

FIGURE 35-6
Menstrual blood loss (MBL) before and after insertion of Progestasert (*arrow*) in menorrhagic women. (Each dot marks a separate patient, and the median value is marked with a line.) (From Bergqvist A and Rybo G: Br J Obstet Gynaecol 90:255, 1983.)

The progesterone-releasing IUD has been found to be effective in the treatment of women with ovulatory DUB. Bergqvist and Rybo inserted this device into 12 women with ovulatory DUB and found their MBL declined from an average of 138 ml to 49 ml in 1 year, a 65% reduction in MBL (Figure 35-6). This device needs to be reinserted annually because of the rapid diffusion of progesterone through polysiloxone.

A levonorgestrol-releasing IUD has been developed that has an effective duration of action of more than 7 years. Milson et al. studied use of this IUD as treatment for menorrhagia and found that at the end of 3 months it caused an average 80% reduction in MBL, which increased to 100% at the end of 1 year. This reduction in MBL was significantly greater than that achieved with either an antifibrinolytic agent or a prostaglandin synthetase inhibitor in studies by the same investigators (Figure 35-7).

Progestin therapy is ultimately the treatment of choice for the majority of patients with anovulatory DUB, as already mentioned. However, progestin therapy usually does not stop the acute bleeding episode as effectively as estrogen and is warranted for long-term treatment of patients only after the acute episode of bleeding has been controlled.

MPA in a dose of 10 mg daily for 10 days each month is a successful therapeutic regimen that produces regular withdrawal bleeding in patients with adequate amounts of endogenous estrogen to cause endometrial growth. Although other progestins have been used, MPA does not alter serum lipids as much as the 19-

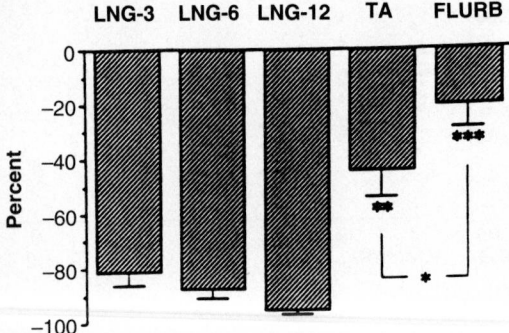

FIGURE 35-7
Reduction in menstrual blood loss (MBL) expressed as percentage of mean of two control cycles for each form of treatment. Significance of difference between treatment with levonorgestrel-releasing IUD (*LNG*) and tranexamic acid (*TA*) and flurbiprofen (*FLURB*) indicated by double asterisks (*P* < 0.01) and triple asterisks (*P* < 0.001) and between treatment with tranexamic acid and flurbiprofen indicated by asterisk (*P* < 0.05). (From Milson I, Andersson K, Andersch B, and Rybo G: Am J Obstet Gynecol 164:879, 1991.)

nortestosterone derivatives and thus may have fewer adverse long-term effects. Progestins are beneficial, since in pharmacologic doses they act as antiestrogens. They diminish the effect of estrogen on target cells by inhibiting estrogen receptor replenishment in the cell and induce the activation of 17-hydroxysteroid dehydrogenase, which converts estradiol to the less active estrone. These findings account for the antimitotic, antigrowth effect of the progestins and support the rationale for its use in the treatment of unopposed estrogen and endometrial hyperplasia.

Adolescent anovulatory patients represent an ideal model for the use of progestins in the treatment of DUB. These patients exhibit immaturity of the hypothalamic-pituitary axis, and progestin therapy for 10 days every month is a reasonable mode of treatment that is highly successful and produces regular cyclic withdrawal bleeding until maturity of the positive feedback system is achieved. This therapy does not interfere with the normal resumption of ovulatory cycles. Although controversial, it is probably best that these patients do not use oral contraceptives, since this therapy prolongs hypothalamic-pituitary inhibition and may delay the maturation of the hypothalamic-pitu-

itary axis. In women of reproductive age who have DUB, long-term use of oral contraceptives is acceptable after the acute bleeding episode is controlled unless the patient wishes to conceive, in which case cyclic treatment with clomiphene citrate should be used.

The major therapeutic use of progestins is to treat anovulatory patients for 10 days each month. However, because progestins have a profound effect on inhibiting endometrial growth and inducing atrophic changes, a therapeutic trial with these agents may be used in patients with menorrhagia who also ovulate.

Nonsteroidal Antiinflammatory Drugs

Nonsteroidal antiinflammatory drugs (NSAIDs) are prostaglandin synthetase inhibitors that inhibit the biosynthesis of the cyclic endoperoxides, which convert arachidonic acid to prostaglandins. In addition, these agents block the action of prostaglandins by interfering directly at their receptor sites.

To decrease bleeding of the endometrium, it would be ideal to block selectively the synthesis of prostacyclin alone, without decreasing thromboxane formation, as the latter increases platelet aggregation. Presently there are no NSAIDs that possess this ability. All NSAIDs are cyclooxygenase inhibitors and thus block the formation of both thromboxane and the prostacyclin pathway. Nevertheless, NSAIDs have been shown to reduce MBL, primarily in patients who ovulate. However, a complete understanding of the mechanisms whereby prostaglandin inhibitors reduce MBL is still undetermined, and their therapeutic action may take place through some as yet undiscovered mechanism. Several NSAIDs have been administered during menses to groups of women with menorrhagia and ovulatory DUB and have been found to reduce effectively mean MBL by about 20% to 50% (Figure 35-8).

Drugs and dosages in studies include mefenamic acid, 500 mg three times a day; ibuprofen, 400 mg three times a day; meclofenamate sodium, 100 mg three times a day; and naproxen sodium, 275 mg every 6 hours after a loading dose of 550 mg, as well as other NSAIDs. These drugs are usually given for the first 3 days of menses or throughout the bleeding episode, and they appear to have a similar level of effectiveness.

Not all women treated have reduction in blood flow, but those without a decrease usually have only a mildly increased amount of MBL with these agents. The greatest amount of MBL reduction occurs in the women with the greatest pretreatment blood loss. Fraser et al. reported that treatment of menorrhagia with mefenamic acid in 36 women for more than 1 year resulted in a significantly sustained reduction in amounts of MBL and a significant increase in serum ferritin. Thus this therapy can be used for long-term treatment because side effects, mainly gastrointestinal, are mild with this intermittent therapy.

To date, there have been very few studies comparing NSAIDs with other treatment modalities. It appears, however, that the beneficial reduction in MBL with NSAIDs occurs primarily in patients who ovulate. Furthermore the degree of reduction of MBL with NSAIDs in noncomparative studies is similar to that reported for the use of either antifibrinolytic agents or oral contraceptives alone.

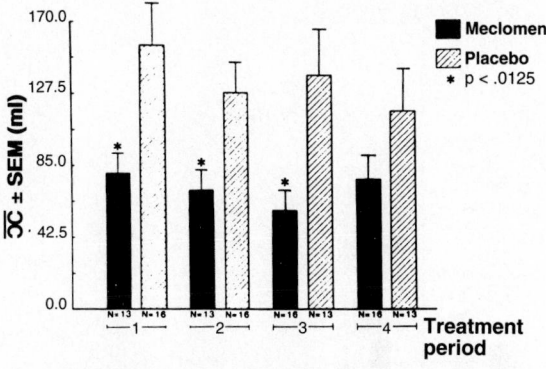

FIGURE 35-8
Menstrual blood loss (MBL) by treatment period and drug. (From Vargyas JM, Campeau JD, and Mishell DA: Am J Obstet Gynecol 157:944, 1987.)

Although NSAIDs are used by themselves to treat patients with MBL who ovulate, they can also be given in combination with oral contraceptives or progestins. With this combined approach, reduction in MBL can be achieved more effectively than with use of any of these agents by themselves.

Antifibrinolytic Agents

Epsilon-aminocaproic acid (EACA), tranexamic acid (AMCA), and para-aminomethylbenzoic acid (PAMBA) are potent inhibitors of fibrinolysis and have, therefore, been used in the treatment of various hemorrhagic conditions. Nilsson and Rybo compared the effect on blood loss of EACA, AMCA, and oral contraceptives in 215 women with menorrhagia. EACA was given in a dose of 18 g per day for 3 days and then 12, 9, 6, and 3 g daily on successive days. The total dose was always at least 48 g. AMCA was administered in a dose of 6 g per day for 3 days followed by 4, 3, 2, and 1 g daily on successive days. The total dose of AMCA was at least 22 g. There was a significant reduction in blood loss after treatment with EACA, AMCA, and oral contraceptives, and use of each of these agents resulted in about a 50% reduction in MBL (Table 35-1). Of interest was the finding that the greatest reduction in blood loss with antifibrinolytic therapy occurred in women who exhibited the greatest MBL. The side effects of this class of drugs in decreasing order of frequency are nausea, dizziness, diarrhea, headaches, abdominal pain, and allergic manifestations. These side effects are much more common with EACA than with AMCA. Other investigators have compared use of AMCA to placebo in double-blind studies and

TABLE 35-1
Mean Menstrual Blood Loss and Reduction with Treatment with EACA, AMCA, Oral Contraceptives, and Methylergobaseimmaleate

	Mean Blood Loss (ml)		% Decrease
	Before Treatment	After Treatment	
EACA	164	87	47
AMCA	182	84	54
Oral contraceptives	158	75	52
Methylergobaseimmaleate	164	164	0

Adapted from Nilsson L and Rybo G: Treatment of menorrhagia, Am J Obstet Gynecol 110:713, 1971.

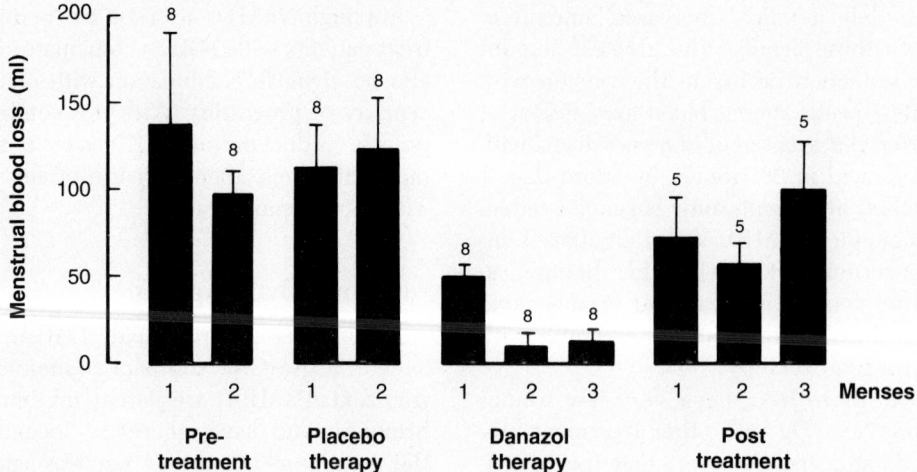

FIGURE 35-9
Mean (±SEM) menstrual blood loss in eight patients with menorrhagia before treatment, with placebo therapy, with 200 mg danazol daily, and after treatment. Number of patients is shown above each histogram. (From Chimbria TH, Anderson ABM, Naish C, et al: Br J Obstet Gynaecol 87:1152, 1980.)

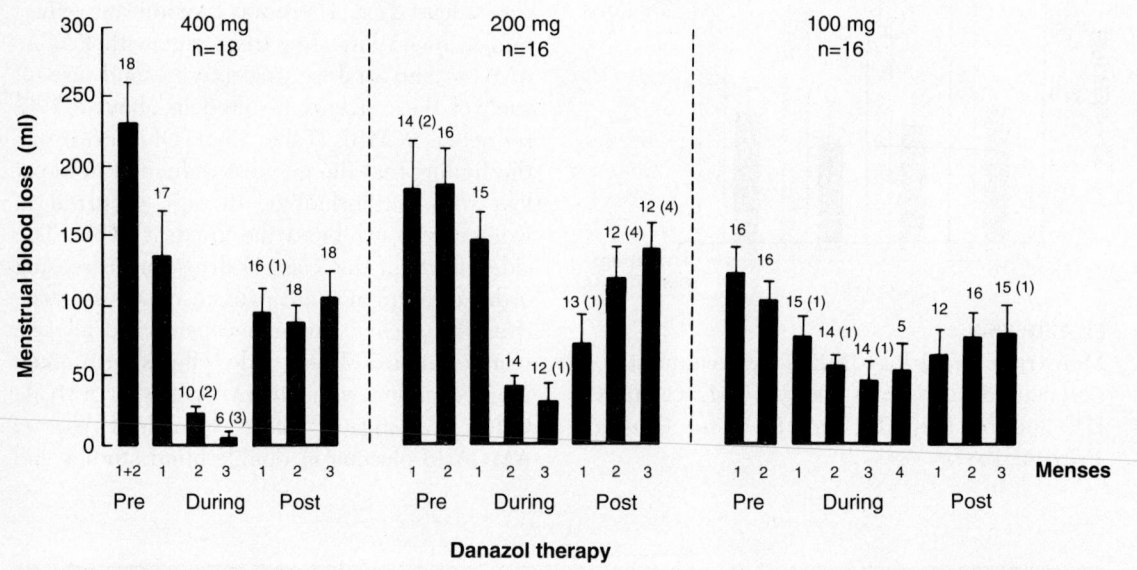

FIGURE 35-10
Mean (±SEM) menstrual blood loss in three groups of patients with menorrhagia treated with 400, 200, or 100 mg danazol daily for 12 weeks. Menstrual blood loss measurements are shown for each group before, during, and after danazol therapy. Number of patients menstruating is shown above each histogram, with number of missing menstrual loss collections in parentheses. (Adapted from Chimbria TH, Anderson ABM, Naish C, et al: Br J Obstet Gynaecol 87:1152, 1980.)

have found no significant differences in the occurrence of side effects. Renal failure and pregnancy are contraindications to the use of antifibrinolytic agents.

Antifibrinolytic agents clearly produce a reduction in blood loss and may be used as therapy for patients with menorrhagia who ovulate. However, their use is somewhat limited by the side effects. Furthermore, as with NSAIDs, they are best combined with another agent such as oral contraceptives for a greater effect on MBL reduction.

Ergot

Ergot derivatives are not recommended for therapy because they are rarely effective and have a high incidence of side effects (nausea, vertigo, abdominal cramps). Nilsson and Rybo demonstrated no reduction in blood loss among 82 women with menorrhagia who were treated with methylergobaseimmaleate (Table 35-1).

Androgenic Steroids (Danazol)

In recent years, the androgenic steroid that has proved most useful in the treatment of DUB is danazol. Danazol has been used by several investigators for the treatment of menorrhagia. Doses of 200 and 400 mg daily have been given over 12 weeks after careful pretreatment observation and evaluation. MBL was markedly reduced in these studies from more than 200 ml to less than 25 ml. Also, there was an increased interval between bleeding episodes (Figure 35-9). The most common side effects of danazol treatment are weight gain and skin disorders such as acne. Reduction of dosage from 400 to 200 mg daily decreased the side effects but did not affect the reduction in blood loss (Figure 35-10). Some patients may ovulate when receiving this dose of danazol. Further reduction to 100 mg daily did not effectively reduce MBL in most patients. Although danazol is effective, it is also expensive and has moderate side effects.

Dockeray et al. treated 40 women with DUB, half with menfenamic acid, 500 mg three times a day for 3 to 5 days of menses, and half with danazol, 100 mg twice a day for 60 days. Danazol was more effective in reducing MBL, 60% compared with 20% for mefenamic acid (Figure 35-11). However, adverse side effects were more severe with danazol and occurred in 75% of patients, compared with side effects in only 30% of patients treated with mefenamic acid.

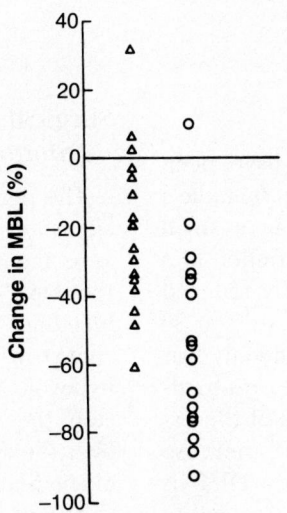

FIGURE 35-11

Percentage change in menstrual blood loss (MBL) between pretreatment cycles 1 and 2 and treatment cycles 3 and 4 shown for individual women treated with (Δ) mefenamic acid or (○) danazol. Mean % change is −22.3% in the mefenamic acid group and −56.0% in the danazol-treated group. (From Dockeray CJ, Sheppard BL, and Bonnard J: Br J Obstet Gynaecol 96:840, 1989.)

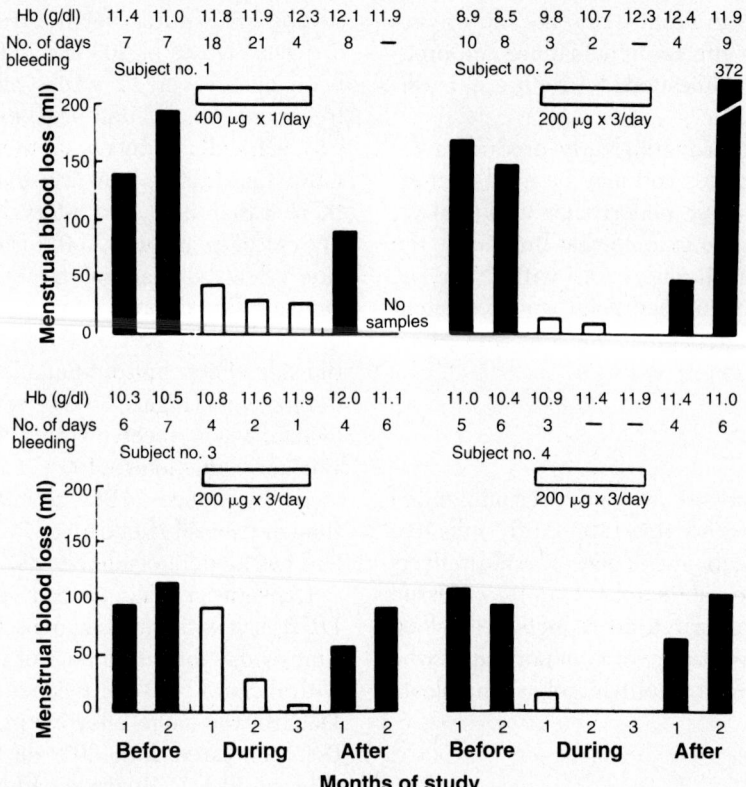

FIGURE 35-12

Alterations in measured monthly menstrual blood losses, number of days of menstrual bleeding, and hemoglobin estimates before, during, and after therapy with intranasal luteinizing hormone–releasing hormone (LHRH) agonist. (From Shaw RW and Fraser HM: Br J Obstet Gynaecol 9:913, 1984.)

GnRH Agonists

Although no large-scale studies have been performed, it is possible to induce a medical menopause with GnRH agonists. In a small study of four women, daily administration of a GnRH agonist for 3 months markedly reduced MBL from 100 to 200 ml per cycle to 0 to 30 ml per cycle. Unfortunately, after therapy was discontinued, blood loss returned to pretreatment levels (Figure 35-12). Because of the expense and side effects of these agents, their use for menorrhagia caused by ovulatory DUB is limited to women with severe MBL who fail to respond to other methods of medical management and wish to retain their childbearing capacity. Use of an estrogen and/or progestin ("add back" therapy) together with the agonist will help prevent bone loss.

Surgical Therapy
Dilation and Curettage

The performance of a D&C can be both diagnostic and therapeutic. For patients with severe menorrhagia who may be hypovolemic, the D&C is the quickest way to stop acute bleeding. Therefore it is the treatment of choice in women with DUB who suffer from hypovolemia. A D&C should also be utilized to stop the acute bleeding episode in patients over the age of 35 when the incidence of pathologic findings increases.

The use of D&C for the treatment of DUB has been reported to be curative in only a minority of patients. Temporary cure of the problem may occur in some patients with chronic anovulation, since the curettage removes much of the hyperplastic endometrium; however, the underlying pathophysiologic cause is unchanged. A D&C has not proved useful for treatment of patients who ovulate and have menorrhagia. More than 1 month after the D&C, Nilsson and Rybo have shown that there was either no difference or an increase in MBL in patients who ovulate.

Therefore D&C is only indicated for patients with acute bleeding resulting in hypovolemia, and for older patients who are at higher risk of having endometrial neoplasia. All other patients, after having an endometrial biopsy and hysteroscopy to rule out organic disease, are best managed by medical therapy as outlined earlier without a D&C.

Endometrial Ablation

Laser photovaporization of the endometrium for treatment of menorrhagia was originally reported by Goldrath et al. in 1981. Photovaporization of the endometrium was performed by use of a neodymium-YAG laser with hysteroscopic visualization. Patients were treated with danazol 800 mg per day for 2 to 3 weeks before the procedure, and an additional 2 weeks of danazol treatment was given afterwards. This procedure was curative in 160 of 180 patients, and follow-up biopsies showed no evidence of inflammation other than foreign body giant cells secondary to the carbon particles left after laser treatment. There was minimum endometrial regeneration. Photovaporization causes varying degrees of uterine contraction, scarring, and adhesion formation, as demonstrated by follow-up hysterosalpingograms and hysteroscopy.

Recently a large prospective 3-year multicenter study with this technique was reported by Garry et al. A total of 859 women with menorrhagia, most with ovulatory DUB, were enrolled. After producing endometrial atrophy with at least 1 month of 600 mg danazol daily or a GnRH agonist, the endometrium was ablated with a Nd-YAG laser inserted through a hysteroscope. Complications were uncommon and minor: 0.4% fluid overload, 0.4% infection, and 0.3% uterine perforation. No major hemorrhage requiring a transfusion or lapartomy occurred. The mean duration of the procedure was 24 minutes. Of the 479 women followed for 6 months, 60% had amenorrhea, 32% had a

TABLE 35-2

Clinical Results Following Endometrial Ablation with Nd-YAG Laser in 479 Menorrhagic Women

Clinical Result	No. (%) of Women
Amenorrhea	288 (60%)
Reduced menses	151 (32%)
First failure	39 (8%)
Subsequent success	26 (5%)
Hysterectomy	13 (3%)

From Garry R, Erian J, and Grochmal SA: Br J Obstet Gynaecol 98:357, 1991.

satisfactorily reduced amount of menses, and 8% had no reduction, requiring a second treatment (Table 35-2). Most of the latter responded to a second treatment, and only 3% required a hysterectomy.

Because the Nd-YAG laser is expensive, others have ablated the endometrium with electrocautery delivered by a urologic resectoscope placed through a hysteroscope. Magos et al. utilized this technique in 16 women and produced amenorrhea in 6 and reduced MBL in the remainder (Figure 35-13).

In 1989 Vancaillie reported that thermal destruction of the endometrium could be accomplished easily and rapidly with electrocautery applied through a ball-end electrode attached to a urologic resectoscope. The ball-end electrode has several advantages compared with the loop electrode. These include a larger contact area, better fit into the cornual area, and because of the rotation, easier contact with the tissue as the ball-end electrode moves (Figure 35-14). Townsend et al. treated 50 patients who had menorrhagia with this technique after thinning the endometrium with either a month of danazol, low-dose combined oral contraceptives, or MPA. The average duration of the procedure, which was performed on an outpatient basis with general or conduction anesthesia, was 25 minutes. None of the patients had a return of menorrhagia, although half received 400 mg doses of MPA at the time of discharge. Of the women not treated with MPA, half were amenorrheic, with the others reporting only light bleeding.

The time to learn the roller-ball technique is

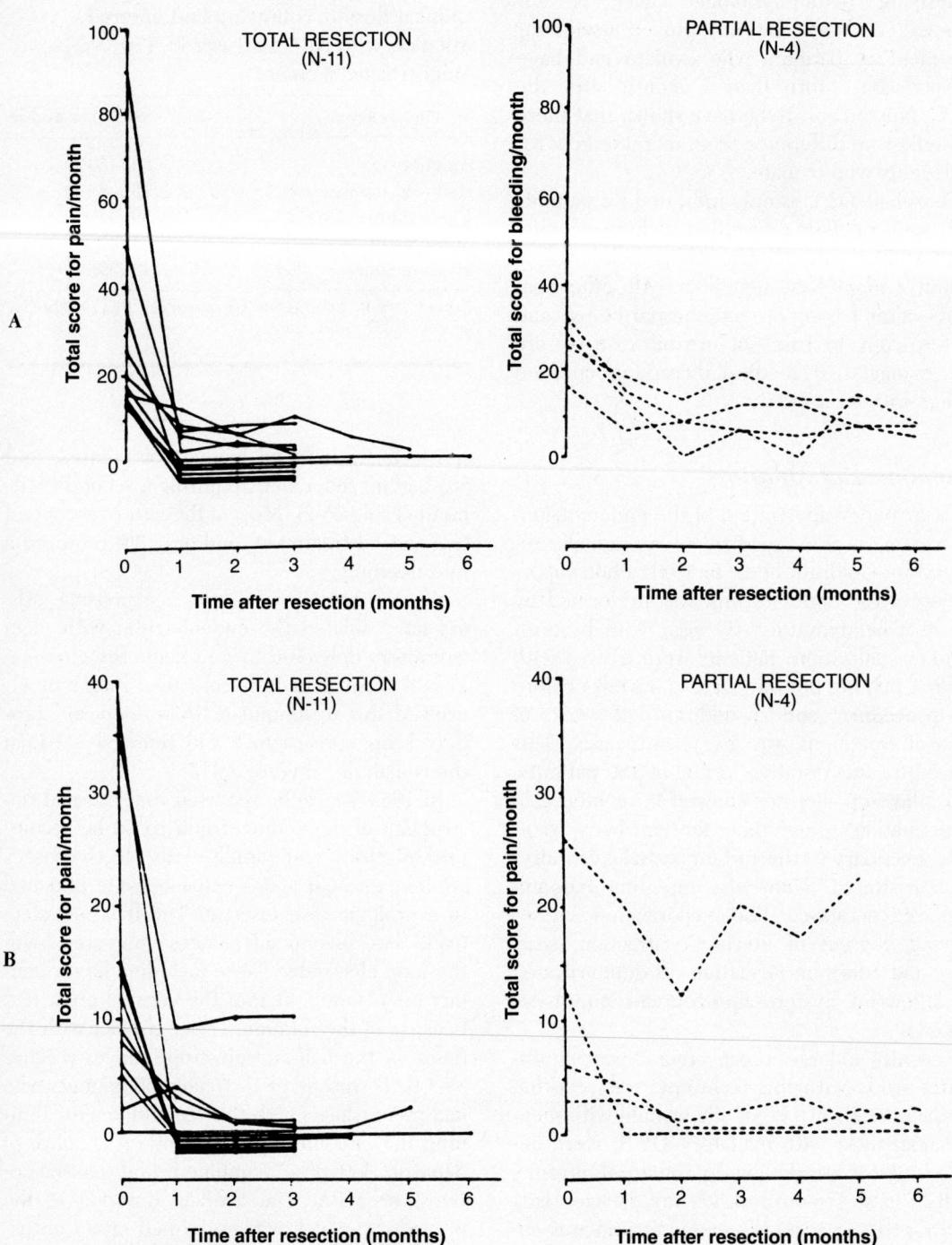

FIGURE 35-13
A, Effect of total and partial endometrial resection on total amount of menstrual bleeding each month. Blood loss was scored daily on scale of 0 to 3 (none to heavy). **B,** Effect of total and partial endometrial resection on total amount of menstrual pain each month. Pain was scored daily on score of 0 to 3 (none to severe). (From Magos AL, Baumann R, and Turnbull AC: Br Med J 298:1209, 1989.)

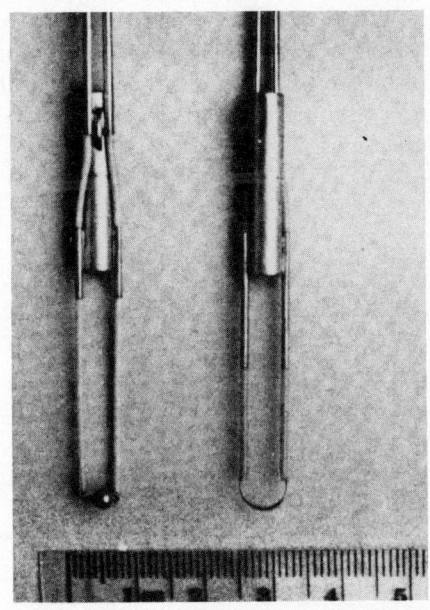

FIGURE 35-14
Ball-end and loop electrodes, side by side. Ball-end electrode is 2 mm in diameter and the loop, 7 mm. (From Vancaillie TG: Obstet Gynecol 74:425, 1989.)

shorter than for the laser and the equipment is less expensive. However, the long-term effects of all techniques of endometrial ablation are not yet known. Nevertheless, the technique is being used with increasing frequency for the treatment of women with menorrhagia but without uterine lesions who are unresponsive to medical therapy, since the cost, mortality, and length of hospitalization is less than with hysterectomy. Endometrial ablation may therefore be used as an alternative to hysterectomy in patients for when other modalities have failed or who have contradictions to their use. Ablation is also useful in treating patients with severe menorrhagia who have medical contraindications against performing a hysterectomy or treating women with ovulatory DUB who do not wish to take medications. Obviously, ablation should not be used in women who wish to maintain their reproductive capacity.

Hysterectomy

Surgical removal of the uterus should be individualized and should usually be reserved for the patient with other indications for hysterectomy, such as leiomyomas or uterine prolapse.

Hysterectomy should only be used to treat persistent ovulatory DUB after all medical therapy has failed and the amount of MBL has been documented to be excessive by direct measurement or by abnormally low serum ferritin levels. With increasing use of endometrial ablation for these individuals, the incidence of hysterectomy for ovulatory DUB should decrease. It has been estimated that as many as half the women over 40 years of age with menorrhagia without uterine lesions are now being treated by hysterectomy and that 20% of all hysterectomies in women of reproductive age are performed for menorrhagia.

Short- and Long-Term Treatment

Patients who are treated for menorrhagia should be divided into those with acute symptoms and signs and those with chronic problems.

Acute bleeding is best controlled with the use of estrogen. A D&C is indicated for patients over the age of 35 who have persistent abnormal bleeding or for patients with bleeding that is sufficiently severe to produce anemia.

After the diagnosis of anovulation is confirmed, long-term therapy should be directed by individual needs in the majority of patients. In the adolescent, 10 mg of MPA for 10 days each month for at least 3 months should be prescribed, and the patient should be observed carefully thereafter. In this group of patients additional diagnostic studies should be performed to detect possible defects in the coagulation process, particularly if bleeding is severe. For the woman of reproductive age, long-term therapy depends on whether the patient requires contraception, induction of ovulation, or treatment of DUB alone. In the last circumstance, MPA is administered, as stated above, monthly for at least 6 months, while oral contraceptives and clomiphene citrate are used for the other indications. In the perimenopausal patient who characteristically has lower amounts of circulating estrogen, use of cyclic MPA alone is frequently not curative. In these patients abnormal bleeding may be treated by the cyclic use of CE (0.625 to 1.25 mg) given for 25 days, with 10 mg of MPA added to the CE from days 15 to 25 after abnormal endometrial histologic findings have been ruled out.

Chronic treatment for ovulatory patients

with menorrhagia constitutes the most difficult problem of DUB. In patients for whom cavity defects have been ruled out, long-term treatment is directed at a reduction in MBL. For these patients NSAIDs, prolonged progestin use, oral contraceptives, danazol, and GnRH analogues are part of the therapeutic armamentarium. A combination of two or more of these agents is often required to obviate the need for hysterectomy.

_____ KEY POINTS _____

- The percentage of blood to total fluid volume of menstrual discharge averages 36%.

- The most precise method to measure menstrual blood loss (MBL) is the alkaline hematin method.

- Average loss of iron in each menses is 16 mg.

- About 70% of total MBL occurs in the first 2 days of menses.

- Menorrhagia occurs in 9% to 14% of healthy women, and most have normal duration of menses.

- The predominant cause of dysfunctional uterine bleeding (DUB) in the postmenstrual and premenopausal years is anovulation. During the rest of the reproductive years, most DUB is associated with ovulation.

- Hemostatic plugs in the endometrium are smaller, have different morphology, and persist for a shorter time than when vessel damage occurs in other tissue.

- There is an increase in the amount of both PGE_2 and $PGF_{2\alpha}$ in the endometrium in the late secretory phase and during menses, with the $PGF_{2\alpha}/PGE_2$ ratio steadily increasing from midcycle to menses.

- There is an inverse correlation between endometrial $PGF_{2\alpha}/PGE_2$ ratio and MBL.

- Anovulatory cycles are usually not associated with dysmenorrhea because of reduced levels of $PGF_{2\alpha}$ in the endometrium.

- Alterations in prostaglandin synthesis and release occur in women with both ovulatory and anovulatory DUB.

- Diagnostic tests in women with menorrhagia include measurement of hemoglobin, serum iron, serum ferritin, HCG, TSH, endometrial biopsy, and hysteroscopy or hysterosalpingography.

- High doses of oral or intravenous estrogen will usually stop acute bleeding episodes caused by anovulatory DUB. Oral estrogen is less expensive and easier to administer than the intravenous form.

- Ergot derivatives do not reduce MBL and should not be used as therapy.

- Anovulatory DUB can be treated by cyclic use of progestins, oral contraceptives, or intermittent clomiphene citrate.

- Patients with ovulatory DUB are best treated with oral contraceptives, NSAIDs (antiprostaglandins), danazol, or progestins during the luteal phase or progesterone or progestins released locally from an IUD.

- NSAIDs administered during menses reduce MBL by 20% to 50% in women with ovulatory DUB.

- The blind technique of dilation and curettage (D&C) misses the diagnosis of uterine lesions in 10% to 25% of patients.

- A D&C should be used to stop the acute bleeding episode in patients with hypovolemia or those over age 35. A D&C only treats the acute episode of excess uterine bleeding, not subsequent episodes.

- Endometrial ablation with laser or electrocautery is a useful technique to control ovulatory DUB in women who do not respond to medical management, have excessive side effects with medical therapy, or have no other indications for hysterectomy.

- Hysterectomy should be used to treat women with ovulatory DUB only after medical therapy has failed and excessive MBL has been documented by objective measurement.

BIBLIOGRAPHY

Adelantado JM, Rees CP, Bernal AL, and Turnbull AC: Increased uterine prostaglandin E receptors in menorrhagic women, Br J Obstet Gynaecol 95:162, 1988.

Bergqvist A and Rybo G: Treatment of menorrhagia with intrauterine release of progesterone, Br J Obstet Gynaecol 90:255, 1983.

Bonney RC, Higham JM, Watson H, et al: Phospholipase activity in the endometrium of women with normal menstrual blood loss and women with proven ovulatory menorrhagia, Br J Obstet Gynaecol 98:363, 1991.

Chimbria TH, Anderson ABM, Naish C, et al: Reduction of menstrual blood loss by danazol in unexplained menorrhagia: lack of effect of placebo. Br J Obstet Gynaecol 87:1152, 1980.

Chimbira TH, Anderson AC, and Turnbull AC: Relation between measured menstrual blood loss and patients' subjective assessment of loss, duration of bleeding, number of sanitary towels used, uterine weight and endometrial surface area, Br J Obstet Gynaecol 87:603, 1980.

Chimbria TH, Cope E, Anderson ABM, et al: The effect of danazol on menorrhagia, coagulation mechanisms, haematological indices and body weight, Br J Obstet Gynaecol 86:46, 1979.

Christiaens GC, Sixma JJ, and Haspels AA: Morphology of haemostasis in menstrual endometrium, Br J Obstet Gynaecol 87:425, 1980.

Claessens EA and Cowell CL: Acute adolescent menorrhagia, Am J Obstet Gynecol 139:277, 1981.

Cole SK, Billwicz WZ, and Thomson AM: Sources of variation in menstrual blood Loss, J Obstet Gynaecol Br Commonwlth 78:933, 1971.

DeCherney AH, Diamond MP, Lavy G, and Polan ML: Endometrial ablation for intractable uterine bleeding: hysteroscopic resection, Am J Obstet Gynecol 155:574, 1986.

DeVore GR, Owens O, and Kase N: Use of intravenous Premarin in the treatment of dysfunctional uterine bleeding: a double-blind randomized control study, Obstet Gynecol 59:285, 1982.

Dockeray CJ, Sheppard BL, and Bonnard J: Comparison between mefenamic acid and danazol in the treatment of established menorrhagia, Br J Obstet Gynaecol 96:840, 1989.

Fraser IS; Menorrhagia due to myometrial hypertrophy: treatment with tamoxifen, Obstet Gynecol 70:505, 1987.

Fraser IS: Treatment of ovulatory and anovulatory dysfunctional uterine bleeding with oral progestogens, Aust NZ J Obstet Gynecol 30:353, 1990.

Fraser IS, McCarron G, and Markham R: A preliminary study of factors influencing perception of menstrual blood loss volume, Am J Obstet Gynecol 149:788, 1984.

Fraser IS, McCarron G, Markham R, and Resta T: Blood and total fluid content of menstrual discharge, Obstet Gynecol 65:194, 1985.

Fraser IS, McCarron G, Markham R, et al: Measured menstrual blood loss in women with menorrhagia associated with pelvic disease or coagulation disorder, Obstet Gynecol 68:630, 1986.

Fraser IS, McCarron G, Markham R, et al: Long-term treatment of menorrhagia with mefenamic acid, Obstet Gynecol 61:109, 1983.

Fraser IS, Pearse C, Shearman RP, et al: Efficacy of mefenamic acid in patients with a complaint of menorrhagia, Obstet Gynecol 58:543, 1981.

Garry R, Erian J, and Grochmal SA: A multi-centre collaborative study into the treatment of menorrhagia by Nd-YAG laser ablation of the endometrium, Br J Obstet Gynaecol 98:357, 1991.

Gimpelson RJ and Rappold HO: A comparative study between panoramic hysteroscopy with directed biopsies and dilatation and curettage, Am J Obstet Gynecol 158:489, 1988.

Goldrath MH, Fuller TA, and Segal S: Laser photovaporization of endometrium for the treatment of menorrhagia, Am J Obstet Gynecol 140:14, 1981.

Granstrom E, Swahn ML, and Lundstrom V: The possible roles of prostaglandins and related compounds in endometrial bleeding, Acta Obstet Gynecol Scand Suppl 113:91, 1983.

Grimes DA: Estimating vaginal blood loss, J Reprod Med 22:190, 1979.

Hahn L and Rybo G: Fibrinogen-fibrin degradation products in menstrual blood from women with normal and excessive menstrual blood losses, Acta Obstet Gynecol Scand 54:119, 1975.

Hall P, Maclachlan N, Thorn N, et al: Control of menorrhagia by the cyclo-oxygenase inhibitors naproxen sodium and mefenamic acid, Br J Obstet Gynaecol 94:554, 1987.

Hallberg L, Högdahl A-M, Nilsson L, and Rybo G: Menstrual blood loss—a population study: variation at different ages and attempts to define normality, Acta Obstet Gynecol Scand 45:320, 1966.

Hallberg L and Nilsson L: Constancy of individual menstrual blood loss, Acta Obstet Gynecol Scand 43:352, 1964.

Hammond RH, Oppenheimer LW, and Saunders PG: Diagnostic role of dilatation and curettage in the management of abnormal premenopausal bleeding, Br J Obstet Gynaecol 96:496, 1989.

Haynes PJ, Hodgson H, Anderson ABM, and Turnbull AC: Measurement of menstrual blood loss in patients complaining of menorrhagia, Br J Obstet Gynaecol 84:763, 1977.

Livio M, Mannucci PM, Vigano G, et al: Conjugated estrogens for the management of bleeding associated with renal failure, N Engl J Med 315:731, 1986.

Loffer FD: Hysteroscopic endometrial ablation with the Nd:YAG laser using a nontouch technique, Obstet Gynecol 69:679, 1987.

Loffer FD: Hysteroscopy with selective endometrial sampling compared with D&C for abnormal uterine bleeding: the value of a negative hysteroscopic view, Obstet Gynecol 73:16, 1989.

Magos AL, Baumann R, and Turnbull AC: Transcervical resection of endometrium in women with menorrhagia, Br Med J 298:1209, 1989.

Makarainen L and Ylikorkala O: Ibuprofen prevents IUD-induced increases in menstrual blood loss, Br J Obstet Gynaecol 93:285, 1986.

Makarainen L and Ylikorkala O: Primary and myoma-associated menorrhagia: role of prostaglandins and effects of ibuprofen, Br J Obstet Gynaecol 93:974, 1986.

March CM: The endometrium in the menstrual cycle. In Mishell DR Jr, Davajan V, and Lobo RA, editors: Infertility, contraception, and reproductive endocrinology, ed 3, Cambridge, Mass, 1991, Blackwell Scientific Publications.

Mencaglia L, Perino A, and Hamou J: Hysteroscopy in perimenopausal and postmenopausal women with abnormal uterine bleeding, J Reprod Med 32:577, 1987.

Milson I, Andersson K, Andersch B, and Rybo G: A comparison of flurbiprofen, tranexamic acid, and a levonorgestrel-releasing intrauterine contraceptive device in the treatment of idiopathic menorrhagia, Am J Obstet Gynecol 164:879, 1991.

Newton J, Barnard G, and Collins W: A rapid method for measuring menstrual blood loss using automatic extraction, Contraception 16:269, 1977.

Nilsson L and Rybo G: Treatment of menorrhagia with an antifibrinolytic agent, tranexamic acid (AMCA): a double-blind investigation, Acta Obstet Gynecol Scand 46:572, 1967.

Nilsson L and Rybo G: Treatment of menorrhagia, Am J Obstet Gynecol 110:713, 1971.

Parmer J: Long-term suppression of hypermenorrhea by progesterone intrauterine contraceptive devices, Am J Obstet Gynecol 149:578, 1984.

Rees MCP, Cederholm-Williams SA, and Turnbull AC: Coagulation factors and fibrinolytic proteins in menstrual fluid collected from normal and menorrhagic women, Br J Obstet Gynaecol 92:1164, 1985.

Rees MCP, Dunnill MS, Anderson ABM, and Turnbull AC: Quantitative uterine histology during the menstrual cycle in relation to measured menstrual blood loss, Br J Obstet Gynaecol 91: 662, 1984.

Rueda R, Falcone T, Hemmings R, and Tulandi T: Dysfunctional uterine bleeding: a reappraisal. In Barbieri RL, Berek JS, Greasy RK, et al: Current problems in obstetrics, gynecology and fertility, vol XIV, St Louis, 1991, Mosby–Year Book.

Rybo G: Plasminogen activators in the endometrium, Acta Obstet Gynecol Scand 45:411, 1966.

Shaw RW and Fraser HM: Use of a superactive luteinizing hormone releasing hormone (LHRH) agonist in the treatment of menorrhagia, Br J Obstet Gynaecol 9:913, 1984.

Sheppard BL, Dockeray CJ, and Bonnar J: An ultrastructural study of menstrual blood in normal menstruation and dysfunctional uterine bleeding, Br J Obstet Gynaecol 90:259, 1983.

Smith SK, Abel MH, Kelly RW, and Baird DT: Prostaglandin synthesis in the endometrium of women with ovular dysfunctional uterine bleeding, Br J Obstet Gynaecol 88:434, 1981.

Smith SK, Abel MH, Kelly RW, and Baird DT: The synthesis of prostaglandins from persistent proliferative endometrium, J Clin Endocrinol Metab 55:284, 1982.

Smith SK, Kelly RW, Abel MH, and Baird DT: A role for prostacyclin (PGI2) in excessive menstrual bleeding, Lancet, March 1981, p 522.

Townsend DE, Ricart RM, Paskowitz RA, and Woolford RE: Rollerball coagulation of the endometrium, Obstet Gynecol 76:310, 1990.

Vancaillie TG: Electrocoagulation of the endometrium with the ball-end resectoscope, Obstet Gynecol 74:425, 1989.

van EijKeren MA, Christiaens GC, Sixma JJ, and Haspels AA: Menorrhagia: a review, Obstet Gynecol Surv 44:421, 1989.

van Eijkeren MA, Scholten PC, Christiaens GC, et al: The alkaline hematin method for measuring menstrual blood loss—a modification and its clinical use in menorrhagia, Eur J Obstet Gynecol Reprod Biol 22:345, 1986.

Vargyas JM, Campeau JD, and Mishell DA: Treatment of menorrhagia with meclofenamate sodium, Am J Obstet Gynecol 157:944, 1987.

Vasilenko P, Kraicer PF, Kaplan R, et al: A new and simple method of measuring menstrual blood loss, J Reprod Med 33:293, 1988.

Wilansky DL and Greisman B: Early hypothyroidism in patients with menorrhagia, Am J Obstet Gynecol 160:673, 1989.

Amenorrhea

———————— **KEY TERMS AND DEFINITIONS** ————————

Amenorrhea. Absence of menses during the reproductive years. It can be either physiologic (pregnancy) or pathologic.

Androgen Insensitivity Syndrome. A genetically transmitted androgen receptor defect in a 46,XY individual with testes and normal male testosterone levels. These individuals have absent uterus, normal female phenotype, and scanty body hair.

Anorexia Nervosa. A psychiatric disease associated with a fear of weight gain or obesity, food aversion, and a distorted body image in which the individual limits caloric intake to starvation levels. In addition to severe weight loss, there is a decreased metabolic rate and amenorrhea.

Chromophobe Adenoma. A non-hormone-secreting pituitary tumor that can disrupt normal pituitary function and thus produce low gonadotrophin levels.

Congenital Absence of Uterus and Vagina. A malformation in a 46,XX individual with normal ovarian function resulting in failure of the uterus and vagina to form. It is also called *uterovaginal agenesis* and *Rokitansky-Kuster-Hauser syndrome.*

Cryptomenorrhea. Menstruation without egress of menses through the introitus.

Delayed Menarche. Onset of menses in women older than 16.5 years who have no reproductive abnormalities.

Functional Hypothalamic Amenorrhea. Amenorrhea caused by nonorganic impairment of normal hypothalamic function with slowing of normal gonadotrophin-releasing hormone (GnRH) pulsatility.

Gonadal Failure. Failure of the gonads to develop. It is also called *gonadal dysgenesis* if the karyotype is abnormal and *gonadal agenesis* if the karyotype is normal.

Gonadal Streaks. Streaks of fibrous tissue in the normal position of the ovaries.

Gonadotrophin-Resistant Ovary Syndrome. Premature ovarian failure in which the ovary contains normal-appearing primordial follicles but no follicular development. It is also called *ovarian hypofolliculogenesis.*

Hypogonadotrophic Hypogonadism. Failure of the ovaries to develop as a result of low amounts of circulatory gonadotrophins. When anosmia is present, the term *Kallmann's syndrome* is used.

Hypothalamic Dysfunction. Secondary amenorrhea caused by an abnormal pattern of GnRH pulsatility and circulatory estradiol levels above 40 pg/ml.

Hypothalamic Failure. Secondary amenorrhea caused by an abnormal pattern of GnRH pulsatility and estradiol levels below 40 pg/ml.

Insulin Tolerance Test. A test of adrenocorticotropic hormone function in which hypoglycemia is produced and cortisol measured.

Intrauterine Adhesions or Synechiae. A condition in which fibrous tissue partially or completely obliterates the uterine cavity. It is also called *Asherman's syndrome.*

Isolated Gonadotrophin Deficiency. The presence of hypogonadotrophic hypogonadism in individuals who do not produce gonadotrophins after prolonged administration of GnRH.

Pituitary Destruction. Damage or necrosis of the pituitary gland caused by anoxia, thrombosis, or hemorrhage. It is called *Sheehan's syndrome* when related to pregnancy and *Simmond's disease* when unrelated to pregnancy.

Polycystic Ovary Syndrome. An endocrinologic disorder characterized by excessive androgen production, inappropriate gonadotrophin secretion, and chronic anovulation. It begins perimenarcheally, and its clinical manifestations include hirsutism and menstrual irregularity (oligomenorrhea or amenorrhea).

Premature Ovarian Failure. Cessation of menstruation caused by depletion of ovarian follicles or failure of primordial follicles to respond to gonadotrophin before the age of 40. It is also called *hypergonadotrophic hypogonadism.*

Primary Amenorrhea. Absence of any spontaneous menses in an individual older than 16.5 years of age.

Pure Gonadal Dysgenesis. Absence of the gonads in an individual with a normal 46,XX or 46,XY karyotype. It is also called *gonadal agenesis.*

Secondary Amenorrhea. Absence of menses for a variable period of time (for at least 3 to 12 months, usually 6 months or longer) in an individual who has previously had spontaneous menstrual periods.

Amenorrhea can be either physiologic, when it occurs during pregnancy and the postpartum period (particularly when nursing), or pathologic, when it is produced by a variety of endocrinologic and anatomic disorders. In the latter circumstance the failure to menstruate is a symptom of these various pathologic conditions. Thus amenorrhea itself is not a pathologic entity and should not be used as a final diagnosis.

Although the absence of menses causes no harm to the body, in a nonpregnant or postpartum woman it is abnormal and thus is a source of concern. For this reason women usually seek medical assistance when the condition occurs. Therefore the clinician needs to know the various etiologies of amenorrhea, how to diagnose the etiology, and how to treat the underlying pathologic condition. This chapter will present the etiology, diagnostic evaluation, and treatment of the various causes of both primary and secondary amenorrhea.

Many individuals with ambiguous external genitalia resulting from various intersex problems are raised as females and never menstruate. The etiology of the intersex problem is usually determined at birth or soon thereafter. Since such disorders are discussed in Chapter 3, they will not be discussed in this chapter. Although women with cryptomenorrhea caused by anatomic disorders interfering with the outflow of menses, such as an imperforate hymen or transverse vaginal septum, have the symptom of amenorrhea, they are actually menstru-

ating. These conditions are discussed in Chapter 9. Severe systemic diseases such as metastatic carcinoma and chronic renal failure can also cause amenorrhea; however, since amenorrhea is not the presenting symptom of these disorders, they will not be discussed in this chapter.

Primary amenorrhea is defined as the absence of menses in a woman who has never menstruated by the age of 16½ years. The incidence of primary amenorrhea is less than 0.1%. Secondary amenorrhea is defined as the absence of menses for an arbitrary time period, usually longer than 6 to 12 months. The incidence of secondary amenorrhea of more than 6 months' duration in a survey of a general population of Swedish women of reproductive age was found by Pettersson et al. to be 0.7%. The incidence was significantly higher in women younger than 25 years of age and those with a prior history of menstrual irregularity.

DELAYED MENARCHE

Before the onset of menses the normal female goes through a progressive series of morphologic changes produced by the pubertal increase in estrogen and androgen production. In 1969 Marshall and Tanner defined five stages of breast development and pubic hair development (Figure 36-1, Table 36-1). These changes sometimes are combined and called *Tanner* or *pubertal stages 1 through 5.* The first sign of puberty is usually the appearance of breast budding followed within a few months by the appearance of pubic hair.

Thereafter the breasts enlarge, the external pelvic contour becomes rounder, and the most rapid rate of growth occurs (peak height velocity). Thus breast budding is the earliest sign of puberty and menarche the latest. The mean ages of occurrence of these events in American women are shown in Table 36-2, and the mean intervals (with standard deviation) between initiation of breast budding and other pubertal events are shown in Table 36-3. The mean interval between breast budding and menarche is 2.3 years, with a standard deviation of about 1 year. Some individuals can progress from breast budding to menarche in 18 months, while others may take 5 years. Thus although the arbitrary age of primary amenorrhea is 16½ years, if a woman 14 years of age or older presents to the clinician with absence of breast budding, diagnostic evaluation should be performed at this time, as it is highly unlikely she will menstruate within the next 2 years.

The mean time of onset of menarche was previously thought to occur when a critical body weight of about 48 kg, or 106 lb, was reached. However, it is now believed that body composition is more important than total

TABLE 36-1

Classifications of Breast Growth and Pubic Hair Growth

Classification	Description
Breast growth	
B1	Prepubertal: elevation of papilla only
B2	Breast budding
B3	Enlargement of breasts with glandular tissue, without separation of breast contours
B4	Secondary mound formed by areola
B5	Single contour of breast and areola
Pubic hair growth	
PH1	Prepubertal: no pubic hair
PH2	Labial hair present
PH3	Labial hair spreads over mons pubis
PH4	Slight lateral spread
PH5	Further lateral spread to form inverse triangle and reach medial thighs

Adapted from Roy S and Brenner PF: Puberty. Reproduced with permission from Infertility, contraception and reproductive endocrinology, ed 2, by Daniel R. Mishell, Jr., M.D., and Val Davajan, M.D. Copyright © 1986 Medical Economics Books, Oradell, N.J. 07649. All rights reserved.

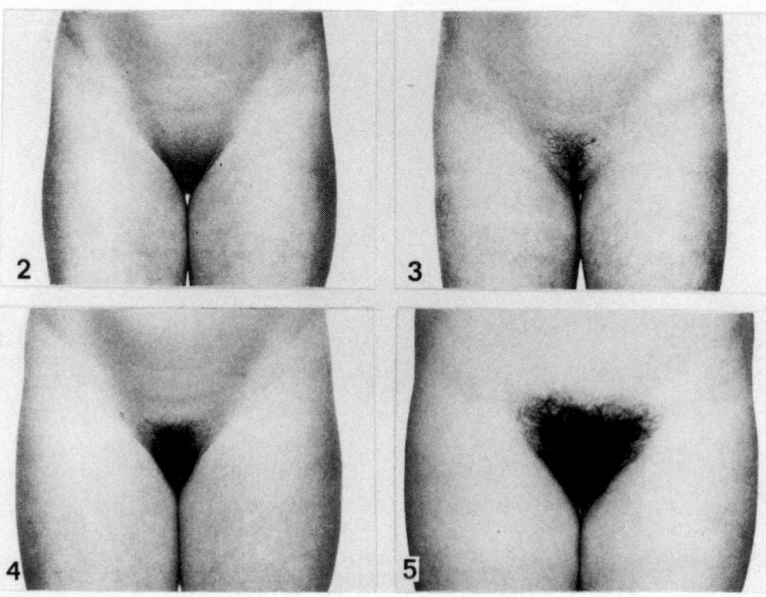

FIGURE 36-1

Standards for pubic hair ratings. (Modified from Tanner JM: Growth and endocrinology of the adolescent. In Gardner L, editor: Endocrine and genetic diseases of childhood, ed 2, Philadelphia, 1975, WB Saunders Co.)   *Continued.*

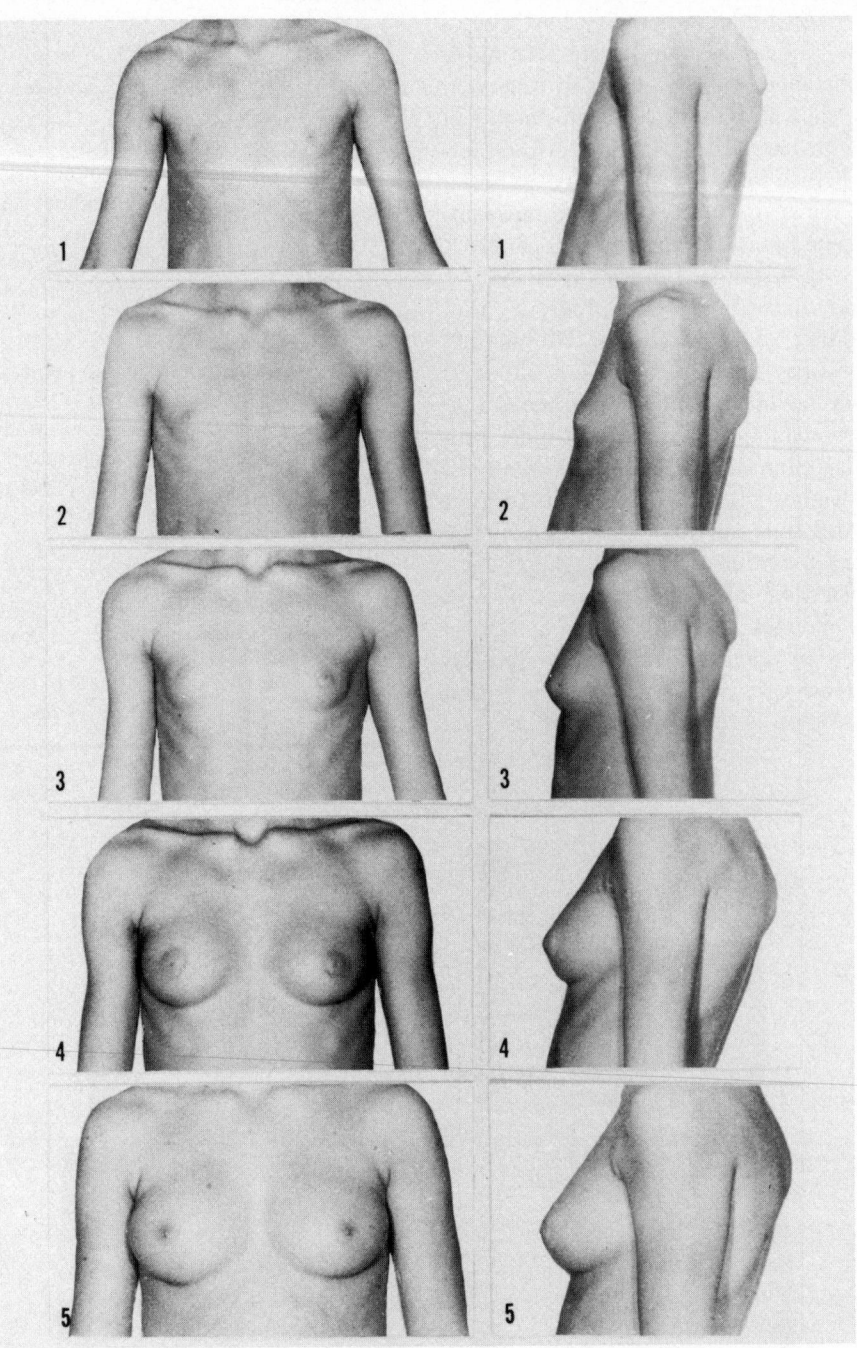

FIGURE 36-1, cont'd
Standards for breast ratings.

TABLE 36-2
Mean Ages of Girls at the Onset of Pubertal Events (United States)

Event	Mean Age ± SD (Years)
Initiation of breast development (B2)	10.8 ± 1.10
Appearance of pubic hair (PH2)	11.0 ± 1.21
Menarche	12.9 ± 1.20

Adapted from Frisch RE and Revelle R: Arch Dis Child 46:695, 1971.

TABLE 36-3
Pubertal Intervals

Interval	Mean Age ± SD (Years)
B2-peak height velocity	1.0 ± 0.77
B2-menarche	2.3 ± 1.03
B2-PH5	3.1 ± 1.04
B2-B5 (average duration of puberty)	4.5 ± 2.04

Adapted from Frisch RE and Revelle R: Arch Dis Child 46:695, 1971.

body weight in determining the time of onset of puberty and menstruation. Thus the ratio of fat to both total body weight and lean body weight is probably the determining factor in the time of onset of puberty and menstruation. Individuals who are moderately obese, between 20% and 30% above the ideal body weight, will have an early onset of menarche. Malnutrition is known to delay the onset of puberty, and well-nourished individuals with prepubertal strenuous exercise programs resulting in less total body fat have also been shown to have a delayed onset of puberty. Warren et al. reported that ballet dancers, swimmers, and runners had menarche delayed to about age 15 if they began exercising strenuously before menarche (Figure 36-2). These investigators also determined that stress is not the cause of the delayed menarche in these exercising girls, as girls of the same age with stressful musical careers did not have a delayed onset of menarche. The girls with strenuous exercise programs have sufficient estrogen to produce some

breast development and thus do not need extensive endocrinologic evaluation if concern arises about lack of onset of menses. Frisch et al. reported that for girls engaged in premenarcheal athletic training, menarche was delayed 0.4 years for each year of athletic training. An endocrinologic diagnostic evaluation is not necessary for these individuals. They should be counseled that they will have a delayed onset of menses, but it is not a health problem; they will have regular ovulatory cycles when they either stop exercising or become older.

Before puberty, circulating levels of luteinizing hormone (LH) and follicle-stimulating hormone (FSH) are low (FSH/LH ratio being greater than 1) because the central nervous system (CNS)-hypothalamic axis is extremely sensitive to the negative feedback effects of low levels of circulating estrogen. As the critical weight or body composition is approached, the CNS-hypothalamic axis becomes less sensitive to the negative effect of estrogen, and gonadotrophin-releasing hormone (GnRH) is secreted in greater amounts, causing an increase in both LH and to a lesser extent FSH. The initial endocrinologic change associated with the onset of puberty is the occurrence of episodic pulses of LH occurring during sleep (Figure 36-3). These pulses are absent before the onset of puberty. After menarche the episodic secretions of LH occur both during sleep and while awake. The last endocrinologic event of puberty is activation of the positive gonadotrophin response to increasing levels of estradiol, which results in the midcycle gonadotrophic response.

PRIMARY AMENORRHEA

It is important that the clinician understand both the sequential endocrinologic and the morphologic chronologic changes taking place during normal puberty in order to make the differential diagnosis between delayed menarche and primary amenorrhea. Although the former condition requires only reassurance, the latter requires an endocrinologic evaluation to establish the etiology of this symptom.

Etiology

Although numerous classifications have been used for the various etiologies of primary amenorrhea, it has been found most clinically useful to group them on the basis of whether

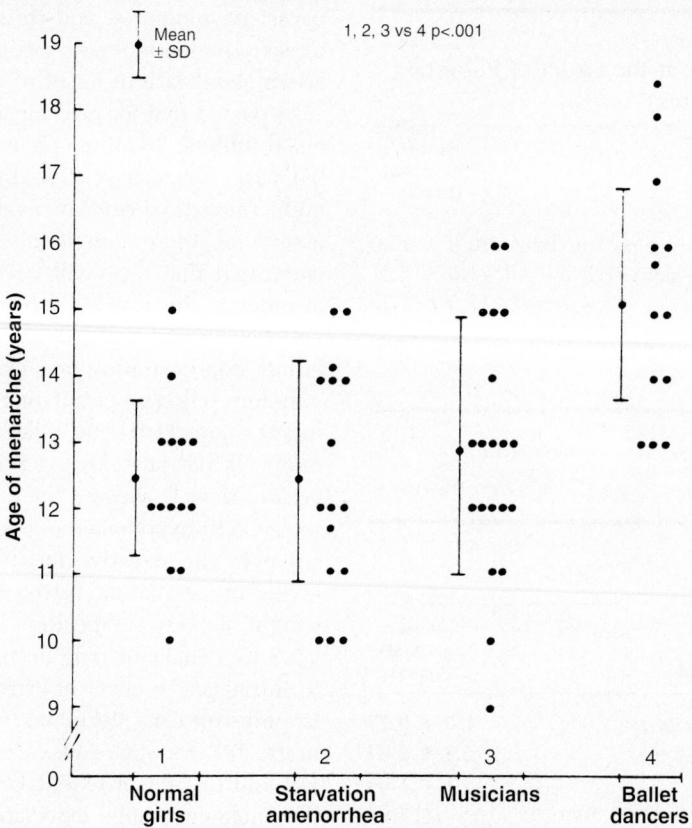

FIGURE 36-2
Ages of menarche in ballet dancers as compared with those of three other groups.
(From Warren MP: J Clin Endocrinol Metab 51:1150, 1980. Copyright © by The
Endocrine Society 1980.)

secondary sexual characteristics (breasts) and
female internal genitalia (uterus) are present or
absent (see box, p. 1107). Thus the findings of
a physical examination can alert the clinician to
possible causes and indicate which laboratory
tests should be performed. In a series of 62 patients reported by Maschchak et al. the largest
subgroup of individuals with primary amenorrhea (29) were those with absent breasts and a
uterus present; the second largest subgroup
(22) had both breasts and uterus; an absent
uterus together with breast development accounted for the third largest category (9); and
absent breasts and uterus were the least common (2).

Breasts Absent and Uterus Present

All individuals with no breast development
and a uterus present have no ovarian estrogen
production as a result of either a CNS hypothalamic-pituitary abnormality or a gonadal disorder. Although the phenotype of these individu-

als is similar, the etiology and prognosis for fertility of these disorders differ; therefore it is
important to establish the exact diagnosis.

**GONADAL FAILURE (HYPERGONADOTRO-
PHIC HYPOGONADISM).** Failure of gonadal
development is the most common cause of primary amenorrhea, occurring in almost half the
patients with this symptom. Gonadal failure is
most frequently due to a chromosomal disorder
or deletion of all or part of an X chromosome,
but it is sometimes due to a genetic defect.
The chromosome disorders are usually due to a
random meiotic or mitotic abnormality (e.g.,
nondisjunction or anaphase lag) and thus are
not inherited. However, if absent gonadal development occurs in the presence of a 46,XX or
46,XY karyotype, called *pure gonadal dysgenesis*, a gene disorder may be present, as it has
been reported to occur in siblings. Reindollar
et al., in the largest single series of patients
with primary amenorrhea, reported that all individuals with gonadal failure and an X chromosome abnormality were less than 63 inches

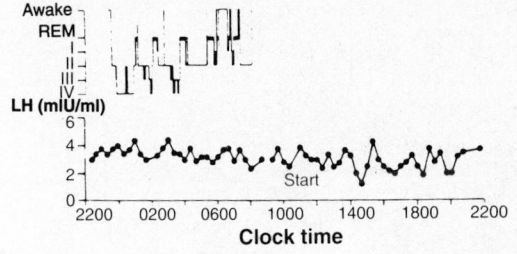

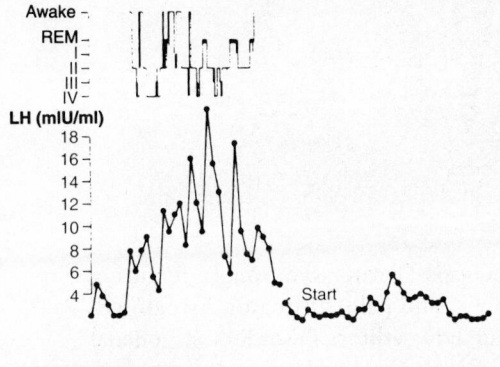

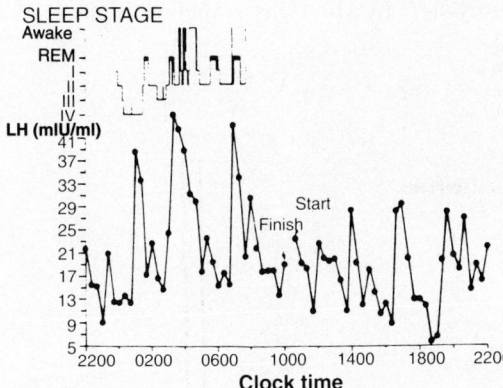

FIGURE 36-3

Plasma LH concentration measured every 20 minutes for 24 hours in normal prepubertal girl *(upper panel)*, early pubertal girl *(center panel)*, and normal late pubertal girl *(lower panel)*. In top and center panels sleep histogram is shown above period of nocturnal sleep. Sleep stages are awake, rapid eye movement (REM), and stages I to IV by depth of line graph. Plasma LH concentrations are expressed as milli–international units per milliliter of Second International Reference Preparation of Human Menopausal Gonadotropin. (Modified from Boyar RM, Katz J, Finkelstein JW, et al: N Engl J Med 291:861, 1974. Reprinted by permission of The New England Journal of Medicine.)

in height. About one third had major cardiovascular or renal anomalies.

Since at least two X chromosomes are neces-

DIFFERENTIAL DIAGNOSIS OF PRIMARY AMENORRHEA WITH NORMAL FEMALE EXTERNAL GENITALIA

I. Primary amenorrhea without breast development and uterus present
  A. Gonadal failure
    1. 45,X
    2. 46,X, abnormal X (e.g., short-arm or long-arm deletion)
    3. Mosaicism (e.g., X/XX, X/XX/XXX)
    4. 46, XX or XY pure gonadal dysgenesis
    5. 17α-Hydroxylase deficiency (with 46,XX karyotype)
  B. CNS-hypothalamic-pituitary disorders
    1. CNS lesion (congenital or acquired)
    2. Hypothalamic failure secondary to inadequate GnRH synthesis and/or release
    3. Isolated gonadotrophin insufficiency
II. Primary amenorrhea with breast development and absent uterus
  A. Congenital absence of uterus (uterovaginal agenesis)
  B. Androgen insensitivity (testicular feminization)
III. Primary amenorrhea with no breast development and absent uterus
  A. 17,20-Desmolase deficiency
  B. Agonadism
  C. 17α-Hydroxylase deficiency (with 46, XY karyotype)
IV. Primary amenorrhea with breast development and uterus present
  A. Hypothalamic causes
  B. Pituitary causes
  C. Ovarian causes
  D. Uterine causes

sary for normal ovarian development, individuals with a 45,X karyotype, mosaicism involving a single X chromosome, or abnormalities of the X chromosome may fail to develop ovaries and usually have only a mass of fibrous tissue present in the normal anatomic position of the ovary. These fibrous bands have been called gonadal streaks (Figure 36-4). Streaks are also present in individuals with pure gonadal dysgenesis. These persons fail to develop breasts

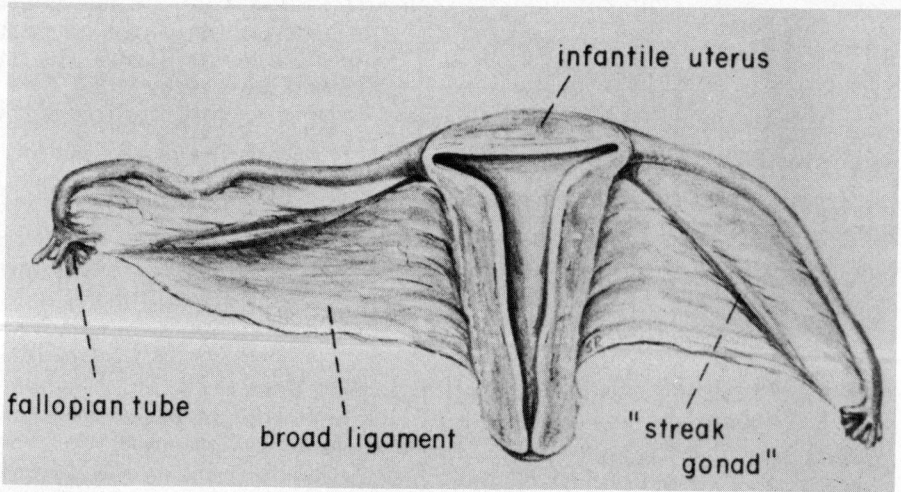

FIGURE 36-4
Internal genitalia of patient with gonadal dysgenesis (Turner syndrome), featuring normal but infantile uterus, normal fallopian tubes, and pale, glistening "streak" gonads in both broad ligaments. (From Federman DD, editor: Disorders of gonadal development: gonadal dysgenesis [Turner syndrome]. In Abnormal sexual development, Philadelphia, 1967, WB Saunders Co.)

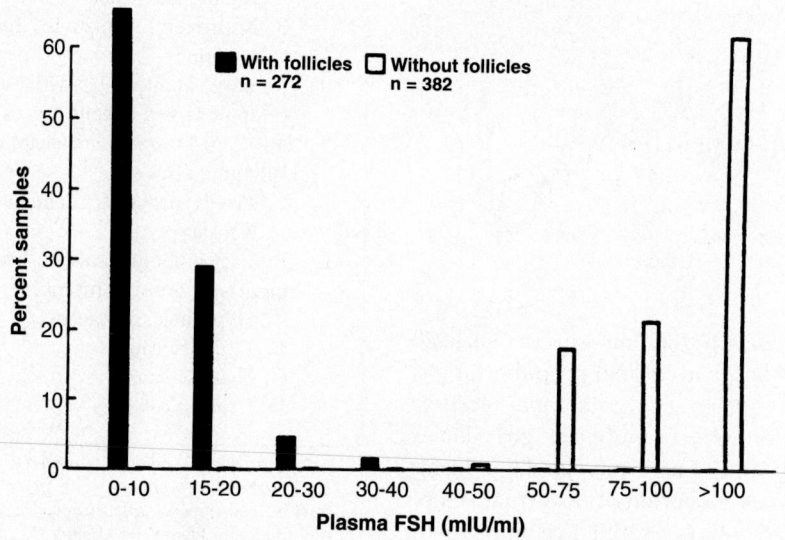

FIGURE 36-5
Distribution of plasma FSH (radioimmunoassay) in samples from women with primary amenorrhea with and without follicles. n = Number of samples. (From Goldenberg RL, Grodin JM, et al: Am J Obstet Gynecol 116: 1003, 1973.

because they have absent or markedly reduced gonadal steroid secretion. With the absence of the negative hypothalamic-pituitary action of estrogen, gonadotrophin levels are markedly elevated. Since estrogen is not necessary for müllerian duct development or wolffian duct regression, the internal and external genitalia are phenotypically normal female.

In a classic paper Goldenberg et al. demonstrated that all individuals with primary amenorrhea and plasma FSH levels greater than 40 mIU/ml had no functioning ovarian follicles in the gonadal tissue. Thus, in women with primary amenorrhea, the dignosis of gonadal failure, hypergonatrophic hypogonadism, can be made if the FSH levels exceed 40 mIU/ml (Figure 36-5).

45,X Anomalies. Turner syndrome occurs in about 1 per 2000 to 1 per 3000 live births but is much more frequent in abortuses. In addition to primary amenorrhea and absent breast development, these individuals have other somatic abnormalities, the most prevalent being short stature (less than 60 inches in height), a web neck, a short fourth metacarpal, and cubitus valgus. Thus the diagnosis is usually made before puberty (Chapter 3).

A wide variety of chromosomal mosaics are associated with primary amenorrhea and normal female external genitalia, the most common being X/XX. In addition, individuals with X/XXX and X/XX/XXX mosaicism have primary amenorrhea. These individuals are generally taller and have fewer anatomic abnormalities than individuals with a 45,X karyotype. In addition, some of them may have a few gonadal follicles, and about 20% have sufficient estrogen production to menstruate. Occasionally ovulation may occur.

Structurally Abnormal X Chromosome. Although individuals with this disorder have a 46,XX karyotype, part of one X chromosome is structurally abnormal. If there is deletion of the long arm of the X chromosome (Xq), normal height has been reported to occur, but in Reindollar's series such individuals were all short. These individuals have no somatic abnormalities. However, if there is deletion of the short arm of the X chromosome (Xp), the individual phenotypically resembles those with a 45,X karyotype (Turner syndrome). A similar phenotype occurs in persons with isochrome of the long arm of the X chromosome. Other X chromosome abnormalities include a ring X and minute fragmentation of the X chromosome.

Pure Gonadal Dysgenesis (46,XX and 46,XY with Gonad Streaks; Gonadal Agenesis). As already mentioned, this abnormality is probably a genetic disorder, as it has been reported in siblings. These individuals have normal stature and phenotype, absence of secondary sexual characteristics, and primary amenorrhea. Some of these individuals have a few ovarian follicles, develop breasts, and may even menstruate spontaneously for a few years. In Reindollar's series nearly all such individuals were taller than 63 inches.

17α-Hydroxylase Deficiency with 46,XX Karyotype. A rare gonadal cause of primary amenorrhea without breast development and normal female internal genitalia is deficiency of the enzyme 17α-hydroxylase in an individual with a 46,XX karyotype. Only a few such individuals have been described in the literature, but it is important for the clinician to be aware of this entity because these individuals, in contrast to those described earlier, have hypernatremia and hypokalemia. Because of decreased cortisol, adrenocorticotropic hormone (ACTH) levels are elevated. The mineralocorticoid levels are also elevated, as 17α-hydroxylase is not necessary for the conversion of progesterone to deoxycortisol or corticosterone. Thus there is excessive sodium retention and potassium excretion, leading to hypertension and hypokalemia. Serum progesterone levels are also elevated because progesterone is not converted to cortisol. In addition to sex steroid replacement, these individuals need cortisol administration.

CNS-HYPOTHALAMIC-PITUITARY DISORDERS. In contrast to individuals with absent secondary sex characteristics and normal female internal genitalia caused by gonad disorders described earlier, these individuals have low gonadotrophin and estrogen levels. The etiology of low gonadotrophin production can be morphologic or endocrinologic.

Lesions. Any anatomic lesion of the hypothalamus or pituitary can be a cause of low gonadotrophin production. These lesions can be congenital (stenosis of aqueduct or absence of sellar floor) or acquired (tumors). Many of these lesions, particularly pituitary adenomas, result in elevated prolactin levels (Chapter 37).

However, non-prolactin-secreting pituitary tumors (chromophobe adenomas) as well as craniopharyngiomas may not be associated with hyperprolactinemia and can rarely be the cause of primary amenorrhea with low gonadotrophin levels. Thus individuals with this symptom complex should have computed tomography (CT) scanning or magnetic resonance imaging (MRI) of the hypothalamic-pituitary region to rule out the presence of a lesion.

Inadequate GnRH Release (Hypogonadotrophic Hypogonadism). Individuals without a demonstrable lesion and a low gonadotrophin level were previously thought to have primary pituitary failure (hypogonadotrophic hypogonadism). However, when they are stimulated with GnRH, there is an increase in FSH and LH, indicating that the basic defect is either hypothalamic with insufficient GnRH or a CNS neurotransmitter defect resulting in inadequate GnRH synthesis or release or both. Although a single bolus of GnRH may not initially cause a rise in gonadotrophin level in these individuals, after 4 days of GnRH administration they will have a rise in gonadotrophins after a single GnRH bolus. Some of these individuals also have anosmia (Kallmann's syndrome), and they should be tested for olfaction with coffee, orange, and cocoa. Kallmann's syndrome is a genetically transmitted disorder and is frequently associated with other anatomic and functional abnormalities.

Isolated Gonadotrophin Deficiency. Rarely individuals with primary amenorrhea and low gonadotrophin levels do not respond to GnRH even after 4 days of administration. These individuals nearly always have an associated disorder such as thalassemia major or retinitis pigmentosa. Occasionally this pituitary abnormality had been associated with prepubertal hypothyroidism kernicterus, or mumps encephalitis.

Breast Development Present and Uterus Absent

In patients with breast development and absent uterus, two disorders can produce primary amenorrhea—androgen insensitivity and congenital absence of the uterus. The former is a genetic inherited disorder, whereas the latter is an accident of development and is only rarely genetically inherited.

ANDROGEN INSENSITIVITY. Androgen insensitivity, originally termed *testicular feminization,* is a genetically transmitted disorder in which there is an absence of androgen receptor synthesis or action. The syndrome is due to absence of an X-chromosomal gene responsible for the cytoplasmic or nuclear testosterone receptor. It is either an X-linked recessive or sex-limited autosomal dominant disorder with transmission through the mother. These individuals have an XY karyotype and normally functioning male gonads that produce normal male levels of testosterone and dihydrotestosterone. However, because of a lack of receptors in the target organs, there is a lack of male differentation of the external and internal genitalia. As occurs in the absence of sex steroids,

the former remain feminine. Wolffian duct development, which normally occurs as a result of testosterone stimulation, fails to take place; however, müllerian duct regression, which is produced by the peptide elaborated by the fetal testes, müllerian inhibiting factor (MIF), occurs normally since steroid receptors are not necessary for its action. Thus individuals with this condition have no female or male internal genitalia, normal female external genitalia, and either a short or absent vagina. Pubic and axillary hair is absent or scanty as a result of a lack of androgenic receptors, but breast development is normal or enlarged due to the fact that there is no androgenic opposition to the stimulation of breast tissue by the small circulating levels of estrogen secreted by the gonads and adrenals as well as the estrogen produced by peripheral conversion of androstenedione. The abnormal gonads are at increased risk of developing a malignancy (gonadoblastoma or dysgerminoma), with an incidence reported to be about 20%. However, these malignancies rarely occur before age 20. Therefore it is usually recommended that the gonads be left in place until after puberty is completed to allow normal sexual maturity. After such time they should be removed. It is probably best that the patient not be informed that the gonads are testes and that they are male because these individuals are phenotypically female and have been raised as such. Instead they should be informed that they are sterile as a result of a missing piece of the X chromosome, and the gonads (not testes) need to be removed because they have a high malignant potential.

CONGENITAL ABSENCE OF THE UTERUS (UTERINE AGENESIS; UTEROVAGINAL AGENESIS; ROKITANSKY-KUSTER-HAUSER SYNDROME). This disorder is the second most frequent cause of primary amenorrhea. It occurs in 1 in 4000 to 5000 female births and accounts for about 15% of individuals with primary amenorrhea. Individuals with complete uterine agenesis have no underlying endocrine abnormality but are amenorrheic because of absence of the end organ. They have normal breast and pubic and axillary hair development but have a shortened or absent vagina in addition to absence of the uterus (Figure 36-6). Congenital renal abnormalities occur in about one third of these individuals and skeletal abnormalities in about 12%. Cardiac and other congenital abnormalities also occur with increased frequency. The overwhelming majority of these

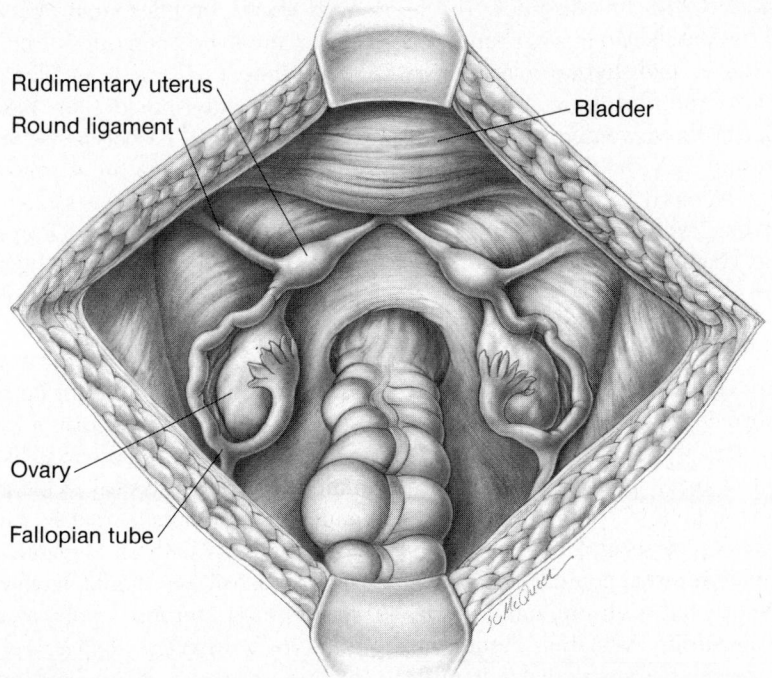

Rudimentary uterus

Round ligament

Bladder

Ovary

Fallopian tube

FIGURE 36-6

Congenital absence of vagina. Laparotomy revealed rudimentary uterus that showed evidence of failure of fusion of müllerian ducts. This is a common finding in this condition and indicates that disorder is more extensive than simple anomaly of vagina. (Redrawn from Jones HW Jr and Scott WW, editors: Hermaphroditism, genital anomalies and related endocrine disorders, ed 2, Baltimore, 1971, Williams & Wilkins Co.)

disorders are due to an isolated developmental defect, but on occasion the condition is genetically inherited. Endocrinologically the ovaries are present and function normally, so that ovulation occurs cyclically. It is usually easy to differentiate these individuals from those with androgen insensitivity by the presence of normal pubic hair, but some individuals with incomplete androgen insensitivity have some pubic hair. However, women with congenital absence of the uterus are endocrinologically normal females, whereas those with androgen insensitivity are endocrinologically male with male testosterone levels and an XY karyotype, so the differential diagnosis is easily made.

Absent Breast and Uterine Development

Persons with no breast or uterine development are rare and have a male karyotype, elevated gonadotrophin levels, and testosterone levels in the normal or below normal female range. Etiologies for this phenotype include

17α-hydroxylase deficiency, 17,20-desmolase deficiency, and agonadism. Individuals with the first disorder have testes present but lack the enzyme necessary to synthesize sex steroids and thus have female external genitalia. Because they have testes, MIF is produced and the female internal genitalia regress; with low testosterone levels the male internal genitalia do not develop. Insufficient estrogen is synthesized for breast development. A similar lack of sex steroid synthesis occurs in males with a 17,20-desmolase deficiency. Individuals with agonadism, sometimes called the *vanishing testes syndrome*, have no gonads present, but since the female internal genitalia are also absent it has been postulated that testicular MIF production occurred during fetal life, but the gonadal tissue subsequently regressed.

Secondary Sex Characteristics and Female Internal Genitalia Present

This is the second largest category of patients with primary amenorrhea, accounting for about one third of patients with this disorder. In the series reported by Maschchak et al., about 25% of these individuals had hyperprolactinemia and prolactinomas. The remaining patients had etiologies similar to those women with secondary amenorrhea and thus should be subcategorized and treated similarly to patients with secondary amenorrhea, which is discussed in the latter half of this chapter.

Differential Diagnosis and Management

After a history is obtained and a physical examination performed, including measurement of height, span, and weight, such patients are placed into one of the four general categories listed in the box on p. 1107, depending on the presence or absence of secondary sex characteristics and female internal genitalia.

If breast development is absent and a uterus is present, the diagnostic evaluation should differentiate between CNS-hypothalamic-pituitary disorders and failure of normal gonadal development. Although individuals with both these disorders have similar phenotypes because of low estradiol levels, a single serum

FSH assay can differentiate between these two major etiologic categories (Figure 36-7). Only those individuals with an elevated FSH level (>40 mIU/ml) should then have a peripheral white blood cell karyotype performed to determine if a Y chromosome is present. If a Y chromosome is present, the streak gonads should be excised, as the incidence of malignancy occurring subsequently, mainly gonadoblastomas, is relatively high. If a Y chromosome is absent, it is not necessary to perform laparoscopy or laparotomy or to remove the gonads; such surgical procedures should not be performed. It is also unnecessary to perform a karyotype on the gonadal tissue to detect mosaicism in the gonad unless there is physical evidence of excessive androgen production, that is, hirsutism.

All patients with an elevated FSH level and an XX karyotype should have electrolyte and serum progesterone levels measured to rule out 17α-hydroxylase deficiency. In addition to hypernatremia and hypokalemia, individuals with 17α-hydroxylase deficiency have an elevated serum progesterone level (>3 ng/ml), a low 17α-hydroxyprogesterone level (<0.2 ng/ml), and an elevated serum deoxycorticoster-

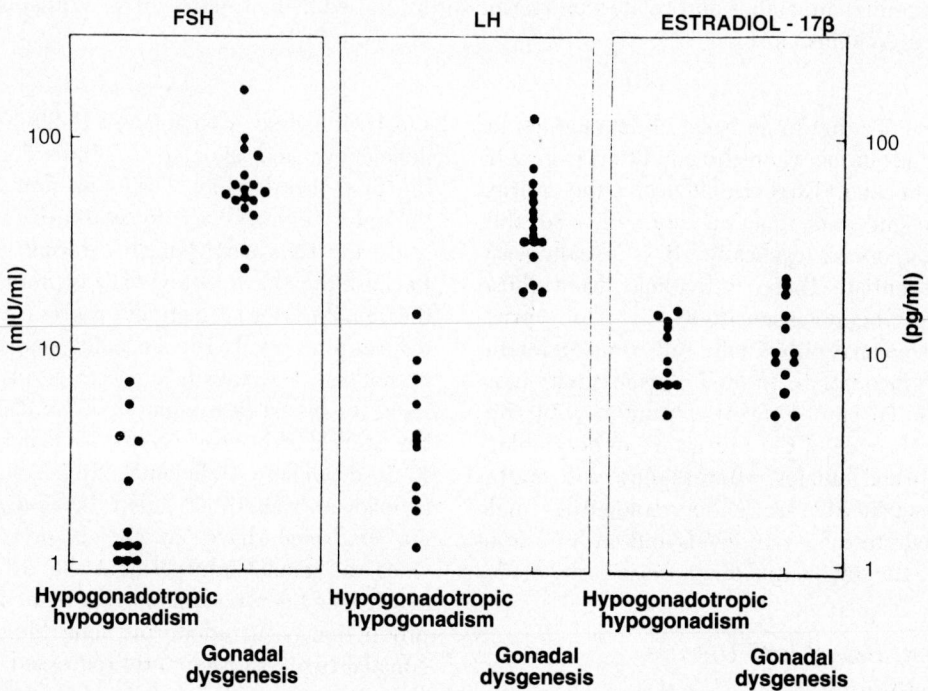

FIGURE 36-7
Levels of serum FSH, LH, and estradiol in patients with primary amenorrhea who have an intact uterus and no breast development. (From Maschchak CA, Kletzky OA, Davajan V, et al: Obstet Gynecol 57:715, 1981. Reprinted with permission from The American College of Obstetricians and Gynecologists.)

one level (>17 ng/100 ml), so the diagnosis is easily established.

All individuals in this category are sterile but need estrogen-progestogen replacement therapy to develop breast tissue and prevent osteoporosis. The progestogen is necessary to decrease the risk of endometrial carcinoma, which may be increased by long-term unopposed estrogen administration. Ingestion of 0.625 mg conjugated estrogen or 1 mg estradiol daily for 25 days per month and 5 to 10 mg medroxyprogesterone acetate daily for the last 12 days of estrogen therapy is sufficient to achieve maximal breast growth and prevent osteoporosis. Larger doses of estrogen will not result in larger breasts. Those rare individuals with 17α-hydroxylase deficiency need to have adequate cortisol replacement in addition to sex steroid treatment.

If the FSH level is low, the underlying disorder is in the CNS-hypothalamic-pituitary region and a serum prolactin measurement should be obtained. Even if the prolactin level is not elevated, all such individuals should have a cranial CT scan or MRI obtained to rule out a lesion in this area. If no tumor is found, it is not necessary to perform a karyotype, as all these individuals are 46,XX. The use of GnRH testing is optional but is expensive and is clinically unnecessary unless GnRH is going to be used for ovulation induction. Such individuals are potentially fertile because their ovaries are normal. Initially they should receive estrogen-progestogen treatment to promote breast growth. When fertility is desired, treatment with human menopausal gonadotrophins or pulsatile GnRH should be administered to induce ovulation.

The differential diagnosis of androgen insensitivity from uterine agenesis can be made by the presence in the latter condition of normal body hair, ovulatory and premenstrual-type symptoms, a biphasic basal temperature, and a normal female testosterone level. Such individuals are sterile but are endocrinologically normal females, and they do not need hormonal therapy or karyotyping. An intravenous urogram or some type of scanning should be performed because of the high incidence of renal abnormalities. They may need surgical reconstruction of an absent vagina (McIndoe procedure), but progressive mechanical dilation with plastic dilators as described by Frank should be tried first.

Individuals with androgen insensitivity have an XY karyotype and male levels of testosterone. After full breast development is obtained and epiphyseal closure occurs, the gonads should be removed because of their malignant potential. Thereafter estrogen-progestogen replacement therapy, as outlined earlier, should be administered.

Those rare individuals with absent breast development and absent internal genitalia should be referred to an endocrine center for the sophisticated type of testing necessary to establish the diagnosis. If gonads are present, they should be removed, because a Y chromosome is present, and replacement female sex steroid therapy should be administered.

SECONDARY AMENORRHEA

Etiology

The symptom of amenorrhea associated with hyperprolactinemia or excessive androgen or cortisol production will not be considered in this chapter as these disorders are discussed in Chapters 37 and 38. If amenorrhea is present without galactorrhea, hyperprolactinemia, or hirsutism, the symptom can result from disorders in the CNS-hypothalamic-pituitary axis, ovary, or uterus. In a review of 262 patients presenting with secondary amenorrhea during a 20-year period at a tertiary medical center, Reindollar et al. (1986) reported that 12% of cases resulted from a primary ovarian problem, 62% from a hypothalamic disorder, 16% from a pituitary problem (including prolactinomas), and 7% from a uterine disorder. The uterine cause of amenorrhea is the only one in which the patient has normal endocrinologic function and will be discussed first.

Uterine Cause

Intrauterine adhesions (IUAs) or synechiae (Asherman's syndrome) can obliterate the endometrial cavity and produce secondary amenorrhea. Rarely, a missed abortion or endometrial tuberculosis can also cause endometrial destruction. The most frequent antecedent factor of IUAs is endometrial curettage associated with pregnancy—either evacuation of a normal-gestation fetus by mechanical means or postpartum or postabortal curettage. Curettage for a missed abortion results in a high (30%) incidence of IUA formation. IUAs may also occur after diagnostic dilation and curettage (D&C) in a nonpregnant individual, so this procedure

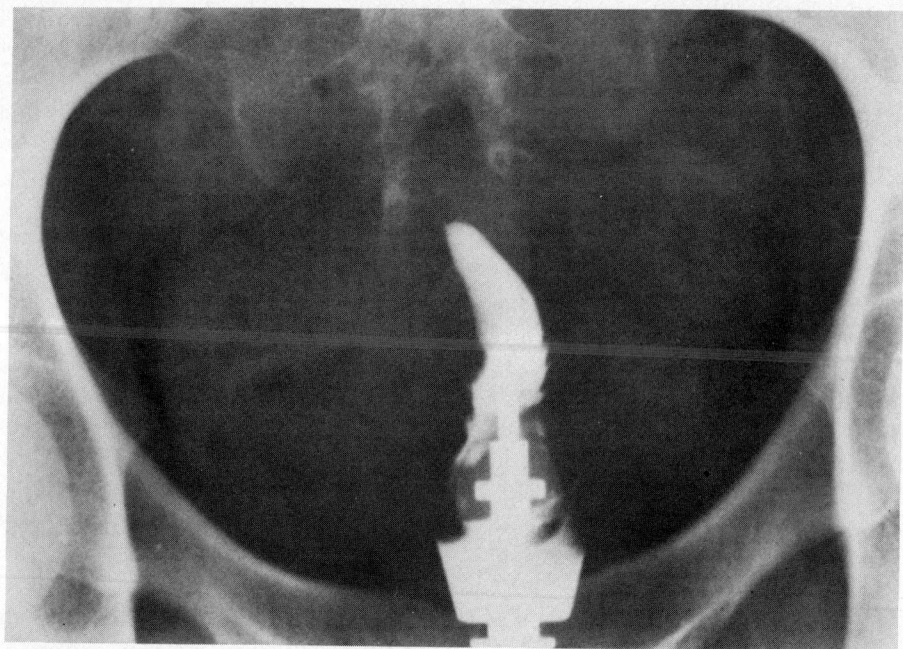

FIGURE 36-8

X-ray film of patient with Asherman's syndrome. Patient (33 years, gravida 3, para O, abortus 3) had been amenorrheic for 6 months after D&C for most recent therapeutic abortion (TAB). Filling of endocervical canal and nonvisualization of endometrial cavity are consistent with complete obliteration of cavity by adhesions or with obstruction at internal os level by adhesions in lower endometrial cavity. This appearance may also be seen with advanced endometrial tuberculosis. (From Richmond JA: Hysterosalpingography. Reproduced with permission from Infertility, contraception and reproductive endocrinology, ed 2, by Daniel R. Mishell, Jr., M.D., and Val Davajan, M.D. Copyright © 1986 by Medical Economics Books, Oradell, N.J. 07649. All rights reserved.)

should be performed only when indicated and not routinely at the time of other surgical procedures such as diagnostic laparoscopy. A less common cause of IUA is severe endometritis or fibrosis following a myomectomy, metroplasty, or cesarean section. The etiology should be suspected if there is difficulty or inability to pass a sound into the uterine cavity; this can be confirmed by means of a hysterogram (Figure 36-8) or hysteroscopy. Although some researchers have advocated that sequential administration of estrogen-progestogen be used as the initial diagnostic procedure when IUA is suspected, withdrawal bleeding occurs following administration of the steroids in most patients with IUA, and therefore this test is not definitive for establishing the diagnosis and is unnecessary.

CNS-Hypothalamic Causes

LESIONS. The same anatomic lesions in the brainstem or hypothalamus that can produce primary amenorrhea by interfering with GnRH release can also cause secondary amenorrhea. Hypothalamic lesions include craniopharyngiomas, granulomatous disease (tuberculosis and sarcoidosis), and sequelae of encephalitis. When such uncommon lesions are present, circulating gonadotrophin levels and estradiol levels are low; as a result, uterine bleeding will not occur after progesterone administration.

DRUGS. Phenothiazine derivatives, certain antihypertensive agents, and other drugs listed in Chapter 37 can also produce amenorrhea without galactorrhea, although usually the prolactin levels are elevated. Therefore, every individual with secondary amenorrhea should

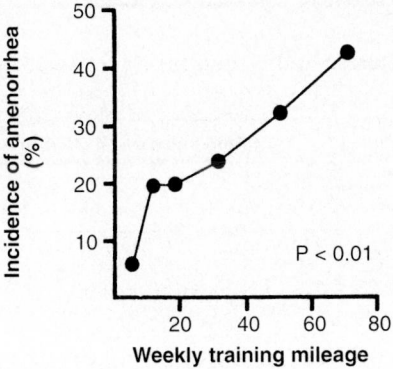

FIGURE 36-9
Correlation between training mileage and amenorrhea. Each point represents average of 21 respondents. Statistical significance of relationship was obtained from point-biserial correlation (1 mile [1.6 km]). (From Feicht CB, Johnson TS, and Matrin BJ: Lancet 2:1145, 1978.)

have a detailed medication history obtained even if galactorrhea is not present. Oral contraceptive steroids inhibit ovulation by acting both on the hypothalamus to suppress GnRH and directly on the pituitary to suppress FSH and LH. Sometimes this hypothalamic-pituitary suppression persists for several months after oral contraceptives are discontinued, producing the syndrome termed "postpill amenorrhea." This oral contraceptive–induced suppression does not last more than 6 months, as it has been reported that the incidence of amenorrhea persisting more than 6 months after discontinuation of oral contraceptives (0.8%) is about the same as the incidence of secondary amenorrhea in the general population (0.7%). Thus the etiology of amenorrhea persisting more than 6 months after discontinuation of oral contraceptives is unrelated to their use, except that the regular withdrawal bleeding produced by oral contraceptives masks the development of this syndrome.

STRESS AND EXERCISE. Stressful situations including a sudden change in environment (e.g., going away to school), a death in the family, or divorce can produce amenorrhea. A high percentage of women who had been placed in concentration camps or those sentenced for execution also became amenorrheic as a result of stress.

It is also now believed that the amenorrhea associated with strenuous exercise is also related to stress. Feicht et al. reported that the incidence of secondary amenorrhea in runners had a positive correlation with the number of miles run per week (Figure 36-9). In a comparison of amenorrheic and eumenorrheic athletes, this group of investigators showed that physical parameters such as age, weight, lean body mass, and body fat were similar. The only significant difference between the two groups was the fact that the amenorrheic athletes ran more miles per week. McArthur et al. reported there was no significant difference in the percentage of body fat in amenorrheic runners compared with runners who were menstruating. In a longitudinal study of competitive swimmers, Russell et al. found that when the training became more strenuous, their LH and FSH levels fell significantly, while levels of beta-endorphin and catechol estrogens rose significantly as compared with levels of these hormones when the swimmers were exercising to a moderate degree (Tables 36-4 and 36-5). Individuals with a low percentage of adipose tissue have a shift in the pathway of estrogen metabolism from 16-hydroxylation, which forms estriol, to 2-hydroxylation, which forms catechol estrogens. It has been postulated that the decreased fatty tissue in individuals who exercise is the reason for the increased levels of catechol estrogens. However, when the swimmers were exercising only moderately, levels of catechol estrogens as well as beta-endorphin were not significantly different from those of a control group of similar body weight and percentage body fat who were not participating in organized physical activity. This group of investigators also reported that another group of swimmers and runners had significantly higher levels of catechol estrogens than a control group of normally menstruating women with a similar weight and low percentage of body fat. Whether catechol estrogens are increased as a result of less fatty tissue, the stress of training, or a combination of both, the increase may be the cause of the amenorrhea. The competition between catecholamine and catechol estrogens for catechol-O-methyltransferase may result in increased levels of dopamine, which in turn suppresses the release of GnRH and thus LH. Adashi et al. showed that infusion or injection of catechol estrogens decreased LH levels in humans.

Carr et al. also reported that physical condi-

TABLE 36-4

Analysis* of Protein Hormones for Swimmers During Moderate and Strenuous Exercise and for Nonexercising Control Subjects

| Hormone | Control Subjects | Swimmers | | Group Comparison (Median Values) | | |
		Moderate (60,000 yards)	Strenuous (100,000 yards)	C vs. 60	C vs. 100	100 vs. 60
No.	6	5	5			
LH (mIU/ml)	23.1[21.4] ± 10.5 (12.3-13.3)	22.9[22.2] ± 5.7 (15.9-30.7)	10.9[11.3] ± 2.8 (7.4-13.6)	P = 0.66	P = 0.02	P = 0.02
FSH (mIU/ml)	10.9[9.6] ± 3.5 (7.1-15.7)	20.2[18.2] ± 5.1 (15.3-27.7)	6.54[6.8] ± 2.1 (4.0-9.5)	P = 0.05	P = 0.04	P ≤ 0.001
Prolactin (ng/ml)	20.8[13.5] ± 15.0 (9.0-47.2)	10.6[10.5] ± 3.6 (5.9-16.1)	1.36[1.0] ± 0.9 (0.7-3.0)	P = 0.18	P = 0.004	P = 0.006

Adapted from Russel JB, Mitchell DE, Musey PI, et al: Fertil Steril 42:690, 1984. Reproduced with permission of the publisher, The American Fertility Society.
*Mean (median) value ± SD with range in parentheses.

TABLE 36-5

Analysis* of Beta-Endorphin Immunoreactivity, Estradiol, and Catechol Estrogens for Swimmers During Moderate and Strenuous Exercise and for Nonexercising Control Subjects

| Hormone | Control Subjects | Swimmers | | Group Comparisons | | |
		Moderate (60,000 yards)	Strenuous (100,000 yards)	C vs. 60	C vs. 100	100 vs. 60
No.	6	5	5			
Estradiol (pg/ml)	264[193] ± 253 (78-759)	61.8[65] ± 16.8 (36-79)	76.8[52] ± 61.9 (36-185)	P = 0.009	P = 0.003	P = 0.68
Catecholestrogens (pg/ml)	35.3[35] ± 7.5 (25-46)	28.6[28] ± 1.2 (26-29)	92.4[88] ± 12.8 (83-115)	P = 0.08	P ≤ 0.001	P ≤ 0.001
Beta-endorphin immunoreactivity (pmol/L)	8.50[2] ± 15.4 (2-40)	4.40[4] ± 2.2 (2-8)	31.2[24] ± 14.3 (18-52)	P = 0.25	P = 0.03	P = 0.01

Adapted from Russel JB, Mitchell DE, Musey PI, et al: Fertil Steril 42:690, 1984. Reproduced with permission of the publisher, The American Fertility Society.
*Mean (median) value ± SD with range in parentheses.

tioning facilitates the exercise-induced secretion of beta-endorphin and its precursor beta-lipoprotein in women. Reid et al. showed that infusion of beta-endorphin into women caused a significant decrease in LH. Beta-endorphin and its analogues inhibit GnRH release, possibly by inhibiting the stimulating effect of norepinephrine on GnRH. Russell et al. (1989) administered the opioid antagonist naloxone to a group of oligomenorrheic and eumenorrheic competive swimmers and noted an increase in baseline LH only in the former group.

Thus the increase in both catechol estrogens and beta-endorphins associated with strenuous exercise appears to be the mechanism whereby LH and probably FSH release is inhibited, most likely by acting on the neurotransmitters responsible for release of GnRH. The decreased gonadotrophin levels produce amenorrhea by failing to stimulate sex steroid production.

It is probable that emotionally stressful situations such as divorce or a sudden change in environment can also cause alterations in beta-endorphin and catechol estrogens. When the stressful situation (whether emotional in origin or related to strenuous exercise) abates, menstruation usually resumes promptly.

WEIGHT LOSS. Both male and female animals who are malnourished have decreased reproductive capacity. Weight loss is also associated with amenorrhea in women and has been classified into two groups: the moderately underweight group includes individuals whose weight is 15% to 25% below ideal body weight; severely underweight women are those whose weight loss is greater than 25% of ideal body weight. Weight loss can occur from excessive dietary restrictions as well as malnutrition. Vigersky et al. have demonstrated that women with amenorrhea associated with simple weight loss have both direct and indirect evidence of hypothalamic dysfunction, while pituitary and end-organ function is normal. Mason and Sagle showed that in contrast to women with normal cycles, a group of women with weight loss amenorrhea had similar mean levels of LH as well as LH pulse amplitude but decreased frequency of LH pulses. Warren et al. however, showed that when women were severely underweight, in addition to hypothalamic dysfunction, pituitary gonadotrophin function was also altered because there was no increase in LH and a decreased response of FSH following GnRH administration. However, these responses could be due to a lack of prolonged GnRH secretion, because the studies were not performed after several days of GnRH priming. Thus the amenorrhea associated with weight loss appears to be due mainly to failure of normal GnRH release, with a possible pituitary disorder also occurring when the weight loss is severe.

A severe psychiatric disorder called *anorexia nervosa* is also associated with severe weight loss and amenorrhea. Anorexia nervosa is not rare, and it is estimated to occur in about 1 in 1000 white women in the United States. It is uncommon in men and rare in blacks and Orientals. This disorder is most frequent in teenagers and is uncommon after the age of 25. It is one of the most important and probably the most common causes of secondary amenorrhea in adolescent women. This disorder is associated with other physical changes, including dry skin, bradycardia, hypotension, constipation, and hypothermia (see box at right). Individuals with anorexia nervosa usually have a normal

CRITERIA FOR DIAGNOSIS OF ANOREXIA NERVOSA

Onset before 25 years of age

Anorexia with accompanying weight loss of at least 25% of original body weight

Distorted, implacable attitude toward eating, food, or weight that overrides hunger, admonitions, reassurance, and threats—for example
  Denial of illness
  Failure to recognize nutritional needs
  Apparent enjoyment in losing weight
  Desired body image of extreme thinness
  Unusual hoarding or handling of food

No known medical illness that could account for the anorexia and weight loss

No other known psychiatric disorder

At least two of the following manifestations:
  Amenorrhea
  Lanugo
  Bradycardia (persistent resting pulse of 60 bpm or less)
  Periods of overactivity
  Episodes of bulimia
  Vomiting (may be self-induced)

From Sherman BM, Halmi KA and Zamudio R: J Clin Endocrinol Metab 41:135, 1975. Copyright © by the Endocrine Society, 1975.

thyroxine (T_4) level and an abnormally low serum triiodothyronine (T_3) level. If the clinician cannot make the differential diagnosis between amenorrhea caused by simple weight loss and that caused by anorexia nervosa on clinical findings alone, measurement of the serum T_3 level is most helpful, as individuals with simple weight loss usually have normal T_3 levels. In patients with anorexia nervosa T_4 levels are normal, T_3 levels are low, and reverse T_3 (an inactive metabolite) levels are increased, indicating that peripheral conversion of T_4 to T_3 is impaired. Patients with anorexia nervosa have a hypothalamic disorder interfering with normal GnRH release, and their amenorrhea frequently occurs at the time of initiation of food restriction before they lose weight. However, after severe weight loss occurs in these individuals and they are less than 65% of ideal body weight, an abnormal gonadotrophin response to GnRH takes place similar to those seen in individuals with severe weight loss caused by dieting. This indicates that pituitary dysfunction also occurs in persons with anorexia ner-

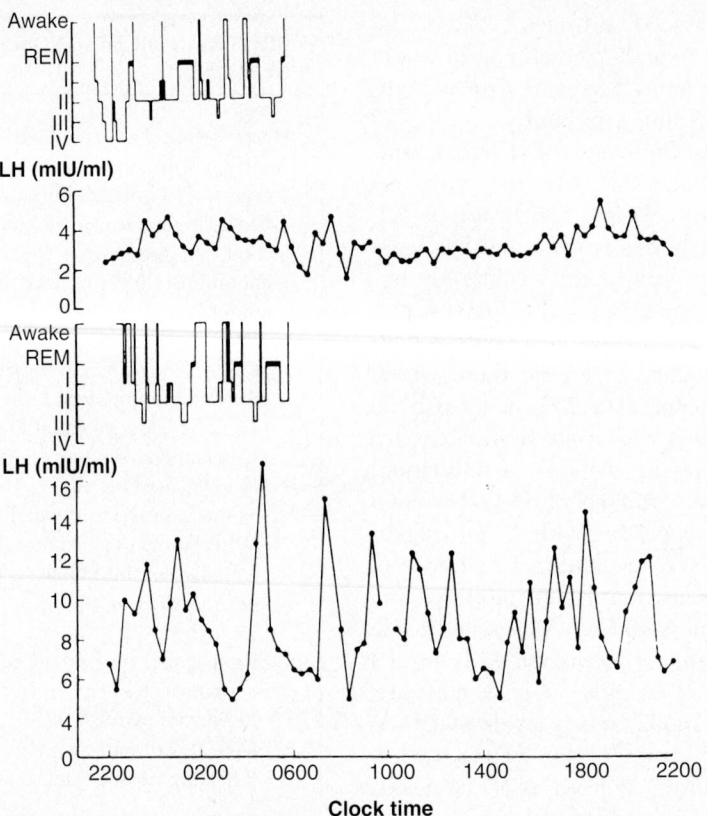

FIGURE 36-10

Plasma LH concentrations every 20 minutes for 24 hours during acute exacerbation of anorexia nervosa *(upper panel)* and after clinical remission with return of body weight to normal *(lower panel)*. (From Boyar RM, Katz J, Finkelstein JW, et al: N Engl J Med 291:861, 1974. Reprinted by permission of The New England Journal of Medicine.)

vosa when the weight loss becomes severe. Boyar et al. have shown that patients with anorexia nervosa have an LH secretion pattern similar to that observed in prepubertal children (absent LH pulses) (Figure 36-10) or pubertal premenarcheal girls (nocturnal LH pulses only). When these individuals gain weight, the normal 24-hour LH pulsatile patterns return. Weight gain in either individuals with anorexia nervosa or those with severe simple weight loss results in their gonadotrophin response to GnRH infusion becoming normal or even exaggerated, with the FSH response resuming in proportion to the weight gain and the LH responsiveness returning only after the individual reaches about 85% of ideal body weight. These progressive endocrine responses are also similar to those occurring during puberty, indicating the importance of body weight in causing maturation of the CNS-hypothalamic-pituitary

axis and providing additional information as to why girls who exercise strenuously before menarche and have less body fat also have a delayed onset of menstruation. Frisch and Revelle reported that undernourished girls reach menarche at an older age but at the same mean weight as well-nourished girls. Treasure et al. using ultrasound scanning, showed that as patients with anorexia nervosa gained weight, changes occurred in ovarian morphology. These changes progressed from small ovaries without follicles, to ovaries of normal size and multiple small cysts, then to the appearance of a dominant cyst. These are similar to the changes in ovarian morphology that occur during normal pubertal development.

Anorexia nervosa is a psychiatric disorder, and patients with this disease should receive appropriate psychiatric treatment. These individuals as well as those with dietary weight loss

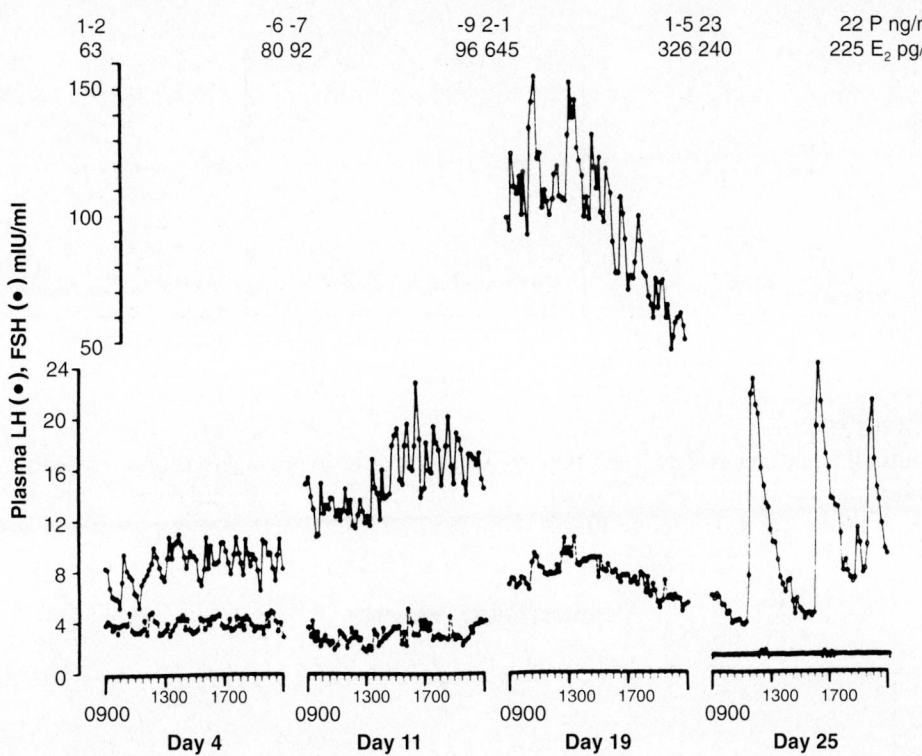

FIGURE 36-11

Serial measurements of plasma LH and FSH in two subjects sampled every 10 minutes at weekly intervals during cycles in which LH surge was observed on one of sampling days. (From Reame NE, Sauder SE, Kelch RP, et al: J Clin Endocrinol Metab 59:328, 1984. Copyright © by The Endocrine Society 1984.)

usually resume ovulatory menstrual cycles when they gain weight and approach their ideal body weight.

POLYCYSTIC OVARY SYNDROME. It is now believed that polycystic ovary syndrome (PCOS) is a CNS-hypothalamic disorder that produces tonically elevated LH levels. Most of the women with these disorders have elevated androgen levels, but not all have clinical evidence of androgen excess (hirsutism). Thus the presence of PCO must be considered in the differential diagnosis of both primary and secondary amenorrhea even if hirsutism is absent. Because most individuals with PCO have signs of androgen excess, this subject is discussed in detail in Chapter 38.

FUNCTIONAL HYPOTHALAMIC AMENORRHEA. There is a group of individuals with secondary amenorrhea who do not ingest drugs, do not engage in strenuous exercise, are not under severe environmental stress, and have not lost weight. No pituitary, ovarian, or uter-

ine abnormalities are present in these individuals. The general term *functional hypothalamic amenorrhea* (FHA) has been used to characterize this disorder. Several investigators, using frequent blood sampling, have shown that LH is secreted in a pulsatile manner that varies in frequency and amplitude throughout the normal ovulatory menstrual cycle, being more rapid in the follicular phase than the luteal phase (Figure 36-11). These investigators have shown that women with amenorrhea due to hypothalamic dysfunction do not exhibit these characteristic cyclic alterations in LH pulsatility. They either have no pulses (Figure 36-12) or have a persistent pattern of pulsatility that is normally found in only one portion of the ovulatory cycle, usually the slow frequency found in the luteal phase, despite having a steroid milieu similar to the follicular phase (Figure 36-13). Since each LH pulse represents a response to a pulse of GnRH, it appears that these individuals have an abnormal-

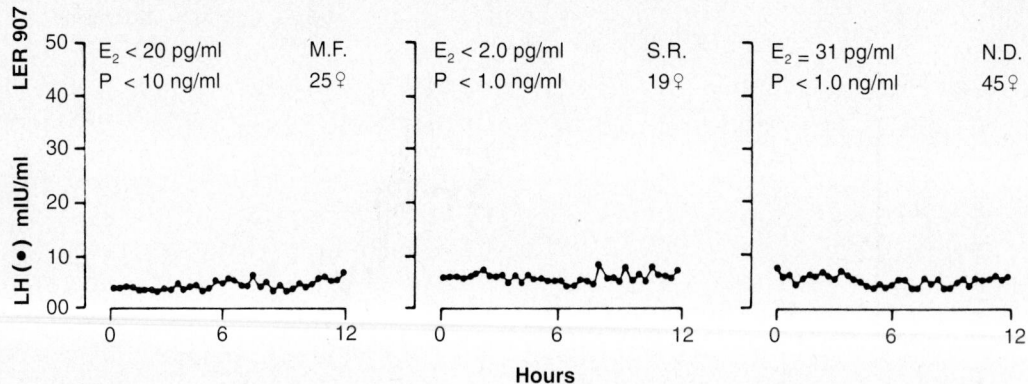

FIGURE 36-12
Apulsatile pattern of LH secretion in women with hypogonadotrophic hypogonadism and hypothalamic amenorrhea. (From Crowley WF Jr, Filicori M, Spratt DI, et al: Rec Prog Hormone Res 41:473, 1985.)

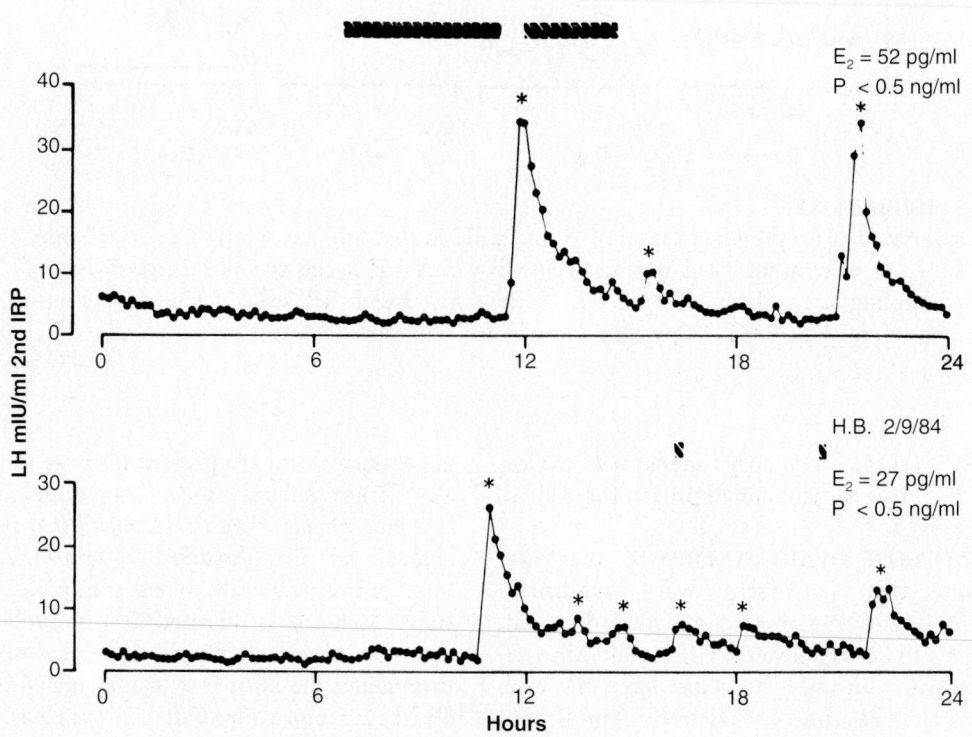

FIGURE 36-13
Defects in frequency of LH secretion episodes in subjects with hypothalamic amenorrhea. (From Crowley WF Jr, Filicori M, Spratt DI, et al: Rec Prog Hormone Res 41:473, 1985.)

ity in the normal cyclic variations of GnRH pulsatility, probably due to an abnormality in the CNS neurotransmitters and possibly produced by increased opioid activity. As reported by Ferin et al. Quigley et al. and Wildt and Leyendecker, administration of the opioid antagonists naloxone and naltrexone to women with

FHA is followed by an increase in frequency of LH pulses as well as induction of ovulation.

Berga et al. measured several pituitary hormones at frequent intervals in a 24-hour period in 10 women with FHA and 10 women with normal cycles. As also reported by others, they found a 53% reduction in LH pulse frequency among the women with FHA; however, the LH pulse amplitude was similar in the two groups. In addition to reduced secretion of LH, there was reduced secretion of FSH, prolactin, and thyroid-stimulating hormone (TSH), as well as altered rhythms of growth hormone (GH) and cortisol with elevated cortisol levels. However, the pituitary response to releasing hormones was unchanged. Thus multiple hormonal alterations occur in FHA as an adaptive central neuroendocrine event.

When sufficient GnRH is produced to stimulate sufficient gonadotrophin production to maintain circulating estradiol levels above 40 pg/ml, the term *hypothalamic-pituitary dysfunction* is used to characterize this disorder. However, when the estradiol levels fall below 40 pg/ml, the term *hypothalamic-pituitary failure* has been used, indicating a more serious disorder. Serum estradiol levels above 40 pg/ml are usually sufficient to stimulate endometrial growth to an extent that sloughing occurs when progesterone levels fall several days after an injection of progesterone in oil is given. The withdrawal bleeding response to progesterone administration has also been used to differentiate between these two diagnostic categories.

Pituitary Causes (Hypoestrogenic Amenorrhea)

NEOPLASMS. Although most pituitary tumors secrete prolactin, some do not and may be associated with the onset of secondary amenorrhea without galactorrhea. Chromophobe adenomas are the most common non-prolactin-secreting pituitary tumors; however, both basophilic (ACTH secreting) and acidophilic (GH secreting) adenomas may be incapable of secreting prolactin. Individuals with the latter types of tumor, although having secondary amenorrhea, frequently have other symptoms produced by these lesions and present to the clinician with symptoms of acromegaly or Cushing's syndrome.

NONNEOPLASTIC LESIONS. Pituitary cells can also become damaged or necrotic as a result of anoxia, thrombosis, or hemorrhage. When pituitary cell destruction occurs as a result of a hypotensive episode during pregnancy, the disorder is called *Sheehan's syndrome*. When the disorder is unrelated to pregnancy, it is called *Simmond's disease*. It is important to diagnose this cause of secondary amenorrhea, because in contrast to the hypothalamic disorders, pituitary damage can be associated with decreased secretion of other pituitary hormones, particularly ACTH and TSH, in addition to LH and FSH. Thus these individuals may have secondary hypothyroidism or adrenal insufficiency that may seriously impair their health, in addition to their decreased estrogen levels.

Ovarian Causes (Hypogonadotrophic Hypogonadism)

The ovaries may fail to secrete sufficient estrogen to produce endometrial growth if the follicles are damaged as a result of infection, interference with blood supply, or depletion of follicles caused by bilateral cystectomies. These individuals may become amenorrheic after a variable period of time has elapsed following medical treatment of bilateral tuboovarian abscess, after bilateral cystectomy for benign ovarian neoplasm, or sometimes after a hysterectomy during which the vascular supply to the ovaries is compromised (sometimes called *cystic degeneration of the ovaries*).

Occasionally the ovaries cease to produce sufficient estrogen to stimulate endometrial growth several years before the age of the physiologic menopause. When this condition occurs before the age of 40, the term *premature ovarian failure* (POF) instead of premature menopause is best used to describe the clinical entity. Coulam et al. estimated that as many as 1% of women under age 40 have hypergonadotrophic amenorrhea, with the incidence steadily increasing from ages 15 to 39. Histologically, individuals with POF have two types of ovarian pathologic findings. In the majority there is generalized sclerosis similar to the findings of a normal postmenopausal ovary (Figure 36-14), whereas in about 30% numerous primordial follicles with no progression past the antrum stage are seen (Figure 36-15). The latter condition has been called the *gonadotrophin-resistant ovary syndrome* or *ovarian hypofolliculogenesis* and is histologically different from the gonadal streak, in which no follicles are seen. Women with this condition may have primary amenorrhea, but usually sufficient estrogen is produced so that they menstruate for several months or even years. POF has also been reported in individuals with steroid hormonal enzyme deficiencies who menstruate temporarily and then have secondary

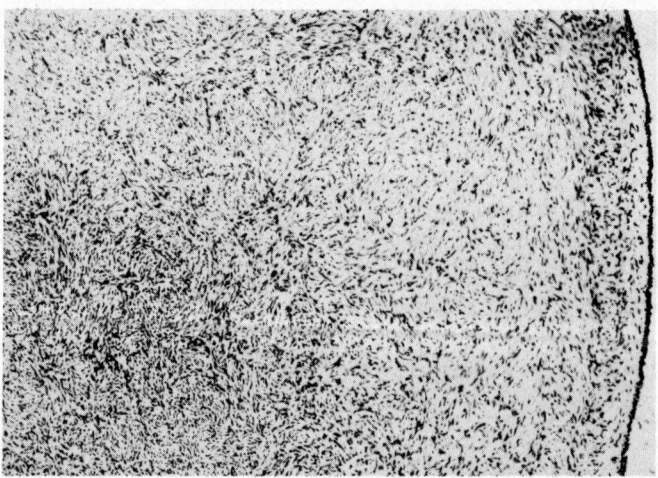

FIGURE 36-14
Representative section of ovary from patient with premature ovarian failure (POF). Cortex of ovary is devoid of follicles. (From Tulandi T and Kinch RAH: Obstet Gynecol Surv 35:521, 1981.)

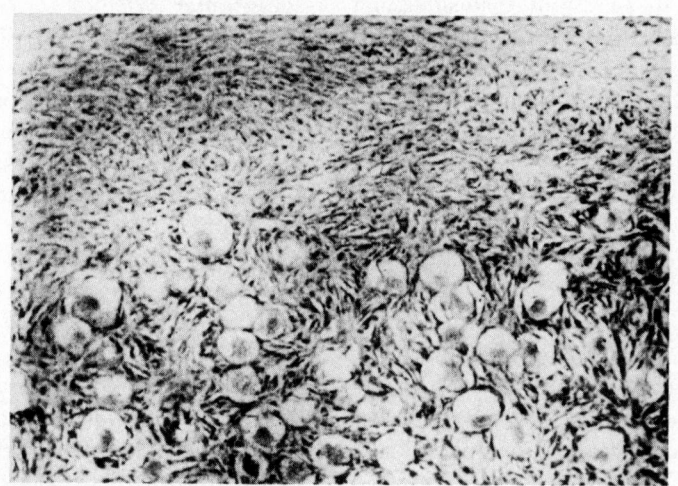

FIGURE 36-15
Representative section of ovary from patient with insensitive ovary syndrome. Numerous primordial follicles are seen. (From Tulandi T and Kinch RAH: Obstet Gynecol Surv 35:521, 1981.)

amenorrhea. Many individuals with POF, particularly those with primordial follicles that appear normal, also have an autoimmune disease such as hypoparathyroidism, Hashimoto's thyroiditis, or Addison's disease. Many individuals with POF who do not have clinical evidence of an autoimmune disease have antibodies to gonadotrophins as well as to several other endocrine organs such as the thyroid and adrenal glands, suggesting an autoimmune etiology. POF can also occur after gonadal irradiation or systemic chemotherapy. In some instances the condition may be transient before permanent ovarian failure; occasionally these individuals may ovulate and conceive.

Alper and Garner estimated that about 30% to 50% of individuals with chromosomally normal POF without a history of irradiation or chemotherapy have an associated autoimmune disease, most commonly thyroid disease, which was present in 85% of the group with an autoimmune disorder. Mignot et al., using sophisticated immunofluorescence techniques, demonstrated that 92% of women with POF had laboratory evidence of autosensitization. About two thirds of these were positive for nonorgan-specific antibodies, mainly antinuclear antibodies and rheumatoid factors. Fifty percent had organ-specific antibodies. Although the majority of these women had no evidence of autoimmune disease, it is recommended that immunologic screening be perfomed on such individuals.

Diagnostic Evaluation and Management

For any patient consulting a clinician for the symptom of secondary amenorrhea, a diagnostic evaluation should be initiated at that visit, even though 6 months may not have elapsed since the last menstrual period. Amenorrhea is a source of concern to the patient, and it will relieve her concern if attempts are made to find the cause of the symptom. The clinician first should perform a detailed history and physical examination to rule out pregnancy as a cause of the amenorrhea. In addition, he or she should determine whether there is the possibility of IUA. Any instrumentation of the endometrial cavity, particularly temporally related to pregnancy, should alert the clinician to the possibility that an IUA is present. The next steps in the evaluation include placing a uterine sound into the uterine cavity and obtaining a hysterogram. The diagnosis can also be confirmed by detecting presumptive evidence of ovulation by means of either a biphasic basal temperature or an elevated serum progesterone level. If an IUA is ruled out, the history should disclose whether medications are currently being used or if oral contraceptives have been recently discontinued. In addition, questions regarding diet, weight loss, stress, and strenuous exercise are pertinent. A history of decreasing breast size or vaginal dryness and physical examination of these organs are helpful in estimating the degree of estrogen deficiency. If the history and physical examination fail to reveal the cause of the amenorrhea, measurement of thyroid function should be performed (T_3, T_4, and TSH) to rule out the uncommon asymptomatic thyroid disorders that produce secondary amenorrhea. A complete blood count, urinalysis, and serum chemistries should be measured to rule out systemic disease.

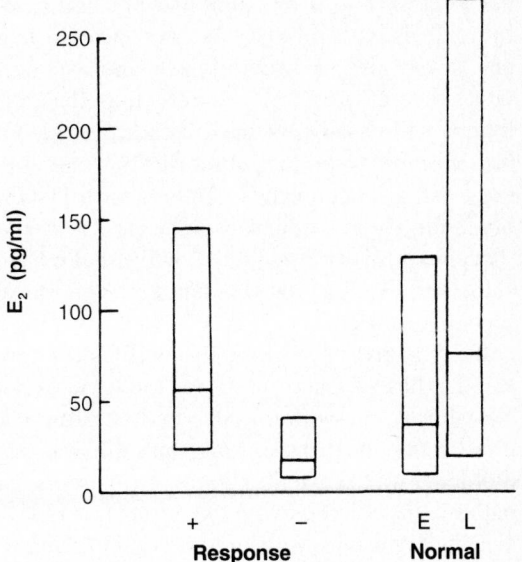

FIGURE 36-16
Estradiol levels in secondary amenorrhea in positive and negative categories. Mean values and 95% confidence limits in both groups are compared with estradiol levels in early and late follicular phase of normal ovulatory cycles. (From Kletzky OA, Davajan V, Nakamura RM, et al: Am J Obstet Gynecol 121:695, 1975.)

If the initial examination fails to reveal the cause of the amenorrhea, progesterone may be administered to determine if sufficient estrogen is present to produce endometrial growth that will slough after the progesterone levels fall (progesterone challenge test). As mentioned earlier, withdrawal bleeding after an intramuscular injection of 100 to 200 mg of progesterone in oil (depending on body weight) usually occurs if the circulating estradiol level is 40 pg/ml or greater (Figure 36-16). If desired, a serum estradiol level can be obtained. Alternatively, oral progestogen (10 mg of medroxyprogesterone acetate [MPA] daily for 5 days) can be administered, but if oral MPA is prescribed, compliance may be a problem. Any type of clinically observed uterine bleeding, even spotting, occurring within 2 weeks after the injection should be considered a positive response. In addition to reassuring the patient that she can menstruate, the observation of withdrawal bleeding after progesterone indicates that estradiol secretion is not markedly decreased and the cause of the amenorrhea is not as serious as if bleeding had not occurred. Individuals with pituitary tumors, ovarian failure, severe dietary weight loss or anorexia nervosa, severe stress, or the rare hypothalamic lesions will usually not have withdrawal bleeding after progesterone administration and hypoestrogenic amenorrhea. Patients with PCOS, moderate stress, exercise weight loss, or hypothalamic-pituitary dysfunction will usually have sufficient estradiol production for withdrawal bleeding to occur.

In a study of 60 women with secondary amenorrhea, Kletzky et al. found that about two thirds had withdrawal bleeding after administration of progesterone, and their estradiol level was above 40 pg/ml. In this group of patients there were two populations of LH levels, high and low, with only one population of FSH levels. Thus it is of value to obtain LH and prolactin measurements in patients with secondary amenorrhea who have withdrawal bleeding after progesterone administration. If the LH level is above 25 mIU/ml, a diagnosis of PCO should be suspected and confirmed by finding an LH/FSH ratio greater than 3. Even if hirsutism is absent, when this endocrinologic evidence of PCO is present, serum testosterone and DHEA-S should then be measured to determine if either or both are elevated.

If withdrawal bleeding occurs, LH and prolactin levels are in the normal range, and a history of drug ingestion, stress, weight loss, or strenuous exercise is not obtained, the patient should be told that hypothalamic-pituitary dysfunction is present and the exact etiology cannot be determined with current technology, as frequent LH sampling is costly and impractical. Hypothalamic-pituitary dysfunction is usually a self-limiting disorder and not a serious threat to health or a cause of untreatable infertility.

If withdrawal bleeding occurs and the prolactin level is elevated, further evaluation to detect the etiology of the hyperprolactinemia should be performed (Chapter 37).

If the patient with secondary amenorrhea fails to bleed after progesterone administration, Kletzky et al. found that the LH values belonged to a single population but the FSH values identified two populations, low and high. Those with low FSH levels had either a pituitary lesion or hypothalamic-pituitary failure, while those with elevated FSH levels (>30 mIU/ml) had POF.

Thus patients who fail to bleed after progesterone administration should have FSH and estradiol measured. Measurement of the actual estradiol level is useful in determining whether exogenous estrogen replacement is necessary. If the patient fails to bleed after progesterone and FSH is not elevated, prolactin should be measured. If severe weight loss, strenuous exercise, or severe stress is not present, a CT scan of the hypothalamic-pituitary region should be performed to rule out a lesion, even if the prolactin level is normal. If a lesion is seen or if there is a history compatible with possible pituitary destruction (hypotension during pregnancy), a test of ACTH reserve should be performed. An insulin tolerance test in which hypoglycemia is induced should normally cause an increase of 6 μg/100 ml of cortisol within 120 minutes and is a satisfactory test of ACTH function. If no lesion is identified, the term *hypothalamic-pituitary failure* may be used as a nonspecific diagnosis. Frequently these individuals resume normal ovarian function without treatment.

If POF is diagnosed because of an elevated FSH level and no cause of ovarian destruction is elicited, the possibility of autoimmune disease should be considered if the patient is less than 35 years of age. In these individuals antithyroid antibodies and antinuclear antibodies should be measured and a 24-hour urine-free cortisol level measured to detect possible Addison's disease. In addition, it is recommended that tests to detect rheumatoid factors be performed, fasting blood sugar, serum calcium, phosphorus, and T_4, and TSH levels should also be measured. To rule out mosaicism, a karyotype should be measured in women with POF who are 25 or younger, but not older. Biopsy of the gonads by laparoscopy or laparotomy is not indicated, because these individuals are usually sterile, although occasionally a follicle may ovulate. Suppression of gonadotrophin levels with estrogen, oral contraceptives, and GnRH analogues has been advocated by some clinicians to induce ovulation. Although gonadotrophins are suppressed by these agents, as shown by Ledger et al. and most other investigators, these techniques are usually ineffective in inducing ovulation. If ovulation occurs following such treatment, it is sporadic event and not a result of the therapy. The systematic evaluation is shown schematically in the box on p. 1125.

DIAGNOSTIC EVALUATION OF SECONDARY AMENORRHEA

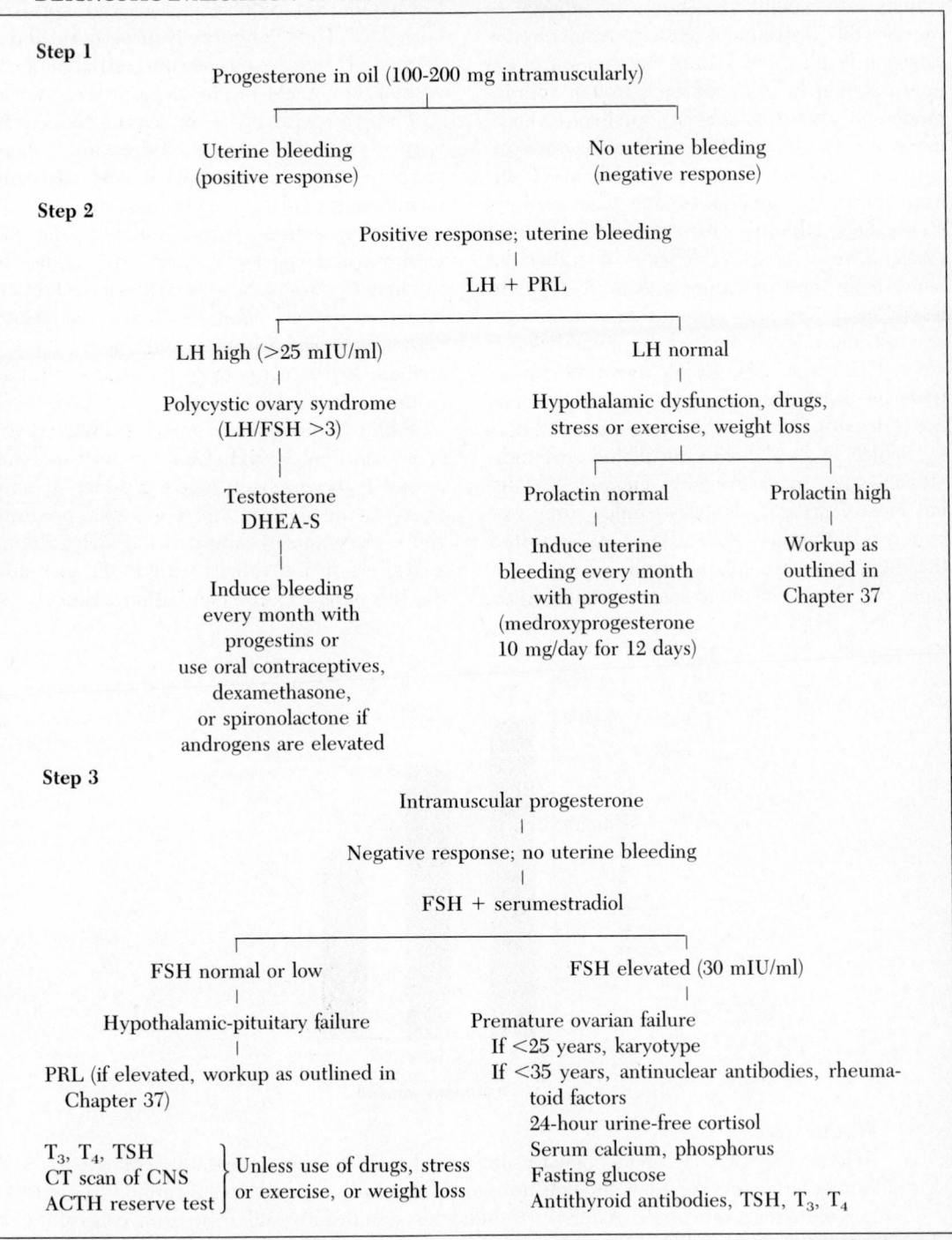

Step 1

Progesterone in oil (100-200 mg intramuscularly)

Uterine bleeding
(positive response)

No uterine bleeding
(negative response)

Step 2

Positive response; uterine bleeding

LH + PRL

LH high (>25 mIU/ml)

Polycystic ovary syndrome
(LH/FSH >3)

Testosterone
DHEA-S

Induce bleeding
every month with
progestins or
use oral contraceptives,
dexamethasone,
or spironolactone if
androgens are elevated

LH normal

Hypothalamic dysfunction, drugs,
stress or exercise, weight loss

Prolactin normal

Induce uterine
bleeding every month
with progestin
(medroxyprogesterone
10 mg/day for 12 days)

Prolactin high

Workup as
outlined in
Chapter 37

Step 3

Intramuscular progesterone

Negative response; no uterine bleeding

FSH + serumestradiol

FSH normal or low

Hypothalamic-pituitary failure

PRL (if elevated, workup as outlined in
Chapter 37)

T_3, T_4, TSH
CT scan of CNS   } Unless use of drugs, stress
ACTH reserve test   or exercise, or weight loss

FSH elevated (30 mIU/ml)

Premature ovarian failure
If <25 years, karyotype
If <35 years, antinuclear antibodies, rheuma-
toid factors
24-hour urine-free cortisol
Serum calcium, phosphorus
Fasting glucose
Antithyroid antibodies, TSH, T_3, T_4

Adapted from Davajan V and Kletzky OA: Secondary amenorrhea. In Mishell DR Jr, Davajan V, and Lobo
RA, editors: Infertility, contraception and reproductive endocrinology, ed 3, Cambridge, Mass. 1991, Blackwell Scientific Publications.

The appropriate treatment depends on the diagnosis and on whether conception is desired. Non-prolactin-secreting pituitary tumors should be surgically excised if possible. Individuals with weight loss should be advised to gain weight. If strenuous exercise results in low estrogen levels (<30 pg/ml), the amount of exercise should be reduced or estrogen supplementation advised to prevent possible development of osteoporosis. Several investigators, including Drinkwater et al. and Lloyd et al., have shown that amenorrheic as well as oligomenorrheic athletes with decreased estradiol levels have decreased density of trabecular bone in the lumbar spine (Figure 36-17). Klibanski et al. also have shown that women with low estradiol levels caused by hypothalamic amenorrhea who have normal nutrition and activity levels have a profound reduction in spinal bone density. In contrast to an earlier report by Schlechte et al., who postulated that individuals with hypoestrogenic amenorrhea did not have decreased bone loss unless they had hyperprolactinemia, Klibanski et al. reported that hyperprolactinemia by itself did not influence the degree of bone loss. In their study bone loss was similar in hyperprolactinemic amenorrheic women with low estrogen levels and women with normal prolactin levels (Figure 36-18). A group of women with hyperprolactinemia and regular menses did not have bone loss. Thus bone loss is directly related to decreased endogenous serum estradiol levels without being affected by hyperprolactinemia.

If women with PCOS or hypothalamic-pituitary dysfunction desire conception, clomiphene citrate administration is very successful in inducing ovulation. If pregnancy is not desired, progesterone withdrawal bleeding with medroxyprogesterone acetate (10 mg/day for the first 12 days of each month) will reduce the increased risk of endometrial cancer associated with unopposed estrogen and should be prescribed. If patients with hypothalamic-pituitary failure desire fertility, ovulation can be induced with human menopausal gonadotrophin (HMG) or intermittent GnRH. Clomiphene is not successful if the estrogen levels are low. If pregnancy is not desired, then estrogen-progestogen replacement is indicated for such patients, as well as all individuals with POF, to reduce the risk of osteoporosis and atherosclerosis.

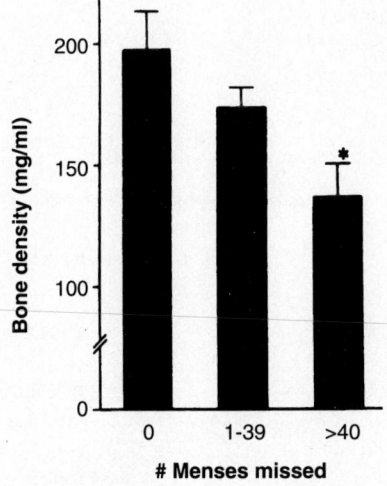

FIGURE 36-17
Relationship between bone density and number of missed menses in collegiate women athletes. For each subject, number of missed menses was determined from her menarche to age 19. Asterisk (*) indicates significantly different from control group. (From Lloyd T, Myers C, et al: Obstet Gynecol 72:639, 1988.)

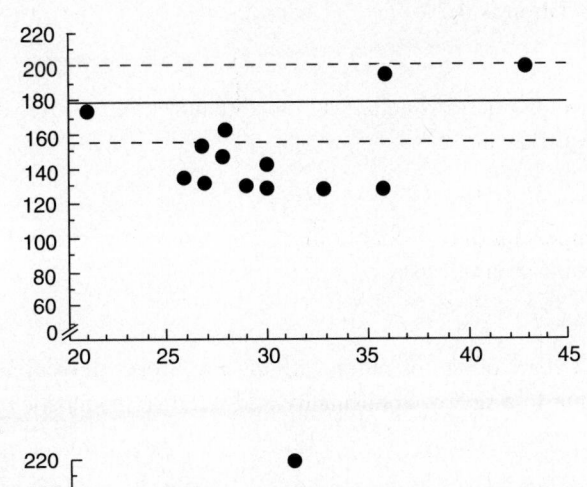

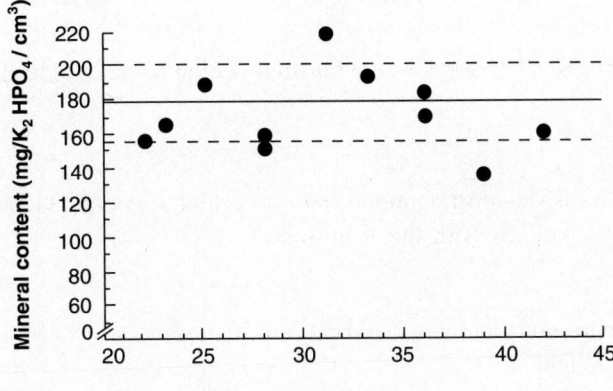

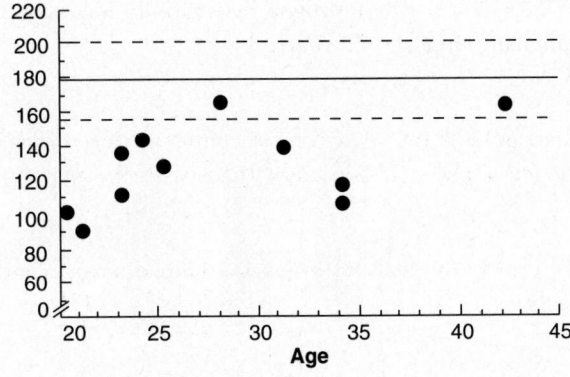

FIGURE 36-18
Spinal bone density in 13 women with hyperprolactinemic amenorrhea *(top panel)*, 12 eumenorrheic hyperprolactinemic women *(middle panel)*, and 11 women with hypothalamic amenorrhea *(bottom panel)*. Mean *(solid lines)* and standard deviation (± SD, *dashed lines*) for 19 normal women are shown. (From Klibanski A, Biller BMK, et al: J Clin Endocrinol Metab 67:124, 1988.)

_____ **KEY POINTS** _____

- The incidence of secondary amenorrhea of more than 6 months' duration in the general population is 0.7%.

- The incidence of amenorrhea lasting more than 6 months after discontinuation of oral contraceptives in 0.8%.

- The most important and probably most common cause of amenorrhea in adolescent girls is anorexia nervosa.

- A woman 13 years of age or older without any breast development has estrogen deficiency due to a severe abnormality and needs a diagnostic evaluation.

- Menarche is delayed about 0.4 year for each year of premenarcheal athletic training.

- Gonadal failure is the most common cause of primary amenorrhea, accounting for nearly half the patients with this syndrome.

- Individuals with gonadal failure and an X chromosome abnormality are less than 63 inches in height.

- The testes of individuals with androgen insensitivity have about a 20% chance of becoming malignant after age 20 years.

- Uterovaginal agenesis is the second most common cause of primary amenorrhea, with an incidence of about 15% of individuals with this symptom.

- About one third of individuals with gonadal failure have major cardiovascular or renal abnormalities.

- Congenital renal abnormalities occur in about one third of women with uterovaginal agenesis.

- The differential diagnosis between estrogen deficiency caused by gonadal failure and hypogonadotrophic hypogonadism is best made with measurement of serum follicle-stimulating hormone (FSH).

- The diagnosis of gonadal failure, or hypergonadotrophic hypogonadism, can be made if the FSH levels exceed 40 mIU/ml.

- Individuals with gonadal failure should have a peripheral karyotype performed to determine if a Y chromosome is present. If it is present, the gonads should be excised to prevent development of malignancy, mainly a gonadoblastoma.

- It is unnecessary to perform laparoscopy or laparotomy on an individual with gonadal failure if no Y chromosome is present in the peripheral karyotype unless the individual has hirsutism.

- Individuals with primary amenorrhea and hypogonatrophic hypogonadism do not need karyotyping but need a cranial computed tomography (CT) scan to rule out a central nervous system (CNS) tumor.

- The most frequent cause of intrauterine adhesion (IUA) is curettage performed during pregnancy or shortly thereafter.

- The amenorrhea associated with strenuous exercise is related to stress, not weight loss, and is most probably caused by an increase in CNS opioids (beta-endorphin) and catechol estrogens, both of which interfere with gonadotrophin-releasing hormone (GnRH) release.

- When women lose weight 15% below ideal body weight, amenorrhea can occur due to CNS-hypothalamic dysfunction. When weight loss drops below 25% of ideal body weight, pituitary gonadotrophin function can also become abnormal.

- Anorexia nervosa occurs in about 1 in 1000 white women. It is uncommon in men and women older than 25 and rare in blacks and Orientals.

- Individuals with anorexia nervosa have impaired peripheral conversion of thyroxine (T_4) to triiodothyronine (T_3), resulting in normal T_4 levels, decreased T_3 levels, and increased reverse T_3 levels.

- The normal cyclic pattern of luteinizing hormone (LH) pulsatility is not present in individuals with hypothalamic dysfunction. Either no pulse or pulses of slow frequency, similar to those in the normal luteal phase, are usually observed.

- The GnRH alterations as reflected in LH pulsatility in persons with severe weight loss and anorexia nervosa are similar to those seen in normal prepubertal girls. When such individuals gain weight, GnRH changes similar to those occurring during puberty take place.

- When uterine bleeding fails to occur after progestin is administered, estradiol levels are usually lower than 40 pg/ml.

- In contrast to hypothalamic disorders, pituitary causes of amenorrhea can be associated with ACTH and TSH deficiency.

- Individuals with premature ovarian failure have two different histologic findings: generalized sclerosis or primordial follicles scattered through the stroma.

- Individuals with premature ovarian failure frequently have antibodies to gonadotrophins and other endocrine organs, indicating an autoimmune etiology.

- A karyotype should be obtained in women with premature ovarian failure younger than 25 but not in those who are older.

- Amenorrhea with low estrogen levels is associated with decreased density of trabecular bone.

- The most frequent cause of amenorrhea is hypothalamic dysfunction.

BIBLIOGRAPHY

Adashi EY, Casper RF, Fishman J, et al: Stimulatory effect of 2-hydroxyestradiol on prolactin release in hypogonadal women, J Clin Endocrinol Metab 51:413, 1980.

Adashi EY, Rakoff J, Divers W, et al: The effect of acutely administered 2-hydroxyestrone on the release of gonadotropins and prolactin before and after estrogen priming in hypogonadal women, Obstet Gynecol Surv 35:363, 1980.

Alper MM and Garner PR: Premature ovarian failure: its relationship to autoimmune disease, Obstet Gynecol 66:27, 1985.

Berga SL, Mortola JF, Girton BS, et al: Neuroendocrine aberrations in women with functional hypothalamic amenorrhea, J Clin Endocrinol Metab 68:301, 1989.

Beumont PJV, George GCW, Pimstone BL, et al: Body weight and the pituitary response to hypothalamic releasing hormones in patients with anorexia nervosa, J Clin Endocrinol Metab 43:487, 1976.

Boyar RM, Katz J, Finkelstein JW, et al: Anorexia nervosa: immaturity of the 24-hour luteinizing hormone secretory pattern, N Engl J Med 291:861, 1974.

Carr DB, Bullen BA, Skrinar GS, et al: Physical conditioning facilitates the exercise-induced secretion of beta-endorphin and beta-lipotropin in women, N Engl J Med 305:560, 1981.

Coulam CB, Adamson SC, and Annegers JF: Incidence of premature ovarian failure, Obstet Gynecol 67:604, 1986.

Crowley WF Jr, Filicori M, Spratt DI, et al: The physiology of gonadotropin-releasing hormone (GnRH) secretion in men and women, Rec Prog Hormone Res 41:473, 1985.

Drinkwater BL, Nilson K, Chestnut III CH, et al: Bone mineral content of amenorrheic and eumenorrheic athletes, N Engl J Med 322:277, 1984.

Federman DD, editor: Abnormal sexual development, Philadelphia, 1967, WB Saunders Co.

Feicht CB, Johnson TS, and Matrin BJ: Secondary amenorrhea in athletes, Lancet 1:1145, 1978.

Ferin M, Van Vugt D, and Wardlaw S: The hypothalamic control of the menstrual cycle and the role of endogenous opioid peptides, Recent Prog Horm Res 40:441, 1984.

Friedman CI, Barrows H, and Kim MH: Hypergonadotropic hypogonadism, Am J Obstet Gynecol 145:360, 1983.

Fries H, Nillius SJ, and Pettersson F: Epidemiology of secondary amenorrhea, Am J Obstet Gynecol 118:473, 1974.

Frisch RE, Gotz-Welbergen AV, McArthur JW, et al: Delayed menarche and amenorrhea of college athletes in relation to onset of training, JAMA 246:1559, 1981.

Frisch RE and Revelle R: Height and weight at menarche and a hypothesis of critical body weights and adolescent events, Science 169:397, 1970.

Frisch RE and Revelle R: Height and weight at menarche and a hypothesis of menarche, Arch Dis Child 46:695, 1971.

Frisch RE, Rose E, Wyshak G, et al: Delayed menarche and amenorrhea in ballet dancers, N Engl J Med 303:17, 1980.

Goldenberg RL, Grodin JM, Aodbard D, and Ross GT: Gonadotropins in women with amenorrhea, Am J Obstet Gynecol 116:1003, 1973.

Griffin JE, Edwards C, Madden JD, et al: Congenital absence of the vagina, Ann Intern Med 85:224, 1976.

Ingram JM: The bicycle stool in the treatment of vaginal agenesis and stenosis: a preliminary report, Am J Obstet Gynecol 140:867, 1981.

Kletzky OA, Davajan V, Nakamura RM, et al: Clinical categorization of patients with secondary amenorrhea using progesterone-induced uterine bleeding and measurement of serum gonadotropin levels, Am J Obstet Gynecol 121:695, 1975.

Klibanski A, Biller BMK, Rosenthal DI, et al: Effects of prolactin and estrogen deficiency in amenorrheic bone loss, J Clin Endocrinol Metab 67:124, 1988.

LaBarbera AR, Miller MM, et al: Autoimmune etiology in premature ovarian failure, Am J Reprod Immunol Microbiol 16:115, 1988.

Ledger WL, Thomas EJ, et al: Suppression of gonadotrophin secretion does not reverse premature ovarian failure, Br J Obstet Gynaecol 96:196, 1989.

Lieblich JM, Rogol AD, White BJ, et al: Syndrome of anosmia with hypogonadotropic hypogonadism (Kallmann syndrome): clinical laboratory studies in 23 cases, Am J Med 73:506, 1982.

Lloyd T, Myers C, et al: Collegiate women athletes with irregular menses during adolescence have decreased bone density, Obstet Gynecol 72:639, 1988.

Marshall WA and Tanner JM: Variations in pattern of pubertal changes in girls, Arch Dis Child 44:291, 1969.

Maschchak CA, Kletzky OA, Davajan V, et al: Clinical and laboratory evaluation of patients with primary amenorrhea, Obstet Gynecol 57:715, 1981.

Mason HD and Sagle M: Reduced frequency of luteinizing hormone pulses in women with weight loss–related amenorrhea and multifollicular ovaries, Clin Endocrinol 280:611, 1988.

McArthur JW, Bullen BA, Beitins IZ, et al: Hypothalamic amenorrhea in runners of normal body composition, Endocr Res Commun 7:13, 1980.

Mignot MH, Schoemaker J, Kleingeld M, et al: Premature ovarian failure. I. The association with autoimmunity, Eur J Obstet Gynecol Reprod Biol 30:59, 1989.

Moraes-Ruehsen M de, Blizzard RM, Garcia-Bunuel R, et al: Autoimmunity and ovarian failure, Am J Obstet Gynecol 112:693, 1972.

Penny R, Goldstein IP, and Frasier SD: Gonadotropin excretion and body composition, Pediatrics 61:294, 1978.

Pettersson F, Fries H, and Nillius SJ: Epidemiology of secondary amenorrhea, Am J Obstet Gynecol 117:80, 1973.

Quigley ME, Sheehan KL, Casper RF, and Yen SSC: Evidence for increased dopaminergic and opioid activity in patients with hypothalamic hypogonadotropic hypogonadism, J Clin Endocrinol Metab 50:949, 1980.

Reame NE, Sauder SE, Case GD, et al: Pulsatile gonadotropin secretion in women with hypothalamic amenorrhea: evidence that reduced frequency of gonadotropin-releasing hormone secretion is the mechanism of persistent anovulation, J Clin Endocrinol Metab 61:851, 1985.

Reame NE, Sauder SE, Kelch RP, et al: Pulsatile gonadotropin secretion during the human menstrual cycle: evidence for altered frequency of gonadotropin-releasing hormone secretion, J Clin Endocrinol Metab 59:328, 1984.

Rebar RW and Connolly HV: Clinical features of young women with hypergonadotropic amenorrhea, Fertil Steril 53:804, 1990.

Rebar RW, Erickson GF, and Yen SSC: Idiopathic premature ovarian failure: clinical and endocrine characteristics, Fertil Steril 137:35, 1982.

Reid RL, Hoff JD, Yen SSC, et al: Effects of exogenous β-endorphin on pituitary hormone secretion and its disappearance rate in normal human subjects, J Clin Endocrinol Metab 52:1179, 1981.

Reindollar RH, Byrd JR, and McDonough PG: Delayed sexual development: a study of 252 patients, Am J Obstet Gynecol 140:371, 1981.

Reindollar RH, Novak M, Tho SPT, and McDonough PG: Adult-onset amenorrhea: a study of 262 patients, Am J Obstet Gynecol 155:531, 1986.

Richmond J: Hysterosalpingography. In Mishell DR Jr and Davajan V, editors: Infertility, reproductive endocrinology and contraception, ed 2, Oradell NJ, 1986, Medical Economics Books.

Russell JB, DeCherney AH, and Collins DC: The effect of naloxone and metoclopramide on the hypothalamic pituitary axis in oligomenorrheic and eumenorrheic swimmers, Fertil Steril 52:583, 1989.

Russell JB, Mitchell D, Musey PI, et al: The relationship of exercise to anovulatory cycles in female athletes: hormonal and physical characteristics, Obstet Gynecol 63:452, 1984.

Russell JB, Mitchell DE, Musey PI, et al: The role of β-endorphins and catechol estrogens on the hypothalamic-pituitary axis in female athletes, Fertil Steril 42:690, 1984.

Schlechte JA, Sherman B, and Martin R: Bone density in amenorrheic women with and without hyperprolactinemia, J Clin Endocrinol Metab 56:1120, 1983.

Sherman BM, Halmi KA, and Zamudio R: LH and FSH response to gonadotropin-releasing hormone in anorexia nervosa: effect of nutritional rehabilitation, J Clin Endocrinol Metab 41:135, 1975.

Treasure JL, King EA, Gordon PAL, et al: Cystic ovaries: a phase of anorexia nervosa, Lancet 28:1379, 1985.

Tulandi T and Finch RA: Premature ovarian failure, Obstet Gynecol Surv 36:521, 1981.

Vigersky RA, Andersen AE, Thompson RG, et al: Hypothalamic dysfunction in secondary amenorrhea associated with simple weight loss, N Engl J Med 297:1141, 1977.

Vigersky RA, Loriaux DL, Andersen AE, et al: Delayed pituitary hormone response to LRF and TRF in patients with secondary amenorrhea associated with simple weight loss, J Clin Endocrinol Metab 43:893, 1976.

Warren MP: The effects of exercise on pubertal progression and reproductive function in girls, J Clin Endocrinol Metab 51:1150, 1980.

Warren MP, Jewelwicz R, Dyrenfurth I, et al: The significance of weight loss in the evaluation of pituitary response to LH-RH in women with secondary amenorrhea, J Clin Endocrinol Metab 40:601, 1975.

Wildt L and Leyendecker G: Indication of ovulation by the chronic administration of naltrexone in hypothalamic amenorrhea, J Clin Endocrinol Metab 64:1334, 1987.

Hyperprolactinemia, Galactorrhea, and Pituitary Adenomas

KEY TERMS

Bromocriptine (2-Br-Alpha-Ergocryptine Mesylate). Semisynthetic ergot alkaloid that is a dopamine receptor agonist and is used to treat hyperprolactinemia.

Computed Tomography (CT). An imaging technique to detect soft tissue abnormalities that uses a computer to integrate differences in x-ray beam attenuation resulting from varying densities in adjacent tissue.

Craniopharyngioma. A rare hypothalamic tumor that can produce hyperprolactinemia.

Empty Sella Syndrome. An intrasellar extension of the subarachnoid space resulting in compression of the pituitary gland and an enlarged sella turcica that may be associated with galactorrhea and hyperprolactinemia.

Galactorrhea. Nonpuerperal secretion from the breast of watery or milky fluid that contains neither pus nor blood.

Hyperprolactinemia. Levels of circulating prolactin above normal (greater than 20 to 25 ng/ml) that can cause galactorrhea or amenorrhea or both.

Hypocycloidal Tomography. Multiple radiographs of the sella turcica at intervals of 2 to 3 mm with a hypocycloidal movement.

Macroadenoma. An uncommon type of prolactin-secreting pituitary adenoma (prolactinoma) greater than 1 cm in diameter, usually with extrasellar extension.

Magnetic Resonance Imaging (MRI) (previously Nuclear Magnetic Resonance [NMR]). Technique of soft tissue imagery using resonance of hydrogen nuclei in static magnetic field exposed to low-frequency radiowaves.

Microadenoma. The more common type of prolactinoma less than 1 cm in diameter.

Prolactin. Polypeptide hormone secreted by anterior pituitary lactotrophs that has mammotrophic and lactogenic functions.

Prolactin-Inhibiting Factor. The neurotransmitter (believed to be dopamine) that inhibits prolactin synthesis and release.

Prolactinoma. The most common pituitary tumor arising from chromophobic cells that secrete prolactin.

Thyrotropin-Releasing Hormone (TRH) Stimulation Test. Provocative response of prolactin following TRH infusion. The normal response is greater than 3 times the baseline of prolactin after infusion of 500 μg of TRH.

$\mathbf{P}$rolactin is a polypeptide hormone containing 198 amino acids and having a molecular weight of 22,000 daltons. It circulates in different molecular sizes—a monomeric (small) form (mol wt 22,000), a polymeric (big) form (mol wt 50,000), and an even larger polymeric (big-big) form (mol wt >100,000). Big prolactin is presumed to be a dimer, and big-big prolactin may represent an aggregation of monomeric molecules. The small form is biologically active, and about 80% of the hormone secreted is in this form. Most immunoassayable prolactin is also in this form; however, the larger forms are also immunoreactive and thus are measurable in prolactin radioimmunoassays. The biologic effects of the polymeric forms are unclear, but in some bioassays the forms are inactive, as they have reduced binding to mammary tissue membranes. Prolactin is synthesized and stored in the pituitary gland in chromophobe cells called *lactotrophs*, which are located mainly in the lateral areas of the gland. In addition, prolactin is synthesized in decidual and endometrial tissue. From these tissues prolactin is secreted into the circulation and, in the event of pregnancy, into the amniotic fluid. Prolactin is normally present in measurable amounts in serum, with mean levels of about 8 ng/ml in adult women. It circulates in an unbound form, has a 20-minute half-life, and is cleared by the liver and kidney. The main function of prolactin is to stimulate the growth of mammary tissue as well as to produce and secrete milk into the alveoli. Thus it has both mammogenic and lactogenic functions. Specific receptors for prolactin are present in the plasma membrane of mammary cells as well as many other tissues.

PHYSIOLOGY

Prolactin synthesis and release from the lactotrophs are controlled by central nervous system neurotransmitters, which act on the pituitary via the hypothalamus. The major control mechanism is inhibition, as pituitary stalk section results in increased prolactin secretion. It appears that the major physiologic inhibitor of prolactin release is the neurotransmitter dopamine, which acts directly on the pituitary gland. There are specific dopamine receptors on the lactotrophs, and dopamine inhibits prolactin synthesis and release in pituitary cell cultures. Thus dopamine appears to be the prolactin-inhibiting factor (PIF), also called *prolactin release–inhibiting factor*. Although a hypothalamic prolactin release factor (PRF) has not been isolated, it is known that both the neurotransmitter serotonin and thyrotropin-releasing factor stimulate prolactin release. Since the latter stimulates prolactin release only minimally unless infused, it appears that serotonin is PRF or is responsible for its secretion. The rise in prolactin levels during sleep appears to be controlled by serotonin.

Prolactin is secreted episodically, and serum levels fluctuate throughout the day and throughout the menstrual cycle, with peak levels occurring at midcycle. Although changes in prolactin levels are not as marked as the pulsatile episodes of luteinizing hormone (LH), Bäckström et al. reported a decline in both basal concentration and pulse frequency of prolactin in the luteal phase of the cycle. Estrogen stimulates prolactin production and release. Under the influence of estrogen, prolactin levels increase in females at the time of puberty.

During pregnancy, as estrogen levels increase, there is a concomitant hypertrophy and hyperplasia of the lactotrophs. The maternal increase in prolactin occurs soon after implantation, concomitant with the increase in circulating estrogen. Circulating levels of prolactin steadily increase throughout pregnancy, reaching about 200 ng/ml in the third trimester, and the rise is directly related to the increase in circulating levels of estrogen. Despite the elevated prolactin levels during pregnancy, lactation does not occur because estrogen inhibits the action of prolactin on the breast, most likely blocking prolactin's interaction with its receptor. A day or two following delivery of the placenta, both estrogen levels and prolactin levels decline rapidly and lactation is initiated. Prolactin levels reach basal levels in nonnursing women in 2 to 3 weeks. Although basal levels of circulating prolactin decline to the nonpregnant range about 6 months after parturition in nursing women, following each act of suckling, prolactin levels increase markedly and stimulate milk production for the next feeding.

Nipple and breast stimulation also increase prolactin levels in the nonpregnant female. Other physiologic stimuli that increase prolactin release are exercise, sleep, and stress. In addition, prolactin levels normally rise following ingestion of the noonday meal. For these reasons prolactin levels normally fluctuate throughout the day, with maximal levels observed during nighttime while asleep and a smaller increase occurring in the early afternoon (Figure 37-1). When the amount measured in the circulation in the nonpregnant woman exceeds a certain level, usually 20 to 25 ng/ml, the condition is called *hyperprolactinemia*. The optimal time to obtain a blood sample for assay to diagnose hyperprolactinemia is during the morning hours. Increases in prolactin levels above the normal range can occur without a pathologic condition if the serum sample is drawn from a patient who has recently awakened, has exercised, or has had recent breast stimulation, such as breast palpation, during a physical examination.

The most frequent cause of slightly elevated

DIURNAL VARIATION OF PROLACTIN

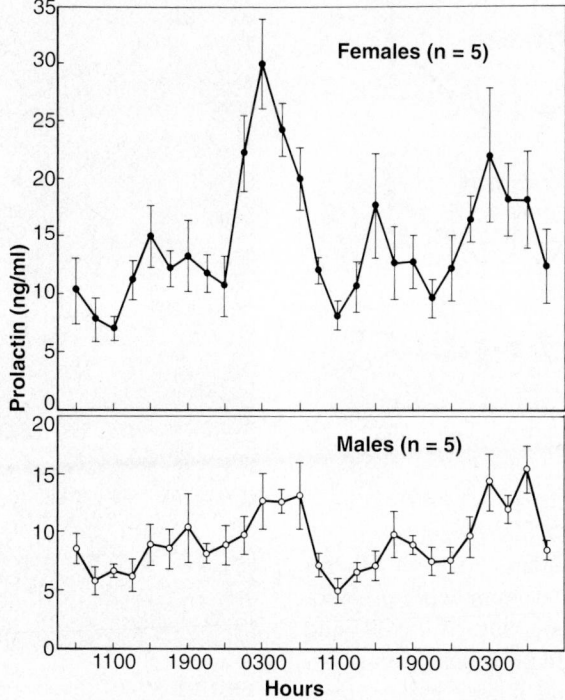

FIGURE 37-1

Hour-to-hour variation of serum prolactin concentration in normal women and men studied throughout 48 consecutive hours. (From Kletzky OA and Davajan V: Hyperprolactinemia: diagnosis and treatment. Reproduced with permission from Infertility, contraception and reproductive endocrinology, ed 2, by Daniel R. Mishell, Jr., M.D., and Val Davajan, M.D. Copyright © 1986 Medical Economics Books, Oradell, N.J. 07649. All rights reserved.)

prolactin levels is stress, particularly the stress caused by visiting the physician's office. An excellent study demonstrating that most mildly elevated prolactin levels are not caused by pathologic hyperprolactinemia was performed by Muneyyirci-Delale et al. These investigators studied 50 women without radiologic evidence of a prolactinoma who had elevated prolactin levels (23 to 156 ng/ml) measured in two consecutive blood samples obtained 1 to 2 weeks apart. When these women had serial blood sampling subsequently performed in a quiet room, 20 had normal prolactin levels in the 1-hour blood sample (Figure 37-2). The initial prolactin levels in these 20 women ranged from 26 to 69 ng/ml. The results of this study indicate that stress-related hyperprolactinemia is a common cause of a mild increase in prolactin. All women with initial prolactin levels less than

70 mIU/ml should have subsequent samples drawn 60 minutes after resting in a quiet room to determine whether true pathologic hyperprolactinemia is present.

Hyperprolactinemia can produce disorders of gonadotrophin–sex steroid function, resulting in menstrual cycle derangement (oligomenorrhea and amenorrhea) and anovulation, as well as inappropriate lactation or galactorrhea. The mechanism whereby elevated prolactin levels interfere with gonadotrophin release has not been completely elucidated, but the major factor appears to be alterations in normal gonadotrophin-releasing hormone (GnRH) release. Women with hyperprolactinemia have abnormalities in the frequency and amplitude of LH pulsations, with a normal or increased gonadotrophin response following GnRH infusion.

This abnormality of normal GnRH cyclicity

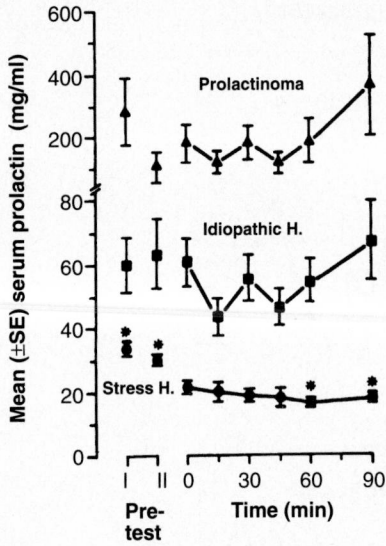

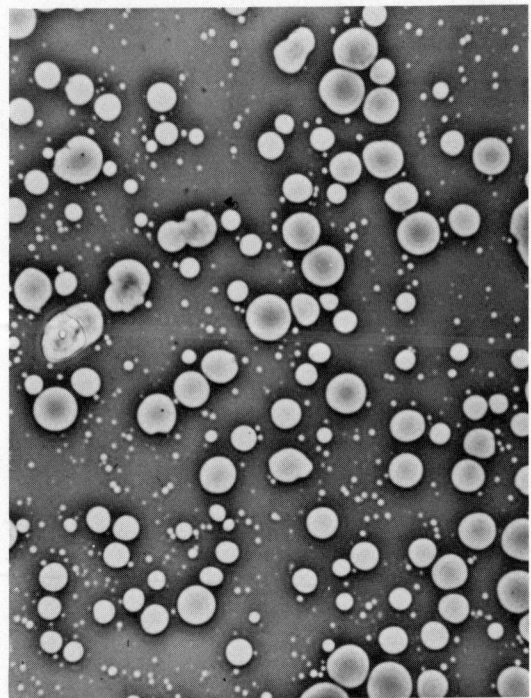

FIGURE 37-2

Mean plus or minus standard error (± SE) serum prolactin levels in women with prolactinoma *(N = 20)* and idiopathic *(N = 30)* and stress-related *(N = 20)* hyperprolactinemia before (pretest I and II) and during hyperprolactinemia test. Differences (* *p<* 0.01) are in relation to time zero values. (Mean prolactin values among groups were also significantly different—*p* < 0.01—at all times.) (From Muneyyirci-Delale O, Goldstein D, Reyes FI, et al: NY State J Med 89:205, 1989.)

FIGURE 37-3

Fat droplets seen under microscope from a patient with galactorrhea. (From Kletzky OA and Davajan V: Hyperprolactinemia: diagnosis and treatment. In Mishell DR, Davajan V, and Lobo RA, editors: Infertility, contraception, and reproductive endocrinology, ed 3, Cambridge, Mass, 1991, Blackwell Scientific Publications.)

thus inhibits gonadotrophin release but not synthesis. The reason for the abnormal secretion of GnRH has not been completely elucidated, but it is hypothesized that the elevated prolactin levels produce a rise in hypothalamic dopamine levels by a short-loop feedback that fails to suppress prolactin but interferes with normal GnRH release, perhaps by altering norepinephrine secretion. In addition, elevated prolactin levels have been shown to interfere with the positive estrogen effect on midcycle LH release. It has also been shown that elevated levels of prolactin directly inhibit basal as well as gonadotrophin-stimulated ovarian secretion of both estradiol and progesterone. However, this mechanism is probably not the primary cause of anovulation, because women with hyperprolactinemia can have ovulation induced with various agents, including pulsatile GnRH. Some patients with moderate hyperprolactinemia as determined by radioimmunoassay have a greater than normal proportion of the big-big forms. Because of this form of prolactin's reduced bioactivity, these individuals can have normal pituitary and ovarian function.

The clinician should measure serum prolactin levels in all patients with galactorrhea, as well as those with oligomenorrhea and amenorrhea without the presence of an elevated level of follicle-stimulating hormone (FSH). Hyperprolactinemia has been reported to be present in 15% of all anovulatory women and 20% of women with amenorrhea of undetermined cause. Galactorrhea is defined as the nonpuerperal secretion from the breast of watery or milky fluid that contains neither pus nor blood. The fluid may appear spontaneously or after palpation. To determine if galactorrhea is present, the clinician should palpate the breast, moving from the periphery toward the nipple in an attempt to express any secretion. The diagnosis of galactorrhea can be confirmed by observing multiple fat droplets in the fluid when it is examined under low-power magnification (Figure 37-3). The incidence of galactorrhea in women with hyperprolactinemia has been reported to range from 30% to 80%, and these differences probably reflect variations in the techniques used to detect mammary excretion. Unless there has been continued breast stimulation after a pregnancy, the presence of galactorrhea serves as a biologic indicator that the prolactin level is abnormally elevated. Davajan et al. reported that 62% of women with galactorrhea have hyperprolactinemia, and some individuals with galactorrhea have normal immunoassayable prolactin levels, indicating they may have elevated levels of biologically active prolactin. The incidence of hyperprolactinemia is higher (88%) in those women with galactorrhea who have amenorrhea and low estrogen levels than in those women with galactorrhea and normal menses, oligomenorrhea, or amenorrhea with normal estrogen levels (49%).

ETIOLOGY

Pathologic causes of hyperprolactinemia, in addition to a prolactin-secreting pituitary adenoma (prolactinoma) and other pituitary tumors that produce acromegaly and Cushing's disease, include hypothalamic disease, various pharmacologic agents, hypothyroidism, chronic renal disease, or any chronic type of breast nerve stimulation, such as may occur with thoracic operation, herpes zoster, or chest trauma.

One of the most frequent causes of galactorrhea and hyperprolactinemia is the ingestion of pharmacologic agents, particularly tranquilizers, narcotics, and antihypertensive agents (see box, upper right). Of the tranquilizers, the phenothiazines and diazepam can produce hyperprolactinemia either by depleting the hypothalamic circulation of dopamine or by blocking its binding sites and thus decreasing dopamine action (Figure 37-4). The tricyclic antidepressants block dopamine uptake, and propranolol, haloperidol, phentolamine, and cyproheptadine block hypothalamic dopamine receptors. The antihypertensive agent reserpine depletes catecholamines, and methyldopa blocks the conversion of tyrosine to dihydroxyphenylala-

PHARMACOLOGIC AGENTS AFFECTING PROLACTIN CONCENTRATIONS

Stimulators

Anesthetics
Psychotropics
    Phenothiazines
    Tricyclic antidepressants
    Opiates
Hormones
    Estrogen
    Oral steroid contraceptives
    Thyrotropin-releasing hormone
Anhtihypertensives
    α-Methyldopa
    Reserpine
Antiemetic
    Sulpiride
    Metoclopramide

Inhibitors

L-Dopa
Dopamine

From Kletzky OA and Davajan V: Hyperprolactinemia. In Mishell DR, Davajan V, and Lobo RA, eds: Infertility, contraception, and reproductive endocrinology, ed 3, Cambridge, Mass, 1991, Blackwell Scientific Publications.

nine (dopa). Ingestion of oral contraceptive steroids can also increase prolactin levels, with a greater incidence of hyperprolactinemia occurring with higher estrogen formulations. Nevertheless, galactorrhea does not usually occur during oral contraceptive ingestion because the exogenous estrogen blocks the binding of prolactin to its receptors.

Patients developing galactorrhea while ingesting oral contraceptives or any of the other drugs just listed should ideally discontinue the medication, and prolactin should be measured 1 month thereafter to determine if the level has returned to normal. If the medication cannot be discontinued, the prolactin level should be measured, and if it is elevated above 100 ng/ml, visualization of the sella turcica should be performed by one of the techniques described below.

Primary hypothyroidism can also produce hyperprolactinemia and galactorrhea because of decreased negative feedback of thyroxine (T_4) on the hypothalamic-pituitary axis. The resulting increase in thyrotropin-releasing hormone (TRH) stimulates prolactin secretion as well as

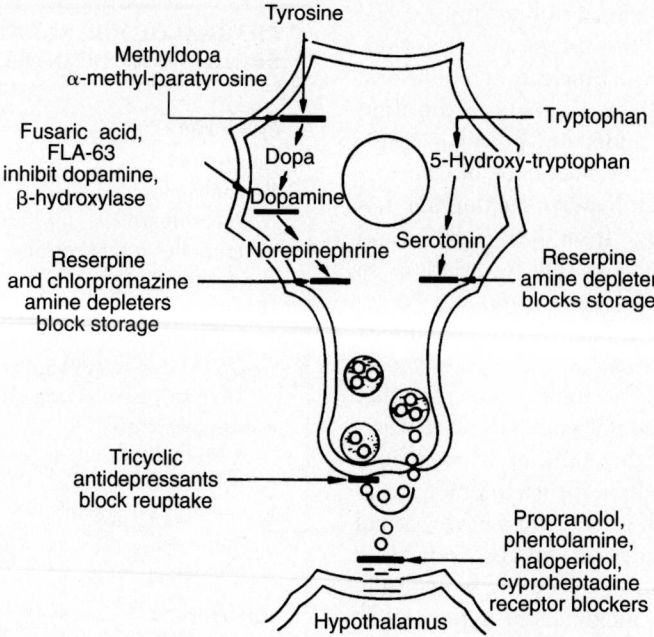

FIGURE 37-4
Schematic representation of inhibitory effects of drugs on synthesis and release of neurotransmitters. (From Kletzky OA and Davajan V: Hyperprolactinemia. In Mishell DR, Davajan V, and Lobo RA, eds: Infertility, contraception, and reproductive endocrinology, ed 3, Cambridge, Mass, 1991, Blackwell Scientific Publications.)

thyroid-stimulating hormone (TSH) secretion from the pituitary. About 3% to 5% of individuals with hyperprolactinemia have hypothyroidism, and thus a TSH assay, the most sensitive indicator of hypothyroidism, should be obtained for all individuals with hyperprolactinemia. If the TSH level is elevated, triiodothyronine (T_3) and T_4 should be measured to confirm the diagnosis of primary hypothyroidism, as occasionally a TSH-secreting pituitary adenoma will be present. Treatment with appropriate thyroid replacement usually returns the TSH and prolactin levels to normal within a short time.

Hyperprolactinemia can occur in patients with abnormal renal disease resulting from decreased metabolic clearance as well as increased production rate. The cause of the latter is not known.

Central Nervous System Disorders

Hypothalamic Causes

Diseases of the hypothalamus that produce alterations in the normal portal circulation of dopamine can result in hyperprolactinemia. Such diseases include craniopharyngioma and infiltration of the hypothalamus by sarcoidosis, histiocytosis, leukemia, or carcinoma. All these conditions are rare, with craniopharyngioma being the most common. These tumors arise from remnants of Rathke's pouch along the pituitary stalk. Grossly they can be cystic, solid, or mixed, and calcification is usually visible on x-ray examination. They are most frequently diagnosed during the second and third decades of life and usually result in impairment of secretion of several pituitary hormones.

Pituitary Causes

Various types of pituitary tumors, lactotroph hyperplasia, and the empty sella syndrome can be associated with hyperprolactinemia. It has been estimated that as many as 80% of all pituitary adenomas secrete prolactin. The most common pituitary tumor associated with hyperprolactinemia is the prolactinoma, arbitrarily defined as a microadenoma if its diameter is less than 1 cm and as a macroadenoma if it is

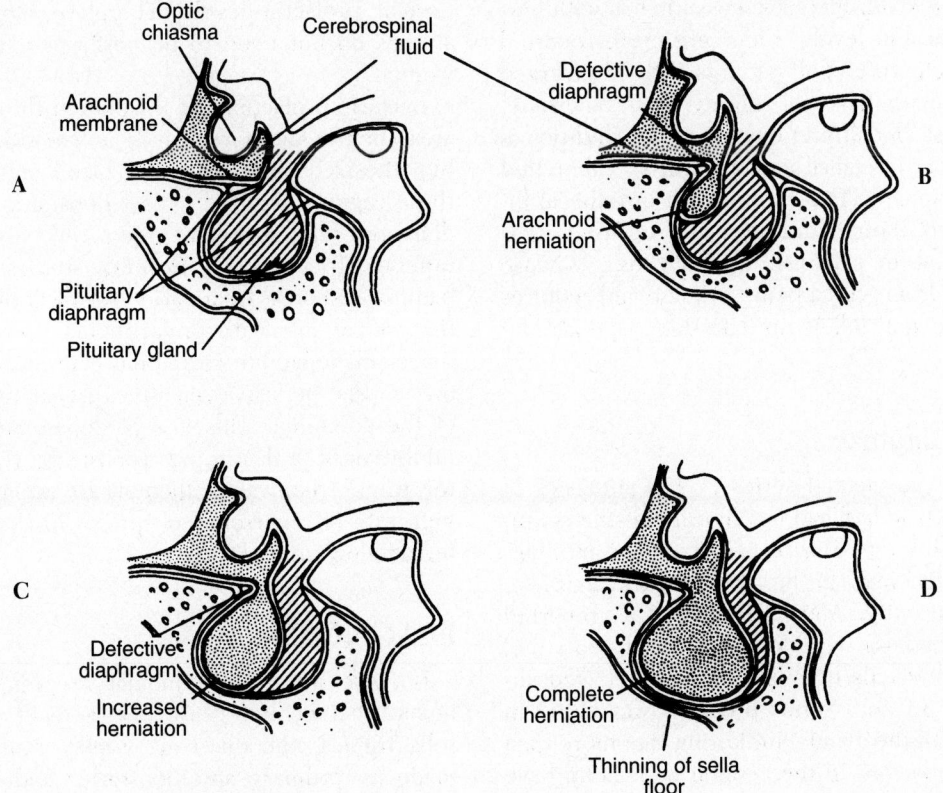

FIGURE 37-5

Diagrammatic representation of empty sella syndrome. **A,** Normal anatomic relationship. **B,C,** and **D,** Progression in development of empty sella syndrome. Note thinning of floor and symmetric enlargement of sella turcica. (From Kletzky OA and Davajan V: Hyperprolactinemia. In Mishell DR, Davajan V, and Lobo RA, eds: Infertility, contraception, and reproductive endocrinology, ed 3, Cambridge, Mass, 1991, Blackwell Scientific Publications.)

larger. Hyperprolactinemia has been reported to occur in about 25% of patients with acromegaly and 10% of those with Cushing's disease, indicating that the pituitary adenomas, which mainly secrete growth hormones and adrenocorticotropic hormone (ACTH), frequently also secrete prolactin. Hyperplasia of lactotrophs has been reported to occur in about 8% of pituitary glands examined at autopsy.

Another cause of hyperprolactinemia is the primary empty sella syndrome. The term *primary empty sella syndrome* describes a clinical situation in which an intrasellar extension of the subarachnoid space results in compression of the pituitary gland and an enlarged sella turcica. The etiology is believed to result from a congenital or acquired (by radiation or surgery) defect in the sella diaphragm that allows the

subarachnoid membrane to herniate into the sella turcica (Figure 37-5). The syndrome is usually associated with normal pituitary function except for hyperprolactinemia. Although some patients with primary empty sella syndrome have a coexistent prolactinoma, Gharib et al. reported a series of 11 patients with an empty sella and hyperprolactinemia who had no histologic evidence of a prolactinoma or hyperplasia of the lactotrophs. They stated that about 5% of individuals with the empty sella have hyperprolactinemia or amenorrhea-galactorrhea or both. It is theorized that in these patients distortion of the infundibular stalk results in decreased levels of dopamine reaching the pituitary to inhibit prolactin. Serum prolactin levels are usually less than 100 ng/ml in patients with this syndrome, and some patients with this syndrome have galactorrhea with normal prolactin levels. Kleinberg et al. reported that about 10% of all patients with an enlarged sella turcica have the empty sella syndrome. The best modality to diagnose this condition is magnetic resonance imaging (MRI). Computed tomographic (CT) scanning with intrathecal injection of metrizamide can also be used. It is important to establish the diagnosis because the syndrome has a benign course and requires less stringent follow-up than does a prolactinemia.

Prolactinomas

In an unselected series of 120 autopsies of persons who had had no clinical evidence of pituitary disease, Burrow et al. found pituitary microadenomas to be present in 32 (27%). More recently, Abd El-Hamid et al. reported that adenomas were found in 78 of 486 (16%) pituitary glands examined after unselected autopsies. In both series prolactin was found in about half the glands, indicating that more than 1 in 10 persons in the general population have a prolactinoma.

Overall about 50% of women with hyperprolactinemia have a prolactinoma. The incidence is higher when the prolactin levels exceed 100 ng/ml, and nearly all individuals with prolactin levels greater than 200 ng/ml harbor a prolactinoma. The vast majority of prolactinomas in women are microadenomas. Kleinberg et al. reported that overall 20% of individuals with galactorrhea and 35% of women with amenorrhea-galactorrhea had radiologic evidence of pituitary tumors. Tumors are also present in about 20% of women with hyperprolactinemia and menstrual irregularities without galactorrhea. The incidence of prolactinoma is greater in those individuals with a more profound disturbance of normal hypothalamic-pituitary-ovarian function. Davajan et al. reported that 70% of women with hyperprolactinemia, galactorrhea, and secondary amenorrhea with low estrogen levels had radiologic evidence of a pituitary adenoma. Evidence of a tumor occurred in only 20% to 30% of those with hyperprolactinemia and normal menses, oligomenorrhea, or secondary amenorrhea who had sufficient estrogen to undergo withdrawal bleeding after progesterone administration. In both these studies no evidence of tumor was found in individuals with normal menses, galactorrhea, and normal prolactin levels. Therefore radiologic studies do not need to be performed in such women.

Because prolactinomas develop in the lateral areas of the pituitary gland, it was originally hypothesized that decreased blood supply to these regions resulted in less dopamine being delivered and resultant increased size and number of lactotrophs. Recently studies of dopamine response by a variety of tests indicate that in patients with prolactinomas there is a defect in dopamine regulation of prolactin secretion that persists even after surgical removal of the adenoma. This loss of dopaminergenic inhibition of prolactin that persists for years after tumor removal is thought to explain the high rate of recurrence of tumors in the long-term follow-up of patients.

DIAGNOSIS

Because most prolactinomas are microadenomas that do not cause enlargement of the sella turcica, the diagnosis usually cannot be made by ordinary anteroposterior and lateral coned x-ray examination of the sella turcica. With the development of more precise radiologic methods of detecting soft tissue pituitary abnormalities, it is now possible to detect even small adenomas.

Initially detection of microadenomas was accomplished by obtaining tomographic radiographic examination of the sella turcica at intervals of 2 to 3 mm in the anteroposterior and lateral projections with a hypocycloidal movement. These are called *hypocycloidal tomograms*. Comparing the results of tomograms with the findings of microadenoma at autopsy, Burrow et al. found that the incidence of both false positive and false negative tomographic findings was about 20% each, with an overall accuracy rate of 61%. Furthermore, radiation exposure with polytomography may be in excess of 20 rads.

Since about 1980 a more accurate diagnostic technique, CT imagery, has been available. After infusion of at least 200 ml of 30% iodinated contrast medium, CT imagery is performed in coronal sections of 1.5 mm. The typical appearance of an adenoma is a region of diminished enhancement in the pituitary gland with a convex upper surface and an abnormal height of 8 mm or greater. With this technique it is possible to assess accurately the presence of a microadenoma 2 mm in diameter or larger as well as the suprasellar and other extrasellar extensions. This technique also will indicate the presence of an empty sella. Radiation exposure in a CT scan is about 3 rads, significantly less than with polytomography. However, this technique mainly provides information about the bony structure of the sella turcia, not the soft tissue lesions, the adenomas themselves.

Recently the technique of MRI has been developed. With this technique accurate soft tissue imagery is obtained without radiation. Instead, hydrogen nuclei in static magnetic fields exposed to radiowaves of specific frequency resonate and depict tissue hydrogen density. This technique provides 1 mm resolution and thus should be able to detect all significant microadenomas. Stein et al. compared results of CT and MRI in 22 patients with suspected pituitary adenomas. MRI was found to be the superior diagnostic modality because of its greater soft tissue contrast (Figure 37-6). Thus MRI should be the diagnostic technique of choice. Since areas with access to MRI are still limited if it is not available, CT scanning is the next best alternative. If neither one is available, hypocycloidal tomography can be used.

Since provocative stimuli of dopamine re-

lease such as insulin-induced hypoglycogenemia and infusion of either chlorpromazine or TRH are abnormal in most individuals with prolactinomas, studies of the use of such stimuli as diagnostic tests to determine whether a tumor is present have been undertaken. Of these tests it appears that administration of TRH in individuals with mild hyperprolactinemia (less than 60 ng/ml) may be beneficial. Shangold et al. found that if prolactin is measured before and 20 minutes after administration of an intravenous bolus of 500 μg of TRH, normal individuals have at least a 200% increase (3 times baseline) of prolactin.

All patients with hyperprolactinemia greater than 60 ng/ml as well as those with prolactin levels of 20 to 60 μg/ml and CT evidence of tumor had less than a threefold increase in prolactin (Figure 37-7). Thus if a normal response to TRH is found in individuals with mild hyperprolactinemia, there is no need to perform a CT scan.

Visual field determination and tests of adrenocorticotropic hormone (ACTH) and thyroid function are not necessary in patients with microadenomas, as these small tumors do not interfere with overall pituitary function and do not extend beyond the sella. However, these

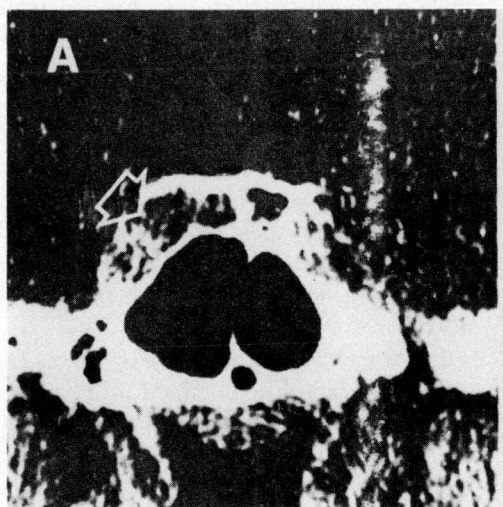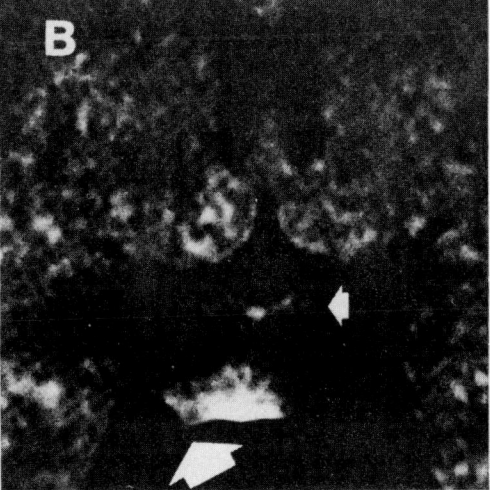

FIGURE 37-6
Images were selected to best demonstrate pathology and do not exactly correspond in level of section through sella turcica. **A,** CT scan (coronal section) showing bony erosion of right sella turcia *(arrow)* with possible soft tissue extension into right cavernous sinus. Height of pituitary gland (not shown) is 9mm. **B,** MRI (coronal section) showing soft tissue mass extending into right cavernous sinus near carotid artery *(large arrow)*. Height of pituitary gland is 9 mm. Normal optic chiasm is seen *(small arrow)*. (From Stein AL, Levenick MN, et al: Obstet Gynecol 73:996, 1989.)

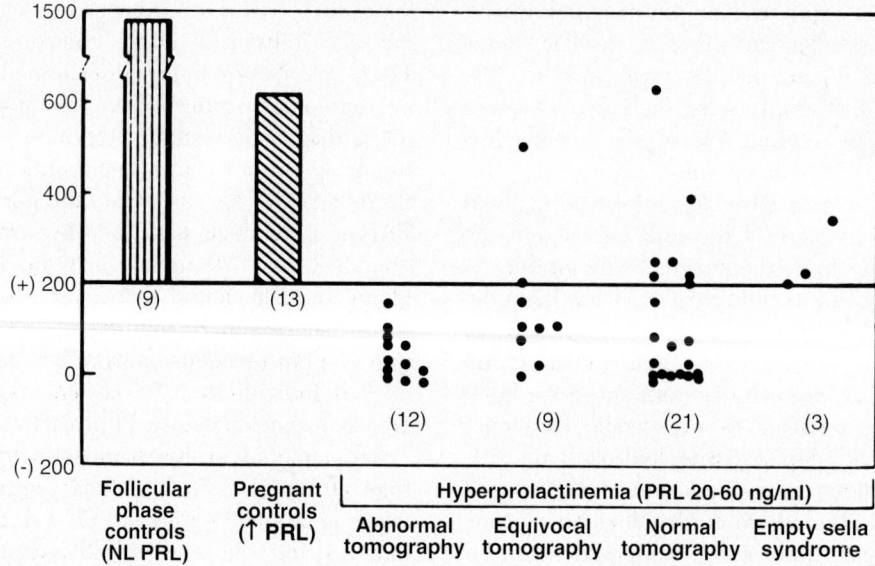

FIGURE 37-7
Individual prolactin (PRL) responses to TRH stimulation in nonpregnant women with mild hyperprolactinemia in relation to tomographic findings. Bars represent 95% confidence limits for follicular phase and pregnancy controls. (From Shangold GA, Kletzky OA, Marrs RP, et al: Obstet Gynecol 63:771, 1984. Reprinted with permission from The American College of Obstetricians and Gynecologists.)

evaluations should be performed in individuals with macroadenomas because suprasellar extension of the tumor may exert pressure on the optic chiasm, resulting in bitemporal visual field defects and interference with vision. The size of these tumors may also affect other aspects of pituitary function. Thus a test of ACTH reserve, such as insulin-induced hypoglycemia (insulin tolerance test), as well as tests of thyroid function, should be performed on all individuals with a macroadenoma.

Recommended Diagnostic Evaluation

It is currently recommended that prolactin levels be measured in all patients with galactorrhea, oligomenorrhea, or amenorrhea who do not have an elevated FSH level. If prolactin is elevated, a TSH assay should be performed to rule out the presence of primary hypothyroidism. If TSH is elevated, T_3 and T_4 should be measured to rule out the rare possibility of a TSH-secreting pituitary adenoma (Figure 37-8). If TSH is elevated, appropriate thyroid replacement should begin, and the prolactin level will usually return to normal. If TSH is

normal and the patient has a normal prolactin level with galactorrhea, no further tests are necessary if she has regular menses (Figure 37-9). Because some patients with galactorrhea, abnormal menstrual function, and normal prolactin levels have been found to have the empty sella syndrome, anteroposterior and lateral coned-down views of the sella should be obtained in such cases (Figure 37-10). If these findings are abnormal, MRI or a CT scan should be obtained to establish the diagnosis.

In patients with a normal TSH level, MRI or a CT scan should be obtained if prolactin is elevated above 60 ng/ml (see Figure 37-8). If the prolactin level is between 20 and 60 ng/ml, TRH should be administered as a bolus intravenously. Prolactin should be measured immediately before and 20 minutes after TRH administration. If a normal (threefold) response of prolactin to TRH is obtained, a repeat test should be performed annually; scans are not necessary. However, anteroposterior and lateral coned-down views of the sella should be obtained to rule out the possibility of an empty sella. If the TRH test results are abnormal,

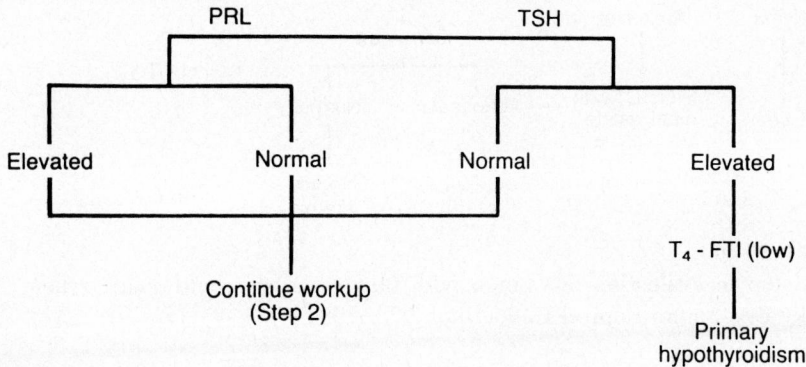

FIGURE 37-8
First step in workup of patients with hyperprolactinemia, evaluation of all those with galactorrhea. FTI = Free thyroxine index. (From Kletzky OA and Davajan V: Hyperprolactinemia: diagnosis and treatment. In Mishell DR, Davajan V, and Lobo RA, editors: Infertility, contraception, and reproductive endocrinology, ed 3, Cambridge, Mass, 1991, Blackwell Scientific Publications.)

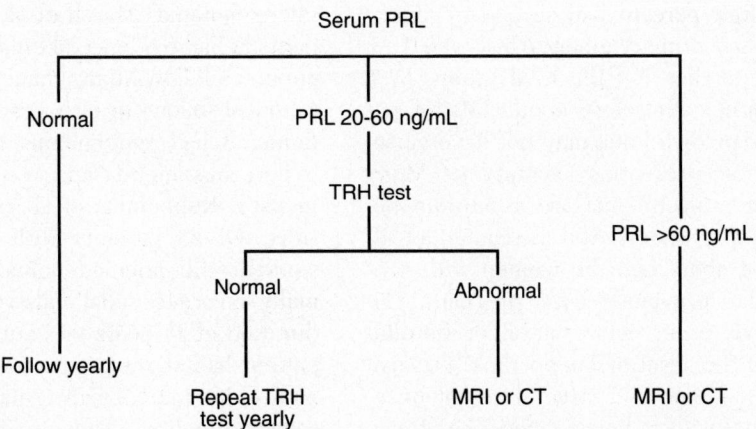

FIGURE 37-9
Second step in workup of patients with hyperprolactinemia. (From Kletzky OA and Davajan V: Hyperprolactinemia: diagnosis and treatment. In Mishell DR, Davajan V, and Lobo RA, editors: Infertility, contraception, and reproductive endocrinology, ed 3, Cambridge, Mass, 1991, Blackwell Scientific Publications.)

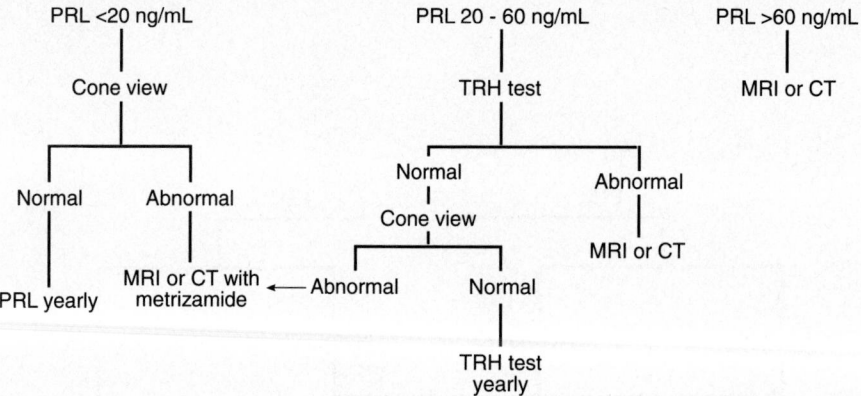

FIGURE 37-10
Third step in evaluation of women with oligomenorrhea and galactorrhea. (From Kletzky OA: Semin Reprod Endocrinol 2:23, 1984.)

MRI or a CT scan should be performed; not all individuals with an abnormal TRH response have radiologic evidence of a microadenoma.

Natural History of Prolactinomas

In a series of 84 women with surgically treated prolactinomas, Randall et al. reported that all had some form of menstrual abnormality. Eighty-four percent had secondary amenorrhea, 6% had primary amenorrhea, and 10% had oligomenorrhea. Of the total group, 87% had galactorrhea; therefore about 13% of patients with a prolactinoma may not have galactorrhea as a presenting symptom. Many women with prolactinemia are asymptomatic. In their autopsy series, Abd El-Hamid et al. reported that about half the women with prolactinomas had previously been pregnant. Galactorrhea may occur before, after, or simultaneously with the onset of amenorrhea. Davajan et al. reported that in a large series of unselected patients with radiologic evidence of prolactinomas the most common clinical findings were galactorrhea and secondary amenorrhea with low estrogen status. Therefore the clinician should suspect that a prolactinoma is present in patients with galactorrhea and amenorrhea who fail to experience withdrawal bleeding after progesterone administration. The diagnosis becomes more likely if the prolactin levels exceed 100 ng/ml. Macroadenomas can enlarge and cause visual field distortion or disturbance of pituitary function. Thus even if these findings are not present when the diag-

nosis of macroadenoma is made, treatment should be initiated to prevent further enlargement of the macroadenoma.

Long-term studies of patients with microadenomas demonstrate that enlargement is uncommon and that some of these tumors can actually regress spontaneously. In a longitudinal retrospective study of 43 untreated patients with hyperprolactinemia and a radiologic diagnosis of microadenoma, March et al. found that only 2 patients had evidence of enlargement of the adenoma (1 following pregnancy) with a mean duration of follow-up of 5 years. Of these 43 patients, 3 had spontaneous regression of their hyperprolactinemia and resumption of normal menses. Koppelman et al. reported similar results. Of 25 patients with prolactinomas (18 women with microadenoma and 7 with minimally enlarged sella) followed up for a mean duration of 11 years without treatment, only 1 patient had slight progression of a sella abnormality. No patient had visual field or other pituitary function changes, 7 resumed normal menses spontaneously, and galactorrhea spontaneously resolved in 6.

The results of these retrospective studies have been confirmed by two prospective studies of untreated microprolactinomas. In a 3- to 7-year prospective longitudinal study of 30 hyperprolactinemic women, Schlechte et al. found that of 13 women with initially abnormal radiographic findings, 4 became normal, 7 did not change, and 2 had evidence of tumor growth. Of 17 women with initially normal radiographic findings, 4 became minimally abnormal. None of the 30 developed a macroadenoma of pituitary hypofunction. In this study, as in the two retrospective studies just reported, more sensitive radiographic techniques (tomograms, followed by CT) were used as the study progressed and could account for the minimal evidence of tumor growth. Sisam et al. overcame this problem by prospectively following a group of 38 patients with hyperprolactinemia and microprolactinomas by serial CT scans performed initially and about every 2½ years thereafter for a mean duration of 50 months. None of these patients had evidence of tumor progression, even in 2 who had a marked increase in prolactin levels. In this group, 9 (25%) had spontaneous improvement of their symptoms. These studies demonstrate the benign course of untreated microadenomas. Therefore treatment may not be necessary if the patient is not bothered by the amenorrhea or galactorrhea unless she appears to be at risk for developing osteoporosis.

MANAGEMENT

Expectant Treatment

Patients with radiologic evidence of a microadenoma who do not wish to conceive may be followed without treatment by measuring prolactin levels once yearly and performing CT scans every 2 years. Many of these patients have deficient estrogen, and low estrogen levels in combination with hyperprolactinemia have been shown to be associated with the early onset of osteoporosis. If the individual has low estrogen levels, treatment involves replacement estrogen-progestin therapy (as is used for postmenopausal women) or bromocriptine. Individuals with hyperprolactinemia with or without microadenomas who have adequate estrogen levels as evidenced by the presence of oligomenorrhea or amenorrhea with progesterone-induced withdrawal bleeding and who do not wish to conceive should be treated with periodic progestin withdrawal (medroxyprogesterone acetate 10 mg per day for 10 days each month) to prevent endometrial hyperplasia. Barrier types of contraception are advised.

Medical Therapy

Currently the treatment of choice for microadenomas as well as the initial treatment for macroadenomas is oral ingestion of a potent dopamine receptor agonist. Bromocriptine, methysergide, and metergoline have been used with success, but only bromocriptine (2-Br-alpha-ergocryptine mesylate) is approved for use in the United States (Figure 37-11). The greatest amount of clinical experience has been with use of this agent. This semisynthetic ergot alkaloid was developed in 1967 to inhibit prolactin secretion. It directly stimulates dopamine receptors, and as a dopamine receptor agonist it inhibits prolactin secretion both in vitro and in vivo. After ingestion, bromocriptine is rapidly absorbed, with peak blood levels reached 1 to 3 hours later. Serum prolactin levels remain depressed for about 14 hours after ingestion of a single dose, after which time the drug is not detectable in the circulation. For this reason the drug is usually given at least twice daily, with initial therapy being started at one half of the 2.5 mg tablet to minimize side effects. The most frequent side effects are orthostatic hypotension (with an incidence of 15%), which can produce fainting and dizziness as well as nausea and vomiting. To minimize these symptoms the initial dose should be taken in bed and with food at nighttime. Less frequent adverse symptoms include headache, nasal congestion, fatigue, constipation, and diarrhea. Most of these reactions are mild, occur early in the course of treatment, and are transient. To reduce the adverse symptoms, the dose should be gradually increased every 1 to 2 weeks until prolactin levels fall to normal. The usual therapeutic dose is 2.5 mg twice or three times a day, but larger doses are sometimes used when a macroadenoma is present.

About 10% of women cannot tolerate oral bromocriptine because of severe side effects. Vermesh et al. reported that the drug was very well absorbed vaginally without the presence of side effects. Furthermore, when the tablet was placed deep in the posterior vaginal fornix, therapeutic blood levels persisted for more than 24 hours, during which time prolactin levels remained suppressed (Figure 37-12). Kletzky and Vermesh subsequently reported that this method of bromocriptine administration was well accepted, effective, and well tolerated in a group of 115 hyperprolactinemic women, several of whom have subsequently conceived. The tablet is placed digitally deep in the vagina nightly at bedtime. A single 2.5 mg dose is usually sufficient to restore normal prolactin levels (Figure 37-13).

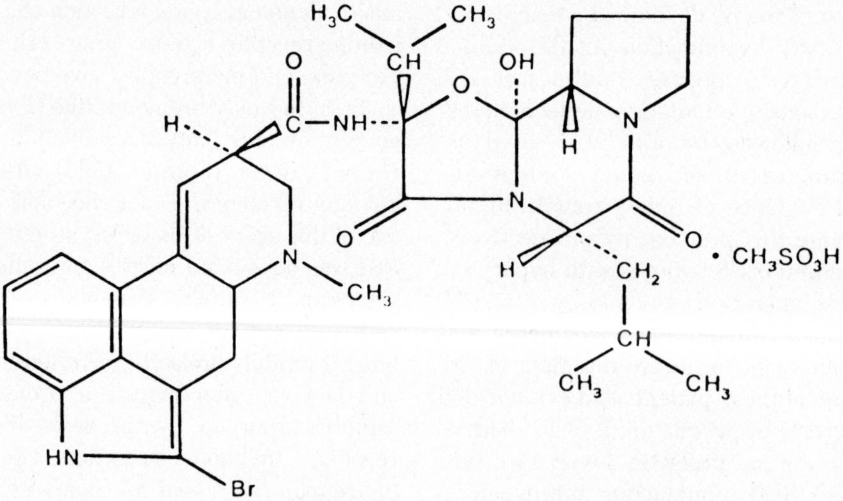

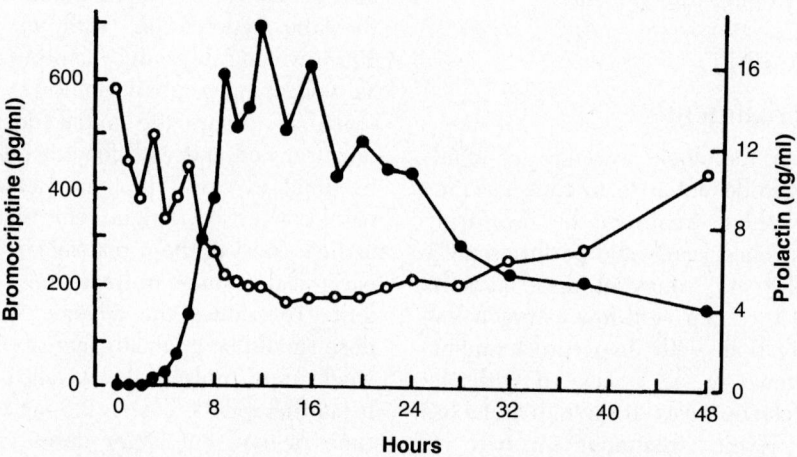

FIGURE 37-11
Formula of bromocriptine.

FIGURE 37-12
Mean (± SEM) plasma levels of bromocriptine *(solid circles)* and prolactin *(open circles)* in a single study, extended to 48 hours, after vaginal bromocriptine (2.5 mg). (From Vermesh M, Fossum GT, et al: Obstet Gynecol 72:693, 1988.)

A long-acting injectable form of bromocriptine that is effective for 1 month has also been developed, but it is not yet available for clinical use. Bromocriptine is approved for treatment of dysfunctions associated with hyperprolactinemia, including amenorrhea with or without galactorrhea, as well as infertility with and without the presence of a prolactin-secreting adenoma. In women without adenomas, prolactin levels return to normal in more than 90%,

fertility is restored in 80%, and galactorrhea is eradicated in 60%. In patients with hyperprolactinemia and microadenoma, similar rates of success have been reported. Therefore bromocriptine is the treatment of choice in patients with microadenoma who desire return of menses and ovulation and disappearance of galactorrhea.

Kletzky et al. reported that patients with hyperprolactinemia without radiologic evidence

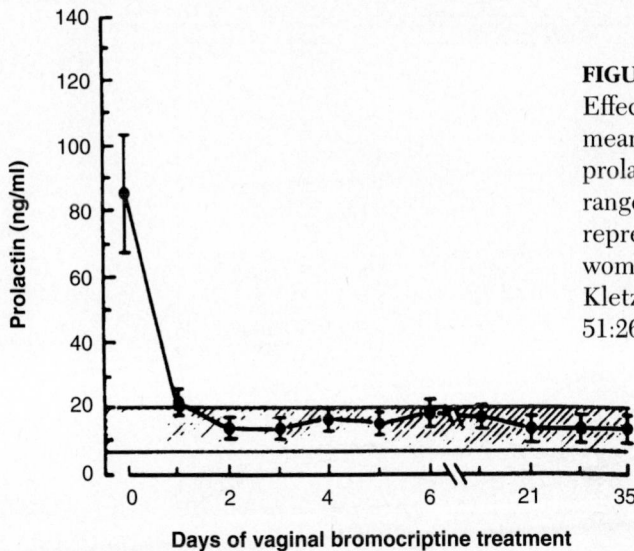

FIGURE 37-13

Effect of 2.5 mg vaginal bromocriptine on mean (± SEM) serum prolactin in 13 hyperprolactinemic women. Normal serum prolactin range is indicated by shaded area. Shaded area represents 95% confidence limits for normal women in follicular phase (*N* = 25). (From Kletzky OA and Vermesh M: Fertil Steril 51:269, 1989.)

TABLE 37-1

Effective Dose of Bromocriptine to Normalize Prolactin or Achieve Pregnancy

Daily Dose (mg)	Adenoma (No. = 19)	No Adenoma (No. = 21)
5.0	9 (47%)	20* (95%)
7.5	5 (47%)	1
10.0	2 (47%)	0
15.0	1 (47%)	0
20.0	2 (47%)	0

From Kletzky OA, Marrs RP, and Davajan V: Am J Obstet Gynecol 147:528, 1983.
*$P < 0.005$.

TABLE 37-2

Duration of Treatment (Weeks) to Correct Symptoms

	Adenoma	No Adenoma
Galactorrhea	11.3* ± 2.1 (No. = 17)	5.6 ± 1.1 (No. = 19)
Amenorrhea	8.7† ± 1.2 (No. = 17)	5.7 ± 0.6 (No. = 15)
Infertility	16.2‡ ± 2.1 (No. = 17)	9.8 ± 1.5 (No. = 12)

From Kletzky OA, Marrs RP, and Davajan V: Am J Obstet Gynecol 147:528, 1983.
*$P < 0.001$.
†$P < 0.01$.
‡$P < 0.02$.

of tumor required a lower dose of bromocriptine than patients with adenomas to reduce prolactin levels to normal (Table 37-1) and less duration of therapy to resume ovulatory cycles, establish pregnancy, and end galactorrhea (Table 37-2).

Despite administration of up to 20 mg of bromocriptine per day, about 10% of patients with microadenomas fail to have prolactin levels return to normal, probably because of individual differences in the sensitivity of lactotrophs to bromocriptine. Nevertheless, despite the persistently elevated prolactin levels, many of these patients ovulate and conceive (Figure 37-14).

If pregnancy is desired and effected, after conception occurs bromocriptine therapy is usually discontinued, although there is no evidence that the drug is teratogenic or adversely affects pregnancy outcome. If pregnancy is not desired, therapy is usually continued for at least 12 months, after which it is discontinued for a few weeks. Most patients with microadenomas have recurrence of hyperprolactinemia, amenorrhea, and galactorrhea, although about 10% to 20% have permanent remission after discontinuing bromocriptine treatment. Moriondo et al. reported that after 1 year of bromocriptine treatment, 11% of women with microadenomas had persistent normalization of prolactin, with return of regular menses after the drug was discontinued (Figure 37-15).

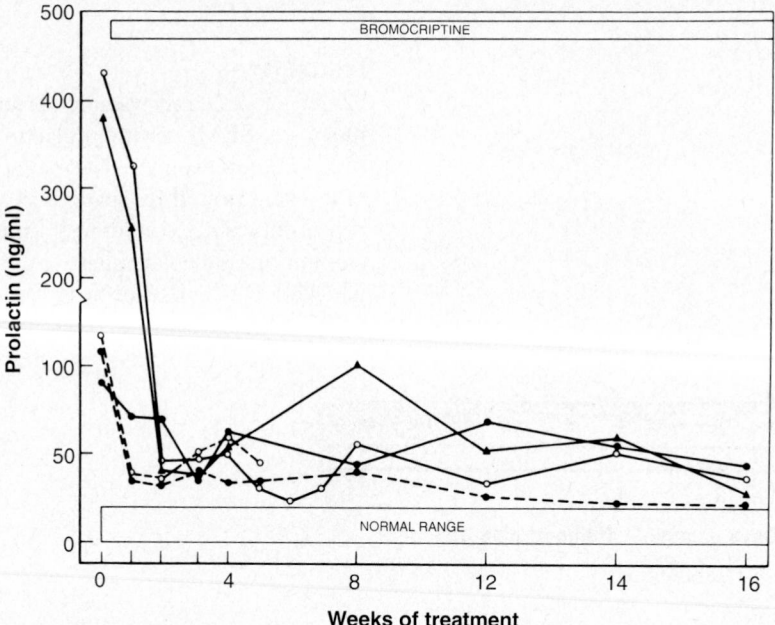

FIGURE 37-14
Mean serum prolactin response to bromocriptine therapy in five patients with radiographic evidence of pituitary adenoma and residual hyperprolactinemia. All five ovulated, and four conceived. (From Kletzky OA, Marrs RP, and Davajan V: Am J Obstet Gynecol 147:528, 1983.)

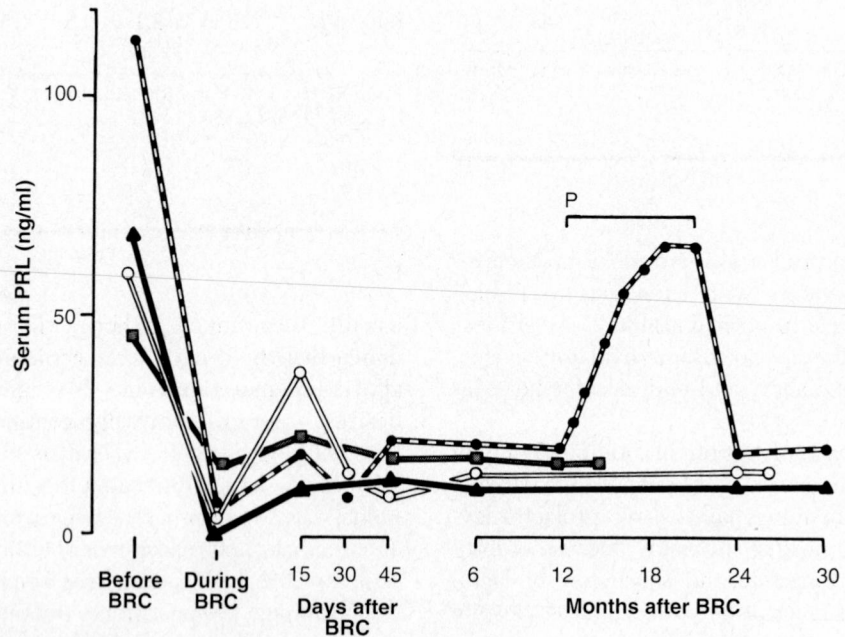

FIGURE 37-15
Serum prolactin levels in four patients who had persistently normal prolactin levels after bromocriptine *(BRC)* treatment for 12 months. *P,* Pregnancy. (From Moriondo P, Travaglini P, Nissim M, et al: J Clin Endocrinol Metab 60:764, 1985. Copyright © by The Endocrine Society 1985.)

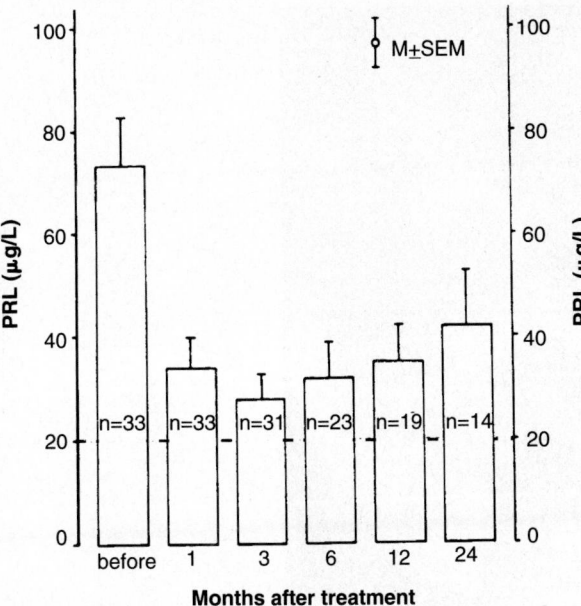

FIGURE 37-16

Geometric mean serum prolactin levels before and after discontinuation of bromocriptine treatment in 33 women with hyperprolactinemic amenorrhea. (From Rasmussen C, Bergh T, and Wide L: Fertil Steril 48:550, 1987.

This incidence of permanent remission reached 22% after 2 years of treatment. A higher rate of permanent remission occurred in patients treated with 10 mg per day than with lower dosages, but higher doses of drug increase the incidence of adverse reactions and cause discontinuation of treatment. These investigators found that after bromocriptine was discontinued, there was a 40% reduction in mean prolactin levels in all patients treated, and about 60% of patients had a greater than 30% reduction from pretreatment prolactin levels after the drug was discontinued. Rasmussen et al. reported the results of discontinuation of long-term (medium of 2 years) bromocriptine therapy in 75 hyperprolactinemic women. In about half the women it was necessary to reinstate treatment because prolactin levels rose. However, in the other half further treatment was unnecessary because mean prolactin levels decreased more than 60% and either returned to normal or were only slightly elevated (Figure 37-16). More than half of these 33 women resumed regular menses without treatment. These data indicate that the remissions were drug related and not spontaneous. Using CT scans before and during bromocriptine therapy, Bonneville et al. found that about 75% of patients with microadenomas had reduction in tumor size during bromocriptine treatment, and in 40% the tumor had disappeared (Figure 37-17). To determine if permanent remission has occurred, the prolactin level should be measured about 6 weeks after discontinuation of treatment because the levels plateau at this time.

Bromocriptine treatment has also been shown to reduce tumor mass in 80% to 90% of individuals with macroadenomas. In addition, visual disturbances, if present, are usually promptly relieved. Following subsequent surgical removal of these bromocriptine-treated tumors, histologic examination revealed a reduction of tumor cell size, with shrinkage of the cytoplasm being greater than the nucleus. In addition, there are modifications of cell structure and morphology as compared with tumors removed without prior medical treatment. The organelles responsible for prolactin synthesis shrink, indicating that bromocriptine impairs prolactin synthesis as well as release. The reduction in size of macroadenomas usually occurs rapidly, within a few weeks after starting treatment, but following withdrawal of drug the tumor size may increase just as rapidly; thus the drug should be withdrawn cautiously. In contrast to the frequent occurrence of pituitary insufficiency, including diabetes insipidus, after surgical or radiologic treatment of large tumors, bromocriptine treatment is not accompanied by any type of pituitary insufficiency.

Because permanent remission rarely occurs following withdrawal of bromocriptine treatment from individuals with large tumors, long-term treatment is usually necessary. The drug has been administered for up to 12 years in some patients without problems, and once biochemical, radiologic, and clinical responses to treatment are established, they are generally maintained over a long-term period. Bromocriptine has also been successfully used to treat patients with failure of, or recurrence after, operation or irradiation therapy.

Molitch et al. reported the results of a 1-year prospective multicenter study of the use of bromocriptine as primary therapy for prolactin-secreting macroadenomas in 27 patients. Bromocriptine dosage ranged from 5 to 12.5 mg daily, with 7.5 mg being the most frequent

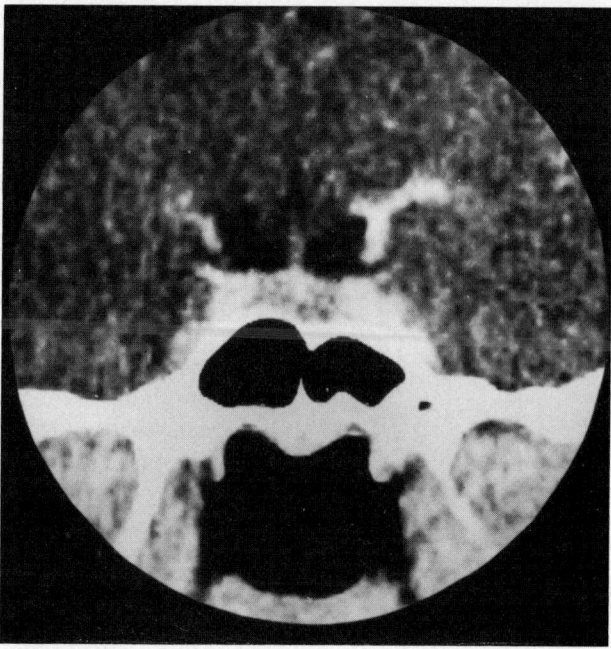

FIGURE 37-17
Coronal CT scan of woman with microadenoma 4 months after bromocriptine therapy (5 mg per day). Clinical and biologic results were excellent; pituitary gland is nearly normal, with reconstruction of sellar floor. (From Bonneville J-F, Poulignot D, Cattin F, et al: Radiology 143:451, 1982.)

dose. Prolactin levels fell in all patients, and to 11% or less of pretreatment values in all but one. Of this group, two thirds had prolactin levels decrease to normal during treatment. Tumor shrinkage was observed in all patients, being reduced by more than 50% in half the patients and by about 50% in an additional 20% of the study group. Visual field impairment disappeared in 9 of the 10 patients with abnormalities. In two thirds of the patients reduction in tumor size occurred by 6 weeks, but in one third it was not evident until 6 months, indicating there were both rapid and slow responses of tumor to drug treatment. Therefore at least a 6-month trial of medical therapy is warranted in patients with a macroadenoma.

Because of these excellent results, the poor initial results of operation, and the high recurrence rates, these investigators concluded that bromocriptine should be used as the initial management of patients with prolactin-secreting macroadenomas. After maximal shrinkage of tumor, medical therapy can be continued or operative treatment used. The cost of continuing bromocriptine treatment is considerable; it is inconvenient to take medication several times a day, and some patients have unpleasant side effects with the higher dosages that may be necessary. Therefore some patients prefer operative treatment. In patients who elect to have an operation, the drug should be continued until the time of operation to prevent tumor expansion. The rates of success after operation are no different in patients who received or did not receive bromocriptine before the operation.

Operative Approaches

Transsphenoidal microsurgical resection of prolactinoma has been widely used for therapy, and numerous reports of large series of patients treated by this technique have been published. In a review of these studies Randall et al. concluded that transsphenoidal operations have minimal risk with a mortality of less than 0.5%, all deaths being reported to occur after treatment of macroadenomas. The risk of temporary postoperative diabetes insipidus is 10% to 40%, but the risk of permanent diabetes insipidus and iatrogenic hypopituitarism is less than 2%. The initial cure rate, with normalization of prolactin levels and return of ovulation, is relatively high for microadenomas (65% to 85%)

and less so with macroadenomas (20% to 40%). Vision can return to normal in 85% of patients with loss of acuity and visual field defects.

The initial cure rate is related to the pretreatment prolactin levels. Those tumors with levels less than 100 ng/ml have an excellent prognosis (85%), and those with levels greater than 200 ng/ml have a poor prognosis (35%). Operative treatment of tumors in patients older than 26 with amenorrhea for more than 6 months carries a poorer prognosis than tumors in younger patients with a shorter duration of amenorrhea. Nevertheless, long-term follow-up of patients after operation indicates that late recurrence of hyperprolactinemia is common. Serri et al. followed 28 patients with microadenomas and 16 with macroadenomas for 6 years after operation. Although prolactin levels normalized and menses resumed in 24 (85%) of those with microadenomas and 5 (31%) of those with macroadenomas who had a good initial postoperative response, hyperprolactinemia recurred in half of those with microadenoma and 4 of the 5 with macroadenomas after a mean period of 4 and 2.5 years, respectively (Figure 37-18). There was no significant difference in recurrence rates for those who conceived and those who did not. Rodman et al. reported a lower postoperative recurrence rate (about 20% for both microadenomas and macroadenomas) following initial cure rates of 85% and 37%, respectively. The risk of recurrence in both series appeared to be related to the immediate postoperative prolactin levels, being greater in persons with a prolactin level greater than 10 ng/ml.

The relatively high rates of late recurrence indicate that these patients have an underlying hypothalamic defect in dopamine regulation that continues after operative removal of the adenoma.

Because of the good results with medical therapy, surgery is recommended only for patients who fail to respond to medical therapy or have poor compliance with this regimen. It is best to reduce the size of macroadenomas maximally with bromocriptine before surgical removal of these extrasellar tumors.

Radiation Therapy

External radiation with cobalt, proton beam, or heavy particle therapy and brachytherapy with yttrium-90 rods implanted in the pituitary

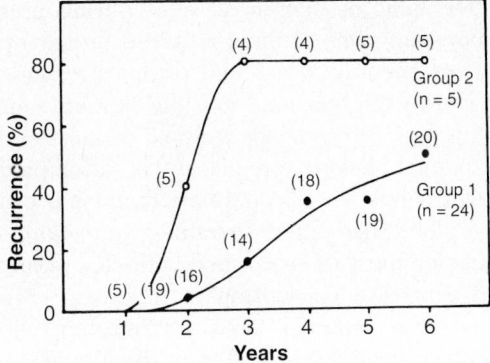

FIGURE 37-18
Cumulative recurrence rate in patients with microprolactinoma (group 1) or macroprolactinoma (group 2) after initially successful operation. Figures in parentheses indicate numbers of patients who were seen at each yearly interval. (From Serri O, Rasio E, Beauregard H, et al: N Engl J Med 309:280, 1983. Reprinted by permission of The New England Journal of Medicine.)

have all been used to treat macroadenomas but are not the primary mode of treatment. Results of such therapy have been inconsistent, and there is a delay of several months between treatment and resumption of ovulation. Furthermore, damage to normal pituitary tissue occurs, frequently leading to abnormal anterior pituitary function as well as diabetes insipidus. Damage to the optic nerves may also occur. Thus radiation therapy should be used only as adjunctive management following incomplete operative removal of large tumors.

Pregnancy

Many women with hyperprolactinemia with or without adenomas wish to become pregnant. A small percentage conceive spontaneously, while most require treatment to induce ovulation. Barbieri and Ryan compiled a literature review of the pregnancy courses of 275 women with adenomas, the majority of whose conceptions had been induced by bromocriptine. They reported that of 215 patients with microprolactinomas, less than 1% had changes in visual fields, radiologic evidence of tumor enlargement, or neurologic signs. About 5% developed headaches during pregnancy. Of 60 patients with macroprolactinomas, 20% developed adverse changes in visual fields and polytomographic or neurologic signs during pregnancy, and some of them required bromocriptine or operative treatment during pregnancy or shortly postpartum. For this reason some authorities recommend excision of macroprolactinomas before pregnancy is attempted. Nevertheless, because pituitary function is usually diminished after operation, induction of ovulation must be performed with complicated and expensive gonadotrophin treatment. Bromocriptine treatment does not interfere with pituitary function and is thus the therapy of choice for patients with macroadenomas who wish to conceive. Some authors advise continuous bromocriptine treatment throughout pregnancy in patients with macroadenomas, because with this therapy visual disturbances are rare. Despite a lowering of prolactin levels, there is no effect on placental hormone production, and pregnancy outcome does not appear to be affected.

Nevertheless, since bromocriptine crosses the placenta and suppresses fetal prolactin levels, its long-term effects on the newborn are unknown. Therefore it is advised that patients with macroadenomas discontinue the drug after conception, as do patients with microadenomas, and have therapy reinitiated if and when symptoms of visual disturbance or severe headaches occur. Most patients who conceive after bromocriptine treatment have ingested the drug for a few weeks after conception. In a review of 1410 such pregnancies compiled by Turkalj et al. there was a spontaneous abortion rate of 11%, ectopic pregnancy rate of 0.7%, and twin pregnancy rate of 1.8%. The incidence of minor (2.5%) and major (1%) congenital defects was similar to pregnancy outcomes in untreated populations of women. The mean amount of drug ingested and duration of postconception treatment were similar in mothers who had normal children and those with defects. Thus ingestion of bromocriptine during pregnancy does not appear to increase the risk of congenital abnormalities, spontaneous abortion, or multiple gestation. Postnatal surveillance of more than 200 children born in this series has revealed no adverse effects to date.

Ruiz-Velasco and Tolis compiled the obstetric histories of nearly 2000 pregnancies occurring in hyperprolactinemic women that have been reported in the literature. Most of these pregnancies were induced with bromocriptine.

There was a term delivery rate of 85%, an abortion rate of 11%, a prematurity rate of 2%, and a multiple pregnancy rate of 1.2%. Although prolactin levels increased during pregnancy, after delivery the levels returned to pretreatment values in about 85%. A postpartum increase over pretreatment levels was uncommon (3%), while prolactin levels returned to normal in 13%. Likewise, in patients who had postpartum radiologic sellar examination, 84% showed no change, 9% improved, and 7% worsened. Thus stopping treatment during pregnancy only occasionally results in tumor growth. It is advised that patients with macroadenoma have monthly visual field examination and neurologic testing during pregnancy, but this is probably unnecessary for patients with microadenoma unless they develop symptoms.

Following delivery, breast-feeding may be initiated without adverse effects on the tumors. Godo et al. reported that use of bromocriptine before conception and during pregnancy did not effect puerperal lactation following discontinuation of nursing. The incidence of menstrual abnormalities and degree of galactorrhea were usually similar to the state that existed before starting bromocriptine therapy. Therefore, following completion of nursing, as well as for women who do not breast-feed at all, bromocriptine should be ingested for 2 to 3 weeks and then discontinued. At that time serum prolactin measurement and repeat MRI or CT scan should be performed and treatment reinstituted according to the findings.

Patients with Hyperprolactinemia Who Do Not Wish to Conceive

For patients who do not wish to conceive and for whom galactorrhea is not a problem, no therapy is necessary unless estrogen levels are low. Thus to prevent osteoporosis in this clinical situation, bromocriptine should be given, regardless of whether an adenoma is present, and a mechanical type of contraceptive should be used. Long-term evaluation of all patients with hyperprolactinemia is important. Unless a macroadenoma is present, measurement of prolactin levels every 6 months and MRI or CT examination every 2 years are advised. If bromocriptine therapy is used, temporary discontinuation of medication every 1 to 2 years is advisable, with prolactin measurement 6 weeks later. If the level is normal, repeat prolactin measurements should be made semiannually. If the level is increased, therapy should be restarted, and if a microadenoma is present, the option of operation should be offered. During medical treatment of macroadenomas, MRI or CT and visual field examination should be performed every 6 months to determine the effect of medication on the tumor. At these intervals a decision about whether to continue long-term bromocriptine treatment or perform an operation can be made.

KEY POINTS

- Estrogen stimulates prolactin release but blocks its action at the receptor in the breast.

- Physiologic stimuli for prolactin release include breast and nipple palpation, exercise, stress, sleep, and the noonday meal.

- The main symptoms of hyperprolactinemia are galactorrhea and amenorrhea, the latter caused by alterations in normal gonadotrophin-releasing hormone (GnRH) release.

- Hyperprolactinemia is present in 15% of all anovulatory women and 20% of women with amenorrhea of undetermined cause.

- About 60% of all women with galactorrhea have hyperprolactinemia, but almost 90% of women with galactorrhea, amenorrhea, and low estrogen levels have hyperprolactinemia.

- Pathologic causes of hyperprolactinemia include pharmacologic agents (tranquilizers, narcotics, and antihypertensive drugs), hypothyroidism, chronic renal disease, chronic neurostimulation of the breast, hypothalamic disease, and pituitary tumors (prolactinoma, acromegaly, Cushing's disease).

- About 3% to 5% of individuals with hyperprolactinemia have hypothyroidism.

- About 80% of all pituitary tumors secrete prolactin.

- About 25% of patients with acromegaly and 10% of those with Cushing's disease have hyperprolactinemia.

- About 10% of patients with an enlarged sella have the empty sella syndrome.

- Autopsy studies reveal that prolactinomas are present in about 10% of the population.

- About 50% of women with hyperprolactinemia will have a prolactinoma, as will nearly all of those with prolactin levels greater than 200 ng/ml.

- About 20% of women with galactorrhea and 35% of those with amenorrhea and galactorrhea have prolactinomas.

- About 70% of women with hyperprolactinemia, galactorrhea, and amenorrhea with low estrogen levels will have a prolactinoma.

- Women with regular menses, galactorrhea, and normal prolactin levels do not have prolactinomas.

- About 13% of women with prolactinomas do not have galactorrhea.

- Most macroadenomas enlarge with time; most microadenomas do not.

- The initial operative cure rate for microadenomas is about 80% and for macroadenomas 30%, but the long-term recurrence rate is at least 20% for each.

- Most frequent side effects of bromocriptine are orthostatic hypotension, nausea, and vomiting.

- In patients with hyperprolactinemia and no macroadenoma, bromocriptine treatment returns prolactin levels to normal in 90%, induces ovulatory cycles in 80%, and eradicates galactorrhea in 60%.

- After 1 year of bromocriptine treatment, prolactin levels remain normal in 11% of women with macroadenomas; after 2 years permanent remission reaches 22%. After longer use, remissions of 50% have been reported.

- Bromocriptine shrinks 80% to 90% of macroadenomas.

- When pregnancy occurs in women with microadenomas, less than 1% have visual field changes, tumor enlargement, or neurologic signs; about 20% of women with macroadenomas have such adverse changes.

- Bromocriptine induction of pregnancy is not associated with an increased risk of congenital abnormalities, spontaneous abortion, or multiple gestation.

- About 85% of patients with prolactinomas have no change in prolactin levels or tumor size after delivery, 10% improve, and 5% worsen.

- The most frequent cause of mildly elevated prolactin levels is stress.

- The best modality to diagnose pituitary adenomas or empty sella syndrome is magnetic resonance imaging (MRI).

- The natural history of nearly all microprolactinomas is to stay the same size, with adverse menstrual problems resolving spontaneously in about one fourth of patients.

- Surgical treatment of prolactinomas is recommended only for patients who fail to respond or do not comply with medical management.

- For patients who develop side effects with oral bromocriptine, vaginal administration usually alleviates the problem.

BIBLIOGRAPHY

Abd El-Hamid MW, Joplin EF, and Lewis PD: Incidentally found small pituitary adenomas may have no effect on fertility, Acta Endocrinol (Copenh) 117:361, 1988.

Bäckström CT, McNeilly AS, Leash RM, et al: Pulsatile secretion of LH, FSH, prolactin oestradiol and progesterone during the human menstrual cycle, Clin Endocrinol 17:29, 1982.

Barbieri RL and Ryan KJ: Bromocriptine: endocrine pharmacology and therapeutic applications, Fertil Steril 39:727, 1983.

Bonneville J-F, Poulignot D, Cattin F, et al: Computed tomographic demonstration of the effects of bromocriptine on pituitary microadenoma size, Radiology 143:451, 1982.

Burrow GN, Wortzman G, Rewcastle NB, et al: Microadenomas of the pituitary and abnormal sellar tomograms in an unselected autopsy series, N Engl J Med 304:156, 1981.

Chapler FK: Hyperprolactinemia. In Pitkin RM and Zlatnik FJ: Yearbook of obstetrics and gynecology, Chicago, 1985, Mosby–Year Book, Inc.

Ciccarelli E, Miola C, Avateneo T, et al: Long-term treatment with a new repeatable injectable form of bromocriptine, Parlodel LAR, in patients with tumorous hyperprolactinemia, Fertil Steril 52:930, 1989.

Davajan V, Kletzky O, March CM, et al: The significance of galactorrhea in patients with normal menses, oligomenorrhea, and secondary amenorrhea, Am J Obstet Gynecol 130:894, 1978.

Gharib H, Frey HM, Laws ER Jr, et al: Coexistent primary empty sella syndrome and hyperprolactinemia: report of 11 cases, Arch Intern Med 143:1383, 1983.

Godo G, Kolosziar S, Szilagyi I, et al: Experience related to pregnancy, lactation, and the after-weaning condition of hyperprolactinemic patients treated with bromocriptine, Fertil Steril 51:529, 1989.

Kleinberg DL, Noel GL, and Frantz AG: Galactorrhea: a study of 235 cases, including 48 with pituitary tumors, N Engl J Med 296:589, 1977.

Kletzky OA: Diagnostic approaches to hyperprolactinemic states, Semin Reprod Endocrinol 2:23, 1984.

Kletzky OA and Davajan V: Hyperprolactinemia: diagnosis and treatment. In Mishell DR Jr and Davajan V, editors: Infertility, reproductive endocrinology and contraception, ed 2, Oradell, NJ, 1986, Medical Economics Books.

Kletzky OA and Davajan V: Hyperprolactinemia. In Mishell DR, Davajan V, and Lobo RA, editors: Infertility, reproductive endocrinology and contraception, ed 3, Cambridge, Mass, 1991, Blackwell Scientific Publications.

Kletzky OA, Marrs RP, and Davajan V: Management of patients with hyperprolactinemia and normal or abnormal tomograms, Am J Obstet Gynecol 147:528, 1983.

Kletsky OA and Vermesh M: Effectiveness of vaginal bromocriptine in treating women with hyperprolactinemia, Fertil Steril 51:269, 1989.

Koppelman MCS, Jaffe MJ, Rieth KG, et al: Hyperprolactinemia, amenorrhea, and galactorrhea: a retrospective assessment of 25 cases, Ann Intern Med 100:115, 1984.

March CM, Kletzky OA, Davajan V, et al: Longitudinal evaluation of patients with untreated prolactin-secreting pituitary adenomas, Am J Obstet Gynecol 139:835, 1981.

Molitch ME, Elton RL, Blackwell RE, et al: Bromocriptine as primary therapy for prolactin-secreting macroadenomas: results of a prospective multicenter study, J Clin Endocrinol Metab 60:698, 1985.

Moriondo P, Travaglini P, Nissim M, et al: Bromocriptine treatment of microprolactinomas: evidence of stable prolactin decrease after drug withdrawal, J Clin Endocrinol Metab 60:764, 1985.

Muneyyirci-Delale O, Goldstein D, Reyes FI, et al: Diagnosis of stress-related hyperprolactinemia: evaluation of the hyperprolactinemia rest test, NY State J Med 89:205, 1989.

Randall RV, Laws ER Jr, Abboud CF, et al: Transsphenoidal microsurgical treatment of prolactin-producing pituitary adenomas, Mayo Clin Proc 58:108, 1983.

Rasmussen C, Bergh T, and Wide L: Prolactin secretion and menstrual function after long-term bromocriptine treatment, Fertil Steril 48:550, 1987.

Rodman EF, Molitch ME, Post KD, et al: Long-term follow-up of transsphenoidal selective adenomectomy for prolactinoma, JAMA 252:921, 1984.

Ruiz-Velasco V and Tolis G: Pregnancy in hyperprolactinemic women, Fertil Steril 41:793, 1984.

Schlechte J, Dolan K, Sherman B, et al: The natural history of untreated hyperprolactinemia: a prospective analysis, J Clin Endocrinol Metab 68:412, 1989.

Serri O, Rasio E, Beauregard H, et al: Recurrence of hyperprolactinemia after selective transsphenoidal adenomectomy in women with prolactinoma, N Engl J Med 309:280, 1983.

Shangold GA, Kletzky OA, Marrs RP, et al: Hyperprolactinemia: comparison of thyrotropic-releasing hormone and tomography, Obstet Gynecol 63:771, 1984.

Sisam DA, Sheehan JP, et al: the natural history of untreated microprolactinomas, Fertil Steril 48:67, 1987.

Stein AL, Levenick MN, et al: Computer tomography versus magnetic resonance imaging for the evaluation of suspected pituitary adenomas, Obstet Gynecol 73:996, 1989.

Turkalj I, Brain P, and Krupp P: Surveillance of bromocriptine in pregnancy, JAMA 247:1589, 1982.

Vermesh M, Fossum GT, et al: Vaginal bromocriptine: pharmacology and effect on serum prolactin in normal women, Obstet Gynecol 72:693, 1988.

KEY TERMS AND DEFINITIONS

Acanthosis Nigricans. Dark, raised hyperpigmentation of the skin, found particularly on the nape of the neck and axilla.

5α-Androstane-3α,17β-diol Glucuronide (3α-diol-G). A metabolite of 5α-reductase conversion of testosterone (T) to dihydrotestosterone (DHT) that can be measured in serum and is the most accurate indicator of peripheral androgen metabolism.

Congenital Adrenal Hyperplasia with Adult Onset. Mild degree of enzymatic deficiency of cortisol biosynthesis (usually 11β-hydroxylase or 21-hydroxylase) that produces signs of androgen excess after puberty without external sexual ambiguity being present at birth.

Cryptic Hyperandrogenism. Elevated levels of circulatory androgens without clinical manifestations of hirsutism or acne. It is usually accompanied by anovulation.

Dehydroepiandrosterone Sulfate (DHEA-S). An androgen secreted nearly exclusively by the adrenal gland. Serum levels are used as a marker of adrenal androgen activity.

Free Androgen Index. Measurement of biologically active testosterone, calculated as follows: total testosterone times 1000 divided by sex hormone–binding globulin (SHBG).

Hilus Cell Tumor. Small testosterone-secreting ovarian tumors that most frequently develop after menopause.

Hirsutism. Presence of hair in locations where it is not normally found in a woman, specifically in the midline of the body.

Hypertrichosis. A generalized increase in the amount of body hair in its normal location.

Idiopathic Hirsutism (Constitutional or Familial Hirsutism). The most common disorder associated with androgen excess. It is due to increased peripheral androgen metabolism and is associated with normal circulating levels of testosterone and DHEA-S but increased levels of 3α-diol-G.

17-Ketosteroids. Urinary metabolites of DHEA, DHEA-S, androstenedione, and testosterone. They consist of DHEA, androsterone, and etiocholanolone.

Late-Onset Congenital Adrenal Hyperplasia/Late-Onset 21-Hydroxylase Deficiency (LOHD). Also called *late-onset hyperplasia, nonclassic congenital adrenal hyperplasia attenuated,* or *acquired adrenal hyperplasia.* Mild degree of enzymatic 21-hydroxylase deficiency of cortisol biosynthesis that produces signs of androgen excess after puberty without external sexual ambiguity being present at birth. This genetically acquired entity can be present in both severe (homozygous) and mild (heterozygous) forms.

Non-SHBG Bound Testosterone. Biologically active testosterone, consisting of free testosterone and albumin-bound testosterone.

Pilosebaceous Unit. Structure in skin from which sebaceous glands and hair are derived. Found in the skin in every area of the body except the palms and soles.

Polycystic Ovarian Syndrome (PCOS). An endocrinologic disorder characterized by excessive androgen production, inappropriate gonadotrophin secretion, and chronic anovulation. It begins perimenarcheally, and its clinical manifestations include hirsutism, menstrual irregularity (oligomenorrhea or amenorrhea), and obesity.

5α-Reductase. The enzyme that converts testosterone to its more active metabolite, dihydrotestosterone (DHT).

Sertoli-Leydig Cell Tumors. Testosterone-secreting ovarian tumors that usually are unilateral and palpably enlarged. They occur most frequently in the second to fourth decades of life.

Spironolactone. An aldosterone antagonist that acts as an antiandrogen by binding to the peripheral androgen acceptor without inducing androgenic activity. It also inhibits steroidogenesis by interfering with ovarian enzymatic activity as well as inhibiting 5α-reductase activity in the pilosebaceous unit.

Stromal Hyperthecosis. An ovarian disorder characterized by nests of luteinized theca cells within the stroma of bilaterally enlarged ovaries. Clinically this condition is associated with slowly but progressively increasing signs of virilization.

Virilization. Presence of signs of masculinization in a woman. These signs include temporal balding, voice deepening, clitoral enlargement, and increased muscle mass.

The clinical signs associated with excessive androgen production in women are hirsutism and virilization, with hirsutism being much more common.

The pilosebaceous unit is composed of a sebaceous component and a pilary component from which the hair shaft arises. There are two types of hair; vellous hair (vellus) is soft, fine, and unpigmentated, whereas terminal hair undergoes cyclic changes. *Anagen* is the growth phase of hair. It is followed by the transitional *catagen* phase and finally by a resting, or *telogen* phase, after which the hair sheds. Androgen is necessary to produce development of terminal hair, and the time spent in anagen is governed by circulating androgen levels.

The level of activity of the enzyme 5α-reductase in the hair follicle influences the degree of androgenic activity on hair growth. With elevated levels of androgen or increased activity of 5α-reductase, terminal hair appears where normally vellous hair is present. In this situation the length of anagen is prolonged and the hair becomes thicker.

The presence of hirsutism without other signs of virilization is associated with relatively mild disorders of androgen production, and circulating testosterone levels are either normal or mildly to moderately elevated (less than 1.5 ng/ml). Hirsutism usually has a gradual onset and if unaccompanied by signs of virilization is not caused by a severe enzymatic defect or a neoplasm. The amount and location of the central hair growth found in women with hirsutism vary. Generally in the milder forms hair is found only on the upper lip and chin, whereas with increasing severity it appears on the cheeks, chest (intermammary), abdomen (superior to the umbilicus), inner aspects of thighs, and lower back and intergluteal areas. The severity of the hirsutism can be roughly quantified by means of the scoring system of Ferriman and Gallwey (Figure 38-1 and Table 38-1). Increased hair growth only on the extremities (hypertrichosis) should not be considered hirsutism, as hair is normally found in this location in women. Women with hirsutism can have normal ovulatory menstrual cycles, oligomenorrhea, or amenorrhea.

Virilization is a relatively uncommon clinical finding, and its presence is usually associated with markedly elevated levels of circulating testosterone (2 ng/ml or greater). In contrast to the gradual development of hirsutism, signs of virilization usually occur over a relatively short period of time. These signs are due to both the masculinizing and the defeminizing (antiestrogenic) action of testosterone and include temporal balding, clitoral hypertrophy, decreased breast size, dryness of the vagina, and increased muscle mass. Women with virilization are nearly always amenorrheic. The presence of androgen-secreting neoplasms should always be suspected in any woman who develops

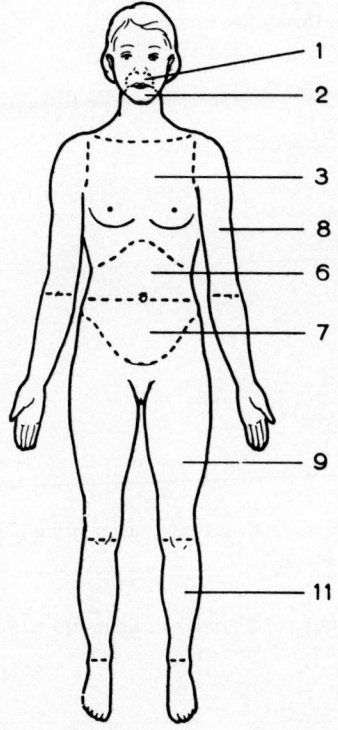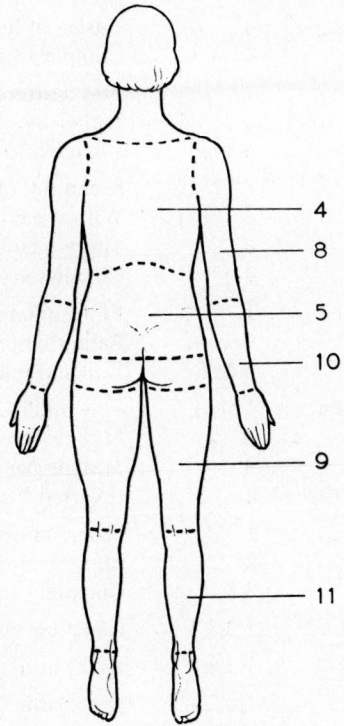

FIGURE 38-1
Demarcation of 11 sites used for numerically grading amount of hair growth—anterior and posterior views. (From Ferriman D and Gallwey JD: J Clin Endocrinol Metab 21:1440, 1961. © by The Endocrine Society, 1961.)

TABLE 38-1

Definition of Hair Gradings at 11 Sites*

Site	Grade	Definition
Upper lip	1	Few hairs at outer margin
	2	Small moustache at outer margin
	3	Moustache extending halfway from outer margin
	4	Moustache extending to midline
Chin	1	Few scattered hairs
	2	Scattered hairs with small concentrations
	3 & 4	Complete cover, light and heavy
Chest	1	Circumareolar hairs
	2	With midline hair in addition
	3	Fusion of these areas, with three-quarters cover
	4	Complete cover
Upper back	1	Few scattered hairs
	2	Rather more, still scattered
	3 & 4	Complete cover, light and heavy
Lower back	1	Sacral tuft of hair
	2	With some lateral extension
	3	Three-quarters cover
	4	Complete cover
Upper abdomen	1	Few midline hairs
	2	Rather more, still midline
	3 & 4	Half and full cover
Lower abdomen	1	Few midline hairs
	2	Midline streak of hair
	3	Midline band of hair
	4	Inverted V-shaped growth
Arm	1	Sparse growth affecting not more than one quarter of limb surface
	2	More than this; cover still incomplete
	3 & 4	Complete cover, light and heavy
Forearm	1,2,3,4	Complete cover of dorsal surface; 2 grades of light and 2 of heavy growth
Thigh	1,2,3,4	As for arm
Leg	1,2,3,4	As for arm

From Ferriman D and Gallwey JD: J Clin Endocrinol Metab 21:1440, 1961. © by The Endocrine Society, 1961.
*Grade 0 at all sites indicates absence of terminal hair.

signs of virilization, particularly if the onset is rapid.

PHYSIOLOGY

The sources of androgen production in the human female are the ovaries and the adrenal glands. The major androgen produced by the ovaries is testosterone and that of the adrenal glands is dehydroepiandrosterone sulfate (DHEA-S). Measurement of the amount of these two steroids in the circulation provides clinically relevant information regarding the presence and source of increased androgen production. In addition to glandular production of androgens, conversion of estrone to androstenedione and DHEA-S to testosterone occurs in peripheral tissue.

The ovaries secrete only about 0.1 mg of testosterone each day, mainly from the theca-stroma cells. Other androgens secreted by the ovary are androstenedione (1 to 2 mg/day) and DHEA (<1 mg/day). The adrenal glands, in addition to secreting large quantities of DHEA-S (6 to 24 mg/day), secrete about the same daily amount of androstenedione (1 mg/day) as the

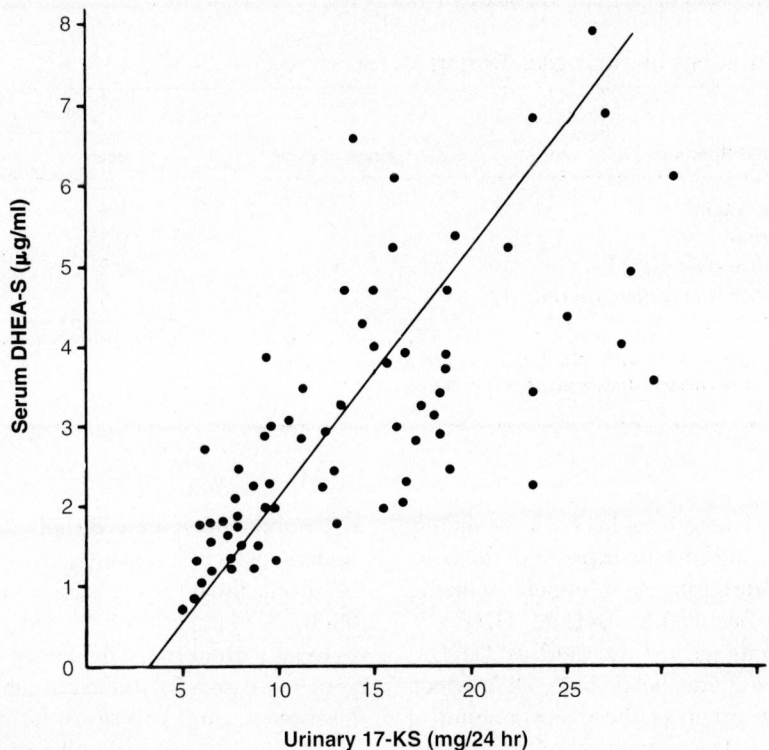

FIGURE 38-2

Correlation between serum dehydroepiandrosterone sulfate *(DHEA-S)* and urinary 17-ketosteroids *(17-KS)* in 71 patients (*r* = 0.7, *P* <0.0005). (From Lobo RA, Paul WL, and Goebelsmann U: Obstet Gynecol 57:69, 1981. Reprinted with permission from The American College of Obstetricians and Gynecologists.)

ovaries and less than 1 mg of DHEA per day. The normal adrenal gland secretes little testosterone, although some uncommon adrenal tumors may secrete testosterone directly.

Androstenedione and DHEA do not have androgenic activity but are peripherally converted at a slow rate to a biologically active androgen, testosterone. Only about 5% of androstenedione and a smaller percentage of DHEA are converted to testosterone. The total daily production of testosterone in women is normally about 0.35 mg. Of this, 0.1 mg comes from direct ovarian secretion, 0.2 mg from peripheral conversion of androstenedione, and 0.05 mg from peripheral conversion of DHEA (Table 38-2). Since the ovary and adrenal gland secrete about equal amounts of androstenedione and DHEA, about two thirds (0.22 mg) of the daily testosterone produced in a woman originates from the ovaries. Thus increased circulating levels of testosterone usually indicate abnormal ovarian androgen production. Nor-

TABLE 38-2
Origin of Testosterone in Women

Origin	Amount
Ovarian secretion	0-1 mg/day
Peripheral conversion	
Androstenedione → testosterone	0.2 mg/day
Dehydroepiandrosterone → testosterone	0.05 mg/day
Total testosterone production	0.35 mg/day

From Lobo RA: Reproductive neuroendocrinology. In Mishell DR Jr, Davajan V, and Lobo RA, editors: Infertility, contraception and reproductive endocrinology, ed 3, Cambridge, Mass, 1991, Blackwell Scientific Publications.

mal circulating levels of these androgens in women of reproductive age are shown in Table 38-3. Only a small amount of testosterone is metabolized to testosterone glucuronide and then excreted in the urine. Testosterone,

TABLE 38-3

Plasma Concentrations of Androgens During Menstrual Cycle

Steroid Hormone	Phase of Cycle	Plasma Concentration	
		Mean	Range
Androstenedione (ng/ml)	*	1.4	0.7-3.1
Testosterone (ng/ml)	*	0.35	0.15-0.55
Dehydroepiandrosterone (ng/ml)	*	4.2	2.7-7.8
Dehydroepiandrosterone sulfate (μg/ml)	*	1.6	0.8-3.4

From Goebelsmann U: Steroid hormones. In Mishell DR Jr and Davajan V, editors: Infertility, contraception and reproductive endocrinology, ed 2, Oradell, NJ, 1986, Medical Economics Books.
*Unspecified; no major changes during menstrual cycle.

which is not a 17-ketosteroid (17-KS), is mainly metabolized to androstenedione and then excreted as androsterone and etiocholanolone, both of which are 17-KS. DHEA, DHEA-S, and androstenedione are excreted as DHEA, androsterone, and etiocholanolone, all of which are 17-KS. The origin of the major amount of urinary 17-KS is the precursor androgen produced in the greatest amounts, DHEA-S. Because DHEA-S has a long half-life in serum, serum levels of DHEA-S correlate well with 17-KS excretion (Figure 38-2). It is much better to measure serum DHEA-S than urinary 17-KS to assess adrenal androgen production. Because some glucocorticoid metabolites are also measured as 17-KS, the amount of creatinine in the urine needs to be determined, and it is difficult to collect a 24-hour urine specimen.

Most testosterone in the circulation (about 85%) is tightly bound to sex hormone–binding globulin (SHBG) and is believed to be biologically inactive. An additional 10% to 15% is loosely bound to albumin, with only about 1% to 2% not bound to any protein (free testosterone). Both the free and albumin-bound fractions are biologically active. Serum testosterone can be measured as the total amount, the amount that is believed to be biologically active (non-SHBG bound), and as the free form.

To exert a biologic effect, testosterone is metabolized peripherally in target tissues to the more potent androgen 5α-dihydrotestosterone (DHT) by the enzyme 5α-reductase. After further 3-keto reduction, DHT is converted to its distal metabolite, 5α-androstane-3α,17β-diol(3α-diol). 3α-Diol is conjugated to

a 5α-androstane-3α,17β-diol glucuronide (3α-diol-G), which is a stable, irreversible product of intracellular 5α-reductase activity (Figure 38-3).

Even with normal circulatory levels of androgen, increased 5α-reductase activity in the pilosebaceous unit will result in increased androgenic activity, producing hirsutism (Figure 38-4). Serafini et al. measured 5α-reductase activity in skin biopsies and found the level of activity correlated very well with the degree of hirsutism present.

Since it is impractical to measure 5α-reductase activity directly, measurement of its metabolite, 3α-diol-G, in serum can be performed. Lobo et al. have shown measurement of this metabolite to be the most accurate indicator of the degree of peripheral androgen metabolism in women. Horton et al. have shown that although serum levels of total testosterone are similar in normal and hirsute women, there are significant differences in the amounts of non-SHBG bound testosterone as well as 3α-diol-G (Figure 38-5). Non-SHBG bound testosterone is elevated in about 60% to 70% of hirsute women, but 3α-diol-G is elevated in more than 80% of such individuals. Thus increased levels of non-SHBG bound testosterone indicate increased ovarian production. If levels of non-SHBG bound testosterone are normal and levels of 3α-diol-G are elevated, testosterone production is not increased, but peripheral conversion of testosterone to its active metabolite is increased above normal. Either of these processes can cause symptoms and signs of androgen excess. Thus there are three markers of androgen production in serum, one for each

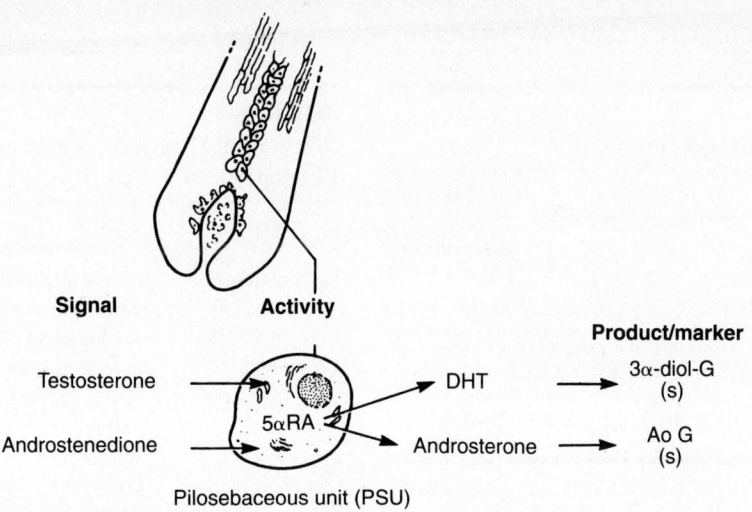

Signal   **Activity**   **Product/marker**

Testosterone → 5αRA → DHT → 3α-diol-G (s)

Androstenedione → 5αRA → Androsterone → Ao G (s)

Pilosebaceous unit (PSU)

FIGURE 38-3

Peripheral androgen metabolism and markers of this activity. *5α RA,* 5α-Reductase; *DHT,* dihydrotestosterone. (From Lobo RA: Reproductive neuroendocrinology. In Mishell DR Jr, Davajan V, and Lobo RA editors: Infertility, contraception, and reproductive endocrinology, ed 3, Cambridge, Mass, 1991, Blackwell Scientific Publications.)

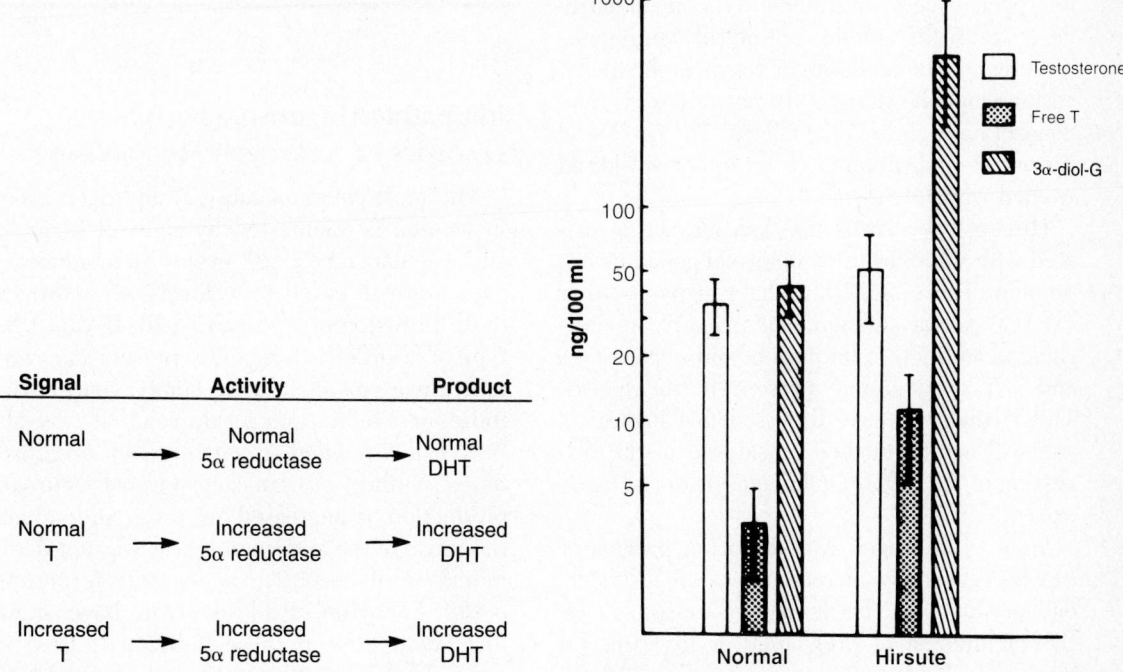

Signal	**Activity**	**Product**
Normal	Normal 5α reductase	Normal DHT
Normal T	Increased 5α reductase	Increased DHT
Increased T	Increased 5α reductase	Increased DHT

FIGURE 38-4

Influence of androgen substrate (signal, e.g., testosterone or androstenedione) and 5α-reductase activity (in pilosebaceous units) on local production of biologically active androgens. *T,* Testosterone; *DHT,* dihydrotestosterone. (From Lobo RA: Reproductive neuroendocrinology. In Mishell DR Jr, Davajan V, and Lobo RA editors: Infertility, contraception, and reproductive endocrinology, ed 3, Cambridge, Mass, 1991, Blackwell Scientific Publications.)

FIGURE 38-5

Plasma total testosterone, unbound testosterone *(free T)* and 5α-androstane-3α, 17β-diol glucuronide *(3α-diol-G)* in normal and hirsute women. Note insignificant elevation with overlap for testosterone and free T testosterone and highly significant increase in *3α-diol-G* without overlap between two groups of women. (Reproduced from Horton R, Hawks D, and Lobo RA: J Clin Invest 69:1203, 1982. By Copyright permission of The American Society for Clinical Investigation.)

TABLE 38-4
Markers of Androgen Production

Source	Marker
Ovary	Testosterone
Adrenal gland	DHEA-S
Periphery	3α-diol-G

From Lobo RA: Reproductive neuroendocrinology. In Mishell DR Jr, Davajan V, and Lobo RA editors: Infertility, contraception and reproductive endocrinology, ed 3, Cambridge, Mass, 1991, Blackwell Scientific Publications.

TABLE 38-5
Differential Diagnosis of Hirsutism and Virilization*

Source	Diagnosis
Nonspecific	Exogenous/iatrogenic
	Abnormal gonadal or sexual development
Pregnancy	Androgen excess in pregnancy: luteoma or hyperreactio luteinalis
Periphery	"Idiopathic" hirsutism
Ovary	"Polycystic ovary syndrome"
	Stromal hyperthecosis
	Ovarian tumors
Adrenal gland	Adrenal tumors
	Cushing's syndrome
	Adult-onset congenital adrenal hyperplasia

*Idiopathic hirsutism and polycystic ovary sydrome do not present with virilizations.

compartment where androgens are produced (Table 38-4).

ETIOLOGY

There are 10 currently recognized causes of androgen excess in women. One main iatrogenic cause is administration of androgenic medication. In addition to testosterone itself, various anabolic steroids, 19-norprogestins, and danazol have androgenic effects. Thus a careful history of medication intake is important for all women with hirsutism.

Hirsutism or virilization can also be associated with some forms of abnormal gonad development. These individuals have signs of either external sexual ambiguity or primary amenorrhea, in addition to findings of androgen excess and a Y chromosome present in the gonad. These conditions are discussed in Chapter 36 and will not be further considered in the discussion of the differential diagnosis of androgen excess.

Signs of androgen excess during pregnancy can be caused by increased ovarian testosterone production. This is usually caused by either a luteoma of pregnancy or hyperreactio luteinalis. The former is a unilateral or bilateral solid ovarian enlargement, whereas the latter is bilateral cystic ovarian enlargement. After pregnancy the androgenic characteristics regress.

A diagnosis of these three causes of androgen excess can usually be easily made by means of a careful history and physical examination. The remaining causes of androgen excess, together with the origin of hyperandrogenism, are listed in Table 38-5. These causes will be discussed according to their approximate frequency.

Idiopathic Hirsutism (Peripheral Disorder of Androgen Metabolism)

The most common cause of androgen excess in women is manifested by signs of hirsutism and regular menstrual cycles in conjunction with normal circulatory levels of androgens (both testosterone and DHEA-S). Because this type of disorder is frequently present in several individuals in the same family, particularly those of Mediterranean descent, it has also been called *familial* or *constitutional hirsutism.* Since neither ovarian nor adrenal androgen production is increased in these individuals, the cause of the androgen excess was not determined until recently, hence the term *idiopathic hirsutism.* Paulson et al. have shown that about 80% of these individuals have increased levels of 3α-diol-G, indirectly indicating that the cause of hirsutism is increased 5α-reductase activity (Figure 38-6). These investigators have directly measured the percent conversion of testosterone to DHT in genital skin as an assessment of 5α-reductase activity in the skin of women with idiopathic hirsutism. The amount of 5α-reductase activity was increased in hirsute women as compared with normal women and correlated well with both the degree of hirsutism and serum levels of 3α-diol-G (Figure 38-7). Thus idiopathic hirsutism is in fact a disorder of peripheral androgen metabolism in the pilosebaceous apparatus of the skin and is possibly genetically determined. The condition should probably be renamed *abnormal peripheral androgen metabolism.* Antiandrogens that block peripheral testosterone action or interfere with 5α-reductase activity are effective therapeutic agents for this disorder. Such antiandrogens include spironolactone, cimetidine, and cyproterone acetate.

Polycystic Ovarian Syndrome

Polycystic ovarian syndrome (PCOS) was originally described in 1905 by Stein and Leventhal as a syndrome consisting of amenorrhea, hirsutism, and obesity in association with enlarged polycystic ovaries. It is now realized that this relatively common syndrome is an endocrinologic disorder that begins soon after menarche and consists of inappropriate gonadotrophin secretion associated with increased gonadotrophin-releasing hormone (GnRH) pulse amplitude and tonically elevated levels of luteinizing hormone (LH) (Figure 38-8). In some studies GnRH pulse amplitude is increased, whereas in others it is not. However,

after a bolus of GnRH, there is an exaggerated response of LH, but not follicle-stimulating hormone (FSH), in patients with PCOS (Figure 38-9). In addition, there are increased circulatory levels of androgens produced by both the ovaries and the adrenal glands (Figure 38-10). Thus, as stated by Lobo, PCOS is really a syndrome of hyperandrogenic chronic anovulation. If they are elevated, serum testosterone levels are usually between 70 and 120 ng/dl, and androstenedione levels are usually between 3 and 5 ng/ml. In addition, about half the women with this syndrome have elevated levels of DHEA-S. In 1963 Goldzieher and Axelrod compiled the incidence of the various symptoms associated with PCOS that had been reported in the literature (Table 38-6). From these and other data it has been estimated that about 30% of women with PCOS do not have hirsutism, even though DeVane et al., as well as others, have reported that nearly all of them have elevated levels of circulating androgens. Lobo et al. found that the presence or absence of hirsutism depends on whether those androgens are converted peripherally by 5α-reductase to the more potent androgen DHT and 3α-diol-G, as reflected by increased levels of 3α-diol-G (Figure 38-11).

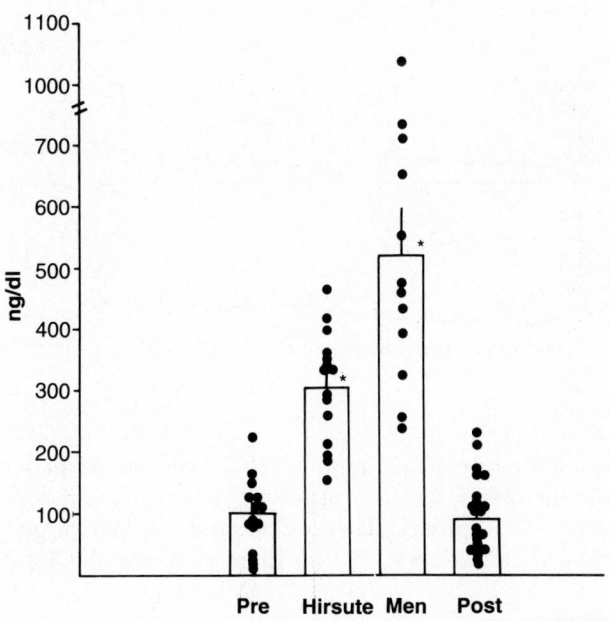

FIGURE 38-6
Serum 3α-diol-G in premenopausal nonhirsute women *(PRE)*, hirsute women, normal men, and postmenopausal nonhirsute women *(POST)*. The asterisks denote *P*<0.05, as compared with PRE. (From Paulson RJ, Serafini PC, Catalino JA, and Lobo RA: Fertil Steril 42:422, 1986.)

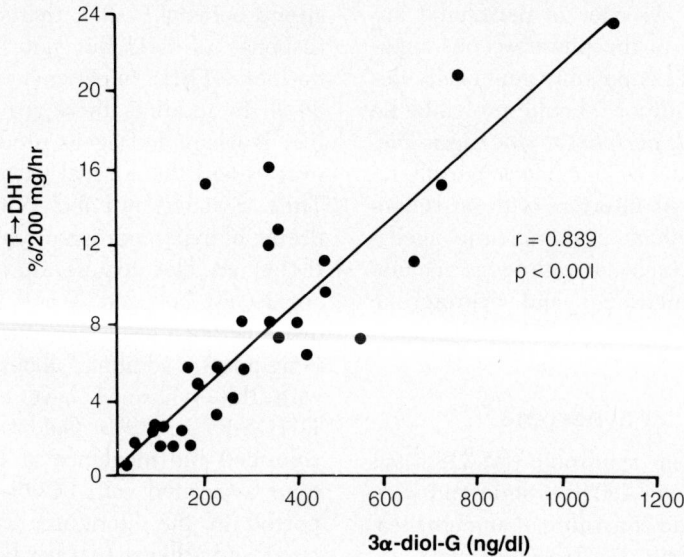

FIGURE 38-7

5α-Reductase expressed as percent conversion of testosterone *(T)* to DHT per 200 mg genital skin per hour, correlated with 5α-androstane-3α,17β-diol glucuronide *(3α-diol-G)*. Correlation is highly significant: (r = 0.839, P <0.001). (From Paulson RJ, Serafini PC, Catalino JA, and Lobo RA: Fertil Steril 46:222, 1986. Reproduced with permission of the publisher, The American Fertility Society.)

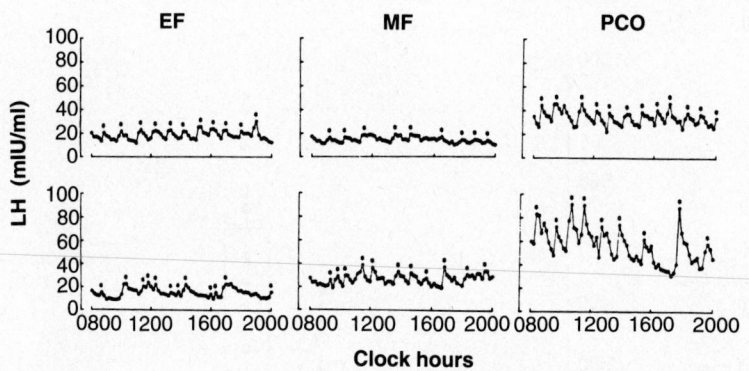

FIGURE 38-8

Patterns of pulsatile luteinizing hormone *(LH)* secretion in patients with polycystic ovarian syndrome *(PCO)* and in control subjects with normal early follicular *(EF)* and midfollicular *(MF)* phases. The asterisks indicate significant pulses. (From Kazer AR, Kessel B, and Yen SSC: J Clin Endocrinol Metab 65:233, 1987.)

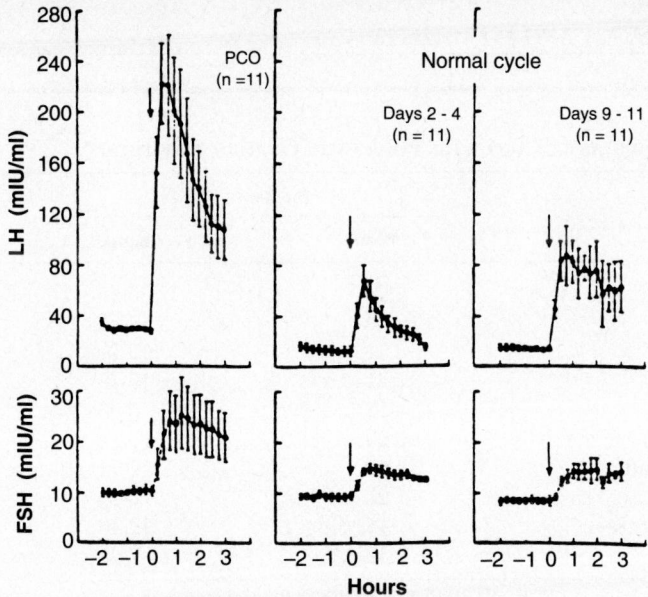

FIGURE 38-9

Comparison of quantitative luteinizing hormone *(LH)* and follicle-stimulating hormone *(FSH)* release in response to a single bolus of 150 μg of GnRH in patients with polycystic ovarian syndrome *(PCO)* and in normal women during low-estrogen (early follicular) and high-estrogen (late follicular) phases of their cycles. (From Rebar R, Judd HL, Yen SSC, et al: J Clin Invest 57:1320, 1976.)

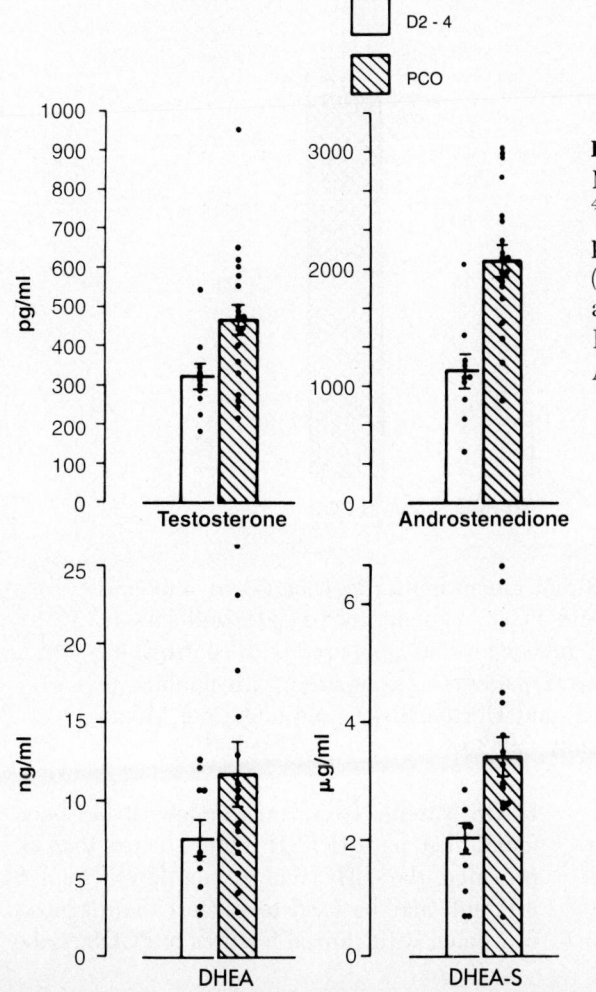

FIGURE 38-10

Mean (±SD) concentrations of testosterone, Δ⁴-androstenedione, DHEA, and DHEA-S in 19 patients with polycystic ovarian syndrome *(PCO)* and 10 normal subjects between days 2 and 4 *(D2-4)* of their menstrual cycles. (From DeVane GW, Czekala NM, Judd HL, et al: Am J Obstet Gynecol 121:496, 1975.)

TABLE 38-6
Incidence of Symptoms Associated with Polycystic Ovarian Syndrome*

| | Incidence (%) | | No. of Usable |
Symptom	Mean	Range	Cases†
Infertility	74	35-95	596
Hirsutism	69	17-83	819
Amenorrhea	51	15-77	640
Obesity	41	16-49	600
Functional bleeding	29	6-65	547
Dysmenorrhea	23	—	75
Corpus luteum at operation	22	0-71	391
Virilization	21	0-28	431
Biphasic body temperature	15	12-40	288
Cyclic menses	12	7-28	395

From Goldzieher JW and Axelrod LR: Fertil Steril 14:631, 1963. Reproduced with permission from The American College of Obstetricians and Gynecologists.
*Tabulated from 187 references with a total of 1079 cases.
†Indicates how many of the 1079 total cases could be evaluated for the presence or absence of a particular symptom.

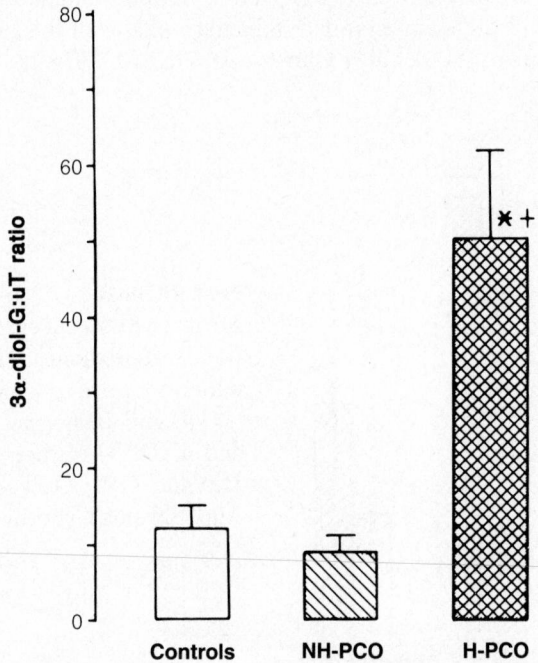

FIGURE 38-11
Ratios of serum 5α-androstane-3α,17β-diol glucuronide *(3α-Diol G)* to unbound testosterone *(uT)* in controls, nonhirsute PCOS patients *(NH-PCO)*, and hirsute PCOS patients *(H-PCO)*. *,Significantly higher level as compared with controls; +, significantly higher level in hirsute PCOS patients as compared with nonhirsute ones. (From Lobo RA, Goebelsmann U, and Horton R: J Clin Endocrinol Metab 57:393, 1983. © by The Endocrine Society, 1983.)

Thus nonhirsutic women with PCOS have elevated circulatory levels of testosterone or DHEA-S or of both but not of 3α-diol-G. The tonically elevated levels of LH are usually above 20 mIU/ml. Because FSH levels in PCOS patients are normal or low, it has been found that an LH-FSH ratio greater than 3, provided the LH level is not lower than 8 mIU/ml, may be used to suggest the diagnosis in women with clinical features of PCOS. Lobo et al. reported that about 70% of women with PCOS had either an elevated level of immunologic LH or an immunologic LH-FSH ratio greater than 3 but that all but one woman with PCOS had elevated serum levels of biologically active LH (Figure 38-12).

Hoffman et al. reported that about one-half the women with PCOS have elevated levels of DHEA-S, with one third of them having levels greater than 4 ng/ml. Although Chang et al. have shown that adrenocorticotropic hormone (ACTH) levels in these women are normal, they found that infusions of ACTH produce an exaggerated response of DHEA-S, indicating that the zona reticularis of the adrenal gland in some patients with PCOS has increased sensitivity to ACTH and that the adrenal gland may be involved in the pathogenesis of this syndrome.

In addition to increased levels of circulatory androgens, Lobo et al. found that women with PCOS had increased levels of biologically active (non-SHBG bound) estradiol, although total circulating levels of estradiol were not increased (Figure 38-13). The increased amount of non-SHBG bound estradiol is caused by a decrease in SHBG levels, which is produced primarily by the increased levels of androgens and secondarily by the obesity present in many of these women. The tonically increased levels of biologically active estradiol may stimulate increased GnRH pulsatility and produce tonically elevated LH levels and anovulation. In addition, the lowered SHBG level increases the biologically active fractions of the elevated androgens in the circulation. The importance of the decreased levels of SHBG is shown schematically in Figure 38-14.

About 20% of women with PCOS also have mildly elevated levels of prolactin (20 to 30 ng/ml), possibly related to increased pulsatility of GnRH or to a relative dopamine deficiency or to both. In addition, many women with this syndrome have mild degrees of hyperinsulinism and insulin resistance.

Dunaif et al. studied a group of hyperandrogenic women with and without PCOS and obesity with glucose tolerance tests and insulin levels. They found that hyperinsulinemia occurred only in the women with PCOS, whether or not they were obese, but only the obese women with PCOS had impaired glucose tolerance. Thus the negative impact of obesity and PCOS on insulin resistance is additive. Acanthosis nigricans (AN) was found in about 30% of

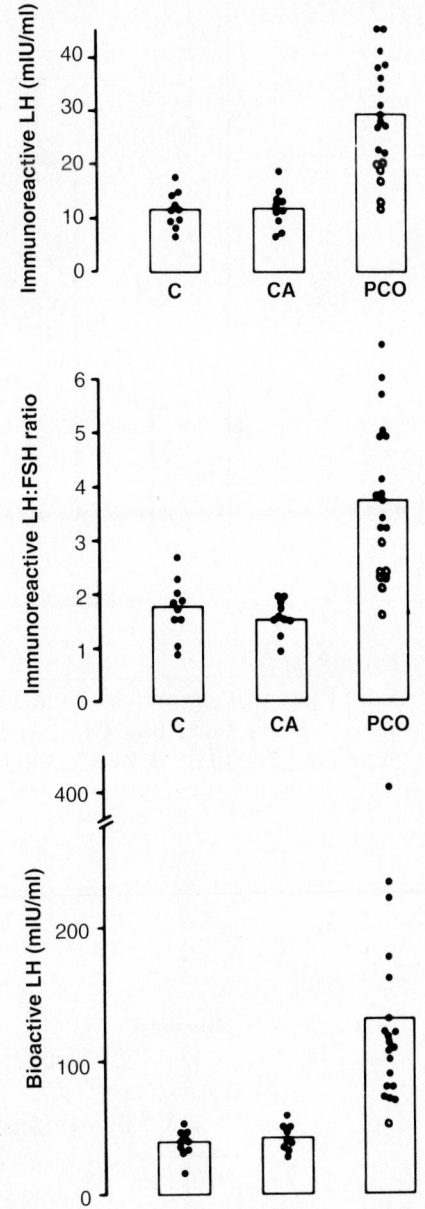

FIGURE 38-12
Serum measurements of immunoreactive LH, immunoreactive LH:FSH ratios, and bioactive LH in control subjects *(C)*, women with chronic anovulation *(CA)*, and women with PCOS *(PCO)*. Boxes represent the mean ±3 standard deviation (SD) of control levels. (From Lobo RA, Kletzky OA, Campeau JD, et al: Fertil Steril 39:674, 1983. Reproduced with permission of the publisher, The American Fertility Society.)

the hyperandrogenic women, particularly if they were obese and had PCOS. About half of the latter group had AN. Although it has been suggested that the presence of *hyperandro-*

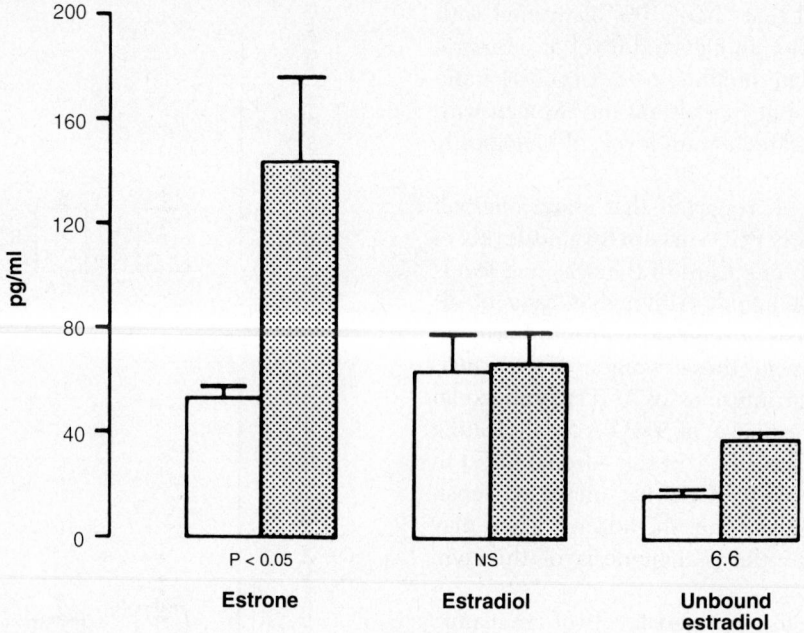

FIGURE 38-13
Serum estrogen concentrations in 13 normal women and 22 PCOS patients (*shaded areas*). (From Lobo RA, Granger L, Goebelsemann U, et al: J Clin Endocrinol Metab 52:156, 1981. © by The Endocrine Society, 1981.)

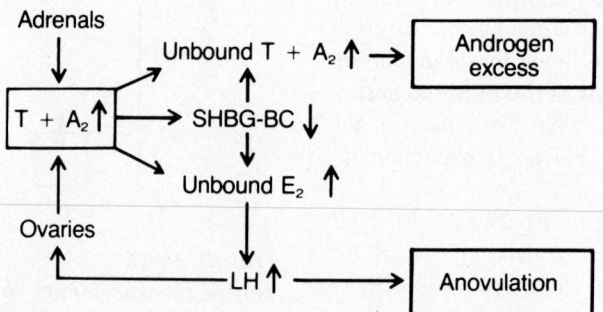

FIGURE 38-14
Scheme depicting the possible role of adrenal-derived androgen (T, testosterone; A_2, androstanediol) in initiating androgen excess and anovulation. (From Lobo RA and Goebelsmann U: Am J Obstet Gynecol 142:394, 1982.)

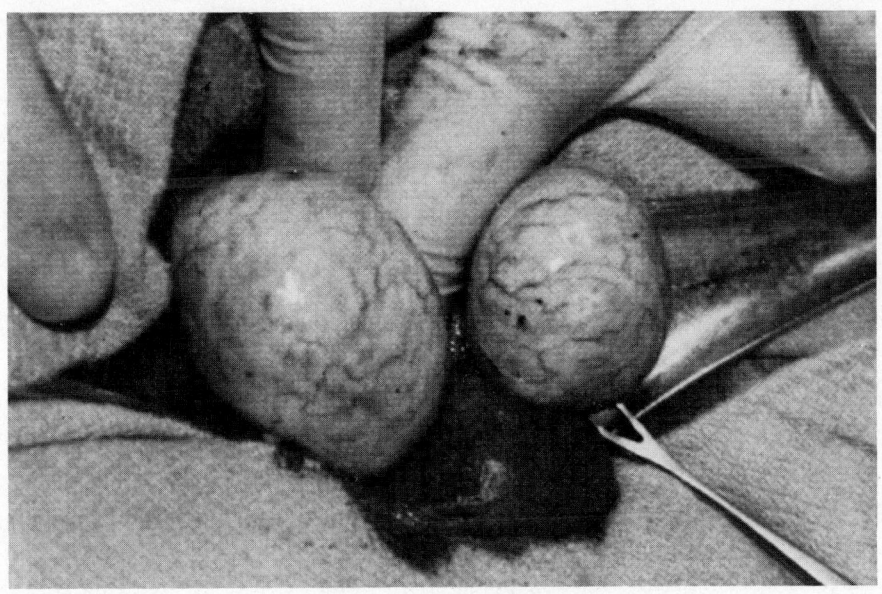

FIGURE 38-15
Gross characteristics of polycystic ovaries. Bilateral enlarged ovaries with smooth and thickened capsule. (From Yen SSC: Chronic anovulation caused by peripheral endocrine disorders. In Yen SSC and Jaffe RB, editors: Reproductive endocrinology, ed 2, Philadelphia, 1986, WB Saunders Co.)

genism insulin resistance, and AN constituted a special syndrome, the HAIR-AN syndrome, most investigators believe women with PCOS who have AN are a subgroup of those with PCOS and do not have a distinct endocrine disorder. No causal relation among PCOS, obesity, insulin resistance, and hyperandrogenism has been elucidated to date. Although some investigators have suggested that hyperandrogenism causes insulin resistance, Lobo et al. have presented data indicating that the reverse is true: hyperinsulinemia produces hyperandrogenism in women with PCOS.

The ovaries of most women with PCOS are enlarged, being as much as 5 cm in diameter. The capsules are smooth, white, and thickened (Figure 38-15). Beneath the capsules are numerous small cysts (Figure 38-16). These anatomic findings are not pathognomonic for PCOS, because they also have been noted in some women with Cushing's syndrome or congenital adrenal hyperplasia and in association with certain adrenal tumors. Although the ovaries of women with PCOS produce excessive amounts of androgen, particularly androstenedione, there is no inherent endocrinologic abnormality in the ovaries. The tonically elevated levels of LH cause the stromal tissue to produce more androstenedione and

other androgens, which in turn produces premature follicular atresia. Furthermore, the ovaries are deficient in aromatase, probably because of the low FSH levels, and this deficiency results in less conversion of androstenedione to estrogen in the ovary. The polycystic ovary does not secrete increased amounts of estrogen or estradiol, but the increased levels of androstenedione are peripherally converted to estrone, causing increased circulating estrone levels.

The etiology of this endocrinologic abnormality has not been determined. It has been suggested that heredity, central catecholamine abnormalities, psychological stress, insulin resistance, and obesity may be involved (see box on p. 1172). The evidence for a genetic cause is suggestive but not clearly established. Data suggesting an abnormality in central nervous system catecholamine metabolism are more convincing but not yet conclusive. Although women with PCOS have more psychological stress than do control subjects, the stress may be a result, not the cause, of the syndrome. Obesity probably enhances the syndrome because of the decrease in SHBG but is probably not important in its pathogenesis, because the syndrome occurs in some thin women and because many obese women do not have PCOS.

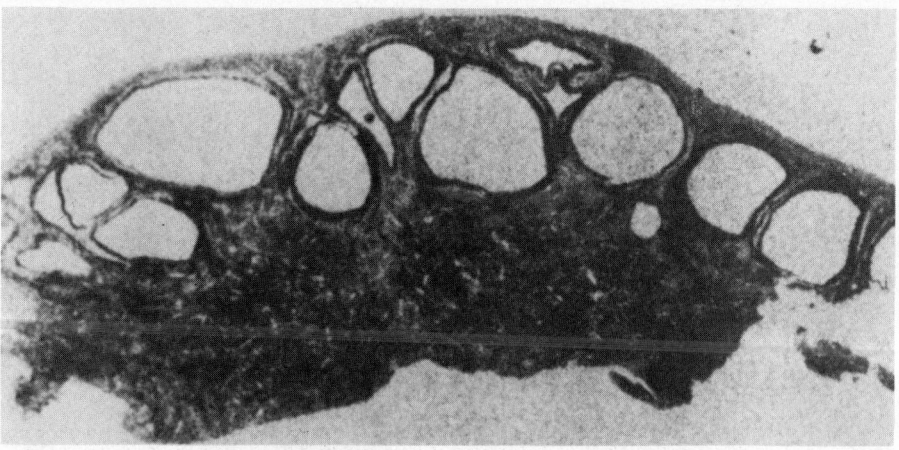

FIGURE 38-16
Sagittal section of typical Stein-Leventhal type of polycystic ovary illustrating large number of follicular cysts. (From Wilroy RS Jr, Givens JR, Wiser WL, et al: Hyperthecosis: an inheritable form of polycystic ovarian disease. In Bergsma D, editor: Genetic forms of hypogonadism, Miami: Symposia Specialists for the National Foundation-March of Dimes, BD:OAS XI(4):81, 1975, with permission.)

HYPOTHESES ON THE PATHOGENESIS OF PCOS

Genetic
Psychological stress and hypothalamic distur-
  bances
    Catecholamine
    Opioid
    Others
Ovarian defect
Insulin resistance
Obesity and decreased SHBG
Combinations of the above

From Lobo RA: Syndrome of hyperandrogenic chronic anovulation. In Mishell DR Jr, Davajan V, and Lobo RA, editors: Infertility, contraception and reproductive endocrinology, ed 3, Cambridge, Mass, 1991, Blackwell Scientific Publications.

Whatever the etiology, the endocrinologic effects of PCOS produce a vicious cycle of events, as shown by Yen et al. (Figure 38-17). The increased pulsatility of GnRH produces tonically elevated LH levels and increased ovarian androgen production. Peripheral conversion of androstenedione to estrone in conjunction with the decreased SHBG levels causes tonic hyperestrogenism, which increases the pituitary sensitivity to GnRH and leads to increased LH release.

Stromal Hyperthecosis

Stromal hyperthecosis is an uncommon benign ovarian disorder in which the ovaries are bilaterally enlarged, being about 5 to 7 cm in diameter, and histologically have nests of luteinized theca cells within the stroma (Figure 38-18). The capsules of these ovaries are thick and similar to those found in women with PCOS, but unlike PCOS, subcapsular cysts are uncommon. The theca cells produce large amounts of testosterone as determined by retrograde ovarian vein catheterization. Like PCOS, this disorder has a gradual onset and is initially associated with anovulation or amenorrhea and hirsutism. However, unlike PCOS, with increasing age the ovaries secrete steadily increasing amounts of testosterone. Thus when women with this disorder reach the fourth decade of life, the severity of the hirsutism increases and signs of virilization, such as temporal balding, clitoral enlargement, deepening of the voice, and decreased breast size, appear and gradually increase in severity. By this time serum testosterone levels are usually in excess of 2 ng/ml, similar to levels found in ovarian and adrenal testosterone-producing tumors. However, with the latter conditions the symptoms of virilization appear and progress much more rapidly than with ovarian hyperthecosis, in which symptoms progress gradually over many years.

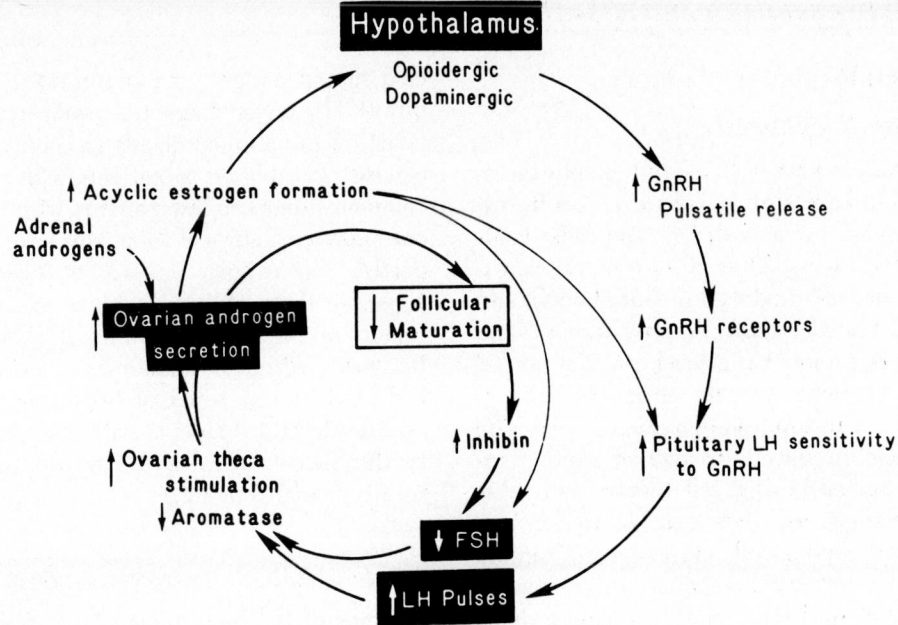

FIGURE 38-17
The interdependent event of high LH-FSH ratio occasioned by an increased GnRH secretion as a consequence of reduced hypothalamic inhibition. This setting induces an increased ovarian androgen production by the theca cells and acyclic estrogen feedback system in maintenance of chronic anovulation in PCOS. (Modified from Yen SSC, Chaney C, and Judd HL: Functional aberrations of the hypothalamic-pituitary system in polycystic ovary syndrome: a consideration of the pathogenesis. In James VHT, Serio M, and Guisti G, editors: The endocrine function of the human ovary, New York, 1976, Academic Press.)

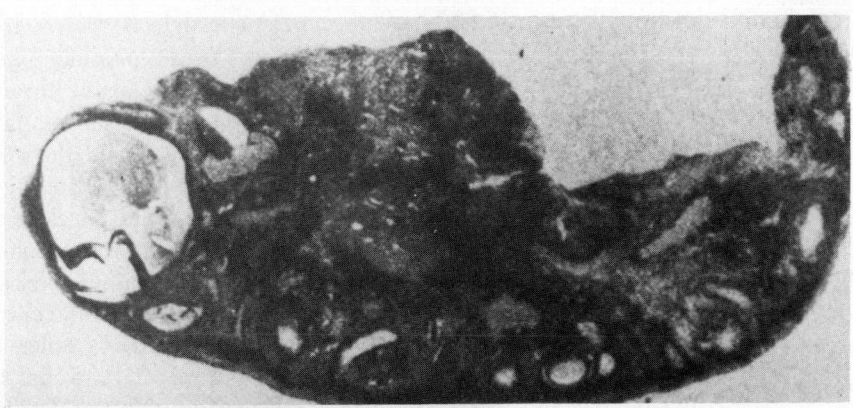

A

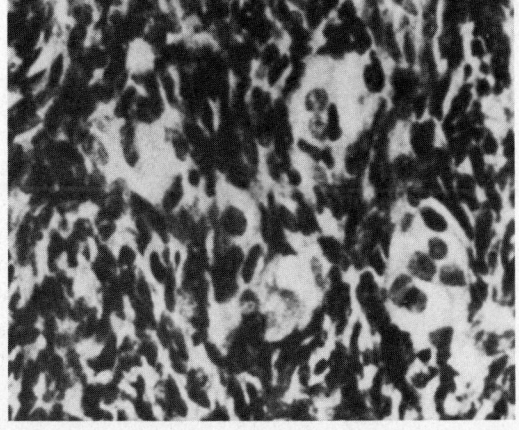

B

FIGURE 38-18
A, Sagittal section of typical hyperthecotic ovary illustrating small number of follicular cysts and massive amount of stromal hyperplasia. **B,** Islands of luteinized thecalike cells deep in stroma of ovary in hyperthecosis. (From Wilroy RS Jr, Givens JR, Wiser WL, et al: Hyperthecosis: an inheritable form of polycystic ovarian disease. In Bergsma D, editor: Genetic forms of hypogonadism, Miami: Symposia Specialists for the National Foundation-March of Dimes, BD:OAS XI(4):81, 1975, with permission.)

Androgen-Producing Tumors

Ovarian Neoplasms

It is possible for nearly every type of ovarian neoplasm to have stromal cells that secrete excessive amounts of testosterone and cause signs of androgen excess. Thus on rare occasions excess testosterone produced by both benign and malignant cystadenomas, Brenner tumors, and Krukenberg tumors has caused hirsutism or virilization or both. Certain germ cell tumors contain many testosterone-producing cells. The testosterone produced by two of these neoplasms—Sertoli-Leydig cell tumors and hilus cell tumors—nearly always causes virilization. In addition, lipoid cell (adrenal rest) tumors can produce increased amounts of testosterone or DHEA-S or both. Rarely granulosa-theca cell tumors can also produce testosterone in addition to increased levels of estradiol.

Androgen-producing ovarian tumors usually produce rapidly progressive signs of virilization. Sertoli-Leydig cell tumors usually develop during the reproductive age (second to fourth decades), and by the time they produce detectable signs of androgen excess, the tumor is nearly always (more than 85% of the time) palpable during bimanual examination. These tumors are uncommon. Less than 1% of solid ovarian neoplasms are Sertoli-Leydig cell tumors. Hilus cell tumors most often occur after menopause. They are usually small and not palpable during bimanual examination; however, the history of rapid development of signs of virilization and the presence of markedly elevated levels of testosterone (more than 2½ times the upper limits of the normal range) with normal levels of DHEA-S usually facilitate the diagnosis.

Adrenal Tumors

Nearly all the androgen-producing adrenal tumors are adenomas or carcinomas that generate large amounts of the C_{19} steroids normally produced by the adrenal gland: DHEA-S, DHEA, and androstenedione. Although these tumors do not usually directly secrete testosterone, testosterone is produced by extraglandular conversion of DHEA and androstenedione. Patients with these tumors usually have markedly elevated serum levels of DHEA-S (>8 µg/ml), as well as urinary excretion of 17-KS. Patients with these laboratory findings and a history of rapid onset of signs of androgen ex-

cess should undergo a computerized tomography (CT) scan or magnetic resonance imaging (MRI) of the adrenal glands to confirm the diagnosis. In addition to patients with these uncommon tumors, a few patients with testosterone-producing adrenal adenomas have been reported. The cellular patterns of these tumors resemble those of ovarian hilus cells, and the tumors secrete large amounts of testosterone. Because adrenal adenomas also secrete DHEA-S, the presence of such tumors should be considered in patients with DHEA-S levels greater than 8 ng/ml and a testosterone level greater than 1.5 ng/ml.

Late-Onset 21-Hydroxylase Deficency

Congenital adrenal hyperplasia (CAH) is an inherited disorder caused by an enzymatic defect (usually 21-hydroxylase [21-OHase] or less often 11β-hydroxylase), resulting in decreased cortisol biosynthesis. As a consequence, ACTH secretion increases and adrenal cortisol precursors produced proximal to the enzymatic block accumulate and are converted mainly to DHEA and androstenedione. These C_{19} steroids are in turn peripherally converted to testosterone, which produces signs of androgen excess.

Because the enzymatic defects are congenital, the classic severe form (complete block) usually becomes manifest in fetal life through masculinization of the female external genitalia. Importantly, this form of CAH is the most common cause of sexual ambiguity in the newborn. The more attenuated (mild) block of 21-OHase activity usually does not produce physical signs associated with increased androgen production until after puberty. Thus the entity, called late-onset 21-hydroxylase deficiency (LOHD) or late-onset congenital adrenal hyperplasia, may be associated with the development of hirsutism or virilization or both in a woman in the second or early third decade of life.

Although the incidence of classic CAH is only 1 per 14,500 live births worldwide, Speiser et al., using HLA-B genotyping of families with LOHD-affected individuals, concluded that LOHD varied in incidence among different ethnic groups but overall was probably the most frequent autosomal genetic disorder in humans. The incidence of LOHD was estimated to be 0.1% among a diverse white population; among Yugoslavians, Hispanics,

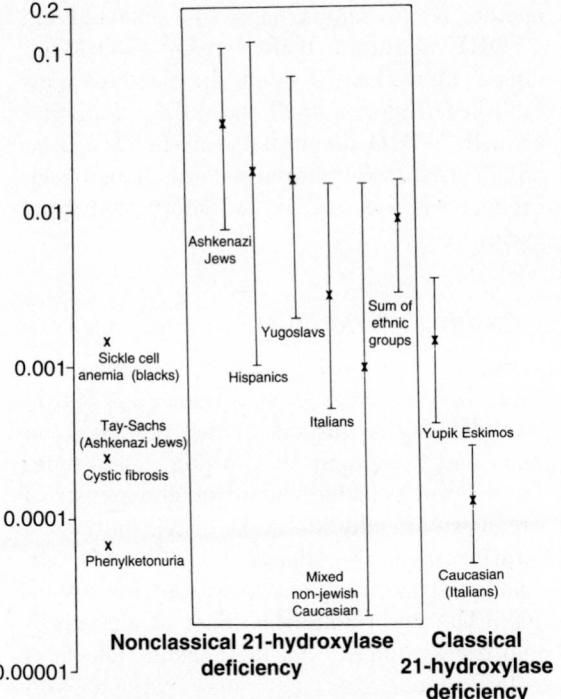

FIGURE 38-19
Relative frequencies of nonclassic 21-hydroxy-
lase deficiency, classic 21-hydroxylase deficiency, and other autosomal recessive disorders. (From Speiser PW, Dupont B, Rubenstein P, et al: Am J Hum Genet 37:650, 1985.)

and Ashkenazi Jews, however, the incidence
was 1.6%, 1.9%, and 3.7% respectively (Figure
38-19). Both classic CAH and LOHD are transmitted in an autosomal recessive manner at the
CYP21B locus and are linked to the HLA-B locus.

The molecular basis of the disease is complex. Depending on the population, one fourth
to one fifth of patients with classic CAH have a
deletion of the CYP21B locus, as detected by
restriction endonuclease digestion and the
Southern blot test. In other families the gene
defect is caused by a point or frame shift mutation that alters the protein product, greatly impairing its function. Thus a spectrum of mutations results in the enzymatic defects, as shown
in Table 38-7.

LOHD is a phenotype that is symptomatic
after adolescence and does not define the gen-
otype. Affected individuals may be homozygous for alleles, yielding mildly abnormal enzymatic activity, or compound heterozygotes with
a combination of defective alleles. The so-
called cryptic 21-OHase deficiency, on the
other hand, represents mild or asymptomatic
individuals with biochemically identified defects that, with the advent of molecular diagnostic techniques, have been redefined into
several different clinical presentations.

TABLE 38-7
Genotypic Characterization of the Forms of 21-Hydroxylase Deficiency

Form of 21-Hydroxylase Deficiency	Clinical Phenotype	Hormonal Phenotype (in Response to ACTH)	Genotype
Classic (CAH)	Prenatal virilization, fully symptomatic	Marked elevation of precursors (serum 17-hydroxyprogesterone and Δ-androstenedione)	21-OH-def^{severe} / 21-OH-def^{severe}
Nonclassic (LOHD)	Symptomatic: later development of virilization; milder symptoms / Asymptomatic: no virilization or other symptoms	Moderate elevation of precursors	21-OH-def^{severe} / 21-OH-def^{mild} ; 21-OH-def^{mild} / 21-OH-def^{mild}
Carrier	Asymptomatic	Precursor level greater than normal	21-OH-def^{severe} / 21-OHase (normal) ; 21-OH-def^{mild} / 21-OHase (normal)
Normal	(Asymptomatic)	Lowest levels—some overlap seen with carriers	21-OHase (normal) / 21-OHase (normal)

From New MI, White PC, et al: The adrenal hyperplasias. In Scriver CR, Beaudet AL, Sly S, and Valle D: Metabolic basis
of inherited diseases, ed 6, New York, 1989, McGraw-Hill Book Co.

New et al. have proposed a schema for identifying and classifying the clinical spectrum of disease shown in Table 38-7. Since there are three possible manifestations of CYP21Y alleles (normal, mildly defective, or severely defective), there are six possible genotypes representing three clinical phenotypes (asymptomatic, LOHD, and classic CAH). Patients with LOHD may be compound heterozygotes, with one mildly and one severely defective allele, or homozygous, with two mildly defective alleles. Although biochemical differences in the hormonal response to ACTH have been shown between these two genotypes, their phenotypes are similar. Carriers can be identified among family members who are heterozygous with one normal allele. These individuals have normal basal 17-hydroxyprogesterone (17-OHP) levels, a milder degree of hirsutism, if present, and smaller increases of 17-OHP after ACTH stimulation, usually between 3.5 and 10 ng/ml.

LOHD is also usually associated with menstrual irregularity. It has been hypothesized that the mechanism for anovulation is similar to that occurring with PCOS. The increased levels of androgen lower SHBG levels, thus increasing the amount of biologically active circulating estradiol. The increased estradiol stimulates tonic LH release, which increases ovarian androgen production and locally inhibits follicular growth and ovulation. Thus women with this disorder present with postpubertal onset of hirsutism and oligomenorrhea or amenorrhea, similar to women with PCOS. However, women with LOHD, unlike those with PCOS, may have a history of prepubertal accelerated growth (ages 6 to 8 years) with later decreased growth and a short ultimate height. This growth pattern, a family history of postpubertal onset of hirsutism, findings of mild virilization, and DHEA-S levels greater than 5 μg/ml all indicate that CAH may be present.

To differentiate LOHD from PCOS, measurement of basal (early morning) serum 17-OHP levels should be performed. This test has replaced the less precise measurement of the 17-OHP urinary metabolite, pregnanetriol. If basal levels of 17-OHP are greater than 8 ng/ml, the diagnosis of LOHD is established. If 17-OHP is above normal (2.5 to 3.3 ng/ml) but less than 8 ng/ml, an ACTH stimulated test should be performed. A baseline 17-OHP should be measured and 25 μg of synthetic ACTH infused as a single bolus. One hour later another serum sample should be obtained and 17-OHP measured. If the level of 17-OHP increases more than 10 ng/ml, the diagnosis is established (Figures 38-20 and 38-21). Individuals with LOHD should be treated with continuous corticosteroids to arrest the signs of androgenicity and restore ovulatory menstrual cycles.

Cushing's Syndrome

Excessive adrenal production of glucocorticoids due to increased ACTH secretion (Cushing's disease) or adrenal tumors produces the signs and symptoms of Cushing's syndrome. These findings include hirsutism and menstrual irregularity in addition to the classic findings of centripetal obesity, dorsal neck fat pads, abdominal striae, and muscle wasting and weakness. The latter catabolic effect of glucocorticoid excess differs from the anabolic effects of testosterone excess, but some patients with PCOS may have other clinical findings that are similar to those found with Cushing's syndrome. In such instances Cushing's syndrome can be easily excluded by performing an overnight dexamethasone suppression test. Dexamethasone, 1 mg, is ingested at 11 PM, and plasma cortisol is measured the following morning at 8 AM (Figure 38-22). If the cortisol level is less than 5 μg/100 ml, Cushing's syndrome is ruled out. If the cortisol level fails to suppress to this degree, the diagnosis of Cushing's syndrome is not established. It is necessary to perform a complete dexamethasone suppression test (Liddle's test) or measurement of urinary free cortisol and plasma ACTH to determine whether Cushing's syndrome exists.

DIFFERENTIAL DIAGNOSIS

The differential diagnosis of the causes of androgen excess just presented can usually be made without difficulty by means of a complete history, a careful physical examination, and measurement of serum levels of testosterone and DHEA-S to determine if there is an ovarian or adrenal source of excess androgen production.

Measurement of total testosterone, free testosterone, the free androgen index, and non-SHBG bound testosterone (unbound testosterone) have all been advocated to assist in the diagnosis of hyperandrogenism. Loric et al. mea-

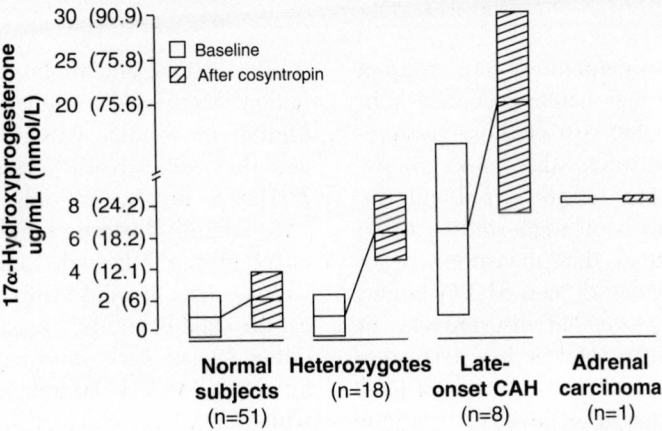

FIGURE 38-20
Means and ranges of 17α-hydroxyprogesterone levels before and after cosyntropin administered intramuscularly in normal subjects, suspected heterozygotes, patients with late-onset congenital adrenal hyperplasia *(CAH)*, and one patient with adrenal carcinoma. (From Baskin HJ: Arch Intern Med 147:847, 1987.)

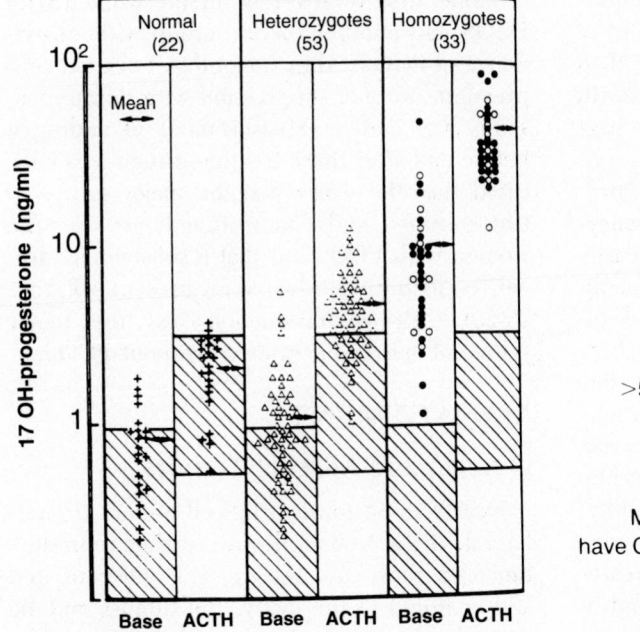

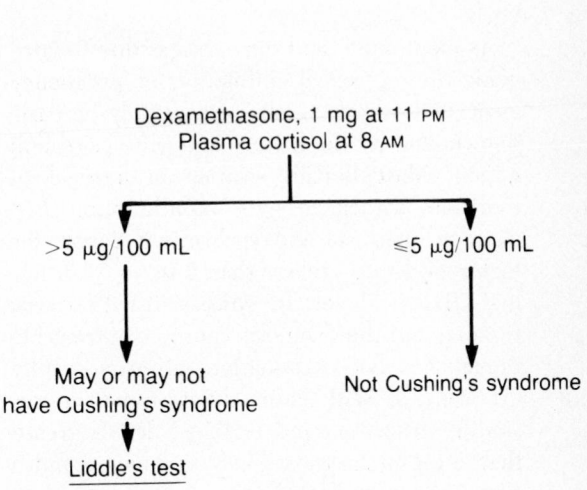

FIGURE 38-21
Basal and ACTH-stimulated levels of 17-hydroxyprogesterone in patients and their families. All subjects were divided into three groups: group 1, the 24 propositi (●) and 9 siblings (○) having the same two HLA haplotypes as the propositus (homozygotes); group 2, 53 parents and siblings with only one HLA haplotype identical to that of the propositus (heterozygotes); and group 3, 22 siblings having no HLA haplotype identical to that of the propositus (normal). Hatched areas indicate normal ranges. (To convert nanograms per milliliter to nanomoles per liter, multiply by 3.025.) (From Kuttenn F, Couillin P, Girard F, et al: N Engl J Med 313:224, 1985.)

FIGURE 38-22
Outline of overnight dexamethasone suppression test. (From Goebelsmann U and Lobo RA: Androgen excess. In Mishell DR Jr, Davajan V, and Lobo RA, editors: Infertility, contraception and reproductive endocrinology, ed 3, Cambridge, Mass, 1991, Blackwell Scientific Publications.

sured all these serum parameters in a group of hirsute women and age-matched control subjects. Slopes of the first two of these parameters overlapped between the two groups, whereas no overlap of values occurred with the last two assays. It has been suggested by these and other investigators that measurement of the free androgen index or non-SHBG bound testosterone is a more specific discriminator of hyperandrogenism than total or free testosterone. Clinically, however, measurement of total testosterone is all that is necessary. It is not clinically important whether a hirsute woman has a total testosterone level in the highest portion of the normal range or a mildly elevated level of non-SHBG bound testosterone. Schwartz et al. reported that when total testosterone levels are elevated, there is an excellent correlation with free testerone levels. Thus, to determine the magnitude of elevated androgens, as well as their source, measurement of total testosterone is more cost-effective than the other assays and provides the clinician with the information necessary to establish the diagnosis.

As mentioned, androgen excess due to iatrogenic causes, sexual ambiguity, or pregnancy-associated ovarian tumors can usually be easily determined by the history and physical examination. Masculinizing ovarian or adrenal tumors are associated with rapidly progressive signs of hirsutism and virilization. Serum testosterone levels greater than 2 ng/ml with normal DHEA-S levels are consistent with ovarian tumors, and the diagnosis can be confirmed by bimanual pelvic examination, ultrasonography, CT scans, or MRI. Patients with rapid progression of virilization and DHEA-S levels greater than 8 μg/ml are most likely to have an androgen-producing adrenal adenoma, and the diagnosis can be confirmed by CT scan or MRI. A long history of gradually increasing hirsutism, even if accompanied by virilization, is not consistent with the diagnosis of adrenal or ovarian tumors. The diagnosis of ovarian stromal hyperthecosis should be suspected for individuals with these signs and testosterone levels greater than 1.5 ng/ml. Patients with physical findings consistent with Cushing's syndrome should have the diagnosis ruled out or confirmed by an overnight dexamethasone suppression test followed by Liddle's test if necessary. The remaining three diagnoses—PCOS, LOHD and idiopathic hirsutism—may be associated with a similar history and findings at physical examination. Menstrual irregularity is an uncommon finding in women with idiopathic hirsutism, and they will have a normal testosterone and DHEA-S levels. Patients with LOHD may have a family history of androgen excess, early onset of rapid growth, and short stature, as well as signs of mild virilization. The diagnosis can be established by measurement of 17-OHP either by an early-morning serum sample or following ACTH stimulation. Most patients with PCOS have elevated LH levels and mildly increased testosterone or DHEA-S levels, whereas women with idiopathic hirsutism have normal levels of these hormones. Treatment of hirsutism depends on whether the androgen excess is ovarian, adrenal, or peripheral.

Rittmaster and Thompson suppressed ovarian function with a GnRH analogue in a group of moderately or severely hirsute women with PCOS and another hirsute group without evidence of PCOS. After 6 months of ovarian suppression, adrenal suppression with dexamethasome was added. Measurement of androgen before and after these treatment regimens indicated that the ovary was the major source of testosterone and androstenedione in the women with PCOS but that a substantial adrenal contribution also was present (Figure 38-23). Adrenal production was the major source of androgens in those without PCOS.

MANAGEMENT

Ovarian and Adrenal Tumors

Nearly all Sertoli-Leydig cell tumors are unilateral. If the woman desires further reproduction and these tumors are well differentiated and confined to the ovary, the tumors may be treated by unilateral salpingo-oophorectomy. Since most hilus cell tumors occur after menopause, they are best treated by bilateral salpingo-oophorectomy and total abdominal hysterectomy. Adrenal adenomas and carcinomas also should be treated by operative removal. Adrenal carcinomas frequently have metastasized to the liver by the time the androgenic signs have developed. Despite chemotherapy the prognosis is poor after metastases have occurred. Stromal hyperthecosis is also best treated by bilateral salpingo-oophorectomy together with total abdominal hysterectomy. After removal of the ovaries of patients with stromal hyperthecosis or any of the androgen-pro-

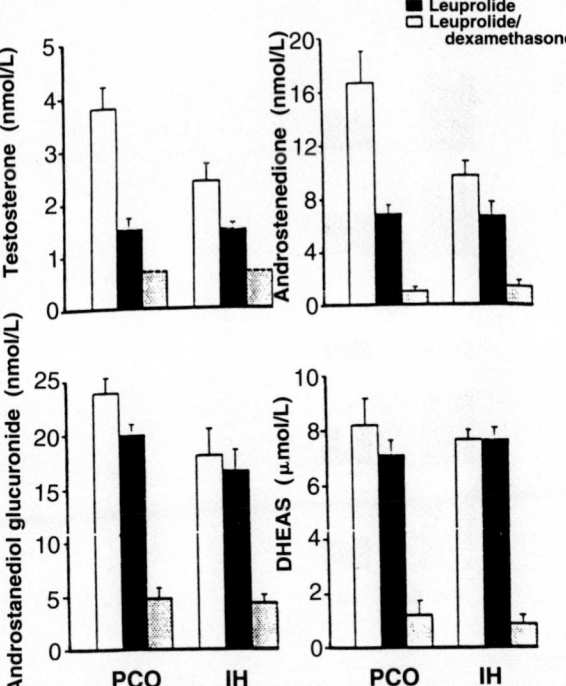

FIGURE 38-23

Hormone levels in women with polycystic ovary syndrome *(PCO)* and idiopathic hirsutism *(IH)* at baseline, after leuprolide alone, and after the combination of leuprolide and dexamethasone. Testosterone levels (**A**) after leuprolide and dexamethasone were undetectable; the detection limit of the assay is shown. (From Rittmaster RS and Thompson DL: J Clin Endocrinol Metab 70:1096, 1990.)

ducing tumors, the acne and oiliness of the skin disappear, breast size increases, and clitoral size decreases. The excess central hair becomes finer and grows less rapidly but does not disappear. Electrolysis can remove the facial hair, and depilatories, bleaches, or shaving can be used to treat the body hair.

Late-Onset 21-Hydrolase Deficiency

Patients with late-onset of CAH (LOHD) should be treated daily with glucocorticoids such as hydrocortisone (15 to 20 mg), prednisone (5 to 7.5 mg), or dexamethasone (0.5 to 0.75 mg) in divided doses. Sometimes lower doses of these agents may be sufficient to suppress ACTH and decrease adrenal androgen production. The aim of treatment is to suppress androstenedione and 17-OHP levels to the normal range. Signs of androgen excess lessen

over a few months. Ovulation usually resumes within a few weeks.

Polycystic Ovarian Syndrome

The treatment of PCOS depends on which aspect of the disorder—hirsutism, infertility, or irregular prolonged menses (dysfunctional uterine bleeding)—is of greatest concern to the patient. The best treatment for PCOS, unless pregnancy is desired, is oral steroid contraceptives, because these agents inhibit LH, decrease circulating testosterone levels, and increase levels of SHBG and thus bind and inactivate more of the testosterone in the circulation (Figure 38-24). It is best to use an oral contraceptive formulation that contains less than 50 µg estrogen and a progestin other than norgestrel, because norgestrel is the most androgenic progestin in current use. As reported by Wild et al. and Klove et al., oral contraceptives also decrease serum DHEA-S. If the levels are only mildly elevated, oral contraceptives alone will reduce them to normal. If DHEA-S levels are moderately elevated (>4 µg/ml), dexamethasone (0.25 to 0.5 mg at bedtime) should be given together with the oral contraceptive to reduce DHEA-S to normal. Silver et al. have shown that if hirsutism continues to be a problem, spironolactone (50 to 100 mg twice daily) causes regression of the hirsutism in women with PCOS by decreasing androgenic action in the target organs.

GnRH analogues have been shown by several investigators to treat effectively ovarian sources of hyperandrogenism. Since in many women with PCOS there is also an adrenal source, using these agonists together with oral contraceptives should also reduce adrenal androgen production, increase SHBG, as well as prevent the hypoestrogenic side effects associated with GnRH agonist therapy. GnRH agonists are expensive, and their use should be reserved for women whose treatment does not improve with combinations of oral contraceptives and spironolactone and wish to preserve ovarian function. Williams et al. have shown that treatment with GnRH analogues does not permanently alter the pathophysiology of PCOS. A few months after analogue treatment is discontinued, gonadotrophin and androgen levels return to pretreatment concentrations.

Although ovarian wedge resection was advocated in the past for treatment of androgen ex-

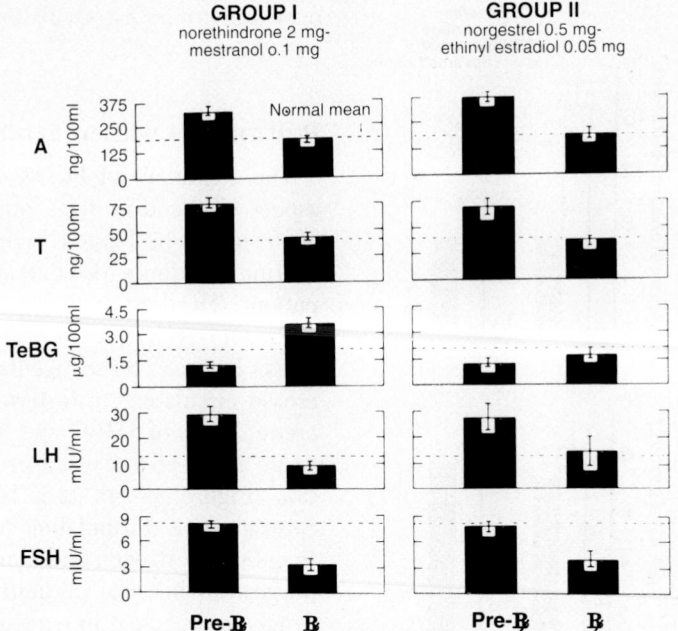

GROUP I
norethindrone 2 mg-
mestranol o.1 mg

GROUP II
norgestrel 0.5 mg-
ethinyl estradiol 0.05 mg

FIGURE 38-24

Mean pretreatment *(Pre-℞)* and treatment *(℞)* plasma levels of Δ^4-androstenedione *(A)*, testosterone *(T)*, testosterone-estrogen-binding globulin *(TeBG)* capacity, LH, and FSH of hirsute women. Bars define standard errors of means. (From Givens JR, Andersen RN, Wiser WL, et al: Am J Obstet Gynecol 124:333, 1976.)

cess, the decrease in circulating androgens occurred for only a short period of time, and thus this therapy should no longer be used.

However, laparoscopic cauterization of multiple sites on the ovary has been reported by Aakvaag and Gjønnaess to reduce serum androgen levels in most patients for 12 months as well as induce ovulation.

For the woman over 35 who does not desire future childbearing and who has excess ovarian androgen production due to PCOS, bilateral salpingo-oophorectomy and hysterectomy may be a desirable method of alleviating the problem.

Although it was suggested in the past that bromocriptine may be of value in the treatment of PCOS, more recent studies by Chapman et al., Murdoch et al., and the double-blind placebo-controlled study of Buvat et al. concluded that no evidence indicates the efficacy of bromocriptine in the treatment of PCOS.

Women with PCOS who desire fertility should be treated with agents that stimulate ovulation, starting with clomiphene citrate and, if the condition is unresponsive, proceeding to human menopausal gonadotrophin (HMG) or GnRH. If women with PCOS do not have hirsutism but have dysfunctional bleeding or oligomenorrhea, regular withdrawal bleeding should be induced with monthly progestins such as oral medroxyprogesterone acetate 10 mg daily for the first 10 days of the month. Progestins should be administered to prevent development of endometrial hyperplasia due to unopposed menopausal estrogen.

Idiopathic Hirsutism

Although hirsutism is a benign condition, it is frequently of great concern to the patient. Women with idiopathic hirsutism have normal circulating levels of testosterone and DHEA-S. Nearly all those individuals with symptomatic hirsutism who have normal testosterone and DHEA-S levels have elevated levels of α-diol-G indicative of increased peripheral androgen activity. It is not necessary to measure α-diol-G in patients with hirsutism without elevated circulating androgen levels, because the presence of hirsutism is itself evidence of increased peripheral androgen activity. An agent that inhibits peripheral androgen activity should be ad-

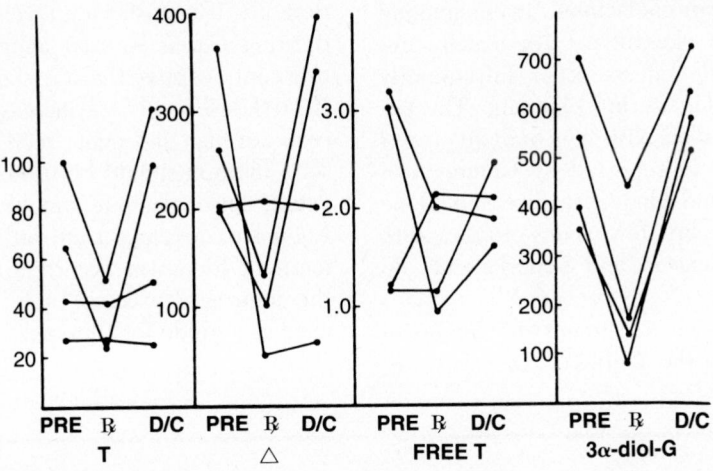

FIGURE 38-25
Serum testosterone *(T)*, $\triangle^4$-androstenedione *(△)*, free testosterone *(free T)*, and 5α-androstane-3α,17B-diol glucuronide *(3α diol G)* levels in four hirsute women before, during, and after therapy. Each had improved clinically during therapy with prednisone or spironolactone, and each noted increased hirsutism after it was discontinued. The treatment (Ɍ) results were obtained after 5 to 12 months of therapy, and the *D/C* results 1 to 6 months after therapy was discontinued. *PRE*, Pretreatment levels. (From Kirschner MA, Samojlik E, and Szmal E: J Clin Endocrinol Metab 65:597, 1987.)

ministered to women with these findings.

Because of the length of the hair growth cycle, responses to treatment should not be expected within the first 3 months. Objective methods of assessing changes of hair growth, such as photographs, are useful. With use of the agents listed in Table 38-8, a successful response should occur in about 70% of patients with 1 year of therapy. Remaining excess hair can be removed by electrolysis. Treatment can be continued for 2 years and then stopped to determine if hirsutism recurs. If so, therapy can be reinitiated.

Kirschner et al. measured 3α-diol-G in 29 women with idiopathic hirsutism and found it was elevated in all but one woman. After treatment with spironolactone, oral contraceptives, or dexamethasone, the women showed good clinical response. This response correlated much better with 3α-diol-G levels than levels of total or free testosterone or androstenedione (Figure 38-25). Responses to therapy are generally judged clinically, but in some instances it may be useful to measure serum 3α-diol-G levels.

Ketoconazole, which blocks adrenal and gonadal steroidogenesis by inhibiting cytochrome P-450–dependent enzyme pathways, has been used by Venturoli et al. in dosages of 200 mg twice a day to treat women with hyperandrogenism associated with PCOS and idiopathic hirsutism. This potent drug effectively decreased hair growth and acne, but major side effects and complications (including hepatitis) occurred in most patients. These problems limit the use of ketoconazole to very select patients, who require careful monitoring.

Antiandrogens include spironolactone, an aldosterone antagonist, a C_{21} progestin, or cyproterone actate. The latter drug is available in Europe but not in the United States. Spironolactone has been used and studied extensively and should be considered the treatment of choice in the United States for women with idiopathic hirsutism (as well as some with PCOS). Various dosages from 50 to 200 mg daily have been used. Lobo et al. reported that a dose of 200 mg/day of spironolactone is more effective than 100 mg/day. Barth et al. found a clinically evident response of decreased hair after 3 months of 200 mg spironolactone daily. After 1 year of treatment a 15% to 25% reduction occurred in both hair shaft diameter and linear growth rate at all body sites. With the higher dose of spironolactone, liver function tests and plasma electrolytes are usually unchanged, and side effects occur infrequently except for irregular uterine bleeding. The latter can be controlled with concomitant use of oral contractives, as reported by Chapman et al. Electrolytes and blood pressure should be monitored for the first few weeks of therapy to be certain hypotension and hyperkalemia do not occur.

In summary, the treatment of hirsutism should depend on the source of the excess androgens. If testosterone levels are elevated, indicating excess ovarian androgen production, oral contraceptive therapy should be instituted. If DHEA-S levels are increased, indicating excess adrenal androgen secretion, dexamethasone therapy should be used. If neither is elevated, spironolactone should be administered. Lobo has developed an outline for the treatment of hirsutism according to the source of the androgen excess (Table 38-8). It can be used as a guide for therapy.

TABLE 38-8

Treatment of Hirsutism According to Source of Androgen Excess

Androgen	Treatment
↑ Testosterone	Oral contraceptives
↑ DHEA-S (<5 µg/ml)	Oral contraceptives
↑ DHEA-S (>5 µg/ml)	Dexamethasone
↑ Testosterone, ↑ DHEA-S (>5 µg/ml)	Oral contraceptives + dexamethasone
Normal Testosterone, normal DHEA-S	Spironolactone*
3α-diol-G	

From Mishell DR Jr, Davajan V, and Lobo RA, editors: Infertility, contraception and reproductive endocrinology, ed 3, Cambridge, Mass, 1991, Blackwell Scientific Publications.
*Spironolactone may also be substituted for any of the above regimens if no improvement is noted after 3 to 4 months of treatment.

_____ KEY POINTS _____

- The three cyclic changes of hair development include a growth phase called anagen, followed by transitional phase called catagen and a resting phase called telogen.

- Testosterone levels in women with hirsutism without virilization are lower than 1.5 ng/ml.

- Circulating testosterone levels in the presence of virilization are usually greater than 2 ng/ml.

- The major androgen provided by the ovaries is testosterone and that of the adrenal glands, DHEA-S.

- Total daily testosterone production is 0.35 mg: 0.1 mg from ovarian secretion, 0.2 mg from peripheral conversion of androstenedione, and 0.05 mg from peripheral conversion of DHEA.

- About two thirds of the daily testosterone production in a woman originates in the ovaries.

- Serum levels of DHEA-S correlate well with daily urinary 17-KS excretion.

- There are three markers of androgen production, one for each compartment where androgens are produced. In the ovary it is testosterone; in the adrenal gland, DHEAS; and in the periphery, 3α-diol-G.

- About 85% of testosterone is bound to SHBG and is biologically inactive, 10% to 15% is bound to albumin, and 1% to 2% is not bound. Both of the latter fractions are biologically active.

- Non-SHBG bound testosterone is elevated in about 60% to 70% of women with hirsutism, and 3α-diol-G is elevated in about 98%.

- About 80% of individuals with idiopathic hirsutism have elevated levels of 3α-diol-G.

- Individuals with idiopathic hirsutism show increased 5α-reductase activity.

- Women with PCOS have testosterone levels between 70 and 120 ng/dl and androstenedione levels of 3 to 5 ng/ml; about half have elevated levels of DHEA-S.

- About 30% of women with PCOS do not have hirsutism.

- About 70% of women with PCOS have elevated levels of immunologic LH or an immunologic LH-FSH ratio greater than 3, and nearly all have elevated levels of biologically active LH and biologically active estradiol.

- A high percentage of women with PCOS have hyperinsulinemia and impaired glucose tolerance.

- Acanthosis nigricans is a common finding in obese women who have PCOS. It is generally unnecessary to measure free testosterone, free androgen, free androgen index, or non-SHBG bound testosterone in clinical situations. Measurement of total testosterone is all that is necessary.

- Patients with PCOS syndrome have increased amplitude of GnRH pulses.

- Patients with ovarian neoplasms have testosterone levels more than 2½ times the upper limits of the normal range.

- The diagnosis of LOHD is established if the basal (early morning) serum 17-hydroxyprogesterone (17-OHP) levels are greater than 8 ng/ml or if the level at 1 hour after infusion of ACTH is more than 10 ng/ml.

- Women with LOHD have a block in cortisol biosynthesis of 11β-hydroxylase or 21-hydroxylase resulting in increased circulating levels of 17-OHP.

- The incidence of LOHD varies among different population groups, being highest in Ashenazi Jews.

- The incidence of LOHD varies from 1% to 6% in different series. The incidence of heterozygous carrier form is usually two to three times higher.

- Because of the length of the hair growth cycle, response should not be expected until after 3 months of therapy has been used. Successful responses should occur in about 70% of those patients treated.

- If after an overnight dexamethasone suppression test serum cortisol levels are lower than 5 μg/100 ml, Cushing's syndrome is ruled out.

- The best treatment for hirsutism due to increased peripheral androgen metabolism is the antiandrogen spironolactone.

- Women with PCOS who desire fertility should be treated with agents that stimulate ovulation, starting with clomiphene citrate and, if the condition is unresponsive, proceeding to HMG or GnRH.

- The treatment of hirsutism should depend on the source of the excess androgens. If testosterone levels are elevated, indicating excess ovarian androgen production, oral contraceptive therapy should be instituted. If DHEA-S is increased, indicating excess adrenal androgen secretion, dexamethasone therapy should be used. If neither is elevated, spironolactone should be administered.

- Spironolactone, an aldosterone antagonist, is the most effective treatment for idiopathic hirsutism. The major side effect is abnormal bleeding. It should be administered in a dose of 200 mg/day.

- Bromocriptine is of no therapeutic value in the treatment of PCOS.

BIBLIOGRAPHY

Aakvaag A and Gjønnaess H: Hormonal response to electrocautery of the ovary in patients with polycystic ovarian disease, Br J Obstet Gynaecol 92:1258, 1985.

Anderson DC: Sex hormone-binding globulin, Clin Endocrinol 3:69, 1981.

Andreyko JL, Monroe SE, Jaffe RB, et al: Treatment of hirsutism with a gonadotrophin-releasing hormone agonist (nafarelin), J Clin Endocrinol Metab 63:854, 1986.

Azziz R and Zacur HA: 21-Hydroxylase deficiency in female hyperandrogenism: screening and diagnosis, J Clin Endocrinol Metab 69:577, 1989.

Barth JH, Cherry CA, Wojnarowska F, and Dawber RPR: Spironolactone is an effective and well tolerated systematic antiandrogen therapy for hirsute women, J Clin Endocrinol Metab 68:966, 1989.

Baskin HJ: Screening for late-onset congenital adrenal hyperplasia in hirsutism or amenorrhea, Arch Intern Med 147:847, 1987.

Behrman SJ and Scully RE: Case records of the Massachusetts General Hospital: infertility and irregular menses in a 27-year-old woman, N Engl J Med 287:1192, 1972.

Benjamin F, Deutsch S, Saperstein H, and Seltzer VL: Prevalence of and markers for the attenuated form of congenital adrenal hyperplasia and hyperprolactinemia masquerading as polycystic ovarian disease, Fertil Steril 46:215, 1986.

Boyers P, Buster JE, and Marshall JR: Hypothalamic-pituitary-adrenocortical function during long-term low-dose dexamethasone therapy in hyperandrogenized women, Am J Obstet Gynecol 142:330, 1982.

Burger CW, Korsen T, van Kessel H, et al: Pulsatile luteinizing hormone patterns in the follicular phase of the menstrual cycle, polycystic ovarian disease (PCOD) and non-PCOD secondary amenorrhea, J Clin Endocrinol Metab 61:1126, 1985.

Buvat J, Buvat-Herbaut M, Marcolin G, et al: A double blind controlled study of the hormonal and clinical effects of bromocriptine in the polycystic ovary syndrome, J Clin Endocrinol Metab 63:119, 1986.

Carlstrom K, Gershagen S, Marcolin G, et al: Free testosterone and testosterone/SHBG index in hirsute women: a comparison of diagnostic accuracy, Gynecol Obstet Invest 24:256, 1987.

Casey J: Chronic treatment regimens for hirsutism in women: effect on blood production rates of testosterone and on hair growth, Clin Endocrinol 4:313, 1975.

Chang RJ, Mandel FP, Wolfsen AR, et al: Circulating levels of plasma adrenocorticotropin in polycystic ovary disease, J Clin Endocrinol Metab 54:1265, 1982.

Chapdelaine A, Desmarias J-L, & Derman RJ: Clinical evidence of the minimal androgenic activity of norgestimate, Int J Fertil 34:347, 1989.

Chapman AJ, Wilson M, Obhrai M, et al: Effect of bromocriptine on pulsatility in the polycystic ovary syndrome, Clin Endocrinol 27:571, 1987.

Chapman G, Dowsett M, Dewhurst CJ, and Jeffocate SL: Spironolactone in combination with an oral contraceptive: an alternative treatment for hirsutism, Br J Obstet Gynaecol 92:983, 1985.

Chez RA: Clinical aspects of three new progestogens: desogestrel, gestodene, and norgestimate, Am J Obstet Gynecol 160:1296, 1989.

Cumming DC and Wall SR: Non–sex hormone–binding globulin–bound testosterone is a marker for hyperandrogenism, J Clin Endocrinol Metab 61:873, 1985.

Cumming D, Yang JC, Rebar RW, et al: Treatment of hirsutism with spironolactone, JAMA 247:1295, 1982.

Daly L and Bonnar J: Comparative studies of 30-μg ethinyl estradiol combined with gestodene and desogestrel on blood coagulation, fibrinolysis, and platelets, Am J Obstet Gynecol 163:430, 1990.

DeVane GW, Czekala NM, Judd HL, Sainsard C, et al: Circulating gonadotropins, estrogens, and androgens in polycystic ovarian disease, Am J Obstet Gynecol 121:496, 1975.

Dewailly D, Vantyghem-Haudiquet MC, Sainsard C, et al: Clinical and biological phenotyopes in late-onset 21-hydroxylase deficiency, J Clin Endocrinol Metab 63:418, 1986.

Dibbelt L, Knuppen R, Jutting G, et al: Group comparison of serum ethinyl estradiol, SHGB and CBG levels in 83 women using 2 low-dose combination oral contraceptives for 3 months, Contraception 43:1, 1991.

Dunaif A, Graf M, Mandeli J, et al: Characterization of groups of hyperandrogenic women with acanthosis nigricans, impaired glucose tolerance, and/or hyperinsulinemia, J Clin Endocrinol Metab 65:499, 1987.

Ferriman D and Gallwey JD: Clinical assessment of body hair growth in women, J Clin Endocrinol Metab 21:1440, 1961.

Filicori M, Flamigni C, Campaniello E, et al: The abnormal response of polycystic ovarian disease patients to exogenous pulsatile gonadotropin-releasing hormone: characterization and management, J Clin Endocrinol Metab 69:825, 1989.

Gillmer MDG: Progestogen potency in oral contraceptive pills, Am J Obstet Gynecol 157:1048, 1987.

Givens JR, Andersen RN, Wiser WL, et al: The effectiveness of two oral contraceptives in suppressing plasma androstanedione, testosterone, LH and FSH, and stimulating plasma testosterone-binding capacity in hirsute women, Am J Obstet Gynecol 124:333, 1976.

Givens JR, Andersen RN, Wiser WL, et al: A gonadotropin responsive adrenocortical adenoma, J Clin Endocrinol Metab 38:126, 1974.

Godsland IF, Crook D, Simpson R, et al: The effects of different formulations of oral contraceptive agents on lipid and carbohydrate metabolism, N Engl J Med 323:1375, 1990.

Goebelsmann U: Steroid hormones. In Mishell DR and Davajan V, editors: Infertility, contraception and reproductive endocrinology, ed 2, Oradell, NJ, 1986, Medical Economics Books.

Goebelsmann U and Lobo RA: Androgen excess. In Mishell DR, and Davajan V, editors: Infertility, contraception and reproductive endocrinology, ed 2, Oradell, NJ, 1986, Medical Economics Books.

Goldzieher JW: Polycystic ovarian syndrome, Fertil Steril 35:371, 1981.

Goldzieher JW and Axelrod LR: Clinical and biochemical features of polycystic ovarian disease, Fertil Steril 14:631, 1963.

Hahn DW, Allen GO, & McGuire JL: The pharmacological profile of norgestimate, a new orally active progestin, Contraception 16:541, 1977.

Helfer EL, Miller JL, & Rose LI: Side-effects of spironolactone therapy in the hirsute woman, J Clin Endocrinol Metab 66:208, 1988.

Hensleigh PA, Woodruff JD: Differential maternal-fetal response to androgenizing luteoma or hyperreactio luteinalis, Obstet Gynecol Surv 33:262, 1978.

Hoffman D, Klove K, Lobo RA: The prevalence and significance of elevated dehydroepiandrone sulfate levels in anovulatory women, Fertil Steril 42:76, 1984.

Horton R, Hawks D, and Lobo RA: 3α,17β-androstanediol glucuronide in plasma: a marker of androgen action in idiopathic hirsutism, J Clin Invest 69:1203, 1982.

Horton R and Lobo RA: Peripheral androgens and the role of androstanediol glucuronide, Clin Endocrinol Metab 15:293, 1986.

Humpel M, Tauber U, Kuhnz W, et al: Protein binding of active ingredients and comparison of serum ethinyl estradiol, sex hormone-binding globulin, corticosteroid-binding globulin, and cortisol levels in women using a combination of gestodene/ethinyl estradiol (Femovan) or a combination of desogestrel/ethinyl estradiol (Marvelon) and single-dose ethinyl estradiol bioequivalence from both oral contraceptives, Am J Obstet Gynecol 163:329, 1990.

Ireland K and Woodruff JD: Masculinizing ovarian tumors, Obstet Gynecol Surv 31:83, 1976.

Jespersen J, Petersen KR, and Skouby SO: Effects of newer oral contraceptives on the inhibition of coagulation and fibrinolysis in relation to dosage and type of steroid, Am J Obstet Gynecol 163:396, 1990.

Judd HL, Rigg LA, Anderson DC, et al: The effects of ovarian wedge resection on circulating gonadotropin and ovarian steroid levels in patients with polycystic ovary syndrome, J Clin Endocrinol Metab 43:347, 1976.

Judd HL, Scully RE, Herbst AL, et al: Familial hyperthecosis: comparison of endocrinologic and histologic findings with polycystic ovarian disease, Am J Obstet Gynecol 117:976, 1973.

Klove KL, Roy S, and Lobo RA: The effect of different contraceptive treatments on the serum concentration of dehydroepiandrosterone sulfate, Contraception 29:319, 1984.

Jung-Hoffman C and Kuhl H: Interaction with the pharmacokinetics of ethinylestradiol and progestogens contained in oral contraceptives, Contraception 40:299, 1989.

Kazer AR, Kessel B, and Yen SSC: Circulating luteinizing hormone pulse frequency in women with polycystic ovary syndrome, J Clin Endocrinol Metab 65:233, 1987.

Kirschner MA, Samojlik E, and Szmal E: Clinical usefulness of plasma androstanediol glucuronide measurements in women with idiopathic hirsutism, J Clin Endocrinol Metab 65:597, 1987.

Kjaer A, Lebech A-M, Borggaard B, et al: Lipid metabolism and coagulation of two contraceptives: correlation to serum concentrations of levonorgestrel and gestodene, Contraception 40:665, 1989.

Klove KL, Roy S, and Lobo RA: The effect of different contraceptive treatments on the serum concentration of dehydroepiandrosterone sulfate, Contraception 29:319, 1984.

Kohn B, Levine MS, Pollack MS, et al: Late-onset steroid 21-hydroxylase deficiency: a variant of classical congenital adrenal hyperplasia, J Clin Endocrinol Metab 55:817, 1982.

Kuttenn F, Couillin P, Girard F, et al: Late-onset adrenal hyperplasia in hirsutism, N Engl J Med 313:224, 1985.

Lobo RA and Goebelsmann U: Adult manifestation of congenital adrenal hyperplasia due to incomplete 21-hydroxylase deficiency mimicking polycystic ovarian disease, Am J Obstet Gynecol 138:720, 1980.

Lobo RA and Goebelsmann U: Effect of androgen excess on inappropriate gonadotropin secretion as found in polycystic ovary syndrome, Am J Obstet Gynecol 142:394, 1982.

Lobo RA and Goebelsmann U: Evidence for reduced 3β-ol-hydroxysteroid dehydrogenase activity in some hirsute women thought to have polycystic ovary syndrome, J Clin Endocrinol Metab 53:394, 1981.

Lobo RA, Goebelsmann U, and Horton R: Evidence for the importance of peripheral tissue events in the development of hirsutism in polycystic ovary syndrome, J Clin Endocrinol Metab 57:393, 1983.

Lobo RA, Granger L, Goebelsmann U, et al: Elevation in unbound serum estradiol as a possible mechanism for inappropriate gonadotropin secretion in women with PCO, J Clin Endocrinol Metab 52:156, 1981.

Lobo RA, Granger LR, Paul WL, et al: Psychological stress and increases in urinary norepinephrine metabolites, platelet serotonin and adrenal androgens in women with polycystic ovary syndrome, Am J Obstet Gynecol 145:496, 1983.

Lobo RA, Kletzky OA, Campeau JD, et al: Elevated bioactive luteinizing hormone in women with the polycystic ovary syndrome, Fertil Steril 39:674, 1983.

Lobo RA, Paul WL, and Goebelsmann U: Dehydroepiandrosterone sulfate as an indicator of adrenal androgen function, Obstet Gynecol 57:69, 1981.

Lobo RA, Paul WL, and Goebelsmann U: Serum levels of DHEA-S in gynecologic endocrinopathy and infertility, Obstet Gynecol 57:607, 1981.

Lobo RA, Shoupe D, Serafini P, et al: The effects of two doses of spironolactone on serum androgens and anagen hair in hirsute women, Fertil Steril 43:200, 1985.

Loric S, Guechot J, Duron F, et al: Determination of testosterone in serum not bound by sex-hormone-binding globulin: diagnostic value in hirsute women, Clin Chem 34:1826, 1988.

Luciano AA, Chapler FK, and Sherman BM: Hyperprolactinemia in polycystic ovary syndrome, Fertil Steril 41:719, 1984.

Mandel FP, Chang RJ, Dupont B, et al: HLA genotyping in family members and patients with familial polycystic ovarian disease, J Clin Endocrinol Metab 56:862, 1983.

Marz W, Jung-Hoffman C, Heidt F, et al: Changes in lipid metabolism during 12 months of treatment with two oral contraceptives containing 30 μg ethinylestradiol and 75 μg gestodene or 150 μg desogestrel, Contraception 41:245, 1990.

Miccoli R, Orlandi MC, Fruzzetti MD, et al: Metabolic effects of three new low-dose pills, Contraception 39:643, 1989.

Milewicz A, Silber D, and Kirschner MA: Therapeutic effects of spironolactone in polycystic ovary syndrome, Obstet Gynecol 61:429, 1983.

Mornet E, Crete P, Kuttenn F, et al: Distribution of deletions and seven point mutations on CYP21-genes in three clinical forms of steroid 21-hydroxylase deficiency, Am J Hum Genet 48:79, 1991.

Murdoch AP, McClean KG, Watson MJ, et al: Treatment of hirsutism in polycystic ovary syndrome with bromocriptine, Br J Obstet Gynaecol 94:358, 1987.

New MI, Lorenzen F, Lerner AJ, et al: Genotyping steroid 21-hydroxylase deficiency: hormonal reference data, J Clin Endocrinol Metab 57:320, 1983.

New MI, White PC, Pang S, et al: The adrenal hyperplasias. In Scriver CR, Beaudet AL, Sly S, and Valle D: Metabolic basis of inherited diseases, ed 6, New York, 1989, McGraw-Hill Book Co.

Omsjo IH, Oian P, Maltau JM, and Osterud B: Effects of two triphasic oral contraceptives containing ethinylestradiol plus levonorgestrel or gestodene on blood coagulation and fibrinolysis, Acta Obstet Gynecol Scand 68:27, 1989.

Pang S, Wallace MA, Hofman L, et al: Worldwide experience in newborn screening for classical congenital adrenal hyperplasia due to 21-hydroxylase deficiency, Pediatrics 81:866, 1988.

Paulson RJ, Serafini PC, Catalino JA, and Lobo RA: Measurements of 3α,17β-androstanediol glucuronide in serum and urine and the correlation with skin 5α-reductase activity, Fertil Steril 46:222, 1986.

Phillips A, Demarest K, Wong F, and McGuire JL: et al: Progestational and androgenic receptor binding affinities and in vivo activites of norgestimate and other progestins, Contraception 41:399, 1990.

Plymate SR, Fariss BL, Bassett ML, et al: Obesity and its role in polycystic ovary syndrome, J Clin Endocrinol Metab 52:1246, 1981.

Pollow K, Juchem M, Grill H-J, et al: Gestodene: a novel synthetic progestin—characterization of binding to receptor and serum proteins, Contraception 40:325, 1989.

Raj SG, Thompson IE, Berger MJ, et al: Clinical aspects of the polycystic ovary syndrome, Obstet Gynecol 49:552, 1977.

Rebar R, Judd HL, Yen SSC, et al: Characterization of the inappropriate gonadotropin secretion in polycystic ovary syndrome, J Clin Invest 57:1320, 1976.

Rittmaster RS: Differential suppression of testosterone and estradiol in hirsute women with the superactive gonadotropin-releasing hormone agonist leuprolide, J Clin Endocrinol Metab 67:651, 1988.

Rittmaster RS and Thompson DL: Effect of leuprolide and dexamethasone on hair growth and hormone levels in hirsute women: the relative importance of the ovary and the adrenal in the pathogenesis of hirsutism, J Clin Endocrinol Metab 70:1096, 1990.

Rittmaster RS, Loriaux DL, and Cutler GB: Sensitivity of cortisol and adrenal androgens to dexamethasone suppression in hirsute women, J Clin Endocrinol Metab 61:462, 1985.

Runnebaum B and Rabe T: New progestogens in oral contraceptives, Am J Obstet Gynecol 157:1059, 1987.

Schwartz U, Moltz L, Brptherton J. and Hammerstein J: The dianostic value of plasma free testosterone in nontumorous and tumorous hyperandrogenism, Fertil Steril 40:66, 1983.

Serafini P, Ablan R, and Lobo RA: 5α-Reductase activity in the genital skin of hirsute women, J Clin Endocrinol Metab 60:349, 1985.

Shoupe D and Lobo RA: Prolactin responses after gonadotropin releasing hormone in polycystic ovary syndrome, Fertil Steril 43:549, 1985.

Speiser PW, Dupont B, Rubenstein P, et al: High frequency of nonclassical steroid 21-hydroxylase deficiency, Am J Hum Genet 37:650, 1985.

Speiser PW, New MI, and White PC: Molecular genetic analysis of nonclassic steriod 21-hydroxylase deficiency associated with HLA-B14, DR1, N Engl J Med 319:19, 1988.

Van der Vange N, Kloosterboer HJ, & Haspels AA: Effect of seven low-dose combined oral contraceptive preparations on carbohydrate metabolism, Am J Obstet Gynecol 156:918, 1987.

Venturoli S, Fabbri R, Dal Prato L, et al: Ketoconazole therapy for women with acne and/or hirsutism, J Clin Endocrinol Metab 71:335, 1990.

Vigersky RA, Mehlman I, Glass AR, et al: Treatment of hirsute women with cimetidine, N Engl J Med 303:1042, 1980.

Wild RA, Umstot ES, Andersen RN, et al: Adrenal function in hirsutism. II. Effect of an oral contraceptive, J Clin Endocrinol Metab 54:676, 1981.

Williams IA, Shaw RW, and Burford G: An attempt to alter the pathophysiology of polycystic ovary syndrome using a gonadotrophin hormone releasing hormone agonist—nafarelin, Clin Endocrinol 31:345, 1989.

Wilroy RS Jr, Givens JR, Wiser WL, et al: Genetic forms of hypogonadism, Birth Defects 11(4), 1975.

Yen SSC: Chronic anovulation caused by peripheral endocrine disorders. In Yen SSC and Jaffe RB, editors: Reproductive endocrinology, ed 2, Philadelphia, 1986, WB Saunders Co.

Yen SSC, Chaney C, and Judd HL: Functional aberrations of the hypothalamic-pituitary system in polycystic ovary syndrome: a consideration of the pathogenesis. In James VHT, Serio M, and Guisti G, editors: The endocrine function of the human ovary, New York, 1976, Academic Press.

CHAPTER 39 — Infertility

KEY TERMS AND DEFINITIONS

Artificial Insemination. Method to place sperm in the female reproductive tract by means other than sexual intercourse. If the sperm are from the husband, the technique is called *artificial insemination husband* (AIH). If the sperm are from another man, the method has been called *artificial insemination donor* (AID). Other terms are donor insemination and therapeutic donor insemination (TDI).

Asthenospermia. Greater-than-normal incidence of sperm with decreased motility in semen analysis.

Azoospermia. Absence of sperm in the semen.

Clomiphene Citrate. Weak estrogenic compound given orally to induce ovulation in anovulatory women with a sufficient amount of circulating estrogen (>40 pg/ml).

Fecundability. Probability of conception occurring in a population of couples in a given period of time, usually 1 month.

Fimbrioplasty. Surgical technique of removing adhesions between fimbrial fronds of the partially occluded distal end of the oviduct.

Gamete Intrafallopian Transfer (GIFT). Placement of human ova and sperm into the distal end of the oviduct.

Hamster Egg Penetration Assay (Sperm Penetration Assay). Test of the fertilizing ability of human sperm based on penetration of zona-free hamster ova by the sperm.

Human Menopausal Gonadotrophin (HMG). Formulation made up of equal amounts of follicle-stimulating hormone (FSH) and luteinizing hormone (LH) derived from urine obtained from menopausal women. The injectable agent is used to stimulate follicular development.

Hysterosalpingogram (HSG). Fluoroscopic and x-ray visualization of the interior of the female upper genital tract after instillation of radiopaque dye.

Infertility. Inability of couples of reproductive age to establish a pregnancy by having sexual intercourse within a certain period of time, usually 1 year. Infertility is considered primary if the woman has never been pregnant and secondary if it occurs after one or more pregnancies.

In Vitro Fertilization. Fertilization of human ova by sperm in a laboratory environment.

Luteal Phase Deficiency (Inadequate Luteal Phase). Deficient progesterone secretion or action resulting in a lag of normal endometrial development.

Microsurgery. Operative technique using magnification and fine, nonreactive suture material. Fine electrocoagulation and saline irrigation are also used.

Oligozoospermia (Oligospermia). Presence of fewer than 20 million sperm per milliliter of semen.

Ovarian Hyperstimulation. Enlargement of many ovarian follicles causing gross enlargement of the ovary. It is sometimes accompanied by ascites and hemoconcentration.

Postcoital Test. Microscopic examination of the sperm present in a cervical mucus specimen obtained from a woman several hours after sexual intercourse.

Pronuclear Stage Tubal Transfer (PROST) or Zygote Intrafallopian Transfer (ZIFT). In vitro fertilization with transfer of the zygote to the oviducts by transabdominal cannulation.

Salpingitis Isthmica Nodosa. Diverticula of the endosalpinx in the muscularis of the isthmic portion of the oviduct.

Salpingolysis. Removal of adhesions attached to an oviduct that appears normal on gross inspection.

Salpingostomy. Surgical creation of a new opening of a completely occluded distal end of the oviduct.

Semen Analysis. Quantitation of various parameters of a semen specimen analyzed after liquefaction has occurred.

Spinnbarkeit. Property of elasticity (distensibility) of cervical mucus.

Teratozoospermia. Greater-than-normal (50%) incidence of abnormal forms of sperm in semen analysis.

Treatment-Independent Pregnancy. Infertile women conceiving without use of infertility therapy.

Tubal Embryo Transfer (TET) or Tubal Embryo Stage Transfer (TEST). Same as ZIFT, except additional incubation to embryo stage occurs before transfer to the oviducts.

Washed Intrauterine Insemination. Technique of separating sperm from the semen in an electrolyte solution and then placing the sperm directly into the uterine cavity.

The term *infertility* is generally used to indicate that a couple has a reduced capacity to conceive as compared with the mean capacity of the general population. In a group of normal fertile couples, the monthly conception rate, or fecundability, is about 20%. Couples with infertility are grouped into two categories: (1) those with low fecundability who are hypofertile and eventually are able to conceive without treatment and (2) those who are never able to conceive without therapy and are therefore sterile. Examples of the first group include couples whose male partner has oligospermia or female partner has mild endometriosis. Examples of the second group include couples with male partners who have azoospermia and those with female partners who have complete occlusion of the oviducts.

INCIDENCE OF INFERTILITY

Information from a national survey conducted by the National Center for Health Statistics in 1988 indicated that about 8.4% of all U.S. couples with wives in the reproductive age group, 15 to 44 years, were infertile. Thus in 1988 about 4.9 million married couples in the United States were infertile. About 2.2 million of these couples had no children and thus had primary infertility, whereas 2.7 million had

at least one child and thus had secondary infertility. Between 1965 and 1982 the incidence of primary infertility increased in the United States, probably because of an increased incidence of genital infection with gonorrhea and chlamydia, which produces tubal blockage. However, between 1982 and 1988 the incidence of primary infertility did not change. Nevertheless, because of an increased number of women in the reproductive age group between 1982 and 1988, there were many more infertile women in the United States in 1988 compared with 1982. It has been estimated that about one half of the couples with primary infertility and one fifth of those with secondary infertility seek medical treatment and that physician office visits for infertility services in the United States increased from about 600,000 in 1968 to about 1.6 million in 1984. Overall it is estimated about 2.3% of women of reproductive age, 1.26 million, seek advice or treatment for infertility in the United States each year.

INFERTILITY AND AGE

Data from both older and more recent studies indicate that the percentage of infertile couples increases with increasing age of the female partner. Analysis of data from three national surveys in the United States revealed that the percentage of presumably fertile married women not using contraception who failed to conceive in 1 year steadily increased from ages 25 to 44 (Table 39-1). Data from a study of presumably fertile nulliparous women married to

Portions of this chapter adapted from Mishell DR Jr, Davajan V, and Lobo RA, editors: Infertility, contraception and reproductive endocrinology, ed 3, Cambridge, Mass, 1991, Blackwell Scientific Publications.

TABLE 39-1

Percentage of Married Women Who Are Infertile, by Age, from Three National U.S. Surveys

Age	Infertile (%)
20-24	7.0
25-29	8.9
30-34	14.6
35-39	21.9
40-44	28.7

From Menken J, Trussell IJ, and Larsen U: Science 23:1389, 1986.

TABLE 39-2

Percentage of Pregnancy Rates by Age at 1 Year in Normal Women with Azoospermatic Husbands After Donor Insemination

Age	Pregnancy Rate (%)
<25	73.0
26-30	74.1
31-35	61.5
36-40	55.8

From Schwartz D and Mayaux MJ: N Engl J Med 306:404, 1982.

husbands with azoospermia who underwent donor artificial insemination revealed that the percentage who conceived after 12 cycles of insemination declined substantially after age 30 (Table 39-2). In general terms, about one in seven couples are infertile if the wife is 30 to 34 years of age, one in five are infertile if she is 35 to 40, and one in four are infertile if she is 40 to 44. Another way to interpret these data is to state that as compared with women aged 20 to 24, fertility is reduced by 6% in the next 5 years, by 14% when she is 30 to 34, by 31% when she is 35 to 39, and to a much greater extent after age 40.

Because human reproduction is an inefficient process, it takes time to become pregnant. Therefore, because a woman's reproductive life span is limited to a certain number of years, if couples intend to have children, they should be counseled to maximize the length of time during which they attempt to conceive. Because the percentage of couples with decreased rates of fecundability increases with age of the

female partner, couples should be informed that the probability of conception is substantially reduced by delaying childbearing until later in life. This reduction is caused by two factors: (1) the incidence of infertility increases with increasing age of the woman and (2) the total length of time during which conception is possible is less in older women. Because the occurrence of monthly ovulation decreases greatly after age 45, as a woman becomes older, a corresponding decrease occurs in the total duration of time during which she may conceive.

FECUNDABILITY

Analysis of data from presumably fertile couples who stop using contraception in order to conceive reveals that about only half the couples will conceive in 3 months, three fourths will conceive in 6 months, and by 1 year about 90% will have conceived (Figure 39-1). Statistical analysis of these data indicate that the normal monthly fecundability rate is about 0.2.

This information is extremely important when analyzing data concerning the results of various treatment methods applied to a group of infertile couples. This group includes those with hypofertility due to presumed causes (e.g., mild endometriosis) as well as those with idiopathic (unexplained) infertility. For example, Leridon and Spira estimated that if the mean fecundability of the population is 0.2, 14% of the couples will not have conceived after 12 months; during the following year, however, 69% of the nonsterile couples in this population will conceive without treatment (Table 39-3). Analysis of these statistical tables reveals that after 2 years of trying to conceive, about 4% of these couples will not have done so. Their mean fecundability is about 0.08, and 57% will conceive in the next year. Of the 2% still not pregnant at this time, 3 years after trying to conceive, the fecundability rate drops to about 0.06, 0.05, and 0.04 in the next 3 years, respectively. Thus in the fourth, fifth, and sixth years of attempting to conceive, 48%, 42%, and 37% of the nonpregnant women should conceive without treatment. Infertility is usually defined as inability to conceive in 1 year. When so defined, the group of infertile couples includes those who have difficulty in conceiving quickly (hypofertile) as well as those who will never be able to conceive (sterile).

In the past decade, several estimates have

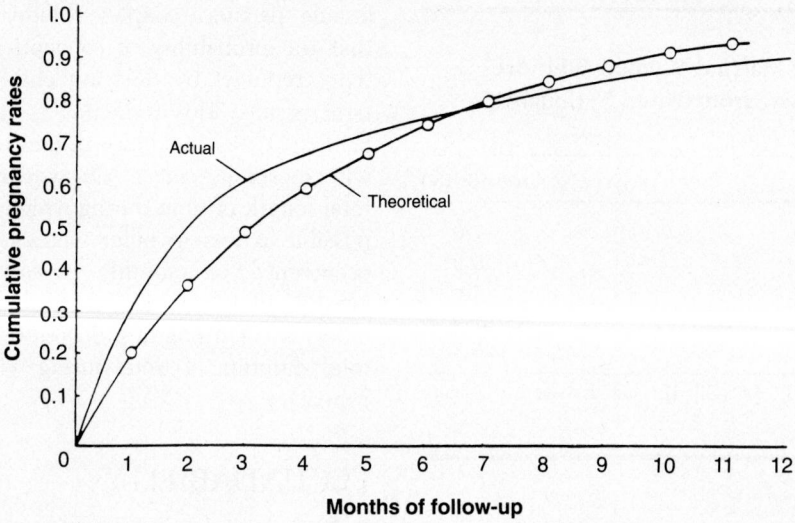

FIGURE 39-1

Curve of theoretic time to pregnancy in women with a monthly fecundability rate of 0.2 *(open circles)* and curve of actual time to pregnancy in fertile women discontinuing contraception *(solid line)*. (Open-circle data from Hull MGR, Glazener CMA, Kelly NJ, et al: Br Med J 291:1693, 1985; and solid-line data from Murray DL, Reich L, and Adashi EY: Fertil Steril 51:35, 1989.)

TABLE 39-3

Incidence of Conception Over Time Among Nonsterile Couples with Mean Fecundability of 0.2

No. of Months Without Conception	Proportion (%) of Couples Not Yet Having Conceived	Mean Fecundability of Couples Not Yet Having Conceived	Proportion (%) of Couples Who Will Conceive Within 12 Months Among Couples Not Yet Having Conceived
0	100.0	0.20	86.0
6	31.9	0.14	77.0
12	14.0	0.11	69.2
24	4.3	0.08	57.0
36	1.9	0.06	48.2
48	1.0	0.05	41.7
60	0.6	0.04	36.7

Adapted from Leridon H and Spira A: Fertil Steril 41:580, 1984.

been made of the actual incidence of infertile couples without diagnosed causes of infertility who will be able and unable to conceive over time without treatment. Four recently published long-term studies investigated fertility rates among couples with unexplained infertility of at least 1 year's duration who had not received any treatment. The evaluation consisted of documentation of ovulation, the presence of a normal semen analysis, and evidence of tubal patency. In three of the four studies, a normal postcoital test and normal laparoscopic evaluation of the pelvis were also present. Thus the five initial fundamental steps of the infertility evaluation were normal in the majority of these individuals. Pregnancy rates at the end of 2 to 7 years without any treatment ranged from 43% to 87% (Figure 39-2).

Thus, in order to determine that any method of treatment of infertility is superior to no treatment, statistical analysis of the treatment results on the incidence of pregnancy over time

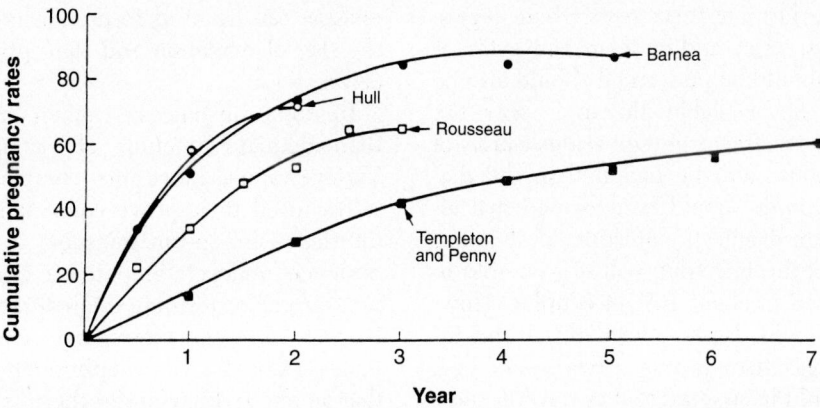

FIGURE 39-2
Pregnancy rates over time in untreated couples with normal basic (five-step) infertility investigation—results of four studies. (Adapted from Barnea ER, Holford TR, and McInnes DRA: Obstet Gynecol 66:24, 1985; Hull MGR, Glazener CMA, Kelly NJ, et al: Br Med J 291:1963, 1985; Rousseau S, Lora J, Lepage Y, and Van Campenhout J: Fertil Steril 40:768, 1983; and Templeton AA and Penney GC: Fertil Steril 37:175, 1982.)

needs to be performed. Ideally, these results should be compared with a nontreated control group. At the least, these pregnancy rates should be compared with the rates of the non-treated women reported in the four studies mentioned. Various statistical formulas for performing such analysis based on life-table analysis have been described. As stated by Cooke et al., this statistical approach is necessary to determine if treatment methods are indeed beneficial, since data from uncontrolled studies can be erroneous. These formulas provide techniques to determine the monthly probability of conception and the cumulative conception rate.

After using these techniques of analysis, therapy should be offered to the couple only if it is found that such therapy hastens the time in which conception will take place as compared with untreated controls or couples with a similar duration of infertility and a normal basic infertility evaluation. Furthermore, couples should be counseled that with sufficient time the likelihood of eventually conceiving without empiric treatment (and its associated expense) may be similar to that with use of such therapy.

CAUSES OF INFERTILITY

The exact incidence of the various factors causing infertility varies among different populations and cannot be precisely determined. In general, however, 10% to 15% of infertility results from anovulation; 30% to 40% is caused

by pelvic factors, such as adhesions from endometriosis or infection or tubal occlusion that interferes with normal ovum transport; about 30% to 40% is associated with abnormalities in the male reproductive system, which are associated with either oligozoospermia, high viscosity of semen, low sperm motility, or low volume of semen (male factor); and an additional 10% to 15% of infertility is associated with abnormal sperm–cervical mucus penetration (cervical factor). Whether other abnormalities, such as antisperm antibodies, luteal phase deficiency, subclinical genital infection, or subclinical endocrine abnormalities such as hypothyroidism, cause infertility has not been accurately determined. If any of these entities do cause infertility, they do so infrequently. With current techniques of investigation, it is impossible to diagnose the cause of infertility in about 10% of couples, and they are considered to have idiopathic or unexplained infertility. However, as explained earlier, most of these couples are hypofertile and eventually are able to conceive without treatment.

DIAGNOSTIC EVALUATION

The diagnostic evaluation of infertility should be thorough and completed as rapidly as possible. At the initial interview the various tests in the diagnostic evaluation and the reasons why they are performed should be thoroughly explained to the couple. In addition, the sequence of performing these tests, their degree of discomfort, cost, and time in the cycle at which they should be performed should also be discussed. The available therapies and the prognosis for treatment of the various causes of infertility should also be included in the dialogue. The couple should be informed that after a complete diagnostic infertility evaluation, the cause for the infertility will not be able to be determined in about 10% of couples. However, they should also be informed that this incidence is less than it was a few years ago. Couples should be assured that as new diagnostic tests are developed, physicians have the responsibility to make the new advances available to their patients.

Laboratory Tests

All patients should have a complete history taken, including a sexual history and physical examination. The initial laboratory tests should include a complete blood count, urine analysis, cervical cytology, and a fasting blood-glucose determination. Routine measurement of thyroid-stimulation hormone (TSH) and prolactin in asymptomatic patients at the time of the initial visit is not cost-effective. These tests are usually normal, and even if abnormalities are found in these tests in couples with regular ovulating cycles, they are not associated with infertility. Treatment with thyroid replacement therapy and bromocriptine has not been shown to increase the chance of conception in women with ovulatory cycles as compared with no therapy. Each couple should be instructed about the optimal time in the cycle for conception to occur and should be encouraged to have coitus on the day before ovulation.

Unless the husband has oligospermia, daily intercourse for 3 consecutive days at midcycle should be encouraged. Since the egg disintegrates within a few hours after it reaches the ampulla of the oviduct, it is best that sperm be present in this area when the egg arrives so that fertilization can occur. Sperm transport to the oviduct from the cervix normally occurs from 5 minutes to more than 1 day after coitus. Therefore coitus should occur before ovulation. Since the day of ovulation usually occurs 1 to 3 days after the basal body temperature (BBT) nadir, which cannot be determined prospectively, as well as 1 day after the day of the urinary luteinizing hormone (LH) peak, measurement of the urinary LH surge by rapid immu-

noassay can be used to predict more precisely the day of ovulation and the optimal time for coitus.

In some instances, women produce less-than-adequate amounts of vaginal lubricant. Various vaginal lubricants, chemicals as well as saliva, used to improve coital satisfaction may interfere with sperm transport. Some men experience midcycle impotence because of the pressure of performing intercourse on demand. In such cases the intercourse schedule should be less rigorous. The couple should also be told that among fertile couples there is only about a 20% chance of conceiving in each ovulatory cycle even with optimally timed coitus, and that it takes time to become pregnant. Thus the two terms *time* and *timing* should be emphasized during the initial counseling session. Couples should also be advised to cease smoking cigarettes and drinking caffeinated beverages, if they do so, since both cigarette smoking and possibly caffeine consumption have been shown independently to decrease the chances of conception.

Primary Evaluation

The five diagnostic steps to be followed in the workup of the infertile couple are best performed in the following order: (1) presumptive documentation of ovulation, (2) semen analysis, (3) fractional postcoital test, (4) hysterosalpingography, and (5) laparoscopy. These tests are most revealing when performed at certain times during the menstrual cycle. This initial infertility evaluation should be performed over 3 months and not prolonged unnecessarily. The following is a description of how and when to perform these tests.

Documentation of Ovulation

Preliminary information that the woman is ovulatory is provided by a history of regular menstrual cycles. If the woman is having regular menstrual cycles, a serum progesterone level should be measured in the midluteal phase to provide indirect evidence of ovulation as well as normal luteal function. Although in the normal luteal phase progesterone levels in blood vary in a pulsatile manner, a serum progesterone level above 10 ng/ml indicates adequate luteal function. Progesterone levels of 10 ng/ml or higher have been measured during at least 1 day of the luteal phase of normal ovula-

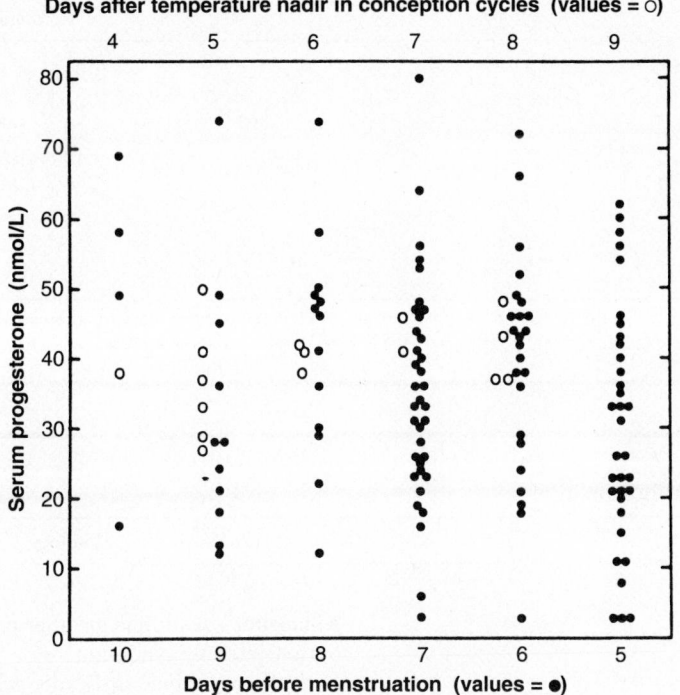

Days after temperature nadir in conception cycles (values = ○)

FIGURE 39-3

Midluteal serum progesterone concentration in untreated conception *(open circles)* and nonconception *(closed circles)* cycles related, respectively, to time elapsed since presumed ovulation or to time before the following menses. (1 ng/ml = 3.18 nmol/L.) (From Hull MGR, Savage PE, Bromham DR, et al: Fertil Steril 37:355, 1982.)

tory cycles in which conception occurred (Figure 39-3). Measurement of daily BBT also provides indirect evidence that ovulation has taken place. The BBT graph also provides information concerning the approximate day of ovulation and duration of the luteal phase.

Women with oligomenorrhea (menses at intervals of 35 days or longer) or amenorrhea who wish to conceive should be treated with agents that induce ovulation regardless of whether they have occasional ovulatory cycles. Therefore for such women direct or indirect measurement of progesterone is unnecessary until after therapy is initiated.

Semen Analysis

While information about ovulation is being obtained, the male partner's reproductive system should be evaluated by means of semen analysis. The male partner should be advised to abstain from coitus for 2 to 3 days before collection of the semen sample, because frequent ejaculation lowers the sperm count in some in-

dividuals. It is best to collect the specimen in a clear (not necessarily sterile), wide-mouthed jar after masturbation. It is important that the entire specimen be collected, because the initial fraction contains the greatest density of sperm. Ideally, collection should take place in the location where the analysis will be performed. The degree of sperm motility should be determined as soon as possible after liquefaction, which usually occurs 15 to 20 minutes after ejaculation. Sperm motility begins to decline 2 hours after ejaculation, and it is best to examine the specimen within this period. Semen should not be exposed to marked changes in temperature, and if collected at home during cold weather, the specimen should be kept warm during the trip to the laboratory.

Parameters of semen that should be evaluated include volume, viscosity, sperm density, sperm morphology, and sperm motility. The last parameter should be evaluated in terms of percent of total motile sperm as well as quality of motility (rapidity of movement and amount of progressive motility). There are no absolute

TABLE 39-4
Recommended Standards for Semen Analysis

Parameter	Recommended Normal Value
Volume	2.0 ml or more
pH	7.2–7.8
Sperm density	$\geq 20 \times 10^6$/ml
Total sperm count	$\geq 40 \times 10^6$/ml
Sperm motility	$\geq 50\%$ with progressive motility
Vital staining	$\geq 50\%$ live (exclude dye)
Sperm morphology	$\geq 50\%$ or more
White cell count	$< 10^6$/ml

Modified from Aitken RJ, Comhaire FH, Eliasson R, et al: WHO laboratory manual for the examination of human semen and semen–cervical mucus interaction, Cambridge, 1987, Cambridge University Press.

TABLE 39-5
Causes of Semen Abnormalities

Finding	Etiology
Abnormal count	
Azoospermia	Klinefelter's syndrome or other genetic disorders
	Sertoli-cell-only syndrome
	Seminiferous tubule or Leydig cell failure
	Hypogonadotrophic hypogonadism
	Ductal obstruction, including Young's syndrome
	Varicocele
	Exogenous factors
Oligozoospermia	Genetic disorder
	Endocrinopathies, including androgen receptor defects
	Varicocele and other anatomic disorders
	Maturation arrest
	Hypospermatogenesis
	Exogenous factors
Abnormal volume	
No ejaculate	Ductal obstruction
	Retrograde ejaculation
	Ejaculatory failure
	Hypogonadism
Low volume	Obstruction of ejaculatory ducts
	Absence of seminal vesicles and vas deferens
	Partial retrograde ejaculation
	Infection
High volume	Unknown factors
Abnormal motility	Immunologic factors
	Infection
	Varicocele
	Defects in sperm structure
	Metabolic or anatomic abnormalities of sperm
	Poor liquefaction of semen
Abnormal viscosity	Etiology unknown
Abnormal morphology	Varicocele
	Stress
	Infection
	Exogenous factors
	Unknown factors
Extraneous cells	Infection or inflammation
	Shedding of immature sperm

From Mishell DR Jr, Davajan V, and Lobo RA, editors: Infertility, contraception and reproductive endocrinology, ed 3, Cambridge, Mass, 1991, Blackwell Scientific Publications.

TABLE 39-6

Indications for Various Types
of Diagnostic Tests

Findings	Recommended Tests
Most patients	General laboratory evaluation
Sperm count <40 × 10⁶/ml	Endocrine evaluation
Sperm count <20 × 10⁶/ml	Genetic studies
Teratozoospermia	
Partner has recurrent abortion	
Sperm agglutination	Immunologic studies
Poor motility	Microbiologic studies
Poor cervical mucus penetration	
Inflammatory or red blood cells in semen	Bacteriologic studies

Modified from Eliasson R: Semen analysis and laboratory work-up. In Cockett ATK and Urry RL, editors: Male infertility: Work-up, treatment, and research, New York, 1977, Grune & Stratton.

standards for determining the normality of a semen sample, but recommended guidelines are shown in Table 39-4. It is beyond the scope of this text to fully discuss the etiology and diagnostic evaluation of men with semen abnormalities. The various etiologies of semen abnormalities are cited in Table 39-5, and the indications for performing the various types of additional diagnostic tests are listed in Table 39-6. However, as reported by Barratt et al., when semen analyses were performed on a group of men whose wives had conceived within the past 4 months, about 75% had at least one abnormal characteristic and 25% had two abnormalities (Table 39-7). These results indicate that there is normally a wide variability in the parameters used to characterize semen. Second, the criteria used to establish morphology may be too stringent. Third, it is probably more important to consider the number of abnormal parameters instead of an abnormality in a single parameter when interpreting a semen analysis. Finally, because the characteristics of semen analysis will vary over time, if an abnormality is found, it is best to repeat the test on two or three occasions at least a month apart.

TABLE 39-7

Semen Characteristics (Mean, Fifth, and 95th Percentiles)

Characteristic	No. of men	Mean	5th Percentile	95th Percentile
Density (×10⁶/ml)	48	73.0	6.0	194.0
Volume (ml)	49	3.1	1.0	7.0
pH	33	7.8	7.4	8.5
Motility (%)				
I	49	30.0	0.1	67.8
II	49	17.2	3.0	34.8
III	49	11.4	1.1	28.7
IV	49	36.0	11.2	87.4
Morphology (%)				
Ideal	44	53.3	18.0	80.6
Head defects	44	31.0	9.9	74.2
Midpiece defects	44	2.1	0.3	21.7
Tail defects	44	4.1	0.9	18.7
Total germinal cells (×10⁶/ml)	43	0.4	0.1	6.3
Total white blood cells (×10⁶/ml)	43	0.1	0.1	2.8
MAR (% positive)	42	1.4		
Viability (%)	39	76.0	18.2	82.4
Peroxidase-positive cells (%)	40	1.4	49.0	87.6

From Barratt CIR, Dunphy BC, Thomas EJ, and Cooke ID: Andrologia 20:264, 1988.

Postcoital Test

Although there are various in vitro tests to evaluate sperm–cervical mucus interaction, it is best to perform an in vivo postcoital test (PCT), as this is the only in vivo test that provides information from both partners. The quality and quantity of cervical mucus are optimal when there is maximal estrogen stimulation unopposed by any progesterone, and this hormone profile occurs on the day before ovulation. Therefore during the cycle in which the PCT is scheduled, the woman should measure her BBT daily to determine the approximate day of ovulation and ensure that the test is performed at the optimal time of the cycle. If the mucus is scanty or viscid, the test should be repeated every 2 days until there is a shift in the BBT. It is best to perform the PCT 2 to 3 hours after coitus, because as has been shown, the number of sperm in the mucus is maximal at this time.

Although various techniques have been described for performing postovulatory testing, the fractional PCT as described by Davajan is easily performed and interpreted. After the cervix has been cleansed with a saline-moistened sponge, the cervical mucus is aspirated through a portion of polyethylene tubing attached to a syringe. The tubing size should allow easy passage into the cervical canal, and the distal end should be beveled with scissors. The tubing should be stabilized by grasping it with an incompletely closed, large Allis clamp about 2.5 cm from the tip. As the tubing is advanced into the cervical canal, maintaining a constant negative pressure allows the mucus to be withdrawn into the tubing (Figure 39-4). After the level of the internal os is reached, the clamp is closed and the tubing slowly withdrawn from the cervical canal. The trailing edge of mucus is cut at the level of the external os, and the mucus in the tubing is taken for ex-

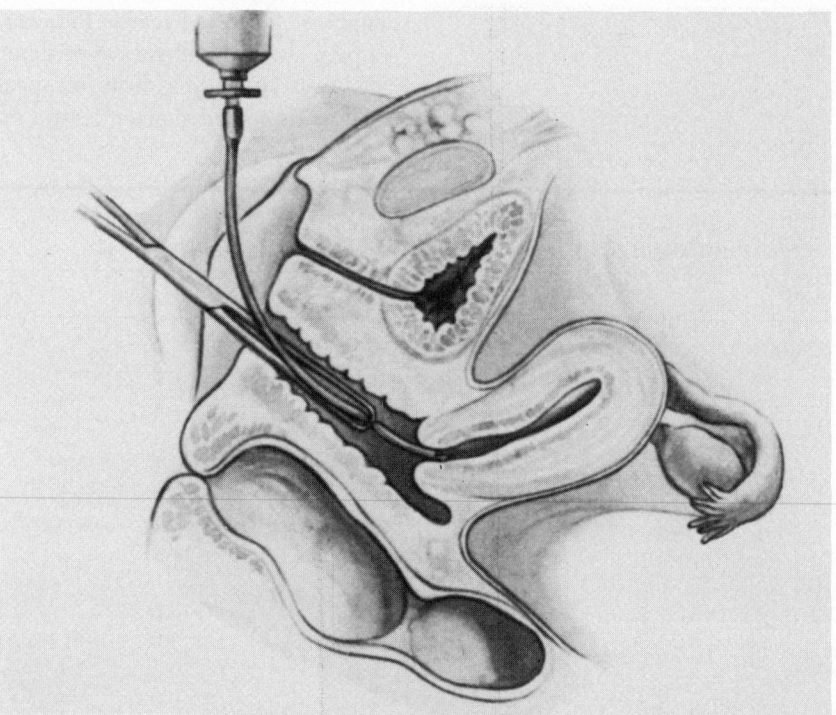

FIGURE 39-4
Syringe attached to polyethylene suction catheter is used in aspiration of cervical mucus. Tubing is stabilized by grasping it 2.5 cm from the distal end with a clamp. Handle of clamp should be adjusted so that when clamp is set at first ratchet, tube is partially but not totally occluded. Aspiration must be initiated just as tip of catheter is inserted into external os. (From Mishell DR Jr, Davajan V, and Lobo RA, editors: Infertility, contraception and reproductive endocrinology, ed 3, Cambridge, Mass, 1991, Blackwell Scientific Publications.)

amination (Figure 39-5). The tubing is then cut into three segments, and the mucus within the distal segment, representing the mucus at the internal os level, is placed on a slide, covered with a coverslip, and examined under low- and high-power ($\times 400$) magnification. A portion of the vaginal fluid should also be placed on a slide and examined to be certain that sperm were deposited in the vagina. The mucus from the proximal segment can be evaluated for spinnbarkeit and then dried to observe whether a fern leaf pattern is present.

Normal midcycle cervical mucus is clear and watery with a spinnbarkeit of at least 6 cm and a normal fern pattern. For a PCT result to be considered normal at least five motile sperm should be observed per high-power field in the mucus obtained from the level of the internal os. An abnormal PCT result can be due to anatomic defects of the cervix, abnormal cervical mucus, and abnormalities of the sperm in normal cervical mucus. The etiologies of these types of abnormal PCT results are listed in the box on the right.

Hysterosalpingogram

It is best to schedule the hysterosalpingogram (HSG) during the week following the end of menses to avoid irradiating a possible preg-

nancy. Before the procedure a bimanual pelvic examination should be performed, and if adnexal tenderness is present the procedure should be postponed until antibiotic therapy has been administered and the tenderness has

---

CAUSES OF ABNORMAL POSTCOITAL TEST RESULTS

Anatomic Defects

Cervical stenosis
Varicosities of hypoplastic endocervical canal

Abnormal Cervical Mucus

Poor quality
Low quantity

Abnormal PCT with Normal Cervical Mucus

Faulty coital technique
Vaginal factor or weak sperm factor
Oligospermia or low motility or both
Low semen volume
Immobilized sperm in endocervical canal
Large semen volume
Highly viscous semen

From Mishell DR Jr, Davajan V, and Lobo RA, editors: Infertility, contraception and reproductive endocrinology, ed 3, Cambridge, Mass, 1991, Blackwell Scientific Publications.

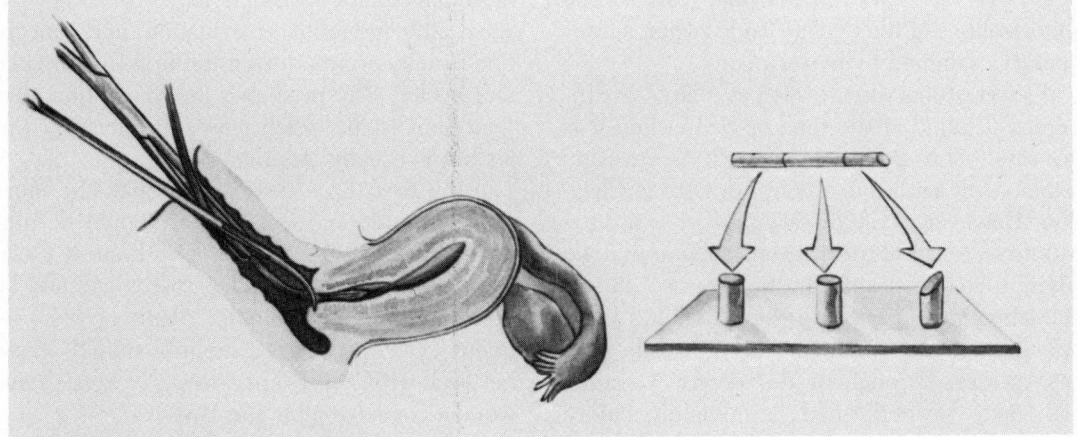

FIGURE 39-5
Catheter should be gently withdrawn and trailing mucus cut away with scissors. Catheter segment is then cut into three smaller segments. Distal segment (beveled end) contains mucus collected from internal os level, and most proximal segment contains mucus collected from level of external os. (From Mishell DR Jr, Davajan V, and Lobo RA, editors: Infertility, contraception and reproductive endocrinology, ed 3, Cambridge, Mass, 1991, Blackwell Scientific Publications.)

resolved. This technique reduces the risk of causing an episode of acute recurrent salpingitis. Some authorities recommend that antibiotic prophylaxis (such as doxycycline 100 mg twice a day for 5 days starting 2 days before the procedure) be given to all women who have an HSG. The examination should be performed with use of a water-soluble contrast medium and image-intensified fluoroscopy. A water-soluble contrast medium enables better visualization of the tubal mucosal folds and vaginal markings than does an oil-based medium. It is important to be able to evaluate the appearance of the intratubal architecture to determine the extent of damage to the oviduct. Although some studies have shown an increased pregnancy rate after use of an oil-based contrast medium, a recent randomized prospective study by Alper et al. has not confirmed this finding. The HSG not only will determine whether the tubes are patent but also, if disease is present, will help to determine the magnitude of the disease process as well as give information about the lining of the oviduct and uterine cavity that cannot be obtained by laparoscopic visualization. It can also determine whether salpingitis isthmica nodosa is present in the interstitial portion of the oviduct. The finding of a normal endometrial cavity at the time of HSG obviates the need for hysteroscopy. Fayes et al. reported that patients with infertility and a normal HSG had no abnormalities of the uterine cavity when subsequently examined by hysteroscopy.

If severe tubal disease such as a large hydrosalpinx is found at the time of HSG, then it is not essential to perform diagnostic laparoscopy if the couple wishes to attempt in vitro fertilization. However, if the disease process is not too extensive, surgical tubal reconstruction may be advised, and then a diagnostic laparoscopic examination should precede the scheduled tubal operation to determine the extent of the disease process throughout the pelvis. Laparoscopy may be performed immediately before laparotomy, or the two procedures can be performed separately to allow time to explain the prognosis of tubal surgery to the patient.

Diagnostic Laparoscopy

If the HSG reveals no abnormalities, the fifth step in the infertility evaluation—diagnostic laparoscopy—should be scheduled to take place in the follicular phase of a menstrual cycle to determine whether peritoneal or peritubal pelvic disease, such as endometriosis or pelvic adhesions, is present. At the time of laparoscopy following a normal HSG, neither a D&C (dilation and curettage) nor a hysteroscopy should be routinely performed. Neither procedure will provide additional information or therapy, and the curettage may further impede future fertility by producing intrauterine adhesions. At the time of laparoscopy, indigo carmine should be introduced through the cervix into the peritoneal cavity to confirm tubal patency. Performing the laparoscopy in the follicular phase of the cycle before maximal endometrial growth enables the dye to pass into the oviducts with less chance of obstruction.

• • •

If an abnormality is found in one of the first three noninvasive diagnostic procedures (documentation of ovulation, semen analysis, postcoital test), that abnormality should be treated before proceeding with the more costly and invasive procedures. For example, if the woman has oligomenorrhea and does not ovulate each month, after a semen analysis, ovulation should be induced with clomiphene citrate before performing the other diagnostic measures. Provided no other infertility factors are present, most anovulatory women (80% to 90%) conceive after induction of ovulation, and conception usually occurs during the first three ovulatory cycles. The prognosis for conception after treatment of the other causes of infertility varies but is usually less than 30%.

If the first three tests are normal, the more uncomfortable and costly HSG should be performed in the follicular phase of the next cycle. If the HSG is normal, a laparoscopy should be performed in the follicular phase of a subsequent cycle. At least 3 months should elapse between HSG and laparoscopy because some women conceive after the HSG.

Secondary Evaluation

If the results of all five tests just described are normal, the following additional laboratory procedures have been advocated by some to assist in determining the cause of the infertility: (6) immunologic test(s); (7) bacteriologic cultures of the cervical mucus and semen; (8)

measurement of serum TSH and prolactin; (9) luteal phase endometrial biopsy; and (10) hamster egg penetration test.

If abnormalities are discovered in any of the initial five steps of the infertility evaluation, treatment has been found to increase the incidence of pregnancy significantly as compared with no treatment, particularly anovulation or total tubal obstruction. Treatment of abnormalities found in the last five diagnostic steps has not been documented to be more effective than withholding therapy. Therefore the necessity and cost-effectiveness of performing these secondary tests and correcting the abnormalities found by them have not been demonstrated. Until it is demonstrated conclusively that treatment of abnormalities diagnosed in the last five steps of the infertility investigation results in a significantly better pregnancy rate than placebo or no treatment, the advisability of continuing the diagnostic evaluation beyond the first five steps remains uncertain.

PROGNOSIS

All infertile couples should be informed of the prognosis for curing their particular cause of infertility. The highest chance of conception occurs among couples in whom anovulation is the only abnormality, with substantially lower chances if other causes of infertility are diagnosed (Figure 39-6). Among a group of infertile couples with unexplained infertility who were followed for 2 years after the evaluation was completed, it was found that the chances of becoming pregnant were greater in women younger than 35 (about 75%) than in women older than 35 (50%) (Figure 39-7). In the same study the conception rate was much greater in couples who had tried to conceive for less than 3 years before evaluation (about 80%) than in those who had tried for 3 to 5 years (about 55%) or 5 years or longer (about 20%) (Figure 39-8). Among couples with unexplained infertility it is important to emphasize the principles of *time* and *timing*. In three of the four studies

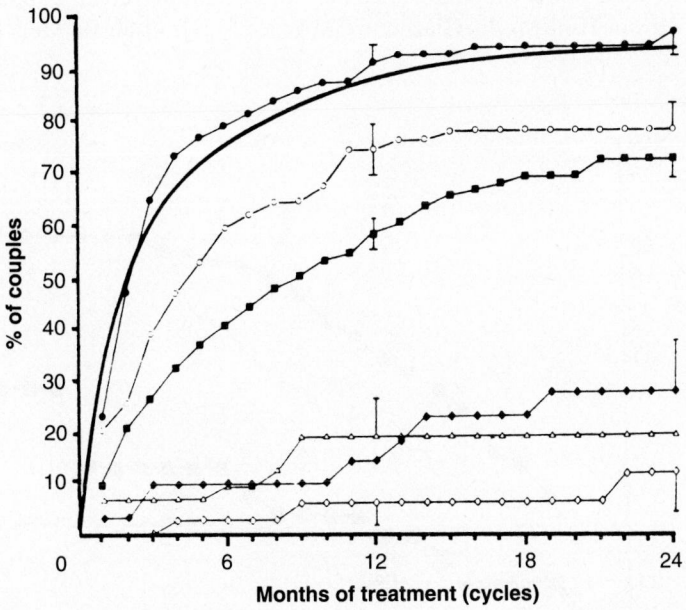

FIGURE 39-6
Cumulative rates of conception in couples with a single cause of infertility treated appropriately, excluding use of donor insemination or in vitro fertilization, as compared with normal rates (highest rates reported in couples with proved fertility). Rates for couples with each cause shown as *solid line,* normal; *solid circles,* amenorrhea; *open circles,* oligomenorrhea; *solid squares,* unexplained infertility; *open triangles,* tubal damage (moderate or severe); *solid triangles,* failure of sperm penetration of mucus (normal semen); *open squares,* oligospermia and failure to penetrate mucus. Standard errors of proportions are given at 12 and 24 months. (From Hull MGR, Glazener CMA, Kelly NJ, et al: Br Med J 291:1693, 1985.)

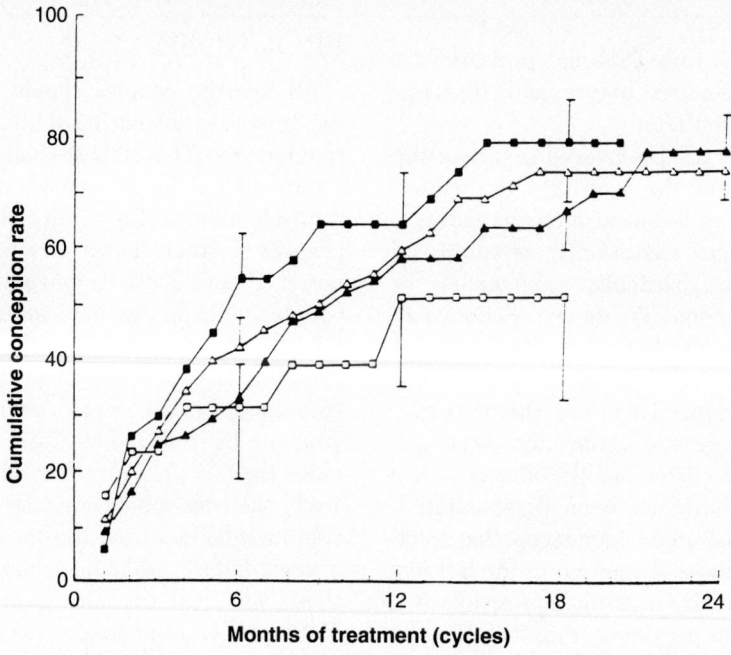

FIGURE 39-7
Cumulative rates of conception from first attendance at clinic in couples with unexplained infertility related to age of woman. Rates for each age group are shown as *solid squares*, <25 years; *open triangles*, 25-29 years; *solid triangles*, 30-34 years; *open squares*, ≥35 years. Standard errors of proportions are given at 6, 12, 18, and 24 months. (From Hull MGR, Glazener CMA, Kelly NJ, et al: Br Med J 291:1693, 1985.)

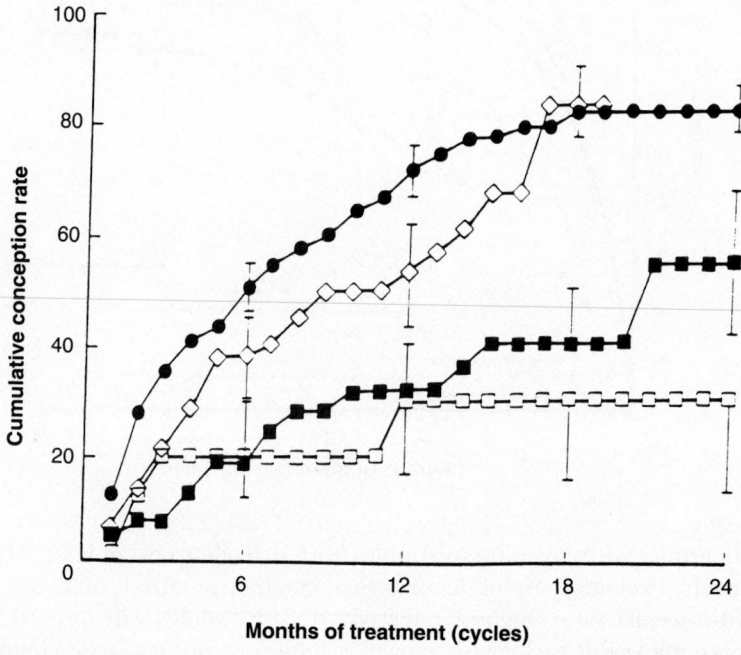

FIGURE 39-8
Cumulative rates of conception in couples with unexplained infertility related to duration of infertility at first attendance at clinic. Rates shown as *solid circles*, *1-2 years*; *open diamonds*, 2-3 years; *solid squares*, 3-5 years; *open squares*, ≥5 years. Standard errors of proportions are given at 6, 12, 18, and 24 months. (From Hull MGR, Glazener CMA, Kelly NJ, et al: Br Med J 291:1693, 1985.)

mentioned earlier, more than half the couples that eventually conceived did so in the first year after completing the infertility evaluation, and the vast majority of those who conceived, which was greater than 50% of the entire group, did so within 2 years. However, in the fourth study more than half the couples who conceived did so more than 2 years after their evaluation was complete (see Figure 39-2). Thus infertile couples with no demonstrable cause of infertility have a good prognosis for conception without treatment for about 2 years after laparoscopy is performed and the initial infertility evaluation is completed, but they have a relatively poor prognosis thereafter. To increase their chances of conception or to shorten the time interval until conception takes place, various treatment methods have been advocated.

Both *in vitro fertilization* (IVF) and *gamete intrafallopian transfer* (GIFT) have been used to treat couples with unexplained infertility. Although with each of these techniques monthly fecundability rates approach normal, 0.20, these methods are invasive, time consuming, costly, and uncomfortable.

Byrd et al. reported that treatment of women with unexplained infertility for up to six cycles with washed intrauterine insemination (IUI) resulted in a pregnancy rate of nearly 40%. Weiner et al. reported that stimulation of multiple follicles with human menopausal gonadotrophin (HMG) resulted in significantly higher pregnancy rates among couples with unexplained infertility than no treatment, and it compared favorably with the pregnancy rate after subsequent in vitro fertilization. Results of a large, double-blind, randomized prospective trial of treatment and no treatment in couples with unexplained infertility by Fisch et al. indicated that 4 consecutive months of clomiphene citrate therapy resulted in significantly greater pregnancy rates than no treatment. Thus both ovarian stimulation and washed IUI have resulted in greater pregnancy rates than no treatment during short time intervals.

There also have been studies in which a combination of superovulation and washed IUI has been used to treat couples with unexplained infertility. Dodson et al. reported that use of HMG and IUI resulted in a cycle fecundity rate of 0.19, similar to that of normal couples and similar to or greater than that of IVF or GIFT. Serhal et al. reported a per-cycle

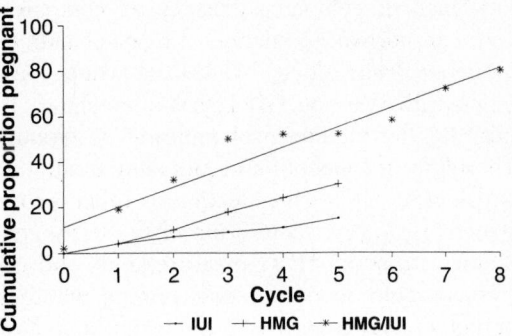

FIGURE 39-9
Overall cumulative proportion of pregnant patients comparing HMG, IUI, and combined HMG/IUI therapies. Life-table analysis was calculated by the method of Cramer et al., and the curves were fitted by computer analysis of the individual data points. (From Chaffkin LM, Nulsen JC, Luciano AA, and Metzger DA: Fertil Steril 55:252, 1991.)

pregnancy rate of 0.26 and Chaffkin et al. reported a cycle fecundity rate of 0.32 with the use of HMG plus washed IUI among 22 couples with unexplained infertility. This rate was significantly higher than that achieved with either HMG or washed IUI alone in the same studies (Figure 39-9). Their data indicate that for couples with a prolonged duration of idiopathic infertility, treatment with HMG plus washed IUI should be initiated to hasten the occurrence of conception. Gagliandi recently reported that the addition of a gonadotrophin-releasing hormone (GnRH) agonist to treatment with HMG and IUI for women with persistent infertility increased the pregnancy rate per cycle from 16% to 26.5%. Randomized prospective studies need to be done to determine whether this approach is as successful as IVF or GIFT, as well as to determine the incidence of pregnancy with either of these latter two techniques when 6 months of treatment with HMG plus IUI has not resulted in conception.

OUTCOME OF PREGNANCY

Several studies have followed the pregnancy outcome of women with longstanding infertility who conceive after treatment. The use of ovulation-inducing drugs as well as reconstructive tubal surgery have each independently been shown to be associated with an increased incidence of ectopic pregnancy as compared with the normal population. Use of ovulation-inducing drugs alone, as well as when combined with IVF and GIFT, has been shown to increase the incidence of multiple gestations. Therefore, if conception occurs after treatment with either ovulation induction or tubal reconstructive surgery, monitoring of the early gestation with serial HCG measurements and ultrasonography assists in determining whether or not the pregnancy is intrauterine and how many gestational sacs are present. Varma et al. reported that infertile couples who conceive do not have a higher rate of spontaneous abortion or perinatal mortality than occurs in normal couples.

MANAGEMENT OF THE CAUSES OF INFERTILITY

The management of the various causes of infertility will be presented in the order generally followed in an infertility investigation. Management of primary infertility factors are presented first, followed by management of secondary factors.

Anovulation

Therapeutic agents currently available to induce ovulation are clomiphene citrate, HMG, pure follicle-stimulating hormone (FSH) and GnRH. In addition, as discussed in Chapter 37, if anovulation is due to hyperprolactinemia, bromocriptine is an effective means to induce ovulation. Also, as noted in Chapter 38, women with congenital adrenal hyperplasia or anovulation accompanied by excessive production of adrenal androgens resulting from other causes can have ovulation induced by corticosteroid therapy.

Clomiphene Citrate

Clomiphene citrate is the pharmacologic agent of choice for women with oligomenorrhea as well as those with amenorrhea and evidence of sufficient ovarian follicular function to raise circulating estradiol levels above 40 pg/ml and thus have uterine withdrawal bleeding induced after progesterone administration. This synthetic, weak estrogen acts by competing with endogenous circulating estrogens for estrogen binding sites in the hypothalamus and blocking

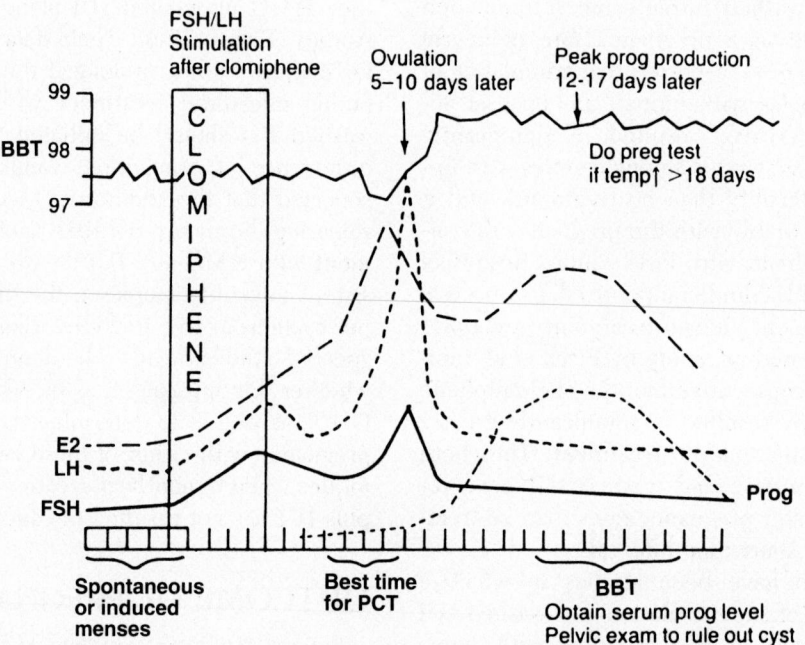

FIGURE 39-10
LH, FSH, estradiol (E_2), and progesterone *(prog)* levels before, during, and after successful treatment with clomiphene citrate. (From Mishell DR Jr, Davajan V, and Lobo RA, editors: Infertility, contraception and reproductive endocrinology, ed 3, Cambridge, Mass, 1991, Blackwell Scientific Publications.)

the negative feedback of endogenous estrogen. Thus GnRH is then released in a normal manner, stimulating FSH and LH, which in turn cause oocyte maturation with increased estradiol production. The drug is usually given daily for 5 days beginning 5 days after the onset of spontaneous menses or withdrawal bleeding induced with progesterone in oil or an oral progestin.

During the days the drug is ingested, serum levels of LH and FSH rise, accompanied by a steady increase in serum estradiol (Figure 39-10). Following ingestion of clomiphene, estradiol levels continue to increase, and the negative feedback on the hypothalamic-pituitary axis causes a decrease in FSH and LH, similar to the change seen in the late follicular phase of a normal ovulatory cycle. About 5 to 9 days (mean 7 days) after the last clomiphene tablet has been ingested, the exponentially rising level of estradiol from the dominant follicle has a positive feedback effect on the hypothalamus, producing a surge in LH and FSH, which usually results in ovulation and luteinization of the follicle.

Presumptive evidence of ovulation can be obtained by observation of a sustained rise in BBT or measurement of an elevation of serum progesterone. It is best to obtain the serum sample for progesterone measurement about 2 weeks after the last clomiphene tablet has been ingested, because this will usually be in the middle of the luteal phase, about 1 week after ovulation. A rise in serum progesterone level above 3 ng/ml correlates well with the finding of secretory endometrium on an endometrial biopsy sample, but Hull et al. have reported that maximal midluteal progesterone levels in clomiphene-induced ovulatory conception cycles are consistently above 15 ng/ml (Figure 39-11). These levels are higher than the 10 ng/ml found in spontaneous ovulatory conception cycles because following artificial ovulation induction, more than one follicle usually matures and undergoes luteinization.

Various treatment regimens have been advocated for the use of clomiphene citrate. Most start with an initial dosage of 50 mg per day for 5 days beginning on the fifth day of spontaneous or induced menses. If presumptive evidence of ovulation occurs with this dosage, clomiphene is continued in subsequent cycles until conception occurs. If ovulation fails to occur with the initial dosage, a sequential, graduated

dosage regimen has proven to be effective with a minimum of side effects. With this regimen if ovulation does not occur with the 50 mg dosage, the dosage of clomiphene is increased in the next treatment cycle to 100 mg per day for 5 days. If ovulation does not occur with 100 mg per day in subsequent cycles, the dosage is sequentially increased to 150 mg, 200 mg, and finally 250 mg for 5 days. If ovulation is induced with any of these dosages, the patient is maintained on her individualized ovulatory dosage until conception occurs. If ovulation does not occur with 250 mg, in the next cycle 250 mg is given daily for 5 days, and 1 week after the last tablet has been ingested, 5000 IU of human chorionic gonadotrophin (HCG) is given to increase the chances of inducing ovulation by simulating the LH surge. In the 10 years' experience reported by Gysler et al. about half the patients who ovulated and those who conceived did so following treatment with the 50 mg per day regimen, and an additional one fifth did so with the 100 mg per day dosage. However, about one fourth of all women who ovulated or conceived did so following treatment with a higher dosage regimen, indicating the value of the individualized sequential treatment regimen.

With this dosage regimen of clomiphene citrate more than 90% of women with oligomenorrhea and 66% with secondary amenorrhea and progesterone-induced withdrawal bleeding (estradiol levels of 40 pg/ml or higher) will have presumptive evidence of ovulation (Table 39-8). Although only about half the patients who ovulate with this treatment will conceive, Gysler et al. reported that 85% of those with no other causes of infertility conceived after such treatment. Hammond et al., by calculating the fecundability index, reported that if ovulation is induced with clomiphene citrate and no other causes of infertility are present, conception rates over time are similar to those of a normal fertile population who stop using barrier methods of contraception in order to conceive (Figure 39-12). Using life-table analysis these investigators reported that the monthly pregnancy rate (fecundability) of patients treated with clomiphene who had no other infertility factor was 22%, as compared with 25% calculated for women discontinuing diaphragm use. The monthly fecundability remained constant throughout treatment. Nearly all of the anovulatory women without other in-

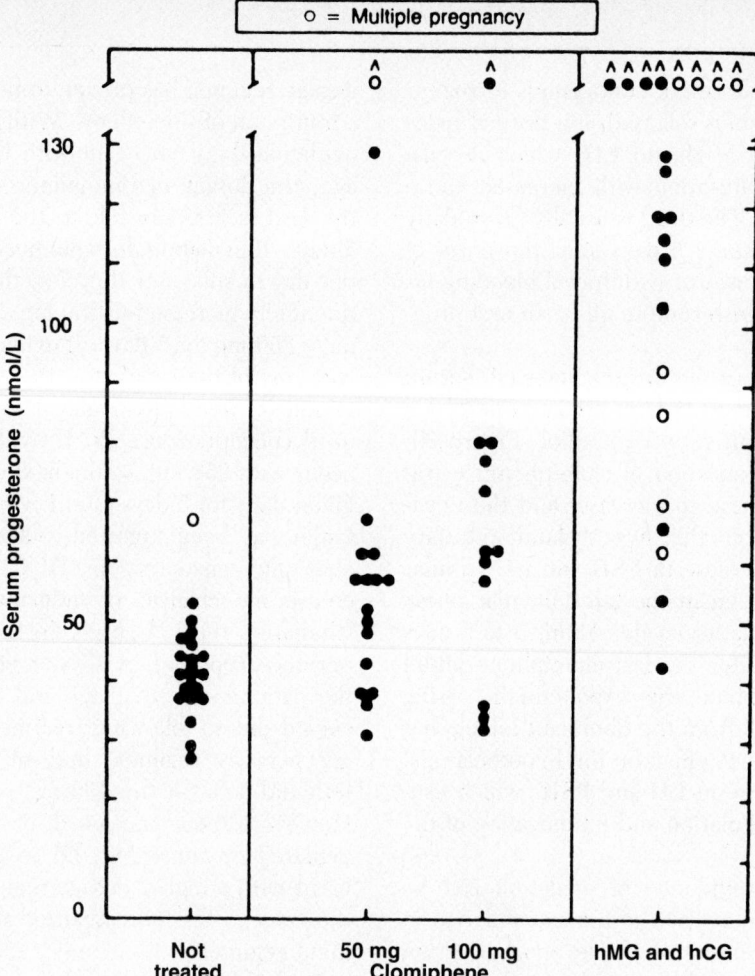

FIGURE 39-11

Midluteal serum progesterone concentration in conception cycles after treatment with clomiphene, in two different daily doses, or with gonadotrophins, compared with untreated conception cycles. (1 ng/ml = 3.18 nmol/L.) (From Hull MGR, Savage PE, Bromham DR, et al: Fertil Steril 37:355, 1982.)

TABLE 39-8

Response to Clomiphene Citrate

Category	Total	Ovulated		Conceived	
		No.	%	No.	%
Oligomenorrhea	330	307	93.0	157	51.1
Amenorrhea					
Polycystic ovary disease	29	18	62.1	12	66.7
Hypothalamic-pituitary dysfunction	39	30	76.9	9	30.0
Hypothalamic-pituitary failure	10	0	0	0	0
Amenorrhea/galactorrhea					
Progesterone (+)*	10	9	90	5	55.6
Progesterone (−)†	10	1	10	0	0
All amenorrheic patients	98	58	59.1	26	44.8
Total	428	365	85.3	183	50.1

Modified from Gysler M, March CM, Mishell DR Jr, et al: A decade's experience with an individualized clomiphene treatment regimen including its effect on the post-coital test, Fertil Steril 37:161, 1982.
*Withdrawal bleeding after intramuscular progesterone.
†No progesterone-induced uterine bleeding.

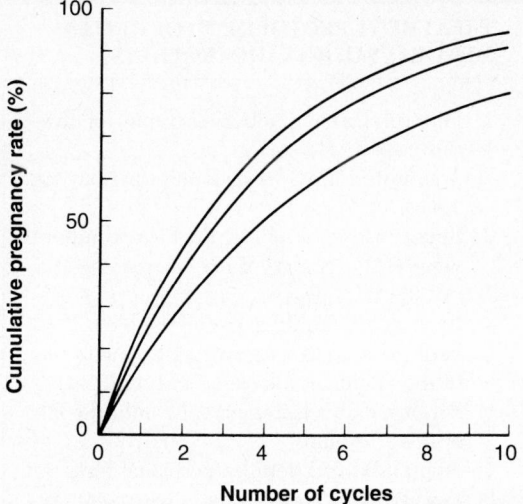

FIGURE 39-12
Cumulative pregnancy rates in patients undergoing ovulation induction as compared with patients discontinuing diaphragm use. Top curve: diaphragm (monthly fecundability = 0.247); middle curve: clomiphene, pure (monthly fecundability = 0.22); bottom curve: clomiphene, all (monthly fecundability = 0.157). (Modified from Hammond G, Halme JK, and Talbert LM: Obstet Gynecol 62:196, 1983.)

fertility factors in this series as well as other women with correctable infertility factors had conceived after 10 cycles of treatment. Therefore therapy should be continued for at least 10 to 12 cycles to improve the chance of conception. These data indicate that patient discontinuation of therapy is the major reason for the reported difference in ovulation and conception rates in anovulatory women treated with clomiphene. Clomiphene citrate does not itself cause infertility, as has been stated in some reports. If other causes of infertility are found, they should be treated and clomiphene continued.

When conception occurs after ovulation has been induced with this drug, the incidence of multiple gestation is increased to about 5%, with nearly all being twin gestations. The incidence of clinical spontaneous abortion ranges between 15% and 20%, similar to the rate in the general population. The rates of ectopic gestation, intrauterine fetal death, and congenital malformation are also not significantly increased. Animal data indicate that if the drug is given in high dosages during the time of embryogenesis, there is an increased incidence of

fetal anomalies. However, limited human data indicate that if the drug is ingested during the first 6 weeks after conception has occurred, the incidence of fetal malformation, although higher (5.1%) than normal, is not significantly increased. Although no definitive data show that the drug is teratogenic in humans, it is best that the woman be reexamined before each course of treatment to be certain that she is not pregnant. It is also important to determine that the ovaries have not become enlarged, because formation of ovarian cysts is the major side effect of clomiphene treatment.

If cysts are present, they will regress spontaneously without therapy, but if clomiphene is given and further gonadotrophin release is induced, stimulation and further enlargement of the cyst may occur. Clinically palpable ovarian cysts occur in about 5% of patients treated with clomiphene but in less than 1% of treatment cycles. The cysts usually range in size from 5 to 10 cm and do not require operation. Cysts can occur in any treatment cycle with any dosage, and the incidence is not increased with the higher dosages of drug. Recurrence of cyst formation with the same dosage is uncommon. Other side effects, which occur in less than 10% of women treated with this drug, include vasomotor flushes, blurring of vision, abdominal pain or bloating, urticaria, and a slight degree of hair loss.

About 5% to 10% of women treated with the individually graduated, sequential regimen of clomiphene citrate fail to ovulate with the highest dosage. Because treatment with HMG and GnRH is expensive and time consuming, other treatment regimens have been used with success. For the patient with evidence of adrenal hyperplasia as determined by the finding of an elevation of dehydroepiandrosterone sulfate (DHEA-S) (>2.8 mg/ml), Lobo et al. report an ovulation rate of approximately 50% when clomiphene is given after adrenal suppression has been achieved by administration of 0.5 mg dexamethasone nightly for 2 weeks. Withdrawal bleeding is then induced with 100 mg progesterone in oil given intramuscularly. Dexamethasone is continued nightly, and the high dose of clomiphene (250 mg per day) is given for 5 days, followed 1 week later by 5000 IU of HCG. In patients with normal DHEA-S levels, Lobo et al. reported that ovulation can sometimes be induced if clomiphene is given at a dosage of 250 mg per day for 8 days instead of

TABLE 39-9

Typical Overall Results After Clomiphene Citrate Therapy

Result	Percentage
Ovulation	
Oligomenorrhea	>90
Secondary amenorrhea	67
Pregnancy (overall)	50
Pregnancy (no other infertility factors)	85
Twins	5
Abortion	20
Other side effects	13
Teratogenicity	No increase

From Mishell DR Jr, Davajan V, and Lobo RA, editors: Infertility, contraception and reproductive endocrinology, ed 3, Cambridge, Mass, Blackwell Scientific Publications.

TREATMENT PROTOCOL WITH HUMAN MENOPAUSAL GONADOTROPHINS

1. Perform baseline ultrasonography of ovaries.
2. Administer HMG, two ampules per day for 3 days.
3. Repeat estradiol. If it is doubled, continue same HMG dosage; if not, increase HMG by 50% for 3 days.
4. Repeat step 3 until estradiol doubles.
5. Perform ovarian scan every 2 to 3 days until the dominant follicle is ≥14 mm.
6. Perform daily ultrasonography until the follicle is ≥16 mm.
7. Stop HMG and perform postcoital test.
8. Twenty-four hours later give 5000 IU HCG. If the PCT result is poor, use artificial insemination husband (AIH).
9. Administer 3000 IU HCG 7 days later if ovaries are not enlarged and not tender.

5 days, followed 1 week later by HCG. Others, such as O'Herlihy et al., have recommended that the higher dosage of clomiphene be administered daily until the diameter of the largest follicle measured by ultrasound reaches 1.8 cm, at which time HCG is given. The overall results achieved with clomiphene citrate therapy are shown in Table 39-9.

HMG and GnRH

Anovulatory women with adequate estrogen who fail to respond to these regimens, as well as amenorrheic women with low estrogen levels, need to be treated with either HMG or GnRH. Both these methods of ovulation induction are more complicated, time consuming, and expensive than treatment with clomiphene citrate. The incidence of side effects is greater and the type of side effect is more serious than occurs with clomiphene. These side effects include superovulation, multiple pregnancy, and the hyperstimulation syndrome, which includes ascites, pleural effusion, and possibly thrombosis secondary to hemoconcentration.

Because each patient responds individually to the dosage of HMG—even the same patient in different treatment cycles—it is essential to monitor treatment carefully with frequent measurement of estrogen levels and ovarian ultrasonography. Monitoring needs to take place daily, because there is little difference between the minimal degree of ovarian follicular development necessary to induce ovulation and the

amount of follicular development that results in hyperstimulation. When urinary estrogen alone was used to determine the optimal time to induce ovulation with HCG, a level between 50 and 100 μg per day was used, equivalent to serum estrogen levels of 500 to 1000 pg/ml. With ultrasound monitoring, HCG is administered when the follicle reaches a diameter of at least 1.6 cm. A treatment protocol for HMG monitoring is shown in the box above.

This regimen should be able to consistently induce ovulation with an overall pregnancy rate of about 60%. The pregnancy rate per cycle is similar to that following clomiphene therapy— 22%. Therefore, with sufficient duration of treatment and no other infertility factors, pregnancy rates should be greater than 90%. Lam et al. reported that the cumulative pregnancy rate after nine cycles of HMG therapy was 77%. The incidence of spontaneous abortion after HMG therapy is high (25% to 35%), and despite monitoring, clinically detectable ovarian enlargement occurs in about 5% to 10% of treatment cycles. There is no evidence of an increase in fetal malformation rates after HMG treatment.

Gonadotrophin-Releasing Hormone

An alternative to administration of HMG is GnRH treatment. Because continuous adminis-

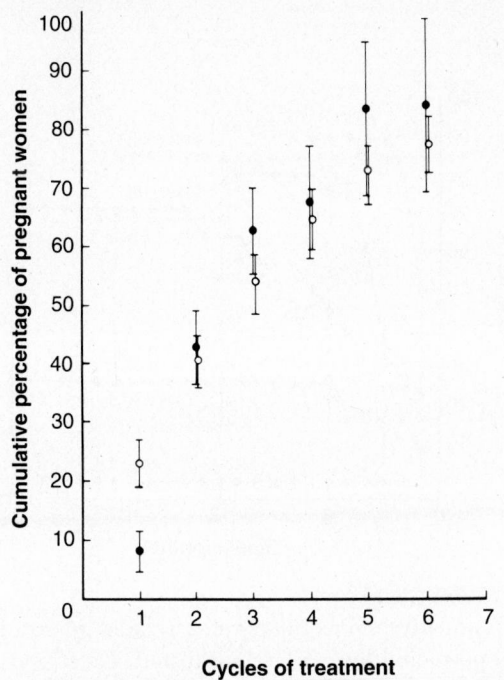

FIGURE 39-13
Comparison of therapy with gonadotrophin-releasing hormone (●) to that with human pituitary gonadotrophin (○) (mean ± SE). (From Kovacs GT, Phillips S, Healy DL, and Burger HG: Med J Aust 151:21, 1989.)

tration of GnRH will saturate the receptors and thus inhibit gonadotrophin release, GnRH should be administered in a pulsatile manner at intervals of 1 to 2 hours. Because GnRH is a peptide, it cannot be administered orally, and the two routes of administration in current use are intravenous and subcutaneous. A greater amount of drug must be administered by the subcutaneous route than by the intravenous route; however, the subcutaneous route avoids use of an intravenous catheter with its accompanying problems. The medication is administered by means of a small portable pump, which is usually worn attached to an article of clothing. Ovulation rates of about 75% to 85% per treatment cycle have been reported. Kovacs et al. and Bratt et al. administered pulsatile GnRH by subcutaneous route and intravenous route to 41 and 49 anovulatory women, respectively. Each reported that the conception rate per cycle of treatment was 22%. The cumulative pregnancy rate at the end of six cycles of treatment was 85% in the first study and 78% in the second. These pregnancy rates are similar to that reported with use of HMG (Fig-

ure 39-13). One advantage of GnRH is that hyperstimulation occurs less often with it than with HMG and therefore less monitoring is required. However, many women find wearing the pump, which is needed for intermittent pulsing, to be inconvenient. Therefore the patient can choose whether she wishes to receive HMG or GnRH.

• • •

In 1985 Hull et al. reported that of all the causes of infertility, treatment of anovulation results in the greatest success. In their study treatment of women with anovulation accompanied by amenorrhea (excluding ovarian failure) by one of the methods just discussed resulted in a 96% pregnancy rate after 2 years, with a fecundability curve nearly identical to the rates of normal fertile couples (see Figure 39-6). In a group of women with oligomenorrhea the 2-year pregnancy rate was 78%—significantly lower, mainly because of failure of ovulation induction in some women with polycystic ovarian syndrome. Newly developed gonadotrophin preparations that contain three to nine times as much FSH as LH have not proved to be more successful for such patients. However, pretreatment with GnRH analogues followed by either HMG or GnRH has resulted in higher pregnancy rates.

Fleming et al. reported that use of this combination treatment in women with polycystic ovaries who had not ovulated after treatment with clomiphene citrate or HMG resulted in a cumulative pregnancy rate of 77% after six cycles of treatment (Figure 39-14). Dodson et al. reported that in a small group of anovulatory women with polycystic ovaries use of HMG alone resulted in a cycle fecundity of 0.16, but with a GnRH agonist together with HMG the cycle fecundity was 0.27. Thus use of a GnRH agonist together with HMG may result in conception in those women with polycystic ovary syndrome who fail to respond to HMG alone.

Because these medications are expensive, partial ovarian destruction has been advocated by several groups of investigators to treat women with polycystic ovaries who do not ovulate with clomiphene citrate. Ovarian wedge resection was previously used to induce ovulation in those women before ovulatory-inducing drugs became available. However, severe postoperative adhesion formation often occurred, and this technique should no longer be used.

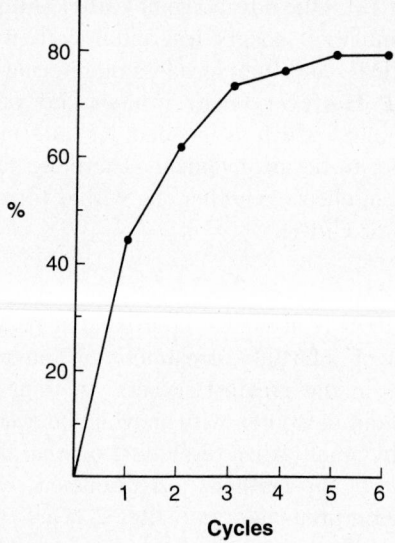

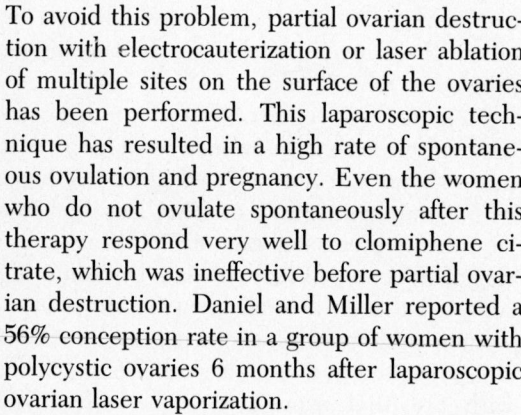

FIGURE 39-14
Cumulative pregnancy rates in patients with polycystic ovary syndrome receiving combined gonadotrophin and HMG therapy. (Modified from Fleming R, Haxton MJ, Hamilton MPR, et al: Am J Obstet Gynecol 159:376, 1988.)

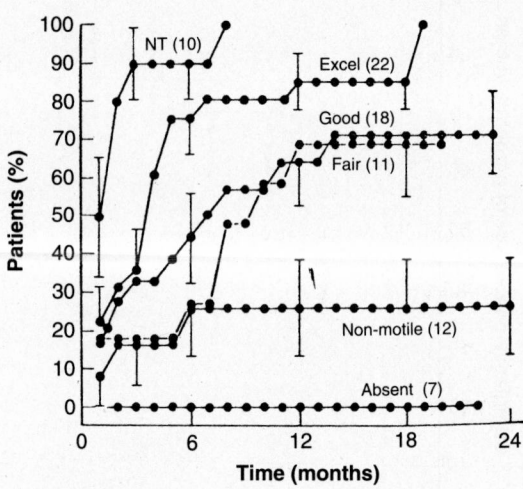

FIGURE 39-15
Cumulative conception rates related to result of postcoital test. *NT* = not tested. *Excel* = excellent. Standard error bars are shown. (From Hull MGR, Savage PE, and Bromham DR: Br J Obstet Gynecol 89:299, 1982.)

To avoid this problem, partial ovarian destruction with electrocauterization or laser ablation of multiple sites on the surface of the ovaries has been performed. This laparoscopic technique has resulted in a high rate of spontaneous ovulation and pregnancy. Even the women who do not ovulate spontaneously after this therapy respond very well to clomiphene citrate, which was ineffective before partial ovarian destruction. Daniel and Miller reported a 56% conception rate in a group of women with polycystic ovaries 6 months after laparoscopic ovarian laser vaporization.

Abnormal Postcoital Test

Although some authorities have questioned the clinical validity of the prognostic value of the PCT, a 1982 study by Hull et al. using life-table analysis demonstrated a highly significant difference in cumulative conception rates between couples with a normal PCT and couples with an abnormal PCT (Figure 39-15). At the end of 2 years, 84% of the couples with a normal PCT had conceived, but only 16% of the couples with an abnormal PCT had become pregnant. Eggert-Kruse et al. reported that pregnancy rates after 6 months with good

sperm cervical mucus penetration was 29.1% compared with only 2.3% in couples with a poor test. Thus an abnormal PCT, without treatment, represents a poor prognosis for conception.

Treatment initiated because of an abnormal PCT depends on the cause. If the amount of mucus is small or the mucus is not thin and watery with good spinnbarkeit, some success has been achieved by administration of low-dose estrogen (diethylstilbestrol [DES] 0.1 mg or estrone sulfate 0.3 mg) daily from day 5 of the cycle for 10 to 12 days. This problem can also be treated by means of intrauterine insemination of sperm following their separation from the semen by centrifugation, a technique called *washed intrauterine insemination*. If the mucus is adequate in amount and quality but no sperm are found in the semen, it is essential to determine that sperm are being deposited in the vagina. If they are not, sexual counseling is warranted. If sperm are found in the vagina but not in the mucus, or if sperm are found in the mucus but they are nonmotile or do not exhibit good forward motility, either cervical insemination with a plastic cup or washed intrauterine insemination should be performed. Intrauterine insemination is also of benefit to women

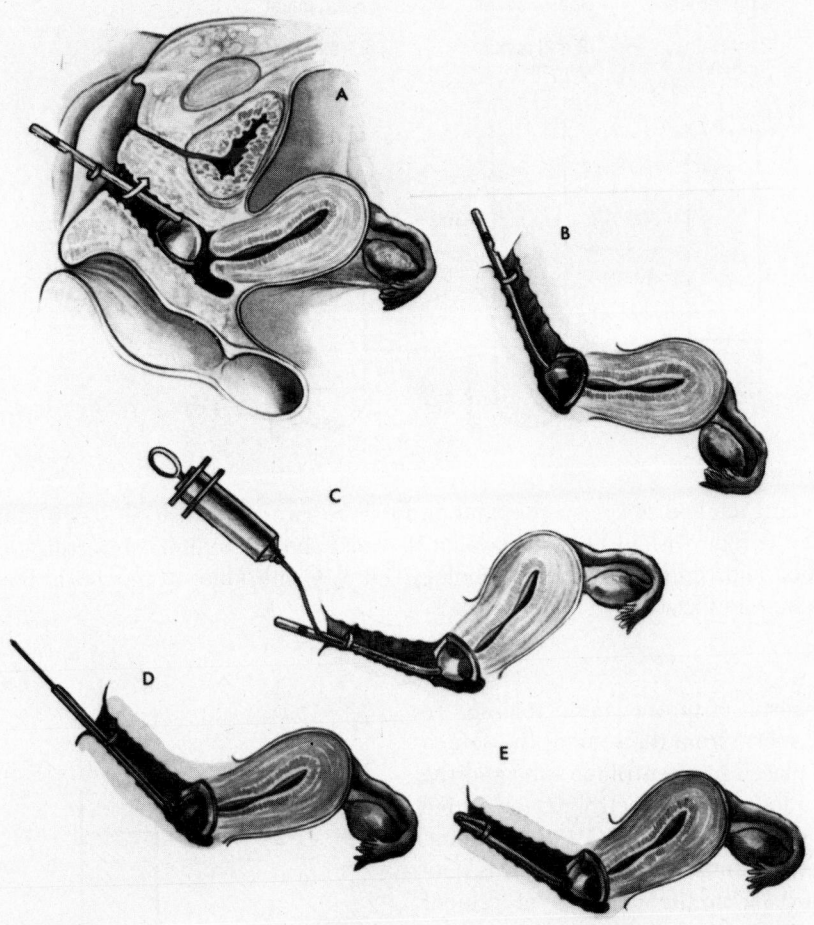

FIGURE 39-16

Use of Milex cervical cup for insemination. **A,** Before insertion of cervical cup into vagina, ball valve must be pushed past aperture to distal segment of stem. Cup is introduced into vagina with dome up. **B,** Cup is then turned 180 degrees and applied to cervix with dome pointing dorsally. **C,** Semen is injected through aperture in stem. **D,** After injection of semen, ball valve is pushed down stem to its junction with cup. **E,** Stem is folded into vagina. (From Mishell DR Jr, Davajan V, and Lobo RA, editors: Infertility, contraception and reproductive endocrinology, ed 3, Cambridge, Mass, 1991, Blackwell Scientific Publications.)

with cervical stenosis, such as that sometimes found following cervical conization. This technique is also useful for men with oligospermia or those whose volume of semen is small (<2 ml) or large (>8 ml) or whose semen has a high viscosity. Ideally, insemination should take place 1 or 2 days before ovulation. If timing is done by the calendar or BBT, it may be necessary to repeat the procedure at 2-day intervals until the BBT increases. Urinary LH enzyme-linked immunosorbent assay (ELISA) kits provide a more precise method to determine the optimal date to perform insemination.

The technique of cervical cup insemination with the husband's sperm is illustrated in Fig-

ure 39-16. The semen sample should be placed into the woman as soon as possible after it liquefies. The cup should be left on the cervix for 2 to 3 hours, after which the woman can remove it herself. Following the first cup insemination, another PCT should be done at the time the cup is removed to determine whether the technique has improved the mucus penetration by sperm. If improvement is observed, the insemination should be repeated in subsequent cycles until conception occurs.

The technique of washed intrauterine insemination allows insemination of only sperm into the uterine cavity. Intrauterine insemination of seminal fluid can produce severe uterine

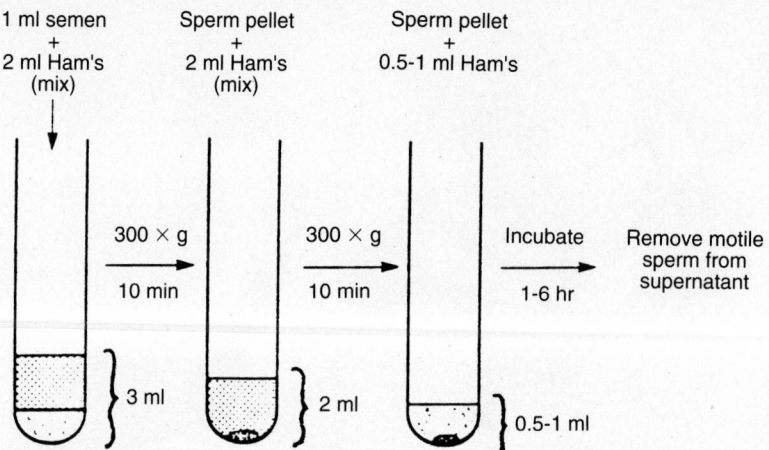

FIGURE 39-17
Standard method of sperm preparation for IVF: two-step wash plus swim-up technique. (From Mishell DR Jr, Davajan V, and Lobo RA, editors: Infertility, contraception and reproductive endocrinology, ed 3, Cambridge, Mass, 1991, Blackwell Scientific Publications.)

cramps as a result of prostaglandin release. To separate the sperm from the semen, the semen specimen is placed in a centrifuge tube and the volume is tripled with an electrolyte and amino acid solution such as Ham's F-10. After being mixed on a vortex mixer, the specimen is centrifuged twice, with the addition of diluent each time.

Various techniques are used to separate the sperm with the greatest motility from the remainder of sperm in the specimen, so that only the highest-quality sperm are used for insemination. Layering a solution of Ham's F-10 over the sperm pellet, incubating the mixture for a few hours, and inseminating the supernate (the swim-up technique) has been utilized (Figure 39-17). Separation of mobile sperm with various gradients such as Percoll or albumin has also been utilized (Figure 39-18).

McGovern et al. reported that the prognosis for pregnancy after intrauterine insemination was significantly greater if the original semen analysis had greater than 30% motility and after washing and swim-up there was a motility rate greater than 70%. Lalich et al. performed a life-table analysis of couples with cervical factor infertility treated with washed intrauterine insemination utilizing the swim-up technique. The cumulative pregnancy rate after six cycles of treatment was 29%, which increased to 43% after 12 cycles

Te Velde et al. compared the effect of natural intercourse and intrauterine insemination

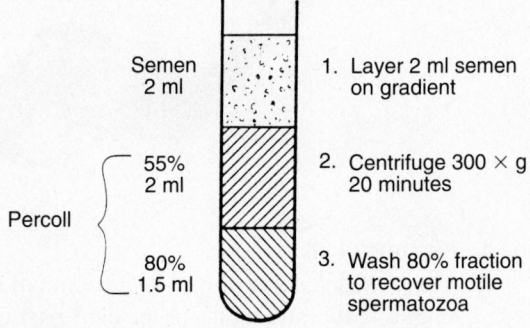

FIGURE 39-18
Percoll-column separation method of sperm preparation. (From Mishell DR Jr, Davajan V, and Lobo RA, editors: Infertility, contraception, and reproductive endocrinology, ed 3, Cambridge, Mass, 1991, Blackwell Scientific Publications.)

by alternating these technique in successive cycles in couples with a poor PCT. No woman conceived after natural intercourse, whereas conception occurred in 16% of cycles after washed intrauterine insemination was performed. This study establishes the benefit of this therapy in a randomized trial.

Male Factor Infertility

Most gynecologists who care for infertile couples should understand how to interpret a semen analysis as well as how to offer a prognosis for a disorder of abnormal semen. Although gynecologists usually do not perform a diagnostic evaluation or treat the male with a reproductive disorder, they should be able to provide counsel regarding the use of artificial insemination with either the husband's (AIH) or a donor's (AID) semen.

AIH has been used to treat oligospermia as well as abnormalities of semen volume or viscosity. Pregnancy rates following either cervical cup insemination or intrauterine insemination have been reported to be in the 25% to 35% range in various series. Cruz et al. reported that in a group of infertile couples whose male partner had oligoasthenospermia, the pregnancy ratio was significantly greater with intrauterine inseminations, 14.3%, than with intracervical inseminations, 2.0%, of their husband's semen.

In the study by Te Velde et al., however, in which natural intercourse was randomized with intrauterine insemination, in couples with male subfertility, the pregnancy rate per cycle was low and not significantly different with the two techniques, 2.7% and 2.2% per cycle. In the series of Lalich et al. only 6% of 55 women treated with washed intrauterine insemination of sperm conceived, for a cumulative pregnancy rate of only 0.095 after three cycles of treatment, increasing to only 0.167% after six cycles of treatment. However, in a study performed by Martinez et al., 4 of 24 couples with male factor infertility conceived after intrauterine insemination, and none conceived after timed intercourse. Thus the technique of IUI may offer some slight benefit for AIH.

Couples who fail to conceive with AIH because of azoospermia, oligospermia, or other semen abnormalities may elect to utilize donor semen insemination. The attitudes of both partners regarding AID and the stability of the marriage need to be thoroughly discussed before the procedure is performed. Donors must be carefully screened to be certain that they are in good health, do not have a potentially inherited disorder, and will not transmit an infectious agent in the semen. Thus laboratory screening for syphilis, serum hepatitis B, *Neisseria gonorrhoeae*, and *Chlamydia trachomatis* must be performed. Since cultures for the AIDS retrovirus (human immunodeficiency virus—HIV) may not become positive for 2 to 3 months after the disease has been acquired, some authorities recommend that only frozen

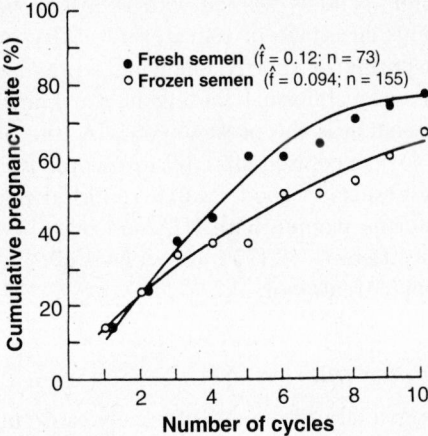

FIGURE 39-19
Cumulative fecundability curves for fresh or frozen semen (fresh: f = 0.12, n = 73; frozen: f = 0.094, n = 155). (From Hammond MG, Jordan S, and Sloan CS: Am J Obstet Gynecol 155:480, 1986.)

semen of at least 6 months' storage be used for AID, at which time an antibody test for the AIDS virus can be performed on the donor. A set of guidelines for semen donor insemination was published by the American Fertility Society. These guidelines provide information regarding indications for AID as well as suggested procedures for selection and screening of possible semen donors.

Most centers using frozen semen for insemination report that the pregnancy rate per cycle is less than with fresh semen; however, in the report by Hammond et al. only a slight, insignificantly decreased pregnancy rate was found with frozen semen. It should be noted that a 50% cumulative pregnancy rate was only reached after 6 months of treatment, and the monthly fecundity rate was only 9% (Figure 39-19). However, in the study by Gillett et al. the monthly fecundity rate was 18%, with a 45% cumulative pregnancy rate at 3 months. Thus the pregnancy rate with frozen sperm varies from center to center, and the couple should be appropriately counseled.

Uterine Causes of Infertility

Intrauterine Adhesions

In addition to menstrual abnormalities and recurrent abortion, some women may not be able to conceive because of the presence of intrauterine adhesions (IUA). As mentioned in

Chapter 15, most women with IUA have had a previous curettage of the uterine cavity, most often during or shortly following a pregnancy. If the only abnormal finding in the infertility investigation is the presence of IUA, the prognosis for conception after hysteroscopic lysis of the adhesions is good. March reported that of 69 infertile women with IUA and no other infertility factors, 52 (75%) conceived after hysteroscopic treatment.

Leiomyoma

Congenital uterine defects rarely cause infertility, and the uterine anomalies associated with maternal ingestion of DES have not been shown in randomized studies to be a cause of infertility. It is also difficult to assess the effect of leiomyomas on conception, since so many women with leiomyomas have no difficulty conceiving. Nevertheless, it is plausible that cervical myomas cause distortion of the endocervix, interfering with normal sperm transport, and that some submucous leiomyomas may interfere with sperm transport or normal implantation of the blastocyst. Large intrauterine leiomyomas can also occlude the interstitial portion of the oviduct and prevent normal sperm transport. If no other cause of infertility is found and myomas of moderate size and position that may interfere with sperm transport are found, then a myomectomy is justified. Malone and Ingersol reported that about half of 75 infertile women with myomas conceived after myomectomy.

Tuberculosis

If the HSG reveals findings consistent with pelvic tuberculosis, then endometrial biopsy and culture should be performed to confirm the diagnosis. The radiographic features of pelvic tuberculosis that are virtually diagnostic of the disease include (1) calcified lymph nodes or granulomas in the pelvis, (2) tubal obstruction in the distal isthmus or proximal ampulla, sometimes resulting in a "pipe-stem" configuration of the tube proximal to the obstruction, (3) multiple strictures along the course of the tube, (4) irregularity to the contour of the ampulla, and (5) deformity or obliteration of the endometrial cavity without a previous curettage (Figure 39-20). Appropriate chemotherapy should be initiated, but women with pelvic tu-

berculosis should be considered sterile, as pregnancies after chemotherapy are rare. Therefore no tubal reconstructive surgical procedures should be attempted.

Tubal Causes of Infertility

During the past decade the incidence of infertility caused by damage to the oviduct has increased because of an increased incidence of salpingitis. Obstructions occur at either the distal or proximal portion of the oviduct and sometimes in both regions. The prognosis for fertility after surgical tubal reconstruction depends on the amount of damage to the oviduct as well as the location of the obstruction. If there is extensive damage, the chances for conception after tubal reconstruction are almost nil. These women have a greater chance of conceiving with an in vitro fertilization procedure, and thus the extent and location of the intrinsic and extrinsic tubal disease must be ascertained by both hysterosalpingography and laparoscopy in an effort to determine whether tubal reconstruction or in vitro fertilization offers the better prognosis. If both proximal and distal obstructions of the oviduct exist, the damage to the oviduct is usually so extensive that the oviduct can never function normally. Therefore, although it is possible to achieve tubal patency after surgical repair of a tube with both proximal and distal blockage, subsequent intrauterine pregnancy is uncommon. Therefore, surgical reconstruction should not be performed in such instances.

Distal Tubal Disease

The HSG will determine whether the tubal obstruction is complete or partial, the size of the distal sacculation, and the appearance of the mucosal folds and rugal pattern of the endosalpinx (Figure 39-21). Laparoscopy will assist in determining the size of the hydrosalpinx, the amount of muscularis, and the thickness of the wall of the oviduct after distention with dye. Laparoscopic examination will determine whether pelvic adhesions are present and the extent of such adhesions. Women with fimbrial obstruction are not a homogeneous group, and the prognosis for intrauterine pregnancy following distal tubal reconstruction is related to the extent of the disease process. Therefore, it is important to perform both hysterosalpingog-

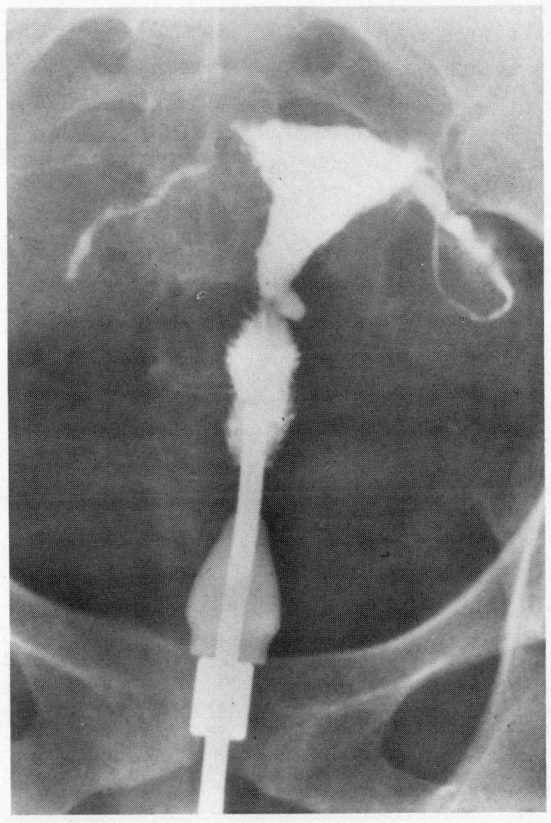

FIGURE 39-20
Tuberculous salpingitis in 37-year-old nulligravida with primary infertility for 15 years. Right tube is obstructed in zone of transition between isthmus and ampulla. Arrows indicate multiple strictures in both tubes. Nodular contour of endometrial cavity may also be related to tuberculosis and is analogous to pattern that has been found in ampulla in other cases. Small diverticulum near internal os probably represents adenomyosis. Diagnosis of tuberculosis was confirmed by endometrial culture. (From Mishell DR Jr, Davajan V, and Lobo RA, editors: Infertility, contraception and reproductive endocrinology, ed 3, Cambridge, Mass, 1991, Blackwell Scientific Publications.)

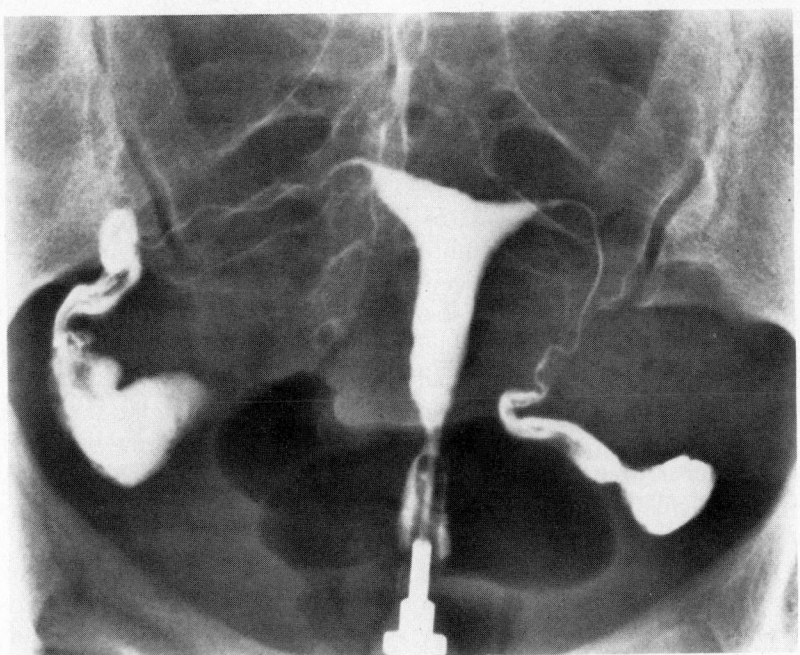

FIGURE 39-21
HSG showing bilateral hydrosalpinges with dilation, clubbing, and obstruction at fimbriated ends. Patient was 32-year-old woman with 10-year history of primary infertility. (From Mishell DR Jr, Davajan V, and Lobo RA, editors: Infertility, contraception and reproductive endocrinology, ed 3, Cambridge, Mass, 1991, Blackwell Scientific Publications.)

TABLE 39-10

Comparison of Pregnancy Outcome After Terminal Neosalpingostomy Using Careful Conventional Techniques (1978) Versus Microsurgical Techniques (1989)

	1978	1989
Mild	15	10
Pregnant*	13 (86)	7 (70)
Ectopic†	1 (7/8)	1 (10/14)
Moderate	30	29
Pregnant*	9 (30)	9 (31)
Ectopic†	4 (13/44)	4 (14/44)
Severe	42	56
Pregnant*	2 (5)	9 (16)
Ectopic†	0 (0/0)	2 (4/22)
Total	87	95
Pregnant*	24 (28)	26 (27)
Ectopic†	5 (6/21)	7 (7/27)

From Schlaff WD, Hassiakos DK, Damewood MD, and Rock JA: Fertil Steril 54:984, 1990.
*Values in parentheses are percentages.
†Values in parentheses are percentages of total patients in the category/percentages of only those patients in the category who became pregnant.

raphy and laparoscopy before surgical reconstruction to provide an individualized prognosis.

If the fimbriae of the distal end of the oviduct are relatively normal with only partial occlusion by adhesions or fimbrial bridges, removal of these adhesions by means of a fimbrioplasty procedure will result in higher conception rates (in the range of 60%) than if the distal end is completely occluded and a cuff salpingostomy procedure is required. Overall conception rates following salpingostomy are in the 30% range, with a high percentage (about one fourth) being tubal pregnancies, as reported by Schlaff et al. With the use of microsurgical techniques for the treatment of distal tubal disease the intrauterine pregnancy rate has not increased as compared with the results following conventional macrosurgery, but the rate of ectopic pregnancy appears to be somewhat greater following microsurgery (Table 39-10). The incidence of ectopic pregnancy after surgical reconstruction for distal tubal disease is directly related to the amount of tubal damage existing before the operative procedure.

Boer-Meisel et al. correlated the results of tubal reconstruction with the degree of tubal damage according to the severity of five factors: (1) extent of adhesions, (2) nature of adhesions, (3) diameter of the hydrosalpinx, (4) appearance of the endosalpinx, and (5) thickness of the tubal wall. Utilizing these criteria they developed three prognostic categories: good—with a cumulative pregnancy rate of about 75%; intermediate—about 20%; and poor—less than 5%. In the good category, only 1 of 22 pregnancies was ectopic, but in the intermediate group half the pregnancies were tubal, and in the poor prognostic group six of seven pregnancies were ectopic. They concluded that if there were fixed adhesions with absent rugal folds and a thick, fixed tubal wall, distal tubal operation should not be performed.

Donnez and Casanas-Roux classified the degree of distal tubal occlusion into four categories on the basis of hysterosalpingography (see Figure 39-22). Following microscopic tubal reconstruction the cumulative pregnancy rate was directly related to the degree of occlusion. If the distal tubal ostium was completely normal but peritubal adhesions were present, lysis of these adhesions by a procedure called salpingolysis resulted in a 64% intrauterine pregnancy rate, similar to that obtained with a fimbrioplasty for partial obstruction. About half the women who underwent salpingostomy for degree II occlusion conceived, with no ectopic pregnancies, but only about one fourth of those with degree III or IV occlusions had subsequent intrauterine pregnancies, and the ectopic pregnancy rate was about 10% (Figure 39-23 and Table 39-11). Thus following operation for more extensive distal tubal disease, nearly one third of the pregnancies that occurred were ectopic.

In both these studies the best prognostic factor was thickness of the tubal wall. If there was a hydrosalpinx greater than 2 cm in diameter with a thick tubal wall, the prognosis for a term pregnancy following distal tubal reconstruction was extremely poor. Hulka reported that when more than one half of the ovary was involved with adhesions, no patient had a term pregnancy following salpingostomy.

Rock et al. classified patients with distal fimbrial occlusion into three categories based on the extent of tubal disease (see the box on p. 1218). Schlaff et al. thus performed a life-table analysis of couples in these three categories with no other causes of infertility whose female

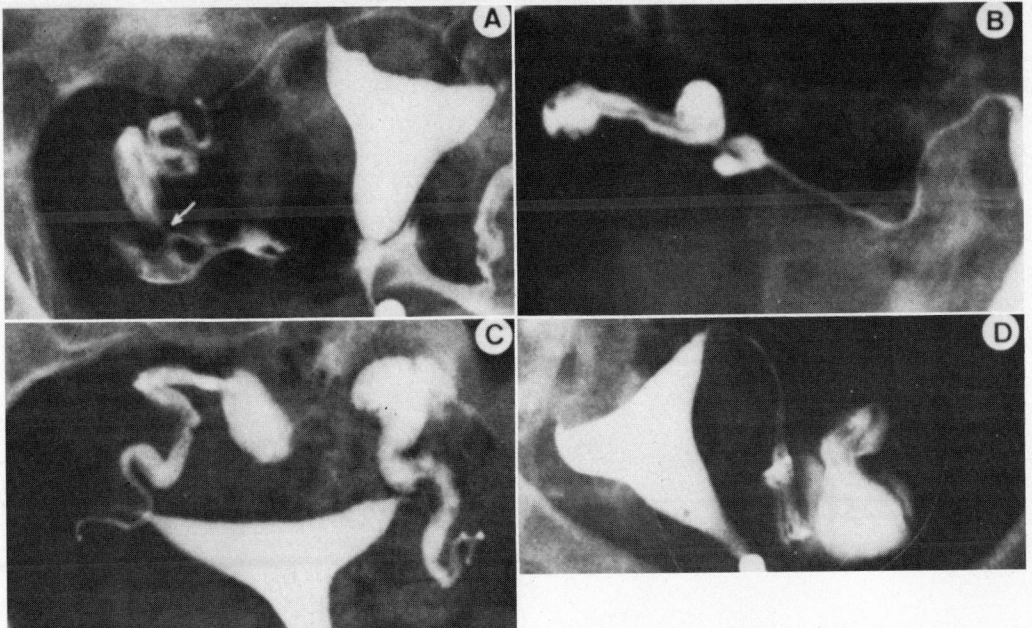

FIGURE 39-22

Classification of distal tubal occlusion based on degree of dilation seen on HSG. **A,** Degree I—conglutination of the fimbrial folds *(arrow)* with tubal patency. **B,** Degree II—complete distal occlusion with normal ampullary diameter. **C,** Degree III— complete distal occlusion with ampullary dilation 15 to 25 mm in diameter. **D,** Degree IV—occlusion with ampullary distension greater than 25 mm. (From Donnez J, and Casanas-Roux F: Fertil Steril 46:200, 1986.)

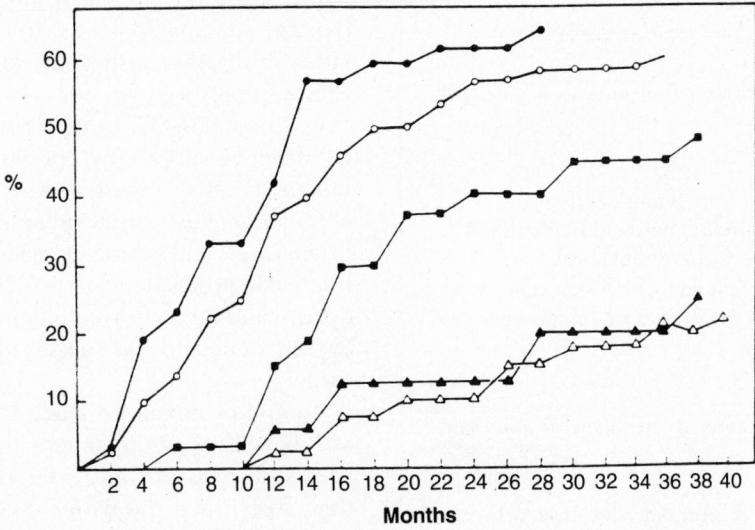

FIGURE 39-23

Classification of distal tubal disease based on the degree of dilation noted on HSG. **A,** Degree I—conglutination of the fimbrial folds *(arrow)* with tubal patency. **B,** Degree II—distal occlusion with normal ampullary diameter. **C,** Degree III—distal occlusion with ampullary dilation of 15 to 25 mm diameter. **D,** Degree IV— distal occlusion with dilation >25 mm. Cumulative pregnancy rates following microsurgical repair of these lesions are depicted in **E,** (● = salpingolysis; ○ = fimbrioplasty; ■ = salpingostomy (degree II); ▲ = salpingostomy (degree III); △ = salpingostomy (degree IV). (From Donnez J and Casanas-Roux F: Fertil Steril 46:200, 1986.)

TABLE 39-11

Pregnancy Rate After Microsurgery and Ciliated Cell Percentage in Cases of Distal Tubal Occlusion

Type of Operation	No. Patients	No. Intrauterine Pregnancies	No. Ectopic Pregnancies
Fimbrioplasty			
Occlusion of degree I	132	79 (60%)	2 (2%)
Salpingostomy			
Occlusion of degree II	27	13 (48%)	0
Occlusion of degree III	16	4 (25%)	1 (6%)
Occlusion of degree IV	40	9 (22%)	5 (12%)
TOTAL	83	26 (31%)	6 (7%)
Salpingolysis	42	27 (64%)	1 (2%)

Modified from Donnez J and Casanas-Roux F: Prognostic factors of fimbrial microsurgery, Fertil Steril 46:200, 1986.

CLASSIFICATION OF THE EXTENT OF TUBAL DISEASE WITH DISTAL FIMBRIAL OBSTRUCTION

Mild

Absent or small hydrosalpinx less than 15 mm diameter

Inverted fimbria easily recognized when patency achieved

No significant peritubal or periovarian adhesions

Preoperative hysterogram reveals a rugal pattern

Moderate

Hydrosalpinx 15 to 30 mm diameter

Fragments of fimbria not readily identified

Periovarian and/or peritubular adhesions without fixation, minimal cul-de-sac adhesions

Absence of a rugal pattern on preoperative hysterogram

Severe

Large hydrosalpinx greater than 30 mm diameter

No fimbria

Dense pelvic or adnexal adhesions with fixation of the ovary and tube to either the broad ligament, pelvic sidewall, omentum, and/or bowel

Obliteration of the cul-de-sac

Frozen pelvis (adhesion formation so dense that limits of organs are difficult to define)

From Rock JA, Katayama P, Martin EJ, et al: Obstet Gynecol 52:591, 1978.

partner underwent neosalpingostomy. They found that 80% of those women with mild tubal disease conceived, whereas only 31% of those with moderate disease and 16% of those with severe disease conceived (Figure 39-24). The ectopic pregnancy rate was higher in the latter two categories. Thus this information should be presented to the woman when she is counseled, and if the prognosis for term pregnancy is poor, she should be advised to undergo in vitro fertilization instead of surgical tubal reconstruction.

It is now possible to perform distal tubal reconstructive surgery by operative laparoscopy. Dubuisson et al. reported the results of a series of 65 consecutive distal tuboplasties, both fimbrioplasties and neosalpingostomies. The intrauterine pregnancy rate was 26% after fimbrioplasty and 29% after neosalpingostomy (Table 39-12), similar to the success rate after microsurgery.

An argument can be made that if the extent of tubal disease is so severe that it cannot be treated by laparoscopic surgery on an outpatient basis, then the patient should not have a laparotomy but be treated by one or more cycles of in vitro fertilization.

Proximal Tubal Blockage

If no dye reaches the oviduct during an HSG, the diagnosis of proximal tubal blockage should be considered. However, since spasm of the intrauterine portion of the oviduct can occur, the diagnosis should be confirmed during

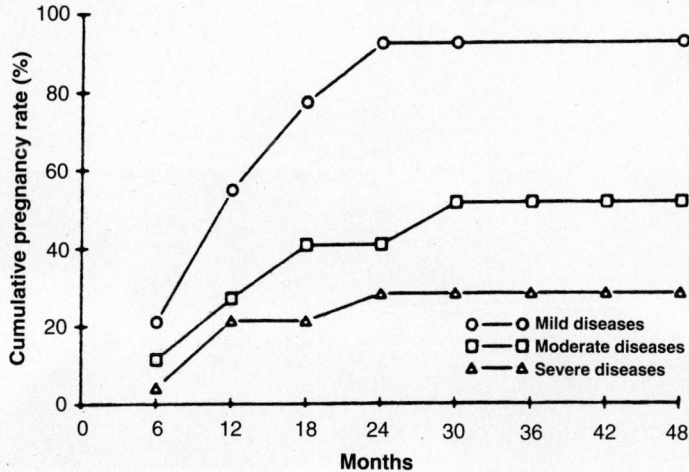

FIGURE 39-24

Life-table analysis of pregnancy outcome after neosalpingostomy by extent of disease. (From Schlaff WD, Hassiakos DK, Damewood MD, and Rock JA: Fertil Steril 54:984, 1990.)

TABLE 39-12
Reproductive Outcome After Distal Tuboplasties*

	Total	Fimbrioplasties	Neosalpingostomies
No. of patients	65	31	34
Total pregnancies	22 (33.8)†	11 (35.5)	11 (32.4)
Intrauterine pregnancies	18 (27.7)	8 (25.8)	10 (29.4)
Ectopic pregnancies	4±1‡ (7.7)	3±1‡	1

From Dubuisson JB, Bouquet de Joliniere J, Zubriot FX, et al: Fertil Steril 54:401, 1990.
*Follow-up of 18 months.
†Values in parentheses are percentages.
‡Abortion followed by ectopic pregnancy.

laparoscopy performed with the patient under general anesthesia. Laparoscopy also allows examination of the distal portion of the oviduct. Proximal tubal blockage is most commonly due to residual damage after infection, but it can occasionally be due to endometriosis. Frequently, tubal diverticula, also called salpingitis isthmica nodosa (SIN), are present.

Unlike the results of distal tubal reconstruction, the use of microsurgery has improved intrauterine rates for proximal tubal disease. Before the use of microsurgery, tubal intrauterine blockage was treated by reimplantation of the patent portion of the oviduct into the endometrial cavity. Term pregnancy rates following tubocornual implantation were in the 30%

range. This procedure has now been replaced by a microsurgical tubocornual reanastomosis procedure in which the diseased portion of oviduct is excised and the patent distal oviduct is reanastomosed to the portion of the interstitial segment of the oviduct that is patent. With this technique various authors have reported term pregnancy rates of about 50%, with ectopic pregnancy rates of less than 10%.

Donnez and Casanas-Roux reported that the pregnancy rate following tubocornual reanastomosis was related to the extent of preexisting disease as determined at the time of HSG (Figure 39-25). The best pregnancy rate—55%—was obtained when the interstitial portion of the oviduct was not damaged and less than 1.5

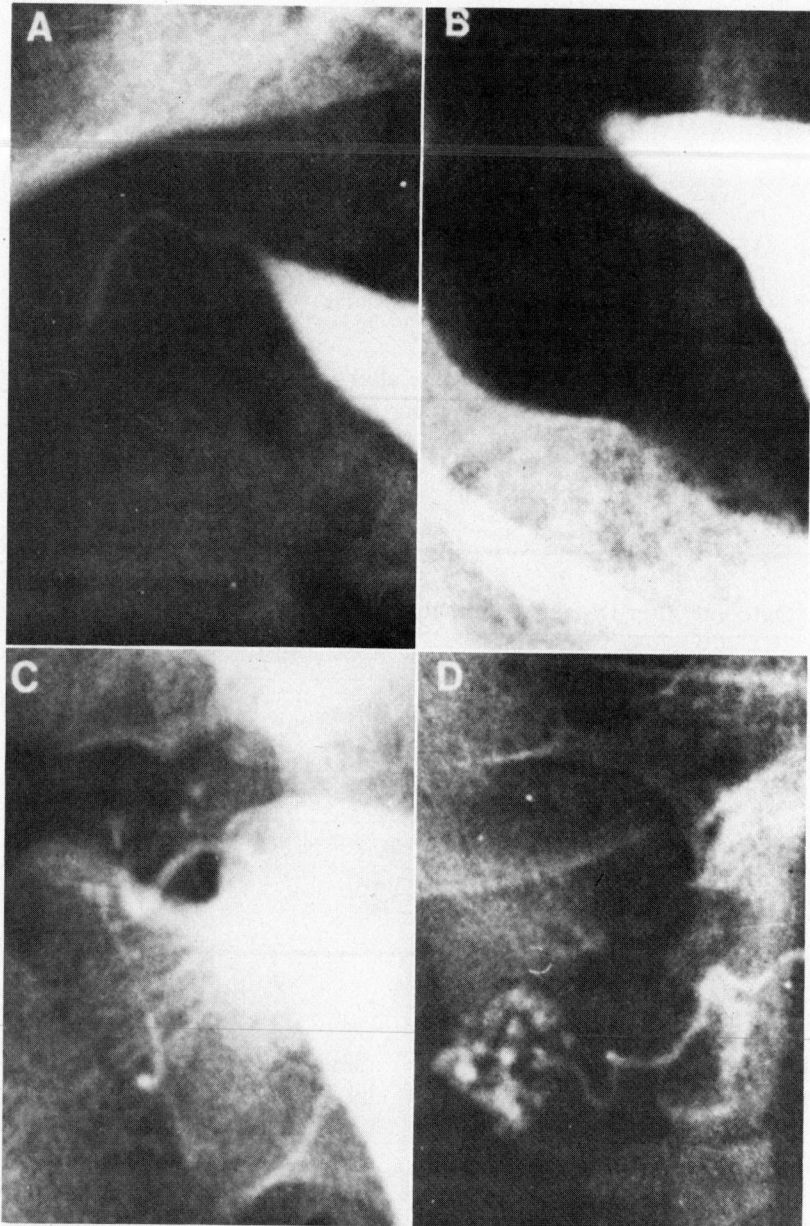

FIGURE 39-25
Types of occlusion following HSG. **A,** Undamaged intramural portion. **B,** Occluded intramural portion. **C,** Cornual occlusion with contrast extravasation in tubal wall. **D,** Occlusion with numerous diverticular lesions. (From Donnez J and Casanas-Roux F: Fertil Steril 46:1089, 1986.)

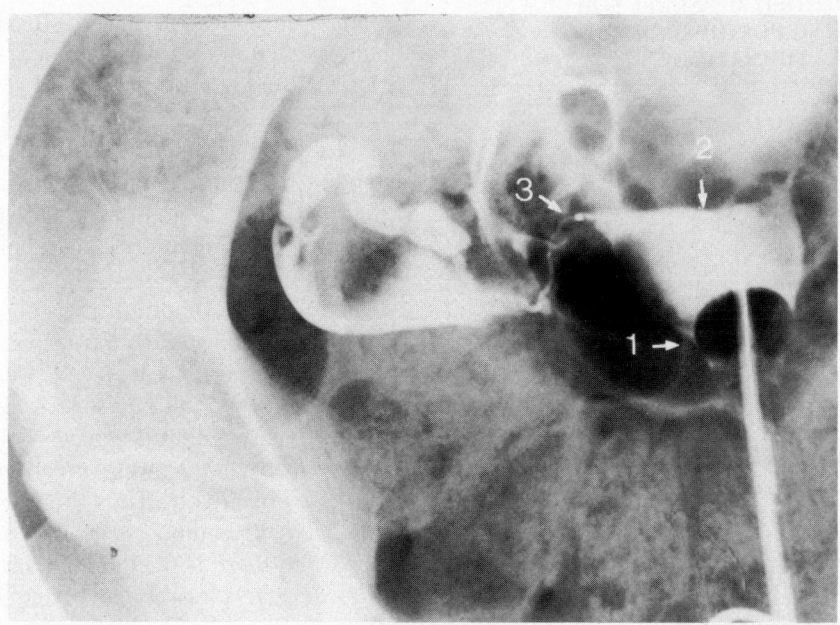

FIGURE 39-26
Hysterosalpingogram demonstrating transcervical balloon tuboplasty system in place following successful balloon dilation of a cornual occlusion. Two tandem balloons of the introductory catheter are inflated in lower uterine segment and in the endocervical canal (*1*). The selective salpingography catheter is wedged into the cornual angle (*2*). Balloon marker of the transcervical balloon tuboplasty catheter is shown (*3*). Injection of contrast medium through transcervical balloon tuboplasty catheter demonstrates tubal patency and peritoneal spillage. (From Confino E, Tur-Kaspa I, DeCherney A, et al: JAMA 264:2079, 1990.)

cm of occluded tube needed to be removed. The pregnancy rate declined to 33% when the interstitial portion of the tube was occluded and still further with the presence of some (25%) or numerous (16%) diverticular lesions. The overall ectopic pregnancy rate was 7%. Thus of patients who conceived, 15% had an ectopic pregnancy.

Several investigators have recently reported the results of treating proximal tubal obstruction by transcervically placed probes, catheters, or balloons, which are usually placed under fluoroscopic guidance in an outpatient setting (Figure 39-26). Preliminary results reveal that this outpatient procedure, provided it is performed by well-trained capable individuals, yields patency and pregnancy rates similar to those achieved by microsurgical reanastomosis, which requires a laparotomy. When sufficient individuals are trained in the technique of transvaginal tubal catheterization, this technique will become the treatment of choice for proximal tubal obstruction.

Adjunctive Therapy

Adjunctive procedures for surgical tubal reconstruction include prophylactic antibiotics, postoperative hydrotubation, placement of tubal stents, and methods to reduce postoperative adhesion formation, such as intraoperative instillation of high-molecular-weight dextran, heparin corticosteroids, or combinations of these, as well as systemic postoperative corticosteroid treatment. No prospective studies have shown postoperative hydrotubation to be of value, and tubal stents should not be used because they may cause mucosal damage. Intraperitoneal dextran is widely used, and some studies indicate that it may reduce adhesion formation. No randomized studies have shown that prophylactic antibiotic treatment or postoperative corticosteroid treatment is of any value, but each is widely used. Jansen et al., in separate randomized prospective studies, reported that intraperitoneal dilute heparin, dextran, and corticosteroids were of no value in reducing adhesion formation. Some preliminary

RECOMMENDED MEASURES FOR PREVENTING POSTOPERATIVE ADHESION FORMATION

Minimize Tissue Injury

Moisten tissues; use constant irrigation
Avoid clamping and coagulating
Limit abdominal packing
Use tapered needles
Employ magnification (microscope or loupes)

Decrease Inflammation

Use fine-caliber, nonreactive sutures
Administer prophylactic antibiotics
Minimize suturing

Prevent Raw Surface Apposition and Fibrin Deposition (efficacy unproven)

Intraperitoneal dextran 70
Oxidized cellulose
Heparinized lactated Ringer's irrigants

Extirpate Existing Adhesions

From Sauer MV: Tubal surgery. In Mishell DR Jr, Davajan V, and Lobo RA, editors: Infertility, contraception and reproductive endocrinology, ed 3, Cambridge, Mass, 1991, Blackwell Scientific Publications.

data indicate that oxidized cellulose may be of value in reducing adhesion formation postoperatively. Probably the most important way to reduce adhesion formation is meticulous surgical technique, including atraumatic tissue handling and small-caliber, nonreactive suture method. Continuous irrigation throughout the surgical procedure keeps the serosa moist and should retard adhesion formation (see the box above).

Tulandi et al., in a randomized prospective study, demonstrated that second-look laparoscopy 1 year after failure of terminal salpingostomy or salpingo-ovariolysis was not beneficial in achieving higher pregnancy rates. The benefit of second-look laparoscopy performed within a few weeks or months after tubal reconstructive surgery has also not been demonstrated in a prospective randomized trial. Thus a second-look laparoscopy after tubal reconstructive surgery is not cost-effective.

Conception should not be attempted for 8 weeks after tubal reconstruction. If pregnancy does not occur within 6 to 12 months, another HSG should be performed. If tubal obstruction has recurred, a repeat surgical procedure is not advised because pregnancy rates are less than 10%.

Endometriosis

Some investigators have estimated that as many as 40% of infertile women have endometriosis. If endometriosis is found at the time of laparoscopy, the extent of the disease should be classified according to the stages recommended by the American Fertility Society (Figure 39-27). The etiology, diagnosis, and treatment of endometriosis are presented in detail in Chapter 18.

Olive et al. reported that about 65% of women with mild endometriosis and no other cause of infertility conceived without treatment. With moderate or severe disease these authors reported that pregnancy rates with expectant management were much lower—25% and 0%, respectively. Thus the causal relationship between endometriosis and infertility is clear when there is moderate or severe disease with extensive adhesions involving the oviducts and interfering with their normal motility. However, evidence showing that minimal or mild endometriosis is a cause of infertility, instead of a result of not being pregnant, has not been established.

Mild Endometriosis

It has been postulated that there is an increase in intraperitoneal macrophages in women with mild endometriosis, and these cells may enter the lumen of the oviducts and phagocytose sperm. However, medical or surgical treatment of mild endometriosis does not result in significantly increased pregnancy rates as compared with no treatment. Overall pregnancy rates for women with mild endometriosis, with or without treatment, are in the 60% to 75% range. In a prospective randomized study, Bayer et al. reported that the pregnancy rate of a group of women with mild endometriosis was not increased following a course of danazol therapy as compared with those receiving no medical treatment (Figure 39-28). Schenken and Malinak as well as Garcia and David reported that pregnancy rates following conservative surgical treatment of mild endometriosis were nearly identical to the rates of groups of women in the same institution who had no surgical corrective treatment. These studies indicate that mild endometriosis most likely is not a cause of infertility, and there is no proven efficacy of therapy. Endometriosis may be a result of infertility, and women with

Patient's Name _____ Date_____

Laparoscopy_____ Laparotomy_____ Photography_____
Recommended Treatment_____
_____
Prognosis_____

Stage I (Minimal) - 1-5
Stage II (Mild) - 6-15
Stage III (Moderate) - 16-40
Stage IV (Severe) - >40
Total_____

PERITONEUM	ENDOMETRIOSIS	<1cm	1-3cm	>3cm
	Superficial	1	2	4
	Deep	2	4	6
OVARY	R Superficial	1	2	4
	Deep	4	16	20
	L Superficial	1	2	4
	Deep	4	16	20

POSTERIOR CULDESAC OBLITERATION	Partial	Complete
	4	40

	ADHESIONS	<1/3 Enclosure	1/3-2/3 Enclosure	>2/3 Enclosure
OVARY	R Filmy	1	2	4
	Dense	4	8	16
	L Filmy	1	2	4
	Dense	4	8	16
TUBE	R Filmy	1	2	4
	Dense	4*	8*	16
	L Filmy	1	2	4
	Dense	4*	8*	16

*If the fimbriated end of the fallopian tube is completely enclosed, change the point assignment to 16.

FIGURE 39-27

American Fertility Society classification of endometriosis. (From Andrews WC, Buttrom VC, Behrman SJ, et al: Fertil Steril 43:351, 1985.)

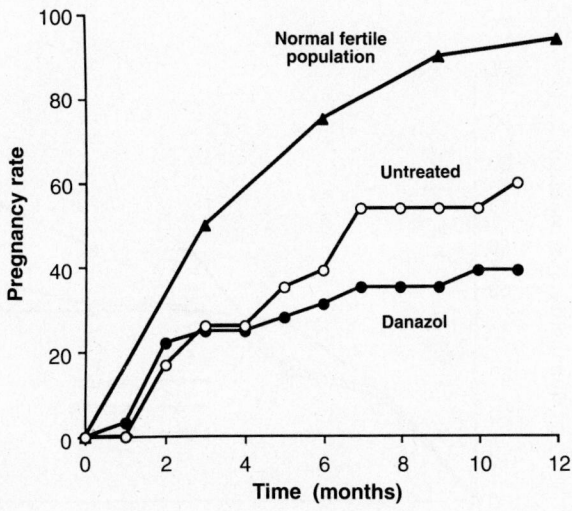

FIGURE 39-28

Cumulative pregnancy rates in danazol-treated and untreated groups over a 12-month period. Cumulative pregnancy rate in an ideal fertile population is also shown for comparison. (Adapted from Cooke ID, Sulaiman RA, Lenton EA, and Parsonos RJ: Clin Obstet Gynecol 8:531, 1981; and Bayer SR, Seibel MM, Saffan DS, et al: J Reprod Med 33:179, 1988.)

endometriosis are a subfertile population. Thus if only mild endometriosis is found at the time of laparoscopy and no other cause of infertility is present, then it is advisable to wait at least 12 months, with intercourse timed to occur just before ovulation, before treating the patient medically or surgically if such therapy is going to be used.

Moderate Endometriosis

If pelvic adhesions that cannot be lysed at the time of laparoscopy or ovarian endometriomas larger than 1 cm in diameter are present, medical therapy will not cause sufficient regression to improve fertility rates, and surgical treatment should be undertaken. For patients with moderate disease without ovarian endometriomas and minimal adhesions that can be cut at the time of laparoscopy, no evidence indicates that medical treatment improves fertility rates compared with no treatment.

The use of danazol, GnRH agonists, progestins, or oral contraceptives has not been shown to increase fertility rates compared with observation without treatment.

Hull et al. compared the use of oral medroxyprogesterone acetate (MPA), (30 mg daily), danazol (600 to 800 mg daily), and no treatment in a group of infertile women with mild or moderate endometriosis without adhesions or tubal obstruction who were not treated at the time of the diagnostic laparoscopy. After 30 months, pregnancy rates were highest for the MPA group, 71%, lowest for the danazol group, 46%, and intermediate for controls, 55% (Figure 39-29). However, there was no difference in pregnancy rates between individuals with stage I or stage II endometriosis (Figure 39-30). The mean monthly conception rate was low in each treatment category, 3.1% to 3.5%.

Telimaa performed a similar study in 49 women, but 22 of them had previous conservative surgery for endometriosis. The results were similar, with no significant differences in conception rates among the three groups (Figure 39-31).

Fedele et al. performed a similar study comparing a GnRH agonist and danazol in a group of women with primarily stage I and stage II endometriosis. They reported similar pregnancy rates to those noted by Hull et al. with 18-month cumulative rates of 48% and 43% for the GnRH and danazol groups, respectively, an insignificant difference (Figure 39-32).

The results of these studies provide additional evidence for the belief that unless the extent of the endometrial disease is severe enough to produce adhesions that interfere with oviduct motility, endometriosis itself is a result and not a cause of infertility. In these

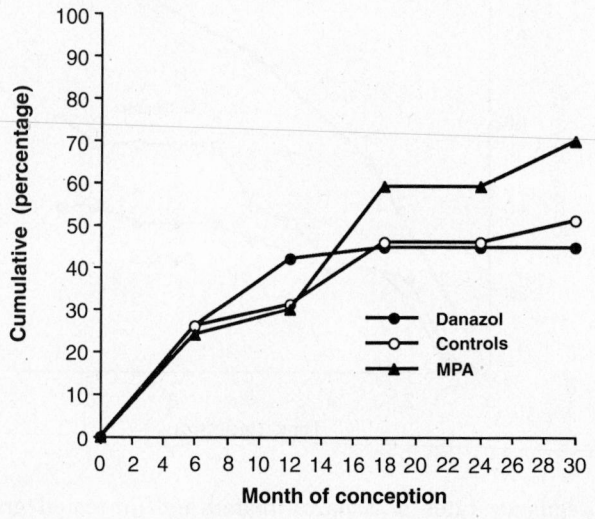

FIGURE 39-29
Cumulative pregnancy rates for three groups of women with endometriosis receiving medroxyprogesterone acetate (MPA), danazol, or no treatment. (From Hull ME, Moghissi KS, Magyar DF, and Hayes MF: Fertil Steril 47:40, 1986.)

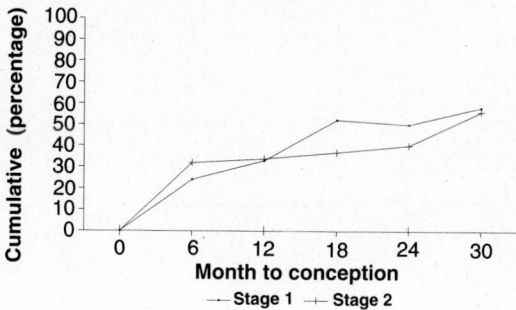

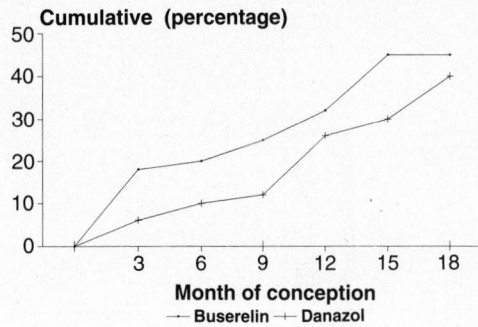

FIGURE 39-30
Cumulative pregnancy rates for three groups of women with stage I or stage II endometriosis receiving MPA, danazol, or no treatment. (From Hull ME, Moghissi KS, Magyar DF, and Hayes MF: Fertil Steril 47:40, 1986.)

FIGURE 39-32
Cumulative pregnancy rates for two groups of women with endometriosis receiving GnRH agonist (buserelin) or danazol therapy. (From Fedele L, Bianchi S, Arcaini L, et al: Am J Obstet Gynecol 161:871, 1989.)

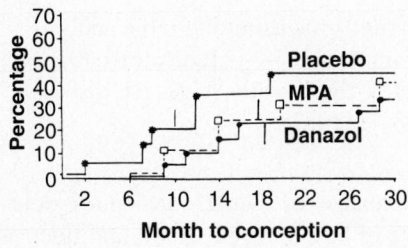

FIGURE 39-31
Cumulative pregnancy rates in groups given danazol (*filled circles*), MPA (*open squares*), or placebo (*asterisks*). Vertical lines indicate the mean intervals to fecundation. (From Telimaa S: Fertil Steril 50:872, 1988.)

studies all patients with tubal occlusion were excluded, as were those who still had adhesions and endometriosis at the time of second-look laparoscopy after conservative surgical treatment. However, the low cumulative fertility rates 30 months later confirm that women with endometriosis have impaired fertility. Furthermore, because danazol, MPA, or a GnRH agonist each causes regression of endometriosis, the fact that pregnancy rates are no greater in women receiving treatment than in those receiving no therapy confirms the belief that the residual endometriosis does not cause infertility. Regression of the disease does not result in higher conception rates.

Women with severe endometriosis have no endocrinologic abnormalities but may have a yet-to-be-defined disorder that inhibits normal endometrial implantation of the human embryo. Perhaps this implantation-inhibitory factor prevents pregnancy in certain women and allows endometriosis to develop and progress until it causes tubal damage.

Seiler et al. reported the rates of pregnancy to be similar in women with moderate endometriosis whose treatment was randomized between danazol and electrocauterization performed at the time of laparoscopy. Each group had pregnancy rates of about 50% within 7 months after therapy. The use of laparoscopic electrocautery at the time of the diagnostic evaluation for infertility appears warranted and avoids the expense and problems of medical suppressants.

Severe Endometriosis

Conservative operative resection of endometriosis should be performed for patients with infertility and moderate or severe disease with adhesions that cannot be cauterized or lysed at the time of laparoscopy or patients with endometriomas more than 1 cm in diameter. Preoperative treatment with danazol or GnRH agonists for 6 weeks to 3 months is advised by some authorities to facilitate the surgical resection, but there appears to be no benefit from postoperative danazol or GnRH agonist treatment. Conception rates for women treated operatively have been reported to be in the 50% to 60% range for those with moderate disease

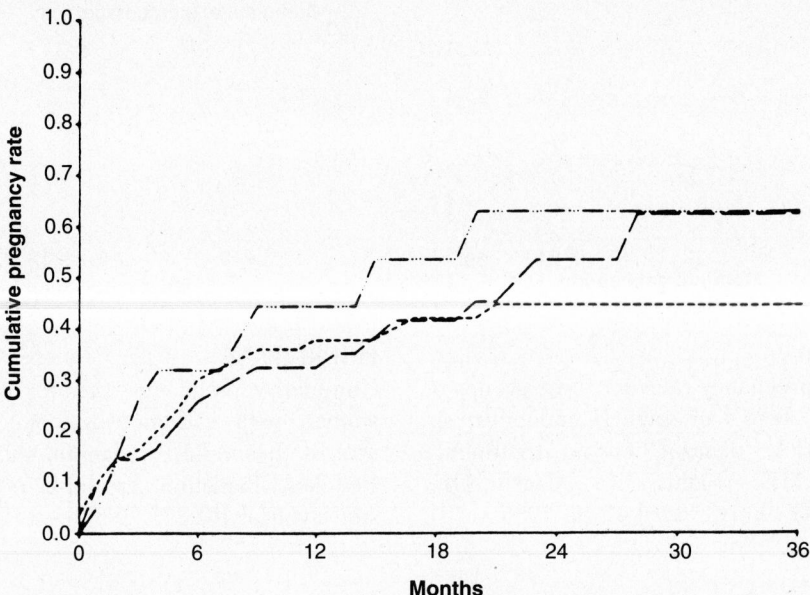

FIGURE 39-33
Cumulative pregnancy rates for women with endometriosis using life-table analysis. The --- line indicated patients with stage I endometriosis, ––– indicates patients with stage II endometriosis, and —...— indicates those with stage III disease. (From Olive DL, and Martin DC: Fertil Steril 48:18, 1987.)

and 30% to 40% for those with severe disease. These rates are better than those reported for expectant management of women with this degree of disease.

Of the women who do conceive after surgical reconstruction, about half will do so in the first 6 months, and nearly all in the first 15 months after the operative procedure, similar to what occurs after discontinuation of medical therapy.

Olive and Martin reported that patients with severe endometriosis had a 50% pregnancy rate after being treated with carbon dioxide laser laparoscopy, similar to the results of those treated with laparotomy (Figure 39-33). If patients have such severe disease that it cannot be treated with laparotomy, perhaps in vitro fertilization should be utilized instead of performing a laparotomy, similar to the approach some have proposed for severe distal tubal disease. Pregnancy rates following in vitro fertilization for endometriosis are about 20% per treatment cycle. Therefore both treatment options should be offered to individual patients with severe endometriosis.

The therapeutic options available to the clinician and patient at the time of diagnostic laparoscopy are listed in Figure 39-34. However, one must remember that inhibition of ovulation with danazol or GnRH analogues delays the chance of becoming pregnant and does not improve fertility.

Operative treatment of endometriosis has for many years included the use of electrocautery as well as microsurgical techniques. In the past 10 years argon and carbon dioxide lasers have been used to vaporize adhesions and endometrial implants. Studies in animals and humans have shown no difference in the results of treatment of periadnexal adhesions with carbon dioxide laser or electrocautery. In a prospective randomized study Tulandi reported that pregnancy rates were similar following the use of each of these two techniques for lysis of periadnexal adhesions. The duration of operating time may be reduced with the laser, but the technique has the disadvantages of higher cost and necessity for additional training, because it is more difficult to use the laser than electrocautery.

Secondary Infertility Factors

As mentioned previously, unlike treatment of the five primary infertility factors, there is no evidence that treatment of the five secondary infertility factors significantly improves pregnancy rates as compared with withholding

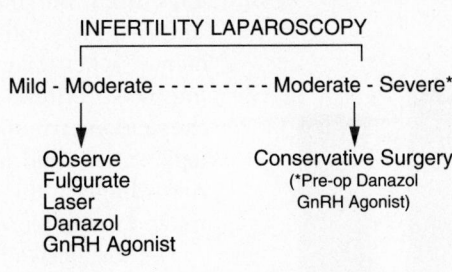

INFERTILITY LAPAROSCOPY

Mild - Moderate - - - - - - - - - Moderate - Severe*

Observe
Fulgurate
Laser
Danazol
GnRH Agonist

Conservative Surgery
(*Pre-op Danazol
GnRH Agonist)

FIGURE 39-34
Therapeutic options for the infertile patient. *GnRH*, Gonadotropin-releasing hormone. (From Mishell DR Jr, Davajan V, and Lobo RA, editors: Infertility, contraception and reproductive endocrinology, ed 3, Cambridge, Mass, 1991, Blackwell Scientific Publications.)

therapy. There are few randomized trials of therapy for these factors, such as has been done for mild endometriosis. In a 2- to 7-year follow-up of 1145 infertile couples, Collins et al. reported that the conception rate was 41% for the 517 couples treated for infertility and 35% for the 548 couples who received no treatment. The majority of pregnancies occurred independent of therapy for infertility. In the 1985 report of Hull et al. no further diagnostic evaluation was performed after the five primary steps of the infertility workup were completed. Among the group of couples in whom no abnormality was found in these primary five diagnostic categories and no therapy was initiated, the conception rate was 72% after 2 years (see Figure 39-6). The conception rate in this group did not vary according to age unless the woman was older than 35 years (Figure 39-7). Conception rates varied markedly according to the duration of infertility, being significantly less when the duration of infertility was 3 to 5 years (about 50%) and decreasing to about 25% when the duration was 5 years or longer. These fertility rates observed with no treatment need to be compared with fertility rates after treatment of the secondary infertility factors in prospective randomized studies.

Subclinical Hypothyroidism and Hyperprolactinemia

It is unusual to find an elevation of either TSH or prolactin in women with regular ovulatory cycles and no galactorrhea. However, if such a finding is confirmed, it seems reason-able to treat subclinical hypothyroidism with thyroid replacement and subclinical hyperprolactinemia with bromocriptine, because clinical hypothyroidism and hyperprolactinemia are both associated with subfertility.

Luteal Deficiency

The incidence of luteal deficiency in infertile couples is less than 5%. As with the other secondary infertility factors, it has not been established that luteal phase defects of progesterone production or action cause infertility. The evidence is more convincing that luteal deficiency is a cause of recurrent abortion. The degree of luteal deficiency can be determined by finding serum progesterone levels consistently below 10 ng/ml in the luteal phase of the cycle, indicating a deficit in progesterone production, or finding histologic evidence of a delay in development of the normal secretory endometrial pattern, indicating an inadequate effect of normal progesterone production on the endometrium. To establish the latter diagnosis the normal secretory endometrial development must lag 3 *days* or more behind the expected pattern for the time of the cycle originally described by Noyes et al. Furthermore, this finding must be consistent and found in *at least two cycles*. The luteal phase dating of the biopsy specimen must be calculated on the basis of the onset of the subsequent menses, not the previous menses, because of the greater normal variability at the follicular phase of the cycle. Dating should be calculated by use of indicators that will detect the day of the urinary LH surge or shift in BBT as an aid in identifying the day of

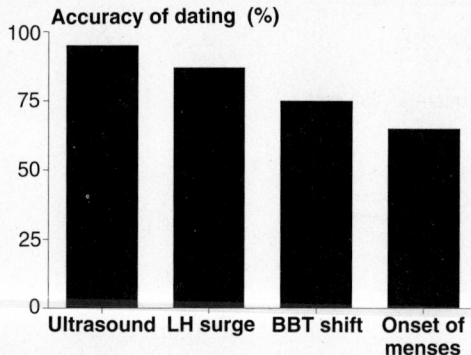

Accuracy of dating (%)

FIGURE 39-35

Percentage of endometrial biopsy interpretations that correlated within 2 days using four different methods of ovulation prediction. Onset of menses: $P < 0.05$ compared with ultrasonography. (From Shoupe D, Mishell DR Jr, LaCarra M, et al: Obstet Gynecol 73:88, 1988.)

ovulation, not by substracting 14 days.

Because the onset of the next menses is the least accurate parameter (Figure 39-35), the diagnosis of this entity probably occurs more frequently than the condition exists; the histologic dating of the endometrium is not a precise measurement.

Li et al. reported that a 10% disagreement of more than 2 days occurred when the same observer dated the specimens on two separate occasions. Scott et al. reported that there was great interobserver variation in dating endometrial biopsy specimens, even when performed by five experienced pathologists. Davis et al. reported that the incidence of luteal phase defect in normal fertile women, as determined by serial endometrial biopsies, was 31.4% if a single biopsy was three or more days out of phase and 6.6% if sequential biopsies were analyzed.

The data from these and other studies indicate that the diagnosis of luteal phase inadequacy by the use of subjective histologic observations of endometrial biopsy specimens is imprecise, and when used, the incidence of this entity is similar in fertile and infertile populations. The frequency of this abnormality is related to several variables. These include the criteria used for diagnosis (more than 1 or 2 days' lag), its presence in at least one or more cycles, and whether dating is done according to days postovulation, as determined by daily ultrasonic examination of the ovaries or serial LH measurements, or calculated by subtracting 14

days from the onset of subsequent menses. These results indicate that luteal phase deficiency, when diagnosed by the currently used imprecise criteria of histologic maturation of the endometrium, is probably a normal biologic variant and not a true cause of infertility. Accordingly, this entity is diagnosed and treated much more often than it actually exists.

The diagnosis of luteal phase deficiency cannot be made by observation of the BBT curve alone, but analysis of the BBT allows the clinician to obtain the sample of endometrium at the optimal time—12 days after the temperature shift, about 2 days before the next expected menses (Figure 39-36). At this time the appearance of the endometrium will reflect the maximal effect from the sex steroids produced by the corpus luteum.

Inadequate progesterone production can be caused by hypothalamic-pituitary defects, particularly those resulting in inadequate FSH production in the follicular phase of the cycle. In addition, deficient progesterone production by the corpus luteum has been reported to occur with hyperprolactinemia. It is possible that the ovary will fail to produce sufficient progesterone with normal gonadotrophin levels because of a defect in gonadotrophin receptors. It has also been postulated that the endometrium may not respond normally to adequate levels of progesterone as a result of a defect in its steroid receptors.

The main treatment of luteal phase defects has consisted of progesterone suppositories, 25 mg twice daily, or 12.5 mg progesterone in oil given intramuscularly daily, beginning the day after the BBT shift and continuing until menstruation occurs or, if conception takes place, until 10 to 12 weeks of gestation. In addition, clomiphene citrate (50 to 100 mg per day for 5 days beginning on day 2 of the cycle), luteal phase HCG injections (2500 to 5000 IU every other day), and follicular phase HMG have all been used to treat luteal deficiency. If there is an elevation of serum prolactin, bromocriptine therapy is the treatment of choice. March has suggested that the agent should be selected based on the type of abnormality that is present (Table 39-13). Conception rates as high as 75% have been reported by certain investigators, but there are no randomized, placebo-controlled trials to indicate that the conceptions are a result of the treatment utilized.

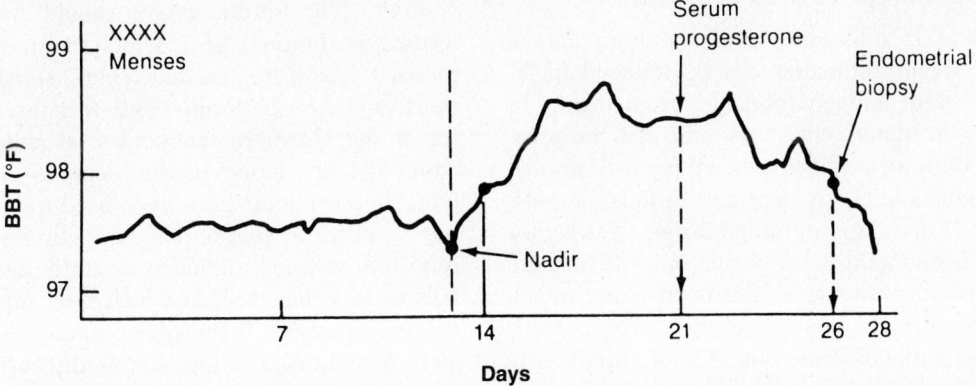

FIGURE 39-36
Method of evaluating luteal phase function in patients with biphasic BBT. Serum progesterone level is measured 7 days after temperature shift, and endometrial biopsy is performed 5 days after measurement of progesterone level. (From Mishell DR Jr, Davajan V, and Lobo RA, editors: Infertility, contraception and reproductive endocrinology, ed 3, Cambridge, Mass, 1991, Blackwell Scientific Publications.)

TABLE 39-13
Selection of Treatment for Luteal Phase Defect

Abnormality*	Treatment	Follow-up†
Low prog. Normal PRL Endometrium in phase	Clomiphene citrate	Prog.
Low prog. Normal PRL Retarded endometrium	Clomiphene citrate	Prog. EMB
Low prog. ↑ PRL Endometrium in phase	Bromocriptine	PRL Prog.
Low prog. ↑ PRL Retarded endometrium	Bromocriptine	PRL Prog. EMB
Retarded endometrium ↑ PRL Normal prog.	Bromocriptine	PRL EMB
Retarded endometrium Normal prog. Normal PRL	Progesterone	EMB

From Mishell DR Jr, Davajan V, and Lobo RA, editors: Infertility, contraception and reproductive endocrinology, ed 3, Cambridge, Mass, 1991, Blackwell Scientific Publications.
Prog., Progesterone; *PRL*, prolactin; *EMB*, endometrial biopsy.
*Low progesterone = peak serum progesterone level <10 ng/ml; "retarded" = more than 2 days out of phase.
†Follow-up peak serum progesterone levels should be ≥15 ng/ml. Combination therapy may be necessary in some patients.

Immunologic Causes of Infertility

There is substantial evidence from animal studies that antibodies can be induced in females from antigens obtained from organs in the male reproductive tract and that the presence of these antibodies interferes with normal reproduction. Both sperm-agglutinating antibodies and sperm-immobilizing antibodies have been found in the serum of some infertile women, but they have also been found in the serum of fertile control subjects. The agglutinating antibodies are found more frequently than immobilizing antibodies in most series, and agglutinating antibodies occur more frequently in fertile control subjects. In some series the incidence of sperm-agglutinating antibodies in infertile women is similar to that of the control group. Even with the finding of sperm agglutination or immobilization in serum, it has not been demonstrated that a similar degree of sperm inactivation occurs in the lower genital tract. Thus there is no definitive evidence that sperm agglutination or immobilization in the serum of infertile women is the cause of their infertility. One of the reasons for this discrepancy is the fact that both the serum assays—agglutination and immobilization—measure mainly IgM and IgG antibodies but the antibodies locally produced in the genital tract are mainly IgA. For this reason some investigators have measured antisperm antibodies in cervical mucus and found a correlation between the presence of such antibodies and infertility.

There are several tests to detect agglutinating antibodies in serum, including the Franklin-Dukes test, the Friberg microsurgical agglutination test, and the gelatin agglutination test described by Kibɪ   The Kibrick test, which identifies macroagglutinating antibodies, appears to have fewer false positive results than the other two microagglutination tests. The complement-dependent sperm immobilization antibody test described by Isojima et al. is specific and has few false positive results. Clarke et al. have described a test that is able to detect IgA, IgM, and IgG antibodies bound to sperm membranes. This test, called the *immunobead test*, is less sensitive than the tests to detect sperm-agglutinating or sperm-immobilizing antibodies in serum, but it may be more specific.

If any of these assays is used, it is important to utilize appropriate positive and negative controls. The serum assays should be performed at dilutions of 1:4 for screening purposes. If a positive reaction occurs, serial dilutions should be performed to determine the titer of the antisperm antibodies. If antisperm antibodies are found in the woman's circulation, then condoms have been used to prevent her exposure to sperm. The antibody tests are repeated at 3-month intervals until the titer falls to less than 1:4, at which time midcycle coitus is advised. If the titer remains elevated after 6 months, condom use is discontinued. Pregnancy rates as high as 50% have been reported after such treatment as well as after corticosteroid immunosuppressive therapy, but no prospective randomized controlled studies have demonstrated the validity of either type of therapy.

No data demonstrate conclusively that the finding of antibodies against sperm in either the male or the female partner is a cause of infertility. A retrospective analysis of corticosteroid therapy and no treatment was performed by Smarr et al. in women with high titers of antisperm antibodies. Even though the analysis was retrospective and therapy was administered in a nonrandomized manner, the results are in agreement with those of a recently published randomized study in males indicating that corticosteroid treatment does not produce a significantly increased pregnancy rate. More randomized prospective studies with precise diagnostic techniques need to be performed to determine if corticosteroid administration has a place in the treatment of certain infertile couples.

Autoimmunity to sperm in both semen and serum has been found in some infertile men, particularly those who have had testicular infection, injury, or a surgical procedure such as vasectomy reversal. Men with these antibodies have been treated with corticosteroid therapy as well as sperm-washing techniques. The effectiveness of such treatment remains to be established, since a study by Haas et al. failed to show that corticosteroid therapy resulted in significantly greater pregnancy rates.

Infection

Some researchers have suggested that asymptomatic, or occult, infection of the upper female genital tract and the male genital tract is a cause of infertility. Friberg and Gnarpe suggested in 1973 that infection with what was then called T mycoplasma in the male could interfere with normal sperm function, and infection of the female reproductive tract could interfere with normal sperm transport. The current name now used for those organisms is *Ureaplasma urealyticum*. Two other microscopic organisms of the genus *Mycoplasma* that are found in the female genital tract are *Mycoplasma hominis* and *Mycoplasma fermentans*. Although Friberg and Gnarpe and others have reported that treatment of infertile couples with antibiotics that eradicate these organisms, such as tetracycline or doxycycline, resulted in high pregnancy rates, controlled studies have reported no difference in pregnancy rates between couples treated with antibiotics and those not treated. Harrison et al. studied 88 infertile couples with no demonstrable cause of infertility. One third were treated with doxycycline, one third received placebo, and one third received no treatment. T mycoplasma was isolated from about two thirds of the couples in each group and was eradicated only in the group treated with doxycycline. Nevertheless, conception rates were similar in each group. Matthews et al. performed a similar study and obtained similar results (Table 39-14). Other investigators have suggested that asymptomatic *C. trachomatis* infection may also cause infertility, but the dosage of doxycycline used in these randomized studies would also have eradicated these organisms. Thus there is no evidence that asymptomatic infection of the genital tract of the human male or female can cause infertility. Nevertheless, some authorities suggest that cultures of the semen and endocervix be performed in an attempt to isolate *U. urealyticum*, *M. hominis*,

and *C. trachomatis* in couples with otherwise unexplained infertility. If any of these organisms is detected, these individuals suggest treating both the husband and wife with doxycycline at a dosage of 100 mg twice daily from the seventh through the sixteenth day of the wife's menstrual cycle.

Fertilization Abnormality: Zona-Free Hamster Egg Penetration Test

The last step of the infertility investigation is a test developed to predict the fertilizing ability of sperm. This assay—the zona-free hamster egg penetration test originally described by Yanagimachi et al.—provides an additional, more sensitive parameter to assess sperm function than the routine semen analysis. Many variable factors affect the test results (see the box below). For this reason it is important to use positive and negative controls in each assay and to establish the threshold value of the assay. The threshold value, usually about 10% of

---

FACTORS INFLUENCING OUTCOME OF SPERM PENETRATION ASSAY

Time of sperm preincubation
Time of incubation of sperm with ova
Sperm concentration
Time sperm reside in seminal plasma before first washing
Presence of leukocytes in semen

From Mishell DR Jr, Davajan V, and Lobo RA, editors: Infertility, contraception and reproductive endocrinology, ed 3, Cambridge, Mass, 1991, Blackwell Scientific Publications.

TABLE 39-14
Controlled Studies of Outcome of Therapy of Couples with Unexplained Infertility and *U. urealyticum* Infections

Authors	Treatment	No. of Couples	No. of Pregnancies	Conceptions (%)
Harrison et al.	Doxycycline	30	5	17
	Placebo	28	4	14
	None	30	5	17
Matthews et al.	Treated	51	10	20
	None	18	4	22

From Mishell DR Jr, Davajan V, and Lobo RA, editors: Infertility, contraception and reproductive endocrinology, ed 3, Cambridge, Mass, 1991, Blackwell Scientific Publications.

eggs penetrated, can be used to distinguish between a positive and negative response. Since variation in the results of the same individual over time have been observed, the results of a single assay are not definitive. Thus if a negative sperm penetration test result is obtained, the assay should be repeated at several intervals with sperm separation techniques in an attempt to improve penetration before the couple is advised that the husband has a defect in his sperm that will most probably prevent conception.

Vazquez-Levin et al. reported that this test did not correlate well with in vitro fertilization of human eggs. Mao and Grimes surveyed the literature about this test and concluded the sensitivity and specificity of the sperm penetration assay are too low to justify its routine use as part of the infertility investigation.

The value of performing the zona-free hamster egg–human sperm penetration test as part of the evaluation of the infertile couple has not been satisfactorily demonstrated. Therefore, it is not cost-effective to perform this expensive assay as part of the routine infertility evaluation.

In Vitro Fertilization

The technique of in vitro fertilization (IVF) with embryo transfer is now being widely used to treat infertile couples. Although the method was originally restricted to women who had no functioning oviducts as a result of severe tubal disease, it is now being used for women with severe endometriosis and couples with male factor or unexplained infertility. Since the rate of pregnancy following IVF is related to the number of embryos placed in the uterine cavity, nearly all IVF clinics currently utilize some form of ovarian hyperstimulation to increase the number of oocytes obtained at the time of follicle aspiration. Stimulation protocols utilizing clomiphene citrate, HMG, or a combination of the two are being used. Monitoring of follicle growth is usually performed by both daily ultrasonography and estrogen measurement.

Recently there have been reports of similar success with in vitro fertilization performed by both daily ultrasonography and estrogen measurement. There are two main advantages for performing IVF with eggs collected from the dominant follicle in a normal, unstimulated ovulatory cycle. First, the substantial cost of administering HMG and additional days of monitoring that are necessary in stimulated cycles are avoided. Second, more aspiration cycles can be performed in the same time period. Thus aspirating eggs from unstimulated cycles is both cost efficient and time efficient. In addition, the problems associated with multiple gestation, which is necessary to perform cryopreservation of excess embryos, are also avoided. Foulet et al. reported a similar pregnancy rate, 22.5% per cycle, with this technique as others have with hyperstimulation.

Originally oocyte retrieval was done by laparoscopic visualization, but with the use of high-resolution ultrasound equipment and the recently developed vaginal ultrasound probe, follicle aspiration is now being done routinely with the use of ultrasound-directed needle placement. These needles are directed into the ovaries through the vagina into the cul-de-sac. The number of oocytes retrieved per follicle aspirated is similar with these ultrasound techniques and laparoscopy. Although an operating room and general anesthesia are required for laparoscopy, neither is necessary for ultrasound-guided ovarian follicle aspiration.

Following aspiration of the oocytes they are cultured in a rigidly controlled, sterile laboratory environment. Various culture media are used in different clinics. The media are freshly prepared at frequent intervals, and sterility is ensured. The eggs are incubated in an atmosphere of 5% carbon dioxide and high humidity.

After 6 to 12 hours of preincubation, sperm prepared by a washing procedure are added to the culture medium. About 18 hours later the oocytes are observed to determine if fertilization has occurred. The oocytes that are fertilized are then cultured for about another 24 hours, and from one to four normally cleaving embryos are then placed into the uterus of the patient in a sterile environment without the use of general anesthesia. Embryo placement is performed through a small catheter placed through the cervical canal. Some centers are freezing some of the embryos and transferring them in subsequent spontaneous ovulatory cycles, but the success rate of the technique is not high.

Pregnancy rates with IVF vary among different centers, and one of the reasons for the variability is the lack of standardization of the definition of pregnancy rate. If women who exhibit

TABLE 39-15

Outcome According to Infertility Diagnosis and Treatment

				IVF			GIFT	
Infertility Diagnosis*	Stimulation Cycles	Canceled Cycles†	ETs	Clinical Pregnancies‡	All Deliveries§	Transfer Cycles	Clinical Pregnancies‖	All Deliveries¶
Tubal disease/problem#	3779	709 (19)	2348	468 (20)	333 (14)	335	82 (24)	58 (17)
Female unexplained	1042	207 (20)	247	58 (23)	50 (20)	378	126 (33)	99 (26)
Female immune	351	62 (18)	150	36 (24)	21 (14)	81	28 (35)	19 (23)
Endometriosis	2417	453 (19)	904	180 (20)	129 (14)	704	229 (33)	177 (25)
Male factor	2322	424 (18)	807	162 (20)	121 (15)	578	180 (31)	146 (25)

*Represents cycle with specific diagnosis indicated. Patient may be represented in more than one category.
†A cycle is defined as canceled if no retrieval is performed.
‡Clinical pregnancy rates are expressed as a percentage of embryo transfer (ET) cycles.
§Delivery rates (live) are expressed as a percent of ET cycles.
‖Clinical pregnancy rates are expressed as a percentage of gamete intrafallopian transfer (GIFT) cycles.
¶Delivery rates (live) are expressed as a percentage of GIFT transfer cycles.
#Tubal disease or problem including previous tubal surgery, tubal ligation, and absence of tube(s).
**Values in parenthesis are percentages.

a transitory rise of HCG following embryo transfer but who have no clinical or ultrasound-demonstrated evidence of pregnancy are defined as pregnant, then the size of the numerator will be increased. The denominator will be highest if all women starting the process are included, but most centers report pregnancy rates per number of women with follicle aspiration or number of women with embryo transfer. Use of the latter two categories will decrease the size of the denominator and thus increase the pregnancy rates reported.

The Society for Assisted Reproductive Technology (SART) performs annual surveys of the various techniques of assisted reproduction. These annual surveys provide useful information for infertile couples who wish to consider use of assisted reproductive technology to conceive. However, those using these surveys must remember that transmission of data to the national registry is voluntary, not compulsory, and reports are not audited for accuracy. Therefore the final results may be more optimistic than what actually occurs in each IVF clinic. The data in Table 39-15 are particularly important because the etiology of infertility varies. Because of the low rate of embryo transfer per stimulation cycle in couples with endometriosis or male factor infertility, the delivery rate per stimulation cycle varies from a high of 9% for infertility caused by tubal disease to lows of 5% for female unexplained endometriosis and male factor etiology. In other words, 1 of 10 women initiating an IVF cycle

for tubal blockage will deliver an infant, whereas only 1 in 20 women with other diagnoses will do so. Patients should be informed of these data at the onset of counseling.

When preclinical abortions were excluded from the numerator and all cycles in which oocyte aspiration was attempted were used as the denominator, two large centers (one in the United States and one in Australia) reported similar pregnancy rates—about 13% in the first IVF treatment cycle. Both these centers have sufficient experience with couples undergoing several IVF procedures if conception did not occur with the first procedure. Using life-table analysis they each reported that the pregnancy rate per cycle remained relatively constant, and after six cycles the cumulative pregnancy rate was about 60% (Table 39-16).

The cumulative pregnancy rate after three cycles was similar for couples with a diagnosis of tubal disease, endometriosis, and unexplained infertility but was lower for those with a male factor etiology. Couples with a sperm problem have a reduced chance of fertilization. An important factor when counseling patients about IVF concerns the pregnancy outcome. When IVF or any form of treatment of the infertile couples results in a singleton gestation advancing to the second trimester, perinatal outcome, gestational age, mean birth weight, congenital malformations, and complications of pregnancy or labor are no different than in the normal fertile population. Therefore viable singleton pregnancies occurring after IVF (or

TABLE 39-16

Life-Table Data of Cumulative Pregnancy Rate with IVF Following 1775 Laparoscopies

	Cycle No.							
	1	**2**	**3**	**4**	**5**	**6**	**7**	**8**
Laparoscopies	885	446	224	110	56	36	14	4
Pregnancies	114	60	30	11	7	4	2	1
Percentage conceiving per cycle	12.9%	13.5%	13.4%	10.0%	12.5%	11.1%	14.3%	25.0%
Cumulative percentage pregnant (P%)	12.9%	24.6%	34.7%	41.2%	48.6%	54.3%	60.8%	70.6%
Standard error of P%	1.1	1.8	2.6	3.6	4.8	5.6	8.2	12.3

From Kovacs GR, Rogers P, Leeton JF, et al: In-vitro fertilization and embryo transfer, Med J Aust 144:682, 1986.

GIFT) should not be considered to be high-risk pregnancies. However, there is an increased risk of spontaneous abortion and preterm delivery among women with multiple gestations conceived by IVF. IVF with embryo transfer is followed by a relatively high incidence of multiple gestations. Furthermore, there is an increased frequency of ectopic and combined ectopic and intrauterine pregnancies after IVF. Therefore such pregnancies need to be closely monitored.

A modification of in vitro fertilization, called *gamete intrafallopian transfer* (GIFT), is used if the infertile woman has functioning oviducts. This technique consists of placement of both oocytes and sperm into the oviduct through a catheter at the time of laparoscopy or minilaparotomy. Although in vitro fertilization, embryo culturing, and embryo transfer into the uterus are avoided by this technique, ovarian hyperstimulation and laparoscopy are still required. Modifications of GIFT include zygote intrafallopian transfer (ZIFT) and tubal embryo stage transfer (TEST). The 1989 SART survey reported that the live delivery rate per embryo transfer for IVF was 14% but was 23% for GIFT and 17% for ZIFT. Many women treated with GIFT have no abnormalities found that could cause infertility and therefore may have a similar conception rate if treated by hyperstimulation and washed intrauterine insemination. Randomized studies comparing these techniques are needed.

FINAL COUNSELING

If treatment of the infertile couple fails to result in conception after 2 years or the couple with unexplained infertility fails to conceive 3

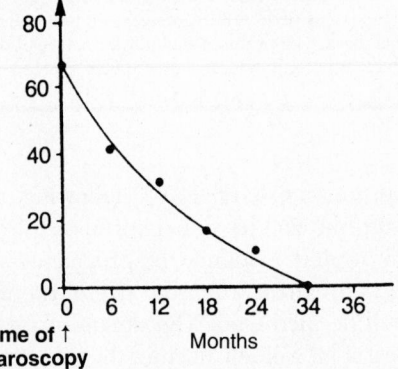

FIGURE 39-37

Expectation of pregnancy in study population following laparoscopy. (From Rousseau S, Lord J, Lepage Y, et al: Fertil Steril 40:768, 1983.)

years after laparoscopy, the couple should be informed that the chances for conception are remote. In the study by Rousseau et al. in which no cause for infertility could be determined after the laparoscopy was performed, no couple conceived beyond 30 months after the procedure (Fig. 39-37). It is best to inform the couple of the prognosis for fertility and the duration beyond which conception should not be expected at the time of the initial consultation, and this information should be restated at subsequent visits. When the period during which conception should be expected has been exceeded, the couple should be informed that further testing and treatment are not warranted and other alternatives such as adoption should be considered.

Finally, it is important for the couple to consider psychological counseling, because the prospect of permanent infertility can cause severe mental trauma.

KEY POINTS

- In 1982 about 8.5% of all U.S. couples with wives in the reproductive age group were infertile. This index was estimated to be 2.4 million couples.

- The incidence of infertility gradually increases in women after age 30.

- Among fertile couples who have coitus shortly before ovulation, there is only about 20% (monthly fecundability rate of 0.2) chance of developing a clinical pregnancy in each ovulatory cycle.

- About half of fertile couples attempting to conceive will become pregnant in 3 months, 75% in 6 months, and 90% at the end of 1 year.

- Infertile couples who conceive do not have higher rates of spontaneous abortion or perinatal mortality than age-matched control subjects.

- In the United States approximately 10% to 15% of cases of infertility are caused by anovulation, 30% to 40% by an abnormality of semen production, 30% to 40% by pelvic disease, 10% to 15% by abnormalities of sperm transport through the cervical canal, and about 5% by uncommon causes.

- The five primary tests for infertility are documentation of ovulation, semen analysis, postcoital test, hysterosalpingogram, and diagnostic laparoscopy.

- The basal body temperature (BBT) increases when circulating levels of progesterone increase, and a sustained increase of BBT occurs following ovulation.

- A sustained rise in BBT or a serum progesterone level greater than 5 ng/ml is presumptive evidence of ovulation.

- A serum progesterone level above 10 ng/ml is an indication of adequate luteal function.

- A high percentage of fertile men will have at least one abnormal parameter in their semen analysis.

- It is best to perform the postcoital test (PCT) on the day before ovulation. A normal postcoital test is the presence of more than five motile sperm per high-power field.

- In women with a normal hysterosalpingogram, a hysteroscopy is unnecessary because it will not detect additional abnormality.

- The five secondary tests for infertility are measurement of serum prolactin and TSH; a late luteal phase endometrial biopsy; immunologic tests to detect sperm antibodies; bacterial culture of cervical mucus and semen; and zona-free hamster egg penetration test by husband's sperm.

- There is no evidence that treatment after five secondary infertility factors significantly improves pregnancy rates compared with withholding therapy.

- Of all the causes of infertility, treatment of anovulation results in the greatest success.

- When ovulation is induced with clomiphene citrate and no other causes of infertility are present, conception rates over time are similar to those of a normal fertile population.

- Patient discontinuation of therapy is the major reason for the reported difference in ovulation and conception rates in anovulatory women treated with clomiphene.

- More than 90% of women with oligomenorrhea and 66% with secondary amenorrhea and estradiol levels of 40 pg/ml or higher will have presumptive evidence of ovulation following clomiphene therapy.

- When conception occurs after clomiphene treatment, the incidence of multiple gestation is increased to about 5%, with nearly all of them being twin gestations. The incidences of clinical spontaneous abortion, ectopic gestation, intrauterine fetal death, and congenital malformation are not significantly increased.

- Formation of ovarian cysts is the major side effect of clomiphene treatment.

- About 5% to 10% of women treated with the individualized, graduated, sequential regimen of clomiphene citrate fail to ovulate with the highest dosage.

- Treatment of anovulation with HMG effects an ovulatory rate of about 100% and an overall pregnancy rate of about 60%.

- The pregnancy rate per cycle with HMG treatment is similar to that following clomiphene therapy—22%.

- The incidence of spontaneous abortion after HMG therapy is high—25% to 35%—and clinically detectable ovarian enlargement occurs in about 5% to 10% of treatment cycles.

- For ovulation induction GnRH should be administered in a pulsatile manner at intervals of 1 to 2 hours.

- Pregnancy rates per cycle with pulsatile GnRH are similar to those with HMG, but hyperstimulation occurs less frequently.

- For women with polycystic ovaries who do not ovulate following administration of clomiphene citrate, partial ovarian destruction by electrocautery or laser through the laparoscope is effective in inducing ovulation.

- Pregnancy rates for oligospermia following either cervical cup insemination or intrauterine insemination are in the 25% to 35% range.

- The prognosis for pregnancy after intrauterine insemination is significantly greater if the motility rate is 30% or more in the pretreatment semen analysis and more than 70% after washing and the swim-up technique.

- Semen donors need to be carefully screened to be certain that they are in good health, do not have a potentially inherited disorder, and will not transmit an infectious agent in the semen.

- Because antibodies to HIV may not develop for several months after infection, it is now recommended that all donor insemination be performed with frozen sperm that has been stored for 6 months.

- The prognosis for fertility after tubal reconstruction depends on the amount of damage to the oviduct as well as the location of the obstruction.

- If both proximal and distal obstructions of the oviduct exist, intrauterine pregnancy is uncommon, and operative reconstruction should not be performed.

- Women with pelvic tuberculosis should be considered sterile, and no tubal reconstructive procedures should be attempted.

- Overall conception rates following salpingostomy are in the 30% range with a high percentage—about one fourth—being tubal pregnancies.

- The pregnancy rate after salpingolysis and fimbrioplasty for partial obstruction is about 65%.

- Unlike the results of distal tubal reconstruction, the use of microsurgery has improved intrauterine pregnancy rates for proximal tubal disease.

- With tubocornual reanastomosis for proximal tubal blockage, term pregnancy rates of about 50% have been reported, with ectopic pregnancy rates less than 10%.

- Proximal tubal obstruction can now be treated by fluoroscopically placed transuterine probes in an outpatient setting.

- The benefit of second-look laparoscopy after tubal surgery has not been established.

- Evidence that minimal or mild endometriosis is a *cause* of infertility has not been established.

- No medical therapy for endometriosis has proved to increase pregnancy rates compared with no treatment.

- Overall pregnancy rates for women with mild endometriosis, with or without treatment, are in the 60% to 75% range.

- About 65% of women with mild endometriosis and no other cause of infertility conceive without treatment. With moderate or severe disease, pregnancy rates with expectant management are 25% and 0%, respectively.

- Conception rates for women treated surgically have been reported to be in the 50% to 60% range for those with moderate endometriosis and 30% to 40% for those with severe endometriosis.

- About half of infertile women with myomas conceive after myomectomy.

- Luteal phase deficiency, as currently diagnosed histologically, is probably a normal biologic variant and not a true cause of infertility.

- No data conclusively demonstrate that the finding of antisperm antibodies in either member of the couple is a cause of infertility.

- In women with unexplained infertility the combination of intrauterine insemination and superovulation yields monthly fecundability rates of 0.2 or higher and may be as successful as IVF or GIFT.

- Pregnancy rates following in vitro fertilization with stimulated and unstimulated cycles are similar.

- The delivery rate per embryo transfer for IVF is about 14%, whereas for GIFT it is about 23%.

- The rate of pregnancy following in vitro fertilization is related to the number of embryos placed in the uterine cavity.

- The delivery rate following IVF for tubal disease is about 9% per transfer cycle, whereas for endometriosis, male infertility, and female unexplained infertility, it is only 5%.

- The pregnancy rate is about 13% in the first in vitro fertilization treatment cycle.

- The pregnancy rate per cycle of in vitro fertilization remains relatively constant, and after six cycles the cumulative pregnancy rate is about 60%.

- There is a high spontaneous abortion rate (about 30%) for pregnancies after in vitro fertilization.

- If an infertile couple fails to conceive after 2 years or with unexplained infertility 3 years after laparoscopy, they should be informed the chances for conception are remote.

BIBLIOGRAPHY

Aitken RJ, Comhaire FH, Eliasson R, et al: WHO laboratory manual for the examination of human semen and semen-cervical mucus interaction, Cambridge, 1987, Cambridge University Press.

Alper MM, Garner PR, Spence JEH, et al: Pregnancy rates after hysterosalpingography with oil- and water-soluble contrast media, Obstet Gynecol 68:6, 1986.

Andrews WC, Buttram VC, Behrman SJ, et al: Revised American Fertility Society classification of endometriosis: 1985, Fertil Steril 43-351, 1985.

Armar NA, McGarrible HHG, Honour J, et al: Laparoscopic ovarian diathermy in the management of anovulatory infertility in women with polycystic ovaries: endocrine changes and clinical outcome, Fertil Steril 53:45, 1990.

Barnea ER, Holford TR, and McInnes DRA: Long-term prognosis of infertile couples with normal basic investigations: a life-table analysis, Obstet Gynecol 66:24, 1985.

Barratt CIR, Dunphy BC, Thomas EJ, and Cooke ID: Semen characteristics of 49 fertile males, Andrologia 20:264, 1988.

Bauer O, Van der Ven H, Diedrich K, et al: Preliminary results on transvaginal tubal embryo stage transfer (TV-TEST) without ultrasound guidance, Hum Reprod 5:553, 1990.

Bayer SR, Seibel MM, Saffan DS, et al: Efficacy of danazol treatment for minimal endometriosis infertile women: a prospective randomized study, J Reprod Med 33:179, 1988.

Berger T, Marrs RP, and Moyer DL: Comparison of techniques for selection of motile spermatozoa, Fertil Steril 43:268, 1984.

Bernstein GS: Male factor in infertility. In Mishell DR Jr, Davajan V, and Lobo RA, editors: Infertility, contraception and reproductive endocrinology, ed 3, Cambridge, Mass, 1991, Blackwell Scientific Publications.

Bernstein GS: Occult genital infection. In Mishell DR Jr, Davajan V, and Lobo RA, editors: Infertility, contraception and reproductive endocrinology, ed 3, Cambridge, Mass, 1991, Blackwell Scientific Publications.

Boer-Meisel ME, te Velde ER, Habbema JDF, et al: Predicting the pregnancy outcome in patients treated for hydrosalpinx: a prospective study, Fertil Steril 45:23, 1986.

Braat DDM, Schoemaker R, and Schoemaker J: Life table analysis of fecundity in intravenously gonadotropin releasing hormone–treated patients with normogonadotropic and hypogonadotropic amenorrhea, Fertil Steril 55:266, 1991.

Buttram VC Jr: Evolution of the revised American Fertility Society classification of endometriosis, Fertil Steril 43:347, 1985.

Byrd W, Guzick DS, Ackerman GE, et al: Treatment of refractory infertility by transcervical intrauterine insemination of washed spermatozoa, Fertil Steril 48:921, 1987.

Chaffkin LM, Nulsen JC, Luciano AA, and Metzger DA: A comparative analysis of the cycle fecundity rates associated with combined human menopausal gonadotropin (HMG) and intrauterine insemination (IUI) versus either MHG or IUI alone, Fertil Steril 55:252, 1991.

Clarke GN, Lopata A, and Johnston WIH: Effect of sperm antibodies in females on human in vitro fertilization, Fertil Steril 46:435, 1986.

Collins JA, Wrixon W, Janes LB, et al: Treatment-independent pregnancy among infertile couples, N Engl J Med 309:1201, 1983.

Confino E, Tur-Kaspa I, DeCherney A, et al: Transcervical balloon tuboplasty: a multicenter study, JAMA 264:2079, 1990.

Congressional Board of the 100th Congress, Office of Technology Assessment: Infertility: medical and social choices, pub no 20510-8025, Washington, DC, 1988, US Government Printing Office.

Cooke ID, Sulaiman RA, Lenton EA, and Parsonos RJ: Fertility and infertility statistics: their importance and application, Clin Obstet Gynecol 8:531, 1981.

Cramer DW, Walker AM, and Schiff I: Statistical methods in evaluating the outcome of infertility therapy, Fertil Steril 32:80, 1979.

Cruz RI, Kemmann E, Brandeis VT, et al: A prospective study of intrauterine insemination of processed sperm from men with oligoasthenospermia in superovulated women, Fertil Steril 46:673, 1986.

Daly DC, Walters CA, Soto-Albors CE, et al: A randomized study of dexamethasone in ovulation induction with clomiphene citrate, Fertil Steril 41:844, 1984.

Daniell JF and Herbert CM: Laparoscopic salpingostomy utilizing the CO_2 laser, Fertil Steril 41:558, 1984.

Daniell JF and Miller W: Polycystic ovaries treated by laparoscopic laser vaporization, Fertil Steril 51:232, 1989.

Davajan V: Postcoital testing: the cervical factor as a cause of infertility. In Mishell DR Jr, Davajan V, and Lobo RA, editors: Infertility, contraception and reproductive endocrinology, ed 3, Cambridge, Mass, 1991, Blackwell Scientific Publications.

Davajan V, Mishell DR Jr: Evaluation of the infertile couple. In Mishell DR Jr, Davajan V, and Lobo RA, editors: Infertility, contraception and reproductive endocrinology, ed 3, Cambridge, Mass, 1991, Blackwell Scientific Publications.

Davis OK, Berkeley AS, Naus GJ, et al: The incidence of luteal phase defect in normal, fertile women, determined by serial endometrial biopsies, Fertil Steril 51:582, 1989.

Dodson WC, Hughes CL, Yancy SE, and Haney AF: Clinical characteristics of ovulation induction with human menopausal gonadotropins with and without leuprolide acetate in polycystic ovary syndrome, Fertil Steril 42:915, 1989.

Dodson WC, Whitesides DB, Hughes CKL, et al: Superovulation with intrauterine insemination in the treatment of infertility: a possible alternative to gamete intrafallopian transfer and in vitro fertilization, Fertil Steril 48:441, 1987.

Donnez J and Casanas-Roux F: Prognostic factors influencing the pregnancy rate after microsurgical cornual anastomosis, Fertil Steril 46:1089, 1986.

Donnez J and Casanas-Roux F: Prognostic factors of fimbrial microsurgery, Fertil Steril 46:200, 1986.

Dubuisson JB, Bouquet de Joliniere J, Zubriot FX, et al: Terminal tuboplasties by laparoscopy: 65 consecutive cases, Fertil Steril 54:401, 1990.

Eggert-Kruse W, Leinhos G, Gerhard I, et al: Prognostic value of in vitro sperm penetration into hormonally standardized human cervical mucus, Fertil Steril 51:317, 1989.

Fayes JA, Mutie G, and Schneider PJ: The diagnostic value of hysterosalpingography and hysteroscopy in infertility investigation, Am J Obstet Gynecol 156:558, 1987.

Fedele L, Bianchi S, Arcaini L, et al: Buserelin versus danazol in the treatment of endometriosis-associated infertility, Am J Obstet Gynecol 161:871, 1989.

Filmar S, Gomel V, and McComb P: The effectiveness of CO_2 laser and electromicrosurgery in adhesiolysis: a comparative study, Fertil Steril 45:407, 1986.

Fisch P, Collins JA, Casper RF, et al: Unexplained infertility: evaluation of treatment with clomiphene citrate and human chorionic gonadotropin, Fertil Steril 51:441, 1987.

Fleming R, Haxton MJ, Hamilton MPR, et al: Combined gonadotropin-releasing hormone analog and exogenous gonadotropins for ovulation induction in infertile women: efficacy related to ovarian function assessment, Am J Obstet Gynecol 159:376, 1988.

Forster MS, Smith W, Lee WI, et al: Selection of human spermatozoa according to their relative motility and interaction with zona free hamster eggs, Fertil Steril 40:655, 1983.

Foulet H, Ranoux C, Dubuisson JB, et al: In vitro fertilization without ovarian stimulation: a simplified protocol applied in 80 cycles, Fertil Steril 52:617, 1989.

Friberg J and Gnarpe H: Mycoplasma and human reproductive failure. III. Pregnancies in "infertile" couples treated with doxycycline for T-mycoplasmas, Am J Obstet Gynecol 116:23, 1973.

Gadir AA, Mowafi RS, Alnaser HMI, et al: Ovarian electrocautery versus human menopausal gonadotrophins and pure follicle stimulating hormone therapy in treatment of patients with polycystic ovarian disease, Clin Endocrinol 33:585, 1990.

Gagliardi CL, Emmi AM, Weiss G, and Schmidt CL: Gonadotropin-releasing hormone agonist improves the efficiency of controlled ovarian hyperstimulation/intrauterine insemination, Fertil Steril 55:939, 1991.

Garcia CR and David SS: Pelvic endometriosis: infertility and pelvic pain, Am J Obstet Gynecol 129:740, 1977.

Gillett WR, Cameron MC, MacKay-Duff M, and Seddon RJ: Pregnancy rates with artificial insemination by donor: the influence of the cryopreservation method and coexistent fertility factors, NZ Med J 99:891, 1986.

Glazener CMA, Kelly NJ, and Hull MGR: Prolactin measurement in the investigation of infertility in women with a normal menstrual cycle, Br J Obstet Gynaecol 94:535, 1987.

Gorus FK and Piplers DG: A rapid method for the fractionation of human spermatozoa according to their progressive motility, Fertil Steril 35:662, 1981.

Guzick DS, Wilkes C, and Jones HW Jr: Cumulative pregnancy rates for in vitro fertilization, Fertil Steril 46:663, 1986.

Gysler M, March CM, Mishell DR Jr, et al: A decade's experience with an individualized clomiphene treatment regimen including its effect on the postcoital test, Fertil Steril 37:161, 1982.

Haas GG Jr and Beer AE: Immunologic influences on reproductive biology: sperm gametogenesis and maturation in the male and female genital tracts, Fertil Steril 46:753, 1986.

Hammond MG: Monitoring techniques for improved pregnancy rates during clomiphene ovulation induction, Fertil Steril 42:499, 1984.

Hammond MG, Halme JK, and Talbert LM: Factors affecting the pregnancy rate in clomiphene citrate induction of ovulation, Obstet Gynecol 62:196, 1983.

Hammond MG, Jordan S, and Sloan CS: Factors affecting pregnancy rates in a donor insemination program using frozen semen, Am J Obstet Gynecol 155:480, 1986.

Hammond MG and Talbert LM: Clomiphene citrate in the management of infertile women with low luteal phase progesterone levels, Am J Obstet Gynecol 59:275, 1982.

Harrison RF, DeLouvois J, Blades M, et al: Doxycycline treatment and human infertility, Lancet 1:605, 1975.

Hendershot GE, Mosher WD, and Pratt WF: Infertility and age: an unresolved issue, Fam Plann Perspect 14:287, 1982.

Hill GA, Bryan S, Herbert CM III, et al: Complications of pregnancy in infertile couples: routine treatment versus assisted reproduction, Obstet Gynecol 75:790, 1990.

Holst N, Maltau JM, Forsdahl F, and Hansen LJ: Handling of tubal infertility after introduction of in vitro fertilization: changes and consequences, Fertil Steril 55:140, 1991.

Holtz G, Kling OR: Effect of surgical technique on peritoneal adhesion reformation after lysis, Fertil Steril 37:494, 1982.

Homburg R, Eshel A, Kilborn J, et al: Combined luteinizing hormone releasing hormone analogue and exogenous gonadotrophins for the treatment of infertility associated with polycystic ovaries, Hum Reprod 5:32, 1990.

Howe G, Westhoff C, Vessey M, et al: Effects of age, cigarette smoking, and other factors on fertility: findings in a large prospective study, Br Med J 290:1697, 1985.

Howe RS, Sayegh RA, Durinzi KL, and Tureck RW: Perinatal outcome of singleton pregnancies conceived by in vitro fertilization: a controlled study, J Perinatol 10:261, 1990.

Hulka JF: Adnexal adhesions: a prognostic staging and classification system based on a five-year survey of fertility surgery results at Chapel Hill, North Carolina, Am J Obstet Gynecol 144:141, 1982.

Hull ME, Moghissi KS, Magyar DF, and Hayes MF: Comparison of different treatment modalities of endometriosis in infertile women, Fertil Steril 47:40, 1986.

Hull MGR, Glazener CMA, Kelly NJ, et al: Population study of causes, treatment, and outcome of infertility, Br Med J 291:1984, 1985.

Hull MGR, Savage PE, and Bromham DR: Prognostic value of the postcoital test: prospective study based on time-specific conception rates, Br J Obstet Gynecol 89:299, 1982.

Hull MGR, Savage PE, Bromham DR, et al: The value of a single serum progesterone measurement in the mid-luteal phase as a criterion of a potentially fertile cycle ("ovulation") derived from treated and untreated conception cycles, Fertil Steril 37:355, 1982.

Isojima S, Li TS, and Ashitaka Y: Immunologic analysis of sperm-immobilizing factor found in sera of women with unexplained sterility, Am J Obstet Gynecol 101:677, 1968.

Jansen RPS: Failure of intraperitoneal adjuncts to improve the outcome of pelvic operations in young women, Am J Obstet Gynecol 153:363,1985.

Jones WR: Immunologic infertility: fact or fiction? Fertil Steril 33:577, 1980.

Kovacs GT, Rogers P, Leeton JF, et al: In-vitro fertilization and embryo transfer, Med J Aust 144:682, 1986.

Kovacs GT, Phillips S, Healy DL, and Burger HG: Induction of ovulation with gonadotrophin-releasing hormone—life-table analysis of 50 courses of treatment, Med J Aust 151:21, 1989.

Kurachi K, Aono T, Minagawa J, et al: Congenital malformations of newborn infants after clomiphene-induced ovulation, Fertil Steril 40:187, 1983.

Lalich RA, Marut EL, Prins GS, and Scommegna A: Life table analysis of intrauterine insemination pregnancy rates, Am J Obstet Gynecol 158:980, 1988.

Lam S-Y, Baker G, Pepperell R, and Evans JH: Treatment-independent pregnancies after cessation of gonadotropin ovulation induction in women with oligomenorrhea and anovulatory menses, Fertil Steril 50:26, 1988.

Lang EK, Dunaway HE, and Roniger WE: Selective osteal salpingography and transvaginal catheter dilatation in the diagnosis and treatment of fallopian tube obstruction, AJR 154:735, 1990.

Larsen T, Larsen JF, Schioler V, et al: Comparison of urinary human follicle-stimulating hormone and human menopausal gonadotropin for ovarian stimulation in polycystic ovarian syndrome, Fertil Steril 53:426, 1990.

Lauritsen JG, Pagel JD, Vangsted P, et al: Results of repeated tuboplasties, Fertil Steril 37:68, 1982.

Leeton J, Healy D, Rogers P, et al: A controlled study between the use of gamete intrafallopian transfer (GIFT) and in vitro fertilization and embryo transfer in the management of idiopathic and male infertility, Fertil Steril 48:605, 1987.

Lenton EA, Sobowale OS, and Cooke ID: Prolactin concentrations in ovulatory but infertile women: treatment with bromocriptine, Br Med J 2:1179, 1977.

Lenz S and Lauritsen JG: Ultrasonically guided percutaneous aspiration of human follicles under local anesthesia: a new method of collecting oocytes for in vitro fertilization, Fertil Steril 38:673, 1982.

Leridon H and Spira A: Problems in measuring the effectiveness of infertility therapy, Fertil Steril 41:580, 1984.

Lessing JB, Amit A, Barak Y, et al: The performance of primary and secondary unexplained infertility in an in vitro fertilization—embryo transfer program, Fertil Steril 50:903, 1988.

Lewin A, Laufer N, Rabinowitz R, et al: Ultrasonically guided oocyte collection under local anesthesia: the first choice method for in vitro fertilization—a comparative study with laparoscopy, Fertil Steril 46:257, 1986.

Li TC, Dockery P, Rogers AW, and Cooke ID: How precise is histologic dating of endometrium using the standard dating criteria? Fertil Steril 51:759, 1989.

Lipshultz LI and Howards SS, editors: Infertility in the male, New York, 1983, Churchill Livingstone Inc.

Lobo RA, Granger LR, Davajan V, et al: An extended regimen of clomiphene citrate in women unresponsive to standard therapy, Fertil Steril 37:762, 1982.

Lobo RA, Paul W, March CM, et al: Clomiphene and dexamethasone in women unresponsive to clomiphene alone, Obstet Gynecol 60:497, 1982.

Luciano AA, Hauser KS, and Benda J: Evaluation of commonly used adjuvants in the prevention of postoperative adhesions, Am J Obstet Gynecol 146:88, 1983.

Luciano AA, Turksoy RN, and Carleo J: Evaluation of oral medroxyprogesterone acetate in the treatment of endometriosis, Obstet Gynecol 72:323, 1988.

Malone MJ and Ingersol FM: Myomectomy in infertility. In Behrman SJ and Kistner RW, editors: Progress in infertility, ed 2, Boston, 1975, Little, Brown & Co.

Mao C and Grimes DA: The sperm penetration assay: can it discriminate between fertile and infertile men? Am J Obstet Gynecol 159:279, 1988.

March CM: Luteal phase defects. In Mishell DR Jr, Davajan V, and Lobo RA, editors: Infertility, contraception and reproductive endocrinology, ed 3, Cambridge, Mass, 1991, Blackwell Scientific Publications.

March CM: Improved pregnancy rates with monitoring of gonadotropin therapy by three modalities, Am J Obstet Gynecol. In press.

March CM and Israel R: Gestational outcome following hysteroscopic lysis of adhesions, Fertil Steril 36:455, 1981.

March CM and Mishell DR Jr: Induction of ovulation. In Mishell DR Jr, Davajan V, and Lobo RA, editors: Infertility, contraception and reproductive endocrinology, ed 3, Cambridge, Mass, 1991, Blackwell Scientific Publications.

Martinez AR, Bernardus RE, Voorhorst FJ, et al: Intrauterine insemination does and clomiphene citrate does not improve fecundity in couples with infertility due to male or idiopathic factors: a prospective, randomized, controlled study, Fertil Steril 53:847, 1990.

Matthews CD, Clapp KH, Tansing JA, et al: T-mycoplasma genital infection: the effect of doxycycline therapy on human unexplained infertility, Fertil Steril 30:98, 1978.

McFaul PB, Traub AI, and Thompson W: Treatment of clomiphene citrate–resistant polycystic ovarian syndrome with pure follicle-stimulating hormone or human menopausal gonadotropin, Fertil Steril 53:792, 1990.

McGovern P, Quagliarello J, and Arny M: Relationship of within-patient semen variability to outcome of intrauterine insemination, Fertil Steril 51:1019, 1989.

Menken J, Trussell IJ, and Larsen U: Age and infertility, Science 23:1389, 1986.

MRC Working Party on Children Conceived by In Vitro Fertilisation: Births in Great Britain resulting from assisted conception, 1978-1987, Br Med J 300:1299, 1990.

Moghissi KS, Sacco AG, and Borin K: Immunologic infertility. I. Cervical mucus antibodies and postcoital tests, Am J Obstet Gynecol 136:941, 1980.

Murray DL, Reich L, and Adashi EY: Oral clomiphene citrate and vaginal progesterone suppositories in the treatment of luteal phase dysfunction: a comparative study, Fertil Steril 51:35, 1989.

Noyes RW, Hertig AT, and Rock J: Dating the endometrial biopsy, Fertil Steril 39:277, 1983.

O'Herlihy C, Pepperell JR, Brown JB, et al: Incremental clomiphene therapy: a new method for treating persistent anovulation, Obstet Gynecol 58:535, 1981.

Olive DL and Martin DC: Treatment of endometriosis-associated infertility with CO_2 laser laparoscopy: the use of one- and two-parameter exponential models, Fertil Steril 48:18, 1987.

Olive DL, Stohs GF, Metzger DA, et al: Expectant management and hydrotubations in the treatment of endometriosis-associated infertility, Fertil Steril 44:35, 1985.

Patton GW Jr: Pregnancy outcome following microsurgical fimbrioplasty, Fertil Steril 37:150, 1982.

Patton PE, Williams TJ, and Coulam CB: Microsurgical reconstruction of the proximal oviduct, Fertil Steril 47:35, 1986.

Paulson RJ: Human in vitro fertilization and related assisted reproductive techniques. In Mishell DR Jr, Davajan V, and Lobo RA, editors: Infertility, contraception and reproductive endocrinology, ed 3, Cambridge, Mass, 1991, Blackwell Scientific Publications.

Quagliarello J and Arny M: Intracervical versus intrauterine insemination: correlation of outcome with antecedent postcoital testing, Fertil Steril 46:870, 1986.

Richmond JA: Hysterosalpingography. In Mishell DR Jr, Davajan V, and Lobo RA, editors: Infertility, contraception and reproductive endocrinology, ed 3, Cambridge, Mass, 1991, Blackwell Scientific Publications.

Risquez F, Boyer P, Rolet F, et al: Retrograde tubal transfer of human embryos, Hum Reprod 5:185, 1990.

Rock JA, Katayama P, Martin EJ, et al: Factors influencing the success of salpingostomy techniques for distal fimbrial obstruction, Obstet Gynecol 52:591, 1978.

Rousseau S, Lord J, Lepage Y, and Van Campenhout J: The expectancy of pregnancy for "normal" infertile couples, Fertil Steril 40:768, 1983.

Sauer MV: Tubal surgery. In Mishell DR Jr, Davajan V, and Lobo RA, editors: Infertility, contraception and reproductive endocrinology, ed 3, Cambridge, Mass, 1991, Blackwell Scientific Publications.

Schenken RS and Malinak LR: Conservative surgery versus expectant management for the infertile patient with mild endometriosis, Fertil Steril 37:183, 1982.

Schlaff WD, Hassiakos DK, Damewood MD, and Rock JA: Neosalpingostomy for distal tubal obstruction: prognostic factors and impact of surgical technique: Fertil Steril 54:984, 1990.

Scholtes MCW, Roosenberg BJ, Alberda AT, and Zeilmaker GH: Transcervical intrafallopian transfer of zygotes, Fertil Steril 54:283, 1990.

Schwarz D and Mayaux MJ: Female fecundity as a function of age: results of artificial insemination in 2193 nulliparous women with azoospermic husbands, Fédération des Centres d'Etude et de Conservation du Sperme Humain, N Engl J Med 306:404, 1982.

Scott JZ, Nakamura RM, Mutch J, et al: The cervical factor in infertility: diagnosis and treatment, Fertil Steril 28:1289, 1977.

Scott RT, Snuder RR, Strickland DM, et al: The effect of interobserver variation in dating and endometrial histology on the diagnosis of luteal phase defects, Fertil Steril 50:888, 1988.

Seibel MM, Berger MJ, Weinstein FG, et al: The effectiveness of danazol on subsequent fertility in minimal endometriosis, Fertil Steril 38:534, 1982.

Seiler JC, Gidwani G, and Ballard L: Laparoscopic cauterization of endometriosis for fertility: a controlled study, Fertil Steril 46:1098, 1986.

Serhal PF, Katz M, Little V, and Woronowski H: Unexplained infertility—the value of Pergonal superovulation combined with intrauterine insemination, Fertil Steril 49:602, 1988.

Settlage DSF, Motoshima M, and Tredway DR: Sperm transport from the external cervical os to the fallopian tubes in women: a time and quantitation study, Fertil Steril 24:655, 1973.

Siegler AM and Kontopoulos V: An analysis of macrosurgical and microsurgical techniques in the management of the tuboperitoneal factor in infertility, Fertil Steril 32:377, 1979.

Shoupe D, Mishell DR Jr, LaCarra M, et al: Correlation of endometrial maturation with four methods of estimating day of ovulation, Obstet Gynecol 73:88, 1988.

Smarr SC and Hammond MG: Effect of therapy on infertile couples with antisperm antibodies, Am J Obstet Gynecol 158:969, 1988.

Stumpf PG and March CM: Febrile morbidity following hysterosalpingography: identification of risk factors and recommendations for prophylaxis, Fertil Steril 33:487, 1980.

Sumioki H, Utsunomyiya T, Matsuoka K, et al: The effect of laparoscopic multiple punch resection of the ovary on hypothalamo-pituitary axis in polycystic ovary syndrome, Fertil Steril 4:567, 1988.

Telimaa S: Danazol and medroxyprogesterone acetate inefficacious in the treatment of infertility in endometriosis, Fertil Steril 50:872, 1988.

Templeton AA and Penney GC: The incidence, characteristics, and prognosis of patients whose infertility is unexplained, Fertil Steril 37:175, 1982.

Te Velde ER, Van Kooy RJ, and Waterreus JJH: Intrauterine insemination of washed husband's spermatozoa: a controlled study, Fertil Steril 51:182, 1989.

Thurmond AS and Rosch J: Nonsurgical fallopian tube recanalization for treatment of infertility, Radiology 174:371, 1990.

Tulandi T: Salpingo-ovariolysis: a comparison between laser surgery and electrosurgery, Fertil Steril 45:489, 1986.

Tulandi T and Guralnick M: Treatment of tubal ectopic pregnancy by salpingotomy with or without tubal suturing and salpingectomy, Fertil Steril 55:53, 1991.

Varma TR, Patel RH, and Bhathenia RK: Outcome of pregnancy after infertility, Acta Obstet Gynecol Scand 67:115, 1988.

Vazquez-Levin M, Kaplan P, Sandler B, et al: The predictive value of zona-free hamster egg sperm penetration assay for failure of human in vitro fertilization and subsequent successful zona drilling, Fertil Steril 53:1055, 1990.

Vermesh M, Kletzky OA, Davajan V, and Israel R: Monitoring techniques to predict and detect ovulation, Fertil Steril 147:259, 1987.

Weiner S, DeCherney AH, and Polan ML: Human menopausal gonadotropins: a justifiable therapy in ovulatory women with long-standing idiopathic infertility, AM J Obstet Gynecol 158:111, 1988.

Wilcox A, Westhoff C, Vessey M, et al: Effects of age, cigarette smoking, and other factors on fertility: findings in a large prospective study, Br Med J 290:1697, 1985.

Winston RM: Microsurgical tubocornual anastomosis for reversal of sterilization, Lancet 1:284, 1977.

Winston RM: Microsurgery of the fallopian tube: from fantasy to reality, Fertil Steril 34:521, 1980.

Yanagimachi R, Yanagimachi H, and Rogers BT: The use of zona-free animal ova as a test system for the assessment of the fertilizing capacity of human spermatozoa, Biol Reprod 15:471, 1976.

CHAPTER 40 | Menopause

KEY TERMS AND DEFINITIONS

Atrophic Vaginitis. Inflammation of the vaginal mucosa due to atrophy secondary to decreased estrogen level.

Climacteric. The physiologic period in a woman's life during which there is regression of ovarian function.

Cortical Bone. Bone in the limbs (axial skeleton). It is more slowly affected by estrogen deficiency than trabecular bone.

Hot Flush. Pathognomonic symptom of the menopause; a sudden, explosive physiologic phenomenon lasting 3 to 4 minutes accompanied by increased digital perfusion and increased peripheral skin temperature.

Menopause. Permanent cessation of menstruation caused by failure of ovarian follicular development in the presence of adequate gonadotrophin stimulation.

Osteoporosis. Asymptomatic reduction in the mass-per-unit bone volume (density) so that there is a significantly increased risk of fracture in the absence of trauma.

Premature Ovarian Failure. Cessation of menstruation due to depletion of ovarian follicles before the age of 40. It is also called premature menopause.

Trabecular Bone. Bone in the spinal column and distal radius. It is more rapidly affected by estrogen deficiency than cortical bone.

The decline of ovarian function occurs gradually, and the cessation of menses is only one facet of the climacteric process. In practice the terms *menopause* and *climacteric* are used interchangeably. The mean age of menopause in the United States is about 51 years, with a normal distribution curve and 95% confidence limits between ages 45 and 55 years (Figure 40-1). If a woman stops menstruating before age 40, the condition should be called premature ovarian failure instead of premature menopause because of the severe psychologic connotations of the latter term. If a woman continues to menstruate after the age of 55, there is an increased possibility that the endometrium will be hyperplastic or malignant. Therefore, it is advisable to biopsy the endometrium of any woman who continues to menstruate after the age of 55.

The age at which the menopause occurs is genetically predetermined, unlike the age of menarche, which is related to body mass. The age at menopause is not related to the number of prior ovulations, that is, is not affected by pregnancy, lactation, use of oral contraceptives, or failure to ovulate spontaneously. It is also not related to race, socioeconomic conditions, education, height, weight, age at menarche, or age at the last pregnancy. The age at menopause may be affected by smoking, as it has been reported that cigarette smokers experience an earlier spontaneous menopause than do nonsmokers. About 100 years ago the mean age of the menopause was approximately 40 years, but now it is about 50 years because women are living longer, and those who genetically would have a later menopause are now living past that age (Figure 40-2).

In the United States the average life expectancy for a woman is about 78 years. About 28 years, or more than one-third of a woman's life, will be spent after the menopause, a time when many women will be seeking medical

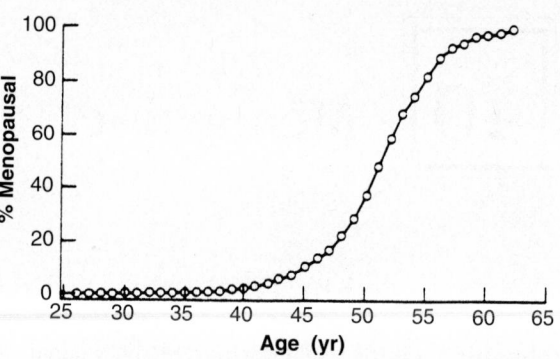

FIGURE 40-1
Cumulative proportion of women experiencing natural menopause, according to age. (From Stanford JL, Hartge P, Brinton LA, et al: J Chronic Dis 40:995, 1987.)

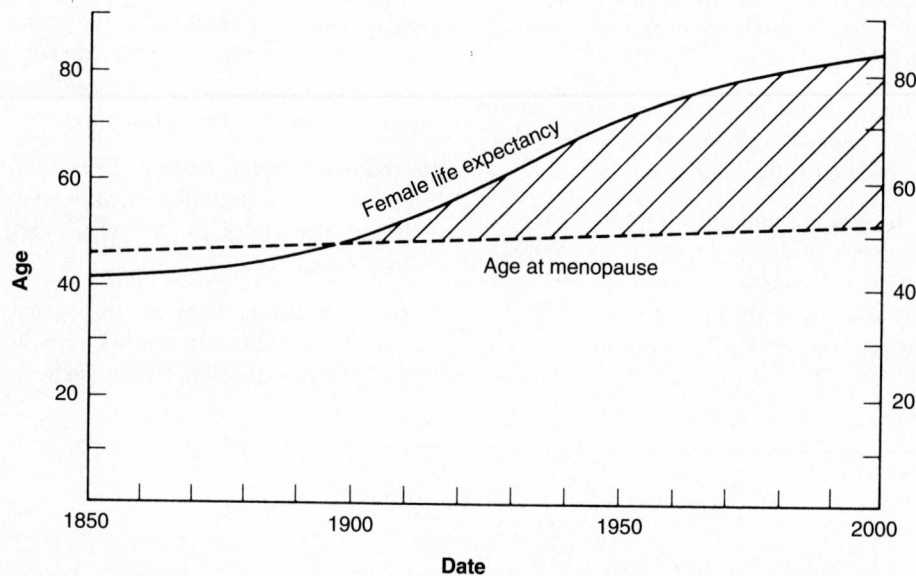

FIGURE 40-2
Female life expectancy. (From Cope E: Physical changes associated with the postmenopausal years. In Campbell S, editor: Management of the menopause and postmenopausal years, Lancaster, England, 1976, MTP Press Ltd.)

care. Thus a large proportion of all physicians' time (gynecologists, internists, and family practitioners) will be spent taking care of postmenopausal women. In 1990 there were 127 million women in the United States, with more than 35 million women over 50 years of age. The population of women overall as well as that of postmenopausal women have been steadily increasing in the United States and worldwide.

ENDOCRINOLOGY

The basic feature of menopause is depletion of ovarian follicles with degeneration of the granulosa and theca cells. As theca cells degenerate, they fail to react to endogenous gonadotrophins. As a result less estrogen is produced, and there is a decrease in the negative feedback on the hypothalamic-pituitary axis. With less inhibition, gonadotrophin production increases in an attempt to stimulate the ovary. After menopause, circulating estradiol levels generally less than 15 pg, wheras follicle-stimulating hormone (FSH) levels are greater than 40 mIU/ml and luteinizing hormone (LH) levels are also increased. Administration of large amounts of oral or parenteral estrogen will not cause FSH levels to return to premenopausal

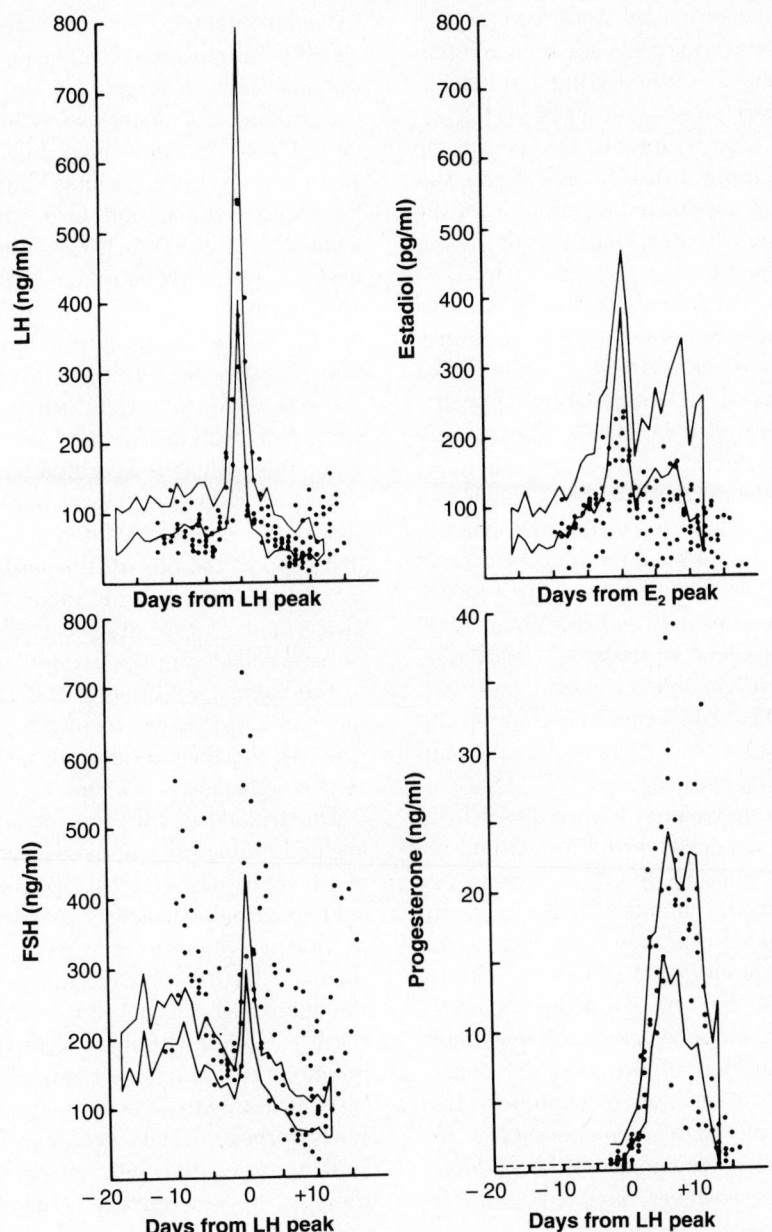

FIGURE 40-3
Serum concentrations of LH, FSH, estradiol, and progesterone in eight cycles from perimenopausal women. Mean values (±2 SEM) in 10 normal ovulatory cycles from women under 30 years are in enclosed area. (From Sherman BM, West JH, and Korenman SG: J Clin Endocrinol Metab 42:629, 1976. © by The Endocrine Society, 1976.)

concentrations, since FSH release is mainly controlled by circulating inhibin levels. Since inhibin levels decline with absent ovarian follicular activity, FSH will remain elevated even when estrogen replacement is given.

As reported by Sherman et al., this process begins about 5 years before the actual menopause. At this time, FSH levels increase and estradiol levels decrease whereas LH and progesterone levels remain unchanged, indicating that the cycles probably remain ovulatory (Figure 40-3). As estrogen concentrations decline, there is an associated decrease in prolactin levels. The decrease in estradiol before the actual menopause accounts for the fact that some women will have hot flushes during the 5 years or so before menstruation stops completely. Patients over 40 who are having regular menstrual cycles and are also having hot flushes should be treated with low doses of oral estrogen to relieve these symptoms, that is, 0.3 mg of conjugated equine estrogen or estrone sulfate or 0.5 mg of micronized estradiol from the fifth day after menstruation begins until the onset of the next menses.

In contrast to the follicular cells, the stromal cells of the ovary continue to produce androgens, androstenedione and testosterone, as the result of increased LH stimulation after the menopause. The adrenal glands also secrete these two androgens at the same rate after menopause as before menopause. The physiologic process of a decrease in the estrogen-androgen ratio is the cause of the increased facial hair growth that frequently occurs after menopause. In postmenopausal women about 3000 μg of androstenedione is produced each day— 95% of adrenal origin and 5% of ovarian origin. Androstenedione is converted to estrone in the peripheral body fat, and its rate of conversion increases as individuals age.

In a slim postmenopausal woman about 1.5% of androstenedione is converted to estrone, resulting in production of 40 μg of estrone per day. With a greater amount of body fat, more estrone is produced. An obese woman converts as much as 7% of androstenedione to estrone, producing about 200 μg of estrone per day. For this reason obese women are less likely to develop symptoms of estrogen deficiency, are less likely to develop osteoporosis, and are also more likely to develop endometrial hyperplasia and adenocarcinoma of the endometrium. Slimness, however, is a risk factor for both osteoporosis and hot flushes.

PHYSIOLOGIC ALTERATIONS

Because of the marked and persistent decrease in circulating estrogen levels, adverse effects occur in many body tissues. Unless these problems associated with this generalized condition of hypoestrogenism are corrected by estrogen replacement, adverse symptoms and an increased mortality from acceleration of atherosclerosis will occur.

Genitourinary Changes

There are a number of changes in a woman's body after the menopause. The lack of ovarian follicular function produces amenorrhea and sterility. In addition, decreasing estrogen production leads to atrophy of the vagina, which can produce the distressful symptoms of senile vaginitis or atrophic vaginitis. This type of vaginitis can cause itching, burning, discomfort, dyspareunia, and also vaginal bleeding when the epithelium thins. Senile vaginitis is best treated with estrogen replacement therapy. Local therapy can be used for the first few weeks. However, because vaginal administration of estrogen results in irregular systemic absorption, for long-term prevention of vaginal atrophy as well as osteoporosis and atherosclerosis, the patient is best treated with systemic estrogen. Estrogen deprivation may also decrease the collagen content of the structures that support the uterus, the cardinal and uterosacral ligaments, causing them to lose their tonicity, and uterine descensus may occur. Decreased collagen in the endopelvic fascial tissue in the vaginal wall may result in the development of a cystocele, rectocele, and/or enterocele. All these conditions are more often found in postmenopausal women.

The trigone of the bladder and the urethra are embryologically derived from estrogen-dependent tissue, and estrogen deficiency can lead to atrophic changes in their epithelium, producing symptoms of urinary urgency, incontinence, dysuria, and urinary frequency. With the decreased collagen in the endopelvic fascia, there is lessened support of the urethrovesical junction; with increased intraabdominal pressure, urinary stress incontinence can develop. Each of these urinary symptoms can be alleviated or prevented with estrogen replacement therapy. Several groups of investigators have reported that estrogen replacement results in subjective improvement of the symptoms of stress urinary incontinence in more than half the women receiving such therapy. It is also advisable for postmenopausal women to perform pelvic floor exercises routinely to reduce their likelihood of developing severe stress urinary incontinence.

Skin and Body Mass

Most of the subepithelial portion of the skin is composed of the protein collagen. With postmenopausal estrogen deficiency the amount of collagen in the dermis progressively diminishes, the skin becomes thin, and wrinkling occurs. In a long-term study of the effect of estro-

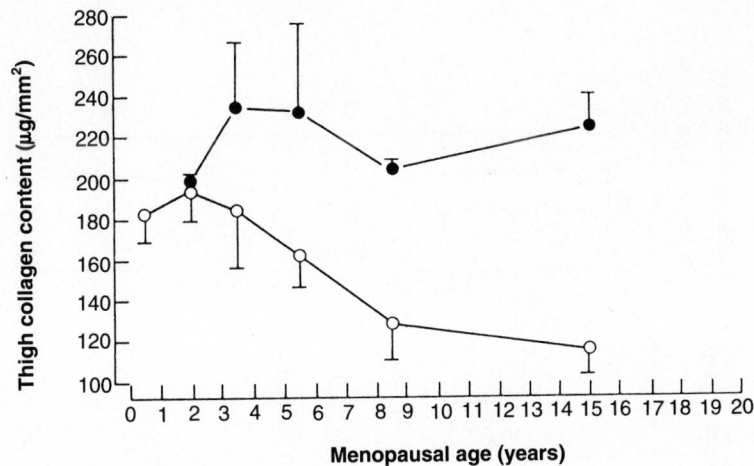

FIGURE 40-4
Relation between thigh skin collagen content and menopausal age in 52 patients treated with sex hormone implants *(closed circles)* and in 77 untreated patients *(open circles)*. (From Brincat M, Moniz CJ, Studd JWW, et al: Br J Obstet Gynaecol 92:256, 1985.)

gen on skin, Brincat et al. found that postmenopausal estrogen users had significantly thicker skin and a greater amount of collagen in the dermis than had nonestrogen users (Figure 40-4). The difference became significant more than 3 years after the menopause. Estrogen users maintained their premenopausal skin thickness, whereas the nonusers had progressively thinner skin with less collagen in the dermis as they aged. This study indicates that systemic estrogen use can retard wrinkling of the skin postmenopausally.

In a prospective study, Hassager and Christiansen reported that estrogen also prevented the 1 to 2 kg increase in fat mass of the body as well as in total body weight that occurred postmenopausally in untreated women (Figure 40-5). More studies are needed to confirm this finding.

Hot Flushes

In addition to these changes in the urogenital tract and in skin and body mass, several systemic effects may occur after menopause. The pathognomonic symptom of menopause is the hot flush or flash, which is caused by a decrease in circulating estrogen levels. Individuals who have low estrogen levels throughout their life, such as those without gonads, will not have hot flushes. If these patients receive estrogen therapy that is subsequently discontinued, they may also experience menopausal symptoms when the estrogen is stopped. The change in estrogen levels leads to alterations in the hypothalamus that are probably mediated through the central nervous system. When the change in estrogen levels is not gradual but sudden, such as occurs after castration, the individual is more likely to develop symptomatic hot flushes.

About 75% of all women going through menopause develop hot flushes. Obese individuals are less likely to develop flushes, as they do not have as great a decrease in estrogen levels. Erlik et al. have shown that postmenopausal women with hot flushes have lower circulating estrone and estradiol levels as well as less sex hormone–binding globulin (SHBG) bound estradiol than postmenopausal women without hot flushes (Figure 40-6). These investigators reported that women with hot flushes had less total body weight and a lower percentage of ideal body weight as compared with those without hot flushes. About one third of women with hot flushes have sufficiently severe symptoms to require medical assistance. About one half of the patients with flushes have at least one a day, and about 20% have more than one a day. These flushes frequently occur at night, awaken the individual, and then produce insomnia (Figure 40-7). Hot flushes do not persist in most women for more than 2 to 3 years, and it is uncommon for a woman to have hot flushes that last more than 5 years after menopause. A hot flush is a sudden, explosive

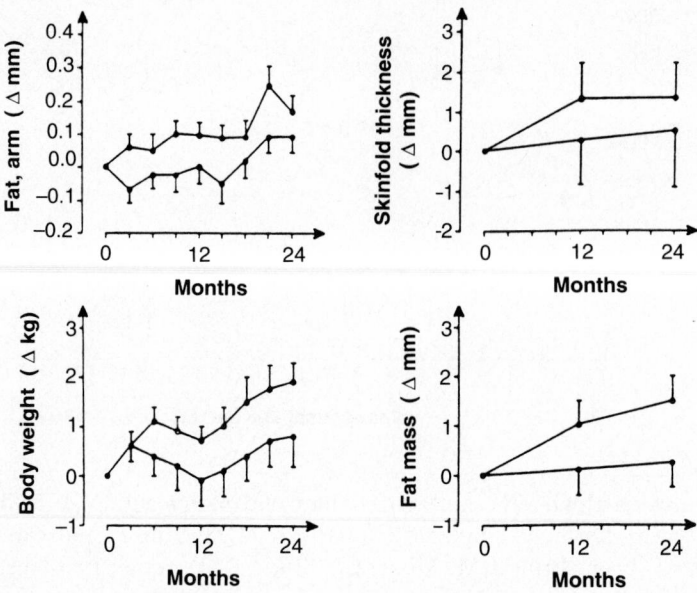

FIGURE 40-5
Course of forearm fat content (**Fat**), fat mass, skinfold thickness, and body weight in women taking oral estrogens. Values are given as difference from initial values. Circles indicate placebo group; traingles, hormone therapy group. (From Hassager C and Christiansen C: Metabolism 38:662, 1989.)

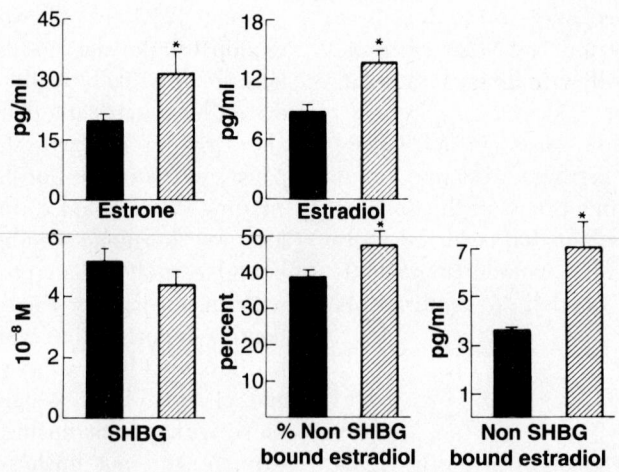

FIGURE 40-6
Mean ± SE levels of estrone, estradiol, sex hormone–binding globulin *(SHBG)*, percent non-SHBG-bound estradiol, and non-SHBG-bound estradiol in 24 women with hot flashes *(solid bars)* as compared with levels in 24 asymptomatic subjects *(striped bars)*. *, Significantly different from asymptomatic subjects. (From Erlik Y, Meldrum DR, and Judd HL: Obstet Gynecol 59:403, 1982. Reprinted with permission from The American College of Obstetricians and Gynecologists.)

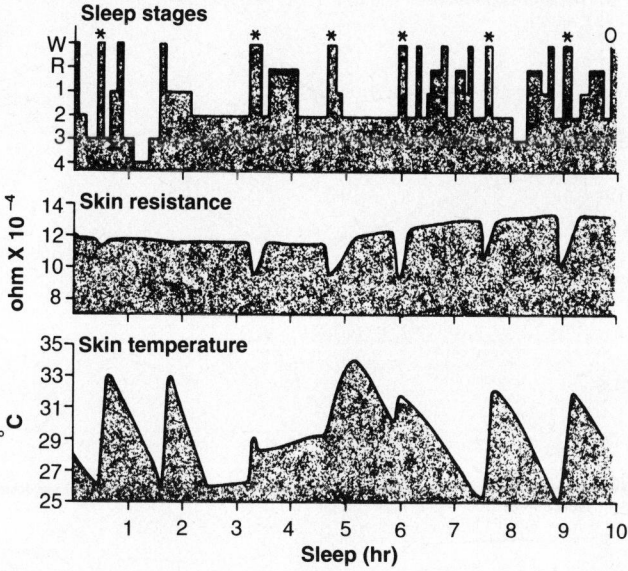

FIGURE 40-7
Sleepgram and recordings of skin resistance and temperature in postmenopausal subject with severe hot flushes. Asterisk indicates an objectively measured hot flush. (From Erlik Y, Tataryn IV, Meldrum DR, et al: JAMA 245:1741, 1981. Copyright 1981, American Medical Association.)

systemic physiologic phenomenon that takes place over a period of 30 seconds to 5 minutes. The flush is preceded by an increase in digital perfusion, which is followed by increases in peripheral skin temperature, circulating norepinephrine and LH levels, and heart rate (Figure 40-8). With each flush there are increases in LH, adrenocorticotropic hormone (ACTH), and cortisol but not FSH or estradiol. The LH increase is an effect of the change in the hypothalamic-pituitary axis and not a cause of the hot flush, because patients without a pituitary gland also have hot flushes.

The most effective treatment for the hot flush is estrogen, as Coope demonstrated in an excellent randomized, double-blind crossover study with estrogen and placebo. Women with hot flushes initially received either a placebo or estrogen and after 3 months crossed over to the other therapy. Although the placebo diminished the frequency of hot flushes, when the patients receiving placebo were crossed over to estrogen therapy, their hot flushes disappeared (Figure 40-9). Those who were treated with estrogen first had a marked diminution of hot flushes, significantly more than with the placebo, and when they were crossed over to placebo, the incidence of hot flushes returned to prestudy levels. This study demonstrates that

for treatment of hot flushes, estrogen is more effective than placebo. Since so many of the hot flushes occur at night, it is advisable for the patient to ingest the estrogen tablet before bedtime.

Initially, a dosage equivalence of 0.625 mg of conjugated estrogen or estrone sulfate or 1 mg estradiol should be tried orally, but frequently a higher dose is needed to relieve the symptoms of hot flushes. Occasionally a patient may need parenteral estrogen to relieve her symptoms.

Some patients, such as those with a history of cancer of the breast or a recent (less than 2 years) cancer of the endometrium, should not take estrogen. The next best therapy is a progestogen. Schiff et al. showed in a randomized, double-blind, crossover study that oral medroxyprogesterone acetate (MPA) in a dosage of 20 mg per day relieves hot flushes significantly more effectively than placebo (Figure 40-10). Unfortunately, MPA does not prevent vaginal or urethral atrophy, but it will diminish hot flushes in patients who cannot take estrogen. Oral MPA 20 mg per day is expensive. Several investigators have shown that injections of Depo-Provera (DMPA) in a dosage of 150 mg once every 3 months relieves hot flushes very well. Lobo et al. compared DMPA

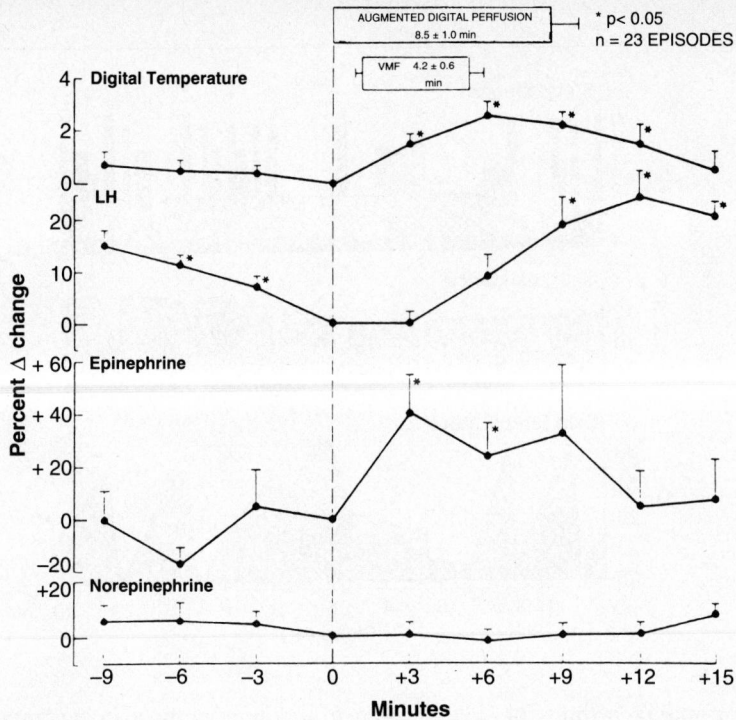

FIGURE 40-8

Composite graph of objective parameters obtained in five symptomatic postmenopausal women. Data are normalized to beginning of augmented digital perfusion (*0 time*). (From Mashchak CA, Kletzky OA, Artal R, and Mishell DR Jr: Maturitas 6:301, 1984.)

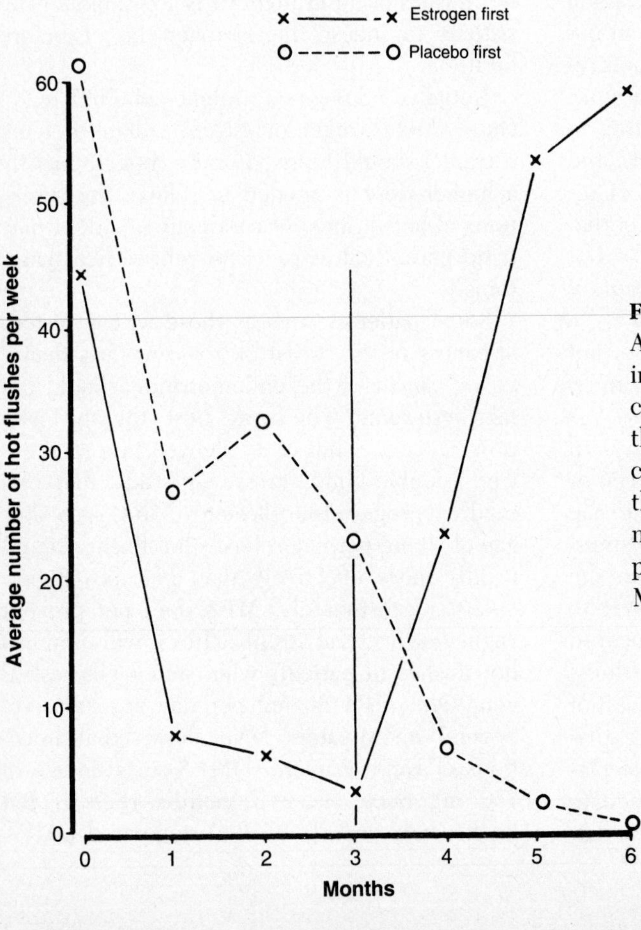

x ———— x Estrogen first
O – – – – O Placebo first

FIGURE 40-9

Average number of hot flushes per week in randomized, double-blind, 6-month crossover study of estrogen and placebo therapy. (From Coope J: Double-blind crossover study of estrogen replacement therapy. In Campbell S, editor: Management of the menopause and post-menopausal years, Lancaster, England, 1976, MTP Press Ltd.)

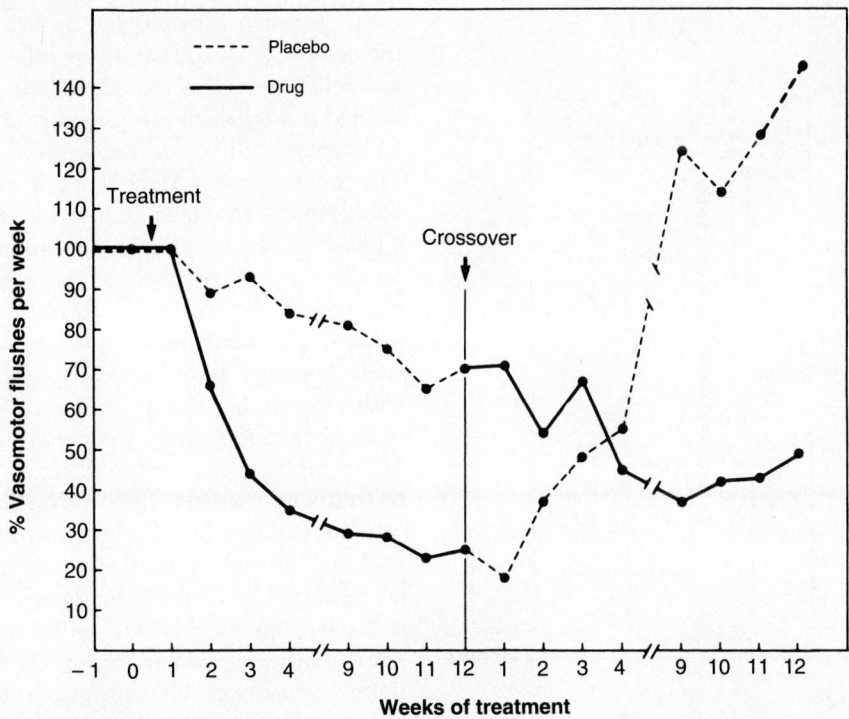

FIGURE 40-10
Mean number of vasomotor flushes as percentage change from pretreatment. Change of treatment regimen (crossover) occurred at 12 weeks. (From Schiff I, Tulchinsky D, Cramer D, and Ryan KJ: JAMA 244:1443, 1980. Copyright 1980, American Medical Association.)

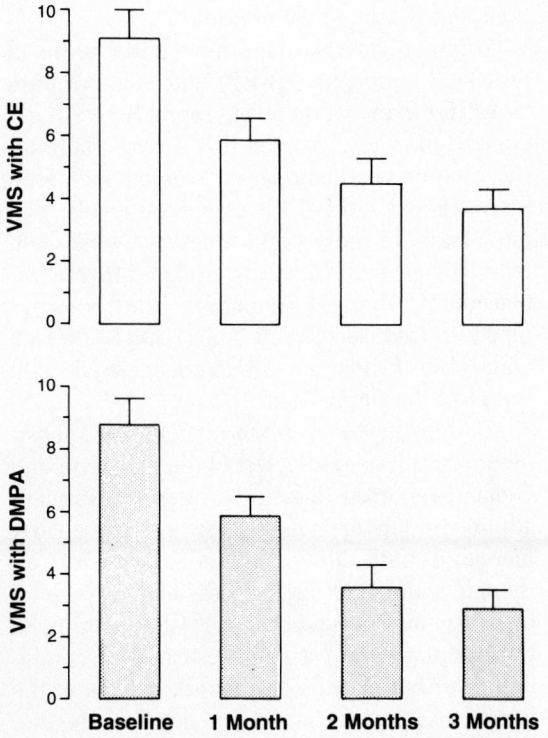

FIGURE 40-11
Vasomotor symptoms (mean ± SE) experienced before treatment (baseline) and after 1, 2, and 3 months of treatment in 23 women receiving conjugated estrogens (*open bars*) and 21 women treated with depomedroxyprogesterone acetate (DMPA; *shaded bars*). (From Lobo RA, McCormick W, Singer F, and Roy S: Obstet Gynecol 63:1, 1984. Reprinted with permission from The American College of Obstetricians and Gynecologists.)

with conjugated equine estrogens in the treatment of hot flushes and found that DMPA was as effective as estrogens in relieving the symptoms of the hot flush (Figure 40-11). In addition, DMPA decreased markers of bone resorption—urinary calcium and hydroxyproline urinary excretion—to an extent similar to that when 0.625 mg of conjugated equine estrogen

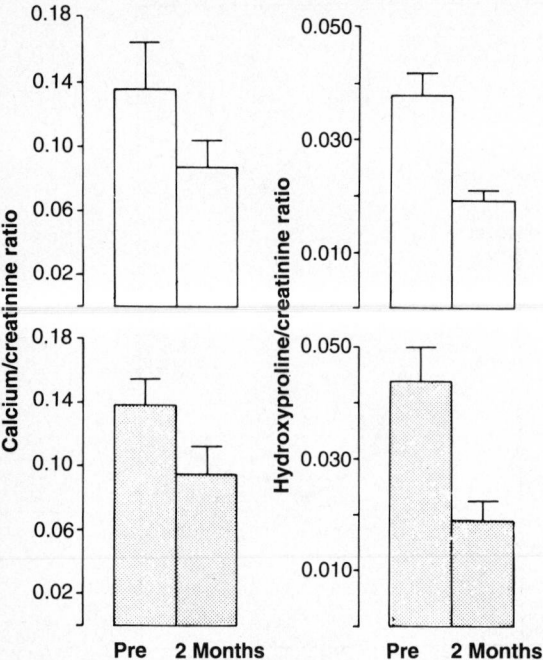

FIGURE 40-12

Calcium-creatinine and hydroxyproline-creatinine ratios (mean ± SE) before and after 2 months of treatment with either conjugated estrogens *(open bars)* or depomedroxyprogesterone acetate (DMPA; *shaded bars*). (From Lobo RA, McCormick W, Singer F, and Roy S: Obstet Gynecol 63:1, 1984. Reprinted with permission from The American College of Obstetricians and Gynecologists.)

(Figure 40-12) was given. Other agents shown to significantly reduce hot flushes include clonidine, naloxone, and methyldopa (Aldomet), but these drugs are not usually prescribed for this purpose.

Bellergal, composed of ergotamine tartrate, levorotatory alkaloids, and phenobarbital, has been used to treat women with postmenopausal hot flushes. However, in a double-blind, placebo-controlled study by Bergmans et al, Bellergal was found to be more effective than a placebo in relieving climacteric complaints only for the first 4 weeks of therapy. After 8 weeks of treatment, relief of hot flushes with Bellergal was no better than with the placebo.

Other Systemic Symptoms

Symptoms such as anxiety, depression, irritability, and fatigue increase after menopause. Controversy exists as to whether estrogen relieves these symptoms directly or whether be-

cause estrogen prevents hot flushes and allows the patient to sleep better, the other symptoms are relieved indirectly. Campbell et al. performed a double-blind placebo study involving 64 women with severe menopausal symptoms. The subjects were treated for 4 months in a double-blind crossover study with estrogen and a placebo. The frequency of symptoms was determined, and psychologic testing was performed. Of the women in this group with hot flushes, the following symptoms had a significantly greater reduction with estrogen than with placebo: hot flushes, insomnia, irritability, headaches, and urinary frequency. The following symptoms were significantly more improved with estrogen than with placebo in the women without hot flushes as well as those with hot flushes: vaginal dryness, poor memory, anxiety, and worry about self. In addition, there was an increase in optimism and good spirits with psychologic testing. Thus estrogen improves many psychologic symptoms in addition to relieving the hot flush and allowing the patient to sleep better. Nevertheless, estrogen is not a panacea for all the problems of aging. The Campbell et al. study found that there was no significant difference between the improvement of some symptoms with this short-term use of estrogen and with the placebo. These symptoms included arthralgias, backache, skin conditions, vaginal discomfort, coital satisfaction, and frequency of orgasm.

Postmenopausal women have lower levels of plasma β-endorphin (β-EP) and β-lipotrophin (β-LPH) than women of reproductive age. Genazzani et al. reported that estrogen administration to postmenopausal women increased plasma β-EP and β-LPH to normal levels. The modulation of these peptide levels by estrogen may be one mechanism whereby estrogen replacement therapy improves the woman's mood and sense of well-being, since lowered endorphin levels have been associated with symptoms of depression.

Another problem often encountered postmenopausally is decreased libido. Sherwin and Gelfand reported that, in addition to estrogen, administration of testosterone intramuscularly increased both libido and coital activity, although some androgenic side effects such as hirsutism also occurred. Myers et al. compared the use of an oral estrogen-testosterone combination with a placebo and found that use of the hormonal preparation did not significantly alter sexual activity or measurements of sexual arousal. The potential deleterious effect of testosterone on lipids also has to be considered. Therefore, whether to advocate the use of testosterone for this troublesome complaint remains controversial, and its use should be curtailed until more studies are performed.

OSTEOPOROSIS

Bone mass is increased in black, obese, and tall women and is decreased in short, frail, thin-skinned, sedentary women. Thus, women in the former group usually do not develop osteoporosis, whereas women in the latter group are at greater risk for developing the disorder and may lose about 1% to 1.5% of bone mass each year after menopause. Factors known to increase the risk of osteoporosis are as follows:

- Race: white or Oriental
- Reduced weight for height
- Early spontaneous menopause
- Early surgical menopause
- Family history of osteoporosis
- Diet: low calcium intake, low vitamin D intake, high caffeine intake, high alcohol intake, and high protein intake
- Cigarette smoking
- Endocrine disorders such as diabetes mellitus, hyperthyroidism, and Cushing's disease
- Sedentary life-style

Osteoporosis is an asymptomatic disease, and its presence usually is not detected until a fracture occurs many years later. In women undergoing a normal menopause, fractures begin to occur about age 60 in structures composed mainly of trabecular bone, such as the vertebral spine. By age 60, 25% of white and Oriental women develop spinal compression fractures. Loss of bone mass in cortical bone occurs at a much slower rate, so osteoporotic fractures of the femur usually do not begin to occur until about age 70 or 75 (Figure 40-13). By age 80, 20% of all white women will develop hip fractures, and about 15% will die from the fracture itself or from complications within 6 months. In the United States it has been estimated that annually there are about 300,000 hip fractures, about 100,000 radius fractures, and about 400,000 other fractures (mainly thoracic vertebral fractures). About 15,000 women die of osteoporosis or its complications annually in the United States, and femoral neck fractures are the twelfth leading cause of death in women in the United States. The total annual acute health care cost from osteoporosis is in excess of $4 billion. An additional $2 billion is spent for long-term convalescent care for women who have suffered a hip fracture.

At least 25% of the bone needs to be lost before osteoporosis is diagnosed by routine x-ray examination. At present the methods now available for establishing the early diagnosis of osteoporosis in trabecular bone, specifically bone density studies and computed tomography (CT) scans, are complicated and expensive. Although dual-photon absorptiometry and CT scans effectively measure bone density in trabecular bone, the equipment necessary to perform these procedures is expensive and needs

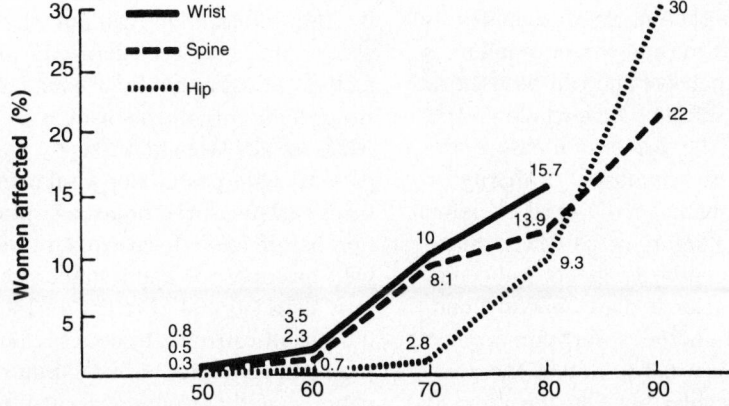

FIGURE 40-13
Cumulative incidence of osteoporosis fractures in women. (From Ettinger B: Symposium proceedings, Int J Fertil, San Francisco, April 1985, p 18.)

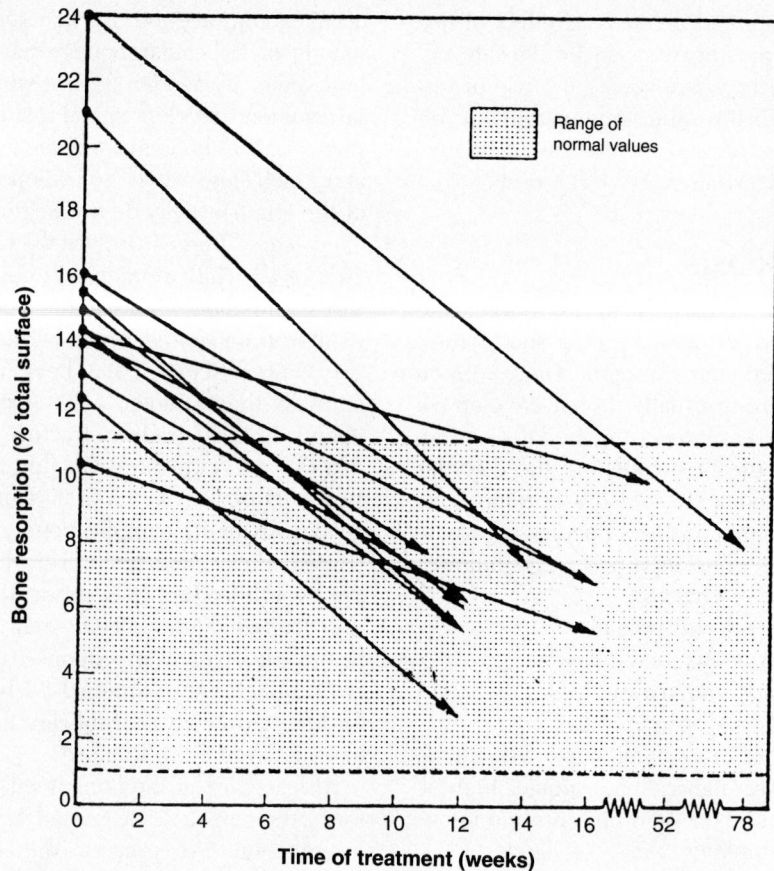

FIGURE 40-14
Effect of sex hormone on bone resorption. (From Riggs BL, Jowsey J, Kelley PJ, et al: J Clin Invest 48:1065, 1969. Copyright 1969, The American Society for Clinical Investigation.)

to be located in institutions. Dual-energy x-ray absorptiometry (DEXA) is a new method of measuring bone density that has greater precision and can be completed in a shorter time than CT or dual-photon absorptiometry. The technique of single-photon absorptiometry is much easier to perform, and the equipment is portable and less expensive and can be used in an office or clinic setting. Nevertheless, this technique can only be used to measure the density of structures composed primarily of cortical bone—the bone in the axial skeleton such as the radius, femur, or os calcis. Since postmenopausal osteoporosis affects trabecular bone more rapidly than it does cortical bone, utilization of single-photon absorptiometry on bones in the limbs can fail to detect the presence of loss of trabecular bone in the thoracic spine because the density of the bone being measured may remain within the normal range. Thus, as stated in a review by Davis,

neither of the photon absorptiometry techniques should be utilized for routine screening of postmenopausal women. Lindsay has stated that bone mass measurements are indicated only when clinical decisions will be influenced by the information gained, that is, when a woman will take estrogen only if there are objective measurements of bone loss. Data in support of this mechanism were provided by Riggs et al., who took biopsy specimens from patients with postmenopausal osteoporotic fractures and measured bone resorption and formation before and after estrogen therapy. Patients with osteoporosis had a higher bone resorption rate than normal (Figure 40-14). With a few months of estrogen treatment, bone resorption rates returned to normal. Bone formation in patients with osteoporosis was normal before and after the estrogen therapy.

Human osteoblast cells have estrogen receptors, and it may be through a receptor phe-

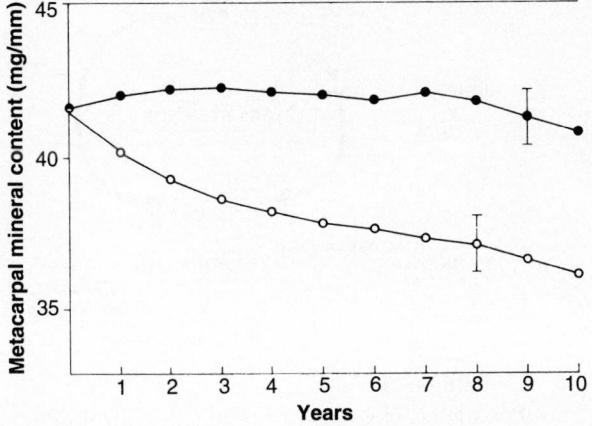

FIGURE 40-15
Bone mineral content ($\pm$ maximum SE) in those treated with estrogen *(upper line)* and placebo *(lower line)*. (From Lindsay R, Hart DM, Forrest C, and Baird C: Lancet 2:1151, 1980.)

FIGURE 40-16
Effects of withdrawal of estrogen therapy on bone mineral content after 4 years of active treatment. (From Lindsay R, Hart DM, Mac-Lean A, et al: Lancet 1:1325, 1978.)

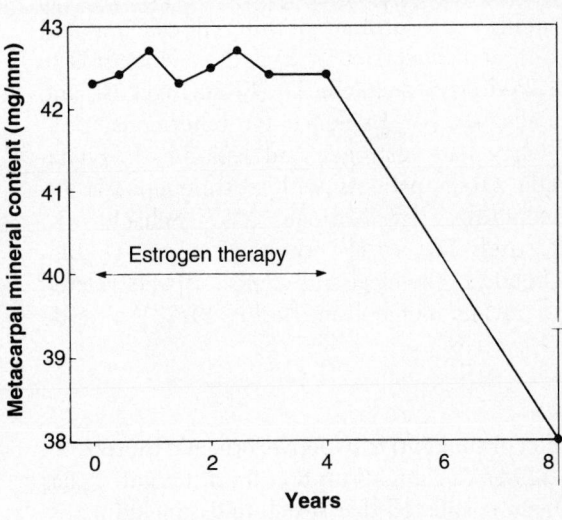

nomenon that estrogen therapy decreases bone loss. Estrogen also increases calcitonin levels, and calcitonin prevents bone resorption. Therefore there may be several mechanisms whereby estrogen prevents bone loss. The best way to prevent loss of calcium from bone in postmenopausal women or castrated women is to administer exogenous estrogens.

Both prospective (cohort) and several retrospective (case-control) studies have shown that estrogen therapy reduces the amount of postmenopausal bone loss as well as the incidence of fracture. Lindsay et al. studied a group of young Scottish women who had undergone oophorectomy. Half of them were treated with 20 μg of mestranol and half with placebo; bone density was measured at yearly intervals. After 10 years the group receiving estrogen had no decrease of bone density, whereas those who received the placebo had a steady decline in bone density (Figure 40-15), and some in this group developed loss of anterior vertebral height, indicating that compression fractures had occurred. One group of women received the estrogen for 4 years and then stopped taking it. Although they did not lose bone mass in the 4 years they took estrogen, once they stopped taking it, they started losing bone at the same rate as the placebo group (Figure 40-

16). These data indicate that estrogen replacement therapy should be maintained as long as the woman is ambulatory in order to prevent osteoporosis.

Although the mechanism whereby estrogen prevents a decrease in bone density is not precisely known, it has been determined that postmenopausal serum levels of calcium and phosphorus are slightly increased and serum levels of parathyroid hormone and the active form of vitamin D (1,25-dihydroxyvitamin D) are decreased, as is calcium absorption. In addition, calcitonin levels are lowered. Serum calcium levels are maintained within a fairly narrow range and regulated in part by parathyroid hormone production. Parathyroid hormone increases serum calcium levels by three mechanisms: bone resorption, tubal resorption of calcium in the kidney, and production of an enzyme (1-alpha-hydroxylase) that changes vitamin D from its inactive form (which occurs in the

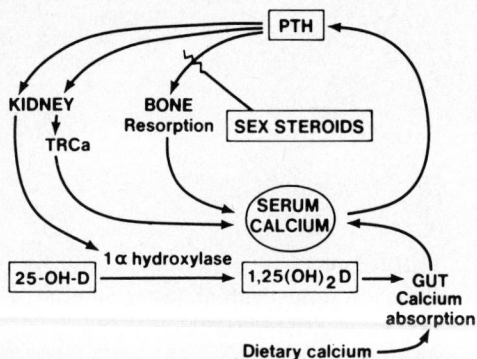

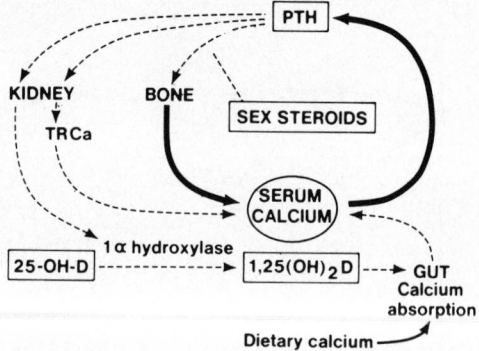

FIGURE 40-17

Hormonal control of calcium hemostasis in normal premenopausal women. Parathyroid hormone *(PTH)* increases bone resorption, renal tubular reabsorption of filtered calcium *(TR Ca)*, and conversion of 25-hydroxyvitamin D to 1,25-dihydroxyvitamin D. (From Riggs BL and Gallagher JC: Evidence for bihormonal deficiency state [estrogen and 1,25-dihydroxyvitamin D] in patients with postmenopausal osteoporosis. In Norman AW, Schaefer K, Herrath Dv, et al, editors: Vitamin D: biochemical, chemical and clinical aspects related to calcium metabolism, Berlin, 1977, Walter de Gruyter & Co.)

FIGURE 40-18

Postulated changes in hormonal control of calcium hemostasis in postmenopausal women with osteoporosis. Bone-resorbing cells have increased sensitivity to parathyroid hormone *(PTH)* action. Bone resorption increases despite decreased PTH. Decreased PTH results in decreased production of 1,25-dihydroxyvitamin D, leading to increased intestinal calcium absorption. (From Riggs BL and Gallagher JC: Evidence for bihormonal deficiency state [estrogen and 1,25-dihydroxyvitamin D] in patients with postmenopausal osteoporosis. In Norman AW, Schaefer K, Herrath Dv, et al, editors: Vitamin D: biochemical, chemical and clinical aspects related to calcium metabolism, Berlin, 1977, Walter de Gruyter & Co.)

diet or sunlight) to its active form and thereby increases calcium absorption from the gut. It has been postulated that sex steroids, including estrogen, androgens, and progestins, block the action of parathyroid hormone on bone, reducing the amount of calcium resorbed from bone (Figure 40-17). After menopause, as estrogen levels decline, there is less inhibition of the action of parathyroid hormone on bone resorption, so serum calcium levels increase, serum parathyroid hormone levels decrease, and there is less tubular reabsorption of calcium. There is less formation of 1-alpha-hydroxylase, reducing the amount of active vitamin D and leading to less absorption of dietary calcium from the gut (Figure 40-18). Most of the serum calcium is then derived from bone, which causes the steady loss of about 1.5% of bone mass each year after menopause.

Al-Azzawi and Rindsay used dual-photon absorptiometry to measure bone mass in the lumbar spine and the femoral neck in a group of women 15 years after oophorectomy. Long-term estrogen treatment resulted in a greater bone mineral density in these two sites, one cortical and the other trabecular bone, in the

estrogen users as compared with the placebo group. This prospective study indicates that estrogen replacement therapy protects against the loss of cortical bone as well as trabecular bone.

Ettinger performed a cohort study among postmenopausal women who used estrogen and found a significantly reduced risk of wrist and vertebral fractures among the group using estrogen. The number of fractures in both groups increased with the number of postmenopausal years (Figure 40-19).

In addition to these prospective and cohort studies, several retrospective epidemiologic studies have shown that estrogens reduce the incidence of fractures. Weiss et al. reported that a reduction in fractures occurred mainly in those women who had taken estrogen for more than 5 years (Table 40-1). In this study, women who took estrogen for more than 5 years had less than half the number of fractures as the control subjects. Paganini-Hill et al. reported similar results among women undergoing a nat-

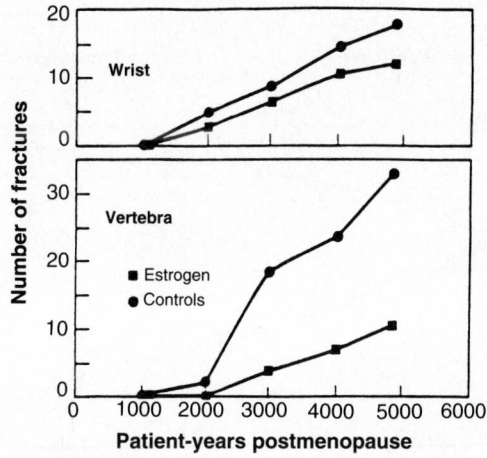

FIGURE 40-19
Cumulative wrist and vertebral fractures according to postmenopausal patient-years at risk. (From Ettinger B: Estrogen replacement therapy. In symposium Proceedings, Int J Fertil, San Francisco, April 1985.)

TABLE 40-1
Menopausal Estrogen Use and Osteoporotic Fractures

Duration of Use (Years)	Cases (%)	Controls (%)	Relative Risk*	95% Confidence Limit†
None‡	66	48	1.0	—
1-2	10	9	0.84	0.51-1.4
3-5	9	10	0.89	0.54-1.4
6-9	5	12	0.38	0.22-0.66
≥10	11	21	0.46	0.30-0.69

From Weiss NS, Ure CL, Ballard JH, et al: Decreased risk of fractures of the hip and lower forearm with postmenopausal use of estrogen, N Engl J Med 303:1195, 1980. Reprinted by permission of The New England Journal of Medicine.
*Standardized for age group (50 to 59, 60 to 69, and 70 to 74 years), history of hysterectomy, and current use versus past use of estrogens, by the method of Mantel and Haenszel.
†Approximate values, by the method of Miettinen.
‡Includes women using estrogens for less than 1 year.

ural menopause. After 5 years of ingesting estrogen, the users had less than half the risk of developing a hip fracture as did nonusers. Even less than 5 years' use of estrogen reduced the risk of hip fractures in women who had had a premenopausal oophorectomy, and more than 5 years of use resulted in a 90% lower incidence of fracture compared with nonusers.

Studies in which bone density was measured have shown the minimal dosage of estrogen needed to prevent osteoporosis is 0.625 mg of conjugated equine estrogens or estrone sulfate. One milligram of micronized estradiol appears to be equivalent to two dosages of conjugated estrogen for preventing bone loss. In addition, estrogen administered by subdermal pellets, transdermal patch, or transdermal gel has been shown to decrease the urinary calcium/creatinine ratio. These data provide indirect evidence that these parenteral routes of administration of estrogen should also decrease the loss of bone mass.

Therefore, indirect evidence suggests that progestins by themselves also reduce the rate of bone reabsorption because they decrease the amount of urinary calcium excretion. Addition of a progestin to estrogen replacement therapy does not inhibit the beneficial effect of estrogen

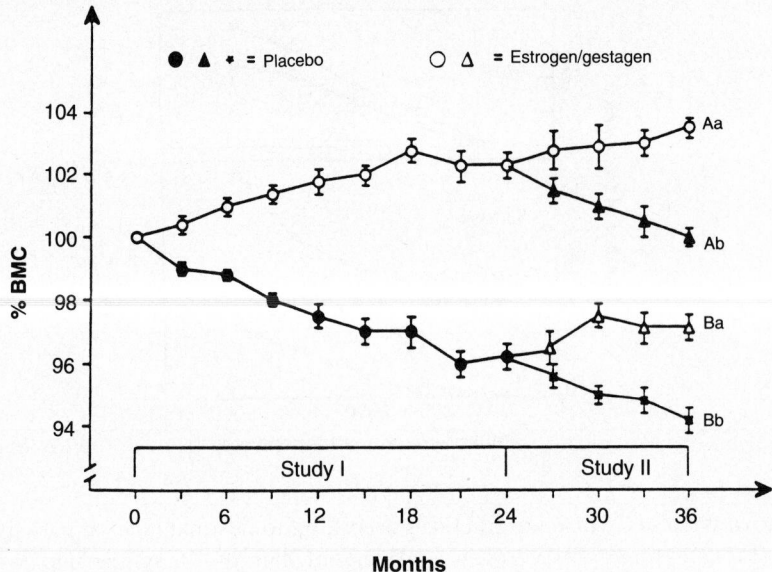

FIGURE 40-20
Bone mineral content as a function of time and treatment in 94 (study I) and 77 (study II) women soon after menopause. (From Christiansen C, Christiansen MS, and Transbol I: Lancet 1:459, 1981.)

in reducing the rate of bone reabsorption. Studies by Munk-Jensen et al., Riis et al., and Christiansen et al. have all demonstrated that both the sequential and the continuous administration of a progestin with an estrogen prevents loss of bone density and may actually increase bone density slightly, suggesting a synergistic action of the progestin with the estrogen (Figure 40-20).

Several investigators have shown that dietary calcium supplementation without estrogen does not prevent postmenopausal bone loss. Riis et al. and Ettinger et al., among others, have shown that 2 years' ingestion of 1500 or 2000 mg calcium daily (without estrogen) by postmenopausal women resulted in a similar decrease in density of trabecular bone as occurred in women receiving no calcium supplementation (Figure 40-21).

Ingesting the recommended daily intake of dietary calcium (800 to 1000 mg/day) during the adolescent years results in greater peak adult bone mass than occurs if insufficient calcium is ingested. Thus postmenopausally, with steady loss of bone, women ingesting the recommended intake are less likely to have sufficient reduction in bone density to cause fractures than those ingesting insufficient calcium (Figure 40-22).

Controversy exists whether calcium supplementation is advisable in postmenopausal women receiving estrogen replacement. Stevenson et al. reported that no significant differences in the changes in bone density occurred among a group of postmenopausal women with and without estrogen treatment who ingested a mean of 500 mg of calcium daily compared with those who ingested a mean of 1600 mg daily. However, Dawson-Hughes et al. reported that postmenopausal women with a daily calcium intake of only 400 mg could significantly reduce bone loss by increasing their calcium intake to 800 mg/day by ingesting 500 mg calcium citrate malate daily. It thus appears that in postmenopausal women ingesting an adequate amount of calcium in their diet, more than 400 mg daily, calcium supplementation is of no benefit, especially if they are also receiving estrogen. Calcium supplementation is only of benefit for those women who have an inadequate daily ingestion of calcium. It is preferable to maintain adequate intake of calcium by eating foods containing this mineral than by supplemental calcium sources. Foods rich in calcium are shown in Table 40-2.

Exercise in the premenopausal years increases bone density. However, weight-bearing exercise alone will not prevent postmeno-

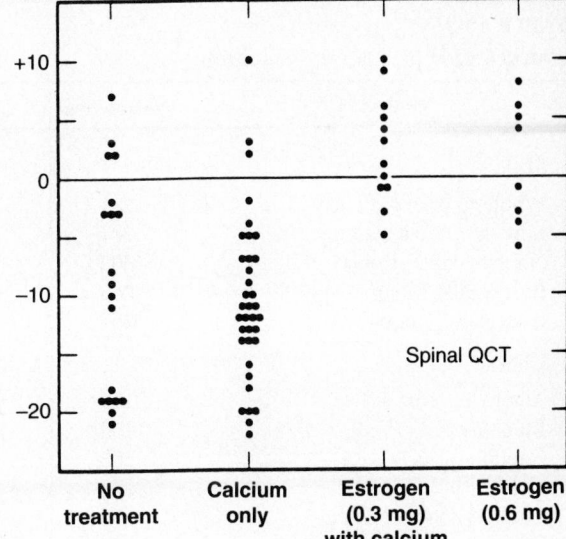

FIGURE 40-21
Skeletal changes in women after 2 years of calcium ingestion, expressed as a percentage of baseline values. (From Ettinger B, Genant HK, and Cann CE Ann Intern Med 106:40, 1987.)

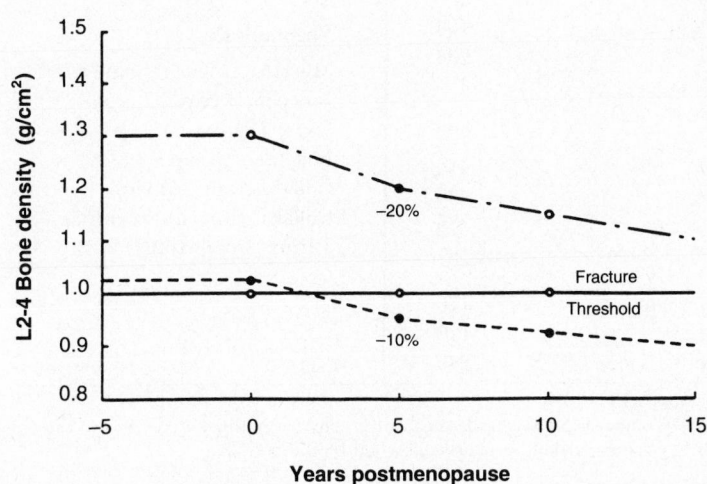

FIGURE 40-22
Effect of peak bone mass. Upper line represents bone density in woman with high peak bone mass who loses 20% of bone density after menopause. Lower line represents bone density in woman with low peak bone mass who loses only 10% of bone density postmenopausally but becomes osteoporotic. (From Stevenson JC: Obstet Gynecol 175:36S, 1990.)

pausal bone loss. Studies by Cavanaugh et al. and Sinaki et al. reported that neither a program of brisk walking nor nonloading back exercise altered the rate of trabecular bone loss postmenopausally. Thus calcium alone and a moderate exercise program apparently cannot prevent the loss of bone mass in the early postmenopausal woman, but exercise is beneficial for the woman's overall health.

It is not necessary for postmenopausal women to receive vitamin D, because Riggs and Gallagher showed that women with osteoporosis treated with various regimens with and without vitamin D had no difference in incidence of osteoporotic fractures.

In summary, estrogen increases calcium absorption and reduces the rate of bone reabsorption. It will not stimulate new bone growth but will stabilize osteoporosis if it is present and, most important, will prevent osteoporosis if therapy is started at the time of menopause. For women at risk to develop osteoporosis, specifically nonobese white or Oriental women, estrogen replacement is the keystone to the

TABLE 40-2
Sources of High Dietary Calcium

Product	Calcium (mg)	Product	Calcium (mg)
Milk		**Fruit juice**	
Whole (3.3% fat), 1 cup	291	Orange (calcium fortified), 8 oz	300
Low fat (2% fat), 1 cup	297		
Nonfat (skim), 1 cup	302	**Seafood**	
Buttermilk, 1 cup	285	Sardines (with bones), 4 oz	496
Chocolate, 1 cup	284	Salmon (pink, canned), 6 oz	333
Cheese		Oysters (fresh, raw), 8 oz	213
American, 1 oz	163	Shrimp (canned), 3 oz	98
Blue, 1 oz	150	Lobster, 3 oz	55
Cheddar, 1 oz	205	**Nuts**	
Swiss, 1 oz	273	Almonds, ½ cup	152
Cottage, low fat, ½ cup	77	Peanuts (roasted), 1 cup	104
Edam, 1 oz	208	Brazil nuts (shelled), ½ cup	130
Feta, 1 oz	140	Soybean nuts, ½ cup	75
Gruyere, 1 oz	287	**Vegetables***	
Mozzarella, part skim, 1 oz	183	Mustard greens, 1 cup	193
Muenster, 1 oz	204	Broccoli, 1 cup	136
Yogurt		Okra, 1 cup	147
Whole, plain, 8 oz	274	Bokchoy, ½ cup	126
Low fat, plain, 8 oz	415	Collards (raw), ½ cup	179
Nonfat, plain, 8 oz	452	Collards (frozen), ½ cup	149
Flavored, low fat, 1 cup	389	Turnip greens (raw), ½ cup	126
Frozen dairy			
Ice cream, vanilla, 1 cup	176		
Ice milk, vanilla, 1 cup	176		
Frozen yogurt, vanilla, 1 cup	249		

From Menopause Managment 3:15, 1990
*High calcium foods such as spinach, Swiss chard, and beet greens are not included because they have a high content of oxalic acid, which binds to calcium, making it poorly absorbed by the body.

triad approach of estrogen, calcium supplementation, and weight-bearing exercise as a method to prevent this debilitating and painful disease.

ATHEROSCLEROSIS

Under the age of 50, men have about a threefold greater incidence of myocardial infarction (MI) than women. In both sexes the incidence increases as persons age, but the rate of increase is greater in women after age 50 than in men. As a result, the ratio of MI in women to men after age 50 decreases to 2:1 by age 65 and 1:1 by age 80.

Although no randomized prospective studies have been performed to date, an abundance of epidemiologic data indicates that estrogen replacement therapy retards the development of atherosclerosis in postmenopausal women and reduces their risks of developing MI and cerebrovascular accident (CVA, stroke). Several retrospective case-control studies have demonstrated a reduction in risk of coronary heart disease in estrogen users (Table 40-3).

In addition, many prospective studies have also demonstrated that approximately a 50% reduction in MI occurs in estrogen users (Table 40-4). The only study that found an increased risk of MI in postmenopausal estrogen users, by Wilson et al., used a small cohort of women and adjusted the risk ratio with statistical techniques that corrected for the changes in lipids produced by estrogen.

TABLE 40-3

Case-Control Studies of Estrogen Replacement Therapy and Coronary Heart Disease

Investigator/Year	Data Source	Endpoint*	Crude Relative Risk		"Adjusted" Relative Risk	
			Ever Use	Current Use	Ever Use	Current Use
Rosenberg et al., 1976	Interviews	Nonfatal MI	Not reported	0.5	Not reported	1.0
Pfeffer et al., 1978	Pharmacy records	Fatal or nonfatal MI	0.9	0.6	0.9	0.7
Jick et al., 1978	Interviews	Nonfatal MI	Not reported	4.2	Not reported	Not reported
Rosenberg et al., 1980†	Interviews	Nonfatal MI	0.7 1.5	0.5 0.9	Not reported	Not reported
Ross et al., 1981‡	Medical records	Fatal IHD	0.4 0.6	Not reported	0.4 0.6	Not reported
Bain et al., 1981	Mailed survey	Nonfatal MI	0.9	0.7	0.8	0.7
Adam et al., 1981	Physicians	Fatal MI	0.6	0.8	0.6	0.8
Szklo et al., 1984	Interviews	Nonfatal MI	0.5	0.4	0.4	0.4

From Ross RK, Paganini-Hill A, Mack TM, and Henderson BE: Estrogen use and cardiovascular disease. In Mishell DR Jr, editor: Menopause: physiology and pharmacology, Chicago, 1987, Mosby–Year Book, Inc.
*MI, Myocardial infarction; IHD, ischemic heart disease.
†Rosenberg et al. reported the data on women aged 30 to 44 years (top) separately from those on women aged 45 to 49 years. "Adjusted" relative risks for postmenopausal women only were not reported.
‡Ross et al. used two control groups for comparison: living controls (top) and decreased controls.

TABLE 40-4

Risk of Coronary Heart Disease in Cohort (Prospective) Studies of Estrogen Replacement Therapy

Investigator/Year	No. of Women	Description of Postmenopausal Group	Endpoint*	Relative Risk
Criqui et al., 1988	1,868	Planned community	Fatal CHD	0.7
Henderson et al., 1988	8,041	Retirement community	Fatal MI	0.6
Bush et al., 1987	2,270	White women	Fatal CHD	0.3
Petitti et al., 1986	16,638	Prepaid health plan	Fatal CHD†	0.5
Stampfer et al., 1985	32,317	Nurses	CHD	0.5
Wilson et al., 1985	1,234	Residents	CHD	1.9
Bush et al., 1983	2,269	White women	Fatal CHD	0.4
Hammond et al., 1974	610	Hypoestrogenic	CHD	0.3
Burch et al., 1974	737	Hysterectomized	CHD	0.4

From Bush TL, Barrett-Connor E, Cowan LD, Cowan LD, et al: Cardiovascular mortality and noncontraceptive use of estrogen in women: results from the Lipid Research Clinics Program follow-up study, Circulation 75:1102, 1987.
*CHD, Coronary heart disease; MI, myocardial infarction.
†Nonfatal CHD: relative risk, 1.0.

In the prospective cohort study of Bush et al. in every 10-year age category over the age of 50 years, the estrogen users had significantly lower cardiovascular mortality rates than the nonusers of estrogen. After adjustment for age the relative risk of death from cardiovascular disease in the estrogen users compared with the nonusers was 0.34 (95% confidence interval, 0.12 to 0.81) (Table 40-5). The difference in fatal cardiovascular disease in the two groups resulted in lower rates than expected in the women receiving estrogen rather than exces-

TABLE 40-5
Cardiovascular Disease Death Rates (per 10,000) According to Estrogen Use*

	Estrogen Use	
Age at risk	Nonuser (N = 1677)	User (N = 593)
40-49	0.0	0.0
50-59	16.2	4.5
60-69	39.1	11.8
70-79	150.8	61.7
Crude Rate	30.9	11.7
Age-adjusted rate	38.1	13.1
Relative risk (95% confidence interval)		0.34 (0.12-0.81)

From Bush TL, Barrett-Connor E, Cowan LD, Cowan LD, et al: Cardiovascular mortality and noncontraceptive use of estrogen in women: results from the Lipid Research Clinics Program follow-up study, Circulation 75:1104, 1987.

sively high rates in the nonusers. Estrogen use also significantly reduced the risk of death from cardiovascular disease in postmenopausal women who were current smokers and in women in whom clinical cardiovascular disease was already present.

Henderson et al. prospectively followed 8841 women residing in a retirement community and found a significant reduction of deaths from acute MI among estrogen users than nonusers (relative risk, 0.59). Current estrogen users had the greatest protection from death from coronary artery disease, with a relative risk of 0.47, and former estrogen recipients had a relative risk of 0.62 when compared with those who had never used estrogen. Adjustment for the presence of known risk factors for cardiovascular disease, including a history of high blood pressure, a history of angina or acute MI, and smoking, did not alter the protection of the cardiovascular system derived from estrogen therapy for postmenopausal women.

Additional evidence from studies of women undergoing coronary artery angiography supports the belief that estrogen use retards the development of atherosclerosis. In a retrospective study of women undergoing coronary angiography, Gruchow et al. reported that the degree of coronary artery occlusion did not increase after age 60 among estrogen users,

whereas it did among nonusers (Figure 40-23).

McFarland et al. reported that among 345 women undergoing coronary artery catheterization for suspected MI, estrogen users were only half as likely as nonusers to have severe coronary artery disease (more than 70% occlusion). Sullivan et al. performed a retrospective 10-year follow-up of 2268 women who had coronary angiography. Survival rates at 10 years were significantly higher among estrogen users with both mild to moderate as well as severe degrees of coronary artery occlusion. Survival was only 60% among estrogen nonusers whereas it was 97% among estrogen users (Figure 40-24). After appropriate adjustment for other risk factors, estrogen was found to have a significant independent effect on survival. These data indicate that estrogen prevents worsening of existing atherosclerosis and that prior cardiovascular disease is not a contraindication to estrogen replacement.

Paganini-Hill et al. showed in a cohort study that postmenopausal estrogen use significantly reduced the risk of death from CVA (stroke) among women 75 to 85 years of age (Table 40-6). Thus estrogen use protects against the development of cerebral artery atherosclerosis as well as coronary artery atherosclerosis. Since cardiovascular disease is the major cause of death among women over 50, many studies have shown that estrogen reduces the risk of overall mortality among postmenopausal women (Table 40-7).

In the study by Henderson et al. the relative risk of overall mortality steadily decreased with increasing duration of estrogen use. Thus estrogen replacement increases a woman's life span.

Probably the main mechanism whereby oral estrogen replacement retards atherosclerosis postmenopausally is prevention of the adverse alterations in endogenous circulating lipid levels that normally occur after the menopause. In longitudinal studies, Matthews et al. and Jensen et al. found that total serum cholesterol, low-density lipoprotein (LDL) cholesterol, and triglyceride levels increased postmenopausally, whereas high-density lipoprotein (HDL) cholesterol levels declined (Figure 40-25). Several investigators have reported that ingestion of various oral estrogen formulations postmenopausally prevents these unfavorable alterations in the lipid profile. As summarized by Bush and Miller, numerous studies have shown that administration of oral conjugated equine estro-

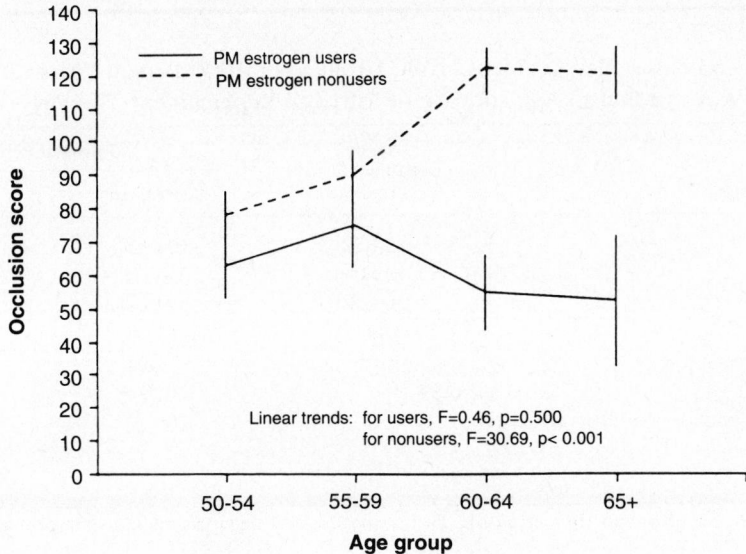

FIGURE 40-23
Occlusion scores by age groups for postmenopausal (**PM**) estrogen users and nonusers. Numbers of users/nonusers in each age group are 48/174 (50 to 54 years), 47/224 (55 to 59 years), 35/203 (60 to 64 years), and 24/178 ($\geq$ 65 years). (From Gruchow HW, Anderson AJ, Barboriak JJ, and Sobocinski KA: Am Heart J 115:954, 1988.)

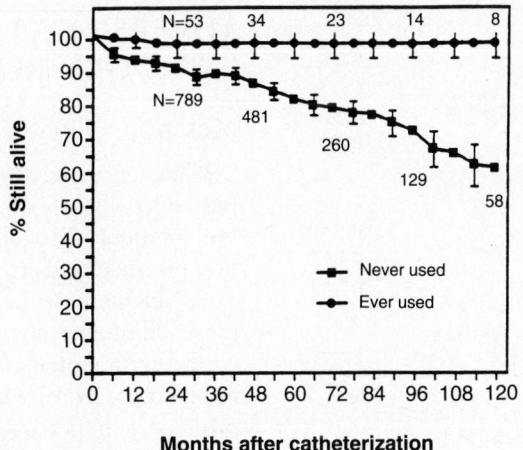

FIGURE 40-24
Ten-year survival of patients with left main coronary stenosis of 50% or greater or other stenosis of 70% or greater. (From Sullivan JM, Vander Zwaag R, Hughes JP, et al: Arch Intern Med 150:2557, 1990.)

gens as well as other oral estrogens raises triglyceride and serum HDL cholesterol levels and lowers LDL cholesterol levels, with minimal changes in total cholesterol levels (Figure 40-26). Data regarding parenteral administration of estrogen fail to show similar consistent significant lipid changes, indicating the first pass of the oral estrogen through the liver has a major influence on lipid metabolism.

The effects of combinations of estrogens and

TABLE 40-6

Mortality from Cerebrovascular Accident (CVA, Stroke) per 1000 Person-Years (and Numbers of Deaths) from CVA According to Age and Use of Estrogen Replacement Therapy

Age	No. of Follow-up Years	Estrogen Replacement	
		Never Used	Ever Used
<75	16,872	0.4 (2)	0.4 (4)
75-79	10,806	1.5 (7)	0.3 (2)
80-84	8,423	3.2 (14)	1.0 (4)
≥85	4,682	6.8 (20)	5.7 (10)
No. of follow-up years		17.624	23.159
Age adjusted		2.0 (43)	1.1 (20)
Relative risk (95% confidence interval)		1.00	0.53 (0.31-0.91)
Two-sided P value			0.02

From Paganini-Hill A, Ross RK, and Henderson BE: Postmenopause oestrogen treatment and stroke: a prospective study, Br Med J 297:519, 1988.

TABLE 40-7

Relative Risk Estimates from Cohort Studies of Use of Estrogen Replacement Therapy and All Causes of Mortality

Investigator/Year	Relative Risk AC
Burch et al., 1974	0.4*
Stampfer et al., 1985	0.5†
Wilson et al., 1985	0.97
Henderson et al., and Paganini-Hill et al., 1988	0.8*
Pettiti et al., 1986	0.7*
Bush et al., 1987	0.5*
Hunt et al., 1988	0.6*
Criqui et al., 1988	0.7*
Henderson et al., 1991	0.8*

*$P<0.05$.
†RR=0.9 after eliminating that part of the cohort with cancer or coronary heart disease at baseline ($P= 0.42$).

progestins for postmenopausal women on lipid metabolism depend on the doses and the potencies of both the estrogen and the progestin used in the regimen. In most studies, the beneficial changes with estrogen alone are reduced or eliminated with the addition of a synthetic progestin.

Nevertheless, estrogen may have other actions, including a direct effect on the coronary arteries, to prevent atherosclerosis. Additional studies are currently being performed to determine whether parenteral estrogen and various estrogen-progestin combinations will also prevent atherosclerosis.

ADVERSE EFFECTS OF ESTROGEN REPLACEMENT

Metabolic Effects

With any drug there is a benefit-risk ratio, but the risks of estrogen replacement therapy are minimal. Exogenous estrogen administration produces effects on serum proteins, specifically an increase in serum globulins. One of these globulins, angiotensinogen, can be converted to angiotensin and produce an increase in blood pressure, whereas other globulins may produce a hypercoagulable state and possibly thrombosis. In addition, exogenous estrogens may alter lipid levels and other metabolic processes. However, these metabolic changes are related to the dosage and type of estrogen administered, and the dose and type of estrogen given for postmenopausal hormone replacement therapy are much less potent than those used in oral contraceptives. For prevention of osteoporosis, bone density studies have shown that at least the equivalent of 0.625 mg of conjugated equine estrogen needs to be ingested. Patients with hot flushes sometimes need to receive a higher dose, the equivalent of 1.25 mg

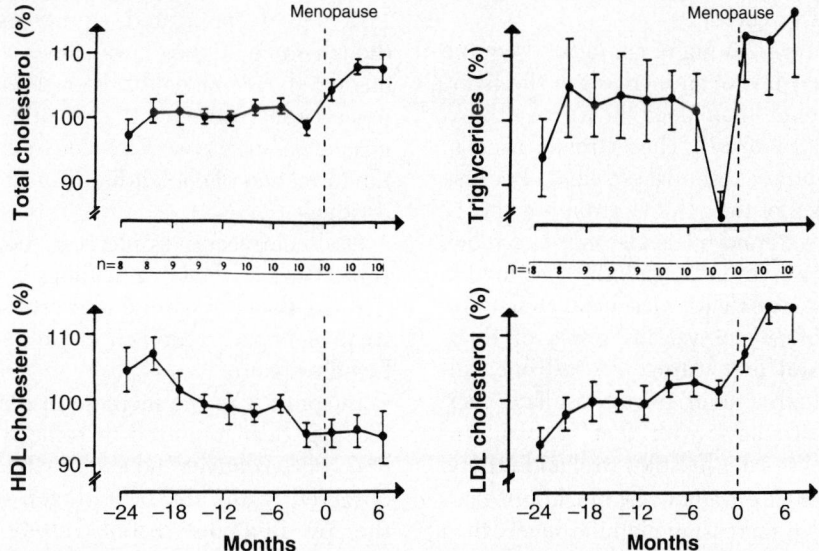

FIGURE 40-25
Time course of menopause-related changes in serum lipids and lipoproteins in 10 women who underwent natural menopause during study and number at each examination. (Values are expressed as percentages of mean during premenopausal period and are given as mean± SEM for every two examinations performed.) **H/LDL**, High-low-density lipoprotein. (From Jensen J, Nilas L, and Christiansen C: Maturitas 12:321, 1990.)

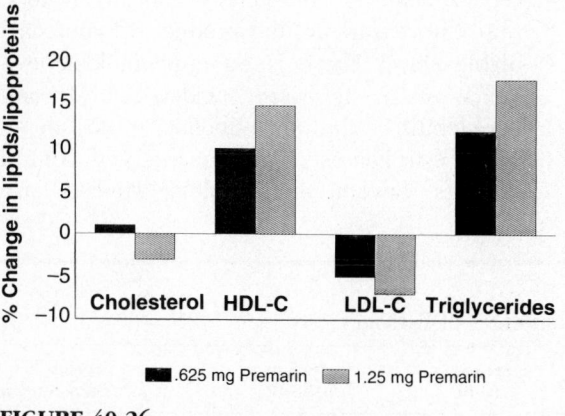

FIGURE 40-26
Percent change in lipid lipoproteins by dose or premarin. (From Bush TL and Miller VT: Effects of pharmacologic agents used during menopause: impact on lipids and lipoproteins. In Mishell DR Jr, editor: Menopause: physiology and pharmacology, Chicago, 1987, Mosby–Year Book Inc.)

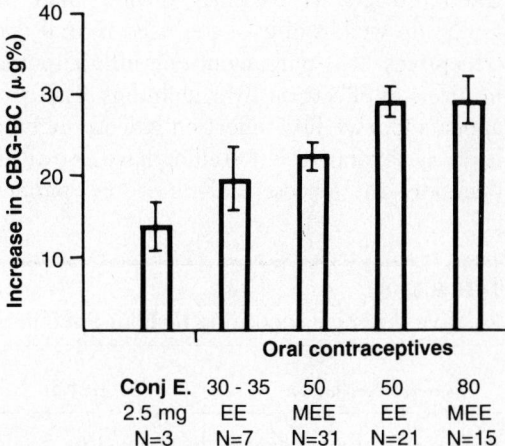

FIGURE 40-27
Increase in corticosteroid-binding globulin–binding capacity (CBG-BC) (μg/dl) in relation to dose of synthetic estrogen. *Conj E*, Conjugated equine estrogen; *EE*, ethinyl estradiol; *MEE*, mestranol. (From Moore DE, Kawagoe S, Davajan V, et al: Am J Obstet Gynecol 130:482, 1978.)

of conjugated equine estrogen or greater, for relief of these symptoms.

However, even 2.5 mg of conjugated equine estrogen causes less of an increase in the liver-binding globulins than does 30 μg of ethinyl estradiol (Figure 40-27). The estrogen used in oral contraceptives, ethinyl estradiol, because of the presence of the ethinyl group on the 17 position of the steroid molecule, causes a much greater increase in liver globulin production than does estrone sulfate. Mashchak et al. compared the potency of various doses of three types of natural oral estrogens—estrone sulfate, conjugated equine estrone sulfate, and micronized estradiol—with that of two synthetic estrogens—diethylstilbestrol and ethinyl estradiol. Ethinyl estradiol was much more potent in terms of increasing globulin levels than any of the natural estrogens. In terms of equivalent weight, when an increase in liver globulins was used as the parameter of estrogenic activity, ethinyl estradiol was found to be about 90 times as potent as conjugated equine estrogen and about 200 times as potent as estrone sulfate (Table 40-8). Thus 30 or 35 μg of ethinyl estradiol, which is the dosage of estrogen in most of the currently used oral contraceptive formulations, is the equivalent of about 2.5 mg of conjugated equine estrogens. Therefore, although the usual dosage of 0.625 mg of conjugated estrogen is 20 times greater than the minimum weight of estrogen used in oral contraceptives, it is only about one-fifth as potent in terms of effects on liver globulins. Estrogen appears to have little effect on glucose metabolism, as several recent studies have shown no decrease in glucose tolerance in patients treated with doses of estrogen equivalent to 1.25 mg of conjugated equine estrogen. Although some studies have shown a statistically increased risk of gallbladder disease in postmenopausal estrogen users, others have reported no such risk. Estrogens may accelerate the formation of cholelithiasis in susceptible individuals.

Oral contraceptives increase the blood pressure of some women, but there is no evidence that the doses of natural oral estrogens used to treat menopausal women cause an increase in blood pressure.

In contrast to the increase in blood pressure that has been reported in some women using oral contraceptives, no such increase has been observed with use of estrogen replacement therapy. In a cross-sectional study reported by Barrett-Connor et al., although mean systolic and diastolic blood pressure increased with age, there was no significant difference between estrogen users and nonusers (Table 40-9). In a longitudinal prospective study Wren and Routledge reported that women ingesting piperazine estrone sulfate actually had a significant decrease in systolic and diastolic blood pressure, whether or not they were receiving antihypertensive therapy (Table 40-10).

In addition, Aylwood showed that the natural estrogens in the dosages used for hormonal replacement do not increase clotting factors, but ethinyl estradiol did produce a hypercoagulable state. There is no epidemiologic evidence of an increased incidence of thrombophlebitis or thromboembolism in postmenopausal estrogen users as compared with control subjects. Several epidemiologic studies have

TABLE 40-8
Relative Potency According to Four Specific Parameters of Estrogenicity

Estrogen Preparation	Serum FSH	Serum CBG-BC	Serum SHBG-BC	Serum Angiotensinogen
Piperazine estrone sulfate	1.0	1.0	1.0	1.0
Conjugated estrogens	1.4	2.5	3.2	3.5
Micronized estradiol	1.3	1.9	1.0	0.7
Diethylstilbestrol	3.8	70.0	28.0	13.0
Ethinyl estradiol	(80-200)*	(1000)*	614	232

From Mashchak CA, Lobo RA, Dozono-Takano R, et al: Comparison of pharmacodynamic properties of various estrogen formulations, Am J Obstet Gynecol 144:511, 1982.
FSH, Follicle-stimulating hormone; *CBG-BC*, corticosteroid-binding globulin–binding capacity; *SHBG-BC*, sex hormone–binding globulin–binding capacity.
*Estimate in absence of parallelism.

TABLE 40-9

Systolic and Diastolic Blood Pressure According to Age and Postmenopausal Estrogen Use*

Age	Systolic Blood Pressure (mm Hg)		Diastolic Blood Pressure (mm Hg)	
	Users	Nonusers	Users	Nonusers
55-59	130.8 ± 18.8	135.0 ± 25.1	79.4 ± 9.6	81.3 ± 12.0
60-64	134.1 ± 18.9	136.5 ± 19.2	79.4 ± 9.4	81.6 ± 9.8†
65-69	139.3 ± 20.3	140.4 ± 21.4	81.9 ± 10.8	82.6 ± 12.2
70-74	147.9 ± 25.9	147.8 ± 20.9	82.0 ± 10.3	83.8 ± 22.7

From Barrett-Connor E, Brown WV, Turner J, et al: Heart disease risk factors and hormone use in postmenopausal women, JAMA 241:2167, 1979. Copyright 1979, The American Medical Association.
*All data adjusted for obesity. Means and standard deviations are given.
†$P \leq 0.05$.

TABLE 40-10

Piperazine Estrone Sulfate—Women Taking and Not Taking Antihypertensives

	Mean	SD	t*	P	N
Taking antihypertensives (N = 34)					
Systolic visit 1	151.26	22.75	—	—	34
Systolic visit 2	143.03	16.45	—	—	34
Mean change	−8.23	17.21	2.79	< 0.01	34
Diastolic visit 1	91.82	9.69	—		34
Diastolic visit 2	86.53	10.72	—		34
Mean change	−5.29	9.29	3.32	< 0.01	34
Not Taking antihypertensives (N = 150)					
Systolic visit 1	134.77	16.35	—	—	150
Systolic visit 2	130.41	15.42	—	—	150
Mean change	−4.36	15.35	3.48	< 0.001	150
Diastolic visit 1	84.37	9.83	—	—	150
Diastolic visit 2	81.08	9.32	—	—	150
Mean change	−3.29	9.49	4.25	< 0.001	150

From Wren BG, Routledge AD: The effect of type and dose of oestrogen on the blood pressure of post-menopausal women, Maturitas 5:135, 1983.
*Student's *t* test.

reported no increased incidence of these disorders in postmenopausal women taking estrogen in comparison to the increased incidence found in oral contraceptive users. Furthermore there is no evidence that postmenopausal women with a past history of thrombophlebitis have an increased incidence of thrombophlebitis with estrogen replacement therapy.

Hassager and Christiansen reported on a series of double-blind, placebo-controlled studies of long-term estradiol given to early (6 months to 3 years) and to late (14 to 20 years) healthy, normotensive postmenopausal women. There was no difference in systolic blood pressure in the estrogen-treated group as compared with those receiving a placebo. There were lower diastolic blood pressure recordings in the hormonal treatment group as compared with the women using a placebo, although the decrease was statistically significant only in the early postmenopausal women (Figure 40-28). The effect of estrogen replacement therapy on blood pressure is neutral or may even be beneficial.

These data indicate that it is safe to prescribe estrogen replacement for postmenopausal women with hypertension, and if blood pressure increases while they are receiving this treatment, it is unlikely that the estrogen is the cause of the blood pressure elevation.

Neoplastic Effects

Much concern has been raised about the neoplastic risks of postmenopausal estrogen replacement therapy, particularly breast and endometrial cancer, since these areas are estrogen target tissues. The possibility exists that estrogen can stimulate a nonpalpable breast cancer, and carcinoma of the breast may exist in the preclinical state for as long as 8 years before it is palpable. Therefore it is advisable to obtain a mammogram to rule out subclinical breast cancer on all patients before initiating estrogen therapy and annually thereafter.

Many epidemiologic studies have investigated the relation between exogenous estrogen and the incidence of breast cancer. In 1988 Armstrong used metaanalysis to determine the effect of estrogen replacement therapy on the

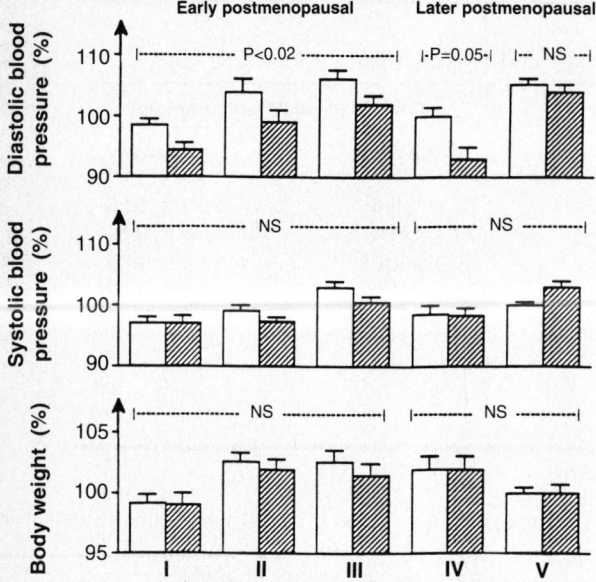

FIGURE 40-28
Cumulative blood pressure and body weight responses (as percentages of initial values) during hormone (**shaded bars**) and placebo (**open bars**) treatment in five trials. (From Hassager C and Christiansen C: Maturitas 9:315, 1988.)

risk of breast cancer. Metaanalysis is the process whereby the results of multiple studies are combined for statistical evaluation. Armstrong reviewed the results of all 23 studies of estrogen use and breast cancer published before 1987. He concluded that the use of estrogen does not significantly alter the risk of breast cancer (relative risk, 1.01; 95% confidence interval, 0.95 to 1.08) (Table 40-11).

A more recent metaanalysis by Steinberg et al. also found no increase in breast cancer among estrogen users unless they had used the hormone for more than 5 years, at which time the relative risk of breast cancer increased slightly. After 15 years of estrogen use the relative risk of developing breast cancer increased significantly (relative risk, 1.3; confidence interval, 1.2 to 1.6) to 30%. The increased risk occurred mainly among premenopausal estrogen users or women who received an estradiol formulation.

Thus the epidemiologic data are conflicting, but most studies show no increased risk of development of breast cancer among postmenopausal estrogen users, with the possibility of a slightly increased risk with long-term use.

The effect of the administration of a progestin to postmenopausal women on the risk of breast cancer has not been determined. One epidemiologic study by Gambrell suggested that a combination estrogen-progestin menopausal hormonal regimen protects the breast in a manner similar to the way it protects the endometrium, with a decreased risk of breast cancer. However, since mitotic activity in breast tissue increases during the luteal phase of the menstrual cycle and in vitro studies demonstrate increased mitotic activity in breast tissue with progestin exposure, a deleterious effect of progestin on the human breast is suggested. In support of this hypothesis, Bergkvist et al. reported that postmenopausal women using estrogen and a progestin had a 4.6-fold increased risk of breast cancer, although this increase was not statistically significant. At present, it is not clear what effect the addition of a progestin to estrogen replacement therapy has on the risk of breast cancer.

Many epidemiologic studies have reported that there is a significantly increased risk of developing endometrial cancer in postmenopausal women who are ingesting unopposed estrogen as compared with nonestrogen users. The risk increases with increasing duration of use of estrogen as well as with increasing dosage (Table 40-12). In a population-based case-control study, the Cancer and Steroid Hormone Study, Rubin et al. reported that the increased risk of endometrial cancer associated with the use of unopposed estrogen for 2 years or longer persisted for 6 years or more after the estrogen therapy was discontinued. However, these investigators reported that those women who used low doses of estrogen, 0.625 mg of conjugated equine estrogen or less, had only a mild, insignificant increase in the risk of endometrial cancer. These investigators also reported that prior oral contraceptive use of 1 year or longer negated the increased risk of endometrial cancer in postmenopausal women who were receiving only estrogen.

The endometrial cancer that develops in estrogen users is nearly always well differentiated and is usually cured by performing a simple hysterectomy. Collins et al. showed that women who had endometrial cancer and were not receiving estrogen had a 10-year survival rate of about 50%, and a control population without cancer matched for age and lack of estrogen had about an 80% survival rate at the

TABLE 40-11
Estrogen Therapy and Relative Risk of Breast Cancer

Set of studies	No. of Studies	Summary Relative Risk		P Value for Heterogeneity*
		Point Estimate	95% Confidence Interval	
All studies	23	1.01	0.95-1.08	0.006
All studies with adjusted results†	12	1.05	0.97-1.14	0.006
All studies of postmenopausal women	12	0.96	0.89-1.05	0.07
Studies of postmenopausal women with adjusted results†	7	0.99	0.90-1.08	0.04

Armstrong BK: Oestrogen therapy after the menopause—boon or bane? Med J Aust 148:213, 1988.
*P value for heterogeneity among the individual relative risks that contribute to the summary relative risk of breast cancer.
†Results adjusted for type of menopause, whether natural or artificial, or age at menopause, or both.

end of 10 years (Figure 40-29). A group of patients who had endometrial cancer and were also taking estrogen had a survival rate about the same as a control population taking estrogen (90%), indicating that the well-differentiated endometrial carcinoma occurring with estrogen treatment can be adequately treated by performing a hysterectomy and is usually not lethal. The risk of developing endometrial carcinoma for women receiving estrogen replacement can be markedly reduced by giving the patient progestogens. Estrogen acts only if a specific receptor is present within the target cell. The estrogen receptor complex activates messenger RNA, which then changes DNA to produce cell division and also synthesize new estrogen receptors. Progesterone, which normally is produced in the last half of the normal menstrual cycle, blocks receptor synthesis so no new receptors are formed. Therefore the endometrium does not proliferate in the latter half of the menstrual cycle because progesterone prevents receptor synthesis and further growth and division of the cells despite continued estrogen production. To summarize, estrogen increases the synthesis of both estrogen and progesterone receptors in the endometrium; progesterone and synthetic progestins decrease the synthesis of both these receptors and thus have an antiproliferative action.

Progestins have been shown to prevent endometrial hyperplasia. Sturdee et al. performed endometrial biopsies annually in women receiving sex steroids. Twenty-three

TABLE 40-12
Risk Estimates from Case-Control Studies of Estrogen Replacement Therapy and Endometrial Cancer

Study		Relative Risks*	
Author	Year	Ever Users	Long-Term Users
Smith	1975	4.5	—
Ziel	1975	7.6	13.9
Mack	1976	5.6	8.8
Gray	1977	3.1	11.6
McDonald	1977	2.0	7.9
Wigle	1978	2.2	5.2
Horwitz	1978	12.0	—
Hoogerland	1978	2.2	6.7
Antunes	1979	6.0	15.0
Weiss	1979	7.5	8.2
Hulka	1980	—	4.2
Shapiro	1980	3.9	6.0
Jelovsek	1980	2.4	4.8
Spengler	1981	3.2	8.6
Stavraky	1981	4.2	14.4
Kelsey	1982	—	8.2
LaVecchia	1982	2.7	—
Henderson	1983	1.4	3.1

From Peterson HB, Lee MC, Rubin GL: Genital neoplasia. In Mishell DR Jr, editor: Menopause: physiology and pharmacology, Chicago, 1987, Mosby–Year Book, Inc.
*Risk relative to never users.

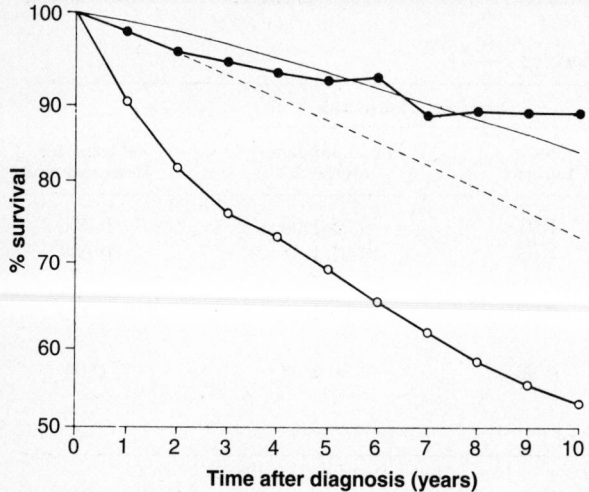

FIGURE 40-29

Survival of women with endometrial cancer and history of estrogen use *(solid circles)* compared with estrogen-user controls (age-adjusted mortality) *(solid line)*, with women with endometrial cancer who were not estrogen users *(open circles)*, and with non-estrogen-user controls (age-adjusted mortality) *(dashed line)*. (From Collins J, Donner A, Allen LH, and Adams O: Lancet 2:961, 1980.)

TABLE 40-13

Effect on Endometrial Cancer of Adding Progestogen (Progestin) to Estrogen Treatment

Investigator/Year	Untreated	Incidence / 1000 Patient-Years		
		Estrogen Alone	Estrogen and Progestogen	
Hammond et al., 1979	0.5	6.5	0	
Nachtigall et al., 1979	1.2	—	0	
Gambrell et al., 1987	2.5	3.9	0.5	
Persson et al., 1989	1.4	1.8	0.9	

From Mishell DR Jr, Davajan V, and Lobo RA, editors: Infertility, contraception and reproductive endocrinology, ed 3, Cambridge, Mass, 1991, Blackwell Scientific Publications.

percent of the women receiving continuous estrogen alone and 12% of patients taking cyclic estrogen alone developed endometrial hyperplasia. When progestins were added for 5 days each month in addition to estrogen, the incidence of hyperplasia decreased to 8%. When progestins were added to treatment for more than 10 days each month for more than 200 women for 4 years, no hyperplasia developed. These and other studies have shown that the duration of progestin therapy is more important than the dosage. Small amounts of progestin administered for more than 10 days each month have also been shown to reduce the incidence of endometrial carcinoma in several studies (Table 40-13).

Thus there is evidence that use of progestins lowers the chances of postmenopausal estrogen users' developing cancer of the endometrium,

and therefore progestins should be given to postmenopausal women receiving estrogen if they have a uterus. The addition of a progestin to estrogen therapy does not appear to cause an increase of any other systemic disease and acts synergistically with estrogen to cause a slight increase in bone density. The use of synthetic progestins may reverse the beneficial effect of estrogen upon serum lipids. Ottoson et al. reported that daily ingestion of 10 mg of MPA in addition to the estrogen reduced HDL cholesterol levels to those present prior to the ingestion of estrogen. The epidemiologic data showing a reduction in heart attacks in estrogen users was derived from women taking estrogen without a progestin. Whether the addition of a progestin to the regimen will reverse the beneficial action of estrogen on cardiovascular disease remains to be determined. Nevertheless, it would appear prudent to use the lowest dose of progestin that will prevent the endometrial proliferation produced by estrogen.

TREATMENT REGIMENS

Estrogen therapy for postmenopausal women should be given in the lowest possible dose that relieves vasomotor symptoms, prevents vaginal-urethral epithelial atrophy, maintains the collagen content of the skin, reduces the rate of bone resorption, and prevents acceleration of atherosclerosis. Estrogen therapy given to postmenopausal women should result in physiologic and not pharmacologic circulating levels of estrogen, so that the risk of hypertension and thromboembolic disease are not increased. This dose of estrogen, termed the *physiologic replacement dose*, is 0.625 mg of conjugated equine estrogen or estrone sulfate or 1 mg of micronized estradiol. The long-term effects of transdermal estradiol have not yet been determined, but it appears the 0.05 mg skin patch provides physiologic estrogen replacement. Higher doses of estrogen may be needed for 1 or 2 years to relieve hot flushes. Vaginal administration of estrogen may be used initially to relieve atrophic vaginitis, but it is best to use other routes for long-term use because vaginal estrogen absorption is greatly variable.

If a progestin is added to the regimen to protect the endometrium, it does not negate the beneficial effects of estrogen on vasomotor symptoms or on bone density. The progestin may have an adverse effect on the vaginal and urethral mucosa and may produce undesired central nervous system (CNS) symptoms and adversely affect mood and sense of well-being. Depending on the dose and biologic activity of the specific progestin, the favorable antiatherogenic lipid profile produced by estrogen may be altered and may result in a partial or complete loss of the cardiovascular protective effect of unopposed estrogen. Finally, a hormonal regimen should be selected that produces the least amount of uterine bleeding.

Hemminki et al. reported that estrogen use declined in the United States from 1973 to 1980, most likely because of the studies that demonstrated an increase of endometrial cancer associated with unopposed estrogen. Since 1980, estrogen therapy for postmenopausal women has increased as the long-term benefits of this therapy has been verified. Concomitant use of estrogen and progestin has increased since 1982. Although the benefits of estrogen replacement therapy far exceed any possible risk, it is estimated that only 10% to 15% of postmenopausal American women are currently taking estrogen. One quarter of American women who are given prescriptions for estrogen therapy never have them filled, and another quarter start the estrogen therapy but discontinue it within 12 months. Ferguson et al. reported that the primary reason that postmenopausal women decide not to use estrogen or discontinue its use is the occurrence of uterine bleeding. For this reason, combination instead of sequential estrogen-progestin regimens are being increasingly prescribed.

The benefit of including a progestin in the estrogen replacement regimen is protection of the endometrium. Unfortunately, this benefit is accompanied by an increase of CNS symptoms and changes in mood and a sense of well-being. Magos et al., in a double blind, placebo-controlled study, demonstrated a dose-related deleterious effect of norethindrone on CNS symptoms, especially depression, anxiety, and irritability. Holst et al. reported that fatigue, tension, irritability, and depression were increased during the interval of progestin administration. Women who have undergone a hysterectomy are no longer at risk for endometrial cancer. Until other significant benefits of progestin therapy for menopausal women are established, an unopposed estrogen regimen, cyclic or continuous, is recommended for postmenopausal women who no longer have a uterus.

For postmenopausal women who have not had a hysterectomy, many treatment regimens are used. An estrogen-only regimen may be used to optimize protection from cardiovascular disease, in conjunction with an annual endometrial biopsy or vaginal ultrasonography to measure the endometrial thickness.

Granberg et al. studied 205 women with postmenopausal uterine bleeding by endovaginal sonography followed by uterine curettage. Of the 18 who had endometrial cancer, none had endometrial thickness less than 8 mm (Table 40-14). All women with endometrial thickness of 5 mm or less had a histologic diagnosis of atrophic endometrium. Thus, if confirmed by others, this technique may be used instead of annual biopsy to screen postmenopausal

TABLE 40-14
Histologic Diagnosis as Related to Endometrial Thickness Obtained by Endovaginal Scanning

| | Final Histologic Diagnosis | | | | |
	Atrophy	Polyp	Hyperplasia	Cancer	Other
Women (no.)	157*	13	13	18	4
Mean age (years)	65.3	69.5	62.0	68.0	76.0
Thickness (mm, mean ± SD)	3.4 ± 1.2	10.8 ± 4.7	9.7 ± 2.5	18.2 ± 6.2	20.0 ± 7.9
Range (mm)	2-11	6-24	6-13	9-35	12-35

From Granberg S, Wikland M, Karlsson B, et al: Endometrial thickness as measured by endovaginal ultrasonography for identifying endometrial abnormality, Am J Obstet Gynecol 164:47, 1991.
*Thirty of these women were receiving a regimen of estrogen therapy.

women with a uterus who receive estrogen without a progestin or those who bleed and receive a continuous combined estrogen-progestin regimen.

Currently in clinical practice, physicians more often include a progestin in the hormonal replacement regimen for postmenopausal women who have a uterus. Various regimens, both sequential and continuous combined, have been used. The hormones are usually administered in a cyclic manner, with a daily dose of estrogen given the first 21 to 25 days each month and a daily dose of progestin administered concomitantly with the last 10 to 13 days of the estrogen. The estrogen may be given every day of the month in a continuous fashion and the progestin given daily for the first 10 to 13 days of the month with the combined regimen. Both the estrogen and the progestin may be administered every day of the month or 5 out of 7 days each week. The cyclic regimens usually result in monthly withdrawal bleeding, which may lessen with continued use. The continuous regimen frequently results in breakthrough bleeding during the first 6 months, but with longer use nearly all women remain amenorrheic.

The minimal dosage and type of progestin necessary to prevent endometrial cancer have not been determined. Fraser et al. showed that, in patients receiving 0.625 mg of conjugated equine estrogens, as little as 350 μg of norethindrone and 150 μg of norgestrel were sufficient to decrease the receptor and DNA activity in the endometrial cells to a level similar to that of the secretory phase of the normal

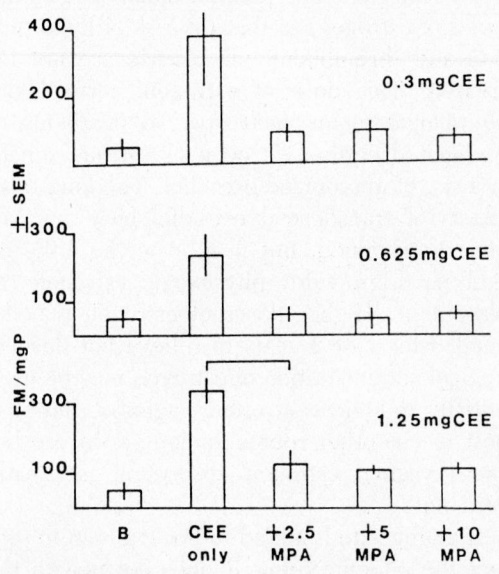

FIGURE 40-30
The concentrations of nuclear estrogen receptor in three groups of postmenopausal women receiving no therapy (B), estrogen only (CEE), and estrogen plus various doses of medroxyprogesterone acetate (MPA). * = $P < 0.001$. (From Gibbons WE, Moyer DL, Lobo RA, et al: Am J Obstet Gynecol 154:456, 1986.)

cycle. Gibbons et al. demonstrated that for postmenopausal women receiving 0.625 mg of conjugated equine estrogen, 2.5 mg of MPA reduced nuclear and cytosol estrogen receptor levels to those found before estrogen administration (Figure 40-30). With a daily dose of 1.25 mg of conjugated equine estrogen, 5 mg of MPA was necessary to decrease receptor synthesis to the same degrees. Since the side effects of progestin therapy are dose related, any reduction in the dose of progestin that still protects the endometrium may lead to improved patient compliance.

Weinstein et al. studied the use of daily conjugated equine estrogen (0.625 mg) with either 2.5 or 5.0 mg of MPA for 1 year in a group of 92 postmenopausal women. The investigators found that both regimens provided an atrophic endometrium, a favorable lipid profile, and a steadily decreased incidence of uterine bleeding with 82% of the women who were amenorrheic during the last 3 months of the study.

A routine pretreatment endometrial biopsy is unnecessary because it is not cost-effective. Also, routine annual biopsies are not necessary. If breakthrough bleeding, but not regular withdrawal bleeding, occurs, the lining of the uterine cavity should be sampled. Annual mammography should be recommended for all women aged 50 years or older, regardless of whether they are receiving estrogen therapy. Contraindications to estrogen therapy occur infrequently. These include a history of breast cancer and thromboembolic disease associated with oral contraceptive use or pregnancy. Although no data support these contraindications, they have become the standard of practice. The Centers for Disease Control have reported that women with a positive family history of breast cancer involving either a second-degree or a first-degree relative may use estrogen replacement therapy without an increased risk of breast cancer. Women with active liver disease should avoid the oral administration of estrogen.

Estrogen is the first treatment of choice in the relief of vasomotor symptoms and symptoms caused by vaginal and urethral mucosa atrophy. In addition, estrogen therapy maintains the integument, improves mood, prevents postmenopausal osteoporosis, and above all, significantly reduces the morbidity and mortality associated with cardiovascular disease. Nearly all postmenopausal women can derive a substantial benefit from the use of estrogen replacement therapy.

KEY POINTS

- The mean age of menopause is about 51 years.

- Age at menopause is genetically predetermined and is not related to the number of ovulations, race, socioeconomic conditions, education, height, weight, age at menarche, or age at last pregnancy.

- The basic feature of menopause is depletion of ovarian follicles with degeneration of the granulosa and theca cells while stromal cells continue to produce the androgens androstenedione and testosterone.

- Androstenedione is converted to estrone in the peripheral body fat, and its rate of conversion increases as women age.

- Postmenopausal women with hot flushes have lower circulating estrone and estradiol levels, less total body weight, and a lower percentage of ideal body weight as compared to those without hot flushes.

- About 1% to 1.5% of bone mass is lost each year after menopause in nonobese white and Oriental women. Fractures begin to occur about age 60 to 65 in trabecular bone, such as the vertebral spine, and by age 60, 25% of these women develop spinal compression fractures.

- By age 80, 20% of all white women will develop hip fractures, and 15% of these fractures are fatal within 6 months. In the United States each year osteoporosis causes about 300,000 hip fractures, 100,000 radius fractures, and 400,000 other fractures. About 15,000 women die of osteoporosis or its complications annually in the United States.

- Patients with postmenopausal osteoporosis have a higher bone resorption rate than normal, while bone formation in patients with osteoporosis is normal.

- After menopause, 800 mg of elemental calcium should be ingested daily.

- For prevention of osteoporosis, at least the equivalent of 0.625 mg of conjugated equine estrone, 0.625 mg of estrone sulfate, or 1 mg of micronized estradiol needs to be ingested.

- In terms of equivalent weight, when an increase in liver globulins is used as the parameter of estrogenic activity, ethinyl estradiol is about 90 times as potent as conjugated equine estrogen.

- Levels of LDL cholesterol have a positive correlation with coronary heart disease, while levels of HDL cholesterol have an inverse relation to coronary heart disease. Postmenopausal estrogen users have decreased levels of LDL cholesterol as well as increased levels of HDL cholesterol as compared with postmenopausal nonestrogen users.

- The risk of developing endometrial cancer is 3 to 7 times greater in postmenopausal women who are ingesting estrogen without progestins as compared with nonestrogen users. The risk is increased with higher dosages and prolonged use.

- Estrogen increases the synthesis of both estrogen and progesterone receptors in the endometrium; progesterone and synthetic progestins decrease the synthesis of both these receptors and thus have an antimitotic, antiproliferative action.

- Indications for estrogen therapy in menopause include the presence of vasomotor symptoms as well as prevention of atrophic vaginitis, atrophic urethritis, and osteoporosis.

- Before estrogen therapy is instituted, a pretreatment mammogram should be performed.

- At least 25% of bone needs to be lost before osteoporosis can be diagnosed by routine x-ray examination.

- Dual-energy x-ray absorptiometry (DEXA) is the most accurate method to measure bone denisty.

- Bone mass measurements are indicated only when clinical decisions will be influenced by the information gained.

- To prevent development of osteoporosis, estrogen replacement should be given as long as the woman is ambulatory.

- Addition of a progestin to estrogen replacement does not inhibit the beneficial effect of estrogen on reducing the rate of bone reabsorption.

- Calcium supplementation and/or weight-bearing exercise without estrogen does not prevent postmenopausal osteoporosis.

- Calcium supplementation is unnecessary for postmenopausal women taking estrogen and having adequate daily calcium intake.

- Estrogen increases calcium absorption and reduces the rate of bone reabsorption postmenopausally. It does not stimulate bone formation.

- Estrogen users have about a 50% reduction in risk of developing myocardial infarction or stroke under the age of 85.

- Angiographic studies indicate estrogen retards the development of coronary atherosclerosis.

- Estrogen therapy improves survival rates in women with existing coronary atherosclerosis.

- Oral estrogen replacement does not raise systolic or diastolic blood pressure.

- Nearly all epidemiologic studies indicate that estrogen replacement does not increase the risk of developing breast cancer. Those that suggest an increased risk are based on long-term usage.

- The effect of progestins on risk of developing breast cancer has not been determined to date.

- The endometrial cancer that develops among estrogen users is usually well differentiated and nearly always cured by hysterectomy.

- It is estimated that currently only 10% to 15% of postmenopausal American women use estrogen replacement.

- Estrogen without a progestin is recommended for postmenopausal women who have had a hysterectomy.

- Progestins can be given cyclically or continuously. Bleeding is more common with the cyclic regimen.

BIBLIOGRAPHY

Al-Azzawi F and Rindsay R: Long term effect of oestrogen replacement therapy on bone mass as measured by dual photon absorptiometry, Br Med J 294:1261, 1987.

Armstrong BK: Oestrogen therapy after the menopause—boon or bane? Med J Aust 148:213, 1988.

Aylwood M, Maddock J, Lewis PA, et al: Oestrogen replacement therapy and blood clotting, Curr Med Res Opin 4(suppl 3):83, 1971.

Barrett-Connor E, Brown WV, Turner J, et al: Heart disease risk factors and hormone use in postmenopausal women, JAMA 241:2167, 1979.

Barrett-Connor E, Wingard DL, and Criqui MH: Postmenopausal estrogen use and heart disease risk factors in the 1980s: Rancho Bernardo, California, revisited, JAMA 261:2095, 1989.

Boston Collaborative Drug Surveillance Program: Surgically confirmed gallbladder disease, venous thromboembolism and breast tumors in relation to postmenopausal estrogen therapy, N Engl J Med 290:15, 1974.

Bergkvist L, Adami H-O, Persson I, et al: The risk of breast cancer after estrogen and estrogen-progestin replacement, N Engl J Med 321:293, 1989.

Bergkvist L, Adami H-O, Persson I, et al: Prognosis after breast cancer diagnosis in women exposed to estrogen and estrogen-progestogen replacement therapy, Am J Epidemiol 130:221, 1989.

Bergmans MGM, Merkus JMWM, Corbey RS, et al: Effect of Bellergal retard on climacteric complaints: a double-blind, placebo controlled study, Maturitas 9:227, 1987.

Bhatia NN, Bergman A, and Karram MM: Effects of estrogen on urethral function in women with urinary incontinence, Am J Obstet Gynecol 160:176, 1989.

Brincat M, Moniz CJ, Studd JWW, et al: Long-term effects of the menopause and sex hormones on skin thicknes, Br J Obstet Gynaecol 92:256, 1985.

Bush TL, Barrett-Connor E, Cowan LD, et al: Cardiovascular mortality and noncontraceptive use of estrogen in women: results from the Lipid Research Clinics Program follow-up study, Circulation 75:1102, 1987.

Bush TL and Miller VT: Effects of pharmacologic agents used during menopause: impact on lipids and lipoproteins. In Mishell DR Jr, editor: Menopause: physiology and pharmacology, Chicago, 1987, Mosby–Year Book.

Campbell S, Beard RJ, McQueen J, et al: Double blind psychometric studies on the effects of natural estrogens on post-menopausal women. In Campbell S, editor: Management of the menopause and post-menopausal years, Lancaster, England, 1976, MTP Press Ltd.

Cauley JA, Gutai JP, Kuller LH, et al: Endogenous estrogen levels and calcium intakes in postmenopausal women, JAMA 260:3150, 1988.

Cavanaugh DJ, Cann CE, Dallal GE, et al: Brisk walking does not stop bone loss in postmenopausal women, Bone 9:201, 1988.

Christiansen C, Christiansen MS, and Transbol I: Bone mass in postmenopausal women after withdrawal of oestrogen/gestagen replacement therapy, Lancet 1:459, 1981.

Collins J, Donner A, Allen LH, and Adams O: Oestrogen use and survival in endometrial cancer, Lancet 2:961, 1980.

Coope J: Double-blind cross-over study of estrogen replacement therapy. In Campbell S, editor: Management of the menopause and post-menopausal years, Lancaster, England, MTP Press Ltd., 1976, p. 167.

Davis MR: Screening for postmenopausal osteoporosis, Fertil Steril 156:1, 1987.

Dawson-Hughes B, Dallal GE, Krall EA, et al: A controlled trial of the effect of calcium supplementation on bone density in postmenopausal women, N Engl J Med 323:878, 1990.

Egeland GM, Kuller LH, Matthews KA, et al: Hormone replacement therapy and lipoprotein changes during early menopause, Obstet Gynecol 76:776, 1990.

Erlik Y, Meldrum DR, and Judd HL: Estrogen levels in postmenopausal women with hot flashes, Obstet Gynecol 59:403, 1982.

Erlik Y, Tataryn IV, Meldrum DR, et al: Association of waking episodes with menopausal hot flushes, JAMA 245:1741, 1981.

Ettinger B: Estrogen replacement therapy. In Symposium proceedings, Int J Fertil, San Francisco, April, 1985.

Ettinger B, Genant HK, and Cann CE: Long-term estrogen replacement therapy prevents bone loss and fractures, Ann Intern Med 102:319, 1985.

Ettinger B, Genant HK, and Cann CE: Postmenopausal bone loss is prevented by treatment with low-dosage estrogen with calcium, Ann Intern Med 106:40, 1987.

Farish E, Fletcher CD, Hart DM, et al: The effects of conjugated equine oestrogens with and without a cyclic progestogen on lipoproteins and HDL subfractions in postmenopausal women, Acta Endocrinol 113:123, 1986.

Ferguson KJ, Hoegh C, and Johnson S: Estrogen replacement therapy: a survey of women's knowledge and attitudes, Arch Intern Med 149:133, 1989.

Fraser DI, Parsons A, Whitehead MI, et al: The optimal dose of oral norethindrone acetate for addition to transdermal estradiol: a multicenter study, Fertil Steril 53:460, 1990.

Gambrell RD Jr: Use of progestogen therapy, Am J Obstet Gynecol 156:1304, 1987.

Gambrell RD Jr, Massey FM, Castaneda TA, et al: Reduced incidence of endometrial cancer among postmenopausal women treated with progestogens, J Am Geriatr Soc 27(9):389, 1979.

Genant HK, Baylink DJ, Gallagher JC, et al: Effect of estrone sulfate on postmenopausal bone loss, Ob Gyn 76:759, 1990, Fig 1.

Genazzani AR, Petraglia F, et al: Steroid replacement treatment increases β-endorphin and β-lipotropin plasma levels in postmenopausal women, Gynecol Obstet Invest 294:1261, 1988.

Gibbons WE, Moyer DL, Lobo RA, et al: Biochemical and histologic effects of sequential estrogen/progestin therapy on the endometrium of postmenopausal women, Am J Obstet Gynecol 154:456, 1986.

Granberg S, Wikland M, Karlsson B, et al: Endometrial thickness as measured by endovaginal ultrasonography for identifying endometrial abnormality, Am J Obstet Gynecol 164:47, 1991.

Gruchow HW, Anderson AJ, Barboriak JJ, and Sobocinski KA: Postmenopausal use of estrogen and occlusion of coronary arteries, Am Heart J 115:954, 1988.

Hammond CB, Jelovsek FR, Lee KL, et al: Effects of long-term estrogen replacement therapy. I. Metabolic effects, Am J Obstet Gynecol 133:525, 1979.

Hammond CB, Jelovsek FR, Lee KL, et al: Effects of long-term estrogen replacement therapy. II. Neoplasia, Am J Obstet Gynecol 133:537, 1979.

Harris RB, Laws A, Reddy VM, et al: Are women using postmenopausal estrogens? A community survey, Am J Public Health 80:1266, 1990.

Hassager C and Christiansen C: Blood pressure during oestrogen/progestogen substitution therapy in healthy postmenopausal women, Maturitas 9:315, 1988.

Hassager C and Christiansen C: Estrogen/gestagen therapy changes soft tissue body composition in postsmenopausal women, Metabolism 38:662, 1989.

Hassager C, Riis BJ, and Strom V: The long-term effect of oral and percutaneous estradiol on plasma renin substrate and blood pressure, Circulation 76:753, 1987.

Hemminki E, Kennedy DL, Baum C, and McKinlay SM: Prescribing of noncontraceptive estrogens and progestins in the United States, 1974-86, Am J Public Health 78:1479, 1988.

Henderson BE, Paganini-Hill A, and Ross RK: Estrogen replacement therapy and protection from acute myocardial infarction, Am J Obstet Gynecol 159:312, 1988.

Henderson BE, Paganini-Hill A, and Ross RK: Decreased mortality in users of estrogen replacement therapy, Arch Intern Med 151:75, 1991.

Henderson BE, Ross RK, Paganini-Hill A, Mack TM: Estrogen use and cardiovascular disease, Am J Obstet Gynecol 154:1181, 1986.

Holst J, Backstrom T, Hammarback S, and von Schoultz B: Progestogen addition during oestrogen replacement therapy—effects on vasomotor symptoms and mood, Maturitas 11:13, 1989.

Hovik P, Sundsbak HP, Gaasemyr M, and Sandvik L: Comparison of continuous and sequential oestrogen-progestogen treatment in women with climacteric symptoms, Maturitas 11:75, 1989.

Jensen J, Nilas L, and Christiansen C: Cyclic changes in serum cholesterol and lipoproteins following different doses of combined postmenopausal hormone replacement therapy, Br J Obstet Gynaecol 93:613, 1986.

Jensen J, Nilas L, and Christiansen C: Influence of menopause on serum lipids and lipoproteins, Maturitas 12:321, 1990.

Jensen J, Riis BJ, Strom V, and Christiansen C: Continuous oestrogen-progestogen treatment and serum lipoproteins in postmenopausal women, Br J Obstet Gynaecol 94:130, 1987.

Jensen J, Riis BJ, Strom V, and Christiansen C: Long-term comparison of normal estradiol delivery in postmenopausal women, Am J Obstet Gynecol 159:1540, 1988.

Lindsay R: The menopause: sex steroids and osteoporosis, Clin Obstet Gynecol 30:847, 1987.

Lindsay R, Hart DM, Forrest C, and Baird C: Prevention of spinal osteoporosis in oophorectomized women, Lancet 2:1151, 1980.

Lindsay R, Hart DM, MacLean A, et al: Bone response to termination of oestrogen treatment, Lancet 1:1325, 1978.

Lindsay R and Tohme JF: Estrogen treatment of patients with established postmenopausal osteoporosis, Obstet Gynecol 76:290, 1990.

Lobo RA, McCormick W, Singer F, et al: Depomedroxyprogesterone acetate compared with conjugated estrogens for the treatment of postmenopausal women, Obstet Gynecol 63:1, 1984.

Magos AL, Brewster E, Singh R, and O'Dowd T: The effects of norethisterone in postmenopausal women on oestrogen replacement therapy: a model for the premenstrual syndrome, Br J Obstet Gynaecol 93:1290, 1986.

Mashchak CA, Kletzky OA, Artal R, and Mishell DR Jr: The relation of physiological changes to subjective symptoms in postmenopausal women with and without hot flushes, Maturitas 6:301, 1984.

Mashchak CA, Lobo RA, Dozono-Takano R, et al: Comparison of pharmacodynamic properties of various estrogen formulations, Am J Obstet Gynecol 144:511, 1982.

Matthews KA, Meilahn E, and Kuller LH: Menopause and risk factors for coronary heart disease, N Engl J Med 321:641, 1989.

McFarland KF, Boniface ME, Hornung CA, et al: Risk factors and noncontraceptive estrogen use in women with and without coronary disease, Am Heart J 117:1209, 1989.

Mishell DR Jr, editor: Menopause: physiology and pharmacology, Chicago, 1987, Mosby–Year Book, Inc.

Mishell DR Jr, Davajan V, and Lobo RA, editors: Infertility, contraception and reproductive endocrinology, ed 3, Cambridge, Mass, 1991, Blackwell Scientific Publications.

Moore DE, Kawagoe S, Davajan V, et al: An in vivo system in man for quantitation of estrogenicity. II. Pharmacologic changes in binding capacity of serum corticosteroid–binding globulin induced by conjugated estrogens, mestranol, and ethinyl estradiol, Am J Obstet Gynecol 130:482, 1978.

Munk-Jensen N, Nielsen SP, Obel EB, and Eriksen PB: Reversal of postmenopausal vertebral bone loss by oestrogen and progestogen: a double blind placebo controlled study, Br Med J 296:1150, 1988.

Myers LS, Dixen J, Morrissette D, et al: Effects of estrogen, androgen, and progestin and sexual psychophysiology and behavior in postmenopausal women, J Clin Endocrinol Metab 70:1224, 1990.

Nachtigall LE, Nachtigall RH, Nachtigall RB, and Beckman EM: Estrogen replacement. II. A prospective study in the relationship to carcinoma and cardiovascular and metabolic problems, Obstet Gynecol 54:74, 1979.

Nagamani M, Kelver ME, and Smith ER: Treatment of menopausal hot flashes with transdermal administration of clonidine, Am J Obstet Gynecol 156:561, 1987.

Notelovitz M, Kitchens C, Ware M, et al: Combination estrogen and progestogen replacement therapy does not adversely affect coagulation, Obstet Gynecol 62:596, 1983.

Ottosson UB, Carlstrom K, Johansson BG, and Von Schoultz B: Estrogen induction of liver proteins and high-density lipoprotein cholesterol: comparison between estradiol valerate and ethinyl estradiol, Gynecol Obstet Invest 22:198, 1986.

Ottosson UB, Johansson BG, and Von Schoultz B: Subfractions of high-density lipoprotein cholesterol during estrogen replacement therapy: a comparison between progestogens and natural progesterone, Am J Obstet Gynecol 151:746, 1985.

Paganini-Hill A, Ross RK, Gerkins VR, et al: A case control study of menopausal estrogen therapy and hip fractures, Ann Intern Med 95:28, 1981.

Paganini-Hill A, Ross RK, and Hendersen BE: Postmenopausal oestrogen treatment and stoke: a prospective study, Br Med J 297:519, 1988.

Persson I, Adami H-O, Bergkvist L, et al: Risk of endometrial cancer after treatment with oestrogens alone or in conjunction with progestogens: results of a prospective study, Br Med J 298:147, 1989.

Peterson HB, Lee NC, and Rubin GL: Genital neoplasia. In Mishell DR Jr, editor: Menopause: physiology and pharmacology, Chicago, 1987, Mosby–Year Book, Inc.

Quigley MET, Martin PL, Burnier AM, and Brooks P: Estrogen therapy arrests bone loss in elderly women, Am J Obstet Gynecol 156:1516, 1987.

Riggs BL and Gallagher JC: Evidence for bihormonal deficiency state (estrogen and 1,25 dihydroxyvitamin D) in patients with postmenopausal osteoporosis. In Norman AW, Schaefer K, Herrath Dv, et al, editors: Vitamin D: biochemical, chemical and clinical aspects related to calcium metabolism, Berlin, 1977, Walter de Gruyter & Co.

Riggs BL, Jowsey J, Kelley PJ, et al: Effects of sex hormones on bone in primary osteoporosis, J Clin Invest 48:1065, 1969.

Riis BJ, Johansen J, and Christiansen C: Continuous oestrogen-progestogen treatment and bone metabolism in post-menopausal women, Maturitas 20:15, 1988.

Riis B, Thomsen K, and Christiansen C: Does calcium supplementation prevent postmenopausal bone loss? N Engl J Med 326:173, 1987.

Ross RK, Paganini-Hill A, Mack TM, Henderson BE: Estrogen use and cardiovascular disease. In Mishell DR Jr, editor: Menopause: physiology and pharmacology, Chicago, 1987, Mosby–Year Book, Inc.

Rubin GL, Peterson HB, Lee NC, et al: Estrogen replacement therapy and the risk of endometrial cancer: remaining controversies, Am J Obstet Gynecol 162:148, 1990.

Samsioe G, Jansson I, Mellstrom D, and Svanborg A: Occurrence, nature and treatment of urinary incontinence in a 70-year-old female population, Maturitas 7:335, 1985.

Schiff I, Tulchinsky D, Cramer D, and Ryan KJ: Oral medroxyprogesterone in the treatment of postmenopausal symptoms, JAMA 224:1443, 1980.

Sherman BM, West JH, and Korenman SG: The menopausal transition: analysis of LH, FSH, estradiol, and progesterone concentrations during menstrual cycles of older women, J Clin Endocrinol Metab 42:629, 1976.

Sherwin BB and Gelfand MM: The role of androgen in the maintenance of sexual functioning in oophorectomized women, Psychosom Med, 49:397, 1987.

Sherwin BB and Gelfand MM: A prospective one-year study of estrogen and progestin in postmenopausal women: effects on clinical symptoms and lipoprotein lipids, Obstet Gynecol 73:759, 1989.

Sinaki M, Wahner HW, Offord KP, and Hodgson SF: Efficacy of nonloading exercises in prevention of vertebral bone loss in postmenopausal women: a controlled trial, Mayo Clin Proc 64:762, 1989.

Stanczyk FZ, Shoupe D, Nunez V, et al: A randomized comparison of normal estradiol delivery in postmenopausal women, Am J Obstet Gynecol 159:1540, 1988.

Stanford JL, Hartge P, Brinton LA, et al: Factors influencing the age at natural menopause, J Chron Dis 40:995, 1987.

Steinberg KK, Thacker SB, Smith J, et al: A meta-analysis of the effect of estrogen replacement therapy on the risk of breast cancer, JAMA 265:2985, 1991.

Stevenson JC: Pathogenes, prevention, and treatment of osteoporosis, Obstet Gynecol 175:36S, 1990.

Stevenson J, Whitehead MI, Padwick M, et al: Dietary intake of calcium and postmenopausal bone loss, Br Med J 297:15, 1988.

Sturdee DW, Wade-Evans T, Paterson ME, et al: Relations between bleeding pattern, endometrial histology, and oestrogen treatment in menopausal women, Br Med J 1(6127):1575, 1978.

Sullivan JM, Vander Zwaag R, Hughes JP, et al: Estrogen replacement and coronary artery disease, Arch Intern Med 150:2557, 1990.

Wahl P, Walden C, Knopp R, et al: Effect of estrogen/progestin potency on lipid/lipoprotein cholesterol, N Engl J Med 308:862, 1983.

Wahner HW, Dunn WL, Brown ML, et al: Comparison of dual energy x-ray absorptiometry for bone mineral measurements of the lumbar spine, Mayo Clin Proc 63:1075, 1988.

Weinstein L, Bewtra C, Gallager JC, et al: Evaluation of a continuous combined low-dose regimen of estrogen-progestin for treatment of the menopausal patient, Am J Obstet Gynecol 162:1534, 1990.

Weiss NS, Ure CL, Ballard JH, et al: Decreased risk of fractures of the hip and lower forearm with postmenopausal use of estrogen, N Engl J Med 303:1195, 1980.

Wilson PWF, Garrison RJ, and Castelli WP: Postmenopausal estrogen use, cigarette smoking, and cardiovascular morbidity in women over 50, N Engl J Med 313:1038, 1985.

Wren BG and Routledge AD: The effect of type and dose of oestrogen on the blood pressure of post-menopausal women, Maturitas 5:135, 1983.

Index